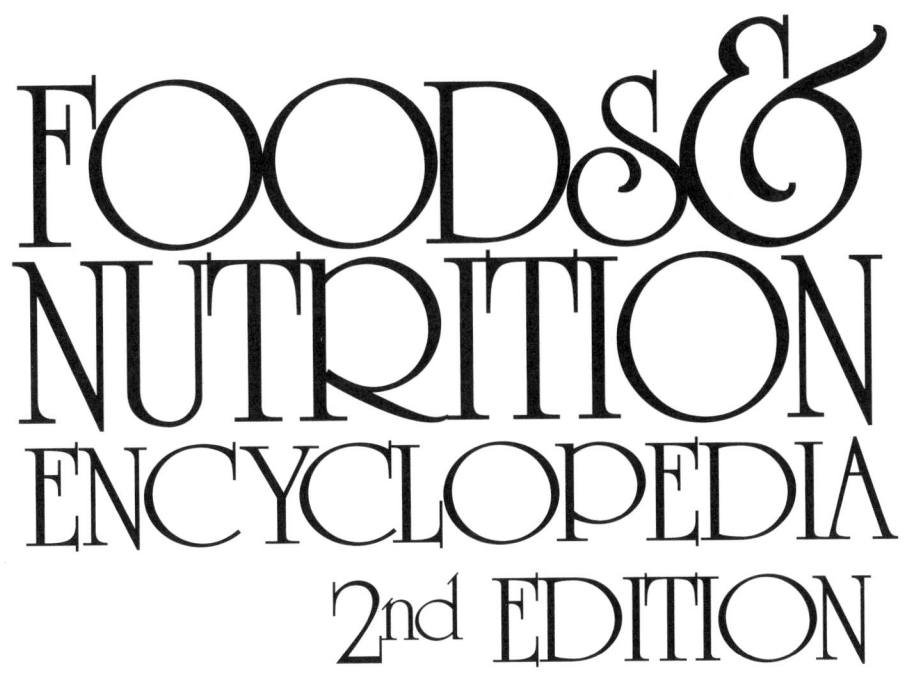

FOODS& NUTRITION ENCYCLOPEDIA 2nd EDITION

Volume 2
I-Z

Audrey H. Ensminger
M. E. Ensminger
James E. Konlande
John R. K. Robson

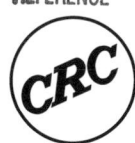

CRC Press

Boca Raton   Ann Arbor   London   Tokyo

Library of Congress Cataloging-in-Publication Data

Foods & nutrition encyclopedia / Audrey H. Ensminger ... [et al.]. --
   2nd ed.
        p.   cm.
    Includes bibliographical references and index.
    ISBN 0-8493-8980-1 (set). -- ISBN 0-8493-8981-X (v. 1). -- ISBN
0-8493-8982-8 (v. 2)
    1. Nutrition--Encyclopedias. 2. Food--Encyclopedias.
I. Ensminger, Audrey. II. Title: Foods and nutrition encyclopedia.
TX349.F575   1993
641′.03--dc20

93-36692
CIP

This book contains information obtained from authentic and highly regarded sources. Reprinted material is quoted with permission, and sources are indicated. A wide variety of references are listed. Reasonable efforts have been made to publish reliable data and information, but the author and the publisher cannot assume responsibility for the validity of all materials or for the consequences of their use.

Neither this book nor any part may be reproduced or transmitted in any form or by any means, electronic or mechanical, including photocopying, microfilming, and recording, or by any information storage or retrieval system, without prior permission in writing from the publisher.

CRC Press, Inc.'s consent does not extend to copying for general distribution, for promotion, for creating new works, or for resale. Specific permission must be obtained in writing from CRC Press for such copying.

Direct all inquiries to CRC Press, Inc., 2000 Corporate Blvd., N.W., Boca Raton, FL 33431.

Dedicated to—

improved food and nutrition for all people
in a world broken by unshared bread

ABOUT THE AUTHORS

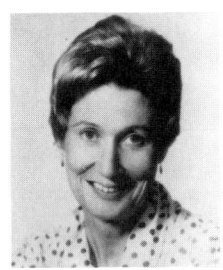 **Audrey H. Ensminger,** whose expertise is human nutrition, is Adjunct Professor, California State University-Fresno. She (1) completed the B.S. degree in Home Economics, University of Manitoba, Canada, and the M.S. degree in Home Economics, Washington State University; (2) taught at the University of Manitoba, the University of Minnesota, and Washington State University; and (3) served as dietitian for the U.S. Air Force, at Washington State University, during World War II. Audrey Ensminger has lectured throughout the world. She is the senior author of the two widely used human nutrition books, *Foods & Nutrition Encyclopedia* and *Food for Health.*

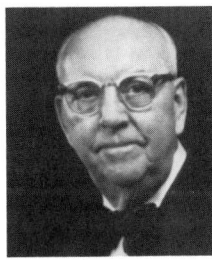 **M. E. Ensminger,** whose field is nutrition and biochemistry, is President, Agriservices Foundation, a nonprofit foundation serving world agriculture. Dr. Ensminger (1) completed B.S. and M.S. degrees at the University of Missouri, and the Ph.D. at the University of Minnesota; (2) served on the staffs of the University of Massachusetts, the University of Minnesota, and Washington State University; and (3) served as Consultant, General Electric Company, Nucleonics Department (Atomic Energy Commission). Dr. Ensminger is the author or co-author of 21 widely used books that are in several languages and used throughout the world. Dr. Ensminger is Adjunct Professor, California State University-Fresno; Adjunct Professor, the University of Arizona-Tucson; and Distinguished Professor, the University of Wisconsin-River Falls.

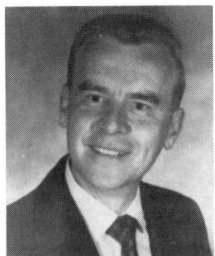 **James E. Konlande** completed the B.A. degree at Brooklyn College, Brooklyn, NY; and the M.S. and Ph.D. degrees at Rutgers University, New Brunswick, NJ, with a major in physiology, biochemistry, and nutrition. Prior to co-authoring FOODS & NUTRITION ENCYCLOPEDIA, he served as (1) Assistant Professor, Nutrition, the University of Michigan School of Public Health, Ann Arbor, Michigan; and (2) Head, Foods and Nutrition, Winthrop College (The University of South Carolina), Rock Hill, South Carolina.

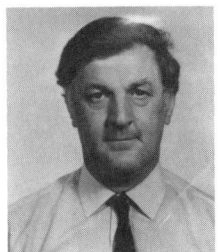 **John R. K. Robson, M.D.** was educated in England. He completed (1) the Bachelor of Medicine (M.B.) and Bachelor of Surgery (B.S.) degrees at Durham University, Kings College Medical School; (2) the Diploma in Tropical Medicine and Hygiene (D.T.M.&H. Edin.), Edinburgh University Medical School; (3) Diploma in Public Health—Special subject Nutrition (D.P.H. London), London University; and (4) the Doctor of Medicine (M.D.) at the University of Newcastle on Tyne, Medical School, and he is a Certified Specialist in Clinical Nutrition, American Board of Nutrition. Dr. Robson has done human nutrition work throughout the world. Also, he served as Professor of nutrition and Director of Nutrition Program, School of Public Health, University of Michigan; and as Professor of Nutrition and Medicine, Medical University of South Carolina, Charleston; and Executive Editor, *Ecology of Food and Nutrition*—and international journal. He is a Fellow of the Royal Society of Tropical Medicine and Hygiene; and a member of the New York Academy of Sciences, the Nutrition Society of Great Britain, the Scientific Council Population Food Fund, and the American Society of Parenteral and Enteral Nutrition.

PREFACE

We never had it so good! For most Americans, the 20th century brought substantial improvements in their standard of living. Greater human productivity and technological advances reduced the six-day, 70-hour work week of the turn of the century to a five-day, 40-hour week. Additionally, most people are able to afford comfortable living quarters, a television set, an automobile, an annual vacation, and educational opportunities for their children. Yet, an uneasy concern hangs over most everyone. They're concerned that their current life-style may be jeopardizing their health. Additionally, the media abound with news about low-level radiation, polluted air and water, and cancer-causing chemicals in our food.

THE GOOD OLD DAYS. The Good Old Days were not so good! Most Americans believe that people were healthier and happier before the advent of nuclear power, pesticides, food additives, and computers. True enough, earlier generations were not concerned about the hazards of technology, but they had a more immediate concern—all-too-frequent early death. In 1900, U.S. life expectancy at birth was only 47.3 years.

Nutritional deficiency diseases were common at the turn of the century. Pellagra, scurvy, beriberi, goiter, rickets, and anemia were major causes of disease, morbidity, and death. Today, these diseases are almost nonexistent, thanks to a better understanding of human nutritional requirements, increased variety of foods, and fortification of foods with minerals and vitamins.

A CENTURY OF PROGRESS. We have been blessed with a century of nutritional progress. The cause and cure of nutritional diseases was not understood until early in the 1900s when the biological approach in experiments—the use of laboratory animals (largely white rats and mice, guinea pigs, chickens, pigeons, and dogs)—was ushered in. Their diets were made up of relatively pure nutrients (proteins, carbohydrates, fats, and minerals)—using casein or albumen, lard, and a pure carbohydrate such as dextrin. Deficiencies followed. Then, it was discovered that dramatic cures resulted when minute amounts of a certain mineral(s) or vitamin(s) were added.

Using the biological approach, the mineral era was ushered in during the 20th century. Phosphorus was found to be essential for people and animals in 1918; copper in 1925; magnesium, manganese, and molybdenum in 1931; zinc in 1934; and cobalt in 1935. But the essentiality of selenium was not discovered until 1957, and of chromium until 1959. Then, as recently as 1972, it was found that fluorine and silicon are essential. Also, using the biological approach, the vitamin era was ushered in during the 20th century. In 1912, Casimir Funk, a Polish scientist working in London, discovered thiamin. The discovery of vitamin A followed in 1913. Since that time, the growth of the vitamin family, the isolation of many vitamins, the partial solution of the puzzle of vitamin functions in the body, the discovery of the amazing therapeutic value of minute quantities of these vitamins in the cure of deficiency diseases, the numerous determinations of food composition with respect to vitamins, and the synthesis of most of them, have had a profound effect in nutrition.

THE BIOTECHNOLOGY ERA. On May 23, 1977, scientists at the University of California-San Francisco reported a major breakthrough as a result of altering genes—turning ordinary bacteria into factories capable of producing insulin, so essential to the survival of diabetics. This feat gave rise to a major scientific revolution, called *biotechnology*. While some aspects of biotechnology are decades away from commercial production, others are near, and still others are here now. The entire food team—producers, processors, and consumers—will benefit from biotechnology, from the greater abundance of high-quality products produced more efficiently.

PUBLIC HEALTH MEASURES. Public health measures, more than any other factor, were responsible for reducing the death rate from infectious diseases—the major killers at the turn of the century. Filtering systems, followed by chlorination, gradually eliminated waterborne bacteria that caused such serious diseases as typhoid fever and cholera. Also, pasteurization of milk reduced the transmission of tuberculosis.

HEALTH MEASUREMENTS. The health of a population is usually measured in the following four ways:

1. **Longevity.** The most common measure of life expectancy is the average number of years that the newborn is expected to live. In 1900, the life expectancy in the United States was 47.3 years. In 1989, 89 years later, it was 75.2 years.

2. **Death rate.** The most dramatic indicator of America's improved health is the declining death rate. It fell from 1,800 deaths per 100,000 people per year in 1900 to 535 deaths per 100,000 people per year in 1988.

3. **Infant mortality.** At the turn of the century, about 100 of every 1,000 infants born in the United States died before their first birthday. In 1988, there were only 10 infant deaths per 1,000 births.

4. **Tooth decay.** At the turn of the century, scientists were just beginning to understand that tooth decay is caused by bacteria-fermenting nutrients in the mouth. Today, we have the methods available virtually to eliminate tooth decay. Yet, dental caries and periodontal disease continue to affect a large proportion of Americans and cause substantial pain, restriction of activity, work loss, and cost.

LEADING CAUSES OF DEATH. The leading causes of death in the United States have changed considerably since 1900.

In 1900, the 10 leading causes of death in descending order were: tuberculosis (accounting for 11% of deaths), pneumonia (accounting for 10%), diarrhea and enteritis, heart diseases, nephritis, accidents and violence, cerebrovascular disease, cancer, bronchitis, and diphtheria.

In 1989, the 10 leading causes of death in descending order were: heart disease, cancer, cerebrovascular disease, accidents and violence, lung diseases, pneumonia and influenza, diabetes mellitus, suicide, liver disease, and nephritis.

It is noteworthy that in 1989 (1) only one of the 10 leading causes of death was an infectious disease (namely, pneumonia and influenza); (2) the leading causes of death were chronic diseases of middle- and old-age; (3) heart disease, stroke, and related disorders accounted for 43% of all deaths; (4) cancer ranked second as cause of death; (5) accidents ranked fourth; and (6) lung diseases (chronic bronchitis, emphysema, and asthma) ranked fifth as cause of death, with cigarette smoking accounting for 80 to 90% of deaths due to lung diseases.

GRAYER BUT HEALTHIER. In 1920, only 4.7% of Americans lived beyond age 65. In 1989, approximately 12.5% lived past 65 and 1.2% lived to be 85 or more.

Although 45% of the elderly must limit their activities somewhat due to heart conditions, arthritis, hearing loss, or visual impairment, the vast majority retain their independence—only 6% of those over 65 are in nursing homes.

PREVENTING PREVENTABLE DEATHS. Each person has the power to reduce significantly his/her chances of dying from such feared killers as heart disease and stroke, cancer, or lung diseases. Here is how:

1. **Preventing heart disease and stroke.** Heredity, male gender, and increasing age are risk factors for heart disease and stroke that cannot be changed. However, the following major risk factors can be controlled: cigarette smoking, high blood pressure, and elevated blood cholesterol.

Cigarette smoking is the major preventable risk factor for heart disease—approximately 30% of all coronary heart disease deaths are attributable to smoking. When people quit smoking, the risk of dying from cardiovascular disease declines rapidly. Ten years after quitting, it is almost the same as that of a lifetime nonsmoker.

High blood pressure (hypertension), which afflicts 15 to 25% of Americans, increases the risk of heart disease (heart attack, congestive heart failure, or stroke) and kidney failure. Fortunately blood pressure may be controlled by proper diet, weight reduction, not smoking, restricted salt intake, exercise, and/or medication.

Blood cholesterol levels are affected by age, gender, genetics, and diet. The ratio of low-density lipoprotein (LDL, or "bad") cholesterol to high-density lipoprotein (HDL, or "good") cholesterol in the blood is also an important determinant of heart disease. The Food and Nutrition Board's Committee on Diet and Health recommends that the fat content of the U.S. diet not exceed 30% of the caloric intake, that less than 10% of the calories should be provided from saturated fatty acids, and that dietary cholesterol should be less than 300 mg/day. When the blood cholesterol is extremely high or diet fails to bring it down sufficiently, medication may be necessary.

Additional measures that may help reduce the risk of heart disease include maintaining a reasonable body weight, eating a nutritionally balanced diet, exercising regularly, and reducing stress.

2. **Preventing cancer.** There are two ways to reduce the risk of dying from cancer:

a. Avoid factors known to cause cancer. This includes (1) avoiding smoking cigarettes, which are re-

sponsible for about 30% of the deaths from cancer; (2) avoiding unprotected exposure to the sun, which is responsible for almost all of the skin cancer that occurs in the United States; and (3) avoiding excessive consumption of any one food (eat a variety of foods), because diet may be responsible for as much as 35% of cancers.

b. Have cancer check-up as part of the regular physical examination, so as to detect cancer early when there is a greater chance of cure.

3. **Preventing lung diseases.** Cigarette smoking is the major cause of lung diseases in the United States among both men and women; it accounts for 80 to 90% of all lung disease deaths.

WE STILL EAT THE WRONG FOODS. Americans are jogging, quitting smoking, buckling seat belts, and installing smoke detectors—all of which will likely help them live longer. But they are risking disease and early death by eating too much of the wrong foods. Cholesterol intake appears to have decreased since the 1980s; but efforts to limit sugar and salt, get enough vitamins, and control weight have slipped. Such trends cannot be ignored because dietary factors are associated with 5 of the 10 leading causes of death, including heart disease, some cancers, and stroke. Next to stopping cigarette smoking and alcohol abuse, choosing the proper diet is the most important action people can take to improve their health and lessen their chances of contracting disease. A recent study also revealed that only 19% of adults maintain their proper weight for their height, age, and sex.

CONCERN ABOUT NUTRITION AT ALL-TIME HIGH. A 1992 survey revealed that 64% of all consumers were concerned about the nutritional content of their food purchases.

Also, this same survey revealed that half of these consumers fretted about the fat in their food—it was their single largest worry.

A NEW FOOD GUIDE PYRAMID. For almost 50 years, the four food groups were arranged on a wheel, which was hung in classrooms all over America. In 1992, the U.S. Department of Agriculture released the *Food Guide Pyramid*, featuring six food groups, designed to reflect the changing eating habits of consumers and giving the department's official recommendations of what is good for you. The *Food Guide Pyramid* and the six food groups are featured in the "F" Section of *Foods & Nutrition Encyclopedia*.

THE PAST IS PROLOGUE. Despite the many advances that typify nutrition, there are many unknowns. So, the search goes on. But the past is prologue! The future promises foods that are tastier, more nutritious, more abundant, and biologically altered. During the next two decades, America's grocery stores will experience the most dramatic transformation since the first supermarket opened in La Habra, California, in 1915 (See *Foods & Nutrition Encyclopedia*, p. 789, Fig. F-40, for a picture of the first supermarket in America). The transformation will not be in new products introduced by food manufacturers, but in the biotechnology wizardry that produced them.

In the decades ahead, consumers will be able to eat cholesterol-free butter, cheese, and eggs; vegetables produced without the use of pesticides and herbicides; disease-resistant crops; foods that prevent cancer; meats in which saturated fats have been converted into unsaturated fats; wheat bread that contains adequate lysine and methionine; food products with improved mineral, vitamin, and fiber content, along with better flavor and longer shelf life; exotic fruits like kiwi, mango, and papaya available the year-round; and a great array of new products designed for microwave cooking. The pace of the biotechnology revolution will depend on two factors: (1) scientific progress, and (2) public acceptance.

BRIDGE THE GAP AND SPEED THE PROCESS. *Foods & Nutrition Encyclopedia* represents the joint effort of four well-known professional nutritionists. It's for consumers all—for everyone who seeks good health, and for those who counsel with them—physicians, dentists, nutritionists, health experts, and others in allied fields. It's for teachers and students. It's for those who produce, process, and market foods. It's for those who wish to know the "why" of foods and nutrition—for those who wish to be educated rather than indoctrinated. It's for those who want the facts—both the pros and cons—on which they may base a judgment. It's for those who wish to know from whence their food comes—from field to table. It's for those who are concerned with getting the most nutrition from their food dollars. It's for those who desire authoritative and pleasurable reading about foods and nutrition, and their relationship to health.

Foods & Nutrition Encyclopedia is not intended as a source of home remedies. Rather, it is the fervent desire of the authors that the enlightened person will institute a health and disease prevention program, call upon the family doctor when ill health strikes, and be better qualified to assist the M.D. in carrying out the prescribed treatment. Most of all, the authors hope that *Foods & Nutrition Encyclopedia* will bridge the gap between awareness and the application of nutrition, and speed the process of buoyant good health.

ACKNOWLEDGMENTS. For Dr. and Mrs. M. E. Ensminger, *Foods and Nutrition Encyclopedia* was their greatest challenge. They, along with a staff of 6 to 8, devoted more than 7 years to the preparation of the first edition; and they have been revising and updating it ever since. It was a team approach; Dr. and Mrs. Ensminger gratefully acknowledge the contributions of all those who assisted them in the preparation of *Foods & Nutrition Encyclopedia*, Second Edition, without whose dedicated efforts the mountainous task could not have been completed. Special appreciation is expressed to the following staff members for their commitment to excellence and a rigid schedule: Joan Wright and Janetta Shumway who deciphered the authors' hieroglyphics and put them through a typewriter; Randall and Susan Rapp, Rapp Publishing & Typographic Services, who typeset the many changes for the second edition; Margo Williams who prepared the new art that enhances the second edition, Jean Nelson who proofread the copy, and Ran Guang Liang who prepared the superb cover design. Also, we shall be ever grateful to Robin Spencer Palmisano, who at the time of preparing the first edition, was Systems Dietitian, University Hospitals, The Ohio State University, Columbus, Ohio, a very special person and dedicated professional, who contributed so much to Table F-36 Food Compositions. (Presently, Robin Spencer Palmisano is a lawyer and a member of the firm of McGlinchey, Stafford, Cellini & Lang, New Orleans, Louisiana.) Further, we are grateful to Ron Bruce, President, Unisoft Systems Associates, 1340 Dublin Road, Columbus, Ohio, 43215, for permission to continue to use Table F-36 Food Compositions. At appropriate places, due acknowledgement and sincere appreciation is expressed to those who responded so liberally to our call for information and pictures. In the preparation of this preface, authoritative information and statistics were secured from *America's Health*, published by American Council of Science and Health, New York. The unnumbered line drawings in *Foods & Nutrition Encyclopedia* were created by Dynamic Graphics, Inc. If *Foods & Nutrition Encyclopedia* will result in people living healthier, happier, and longer—and enjoying buoyant good health—the authors will feel amply rewarded.

A. H. Ensminger
M. E. Ensminger
J. E. Konlande
J. R. K. Robson

Clovis, California   (January, 1994)

INTRODUCTION

(This is an overall view of *Foods & Nutrition Encyclopedia*, and how to use it.)

True to its title, *Foods & Nutrition Encyclopedia*, covers the whole gamut of the three-pronged subject, foods–nutrition–health. A simple definition of each of these terms follows:

A food is any material that is taken or absorbed into the body of an organism for the purpose of satisfying hunger, growth, maintenance, tissue repair, reproduction, work, or pleasure.

Nutrition is the science of food and its nutrients and their relation to health.

Health is the state of complete physical, mental, and social well-being.

Like other sciences, foods and nutrition do not stand alone. They draw heavily on the basic findings of chemistry, biochemistry, physics, microbiology, physiology, medicine, genetics, mathematics, endocrinology, and, most recently, behavior, cellular biology, and genetic engineering. It is noteworthy, too, that much of our knowledge of human foods and nutrition came the animal route. Human nutritionists often use animal subjects for studies, because people usually prove too time-consuming, too costly, too difficult to control, and perhaps undesirable from a medical standpoint.

An overall view of *Foods & Nutrition Encyclopedia* along with instructions on how to use it, is contained in the sections that follow.

AUTHORITY. The authoritativeness of a work is evidenced by the credentials of those who created it. *Foods & Nutrition Encyclopedia* represents the team efforts of four well-known professionals in the field of foods-nutrition-health.

GOALS. At the outset, the authors stated as their objective: To produce the most complete and in-depth foods and nutrition source ever. If they haven't lived up to their objective, it's their fault; and they are willing to let the readers of the encyclopedia make judgments.

(Also see PREFACE.)

SELECTION OF TOPICS. The selection of the topics that are covered in *Foods & Nutrition Encyclopedia* was based on the author's professional experiences and perceptions relative to the needs of consumers, with application to many related fields, including medicine, dentistry, nursing, dietetics, teaching, nutritional science, public health, athletics, homemaking, and food production, processing, distribution and marketing. As the authors selected and treated each of the subjects, they were guided by the simple question: "Is it helpful?" If the answer was in the affirmative, they preceded with the philosophy of "let the chips fall where they may," no matter how complex or how controversial the subject. Also, the authors were ever aware that some contemporary interests are transient; so, they strived to achieve a balance between the timely and timeless.

COMPREHENSIVENESS. *Foods & Nutrition Encyclopedia* covers all aspects of foods–nutrition–health, with adequate historical and interpretive context. Each article includes all relevant aspects of the topic; thus, a few dictionary-type definitions were considered sufficient. Also, the entries reflect the whole gamut of foods–nutrition–health; there are precious few items in any other book on foods and nutrition not found as a subject entry and/or an index entry in *Foods & Nutrition Encyclopedia*.

ILLUSTRATIONS. *Foods & Nutrition Encyclopedia* is profusely illustrated with more than 1,600 pictures and figures, including 16 pages of colored pictures, all of which enhance the work. Each illustration is placed in close proximity to that portion of the subject matter which it clarifies, supplements, or complements. Most of the line drawings were created exclusively for *Foods & Nutrition Encyclopedia* by staff artists.

READABILITY. Writings are like food—both must be used to be of value. In recognition of this fact, the authors made a sincere effort to adhere to the following "musts of good writing":

1. Write as if they were speaking to a college professor, but so that an eavesdropping eighth grader would, quickly and easily, understand what they're saying and get the point.
2. Present human interest and historical events related to the subject.
3. Make events come alive; write with vigor and energy that jumps at the reader.
4. Use a simple, direct style that is easily comprehended.
5. Use words that are easily understood, but use technical terms where needed, with such words defined immediately in the article, thus ensuring understanding.
6. Present both U.S. Customary and Metric Systems of weights and measures.

OBJECTIVITY. To the end that this encyclopedia would be reliable, the authors resolved that the facts and inferences must be accurate and reflect current scholarship. Scholars may and do differ among themselves. Under these circumstances, the authors presented the opposing points of view—the pros and cons, then editorialized.

EASE OF USE. *Foods & Nutrition Encyclopedia* is organized so that readers may quickly and easily find the information that they are seeking. This is achieved through—

1. All topics being arranged alphabetically, using the word-by-word system—the same system that is used in a dictionary or in a library card catalog.

2. Cross referencing to related articles; usually at the end of an article, but within the text of an article when it makes for greater convenience.

3. A comprehensive index, which makes it possible for the reader, easily and quickly, to make a systematic survey of all parts and locations of *Foods & Nutrition Encyclopedia* directly or indirectly pertaining to a given subject. Additionally, where more than one reference page is listed in the index for a given subject, the main section is listed in bold numbers.

ALTERNATE NAMES. Alternate names are used wherever appropriate, with each name indexed, so that the article can be located under any of the alternate names; for example—

Vitamin C (Ascorbic acid)

FOOTNOTING THE NEW AND THE CONTROVERSIAL. The day and age of complete documentation of the literature used as background material for a work of this kind is past—it would be too voluminous. So, *Foods & Nutrition Encyclopedia* is an interpretation, correlation, and application of research findings, based on an extensive review of the literature by the authors. However, literature pertaining to new or controversial material has been documented in footnotes wherever possible.

FOOD COMPOSITION TABLE. Table F-36 Food Compositions is complete; and the edges of the pages are black, thus making for easy and speedy finding. It's without a peer.

(See FOOD COMPOSITIONS.)

PHYSICAL FORMAT. The format of *Foods & Nutrition Encyclopedia* is designed for quick and easy use, including—

1. **Outline.** An outline at the beginning of each major article which gives the reader an overall view of the article and shows the interrelationship of units. For example, four of the selected outline heading of corn follow:

CORN

PROCESSING CORN.

Corn Milling.

WET MILLING.

2. **Dot (bullet) system.** Within a given section, a "dot system" (or "bullet system") is used when it is appropriate, and when it will make for ease of use; for example, under the section of Kinds of Corn, each of the six kinds of corn is made to stand out like dent corn as follows:

• **Dent corn**—This is the most common variety.

3. **Tables.** Tabular presentation, which provides quick answers in concise form, is used wherever possible; for example—

TABLE C–45
CORN PRODUCTS AND USES

Product	Description	Uses	Comments

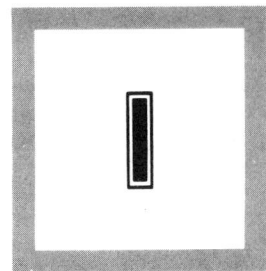

ICELAND MOSS *Cetraria*

This is a lichen, *Cetraria islandica*, which grows in all northern countries. Iceland, Norway, and Sweden export Iceland moss. When it is boiled with water it forms a jelly after cooling. Iceland moss is used like other gums—for foods, cosmetics, and textile sizing. The gum of Iceland moss is a polysaccharide containing uronic acid, galactose, mannose, and glucose.
(Also see GUMS.)

IDIOPATHIC

A condition of spontaneous origin; occurring without known cause.

IDIOSYNCRASY

Characteristic of or peculiar to an individual person.

ILEAL RESECTION

A surgical removal of part of the ileum section of the small intestine.

ILEITIS

Inflammation of the ileum, which is the last two-thirds of the small intestine before joining the large intestine. It may be caused by intestinal infections such as typhoid fever or dysentery, an obstruction, a chronic irritation or a defect in the immune system. Also, like other gastrointestinal disorders, emotional upset seems to contribute to the cause. Sufferers experience loss of appetite, loss of weight, anemia, diarrhea, pain in the lower right of the abdomen, and soreness around the navel. Acute cases are usually self-limiting and respond to bed rest and a change in daily routine. More serious cases may require surgery and medication. Some dietary adjustments may also be necessary. Many persons respond to some degree of fiber restriction. Also vitamin and mineral supplementation are recommended.
(Also see DIGESTION AND ABSORPTION; DISEASES; and MODIFIED DIETS.)

ILEUM

The lower portion of the small intestine extending from the jejunum to the cecum.
(Also see DIGESTION AND ABSORPTION.)

ILEUS

Obstruction of the bowel.

ILLIPE BUTTER

This is oil pressed from the fruits of the *Bassia longifolia* plant, or ilpa, of the East Indies. People of India use it as a butter substitute.

IMMUNOGLOBULINS

A family of proteins found in body fluids which has the property of combining with antigens and, when the antigen is pathogenic, sometimes inactivating it and producing a state of immunity. They are also called antibodies. It is suspected that full protection against disease by these substances depends upon adequate protein nutrition. Colostrum is high in immunoglobulins.
(Also see PROTEIN[S].)

IMPERMEABLE

Not capable of being penetrated.

INBORN ERRORS OF METABOLISM

As often as the genetic code is correctly interpreted and reproduced, mistakes—mutations—do sometimes occur. Mutations result in genetically determined metabolic disorders due to specific defects, present at birth, though not always evident. Inborn errors of metabolism is a phrase coined by Archibald E. Garrod who described only four diseases of a hereditary nature, at the beginning of this century. These disorders may also be referred to as genetic diseases or hereditary molecular diseases. Outwardly, the infant appears normal at birth. However, once it begins to receive nutrition and/or interacts with other environmental factors, some dramatic changes may occur in mental and/or physical development due to abnormal utilization of nutrients by the body. Evidence of other genetic diseases does not appear until later in life. There are two main types of genetic disorders of metabolism: (1) the absence or severe reduction in the activity of an enzyme or enzymes, and (2) a defect in the transport of metabolites across cell membranes. Hence, both types may involve protein molecules whose synthesis is directed by the genetic material of the cells—the DNA. Detrimental effects of these metabolic errors are due to the accumulation of toxic levels of a biochemical and/or the reduced availability of an essential biochemical. Genetic defects vary widely, and may alter the metabolism of amino acids, carbohydrates, lipids, vitamins, and minerals. There are between 100 and 200 genetic disorders. Fortunately, many are extremely rare, while others are harmless and only represent biological variation.

Early diagnosis of inborn errors of metabolism is important so treatment may be initiated before irreversible mental and/or physical damage occurs. In general, some of the approaches to treatment of inborn errors include (1) environmental modification, (2) dietary restriction and/or supplementation, (3) product, enzyme, or cofactor replacement or enhancement, (4) depletion of toxic levels of stored substances, (5) drug avoidance, (6) surgical intervention, and (7) possibly in the future, genetic engineering. For some inborn errors no known therapy is available.

The following tables outline the specific defects, characteristic features, and treatment (particularly dietary management), of some of the more important inborn errors in the metabolism of amino acids, carbohydrates, lipids, and nucleic acids. Also, the last table presents some miscellaneous inborn disorders of metabolism.

(Also see AMINO ACID[S]; CARBOHYDRATE[S]; DIGESTION AND ABSORPTION; DISEASES; ENZYME; FATS AND OTHER LIPIDS; and METABOLISM.)

TABLE I-1
INBORN ERRORS OF AMINO ACID METABOLISM

Disorder	Defect(s)	Characteristic Features	Treatment
Albinism	Insufficient levels of the enzyme tyrosinase.	Inability to form pigment melanin; lack of pigmentation of hair, skin, and eyes.	Protection from sunlight.
Alkaptonuria	Insufficient levels of the enzyme homogentisic acid oxidase.	Incomplete oxidation of tyrosine and phenylalanine; darkening of urine; pigmentation of connective tissue; inflammation of the vertebrae (spondylitis) and joint disease (arthropathy).	Once pigmentation of connective tissue is established, there is no effective treatment. Possible benefit if phenylalanine and tyrosine intake could be limited following early detection; ascorbic acid supplementation.
Argininosuccinic aciduria (Also see UREA CYCLE.)	Insufficient levels of the enzyme argininosuccinase.	Elevated arginosuccinic acid in blood, urine, and spinal fluid; ammonia intoxication; severe mental retardation; seizures; liver dysfunction.	Lowering protein intake to 0.5 to 1.0 g/kg body weight may be effective; frequent feedings.
Citrullinemia (Also see UREA CYCLE.)	Insufficient levels of the enzyme argininosuccinic acid synthetase.	Elevated blood ammonia after eating; nausea; vomiting; mental retardation; elevated blood level of citrulline.	Restriction of dietary protein to 0.5 to 1.0 g/kg per day.
Cystathioninuria (Also see VITAMIN B-6.)	Insufficient levels of the enzyme cystathionase.	Excessive levels of cystathionine in urine, blood and spinal fluid; possibly mental deficiency; seizures.	Marked improvement with vitamin B-6 (pyridoxine) therapy.

(Continued)

TABLE I-1 *(Continued)*

Disorder	Defect(s)	Characteristic Features	Treatment
Cystinuria	Defective membrane transport in kidney and small intestine.	Excessive urinary excretion of cystine, lysine, arginine, and ornithine; formation of cystine kidney stones.	Restriction of dietary methionine; high fluid intake; alkalinizing urine; possible penicillamine to increase solubility of cystine.
Fanconi's syndrome (Also see CALCIUM; and VITAMIN D.)	No specific enzyme; defect in kidney transport mechanism.	Loss of amino acids, glucose, phosphate and bicarbonate in urine; often acidosis; rickets or osteomalacia.	Therapy aimed at replacing losses; control acidosis; infants require vitamin D therapy plus neutral phosphates.
Hartnup disease	Defective membrane transport in kidney and small intestine.	Excretion of the amino acids valine, leucine, isoleucine, threonine, serine, tryptophan, and phenylalanine in urine; pellagra-like skin rash; mental retardation.	Skin and neurological features respond to nicotinamide therapy (50 to 200 mg/day). High protein diet recommended to counter loss in urine; avoidance of undue exposure to sunlight.
Histidinemia	Insufficient levels of the enzyme histidase.	Elevated blood and urine histidine levels; some mental retardation; speech and hearing disorders.	High protein diet in infancy avoided; no claims made for improvement by dietary treatment.
Homocystinuria (Also see AMINO ACID[S]; and PROTEIN.)	Insufficient levels of the enzyme cystathionine synthetase.	High blood levels of methionine and homocysteine; eye problems; bone deformities; mild mental deficiency; common circulatory disorders.	Some types respond to massive vitamin B-6 (pyridoxine); others require low methionine diet with supplemental cystine; soy and gelatin used as protein sources; supplemental synthetic amino acids, fruits, vegetables, breads, cereals, fats supply energy; folic acid supplementation.
Hydroxyprolinemia	Insufficient levels of the enzyme hydroxyproline oxidase.	Hydroxyproline elevated in urine and blood; severe mental retardation in some cases.	Little success with dietary treatment; some cases of hydroxyprolinemia not harmful.
Hyperammonemia	Insufficient levels of the enzyme ornithine transcarbamylase or carbamylphosphate synthetase.	Ammonia intoxication—high blood levels of NH_3; vomiting; lethargy; coma; mental retardation.	Dietary protein restricted to 0.5 to 1.0 g/kg/day.
Hyperlysinemia (lysine intolerance)	Insufficient levels of the enzyme lysine NAD oxidoreductase.	High blood levels of arginine and lysine and sometimes ammonia; vomiting; spacticity; coma; mental retardation.	Dietary protein restricted to 1.5 g/kg/day; no treatment necessary in some cases.
Hyperoxaluria	Insufficient levels of the enzyme 2-oxo-glutarate: glyoxylate carboligase or D-glyceric dehydrogenase.	Increased urinary oxalate, of which ⅓ to ½ originates from glycine, an amino acid; symptoms and signs of kidney stones and advancing kidney failure.	None satisfactory; some use of high phosphate diet; plenty of drinking water; some use of large doses of vitamin B-6 (pyridoxine) and folic acid; possibly restrict dietary sources of oxalate—rhubarb and spinach.

(Continued)

TABLE I-1 (*Continued*)

Disorder	Defect(s)	Characteristic Features	Treatment
Hyperprolinemia	Insufficient levels of the enzyme proline oxidase, or pyrroline-5-carboxylate-dehydrogenase.	Excess urinary excretion of proline, glycine, hydroxyproline, and possibly pyrroline-5-carboxylic acid; fever, diarrhea, convulsions, and possibly mental retardation; one form is without signs or symptoms.	Proline is synthesized by the body. Dietary management probably is difficult. An intermediate restriction of proline (130 mg/kg/day) may be helpful; further study necessary.
Hypervalinemia	Insufficient levels of the enzyme valine trans-aminase.	Elevated urinary and blood valine; growth retardation; mental retardation; vomiting; involuntary rapid eye movements (nystagmus).	Formula diet low in valine.
Isovaleric acidemia	Insufficient levels of the enzyme isovaleryl-CoA dehydrogenase.	Elevated plasma isovaleric acid; incoordination; acidosis; stupor; coma; foul smelling breath.	Management of acidosis; control of acute catabolic stimuli; low protein diet; just sufficient to maintain growth and low in leucine.
Maple syrup urine disease (branched-chain ketoaciduria) (Also see AMINO ACID[S].)	Insufficient levels of the enzyme branched-chain keto acid decarboxylases.	High levels of leucine, isoleucine, valine, and their keto acids in the blood and urine; maple syrup odor of urine; mental retardation; spasticity; seizures; convulsions.	Necessary to begin diet therapy first week of life and run through lifetime; synthetic formula diet; small amounts of milk for growth requirements; some low protein foods identified by their leucine content, for example, low protein cereals, fruits, and vegetables; synthetic formula meets energy, protein, and all other nutrient requirements.
Methionine malabsorption (Oasthouse urine disease)	No specific enzyme; defect in small intestine transport system.	Only a few cases; convulsions and mental retardation; foul odor to urine; large amounts of methionine in urine.	Methionine restriction.
Phenylketonuria (PKU)	Insufficient levels of the enzyme phenylalanine hydroxylase.	Plasma phenylalanine elevated; urinary phenylalanine, phenylpyruvate, phenyllactate, phenylacetate, and O-hydroxy-phenylacetate elevated in urine; "mousy" odor to urine and skin; mental retardation; fair complexion; convulsions; tremors; eczema.	Early detection; "Diaper test," controlled phenylalanine intake; use of commercial preparation, Lofenalac; other foods of known phenylalanine content used to meet requirements for phenylalanine; Lofenalac provides main source of protein and energy; continued adjustment of diet necessary; discontinue at 6 to 8 years of age except during pregnancy.
Tyrosinemia (neonatal tyrosinemia)	Insufficient levels of the enzyme hydroxyphenyl-pyruvic acid oxidase or tyrosine trans-aminase.	Transient condition of newborns; increased levels of tyrosine in blood and urine drop as infant matures; not associated with specific symptoms.	Tyrosine in blood and urine returns to normal as infant matures. Vitamin C helps reduce blood levels. Reduced protein intake beneficial; often occurs in premature babies.
Tyrosinosis	Insufficient levels of the enzyme parahydroxy-phenylpyruvic acid oxidase.	Elevated thyroxin levels in plasma and urine; loss of the amino acids proline, serine, and threonine in urine; kidney damage; liver damage; mental retardation; rickets; may progress so rapid, death results from liver damage.	Diet low in phenylalanine and tyrosine; casein hydrolysate possibly used as source of protein and calories; limited amounts of foods low in phenylalanine and tyrosine.

TABLE I-2
INBORN ERRORS OF CARBOHYDRATE METABOLISM

Disorder	Defect(s)	Characteristic Features	Treatment
Carbohydrate intolerance	Insufficient levels of the enzymes disaccharidases such as maltase, isomaltase, invertase, lactase, and trehalase.	Diarrhea most outstanding feature; abdominal cramps; flatulence.	Dietary elimination of the sugar that is not tolerated; for example, maltose, sucrose, lactose.
Fructose intolerance (fructosemia)	Insufficient levels of the enzyme fructose-1-phosphate aldolase.	Release of glucose from liver blocked by accumulation of fructose-1-phosphate; vomiting; hypoglycemia; death if fructose source not removed from diet.	Exclusion of sucrose and fructose sources from diet; elimination of most fruits; no table sugar; no sorbitol; avoid sweets.
Galactosemia	Insufficient levels of the enzyme galactose-1-phosphate uridyl transferase.	Elevated blood and urine levels of galactose; vomiting; failure to thrive; enlarged liver; mental retardation; cataract formation.	Early diagnosis; complete exclusion of lactose and galactose from diet; use of synthetic milk; milk permanently excluded from diet; supplements of calcium and riboflavin.
Glycogen storage diseases (10 types):			
Type I (von Gierke's disease)	Insufficient levels of the enzyme glucose-6-phosphatase.	Large liver and kidneys; kidney stones; yellowish or orange growth on skin due to lipid deposits (xanthomas); hypoglycemia; convulsions; coma; retarded growth.	High protein diet promoting gluconeogenesis; feedings every 3 to 4 hours; carbohydrate in form of glucose or starch; no sucrose or lactose; feeding medium chain triglycerides for treatment of xanthomas.
Type II (Pompe's disease)	Insufficient levels of the enzyme lysosomal glucosidase.	Massive glycogen infiltration particularly of the heart; cardiac distress; heart failure.	Treatment unavailing.
Type III (limit dextrinosis; Cori's disease; Forbes' disease)	Insufficient levels of the enzyme amylo-1, 6-glucosidase.	Accumulation of glycogen with abnormal chemical structure in liver and muscles; enlarged liver.	High protein, low fat diet; frequent feedings; prompt treatment of infections; prohibition of strenuous exercise.
Type IV (amylopectinosis; brancher glycogenosis; Anderson's disease)	Insufficient levels of the enzyme amylo-1, 4→1,6-transglucosylase.	Abnormally formed glycogen; enlarged spleen; enlarged liver; cirrhosis; liver failure; cardiac failure.	Death before third year; supportive treatment only.
Type V (McArdle's disease)	Insufficient levels of the enzyme muscle phosphorylase.	Accumulation of muscle glycogen; weakness and cramping of muscles on exercise; no rise of blood lactate.	Intravenous glucose; limited exertion; no tight garments; plenty of carbohydrate.
Type VI (liver phosphorylase deficiency; Hers' disease)	Insufficient levels of the enzyme liver phosphorylase.	Liver glycogen accumulation; enlarged liver; cirrhosis.	Avoidance of prolonged fasting; high protein diet; frequent feedings.
Type VII	Insufficient levels of the enzyme phosphofructokinase and phosphoglucomutase.	Muscle pain and stiffness on exercise.	Experience with the value of dietary treatment is limited, due to rare occurrence of diseases.
Type VIII	Insufficient levels of the enzyme liver phosphorylase.	Glycogen accumulation in the liver; enlarged liver; brain degeneration.	
Type IX	Insufficient levels of the enzyme liver phosphorylase kinase.	Enlarged liver.	
Type X	Insufficient levels of the enzyme c-AMP-dependent phosphorylase kinase.	Enlarged liver.	

(Continued)

TABLE I-2 *(Continued)*

Disorder	Defect(s)	Characteristic Features	Treatment
Hemolytic anemia:	Insufficient levels of the following enzymes:		
I	Hexokinase	Enzyme deficiency in red blood cell energy yielding pathway reduces survival time of red blood cells, thus producing anemia. These 10 enzyme deficiencies (I through X) listed, are known to produce hemolytic amemia.	The relationship between abnormalities of the metabolism of glucose in red blood cells and their survival is not completely understood. Splenectomy may or may not be beneficial.
II	Phosphohexose isomerase.		
III	Triosephosphate isomerase.		
IV	Diphosphoglycerate kinase.		
V	Pyruvate kinase.		
VI	Glucose-6-phosphate dehydrogenase.	Most common; requires inducing agent such as aspirin, antimalarial drugs, antibiotics, or fava beans.	Offending foods and chemicals avoided; transfusion may be necessary at times.
VII	6-Phosphoglucomate dehydrogenase.	Most hemolytic anemias due to these enzyme deficiencies are quite rare.	Transfusions may be necessary.
VIII	Glutothione reductase.		
IX	Glutathione peroxidase.		
X	Glutathione synthetase.		
Leucine-induced hypoglycemia	Exact defect unknown.	Apparent 4th month of life; first sign may be convulsions; failure to thrive; possibly some delayed mental development; test dose of leucine produces profound lowering of blood glucose.	Diet low in leucine; diet furnishes minimum requirements of protein for growth; fruits and vegetables added; carbohydrate feeding (10g) 30 to 40 min. after each meal; possible treatment with diazoxide; normal diet by age 5 to 6.
Pentosuria	Insufficient levels of the enzyme xylulose dehydrogenase.	Harmless; large amounts of xylulose—5-carbon sugar (pentose)—excreted in urine; almost exclusively found in Jews.	No treatment necessary.
Renal glycosuria	No specific enzyme; disorder in membrane transport in kidney.	Glucose excreted in urine while blood glucose at normal levels; storage and utilization of carbohydrates normal.	No treatment required providing diagnosis is correct.

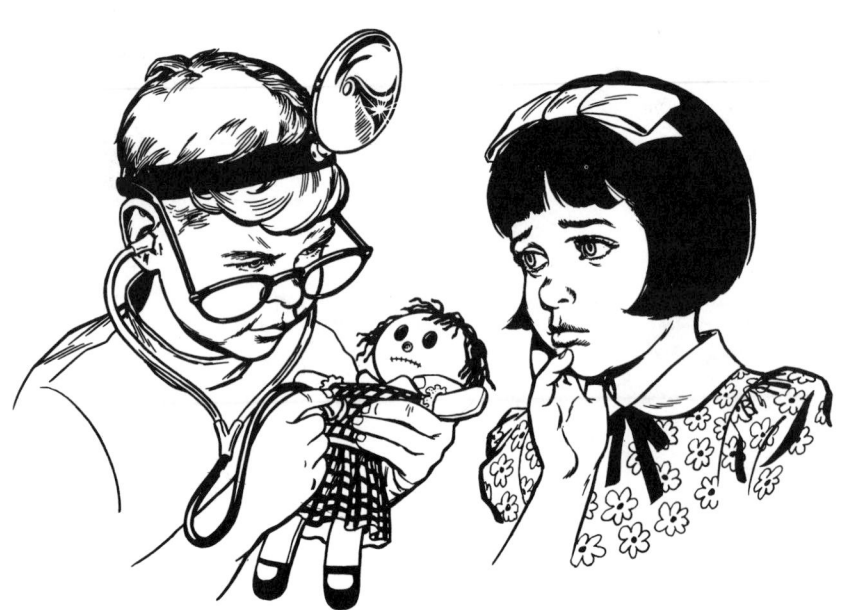

TABLE I-3
INBORN ERRORS OF LIPID METABOLISM

Disorder	Defect(s)	Characteristic Features	Treatment
Abetalipoproteinemia	No specific enzyme defect.	Absence of low density β-lipoprotein (LDL) in blood; steatorrhea (fatty diarrhea); malnutrition; growth retardation; nervous disorders; spiny or thorny shaped red blood cells.	Low fat diet with medium chain triglycerides (MCT) supplementation providing some fat intake; large doses fat-soluble vitamins particularly vitamins A, D, and E may be beneficial.
Angiokeratoma (Fabry's disease; glycolipid liposis)	Insufficient levels of the enzyme ceramide trihexosisidase.	Accumulation of glycolopids in tissues; joint pain; eye disorders; purplish papules on skin; males show progressive kidney failure; some nervous disorders.	Moderate quantities of the drug diphenyhydantion; no dietary therapy.
Familial high-density lypoprotein deficiency (Tangier disease)	No specific enzyme.	Absence of high-density or alpha lipoprotein (HDL); deposition of cholesterol in tonsils; enlarged orange tonsils; peripheral nerves may be affected.	Treatment may not be necessary; sometimes tonsillectomy and splenectomy; no definitive treatment.
Familial hyperlipoproteinemias: Type I (hyperchylomicronemia) (Also see HYPERLIPOPROTEINEMIAS.)	Insufficient levels of the enzyme lipoprotein lipase.	Elevated blood levels of chylomicrons; yellow papules with reddish base develop over skin and mucous membranes (xanthomas); enlarged spleen; enlarged liver; abdominal pain; possible pancreatitis.	Low fat 25–36 g/day; use of medium chain triglycerides; high energy, high protein diet; no alcohol.
Type II (hyperbetalipoproteinemia or hypercholesterolemia) (Also see ATHEROSCLEROSIS; and HYPERLIPOPROTEINEMIAS.)	No specific enzyme defect.	Increased blood levels of beta lipoprotein (LDL) and cholestrol; yellow lipid deposits in skin, tendons, and cornea; accelerated atherosclerosis.	Dietary saturated fat and cholesterol limited sharply; polyunsaturated fats increased; use of the drug cholestryamine.
Type III (broad-beta or floating beta disease) (Also see HEART DISEASE; and HYPERLIPOPROTEINEMIAS.)	No specific enzyme defect.	Elevated blood levels of abnormal prebetalipoproteins (VLDL), cholesterol, and triglycerides; tendon xanthomas; creases in palm of hands show as yellow lines; accelerated atherosclerosis of coronary and peripheral blood vessels; heart disease.	Low cholesterol intake; achieve ideal weight; no concentrated sweets; energy should be 20% from protein, 30% from fat, and 50% from carbohydrates; use of polyunsaturated fats; drug of choice clofibrate.
Type IV (hyperprebetalipoproteinemia) (Also see HEART DISEASE; and HYPERLIPOPROTEINEMIAS.)	No specific enzyme defect.	High blood levels of prebetalipoprotein (VLDL) and triglycerides; cholesterol normal or elevated; accelerated heart disease; glucose intolerance.	Maintenance of ideal weight; controlled carbohydrate intake, about 50% of energy; moderate cholesterol restriction to 300 mg; polyunsaturated fats preferred; no concentrated sweets; drugs of choice clofibrate or nicotinic acid.
Type V (mixed hyperlipidemia) (Also see FATS AND OTHER LIPIDS; and HYPERLIPOPROTEINEMIAS.)	No specific enzyme defect.	Elevated blood levels of chylomicrons, prebetalipoproteins, cholesterol, and triglycerides; eruptive orange yellow deposits of lipid on skin (xanthomas); abdominal pain; lipid in retina of eye; enlarged liver and spleen.	Fat restricted to 30% of energy; high protein diet; maintenance of ideal weight; 300 mg cholesterol daily; no concentrated sweets; possible use of nicotinic acid; no alcohol.
Familial cholesterol ester deficiency	Insufficient levels of the enzyme lecithin: cholesterol acyltransferase (LCAT).	Proteinuria; anemia; corneal opacity; elevated blood levels of triglycerides, lecithin, and unesterified cholesterol.	Low fat diet under trial; none specific.

(Continued)

TABLE I-3 — *(Continued)*

Disorder	Defect(s)	Characteristic Features	Treatment
Glucosyl ceramide lipidosis (Gaucher's disease) (Also see FATS AND OTHER LIPIDS.)	Insufficient levels of the enzyme glucocerebrosidase.	Accumulation of cerebroside in liver, spleen, and bone marrow; enlarged spleen and liver; bone lesions.	Supportive therapy of vitamins and supplemental iron; splenectomy.
Niemann–Pick disease (sphingomyelin lipidosis) (Also see FATS AND OTHER LIPIDS.)	Insufficient levels of the enzyme sphingomyelinase.	Accumulation chiefly of spingomyelin and lecithin in the liver, spleen, and central nervous system; enlarged liver and spleen; mental and physical retardation; cherry red spot on retina of eye.	None of value.
Refsum's disease (phytanic acid storage disease)	Insufficient levels of the enzyme phytanic acid oxidase.	Accumulation of phytanic acid in blood and tissues; vision and hearing disorders; dry skin; bone deformities.	Phytanic acid restriction; diets exclude green vegetables, butter, and ruminant (cattle, sheep, goat) fat; all phytanic acid originates in diet.
Tay–Sachs disease (ganglioside lipidosis)	Insufficient levels of the enzyme hexosaminidase A.	Abnormal glycosphingolipid metabolism; growth retardation; failure to develop coordinated muscular activity; listlessness, blindness with a cherry red spot on retina.	None of value.
Wolman's disease	Insufficient levels of the enzyme acid lipase.	Failure to thrive; vomiting; diarrhea; enlarged spleen and liver; accumulation of cholesterol and triglycerides in liver, lymph nodes, spleen, thymus, intestine and bone marrow; adrenal calcification; death by 6 months of age.	None

TABLE I-4
INBORN ERRORS OF NUCLEIC ACID METABOLISM

Disorder	Defect(s)	Characteristic Features	Treatment
Gout[1] (Also see ARTHRITIS, section headed "Gout [Gouty arthritis]"; and PURINES.)	Insufficient levels of the enzyme hypoxanthine-guanine phosphoribosyltransferase (HPRT).	Uric acid secretion 5 to 6 times greater than normal; gout; severe neurological disorder called Lesch–Nyhan syndrome when there is a complete deficiency of the enzyme; transmitted on sex chromosomes; onset within first year of life; partial deficiency still produces some neurological disorders.	Valium (diazepam) for spasticity and self-mutilating behavior; allopuriol to reduce uric acid formation; adequate nutrition and secure environment beneficial; no treatment prevents neurological disorder.
	Insufficient levels of the enzyme glucose-6-phosphatase (glycogen storage disease, type I).	Over-production of uric acid and under-secretion of uric acid; gout; excessive deposition of glycogen in liver; yellowish or orange growth on skin due to lipid deposits (xanthomas); hypoglycemia; convulsions; coma; acidosis; stunted growth.	Colchicine, phenylbutazone, indomethacin, ACTH, or hydrocortisone for acute attacks; reduction to ideal weight; avoidance of high purine foods, high fluid intake; alkalinized urine.
	Insufficient levels of the enzyme phosphoribosyl-pyrophosphate synthetase.	Accelerated purine biosynthesis; high daily uric acid excretion; problems caused by excessive activity of the enzyme; kidney stones; gout.	
Orotic aciduria	Insufficient levels of the enzyme orotidylic pyrophosphorylase; orotidylic decarboxylase.	Very rare; appears first year or so of life; severe megoblastic anemia resistant to usual treatments; mental and physical retardation; excrete large quantities of ortic acid in urine; needle-shaped crystals in urine.	Dietary supplementation with large doses of uridine improves anemia and mental and physical development. Early diagnosis essential.
Xanthinuria	Insufficient levels of the enzyme xanthine oxidase.	Elevated blood and urine levels of xanthine and hypoxanthine and very low uric acid; a therapeutic xanthinuria accompanies use of allopurinol.	Most cases require no treatment; high fluid intake and restricted purine intake recommended.

[1]Gout that is associated with specific enzyme defects.

TABLE I-5
MISCELLANEOUS INBORN ERRORS OF METABOLISM

Disorder	Defect(s)	Characteristic Features	Treatment
Adrenal hyperplasia (Also see ENDOCRINE GLANDS.)	Insufficient levels of the enzyme 21-hydroxylase.	Most common; overproduction of testosterone; steroid excretion in urine elevated; virilization of the female; derangement of external female genitalia; growth of the penis within the first months of life; accelerated growth; early bone maturation; no sperm production; no ovarian function; sensitive to stress and infection; abnormal, excessive hair growth in unusual places in especially women (hireutism); possibly acne; one form demonstrates a salt-losing (sodium-losing) syndrome.	Daily administration of glucocorticoids; salt-losing form requires fluid replacement; therapy throughout life; prognosis excellent if noted first 2 years of life.
	Insufficient levels of the enzyme 11-hydroxylase.	Clinically indistinguishable from 21-hydroxylase deficit with exception of high blood pressure due to accumulation of 11-deoxycortisol, a steroid.	Daily administration of glucocorticoids; prognosis excellent.
	Insufficient levels of the enzyme 17-hydroxylase.	Accumulation of the steroids progesterone and pregnanediol; no virilization however female fails to mature; sodium retention; potassium wasting; alkalosis; high blood pressure; males fail to mature or have ambiguous external genitalia.	Glucocorticoids correct high blood pressure; sex hormones necessary for sexual maturity.
Congenital lack of intrinsic factor	No intrinsic factor.	Megaloblastic anemia; onset early in life.	Vitamin B-12 therapy
Congenital nonhemolytic jaundice: Type I (Crigler–Najjar syndrome)	Absence of the enzyme glucuronyl transferase.	Jaundice not due to red blood cell bursting; onset of jaundice at birth; serum bilirubin 18 to 50 mg/100 ml; severe neurologic defects; kernicterus (deposition of bile pigments in brain).	Death often in infancy; no response to phenobarbital; albumin infusions; phototherapy; prognosis poor.
Type II	Insufficient levels of the enzyme glucuronyl transferase.	Jaundice not due to red blood cell bursting; onset of jaundice usually at birth; serum bilirubin 6 to 22 mg/100 ml; no intellectual impairment.	Phenobarbital lowers bilirubin; phototherapy (blue light) lowers serum bilirubin.
Hemochromatosis (bronze diabetes or pigment cirrhosis)	Failure of the control mechanism for absorption of iron from the intestine.	Saturation of the plasma iron-binding protein, transferin; excessive deposits of iron in the tissues; enlarged liver; pigmentation of the skin; diabetes mellitus; frequently heart failure.	Once or twice weekly, blood-letting which removes 500 ml of blood and 250 mg of iron for about 2 years; once or twice yearly blood-letting thereafter; supportive treatment of damaged organs.

(Continued)

TABLE I-5 — (Continued)

Disorder	Defect(s)	Characteristic Features	Treatment
Hereditary sphero-cytosis (congenital hemolytic jaundice)	Defect in red blood cells due to excessive permeability to sodium.	Jaundice due to red blood cell bursting; enlarged spleen; increased fragility of red blood cells.	Blood transfusions necessary at times; spelectomy best treatment.
Hypophosphatemia (Also see PHOS-PHORUS; and VITAMIN D.)	Defect in kidney tubules.	Low blood phosphate; blood calcium level normal; rickets and dwarfism; transmitted on the sex chromosomes.	Large doses of vitamin D; oral phosphorus.
Mucopolysaccharid-oses (11 types) (Also see CARBO-HYDRATE[S].)	Deficiency in lyso-somal enzyme important for muco-polysaccharide (complex polysaccharide) degradation.	Depending on the type, nervous disorders from mild to severe; stiff joints to severe bone changes; some forms transmitted on sex chromosomes.	No effective or practical treatment available.
Porphyria: Acute intermittent (Also see METABOLISM.)	Insufficient levels of the enzyme uro-porphyrinogen I synthetase.	Disruption in porphyrin metabolism; urine changes to burgundy wine color on standing; intense abdominal colic with vomiting and nausea; neurotic or psychotic behavior; neuromuscular disturbances; actual lesions of the nerve; course of the disease variable; mortality rate high.	Unpredictable remission and expression of symptoms; no treatment uniformly successful; avoidance of estrogens and barbiturates; drugs for pain, and sedation; best prevention high carbohydrate intake; most effective treatment producing remission is glucose orally or intravenously.
Congenital erythropoietic	Insufficient levels of the enzyme uroporphyrinogen III cosynthetase.	Urinary excretion of large amounts of uroporphyrin I; mutilating skin lesions; photosensitivity; hemolytic (red blood cell bursting) anemia; pink or red urine; symptoms usually appear between birth and 5 years; teeth may turn red to reddish brown.	Avoidance of exposure to sunlight; possibly splenectomy or steroids.
Renal tubular acidosis	Disorder of membrane transport of hydrogen ion and bicarbonate by kidney tubules.	Inability of kidney to excrete an acid urine; persistent metabolic acidosis results; kidney stones; increased urinary calcium and phosphate; osteomalacia; potassium depletion.	Oral administration of sodium bicarbonate or citrate; supplemental potassium and/or calcium until body stores repleted; possibly vitamin D therapy.
Wilson's disease (hepatolenticular degeneration)	Deficient synthesis of ceruloplasmin, the copper-carrying protein of the blood.	Excess copper storage particularly in the liver, kidneys, brain, and cornea of the eye; eventually causing liver, kidney, and brain disorders and a characteristic rusty-brown ring in the cornea known as Kayser–Fleischer ring.	Early diagnosis; administration of the copper-chelating agent, D-penicillamine mobilizes copper in tissue and causes excretion in urine; sulfurated potash with meals prevents copper absorption.

INCAPARINA

A mixture of corn flour, cottonseed flour, torula yeast, minerals, and vitamins developed by the Institute of Nutrition of Central America and Panama (INCAP) with the aid of funds from Central American governments, the Kellogg Foundation, the Rockefeller Foundation, and several other foundations. It has a protein content of about 25%. Incaparina can be used as a cereal for weanling infants and young children. It was test marketed in Nicaragua, El Salvador, Guatemala, and Colombia for the treatment and prevention of protein-energy malnutrition.

(Also see CORN, Table C-45 Corn Products and Uses; MALNUTRITION, PROTEIN[S]; and PROTEIN-ENERGY.)

INCOME, PROPORTION SPENT FOR FOOD

We tend to remember the "good ole days" when a loaf of bread was 25¢ and the Saturday afternoon show was 10¢, while forgetting that our yearly income was proportionately low for the same period. It is true that the price of many things has increased, but so has the average income. Therefore, to gain a better perspective, two important questions are: (1) how long must one labor to put food on the table, and (2) what portion of our income goes for food? The answers to both of these questions determines the money left over for the other necessities and the extras of life—prosperity.

Wage earners in various countries must work longer than their U.S. counterparts to purchase the same foods. Fig. I-1 shows that laborers of North America are in an enviable position. To buy 1 lb (*454 g*) of bread, bacon, steak, pork chops, chicken, tomatoes, and butter, along with 1 dozen oranges and 1 dozen eggs, Canadians and Americans needed to work slightly less than 1½ hours. Laborers of other countries toiled from nearly 2 hours in Australia to as long as 7⅓ hours in Japan.

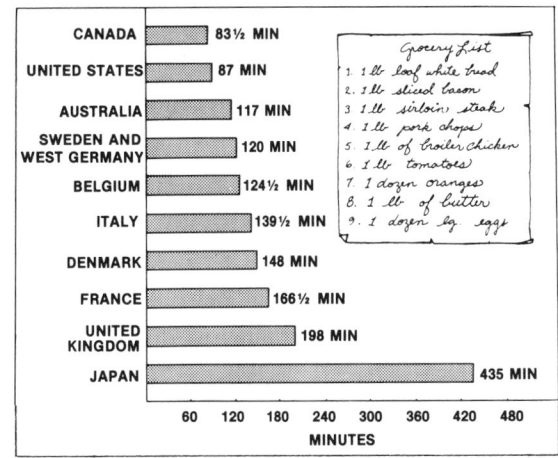

Fig. I-1. The amount of work required in various countries to earn the money necessary to purchase all of the items shown on the grocery list. *Note:* Food prices and wages of laborers in all countries change, but the work/food cost relationship remains about the same within each country. (Source of data: USDA)

As income rises, consumers spend a smaller proportion of their disposable income for food. Fig. I-2 demonstrates this general trend, worldwide.

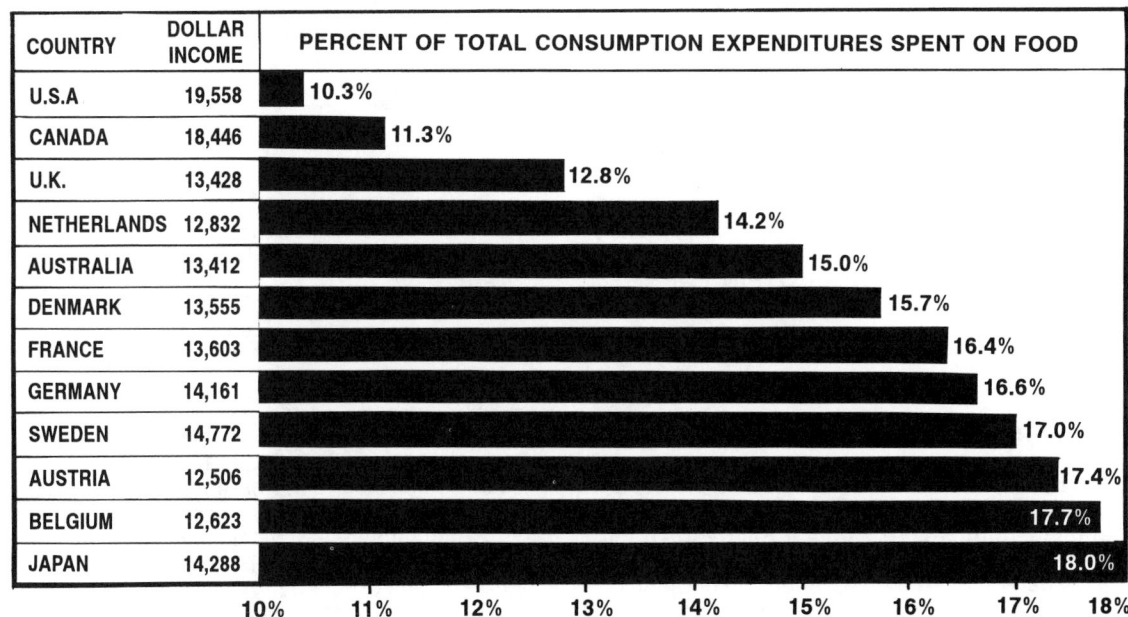

PER CAPITA GROSS DOMESTIC PRODUCT (Purchasing Power Parities)

COUNTRY	DOLLAR INCOME	PERCENT OF TOTAL CONSUMPTION EXPENDITURES SPENT ON FOOD
U.S.A	19,558	10.3%
CANADA	18,446	11.3%
U.K.	13,428	12.8%
NETHERLANDS	12,832	14.2%
AUSTRALIA	13,412	15.0%
DENMARK	13,555	15.7%
FRANCE	13,603	16.4%
GERMANY	14,161	16.6%
SWEDEN	14,772	17.0%
AUSTRIA	12,506	17.4%
BELGIUM	12,623	17.7%
JAPAN	14,288	18.0%

Fig. I-2. Proportion of income spent for food. As income rises, consumers spend a smaller proportion of their wages for food. (*Statistical Abstract of the United States 1991*, p. 843, Table 1450, 1451)

In most low income countries, consumers spend ½ or more of their income for food, whereas in the higher income countries the proportion drops to about ⅕. The data contained in Fig. I-2 shows that consumers spent the following proportion of their income for food: United States, 10.3%; Canada, 11.3%; United Kingdom, 12.8%; Netherlands, 14.2%; Australia, 15.0%; Denmark, 15.7%; France, 16.4%; W. Germany, 16.6%; Sweden, 17.0%; Austria, 17.4%; Belgium, 17.7%; and Japan, 18.0%. Food is still a bargain in some countries, notably the United States and Canada. However, even in the United States, the level of income influences the proportion of income spent for food. Table I-6 shows that within the United States, the trend is the same—the higher the income, the smaller the proportion spent for food.

As shown in Table I-6, there is a wide range in the proportion of income spent on food in the United States.

TABLE I–6
INCOME AND PERCENT OF INCOME
SPENT FOR FOOD IN THE UNITED STATES[1]

Income Group	Food as Percent of Income
Lowest 20%	39.5
Second 20%	21.9
Third 20%	15.7
Fourth 20%	13.2
Highest 20%	9.0

[1]*Statistical Abstract of the United States 1991*, Department of Commerce, p. 446, Table 718.

Worldwide, food preferences, or eating habits, change with income. The hierarchy of preferences, from lowest income to highest income is: lowest for roots and tubers, a little higher for coarse grains (corn, sorghum, etc.) for human consumption, and progressively higher for other cereals (wheat and rice), pulses (the edible seeds of leguminous crops, like peas and beans), fruits and vegetables, and animal products.

Low-income consumers spend a high proportion of their budget for direct cereal grain consumption. High-income consumers spend less of the food budget for cereals and more of it for livestock products. In the United States, consumers spend about 2.5% of their disposable income for red meat and poultry.

(Also see MALNUTRITION; PROTEIN-ENERGY; MEAT[S]; and WORLD FOOD.)

INDIGESTION

The word is rather a catchall label for a variety of disorders associated with eating. Definitions vary between sufferers. Furthermore, a doctor will try to attach a more specific diagnosis to a patient's complaint of indigestion by determining (1) the location and duration of the discomfort; (2) occurrence of the discomfort in relationship to the time of eating; and (3) the relationship of the symptoms to certain food types. Among the disorders which may be referred to as indigestion are: peptic ulcer, gastritis, gastric hyperacidity, heartburn, flatulence (gas), stomach irritation (from corticosteroid drugs, food intolerance, excessive smoking, or alcoholic stimulation), pylorospasm (spasm of the sphincter between the stomach and the small intestine), nervous dyspepsia, bleeding ulcers, colitis, hiccups, hypermotility, diverticulitis, and anxiety.

Where indigestion is caused by emotional or physiological problems rather than by organic or physical diseases or disorders, treatment often includes the following:

1. Eating meals at regular hours.
2. Eating small meals at frequent intervals, rather than large meals less frequently.
3. Eating slowly and in a relaxed atmosphere; avoiding gulping food.
4. Avoiding irritating stimulants, spicy foods, and greasy foods.
5. Drinking a glass of milk between meals.

(Also see ANTACIDS; GASTRITIS; HEARTBURN; and ULCERS, PEPTIC.)

INDISPENSABLE AMINO ACID

This phrase is synonymous to the phrase *essential amino acid*. Both phrases refer to an amino acid which the body cannot synthesize in sufficient amounts to carry out physiological functions and must, therefore, be supplied in the diet. The indispensable amino acids in the human diet are histidine, isoleucine, leucine, lysine, methionine (some used for the synthesis of cysteine), phenylalanine (some used for the synthesis of tyrosine), threonine, tryptophan, and valine.

NOTE WELL: Arginine is not regarded as indispensable for humans, whereas it is for animals; in contrast to human infants, most young mammals cannot synthesize it in sufficient amounts to meet their needs for growth.

(Also see AMINO ACID[S].)

INERT

Relatively inactive.

INFANT ALLERGY

In infants the prime concern is *food* allergies. Symptoms such as wheezing, coughing, running nose, colic, vomiting, diarrhea, constipation, rash, or eczema may suggest an allergy—an unusual or exaggerated response to a particular substance called an allergen. Major food offenders are milk, eggs, wheat, corn, legumes, nuts and seafoods. The offending food, allergen, should be identified and eliminated from the diet. Dietary history, skin test, provocative food test, elimination diets and pulse tests are all useful for identifying the causative food. Fortunately, children tend to outgrow food allergies. Foods known to have caused reactions in infancy may be tried months or years later when perhaps they can be taken with impunity.

(Also see ALLERGIES.)

INFANT ANEMIA

Anemia during infancy, a frequent occurrence, is closely related to the body iron stores at birth. Pregnant women may have an insufficient intake of iron, thus, the newborn infant may develop anemia early in the first year of life. Also, infants (1) born prematurely, (2) of low birth weight, (3) of multiple births, or (4) whose mothers have had several pregnancies are most likely to have inadequate iron reserves at birth. Furthermore, infants are apt to develop iron deficiency anemia because milk has a low iron content and babies are just not born with sufficient iron to meet their needs beyond 6 months. Infant anemia may also be caused by gastrointestinal bleeding due to the ingestion of homogenized milk, infections, diarrhea, or a hemolytic disease.

Clinical features of iron deficiency anemia are the impairment of general health and vitality, paleness of the skin and mucous membranes, and a hemoglobin concentration less than 11g/100 ml of blood.

Appropriate measures should be taken to insure that infants have a daily dietary iron intake of 6 mg from birth to 6 months of age, and of 10 mg from 6 to 12 months of age.

(Also see ANEMIA; and IRON.)

INFANT DIET AND NUTRITION

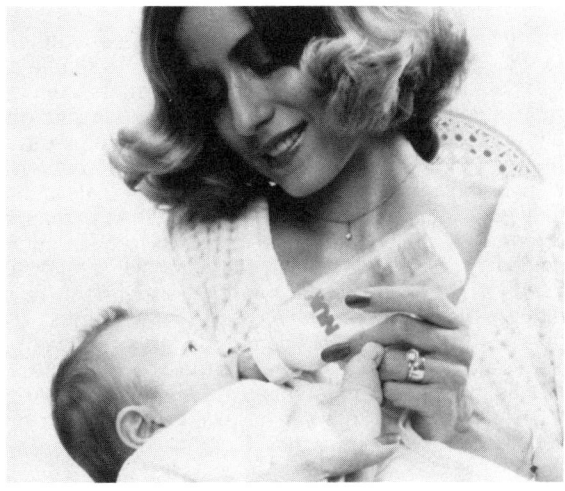

Fig. I-3. Infant being bottle fed. (Courtesy, Gerber Products Company)

The future of each society depends to some extent on how its infants are fed since it is difficult to repair later the damage done by chronic malnutrition in the very young. Furthermore, there are ever increasing numbers of infants in the developing countries which have long had shortages of food. Therefore, economical and efficient infant feeding is a matter of worldwide concern.

HISTORY. It is not known for certain how the breast feeding of infants was supplemented in prehistoric times, since the remains of food found by archaeologists usually tell us what a group of people ate, but they do not always tell how it was allotted to individuals. What is known is that a wide variety of animal and plant foods were obtained by hunting, fishing, and gathering. Furthermore, modern day aborigines, whose modes of living are similar to those of prehistoric nomadic peoples, often eat a larger variety of foods than contemporary subsistence farmers in the developing countries. For example, Australian aborigines wean their babies on honey, turtle eggs, fish, meat, fruits, and vegetables.[1]

On the other hand, the peasants in the densely populated ancient agricultural societies depended mainly on cereal grains, starchy roots and tubers, legumes, vegetables, and only occasionally on some animal foods. Some of the ancient rural peoples may have benefited nutritionally from the raising of livestock, although it is difficult to determine the extent to which eggs, meat, milk, or poultry were used in the feeding of weanling infants. The contemporary counterparts of these early societies rely heavily on products made from cereal grains, such as watery gruels and doughy masses that are literally pushed down an infant's throat.

[1]Robson, J. R. K., "Foods from the Past, Lessons for the Future," *The Professional Nutritionist*, Vol. 8, Spring 1976, pp. 13-15.

In ancient times the failure of a mother to have an adequate supply of breast milk often meant death of her infant unless another lactating female was available as a wet nurse. Occasionally, attempts were made to have infants suckle asses, cows, goats, sheep, dogs, and other animals as evidenced by the story that Romulus and Remus (Romulus was the legendary first King of Rome) were nursed by a she wolf. Of course, the female animals may have been milked and the milk given to babies, but the method of feeding was likely to have been accompanied by contamination with microorganisms that cause deadly diarrheal disease in infants. Furthermore, animal milks differ in composition from human milk. It is noteworthy, that of all the common species of livestock, mares have milk which is closest in characteristics to human milk. The Mongol tribes that roamed the steppes of Central Asia are known to have consumed mare's milk, but it is not known whether it was given to infants.

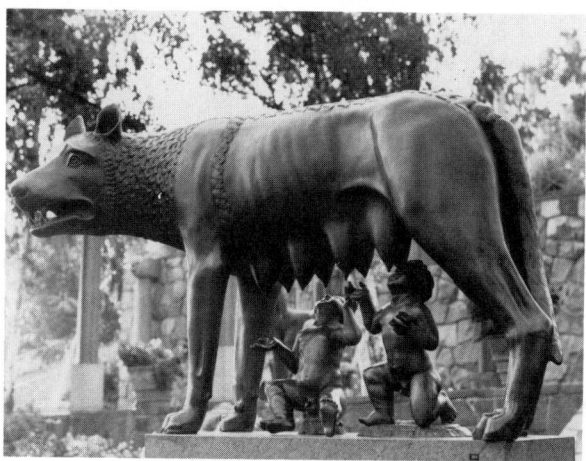

Fig. I-4. She wolf suckling Romulus and Remus. Bronze sculpture by Carl Milles, in Milles Garden, Stockholm, Sweden. (Photo by A. H. Ensminger)

By the beginning of the 19th century, the search for ways to use animals' milks safely in infant feeding became almost desperate, because the practices of wet nurses in the urban societies endangered the health of the infants they fed. Contamination of cow's milk with harmful bacteria had been a problem for ages and the feeding devices (pitchers or pots with long spouts) left much to be desired. However, glass bottles fitted with tanned heifer's teats were introduced in the early 1800s. Nipples made of cork or wood were also used. Another achievement of that era was the development of the first safe canning process by the Frenchman, Nicolas Appert, in 1810. Unfortunately, many years passed and countless

infants died before these inventions were utilized in suitable feeding procedures. There were still great gaps in the knowledge of microbial growth, and of the significant differences in the chemical compositions and physical characteristics of human milk vs cow's milk.

The first major advances in the "humanization" of cow's milk were made around the middle of the 19th century by the great German chemist Justus von Liebig who showed by chemical analyses that cow's milk was considerably higher in protein and lower in carbohydrate than human milk. Shortly thereafter, he developed an infant formula that was a mixture of an extract of malt flour and liquid whole cow's milk. The main shortcoming of this product was that it spoiled readily. It is noteworthy that Nestle of Switzerland started the infant formula industry in 1867, when they produced a dried "milk food" mixture made from milk and malted wheat. Later, William Horlick, who had come to the United States from England, also utilized the principles of Liebig's formula in his invention of malted milk powder, which was patented in 1883.

Meanwhile, other developments for coping with the perishability of fresh milk were (1) the production of sweetened condensed milk, which was invented by Gail Borden in the 1850s; and (2) the pasteurization of milk, a process that had been first used in the 1870s by the French scientist Louis Pasteur to preserve wines from spoilage. The first commercial production of evaporated milk began in 1885 at the Helvetia Milk Condensing Company of Highland, Illinois, which later became the Pet Milk Company. Fourteen years later, evaporated milk was produced on the West Coast by the Pacific Coast Condensed Milk Plant of Kent, Washington—which later became the Carnation Company.

The prevention of the bacterial contamination of milk by pasteurization had its shortcomings in that the vitamin C content became almost negligible and infants developed scurvy. It was not until the late 1920s and early 1930s that the role of vitamin C in the prevention of scurvy was clarified. After that, mothers were told to supplement their infant's diet with orange juice. Rickets was also a common affliction of infants until cod-liver oil was given in the winter months. (Pure vitamin D was isolated in 1932.)

Canning did not become an important means of preserving vegetables until the early 1900s, after researchers at the Massachusetts Institute of Technology devised means of killing heat-resistant bacteria. However, mothers who wished to prepare vegetables for infant feeding had to mash canned or home-cooked items through a pureeing cone or a sieve to remove the fibrous matter which had a laxative effect. Then, in 1928 Dan Gerber started the Gerber Baby Foods Division of the Fremont Canning Company (located in Fremont, Michigan) after his wife asked if canned pureed vegetables could be produced commercially. The birth of the baby food industry led eventually to the production of a wide variety of baked products, cereals, desserts, fruits, meats, and vegetables.

The ready availability of canned evaporated milk led to its extensive use in infant feeding. Usually, it was diluted with water and sweetened with corn syrup, lactose, and/or sugar. Preprepared mixtures called "formulas" came into widespread use in the 1920s, but many mothers found it more economical to prepare the feedings from evaporated milk and store them in nursing bottles in an ice box or a refrigerator. However, commercially prepared formulas became more popular in the 1940s when many mothers went to work to help the war effort.

During World War II, breads, cereals and milk were fortified with essential vitamins and minerals (mainly calcium, iron, vitamin A, vitamin D, thiamin, riboflavin, and niacin). British nutritionists noted that some children developed vitamin D toxicity, and advised the food technologists and government agencies to reduce the amount of vitamin D fortification after the war ended. However, there was a rise in the incidences of rickets in the large cities of northern England and Scotland during the 1950s, which attested to the dangers of inadequate consumption of the vitamin.

Aid to the needy nations of the world was a major part of American foreign policy in the 1950s, as exemplified by the Marshall Plan under President Truman and the Food for Peace program under President Eisenhower. Grains and nonfat dry milk were shipped to various parts of the world for the relief of impoverished people. Vegetable oils were generally used in skim milk formulas to provide the fat that would have been supplied by whole milk. When the cost of nonfat dry milk rose sharply during the 1960s and 1970s, nutritionists developed infant foods that were mixtures of cereal and legume flours fortified with essential minerals and vitamins.

Meanwhile, the cholesterol scare in the United States was one of the factors that led to the growing use of infant formulas containing nonfat dry milk and vegetable oils that were similar to those used in the developing countries. However, it was found that a few premature infants developed severe vitamin E deficiencies when fed the products that were rich in the polyunsaturated fatty acids present in certain oils. Hence, many formulas were fortified with vitamin E and other micronutrients deemed to be essential. Also, formulas based upon soybean substitutes for milk were developed for infants with milk allergies.

Today, there are a large variety of infant formulas that are considered to be nutritionally complete for infants up to age one, although American pediatricians generally recommend that the feeding of supplemental foods start between 3 and 6 months of age. Also, great progress has been made in the widespread application of nutritional and sanitary principles to infant feeding during the 20th century, as evidenced by the sharp drop in infant mortality shown in Fig. I-5.

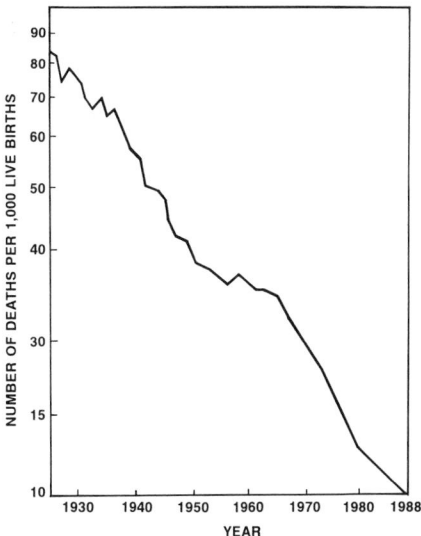

Fig. I-5. Infant mortality in the United States from 1925 to 1988. (Source: *Health, United States*, U.S. Department HEW, p. 345, Table CD. II.1, and *Statistical Abstract of the United States*, 1991, U.S. Department of Commerce, p. 78, Table 114)

GROWTH AND DEVELOPMENT OF INFANTS.

From a nutritional standpoint, a knowledge of normal infant growth and development is useful for gauging the adequacy of nutrient consumption. Growth that is too slow suggests (1) that the diet is nutritionally inadequate, or (2) that there is an impairment(s) in the utilization of food by the body. Excessively rapid growth may lead to obesity, which increases the likelihood of later development of cardiovascular diseases, diabetes, and high blood pressure. However, measurement of growth alone does not tell the whole story, since infants with normal growth may have abnormalities of certain functions due to nutritional deficiencies or excesses, inherited tendencies, congenital defects, or certain illnesses. Some of the most commonly used means of assessing growth and development follow.

Measurement of Growth. Although there are various procedures for determining the growth of bone, fatty tissue, and muscle, the measurement of height and weight is most readily accomplished as follows:

• **Height**—For infants, this measurement is the head to foot length of the subject in the recumbent position, as shown in Fig. I-6.

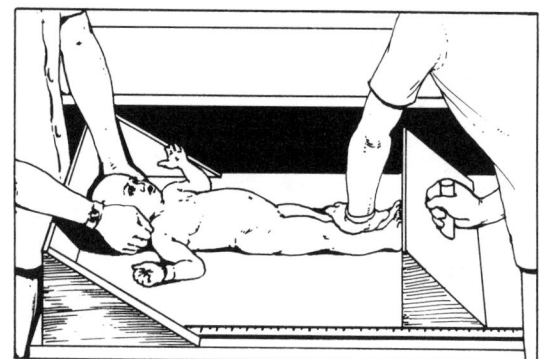

Fig. I-6.   Measurement of an infant's length with the apparatus that is commonly used by pediatricians.

In this procedure, one person holds the infant's head so that its eyes are looking upward and applies gentle traction to bring the top of the head into contact with the fixed headboard. A second person holds the infant's feet, knees, and hips completely extended with the toes pointing upward, and while applying gentle traction, brings the movable footboard to rest against the infant's heels. The length may be read on the scale that runs the length of the apparatus. Measurement of length should be made to the nearest ¼ in. (or *0.5 cm*).

•**Weight**—Measurements of weight of infants are preferably made with the subjects unclothed. Weight should be recorded to the nearest ¼ lb (or *0.1 kg*).

The most recently published standard growth curves for infants are those from the National Center for Health Statistics (NCHS). Data from plotting the curves was obtained in a study conducted by Fels Research Institute of Yellow Springs, Ohio in which 867 children were measured from birth to 3 years of age. The curves are presented in Figs. I-7 through I-10.

To use the growth curves shown in Figs. I-7 through I-10, it is necessary to determine the percentile which corresponds most closely to the data from the infant that was measured. A simple procedure follows:

1.   Locate and mark the height or weight of the infant on the vertical scale in the left margin of the appropriate chart. If the value of the measurement falls between the values marked on the scale, its placement should be estimated as accurately as possible.

2.   With the aid of a ruler draw a light, horizontal line across the chart, starting from the marked value for height or weight.

3.   Using a procedure similar to step 1 (above), locate

²*NCHS Growth Curves for Children, Birth–18 Years, United States*, U.S. Department of HEW.

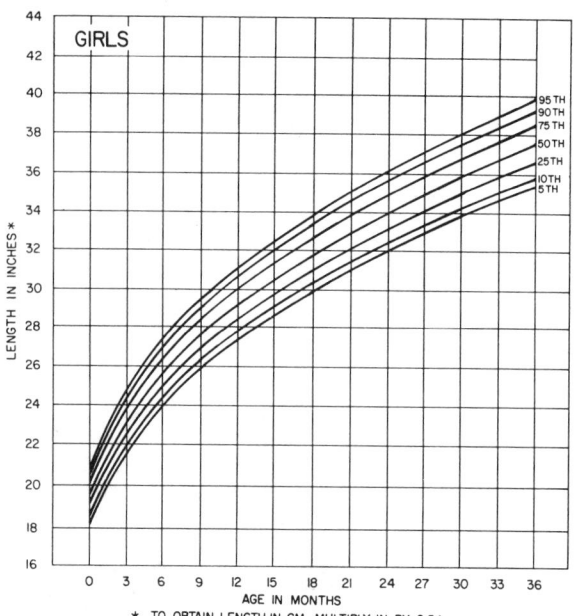

Fig. I-7. Lengths (heights) of girls by age percentiles from birth to 36 months. (Source: *NCHS Growth Curves for Children, Birth–18 Years, United States*, U.S. Department of HEW)

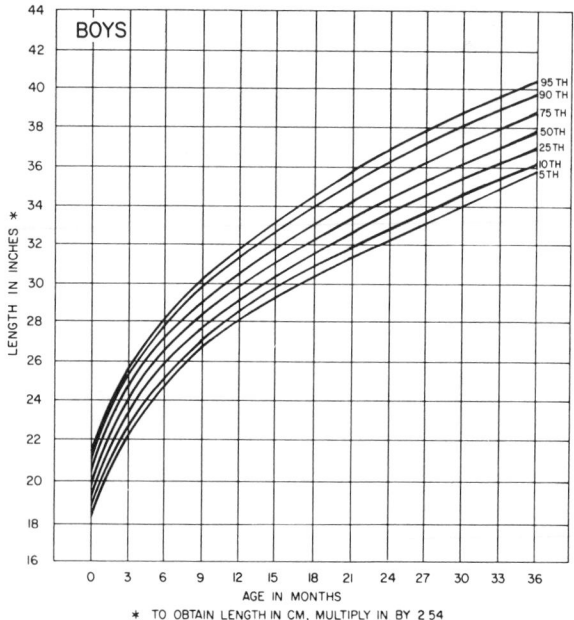

Fig. I-8. Lengths (heights) of boys by age percentiles from birth to 36 months. (Source: *NCHS Growth Curves for Children, Birth–18 Years, United States*, U.S. Department of HEW)

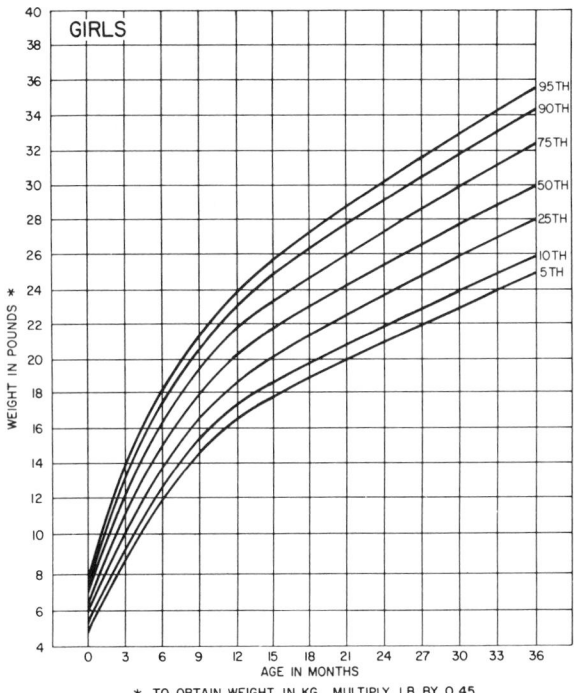

Fig. I-9. Weights of girls by age percentiles from birth to 36 months. (Source: *NCHS Growth Curves for Children, Birth–18 Years, United States*, U.S. Department of HEW)

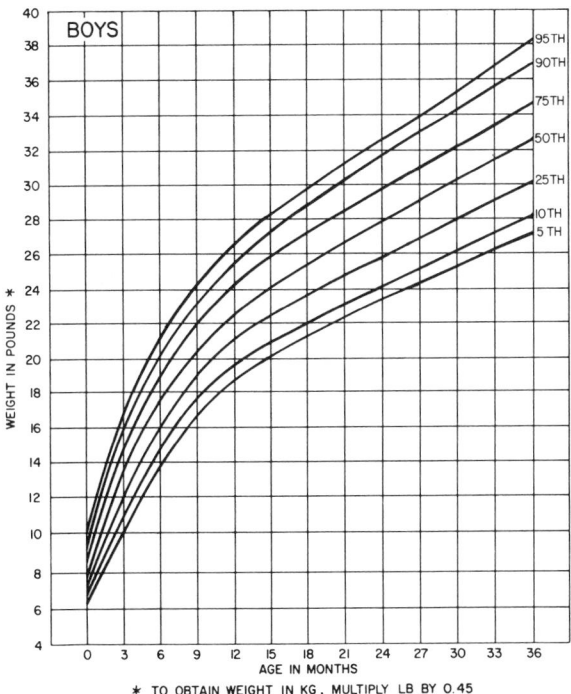

Fig. I-10. Weights of boys by age percentiles from birth to 36 months. (Source: *NCHS Growth Curves for Children, Birth–18 Years, United States*, U.S. Department of HEW)

and mark the age of the child on the horizontal scale at the bottom of the chart.

4. Draw a vertical line on the chart, starting from the marked value for age.

5. Circle the point at which the horizontal and vertical lines intersect on the chart and note the percentile curve which is closest to the intersection.

Values which fall between the 5th and 95th percentiles are considered to be within the normal range. However, there should not be a wide discrepancy between the percentiles for height and weight. Sometimes, a pediatrician will not diagnose and treat an otherwise healthy infant until a clear-cut trend of growth abnormality is indicated by measurements taken at 2 or more consecutive monthly or bimonthly visits. Some typical interpretations of deviant growth measurements follow:

• **Short height for age, or low weight for age or height** —A low value of height for age suggests the possibility of an acute or chronic illness or a nutritional deficiency. This may also be the case when height for age is above the 10th percentile but weight for height is less than the 5th percentile. It is likely that any illness of sufficient severity to cause notable weight loss will result in a decrease in the ratio of weight to height.

When measurements of height (or length) and weight have been made before the time of the current evaluation, they should be analyzed to determine the past rate of growth. When feasible, the child should be followed with sequential measurements so that rate of growth (more sensitive than single measurements in detecting abnormalities) may be recorded.

• **Excess weight for age, or height**—In the case of infants with weight for age or length greater than the 95th percentile, the emphasis should be placed on avoiding further excessive weight gain. With a caloric intake of approximately 40 to 43 kcal/lb/day (*90 to 95 kcal/kg/day*), one may anticipate that gain in fat-free tissue will continue at a normal rate, whereas increase in body content of fat will not occur or will occur only at a slow rate. The major aim should be directed to the correction of any patterns of overeating that may have been associated with the previous abnormal gain in weight.

It is noteworthy that the measurement of weight gain has the weakness of not indicating the composition of the gain. For example, the building up of body protein in muscle is accompanied by 3 to 4 parts of water to 1 of protein, whereas fat deposition is not accompanied by water and is much higher in caloric value than muscle tissue.

Other Means of Assessing Infant Development and Nutritional Status. The measurement of growth is only part of the assessment of infant development. Pediatricians also look for signs of inherited or congenital disorders and nutritional deficiencies. For example, special attention is paid to general features such as pallor, apathy, and irritability. Similarly, the skin is examined carefully for signs of scurvy and the skeletal system for the signs of rickets. These and other telltale signs that a doctor looks for are given in Table I-7.

TABLE I-7
PHYSICAL SIGNS OF GOOD OR POOR NUTRITION IN INFANTS[1]

Area of Body Examined	Normal Appearance of Well-Nourished Babies	Common Signs of Poor Nutrition
Appearance in general	Normal weight for age, sex, and height. Alert and responsive to stimulation. No waterlogging of tissues (edema).	Significant overweight or underweight. Lack of response to stimuli; hyperirritable. Loss or slowness of ankle or knee reflexes. Flesh fails to rebound promptly when pressed in with a finger (pitting edema).
Eyes	Shiny and free from areas of abnormal pigmentation, opacity, bloodshot areas, and dryness.	Paleness, dryness, redness, or pigmentation of membranes (conjunctiva). Foamy patches on conjunctiva (Bitot's spots). Dullness, softness, or bloodshot areas on the cornea. Redness or fissures on eyelids.
Face	Skin is clear and uniform in color, free of all except minor blemishes, and free of swollen or lumpy areas.	Skin has lighter (depigmentation) and darker (over cheeks and under eyes) areas. Greasy scales around nose and lips. Swollen or lumpy areas.
Glands	No swollen areas on face or neck.	Swelling of parotids (enlarged "jowls") or thyroid (front of neck near its base).
Gums	Red, free from bleeding or swelling.	Receded. "Spongy" and bleeding. Swelling of the gingiva.
Hair	Shiny, firmly attached to scalp (not easily plucked without pain to patient).	Dullness, may be brittle and easily plucked without pain. Some areas are lighter in color than others.
Lips	Smooth, not chapped, cracked, or swollen.	Swollen, red, or cracked (cheilosis). Angular fissures and/or scars at the corners of the mouth.
Muscles	Muscles are firm and of normal size.	Wasting and flabbiness of muscle. Bleeding into muscle.
Nails	Firm, pink.	Spoon-shaped nails. Brittle and ridged nails.
Organs, internal	Normal heart rate and rhythm. Normal blood pressure. Internal organs cannot be palpated (except the liver in children).	Racing heartbeat (over 100 beats per minute). Abnormal rhythm of heart. High blood pressure. Palpable enlargement of liver or spleen.
Skeleton	Bones have normal sizes and shapes.	Softening, swelling, or distorted shapes of bones and joints.
Skin	Smooth, free of rashes, swellings, and discoloration.	Roughness (follicular hyperkeratosis), dryness, or flakiness. Irregular pigmentation, black and blue marks, "crazy pavement" lesions. Symmetrical, reddened lesions (like sunburn). Looseness of skin (lack of subcutaneous fat).
Teeth	Enamel is unbroken and unspotted. None or a few small cavities.	Caries. Mottled or darkened areas of enamel.
Tongue	Normal size of papillae (no atrophy or hypertrophy). Color is uniform and deep red. Sense of taste is without impairment.	Atrophy of papillae (the tongue is smooth) or hypertrophy of papillae. Irregularly shaped and distributed white patches. Swollen, scarlet, magenta (purple colored), or raw tongue.

[1]Adapted by the authors from *American Journal of Public Health*, Vol. 63, November 1973 Supplement, p. 19, Table 1.

Any potentially important abnormality that is detected by physical examination usually requires confirmation by laboratory tests, x ray, or other means such as (1) measurement of hemoglobin concentration or hematocrit when anemia is suspected, and (2) x rays of bones if signs of rickets are present.

(Also see BERIBERI; MALNUTRITION; MALNUTRITION, PROTEIN-ENERGY; RICKETS; and SCURVY.)

NUTRIENT REQUIREMENTS. A growing infant usually triples its birth weight within the first year and has high nutrient needs in proportion to its size. Fortunately, much more is now known about infant requirements than was ever known before. Hence, the Food and Nutrition Board of the National Academy of Sciences-National Research Council has established the nutrient allowances for infants that are given in Table I-8.

TABLE I–8
MEAN HEIGHTS AND WEIGHTS AND RECOMMENDED NUTRIENT INTAKES FOR INFANTS[1]

Category	Age	
	(0–6 mo)	(6 mo–1 yr)
Weight . . . . lb *(kg)*	13 *(6)*	20 *(9)*
Height . . . . in. *(cm)*	24 *(60)*	28 *(71)*
Energy . . . . kcal	650	850
Protein . . . . g	13	14
Minerals		
Calcium . . . . mg	400	600
Phosphorus . . . . mg	300	500
Sodium . . . . . . mg	120	200
Chloride . . . . . . mg	180	300
Magnesium . . . . mg	40	60
Potassium . . . . . mg	500	700
Chromium [2,3] . . . . mcg	10–40	20–60
Copper [2,3] . . . . . mg	0.4–0.6	0.6–0.7
Fluoride [2,3] . . . . . mg	0.1–0.5	0.2–1.0
Iodine . . . . mcg	40	50
Iron . . . . mg	6	10
Manganese [2,3] . . . . mg	0.3–0.6	0.6–1.0
Molybdenum [2,3] . . . mcg	15–30	20–40
Selenium [3] . . . . . mcg	10	15
Zinc . . . . mg	5	5
Vitamins, fat-soluble		
Vitamin A . . . . RE	375	375
Vitamin D . . . . . . mcg	7.5	10
Vitamin E . . . mg α TE	3	4
Vitamin K [2,3] . . . . mcg	5	10
Vitamins, water-soluble		
Biotin . . . . mcg	10	15
Folate . . . . mcg	25	35
Niacin . . . . mg	5	6
Pantothenic acid . . mg	2	3
Riboflavin . . . . mg	0.4	0.5
Thiamin . . . . mg	0.3	0.4
Vitamin B-6 . . . . . mg	0.3	0.6
Vitamin B-12 . . . . mcg	0.3	0.5
Vitamin C . . . . . . mg	30	35

[1]*Recommended Dietary Allowances*, 10th ed., 1989, NRC–National Academy of Sciences.
[2]Because there is less information on which to base allowances, these figures are given in the form of ranges of recommended intakes.
[3]Since the toxic levels for many trace elements may be only several times usual intakes, the upper values of the range should not be habitually exceeded.

The allowances shown in Table I-8 were calculated as follows:

• **Birth to 6 months of age**—These values were obtained by estimating the amounts of nutrients received by thriving breast-fed infants of healthy mothers. In certain cases, greater amounts were allowed to cover the infants fed by formulas that contain nutrients in forms that are not as well utilized as those in breast milk.

• **Six months to 1 year**—The values for this age bracket were based upon the assumption that many infants were fed evaporated milk and/or formulas plus increasing amounts of solid foods. Hence, some of the allowances are greater than actual requirements in order to compensate for less than optimal utilization.

It is not expected that mothers will use Table I-8 to make frequent checks on the nutrient compositions of their infants' diets, but rather that they will use it for guidance in selecting (1) fortified infant formulas and cereals, and (2) mineral and vitamin supplements.

(Also see NUTRIENTS: REQUIREMENTS, ALLOWANCES, FUNCTIONS.)

FOODS AND FEEDING. Few subjects outside of politics and religion generate as much controversy as the selection of foods for infant feeding. Hence, the merits and demerits of the various alternatives are noteworthy.

Breast Feeding Vs Bottle Feeding. About 350,000 babies are born around the world daily to face a very uncertain future while the partisans of these feeding systems argue over which one is best.[3] Few people on either side would deny that for the young infant up to age 6 months, breast feeding offers advantages such as (1) convenience for mothers who are able to remain near to their babies, (2) extension of the infertile period between births, (3) partial protection of the infant against diarrheal disease caused by microorganisms such as *Salmonella*, *Shigella*, and pathogenic strains of *E. coli*, and (4) physical and psychological bonding between the mother and infant. These and other benefits are detailed elsewhere.

(Also see BREAST FEEDING.)

INFANT FORMULAS. At this point it should be noted that modern infant formulas represent the latest in a long series of humanitarian efforts to save babies when breast-feeding is not feasible. Some anthropologists believe that in prehistoric nomadic societies, babies that failed to thrive at their mothers' breast were allowed to die.[4] Perhaps it was in the early agricultural societies that the first attempts were made to develop substitutes for breast milk. For example, the Chinese have long used milklike products made from soybeans and a vegetable soup fortified with egg yolk, whereas in 16th-century England orphaned infants were strapped to the bellies of asses so they might suckle.[5]

Excellent results have been obtained with the modern types of mineral and vitamin fortified infant formulas when (1) the prices of the products are affordable by the customers, (2) feedings are prepared with safe water under sanitary conditions according to the manufac-

[3]Edson, L., "Babies in Poverty—The Real Victims of the Breast/Bottle Controversy," *The Lactation Review*, Vol. IV, 1979, pp. 20-38.

[4]Raphael, D., "Of Mothers and Mothering—Remembrances by Margaret Mead," *The Lactation Review*, Vol. IV, 1979, pp. 5-18.

[5]Edson, L. "Babies in Poverty—The Real Victims of the Breast/Bottle Controversy," *The Lactation Review*, Vol. IV, 1979, pp. 20-38.

turer's instructions, and (3) unused portions of formula in opened cans are stored in a refrigerator. Unfortunately, these conditions are not met in certain "poverty pockets" within the developed countries, nor are they likely to be met in many of the Third World countries. Hence, it might be a good idea for the formula companies to develop nonperishable supplements which could be used along with the low cost indigenous foods of each country. Nevertheless, even these products will have limited usefulness unless the educational levels and living conditions of the disadvantaged families are improved.

NOTE: Although many families have fed their infants fresh pasteurized cow's milk, this practice may be harmful because (1) the protein in the milk may not be digested

well, and (2) there is evidence that this type of milk often hastens the development of iron deficiency anemia because it has been found to induce the loss of blood from the gastrointestinal tract in about 50% of the infants who developed anemia. Boiling the milk renders the protein more digestible and reduces the likelihood of blood loss. However, it may be advisable to use either diluted evaporated milk or a commercial formula, rather than fresh homogenized milk, for infant feeding. This matter is still controversial. Therefore, the authors recommend that mothers consult their pediatricians for recommendations regarding the most suitable forms of milk or infant formulas.

Nutrient composition of breast milk, cow's milk, and some typical commercial infant formulas are given in Table I-9.

TABLE I–9
NUTRIENT ALLOWANCES VS. COMPOSITIONS OF SELECTED MILKS AND INFANT FORMULAS

Nutrient	Recommended Intakes for Infants Aged 0 to 6 mo.[1]	Nutrient Composition of Milk or Ready-to-Serve Infant Formula[2]				
		Human Milk[3]	Cow's Milk, Whole, Undiluted[3]	Milk Base Formula[4]	Soy Base Formula[4]	Meat Base Formula[4]
	(per day)	(per qt)	(per qt)	(per qt)	(per qt)	(per qt)
Calories . . . . kcal	650	833	824	645	632	615
Carbohydrates . . . . g	—	66	45	69	64	59
Fats . . . . g	—	36	36	34	32	31
Proteins . . . . g	13	11	31	15	24	27
Macrominerals:						
Calcium . . . . mg	400	322	1,192	484	748	926
Phosphorus . . . . . mg	300	151	936	370	502	615
Sodium . . . . mg	120	142	548	208	398	170
Magnesium . . . . . . mg	40	38	123	39	70	38
Potassium . . . . mg	500	473	1,308	665	700	359
Microminerals:						
Copper . . . . mg	0.4–0.6	0.4	0.3	0.4	0.6	0.4
Iron . . . . .mg	6	2	1.2	11	12	13
Zinc . . . . mg	5	6.2	3.3	5	5	—
Fat-Soluble Vitamins:						
Vitamin A . . . . .mcg RE	375	537	291	711	476	495
Vitamin D . . . . .mcg	7.5	0.5	0.3	9.5	10	11
Vitamin E . . . . mg α TE	3	1.7	0.4	14	10	6
Water-Soluble Vitamins:						
Biotin . . . . .mcg	10	3.8	33	—	51	—
Folate . . . . .mcg	25	2.1	2.7	47	102	25
Niacin . . . . mg	5	1.6	0.8	7	8	7
Pantothenic acid . . mg	2	1.9	3.3	3	3	2
Riboflavin . . . . mg	0.4	0.5	1.5	0.9	0.6	0.9
Thiamin . . . . mg	0.3	0.1	0.4	0.6	0.5	0.6
Vitamin B-6 . . . . . . mg	0.3	0.1	0.4	0.4	0.4	0.8
Vitamin B-12 . . . . .mcg	0.3	0.3	3.8	1.4	1.9	7.6
Vitamin C . . . . mg	30	42	17	52	51	56

[1]*Recommended Dietary Allowances*, 10th rev. ed., 1989, NRC–National Academy of Sciences.
[2]To convert to amount per liter, multiply by 0.95.
[3]Based upon data in Toverud, K. U., *et al., Maternal Nutrition and Child Health, An Interpretive Review*, National Academy of Sciences.
[4]Based upon data from the manufacturers.

It may be noted from Table I-9 that both human milk and cow's milk are low in certain minerals and vitamins, whereas, the commercial infant formulas provide levels of these nutrients that are close to the recommended intakes. Furthermore, cow's milk is exceptionally high in protein and mineral salts, and may stress the ability of the young infant's kidneys to rid the body of the waste products of metabolism. Nevertheless, undiluted cow's milk is a suitable food for infant feeding after supplemental foods have been introduced, provided that the infant receives sufficient water.

Usually, doctors recommend milk base formulas for infants. However, a few infants are allergic to cow's milk, as evidenced by the continuous or frequent occurrence of symptoms such as asthma, colds, colic, constipation, coughing, diarrhea, eczema, poor weight gain, runny nose, spitting up, and vomiting. In such cases, the pediatrician may put the baby on a soy base formula without conducting the usual tests for allergy, since elimination of the symptoms on the substituted formula confirm the diagnosis. Sometimes, babies are also allergic to soy base formulas and are given a meat base formula because the latter type of preparation is the least likely to provoke an allergic response.

Supplemental foods. Some of the advocates of breast feeding have advised against the early introduction of supplemental foods on the grounds that it might tend to discourage the baby from nursing. Therefore, it is noteworthy that the noted anthropologist Margaret Mead observed nursing mothers who fed their infants a wide variety of supplemental foods soon after birth.[6] She

thought that early supplementation (by about 3 months of age) was a good practice because (1) it alleviated some of the physical and emotional strain on the mother when the baby was growing rapidly and developing a large appetite, and (2) the mother was more likely to be able to continue breast-feeding when she was secure in the belief that her infant was contented and doing well. Furthermore, some supplementation is desirable because breast milk is low in protein, minerals, and vitamins.

The supplemental foods that are most commonly utilized in the United States are baby cereals; egg yolks; orange juice; and pureed fruits, meats, and vegetables. Guidelines for using these foods are given in the next section.

Guidelines for Infant Feeding. Mothers who can afford supplemental foods are more likely to err on the side of feeding too much rather than too little. For example, a survey which was conducted during the early 1970s by the research center of a baby foods manufacturer showed that (1) mothers fed their infants about the right amount of calories, and (2) the youngest group of infants was fed an average of 1½ times the recommended protein allowance, and the oldest group was given 2½ times the allowance.[7] However, the dietary content of iron was low because the use of iron-enriched products declined sharply after the infants reached 6 months of age. Hence, the liquids and solid foods fed to infants should be selected carefully in order to avoid giving them too much of some nutrients and too little of others. A typical feeding schedule is given in Table I-10.

[6]Raphael, D., "Margaret Mead—A Tribute," *The Lactation Review,* Vol, IV, 1979, pp. 1-3.

[7]Purvis, G. A., "What Nutrients Do Our Infants Really Get?," *Nutrition Today,* Vol. 8, September-October 1973, pp. 28-34.

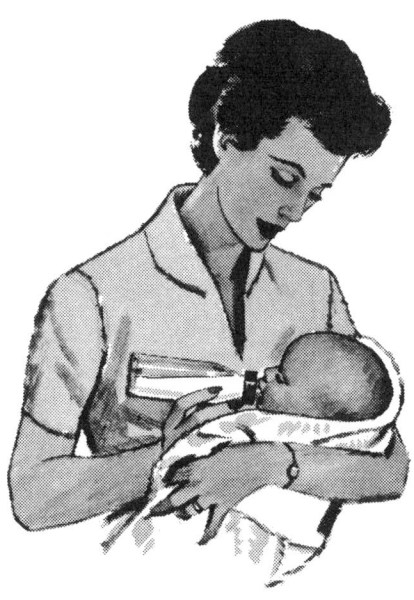

TABLE I-10
SUGGESTED PLAN FOR FEEDING NORMAL, HEALTHY INFANTS DURING THE FIRST YEAR[1]

Time of the Day	1st Month	2nd & 3rd Months	4th & 5th Months	6th & 7th Months	8th & 9th Months	12 Months
2 a.m.	Breast milk or 3 to 4 oz (90 to 120 ml) of formula ----------------▶	—	—	—	—	—
6 a.m.	Breast milk or 3 to 4 oz (90 to 120 ml) of formula ----------------▶		5 to 6 oz (150 to 180 ml) formula[2]	7 to 8 oz (210 to 240 ml) formula[2]	1 cup (240 ml) of whole milk	—
8 a.m.	1 oz (30 ml) orange juice mixed with 3 oz (90 ml) of water. Mineral and vitamin supplement[3] ----------	2 oz (60 ml) orange juice mixed with 2 oz (60 ml) of water.	3 to 4 oz (150 to 180 ml) orange juice or equivalent in vitamin C fortified strained fruit ----------------▶ 2 to 4 oz (60 to 120 ml) of cooled boiled water --------▶			1 cup (240 ml) of whole milk (may be given later). ½ cup (120 ml) fruit or fruit juice. 1 to 2 oz (30 to 60 g) of iron and vitamin enriched bread, dry cereal, muffins, pancakes, toast, or waffles.
10 a.m.	Breast milk or 3 to 4 oz (90 to 120 ml) of formula ----------------▶		5 to 6 oz (150 to 180 ml) formula[2]. ½ to 1 oz (15 to 30 g) infant cereal.	7 to 8 oz (210 to 240 ml) formula[2]. 1 to 2 oz (30 to 60 g) infant cereal, teething biscuits, or toast -▶	1 cup (240 ml) of whole milk	Milk, juice, water,[4] and/or bread or cereal (little or no food is needed if a hearty breakfast was eaten).
12 noon	—	1 to 4 oz (30 to 120 ml) of cooled boiled water (more may be needed in a hot environment) ----▶			½ to 1 cup (120 to 240 ml) water	1 to 2 oz (30 to 60 g) of cottage cheese or yogurt, egg (whole), fish, meat, poultry, or mashed cooked beans or peas. 1 cup (240 ml) of whole milk (may be given later). 1 to 2 oz (30 to 60 g) fruit or vegetable.
2 p.m.	Breast milk or 3 to 4 oz (90 to 120 ml) of formula ----------------▶		5 to 6 oz (150 to 180 ml) formula[2]. 1 to 2 oz (30 to 60 g) strained vegetable ------------	7 to 8 oz (210 to 240 ml) formula[2]. 1 oz (30 g) of cottage cheese, or yogurt, egg yolk, meat, or poultry. --------▶	1 cup (240 ml) of whole milk.	Milk, juice, water,[4] and/or bread or cereal (little or no food is needed if a hearty lunch was eaten).
6 p.m.	Breast milk or 3 to 4 oz (90 to 120 ml) of formula ----------------▶		5 to 6 oz (150 to 180 ml) formula[2]. ½ to 1 oz (15 to 30 g) infant cereal. 1 to 2 oz (30 to 60 g) strained fruit or vegetable --------▶	7 to 8 oz (210 to 240 ml) formula[2]. 1 to 2 oz (30 to 60 g) infant cereal, teething biscuits, or toast -▶	1 cup (240 ml) of whole milk.	1 to 2 oz (30 to 60 g) of cottage cheese or yogurt, egg (whole), fish, meat, poultry, or mashed cooked beans or peas. 1 cup (240 ml) of whole milk (may be given later). 1 to 2 oz (30 to 60 g) of fruit or vegetable.
10 p.m.	Breast milk or 3 to 4 oz (90 to 120 ml) of formula ----------------▶		5 to 6 oz (150 to 180 ml) of formula[2]	Some of the milk from the day's allowance may be given at bedtime (usually at about 8 p.m.)--------▶		

[1]This plan should be modified to meet the particular needs of individual infants. For example, underweight babies might be given more, and overweight ones less food.
[2]Or breast milk. Some mothers who go to work might breast-feed in the morning and evening, but have the sitter give the baby a formula at the other feeding times.
[3]May not be needed if diet contains adequate iron (formula and/or cereal), vitamin D (formula or fortified milk), vitamin C (formula, fruit juice, fruits, and vegetables), and folacin (formula, egg yolks, meats, and vegetables).
[4]Sufficient water should be given between meals so that the total daily intake of fluids is 6 cups (1,440 ml). Additional fluid may be needed in a hot environment.

MILK AND OTHER LIQUIDS. It is very important for mothers who are not breast feeding to recognize that undiluted cow's milk is not suitable for young infants because it contains too much protein and mineral salts and too little carbohydrate. (A calf has very high nutrient requirements because it grows so rapidly that it requires only 47 to 70 days to double its birth weight, whereas, a human infant grows much more slowly and requires about 150 days to double its birth weight.) Therefore, parents who wish to save money by preparing their infant's formula from evaporated milk instead of using a commercial preparation should consult with their pediatrician or local public health nurse or nutritionist for instructions regarding dilution and sweetening of the milk.

NOTE: Evaporated milk is low in iron, vitamin D (unless fortified with the nutrient), folacin, and vitamin C. Hence, babies fed evaporated milk formulas should be given the appropriate nutritional supplements and/or the supplemental beverages or foods that provide the deficient nutrients.

Preparation of Infant Formulas. A typical set of instructions for preparing an infant formula follows:

1. The nursing bottles, caps, and nipples should be washed thoroughly with soap and hot water, then rinsed with boiling water to sterilize them and remove the last traces of soap, and allowed to dry while inverted on a sterilizer rack.

2. A commercially prepared infant formula is poured into clean nursing bottles for feeding, or an evaporated milk formula is prepared from carefully measured amounts of milk, sugar, and water. In the latter case, the filled bottles should be capped, placed on a rack in a sterilizer, and heated in gently boiling water for about 25 minutes. The sterilized bottles of formula should be stored in a refrigerator until used.

NOTE: Sterilized nipples should *not* be handled. Therefore, inserting them into the bottle caps prior to sterilization helps to avoid contamination. Bottles with tapered necks for nipples without caps should *not* be used because (a) the nipples cannot be put on without handling them, and (b) the nipples may come off while the infant is being fed.

3. Evaporated milk formulas should be changed as the infant grows older, according to a schedule such as outlined below.

    a. The formula for the first 2 months should be made from 1 oz of evaporated milk and 2 oz of water for *each* pound (*65 ml evaporated milk + 130 ml water per kg*) of body weight, plus 2 Tbsp (*24 g*) of corn syrup, sugar, or similar sweetener (but *not* honey, because it has been implicated as a source of infant botulism in a very few cases) in the total formula for the day.

    b. During the third, fourth, and fifth months, each day's feeding should consist of one 13 oz (*385 ml*) can of evaporated milk mixed with 19 oz (*565 ml*) of water plus 2 Tbsp (*24 g*) of sweetener.

    c. By the sixth month, the baby can be fed 16 oz (*475 ml*) of evaporated milk diluted with an equal amount of water and sweetened with 3 Tbsp (*36 g*) of sugar or syrup. The sweetener may be reduced or omitted if the infant is receiving supplemental foods and is growing as might be expected.

NOTE: Parents should *not* attempt to force their infants to consume the total feeding for the day, since some infants do well on less than the recommended amounts of formula. Furthermore, obesity that develops at such an early age is difficult to correct later.

The health professional consulted by the parents may also recommend other liquids to supplement the milk formula.

• **Fruit juices**—Fruit juices are usually started between 2 and 4 weeks of age. Use citrus (especially orange and grapefruit) fruit juices that are high in vitamin C, or other fruit juices that have vitamin C added. *Read the label!* Special baby juices have vitamin C added but are usually more expensive. Infants need vitamin C to help build strong healthy gums, strengthen the walls of blood vessels, and aid in healing scratches.

Fresh juice should be strained to remove the pulp. To prepare fruit juice, put a small amount of juice in a sterilized bottle and add cool boiled water. Each day decrease the amount of water and increase the juice until the baby is getting ¾ cup of pure juice daily. Give the infant cool fruit juice. Heating the juice destroys vitamin C. Do not add sugar to juices. This only adds energy (calories)—not nutrients, and it increases an infant's taste for sweets.

• **Water**—In addition to milk and fruit juice, an infant may be given cool, boiled water 2 to 3 times a day. Water is as important to a baby as food. Sugar or other sweeteners should not be added to water.

MINERAL AND VITAMIN SUPPLEMENTS. There is considerable controversy among nutritionists and pediatricians regarding the amounts and types of nutrient supplements that are required by infants, since breast fed infants have long been given little or no supplementation. Furthermore, the need for supplementation depends upon a variety of factors such as (1) status of the infant at birth, since preterm or low birth weight infants have higher nutritional requirements to attain the rates of growth and development of normal infants; (2) type of milk or formula used; (3) affliction of the infant with diarrhea, fever, infection, and/or other stresses; and (4) age at which supplemental foods are introduced. It is noteworthy that even breast milk is low in iron, copper, fluoride, vitamins A, D, and E, and biotin, folacin, niacin, thiamin, and vitamin B-6. Furthermore, diluted evaporated milk is notably inferior to breast milk with respect to the contents of iron, zinc, vitamin A, vitamin E, and vitamin C. Therefore, the need for nutrient supplements should be evaluated by a health professional who is familiar with the diet and the overall health status of the infant.

SOLID FOODS. The time at which solid foods such as cereals, fruits, vegetables, and meats are added to the diet depends on the infant's (1) nutritional needs, (2) digestive tract ability to handle food other than milk, and (3) physical capacity to handle them.

At birth, the infant has strong natural sucking and tongue thrust reflexes. The tongue thrust is a lifesaving reflex. It causes the baby to push solid food or other objects that might cause choking out of his mouth with his tongue. As an infant gets older, the sucking and tongue thrust reflexes are replaced by the swallowing reflex. The swallowing reflex must be learned. When a mother first starts to feed solid food, the young infant may push it out with his tongue. This does not mean that he does not like it. It is due to the tongue thrust reflex. Therefore, some pediatricians believe that solid food should not be given until this tongue thrust reflex disappears at 2½ to 3 months of age. Efforts to force solid food earlier may result in an unhappy feeding experience for mother and baby. All too often doctors advise mothers to start feeding solid food earlier than is necessary. This is usually due to the mother's demands rather than the baby's requirements. Usually, solid foods are introduced in the order which follows:

• **Cereals**—Nutrient-enriched cereals are usually started between 2½ and 3 months of age. Read the label to make certain that the product has been enriched or fortified with iron and other nutrients. Special baby cereal (in a box) is bound to contain the added nutrients, and many other ready-to-eat and cooked products are similarly enriched. Cereal in the jar (wet pack) is usually more expensive than dry cereal.

Use an enriched or fortified cereal each day. Cereal is usually offered at the morning and evening feedings. Try rice cereal first because there is less chance of an infant having an allergic reaction. Then try oat or barley cereals. Wheat cereals may then be added. Mixed cereals should not be started until all of the single-grain cereals have been accepted by the baby without any allergic reaction. Special baby cereals do not need cooking. Just add milk. An infant may be fed cereal cooked for the family, but it should be very soft. Do not add sugar, salt, or fat to cereals.

Begin with 1 tsp (*5 ml*) of cereal made "soupy" with milk. Gradually increase the amount of cereal and thicken it as the infant learns to swallow. Do not add cereal to a baby's bottle. Spoon feeding is important to the development of eating behavior.

• **Fruits**—These foods are usually started between 3 and 4 months. This is a new "sweet taste" for the baby. Fruits supply vitamins and minerals and provide bulk to prevent constipation.

Soft canned fruits such as applesauce, peaches, pears, and peeled apricots can be used if mashed thoroughly. Neither sugar nor syrup from the canned fruit should be used. Sugar only adds extra calories—not nutrients. Home cooked, fresh, and dried fruits may also be used. To prepare dried fruits, soak about 4 hours in water (enough to cover). Cook the fruit in the same water until tender. Mash thoroughly. If commercial strained baby fruits are used, use pure fruits. Avoid fruit mixtures such as fruit with cereal, desserts, cobblers, or pies. These products have less fruit and more calories, usually sugar.

Begin with 1 tsp (*5 ml*) and gradually increase until the infant is getting 2 to 3 Tbsp (*30 to 45 ml*). Do not use raw fruit other than ripe bananas until the infant is older. If the baby's stools become soft and watery, stop the fruit for a few days; then add a small amount gradually.

• **Vegetables**—Mashed, pureed, and/or strained vegetables are usually started between 3 and 4 months of age. They provide vitamins and minerals needed for growing. Dark yellow and leafy green vegetables provide vitamin A which helps keep the eyes and skin healthy. Bulk from vegetables helps to promote regular bowel movements.

Fresh, canned, or frozen vegetables may be used. Cook and mash vegetables thoroughly. At first, you may want to strain the vegetables. Do not add salt, spices, fats, or bacon to the vegetables. Commercial strained baby vegetables may also be used. Choose a pure vegetable rather than a creamed vegetable mixture or dinner. At first, offer the baby mild-tasting vegetables such as green beans, carrots, squash, green peas, and greens.

Begin with 1 tsp (*5 ml*) of vegetable. Gradually increase until the infant is getting 2 or 3 Tbsp (*30 to 45 ml*) a day. Offer the same vegetable for several days before trying a new one. This will give the infant a chance to learn to like the taste of the vegetable. It also gives the mother a chance to see if the baby is allergic to the vegetable. Potato may be added after the baby is eating other vegetables. White potatoes do not take the place of green or yellow vegetables.

Be sure to include a vegetable each day. Remember, that dark yellow and green vegetables are high in vitamin A.

• **Meats**—Easily digested forms of fish, legumes, meats, and poultry are usually started by 6 months of age. These foods supply protein needed to build and repair muscles and other body tissues. They also supply iron needed to prevent the baby from getting anemic and other nutrients needed to keep the body healthy.

Begin with 1 tsp (*5 ml*) of meat and gradually increase to 2 or 3 Tbsp (*30 to 45 ml*) daily. Start with one meat and feed it several days before adding a new flavor. This gives the infant a chance to learn to like the taste. It also gives the mother a chance to see if her baby is allergic to the meat.

"Table" meats such as ground beef, chicken, liver, and fish may be used. Ground beef should be boiled and mashed as it cooks. Fish, chicken, and liver should be finely mashed. Moisten the meat with broth or milk. Do not fry meat. Canned chicken or fish may be finely mashed and used. Remove all bones, fat, and skin.

Commercial strained baby meat may also be used. Use pure meat rather than dinners, meat mixtures, or soups. It takes five jars of meat-vegetable mixture to equal the protein content in one jar of pure meat such as strained chicken. Bacon, fat back, salt pork, broth, and gravy are *not* meat or protein—they are mainly fat.

Dried beans and peas, thoroughly cooked and mashed, may be used in place of part of the meat. Be sure to include milk or a small amount of meat with the beans. Cook beans without bacon, salt pork, lard, or other fats.

Vegetarian diets which contain no meat, eggs, or milk may be harmful for babies. These diets are likely to be lacking in several important nutrients that infants need to grow strong and healthy.

• **Egg yolks**—This food is usually started between 4 and 6 months of age. Egg yolks provide iron needed to make red blood. Begin with 1 tsp (*5 ml*) and gradually increase until the baby is getting one yolk each day. If a rash develops, see your doctor before giving egg yolk again.

(*NOTE:* Egg whites should *not* be used until recommended by your doctor. They may cause the baby to have an allergic reaction.)

Hard cooked egg yolk may be fed to a baby. Use a fresh, uncracked egg. Heat in water until it comes to a boil. Remove from heat. Let the egg set in water for 20 minutes. Crack the shell and remove the yolk. Add warm milk and mash the yolk. Boiling an egg makes it tough.

Special egg yolks in a jar may be used, but they are usually more expensive. Use pure egg yolks rather than egg mixtures such as cereal and egg or bacon-egg dinners. One-third jar of egg yolk is equal to one egg yolk.

SELF FEEDING. At about 5 to 6 months of age, many babies will begin hand-to-mouth movements and chewing movements. These occur at about the same time they begin to cut teeth. It is important that an infant be given the opportunity to develop chewing and self-feeding skills at this time. Chewing strengthens a baby's throat muscles for the development of speech. Dry toast is a good food to develop chewing. To prepare, cut small strips of bread and put in low (200°F [94°C]) oven for 1 hour. Store this hard toast in an air-tight container.

When hand-to-mouth movements begin, the infant is ready to start drinking from a cup and using a spoon. Let the baby play with an empty cup; and teach it how to put the cup to its mouth. Then add a few drops of milk. Increase the amount of milk as he learns to handle the cup.

Choose "child-size" utensils for eating; small spoons with short handles; unbreakable broadmouth and broad-base small cups; dishes with rims that will help the baby push food onto the spoon.

Use of "finger foods" is an excellent way to teach the baby to self-feed. Offer bite-size pieces of meat, vegetables, and fruits that can be picked up with the fingers.

Remember, an infant will be messy while he is learning to feed himself. Don't get upset. Let him do it himself!

Common Problems Encountered in Feeding.

It is always best for parents to consult their pediatrician promptly when feeding problems arise, so that any serious conditions may be diagnosed and treated as soon as possible. However, many parents encounter minor problems that can be remedied by fairly simple measures, which may be recommended by a doctor in a telephone conversation. Therefore, some of the principles that may be applied to the most common problems are presented so that parents may have a better understanding of the physician's recommendations.

LOW BIRTH WEIGHT OR PREMATURITY. Infants that are significantly smaller than average or premature at birth may be given formulas that are more concentrated than usual. (Low birth weight means less than 5½ lb (*2,500 g*) whereas an infant is considered to be premature if born after less than 38 weeks of pregnancy.) This type of problem requires the continuous supervision of the pediatrician, who knows best how to modify the feeding without creating new problems. Usually, special formulas are given to these infants, although in some cases breast-feeding may be adequate. Extremely under-

sized or undermature newborns may require tube feeding or intravenous feeding. Also, they are usually fed every 2 to 3 hours, since the capacity of the stomach is likely to be subnormal.

COLIC. This condition, which is characterized by crying and tensing of the abdomen shorlty after a feeding, is a painful cramping or spasm in the infant's digestive tract that may be caused by (1) feeding too great a quantity of food; (2) overly rapid feeding; (3) conditions which make the infant emotionally tense (tension of the mother, loud noises, family hollering and fighting, etc.) during eating; or (4) a food allergy. Many infants have occasional bouts of colic during the first few months of life. However, frequent occurrences require the attention of a doctor.

DIARRHEA. The passage of loose, watery bowel movements will occur occasionally in almost all infants. However, infant diarrhea should be treated promptly according to a pediatrician's recommendations so that dehydration does not occur. He or she may recommend that the sugar be temporarily eliminated from the formula or that an antidiarrheal agent be given.

NOTE: Parents should *not* give an infant any medication without a doctor's advice at each occurrence of diarrhea, since the condition may have different causes at different times.

CONSTIPATION. This condition, which is characterized by the passage of dry, hard, small infrequent stools, is rarely as serious as diarrhea, unless there is considerable pain (indicated by crying of the baby) while making a bowel movement. The doctor may recommend that a litte extra sugar be added to the formula, or that greater amounts of fruits and vegetables be fed. However, chronic constipation which persists in spite of feeding sufficient bulk may require a medical evaluation to rule out other more serious conditions.

UNDERWEIGHT. Infants vary considerably in their caloric needs, so it is to be expected that some babies will be thinner than others. Nevertheless, a pediatrician will usually want to examine thoroughly any infant that fails to gain at the rate indicated by the growth curve for the 10th percentile of infants of the same age and sex. Some of the most common causes of the failure of infants to gain sufficient weight are (1) underfeeding; (2) frequent vomiting or diarrhea; (3) febrile disease(s); (4) refusal of some or all of the food that is offered; (5) expenditure of above average amounts of energy in crying, kicking, overexcitement, excessive neuromuscular tension, or functioning with various physical handicaps; and (6) digestive or metabolic abnormalities that interfere with the utilization of nutrients. Sometimes, the correction of one or more nutritional deficiencies brings about a normal rate of growth.

OVERWEIGHT AND/OR OBESITY. The presence of excessive body fat (obesity) may be indicated by a weight that is excessive for an infant's age and height. However, overweight and obesity are *not* always equivalent, since a baby with a smaller than normal skeleton and musculature may be of normal weight but obese, whereas a large-boned and heavy-muscled baby may be overweight without being obese. Hence, a doctor or other health professional will most likely measure the thickness of skinfolds on either the triceps or below the shoulder blades, because these measurements are rough indicators of the body fat content. Once obesity has been diagnosed in an infant, the current mode of treatment is to reduce the caloric content of the diet just enough to restrict the rate of additional fat accumulation while allowing the full growth of lean body tissue. Attempts to reduce the amount of fat that is already present may retard the rate of growth for the bones, muscles, and vital organs. Hence, the dietary treatment of obese infants differs significantly from that used for older children or adults.

FOOD ALLERGY (Food Sensitivity). This type of condition is not uncommon in children, especially during the first few months of life. Food allergy may be mild causing only a skin rash, or it may be more severe causing vomiting, diarrhea, and colic.

Cow's milk is a common cause of allergy. Infants with milk allergy can be given a milk-free formula made from soybean or meat. These formulas provide nutrients in amounts similar to those in milk.

Other foods to which infants may be allergic include egg (especially the white), wheat, nuts, chocolate, citrus fruit, tomatoes, strawberries, and fish. Since these foods increase the risk of young infants developing allergy, they are usually left out of the diet for the first few months.

Children tend to become less allergic to food as they grow older, providing that their exposure to the offending food(s) is limited. Food sensitivity is similar to immunity to various diseases in that repeated exposures to the sensitizing agent is like a "booster shot" that stimulates the defense reactions of the body.

(Also see ALLERGIES.)

ANEMIAS. The lack of sufficient red blood cells is considered to be a sign of anemia, although there is still controversy as to the hemoglobin levels that should be characterized as subnormal. Iron-deficiency anemia is the most common one found in infants, although this type of condition may also result from other nutritional deficiencies or certain nonnutritional causes such as slow, but prolonged internal bleeding. Fortunately, there are a variety of iron-fortified infant foods and formulas that may be used to treat mild cases of anemia, and certain forms of medicinal iron may be used in the more severe cases.

(Also see ANEMIA; and IRON.)

Modifications of Infant Diets. Major modifications of the nutrient composition of an infant's diet should be made only under the supervision of a physician or a nutritionist. For example, abnormalities in the metabolism of one or more nutrients may make it necessary to restrict the diet of an infant to special foods or formulas.

These conditions are relatively rare and usually require special diagnostic tests for their detection. Thus, skim milk alone is not suitable for infant feeding, except when prescribed by a doctor for an infant that has an intolerance to dietary fat; normally, it should be used only in formulas or mixtures that contain added fats such as vegetable oils.

(Also see BABY FOODS; BREAST FEEDING; and NUTRIENTS: REQUIREMENTS, ALLOWANCES, FUNCTIONS, SOURCES.)

INFARCTION

Dead tissue caused by blockage of an artery, usually by a blood clot. Infarctions have specific names; for example, the term *myocardial infarction* is used when the area affected is a part of the heart muscle (it is usually the result of a blockage—occlusion—of a coronary artery).

(Also see HEART DISEASE; and MYOCARDIAL INFARCTION.)

INFECTION

A condition that occurs when the body is invaded by disease-producing germs or microorganisms.

(Also see DISEASES.)

INFLAMMATION

A reaction of the tissues of the body to an injury or ailment, characterized by redness, heat, swelling, and pain.

INGEST

To eat or take in through the mouth.

INORGANIC

Denotes substances not of organic origin (not produced by animal or vegetable organisms).

INOSITOL

Inositol, which has been known as a chemical compound since 1850, is widely distributed in foods and closely related to glucose. It was first commonly called "muscle sugar" and given the name inositol from two Greek roots: *inos,* meaning sinews; and *-ose,* the suffix for sugars.

Animal experiments conducted in the 1940s indicated that inositol was an essential nutritional factor and led many investigators to group it with the B vitamins. Today, there is no evidence that humans cannot synthesize all the inositol needed by the body, and its classification as a vitamin is disputed; more properly perhaps, it should be classified as an essential nutrient, rather than a vitamin, for certain species of bacteria and animals. Nevertheless, listing inositol among the B vitamins persists in some books, catalogs, and diet-ingredient lists, and on some labels.

HISTORY.

In 1940, Woolley at the University of Wisconsin demonstrated that inositol could prevent alopecia (patchy-hair, or baldness, condition) in mice. Later studies demonstrated that rats on inositol-deficient diets developed a denuded area around the eyes that imparted a curious "spectacled-eye" appearance. Research has also indicated a need for dietary inositol for chicks, swine, hamsters, and guinea pigs.

CHEMISTRY, METABOLISM, PROPERTIES.

• **Chemistry**—Inositol is a cyclic 6-carbon compound with 6-hydroxy groups, closely related to glucose. It exists in nine forms, but only myo-inositol demonstrates any biological activity.

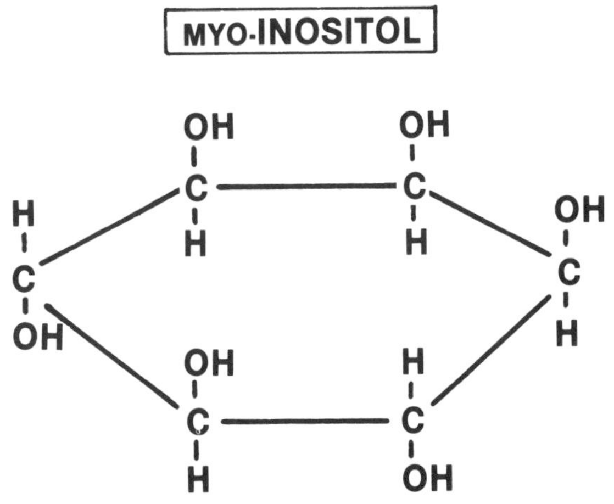

Fig. I-11. Structure of myo-inositol ($C_6H_{12}O_6$).

• **Metabolism**—In addition to food sources of inositol, it is synthesized within the cells. Myo-inositol is present in relatively large amounts in the cells of practically all animals and plants.

In animal cells, it occurs as a component of phospholipids, substances containing phosphorus, fatty acids, and nitrogenous bases. In plant cells, it is found as phytic acid, an organic acid that binds calcium, iron, and zinc in an insoluble complex and interferes with their absorption.

Inositol is stored largely in the brain, heart muscle, and skeletal muscle.

Small amounts of inositol are normally excreted in the urine. Diabetic patients excrete much larger amounts of inositol in their urine than nondiabetics.

• **Properties**—Inositol is a colorless, water-soluble, sweet-tasting crystalline material. It can withstand acids, alkalis, and heat.

MEASUREMENT/ASSAY.

Inositol is measured in milligrams.

Formerly, myo-inositol analysis was by microbiological method only, based on growth of certain yeasts. Later, a time-consuming chemical method became available. Today, microbiologic and chemical assays are giving way to chromatographic methods and enzyme assays.

FUNCTIONS.

The functions of inositol are not completely understood, but the following roles have been suggested:

1. It has a lipotropic effect (an affinity for fat, like choline). It promotes body production of lecithin; in turn, lecithin aids in moving fats from the liver to the cells. It follows that inositol aids in the metabolism of fats and helps reduce blood cholesterol.

2. In combination with choline, inositol prevents the fatty hardening of arteries and protects the heart.

3. It appears to be a precursor of the phosphoinosities, which are found in various body tissues, especially in the brain.

DEFICIENCY SYMPTOMS.

Myo-inositol is a "growth factor" for certain yeasts and bacteria, and for several lower organisms up to and including several species of fish.

Earlier experiments indicated that a deficiency of inositol caused retarded growth and loss of hair in young mice (symptoms closely resembling deficiencies of vitamin B-6 or pantothenic acid), and loss of hair around the eyes in rats. But it is now known that these earlier studies were made with diets partially deficient in certain other vitamins; hence, in retrospect, the relationship of inositol to these symptoms is being questioned.

Large amounts of coffee (caffeine) may deplete the body's storage of inositol and result in deficiency symptoms.

RECOMMENDED DAILY ALLOWANCE OF INOSITOL.

The inositol requirement of man is unknown for two reasons: (1) its role in human nutrition is undetermined, and (2) man and other higher animals appear capable of synthesizing all the inositol needed.

So, no recommended daily allowances are given.

Myo-inositol appears to be required in the diet of the mouse, rat, hamster, guinea pig, duck, and pig, but there is still uncertainty as to whether (1) it is merely performing some of the functions of certain B vitamins, or (2) it is an essential metabolic requirement.

• **Inositol intake in average U.S. diet**—It is estimated that the average daily inositol consumption in the United States ranges from 300 to 1,000 mg per day.

TOXICITY.   There is no known toxicity of inositol.

SOURCES OF INOSITOL.   Inositol is abundantly present in nature.

• **Rich sources**—Kidney, brain, liver, yeast, heart, wheat germ, citrus fruits, and blackstrap molasses.

• **Good sources**—Muscle meats, fruits, whole grains, bran of cereal grains, nuts, legumes, milk, and vegetables.

Also, humans synthesize it within the cells. Perhaps it is also synthesized by intestinal bacteria, although this has not been proven.

(Also see VITAMIN[S], Table V-9.)

INSENSIBLE PERSPIRATION

Perspiration that evaporates before it is noticed as sweat on the skin.

INSIDIOUS

Denoting a disease which progresses with few or no symptoms to indicate its seriousness.

INSTITUTE OF FOOD TECHNOLOGY

This is the professional organization for food technologists. The address: Suite 2120, 221 North La Salle St., Chicago, Ill. 60601. The Institute issues two publications: (1) *Food Technology,* in which applied research articles and news of the society appear; and (2) *The Journal of Food Science,* which carries more fundamental research reports.

(Also see FOOD TECHNOLOGY.)

INSULIN

One of two hormones secreted by the pancreas. Insulin stimulates the transport of glucose (blood sugar) into the cells of the body where it is utilized. Without insulin, glucose reaches extremely high levels in the blood. If left unchecked, coma and death may follow. Such is the problem of persons suffering from diabetes mellitus.

In 1921, one of the great advances of modern medicine was made when two Canadian scientists, Frederick G. Banting and Charles Best, isolated and produced insulin in a form which could be used to treat diabetes. Although insulin is no cure for diabetes, it has saved many lives and is now produced cheaply and used extensively by many millions afflicted with this disease.

Depending upon the type of diabetes, insulin may be injected or its release may be stimulated from the pancreas by drugs.

(Also see DIABETES MELLITUS, section headed "Insulin"; and ENDOCRINE GLANDS.)

INTERESTERIFICATION

Fats are mixtures of triglycerides—various fatty acids esterified to glycerol. The process of interesterification is the migration of the various fatty acids between the glycerol molecules giving the fat different physical properties. Heating a fat will cause this process to occur. A major application of this process in the food industry is the production of mono- and diglycerides. In a mixture of triglycerides and glycerol heated to 400°F (*204°C*) in the presence of a sodium hydroxide catalyst, fatty acid molecules migrate from the triglyceride to the free glycerol molecules thus producing a mixture of mono- and diglycerides because there is an excess of glycerol molecules. Mono- and diglycerides have wide use in the food industry as emulsifiers.

(Also see ADDITIVES; ESTER; and TRIGLYCERIDES.)

INTERMEDIATE HYDROGEN CARRIER

The body utilizes a series of biological oxidations to form energy from foods. Oxidation refers to the loss of electrons—hydrogen—by a compound. For example, lactic acid is dehydrogenated to form pyruvic acid. This hydrogen is then passed to the intermediate hydrogen carriers, nicotinamide adenine dinucleotide (NAD) and flavin adenine dinucleotide (FAD), which, in turn, pass hydrogen to a system known as the electron transport chain, a series of intermediate hydrogen carriers. As the hydrogen is passed down this chain, energy is released. At the end of the chain, the hydrogen combines with the ultimate hydrogen carrier, oxygen, and water is formed.

(Also see METABOLIC WATER; and METABOLISM.)

INTERNATIONAL UNIT (IU)

A standard unit of potency of a biologic agent (e.g., a vitamin, hormone, antibiotic, antitoxin) as defined by the International Conference for Unification of Formulae. Potency is based on bioassay that produces a particular effect agreed on internationally. Also called a USP unit.

INTERSTITIAL (FLUID)

Situated in spaces between tissues.

INTESTINAL FLORA

Relating to the various bacterial and other microscopic forms of plant life in the intestinal contents.

INTESTINAL JUICE

A clear liquid secreted by glands in the wall of the small intestine. It contains the enzymes lactase, maltase, and sucrase, and several peptidases.
(Also see DIGESTION AND ABSORPTION.)

INTESTINE, LARGE

The tubelike part of the digestive tract lying between the small intestine and the anus. It is larger in diameter but shorter in length than the small intestine.
(Also see DIGESTION AND ABSORPTION.)

INTESTINE, SMALL

The long, tortuous, tubelike part of the digestive tract leading from the stomach to the cecum and large intestine. It is smaller in diameter but longer than the large intestine.
(Also see DIGESTION AND ABSORPTION.)

INTOLERANCE

Sensitivity or allergy of certain foods, drugs, or other substances.
(Also see ALLERGIES.)

INTRA-

Prefix meaning within.

INTRACELLULAR

Within the cell.

INTRAMURAL NERVE PLEXUS

A network of interwoven nerve fibers within a particular organ. The smooth muscle layers of the gastrointestinal wall are controlled by such a network of nerve fibers.

INTRAVENOUS FEEDING

At times it becomes necessary to correct acute losses of fluids, salts, vitamins, and other nutrients by application directly into the bloodstream. This process is intravenous feeding. Most times it is practiced on a short term basis. Often it is used to tide a patient over after injuries or operations involving the face, mouth, esophagus, stomach and small intestine. Nutrient-containing fluids used for this purpose are dripped by gravity into a peripheral vein, often a vein in the arm. A bottle containing the fluid is suspended above the patient and connected to a needle in the vein via a small plastic tube. Long-term use of this procedure in patients who cannot be fed by mouth or a stomach tube is hazardous, expensive, and time consuming. It can, however, be accomplished if the plastic tube is inserted into one of the large central veins of the body. There are available a variety of solutions containing fats, amino acids and glucose that can, if needed, provide complete nutrition for weeks and even years.

• **Total parenteral nutrition (hyperalimentation)**—The basic problem associated with conventional intravenous feeding (i.e., 5 to 10% glucose solutions with electrolytes) is the inability to provide sufficient calories to permit utilization of administered amino acids unless very large volumes of water are infused. So, this type of feeding is incapable of either maintaining the well-nourished for prolonged periods or of improving the already malnourished individual.

The term *hyperalimentation* first appeared in the clinical literature in 1965 relating to supplementary intravenous feeding of fat; and it was popularized as a general term for total parenteral nutrition following publication of the results of the excellent studies on dogs and patients conducted by the University of Pennsylvania group. The aid of parenteral nutrition, like that of diet therapy by oral or tube-fed routes, is the provision of the calories and nutrients required by the specific patient. Thus, the phrases "total parenteral nutrition" and "total parenteral alimentation" appear to be more accurate and inclusive than does the term "hyperalimentation." If the latter term is used, it should refer to the administration of calories appreciably in excess of those usually required.

NOTE WELL: Total parenteral nutrition is a potentially lifesaving and morbidity-reducing procedure, but its use requires great expertise in nutrition, patient care, and equipment.

INTRAVENOUS (PARENTERAL) NUTRITION, SUPPLEMENTARY

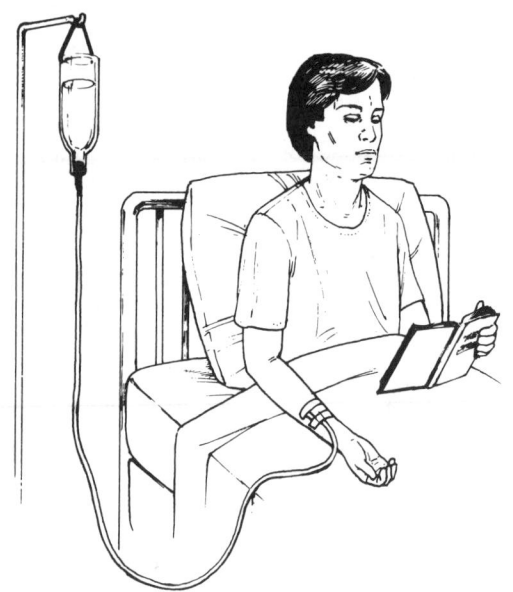

Fig. I-12. Intravenous feeding. This method of providing nutrients and/or medications has long been used to maintain patients when it is inadvisable to attempt to feed them via the mouth and the digestive tract.

This term refers to the temporary provision of supplementary nutrients in a solution that is infused into a vein. When a small vein on the surface of an arm, leg, or the scalp is used, it is called peripheral intravenous feeding, whereas, the infusion of the nutrients into a large vein deep within the body is called central venous feeding. Furthermore, the amounts of nutrients which may be delivered to a peripheral vein is limited because concentrated solutions are likely to cause phlebitis and/or clots (thrombi). On the other hand, rather concentrated nutrient solutions may be infused by central veins because the blood flow is rapid enough to bring about a prompt dilution of the solution so that little irritation to the vein occurs. Therefore, the former procedure is used mainly for providing supplementary nutrients for short periods of time, whereas the latter may supply all of the required nutrients for much longer periods. Only the former type of intravenous feeding is covered in this article, because the details of the latter one are given elsewhere.

(Also see TOTAL PARENTERAL [INTRAVENOUS] NUTRITION [TPN].)

HISTORY. The first experiments on feeding animals and people by intravenous means were conducted shortly after the English physician William Harvey discovered the circulation of the blood in 1616. Among the most notable experiments were (1) those of the English architect Sir Christopher Wren who injected ale, wine, and opium into the veins of a dog by means of a goose quill attached to a pig's bladder; and (2) the attempt of the French physician Jean Baptiste Dennis to transfuse lamb's blood into a man. These and similar experiments were doomed to fail because little was known about the reactions between different types of blood and the need for sterile conditions to prevent the inoculation of the patient with deadly microorganisms. Therefore, almost 2 centuries were to pass before efforts to provide intravenous nutrition met with success.

It appears that the modern era of intravenous nutrition began in 1843, when the renowned French physiologist Claude Bernard injected sugar solutions into a dog. By the end of the 19th century, the intravenous administration of dextrose (glucose) and saline solutions had become a regular practice. During World War II there were many attempts to administer special types of intavenous solutions to wounded military personnel. For example, the Germans tried various synthetic plasma extenders when they ran short of blood for their many casualties near the end of the war. There were also trials of mixtures of dextrose and amino acids in the 1940s, but these solutions were usually sufficiently concentrated to irritate the veins and cause phlebitis and clots (thrombi).

Experiments on dogs in the 1950s suggested that higher levels of calories in intravenous feedings might be provided safely by the use of fat emulsions, which were much less irritating to veins than dextrose and amino acids. Unfortunately, the types of emulsions that were used then produced side effects such as asthma, chills, fever, liver disorders, low back pain and various abnormalities of blood clotting. The reason why these undesirable effects were not detected in the dog experiments was that the emulsions were administered to the dogs on the same body weight basis as the proposed dosages for humans, whereas dogs normally consume about three times the calories per pound of body weight that people consume. Better correlations between the effects of fat emulsions on dogs and on humans were obtained later by Dr. Arvid Wretlind and his co-workers in Sweden when the dogs used in the tests were given the fat emulsions on the basis of their metabolic rates rather than according to body weights. These studies led to the development of a safer fat emulsion in the early 1960s. This product has been used since then in Europe, but only recently in the United States.

Meanwhile, doctors had begun to infuse concentrated solutions of dextrose into the large central veins of patients with kidney failure in order to prevent the wasting of tissues accompanying this condition. However, better means for sustaining these patients came about with the development of improved techniques for dialysis. Nevertheless, a few physicians continued to search for ways of providing more nutritious and safer types of intravenous feedings. The most recent major breakthrough in this field was the development of total parenteral nutrition (TPN) in the mid-1960s by Dr. Stanley Dudrick and his co-workers at the University of Pennsylvania School of Medicine. TPN involves the infusion of a complete and concentrated mixture of nutrients into the vena cava (a large vein that empties directly into the heart) by means of a catheter that is passed down through either the subclavian or jugular veins.

Supplementary parenteral nutrition continues to be used routinely, in spite of the development of TPN, because the latter is a serious surgical procedure, whereas, the former procedure is usually safer and easier to use.

INDICATIONS. Intravenous infusions of glucose solutions through a peripheral vein were once administered routinely to all types of patients who could not take sufficient nourishment by mouth or tube feeding. Salt solutions were administered to correct suspected deficits of water and/or mineral salts, but in some cases may have done more harm than good. However, there is now a wider variety of intravenous solutions that are used selectively for conditions such as acidosis, dehydration, diarrhea, elevated metabolic rate, fever, gastric suction, hemorrhage, malnutrition, N.P.O. (no nourishment may be taken orally), retention of excessive water in the tissues, severe burns, and vomiting.

The major reasons for correcting these conditions intravenously rather than orally are (1) oral treatment may be too slow and uncertain because of disorders of digestion and absorption, (2) inflammation, injury, or surgery of the digestive tract makes it inadvisable to use this route for therapy, (3) the patient may be comatose or paralyzed and subject to aspiration (sucking of material down the windpipe into the lungs) or choking on matter fed orally, and (4) it may not be possible to meet unusually high requirements by oral or tube feeding.

It is noteworthy that supplementary intravenous feeding is almost always a short-term procedure because it is difficult to meet all nutritional requirements by this means. Patients who require long-term intravenous feeding are usually given total parenteral (intravenous) feeding through a central vein. The latter procedure has hazards of its own and should be considered a potentially hazardous procedure that requires a trained team of doctors and nurses for its administration.

Types Of Solutions Used In Peripheral Intravenous Feeding. The selection of the proper solution for treatment of a particular condition may be a matter of life or death for a very ill patient. Descriptions and uses of the major types of intravenous solutions follow:

• **Amino acids and/or protein hydrolysates**—Whole proteins cannot be given intravenously because of the danger of a very strong antigenic reaction. (Blood transfusions are an exception because the proteins present are those which occur naturally in the blood.) Therefore, mixtures of purified amino acids or protein hydrolysates (proteins broken down to amino acids by means of acid, alkaline, and/or enzymatic hydrolysis) are used to meet protein requirements. However, newborn infants can be given only the amino acids, because protein hydrolysates contain more ammonia than their bodies can metabolize readily.

Amino acid solutions may comprise the main source of calories in an intravenous feeding because some doctors believe that this type of therapy is the most effective means of sparing body protein. However, the sparing of protein by these solutions is most likely to be achieved when the patient has sufficient amounts of body fat to furnish the calories lacking in the intravenous solution. Other doctors prefer to administer mixtures of amino acids and glucose, or amino acids and a fat emulsion in the event that the patient utilizes little or none of his or her own body fat.

The different brands of amino acid solutions contain different proportions of the various essential and nonessential amino acids. Therefore, it might be a good idea for doctors ordering these IVs to consult an expert in amino acid metabolism for advice in selecting the most suitable formula.

• **Carbohydrates**—Glucose is most commonly used at a concentration of 5 or 10%, although fructose is sometimes given to diabetics because it does not require insulin for its metabolism. The latter practice is falling into disfavor because the rapid administration of fructose may cause a buildup of lactate in the blood and a corresponding acidosis.

It is noteworthy that each gram of glucose provides 3.4 Calories (kcal) and that 1 liter of 5% glucose supplies 170 Calories (kcal), whereas 1 liter of 10% glucose supplies 340 Calories (kcal). The former is used much more often than the latter because the stronger solution may cause complications such as irritation of the veins, and an excessive buildup of the sugar in the blood that may result in a marked urinary loss of sugar, water, and salt. These complications may lead to dehydration. Most patients can be infused with only 2.5 to 3.0 liter of solution per day, which in the case of 5% glucose, provides only 400 to 500 Calories (kcal). Therefore, it is easy to see why patients maintained on intravenous glucose solutions alone for more than a week or so lose considerable weight and may even become malnourished.

Occasionally, small amounts of alcohol (about 1 oz or 25 ml) have been added to glucose solutions to provide extra calories and a sedative effect. Larger amounts of intravenously administered alcohol are poorly tolerated by many patients.

• **Fat (lipid) emulsions**—These preparations consist of very finely dispersed minute droplets of a vegetable oil in isotonic solutions that contain small amounts of lecithin which help to make the emulsions very stable. (They do not separate into oil and water phases.) For example, the most commonly used product, which was developed by Dr. Wretlind and his co-workers, contains 10% soybean oil, 2.5% glycerol, 1.2% purified egg yolk, and a small amount of phospholipid in an isotonic solution. Each liter of the infusion supplies 1,100 Calories (kcal), which is about 6.5 times as much as a 5% solution of glucose. Also, the fat emulsion is nonirritating to the veins.

Fat emulsions are used alone or in combination with other intravenous solutions to provide extra calories that often mean the difference between the sparing of body protein and the wasting of tissues. A group of patients that was given only glucose and electrolytes after stomach surgery lost from 7 to 9 lb (3 to 4 kg) in a 5 day recovery period, whereas a similar group given a combination of the glucose-electrolyte solution, a protein hydrolysate, and a lipid emulsion lost an average of only 1 lb (0.45 kg). The fats in these preparations are apparently well utilized by most patients, as indicated by a moderately rapid rate of clearance of the infused fats from the blood. Nevertheless, certain highly stressed patients, such as those recovering from burns or fractured bones, also require glucose for optimal sparing of their body protein.

• **Minerals and vitamins**—Generally, doctors are more likely to order the addition of supplementary minerals and vitamins to intravenous solutions infused into central veins (total parenteral feeding) than to those given peripherally (supplementary parenteral feeding) for short periods of time. However, doses of vitamin C as high as one or more grams per day have been utilized in the latter procedure because of the important role of this nutrient in healing.

It is not always necessary to give every essential mineral and vitamin intravenously, since some of these nutrients may be provided in intramuscular or subcutaneous injections made at regular intervals. The present trend appears to be leading in the direction of giving greater mineral and vitamin supplementation than was done in the past.

• **Plasma extenders such as dextran**—These substances are synthetic substances without nutritional value that are used in emergency situations to provide colloid that helps to maintain the water content of the blood. Normally, this function is served by the bloodborne proteins, but these constituents may be at critically subnormal levels when there has been hemorrhage, severe malnutrition, and other serious injuries or disorders.

• **Salt (sodium chloride) and/or other electrolytes**—The most commonly used solution in this category is 0.9% sodium choloride, which is also called "physiological saline" because it has the same solute strength (tonicity) as the body fluids. Some solutions also contain potassium and magnesium salts because these minerals are also highly essential in the maintenance of a variety of vital functions.

Solutions of electrolytes are administered when it is necessary to replace the mineral salts and water that have been lost under circumstances such as dehydration, diarrhea, gastric suction, hemorrhage, moderate to severe burns, and vomiting. For example, sodium bicarbonate is often given to correct acidosis, which occurs in diabetic coma. Also, magnesium sulfate is sometimes given intravenously to correct ventricular fibrillation.

BENEFITS. The leading benefits of intravenous solutions injected into a peripheral vein are as follows:

1. Solutions may be "tailor made" for the patient's needs. For example, patients with abnormal blood levels of certain amino acids (a condition that occurs in septicemia) may be given a solution containing high levels of those that are deficient and low levels of those present in excess.

2. Delivery of the required nutrients directly and rapidly into the bloodstream ensures that they get to where they are needed without being subjected to the uncertainties of a patient's appetite and the ingestion, digestion and absorption of substances given via the digestive tract.

3. Infusion into a peripheral vein may be started by nurses and paramedics, whereas total parenteral feeding via a central vein is a procedure that requires a doctor.

HAZARDS AND PRECAUTIONS. The major hazards of supplementary intravenous feeding via a peripheral vein usually arise from attempting to supply too much, too rapidly, without considering the patient's condition carefully before proceeding. Examples of some common hazards follow:

1. Hypertonic solutions (those that are stronger in solute concentration than the body fluids) are likely to irritate the walls of the veins and may even induce the formation of clots. Therefore, it is preferable to administer a 5% glucose solution plus a lipid emulsion rather than attempting to meet caloric needs with a 10% glucose solution.

2. Intravenous administration of fluids and nutrients may overload the body if the rate of delivery exceeds the rates of utilization and/or excretion. For example, patients who have retained excessive amounts of sodium may develop waterlogged tissues or even congestive heart failure when given a solution containing salt and other electrolytes. Another hazard is the provision of glucose to diabetics who utilize it poorly. They may spill sugar in the urine and pass excessive amounts of water (osmotic diuresis), thereby becoming dehydrated. These hazards may be avoided by keeping accurate records of fluid input and output, and by monitoring the blood sugar of patients known or suspected to suffer from diabetes.

CONTRAINDICATIONS. Intravenous feeding via a peripheral vein should not be used if (1) oral or tube feeding may meet all of the patient's requirements, (2) a long-term intravenous administration of all or most nutrients is required, and total parenteral nutrition is available, or (3) the risks (due to the instability of the patient's condition) outweigh the benefits gained. In the last case, intravenous feedings may be initiated as soon as the patient's condition has been stabilized.

SUMMARY. Supplementary intravenous feeding via a peripheral vein is best suited for meeting short-term needs of patients who are likely to fare poorly without it. It does not require the expertise needed to administer total parenteral nutrition (TPN), but it is more limited with respect to the amounts of nutrients which may be delivered intravenously. Therefore, it is being replaced by TPN in chronic care situations when the capability for administering the latter is present.

(Also see TOTAL PARENTERAL [INTRAVENOUS] NUTRITION.)

INTRINSIC FACTOR

A chemical substance secreted by the stomach which is necessary for the absorption of vitamin B-12. The exact chemical nature of intrinsic factor is not known, but it is thought to be a mucoprotein or mucopolysaccharide. A deficiency of this factor may lead to a deficiency of vitamin B-12, and, ultimately, to pernicious anemia.

(Also see ANEMIA, PERNICIOUS; and VITAMIN B-12.)

INULIN

A polysaccharide found especially in Jerusalem artichokes which yields fructose upon hydrolysis.

INVERSION

The process of splitting table sugar (sucrose) into glucose and fructose—invert sugar. Inversion is carried out by invertase, an enzyme, or by acids. Invert sugar is sweeter than sucrose due to the fructose present. It is often incorporated in products to prevent drying out; thus, it is a humectant. Invert sugar is utilized in the confectionary and brewing industries.

(Also see ADDITIVES.)

INVERTASE (SACCHARASE; SUCRASE)

An enzyme produced by the cells of the small intestine and by yeast. It catalyzes the splitting of table sugar (sucrose) into glucose and fructose.

(Also see DIGESTION AND ABSORPTION.)

INVERTASE (SUCRASE)-ISOMALTASE DEFICIENCY

This is a rare inborn error in the metabolism of carbohydrates. The most common symptom is diarrhea. In this disease the enzymes invertase and isomaltase are missing. Both enzymes are disaccharidases. Invertase splits sucrose (sugar) and isomaltase splits isomaltose, a product of starch digestion. Therefore, sources of sucrose and isomaltose—wheat and potatoes—should be omitted from the diet to control the disease.

(Also see INBORN ERRORS OF METABOLISM.)

INVERT SUGAR

A sugar obtained by splitting sucrose—table sugar—into glucose and fructose. This process—inversion—may be carried out by the enzyme, invertase, or by acids. Invert sugar is sweeter than table sugar due to the presence of fructose. It is a mixture of about 50% fructose and 50% glucose. It is used in foods and confections. In some foods it is used as a humectant to hold moisture and prevent drying. The brewing industry also uses invert sugar. Honey is mostly invert sugar.

(Also see ADDITIVES; CARBOHYDRATE[S]; and SUGAR.)

IODINE (I)

Contents

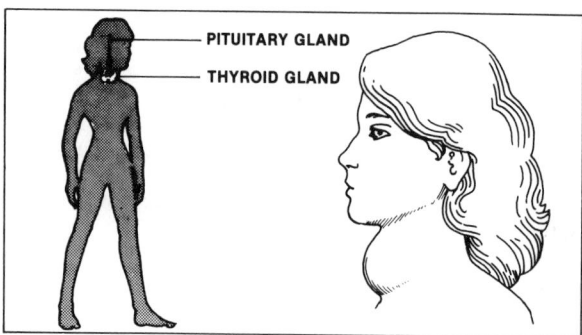

Fig. I-13. When the hormone thyroxin must be made, the pituitary gland sends messages to the thyroid gland. When iodine is lacking in the diet, the thyroid works harder to build more thyroxin. This causes the thyroid to develop a goiter—an enlargement in the neck area.

Iodine is recognized as an essential nutrient for all animal species, including man. The human body contains about 25 mg of iodine, 10 mg of which is in the thyroid gland. It is an integral component of the thyroid hormones, thyroxine and triiodothyronine, both of which have important metabolic roles.

One of the factors affecting the output of thyroid hormones by the thyroid gland is iodine availability. In the absence of sufficient iodine, the gland attempts to compensate for the deficiency by increasing its secretory activity, and this causes the gland to enlarge. This condition is known as simple, or endemic, goiter. Females are consistently more affected than males, because goiter usually develops in periods when metabolic rate is high, such as during puberty and pregnancy. It should be noted that not all goiter is *simple* goiter, due to lack of iodine. Another type of goiter, called *exophthalmic goiter (Graves' disease)*, is due to overactivity of the thyroid gland, which is usually—but not always—enlarged.

Iodine deficiencies are worldwide; wherever foods are grown on iodine-poor soil containing insufficient iodine to meet human needs. The highest incidence has been observed in the Alps, the Pyrenees, the Himalayas, the Thames Valley of England, certain regions of New Zealand, a number of Central and South American countries, and the Great Lakes and Pacific Northwest regions of the United States. Fig. I-14 shows the goiter areas of the world.

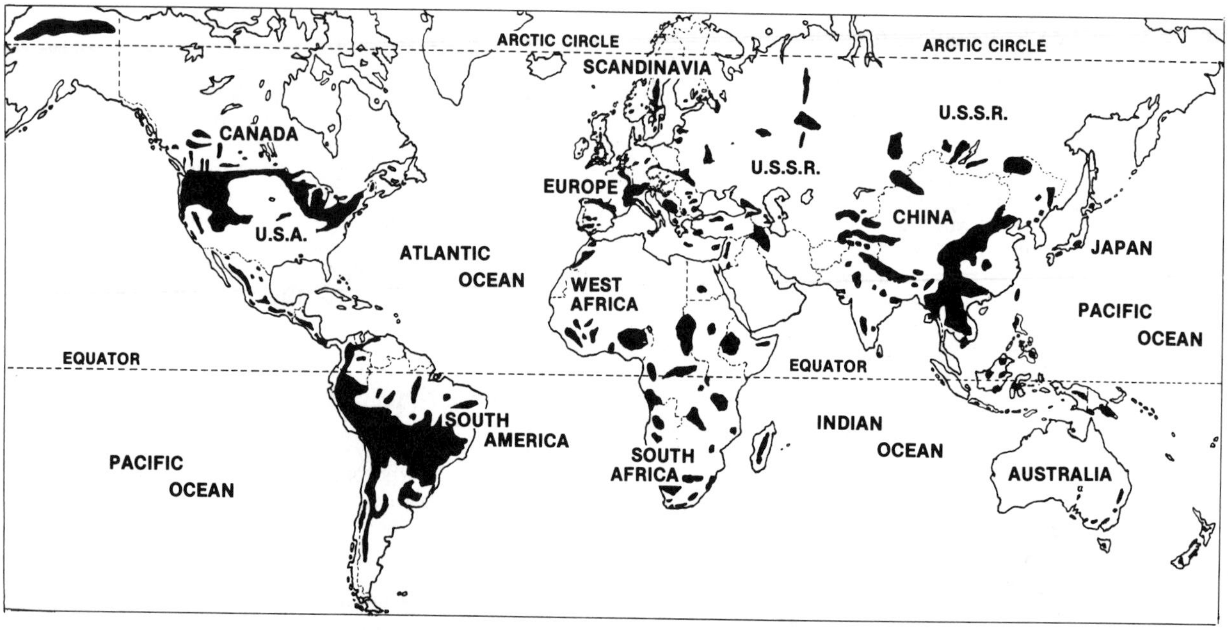

Fig. I-14. Goiter areas of the world. (Map prepared by the authors on the basis of information from the World Health Organization, Geneva, Switzerland)

The incidence of goiter in the United States fell sharply following the introduction of iodized table salt. Nevertheless, some "residual" goiter persists, probably not caused by insufficient iodine intakes, but strongly suggesting causes other than iodine deficiency—such as goitrogens (substances that can cause goiter).

HISTORY. Iodine was the first nutrient to be recognized as essential for humans or animals. As early as 3000 B.C., the Chinese treated goiter by feeding seaweed and burnt sponge. Also, Hippocrates (460 to 370 B.C.), the Greek physician, used the same treatment for enlarged thyroid glands. The name "iodine" is derived from the Greek word *iodes*, meaning violet color, from the color of the fumes of iodine.

In 1811, Bernard Courtois, a French chemist, discovered iodine in seaweed and described some of its basic properties. Five years later, potassium hydriodate was introduced by Prout as a treatment for goiter. However, the widespread appearance of goiter continued in much of the world for many years.

In 1914, Kendall, at the Mayo Clinic, in Minnesota, reported the isolation of a crystalline compound containing 65% iodine from the thyroid gland and named it thyroxin. From this discovery and from other studies, the inclusion of iodine in the diets of man and animals led to a great reduction of goiter in the United States and other developed countries of the world. Kendall received the Nobel Prize for his work on thyroxin and other hormones.

ABSORPTION, METABOLISM, EXCRETION. Most of the iodide present in food is iodine, in which form it is absorbed. Absorption takes place in the small intestine. Following absorption, iodine takes two main pathways within the body. Approximately 30% is removed by the thyroid gland and used for the synthesis of the thyroid hormones; most of the remainder is excreted in the urine, although small amounts are lost in the feces and sweat.

FUNCTIONS OF IODINE. The sole function of iodine is for making the iodine-containing hormones secreted by the thyroid gland, which regulate the rate of oxidation within the cells; and in so doing influence physical and mental growth, the functioning of the nervous and muscle tissues, circulatory activity, and the metabolism of all nutrients.

DEFICIENCY SYMPTOMS. Iodine deficiency is characterized by goiter (an enlargement of the thyroid gland at the base of the neck), coarse hair, obesity, and high blood cholesterol. Simple goiter is prevented by the addition of iodized salt to the diet. The most effective treatment is thyroid hormone, obtained from the glands of animals and prescribed by the physician according to the patient's needs. Surgery may be necessary if the

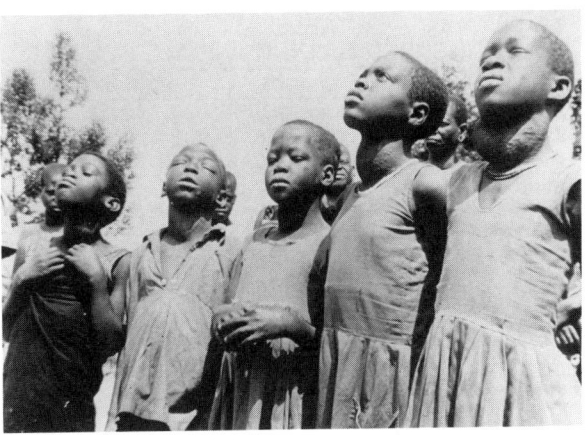

Fig. I-15. Goiter (big neck), caused by iodine deficiency. The enlarged thyroid gland (goiter) is nature's way of attempting to make sufficient thyroxin under conditions where a deficiency exists. (Courtesy, FAO/UN, Rome, Italy)

doctor suspects malignancy or to improve the victim's appearance.

Iodine-deficient mothers may give birth to infants with a type of dwarfism known as cretinism, a disorder characterized by malfunctioning of the thyroid gland, goiter, mental retardation, and stunted growth. Some of these effects may be prevented by diagnosis of the condition right after birth, followed by the administration of thyroid hormones. A similar disorder of the thyroid gland, known as myxedema, may develop in adults.

INTERRELATIONSHIPS. Certain foods (especially plants of the cabbage family—cabbage, kale, turnips, cauliflower, rapeseed, and mustard seed) contain goitrogens, which interfere with the use of thyroxin and may produce goiter. Fortunately, goitrogenic action is prevented by cooking, and an adequate supply of iodine inhibits or prevents it.

Jointly occurring deficiencies of iodine and vitamin A are likely to cause a more severe thyroid disorder than lack of iodine alone.

RECOMMENDED DAILY ALLOWANCE OF IODINE. The daily iodine requirement for prevention of goiter in adults is 50 to 75 mcg, or approximately 1 mcg/kg of body weight. In order to provide an extra margin of safety and to meet increased demands that may be imposed by natural goitrogens under certain conditions, the Food and Nutrition Board of the National Research Council (FNB-NRC) recommends an allowance of 150 mcg per day for adolescents and adults of both sexes, *plus* additional allowances of 25 and 50 mcg per day for pregnant and lactating women, respectively. The FNB-NRC recommended daily iodine allowances are given in Table I-11.

TABLE I–11
RECOMMENDED DAILY IODINE ALLOWANCES[1]

Group	Age	Weight		Height		Iodine
	(yr)	(lb)	(kg)	(in.)	(cm)	(mcg)
Infants	0–0.5	13	6	24	60	40
	0.5–1.0	20	9	28	71	50
Children ..	1–3	29	13	35	90	70
	4–6	44	20	44	112	90
	7–10	62	28	52	132	120
Males	11–14	99	45	62	157	150
	15–18	145	66	69	176	150
	19–24	160	72	70	177	150
	25–50	174	79	70	176	150
	51+	170	77	68	173	150
Females ..	11–14	101	46	62	157	150
	15–18	120	55	64	163	150
	19–24	128	58	65	164	150
	25–50	138	63	64	163	150
	51+	143	65	63	160	150
Pregnant						.175
Lactating						.200

[1]Recommended Dietary Allowances, 10th ed., 1989, NRC–National Academy of Sciences, p. 285.

Iodine intake at the FNB-NRC recommended levels has no demonstrable adverse effects; in fact, an intake in adults between 50 and 1,000 mcg of iodine can be considered safe.

It is recommended that iodized salt be used in households in all noncoastal regions of the United States. In the coastal regions the need is not so great because of the higher iodine concentration in the environment.

It is suggested that all food products designed to provide complete nutrient maintenance of individuals (such as infant formulas and special medical diets) contain iodine in sufficient concentrations to provide their proportion of the recommended dietary allowance.

The FNB-NRC recommends that many added sources of iodine in the American food system, such as iodophors in the dairy industry, alginates, coloring dyes, and dough conditioners, be replaced wherever possible by compounds containing less or no iodine. This recommendation was prompted because the iodine consumed by human beings has increased in recent years, and there is evidence that the quantity of iodine presently consumed in the United States is well above the nutritional requirement. Although there is no direct evidence of an increased human iodine toxicity problem because of the increased intake, there is some concern that if this trend continues, the greater iodine concentration may contribute to an increase in thyroid disorders.

Because iodine content in milk has increased 300 to 500% since about 1965, the Kentucky Agricultural Experiment Station made a study of the factors contributing to this increase. They reported as follows:

Organic iodine additions to the feed supply have contributed large increases in iodine content in milk from some farms, and are considered the main factor contributing to the large increase in iodine content in milk values. Iodine teat dips and udder washes contribute to the increased iodine content of milk, but they generally do not result in increases of more than 150 mcg/liter. Iodine-sanitizing agents used on milking equipment or in milk transfer and storage equipment can contribute large amounts if improperly used, but the frequency of this problem is small. Iodine content in meat does increase with increased iodine intake, but the transfer of iodine to meat is relatively lower than it is in milk.[8]

• **Iodine intake in average U.S. diet**—Studies have estimated the average dietary iodine intake in the United States to range from 64 to 677 mcg per day. Higher intakes are likely in persons subjected to high levels of atmospheric iodine or in those consuming iodine-containing drugs.

TOXICITY. Long-term intake of large excesses of iodine may disturb the utilization of iodine by the thyroid gland and result in goiter. In Tasmania, goiter induced by high dietary iodine intake has been correlated with the introduction of bread fortified with iodine. Also, goiter induced by high iodine intake has been documented in Japan, where seaweeds rich in iodine are habitually consumed. It is unlikely that such adverse effects as those reported in Tasmania and Japan would result in a population with habitual iodine intakes of less than 300 mcg per day.

Therapeutic use of iodine or large intakes of kelp in the diet can be toxic. So, self-treatments with compounds of iodine or concentrates of iodine in dried seaweed over long periods can be hazardous.

It is noteworthy that people with iodine deficiencies have above average susceptibility to the toxic effects of I-131, an atmospheric contaminant produced during the open-air testing of nuclear weapons.

SOURCES OF IODINE. Of the various methods that have been proposed for assuring an adequate iodine intake, especially among populations in iodine-poor regions, the use of iodized salt has thus far proved to be the most successful, and therefore the most widely adopted method. In the United States, iodination is on a voluntary basis, nevertheless slightly more than half of the table salt consumed is iodized. Stabilized iodized salt contains 0.01% potassium iodide (0.0076% I), or 76 mcg of iodine per gram. Thus, the average use of 3.4 g of iodized salt per person per day adds approximately 260 mcg to the daily intake, more than three times the normal requirement.

Iodine may also be provided in bread. But the practice of using iodates (chemicals used as dough conditioners) in bread-making appears to be on the decline.

Among natural foods the best sources of iodine are kelp, seafoods, and vegetables grown on iodine-rich soils. Dairy products and eggs may be good sources if the producing animals have access to iodine-enriched rations. Most cereal grains, legumes, roots, and fruits have low iodine content.

So, for intakes of iodine, man is dependent upon food, soil, and water. The iodine content of foods varies widely, depending chiefly on (1) the iodine content of the soil, (2) the iodine content of the animal feeds (to which iodized salt is routinely added in most countries), and (3) the use of iodized salt in food processing operations. Iodine in drinking and cooking water varies widely in different regions; in some areas, such as near oceans, it is high enough to meet the daily requirement. For these reasons, iodine values in food composition tables should be accepted as indicative, but not precise.

Table I-12 gives the iodine content of some common foods.

(Also see GOITER; and MINERAL[S], Table M-67.)

TABLE I–12
IODINE CONTENT OF SOME COMMON FOODS

Source	Iodine Content
	(mcg / 100 g)
Dried kelp	62,400
Iodized salt	7,600
Saltwater fish (haddock, whiting, herring)	330
Blackstrap molasses	158
Catfish	118
Beans, dried	115
Seafoods	66
Spinach	56
Vegetables	30
Milk and products	14
Eggs	13
Whole grain wheat	9
Whole grain oats	9
Beef	8
Rice polish	7
Wheat bran	7
Rice bran	4
Whole grain barley	4
Rice	4
Fruits	3

IODINE DEFICIENCY (GOITER)

Failure of the body to obtain sufficient iodine from which the thyroid gland can form thyroxin, an iodine-containing compound.

(Also see GOITER; and IODINE.)

IODINE NUMBER

A number which denotes the degree of unsaturation of a fat or fatty acid. It is the amount of iodine in grams which can be taken up by 100 grams of fat.

(Also see FATS AND OTHER LIPIDS, section headed "Fatty Acids"; and OILS, VEGETABLE.)

IODINE 131

The radioactive form of iodine (I). It has a half-life of 8 days. Since its presence can be detected by a Geiger counter or similar instrument, iodine 131 has numerous uses in biology and medicine. Substances can be "tagged" with iodine 131 and then their metabolism, movement or disappearance can be followed in the body. Medical diagnostic and therapeutic uses include: thyroid function, blood volume, location of brain tumors, cancer treatment, and hyperthyroid treatment.

(Also see CANCER.)

IODIZED SALT

Prevention of goiter is usually achieved in the developed countries by the use of iodized salt. For the purpose of iodizing, the FDA allows up to 0.01% of potassium iodide (KI) in table salt. Two grams of iodized table salt per day—most people use more—furnishes about 152 mcg of iodine or slightly more than the Recommended Dietary Allowance for adults.

(Also see GOITER; and IODINE, section headed "Sources.")

IODOPSIN

The main pigment found in the cones of the retina; it contains vitamin A.

(Also see VITAMIN A, section headed "Functions.")

ION

An atom or a group of atoms carrying an electric charge, either positive or negative. They are usually formed when salts, acids, or bases are dissolved in water.

IONIC IRON

Pertaining to an atom of iron, as Fe + + + or Fe + + (ferric and ferrous, respectively).
(Also see IRON.)

IONIZATION

The adding of one or more electrons to, or removing one or more electrons from, atoms or molecules, thereby creating ions.

IONIZED CALCIUM (Ca + +)

This refers to the free, diffusible form of calcium in the blood and other body fluids, amounting to about 1% of the total body calcium. It exerts a profound effect on the function of bone, the heart, and the nervous system.

IRON (Fe)

IRON, needed by the body to build red blood

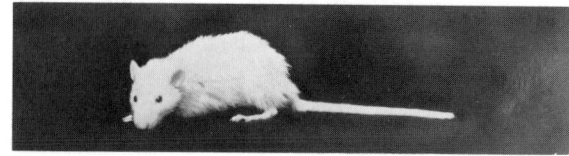

This rat did not have enough iron. It has pale ears and tail. Eight months old, it weighs only 109 g.

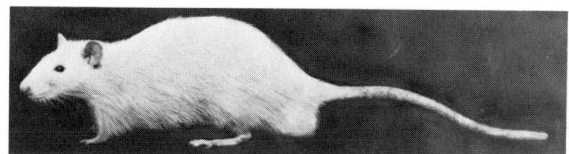

This rat had plenty of iron. Its fur is sleek and its blood has three times as much red coloring as the rat to the left. Though only 5½ months old, it weighs 325 g.

TOP FOOD SOURCES

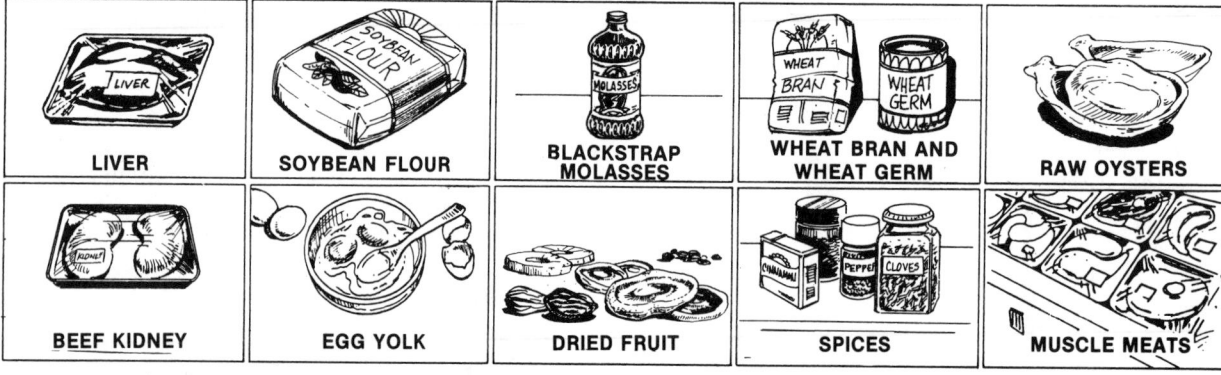

Fig. I-16.   Iron made the difference! *Left*: Rat on iron-deficient diet. *Right*: Rat that received plenty of iron. Note, too, ten top sources of iron. (Adapted from USDA sources)

The human body contains only about 0.004% iron, or only 3 to 4 g in an adult. About 70% of the iron is present in the hemoglobin, the pigment of the red blood cells. Most of the rest (about 30%) is present as a reserve store in the liver, spleen, and bone marrow. Despite the very small amount in the body, iron is one of the most important elements in nutrition and of fundamental importance to life. It is a component of hemoglobin, myoglobin (muscle hemoglobin), the cytochromes, catalase, and peroxidase. As part of these heme complexes and metalloenzymes, it serves important functions in oxygen transport and cellular respiration.

The red blood cells and the pigment within are broken down and replaced about every 120 days, but the liberated iron is not excreted; most of it is utilized to form new hemoglobin.

HISTORY. Elemental iron has been known since prehistoric times. Although how early humans first learned to extract the element from its ores is still debated, scientists are fairly certain that early, highly prized samples of iron were obtained from meteors. Several reference to "the metal of heaven" (thought to be iron) have been found in ancient writings. By approximately 1200 B.C., iron was being obtained from its ores; this achievement marked the beginning of the *Iron Age*.

The early Greeks were aware of the health-imparting properties of iron. Ever since, it has been a favorite health tonic (for better or worse). As early as the 17th century in England, iron was found to be a specific treatment for anemia in man. In 1867, Boussingault, the French chemist, obtained experimental evidence of the essential nature of iron in nutrition.

Although the need for iron was discovered long ago, and although it is the most common and cheapest of all metals, more deficiencies of iron (chiefly in the form of anemia) exist in the United States and in most other developed countries than of any other nutrient. An estimated 10 to 25% of the population is affected. Lack of iron in the diet is attributed primarily to (1) the increased refining and processing of our food supply, and (2) the decreased use of cast-iron cookware.

ABSORPTION, METABOLISM, EXCRETION.
The greatest absorption of iron occurs in the upper part of the small intestine—in the duodenum and jejunum, although a small amount of absorption takes place from the stomach and throughout the whole of the small intestine. Only 10% of the iron present in cereals, vegetables, and pulses, excluding soybeans, is absorb-

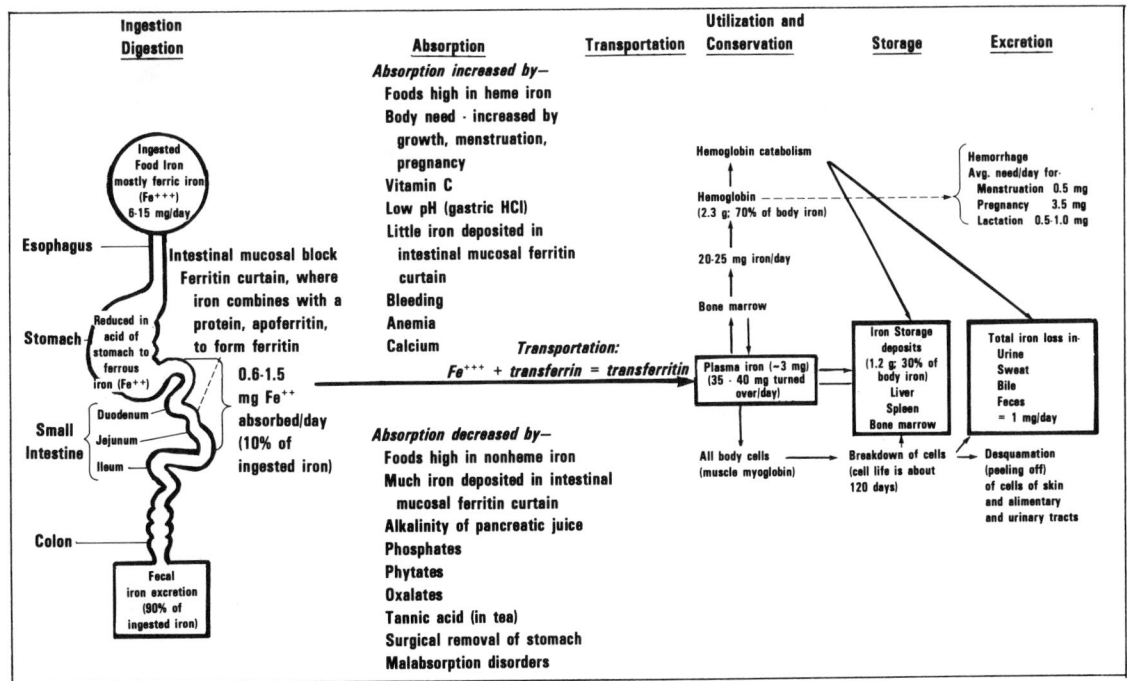

Fig. I-17. Iron absorption, metabolism, and excretion. Note that healthy adults absorb only about 10% of the iron in food, and that about 90% is excreted in the feces. Note, too, the factors that increase and decrease absorption.

ed. Absorption of iron from other foods is slightly higher—for example, 30% from meat, 20% from soybeans, and 15% from fish. For estimating the absorption of iron in diets, a value of 10% is usually taken as the percentage of iron absorbed from mixed foods.

It is noteworthy that there are two forms of food iron—heme (organic) and nonheme (inorganic). Of the two, heme is absorbed from food more efficiently than inorganic iron and is independent of vitamin C or iron-binding chelating agents. Although the proportion of heme iron in animal tissues varies, it amounts to about one-third of the total iron in all animal tissues—including meat, liver, poultry, and fish. The remaining two-thirds of the iron in animal tissues and all the iron of vegetable products are treated as nonheme iron.

Modern knowledge of the existence of two categories of iron-containing foods—heme and nonheme compounds—and of dietary factors influencing their absorption, now makes it possible to replace the estimate of an average 10% absorption of dietary iron by a more precise figure. This concept provides a means for the calculation of absorbable iron in any one meal and for increasing the availability of dietary iron through selection of appropriate food items. The application of this concept gives promise of improving the nutritional status of population groups in need of more iron, and of decreasing the exposure of individuals with excessive iron absorption.

Iron absorption is controlled by the intestinal mucosal block—the ferritin curtain, the exact mechanism of which is not known. It is increased (1) by foods high in heme iron; (2) by body needs—increased by growth, menstruation, and pregnancy; (3) by the presence of vitamin C (ascorbic acid) and gastric HCl, which convert the iron from the ferric ($Fe+++$) to the ferrous ($Fe++$) state; (4) when little iron is deposited in the intestinal mucosal ferritin curtain; (5) when there is increased *hemoglobin* synthesis—for example, following *hemorrhages* (bleeding), or as a result of anemia or *hemopoetic* abnormalities; and (6) by the presence of calcium. Iron absorption is impaired (1) by foods high in nonheme iron; (2) when much iron is deposited in the intestinal mucosal ferritin curtain; (3) by excess phosphates, phytates, oxalates, and tannic acid (in tea), all of which form insoluble compounds that are not readily absorbed—hence, excesses of such substances should be avoided in individuals suffering from severe nutritional anemia; and (4) following surgical removal of the stomach or when there are malabsorption disorders.

Mucosal ferritin delivers ferrous iron ($Fe++$) to the portal blood system. Thence iron is converted back to the ferric ($Fe+++$) state by oxidation. As ferric iron, it combines with protein (transferrin), forming a combination known as transferritin. In this form, iron is transported to the bone marrow where it may be incorporated into newly synthesized hemoglobin molecules; or, alternatively, it may be stored in the liver, spleen, and bone marrow, where it combines with a protein and is deposited as ferritin.

Absorbed iron is lost only by desquamation (shedding or peeling off of cells) from the alimentary, urinary, and respiratory tracts, and by skin and hair losses. The bulk of ingested iron (about 90%) is excreted in the feces. Only neglible amounts of iron are excreted in the urine. The body conserves and reuses iron once it has been absorbed. The combined losses of iron by all routes are of the order of about 1 mg per day for a healthy adult man, and about 1.5 mg per day for a woman during the reproductive period. Added losses of iron of importance occur from blood donation and pathological bleeding (hookworm infections, bleeding ulcers, etc.), and in cases of kidney diseases, particularly nephrosis.

FUNCTIONS OF IRON.   Iron combines with protein to make hemoglobin for red blood cells. *Heme* means iron; *globin* means protein. A small amount of iron (heme) combines with a large protein (globin) to make hemoglobin, the iron-containing compound in red blood cells. So, iron is involved in transporting oxygen. It is also a component of enzymes which are involved in energy metabolism.

DEFICIENCY SYMPTOMS.   A deficiency of iron may cause iron-deficiency (nutritional) anemia, clinically characterized by a decrease in the amount of hemoglobin and by small, pale-red blood cells, depleted iron stores, and a plasma iron content of less than 40 mg per 100 ml. The number of red blood cells may also be reduced, but not as markedly as the hemoglobin content. Iron-deficiency anemia is a medical and public health problem of primary importance, causing few deaths but contributing seriously to the weakness, ill health, and substandard performance of millions of people.

The symptoms of anemia are: paleness of skin and mucous membranes, fatigue, dizziness, sensitivity to cold, shortness of breath, rapid heartbeats, and tingling in the fingers and toes.

An inadequate dietary intake of iron by growing children, by adolescent girls, or by women—especially during pregnancy and in lactation, will produce nutritional anemia.

If a pregnant woman has an insufficient intake of iron, the newborn infant, in turn, will have a relatively low store of iron, causing anemia to develop early in the first year of life. Anemia during infancy, a frequent occurrence, is closely related to the body stores of iron at birth. It is especially common in premature infants and twins, because in such circumstances the body reserves of iron cannot be built up to desirable levels.

Many adolescent girls select a poor diet, to indulge the whims of a freakish appetite or to maintain ill-advised reduction regimens, with resultant anemia. Thus, it is necessary continually to emphasize to them that there is an accelerated demand for iron to satisfy their still-increasing blood volume as well as to compensate for losses through menstruation.

(Also see DEFICIENCY DISEASES, Table D-1 Major Dietary Deficiency Diseases—"Iron Deficiency Anemia.")

INTERRELATIONSHIPS. Iron is associated with hemoglobin and various enzymes. However, the production of hemoglobin in the body also requires protein, copper, vitamin C, vitamin B-6 (pyridoxine), folic acid, and vitamin B-12. An excess of iron in the diet can tie up phosphorus in an insoluble iron-phosphate complex, thereby creating a deficiency of phosphorus.

Free iron ions are very toxic. So, the iron molecule is always transported in combination with protein; 2 atoms of ferric iron are bound to 1 molecule of beta globulin protein called *transferrin*—and the combination forms *transferritin.* When the level of iron ions exceeds the binding capacity of the transferrin, iron toxemia occurs. Normally, the amount of iron in plasma is sufficient to bind only ⅓ of the transferrin—the remaining ⅔ represents the unbound reserve.

Iron overload may occur as a result of metabolic defects, such as idiopathic hemochromatosis—an inherited disease, or from high intakes of iron. The clinical signs and symptoms of iron overload may include hyperpigmentation of the skin, cirrhosis of the liver, diabetes, and myocardial failure. Dr. John R. K. Robson, M.D., one of the coauthors of this book, has observed excessive intakes of iron, characterized by hemosiderosis and cirrhosis of the liver, in the Bantu tribe of South Africa who cook their food in iron pots and ferment their beer in iron utensils—and who have iron intakes of up to 100 mg, or more, per day.

RECOMMENDED DAILY ALLOWANCE OF IRON. There are four situations in which iron intake is frequently inadequate in the United States: (1) in infancy, because of the low iron content of milk and because babies are not born with sufficient iron to meet their needs beyond 6 months; (2) during the periods of rapid growth in childhood and adolescence, because of the need to fill expanding iron stores; (3) during the female reproductive period, because of menstrual iron losses (at least 10% of menstruating women are iron deficient); and (4) in pregnancy, because of the expanding blood volume of the mother, the demands of the fetus and placenta, and blood losses in childbirth. In order to provide for the retention of 1 mg per day in adult males and postmenopausal females, and assuming an average availability of 10% of the food iron, an allowance of 10 mg per day is recommended. Higher recommended allowances are made during the critical periods; in infancy, in childhood and adolescence, during the female reproductive period, and in pregnancy and early lactation.

Recommended daily iron allowances are given in Table I-13.

TABLE I-13
RECOMMENDED DAILY IRON ALLOWANCES[1]

Group	Age	Weight		Height		Iron
	(yr)	(lb)	(kg)	(in.)	(cm)	(mg)
Infants	0–0.5	13	6	24	60	6
	0.5–1.0	20	9	28	71	10
Children ...	1–3	29	13	35	90	10
	4–6	44	20	44	112	10
	7–10	62	28	52	132	10
Males	11–14	99	45	62	157	12
	15–18	145	66	69	176	12
	19–24	160	72	70	177	10
	25–50	174	79	70	176	10
	51+	170	77	68	173	10
Females ...	11–14	101	46	62	157	15
	15–18	120	55	64	163	15
	19–24	128	58	65	164	15
	25–50	138	63	64	163	15
	51+	143	65	63	160	10
Pregnant						30
Lactating						15

[1]*Recommended Dietary Allowances*, 10th ed., 1989, NRC–National Academy of Sciences, p. 285.
[2]The increased requirement during pregnancy cannot be met by the iron content of habitual American diets nor by the existing iron stores of many women; therefore, the use of 30 to 60 mg of supplemental iron is recommended. Iron needs during lactation are not substantially different from those of nonpregnant women, but continued supplementation of the mother for 2 to 3 months after parturition is advisable in order to replenish stores depleted by pregnancy.

• **Iron intake in average U.S. diet**—According to the U.S. Department of Agriculture, there is sufficient iron in foods available for consumption in the United States to provide an average intake of 17.1 mg per person per day. Of this total, the contribution of food groups is as follows: meat, poultry, and fish, 22.1%; flour and cereal products, 42.7%; other vegetables, including tomatoes, 6.9%; sugars and sweeteners, 2.3%; dry beans and peas, nuts, soya flour, and grits, 6.5%; eggs, 2.9%; potatoes, 4.7%; noncitrus fruits, 2.4%; dairy products, 2.4%; dark green and deep yellow vegetables, 1.7%; citrus fruits, 0.6%; and fats and oils, including butter, 0.1%.

Iron fortification of cereals, flour, and bread has added significantly to the total iron intake.

TOXICITY. Approximately 2,000 cases of iron poisoning occur each year in the United States, mainly in young children who ingest the medicinal iron supplements of their parents. The lethal dose of ferrous sulfate for a 2-year-old is about 3 g; for an adult it's between 200 and 250 mg/kg of body weight.

IRON LOSSES DURING PROCESSING AND COOKING. The size of the pieces, the amount of water used, the cooking method, and the length of cooking time affect the extent of mineral loss.

The use of cast-iron cookware increases the iron content of foods, especially those that have an acid reaction, such as applesauce and spaghetti. However, it has not been established that the iron leached from iron cooking utensils is as available to the body as the natural occurring iron in foods.

SOURCES OF IRON.   Milk and milk products are poor sources of iron.

About 20% of the iron in the average U.S. diet comes from fortified products. Enrichment of flour (bread) and cereals with iron (along with thiamin, riboflavin, niacin, and with calcium enrichment optional), which was initiated in 1941, has been of special significance in improving the dietary level of iron in the United States. It is noteworthy that the major iron-enriched foods provide the following quantities of iron:

Food	Iron (mg/100 g)
Wheat flour, all-purpose or family enriched.	2.9
Rice, white, enriched, raw	2.9
Cornmeal, degermed, enriched	2.9
Bread, white, enriched	2.5
Corn flakes, with added nutrients	2.4

Groupings by rank of common food sources of iron follow:

• **Rich sources**—Beef kidneys, blackstrap molasses (there is less iron in molasses processed in modern stainless steel and aluminum vessels than in molasses processed in old-fashioned iron vats and pipes; see MOLASSES, section headed "Food"), caviar, chicken giblets, cocoa powder, fish flour, liver, orange pekoe tea, oysters, potato flour, rice polish, soybean flour, spices, sunflower seed flour, wheat bran, wheat germ, wheat-soy blend flour.

• **Good sources**—Beef, brown sugar, clams, dried fruits, egg yolk, heart, light or medium molasses, lima beans (cooked), nuts, pork, pork and lamb kidneys.

• **Fair sources**—Asparagus, beans, chicken, dandelion greens, enriched bread, enriched cereals, enriched cornmeal, enriched flour, enriched rice, fish, lamb, lentils, mustard greens, peanuts, peas, sausages and luncheon meats, spinach, Swiss chard, turkey, turnip greens, whole eggs.

• **Negligible sources**—Cheese, fats and oils, fresh and canned fruits, fruit juices and beverages, ice cream, milk, most fresh and canned vegetables, sour cream, sugar, yogurt.

• **Supplemental sources**—Dried liver, ferrous gluconate, ferrous succinate, ferrous sulfate, iron fumarate, iron peptonate, seaweed, yeast.

Normal mixed human diets of good quality contain from 6 to 15 mg of iron per day, of which 0.6 to 1.5 mg is absorbed. This amount is adequate for adult males, but it is inadequate for adolescent girls or women on diets of less than 10% calorie content from animal foods; hence, the doctor may recommend iron supplementation for females. It is noteworthy, however, that diets consisting of highly refined foods, such as are common in the United States, contain only 6 to 7 mg of iron, a level that is not high enough to satisfy the requirements. The iron level of such refined food diets can be improved by fortification (through wheat flour and bakery products). The use of ferrous sulfate, one of the most available forms of iron, is recommended. Since too much iron can trigger the hereditary illness called hemochromatosis, iron-rich pills or tonics should be taken only on the advice of a physician or nutritionist.

TOP IRON SOURCES.   The top iron sources are listed in Table I-14.

NOTE WELL: This table lists (1) the top sources without regard to the amount normally eaten (left column), and (2) the top food sources (right column); and the caloric (energy) content of each food.

(Also see ADDITIVES, Table A-3; and MINERAL[S], Table M-67.)

TABLE I-14
TOP IRON SOURCES[1]

Top Sources[2]	Iron (mg/100 g)	Energy (kcal/100 g)	Top Food Sources	Iron (mg/100 g)	Energy (kcal/100 g)
Thyme	123.6	276	Liver, hog, fried in margarine	29.1	241
Parsley, dried	97.9	276	Wheat–soy blend (WSB)/bulgur flour or straight grade wheat flour	21.0	365
Marjoram, dried	82.7	271			
Cumin seed	66.4	375	Molasses, cane, blackstrap	16.1	230
Fish flour from fillet waste	54.0	305	Wheat bran, crude commercially milled	14.9	353
Celery seed	44.9	392	Liver, calf, fried	14.2	261
Dill weed, dried	44.8	253	Kidneys, beef, braised	13.1	252
Oregano	44.0	306	Soybean flour, defatted	11.1	326
Bay leaves	43.0	313	Liver, chicken broiler/fryer, simmered	8.5	165
Basil	42.8	251	Oyster, fried	8.1	239
Coriander leaf, dried	42.5	279	Eggs, raw yolk, fresh	5.5	369
Turmeric	41.4	354	Apricots, dehydrated, sulfured, uncooked	5.3	332
Fish flour from whole fish	41.0	307			
Cinnamon	38.1	261	Sardines, Pacific, canned in brine or mustard, solids/liquid	5.2	186
Savory	37.8	272			
Anise seed	38.0	337	Prunes, dehydrated, uncooked	4.4	344
Fenugreek seed	33.5	323	Peaches, dried, sulfured, uncooked	3.9	340
Tea bag, orange pekoe	33.0	1	Beef, all cuts[3]	3.8	300
Tarragon	32.3	295	Nuts, mixed, dry roasted	3.7	590
Curry powder	29.6	325	Pork, all cuts[3]	3.2	325
			Beans, lima, mature, seeds, dry, cooked	3.1	138
			Rice, white, enriched, raw	2.9	363
			Wheat flour, all-purpose or family, enriched	2.9	365
			Raisins, natural, uncooked	2.8	289

[1]These listings are based on the data in Food Composition Table F–36. Some top or rich food sources may have been overlooked since some of the foods in Table F-36 lack values for iron.

Whenever possible, foods are on an "as used" basis, without regard to moisture content; hence, certain high-moisture foods may be disadvantaged when ranked on the basis of iron content per 100 g (approximately 3½ oz) without regard to moisture content.

[2]Listed without regard to the amount normally eaten.

[3]Values for different cuts range from 3.9 to 2.5 mg/100 g.

IRON-BINDING CAPACITY

The relative saturation of the iron-binding protein transferrin; the amount of transferrin bound to iron in relation to the amount remaining free to combine with iron determines the iron-binding capacity.

(Also see IRON.)

IRRADIATED YEAST

Yeast that has been irradiated. Yeast contains considerable ergosterol, which, when exposed to ultraviolet light, produces vitamin D.

(Also see VITAMIN D.)

IRRADIATION (FOOD)

This refers to the preservation of foods by radiation. It is sometimes referred to as "cold sterilization" because the microorganisms in the food are destroyed or inactivated by nuclear ionization rather than by heat or freezing.

(Also see PRESERVATION OF FOOD; and RADIATION PRESERVATION OF FOOD.)

ISCHEMIA

A local deficiency of blood, chiefly from narrowing of the arteries.

ISCHEMIC HEART DISEASE

A condition in which there is a deficiency of blood supply to the heart muscle due to obstruction or constriction of the coronary arteries.
(Also see HEART DISEASE.)

ISINGLASS

An extremely pure gelatin obtained from the swim bladders of certain species of fish. In the wine and beer industry it is used for clarification. It may also be used as an adhesive and as a lustering and stiffening agent in silks and other fabrics.

ISLETS OF LANGERHANS

The pancreas is a dual purpose organ. It secretes digestive juices to aid the process of digestion, and it secretes the hormones insulin and glucagon which regulate blood glucose levels. These hormones are secreted from the islets of Langerhans which are microscopic patches within the pancreas. In man there are 1 to 2 million islets. Actually, these patches or islands can be further divided into two types of cells: (1) beta cells secreting insulin, and (2) alpha cells secreting glucagon.
(Also see ENDOCRINE GLANDS.)

ISOASCORBIC ACID (ERYTHORBIC ACID)

A form of ascorbic acid, but it has only slight vitamin C activity. Isoascorbic acid is, however, a strong reducing agent and is used in food as an antioxidant and in cured meats to speed up color fixing.
(Also see ADDITIVES; and VITAMIN C.)

ISOCALORIC

Containing an equal number of calories.

ISOENZYME

Proteins with the same enzymatic specificity but which can be made into different molecular forms by physiochemical techniques.

ISOLATED SOYBEAN PROTEIN

Protein obtained from soybeans that can be spun into fibers, flavored, colored, and fabricated into meatlike products, including beef steaks, chicken, pork chops, ham, bacon, lamb chops, or sausage—all difficult to distinguish from the real products.
(Also see SOYBEAN.)

ISOLEUCINE

One of the essential amino acids.

ISOMALTOSE

Two molecules of glucose linked together, but linked between the first carbon of one glucose and the sixth carbon of the other instead of the first and fourth carbon linkage of maltose. Isomaltose and maltose are products of the breakdown of starch.
(Also see CARBOHYDRATE[S]; and DIGESTION AND ABSORPTION.)

ISOMER

Compounds having the same kind and number of atoms but differing in the atomic arrangements in the molecule.

ISOTONIC

Two solutions having the same total osmotic pressure; hence, if two isotonic solutions are separated by a semipermeable membrane, there is no net movement of solutions across the membranes.

ISOTOPE

An element of chemical character identical with that of another element occupying the same place in the periodic table (same atomic number) but differing from it in other characteristics, such as in radioactivity or in the mass of its atoms (atomic weight). Isotopes of the same element have the same number of protons in their nucleus but different numbers of neutrons. A *radioactive* isotope is one with radioactive properties. Such isotopes may be produced by bombarding the element in a cyclotron.

ISOTOPIC LABEL

The marking of a compound by introducing into it an isotope of one of its constituent elements; i.e., using a form of the element with a different atomic mass. For example, the atom mass of carbon (C) is 12; an isotope of carbon has an atomic mass of 14, expressed as ^{14}C.

-ITIS

Suffix denoting inflammation; for example, colitis.

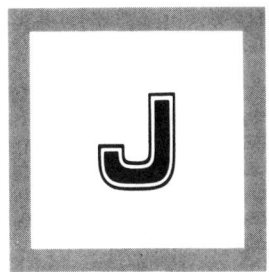

JABOTICABA *Myrciaria cauliflora*

The purple, grapelike fruit from an evergreen tree (of the family *Myrtaceae*) that grows in the tropics of Brazil. Individual fruits within the clusters are about ½ in. (*1.2 cm*) in diameter and contain a seedy pulp that may be eaten raw or made into jam, jelly, juice or wine.

The fruit is fairly low in calories (46 kcal per 100 g) and carbohydrates (12.6%). Also, it is a fair to good source of vitamin C.

JACK BEAN (HORSE BEAN) *Canavalia ensiformis*

This legume, which is sometimes called horse bean, is grown mainly for plowing under to restore soil fertility (as a green manure crop) or for livestock forage or fodder. Occasionally, the immature pods and seeds, or the dried mature seeds, are used as a human food when other items are scarce. Fig. J-1 shows the hardy legume.

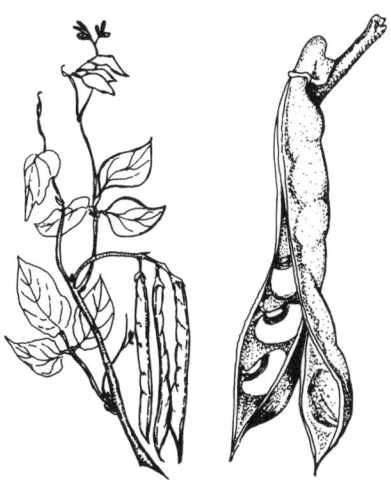

Fig. J-1. The jack bean, a tropical legume.

ORIGIN AND HISTORY. Archaeologists have found the jack bean at various sites in Mexico that are thought to be at least 5,000 years old. The plant appears to be native to Mexico, Central America, and the West Indies. But the earlier explorers of the Americas spread it throughout the tropical areas of the world.

The jack bean is well known to most students of biology because it contains the enzyme urease, which the American biochemist Sumner first extracted, purified, and identified as a protein in 1926. Prior to that time the chemical constitution of enzymes was unknown. (Urease acts to speed up the conversion of urea to ammonia and carbon dioxide.)

PRODUCTION. This legume, which is grown from seeds, is fast-growing and deep-rooted. Also, it is both resistant to drought and tolerant of shade. Hence, it is well suited to a wide range of subtropical and tropical areas. Some jack bean is even grown in the southern United States. When used as a green manure or cattle fodder, yields as high as 16 to 20 tons per acre (*40 to 50 ton/ha*) are obtained, whereas the yield of mature beans is about 1,200 lb per acre (*1,344 kg/ha*).

PROCESSING. In the United States, the jack bean is processed as a livestock feed; there is no commercial processing for human consumption. Where the immature pods are to be used for human food, they are processed similar to snap beans; and where the mature dry beans are to be used for human food, they are processed like mature common beans.

(Also see BEAN, COMMON, section headed "Processing.")

SELECTION AND PREPARATION. One is not likely to see jack beans in a local market, since all of the U.S. crop is used as green manure or forage. However, a few gardeners in the southern part of the United States grow this legume for human food because it requires less care and gives higher yields than some of the more popular beans.

The immature pods and seeds may be used as a green vegetable in ways similar to snap beans. Liberal amounts of seasonings are recommended since the flavor of the beans is not very appealing.

It is essential that the mature seeds be soaked overnight and cooked thoroughly, because (1) the uncooked beans may have a toxic effect, and (2) long boiling may be required to tenderize the seeds which are thick and tough. Therefore, pressure cooking for about an hour may be the most suitable means of cooking. (A tablespoon of fat should be added to prevent foaming which may clog the vent.) The cooked seeds should be well seasoned before serving.

CAUTION: Heat treatment (soaking overnight followed by cooking) renders the seeds and pods harmless. Bean flour should be made from cooked beans only, because the baking of products made from raw bean flour may not reduce the toxicity.

NUTRITIONAL VALUE. Although few North Americans have ever eaten jack beans, they are a potential staple food for people in the developing countries of Africa, Asia, and Latin America. The nutrient composition of jack beans is given in Food Composition Table F-36.

Some noteworthy observations regarding the nutritive value of jack beans follow:

1. Immature jack bean pods are very similar in nutritional value to snap beans, except that they are a much poorer source of vitamins A and C.

2. Dried mature jack beans are very similar in nutrient composition to dried common beans, so the values for cooked beans of the two species might also be expected to be similar. If this is the case, then 1 cup (*240 ml*) of cooked mature jack beans would supply about 14 g of protein, which is the amount present in 2 oz (*57 g*) of cooked lean meat. However, jack beans supply about twice the calories of meat (218 kcal vs 110 kcal).

3. The mature beans contain less than one-half as much calcium as phosphorus, so other foods higher in calcium and lower in phosphorus (such as dairy products and green leafy vegetables) should be consumed along with jack beans to promote optimal utilization of dietary calcium.

4. Both immature and mature jack beans provide ample amounts of iron per calorie.

Protein Quantity And Quality. Some important facts concerning the protein in jack beans follow:

1. One-half cup of cooked beans (about 100 g) supplies about 110 kcal, along with as much protein (7 *g*), as 1¾ oz (*50 g*) of cottage cheese (53 kcal) or 1 large egg (82 kcal).

2. Cooked jack beans furnish from 2 to 4 times as much protein as equal portions of cooked cereals such as corn and rice.

3. The proteins of both beans and cereal grains are deficient in some of the amino acids required by people, but the quality of the protein in combinations of these foods is much higher than that from either one alone. Therefore, jack beans should be eaten with corn, rice, or wheat products.

(Also see BEAN[S], Table B-10 Beans of the World; and LEGUMES, Table L-2 Legumes of the World.)

JAGGERY

Sap obtained from some palm trees contains 10 to 16% sucrose. In processing this sap, it is condensed by heating until the sucrose crystallizes. This product is poured into molds which form small sweet cakes, a product known as jaggery in some areas of the world.

(Also see SUGAR PALM.)

JAMBALAYA

This dish is most often found in the states bordering the Gulf of Mexico because it is usually made with crawfish which abound in the freshwater areas surrounding the gulf. It is made with rice, vegetables, herbs, and either ham, sausage, chicken, shrimp, oysters, or crawfish.

JAPANESE QUAIL (COTURNIX QUAIL, EASTERN QUAIL, PHAROAH'S QUAIL, AND STUBBLE QUAIL)

The Japanese quail (*Coturnix coturnix japonica*) has long been domesticated in Japan. The beginning of Japanese quail breeding can be traced back to 1595. Coturnix were first raised as pets and singing birds, but by 1900 they had become widely used for meat and egg production. Japanese quail develop 3½ times as fast as chickens; at 30 days of age they are almost fully grown. At 6 weeks of age, hens lay their first eggs; thereafter, they proceed, like machines, to lay an egg every 16 to 24 hours for 8 to 12 months.

Japanese quail are also game birds. The breast and legs are considered delicacies.

JAUNDICE

A symptom consisting of a yellow discoloration of both the bodily tissues and the body fluids with bile pigment (bilirubin) in which the skin and whites of the eyes are yellow.

JEJUNUM

The middle portion of the small intestine which extends from the duodenum to the ileum.

(Also see DIGESTION AND ABSORPTION.)

JELLY

A colloidal suspension which contains either gelatin, pectin, or agar. It can be flavored with fruit juice or synthetic flavors and colors. Some jellies are used as spreads on breads, others may be used as an accompaniment to meats.

JERUSALEM ARTICHOKE *Helianthus tuberosus*

This tuber-bearing plant is a member of the daisy family (*Compositae*) and closely related to the sunflower. It is referred to as an artichoke because the tubers have a globe artichokelike flavor. The name Jerusalem is thought to be an English alteration of Ter Neusen, the place in the Netherlands from which the plant was introduced into England. Fig. J-2 shows the plant with its tubers.

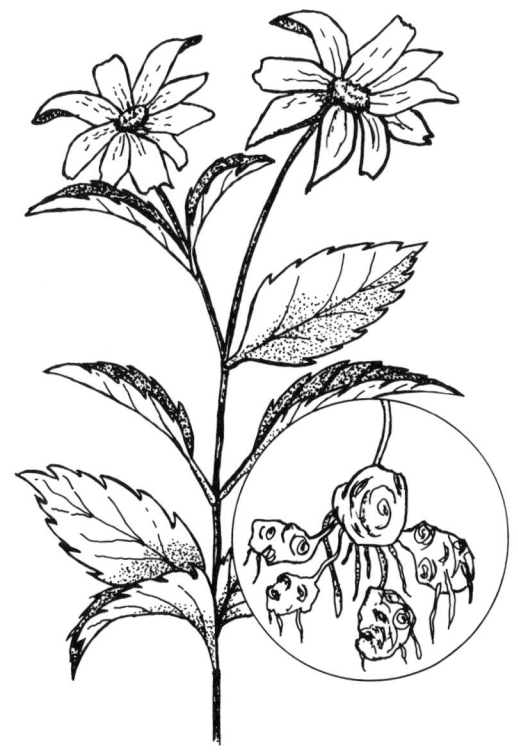

Fig. J-2. The Jerusalem artichoke, source of the edible tubers that are utilized in the preparation of certain dietetic foods.

ORIGIN AND HISTORY. The Jerusalem artichoke is native to a region in eastern North America which extends from the southern United States to southern Canada. It is not known when the plant was first cultivated, but the first settlers of New England noted that the Indians were growing it along the coast of Massachusetts. Shortly thereafter, the tubers were brought to Europe, where they were given names such as artichokes, potatoes, and topinambours. They were relished by the French, who devised various means of preparation. However, interest in Jerusalem artichokes declined with the rise in popularity of the Irish potato, which produced higher yields of tubers. Recently, this trend has been reversed somewhat due to the utilization of Jerusalem artichoke tubers in the production of dietetic flours, breads, and noodles.

PRODUCTION. Data on the commercial production of Jerusalem artichokes are not readily available, but it is known to be grown in Europe, Asia, and the Americas.

The plant is propagated vegetatively by planting (1) pieces of large tubers or (2) whole small tubers, in the fall or early spring. The tubers are quite resistant to frost. A well-drained soil is required since the plant does poorly when the soil is too wet. Little cultivation is needed because the plants outgrow the weeds.

Usually, the tubers are ready to be harvested in the early fall. It is necessary to cut off and remove the woody stems before digging up the tubers. The skin of the tuber is easily damaged, as a result of which moisture is lost readily and shriveling occurs. Therefore, it may be advantageous to leave the tubers in the soil until they can be used. Sometimes the tubers are "hogged off." That is, they are dug and eaten by hogs that have been turned onto the field where the tubers are grown. In this case, people "harvest" the Jerusalem artichoke in the form of pork. Whether the harvesting is performed by man or animal, however, some tubers are almost always left in the ground and will likely sprout during the following spring. Generally the yields of the tubers range from 12,000 to 40,000 lb per acre (*13,440 to 44,800 kg/ha*).

PROCESSING. The most common type of processing is the drying and grinding of the tubers into Jerusalem artichoke flour, a low-calorie product that is used to make dietetic baked goods and pastas. Recently, food technologists have devised means of producing the fructose sugar from the tubers by boiling them in dilute acid.

SELECTION AND PREPARATION. High quality Jerusalem artichokes are fresh looking and firm. Shriveled, wrinkled, or sprouted tubers indicate lack of freshness and are likely to be tough and involve considerable wastage in their preparation.

The tubers should be scrubbed with a vegetable brush, but peeling is not required unless dirt adheres to the skins. Then, the raw vegetable may be grated or thinly sliced and added to salads. Only about 15 minutes of cooking is required to tenderize the whole tubers. Longer cooking may toughen them. The cooked vegetable is very appetizing when served with a well-seasoned cream sauce or white sauce.

NUTRITIONAL VALUE. The nutrient composition of the Jerusalem artichoke is given in Food Composition Table F-36.

Some noteworthy observations regarding the nutrient composition of the Jerusalem artichoke follow:

1. Compared to Irish potatoes, Jerusalem artichokes supply fewer calories, the same amount of protein, more iron, and only about one-quarter as much vitamin C. The caloric content of the Jerusalem artichoke ranges from about 7 kcal per 100 g when freshly harvested to about 75 kcal per 100 g after a long period of storage. During storage the unavailable carbohydrate inulin is broken down to the sugar fructose.

2. Jerusalem artichoke tubers are deficient in calories, minerals, and vitamins. Hence, they should be supplemented with dietary sources of the missing nutrients.

(Also see VEGETABLE[S], Table V-6 Vegetables of the World.)

JICAMA *Exogonium bracteatum*

The large turnip-shaped root of this plant is much esteemed in Mexico and has recently become available in California and in certain large cities in the eastern United States. Jicama is a member of the morning glory family (*Convolvulaceae*), and is related to the sweet potato. (It is noteworthy that Mexicans sometimes apply the name jicama to other edible tubers such as those of the dahlia and the yam bean.)

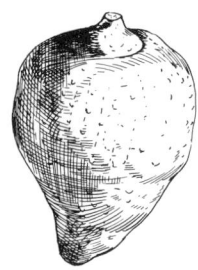

Fig. J-3.   Jicama, a Mexican root vegetable that resembles the water chestnut in texture and flavor.

ORIGIN AND HISTORY.   Jicama is native to Mexico, where it is sometimes called *bejuco blanco,* which means "white vine." It was recently brought to the United States, where certain cooks in Oriental restaurants discovered that it may be substituted for the much more expensive water chestnut. Furthermore, it is now being grown on a small scale in the southern United States by people of Mexican ancestry and is served at the salad bars of certain restaurants.

PRODUCTION.   No production statistics are available for jicama at the present time. However, it might well become an important commercial crop in the future.

This plant requires a long, hot growing season to develop marketable tubers. Hence, it is most suitable for growing in the U.S. "sunbelt." In Mexico, jicama is propagated by planting the tubers in rich, moist soil as soon as the danger of frost has passed and the soil has warmed up. The tubers grow best when the night temperatures remain above 60°F (*16°C*) for at least 5 months. Shorter periods of warm weather result in smaller tubers. Most growers support the vines on trellises, but they should keep them trimmed to a length of 5 ft (*1.5 m*) or less to prevent stunting of the tubers due to overgrowth of the foliage.

The tube. may be dug after the vines have flowered and have started to wither. However, they must be harvested before the first frost, since they are likely to be damaged by freezing.

PROCESSING.   There is little or no processing of jicama tubers at the present time because they are usually used right after harvesting, or after a few weeks of storage. However, they may be canned, dried, or frozen like potatoes and other popular types of starchy roots and tubers, should there be a demand for these products.

SELECTION AND PREPARATION.   High quality jicama tubers are usually heavy in relation to size, and are relatively smooth and firm. Those which are shriveled, soft, extra large, and light in weight for their size are likely to be tough, woody, or hollow.

Jicama may be peeled, diced or sliced, and served raw in relish trays and salads. It may also be used as a substitute for water chestnuts in various Oriental dishes. For example, small cubes of the tubers are good when stir-fried with other vegetables, chopped eggs, fish, meats, or poultry, and various seasonings.

NUTRITIONAL VALUE.   Data on the nutrient composition of jicama is not readily available. Judging from its close resemblance in flavor and texture to both the water chestnut and the yam bean, it seems likely that jicama tubers contain about 85 to 90% water and about 50 Calories (kcal) per 3½ oz (*100 g*) serving. Furthermore, it is probably very low in protein and most other nutrients. Nevertheless, it is a crisp, appetizing item that could be used in abundant amounts by people trying to restrict their calorie intake.

(Also see VEGETABLE[S], Table V-6 Vegetables of the World.)

JOULE

A proposed international unit (4.184j = 1 calorie) for expressing mechanical, chemical, or electrical energy, as well as the concept of heat. In the future, energy requirements and feed values will likely be expressed by this unit.

(Also see WEIGHTS AND MEASURES.)

JUICE

The aqueous substance obtainable from animal or plant tissue by pressing or filtering, with or without the addition of water.

JUJUBE, INDIAN *Zizyphus mauritiana*

The orange-brown egg-shaped fruit of a tree that belongs to the *Rhamnaceae* family and is believed to have originated in India, but is now grown throughout the dry tropics of Asia and Africa. Usually, the fruits are almost 1 in. (*2 to 3 cm*) long and have a tart sweet flavor. They are eaten fresh, candied, dried, or the pulp is made into a refreshing beverage. The dried and fermented pulp may also be used in spice cakes.

Indian jujubes are moderately high in calories (97 kcal per 100 g) and carbohydrates (25%). They are also a good source of fiber and vitamin C. The dried fruit contains approximately 3 times the nutrient levels of the fresh fruit, except that much of the vitamin C is destroyed during drying.

JULEP (MINT JULEP)

• A drink usually consisting of sweet syrup, flavoring, and water.

• A tall drink made from gin, rum, or other alcoholic liquor and sometimes flavored with citrus juice.

• A tall drink consisting of bourbon, sugar, and mint served in a frosted tumbler filled with finely crushed ice—also called a mint julep.

JUNE BERRY (SERVICE BERRY; SUGAR PLUM) *Amelanchier canadensis*

Purplish-red fruits borne by a shrub or small tree (of the family *Rosaceae*) that is native to eastern North America.

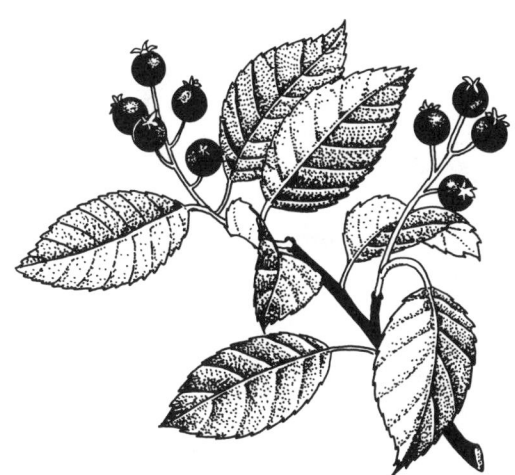

Fig. J-4. June berries, a wild plant of eastern United States and Canada.

June berries resemble blueberries and huckleberries and are used in many of the same ways (fresh, or in pies, puddings, and sauces).

(Also see BLUEBERRY; and HUCKLEBERRY.)

JUNIPER BERRY *Juniperus communis*

The fruit of a shrub or small tree (of the family *Cupressaceae*) that grows wild around the world and is known as the common juniper.

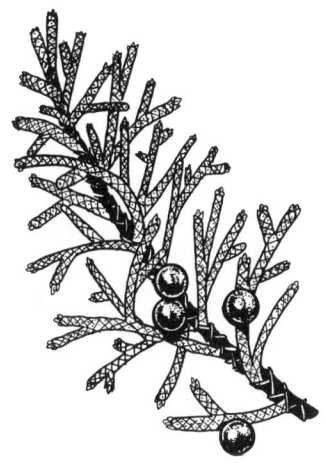

Fig. J-5. Juniper berries.

Juniper berries are a little smaller than wild blueberries and have a blue-black color. They have long been used medicinally for digestive problems and to rid the body of an excess of water (diuretic action). It appears that they were first used in wine and then later to make gin. The berries are also used as a flavoring in herb teas, meat and vegetable dishes, sauces and soups, and in various confections and desserts.

JUNK FOODS

There is no agreement on the definition of a junk food. According to the U.S. Department of Agriculture, a 100-calorie portion of food that does not supply 5% or more of the required daily allowance of one of the eight specified nutrients (protein, vitamin A, ascorbic acid, niacin, riboflavin, thiamin, calcium, and iron) is classified as a food of "minimal nutritional value." However, most people attribute the following characteristics to junk food: high in sugar, fat, calories, salt and/or additives; bad for health; and limited in protein, minerals, and vitamins. But regardless of definition, people eat junk food simply because they like it.

Despite parental concern, most fast foods are not junk foods. Indeed, many of them are very nutritious. Certainly, fast foods are not gourmet meals. Some of them have too few fresh fruits and vegetables. Others have an overabundance of fats and carbohydrates. But most people—whether they are age 6, 16, or 60—can eat today's fast foods that are good—and good for them.

(Also see CONVENIENCE AND FAST FOODS.)

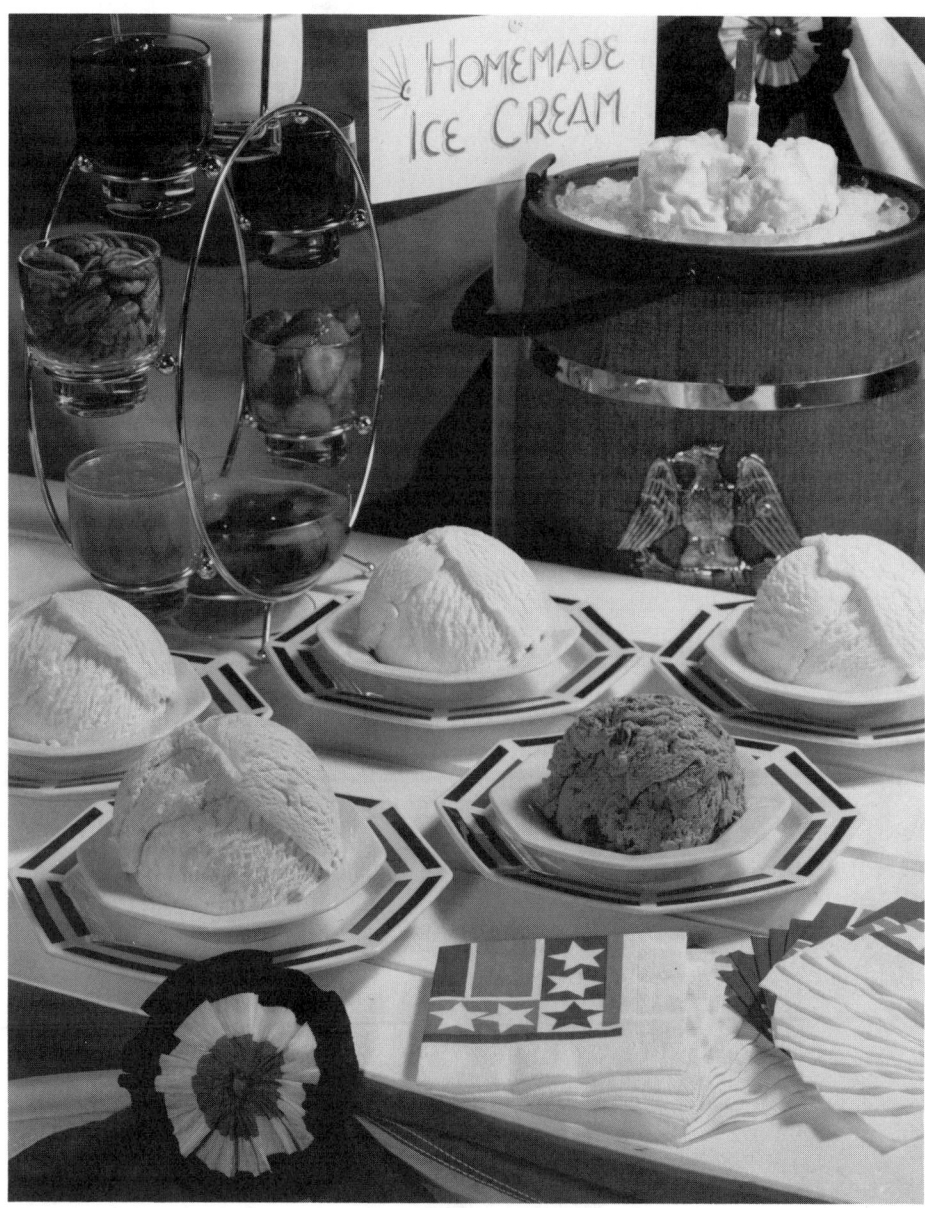

Homemade ice cream made with wholesome cream, eggs, and fresh fruit, and topped with more fresh fruit and nuts. (Courtesy, United Dairy Industry Assn., Rosemont, Ill.)

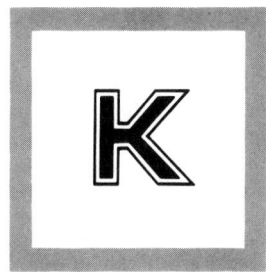

KALE *Brassica oleracea,* variety *acephala*

Most people are unaware that this vegetable is a good to excellent source of a half-dozen essential nutrients because only a small crop is produced in the United States.

Kale is essentially the same vegetable as collards, except that kale has leaves with curly edges and is less tolerant to hot weather. Fig. K-1 shows a typical bunch of kale leaves.

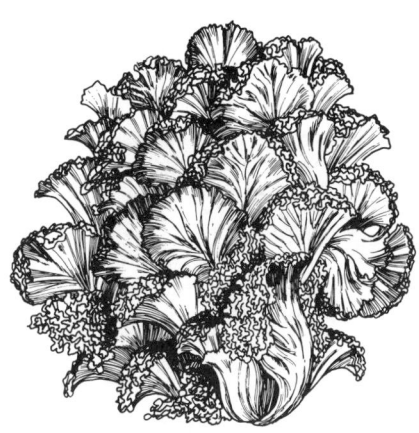

Fig. K-1. Kale, one of the most nutritious vegetables.

ORIGIN AND HISTORY. Kale is more closely related to the wild cabbage than any of the other cabbage vegetables. It was an important crop by the time of the ancient Romans, since it was mentioned in the writings of Cato the Elder (234-149 B.C.). Much of the early domestication of kale appears to have occurred in the Mediterranean region, where it was called "cabbage" in the days before head-forming cabbages were developed.

The popularity of kale as a human food has always been limited by the fact that the mature leaves are fibrous and tough. Hence, many of the early forms of the vegetable were developed for use as animal fodder. Nevertheless, kale eventually became a staple food of the European peasants during the Middle Ages.

Kale was brought to the United States by the English settlers in the 17th century, However, it was eventually replaced by collards in the states south of Virginia, because the latter has a greater tolerance to hot weather.

PRODUCTION. Statistics for the total U.S. production of kale are not readily available, although the American Frozen Food Institute reported that over the past 10 years an average of 4.1 million lb (*1.9 thousand metric tons*) of the crop were frozen each year.[1]

Most of the U.S. kale crop is grown in the vicinity of Norfolk, Virginia, where the mild climate favors its production. It is usually planted in the late summer and early fall because the mature plants do poorly in hot weather. However, it may be planted in the spring in the northern states because (1) it is tolerant to frost, and (2) the spring is sufficiently cool to permit the plants to thrive. The plants require abundant nitrogen, phosphorus, and potassium; hence, almost all soils require some fertilizer.

The plants have to be harvested before the leaves become too tough. Nevertheless, the flavor of the vegetable is improved by frost, so young plants may be left in the ground after freezing temperatures have arrived in the fall.

PROCESSING. In the early days of American agriculture, most of the kale crop was marketed fresh along the East Coast. Now, a large part of the crop is frozen, and some is canned.

SELECTION AND PREPARATION. High quality kale is fresh, young, and tender and ranges in color from blue-green to gray-green. Bunches which show insect injury, coarse stems, dry or yellowing leaves, excessive dirt, or poor development, are usually lacking in quality and may cause excessive waste. Flabby, wilted plants and leaves are generally undesirable.

Kale is rarely eaten raw, because it tends to be tough unless it is tenderized somewhat by freezing temperatures while it is still in the field. Usually, it is boiled briefly, then flavored with bits of crisp bacon, butter, chopped pieces of cooked Polish sausage, cheese sauce, garlic and olive oil, or grated cheese and other seasonings. Kale is also good in soups.

[1]*Agricultural Statistics 1991*, USDA, p. 172, Table 248.

CAUTION: It has been known since the 1950s that cows fed mainly kale will give milk that contains small amounts of goiter-causing (goitrogenic) substances that may interfere with the utilization of iodine by the thyroid gland. However, the significance of this finding in human nutrition is uncertain because (1) the amounts of goitrogens in the milk may be too low to have any effect on people who drink it, (2) people usually eat only small amounts of kale (3 to 6 oz [*85 to 170 g*] at any one meal), so they receive only minute traces of goitrogens from the vegetable itself (cows that are giving milk may eat up to 200 lb [*91 kg*] of kale forage per day), and (3) it appears that the effects of the goitrogens may be counteracted by the consumption of ample amounts of dietary iodine. The best food sources of iodine are iodized salt, ocean fish, seafood, and seaweeds such as kelp.

NUTRITIONAL VALUE.   The nutrient composition of kale is given in Food Composition Table F-36.

Some noteworthy observations regarding the nutrient composition of kale follow:

1.   Cooked kale contains about 90% water. Hence, it is low in calories (40 to 43 kcal per cup [*240 ml*]).

2.   Kale has the highest protein content (6%) of the cabbage vegetables. A 1-cup serving furnishes about 5 g of protein, which is the amount supplied by a cup of cooked corn or rice. However, kale contains only about one-quarter as many calories as the cooked cereals.

3.   The calcium content of kale is high, since a cup of the cooked vegetable supplies as much of the mineral as 5 oz (*150 ml*) of milk. Furthermore, the level of calcium is about three times that of phosphorus, whereas the ratio of calcium to phosphorus is much lower in most other foods. Therefore, kale should be consumed with the other foods in order to obtain a dietary balance between the two minerals.

4.   Kale is a good source of both iron and potassium.

5.   The vitamin A content of kale is very high, and the vitamin C content is moderately high. It is noteworthy that the vitamin C content of cooked fresh kale is double that of the cooked frozen kale. The reason for this difference is that blanching prior to freezing destroys this vitamin.

(Also see VEGETABLE[S], Table V-6 Vegetables of the World.)

KANGAROO MEAT

Australian frontiersmen in remote areas boil or roast the legs of the kangaroo, which look something like ham, and which are especially good when spiked with bacon. Kangaroo tail is used as the base for a rich and heavy soup, which is considered quite a delicacy and is sold commercially. Fearing that the animal might become extinct, in 1973 the Australian Parliament passed a law banning the sale to other countries of live kangaroos or of kangaroo hides or meat.

KANTEN

The name given to agar-agar in Japan.
(Also see AGAR-AGAR.)

KARELL DIET

A special diet for the early stage of victims of congestive heart failure or myocardial infarction. It is a low-calorie fluid diet consisting of only 27 oz (*800 ml*) of milk per day. The milk is given every four hours in 6½ oz (*200 ml*) servings. No other food and little additional fluid is offered for 2 to 3 days.

KCAL

The abbreviation for kilocalorie, a measure of food energy.
(Also see KILOCALORIE.)

KEI-APPLE (UMKOKOLA) *Dovyalis caffra; Aberia caffra*

The fruit of a shrub (of the family *Bixaceae*) that is native to Africa, and is used locally to make jam.

KELP (SEAWEED)

One of the names by which seaweed is known.
(Also see SEAWEED.)

KEMPNER DIET

Used in the treatment of high blood pressure, some kidney disorders, cirrhosis of the liver, and pregnancy toxemia, the Kempner diet is a rice-fruit diet. As such it is low in fat, protein, and sodium. Specifically, it is comprised of 10.5 oz (*300 g*) of raw rice cooked by boiling, or steaming without milk, fat or salt. With this, liberal amounts of canned or fresh fruit may be eaten. Daily fluid intake consists of 1 qt (*700 to 1,000 ml*) of fruit juice, but no additional water.

KERATIN

A sulfur-containing protein which is the primary component of epidermis, hair, wool, hoof, horn, and the organic matrix of the teeth.
(Also see PROTEIN[S].)

KERATINIZATION

A condition occurring in a severe vitamin A deficiency, in which the epithelial cells either slough off or become dry and flattened, then gradually harden and form rough horny scales. The process may occur in the cornea, the respiratory tract, the genitourinary tract, or the skin.

(Also see VITAMIN A, section on "Deficiency Symptoms.")

KERATOMALACIA

A disease resulting from a vitamin A deficiency. It is characterized by softening and perforation of the cornea of the eye. This leads to loss of the lens, infection and scarring of the eye and blindness. Treatment and prevention consist of adequate amounts of vitamin A. In some cases, treatment may occur too late to reverse the effects of the disease.

(Also see BLINDNESS DUE TO VITAMIN A DEFICIENCY; DEFICIENCY DISEASES, Table D-1 major Dietary Deficiency Diseases; and VITAMIN A.)

KERNEL

The whole grain of a cereal. The meats of nuts and drupes (single-stoned fruits).
(Also see CEREAL GRAINS.)

KETO-

A prefix denoting the presence of the carbonyl (CO) group.

KETO-ACID

The amino acid residue after deamination. The glycogenic keto-acids are used to form carbohydrates; the ketogenic keto-acids are used to form fats.

KETOGENESIS

The formation of ketones from fatty acids and some amino acids.

KETOGENIC

Capable of being converted into ketone bodies. The fatty acids and certain amino acids are the ketogenic substances in metabolism.

KETOGENIC AMINO ACID

The amino acids leucine, isoleucine, phenylalanine, tryptophan, and tyrosine are capable of undergoing a metabolic conversion to acetoacetate, a ketone body. Thus, they are said to be ketogenic.
(Also see AMINO ACID[S]; KETOSIS; and METABOLISM.)

KETOGENIC DIET

Diets high in fat and low in carbohydrate are termed ketogenic since they cause the accumulation of ketone bodies in the tissues. These diets eliminate carbohydrate sources such as breads, cereals, fruits, desserts, sweets, and sugar-containing beverages while foods high in fat such as butter, cream, bacon, mayonnaise, and salad dressing are eaten in generous amounts. Ketones are produced from the breakdown (oxidation) of fats. When the ratio of fatty acids to available glucose in the diet exceeds 2:1 ketosis occurs.

A ketogenic diet is considered monotonous and unpalatable. In some cases a ketogenic diet may be prescribed to control epilepsy, if drugs prove ineffective.
(Also see KETOSIS; METABOLISM; and MODIFIED DIETS.)

KETONE

Any compound containing a ketone (CO) grouping.

KETONE BODIES

Acetoacetic acid, acetone, and beta-hydroxybutyric acid.

KETONIC RANCIDITY

Decomposition of fats and oils results in the production of ketones. These ketones give fats or oils an off flavor or odor. The decomposition occurs slowly and spontaneously, however, certain molds of *Aspergillus* and *Penicillium* species may also be responsible.

KETOSIS

Shifting the metabolic machinery of the body to excessive utilization of fats instead of carbohydrates or a balance of fats and carbohydrates results in the buildup of ketone bodies—acetoacetate, beta-hydroxybutyrate, and acetone—in the blood and their appearance in the urine. This condition is referred to as ketosis, and outwardly noted by the sweetish, acetone odor of the breath. Three circumstances can cause ketosis: (1) high dietary intake of fat but low carbohydrate intake as in ketogenic diets; (2) diminished carbohydrate breakdown and high mobilization of fats as in starvation; or (3) disorders in carbohydrate metabolism as in diabetes mellitus. Unless ketosis goes unchecked and results in acidosis, it is a normal metabolic adjustment.
(Also see CARBOHYDRATE[S]; FATS AND OTHER LIPIDS; and METABOLISM.)

KIBBLED

Coarsely ground grain or meal.

KIDNEY DISEASES

Due to their importance, any disorder in the function or structure of the kidneys can have serious consequences, and often require some dietary adjustments. Glomerulonephritis (nephritis), nephrosis, nephroptosis, nephrosclerosis, renal (kidney) failure, kidney stones (nephrolithiasis), pyelitis, and pyelonephritis are all specific diseases which may in general be called kidney diseases.

Before there are any dietary adjustments, the extent of the kidney disease must be evaluated. It may be necessary to restrict sodium and potassium intake, and control the levels of protein and fluid intake. If protein intake is controlled, then it is important that sufficient high caloric but nonprotein food be eaten to meet the body's demand for energy, and to prevent the breakdown of the body's own protein for energy. Those proteins that are eaten should be proteins of high biological value—containing a large number of essential amino acids—like eggs, meat, milk, and milk products.

(Also see AMINO ACID[S]; GLOMERULONEPHRITIS; KIDNEY STONES; MODIFIED DIETS; NEPHROSCLEROSIS; NEPHROSIS; and PROTEIN[S].)

KIDNEYS

They are paired, bean-shaped organs located in the abdominal cavity at the level of the lower ribs next to the back with one on each side of the spine. The kidneys form urine and control the volume and the composition of the blood (extracellular fluid). Each day, the kidneys (1) filter about 50 gal (*190 liter*) of fluid, and (2) remove excesses of substances such as urea and uric acid while conserving needed substances such as water and glucose. Without their cleansing-filtering function, death results in 8 to 14 days. Kidneys also regulate red blood cell production, adrenal secretion of aldosterone, blood pressure, and calcium metabolism.

(Also see CALCIUM; GLOMERULONEPHRITIS; HEMODIALYSIS; and WATER BALANCE.)

KIDNEY STONES (NEPHROLITHIASIS; RENAL CALCULI; URINARY CALCULI; UROLITHIASIS)

Hard concretions primarily composed of calcium oxalate or calcium phosphate which form within the kidney. They vary in size from very small gravel to very large stones. Apparently, a variety of factors may contribute to the formation of kidney stones, and to some extent they may be controlled by diet. Some common contributing factors are (1) a high phosphorus-low calcium diet; (2) a high potassium intake; (3) vitamin A deficiency; (4) high animal protein (meat, fish, poultry) intake; (5) renal infection; (6) urinary tract obstruction; (7) chronic dehydration; (8) long periods of immobilization; (9) hypercalcemia; or (10) heredity. Generally, a kidney stone goes unnoticed until it starts to move out of the kidney and down the ureter. When this occurs there is excruciating pain until the stone is passed or removed surgically or nonsurgically.

Note: Currently, a German-built machine which uses high-energy shock waves to break up kidney stones from outside the body is being tested. The nonsurgical procedure is called extracorporeal shock wave lithotripsy, or stone exploding.

If at all possible the cause and type of kidney stones should be determined since a person forming a kidney stone once is apt to form them repeatedly.

Dietary modification depends on the type of stones formed. The formation of calcium phosphate stones may be lessened by a calcium- and phosphorus-restricted diet, and by aluminum gel which diminishes the absorption of phosphorus. Modification of the urine pH also prevents the formation of kidney stones. An acid urine helps prevent stones of calcium and magnesium phosphate and carbonates, while an alkaline urine helps prevent oxalate and uric acid stones. The diet should support therapy with alkalinizing or acidifying agents by supplying acid-producing or alkaline-producing foods. Also the formation of uric acid stones may be lessened by a purine-restricted diet.

Most importantly, a liberal intake of fluid—3 to 4 qt (*3 to 4 liter*) or more depending upon the environment—is essential to prevent the formation of a concentrated urine which allows the stone-forming salts to precipitate.

(Also see CALCIUM, section headed "Calcium Related Diseases"; MODIFIED DIETS; and URIC ACID KIDNEY STONES.)

KILOCALORIE (kcal)

The amount of energy as heat required to raise the temperature of 1 kilogram of water 1°C (from 14.5 to 15.5°C). It is equivalent to 1,000 calories. In human nutrition, it may also be referred to as a kilogram calorie, k-calorie, kcal, or a "large Calorie." The last designation is spelled with a capital "C" to distinguish it from the "small calorie." However, in some of the literature, the word "calorie" is used, even though it is technically incorrect.

(Also see CALORIE.)

KILOGRAM

A metric measure of weight which is equal to 1,000 g or about 2.2 lb.

(Also see WEIGHTS AND MEASURES.)

KILOJOULE (KJ)

A metric unit of energy, equivalent to 0.239 kcal.

KIM CHEE (KIM CHI)

This is the national dish of Korea. It consists of a vegetable pickle seasoned with garlic, red pepper, and ginger.

KINETIC ENERGY (MECHANICAL ENERGY)

A body, an object, or a molecule in motion which is capable of performing work at once. It possesses kinetic energy, energy of motion.

(Also see ENERGY UTILIZATION BY THE BODY, Section headed "Major Forms of Energy.")

KJELDAHL

Relating to a method of determining the amount of nitrogen in an organic compound. The quantity of nitrogen measured is then multiplied by 6.25 to calculate the protein content of the food or compound analyzed. The method was developed by the Danish chemist, J. G. C. Kjeldahl, in 1883.

(Also see ANALYSIS OF FOOD.)

KOHLRABI *Brassica oleracea,* variety *caulorapo*

The name of this vegetable, which belongs to the mustard family (*Cruciferae*), literally means "cabbage (kohl)-turnip (rabi)." It has both the wild cabbage (*B. oleracea*) and the wild turnip (*B. campestris,* species *rapifera*) as ancestors. Kohlrabi is unlike other cabbage vegetables in that it is comprised of stem tissue, while the rest of these vegetables are buds (sprouts), flowers, and leaves. Fig. K-2 shows a typical kohlrabi.

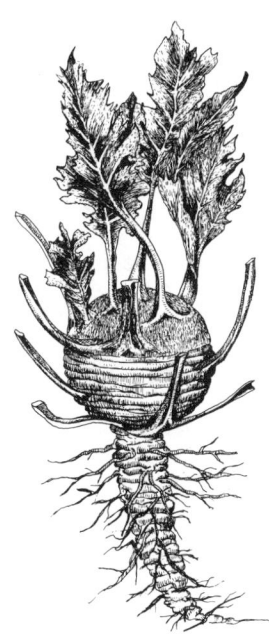

Fig. K-2. Kohlrabi, a vegetable derived from the wild cabbage and the wild turnip.

ORIGIN AND HISTORY. It is not known for certain when the kohlrabi was first developed, because a vegetable described in the writings of the Roman botanist Pliny (1st century, A.D.) had very similar characteristics. However, it is not mentioned in any other writings until after the Middle Ages, when it was a popular vegetable in the central and eastern parts of Europe. Since then, the utilization of kohlrabi has declined to the extent that it is difficult to find in vegetable markets. One of the reasons for the decline in popularity of the vegetable may have been the production of large, tough bulbs the size of softballs, rather than the more tender bulbs that are usually smaller than baseballs.

PRODUCTION. There is little commercial production of the kohlrabi in the United States; hence, statistics on the size of the crop are not available. But per capita consumption is low.

Kohlrabi seeds may be planted as soon as the soil can be cultivated in the spring. The vegetable may also be planted in the summer for harvesting in the fall. A rich soil is needed for high-quality kohlrabi. Therefore, it is often desirable to fertilize with nitrogen, phosphorus, and potassium.

The bulblike vegetables may be harvested when they are between 2 and 3 in. (*5 and 8 cm*) in diameter. It is not wise to let them grow any larger because the edible portion becomes fibrous and tough when it reaches full maturity. The edible portion is the bulbous enlargement of the stem, which like all stems, becomes very woody as it ages.

PROCESSING. It appears that most, or all, of the kohlrabi produced in the United States is marketed fresh, and that very little, if any, is processed.

SELECTION AND PREPARATION. Best quality kohlrabi is from 2 to 3 in. (*5 to 8 cm*) in diameter, and has fresh green tops and a tender rind. Bulbs that are overly large (over 3 in. in diameter), and that have blemishes or growth cracks, are likely to be of poor quality.

Raw kohlrabi may be sliced and added to relish trays and salads. The vegetable is usually cooked by steaming, although the people in the Central European countries may stuff and bake it after scooping out some of the center. Cooked kohlrabi is enhanced by a well-seasoned cheese sauce or cream sauce.

CAUTION: Kohlrabi and other vegetables of the mustard family (*Cruciferae*) contain small amounts of goiter-causing (goitrogenic) substances that may interfere with the utilization of iodine by the thyroid gland. In the quantities normally consumed, this is not a concern. Besides, this effect may be counteracted by the consumption of ample amounts of dietary iodine, a mineral that is abundantly present in iodized salt, ocean fish, seafood, and seaweeds such as kelp.

NUTRITIONAL VALUE. The nutrient composition of kohlrabi is given in Food Composition Table F-36.

Some noteworthy observations regarding the nutrient composition of kohlrabi follow:

1. Kohlrabi is high in water content (over 90%) and low in calories (only about 40 kcal per cup [*240 ml*]).

2. The levels of most nutrients are lower in kohlrabi than in the other cabbage vegetables because it is comprised of stem tissue, whereas, the other vegetables are buds (sprouts), flowers, and leaves. However, kohlrabi is a good source of potassium and vitamin C.

3. Kohlrabi is most comparable to the potato and the other tuberous vegetables that are enlarged stems of plants. On this basis, kohlrabi has about the same amount of protein (2%) as the potato, but contains less then half as many calories, and more than three times as much vitamin C.

(Also see VEGETABLE[S], Table V-6 Vegetables of the World.)

KOJI

A yeast or other starter prepared in Japan from rice inoculated with the spores of the mold *Asperigillus oryzae* and permitted to develop a mycelium. Koji is used for making miso from soybeans, a popular fermented food in Japan.

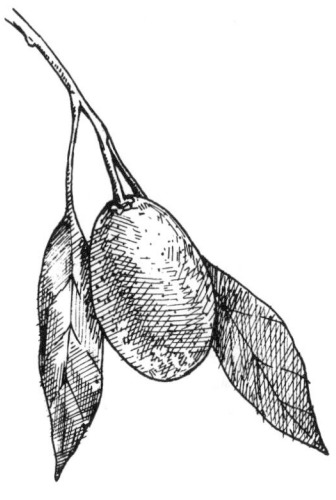

Fig. K-3.   The kumquat, a small orangelike fruit that may be eaten whole, candied, or preserved in syrup.

KORSAKOFF'S SYNDROME (PSYCHOSIS)

A mental disease involving disintegration of the personality or escape from reality. Typical behavior includes confused thinking, making up stories to fill in gaps of memory (confabulation), irresponsibility, and the inability to learn new things. Eventually a stupefied state may result. These effects may be commonly found in chronic alcoholics, semistarved persons such as prisoners of war, and persons suffering from beriberi. Most evidence seems to indicate that the Korsakoff's Syndrome is due to a long-standing thiamin deficiency. Vitamin therapy restores responsiveness and alertness, but some irreversible structural damage to the nervous system may have occurred. Often the early symptoms of a thiamin deficiency—Wernicke's Syndrome—are noted prior to the mental disorders, and the physical and mental symptoms are together called the *Wernicke-Korsakoff Syndrome*.

(Also see ALCOHOLISM; and BERIBERI.)

KUBAN

A type of fermented milk.

KUMQUAT *Fortunella* spp

This fruit resembles a tiny orange and is often grown as an ornamental plant. However, the kumquat belongs to the *Fortunella* genus, rather than the *Citrus* genus. Both genera are closely related, can be crossbred readily, and belong to the rue family (*Rutaceae*).

ORIGIN AND HISTORY.   The kumquat originated in China. It was taken to England in 1846 by a man named Fortune who collected plants for the London Horticultural Society; hence, the genus name *Fortunella*. It was taken from Japan to Florida in 1885.

This fruit is more winter-hardy than the more commonly grown citrus fruits. Hence, it has been crossbred to yield new cold-resistant hybrids such as the limequat and the orangequat.

PRODUCTION.   Statistics on kumquat production are not readily available. However, the major areas in which the fruit is grown are China, southern Japan, and Taiwan. It is also grown on a more limited scale in Florida, where it is marketed in gift packages and specialty jams, jellies, and marmalades for the gourmet and tourist trades.

Kumquat growing is very similar to citrus fruit growing, which is discussed elsewhere.

(Also see CITRUS FRUITS, section headed "Production.")

PROCESSING.   Most people consider the kumquat too sour to be eaten as a fresh fruit. Hence, it is commonly candied or preserved in syrup (the fruit can be eaten whole, including the seeds and the peel) or made into marmalade.

SELECTION AND PREPARATION.   Fresh kumquats are only occasionally found in local stores, but they are readily available by mail order from Florida. However, the tree is more resistant to the cold than most types of citrus fruits and may be grown as an ornamental plant in more northerly states. Those who are able to obtain the fresh fruits can eat them whole with a little honey, or use them to make brandied or candied fruit.

Kumquat jams, jellies, and marmalades are usually sold in gourmet shops, or they may be ordered directly from suppliers in Florida. Stores that carry Oriental exports are likely to have canned or preserved kumquats.

CAUTION: Some people are allergic to one or more constituents of citrus peel, which is very similar in composition to kumquat peel. When such allergies are suspected, it would be wise to avoid consuming kumquat peel unless it is certain that the peel is well tolerated.

NUTRITIONAL VALUE. The nutrient composition of fresh kumquats is given in Food Composition Table F-36.

Some noteworthy observations regarding the nutrient composition of kumquats follow.

Fresh whole kumquats contain 65 Calories (kcal) per 100 g and are high in fiber (nondigestible carbohydrate that helps to promote movement of the bowels and may even help to lower blood cholesterol by binding bile salts). They are also (1) a good source of potassium, vitamin C (ascorbic acid), and (2) a fair source of calcium and vitamin A. Also, kumquats contain the vitaminlike substances, bioflavonoids.

The peels of citrus fruits and certain other closely re-lated species contain citral, an aldehyde that antagonizes the actions of vitamin A. Hence, people should make certain that their dietary supply of this vitamin is adequate before consuming large amounts of kumquat peel.

(Also see FRUIT[S], Table F-47 Fruits of the World.)

KWASHIORKOR

Kwashiorkor is most common in the tropical areas of the world, where it afflicts children from weaning to age 4.

Kwashiorkor results from a severe protein deficiency, and is characterized by changes in pigmentation of the skin and hair, edema, skin lesions, anemia, and apathy. Kwashiorkor differs from marasmus in terms of the greater role of protein deficiency in causing it.

The recommended treatment: Providing 1 to 2 g of high-quality protein per pound of body weight, along with sufficient energy. Cautious replacement of mineral salts may also be needed. In case of severe diarrhea, the protein intake should be temporarily restricted to 0.5 g per pound of body weight.

Prevention consists in feeding children an adequate amount of protein (particularly after weaning) from such sources as fish, legumes, meats, milk, and nuts. (Milk supplies 1 g of protein per oz [*30 ml*].)

(Also see MALNUTRITION, PROTEIN-ENERGY; and PROTEIN[S], section headed "Protein Malnutrition.")

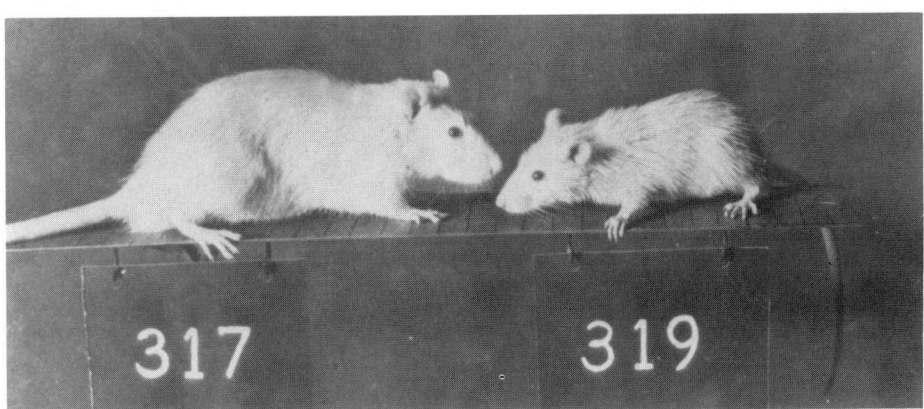

High protein vs low protein diets! The rat on the left had a diet with 18% casein. The other rat's diet consisted of 4% casein. This experiment was conducted by Thomas B. Osborne, of the Connecticut Agricultural Experiment Station and Lafayette B. Mendel, of Yale University, who, in 1911, formed a brilliant partnership and pioneered in studies of protein quality. (Courtesy, The Connecticut Agricultural Experiment Station, New Haven, Conn.)

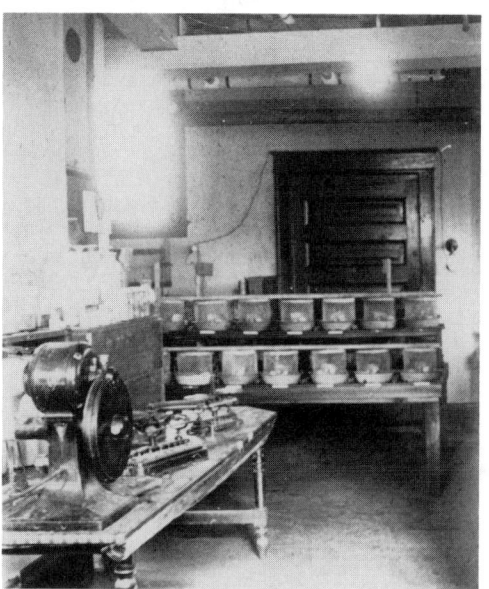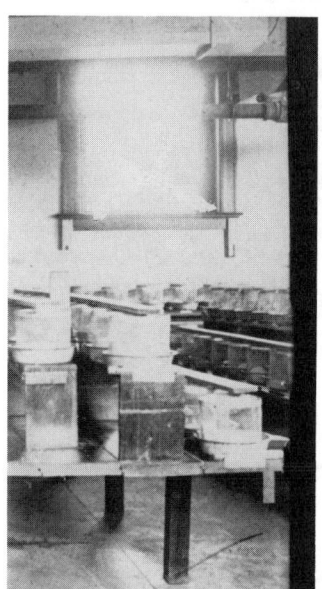

Rat laboratory, 1919, at The Connecticut Agricultural Experiment Station, New Haven, in which Thomas B. Osborne and Lafayette B. Mendel conducted pioneering nutritional experiments. Note the meat grinder in the left foreground. Osborne and Mendel learned how proteins function in living animals, obtained information on the mineral requirements of animals, and discovered a few vitamins. (Courtesy, The Connecticut Agricultural Experiment Station, New Haven, Conn.)

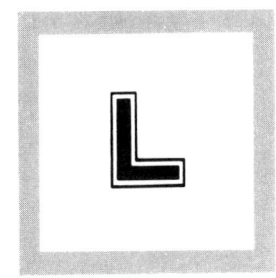

LABELS, FOOD

On November 8, 1990, President Bush signed into law *The Nutrition Labeling and Education Act of 1990*, the most significant revision of the U.S. food labeling law since 1938. The new labeling law requires that the majority of food products under FDA authority carry nutrition labeling, regulates the terms used on labels to describe a food's nutrient content, authorizes and regulates food health claims, and establishes national uniformity by federal preemption for many areas of food labeling other than safety warning statements. In 1992, FDA regulatory authority encompassed about 75% of all food consumed in this country. The remaining foods—mainly meat, poultry, and egg products—are largely under the U.S. Department of Agriculture regulatory authority.

The Nutrition Labeling and Education Act of 1990 (Public Law 101–538–Nov. 8, 1990) amends the Federal Food, Drug, and Cosmetic Act to require the following changes in food labels:

• **Nutrition labeling**—Nutrition labeling is required for all retail food products, including fresh produce, fish, and seafood. *NOTE WELL: Subsequently, President Bush ruled that the law would apply only to packaged foods.*

All foods requiring nutrition labeling must list on a per-serving or unit basis the following information:

Calories	Complex carbohydrates
Calories from fat	Sugars
Total fat	Dietary fiber
Saturated fat	Protein
Cholesterol	Sodium
Total carbohydrates	

The FDA is required to define serving size or other unit of measure of food. Additionally, the food label must state either the total number of servings or unit per container.

The FDA has broad discretion in determining the required listing of minerals, vitamins, and other nutrients on food labels where this information will assist consumers in maintaining healthy dietary practices. Also, the Act required FDA to issue regulations that the mandatory label information be presented on the label in a format which allows the public readily to observe and comprehend information and to understand its relative significance in the context of a total daily diet.

• **Nutrition labeling on fresh produce, fish, and seafood**—For the first time, nutrition labeling is required for fresh produce, fish, and seafood at retail outlets. Under the law, Congress set a strict timetable for implementing the labeling. *NOTE WELL: Before implementing the regulations, on December 2, 1992, President George Bush exempted fresh meat, poultry, fish, and produce.*

• **Education program**—The legislation also instructs the Secretary of the Department of Health and Human Services to carry out activities that educate the public about the availability of nutrition information in the label of food and the importance of that information in maintaining healthy dietary practices.

• **Health claims on food**—The Nutrition Labeling and Education Act permits health claims on foods, provided (1) that such claims are based on scientific evidence (including evidence from well-designed experiments), and (2) that there is significant agreement among experts qualified by scientific training and experience. Under the Act, the FDA is instructed to determine whether claims should be permitted for the relationship between the following initial list of specific food/health claims:

Calcium and osteoporosis
Dietary fiber and cancer
Lipids and cardiovascular disease
Lipids and cancer
Sodium and hypertension
Dietary fiber and cardiovascular disease
Folic acid and neural tube defects
Antioxidant vitamins and cancer
Zinc and immune function in the elderly
Omega-3 fatty acids and heart disease

• **Nutrient content claims**—The FDA is required to define the following nutrient terms as they relate to nutrient content:

Free	Reduced
Low	Less
Light or Lite	High

Further, the Act prohibits a label claim for the absence of a nutrient (e.g., "sodium-free," "no cholesterol") where the nutrient is not normally present in the food.

• **National uniformity**—In the past, state label requirements often hindered interstate commerce. To alleviate this problem, the Act phases in national uniformity for many FDA labeling regulations under a specific timetable. No state or political subdivision can continue existing label requirements or establish new label regulations that are not identical to the label requirements of the new Act. However, the Act does not extend federal preemption to state warning label requirements.

• **Other Amendments to the FD&C Act**—The Act also mandates percentage juice content labeling for beverages containing fruit or vegetable juices that are not pure juices. Also, the Act (1) eliminates the exemption of foods covered by standards of identities from listing all ingredients on the label, and (2) alters the procedural method for issuing new or changing current standards of identity for all foods other than dairy products and maple syrup, thus allowing potentially swifter changes in standards of identity by routine notice.

• **Implementation of food labeling law**—On November 8, 1990, President George Bush signed into law The Nutrition Labeling and Education Act. However, implementation of the law was delayed due to disagreement between the U.S. Secretary of Agriculture and the U.S. Secretary of Health and Human Services relative to certain aspects of food labeling. Finally, on December 2, 1992, President Bush resolved the dispute between the two cabinet secretaries, made some changes in the application of the law, announced that the regulations will be final following their publication in the Federal Register, and ruled that all labels must be on packaged foods by May 1994.

Fig. L-1 shows the format and content of a new food label similar to the type that will be standard on all packaged foods in the future. The label on a carton of yogurt will look just like the label on a can of corn.

Pertinent new food labeling rules which were revealed on December 2, 1992, at the time of implementing the food labeling law, follow.

1. **All packaged foods must be labeled.** The regulations apply to all packaged foods, but not to fresh meat, poultry, fish, and produce.

2. **Percent Daily Value will be used.** Instead of Recommended Daily Allowance (RDA), the new labels will refer to percent of *Daily Value*.

3. **The nutritional value of a food can be compared with daily dietary needs.** The new labels will provide consumers with an opportunity to compare the nutritional value of a food with the daily dietary needs. Thus, the label will show how much fat is in a product, and how much of the daily quotient of fat the consumer will get from one serving of that product. Also, the label provides consumers a way in which to compare the nutrients found in their food with their total daily dietary needs, based on recommended diets of both 2,000 calories and 2,500 calories. Thus, from the label, consumers will be able to compare the percentage of the *Daily Value* of each nutrient contained in a particular product with a chart that shows the total amount of each nutrient that they should be eating.

Nutrition facts

| Serving size | ½ cup (114 g) |
| Servings per container | 4 |

Amount per serving

| Calories 260 | Calories from fat 120 |

		% Daily value*
Total fat	13 g	20%
Saturated fat	5 g	25%
Cholesterol	30 mg	10%
Sodium	660 mg	28%
Total carbohydrate	31 g	11%
Sugars	5 g	
Dietary fiber	0 g	0%
Protein	5 g	

Vitamin A 4% • Vitamin C 2% • Calcium 15% • Iron 4%

* Percents (%) of a Daily Value are based on a 2,000-calorie diet. Your Daily Values may vary higher or lower depending on your calorie needs:

Nutrient		2,000 calories	2,500 calories
Total fat	Less than	65 g	80 g
Saturated fat	Less than	20 g	25 g
Cholesterol	Less than	300 mg	300 mg
Sodium	Less than	2,400 mg	2,400 mg
Total carbohydrate		300 g	375 g
Fiber		25 g	30 g

1 g fat = 9 calories
1 g carbohydrates = 4 calories
1 g protein = 4 calories

Fig. L-1. A new food label.

4. **Serving sizes and descriptive terms will be standardized.** Thus, the serving size in canned soups will be the same, no matter what the brand. Likewise, descriptive phrases like "low-fat" and "light" will be standardized.

5. **Labels must be rewritten and printed.** An estimated 257,000 labels must be rewritten and printed.

6. **Complete nutritional information will be required.** If manufacturers do not report complete nutritional information on their product labels, they will be required to have their products tested.

7. **Calorie information will be given.** The new labels will include information on how many calories are in a gram of fat, in a gram of carbohydrate, and in a gram of protein.

8. **Amounts of essential nutrients, along with the requirements, must be listed.** Every label must list total grams or milligrams, along with required amounts, of fat, saturated fat, cholesterol, sodium, total carbohydrates (sugar and dietary fiber), protein, and essential vitamins and minerals.

• **Basic label and other information to be continued**—In addition to requiring changes in nutrition labeling as detailed above, the following basic information will be continued on food nutrition labels: (1) the name of the product, (2) the net contents or net weight, and (3) the name and place of business of the manufacturer, packer, or distributor. Also, label information may include the following:

• **Grades**—Some food products carry a grade on the label, such as "U.S. Grade A." Grades are set by the U.S. Department of Agriculture, based on the quality levels inherent in a product—its taste, texture, and appearance. U.S. Department of Agriculture grades are not based on nutritional content.

Milk and milk products in most states carry a "Grade A" label. This grade is based on FDA recommended sanitary standards, for the production and processing of milk and milk products, which are regulated by the states.

• **Open dating**—To help consumers obtain food that is fresh and wholesome, many manufacturers date their product. Open dating, as this practice is often called, is not regulated by FDA. Four kinds of open dating are commonly used:

1. **Pack date is the day the food was manufactured or processed or packaged.** In other words, it tells how old the food is at the time of purchase. The importance of this information to consumers depends on how quickly the particular food normally spoils. Most canned and packaged foods have a long shelf life when stored under dry, cool conditions.

2. **Pull or sell date is the last date the product should be sold, assuming it has been stored and handled properly.** The pull date allows for some storage time in the home refrigerator. Cold cuts, ice cream, milk, and refrigerated fresh dough products are examples of foods with pull dates.

3. **Expiration date is the last date the food should be eaten or used.** Baby formula and yeast are examples of products that may carry expiration dates.

4. **Freshness date is similar to the expiration date but may allow for normal home storage.** Some bakery products that have a freshness date are sold at a reduced price for a short time after the expiration date.

• **Code dating**—Many companies use code dating on products that have a long "shelf life." This is usually for the company's information, rather than for the consumer's benefit. The code gives the manufacturer and the store precise information about where and when the product was packaged, so if a recall should be required for any reason the product can be identified quickly and withdrawn from the market.

• **Universal product code**—Many food labels now include a small block of parallel lines of various widths, with accompanying numbers. This is the Universal Product Code (UPC). The code on a label is unique to that product. Some stores are equipped with computerized checkout equipment that can read the code and automatically ring up the sale. The UPC, when used in conjunction with a computer, also can function as an automated inventory system. The computer can tell management how much of a specific item is on hand, how fast it is being sold, and when and how much to order.

• **Symbols**—Food labels can possess a variety of symbols. The letter "R" on a label signifies that the trademark used on the label is registered with the U.S. Patent Office. The letter "C" indicates that the literary and artistic content of the label is protected against infringement under the copyright laws of the United States. Copies of such labels have been filed with the Copyright Office of the Library of Congress. The symbol which consists of the letter "U" inside the letter "O", is one whose use is authorized by the Union of Orthodox Jewish Congregations of America, more familiarly known as the Orthodox Union, for use of foods which comply with Jewish dietary laws. The symbol which consists of the letter "K" inside the letter "O" is used to indicate that the food is "kosher," that is, it complies with Jewish dietary laws, and its processing has been under the direction of a rabbi. None of these symbols is required by, nor under the authority of, any of the laws enforced by the FDA.

(Also see FOOD AND DRUG ADMINISTRATION; and U.S. DEPARTMENT OF AGRICULTURE.)

LABILE

Unstable. Easily destroyed.

LABILE PROTEIN

The reserve protein available in most tissues.

LABRADOR TEA

This term may refer to (1) any of a group of low evergreen shrubs growing in bogs and swamps of the arctic and subarctic regions, or (2) tea made from the leaves of these plants. Labrador tea was popular with miners, mountainmen, and American colonists during the Revolution.

LACTALBUMIN

It is one of the proteins of milk, sometimes called a *whey protein.* During the cheese making process lactalbumin is not precipitated with the protein casein, and thus it appears in the whey. One half, or more, of the protein in human milk is lactalbumin; the rest is casein.

(Also see MILK AND MILK PRODUCTS; and PROTEIN[S].)

LACTASE

An enzyme in intestinal juice which acts on lactose to produce glucose and galactose.
(Also see DIGESTION AND ABSORPTION.)

LACTATION

That process of milk formation common to all mammals for the purpose of nurturing their young. Milk formation occurs in the mammary gland following preparation during pregnancy, and it is initiated near the time of birth. Lactating mothers require more food and more nutritious food than non-lactating females.
(Also see BREAST FEEDING; INFANT DIET AND NUTRITION; and MILK AND MILK PRODUCTS.)

LACTIC ACID ($C_3H_6O_3$)

During strenuous exercise lactic acid is produced in the muscles of the body. Also, this important biochemical forms during some food processes. The fermentation of pickles, sauerkraut, cocoa, tobacco, and silage produces lactic acid. Lactic acid formed by *lactobacillus* bacteria in the fermentation of milk sugar (lactose) is responsible for the sour milk flavor, and for the formation of cottage cheese and yogurt. Furthermore, it is a food additive employed as an acidulant and antimicrobial in cheeses, beverages, and frozen desserts. In addition to the above, lactic acid has some nonfood uses in the tanning, plastic, and textile industries. Commercially, lactic acid is produced by the fermentation of whey, cornstarch, potatoes, or molasses.
(Also see ADDITIVES, Table A-3; METABOLISM; and MILK AND MILK PRODUCTS.)

LACTOBACILLUS ACIDOPHILUS

A lactic-acid forming organism, which occurs as rods sometimes united in short chains; found in intestinal contents of young infants.

LACTOFLAVIN

An obsolete name for riboflavin (vitamin B-2) which described the origin of the isolate in the early days of riboflavin research. Hence, riboflavin isolated from milk was called lactoflavin.
(Also see RIBOFLAVIN.)

LACTOSE (MILK SUGAR)

A disaccharide found in milk having the formula $C_{12}H_{22}O_{11}$. It hydrolyzes to glucose and galactose. Commonly known as milk sugar.
(Also see CARBOHYDRATE[S], and MILK AND MILK PRODUCTS, section headed "Carbohydrates in Milk.")

LAETRILE (VITAMIN B-17, AMYGDALIN, NITRILOSIDES)

NOTE WELL: Laetrile (amygdalin, nitrilosides) has no known value for humans. The authors present this section relative to the controversial compound for informational purposes only. Further, it is listed with the vitaminlike substances because it is sometimes erroneously designated as vitamin B-17. Both the pros and cons relative to Laetrile are given, then the reader may make a judgment.

Laetrile or amygdalin is a natural substance obtained from apricot pits, which its advocates claim to have cancer preventive and controlling effects. Dr. Ernest Krebs, Sr., who was the first to use Laetrile therapeutically in this country, considered it to be an essential vitamin and called it vitamin B-17.

In the United States, Laetrile therapy is not approved by the Food and Drug Administration for treatment of cancer.

In a report before the American Society for Clinical Oncology (the society of cancer specialists) May 1, 1981, Dr. Charles G. Moertel of Mayo Clinic reported on the Laetrile treatment of 156 patients, all with cancers that either had not responded or were not likely to respond to other treatments. Nine months after the beginning of the study in July 1980, 102 of the patients were dead, and the other 54 had seriously "progressive cancer," which did not respond to the Laetrile treatment. The results: Laetrile was not effective; the results were about the same as would be expected had the doctors given the patients either placebos (dummy pills, with no effectiveness), or no treatment at all.

NOTE WELL: This study pertained to the use of Laetrile as a treatment of patients "with cancers that either had not responded or were not likely to respond to other treatments''; and not as a preventive of cancer, or as a treatment of early cancers.

The following statement explains the position of the Soviet Union relative to Laetrile:

"The preparation has never been tested in the Soviet Union. And in our opinion, today there are no grounds to show any interest in it. Why? Because the Soviet medical profession feels that this chemical is a useless preparation. Laetrile does not possess those wonderful properties which are ascribed to it. Moreover, being toxic, Laetrile may actually harm a patient's health.

Soviet specialists in chemotherapy subscribe to the competent opinion of the American Cancer Society and the World Health Organization, who have conducted thorough tests of Laetrile and convincingly proved its quackish nature.''[1]

Despite the above, the advocates of Laetrile advance the following arguments: There is usually a considerable time lag between the scientific validation of a medical treatment and its acceptance. Moreover, the bias against nutrition is frequently deep-seated when it comes to cancer. Then, they make the following statements in support of the use of Laetrile in the prevention and treatment of cancer:

1. It is harmless when not taken in excess amounts all at once.

2. It is low cost.

3. The ancient Chinese got pretty good results using the same treatment (apricot kernels) for cancer.

4. Several distinguished doctors feel that it gives good results.

5. It is manufactured and used legally in about 20 countries throughout the world, including Belgium, Germany, Italy, Mexico, and the Philippines.

HISTORY. Laetrile was first extracted from apricot pits in the early 1900s, and first used as a therapy for cancer in the United States in the 1920s.

CHEMISTRY, METABOLISM, PROPERTIES.

• **Chemistry**—Laetrile or amygdalin is a nitriloside, a simple chemical compound consisting of two molecules of

sugar (glucose), one molecule of benzaldehyde, and one molecule of hydrogen cyanide (HCN) (see Fig. L-2).

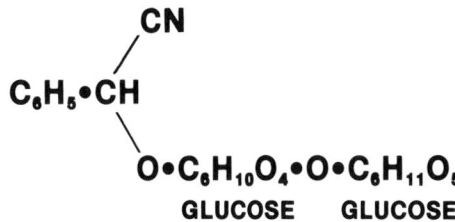

Fig. L-2. Structural formula of Laetrile ($C_{20}H_{27}NO_{11}$).

There are some 20 different nitrilosides occurring in at least 1,200 different plants, many of which were or are used as food, historically or at present. The natural cyanide in such foods, including apricot kernels or bitter almonds, is locked in a sugar molecule, and is released slowly in the digestive tract of man.

• **Metabolism**—Oral doses of Laetrile pass from the stomach into the small intestine, where the substance is acted upon by enzymes. The enzymes break down Laetrile into four components, which are then absorbed into the lymph and portal systems and circulated throughout the body.

• **Properties**—White crystals; bitter taste; soluble in water and alcohol; insoluble in ether.

MEASUREMENT. Laetrile is measured in grams.

FUNCTIONS. Nitrilosides, including apricot kernels and bitter almonds, supply the body a low, but steady, level of HCN. Man and other mammals have an enzyme, rhodanase, which converts the cyanide to thiocyanate.

There are at least three theories as to how the HCN interferes with tumor growth, but all theories relative to the action of nitrilosides recognize the steady low-level supply of HCN as the active agent. The simplest theory postulates that cancer cells do not have rhodanase; instead, they are surrounded by another enzyme, betaglucuronidase, which releases the bound cyanide from the Laetrile at the site of the malignancy. So, Laetrile is believed to attack and destroy only the malignant cells.

The advocates claim that Laetrile is effective in preventing tumor cells from getting a foothold. In support of this thesis, the following epidemiological data has been cited by Dr. James Cason, Professor of Chemistry, University of California, Berkeley, an authority on carcinogenic hydrocarbons:[2]

---

[1]Garbin, Avgust, Professor, Doctor of Science (Medicine), Deputy General, Director of the Oncological Research Center of the USSR Academy of Medical Sciences, "What is the Soviet Attitude Toward Laetrile?," *Soviet Life*, November 1980, p. 30.

[2]Cason, James, "Ascorbic Acid, Amygdalin, and Carcinoma," *The Vortex*, June 1978, pp. 9-23.

1. In a 1958 publication, famed African physician Dr. Albert Schweitzer, stated that for "several decades" his hospital at Lamberene in Gabon did not see a single case of cancer among the cassava-eating tribes. This was attributed to the fact that the natives in the Lamberene area obtain 80 to 90% of their calories from cassava, the tubers of which contain about 0.5% of a nitriloside.

2. Studies by the Loma Linda Hospital and the U.S.C. Medical School on the incidence of cancer in the Los Angeles basin showed that the Seventh-day Adventists had only one-third the incidence of cancer suffered by the rest of the population. For religious reasons, the Adventists' diet is heavily vegetarian; hence, rich in nitrilosides. It is estimated that the Adventists consumed 6 to 8 mg of nitrilosides per person daily, in comparison with an estimated average daily consumption of less than 1 mg per capita by the U.S. population.

3. Among the Hunzakuts (natives of the Himalayan Kingdom of Hunza), it has been estimated that the average daily intake of nitrilosides per capita is more than 100 mg. In addition to being Moslems, a local twist to the religion calls for eating apricot kernels; with the priests seeing that the brethren keep that part of the faith. Moreover, a young woman is not regarded as properly marriageable unless she has at least seven apricot trees in her dowry. After doing a study of morbidity of the Hunzakuts covering 100 years, the World Health Organization reported that not a single death from cancer was recorded.

NOTE WELL: The three reports cited above pertain to the use of Laetrile as a preventive of cancer, and not as a treatment of cancer.

DEFICIENCY SYMPTOMS. The advocates claim that prolonged deficiency of Laetrile or amygdalin may lead to lowered resistance to malignancies.

DOSAGE. The usual dosage is 0.25 to 1.0 g taken at meals. Cumulative daily amounts of more than 3.0 g are sometimes taken, *but more than 1.0 g should never be taken at any one time.*

According to the advocates, 5 to 30 apricot kernels eaten through the day may be effective as a preventive of cancer, but they should not be eaten all at one time.

• **Laetrile intake in average U.S. diet**—It is estimated that the average daily consumption of nitrilosides by the U.S. population is less than 1 mg per person.

TOXICITY. Toxicity levels of Laetrile haven't been established, but one should exercise extreme caution in order to avoid ingesting excessive amounts. *More than 1.0 g should not be taken at any one time.*

SOURCES OF LAETRILE. A concentration of 2 to 3% Laetrile is found in the whole kernels of most fruits, including apricots, apples, cherries, peaches, plums, and nectarines.

SUMMARY. Regardless of the validity of the claims and counter claims pertaining to Laetrile, it is noteworthy that more and more medical authorities are ac-

cepting the nutrition approach in the prevention and treatment of cancer. Although the use of such nutrients as Laetrile, vitamin A (carotene), folic acid, and vitamin C, along with a general supplemental program of minerals and vitamins, is controversial as a cancer treatment, perhaps even more important in the long run is the apparent success of nutrients of many kinds in strengthening the body's immune system—as preventives.

There is evidence that a person's immune capability is enhanced by top physical and mental condition; in turn, physical and mental condition depend heavily on diet. Together, they impart the "fighting spirit" and the "will to live," terms that are often heard in the medical profession.

(Also see VITAMIN[S], Table V-9.)

LAMB AND MUTTON

Contents   *Page*

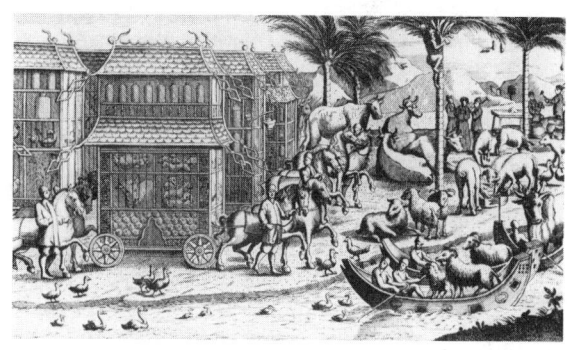

Fig. L-3. Live sheep and other animals sent to Persia and India with an Expeditionary Force in 1670. Until meat preservation was developed, live animals had to be taken along by the explorers. (Courtesy, The Bettmann Archive)

Lamb is the flesh of young sheep; mutton is the flesh of mature sheep. Lamb differs from mutton in both tenderness and flavor.

In general, the packer classes as lamb, all carcasses in which the forefeet are removed at the break-joint or lamb-joint. This joint—which can be severed on all lambs, most yearling wethers, and some yearling ewes (ewes mature earlier than wethers or males)—is a temporary cartilage located just above the ankle. In lambs, the break-joint has four well-defined ridges that are smooth, moist, and red. In yearlings, the break-joint is more porous and dry. In mature sheep, the cartilage is knit or ossified and will no longer break, thus making it necessary to take the foot off at the ankle instead. This makes a round-joint (commonly called spool-joint). All carcasses possessing the round-joint are sold as mutton rather than lamb.

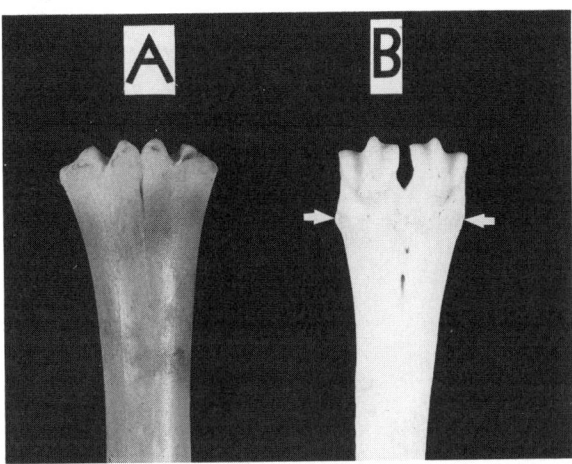

Fig. L-4. The two types of joints of the foreleg of a sheep: A, the break-joint or lamb-joint, and B, the round-joint or spool-joint. Arrow indicates the location of the break-joint or ossification. All carcasses possessing the round-joint are sold as mutton rather than lamb. (Courtesy, Washington State University)

QUALITIES IN LAMB DESIRED BY CONSUMERS. Consumers desire the following qualities in lamb:

1. **Palatability.** First and foremost, people eat lamb because they like it. Palatability is influenced by the tenderness, juiciness, and flavor of the fat and lean. In the United States, this calls for lamb—not mutton.

Lamb flavor is distinctive of the species. Most people find the flavor of the lean very delightful, but they tend to object to the fat flavor. Since lamb fat is highly saturated, it should always be served hot; lamb served hot on a hot plate has a pleasing flavor, and the fat will not stick to the roof of the mouth.

2. **Attractiveness.** The general attractiveness is an important factor in selling lamb to the housewife. The color of the lean, the degree of fatness, and the marbling are leading factors in determining buyer appeal. Most consumers prefer a pinkish-white fat and a light red color in the lean. The muscle meat of mutton is much darker than in lamb.

3. **Maximum muscling; minimum fat.** Maximum thickness of muscling influences materially the acceptability by the consumer. Also, consumer resistance to fat on all meats has been very marked in recent years.

4. **Small cuts.** Most purchasers prefer to buy cuts of lamb that are of a proper size to meet the needs of their respective families. Because the American family has decreased in size, this has meant smaller cuts. This, in turn, has had a profound influence on the type of animals and on market age and weight.

5. **Ease of preparation.** In general, the housewife prefers to select lamb that will give her the greatest amount of leisure time; thus, she selects those cuts that can be prepared with the greatest ease and the least time—often this means lamb chops and leg of lamb.

6. **Tenderness.** Lamb may be aged, but it is not necessary since the meat is tender.

The texture of lamb meat is fine, whereas that of yearling and mutton is coarser.

7. **Repeatability.** The housewife wants to be able to secure a standardized product—meat of the same eating qualities as her previous purchase.

FEDERAL GRADES OF LAMBS, YEARLINGS, AND MUTTON. *The quality grades of lambs, yearlings, and mutton may be defined as a measure of their degree of excellence based on conformation and quality, or eating characteristics of the meat; and the yield, or percent of retail cuts, is based on the thickness of fat over the ribeye.* **Note:** 0.25 in. of fat over the ribeye is considered the line between desirable and somewhat overfat lambs.

From the standpoint of consumers, especially the housewife who buys most of the meat, the grade is important, because (1) in these days of self-service, prepackaged meats there is less opportunity to secure the counsel and advice of the meat cutter when making purchases, and (2) the average consumer is not the best judge of the quality of the various kinds of meats on display in the meat counter.

The current federal grades, which became effective July 6, 1992, on a voluntary basis, call for both quality and yield grading after removal of most of the kidney and pelvic fat, although up to 1.0% of the carcass weight in kidney and pelvic fat is allowed in carcasses.

Federally graded meats are so stamped (with an edible vegetable dye) that the grade will appear on the retail cuts as well as on the carcass and wholesale cuts. The federal quality grades of lambs, yearlings, and mutton are:

Lambs and Yearlings	Mutton
Prime	Choice
Choice	Good
Good	Utility
Utility	Cull

In addition to the quality grades given, there are the following yield grades of lamb, yearling, and mutton carcasses: Yield Grade 1, Yield Grade 2, Yield Grade 3, Yield Grade 4, and Yield Grade 5. The new standards call for both quality and yield grades. Also, the new grades apply to both (1) lamb, yearling, and mutton carcasses; and (2) slaughter (live) lambs, yearlings, and mutton sheep.

The word "quality" infers superiority. It follows that quality grades indicate the relative superiority of carcasses or cuts in palatability characteristics. In turn, palatability is associated with tenderness, juiciness, and flavor. The major quality-indicating characteristics are (1) color and texture of bone, which indicates the age of the animal; (2) firmness; (3) texture; and (4) marbling—the intermixing of fat among the muscle fibers.

Yield grades indicate the *quantity* of meat—the amount of retail, consumer-ready, ready-to-cook, or edible meat that a carcass contains. Yield grade is not to be confused with dressing percent. Dressing percent refers to the amount of carcass from a live animal, whereas yield grade refers to the amount of edible product from the carcass.

LAMB CUTS AND HOW TO COOK THEM. Fig. L-5 illustrates the retail cuts of lamb, and gives the recommended method or methods of cooking each.

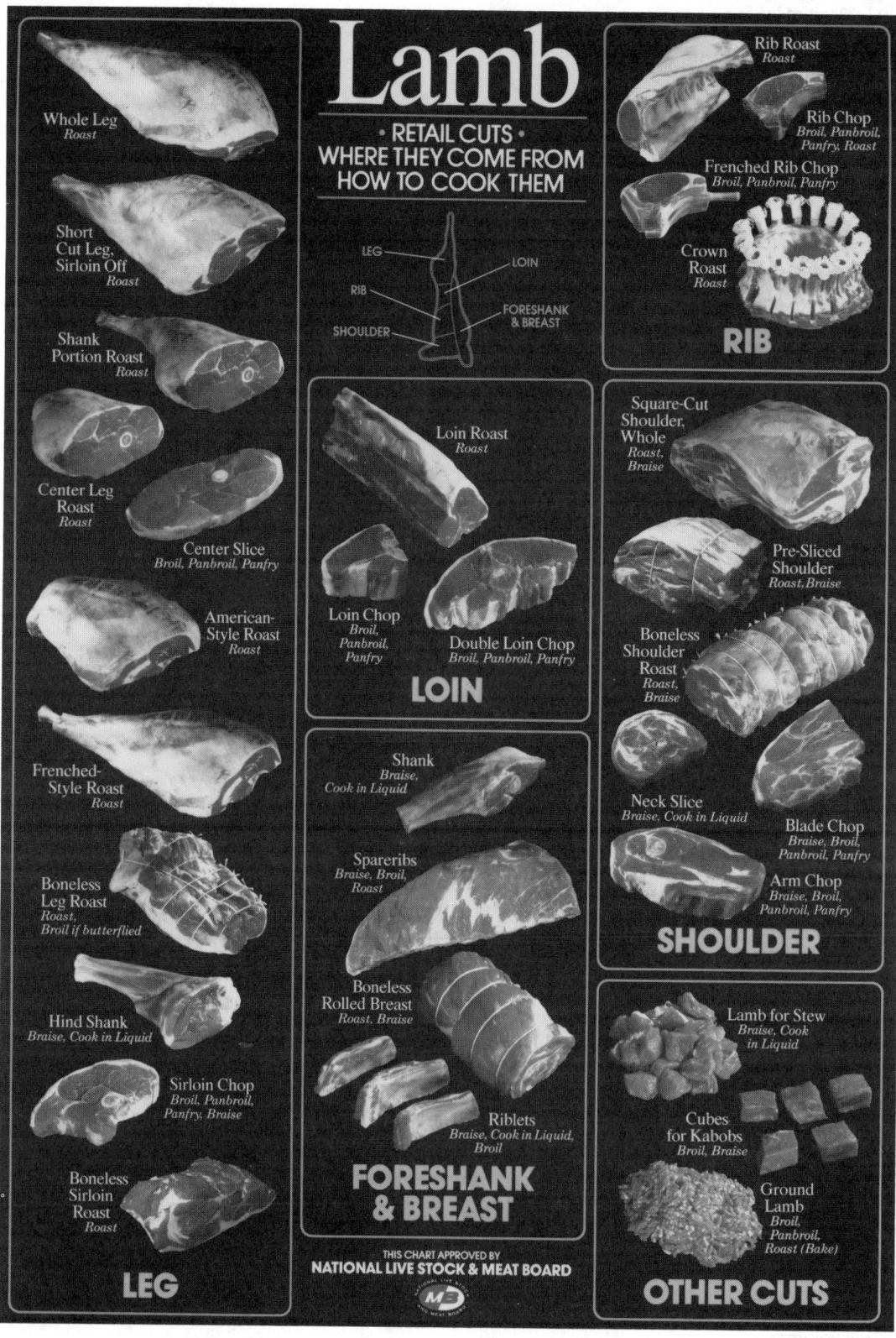

Fig. L-5. The retail cuts of lamb; where they come from and how to cook them. (Courtesy, National Live Stock and Meat Board, Chicago, Ill.)

U.S. LAMB PRODUCTION. In 1990, 362,000,000 lb (*165,000,000 kg*) of lamb and mutton were produced in the United States, which represented only 0.9% of the nation's total meat production. On January 1, 1991, there were 11,200,000 sheep and lambs in the United States.

PER CAPITA LAMB AND MUTTON CONSUMPTION. In 1990, the U.S. per capita consumption of lamb and mutton (and most of it was lamb) was a mere 1.1 lb.

LAMB AND MUTTON AS FOODS.

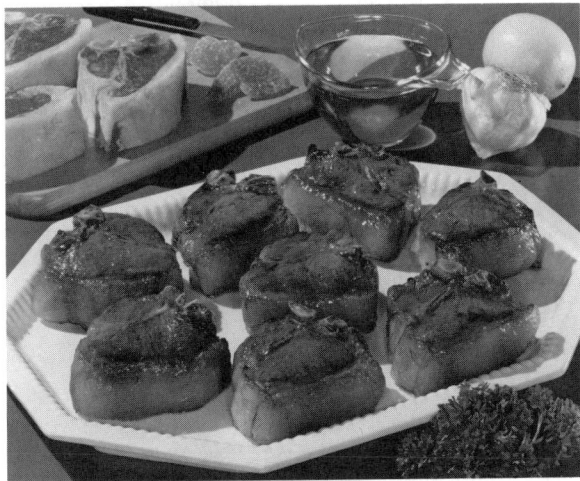

Fig. L-6. Lamb loin chops. (Courtesy, National Live Stock & Meat Board, Chicago, Ill.)

Lamb has long been noted for its delicate flavor and tenderness. In biblical times, frequent reference was made to the desirability of lamb meat. Today, it may be featured for gourmet dining at home and in hotels and restaurants.

Lamb is important in the diet, not for its appetite appeal alone, but for the essential food nutrients that it contains. It is an excellent source of high-quality protein for muscle building and body maintenance. In most cuts of lamb, the fat may be easily separated from the lean; hence, the calories can be adjusted to desired levels. Lamb is one of the best sources of iron, needed for hemoglobin formation; and it is rich in phosphorus, needed for bones and teeth. It is also an excellent source of vitamin B-12, vitamin B-6, biotin, niacin, pantothenic acid, and thiamin. Also, lamb muscle is easily digested, so it is included in the diet of both the young and aged.

In the past, lamb was often considered to be a seasonal meat—spring lamb. Today, it is available the year-round, primarily due to freezer storage and imported lamb. Since lamb will keep frozen for long periods (12 months), large volumes are now marketed as portion-cut, frozen, and ready-to-cook.

LARD

Lard is the fat rendered (melted out) from fresh, fatty pork tissue.

The proportion of live market weight made into lard varies with the type, weight, and finish of the hogs, and the relative price of lard and the cuts of meat. A market weight hog grading U.S. No. 1 yields about 8 lb of lard per 100 lb (*3.6 kg/45 kg*) liveweight, whereas the same weight hog grading U.S. No. 3 yields about 16 lb per cwt (*7.3 kg/45 kg*).

It is noteworthy, too, that lard consumption has steadily declined since 1950. The U.S. per capita consumption of lard in 1950 was 12.6 lb; in 1990, it was only 2.2 lb.

The three most important sources of lard obtained from a hog carcass are: (1) leaf fat, (2) fat trimmings, and (3) fat backs and plates. About 75% of the fat back is rendered for lard, the other 25% is marketed fresh, frozen, or cured.

KINDS OF LARD. Lard is classified according to the part of the animal from which the fat comes and the method of rendering. A brief discussion of each of the kinds of lard follows.

Kettle-Rendered Lard. Steam jacketed kettles with mechanical agitators are used in this method. Leaf fat rendered by this process is known as *open kettle-rendered leaf fat*. It is very white in color, fine textured, and possesses excellent keeping qualities and a pleasing flavor. It is the highest grade of commercial lard outside of the neutral lards or the new processed lards (modern lard). Trimming fats go into kettle-rendered lard.

Steam-Rendered Lard. Steam-rendered lard is made from killing and trimming fats that are rendered in a closed vertical tank or cylinder under steam pressure of from 30 to 50 lb. If it is bleached with fuller's earth and refined, it is known as *refined lard*. Steam-rendered lard is somewhat milder in flavor and odor and lighter in color than lard produced by dry-processed rendering.

Dry-Processed Rendered Lard. Dry-processed rendered lard is made by cooking fats in horizontal steam jacketed tanks under a vacuum. The three kinds of fat may be rendered separately, or all kinds of pork fat may be converted into lard under this process. This method of rendering gives a product that has a fine flavor and excellent keeping quality.

Neutral Lard. Neutral lard is made from leaf or back fats that are rendered in a water jacketed kettle at a very low temperature of about 126°F (*52°C*). Neutral lard is white in color and bland in flavor. It is used almost entirely in the manufacture of butter substitutes.

Lard Substitutes. Lard substitutes, which are sometimes used in place of lard, are made from: (1) lard and other animal fats (lard compound), (2) vegetable oils with animal fats, and (3) hydrogenated vegetable oils, the most prominent of which are cottonseed, soybean, peanut, and coconut oil.

Lard Oil; Stearin. When fat is stored at high temperatures, usually 90° to 100°F (32° to 38°C), the liquid (lard oil) separates from the solid (stearin). Stearin is the white solid material composed of glycerin and stearic acid left after the pressing operation forces out the lard oil. Lard oil, which is made from prime steam lard, consists mainly of olein. Olein is used in the manufacture of margarine, as a burning oil, and as a lubricant for thread-cutting machines.

Modern Lard. During and subsequent to World War II, lard had to meet increasing competition from vegetable shortenings. This necessitated new treatments and an improved product. To meet consumer demands, the manufacturer evolved a new lard. Because the consumer objected to the naturally blue color of lard, the manufacturer decolorized it—he made it white. Because the consumer objected to the odor, he deodorized it. Because lard was too soft at room temperature, he added hydrogenated lard flakes and raised the melting point. In order that it would keep on the shelf as well as in the refrigerator, he gave it stability by adding an antioxidant. Lastly, the manufacturer placed it in a container that would preserve these added qualities.

ANTIOXIDANTS IN ANIMAL FATS. Fats are prone to autoxidation and subsequent rancidity. To curb oxidation, antioxidants are added to fats.

Antioxidants are compounds that prevent oxidative rancidity of polyunsaturated fats. It is important that rancidity of fats be prevented because it may cause destruction of vitamins A, D, and E, and of several of the B-complex vitamins. Also, the breakdown products of rancidity may react with the epsilon amino groups of lysine and thereby decrease the protein and energy values of the diet.

For approval and use in animal fats sold in interstate commerce, antioxidants must be tasteless, odorless, and nontoxic; and must stabilize the fat by retarding rancidity as claimed. To date the following antioxidants have been approved as meeting these requisites: (1) BHA (butylated hydroxyanisole), (2) BHT (butylated hydroxytoluene), (3) glycine, (4) propyl gallate, (5) resin guaiac, and (6) tocopherols.

LARDING

A method of adding fat to lean meat so that it does not dry out during cooking. Narrow strips of fat (as bacon fat) are inserted into the meat with a special larding needle—a large needle with a hollow split end. The strips of fat are called lardoons.

LARK (MEADOWLARK)

Singing and game birds of which there are numerous species, found mostly in Europe, Asia, and northern Africa. The lark has a very delicate flesh and is greatly esteemed by gastronomes.

LATHYRISM

A diseae due to the toxicant found in the Lathyrus seed (*Lathyrus sativus*). The toxin produces an irreversible, gradual weakness, followed by paralysis of both legs (paraplegia). Outbreaks occur in Asia and North Africa mainly during years of poor wheat crops. In these areas, it is common practice to plant Lathyrus with the wheat. If rainfall is adequate, the wheat overgrows the Lathyrus. However, in a year when the rains fail, mainly Lathyrus seed is harvested and it becomes the main dietary energy source; and the symptoms of Lathyrism begin appearing. The disease can affect horses and cattle, too.

LAXATIVE

A food or drug that will induce bowel movements and relieve constipation. Bran and other fibrous foods will soften the stool and encourage more rapid movement through the digestive tract. Numerous laxative drugs are sold, most of which act by increasing the water content of the stool, or by increasing the contraction of the bowel, or by lubricating the lining of the bowel. Persons seeking relief from constipation should exercise care in the choice and use of a laxative; and, when in doubt, consult a doctor.

(Also see CONSTIPATION.)

LEAD (Pb)

Lead poisoning has dogged man for centuries. It is even speculated that it may have caused the decline and fall of the Roman Empire. In recent years, lead poisoning has been reduced significantly with the use of lead-free paints.

(Also see MINERAL[S]; and POISONS, Table P-11 Some Potentially Poisonous [Toxic] Substances.)

LEAVEN

To make light by aerating (adding air) in any of three different methods: (1) by the fermentation of yeast, (2) by the action of baking powder, or (3) by beating air into egg whites.

(Also see BREADS AND BAKING.)

LEBEN

• A type of fermented milk in Egypt.

• A sour milk delicacy of biblical times, made from goat milk.

LEBKUCHEN

A Christmas cookie made with honey, brown sugar, almonds, candied fruit peel and spices.

LECITHIN (PHOSPHATIDYL CHOLINE)

A versatile phospholipid found in all living organisms. It is a mixture of the diglycerides of the fatty acids stearic, palmitic, and oleic combined with the choline ester of phosphoric acid. The body is capable of synthesizing lecithin. In addition, lecithin is found in a wide variety of foods. *At this time, there is no evidence that lecithin has any nutritional significance.*

The commercial source of lecithin is predominately soybeans. It is an FDA approved food additive employed as a stabilizer and emulsifier in margarine, dressings, chocolate, frozen desserts, and baked goods. Furthermore, lecithin is also used in such products as paints, soaps, printing inks, and cosmetics, to name only a few.

(Also see ADDITIVES, Table A-3; CHOLINE; OILS, VEGETABLE; and SOYBEAN, Table S-22 Soybean Products and Uses.)

LEEK *Allium porrum*

This plant is similar to the onion, except that the leaves and stem are eaten rather than the narrow, almost insignificant bulb. The leek, like the other onion vegetables, has long been classified as a member of the Lily family (*Liliaceae*), although some botanists have recently placed this group of vegetables in the *Alliaceae* family. Fig. L-7 shows a typical leek.

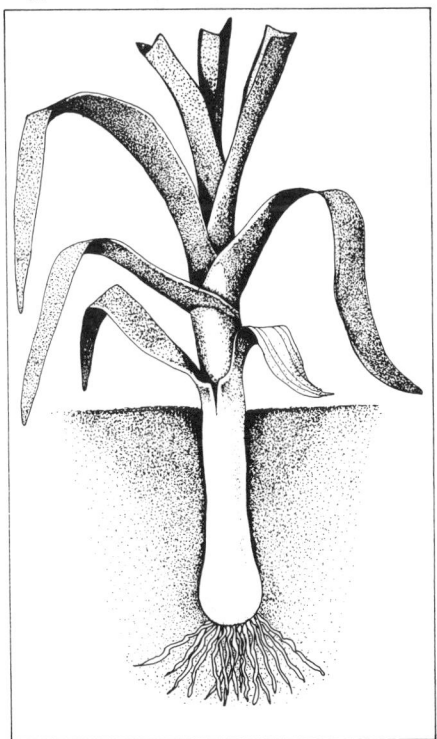

Fig. L-7. The leek, an onionlike vegetable that is the national emblem of Wales.

ORIGIN AND HISTORY. Leeks are native to central Asia. It is believed that the ancient forms of the plant had more of an onionlike bulb than the present day forms.

Egyptian leeks were so highly regarded by the Romans that the Emperor Nero is reported to have consumed leek soup daily in order to strengthen his voice. The Romans introduced the plant into Britain, where it later became the national emblem of Wales. Leeks thrived in Britain because they tolerated cold weather better than onions. Hence, they became an important root crop throughout Europe during the Middle Ages.

Today, leeks are still relished by Europeans, but Americans have not yet acquired a taste for this herb.

PRODUCTION. Much of the commercially grown crop of leeks comes from various European countries,

whereas the smaller U.S. production is grown primarily for people who prepare European style dishes.

Leeks are grown from seeds, which are sometimes planted in a greenhouse or a hotbed. The young plants are transplanted in the field as soon as the danger of a hard frost has passed. It is a common practice to blanch the plants by hilling up the soil around them.

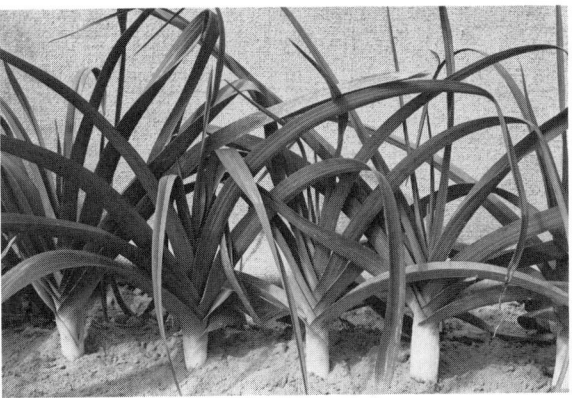

Fig. L-8. Leeks that are ready to be harvested. (Courtesy, USDA)

PROCESSING. There is little or no processing of leeks other than the canning or drying of small amounts in various types of soup preparations. However, frozen chopped leeks could be a profitable item, considering the current market for preprepared ingredients of homemade gourmet-type dishes.

SELECTION AND PREPARATION. High quality leeks have broad dark green solid leaves, and straight, thick white necks with bases about 1 in. (*2.5 cm*) or more in diameter. They have an agreeable mild flavor when they are young, crisp and tender. Yellowing, wilted, or discolored tops may indicate flabby, tough, fibrous necks or other undesirable qualities. Except for appearance, bruised tops are unimportant in utilization.

Leeks should be split lengthwise and washed well to remove any particles of soil that might be caught between the leaves as a result of blanching in the field. The washed raw vegetable may be chopped and mixed with cottage cheese or cream cheese, or it may be added to salads and salad dressings.

Leeks may be cooked in appetizing dishes such as (1) French quiches and Vichyssoise, a cold soup which is rich with heavy cream, chicken broth, and various vegetables—usually potatoes; (2) Scottish Cock-a-Leekie soup, an unusual combination of prunes, beef, chicken, leeks, salt, and pepper; and (3) Welsh chicken-and-leek pie. Finally, the vegetable may be boiled or braised, and served with butter, cheese sauce, or cream sauce.

NUTRITIONAL VALUE. The nutrient composition of leeks is given in Food Composition Table F-36.

Some noteworthy observations regarding the nutrient composition of leeks follow:

1. Leeks have a high water content (85%), and are moderately low in calories (52 kcal per 100 g). They are a good source of iron and potassium, and a fair source of vitamin C.

2.   Europeans have long utilized leeks therapeutically to (a) stimulate the appetite, (b) prevent the growth of disease germs and spoilage organisms, and (c) rid the body of excessive water by stimulation of urination.

(Also see VEGETABLES, Table V-6 Vegetables of the World.)

LEGUMES

Contents

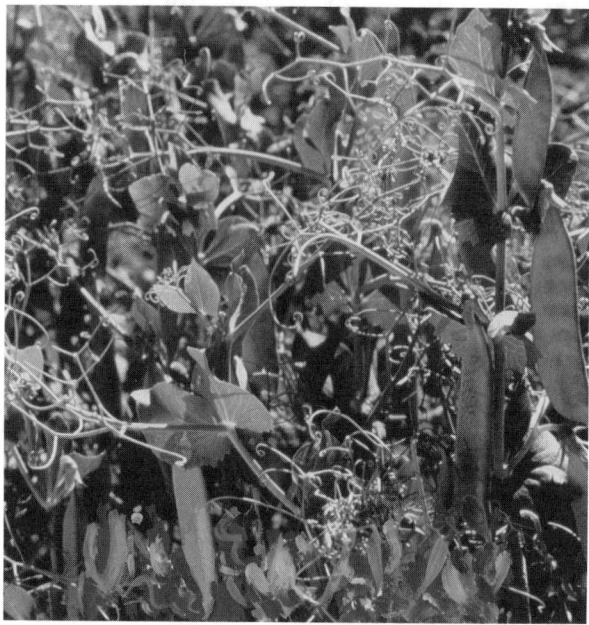

Fig. L-9. Field pea (*Pisum arvense*), showing the seed-bearing pods typical of legumes. (Courtesy, Minnesota Agricultural Experiment Station, University of Minnesota)

This very large family of plants contains about 13,000 species, most of which are distinguished by their seed-bearing pods. These species occur in such diverse forms as short, erect broad-leafed plants; climbing vines; and various types of trees. Legumes rank second only to cereals in supplying calories and protein for the world's population. They supply about the same number of calories per unit weight as the cereals, but they contain from 2 to 4 times more protein. Also, the amino acid patterns of legumes complement those of cereal grains so that combinations of the two foods provide dietary protein that is used much more efficiently by the human body than that from either food alone.

One or more types of edible legumes may be found almost everywhere in the world where the soil is arable and sufficient water is available, because these plants are endowed with certain characteristics which favor their growth and propagation. First, the roots of many legumes harbor bacteria which convert nitrogen gas from the air into nitrogen compounds that may be utilized by the plant. This process is called *nitrogen fixation*. Hence, these plants may grow on soils in which the fixed nitrogen has been exhausted by the growth of other plants such as cereal grains. Also, legumes release their nitrogen compounds upon decaying, so that grains may again grow well on soils that were once depleted. Second, wild legumes have pods that burst open when mature, and scatter their seeds in all directions.

HISTORY.   Historians often express wonder at the apparent wisdom of primitive peoples who produced and utilized legumes and other foods in ways which have only recently received the endorsement of professional agriculturists and nutritionists. Therefore, the history of the use of these foods merits special consideration.

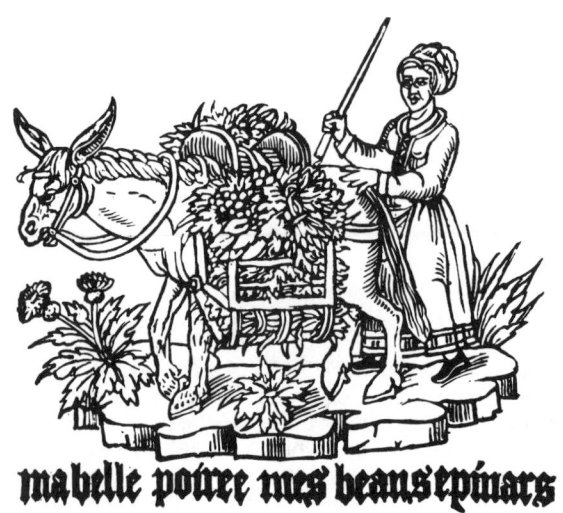

Fig. L-10. French vegetable saleswoman driving a donkey carrying a load of legumes. French Woodcut 18th century. (Courtesy, The Bettmann Archive, Inc., New York, N.Y.)

Ancient times.   By comparing the size of fossilized seed remains at campsites with those of wild species growing in the vicinity, archaeologists have determined that prehistoric peoples domesticated and cultivated certain food legumes. Usually, man has selected and cultivated varieties with large seeds. Furthermore, pods which retain their seeds at maturity have also been selected over those which burst open and scatter. These pieces of evidence, however scanty they might be, have enabled researchers to draw certain conclusions about the origin of agriculture in various parts of the world.

It appears that the first cultivation of legumes occurred in Southeast Asia, rather than in the Middle East, as was originally thought. The recently discovered Spirit Cave near the border between Burma and Thailand contained seeds of beans, peas, and other plants that had been there since about 9750 B.C. (as estimated by radiocarbon dating), and which closely resembled the seeds of today's cultivated plants.

The next oldest sites of agriculture, which date to about 8000 B.C., are those in the Middle East, in the region commonly referred to as the Fertile Crescent, a broad arc of land that curved northward and eastward from the Mediterranean coast of what is now Israel to the Zagros Mountains near the border between Iraq and Iran. This region was probably the place of origin of chickpeas, fava beans, and lentils. Therefore, the following Biblical references to legumes are noteworthy:

• **Genesis 25:29-34**—Esau was so hungry upon his return from a hunting trip that he gave up his birthright to his brother Jacob in exchange for some bread and a bowl of cooked red lentils (sometimes called "pottage.")

• **Ezekiel 4:9**—During the Babylonian captivity of the Jews, the prophet Ezekiel described the making of bread from a variety of grains and legumes (beans, lentils, and vetches).

• **Daniel 1:11-16**—The king of Babylon selected Daniel and other Jewish children that he favored to receive the royal meat and wine, so that they might be healthy and attractive members of his court. However, Daniel refused to eat the king's food, and chose instead a diet of legumes and water. After 10 days on the restricted diet, Daniel appeared fairer than any of the children who ate the king's meat.

Other Biblical references to the leguminous carob pods appear in the narratives about (1) John the Baptist, who ate "locusts" (carob pods, since the carob tree is also called a locust tree); and (2) the prodigal son, when he longed to eat the husks (carob pods) thrown to the swine.

The ancient Greeks and the ancient Romans considered legumes to be "poor man's meat" since most of their poor were lucky to get a little fish, bread, olive oil, and a bowl of *puls* (the Latin word for pottage, which eventually became the English word "pulses," a synonym for legumes). However, the aristocrats among these peoples also disdained legumes because some people became sick after eating them. Many people of Mediterranean and Asian ancestry have an abnormally high susceptibility to a toxic factor present in fava beans, which affirms the truth of the old saying, "One man's meat is another man's poison." Nevertheless, two leading Roman families derived their surnames from the Latin names for legume species. Cicero, from *Cicer arietinum*, or chickpeas; and Fabius, from *Vicia faba*, or fava beans.

Elsewhere, the Egyptians grew grains and legumes, as did the people of Africa, the Americas, Southeast Asia, and China and India. Both the Chinese and Indian peoples were conquered at various times by hordes of nomadic horsemen who rode out of the steppes of Central Asia. Some historians suggest that the largely vegetarian diets of both China and India were attempts by these people to set themselves apart from the nomadic invaders, who subsisted mainly on dairy products and meat. However, the Chinese were forced to eat a predominantly vegetarian diet because they had to feed many people with the food produced on a limited area of land when their conquerors occupied much of what they had previously utilized. Many of the Indian people also became vegetarians, but in their case it resulted from the Hindu teachings against the killing of animals.

The long dependence of these peoples on almost wholly vegetarian diets led to (1) the development of soybean-based imitations of dairy products by the Chinese; and (2) a utilization of legumes for food in India that was unequaled elsewhere in the world. (Lately, the production of legumes in India has declined as a result of the introdution of high-yielding varieties of cereal grains.)

The Middle Ages. Legumes were a staple food of the northern European countries throughout the Middle Ages (a period which lasted from about 476 A.D. to 1450 A.D.) because bad weather often wiped out much of the grain crops. Wheat did not grow well, and rye was susceptible to the poisonous fungus ergot. Hence, the poor often had bread made from mixtures of rye, bean, and pea flours.

Also, legume porridges seasoned with a few scraps of meat, poultry, and/or salt pork kept many of the impoverished from starving to death. Those who were a little better off had sausage, cabbage, lentils, rye bread, and beer. However, this somewhat bleak picture was brightened considerably by the adoption of a system of crop rotations in which plots of land were planted to grain one year, and to legumes the next. This increased food production greatly.

Modern Times. The great expansion of worldwide exploration and trade that occurred in the 15th and 16th centuries resulted in the introduction of various species of legumes to parts of the world where they often displaced native species. For example, the Spanish took peanuts from South America to regions in Africa where they displaced the Bambarra groundnut, a legume that has underground seeds with shells, like the peanut. The peanut was taken to North America by African slaves, who also brought the cowpea. Cowpeas, also called "black-eyed peas," are traditionally served on New Year's Day in southeastern United States.

Apparently, the first cultivation of legumes in the New World occurred around 4000 B.C. in both Peru and Mexico, but the practice gradually spread to other parts of North and South America. Hence, there was much similarity between the American Indian practices observed by the Spanish when they arrived in Latin America and those noted by the English settlers of New England. The Indians of both places planted beans among rows of corn so that the cornstalks might provide convenient supports for the climbing legume vines. This practice eliminated much of the necessity for weeding the crops.

The English colonists also learned from the Indians how to make succotash (a mixture of corn and beans). Boston baked beans were derived from the Indian method of soaking beans until they swelled, then baking them with deer fat and onions in clay pots surrounded by hot stones. The Pilgrims baked their beans on Saturday nights in order to avoid the performance of servile work on Sundays. Later, the custom changed as the strict observance of the Sabbath abated, and baked beans were served on Saturday nights in New England.

During the great westward expansion in the 19th century, the settlers of the southwestern United States adopted many of the Mexican bean dishes such as frijoles (refried beans) and chili. It is believed that the original chili dish was invented by Mexican nuns.

Peanut butter was first used in the United States in the 1890s, although certain South American Indians had used a similar product for centuries. Although this product was originally made by a doctor in St. Louis for people who had poor teeth, it soon became a favorite food of children.

At the present time, food technologists around the world are engaged in testing many new food products made from legumes in the hope that this approach might help to combat protein deficiency. Also, agricultural scientists are conducting experiments designed to (1) improve the per acre yields of legumes, and (2) increase the amount of nitrogen fixed by these plants.

PRODUCTION. In recent years, only modest advances have been made in the production of legumes around the world. This is in marked contrast to the development and promotion of the high-yielding strains of cereals, which have comprised the Green Revolution. There is a great need for improving the yields of legume crops so that the production of these foods may be increased in the densely populated countries where many people are not receiving sufficient dietary protein. Therefore, some of the more important aspects of legume production follow.

Growing Conditions. Returning explorers often brought new legume crops back with them. However, the newly introduced plants did not always grow well because the environmental conditions of the new habitats usually differed vastly from those where the crops had long grown. The major factors that affect the growth of legumes are noteworthy:

• **Amount of sunshine and day length**—Most legumes require considerable sunshine for photosynthesis because large amounts of energy are required for the nitrogen fixation that occurs in the root nodules. Furthermore, many species have patterns of growth, flowering, and setting seed that are quite dependent upon day length. For example, the day length during the summer may be from 2 to 4 hours longer in the northern latitudes

than in the tropics. Generally, the highest yields of legumes are obtained in the temperate zones and the lowest in the humid tropics. Another factor responsible for low yields in the latter areas appears to be the prolonged rainfall and cloudiness, since better yields are obtained in the drier tropical areas.

• **Range of temperatures**—Tropical legumes may be damaged or killed by low temperatures, whereas the species adapted to temperate climates may succumb to high temperatures. For example, cowpeas, mung beans, peanuts, and pigeon peas grow best where the temperatures range between 68°F (20°C) and 104°F (40°C). These conditions usually prevail in a tropical belt lying between 30°N and 30°S latitudes. On the other hand, broad beans, chickpeas, kidney beans, lentils, peas, soybeans, and vetches require temperatures between 50°F (10°C) and 86°F (30°C), which are characteristic of the northern and southern Temperate Zones (between 20° and 40° latitudes). The latter crops may also grow well at high altitudes in lower latitudes (as chickpeas and lentils do in Ethiopia), and in coastal areas between 40°N and 60°N latitudes that are warmed sufficiently by ocean currents.

• **Rainfall and water supply**—Although legumes require adequate moisture for sprouting, growth, and production of seed, too much rainfall may mean too little sunshine and the proliferation of pests. Hence, dry climates favor high yields when irrigation is available.

Nitrogen Fixation by Legumes. Although the ancient Greeks and Romans knew that the growing of leguminous plants somehow restored the fertility of soil previously used to grow grains, it was not until the late 19th century that it was discovered that nitrogen-fixing bacteria reside in nodules on the roots of legumes. Nitrogen fixation refers to the conversion of inert, atmospheric nitrogen gas into compounds which may be utilized by most plants. Fig. L-11 outlines the nitrogen cycle as it occurs in nature.

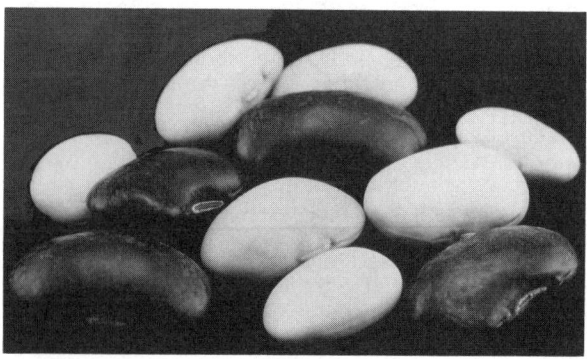

Fig. L-10a. Scarlet runner beans. (Courtesy, Minnesota Agricultural Experiment Station, University of Minnesota)

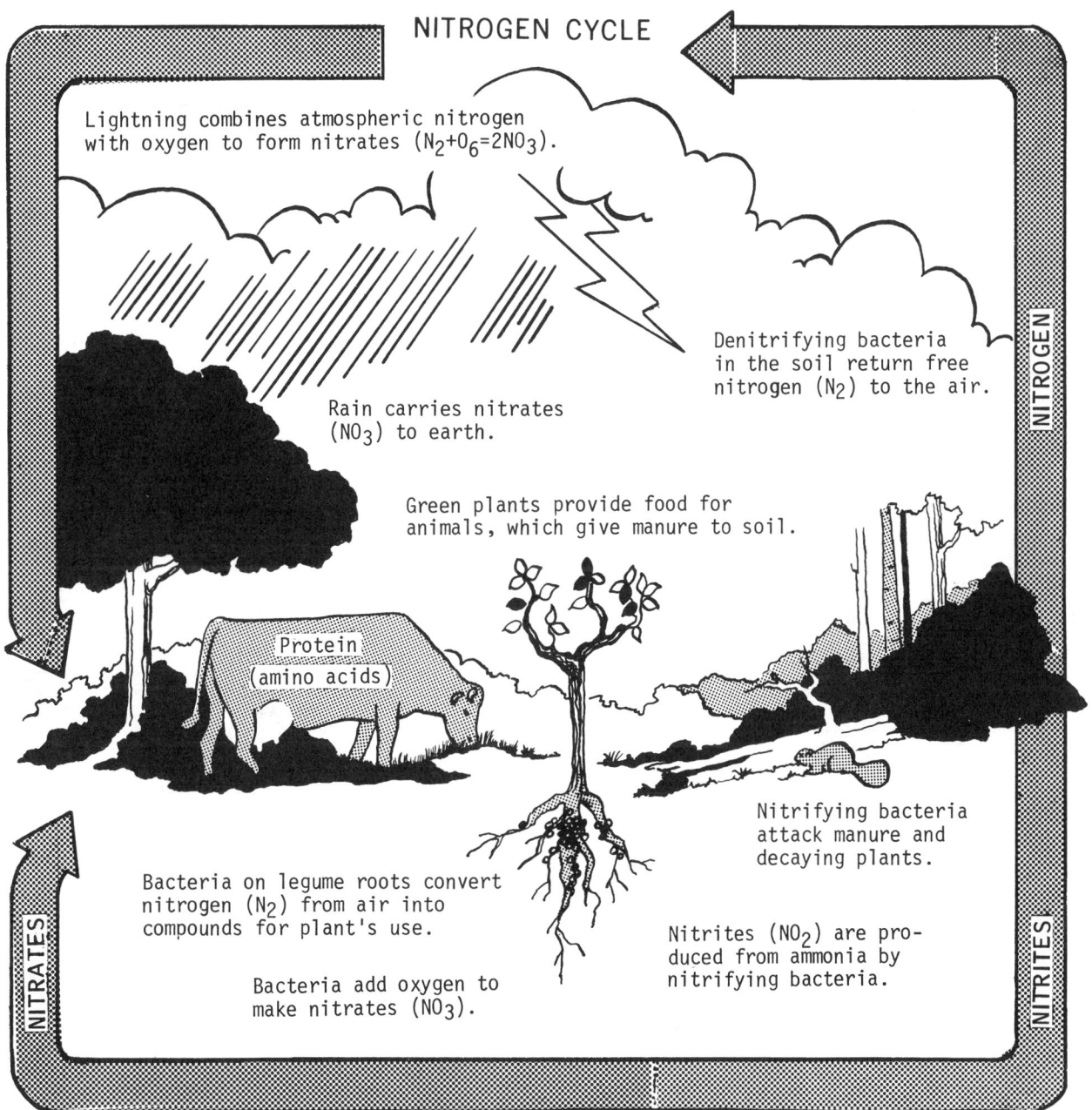

Fig. L-11. The naturally-occurring aspects of the nitrogen cycle. Legumes play a major role in the conversion of nitrogen gas into forms that are much more useful to plants, animals, and people.

It is noteworthy that the conversion of nitrogen gas into ammonia by the bacteria (various species of *Rhyzobia*) in the root nodules of legumes requires considerable chemical energy, which the legume leaves derive from photosynthesis. Hence, the relationship between the legumes and the bacteria which colonize their roots is mutually beneficial, because each organism supplies a vital need of the other. Furthermore, the different species of legumes play host to different species of nitrogen-fixing bacteria. Therefore, it is often necessary to inoculate the seeds of leguminous plants with the appropriate bacterial culture prior to planting, because the organisms present in the soil may not be suitable for the plants.

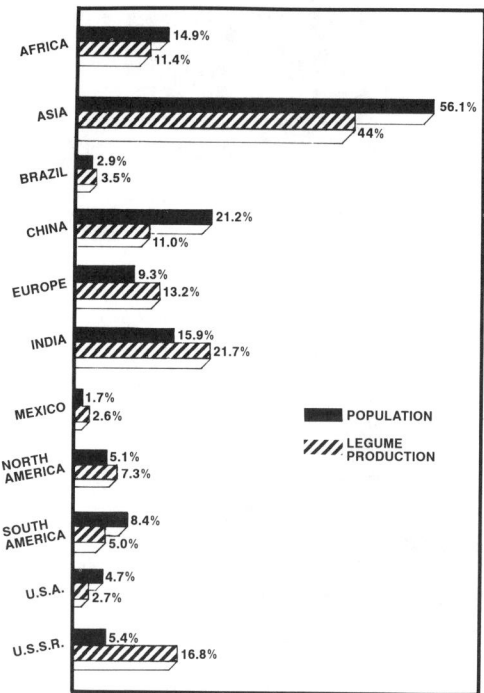

Fig. L-13. Distribution of the world's population vs the world legume production. (Sources: *The World Almanac and Book of Facts, 1991*, p. 773, and *FAO Production Yearbook, 1990*, FAO/UN, Rome, Italy, Vol. 44, p. 98, Table 31)

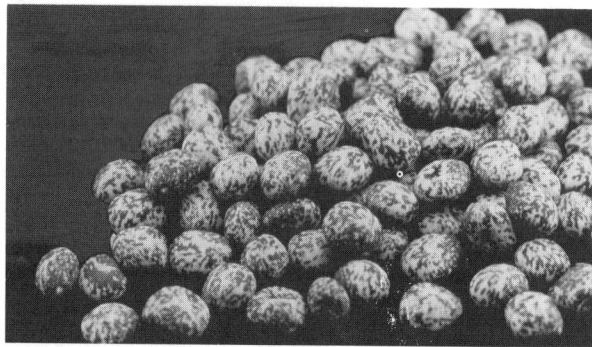

Fig. L-12. Yellow lupines, one of the approximately 100 kinds of lupines. (Courtesy, Minnesota Agricultural Experiment Station, University of Minnesota)

The commercial fixation of nitrogen that is used in the production of synthetic fertilizers also requires considerable energy, most of which is supplied by fossil fuels. Hence, the natural fixation of nitrogen by legumes is likely to become increasingly important to farmers around the world as the supplies of fossil fuels become more scarce and expensive.

World Production. There are now major discrepancies between the food requirements of various peoples and the amounts of legumes that they produce. These discrepancies are shown in Fig. L-13.

It appears that the underdeveloped areas in Africa and Asia may have many people suffering from protein deficiency due to lack of sufficient amounts of legumes. Most of the developed countries with low levels of legume production are sufficiently affluent to import food when it is needed.

Soybeans account for most of the U.S. legume production. Fig. L-14 shows the shares of the world legume production contributed by each of the major U.S. legume crops.

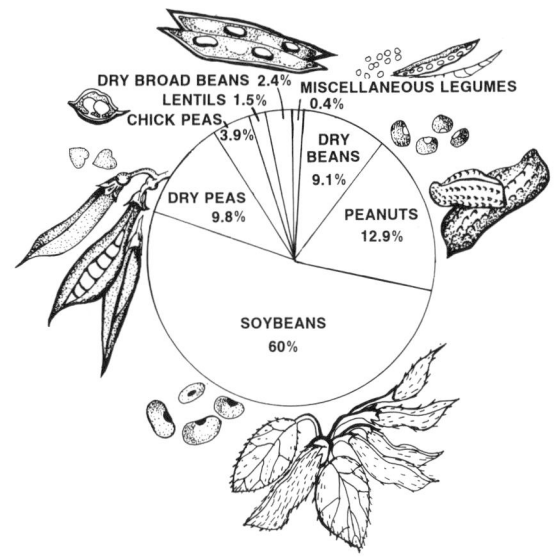

Fig. L-14. Contributions of the U.S. major legume crops to world production. (Based on data from *FAO Production Yearbook*, 1990, FAO/UN, Rome, Italy, Vol. 44)

PREPARATION AND SERVING OF LEGUMES.

Today, many American homemakers work either part time or full time and have little time to boil beans for two or more hours, unless they wish to use a crock pot and start them cooking before they leave for work in the morning. However, long cooking uses a lot of electricity or gas, which are becoming more expensive each day. Therefore, the U.S. Department of Agriculture and various university departments have conducted research to find methods of simplifying the cooking and serving of legumes. Their findings have led to the suggestions which follow:

1. Soaking dry beans cuts cooking time considerably. However, the traditional overnight soaking is not needed if the beans are placed in water, heated to boiling and the boiling maintained for at least 2 minutes, then set aside to soak for at least an hour. The initial boiling rapidly softens the seed coats so that water may penetrate more readily.

2. If hard water is used in cooking, it will take much longer for the legumes to cook because the calcium and magnesium in hard water combine with pectin in the peas or beans and render them tough. The remedy is to add not more than $^1/_8$ to ¼ teaspoon (*0.6 to 1.3 ml*) of baking soda per cup of legumes to the cooking water. Also, such acid ingredients as tomato sauce and vinegar should not be added until the peas or beans have become tender.

3. Most legumes can be made tender by pressure cooking for 10 to 15 minutes, if the pressure is allowed to fall without allowing the steam to escape. Pressure cooking has not usually been recommended because certain legumes generate considerable foam which may plug the vent on the cooker. However, the addition of about a teaspoon or so of oil or melted fat reduces foaming greatly.

4. Whenever feasible, at least small amounts (1 oz or more) of cheese, eggs, fish, meat, milk (1 glass per meal), or poultry should be served with cooked legumes since ½ cup (*120 ml*) or more of the latter are required to furnish an amount of protein equivalent to only 1 oz (*28 g*) of meat. (Adults require a minimum daily protein intake which is equivalent to that in 8 oz of meat.) Most legumes go well with most animal foods when appropriate seasoning is used.

5. Strict vegetarians who eat no animal products (vegans) need to keep track of their protein intake so as to be certain that they get enough, because most plant foods are low in protein. (However, legume flours are high in protein.) Therefore, vegans should eat from 1½ to 2 times as much legumes per meal as a person who eats some animal foods. For example, ¾ cup (*180 ml*) of cooked legumes furnishes about 11 to 13 g of protein. This would need to be supplemented with at least 1½ cups (*360 ml*) of cooked cereal product or 3 to 4 slices of bread to insure that the meal contained sufficient protein. Also, the breads used by vegans should either (1) contain plenty of nuts and/or soy flour; or (2) be eaten with peanut butter or mashed cooked bean spreads (homemade or commercial bean dips are suitable.)

• **Sprouting legume seeds**—Using sprouted seed adds considerably to the dietary intake of vitamins with few added calories because much of the food energy stored in a seed is used up during the growth of the embryonic plant. Also, extra vitamins are synthesized by the seed when the embryo starts to grow. Therefore, it is noteworthy that a dormant seed usually starts sprouting when it has absorbed sufficient water to allow a stepping up of its metabolism. Directions for sprouting seeds follow.

1. Purchase seeds that are guaranteed to sprout. Most health food stores now carry alfalfa seeds for sprouting. Some also sell viable mung bean seeds and soybean seeds. It is not wise to use seeds intended for planting as food because they may have been treated with one or more chemical agents used to prevent fungus diseases.

2. Use only unbroken seeds, and soak them overnight in an amount of water at least four times as great as the seeds. After soaking, drain off water through a strainer. Place seeds in a special sprouter, or in a wide-mouthed jar or a tray. Cover with wet paper toweling. Rinse seeds in a strainer three or four times a day, and replace paper towels. Sprouts should be sufficiently developed for use after 3 to 4 days.

3. Fresh sprouts may be used in salads, sandwiches, soups, stews, casseroles, and baked goods. Generally, seeds yield six or more times their original weight in sprouts. Sprouts have only about ½ the solids content of cooked beans or peas. Hence, one has to eat from 1 to 1½ cups (360 ml) of sprouts to obtain the amount of protein furnished by about ½ cup (120 ml) of cooked dried beans. However, the sprouts furnish fewer calories, but more vitamins per gram of protein.

CAUTION: Deleterious substances of various kinds are present in some legumes eaten by man; among them, the trypsin inhibitor, and the following toxins: cyanogenetic glucosides, saponins, alkaloids, goitrogenic factors, hemagglutinins (substances which agglutinate red cells and destroy them) and the unknown toxic factor which produces lathyrism. Further research on many of these substances is needed. And consumption of certain legumes should be limited to nontoxic species or to those where toxicity can be eliminated or reduced to safe limits by appropriate preparation and cooling. But present knowledge suggests that most of these substances are present only in raw grain and are eliminated by ordinary methods of preparation; e.g., adequate soaking and boiling. There is no existing evidence, for example, that poisoning by cyanogens has ever occurred in human beings as a result of eating cooked legumes, or that goitrogenic substances in legumes have caused goiter. Two toxic substances in certain legumes are, however, of special importance; namely, the factor in lathyrus pea (Lathrus sativus) which causes the disease lathyrism, and the hemolytic factor in broad bean (Vicia faba) associated with the disease favism.

Consumers should be aware of the potentially harmful substances present in certain legumes so that there will be proper preparation. To the latter end, the major antinutritional and toxic factors in certain legumes are presented in Table L-1.

TABLE L-1
ANTINUTRITIONAL AND/OR TOXIC FACTORS WHICH MAY BE PRESENT IN CERTAIN LEGUMES

Type of Factor(s)	Effect of Factor(s)	Method(s) of Counteracting Undesirable Factor(s)	Legumes Containing the Factor(s)
Antivitamin factors:	Interfere with the actions of certain vitamins.		
Antivitamin A	Lipoxidase oxidizes and destroys carotene (provitamin A).	Roasting at 212°F (100°C) or higher.	Soybeans
Antivitamin B-12	Increases requirement for vitamin B-12.	Heating	Soybeans
Antivitamin D	Causes rickets unless extra vitamin D is provided.	Autoclaving (pressure cooking).	Soybeans
Antivitamin E	Damage to the liver and muscles.	Heat treatment (only partially effective).	Alfalfa, Common beans (Phaseolus vulgaris), Peas (Pisum sativum).
Cyanide-releasing glucosides	An enzyme in legumes causes the release of hydrocyanic acid (a cellular poison) from the otherwise inert glucoside. The poison may also be released by an enzyme in E. coli, a normal inhabitant of the human intestine.	Soaking and cooking the beans releases much of the toxic factor. The E. coli population of the human intestine may be reduced by encouraging the growth of Lactobacilli species, which are present in fermented dairy products (sour milk, yogurt, etc.).	All legumes contain at least small amounts of these factors. However, certain varieties of lima beans (Phaseolus lunatus) may contain much larger amounts.

(Continued)

TABLE L-1 *(Continued)*

Type of Factor(s)	Effect of Factor(s)	Method(s) of Counteracting Undesirable Factor(s)	Legumes Containing the Factor(s)
Favism factor	Causes the breakdown of red blood cells in susceptible individuals only (some of the people with ancestors from the Mediterranean, Taiwan, and various parts of Asia). Other people are *not* affected.	Avoidance of fava beans by people who are susceptible to this type of hemolytic anemia. Some of the more sensitive people are even affected by inhalation of the pollen from the bean flower.	Fava beans (*Vicia faba*).
Gas-generating carbohydrates	Certain indigestible carbohydrates are acted upon by gas-producing bacteria in the lower intestine.	**Much of the indigestible carbohydrates may be broken down by (1) soaking and cooking (and discarding the water after each step); (2) acid-treatment followed by incubation; or (3) fermentation and sprouting.**	Many species of mature dry legume seeds, but *not* peanuts. The immature (green) seeds contain much lower amounts.
Goitrogens	Interfere with the utilization of iodine by the thyroid gland. As a result, the thyroid gland becomes enlarged (forms a goiter).	Heat treatment is partially effective. However, it is a good idea to provide extra dietary iodine when large amounts of peanuts and/or soybeans are consumed.	Peanuts and Soybeans.
Inhibitors of trypsin	The inhibitor(s) binds with the digestive enzyme trypsin. As a result, the pancreas may become overworked as it attempts to produce additional enzyme. Normally, the secretion of adequate trypsin acts as a feedback to prevent excessive secretion of pancreatic enzymes.	Heat treatment (soaking, followed by steaming, pressure cooking, extrusion cooking); fermentation; or sprouting.	All legumes contain trypsin inhibitors to some extent.
Lathyrogenic neurotoxins	Consumption of the lathyrogenic legumes in large quantities (1/4 or more of the total diet) for long periods (several months) results in severe neurological disorders.	Dehulling, then soaking overnight and steaming or roasting.	Lathyrus pea (*L. sativus*), which is grown mainly in India. Common vetch (*Vicia sativa*) may also be lathrogenic.
Metal binders	These factors bind certain essential minerals (such as copper, iron, manganese, and zinc) so that they are not well utilized by the body.	Heat treatment.	Soybeans, Peas (*Pisum sativum*).
Red blood cell clumping agents (*hemagglutinins*)	The agents cause the red blood cells to clump together.	Soaking followed by heat treatment.	Occurs in all legumes to some extent.

It may be seen from Table L-1 that various types of heat treatment inactivate most of the antinutritional and toxic factors in legumes. However, heating has no effect on the favism-producing factor in fava beans, or the gas-generating carbohydrates in many legumes. Hence, people troubled with favism should avoid eating the offending beans, whereas those who tolerate gassiness (flatulence) poorly would be better off eating only immature (green) beans or mature beans which have been sprouted.

The most effective detoxifying treatment for the home preparation of beans is soaking until the legumes begin to swell, then cooking them until tender. Also, some researchers have found that pressure cooking prior to grinding them into flour or meal inactivates most of the potentially harmful substances. Finally, it is noteworthy that various types of fermentation, which have been utilized by Asian peoples for centuries, are also means of detoxifying legumes.

NUTRITIONAL VALUE.

Seeds such as those of the common food legumes are good sources of certain nutrients, because they are storehouses of the carbohydrates, fats, proteins, minerals, and vitamins needed to sustain the embryonic plant until it has developed sufficiently to take care of its own needs. The nutritive composition of common legumes is given in Food Composition Table F-36.

Some noteworthy observations regarding the nutrient composition of legumes follow:

1. The items lowest in calories are those with the highest water content. Hence, weight watchers may eat their fill of cooked snap beans (92.4% water and 25 kcal per 100 g), but they should curtail their consumption of roasted peanuts (1.8% water and 589 kcal per 100 g). However, it is noteworthy that the high caloric value of the latter item is also due to a high fat content, since defatted peanut flour is much lower in energy content (371 kcal per 100 g).

2. A 100 g portion (approximately ½ cup) of most types of cooked mature dry beans supplies between 100 and 130 Calories (kcal) and an average of about 7 g of protein, which is about the same as the amount of protein in 1 oz (28 g) of cooked lean meat. However, the quality of protein in legumes is somewhat lower than that of meat and other animal proteins.

3. Sprouted seeds supply more protein per calorie than unsprouted seeds because much of the stored carbohydrate is metabolized for energy during sprouting, whereas little protein is used for this purpose. For example, cooked sprouted soybeans contain 13.9 g of protein per 100 kcal, whereas cooked unsprouted soybeans contain only 8.4 g of protein per 100 kcal.

4. Defatted peanut flour and defatted soybean flour each contain almost 50% protein. Hence, small amounts of these products make major protein contributions when added to cereal flours, which contain only about 8 to 15% protein.

5. The various soybean flours are good sources of calcium and iron, although the beany flavor sometimes limits the amounts which may be used in certain foods.

6. All of the legumes are good to excellent sources of iron, potassium, thiamin, riboflavin, and niacin.

7. Immature cowpea (black-eyed pea) pods and seeds are the best legume sources of vitamins A and C, which are lacking in the mature dry seeds.

8. Cooked hyacinth beans and cooked pigeon peas are high in fiber, which might be beneficial to people bothered with chronic constipation and certain other disorders. Some researchers have reported that the consumption of fibrous legumes lowers blood cholesterol significantly, even when substantial amounts of animal fats are consumed with the legumes.

Additional information on certain nutritional and antinutritional aspects of legumes are given in the sections which follow.

Protein Quantity and Quality. There is much current worldwide interest in the value of legumes as major sources of dietary protein because (1) the prices of meat and other animal products are rising rapidly, and (2) certain densely populated developing countries lack sufficient land to raise large numbers of animals for meat. Therefore, certain facts regarding protein quantity and quality of legumes are noteworthy:

1. Cooked legumes furnish less protein per gram, and per calorie than low and medium fat types of cheeses, eggs, fish, meats, and poultry. For example, 3½ oz (100 g) of cooked common beans supplying 118 calories (kcal) are required to provide the protein in 1 oz (28 g) of cooked lean meat (55 kcal) or medium-fat meat (78 kcal). Also, the protein quality of the legumes is lower than that of the animal foods.

2. The proteins in legumes are moderately deficient in the sulfur-containing amino acids methionine and cystine. However, the importance of this problem has been exaggerated somewhat, because tests of protein quality are usually conducted with rats, which have a higher requirement for these amino acids than people. The feeding of a little extra protein from legumes usually insures that adequate amounts of the deficient amino acids are provided.

3. Mixtures of legumes and cereals have a protein quality which comes close to that of meat, milk, and other animal proteins. The highest protein quality is usually achieved in mixtures comprised of 50% legume protein and 50% cereal protein because the amino acid patterns of the two types of foods complement each other. Some examples of food combinations utilizing this principle are corn tortillas and refried beans, baked beans and brown bread, peanut butter sandwiches, and macaroni products fortified with soy protein.

4. Cooked legumes contain from 2 to 4 times the protein of most cooked cereals. For example, a cup of cooked dried legumes (approximately 200 g) supplies from 10 to 20 g of protein, whereas a cup of cooked cereal (150 g - 250 g) provides from 3 to 7 g of protein. Also, more calories (about 50% more) are supplied by the legumes.

5. Legumes may be used to upgrade the protein quantity and quality of diets based mainly on cereals and/or starchy foods such as bananas, cassava, and sweet potatoes. The latter foods are the mainstays of people in the developing tropical regions. For example, a protein-enriched flour or meal may contain about 15% defatted peanut or soybean flour or meal, and about 85% of cereal product made from corn, rice, or wheat. Highly starchy diets may be upgraded considerably by mixing 20% defatted legume flour with 80% starchy food. For example, one of the first attempts to rehabilitate African children suffering from protein-calorie malnutrition utilized a mixture of soybean flour and bananas.

6. Animal protein foods may be extended by the use of legumes. Some approximate "equations" of protein value follow:

(a) 1 frankfurter + ½ cup cooked beans = 2 frankfurters

(b) 10% legume flour + 5% skim milk powder + 85% cereal flour = 10% skim milk powder + 90% cereal flour

Both examples show that the requirement for expensive animal protein may be halved by the judicious use of legume products. However, it should be noted that the substitution of legumes for animal foods may raise the caloric value of the diet.

CURRENT TRENDS AND FUTURE PROSPECTS FOR LEGUME PRODUCTS.

Although legumes have long been regarded in the western countries of the world as food for poor people, this is not the case in such countries as China and India, where these crops are highly regarded. Actually, legume consumption generally increases with income in India. Perhaps, this occurs because the more affluent people can afford to buy the more highly processed forms of legumes. Recently, it was learned that certain Asiatic methods of processing soybeans enhanced their nutritive value and palatability. Also, the ever increasing demand for peanut and soybean oils has spurred the search for more profitable uses of the residue (press cake) from oil extraction. To date, most of the press cake has been used in livestock feeds. But new legume-based processed foods are being developed for the peoples in both the developed and the developing countries. Some of the recent achievements in this field are noteworthy.

• **Alfalfa leaf protein concentrate**—This product is made by (1) spraying fresh-harvested alfalfa with an antioxidant to preserve vitamins, then extracting the juice by pressing, (2) coagulating the protein in the juice by heating with steam, (3) separating the protein curd from the residual liquid, and (4) drying the curd. The unrefined product is green and has a grassy taste. However, the process has been modified so that two high-protein fractions are produced; one which has the grassy characteristics and is suitable for livestock feeds, and the other which is a whitish, bland-tasting product that may be incorporated into human foods. It is expected that these products may soon be utilized to a greater extent since alfalfa yields more protein per acre than any of the other commonly cultivated green plants.

• **Fermented foods**—These items have long been produced throughout Asia, the Middle East, and Africa. Apparently, fermentation destroys or inactivates most of the antinutritional or toxic factors in legumes. Also, only small amounts of fuel are required for the production of these products. Hence, fermented foods may become increasingly important in the diets of people in the developing countries where even firewood is scarce.

Most Americans are familiar with soy sauce which is used in Oriental cuisine, but few realize that it may be produced by fermentation. There has been so much recent interest among American vegetarians and health food enthusiasts in the soybean products tempeh (mold ripened soybean cake which is fried in deep fat), and tofu (a cheeselike item made from coagulated soybean milk), that they are now being produced in the United States and are sold in some supermarkets.

• **Flours**—Soybean flour has long been used in the United States to make soybean milk (for infants who are allergic to cow's milk) and low gluten baked goods. Similar legume flours have been made from locally grown beans and peas in many countries of the world. At the present time many of these products are being promoted as protein supplements to grain mixtures, in which they augment both the quantity and quality of protein. New types of food additives now make it possible to use considerable amounts of legume flours in yeast-leavened breads without having undesirable effects on the taste and texture of the baked products.

• **Flour fractions (high-protein and high-starch)**—Air classification, which was originally developed for the processing of wheat flour, is now being used experimentally to separate various legume flours into (1) high-protein fractions containing from 29 to 67% protein, 2 to 11% fat, 2 to 3% fiber, and up to 30% starch; and (2) high-starch fractions containing from 12 to 16% protein, 1 to 6% fat, 3 to 11% fiber, and 52 to 68% starch. The high-protein fractions show promise as whipped toppings or foams, whereas the high-starch fractions appear to be useful in baked goods and other items which are presently based mainly upon cereal flours. Also, it is noteworthy that the nutrient compositions of the high starch fractions are similar to those of cereal flours, except that the amino acid patterns of the former products complement those of the latter products.

• **Gums**—Food additive gums are much used by the food industry as emulsifying agents, thickeners, and stabilizers. Four very important food gums which are derived from legumes are carob (locust bean) gum, guar gum, gum arabic, and gum tragacanth. The first two gums are extracted from seeds, whereas the last two are derived from the fluid which exudes from the stems and branches of the plants.

• **Imitation dairy, meat, poultry, and seafood products (analogs)**
—In the latter part of the 19th century, J. H. Kellogg and other Seventh-day Adventists made imitation meat products from wheat gluten for use by vegetarians. However, these products have had only limited success, and are now being replaced to a large extent by the recently developed textured vegetable protein (TVP) products, which are more meatlike in taste and texture. Most of the TVP items are made from soy protein that has been extracted from soy flour and spun into fibrous strands. Some of the more popular items are made from mixtures of soy protein, wheat protein, egg albumin, and various additives.

• **Instant pea soup mixes**—These products are made by (1) cooking dried split peas with various other ingredients, (2) drying and flaking the cooked mixture, (3) mixing the flakes with flavorings and thickening agents, (4) steaming the flaked mixture to cause the ingredients to clump together, and (5) drying the clumps. Instant soup mixes are ready to eat within about a minute after mixing with boiling water.

• **Peanut flakes**—In 1972, a process was patented for making peanut flakes by (1) removing the skins and hearts from fresh peanuts, (2) drying to a low moisture content, (3) grinding to a fine meal, (4) cooking the meal in water, and (5) drying and flaking the cooked meal. The three different types of product are (1) full fat, which contain 51% fat and 29% protein; (2) partially defatted, with 30% fat and 41% protein; and (3) defatted, which contain 1% fat, and 60% protein. Peanut flakes, unlike other legume products, are essentially free of gas-forming carbohydrates. They have been tested experimentally as extenders for cheeses, meats, poultry, and seafood, in which their bland taste makes them virtually undetectable. Also, peanut flakes plus almond flavoring may be used to replace the more expensive almonds in items such as candy bars and marzipan.

• **Precooked beans**—Many busy homemakers are reluctant to prepare beans because of the long cooking time. These products, which have usually been soaked in a tenderizing solution and steamed or pressure cooked, require only about 35 minutes of cooking time in an open pot, or only 5-10 minutes in a pressure cooker.

• **Quick-cooking dried peas**—This convenience food is prepared by soaking the peas in an enzyme solution, followed by steaming and drying. Normally, dried split peas require at least 25 minutes cooking time, but quick-cooking dried peas require only about half as much time.

• **Seedcoat flours**—The recent interest in high fiber foods has spurred attempts to utilize the highly fibrous seedcoats of legumes in baked products. However, items containing substantial amounts of seedcoat flours are usually too heavy and moist. Also, they have beany odors and flavors. These problems have largely been overcome by treating the seedcoats with acid before grinding them into flour.

• **Seed protein concentrates**—These products may contain from 40 to 80% protein, and only small amounts of carbohydrates and fats. They are produced by (1) soaking and dehulling dried beans, (2) drying the dehulled beans and grinding them to a fine powder, (3) suspending the powder in a salt solution and coagulating the protein with steam, (4) separating the protein cake from the starchy liquor by centrifugation, and (5) drying and grinding the protein cake into a meal or a flour. Legume protein concentrates may be used as a means of protein fortification for infant formulas, soft drinks, puddings, cereal flours and meals, macaroni and noodle products, baked goods, and other high-carbohydrate foods.

• **Snack foods**—Crispy bean chips, flakes, or wafers are made from soaked, dehulled beans by (1) blending them with a thickening agent, salt, and vegetable oil, (2) pressure cooking the bean dough, and (3) frying slices of the cooked bean dough in deep fat. Another type of legume snack food is bean dip made from pureed cooked beans mixed with various spices and other ingredients.

• **Soybean infant formulas**—In the early 1900s, these products were made from full fat soybean flour. However, they caused considerable gas and other distress in infants because of the gas-forming carbohydrates which were present. Now, soy products which have had the flatulence-producing substances removed are used. For example, many of the newer products contain soy protein concentrate.

• **Sprouts**—Many supermarkets now carry these items in the fresh produce section. The most popular types of sprouts are made from alfalfa seeds, mung beans, and soybeans. Also, some bean sprouts are canned by the manufacturers of Chinese foods.

LEGUMES OF THE WORLD. About a dozen species account for the greater part of the world's legume production. Additionally, many luguminous food plants with only minor roles in commercial food production at the present time have the potential to become important food crops. Also, most of these lesser known species thrive in subtropical and tropical areas where most of the world's impoverished people live. Table L-2 gives pertinent information relative to the legumes of the world.

TABLE L–2
LEGUMES OF THE WORLD

Popular Name(s); Scientific Name; Origin and History	Importance; Principal Areas of Production; Growing Conditions	Processing; Preparation; Uses	Nutritional Value; Caution[1,2]
Adzuki Bean *Phaseolus angularis* **Origin and History:** It is believed to have originated in Japan and China, where it has been cultivated for centuries. (Also see ADZUKI BEAN.)	**Importance:** Used mainly in eastern Asia. **Principal Areas:** Japan, Korea, China, and Manchuria. **Growing Conditions:** Temperate climate	**Processing:** Usually, the beans are picked when mature. They may be left whole or pounded into a meal. **Preparation:** Whole beans boiled, then mashed. **Uses:** Vegetable dish. Bean flour is used for cakes and various desserts and sweets.	**Nutritional Value:** 100 g of uncooked dried beans supply 324 kcal, 21.1 g protein, 1.0 g fat, 59.5 g carbohydrate, 3.9 g fiber, 82 mg calcium, and 6.4 mg iron. **Caution:** Soaking, followed by cooking, renders potentially harmful agents safe.
Alfalfa (Lucerne) *Medicago sativa* **Origin and History:** Alfalfa was seeded for livestock forage in southwestern Asia long before recorded history. The Persians took it to Greece when they invaded the country in 490 B.C. From Greece it was taken to Italy in the first century A.D., from whence it spread to other parts of Europe. (Also see ALFALFA.)	**Importance:** The most valuable hay plant of the U.S., with an estimated annual production of 70–80 million metric tons. **Principal Areas:** U.S., Argentina, Europe, and Asia. **Growing Conditions:** Temperate climate.	**Processing:** Mature seeds are sprouted. A flour may be made from the dried leaves, and a protein concentrate from the juice of the fresh leaves. **Preparation:** Sprouts may be cooked or left raw. **Uses:** Sprouts, in salads, soups, and sandwiches. Flour may be added in small amounts to various cereal products. Protein concentrate is used mainly in livestock feeds.	**Nutritional Value:** 100 g of sprouted seeds contain 41 kcal, 5.1 g protein, 0.6 g fat, 9.5 g carbohydrate, 1.7 g fiber, 28 mg calcium, and 1.4 mg iron. **Caution:** Usually, only the sprouts are eaten by people. Sprouting counteracts the potentially harmful agents.
Bambarra Groundnut *Voandzeia subterranea* **Origin and History:** Native to tropical Africa. Taken to other parts of Africa, Brazil, and the Orient in the 17th century.	**Importance:** Its use in certain regions of Africa has been replaced to a large extent by the peanut. **Principal Areas:** District of Bambarra in Mali, Zambia, and Madagascar. (All are in Africa.) **Growing Conditions:** Tropical climate.	**Processing:** This plant, like peanuts, must be unearthed for harvesting of the seeds. The hard seeds require soaking and/or breaking up into pieces prior to cooking. **Preparation:** Dry seeds are roasted. Seeds in pods are boiled. **Uses:** Vegetable dish, source of calories and protein.	**Nutritional Value:** 100 g of uncooked dried seeds contain 370 kcal, 16.0 g protein, 6.0 g fat, 65.0 g carbohydrates, 4.8 g fiber, 62 mg calcium, and 12.2 mg iron. **Caution:** Few, if any, studies have been made, since the use of this legume has dropped sharply. Soaking and cooking should be sufficient to make seeds both palatable and wholesome.

Footnotes at end of table

(Continued)

TABLE L–2 *(Continued)*

Popular Name(s); Scientific Name; Origin and History	Importance; Principal Areas of Production; Growing Conditions	Processing; Preparation; Uses	Nutritional Value; Caution[1,2]
Beans: (Adzuki Bean; Broad Bean; Chickpea; Bean, Common; Cowpea; Hyacinth Bean; Jack Bean; Lima Bean; Mung Bean; Scarlet Runner Bean; Soybean, Tepary Bean; Yard-long Bean. For the scientific name refer to the names of the individual beans listed in this table.) **Origin and History:** Various times and places in world history. More details are given under the specific bean names. (Also see BEAN[S].)	**Importance:** Some type of bean is important in most every country or area of the world. These areas or countries are listed under the specific bean names in this table. **Principal Areas:** Largest producers of beans include China, India, Brazil, Mexico, and the U.S. **Growing Conditions:** Temperate climate, modest moisture, various soil types.	**Processing:** Depending on the bean, they may be picked as pods, immature seeds, or mature seeds. Beans can be sold fresh, cooked, canned, frozen, dried, in the form of a flour, or further processed like soybeans. **Preparation:** Depending on personal tastes and their processed form, beans may be boiled, baked, fried, roasted, or sprouted. **Uses:** Beans are consumed primarily as a vegetable in a variety of dishes. Some dishes include soups, bean salads, meat and beans, or beans with cereals. Specific uses are indicated under the individual beans listed in this table.	**Nutritional Value:** The value of beans varies with the type of bean and their processed form—dry, mature, immature, or pods. In general they are a good source of protein, calories, and some minerals and vitamins. **Caution:** Some uncooked mature beans may contain harmful components, but most are harmless following proper preparation and cooking. Details of possible harmful components are listed under the names of specific beans.
Bean: (Common; French Bean; Kidney Bean; Navy Bean; Pea Bean; Pinto Bean; Snap Bean; Stringless Bean; Green Bean) *Phaseolus vulgaris* **Origin and History:** Originated in Mexico and in Peru, where it was grown about 7,000 years ago. It was domesticated independently in each area from a common wild ancestor. Its cultivation was spread northward and southward by American Indians, and it was taken to Europe by Spanish explorers. (Also see BEAN, COMMON.)	**Importance:** The leading nonoilseed legume crop. An estimated 16.3 million metric tons are produced annually, plus about 3.1 million metric tons of green beans. In the U.S. and Canada, the common bean is the most important kind of bean, exclusive of the soybean. **Principal Areas:** The leading producers are India, China, Brazil, and various other countries of Asia, South America, Central America, Africa, and Europe. **Growing Conditions:** Suited to temperate climates where the temperature ranges from 50°F *(10°C)* to 86°F *(30°C)*. Generally, it is grown during the warm season in the cooler parts of the Temperate Zones, and during the cool season in the subtropics and tropics (grown at high altitudes).	**Processing:** May be picked when immature for both pods and seeds (string beans). Both string beans and mature beans (usually dried) are sold fresh, canned, or frozen. **Preparation:** Boil, bake with pork and molasses, or fry (in Mexico). Fresh green beans may be cooked briefly and served with butter and seasonings. **Uses:** Vegetable dish, and in casseroles, soups, and stews.	**Nutritional Value:** There is considerable variation in the composition of the many varieties of the common bean. 3½ oz *(100 g)* of cooked mature beans supply about 118 kcal and about 7.8 g of protein (about as much as 1 oz of lean meat). Green beans are high in water content (90.1%), low in calories (32 kcal/ 100 g), and fair sources of vitamins A and C. **Caution:**[3] Antivitamin E factor (the diet should contain ample vitamin E and selenium). Other potentially harmful substances are rendered safe by (1) soaking and cooking (and discarding the water after each step); (2) acid treatment, followed by incubation; or (3) fermentation and sprouting.

Footnotes at end of table

(Continued)

TABLE L–2 *(Continued)*

Popular Name(s); Scientific Name; Origin and History	Importance; Principal Areas of Production; Growing Conditions	Processing; Preparation; Uses	Nutritional Value; Caution[1,2]
Broad Bean (Fava Bean) *Vicia faba* **Origin and History:** Believed to have originated in northern Africa and in the eastern Mediterranean region. Has been cultivated in various parts of southern and northern Europe (particularly the British Isles) since the Iron Age (1000 B.C.). (Also see BROAD BEAN.)	**Importance:** One of the leading nonoilseed legumes grown in the temperate areas of the world. An estimated 4.3 million metric tons are produced annually. **Principal Areas:** China (over 70% of the world's production), Egypt, Italy, U.K., Morocco, Spain, Denmark, and Brazil. However, it has recently become an important crop in the highlands of Central America. **Growing Conditions:** Thrives under temperatures ranging from 50°F (*10°C*) to 86°F (*30°C*), but is also planted in the British Isles in autumn or early winter, for harvesting in June or in the late summer.	**Processing:** Picked when almost fully mature, shelled, then dried, canned, or quick frozen. **Preparation:** May be boiled, cooked in casseroles, or steamed. Immature pods may be cooked whole or sliced. **Uses:** Vegetable dish, and in casseroles, soups, and stews.	**Nutritional Value:** Mature, uncooked, dried beans are rich in calories (328 kcal per 100 g), proteins (25%) and carbohydrates (56.9%), but low in fat (1.2%). Immature beans and cooked dried beans have a high water content and much lower levels of these nutrients. However, the immature beans are a fair source of vitamin C. **Caution:**[3] Contains a hemolytic anemia factor which triggers favism, but which affects *only* people who have an inherited susceptibility. Other potentially harmful constituents are rendered safe by soaking and cooking, sprouting, or fermentation.
Carob (Locust Bean, St. John's Bread) *Ceratonia siliqua* **Origin and History:** Originated in the eastern Mediterranean region and introduced into tropical areas around the world. (Also see CAROB.)	**Importance:** Appears to be increasing in importance because the seeds yield a valuable gum, and the pods provide a substitute for expensive cocoa. **Principal Areas:** Subtropics and tropics. **Growing Conditions:** Thrives in a hot, dry climate.	**Processing:** First, the pods with seeds are dried in the sun. Then, the pods are ground to a powder. Seeds are crushed, roasted, and boiled in water to extract the gum. **Preparation:** The pod powder may be mixed in hot or cold water or milk to make a drink. **Uses:** Powdered pods are a substitute for cocoa. The seed gum is a food additive.	**Nutritional Value:** 100 g of the dried pod powder supply 380 kcal, 3.8 g protein, 2.0 g fat, 90.6 g carbohydrate, 5.4 g fiber, and 290 mg of calcium per 100 g. **Caution:** The pods are not known to contain any harmful substances, and the seed gum is generally safe in the amounts used. Seeds are rarely prepared and eaten like other legumes.

Footnotes at end of table

(Continued)

TABLE L-2 *(Continued)*

Popular Name(s); Scientific Name; Origin and History	Importance; Principal Areas of Production; Growing Conditions	Processing; Preparation; Uses	Nutritional Value; Caution[1,2]
Chickpea (Garbanzo Bean) *Cicer arietinum* **Origin and History:** Most likely originated in the Near East. From there its cultivation spread eastward to India, and westward throughout the countries of north Africa and southern Europe. (Also see CHICKPEA.)	**Importance:** A leading non-oilseed legume in India and the Middle East. An estimated 6.9 million metric tons are produced annually. **Principal Areas:** Over 87% of the crop is produced in India and Pakistan. Most of the remainder is grown in Mexico, Turkey, and Ethiopia. **Growing Conditions:** Grows best in areas where the temperature ranges from 36°F (2°C) to 86°F (30°C). Hence, it may be grown during the warm season in northern India, and during the cool season in the dry tropics.	**Processing:** Dehulling, then drying. In India, the dried seeds are sometimes ground into a flour. **Preparation:** Boil, fry, or roast. **Uses:** Snack, vegetable dish, and in soups, salads, and stews. In India, the flour is used to make various confections.	**Nutritional Value:** Similar to the various beans in nutritional value. Hence, chickpeas are a good source of calories and protein; 100 g, or about ½ cup of cooked beans supplies about 179 kcal, and 10.2 g of protein. Also, they are a good source of phosphorus and iron. **Caution:** Soaking, followed by cooking (and discarding the water after each step) will alleviate most of the undesirable effects and render them wholesome.
Cowpea (Black-eyed Pea) *Vigna sinensis; V. unguiculata* **Origin and History:** Originated in central Africa. Brought to the West Indies and to the southeastern U.S. by African slaves. Its cultivation also spread northward to the Mediterranean and eastward to China and India. (Also see COWPEA.)	**Importance:** A valuable crop in the subtropical and tropical areas of the world. **Principal Areas:** Africa, India, China, West Indies, and southeastern U.S. **Growing Conditions:** 68°F (20°C) to 95°F (35°C). Hence, the growing season is not long enough in northern U.S. to produce mature beans. However, the immature green pods are very tasty and are much appreciated by the Chinese.	**Processing:** May be picked early for immature pods. Mature beans are dried, canned, and frozen. In Africa, the dried seed may be ground before cooking. **Preparation:** Mature dried beans may be boiled or baked. Immature pods and seeds may be chopped and stir-fried with meats and other foods. **Uses:** Vegetable dish, with or without cooked pork; an ingredient of casseroles, salads, soups, and stews.	**Nutritional Value:** 3½ oz (100 g, or about ⅔ cup) of the cooked mature beans supply 76 kcal and 5.1 g of protein. Compared with cooked, mature beans, the cooked immature seeds contain more calories (108 kcal per 100 g), protein (8.1%), iron (50% more), and vitamins A and C.
Fenugreek *Trigonella foenum-graecum* **Origin and History:** Originated in the Mediterranean region.	**Importance:** Widely used spice. **Principal Areas:** Southern Europe, north Africa, Egypt, and India. **Growing Conditions:** Subtropical climate.	**Processing:** Dried seeds are often ground into a powder. **Preparation:** Pods may be cooked. **Uses:** Pods as a vegetable. Powdered seeds as a condiment.	**Nutritional Value:** 100 g of uncooked dried seeds contain 323 kcal, 23 g protein, 8.1 g fat, 58.4 g carbohydrate, 10.1 mg fiber, 176 mg calcium, and 33.53 mg iron. **Caution:** None.

Footnotes at end of table

TABLE L-2 (Continued)

Popular Name(s); Scientific Name; Origin and History	Importance; Principal Areas of Production; Growing Conditions	Processing; Preparation; Uses	Nutritional Value; Caution[1,2]
Field Pea *Pisum arvense* **Origin and History:** Thought to have originated in central Asia and Europe, with possibly secondary developments in the Near East and north Africa. (Also see PEA, FIELD.)	**Importance:** Less important for human food than garden peas (*Pisum sativum*). Used mainly for green manure and feeding livestock, except in Africa, where it has long been used as a human food. **Principal Areas:** Africa, Asia, and central and northern Europe. **Growing Conditions:** Grows best at temperatures between 50°F (*10°C*) and 86°F (*30°C*). However, they may also be grown in some parts of Africa and Europe as a cold season crop. Field peas are more hardy than garden peas.	**Processing:** Shelling, followed by drying. Entire plant may be plowed under as green manure, or used as a forage. **Preparation:** Boil or bake, with or without meat. Field peas do not become soft like garden peas. **Uses:** Vegetable dish, livestock feed.	**Nutritional Value:** The nutrient content of field peas is given in Food Composition Table F-36. A 3½ oz (*100 g*) serving (about ½ cup) of cooked field peas provides about 117 calories (kcal) and 7.2 g of protein. This is about double the caloric value and approximately equal to the protein value of 1 oz of cooked lean meat. Field peas contain less than half as much calcium as phosphorus. Peas are a good source of iron and potassium. **Caution:** Antivitamin E factor (the diet should contain ample vitamin E and selenium). Metal-binding factor(s). Pressure cooking[4] is more certain to eliminate this problem than boiling at normal pressure.
Garden Pea *Pisum sativum* **Origin and History:** Thought to have originated in central Asia and Europe, with possibly secondary developments in the Near East and north Africa. It appears that the Chinese were the first to eat the immature seeds. Later, Louis XIV popularized this custom in Europe. (Also see PEA, GARDEN.)	**Importance:** Accounts for the crop of all types of peas, for which there is an estimated annual production of 4.8 million metric tons. **Principal Areas:** The U.S. produces 25% of the world production. **Growing Conditions:** Requires temperatures between 50°F (*10°C*) and 86°F (*30°C*). Hence, it is produced mainly in the temperate zones and at the higher elevations in the subtropics and tropics.	**Processing:** Usually picked when immature. In the U.S. they are harvested mechanically by viners. Then, they may be sold fresh, frozen, cooked, or canned. (Same for immature pods.) Mature seeds are usually dried whole or after splitting. **Preparation:** Dried mature seeds or split peas are sometimes ground into flour. But most of them are prepared by boiling. Immature (green) peas, fresh or frozen, are boiled briefly. **Uses:** Vegetable dish, in casseroles, soups, and stews.	**Nutritional Value:** Cooked mature peas are similar in nutritive value to the various types of mature beans (78% water, 84 kcal/ 100 g, and 6.3% protein). In comparison with mature peas, cooked immature (green) peas contain more water (81.5%), fewer calories (71 kcal/100 g); and less protein (5.4%). However, they are better sources of vitamins A and C. **Caution:**[3] Same as those for field pea.
Guar (Cluster Bean) *Cyanopsis tetragonoloba* **Origin and History:** Originated in India. (Also see GUMS.)	**Importance:** Source of a valuable gum. **Principal Areas:** Southeast Asia, India, Indonesia, Burma, and the U.S. **Growing Conditions:** Subtropical climate.	**Processing:** In Asia, immature pods and seeds are picked. In the U.S., the mature seeds are harvested and the gum is extracted. **Preparation:** In Asia, pods are cooked for eating. **Uses:** As a food and livestock feed in Asia. As a source of a food additive in the U.S.	**Nutritional Value:** Data not available. Most likely the composition of the immature pods and seeds is similar to that of other legumes. **Caution:**[3] The mature seeds are used almost exclusively for extraction of the gum, which is a safe food additive. However, the residue from extraction requires detoxification.

Footnotes at end of table

(Continued)

TABLE L–2 *(Continued)*

Popular Name(s); Scientific Name; Origin and History	Importance; Principal Areas of Production; Growing Conditions	Processing; Preparation; Uses	Nutritional Value; Caution[1,2]
Hyacinth Bean (Lablab Bean) *Dolichos lablab* **Origin and History:** Originated in India. Cultivated for many centuries as a food plant, and lately as an ornamental plant. (Also see HYACINTH BEAN.)	**Importance:** Its drought resistance makes it valuable in the developing countries, but it is little known in the developed countries. **Principal Areas:** Southern and eastern Asia and parts of Africa. It is an important crop of India. **Growing Conditions:** Dry, tropical climate.	**Processing:** Picked when immature or mature for human consumption. In India, the mature beans are dried and sometimes split. **Preparation:** The whole beans or the split beans are cooked. The immature pods and seeds may be prepared as a green vegetable. **Uses:** The mature beans are used primarily as cooked whole beans or cooked split seeds. The immature pods and seeds may be used like snap beans.	**Nutritional Value:** 100 g of uncooked, dried whole mature seeds supply 334 kcal, 21.5 g protein, 1.2 g fat, 61.4 g carbohydrate, 6.8 g fiber, 98 mg calcium, and 3.9 mg iron. **Caution:**[3] Much of the gassiness of the beans may be alleviated by (1) soaking and cooking (and discarding the water after each step); (2) acid treatment followed by incubation; or (3) fermentation and sprouting.
Jack Bean (Horse Bean) *Canavalia ensiformis* **Origin and History:** Native to Mexico, Central America, and the West Indies. (Also see JACK BEAN.)	**Importance:** A minor crop grown mainly for green manure or forage. However, the dried seeds and the immature pods and seeds are eaten at times of food scarcity. **Principal Areas:** Tropical regions around the world, including the southern U.S. **Growing Conditions:** Dry, tropical climate.	**Processing:** Immature pods or mature beans may be harvested. **Preparation:** Seeds require prolonged soaking and boiling with several changes of water to soften. Immature pods are cooked in water. **Uses:** Human food, cattle fodder, green manure. During times of food scarcity, both the immature pods and seeds and the mature seeds are used for human food.	**Nutritional Value:** 100 g of uncooked dried beans contain 348 kcal, 21.0 g protein, 3.2 g fat, 61.0 g carbohydrate, 7.6 g fiber, 134 mg calcium, and 8.6 mg iron. The immature beans are similar in nutrient composition to snap beans, but they are poorer sources of vitamins A and C. **Caution:** They may contain more antinutritional factors than occur in most legumes. Hence, prolonged soaking and thorough cooking[4] are required.
Lathyrus Pea (Grass Pea) *Lathyrus sativus* **Origin and History:** Native to India and the Middle East. Excessive consumption of seeds, which occurs in time of famine, can cause a paralyzing disease known as lathyrism. (Also see LATHYRISM.)	**Importance:** An emergency food used by the impoverished and during famines because it grows well on poor soils and is drought resistant. **Principal Areas:** India, southern Europe, and South America. **Growing Conditions:** Semi-tropical climate.	**Processing:** Dehusked seeds may be soaked in water, dried in the sun, then ground into a flour. Sometimes the seeds are steamed and/or roasted to remove a highly toxic constituent which causes the disease lathyrism. **Preparation:** Whole seeds cooked as other legumes. Flour made into thin, unleavened cakes (chapatis) and baked. **Uses:** Human food, livestock feed, green manure.	**Nutritional Value:** 100 g of uncooked, dried whole seeds supply 348 kcal, 27.4 g protein, 1.1 g fat, 59.8 g carbohydrate, 7.3 g fiber, 127 mg calcium, and 10.0 mg iron. **Caution:** Lathyrogens, in addition to factors found in other legumes. Toxicity is counteracted by overnight soaking and thorough cooking.[4] It is *not* sufficient to bake uncooked flour products.

Footnotes at end of table

(Continued)

TABLE L–2 (Continued)

Popular Name(s); Scientific Name; Origin and History	Importance; Principal Areas of Production; Growing Conditions	Processing; Preparation; Uses	Nutritional Value; Caution[1,2]
Lentil *Lens esculenta* **Origin and History:** One of the oldest cultivated legumes. It came from the Middle East. Long used as a Lenten food in Catholic countries. Recently, production has declined in favor of higher-yielding crops. (Also see LENTILS.)	**Importance:** Not as important as other leguminous crops because it has lower yields. An estimated 1.3 million metric tons are produced annually. **Principal Areas:** India, Syria, Turkey, Ethiopia, U.S.S.R., Spain, Iran, Bangladesh. **Growing Conditions:** Tolerates temperatures between 36°F (2°C) and 86°F (30°C), which makes it useful as a cool season crop in the subtropics and tropics.	**Processing:** Seeds are picked only when completely mature. They may be left whole or dehulled, then they are usually dried. Sometimes they are ground into a flour. **Preparation:** Boil or stew. **Uses:** Vegetable dish, soups, stews. Flours may be mixed with cereal flours to make foods for infants and children in the developing countries.	**Nutritional Value:** Has a nutritive value that is about the same as the other cooked immature legumes (106 kcal per 100 g and 7.8% protein). Also, a good source of iron; but low in calcium. **Caution:** Soaking followed by cooking (and discarding the water after each step) will alleviate most of the undesirable effects and render them wholesome.
Lima Bean (Butter Bean) *Phaseolus lunatus* **Origin and History:** First cultivated in Peru 7 to 8 thousand years ago. Spread throughout the Americas and the West Indies by the Indians. Brought to Europe by Spanish explorers. (Also see LIMA BEAN.)	**Importance:** Among the top two dozen vegetable crops in the U.S. **Principal Areas:** Temperate, subtropical, and tropical areas around the world. **Growing Conditions:** Large-seeded types require at least 4 months without frost and a considerable amount of warm weather. Other types tolerate a wider range of temperature.	**Processing:** May be picked while still immature, or when fully mature. They may be sold fresh, cooked and canned, frozen, dried, or in the form of a flour. **Preparation:** Boil or bake. **Uses:** Vegetable dish, casseroles, soups, stews.	**Nutritional Value:** 3½ oz (100 g) of cooked mature beans supply 133 kcal and about 8.2 g of protein. Lima beans are also a good source of phosphorus and iron. Immature (baby or green) limas contain more water than the mature beans. Hence, they supply only about 75% as much energy (calories) and protein as mature limas. **Caution:**[3] Cyanide-releasing glucosides (varieties grown in U.S. contain negligible amounts). Overnight soaking followed by cooking ensures that these and other potentially harmful substances are rendered safe.
Lupines *Lupinus genus* **Origin and History:** There are about 100 kinds of lupines. Some of these originated in the Mediterranean area, whereas others came from North America or South America.	**Importance:** Mainly as an emergency food because the species grows in poor soils. **Principal Areas:** Southern Europe, northern Africa, and North and South America. **Growing Conditions:** Temperate to subtropical climate, depending upon species.	**Processing:** Seeds may be treated as most other legumes, or they may be roasted and ground to make a coffee substitute. **Preparation:** Seeds are soaked in water, then boiled. **Uses:** Vegetable dish, coffee substitute, livestock feed, green manure.	**Nutritional Value:** 100 g of uncooked dried seeds furnish 407 kcal, 44.3 g protein, 16.5 g fat, 28.2 g carbohydrate, 7.1 g fiber, 90 mg calcium, and 6.3 mg iron. **Caution:** Some varieties contain a toxic alkaloid which is removed by soaking in water. It might also be a good idea to rinse the beans after thorough cooking,[4] and to discard the cooking water.

Footnotes at end of table

(Continued)

TABLE L–2 *(Continued)*

Popular Name(s); Scientific Name; Origin and History	Importance; Principal Areas of Production; Growing Conditions	Processing; Preparation; Uses	Nutritional Value; Caution[1,2]
Mesquite *Prosopis* genus **Origin and History:** Most species probably originated in the tropical areas of the Americas, where they were long used by the Indians.	**Importance:** These wild plants are usually grazed by livestock, but occasionally serve as human food. Some species grow on poor soils and withstand severe droughts. **Principal Areas:** South, Central, and North America; Africa; and other subtropical areas. **Growing Conditions:** Subtropical to tropical climate.	**Processing:** Depending upon the species, either the pods and/or the seeds may be used. Sometimes, the dried seeds may be ground into a flour. **Preparation:** Pods and/or seeds may be boiled or steamed. **Uses:** Human food, livestock feed.	**Nutritional Value:** 100 g of uncooked dried seeds contain 347 kcal, 15.4 g protein, 1.6 g fat, 75.5 g carbohydrate, 7.3 g fiber, and 421 mg of calcium. **Caution:** The pods and pod pulp contain large amounts of indigestible carbohydrates (fiber) which may interfere with the utilization of various nutrients. However, soaking and thoroughly cooking[4] the mature seeds should render them wholesome.
Mung Bean (Golden Gram; Green Gram) *Phaseolus aureus* **Origin and History:** Probably originated in India. (Also see MUNG BEAN.)	**Importance:** Important food in India and Pakistan. Used mainly for sprouting in China and U.S. **Principal Areas:** India and Pakistan. **Growing Conditions:** Does well in temperatures between 68°F (*20°C*) and 113°F (*45°C*).	**Processing:** Picked when fully mature. **Preparation:** Boil, or sprout, for eating raw or cooked. **Uses:** Cooked beans as a vegetable dish. Sprouts in salads, soups, sandwiches, etc. In Chinese cooking, the sprouts may be stir-fried with green onions and seasoned with soy sauce.	**Nutritional Value:** 3½ oz (*100 g*) of the raw, sprouted beans supply 28 kcal, 4.3 g of protein, and 16 mg of vitamin C. **Caution:** Soaking followed by cooking (and discarding the water after each step) will alleviate most of the undesirable effects and render wholesome.
Peanut (Groundnut) *Archis hypogaea* **Origin and History:** Native to South America, the plant was introduced to Africa by European explorers and reached North America with the slave trade. Early in the 20th century, G. W. Carver in the U.S. developed hundreds of new uses for the peanut. (Also see PEANUTS.)	**Importance:** The second leading legume crop in the world (the first is soybeans) with an estimated annual production of 17.7 million metric tons. **Principal Areas:** India, China, U.S., the Sudan, Senegal, Indonesia, Argentina, and Burma. **Growing Conditions:** Requires temperatures between 68°F (*20°C*) and 95°F (*35°C*).	**Processing:** The vines are harvested by machine in the U.S., and by hand elsewhere. Then, they are shelled and blanched. Much of the U.S. crop is ground into peanut butter. Oil may be expressed, and/or otherwise extracted, after which the press cake may be ground into defatted flour. **Preparation:** Boil or roast whole nuts with or without shell. **Uses:** Snack food, main dish (in Africa). Flour is added to cereal mixtures for infants and children.	**Nutritional Value:** Rich in calories (564 per 100 g), and protein (26%). Compared to other legumes, fat content (47.5%) is very much higher, and carbohydrate content (18.6%) is very much lower. **Caution:** Peanuts contain small amounts of goitrogens. (See GOITROGENS.)

Footnotes at end of table

(Continued)

TABLE L-2 (Continued)

Popular Name(s); Scientific Name; Origin and History	Importance; Principal Areas of Production; Growing Conditions	Processing; Preparation; Uses	Nutritional Value; Caution[1,2]
Pigeon Pea *Cajanus cajan* **Origin and History:** Probably native to Africa; now widely grown in tropical and subtropical countries particularly India, equatorial Africa, the East Indies, and the West Indies. African slaves took it to the Caribbean.	**Importance:** A valuable drought-resistant tropical food crop. However, the tightly adhering seed coat has an acrid taste, which reduces its acceptability in certain areas. **Principal Areas:** India, Africa, Burma, Dominican Republic, Malawi. **Growing Conditions:** Tropical climate that is moderately dry.	**Processing:** Either immature pods with seeds or mature seeds may be harvested. The latter are canned in the West Indies. In India, the seed coats are removed before preparation. **Preparation:** Cooked like other legumes. **Uses:** Human food, forage plant.	**Nutritional Value:** 100 g of uncooked dried beans furnish 342 kcal, 20.4 g protein, 1.4 g fat, 63.7 g carbohydrate, 7.0 mg fiber, 107 mg calcium, and 8.0 mg iron. **Caution:**[3] Much of the gassiness may be alleviated by (1) soaking and cooking (and discarding the water after each step); (2) acid treatment, followed by incubation; or (3) fermenting and sprouting.
Scarlet Runner Bean *Phaseolus coccineus* **Origin and History:** Originated in Central America or Mexico. (Also see SCARLET RUNNER BEAN.)	**Importance:** Popular in U.K., Asia, and Africa for its immature pods and seeds. Mature seeds used mainly in Central America. **Principal Areas:** Temperate climatic areas of Europe, Asia, Africa, and Central America (grown in the highlands). **Growing Conditions:** Needs a mild climate.	**Processing:** Immature pods and seeds are picked and cut into string beans. May be sold fresh, cooked and canned, or frozen. **Preparation:** Cook briefly in water and serve with butter or margarine. Toss with hot oil and chopped garlic (Italian style). Dried seeds are prepared like dried kidney beans. **Uses:** Vegetable dishes, casseroles, salads, soups, and stews.	**Nutritional Value:** The immature pods and beans contain over 90% water. Hence, the nutrient levels are much lower than those for mature beans. The immature pods and seeds are fair to good sources of vitamins A and C. The dried seeds are deficient in the amino acids cystine and methionine, and deficient in calcium. **Caution:** Mature beans—same as for chickpea (garbanzo bean).
Soybean *Glycine max* **Origin and History:** Originated in northeast China where it has been used for at least 3,000 years. It came to the U.S. by way of Europe in the early 19th century. However, most of the American advances in its production and utilization were made in the 20th century. (Also see SOYBEAN[S].)	**Importance:** The world's leading leguminous crop with an estimated annual production of nearly 100 million metric tons. **Principal Areas:** U.S., China, and Brazil. **Growing Conditions:** Thrives when temperature ranges from 50°F (*10°C*) to 95°F (*35°C*). Hence, it is usually grown between 20°N and 40°N latitudes, at high elevations in lower latitudes, or near to coasts warmed by the ocean in higher latitudes.	**Processing:** May be picked while still immature or after fully mature. Immature seeds sold fresh or cooked and canned. Oil may be expressed or otherwise extracted, after which the press cake may be ground into a defatted flour. Also, mature seeds may be roasted and salted like peanuts. Many other types of processing are utilized in Asia. **Preparation:** Cook immature seeds. Usually mature seeds have been processed. If not, they must be cooked in order to alter various toxic factors. **Uses:** Vegetable dish, main dish, protein supplement.	**Nutritional Value:** Rich in calories (335 per 100 g) and very rich in protein (38%). Compared to other legumes, fat content (18%) is much higher, and carbohydrate content (31.3%) is much lower. **Caution:** Antivitamins A, B-12, and D; goitrogens; metal binders; and other factors common to most legumes. Hence, these beans *always* require thorough processing by soaking and cooking (pressure cooking[4] would be most desirable). Sprouting or fermentation of the uncooked beans also makes them wholesome. (Also see Table L-1)

Footnotes at end of table

(Continued)

TABLE L–2 *(Continued)*

Popular Name(s); Scientific Name; Origin and History	Importance; Principal Areas of Production; Growing Conditions	Processing; Preparation; Uses	Nutritional Value; Caution[1,2]
Tamarind Tree *Tamarindus indica* **Origin and History:** Native to India. Brought to many other tropical areas of the world.	**Importance:** For a very long time, it was of limited local importance, but it may be increasing due to exporting of such products as tamarind juice. **Principal Areas:** India, Arabic countries, East Indies, and countries in the Caribbean. **Growing Conditions:** Tropical climate.	**Processing:** Pulp from ripened pods is made into juice, fruit paste and other products. Seeds may be roasted or boiled, dehulled and ground into a meal. **Preparation:** The pulp is usually mixed with other fruit products, because its strong flavor and acidity accentuate fruity tastes. **Uses:** Consumed fresh where produced, and exported in preserved forms (juices, pastes, etc.)	**Nutritional Value:** 100 g of dried pod pulp furnish 270 kcal, 5.0 g protein, 0.6 g fat, 70.7 g carbohydrate, 166 mg calcium, and 2.2 mg iron. **Caution:** The seeds should be soaked overnight and cooked thoroughly[4] like other mature legume seeds.
Tepary Bean *Phaseolus acutifolius* **Origin and History:** Probably originated in Central Mexico, where it was cultivated by the Mexican Indians 5,000 years ago. (Also see TEPARY BEAN.)	**Importance:** Not grown commercially, but still cultivated by various Indian tribes in U.S. and Mexico. It grows in areas of little rainfall. Less gas-forming than other beans. **Principal Areas:** Western Mexico and southwestern U.S. **Growing Conditions:** Hot, dry climate.	**Processing:** Shelling, drying. **Preparation:** Cook as other legumes. However, tepary beans absorb more water than other beans during soaking and require longer cooking time. **Uses:** Vegetable dish, in mixed meat and bean dishes.	**Nutritional Value:** 100 g of uncooked dried beans contain 353 kcal, 19.3 g protein, 1.2 g fat, 67.8 g carbohydrate, and 4.8 g fiber. **Caution:** Tepary beans contain less gas-forming carbohydrates than most other mature beans. Nevertheless, it is best to soak and cook and discard water at each step.
Yard-Long Bean; Asparagus Bean *Vigna unguiculata; V. sesquipedalis; Dolichos sesquipedalis* **Origin and History:** Thought to have originated somewhere in tropical Asia. (Also see YARD-LONG BEAN.)	**Importance:** Mainly used as a food where grown. Green pods are much liked in Asia and the Americas. **Principal Areas:** Tropical parts of Asia. **Growing Conditions:** Semi-tropical climate.	**Processing:** Much of the crop is sold as a fresh vegetable, but some is also canned or frozen. **Preparation:** Brief cooking in water. **Uses:** Vegetable dish; served in the same ways as snap beans.	**Nutritional Value:** The immature pods and seeds have a high water content (88.3%). Hence, a 100 g portion supplies only 37 kcal, 3.0 g protein, 0.2 g fat, 7.9 g carbohydrate, 44 mg calcium, and 0.7 mg iron. **Caution:**[3] The mature seeds should be treated the same as other mature beans.

[1]Refers to substances other than gas-generating carbohydrates, which are present in almost all types of mature legume seeds other than peanuts. The seeds are rendered less gassy by sprouting or fermentation.

[2]Additional details on specific antinutritional and/or toxic factors are given in the section of this article, "Caution," and Table L-1.

[3]Immature pods with seeds do not appear to contain the antinutritional factors found in the mature seeds of the same species. Hence, the green pods need only be cooked briefly.

[4]Time may be saved by pressure cooking. However, oil or melted fat should always be added to beans before cooking in a pressure cooker so that foaming is reduced. Foaming may result in the plugging of the safety valve and a building up of pressure which may cause the counterweight to be blown off.

LEGUMINOUS

The adjective for legume.

LEMON *Citrus limon*

Contents   *Page*

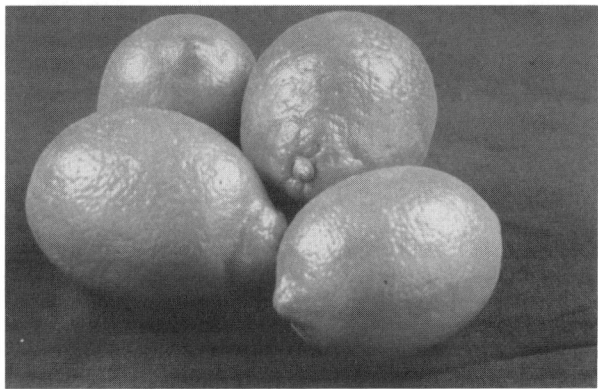

Fig. L-15. The lemon, a tangy-flavored fruit that is used to enhance the flavors of many beverages and foods. (Courtesy, USDA)

A small, yellow, oval-shaped citrus fruit. Although it is too sour to be eaten like other citrus fruits, it imparts an excellent flavor to a wide variety of beverages and other preparations. The lemon is a member of the rue family (*Rutaceae*).

ORIGIN AND HISTORY. The lemon originated somewhere in Southeast Asia between India and south China. Some botanists suspect that it arose as a result of a natural cross between the citron and an unidentified, but closely related species of citrus fruit. Furthermore, its history is clouded because it was often confused with the citron, which has a similar appearance. For example, both lemons and citrons were called "Persian apples" by the ancient Greeks.

Lemons may have been grown in Italy as early as the 1st century A.D. because they are depicted in certain Roman artworks of that period. Furthermore, the citron, which is quite similar in its cultural requirements, was definitely grown there. However, the invasions of Italy by the barbarians which began around the end of the 4th century resulted in the destruction of the estates where the citrus fruits were grown. There is no evidence that the Italians grew lemons after the 5th century, although it is known that citrons were grown without interruption on a small scale in southern Italy. Perhaps, citron production continued after lemon production ceased because the former was used by the European Jews in their Feast of the Tabernacles.

It does not appear that the lemon was grown again in Europe until after it was introduced into Spain by the Arabs in the 11th century. Various citrus fruits were grown by the Persians and Arabs in pre-Christian time, but their production did not travel very far westward from Arabia until after the Islamic religion was founded by the prophet Mohammed in the 6th century and the Arab tribes united under the banner of Islam to expand their empire across North Africa to the Atlantic Ocean.

Columbus took lemon seeds to Haiti in 1493. Shortly thereafter, the Spanish explorers planted lemons on other islands in the Caribbean and the Portuguese introduced the fruit into Brazil. It seems likely that lemon trees were also planted at St. Augustine, Florida by Ponce de Leon when he explored the area in 1513.

By 1600, some of the naval physicians of the major world powers were aware that daily rations of lemon juice would prevent outbreaks of scurvy amoung sailors on long sea voyages. Lemons were used because they remained in good condition for 6 months or more, whereas fresh oranges usually spoiled within 3 weeks. For example, it is recorded that in 1601 an outbound ship on its maiden voyage for the English East India Company stopped at Madagascar to take on lemons. However, the issuance of lemon juice to British sailors was rarely done on a regular basis until near the end of the 18th century, when it was required by the British Admiralty.

The settlers who went to Florida after Spain ceded the territory to the United States in 1821 found many wild citrus trees that were apparently the descendants of those planted by the Spanish almost 3 centuries earlier. However, the predominant citrus species was the sour orange because it was much more resistant to frost damage than either the sweet orange or the lemon. Lemon seedlings were planted in Florida in 1839, but the newly established groves did not last long because hard frosts killed the trees. Another attempt to start a Florida lemon industry was made in 1870, when lemon seeds imported from Sicily were planted. Lemon trees raised from seeds are more resistant to frost than those propagated by grafting lemon buds onto various rootstocks. However, killer frosts struck in the 1890s and once again the growers were forced to abandon their groves. It was not until 1953 that a limited production of lemons for processing was resumed in Florida.

Meanwhile, the California lemon industry began shortly after the gold rush of 1849 when many prospectors and miners developed scurvy due to the lack of fresh fruits and vegetables. The few lemons that were available sold for very high prices because many of the Fortyniners knew that daily rations of lemon juice prevented scurvy. By 1880, the production of lemons was well established in southern California. Shortly thereafter, the growth of the industry was stimulated greatly by the construction of the transcontinental railway system which made it possible to ship the fruit to populous eastern cities. From 1940 to 1965, lemon production in California exceeded that of Italy, which up to then was the world's leading producer of the fruit. Since then, Italy has regained her leadership while California production has declined somewhat.

PRODUCTION. Lemons and limes together, with a worldwide production of about 6.6 million metric tons, rank among the top dozen fruit crops. (The FAO of the UN gives statistics for lemons and limes combined.)

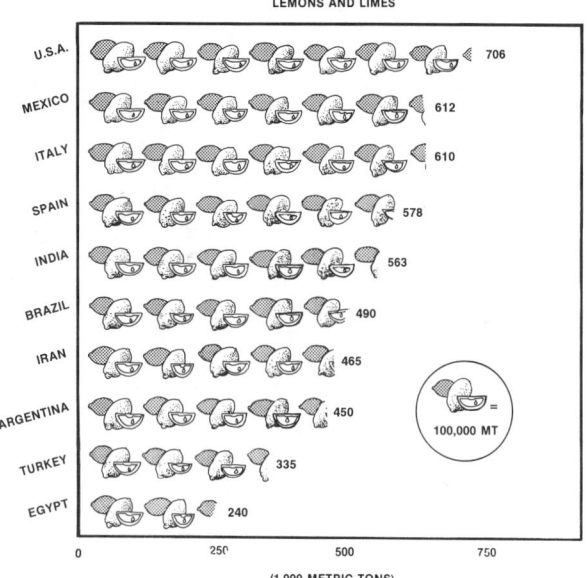

LEMONS AND LIMES

U.S.A.	706
MEXICO	612
ITALY	610
SPAIN	578
INDIA	563
BRAZIL	490
IRAN	465
ARGENTINA	450
TURKEY	335
EGYPT	240

= 100,000 MT

0   250   500   750
(1,000 METRIC TONS)

Fig. L-16. The leading lemon and lime-producing countries of the world. (Based on data from *FAO Production Yearbook*, 1991, FAO/UN, Rome, Italy, Vol. 44, p. 163, Table 71)

In the United States, lemons are the eighth leading fruit crop, with most of the production in California and Arizona.

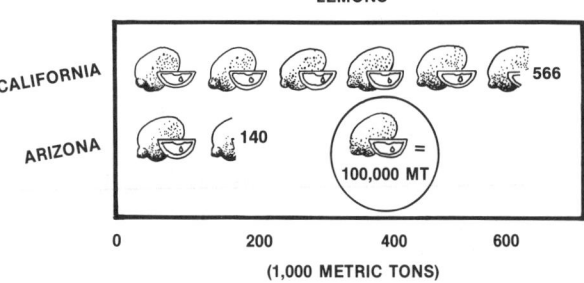

LEMONS

CALIFORNIA	566
ARIZONA	140

= 100,000 MT

0   200   400   600
(1,000 METRIC TONS)

Fig. L-17. The leading lemon-producing states of the United States. (Based upon data from *Agricultural Statistics*, 1991, USDA, p. 189, Table 278)

Lemon trees are more sensitive to freezing temperatures than the other citrus trees. Therefore, it is noteworthy that the severe winter frosts which occurred several times in Florida during the 1890s and the early 19th century wiped out the lemon industry in that state. Lemon trees raised from seeds are more cold resistant than trees produced by grafting buds onto rootstocks, but the former do not bear fruit as soon as the latter.

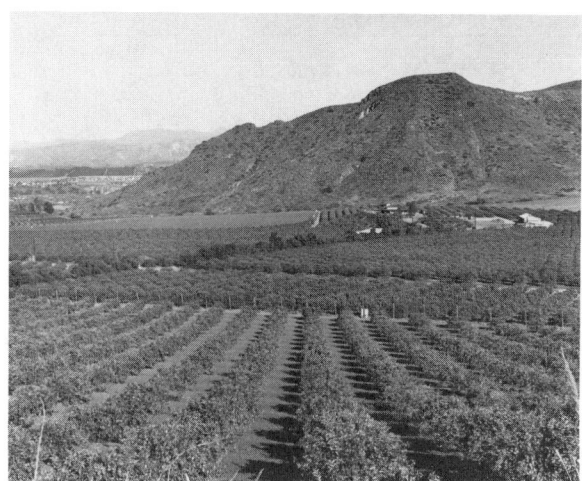

Fig. L-18. Lemon groves (foreground) and orange groves (background) in Ventura County, California. (Courtesy, Union Pacific Railroad Company, Omaha, Nebr.)

Details of growing citrus fruit trees are given elsewhere. However, lemon trees are unlike the other major citrus trees in that they bear fruit continuously. Lemons keep the longest when they are picked before they are fully mature.

Hence, the freshly harvested fruits are likely to be (1) green to yellow green in color, (2) firm and turgid with thick and fleshy rinds, and (3) 2¼ in. (*5.7 cm*) or more in diameter because the pickers take only the fruits that are too large to pass through a ring of that diameter. During

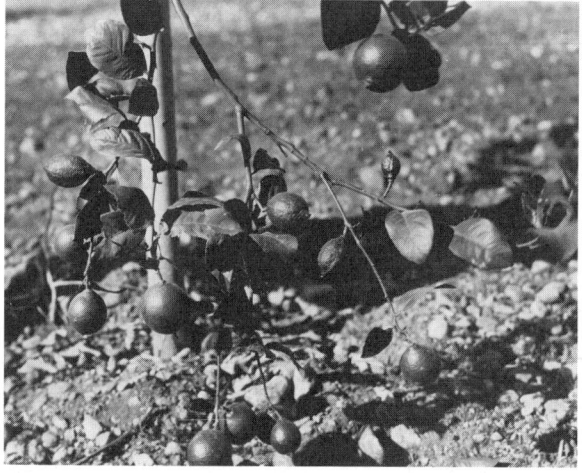

Fig. L-19. A branch of a lemon tree bearing green fruit of various sizes and shapes. (Courtesy, USDA)

storage, the rind dries out and becomes lighter in color, thinner, tougher, leathery, and very resistant to injury. The process which produces these changes is called curing and may be accelerated by exposing the fruit to ethylene gas in a warm room. Ethylene gas is produced naturally by many fruits during ripening.

(Also see CITRUS FRUITS, section headed "Production.")

PROCESSING. More than half of the U.S. lemon crop is processed. A major portion of the processed lemons are converted into lemon juice and related products such as frozen lemon juice concentrates, lemonade, frozen lemonade concentrates, and lemon flavored soft drinks. The peel, pulp, and seeds are used to make lemon oil, lemon essence, pectin, bioflavonoids (vitaminlike substances), and cattle feed ingredients. Details regarding these and other products are given elsewhere.

(Also see CITRUS FRUITS, section headed "Processing.")

SELECTION. Fresh lemons that have a fine-textured skin and are heavy for their size are generally of better quality than those that are coarse-skinned and light in weight. Deep-yellow-colored lemons are usually relatively mature and are not so acid as those of the lighter or greenish-yellow color; they are also generally thinner skinned and may have a relatively larger proportion of juice but they are not so desirable since lemons are wanted for their acid flavor.

When present, decay appears either as a mold or as a discolored soft area at the stem end. Fruits that have been mechanically injured are more or less subject to mold. Shriveled or hard-skinned fruits, or those which are soft or spongy to the touch are not desirable. They may be aged, dried out, mechanically injured, or affected by a rot at the center of the fruit.

Criteria for the selection of processed lemon products are given elsewhere.

(Also see CITRUS FRUITS, section headed "Selection and Preparation.")

PREPARATION. Fresh lemons are available year long. Also they may be stored for much longer than other major citrus fruits. Lastly, lemon juice, peel, and pulp are strongly flavored so that small amounts of each of these items may be used to enhance relatively large amounts of food. Therefore, it would be worthwhile for most homemakers to use the fruit more often in their preparations. Some suggestions follow:

1. Lemon juice may be used instead of vinegar in salad dressings and sauces.
2. Squirt a little lemon juice on the cut surfaces of fresh fruits and vegetables in order to prevent them from darkening.
3. Mixtures of herbs and lemon juice may be substituted for oily, salty, and/or sugary dressings when certain types of restricted diets must be followed.
4. Lemon juice, peel, and pulp may be used to make

homemade items such as candied peel, ice cream, ices, pie fillings, puddings, punches, and sherbets.

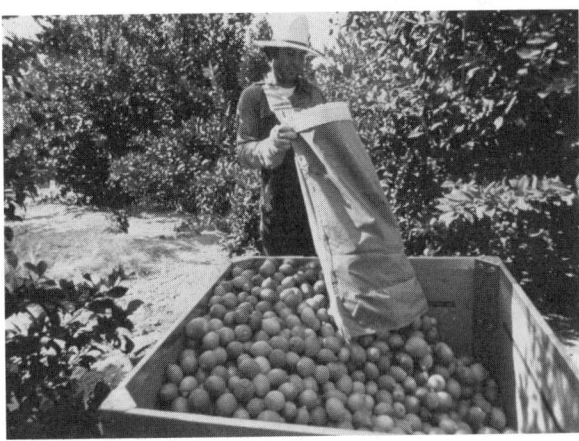

Fig. L-20. Lemon harvest. (Courtesy, USDA)

CAUTION: Some people are allergic to one or more constituents of citrus peel. When such allergies are suspected, neither the peel nor the products containing it should be consumed, and fruit juice should be extracted gently to avoid squeezing the oil and other substances from the peel into the juice. It is noteworthy that some of the commercially prepared lemon juices and lemon drinks may contain peel and/or substances extracted from it, but that prepared citrus juice products for infants contain little or none of the peel constituents.

NUTRITIONAL VALUE. The nutrient compositions of various forms of lemons and lemon products are given in Food Composition Table F-36.

Some noteworthy observations regarding the nutrient composition of these items follow:

1. Fresh lemons are very low in calories (27 kcal per 100 g), and they are a good source of potassium, vitamin C, and bioflavonoids.
2. Bottled, canned, and fresh lemon juice are approximately equal to fresh lemons, except that the bioflavonoid levels may be much lower in the juices than in the fruit because most of the latter nutrient is found in the peel and the membranes of the fruit.
3. Frozen lemon juice concentrate has four times the caloric and nutrient levels of bottled, canned, or fresh lemon juice. Hence, it may make a significant nutritional contribution when added undiluted to drinks, salad dressings, and sauces. However, additional caloric or noncaloric sweetener may be needed because the pure juice concentrate is very tart.
4. Frozen lemonade concentrate contains considerable added sweetener and is 68% higher in calories (it contains 195 kcal per 100 g [3½oz]) than unsweetened frozen lemon juice concentrate. Furthermore, the lemonade concentrate contains much lower levels of potassium and vitamin C.

5. Candied lemon peel is high in calories (316 kcal per 100 g) and is low in almost all nutrients other than carbohydrates and fiber. However, it may contain significant amounts of bioflavonoids (data on the levels of these vitaminlike substances in candied peel are not readily available.)

6. Lemon-flavored carbonated drinks contain little but water, sugar, and imitation or natural flavoring(s).

7. Lemon peel contains considerable amounts of citral, an aldehyde which antagonizes the actions of vitamin A . Hence, people should make certain that their dietary supply of vitamin A is adequate before consuming large amounts of lemon peel.

(Also see BIOFLAVONOIDS; CITRUS FRUITS; FRUIT[S], Table F-47 Fruits of the World; POTASSIUM; and VITAMIN C.)

LENHARTZ DIET

Initially, patients suffering from a bleeding peptic ulcer may be offered this type of diet. It is mainly fluid; it consists of raw eggs or milk and vegetable purees fed frequently throughout the day.

(Also see MODIFIED DIETS; SIPPY DIET; and ULCERS, PEPTIC.)

LENTIL *Lens esculenta*

This appetizing legume is one of the oldest cultivated plants in the world. Fig. L-21 shows a close-up of the seed.

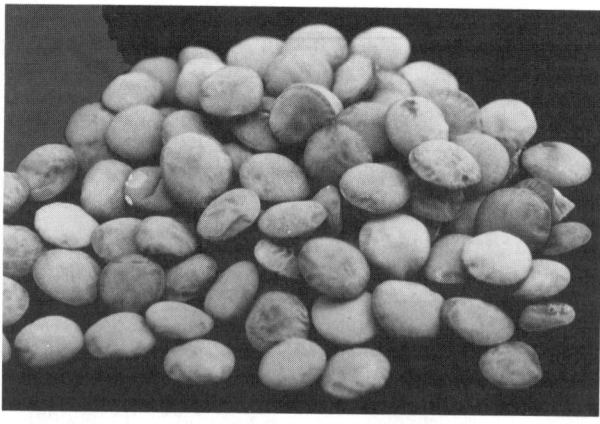

Fig. L-21. Lentils, an ancient food. (Courtesy, Minnesota Agricultural Experiment Station, University of Minnesota)

ORIGIN AND HISTORY. Archaeologists have found lentil seeds at the sites of Near Eastern farming villages that existed about 8,000 years ago. It appears that the legume seeds were consumed with barley and wheat, which were also native to the area. The three foods were taken along when the ancient peoples migrated to Europe and Africa. (These foods were used in Greece and Bulgaria by about 6000 B.C., and a little later in Ethiopia.)

Lentils were introduced into India in pre-Christian times. (At the present time, the Indian subcontinent produces the major part of the world crop.)

There are two noteworthy references to lentils in the *Old Testament.* The first one is depicted in Fig. L-22.

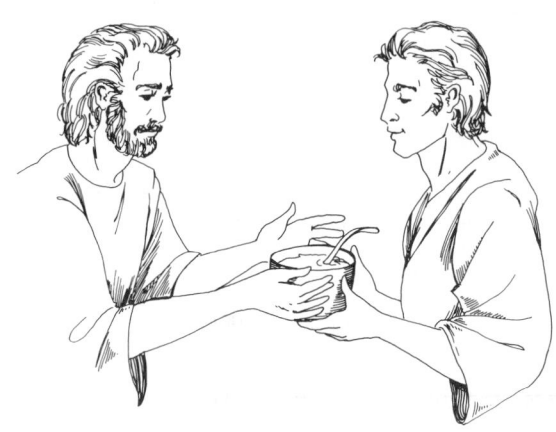

Fig. L-22.   Esau sells his birthright to Jacob for some red lentils. (Genesis 25:29-34)

The other reference describes the making of bread from grains, beans, lentils, and vetches during the Babylonian captivity of the Jews (Ezekial 4:9).

PRODUCTION.   Fig. L-23 shows the estimated annual production of lentils in the leading countries.

From 3½ to 6 months of frost-free weather are required for the production of mature seeds. Furthermore, lentils grow best when the highest temperature does not exceed 86°F (30°C). Hence, most of the crop is grown during the cool season in the subtropics and tropics, or in the warm season in mild temperate areas such as the Pacific Northwest of the United States. Some lentils are also grown at the cooler high altitudes in the tropics. However, the crop does poorly in wet, tropical areas.

In India, lentils may be grown in mixed cultivation with rice. Yields ranging from 400 to 600 lb per acre (*448 to*

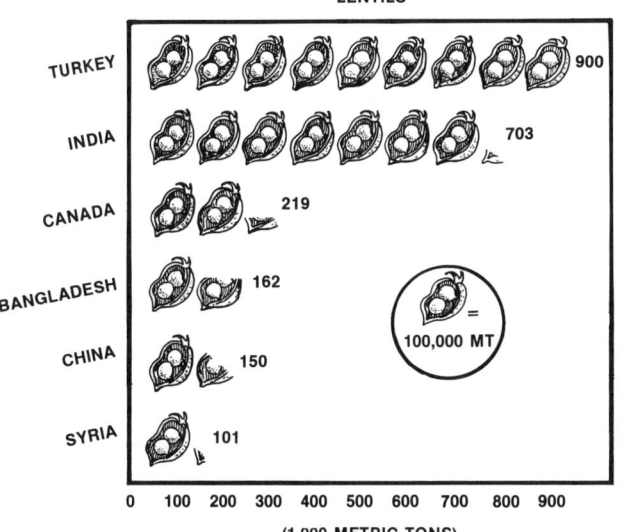

LENTILS

TURKEY 900

INDIA 703

CANADA 219

BANGLADESH 162

CHINA 150

SYRIA 101

= 100,000 MT

0 100 200 300 400 500 600 700 800 900

(1,000 METRIC TONS)

Fig. L-23. Leading lentil-producing countries of the world. (*FAO Production Yearbook*, 1990, FAO/UN, Rome, Italy, Vol. 44, p. 106, Table 36)

672 *kg/ha*) are obtained when the crop is grown in unirrigated dry areas, but as much as 1,500 lb (*1,680 kg/ha*) may be obtained with irrigation.

PROCESSING. Lentils may be marketed as whole dried seeds, split dried seeds, or as an ingredient of canned soups. Occasionally, the legume is ground into a flour and combined with cereal flour to make a protein supplement for children in the developing countries of North Africa and the Middle East.

SELECTION AND PREPARATION. Canned lentil soup is available in most supermarkets. However, this is a rather expensive form of the cooked legume in that (1) the soup contains much water, and (2) a pound (*454 g*) of dried lentils cooks up to over 3 lb of cooked legume.

Previously soaked lentils require only 20 minutes of pressure cooking, providing that the pressure is allowed to drop without opening the cooker, once the heating has been stopped.

NOTE: About a tablespoon of melted fat or oil should be added to the mixture in the pressure cooker to prevent foaming which may clog the vent. Also, about 4 cups (*950 ml*) of water are required per cup of uncooked lentils.

Cooked lentils go well with most other vegetables in casseroles, soups, and stews. Also, they may be used as substitutes for part or all of the more expensive animal foods such as cheeses, eggs, fish, meats, and poultry.

NUTRITIONAL VALUE. The nutrient composition of lentils is given in Food Composition Table F-36.

Some noteworthy observations regarding the nutrient compositon of lentils follow:

1.   A 3½ oz (*100 g*) serving (about ½ cup) of cooked lentils is equivalent in protein value to 1 oz of cooked lean meat, but the legume supplies about twice as many calories.

2.   Lentils are a good source of iron, but they contain less than one-fourth as much calcium as phosphorus. Therefore, foods richer in calcium and lower in phosphorus (such as dairy products and green leafy vegetables) should be consumed to improve the dietary calcium to phosphorus ratio.

Protein Quantity and Quality. Many of the people in India are vegetarians, so they rely heavily upon grains, lentils, and other legumes to supply much of their protein needs. (Milk and other dairy products may also be utilzied, but the supply of these foods is limited.) Hence, certain facts regarding the quantity and quality of lentil protein are noteworthy:

1.   The grams of protein per 100 Calories (kcal) provided by lentils compared to other selected foods follow:

Food	Grams of Protein per 100 Calories (kcal) (g)
Lentils	7.8
Cottage cheese	13.7
Lean meat	12.7
Eggs	12.8
Sweet corn	3.3
Brown rice	2.5

As noted, the substitution of lentils for animal protein foods on an equal protein basis usually results in an increase in the number of calories, whereas the replacement of cereal grains by lentils results in an increase in the amount of protein supplied per calorie.

2.   The protein in lentils is quite deficient in the amino acids methionine and cystine, which are supplied amply by the protein in cereal grains. Furthermore, the grains are short of lysine, an amino acid that is present more abundantly in lentils. Therefore, the amino acid patterns of lentils and grains complement each other so that mixtures of the two foods contain higher quality protein than either one alone.

(Also see LEGUMES, Table L-2 Legumes of the World; and VEGETABLE[S], Table V-6 Vegetables of the World.)

LETHARGY

Drowsiness and lack of energy.

LETTUCE *Lactuca sativa*

This vegetable is the major salad crop of the United States. (Although the U.S. production of tomatoes is more than triple that of lettuce, less than one-sixth of the tomato crop is consumed fresh, whereas all of the lettuce crop is utilized as a raw, fresh vegetable.) Lettuce belongs to the Sunflower family (*Compositae*) Fig. L-24 shows a typical head of lettuce.

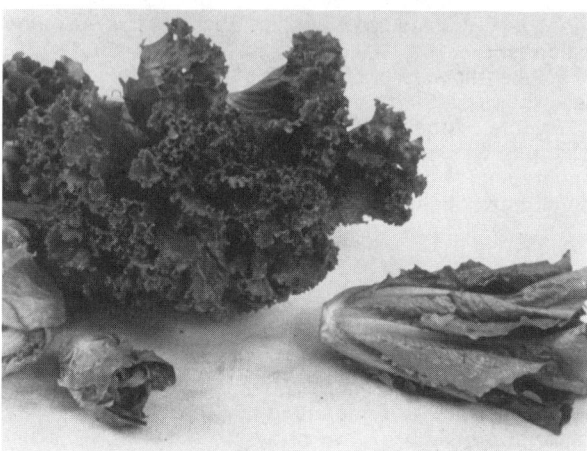

Fig. L-24. Lettuce. (Courtesy, USDA)

ORIGIN AND HISTORY. It is believed that the growing of lettuce may date as far back as 4500 B.C., because depictions of lettucelike leaves were found in ancient Egyptian tombs. However, some authorities suspect that if lettuce was grown in such early times, it was probably for the oil in its seeds, rather than for its leaves. Hence, it is uncertain when people first ate lettuce leaves. Nevertheless, it is well established that the Persian royalty consumed this vegetable in the 6th century B.C.

The ancient Greeks and Romans had a high esteem for lettuce as evidenced by (1) Hippocrates' praise of the vegetable for its medicinal value, and (2) the erection of an altar and a statue in honor of lettuce by Augustus Caesar, who believed that it had brought about his recovery from an illness. In the years that followed, the Roman legions introduced the plant to the European lands they conquered. It is not certain how lettuce was brought to China, but there is evidence that it was grown there by the 5th century A.D.

Columbus brought lettuce seeds with him on his second voyage to the Caribbean, where the early cultivation of this crop led to the development of the Puerto Rican variety that was grown later by the first American colonist. The first lettuce planted in California was taken there by Spanish padres. However, commercial lettuce production did not get underway in the western United States until a few acres were planted near the Salinas-Watsonville area of California, which is now the "Lettuce Capital" of the nation. The rapid growth of lettuce production during the present century was due largely to the development of refrigerated railroad cars and storage facilities that made it possible to distribute the fresh vegetable across the country. Today, certain produce wholesalers in the eastern United States would rather pay a premium price for a steady supply of western lettuce than to pay less for the eastern crop, which is much more likely to be in short supply due to unfavorable weather.

PRODUCTION. Approximately 3.3 million metric tons of lettuce were produced in the United States during 1990. Fig. L-25 shows the states that contributed most of this production.

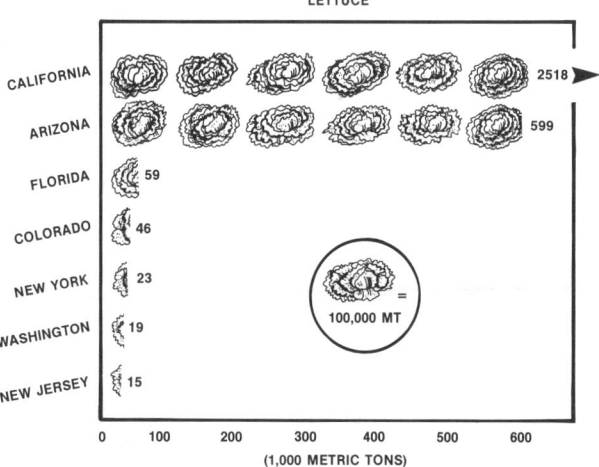

Fig. L-25. The leading lettuce-producing states. (Based upon data from *Agricultural Statistics*, 1991, USDA, p. 155, Table 219)

It is noteworthy that over three-fourths of the U.S. lettuce crop is produced in California.

Growing in the Field. Lettuce requires cool, mild weather for optimal growth. Hence, much of the U.S. production of this vegetable comes from the Salinas-Watsonville area near the central coastal section of California, where the average temperature ranges from 55 to 60°F (*13 to 16°C*). However, lettuce is also grown in many other parts of the United States, but its production in these places is limited to the seasons when the temperature range is favorable. In the New York-New Jersey area, it is planted in the early spring for harvesting in the summer. In the southwestern desert areas, it is planted in the fall for picking in the winter. (Watsonville-Salinas plantings are made throughout the period extending from late fall to late summer, and harvesting is

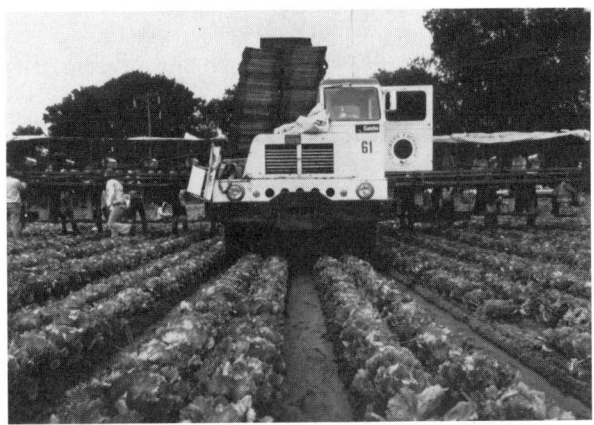

Fig. L-26. Harvesting iceberg lettuce in California. (Courtesy, California Iceberg Lettuce Commission, Monterey, Calif.)

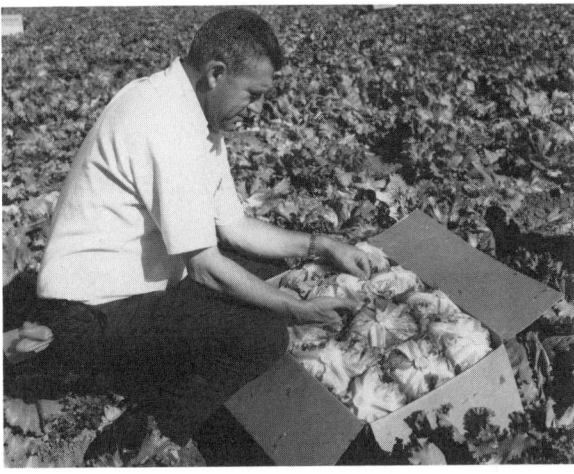

Fig. L-27. Lettuce inspection. Quality control and guaranteed good arrival standards for lettuce are set by law. Government inspection programs are carried on both at shipping and arrival points. Lettuce failing to make grade standards is not allowed to be shipped. (Courtesy, California Iceberg Lettuce Commission, Monterey, Calif.)

done from spring to late fall.) Seeds are planted directly in the field in the warm areas with long growing seasons, but in the cooler areas, seedlings are grown in greenhouses or hotbeds, then transplanted in the field when the weather is sufficiently warm.

Highly acid soils may require the addition of some lime, but it should be used cautiously, because over-alkalinization of the soil may render certain trace minerals unavailable to the plants. Many growers also fertilize the soil with nitrogen, phosphorus, and potassium. A large part of the U.S. lettuce crop is grown in areas where irrigation is required. In the very warm areas, such as the Imperial Valley in California, watering also serves the purpose of cooling the soil so that the lettuce seeds may germinate more readily. It is noteworthy that the optimal temperature range for the germination of lettuce seed is 64 to 70°F (*18 to 21°C*), whereas, the soil temperature in the Imperial Valley may be as high as 104°F (*40°C*) at planting time.

Lettuce grown in warm weather may be ready for harvesting in as little as 60 days after planting, but as many as 120 days may be required for the production of this crop during the winter in the southwestern United States. The average U.S. yield of lettuce is 25,200 lb per acre (*28,224 kg/ha*), but yields as high as 32,000 lb per acre (*35,840 kg/ha*) have been obtained in California. In California, lettuce is usually picked and packed in boxes in the field. Therefore, the inspection and grading of the vegetable is done in the field while the boxes are being packed for shipment.

The packed boxes of lettuce are then loaded into a refrigerated truck which carries them to a vacuum cooler. Prompt cooling of freshly harvested lettuce reduces the likelihood of overripening during shipment or storage. Most of the U.S. lettuce crop is now shipped in refrigerated trucks to its final destination.

Greenhouse Culture. This type of lettuce production is much more common in England, France, and the Netherlands than in the United States; in the U.S., it is limited to a few midwestern states. Although the cost of indoor production is considerably greater than that of field production, well-organized operations are profitable when located near large urban centers that have cold winters, because the only other lettuce available has to be shipped long distances from warmer areas. Furthermore, the greenhouse production of lettuce may be coordinated with the indoor production of cucumbers, tomatoes, and ornamental plants that are grown in the same facilities.

PROCESSING. Lettuce is processed to a very limited extent, since it cannot be frozen or heated without becoming limp and losing much of its appeal. However, the demand for ready-to-use shredded lettuce by many food service establishments has led to the production of prepacked shredded lettuce. This product is made from the freshly harvested vegetable by coring, shredding, cooling, and washing. The shredded lettuce is then packed in plastic bags that are shipped in styrofoam containers to prevent damage during transit.

SELECTION. Consumers are more likely to get the best buy if they know something about (1) the types of lettuce marketed in their locality, and (2) the indicators of quality.

Types of Lettuce. Most of the varieties of lettuce sold in the United States fall into one of the types shown in Fig. L-28.

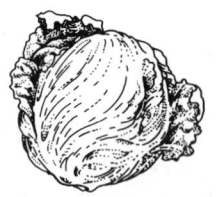
CRISP-HEAD LETTUCE

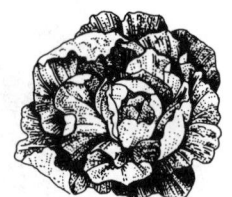
BUTTERHEAD LETTUCE

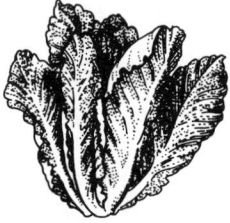
ROMAINE LETTUCE

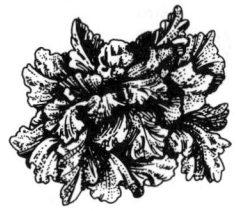
LOOSE-LEAF LETTUCE

Fig. L-28. The four main types of lettuce grown in the United States.

• **Crisp-headed (Iceberg)**—Heads of this type are relatively large and solid, with large, medium-green fringed outer leaves and crisp, blanched inner leaves, which are folded into a dense mass. A very large majority of commercial lettuce shipments are of the crisp-head type.

• **Butterhead**—Varieties of this type, such as Bibb, Big Boston, and White Boston, produce small, rosettelike heads with leaves relatively smooth, fairly light colored, soft, tender, and succulent. The butterhead varieties bruise and tear easily when handled. Hence, they are likely to be grown only for local markets.

• **Cos (Romaine)**—These varieties are distinguished by the tall cylindrical shape and long, folded, very dark-green leaves. Romaine lettuce ships well and is becoming increasingly popular for its distinctive flavor and high nutritional value.

• **Loose-leaf**—Leaves of this nonhead-forming type range from very light yellowish-green to dark green or reddish green. Loose-leaf varieties are not suitable for long distance shipping, but are grown mainly for local markets.

Indicators of Quality. Good quality crisp-head lettuce should be clean, crisp and tender, with heads that are fairly firm to firm. Heads should be free from rusty appearance, decay, and excessive outer leaves. Lettuce with excessive "tipburn"—which usually appears on inner leaves as small, ragged, brown areas—is undesirable. Occasionally lettuce containing advanced seedstem growth may be found in markets. Such heads may have a slightly bitter flavor, and the removal of the seedstem may cause excessive waste. Heads with seedstems can often be detected by wide spaces between the base portions of the outer leaves and an abnormal swelling of one side of the top of the head. Sometimes the relatively hard seedstem growth can be felt at the point of the swelling. Decay, which may be indicated by water-soaked or discolored areas on outer leaves, sometimes deeply penetrates the interior of a head of this type.

Butterhead, romaine, and loose-leaf types should be clean, fresh, and tender. Usually such lettuce can be fully examined for discoloration or other defects.

PREPARATION. The enjoyment of lettuce dishes may be enhanced by taking a few simple measures to ensure that the lettuce is kept as fresh as possible until it is served. These measures are illustrated in Fig. L-29.

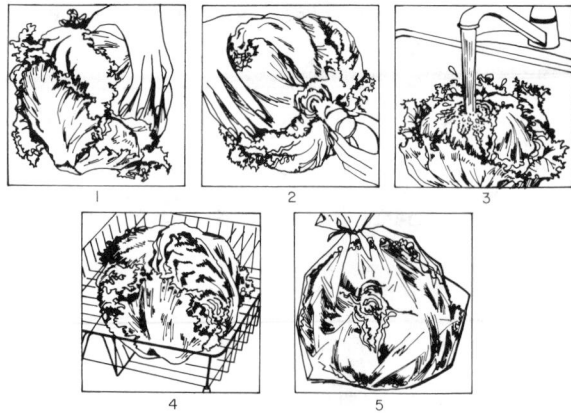

Fig. L-29. Steps for proper lettuce care: 1. SELECT heads that give slightly when gently squeezed. A firm, but not hard, head is a perfectly "mature" head. 2. CORE by holding head core-end down, whack it onto a counter, then lift or twist out the core with fingers. Or, you may cut it with a stainless steel knife; cut edges discolor sooner. 3. RINSE by holding head cored-end up under running tap water allowing water to run all through the head to refresh it. 4. DRAIN the rinsed head *thoroughly* with cored-end down in rack or on drainboard. 5. STORE in refrigerator in a tightly-closed plastic bag or special lettuce crisper. (Courtesy, California Iceberg Lettuce Commission, San Rafael, Calif.)

The California Iceberg Lettuce Commission also suggests serving crisp-head (Iceberg) lettuce as follows:

• **Chunks**—For about 4 cups (*950 ml*) of bite-size chunks, slice a medium head into rafts, then cut them lengthwise and crosswise.

• **Rafts**—Cut head crosswise into slices about 1-in. thick. A medium-sized head yields 3 or 4 rafts. (Store end pieces in a disposable plastic bag for later use.)

• **Shredded**—Cut head lengthwise into halves, then place cut-sides down on board and slice crosswise with a thin-bladed knife. About 4 cups (*950 ml*) shredded lettuce will be obtained from one head of medium size.

• **Wedges**—Using a sharp, stainless steel knife, cut head lengthwise into halves. Place cut-sides down and cut each half-head into halves or thirds. For easier eating, cut wedges into halves crosswise.

Maximum meal pleasure and nutritional benefits may be obtained by utilizing the principles that (1) lettuce is a low-calorie food which goes well with cheese, eggs, fish and seafood, grains and cereal products, legumes, meats, nuts, poultry, and other vegetables; and (2) the larger the quantity of lettuce used, the more likely it will be that hunger will be satisfied and the digestive system stimulated to optimal functioning by the abundant water and gentle bulk provided by this vegetable. Figs. L-30 through L-33 show some appetizing and nutritious lettuce dishes.

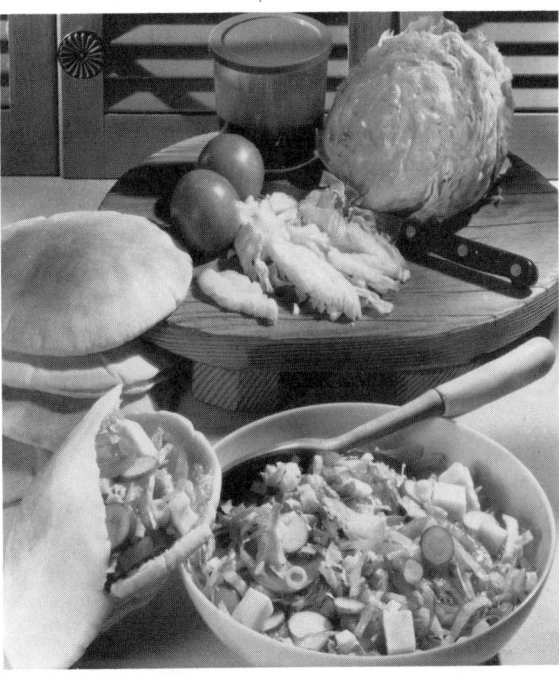

Fig. L-31. "Pocket bread saladwiches." The custom of stuffing delectable morsels into "pocket bread" originated in the Middle East. An Americanized version may utilize fillings containing shredded lettuce, sliced cheese, sliced tomatoes, diced green peppers, sliced onions, sliced radishes, and a well seasoned dressing which is drizzled over the filling. (Courtesy, California Iceberg Lettuce Commission. San Rafael, Calif.)

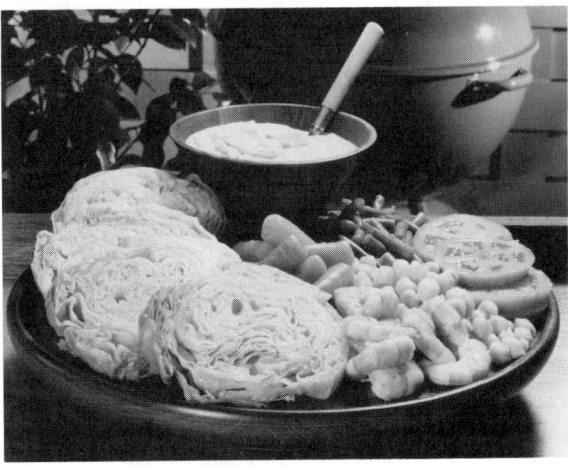

Fig. L-30. "Top-your-own-salads." A busy host may save some time by allowing each guest to make his or her own salad from an assortment of precut lettuce rafts plus canned carrots and green beans; cheeses; cooked dried beans; eggs, fish, meats, poultry, or seafood; tomato slices; and one or more dressings. (Courtesy, California Iceberg Lettuce Commission, San Rafael, Calif.)

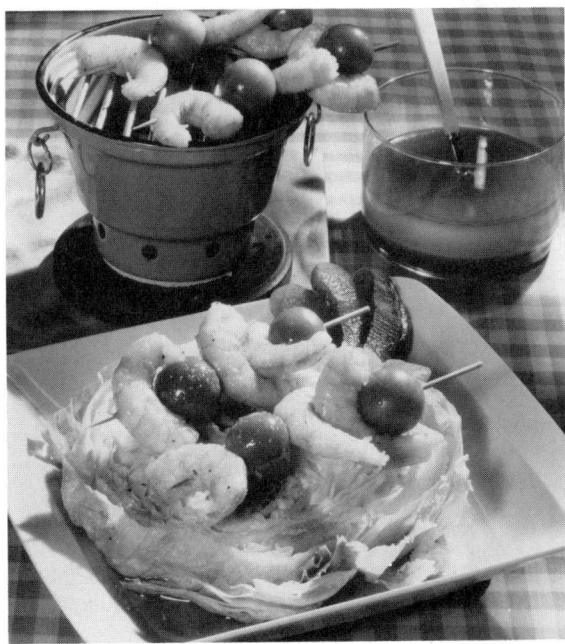

Fig. L-32. "Prawns on a raft." The lettuce raft is topped with twin skewers bearing broiled prawns and cherry tomatoes; and a "chili-lemon dressing" made from salad oil, lemon juice, salt, sugar, onion powder, celery salt, chili powder, lemon pepper and garlic powder. (Courtesy, California Iceberg Lettuce Commission, San Rafael, Calif.)

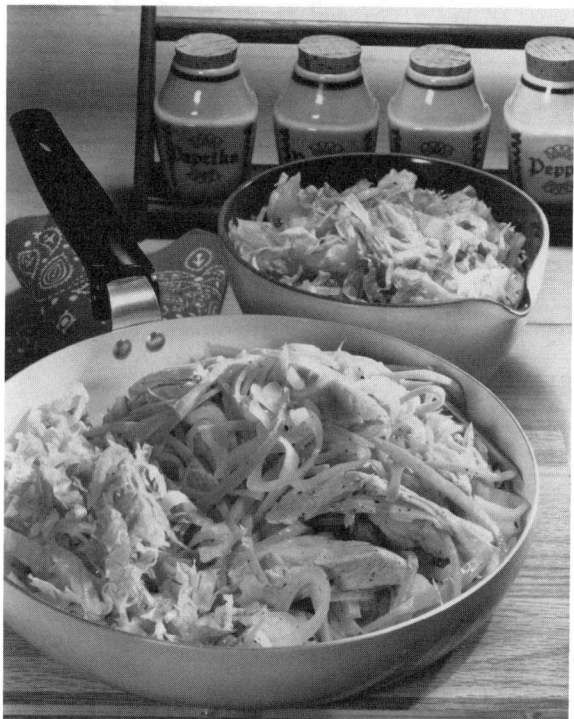

Fig. L-33. "Iceberg holiday stir-fry." Stir-frying was developed to a fine art by the Chinese. Their techniques are utilized in the preparation of this dish which contains shredded lettuce, strips of cooked ham or turkey, julienne carrots, crushed garlic, butter, lemon juice, cornstarch, basil, and sugar. The lettuce retains its crispness because it is stirred in at the end of the brief cooking period. (Courtesy, California Iceberg Lettuce Commission, Monterey, Calif.)

Some other appetizing ways of serving lettuce are: (1) as a wilted salad in which a hot dressing is poured over the raw vegetable, and (2) in cream of lettuce and minestrone soups.

NUTRITIONAL VALUE. The nutrient composition of the major types of lettuce are given in Food Composition Table F-36.

Some noteworthy observations regarding the nutrient composition of lettuce follow:

1. All types of lettuce have a high water content (94 to 96%) and are low in calories (13 to 18 kcal per 100 g). Therefore, a 1-lb (454 g) head of iceberg lettuce furnishes only about 56 Calories (kcal). Hence, people trying to cut their caloric intake in order to lose weight may assuage their hunger pangs by eating large quantities of this vegetable.

2. The darker the green color of lettuce, the richer it is likely to be in nutrients. For example, the butterhead, loose-leaf, and romaine types contain significantly more iron and vitamin A than the crisphead type. Also, it is noteworthy that romaine lettuce contains about 10 times as much folic acid as the other types. Although each of the four types is only a fair source of vitamin C, lettuce may make a significant contribution of this vitamin to the diet if sufficiently large quantities are consumed.

(Also see VEGETABLE[S], Table V-6 Vegetables of the World.)

LEUCINE

One of the essential amino acids.
(Also see AMINO ACID[S].)

LEUKEMIA

A malignant condition, a blood cancer, wherein there is uncontrolled production of abnormal white blood cells, leukocytes. These are produced in the bone marrow, spleen, and lymph tissues. Blood concentrations of leukocytes may increase a hundredfold. There are several forms of the disease, the exact causative factors of which are unknown. However, excessive radiation, certain chemicals, heredity, and hormonal abnormalities have been implicated. New techniques employed to combat leukemia have greatly increased a patient's chances of complete remission. During treatment, a supportive diet should be given which is higher than normal in energy and nutrient content and which is acceptable and appetizing.

(Also see CANCER.)

LEVULOSE

It is another name for fructose, fruit sugar. It is levoratatory (turning to the left) to polarized light; hence, the name levulose. Levulose, which is much sweeter than cane sugar, is found in honey, ripe fruits, and some vegetables.

(Also see CARBOHYDRATE[S]; and FRUCTOSE.)

LICORICE

Licorice is a herb, the root of which produces a flavoring that is used to flavor candy, chewing gum, and soft drinks.

Caution: Licorice raises the blood pressure of some people dangerously high, due to the retention of sodium.

(Also see FLAVORINGS AND SEASONINGS, Table F-22; and MEDICINAL PLANTS, Table M-3.)

LIEBERKUHN'S CRYPT

Tubular glands located in the mucous membrane of the small intestine, named after Johann Lieberkuhn, German anatomist, who first described them. Now they are simply called intestinal glands. They secrete intestinal juices.

(Also see DIGESTION AND ABSORPTION.)

LIFE EXPECTANCY AND NUTRITION

Contents	Page

Experiments with Laboratory Animals.

In the early 1930s, Dr. Clive McKay of Cornell University succeeded in doubling the life expectancy of laboratory rats by drastically restricting their diets from after weaning to death. Furthermore, the incidence of tumors in the restricted rats was much lower than normal. However, the rats given the stringent diets failed to grow and develop at the normal rate and had an increased susceptibility to diseases and death early in their lifespan. These drawbacks make it unlikely that similar measures will be applied deliberately to people, although it has been suggested that very rigorous conditions of life in certain parts of the world have similar effects on human populations. That is, the more vulnerable people die young, while those with unusually strong constitutions live to ripe old ages.

Observations of Human Populations.

The longest-lived peoples of the world are believed to be those that live in the geographic areas depicted in Fig. L-35.

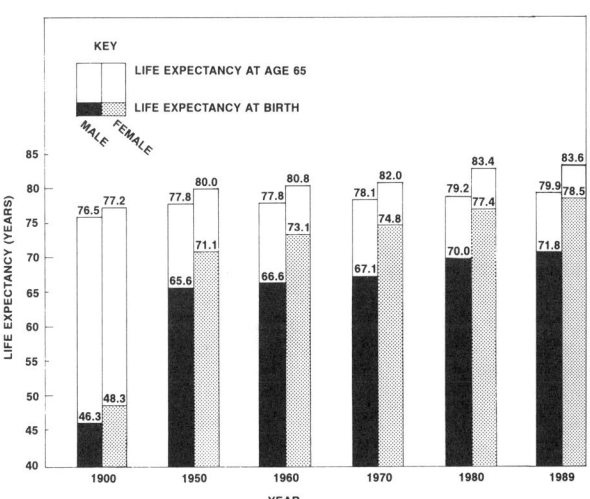

Fig. L-34. Life expectancies in the United States from 1900 to 1989. (Source: *Health, United States 1979*, U.S. Dept. HEW, p. 90, Table 9; and *Statistical Abstract of the United States 1991*, p. 73)

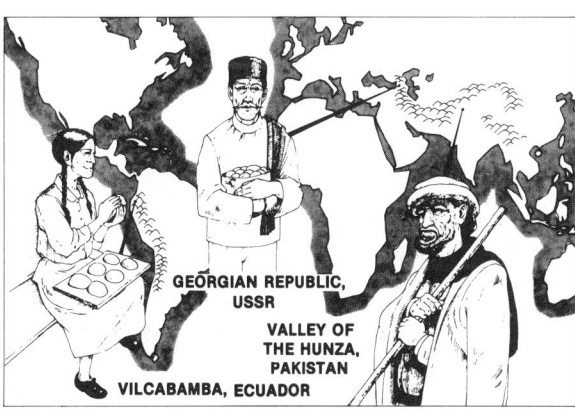

Fig. L-35. The locations where some people of apparently great longevity are found.

The great increase in life expectancy at birth shown in Fig. L-34 was due mainly to the control of many of the infectious diseases that formerly killed many infants and children.

In recent years, researchers have been successful in identifying the factors that increase the life expectancies of older people. As a result, life expectancy at age 65 has increased dramatically, as shown in Fig. L-34.

WELL-KNOWN STUDIES OF HEALTH AND LONGEVITY.

Certain studies are referred to frequently in the popular and scientific literature on longevity. Hence, details of some of the better known observations follow.

Descriptions of the people shown in Fig. L-35 follow:

• **Ecuadorians of Vilcabamba**—These people live in a village that is located at an elevation of 4,600 ft (*1,400 m*) in the Andes mountains of southern Ecuador. They are reputed to live as long as 125 years, although this belief is now being questioned due to the fact that many people take the names of their parents and other close relatives. Hence, it is difficult to determine whether the names listed in the baptismal records of the local church are those for people that are now alive, or those that are deceased. Nevertheless, the older people in this village appear to be sufficiently vigorous and healthy to engage in a primitive type of farming. Furthermore, they have to contend with a mountainous terrain that makes getting about a test of physical fitness. Their caloric intake is low and they eat mainly vegetables because animal foods are scarce in their region. Most Vilcabambans drink moderate amounts of a rumlike alcoholic beverage called zuhmir, and smoke.

• **Georgians of the Soviet Union**—Gerontologists have long thought that these people had the longest lives known to man, since some were once thought to be at least 150 years old. However, the Russian gerontologist Zhores Medvedev believes that the advanced ages may be gross exaggerations which started in the early 1900s as a means of avoiding military service under the Czars. Also, the Soviets may have felt that the reports had propaganda value, since Josef Stalin was born in the Georgian Republic. Even if the reports of the advanced ages prove to be false, the fitness of the people and the scarcity of degenerative diseases in this region provide ample testimony to the benefits of a varied diet and strenuous exercise. The Georgians eat dairy products, meats, plenty of vegetables, and some sweets such as halvah. Many also drink and smoke. Apparently, the potential ill effects of the latter vices are offset by the heavy work on the farms.

• **Hunzas of Pakistan**—There are few American enthusiasts for health foods who have not heard of these people in the Karakorum Mountains (the western end of the Himalayas) in the northeastern part of Pakistan. Now, it appears that the reports of exceptional health and longevity of these people have been less than accurate, since a Japanese medical team found many cases of cancer, heart disease, and tuberculosis, and little evidence to confirm exceptional longevity.[3] Furthermore the death rates for the younger generations are quite high, since 30% of the children died before age 10, and 10% of the survivors died before 40. Therefore, it appears that the sprightly Hunza oldsters observed by the seekers of the secrets of longevity represented the hardiest of the group, who were endowed with exceptional ability to adapt to primitive conditions.

Even if it should be impossible to extend the human lifespan much beyond 100 years, it would still be a great achievement to cut the incidences of the major degenerative diseases drastically, so that more people might live healthier and longer lives. Hence, the groups of people who have lower-than-normal rates of these diseases are noteworthy.

• **Bulgarians**—In the early 1900s, the Russian microbiologist Elie Metchnikoff promoted the consumption of the yogurt bacteria *Lactobacillus bulgaricus* because he observed that the yogurt-consuming Bulgarians appeared to have healthier and more long-lived people than the other groups he studied. Furthermore, he theorized that the *Lactobacillus* organisms prevented the growth of undesirable toxin-producing species of bacteria in the intestine. Many other scientists of that era scoffed at Metchnikoff's ideas, but re-

cent studies have yielded evidence that supports some of his concepts.[4] For example, the feeding of *Lactobacilli* has been beneficial to (1) infants afflicted with diarrhea induced by pathogenic microorganisms, and (2) people suffering from ammonia toxicity due to liver failure. In the latter case, intestinal bacteria convert urea that is present in digestive secretions to ammonia which is then absorbed into the blood. Normally, the liver converts excess ammonia to urea, but in liver failure the ammonia accumulates in toxic amounts. *Lactobacilli* reduce the buildup of ammonia.

• **Longshoremen in San Francisco**—A 22-year study (from 1951 to 1972) of 3,686 longshoremen revealed that those who performed heavy work (that requiring an average of 1,876 Calories [kcal] per day above the BMR) had a much lower risk of a fatal heart attack than those who performed light work which required an expenditure of about 1,066 Calories (kcal) per day over the BMR.[5]

• **Masai tribesmen of Africa**—The males of this tribe, who consume liberal amounts of cow's blood, milk, and meat, do not develop heart disease as they grow older even though atherosclerotic plaques form in their coronary arteries, because the exercise of walking about 11 miles (*18 km*) per day results in compensatory enlargement of the arteries.[6]

• **Mormons**—Various studies of these people have shown them to have a cancer death rate that is about 1/3 lower than the national average, and from 1/3 to 1/2 fewer deaths from heart attacks.[7] Furthermore, many elderly Mormons stay active in businesses, farming, and church affairs well into their 80s and 90s. Their superior health and longevity is thought to result from factors such as (1) abstinence from alcoholic beverages, coffee and tea, habit-forming drugs, and smoking; (2) consumption of liberal amounts of whole grains, fruits and vegetables, and only moderate amounts of meat; (3) adequate physical activity and sufficient rest and recreation; (4) family unity; (5) extensive participation of the laity in church affairs; and (6) striving for high levels of occupational achievement.

• **Seventh-day Adventists**—Adventists men live an average of 6 years longer than other American men, and the women live 3 years longer than their counterparts.[8] Furthermore, the death rates of cancer, heart disease, and stroke for Adventists are only about 50 to 60% of

[3]Jarvis, W. T., "The Myth of the Healthy Savage," *Nutrition Today*, March-April 1981, pp. 14-22.

[4]"Interrelationships of Diet, Gut Microflora, Nutrition, and Health," *Dairy Council Digest*, July-August 1976, pp. 19-24.

[5]Paffenbarger, R. S., Jr., *et al.*, "Work-Energy Level, Personal Characteristics, and Fatal Heart Attack: A Birth-Cohort Effect," *American Journal of Epidemiology*, Vol. 105, 1977, pp. 200-213.

[6]Mann, G. V., Testimony in the hearings of the U.S. Senate Select Committee on Nutrition and Human Needs, March 24, 1977.

[7]Davidson, B., "What Can We Learn About Health from the Mormons?", *Family Circle*, July 1976.

[8]Walton, L. R., *et al.*, *How You Can Live Six Extra Years*, Woodbridge Press Publishing Company, Santa Barbara, Calif., 1981, pp. 4-7.

that of other Americans. It appears that the reduced susceptibility of Adventists to degenerative diseases results from (1) abstinence from alcoholic drinks, caffeine-containing beverages, drugs, and smoking; (2) consumption of strict vegetarian (vegan) diets or lacto-ovo-vegetarian diets (those which contain milk and eggs, but no meat); (3) exercising on a regular basis; and (4) participation in the activities of their church.

PRACTICAL APPLICATIONS.
The observations of the various groups of people who live full lives here and abroad provide some lessons regarding the types of health practices that promote longevity. First of all, the healthiest people usually eat a wide variety of fresh, minimally-processed foods such as meats and fish, dairy products, fruits and vegetables, and whole grain breads and cereals; and they may limit their consumption of potentially harmful items such as strong alcoholic drinks, caffeine-containing beverages, and refined fats, starches, and sugars. Furthermore, the quantities of foods consumed are sufficient to promote health and vitality, but not enough to bring on life-threatening obesity. Finally, the winners in the game of survival have harmonious relationships with their families and neighbors, and engage in moderate to vigorous levels of physical activity on a regular basis.

Suggestions For Selecting Foods And Planning Meals.
Details regarding the nutritional allowances and optimal food patterns for each of the major age groups are given elsewhere. Hence, only general outlines of food selection and meal planning are presented in the sections that follow.

(Also see ADULT NUTRITION; CHILDHOOD AND ADOLESCENT NUTRITION; DIETS OF THE WORLD; FOOD GROUPS; GERONTOLOGY AND GERIATRIC NUTRITION; INFANT DIET AND NUTRITION; NUTRIENTS: REQUIREMENTS, ALLOWANCES, FUNCTIONS, SOURCES; PREGNANCY AND LACTATION NUTRITION; and RELIGIONS AND DIETS.)

SELECTING FOODS.
The food groups which comprise the framework of the daily food plan are: (1) bread, cereal, rice, and pasta group; (2) vegetable group; (3) fruit group; (4) milk, yogurt, and cheese group; (5) meat, poultry, fish, dry beans, eggs, and nuts group; and (6) fats, oils, and sweets. The minimum quantities indicated in the food groups form a foundation for an adequate diet, safeguarding the quantity and proportion of minerals, vitamins, and other nutrients. Many people will use more than the minimum number of servings suggested in each food group; and everyone will add some sugars, fats, and oils during food preparation and at the table. Perhaps a third to a half of the day's calories will come from such additions to the minimal number of servings. However, people who are overweight would be wise to limit their food selections to the basic foods in each group, and to restrict drastically their intake of sugars, fats, and oils.

• **Meats, poultry, fish, eggs, legumes, and nuts**—Two or more servings of beef, veal, pork, lamb, poultry, fish, eggs, dry beans, peas, and nuts.

• **Milk and cheeses**—Two or more servings as follows:
Children.....................3 to 4 cups
Teenagers.................4 or more cups
Adults.....................2 or more cups
Pregnant women...........4 or more cups
Nursing mothers...........6 or more cups
Cheese and ice cream can replace part of the milk.

• **Vegetables and fruits**—Four or more servings, including a dark-green or deep-yellow vegetable that supplies vitamin A—at least every other day; a citrus fruit or other fruit or vegetable rich in vitamin C—daily; and other fruits and vegetables including potatoes.

• **Breads and cereals**—Four or more servings of bread or cereals—whole grain, enriched, and/or fortified.

Additional servings of any of the foods in the foundation plan and additional energy foods when needed will help to meet the daily nutrient requirements of each member of the family.

Preschool children between the ages of 1 and 3 years need more body-building foods in proportion to their size, even though their total intake of food is less than their older brothers and sisters or their parents. Foods rich in iron are essential for this age group. Appetites can be expected to slow down at about 3 years of age as growth slows down. Studies of nursery school children show that when nutritious snacks are eaten reasonably far ahead of mealtime, the appetite for lunch or supper remains good. In fact, if a child is allowed to become too hungry or too tired before a meal, he may become so irritable that he fails to eat at mealtime.

In general, young school children need smaller servings, whereas older children, up to their teens, need average servings.

Teenagers can be expected to eat considerably more food. Because of their higher nutrient requirements, they usually need an additional or larger serving in the meat group and the vegetable-fruit group as well as the increase recommended in dairy foods. Unless weight control is a problem, teenagers will need more food for energy from "seconds" or additional food. Teenage boys need more protein and calcium and greater amounts of almost all nutrients than at any time during their lives because they are experiencing their most rapid growth rate other than in infancy. Energy needs are high. Between-meal snacks are usually needed and should be chosen frequently from the four food groups. Girls' nutrient needs are higher during the teenage years than at any other time in life except during infancy, pregnancy, and lactation. The increasing number of teenage marriages makes nutrition doubly important for the girls. Pregnancy puts an extra stress on the teenage mother-to-be since she must provide nutrients for her own continued development as well as for the baby.

The pregnant and nursing woman requires more or larger servings in dairy foods, in vegetables and fruits, and, usually, in the meat group to meet increased nutrient needs.

Since women generally eat less food than men, women need to choose most of their "additional foods" from the four groups to ensure ample protein, calcium, iron, and B vitamins. Mothers are prone to neglect their own meals, partially because of their attention to the food needs of their family, or perhaps they have become figure-conscious without understanding figure control.

Older adults, who have become less active, need fewer calories than when they were younger. Therefore, it is doubly important that their meals be made up largely of the protective foods in the four groups. Excessive starches and sweets should not replace foods which are sources of needed nutrients.

PLANNING MEALS. The total food eaten during the day is the important key to good nutrition. A meal, however, may mean more than just food—it can mean relaxation and refreshment of spirit and body. Many people seem to feel better and function better if they eat three meals daily. This may be because the body seems to work more efficiently if it receives nourishment at regular intervals—or it may be, in part, because of mealtime relaxation.

Some people find that four or even five meals a day are better suited to their appetites and situations. The "extra meal" may be a hearty snack, and, if eaten, should count toward the day's nutrients. The relation of calories in the extra meal or snack to overweight may be a significant one. Currently, research studies are being carried out to determine what, if any, relation exists between spacing of meals and overweight. There is not yet sufficient evidence to support a recommendation that the generally accepted custom of three meals a day should be markedly altered.

Whatever the family eating pattern is, the homemaker needs to develop a basic pattern that suits both the family members' schedules and their nutritional needs.

The following is an accepted pattern for three daily meals:

• **Breakfast**—This meal should include fruit or fruit juice (preferably high in vitamin C); cereal and milk and/or other protein-rich food; bread with butter, margarine, or other spread; milk, and another beverage if desired.

• **Lunch**—When feasible, this meal should include a protein-rich food (meat, fish, poultry, eggs, cheese, or an alternate); a vegetable or fruit, or both; bread with butter, margarine, or other spread; dessert, if desired; and milk.

• **Supper**—This meal should include a protein-rich food (meat, fish, poultry, eggs, cheese, or an alternate); two vegetables—potato or other starchy vegetable plus a dark green or yellow vegetable; bread with butter, margarine, or other spread; dessert; milk, or other beverage, if desired.

Physical Activity. Regular physical activity helps to utilize dietary calories and prevent obesity, and imparts a good feeling. It is also useful in preventing degenerative diseases and for rehabilitating people who contract them. For example, patients with heart disease have had their health and physical capacity improved by physical training.[9] Also, moderate to strenuous exercise performed on a regular basis helps to retard the loss of bone calcium that occurs with aging. The exercise is most effective in conjunction with adequate amounts of dietary calcium, phosphorus, and vitamin D.

CAUTION: It is wise to consult a doctor before starting strenuous activities that have not been performed recently.

LIGHT OFF-FLAVOR

In some foods, exposure to a light source creates an off-flavor. Light provides the energy for a chemical change which creates the undesirable odor. These chemical changes due to light are known to occur in fats, milk, and beer, and, depending upon the product, they may have a special name such as light-struck flavor in milk and sunlight off-flavor or skunky in beer.

LIGNIN

A practically indigestible compound which along with cellulose is a major component of the cell wall of certain plant foods, such as very mature vegetables.
(Also see FIBER.)

LIMA BEAN (BUTTER BEAN)
Phaseolus lunatus

This bean is believed to have been named after Lima, Peru, the area where it was first cultivated. It belongs to the family *Leguminosae*. The beans may be picked while still immature and green for use as "baby" limas, or when fully mature. Fig. L-36 shows lima beans.

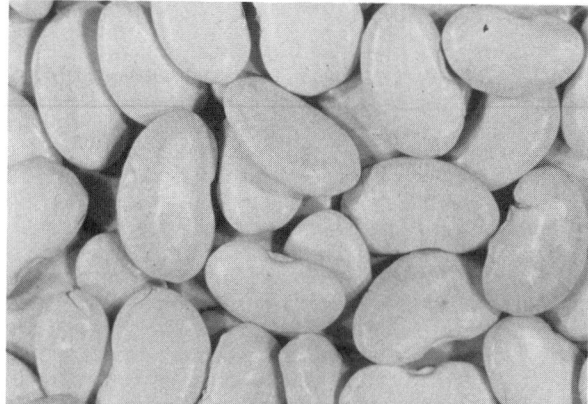

Fig. L-36. Lima beans. (Courtesy, USDA)

[9]Redwood, D. R., *et al.*, "Circulatory and Symptomatic Effects of Physical Training in Patients with Coronary-Artery Disease and Angina Pectoris," *The New England Journal of Medicine*, Vol. 286, May 4, 1972, pp. 959-965.

ORIGIN AND HISTORY. Archaeological evidence shows that large seeded limas were first cultivated in Peru between 7,000 and 8,000 years ago, and that small seeded types were first grown in Mexico much later (1,400 to 1,800 years ago). However, it seems that the two types of lima beans might have been domesticated from a common wild species. The Spanish explorers who came after Columbus discovered America found various types of lima beans growing throughout the Caribbean, Central America, and South America.

PRODUCTION. A long frostfree growing season is required for the production of dried, mature lima beans. Most of the U.S. production is in California, where the beans may be dried in the field with only a very slight chance of rain spoiling the crop. Dry limas account for only about 6% of the dried beans produced in the United States. (Most of the remainder of the dried beans are different varieties of common beans.)

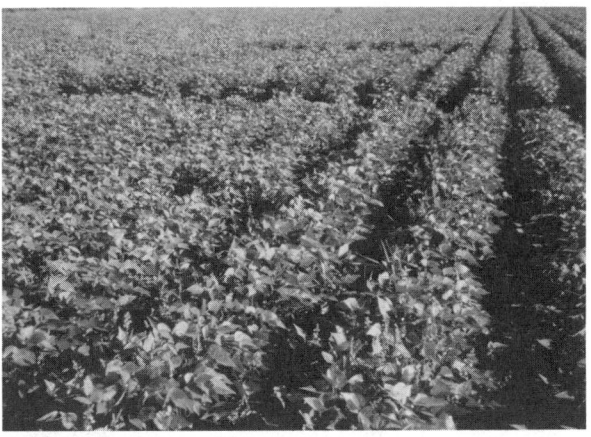

Fig. L-37. A field of lima beans. (Courtesy, Steven R. Temple, Extension Agronomist, University of California, Davis)

Propagation And Growing. Lima beans should not be planted until the danger of frost is past and the soil has reached a temperature of 60°F (*15°C*) or higher, otherwise the seeds may rot before they germinate. The larger varieties of limas require (1) that there be a frostfree growing season of at least 4 months, and (2) that the pods be set ahead of the arrival of prolonged hot weather, because extended high temperature may cause the

flowers to drop. Due to these exacting climatic requirements, large limas are grown commercially only along the coastal areas of California and on the island of Madagascar, off the east coast of Africa—two areas that are far removed from each other, yet have similar marine climates that are mild.

The small types of limas tolerate hot, dry weather better than the large-seeded ones, and they have a shorter growing season. Hence, they may be grown in states other than California. It is noteworthy that the climbing varieties of beans are grown without supports in California, because the dry climate lessens the danger of damage to the plants which lie on the soil.

Harvesting. The beans which are to be sold fresh as green limas are often picked by hand while the pods are still green because (1) under such conditions, the plants will continue to bear and there may be repeated pickings; and (2) mechanical harvestors can only be used for the last harvest of the season, because most of the foliage is stripped from the plants by the machines. However, the cost of labor for hand picking is very high and it may be more profitable to have a single mechanical harvesting operation, even though smaller yields of beans per acre are obtained. The average yield of green beans per acre in the United States is 2,400 lb (*2,688 kg/ha*), but yields as high as 3,000 lb (*3,360 kg/ha*) are obtained in California.

Dried limas are not harvested until the pods start to turn yellow. After cutting, the plants are dried in windrows for about 10 days, then they are threshed to obtain the seeds. The maximum yield of dried beans is about 1,200 lb per acre (*1,344 kg/ha*).

Although the yield of dry lima beans per acre is usually less than half the yield of green limas, the dry beans are generally profitable for growers because (1) labor costs for harvesting are much lower, since the single picking may be done mechanically; (2) they keep well for long periods without the need for refrigeration; and (3) the crop may be stored, then marketed when it is most profitable.

PROCESSING. Only a very small part of the green lima beans grown in the United States is marketed fresh; most of the crop is processed. About 30% of the processed beans is canned and 70% is frozen.

Dried lima beans store well without refrigeration, as long as they are kept under dry conditions and protected from pests. Therefore, they are usually stored after harvesting and either marketed or sent to processors at the most profitable time. Most of the dried beans which are processed are cooked and canned, but small amounts are also ground into flour.

SELECTION AND PREPARATION. Fresh green limas are often marketed in their pods. Hence, the suggestions which follow are noteworthy.

The pods of good quality unshelled lima beans are well filled, clean, bright, fresh, and dark green in color. Dried, shriveled, spotted, yellowing, or flabby pods indicate age or disease. Usually beans from such pods are tough and poor in flavor. Decay may appear on pods as irregular sunken areas, often with accompanying mold.

Shelled lima beans should be plump, have tender skins, and be green or greenish-white in color. Shelled beans are extremely perishable. They deteriorate quickly and soon become moldy or slimy at ordinary temperatures. Shelled limas should be examined closely for mold or breakdown and tested for tenderness by puncturing the skin. Hard, tough skins indicate overmaturity and lack of desirable flavor.

Green limas may be prepared and served in the same ways as green peas—in casseroles, salads, soups, and stews. Usually, they are made tender by 25 to 30 minutes of cooking.

Dry limas have a mild flavor which allows them to mix well with many other foods. Also, their ample protein content makes them nutritionally valuable for extending more expensive animal protein foods such as cheeses, eggs, fish, meats, and poultry. Some ideas for tasty lima bean combinations are presented in Figs. L-38 through L-42.

CAUTION: Many foods contain components which may be harmful under certain circumstances, especially if they have not been improved through breeding, and/or if they are not processed properly; and lima beans are no exception.

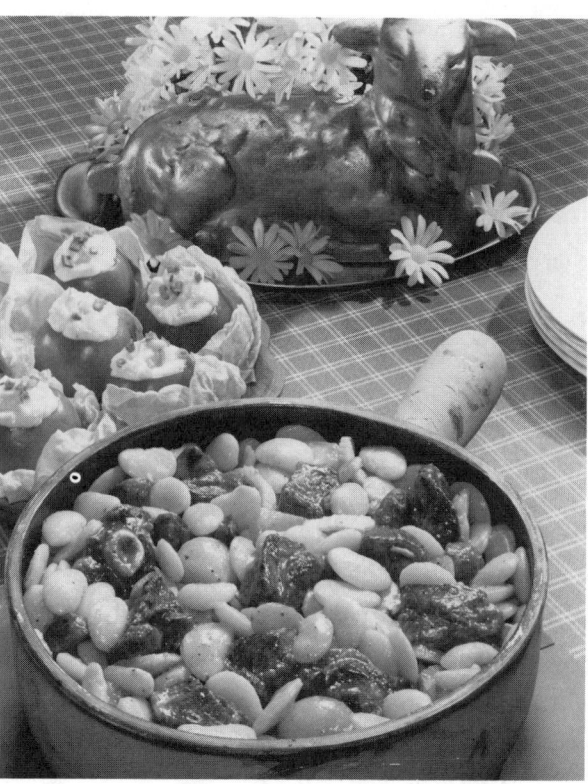

Fig. L-39. Golden limas and lamb. This casserole dish features large limas, lean lamb stew meat, celery, small white onions, carrots, fresh mushrooms, and a variety of delectable seasonings (butter or oil, garlic salt, chicken soup stock, onion salt, tumeric, white pepper, and a dash of brandy or Cognac). (Courtesy, The California Dry Bean Advisory Board, Dinuba, Calif.)

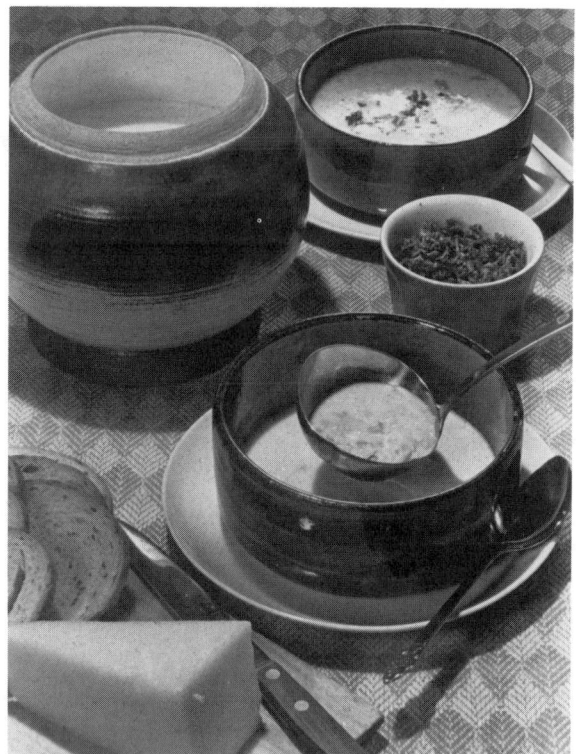

Fig. L-38. Lima-clam chowder. A hearty soup which contains limas, minced clams, evaporated milk, onion, butter or margarine, salt, and pepper. (Courtesy, The California Dry Bean Advisory Board, Dinuba, Calif.)

Some varieties of lima beans, such as those that are native to the Caribbean region—and which are usually colored, contain harmful levels of cyanide-releasing glucosides. In such lima seeds, an enzyme in the legume causes the release of hydrocyanic acid (a cellular poison) from the otherwise inert glucoside. The poison may also be released by the enzyme in *E. coli* bacteria, a normal inhabitant of the human intestine. Fortunately, soaking and cooking the beans releases much of the toxic principle. Also, the *E. coli* population of the human intestine may be reduced by encouraging the growth of *Lactobacilli* species, which are present in fermented dairy products (sour milk, yogurt, etc.). Nevertheless, travelers in the Caribbean region should be wary of eating colored limas.

The varieties of limas grown in the United States contain only negligible amounts of cyanide. Besides, U.S. law prohibits the marketing of lima beans that contain harmful amounts of this toxic factor.

Lima beans also contain inhibitors of trypsin, which bind the digestive enzyme trypsin; and red blood cell clumping agents (hemagglutinins), which cause the red

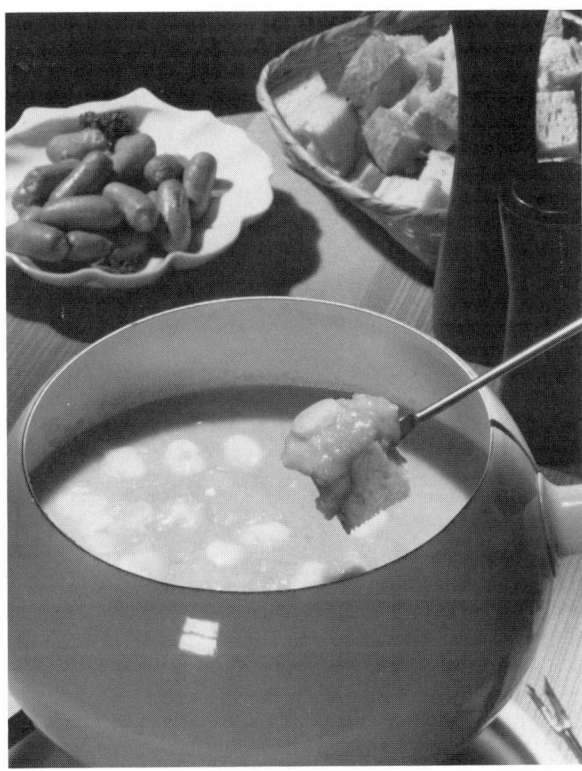

Fig. L-40. Bean and cheese fondue. A rich combination of baby limas, sharp cheese, tomato sauce, green chili salsa, onion, garlic, butter or margarine, and Tabasco sauce. (Courtesy, The California Dry Bean Advisory Board, Dinuba, Calif.)

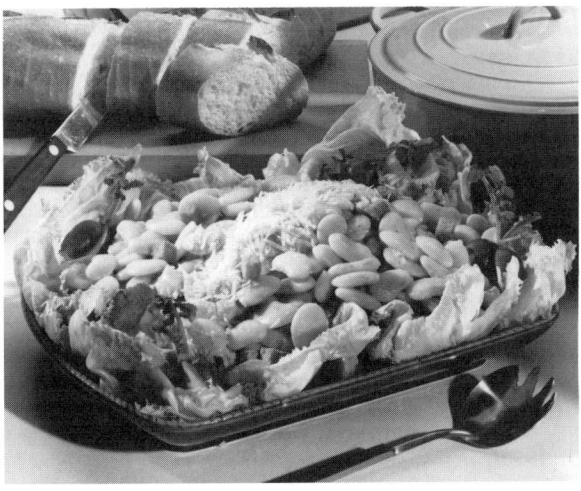

Fig. L-41. California potluck salad. An appetizing dish made from large limas, lettuce, celery, green pepper and pimiento strips, mayonnaise, pickle relish, mustard, dried dill weed, and fresh ground black pepper. (Courtesy, The California Dry Bean Advisory Board, Dinuba, Calif.)

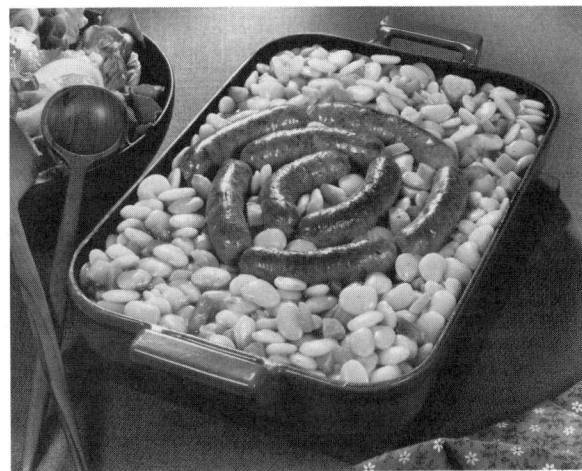

Fig. L-42. Sausage bake with baby limas. This baked casserole presents sausage links on a bed of baby limas, carrot chunks, chopped onion, and pieces of green peppers. (Courtesy, The California Dry Bean Advisory Board, Dinuba, Calif.)

blood cells to clump together. Soaking followed by cooking (steaming, pressure cooking, extrusion cooking), fermentation, or sprouting greatly reduce the effects of trypsin inhibitors and blood cell clumping agents.

Lima beans, in common with most other mature beans, also contain gas-generating carbohydrates—certain indigestible carbohydrates which are acted upon by gas-producing bacteria in the lower intestine. Much of the indigestible carbohydrate may be broken down by incubation of the raw beans in a mildly acid solution for 1 to 2 days. However, people who are greatly troubled with gassiness (flatulence) are admonished not to eat lima beans.

NUTRITIONAL VALUE. The nutrient composition of lima beans is given in Food Composition Table F-36.

Some noteworthy observations regarding the nutritive value of lima beans follow:

1. Cooked mature limas furnish considerably more calories, protein, carbohydrate, phosphorus, iron, and potassium than cooked immature beans ("green limas"). However, the latter are much higher in vitamins A and C. Both types of limas are low in fat.

2. One cup (240 ml) of cooked mature beans contains about the same amount of protein (about 13.9 g) as 2 oz (57 g) of lean meat, but the beans supply more than two times as many calories (233.2 kcal vs 110 kcal).

3. Lima beans, like most other legume seeds, contain much less calcium than phosphorus. Hence, they should be eaten with foods such as milk and green leafy vegetables which have more favorable calcium to phosphorus ratios. An excessively low ratio of dietary calcium to phosphorus will result in poor utilization of

calcium by the body.

4.   Lima bean flour is a concentrated source of both calories and protein.

Protein Quantity And Quality.

Various types of beans are being used all over the world as protein supplements because many people consume only small amounts of animal protein. Lima beans are more acceptable in mixed dishes than many other beans because limas have a milder taste and a lighter color. Therefore, certain facts concerning the quantity and quality of protein in lima beans are noteworthy:

1.   Cooked limas furnish less protein per gram of food, and per calorie than low and medium fat types of cheeses, eggs, fish, meats, milk, and poultry. For example, 3½ oz (100 g) of cooked green lima beans supplying 110 Calories (kcal) are required to provide the amount of protein (about 7 g) in 1¾ oz (50 g) of cottage cheese (53 kcal) or 1 large egg (82 kcal). It is noteworthy, too, that only 3 oz (85 g) of cooked mature limas are equivalent in calorie and protein values to 3½ oz (100 g) of cooked green limas.

2.   Measure for measure, cooked lima beans contain from 2 to 3 times the protein of most cooked cereals. Similarly, lima bean flour provides twice as much protein per calorie as wheat flour.

3.   The protein in lima beans is moderately deficient in the sulfur-containing amino acids methionine and cystine, but it contains ample amounts of lysine, which is deficient in cereal grains. Furthermore, the grains are good sources of methionine and cystine. Therefore, mixtures of the beans with cereal products have a higher quality of protein than either food alone. A good example of this type of mixture is succotash, a combination of lima beans and corn.

4.   Bread made from 70% wheat flour and 30% lima bean flour contains about 40% more protein than bread made from wheat flour alone.[10]

(Also see FLOURS, Table F-26 Special Flours.)

5.   Expensive animal protein foods may be extended by replacing approximately half of the animal protein with an equivalent amount of protein from lima beans, without any significant reduction in the utilization of the dietary protein by the body. Some approximate "equations" of protein value follow:

a.   1 frankfurter + ½ cup cooked beans = 2 frankfurters

b.   10% lima bean flour + 5% skim milk powder + 85% cereal flour = 10% skim milk powder + 90% cereal flour.

However, the substitution of lima beans for protein rich animal foods usually results in the consumption of considerably more calories.

(Also see BEAN[S], Table B-10 Beans of the World; LEGUMES, Table L-2 Legumes of the World; and VEGETABLE[S], Table V-6 Vegetables of the World.)

[10]Luh, B. S., et al., "Biological Quality and Functional Properties of Lima Bean Protein for Bread Enrichment," *Protein Nutritional Quality of Foods and Feeds—Part 2*, edited by M. Friedman, Marcel Dekker, Inc., New York, N.Y., 1975, p. 152, Table 6.

LIME *Citrus aurantifolia*

A rounded fruit that is pointed at both ends and greener than the lemon. The juice of this fruit is used in various refreshing beverages. Limes, like the other citrus fruits, belong to the rue family (*Rutaceae*).

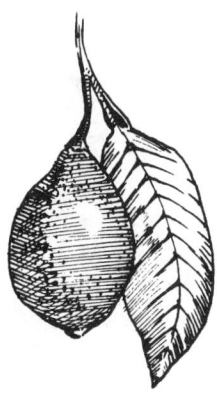

Fig. L-43.   The lime, one of the fruits used to protect sailors against scurvy. The fruit is small (diameter 1½ to 2½ in.; *3 to 6 cm*).

ORIGIN AND HISTORY.

The lime originated somewhere in Southeast Asia between northeastern India and Malaysia. It is not certain when Arab traders first took the fruit to Arabia, but it was before 900 A.D., which was about when they introduced it into Egypt. In the centuries that followed, the lime was grown in the Arab lands of North Africa, and it was introduced into Spain by the 13th century. The fruit was also introduced into Europe by the Crusaders who took it from the Holy Land to France and Italy.

Columbus took lime seeds to Haiti during his second voyage to the New World in 1493. In a short time, lime trees were grown on many of the islands in the Caribbean. As a result, the small, cold-sensitive variety that was grown in this region came to be known as the West Indian lime. It is noteworthy that limes are better adapted than lemons to the hot, humid tropics. The ready availability of limes from their colonies in the West Indies was a major reason for the substitution of lime juice for the lemon juice that as given to British sailors to prevent scurvy. After that, British sailors were called "limeys."

Spanish explorers introduced the West Indian lime into Mexico and the Florida Keys during the 16th century. Since then, this fruit has also been known as Mexican lime and Key lime. Florida was ceded to the United States by Spain in 1821. The early settlers of this territory found a few wild lime trees and planted some new trees in the Florida Keys, where the climate was the most suitable for this fruit. Key limes were produced on a small scale in Florida for almost 100 years until many of the trees were destroyed by the hurricane of 1926.

The West Indian lime was planted in California by Spanish padres during the 17th century, but this variety grew poorly in that location and attempts to produce the fruit were abandoned. Later, the gold rush of 1849 created a demand for lemons and limes because it was well known by then that these fruits prevented scurvy. Fresh fruits and vegetables were scarce in California, and many prospectors and miners came down with scurvy. Hence, limes were imported from Mexico and Tahiti. Also, some Tahiti lime trees were planted in southern California, but after 1880 they were replaced by lemon trees because the latter fruit was more profitable to growers. It is noteworthy that the Tahiti lime, which is sometimes erroneously called the Persian lime, is larger and grows better in cool weather than the West Indian lime.

The Florida lime industry gradually recovered after its destruction by the hurricane of 1926. However, the greatest increase in production occurred in the 1950s, when the frozen citrus juice concentrates were first marketed. Most of the Florida lime trees are now of the Tahiti variety, which grows well on the mainland, as well as on the Florida Keys.

PRODUCTION. In recent years, the annual world production of lemons and limes has been about 6.6 million metric tons. About one-tenth of the world's crop comes from Florida, where the larger (lemon size) and more cold resistant Tahiti and Bearss (a mutant variety of the Tahiti lime) limes are grown. Small amounts of these varieties are also grown in California and Arizona. The rest of the world crop consists mainly of the very cold-sensitive, walnut-size West Indian or Mexican lime which is grown in India, Mexico, Egypt, West Indies and other tropical areas.

Details regarding the growing of citrus fruits are given elsewhere.

(Also see CITRUS FRUITS, section headed "Production.")

PROCESSING. A little more than half of the U.S. lime crop is utilized fresh, and the rest is processed into lime juice, limeades and similar beverages, soft drinks, marmalades, syrups, and lime oil. Descriptions of these and other products are given elsewhere.

(Also see CITRUS FRUITS, section headed "Processing.")

SELECTION. Fresh limes that are green in color and heavy for their size are the most desirable. Deep-yellow-colored fruits do not have the desired acidity.

Decay and mold may affect limes in the same manner that they affect lemons. Limes often become spotted with purple-to-brown colored and irregular-shaped spots. Sometimes the whole fruit turns brown. This is the result of a defect known as scald. Such fruit has a poor appearance and brings a lower price than sound fruit, but in many cases the flesh is unaffected, although occasionally a tainted, moldy taste can be detected immediately below the spots.

Guidelines for the selection of processed lime products are given elsewhere.

(Also see CITRUS FRUITS, section headed "Selection and Preparation.")

PREPARATION. Many adult Americans have used alcoholic drinks made with lime juice. It is commonly used in the "coolers" served in hot weather. However,

there are other good uses for fresh limes and lime juice. For example, the whole fruit makes excellent marmalade after slicing and removing the seeds. Also, the freshly squeezed juice imparts a superb flavor to fish and seafood dishes, fruits and fruit juices, meats, pie fillings, puddings, salad dressings, and sauces.

CAUTION: Some people are allergic to one or more constituents of citrus peel. When such allergies are suspected, neither the peel nor the products containing it should be consumed, and fruit juice should be extracted gently to avoid squeezing the oil and other substances from the peel into the juice. It is noteworthy that some of the commercially prepared lime juices and lime drinks may contain peel and/or substances extracted from it, but that prepared citrus juice products for infants contain little or none of the peel constituents.

Suggestions for preparing dishes from processed lime products are given elsewhere.

NUTRITIONAL VALUE. The nutrient compositions of various forms of limes are given in Food composition Table F-36.

Some noteworthy observations regarding the nutrient composition of limes follow:

1. Fresh limes are low in calories (28 kcal per 100 g). they are good sources of potassium, vitamin C, and bioflavonoids.
2. Fresh lime juice is similar to fresh limes in caloric and nutrient levels, except that the juice is likely to be much lower in bioflavonoids, which are found mainly in the peel and the membranes within the fruit.
3. Reconstituted frozen limeade concentrate contains about 50% more calories, but is much lower in nutrients than fresh lime juice.
4. Bottled lime juice contains only about two-thirds as much vitamin C as fresh lime juice.
5. Citrus peel contains citral, an aldehyde which antagonizes the effects of vitamin A. Hence, people should make certain that their dietary supply of this vitamin is adequate before consuming large amounts of lime peel.

(Also see BIOFLAVONOIDS; CITRUS FRUITS; FRUIT[S], Table F-47 Fruits of the World; POTASSIUM; and VITAMIN C.)

LIMITING AMINO ACID

The essential amino acid of a protein which shows the greatest percentage deficit in comparison with the amino acids contained in the same quantity of another protein selected as a standard.

(Also see AMINO ACID[S]; and PROTEIN.)

LIMONIN

The chemical responsible for the bitter principle of lemons. It is contained in the white spongy inner part of the rind. Too much limonin released into the juice during extraction produces bitter juice.

LINGONBERRY (COWBERRY) *Vacinnium vitis-idaea*

The fruit of a vine (of the family *Ericaceae*) that grows wild throughout the cool, temperate regions of North America and Europe. Lingonberries, which are much esteemed in the Scandinavian countries, closely resemble their nearest relative, the cranberry, and are about the same size. They are too tart to be eaten raw, but they make excellent jams and jellies.

LINOLEIC ACID

An 18-carbon unsaturated fatty acid having two double bonds. It is one of the essential fatty acids.
(Also see FAT; and FATTY ACIDS.)

LINOLENIC ACID

An 18-carbon unsaturated fatty acid having three double bonds.
(Also see FAT; and FATTY ACIDS.)

LIPASE

A fat-splitting enzyme, present in gastric juice and pancreatic juice. It acts on fats to produce fatty acids and glycerol.
(Also see DIGESTION AND ABSORPTION; and ENZYME.)

LIP, CLEFT (HARELIP)

Usually infants born with a cleft palate (roof of the mouth) also have a cleft lip. These are congenital defects characterized by a gap in the palate and a gap in the upper lip. The condition may be bilateral—occurring on both sides of the face under each nostril. Infants with a cleft palate and/or lip have difficulty sucking, drinking, eating and swallowing. Hence, they require some special feeding techniques, depending upon the degree of the defect. Fortunately new plastic surgery methods have been developed and may be employed as early as the third month of life. Nevertheless, afflicted infants must build up their reserves for surgery; hence, the following suggestions will help to cope with feeding problems:

1. Sucking difficulties can be overcome by using a nipple with an enlarged opening, a medicine dropper, or a 10-20 cc syringe with a 2-in. (*5 cm*) piece of rubber tubing.
2. The tendency to choke should be countered by offering liquids slowly and in small amounts.
3. Frequent burpings are necessary as large amounts of air may be swallowed.
4. Irritating food such as spicy and acid foods should be avoided.
5. Foods such as peanut butter, nuts, leafy vegetables and creamed dishes may adhere to the palate.

6. Pureed foods may be given from a bottle with a large nipple opening if diluted with milk, fruit juice or broth.
7. Extra time should be allowed for feeding, and possibly five or six small meals may be better than three larger ones.
8. Supplementing the diet with the proper amounts of vitamins will insure optimal health and growth.

LIPIDES

An alternate, less used spelling of lipids.
(Also see LIPIDS.)

LIPIDS

An all-embracing term referring to any compound that is soluble in chloroform, benzene, petroleum or ether. Included are fats, oils, waxes, sterols and complex compounds such as phospholipids and sphingolipids. There are three basic types of lipids—simple lipids, compound lipids, and derived lipids. When fatty acids are esterified with alcohols, simple lipids result. If compounds such as choline or serine are esterified to alcohols in addition to fatty acids, compound lipids result. The third type of lipid, derived lipids, result from the hydrolysis of simple and compound lipids. The sterols and fatty acids are derived lipids.
(Also see FATS AND OTHER LIPIDS; and OILS, VEGETABLE.)

LIPOGENESIS

The formation of fat.

LIPOIC ACID

Lipoic acid is a fat-soluble, sulfur-containing substance. It is not a true vitamin because it can be synthesized in the body and is not necessary in the diet of animals. However, it functions in the same manner as many of the B-complex vitamins.

HISTORY. The continuing study of thiamin as a coenzyme in carbohydrate metabolism revealed that this metabolic system required other coenzyme factors in addition to thiamin. In work with lactic acid bacteria, Reed discovered, in 1951, that one of these factors is a fat-soluble acid which he named lipoic acid (after the Greek *lipos* for fat).

FUNCTIONS. Lipoic acid functions as a coenzyme. It is essential, together with the thiamin-containing enzyme, pyrophosphatase (TPP), for reactions in carbohydrate metabolism which convert pyruvic acid to acetyl-coenzyme A. Lipoic acid, which has two sulfur bonds of high-energy potential, combines with TPP to reduce pyruvate to active acetate, thereby sending it into the final energy cycle. It joins the intermediary products of protein and fat metabolism in the Krebs cycle in the reactions involved in producing energy from these nutrients. A metal ion (magnesium or calcium) is involved in this oxidative decarboxylation, along with lipoic acid and four vitamins: thiamin, pantothenic acid, niacin, and riboflavin. Thus, this underscores the concept of the interdependent relationships among the vitamins.

RECOMMENDED DIETARY ALLOWANCE OF LIPOIC ACID.
Because the body can synthesize the needed lipoic acid, no dietary requirement for humans or animals has been established.

SOURCES OF LIPOIC ACID.
Lipoic acid is found in many foods. Yeast and liver are rich sources. (Also see VITAMIN[S], Table V-9.)

LIPOLYSIS

The hydrolysis of fats by enzymes, acids, alkalis, or other means to yield glycerol and fatty acids.

LIPOLYTIC RANCIDITY

Food spoilage that is caused by the enzymatic breakdown of fats by lipases. Lipases are produced by some microorganisms, and are present in tissues. Heating destroys the lipases, preventing this type of spoilage.

(Also see FATS AND OTHER LIPIDS; PRESERVATION OF FOOD; and RANCIDITY.)

LIPOPROTEIN

A lipid-protein complex that is water soluble. Hence, it is involved in the transport of lipids in the blood. Four types of lipoprotein circulate in the blood, all of which contain the lipids, triglycerides, cholesterol and phospholipid in varying proportions. The four types of lipoprotein are (1) chylomicrons—lowest density; (2) very low density, VLDL; (3) low density, LDL; and (4) high density, HDL.

(Also see CHOLESTEROL; DIGESTION AND ABSORPTION; and FATS AND OTHER LIPIDS.)

LIPOTROPIC (FACTOR)

A substance that prevents accumulation of fat in the liver. Choline is probably the most important of the lipotropic factors. So, any substance capable of contributing methyl groups for choline synthesis is lipotropic. (Also see CHOLINE, section headed "Functions.")

LIQUID DIETS

Contents   Page

This term covers a wide variety of dietary preparations that range from clear liquids which provide little in the way of nourishment to nearly complete diets in liquid form. For example, an infant formula is one type of liquid diet, whereas tube feedings are another.

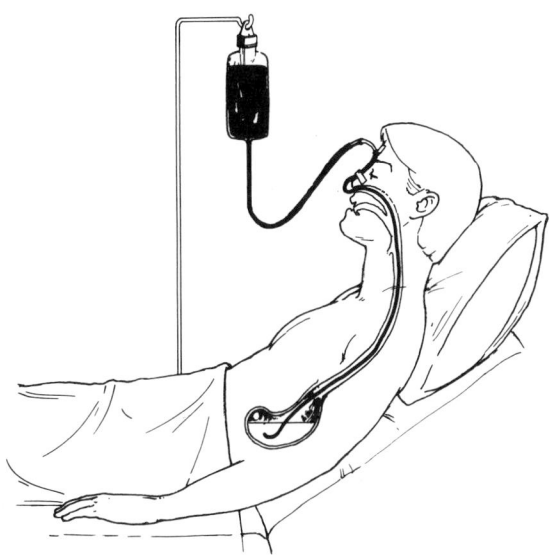

Fig. L-44. A hospital patient being tube fed a liquid diet. This type of feeding may be a lifesaver for people who are unable to eat in the normal way.

The use of liquid diets is growing rapidly, as evidenced by the various types of canned products that may be found in supermarkets and pharmacies. Some time ago, a leading New York department store installed a vending machine which dispensed a liquid dietary formula in paper cups so that workers in the vicinity could gulp their lunch down quickly and spend most of their lunch hour shopping.

TYPES OF LIQUID DIETS. The major types of liquid diets are described in Table L-3.

NOTE: Liquid diets should be used only after consulting a doctor. This caution also applies to liquid reducing diets.

TABLE L-3
MAJOR TYPES OF LIQUID DIETS

Diet	Composition		Uses	Comments
	Foods[1] Included	Foods Excluded		
Clear liquid	Only clear liquids such as tea; coffee; carbonated beverages; cereal beverages (coffee substitutes); flavored gelatin; ices made from strained fruit juices; fruit juices and drinks without pulp; fat-free fish, meat, and poultry broths; consomme; bouillon; sugar; clear syrups; and honey.	All others.	To maintain the body's water balance when other foods and beverages cannot be taken by mouth, or when it is necessary to clear the colon of residue (in preparation for x rays; prior to, and following surgery on the digestive tract; during diarrheal disease; or as an initial oral feeding during the recovery of a critically ill patient).	This diet should be used for only a few days because it is deficient in almost all of the essential nutrients. Elemental diets serve most of the same purposes and are much more suitable for long-term use.
Elemental (semisynthetic liquid diet) (Also see ELEMENTAL DIETS.)	Formula powders that are mixed with water and/or carbonated or noncarbonated fruit drinks that are free of fibrous residues, or bouillon. Essential nutrients are provided in the following forms: Carbohydrates as sugars and other well absorbed, rapidly utilized saccharides. Fat (usually only 0 to 10% of the diet) as a vegetable oil. (1) Amino acids as chemically pure crystalline powders; or (2) A protein hydrolysate such as digested casein; or (3) Egg albumin. Mineral salts and vitamins in chemically pure forms.	All others, unless allowed by a doctor, or a dietitian.	To promote ease of digestion and absorption and minimize food residue in the colon, while providing nearly all of the required nutrients, prior to and following surgery on the digestive tract; during diarrheal disease, infections, or inflammatory conditions; for the rehabilitation of severely injured and/or malnourished patients; minimizing nausea due to chemotherapy and/or radiation treatments; or as an initial oral feeding during the recovery of a critically ill patient. May also be used in tube feeding.	None of the products now available contain the essential trace minerals chromium and selenium, and only some brands contain vitamin K. Therefore, these nutrients must be provided by other means if an elemental diet is the sole means of nourishment for more than a few weeks. Patients have been maintained in good condition on elemental diets for as long as a year or more.
Full liquid	Liquids and liquified solid foods (most homemade preparations are made in a blender)[2] as follows: Finely homogenized and strained fish, meat, or poultry (visible fat should be removed before homogenization) Any type or kind of milk or cream (if dietary fat is not restricted)[3,4]	All other forms of fish, meat, or poultry. None, unless dietary fat is restricted[3,4].	For patients who are unable to chew and/or swallow foods due to circumstances such as surgery on the face, oral cavity, neck, or throat; fractures of the jaw; esophageal strictures; partial paralysis; or unconsciousness[5]. As nutritional supplements for people who find it difficult to eat sufficient amounts of ordinary foods. By athletes prior to, and/or during sporting events because liquids leave the stomach more rapidly than solid foods. Weight reduction, when a liquid diet is used at one or more daily meals in place of foods that supply more calories.	The daily allotment is usually divided into 6 oral or tube feedings[5]. Milk, milk drinks, and strained fruit or vegetable juices may be served between meals.[4] Underweight patients may need supplemental feedings (commonly called "nourishments") that are rich in calories from foods such as melted butter or margarine (added to hot liquids), or honey, sugar, or syrups (added to fruit juices).
	Strained cottage cheese[4].	All other forms of cheese.		
	Eggs in cooked foods such as puddings and soft custards.	All other forms of eggs.		
	Strained fruit juices, pureed and strained fruits.	Berries containing small seeds.		

Footnotes at end of table

(Continued)

TABLE L-3 *(Continued)*

Diet	Composition		Uses	Comments
	Foods[1] Included	**Foods Excluded**		
Full liquid *(Continued)*				
	Strained vegetable juices, pureed and strained mild flavored vegetables such as asparagus, beans (green and wax), beets, carrots, peas, potatoes, spinach, squash, sweet potatoes, and tomatoes.	Strong flavored vegetables.		Liquid diets are usually deficient in certain nutrients. Hence, the doctor or dietitian may recommend certain mineral and vitamin supplements if the diet is to be used for more than a week or so.
	Cereal gruels made from enriched refined cooked cereals.	All prepared or dry cereals, and all whole-grain cooked cereals. All forms of bread.		
	Moderate amounts of butter, margarine, oil, or cream[3].	All other forms of fat.		
	Cream or broth-type soups made with pureed vegetables, strained meats or poultry, broth, bouillon, or consomme.	Highly seasoned soups or those containing pieces of vegetables, meats, or poultry.		
	Sugar, honey, syrups, jelly, and plain sugar candy.	Jams and marmalades.		
	Plain ice cream, sherbets, ices, puddings, junket preparations, soft custard, tapioca, and plain dessert gels.	Desserts that contain nuts, fruit, coconut, or other solids.		
	Coffee, tea, carbonated beverages, cocoa, and cereal beverages (coffee substitutes).	All other beverages.		
	Salt, mild spices, and vanilla and other mild flavorings in moderate amounts.	All other types of condiments, flavorings, seasonings, and spices.		

Footnotes at end of table

(Continued)

TABLE L-3 (*Continued*)

Diet	Composition — Foods[1] Included	Composition — Foods Excluded	Uses	Comments
Infant formulas (Also see BABY FOODS; BREAST FEEDING; and INFANT DIET AND NUTRITION.)	Commercially produced infant formulas based mainly on milk or a milk substitute (usually soy protein isolates or pureed beef or lamb) that may contain added vegetable oil, sweetener, mineral salts, and/or vitamins. Homemade formulas prepared from diluted cow's milk with or without an added sweetener.	Homogenized cow's milk is not considered suitable for infants younger than 6 months, but evaporated milk is usually tolerated well.	In lieu of breast feeding young infants, and for older infants who do not tolerate cow's milk well. May be used by older children and adults who require liquid diets, when the latter is not available. Special modified types of infant formulas are available for children who have intolerances to certain foods and nutrients, but should be used only after consulting a doctor.	Some formulas furnish all of the nutrients required by infants, whereas, others should be supplemented by mineral and vitamin preparations. Infants aged 6 months and older should receive other foods besides a formula, in order to develop good eating habits.
Special dietary products	Liquid or powdered (for mixing with water, milk, or other suitable liquid) dietary preparations that are designed to meet the special needs of patients placed on certain modified diets. Most of the products contain the appropriate types of carbohydrates, fats, amino acids or proteins, mineral salts and vitamins; but some furnish only supplementary nutrients for meeting unusual requirements.	Some products may contain little or no allergens, cholesterol, electrolytes, lactose, milk protein, protein in general, saturated fat, sodium, or other substances that are deemed to aggravate the patient's condition.	As a substitute for a normal diet that may be unsuitable in composition for the patient. Provision of calories and/or nutrients in addition to those in the normal diet where patients cannot or will not consume foods that supply the essential nutrients.	The use of these products alone may become very expensive and monotonous for the patient, who may benefit more by consuming homemade items prepared from common foods by modified recipes (when it is feasible for a lay person to prepare them).
Supplemental feedings	Dietary formulations designed to provide extra calories, proteins, and other nutrients in easily digested and readily absorbed forms when the patient is already receiving some, but not all of his or her nutrient requirements from another source. Most products contain sugars, powdered milk or a substitute for milk protein, vegetable oils or their derivatives, added mineral salts and vitamins, and flavorings such as vanilla and chocolate.	Nutrients that are poorly digested or slowly absorbed, such as fiber, and long chain fatty acids.	Supplementation of the normal or therapeutic diets of growing children, athletes, underweight adults, people recovering from debilitating illnesses, injuries, burns, surgery, gastrointestinal disorders, anorexia, and various other conditions in which nutritional needs are likely to be in excess of the nourishment provided by the unsupplemented diets.	Some of the products in this category are called "nourishments" after the traditional dietary practice of providing certain patients with extra feedings between meals. In the past, these feedings often consisted of items such as cream, milk, milk drinks, puddings, custards, and other high-calorie foods.

Footnotes at end of table

(Continued)

TABLE L-3 (*Continued*)

Diet	Composition		Uses	Comments
	Foods[1] Included	**Foods Excluded**		
Tube feedings	Mixtures of liquids, dissolved powders, and/or pureed solid foods of sufficiently fluid consistencies to pass through feeding tubes without clogging them. Some typical ingredients of the common types of feedings are: commercial formulas; whole milk, evaporated milk, strained buttermilk, and/or ice cream; strained pureed meats, hard cooked yolk, fruits, and/or vegetables; fruit juices; sugar, syrup, and/or honey; added mineral salts and vitamins; and flavorings such as vanilla and chocolate.	Foods and nutrients that are poorly digested or slowly absorbed, such as fiber and long chain fatty acids. Substances that are likely to settle out and clog the tube are also excluded, such as pieces of foods, nuts, seeds, chocolate chips, milk curds, solidified fats, and powders that are difficult to dissolve.	Nutritional support of people who are unable to chew and/or swallow ordinary foods due to surgery on the face, oral cavity, neck, or throat; fractures of the jaw; esophageal strictures; injury, inflammation, or surgery affecting one or more parts of the upper digestive tract; partial paralysis, or unconsciousness. Sometimes, tube feedings are used for force feeding people who refuse to eat and become emaciated, such as those with anorexia nervosa or protesters on a "hunger strike."[6] The tube for feeding may be inserted (1) up through the nose and down to the stomach (nasogastric feeding), (2) through the nose and down to the duodenum (nasoduodenal feeding), (3) into an opening on the abdomen leading to the stomach (gastrostomy feeding), or (4) into an opening on the abdomen leading to the jejunen (jejunostomy feeding).	Care has to be taken that tube feedings are not regurgitated and aspirated into the lungs. This may be prevented by giving the initial feeding at only 1/2 strength, keeping the rate of feeding slow; and by allowing the patient to rest in a sitting position after an intermittent feeding of a large volume of formula. It is noteworthy that some tube feeding formulas have a high concentration of dissolved materials (solutes) and may cause dehydration and/or diarrhea unless some additional water is given. Detailed instructions for tube feedings may be obtained from the manufacturers of the formulas and from nursing manuals.

[1]Many liquid diets provide nutrients in highly purified forms rather than in the forms of ordinary foods.

[2]Commercial formulas prepared from liquified solid foods are available from certain suppliers of liquid diets.

[3]When fat must be restricted, use skim milk or buttermilk in place of whole milk or cream; and use no butter, margarine, or other fats or oils in preparing foods.

[4]Some patients who were previously tolerant of milk products develop temporary intolerances to milk sugar. In such cases milk and milk products must be excluded from the diet.

[5]Full liquid diets must be administered by tube feeding when it is likely that the patient is unable to swallow or to ingest liquids without choking or irritating the mouth and esophagus.

[6]Long-term deliberate or unavoidable abstention from the consumption of adequate food may result in a loss of appetite and other abnormalities that often necessitate forced feeding to initiate recovery of the normal eating and digestive functions.

HOMEMADE PREPARATIONS. Considerable money may be saved on certain types of liquid diets when they must be used at home for long periods of time by using homemade preparations rather than commercial formulas. However, good results are ensured only if the following precautions are taken:

1. All food materials are fresh, the preparation and feeding equipment is kept very clean, and good sanitary practices are followed to prevent contamination by infectious microorganisms, unrinsed soap and detergents, and other harmful agents.

2. The types, amounts, and proportions of ingredients are determined after consultation with a doctor and/or a dietitian.

3. Diarrhea and other digestive disorders are reported to the doctor promptly so that the formula and/or method of administration may be changed if necessary.

SUMMARY. Providing most of a patient's nutrient needs by a liquid diet may be done successfully over long periods of time if this means of nourishment is carried out according to the recommendations of a doctor and/or a dietitian.

LITHIASIS

The formation of calculi (stones) of any kind (as in the urinary tract and gallbladder).

LIVETINS

A collective term for the principal water-soluble proteins that are found in egg yolk—an albumin, a glycoprotein and a globulin.

(Also see EGG.)

LOFENALAC

This term is the registered trademark of the commercially prepared protein formula sold by Mead Johnson & Company of Evansville, Indiana. Ninety-five percent of the amino acid phenylalanine is removed from Lofenalac. It provides the basis for dietary management of phenylketonuria (PKU), an inborn error of metabolism. Most proteins contain 4 to 6% phenylalanine and would be detrimental to an infant with PKU. Lofenalac is used to meet the infant's protein and energy needs while the requirement for phenylalanine, an essential amino acid, is just satisfied—no excess—with foods whose phenylalanine content is known.

(Also see INBORN ERRORS OF METABOLISM; and PHENYLKETONURIA.)

LOGANBERRY *Rubus loganbaccus*

A reddish-purple type of blackberry (fruit of the *Rosaceae* family) that was discovered growing in the garden of Judge Logan of Santa Cruz, California in 1881.

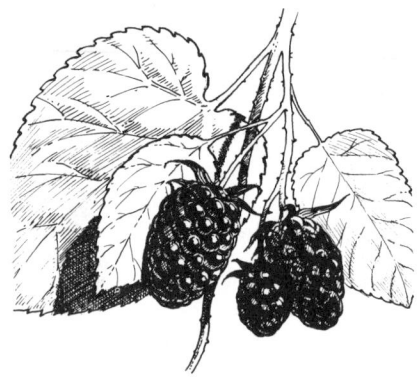

Fig. L-45. Loganberries.

It is believed to have originated as a result of a natural crossbreeding (hybridization) between a western wild blackberry and a domesticated variety of red raspberry.

The loganberry is grown mainly in the central coast region of California, the Willamette Valley of Oregon, and the southwestern part of British Columbia around Vancouver.

Only about 2% of the U.S. crop of loganberries is marketed fresh. The rest is canned, frozen, and made into jam, jelly, juice, and wine. It is noteworthy that the sharp tartness of the fresh berries is improved by cooking.

The nutrient compositions of various forms of loganberries are given in Food Composition Table F-36.

Some noteworthy observations regarding the nutrient composition of loganberries follow:

1. The raw fruit is moderately high in calories (62 kcal per 100 g) and carbohydrates (15%). It is an excellent source of fiber, a good source of potassium, iron, and vitamin C, and only a poor to fair source of vitamin A.

2. Canned loganberries contain about two-thirds of the nutrients of the fresh fruit, except that much of the vitamin C is destroyed during processing. Also, the products containing syrups may be rather high in caloric content.

LOGARITHMIC PHASE (EXPONENTIAL PHASE; LOG PHASE)

Pertaining to bacterial cultures in an adequate medium it is the period of most rapid growth when numbers increase in geometric progression. On a rich medium bacteria can double in numbers every 20 minutes.

LONGAN *Euphoria longana; Nephelium longana*

The fruit of a tree (of the *Sapindaceae* family) that is native to the Asian tropics, and is now grown in some of the other tropical regions of the world. Longans are round, yellowish-brown fruits that contain a white, juicy pulp.

The nutrient compositions of raw and dried longans are given in Food Composition Table F-36.

Some noteworthy observations regarding the nutrient composition of longans follow:

1. The raw fruit is moderately high in calories (62 kcal per 100 g) and carbohydrates (14.9%). It is a good source of iron, but a poor source of vitamin C.

2. Dried longans contain about 5 times the nutrient levels of the fresh fruit. The vitamin C content is apparently retained completely during drying. Hence, the dried fruit is suitable for a nutritious high-calorie (286 kcal per 100 g) snack that contains almost 5% protein, 2% fiber, and is an excellent source of phosphorus and potassium, and a good source of vitamin C.

LONGEVITY

Long-lived.

LOW DENSITY LIPOPROTEIN (LDL)

A lipoprotein with a density of 1.006 to 1.063; composed of about 21% protein; high in cholesterol (free, 8%; ester, 38%).
(Also see BETA-LIPOPROTEINS.)

LUCERNE (ALFALFA) *Medicago sativa*

The plant known as alfalfa (botanically *Medicago sativa*) in the United States is called lucerne in many parts of the world.
(See ALFALFA.)

LUPUS ERYTHEMATOSUS

Recent research indicates that systemic lupus erythematosus is primarily a disease of the immune system in which antigen-antibody complexes cause tissue damage. An early manifestation of the disease is the erosive inflammation of the skin typically in the form of a "butterfly rash" over the nose and cheeks. This rash gave the disease its original name—*lupus erythematosus* or *red wolf*. Besides the rash, other symptoms of lupus include an intermittent fever, severe joint pain, and periods of extreme fatigue. It afflicts about one woman in 500 in the United States, and about one-tenth as many men. Lupus affects not only the skin, but, at different times in different individuals, it may affect the joints, the blood vessels, the heart, the lungs, and the brain—and most significantly the kidneys. The disease probably arises from an interplay of genetics, drugs, hormones and viruses. Methods for early diagnosis have led to improved control of lupus, thereby preventing irreversible tissue damage, particularly to the kidneys.

Part of treatment for lupus may involve cortisone or other steroids to control the inflammation; hence, a sodium-restricted diet may be necessary. Should the kidneys become involved, dietary changes similar to those for kidney diseases may be recommended.
(Also see KIDNEY DISEASES; and MODIFIED DIETS.)

LYCOPENE

A chemical similar to carotene, but it has no vitamin A activity. It is the principal red pigment present in tomatoes, watermelon, pink grapefruit, paprika, rose hips and palm oil.

LYMPH

The slightly yellow, transparent fluid occupying the lymphatic channels of the body. It is derived from the fluid between the cells—interstitial fluid. The chemical makeup of lymph is similar to that of blood plasma. Following a meal, some of the fat from the diet is ab-sorbed into the lymph in the form of chylomicrons.
(Also see BODY FLUIDS; DIGESTION AND ABSORPTION; and LIPOPROTEIN.)

LYMPHATIC SYSTEM

All the vessels and structures that carry lymph from the tissues to the blood.

LYOPHILIZATION (FREEZE DRYING)

A process of rapid freezing followed by drying under a vacuum. The ice sublimes off as water vapor without melting. Freeze drying results in the least damage to foods of all the commercial processes for drying. It can be applied to all foods, both raw and cooked, which can withstand freezing. Freeze drying yields a product that is dried without shrink, and which has a highly porous structure favoring rapid rehydration. After rehydration, freeze-dried foods are often indistinguishable from their commercially frozen counterparts.
(Also see PRESERVATION OF FOOD.)

LYSERGIC ACID

A chemical derived from the hydrolysis (breakdown) of the alkaloids of the fungus ergot. It is thought to be the active component of ergot. Lysergic acid can produce a state resembling psychosis. Also, its diethylamide derivative, LSD, is a potent hallucinogenic drug.
(Also see POISONS, Table P-11 Some Potentially Poisonous [Toxic] Substances—"Ergot.")

LYSINE

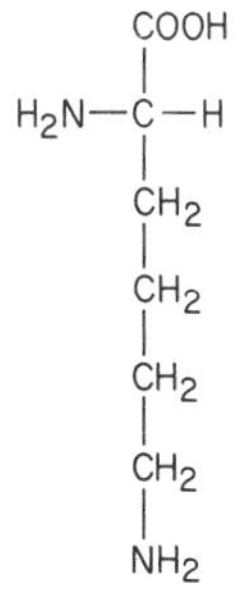

Fig. L-46. The structure of lysine.

Lysine is an essential amino acid. The body requires lysine but cannot synthesize it so it must be provided in the diet. High quality protein foods provide lysine. However, lysine is the limiting amino acid in most cereals—foods for much of the world. It is present in cereal grains, but at low levels. Inadequate lysine in the diet may create a negative nitrogen balance—protein being broken down and excreted. Chemically, lysine is unique among the essential amino acids since it possesses two amino groups (NH_2). This can further affect the availability of lysine when it is in short supply. All other essential amino acids possess one amino group. Since lysine, in the form of lysine monohydrochlorine, can be commercially produced at a reasonable cost, much consideration has been given to the supplementation of cereals with lysine in an effort to improve the nutrition of people who depend largely upon cereal grains.

INVOLVEMENT IN THE BODY. The requirement of lysine for growth is quite high, since tissue proteins contain a high proportion of lysine. Infants require 45 mg/lb (*99 mg/kg*) of body weight per day, and growing children require 20 mg/lb (*44 mg/kg*) of body weight per day, while adults require only 5.5 mg/lb (*12 mg/kg*) of body weight per day. Rats fed diets deficient in lysine grow very little while the addition of lysine to the same diet significantly increases growth. Since protein synthesis—growth of tissue—is an all-or-none phenomenon, it requires that all amino acids necessary for synthesis be present. Otherwise, synthesis will not proceed; hence, growth will be limited. The protein in most cereal grains is poorly utilized by infants and children due to its low lysine content.

SOURCES. Lysine may be obtained from both plant and animal dietary proteins. However, in terms of lysine content, plant proteins and animal proteins are not created equal. In general, plant proteins contain less lysine than animal proteins.

Plant Vs Animal. Protein is a part of all tissue—plant or animal. The seeds of many plants supply protein, hence lysine to mankind; for example, wheat, corn, barley, lentils, peas, rice, and soybeans. Likewise, all animal foods—except pure fats—are good protein sources and, therefore, provide lysine. Table L-4 compares the lysine content of some common protein sources.

Cereal grains—barley, corn, oats, rice, and wheat—are low in lysine as Table L-4 shows, whereas the lysine content of legumes—lentils, peas, and soybeans—is better. The lysine content of animal products is highest.

TABLE L-4
LYSINE CONTENT OF SOME COMMON FOODS[1]

Food	Lysine	
	(mg/100 g)[2]	(mg/g protein)[3]
Beef steak, cooked	2999	98
Chicken, cooked	1830	86
Cheese, cheddar	2072	83
Pork chop, cooked	2044	83
Cod, cooked	2421	83
Sardines, canned	1552	83
Lamb leg, roasted	2081	82
Milk, cow's (2% fat)	264	80
Soybeans, cooked	759	69
Eggs	820	68
Lentils, cooked	476	61
Peas, green, cooked	254	47
Peanuts, roasted	1176	45
Rice, brown, cooked	99	40
Oatmeal, dry	521	37
Wheat, parboiled (bulgur)	217	35
Barley, pearled light, uncooked.	279	34
Corn meal, cooked	29	26

[1]Data from Protein and Amino Acid Content of Selected Foods, Table P-37.
[2]One hundred grams is approximately equal to 3½ oz.
[3]Two grams per kilogram of body weight per day of a protein containing 51 mg of lysine per gram of protein would meet the lysine needs of the infant.

It is a recognized fact that lysine is the limiting amino acid—the essential amino acid most deficient—of the cereal grain proteins. Since cereal grains provide much of the world's food, there have been attempts to increase their lysine content. Plant breeding programs have successfully increased the lysine content of barley, sorghum, and corn as shown in Table L-5. This brings the protein quality of the cereal grains closer to that of animal products.

TABLE L-5
LYSINE CONTENT OF CEREAL GRAINS

Grain	Lysine	
	(mg/100 g)	(mg/g protein)
Barley	435	34
High-lysine barley	1089	56
Corn	290	29
High-lysine corn	491	45
Sorghum	297	27
High-lysine sorghum	611	33

These improved grains have been tested in animal and human trials with good results. However, farmers are reluctant to grow the hybrid varieties because they yield 10 to 15% less grain per acre than the more common varieties.

(Also see CORN, section headed "High-Lysine Corn [Opaque 2, or O_2].")

Other Lysine Sources. Lysine itself may be produced by two processes: (1) the fermentation of carbohydrate materials; and (2) the Toray process, which converts cyclohexene, a by-product of nylon production, to lysine. Following purification procedures, lysine is available as a pure white powder, often as lysine monohydrochlorine. Currently, the cost of producing pure lysine is about $1.50 to $2.00 per pound (*$3.30 to $4.40/kg*).

FACTORS AFFECTING AVAILABILITY. Besides lysine being in short supply in cereal grains, the biological availability—availability to the body once ingested—may be adversely affected. As pointed out, lysine has an extra amino group (NH_2). This amino group can react with other compounds, primarily the aldehyde group of reducing sugars such as glucose or lactose. The reaction yields an amino-sugar complex that is no longer available for use in the body. Digestive enzymes cannot split the amino-sugar complex; hence, it is not absorbed. This reaction—the Maillard reaction—occurs due to extensive heating or prolonged storage. In protein sources such as the cereal grain products where lysine is already in short supply, the reaction can further reduce the lysine content of the diet.

LYSINE SUPPLEMENTATION. Since lysine is the limiting amino acid of cereal grains which make up the diets of a large portion of the world, some scientists propose the enrichment of these grains with pure lysine derived from processes described above. This practice would be similar to that in the United States wherein thiamin, niacin, riboflavin, and iron are added to many cereal products. Indeed, there have been experimental trials with animals and humans demonstrating the beneficial effects of adding lysine. Still, in countries where diets are extremely poor, more may be gained by increasing the food supply in general and providing other protein sources such as legumes which complement the protein of cereal grains. However, some countries have tried lysine supplemented foods. The Japanese school lunch programs fortified bread with lysine and vitamins. Government-controlled bakeries in India produced bread fortified with lysine, vitamins, and minerals. In Guatemala, Incaparina, a new product to increase the quality and quantity of protein, is fortified with lysine. In the United States, Pillsbury test marketed a flour containing added vitamins, minerals, and lysine.

Lysine enrichment is a debatable issue, depending on a variety of factors, primarily the continued availability of major sources of calories and protein. Supplementation is of little value if there is not enough food. But lysine supplementation is a potential tool.

(Also see AMINO ACID[S]; and PROTEIN[S].)

LYSINE AND HERPES INFECTIONS. The Herpes simplex viruses are responsible for cold sores, fever blisters, and genital herpes, while a close relative, Herpes zoster is responsible for chickenpox, shingles, and "infectious mono." In 1979, the Lilly Research Laboratories, a division of Eli Lilly and Company of Indianapolis, released research results showing that supplementary lysine speeded recovery and suppressed recurrences of herpes infections.

Tablets of lysine as the hydrochloride, may be purchased at many general health food stores. Each tablet contains about 300 mg of lysine. A monograph from Lilly Research laboratories recommends the following:

1. When a clearly established herpes infection is present, two lysine tablets should be taken two to four times daily until the infection has cleared.

2. Those individuals who can predict an episode of herpes due to its association with such things as menstruation, exposure to sunlight, eating nuts, or any stressful situation, may take suppressive amounts of lysine—one, two, three, or four tablets daily depending upon the individual. Some individuals may prevent further infection with one tablet daily, while others may require two tablets twice a day.

3. Attacks may be completely aborted if lysine is taken in a dose of two tablets, three times per day for 3 to 5 days as soon as the signs of an attack are noted—a stinging and burning sensation followed by a little reddish nodule.

4. Some individuals can prevent herpes by avoiding known sources of another amino acid—arginine. These sources include: peanut butter, cashews, pecans, almonds, and chocolate. Tissue culture studies have shown that arginine enhances herpes growth.

Supplemental lysine does not produce any undesirable effect nor is it toxic. It is a normal constituent of protein. However, some individuals may not receive adequate amounts, and the needs from individual to individual may vary widely. Hence, to suppress herpes the dose of lysine must be varied.

Some recent work indicates that the continued use of lysine may antagonize (counteract) arginine, another amino acid. Also, drugs and vaccines raise the hope of suppressing the herpes virus. Thus, those who are persistently plagued with herpes are advised to confer with their physician.

LYSOSOMES

Structures of cell cytoplasm that contain digestive enzymes.

LYSOZYME

An enzyme that digests some gram-positive bacteria and certain high molecular weight carbohydrates; present in saliva, tears, and egg white.

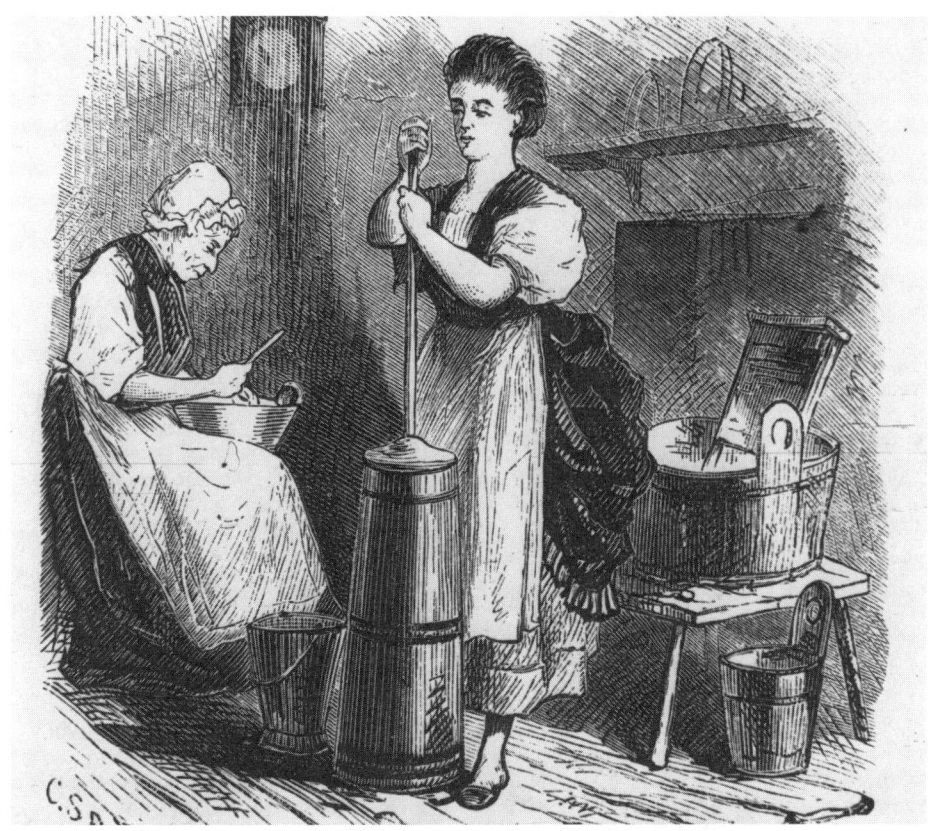

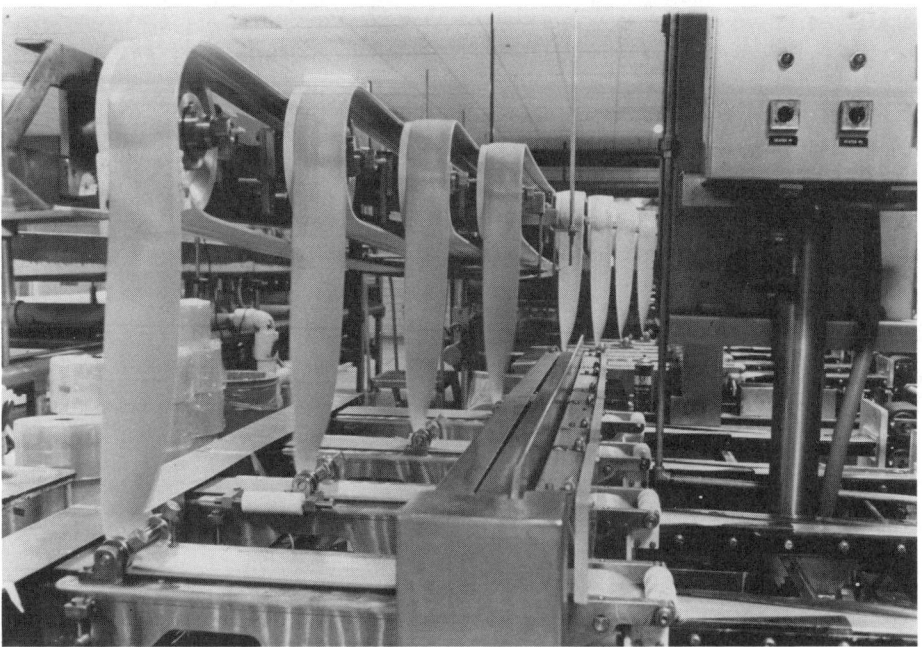

What a difference a "day" makes! Upper sketch depicts the churning of butter in a colonial home. Lower photo shows ribbons of process cheese in the late production stages. Beyond this point, machines cut the ribbons into sandwich-sized portions, wrap each slice individually, then stack and wrap the slices into store-sized packages. (Engraving courtesy The Bettmann Archive, New York, N.Y., photo courtesy of Borden Inc., Columbus, Ohio)

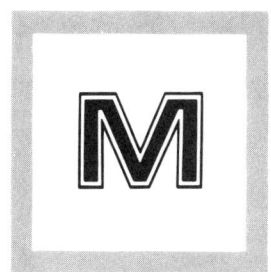

MACARONI AND NOODLE PRODUCTS

Contents   *Page*

These items, which are also called pasta, are pieces of dough that have been formed into various shapes, then dried. In the United States, macaroni products may contain egg as an optional ingredient; but products labeled as noodles must contain a certain minimum amount of egg.[1] The names *macaroni*, *spaghetti*, and *vermicelli* are applied to macaroni products that are cord-shaped and have certain diameters. *Macaroni* has the largest diameter of the macaroni products, while *vermicelli* has the smallest diameter. Fig. M-1 shows some of the more common shapes and sizes of macaroni and noodle products.

It may be noted that some of the products shown in Fig. M-1 have English names, whereas others have Italian names. The former products were adopted by Americans much earlier, when foreign names were frowned upon. Later, the use of foreign names was more acceptable. The consumer shopping for macaroni or noodles should also note that most of the products with different names were likely to have been made from the same type of

---

[1] *Code of Federal Regulations*, Title 21, Revised 4/1/78, Part 139, Sections 139.110 and 139.150.

dough, except in the cases of (1) those containing eggs, and (2) items containing other special ingredients. Therefore, this article will be concerned mainly with (1) the different ingredients which may be used for various types of enriched or fortified pasta, and (2) ways in which the nutritional shortcomings of macaroni and noodles may be offset by accompanying foods.

Macaroni and noodle products are important foods for many peoples around the world because they (1) are easy to make with simple equipment from ingredients that are available in most places, (2) keep well without refrigeration, (3) are bland flavored and mix well with most other foods, and (4) contain sufficient calories and protein to be major dietary sources of these nutrients.

HISTORY. One story has it that the explorer Marco Polo brought pasta to Italy from China in 1295. But this does not appear to be true because certain evidence suggests that forms of pasta were used by the ancient Etruscans (people who settled the upper western coast of the Italian peninsula around 700 B.C.). Also, noodles were made in China as early as 5000 B.C. Hence, it seems likely that primitive pasta products were made for thousands of years by the different people who grew wheat and ground it into meal and flour. Some historians suspect that macaroni and noodle types of pasta were introduced into Italy during the Middle Ages by the Asian slaves who cooked for the affluent Italians, since threadlike noodles were then made in various places across Asia—from China to Arabia.

Perhaps the earliest types of pasta were similar to the present type called *gnocchi*—little balls of dough that are cooked in boiling water. The next stage of refinement might have been the rolling of the dough into sheets which were then cut into strips. Also, some of the peoples who first made pasta probably cooked it right away, instead of drying and storing it. The Chinese, who lived in a damp climate, developed the practice of frying freshly boiled noodles in hot fat to produce the chow mein type of noodle which keeps well.

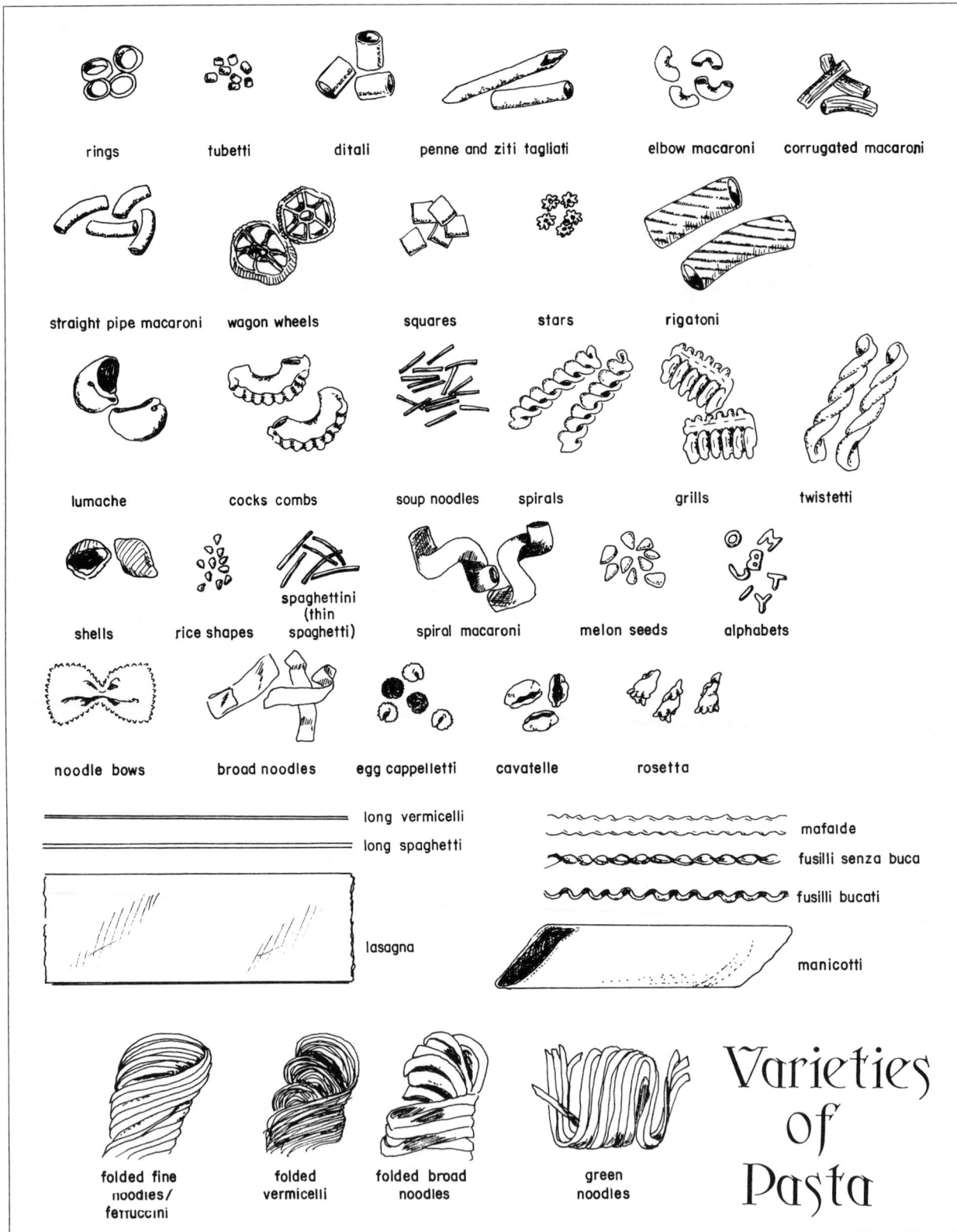

rings   tubetti   ditali   penne and ziti tagliati   elbow macaroni   corrugated macaroni

straight pipe macaroni   wagon wheels   squares   stars   rigatoni

lumache   cocks combs   soup noodles   spirals   grills   twistetti

shells   rice shapes   spaghettini (thin spaghetti)   spiral macaroni   melon seeds   alphabets

noodle bows   broad noodles   egg cappelletti   cavatelle   rosetta

long vermicelli
long spaghetti

lasagna

mafalde
fusilli senza buca
fusilli bucati

manicotti

folded fine noodles/ fettuccini   folded vermicelli   folded broad noodles   green noodles

Varieties of Pasta

Fig. M-1.   Some of the many shapes of pasta.

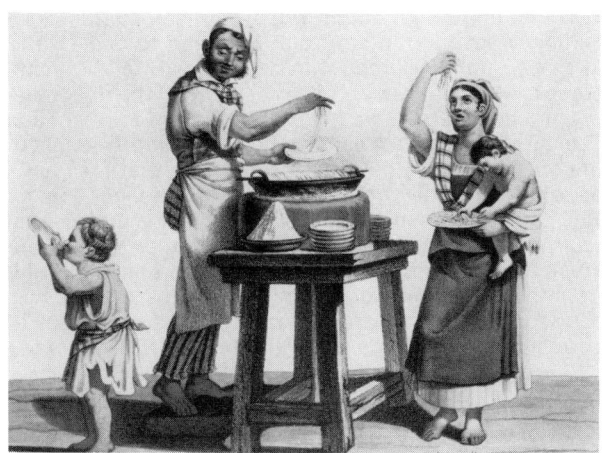

Fig. M-2. The macaroni seller, in Southern Italy. (After a colored lithograph by Muller, courtesy, The Bettman Archive, Inc., New York, N.Y.)

Whatever the origin of pasta, the southern Italians became the masters of its production in Europe, because the northern Italians ate rice in their soups and with their sauces. Also, the warm, dry climate of southern Italy favored the drying of freshly made pasta in the sun. Finally, the southern Italians preferred their pasta firm (*aldente,* which means that it requires chewing), whereas the northern Italians cooked it until it was much more tender. Legend in southern Italy has it that the northerners threw some of their pasta at a nearby wall, and that it was considered sufficiently cooked if it stuck to the wall.

Pasta appears to have spread throughout Europe from Italy, although the peoples in the northern countries apparently preferred flat noodles to the rounded types (macaroni and spaghetti). It is believed that Thomas Jefferson brought pasta to America from France, where he had served as U.S. Ambassador. Later, immigrants from northern Europe brought their own noodle dishes. Still later, Italian immigrants came to America, and for a long time thereafter imported their pasta from Italy.

It is noteworthy that the production of good pasta (that which holds together in boiling water) requires hard wheats with a high gluten content. The Italians obtained most of their wheat from Russia until the Crimean War (1854-1856) cut off their supplies. Shortly thereafter, hard wheats were produced in Canada and the United States. Hence, North America soon became the major source of durum wheat for the pasta industry around the world. However, there was not much production of macaroni or spaghetti in the United States until World War I cut off the supply from Italy.

The production and use of pasta continues to evolve, as new, protein-fortified items are now being used for feeding people in the developing countries. Modern technology makes it possible to use soybean flour and other high protein ingredients in pasta doughs so that the products may serve as major sources of both calories and protein. Furthermore, these fortified items may be stored without refrigeration, which makes them very useful in the growing energy crisis. Nevertheless, preparation by boiling requires considerable fuel, which may be quite scarce in certain areas. One answer to this problem is the instant type of noodles that may be cooked by placing in hot water for a minute or two. Additional information on these and other products is given in the sections which follow.

PRODUCTION. The consumption of macaroni and noodle products in the United States has grown steadily since World War II, even though the total consumption of all types of wheat products declined. It is noteworthy that the production of macaroni utilizes most of the durum wheat grown in North Dakota. Sometimes, it is even necessary to use sprouted durum wheat (a heavy rainfall during the harvest season may cause much of the crop to sprout) to make pasta. However, good macaroni may also be made from weaker flours if certain optional ingredients such as eggs are added. Hence, both commercial products and homemade items may be made from more than wheat and water alone.

Commercial Products. The first machine powered pasta presses were developed around the mid-1800s. Prior thereto, most macaroni was produced in small shops which utilized hand operated equipment. Today, large machines make it possible to turn out large batches of these products. Details of commercial production follow.

INGREDIENTS. The items which follow are the ingredients specified in the U.S. standards of identity for macaroni and noodle products:[2]

• **Semolina, durum flour, farina, flour**—One or more of these wheat products constitute(s) the major ingredient of pasta. Semolina is the coarsely milled endosperm of durum wheat, while durum flour is more finely milled. Farina is similar to semolina, but it is obtained from other than durum wheats, whereas flour is the more finely milled endosperm of nondurum wheats. Each of these four fractions may contain only minimal amounts of branny particles. Generally, pasta makers prefer to use semolina and/or farina since products made from these meals hold up better in cooking than those made from the flours.

• **Water**—This is the usual liquid for making a dough, although it may be replaced completely by fluid milk in certain products. Care is taken that the water is pure and free from undesirable flavors.

• **Eggs**—Egg whites (fresh, frozen, or dried) are optional ingredients for macaroni products, in which they help to strengthen the dough. On the other hand, noodles must contain at least 5½% egg solids from either whole egg or egg yolk. The latter is preferred for the color it imparts to noodles.

• **Disodium phosphate**—Small amounts (0.5 to 1.0%) of this optional additive make pasta cook more quickly.

• **Seasonings and spices**—Onions, celery, garlic, bay leaf, and salt are optional ingredients for macaroni and noodle products. When used, they must be listed on the label.

---

[2]*Ibid,* Sections 139.110 through 139.160.

• **Gum gluten**—Sometimes, this product, which is made from wheat flour by washing out the starch, is added in small amounts to strengthen the dough.

• **Glyceryl monostearate**—Less than 2% of this additive (it is an emulsifying agent) may be used to prevent the formation of clumps of dough.

• **Minerals and vitamins**—Products labeled "enriched" must contain prescribed amounts of iron, thiamin, and riboflavin, which may be (1) added as chemically pure compounds, or (2) supplied by optional ingredients such as dried yeast, dried torula yeast, partly defatted wheat germ, enriched farina, or enriched flour. Certain specified amounts of calcium and vitamin D are optional.

• **Protein supplements**—The sources of extra protein are usually corn flour and other noncereal flours, and soybean flour or meal, although other ingredients such as nonfat dry milk, fish flour, and derivatives of oilseeds (usually peanut, safflower seed, or sunflower seed) also may serve this purpose. These supplements raise both the quantity and quality of protein so that the macaroni and noodle products may be substituted for part of the dietary animal protein.

• **Milk products**—Whole fluid milk may replace completely the water used in making a dough, or the milk ingredient may be concentrated milk, evaporated milk, dried milk, a mixture of butter and skim milk, concentrated skim milk, evaporated skim milk, or nonfat dry milk. In the case of "Milk Macaroni Products," the milk ingredient(s) must supply an amount of milk solids equal to 3.8% of the finished product. Also, the weight of nonfat milk solids cannot be more than 2.275 times the weight of milk fat. This regulation insures uniformity by making all products equivalent to those made with whole milk. It is *not* applicable to items designated as "Macaroni products made with nonfat milk."

• **Carrageenan or its salts**—This optional additive, which is a gum, is used to strengthen products containing greater than average amounts of nonfat dry milk, because the latter ingredient weakens doughs.

• **Vegetable products**—Colorful macaroni and noodle products are produced by the addition of red tomato, artichoke, beet, carrot, parsley, or spinach derivatives. The vegetable ingredient may be fresh, canned, dried, or in the form of a paste or a puree. However, the pasta product must contain at least 3% vegetable solids. Spinach is the most commonly used vegetable ingredient. It is noteworthy that 3% vegetable solids corresponds to a content of about 30% fresh vegetable matter since most fresh vegetables contain about 90% water.

MANUFACTURING PROCEDURES. There must be careful control of each manufacturing stage in order to insure that the product holds up well under (1) handling between the factory and the consumer, and (2) boiling in water. Therefore, the major processes that are utilized in manufacturing of pasta are noteworthy:

1. **Milling of the durum wheat into semolina.** This milling procedure differs from that used to make flour in that a granular product is desired, with a minimum amount of flour. Hence, certain aspects of the flour milling procedure are altered in the production of semolina. The durum wheat is moistened before milling to toughen the outer layers of the wheat kernels so that they may be removed readily from the inner portion (endosperm) which yields the semolina. Then, the wheat is broken into coarse particles by corrugated rolls. Other rolls then crush the grain further and scrape the branny material from the pieces of endosperm. Finally, the particles of endosperm and bran are separated by sifting, and by a stream of air which lifts away the smaller flakes of bran.

2. **Preparation of the pasta dough.** The wheat ingredient may be semolina, durum flour, farina, nondurum flour, or various combinations of these items. About 31 parts of water (by weight) are mixed with about 69 parts of meal and/or flour to make a dough. Then, the dough is mixed well and a vacuum is applied to remove any air that might have been mixed into the dough, because air bubbles weaken the pasta.

3. **Shaping the products.** Macaroni products are given their shapes by a process called extrusion, in which the dough is forced through openings in a die made from bronze or Teflon. An auger (a screwlike shaft shaped like a drill bit) is used to drive the pasta dough through a cylinder leading to the die. The motion of the auger also helps to knead the dough so that is strengthened by the development of strands of gluten (the elastic protein which strengthens wheaten doughs). It is noteworthy that the cylinder through which the dough is forced must be cooled with a water jacket to prevent overheating that may damage the dough. The shaped raw pasta which emerges from the die is cut to the proper length by either a rotating knife (in the case of short products), or by other means.

4. **Drying.** The newly shaped pieces of pasta are carefully dried under strictly controlled conditions to bring the moisture content down to between 12 and 13%. Usually, this involves the passage of the product through several chambers of varying temperatures and humidities so that drying proceeds gradually, and both checking and cracking are avoided.

5. **Packaging.** Most long, cordlike, or tubular macaroni products are packaged in boxes that protect the strands against breakage. However, noodle products are usually packed in plastic bags.

TYPES OF MACARONI AND NOODLES. Many new products have been developed recently by food technologists for use in various parts of the world. However, it could be very confusing for the American consumer if each manufacturer were allowed to make products and label them in an arbitrary manner, since the ingredients and nutritive values might vary widely. Hence, the U.S. Food and Drug Administration, with the cooperation of American pasta manufacturers, has developed names and specifications (standards of identity) for the more common products, which are described in Table M-1.

TABLE M-1
U.S. STANDARDS OF IDENTITY FOR MACARONI AND NOODLE PRODUCTS[1]

Name of Product and Number of Section Where Described	Required Ingredients	Optional Ingredients	Labeling Regulations
Macaroni products[2] (131.110)	Semolina, durum flour, farina, and/or flour; and water.	Egg white, disodium phosphate, onions, celery, garlic, bay leaf, salt, gum gluten,[3] and/or glyceryl monostearate.	The product name[2] and the optional ingredients used must be on the label.
Enriched macaroni products[2] (139.115)	Same as those for *Macaroni products*, except that each pound must also contain 4 to 5 mg of thiamin, 1.7 to 2.2 mg of riboflavin, 27 to 34 mg of niacin, and 13 to 16.5 mg of iron. The required vitamins and iron may be supplied by dried yeast, dried torula yeast, partly defatted wheat germ, enriched farina, enriched flour, or through the direct addition of the specified nutrients.	Same as those for *Macaroni products*, except that each pound may also contain 250 to 1,000 U.S.P. units of vitamin D, 500 to 625 mg of calcium, and/or not more than 5% partly defatted wheat germ.	Same as those for *Macaroni products*, except that "Enriched" must precede the name of the product[4].
Enriched macaroni products[2] with fortified protein (139.117)	Same as those for *Macaroni products*, except that other ingredients must be added so that the protein content is at least 20% and the protein quality is at least 95% that of casein (a protein in milk). Also, each pound must contain 5 mg of thiamin, 2.2 mg of riboflavin, 34 mg of niacin, and 16.5 mg of iron.	Whole wheat flour and/or whole durum wheat flour, flours or meals made from nonwheat cereals or oilseeds, calcium (625 mg per pound, if declared as an enrichment ingredient on the label), color additives, artificial flavorings, artificial sweeteners, chemical preservatives, and/or starches.	Same as those for *Macaroni products*, except that the names of the nonwheat or oilseed materials must be part of the product name.[5] Ingredients that are not part of the product name, but which contribute 10% or more of the protein, must follow the product name in the statement "Made with——" the blank containing the name of the ingredient[6].
Milk macaroni products[2] (139.120)	Same as those for *Macaroni products*, except that milk is used as the sole moistening agent, or water is used with a sufficient quantity of a concentrated form of milk (concentrated milk, evaporated milk, dried milk, a mixture of butter and skim milk, concentrated skim milk, evaporated skim milk, and/or nonfat dry milk) so that the macaroni product contains at least 3.8% milk solids (which contain at least 30% fat).	Onions, celery, garlic, bay leaf, salt, gum gluten,[3] and/or glyceryl monostearate.	Same as those for *Macaroni products*, except "milk" must appear first in the name of the product[7].
Nonfat milk macaroni products[2] (139.121)	Same as those for *Macaroni products*, except that sufficient nonfat dry milk and/or concentrated skim milk is added so that this item contains from 12 to 25% nonfat milk solids.	Onions, celery, garlic, bay leaf, salt, glyceryl monostearate, and/or carrageenan or the salts of carrageenan.	Same as those for *Macaroni products*, except that the product name must be followed by "made with nonfat milk."[8]

Footnotes at end of table

(Continued)

TABLE M-1 (*Continued*)

Name of Product and Number of Section Where Described	Required Ingredients	Optional Ingredients	Labeling Regulations
Enriched nonfat milk macaroni products[2] (139.122)	Same as those for *Nonfat milk macaroni products*, except that each pound must also contain the amounts of vitamins and iron specified for *Enriched macaroni products*.	Same as those for *Nonfat milk macaroni products*, except that the product may contain up to 5% partly defatted wheat germ.	Same as those for *Macaroni products*, except that the product name must be preceded by "Enriched" and followed by "made with nonfat milk."[9]
Vegetable macaroni products[2] (139.125)	Same as those for *Macaroni products*, except that the product contains at least 3% of vegetable solids from red tomato, artichoke, beet, carrot, parsley, or spinach. The vegetable ingredient may be fresh, canned, dried, or in the form of puree or paste.	Onions, celery, garlic, bay leaf, salt, gum gluten,[3] and/or glyceryl monostearate.	Same as those for *Macaroni products*, except that the name of the vegetable ingredient must precede the name of the product.[10]
Enriched vegetable macaroni products[2] (139.135)	Same as those for *Vegetable macaroni products*, except that each pound must contain the amounts of vitamins and iron specified for *Enriched macaroni products*.	Same as those for *Vegetable macaroni products*, except that each pound may also contain the amounts of optional enriching ingredients specified for *Enriched macaroni products*.	Same as those for *Vegetable macaroni products*, except that "Enriched" must precede the name of the vegetable ingredient.[11]
Whole wheat macaroni products[2] (139.138)	Same as those for *Macaroni products*, except that the wheat ingredient(s) consists solely of whole wheat flour and/or whole durum wheat flour.	Onions, celery, garlic, bay leaf, salt, and/or glyceryl monostearate.	Same as those for *Macaroni products*, except that "Whole wheat" must precede the name of the product.[12]
Wheat and soy macaroni products[2] (139.140)	Same as those for *Macaroni products*, except that soy flour (made from heat processed, defatted or undefatted, dehulled soybeans) is added in an amount not less than 12.5% of the combined weight of wheat and soy ingredients.	Onions, celery, garlic, bay leaf, salt, gum gluten,[3] and/or glyceryl monostearate.	Same as those for *Macaroni products*, except that "Wheat and soy" or "Wheat and soybean" must precede the name of the product[13].
Noodle products[14] (139.150)	Same as those for *Macaroni products*, except that these products contain at least 5.5% of solids of egg or egg yolk, which may be supplied by liquid eggs, frozen eggs, dried eggs, egg yolks, frozen yolks, and/or dried yolks.	Onions, celery, garlic, bay leaf, salt, gum gluten,[3] and/or glyceryl monostearate.	The product name[14] and the optional ingredients used must be printed on the label.
Enriched noodle products[14] (139.155)	Same as those for *Noodle products*, except that each pound must also contain the amounts of vitamins and iron specified for *Enriched macaroni products*.	Same as those for *Noodle products*, except that each pound may also contain the optional enriching ingredients specified for *Enriched macaroni products*.	Same as those for *Noodle products*, except that "Enriched" must precede the name of the product.[15]

Footnotes at end of table

(Continued)

TABLE M-1 (*Continued*)

Name of Product and Number of Section Where Described	Required Ingredients	Optional Ingredients	Labeling Regulations
Vegetable noodle products[14] (139.160)	Same as those for *Noodle products*, except that these products must also contain a vegetable ingredient as specified for *Vegetable macaroni products*.	Same as those for *Noodle products*.	Same as those for *Noodle products*, except that the name of the vegetable ingredient must precede the name of the product.[16]
Enriched vegetable noodle products[14] (139.165)	Same as those for *Vegetable noodle products*, except that carrot is not allowed.[17] Also, each pound must contain the amounts of vitamins and iron specified for *Enriched macaroni products*.	Same as those for *Enriched noodle products*.	Same as those for *Vegetable noodle products*, except that "Enriched" must precede the name of the vegetable ingredient.[18]
Wheat and soy noodle products[14] (139.180)	Same as those for *Noodle products*, except that these products contain soy flour as specified for *Wheat and soy macaroni products*.	Same as those for *Noodle products*.	Same as those for *Noodle products*, except that "Wheat and soy" or "Wheat and soybean" must precede the name of the product.[19]

[1]As specified in *Code of Federal Regulations*, Title 21, Revised 4/1/78, Chapter 1, Part 139.

[2]Alternative names for "Macaroni products" are: "Macaroni" (more than 0.11 in., but not more than 0.27 in. diameter), "Spaghetti" (more than 0.06 in., but not more than 0.11 in. diameter), and "Vermicelli" (not more than 0.11 in. diameter).

[3]Quantity is limited so that the total protein from wheat products does not exceed 13% of the weight of the food.

[4]"Enriched macaroni product," or alternatively, "Enriched macaroni," "Enriched spaghetti," or "Enriched vermicelli"

[5]For example, "Wheat Soy Macaroni Product with Fortified Protein" (Where applicable, the names "Macaroni," "Spaghetti," or "Vermicelli" may be substituted for "Macaroni Product.")

[6]For example, "Wheat Macaroni with Fortified Protein Made with nonfat milk"

[7]"Milk Macaroni Product," or where applicable, "Milk macaroni," "Milk spaghetti," or "Milk vermicelli"

[8]"Macaroni product made with nonfat milk" (Where applicable, the names "Macaroni," "Spaghetti," or "Vermicelli" may be substituted for "Macaroni product.")

[9]"Enriched macaroni product made with nonfat milk," or similar names utilizing the words "macaroni," "spaghetti," or "vermicelli."

[10]For example, "Spinach macaroni product," "Spinach macaroni," "Spinach spaghetti," etc.

[11]For example, "Enriched spinach macaroni product," etc.

[12]"Whole wheat macaroni product," "Whole wheat macaroni," "Whole wheat spaghetti," etc.

[13]"Wheat and soy macaroni product," "Wheat and soybean macaroni product," etc.

[14]"Noodle product," "Egg noodle product," "Noodles," "Egg noodles," (Where applicable, the names "Egg macaroni," "Egg spaghetti," or "Egg vermicelli" may be used.)

[15]"Enriched noodle product," "Enriched egg noodle product," "Enriched noodles," etc.

[16]For example, "Spinach noodle product," "Spinach egg noodle product," "Spinach noodles," etc.

[17]Carrots are not allowed in enriched vegetable noodle products because they are apt to impart an egg-yolk color which might suggest a higher egg content than that present.

[18]"Enriched spinach noodle product," "Enriched spinach egg noodle product," etc.

[19]"Wheat and soy noodle product," "Wheat and soybean noodle product," etc.

Homemade Noodles. American farm families have long made their own noodles by (1) making a dough from flour, eggs, and a pinch of salt; (2) kneading the dough, then rolling it into a thin sheet; (3) cutting the sheet of dough into narrow strips (noodles); and (4) cooking the noodles in boiling water. Similarly, people of Italian descent have made homemade ravioli and other types of macaroni products. Usually, homemade pasta is cooked right after its preparation, because drying the dough to obtain a durable, nonperishable product is a difficult job for amateurs. Therefore, this section is concerned solely with noodles rather than pasta products in general, because it is best that homemade items be made with eggs, which impart strength to the dough, particularly in cases where high quality durum semolina or durum flour may not be available.

It is noteworthy that various tyes of hand operated noodle machines and pasta presses may be obtained from certain mail order houses. However, most homemakers prefer to rely on good eyesight and a steady hand for shaping their pasta.

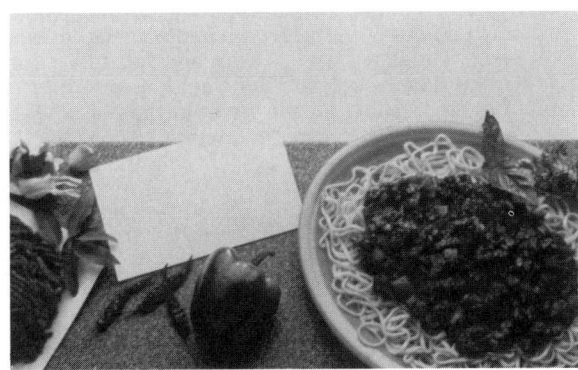

Fig. M-3. Pasta with meat sauce. (Courtesy, USDA)

People who belong to the younger generation may question why those in the older generation go to the trouble of making their own noodles, when they may be obtained for reasonable prices at most supermarkets. The answer is that making homemade noodles allows the cook to incorporate ingredients as desired, within the limits of good culinary practices. Therefore, guidelines for utilizing various ingredients follow:

NOTE: The authors have decided not to provide detailed recipes, but rather to give general guidelines for those who might wish to develop their own recipes by experimentation.)

• **Basic ingredients**—Commercial pasta production generally utilizes a dough containing about 70% solids and 30% water (measured by weighing), which is a good general guideline for the maximum amount of liquid needed for a given amount of meal or flour. This works out to one egg per cup of sifted flour. Usually, about ¼ tsp (*1.25 ml*) of salt is also added for each cup (*240 ml*) of flour.

• **High-protein noodles**—The quantity and quality of protein in noodles may be increased considerably by the addition of certain ingredients. For example, the substitution of defatted soy flour for only one-eighth of the wheat flour raises the quantity of protein by about 40%, and makes the protein quality almost equal to that of animal protein. It is best not to add nonfat dry milk, because this ingredient weakens doughs. Professional pasta makers get around this problem by adding carrageenan (a gum) to strengthen the dough.

• **Seasonings and spices for noodle doughs**—These should be added as fine, dry powders, because larger particles may weaken the noodles. About ¼ tsp (*1.25 ml*) of seasoning per cup of flour is sufficient. Some typical seasonings that might be used are basil, bay leaf, garlic, onion, oregano, sage, and thyme.

• **Vegetable ingredients**—Purees made from deeply colored vegetables add considerable color to noodles. However, only limited amounts of purees can be used without adding excessive water. It might be wise to experiment first by adding small amounts of baby food purees such as beets, carrots, creamed spinach, green beans, peas, squash, sweet potato, and tomato soup. However, the ratio of egg to flour would have to be reduced in order to allow for the water in the puree. For example, a typical mixture might contain 1 Tbsp (*15 ml*) vegetable puree and one-half egg (or only the white of one egg) per cup (*240 ml*) of flour. Usually, concentrated vegetable pastes or powders are used in commercial pasta production.

NUTRITIVE VALUES OF MACARONI AND NOODLE PRODUCTS.

People with low incomes have long relied on pasta dishes to supply most of their dietary calories and other nutrients. Furthermore, these dishes are served regularly in the school lunch programs around the United States. Therefore, it is noteworthy that the nutritive values of these foods vary widely, depending upon the type of macaroni or noodle product and the other items that might be served with them. The nutrient compositions of macaroni, noodles, pastinas, spaghetti, and some of the most common dishes prepared with these products are given in Food Composition Table F-36.

Some of the more noteworthy observations regarding the products listed in Food Composition Table F-36 are as follows:

1.   A cup of a plain, tender cooked macaroni product contains about 5 oz (*140 g*) of food, 155 Calories (kcal), and 4.8 g of protein, whereas a cup of noodles supplies 5⅔ oz (*160 g*) of food, 200 Calories (kcal), and 6.6 g of protein. The superior nutritive values of the noodles are due mainly to the egg content.

2.   Enriched macaroni and noodles supply fair amounts of iron, thiamin, riboflavin, and niacin, but only negligible amounts of calcium, phosphorus, vitamin A and vitamin C.

3.   The addition of cheese to macaroni provides considerable extra calories, protein, calcium, phosphorus, and vitamin A. Similarly, the addition of tomato sauce plus cheese or meat to spaghetti enhances the nutritive value of a pasta dish.

4.   Chow mein noodles are a concentrated source of calories and protein because they contain almost no water. However, the ratio of protein to calories (2.7 g per 100 kcal) is less than those for either macaroni (3.1 g per 100 kcal) or noodles (3.3 g per 100 kcal), because the frying of the Chinese noodles raises the fat content without increasing the protein.

5.   Another important observation regarding macaroni and noodles, which is not apparent from the data presented in Food Composition Table F-36, is that the protein in these products is deficient in the amino acid lysine, which is critical for the growth of infants and children. This defect is offset partly by the high quality of the protein in the eggs that are added to noodles.

There is a great need for supplementing the nutritive contributions of pasta products, when they are used as staple foods for infants and children. (Tiny egg noodles called pastina are used as a baby food in Italy.) Therefore, the current enrichment and fortification practices that are utilized in macaroni and noodle products merit some discussion.

Enrichment.   The most common practice is to add the specified amounts of iron, thiamin, riboflavin, and niacin in chemically pure form. However, the restoration of iron and three vitamins replaces only a few of the 2 dozen or more essential nutrients that are removed in substantial amounts during the conversion of whole wheat kernels into semolina or flour.

Better, but more expensive, means of enrichment are permitted by the standards of identity for enriched macaroni products and enriched noodle products.[3] It consists of providing the specified amounts of iron and the B vitamins through the addition of the highly nutritive ingredients dried yeast, dried torula yeast, and/or partly defatted wheat germ. The use of these ingredients adds extra protein, minerals, and B vitamins that are not provided by the usual means of enrichment.

The federal standards of identity also provide for the optional calcium and vitamin D enrichment of both macaroni and noodles. These nutrients are rarely added, although they would be very beneficial for people who drink little milk or who receive limited amounts of sunshine.

Fortification.

The low quality of the wheat protein in macaroni and noodles is of considerable concern to nutritionists, because these foods are popular with children around the world. This concern led to the development of new products by food companies, which in turn led to the establishment of a standard of identity for "Enriched macaroni products with fortified protein."[4]

These products must contain at least 20% protein with a quality at least 95% that of casein (a major protein in cow's milk). The supplemental protein may be supplied by flours or meals made from nonwheat cereals or oilseeds such as soybeans, peanuts, sunflower seeds, and cotton seeds. Many of these types of macaroni have been developed, but most are currently marketed in other countries where the need for protein is greater than in the United States.

Similar protein fortified products are specified under the standards of identity for "Wheat and soy macaroni products" and for "Wheat and soy noodle products."[5] The quantities of protein in these items are at least 50% greater than those in similar items made from wheat flour alone. They are often sold in health food stores. However, products labeled "imitation soy macaroni" and "imitation soy noodles" may not contain as much protein because the word "imitation" denotes products which do *not* conform to a federal standard of identity.

Finally, "Nonfat milk macaroni products" contain between 12 and 25% nonfat milk solids.[6] These items contain from 36 to 75% more protein than is present in similar products made from wheat flour alone. A cup (*240 ml*) of cooked macaroni would also furnish from 89 to 175 mg of calcium, and from 131 to 197 mg of phosphorus.

---

[3]*Ibid.,* Sections 139.115 and 139.155.

[4]*Ibid.,* Section 139.117.

[5]*Ibid.,* Sections 139.140 and 139.180.

[6]*Ibid,* Section 139.121.

Unfortunately, this type of fortified product does not appear to be available at the present time.

PREPARATION AND SERVING OF PASTA.

Macaroni and noodle dishes may be utilized as main courses, appetizing side dishes, or as substitutes for starchy vegetables such as corn, potatoes, or rice. In whatever ways they are used, it is important to consider certain culinary principles, if one is to serve tasty, nutritious pasta rather than an overcooked mass of mushy matter that provides mainly empty calories. Therefore, some suggestions for preparing and serving these dishes follow:

1. Uncooked pasta should be placed in a sufficient amount of vigorously boiling, salted water (containing about 1 Tbsp [*15 ml*] of salt per pound [*454 g*] of uncooked pasta) so that boiling resumes shortly after the addition of the pasta. This means that about 4 qt of water should be used for each pound of pasta (*about 4 liter for each 500 g*).

2. Pasta should be cooked only until tender, and no longer. Therefore, the cook should sample items being cooked for the first time, in order to avoid overcooking. When it is done, it should be (a) placed in a collander so that the water drains off, or (b) removed from the pot of water with a slotted spoon. Experienced cooks are usually able to pour off most of the water, leaving just enough to prevent the pasta from sticking to the pan.

3. Sometimes, the cooked item is rinsed with cold water to stop it from cooking further and becoming pasty. Then, it may be tossed with a little warmed oil, salad dressing, or melted butter to prevent sticking.

4. Sauces should complement, but not overwhelm, the flavor of macaroni or noodles. Also, the best sauces usually have a blend of several flavors. Hence, herbs and spices such as basil, bay leaf, chives, garlic, onions, oregano, and parsley should be used sparingly. Fresh spices are much more flavorful than dried items. Also, high quality protein foods such as cheese, chopped eggs, fish, meat, nuts, and/or poultry should be used frugally, since one of the functions of macaroni or noodles is to extend more expensive foods. Therefore, the cook need allow only a total of from 2 to 3 oz (*57 to 85 g*) of one or more of these items per person, since that is sufficient to complement the pasta protein considerably. Larger amounts of cooked legumes or vegetables may be used because these items usually have high water contents, and only moderate amounts of calories and protein.

5. Pasta dishes should usually be served hot. Hence, some hosts preheat the serving dishes when there are unavoidable delays between cooking and serving. However, reheating the pasta may overcook it. Similarly, macaroni and noodles which are boiled prior to being baked in casserole dishes should be undercooked in the boiling step.

6.   Only a limited amount of sauce should be placed on the pasta by the host. The remaining sauce should be served in a separate dish so that each diner may use only as much as desired. Similarly, only small amounts of grated cheese should be added by the host.

7.   The best flavored grated cheeses (usually Parmesan and/or Romano) are those which have been purchased in ungrated blocks, then grated fresh when the meal is served; because some of the flavor may be lost or chemically altered by oxidation when pregrated cheese is stored for long periods.

8.   Cooked pasta does not always have to be served hot. Instead, it may be allowed to cool, then mixed in a salad.

RECENT DEVELOPMENTS IN MACARONI AND NOODLE TECHNOLOGY. The use of pasta products around the world is growing steadily because they are convenient items which go well with almost every other type of food. Also, food scientists and nutritionists are busy developing and promoting special fortified products for use by people everywhere. Therefore, some recent developments in this field are noteworthy:

• **Instant Ramen (Oriental instant-cooking noodles)**— This type of product, which has become very popular in the United States, is made from wheat flour, water, potassium carbonate, and sodium carbonate. The dough is (1) cut into long narrow strips, (2) steamed, (3) sprayed with monosodium glutamate, and (4) fried in vegetable oil. These noodles, which are usually sold with packets of flavorings, are cooked by standing for only a few minutes in boiling hot water.
Similar quick-cooking noodle products are mixed with seasonings and dehydrated cheese, fish, meat, poultry, and/or vegetables.

• **Macaroni made from corn, soy, and wheat**—These products have been test marketed in the United States and South America. They contain over 20% protein, the quality of which is on a par with milk protein.

• **Noodles containing fish flour**—The addition of only 10% fish flour (also known as fish protein concentrate or FPC) raises the protein content of noodles from about 14% to 20% or more, while also increasing the quality of protein to a great extent. This type of product was found to promote good growth in malnourished Peruvian children.

• **Use of protein-fortified pasta as a meat substitute**—Institutional food service managers are often caught in a tight squeeze between budgetary limitations and rising costs for foods and personnel. This is particularly true for those in charge of feeding children in schools around the United States because the supplies of low cost surplus foods are nearly exhausted. Hence, the U.S. Department of Agriculture now permits protein-fortified pasta products to be used as partial substitutes for meat products in the national school lunch program.

MACEDOINE

A French word meaning a mixture of fruits or vegetables which are chopped and mixed with a dressing, or put into a gelatin. A macedoine can be served as a salad or as a dessert.

MACROBIOTICS, ZEN

This term encompasses both a diet and a philosophy of life. Zen refers to meditation, and macrobiotic suggests a tendency to prolong life.
(Also see ADZUKI BEAN, section on "Zen Macrobiotic Diets"; and ZEN MACROBIOTIC DIET.)

MACROCYTE

An exceptionally large red blood cell occurring chiefly in anemias.

MACRO (OR MAJOR) MINERALS

The major minerals—calcium, phosphorus, sodium, chlorine, magnesium, potassium, and sulfur.
(Also see MINERAL[S].)

MACRONUTRIENT

These are nutrients that are present in the body and required by the body in amounts ranging from a few tenths of a gram to one or more grams. Macronutrients include fat, water, protein, calcium, phosphorus, sodium, chlorine, magnesium, potassium, and sulfur.
(Also see MINERAL[S].)

MAGMA

• A suspension that is comprised of finely divided insoluble or nearly insoluble material in water; for example, magnesia magma (milk of magnesia).

• A crude organic mixture that is in the form of a paste; for example, the mixture of sugar syrup and sugar crystals produced during the refining process.

MAGNESIUM (Mg)

TOP FOOD   SOURCES

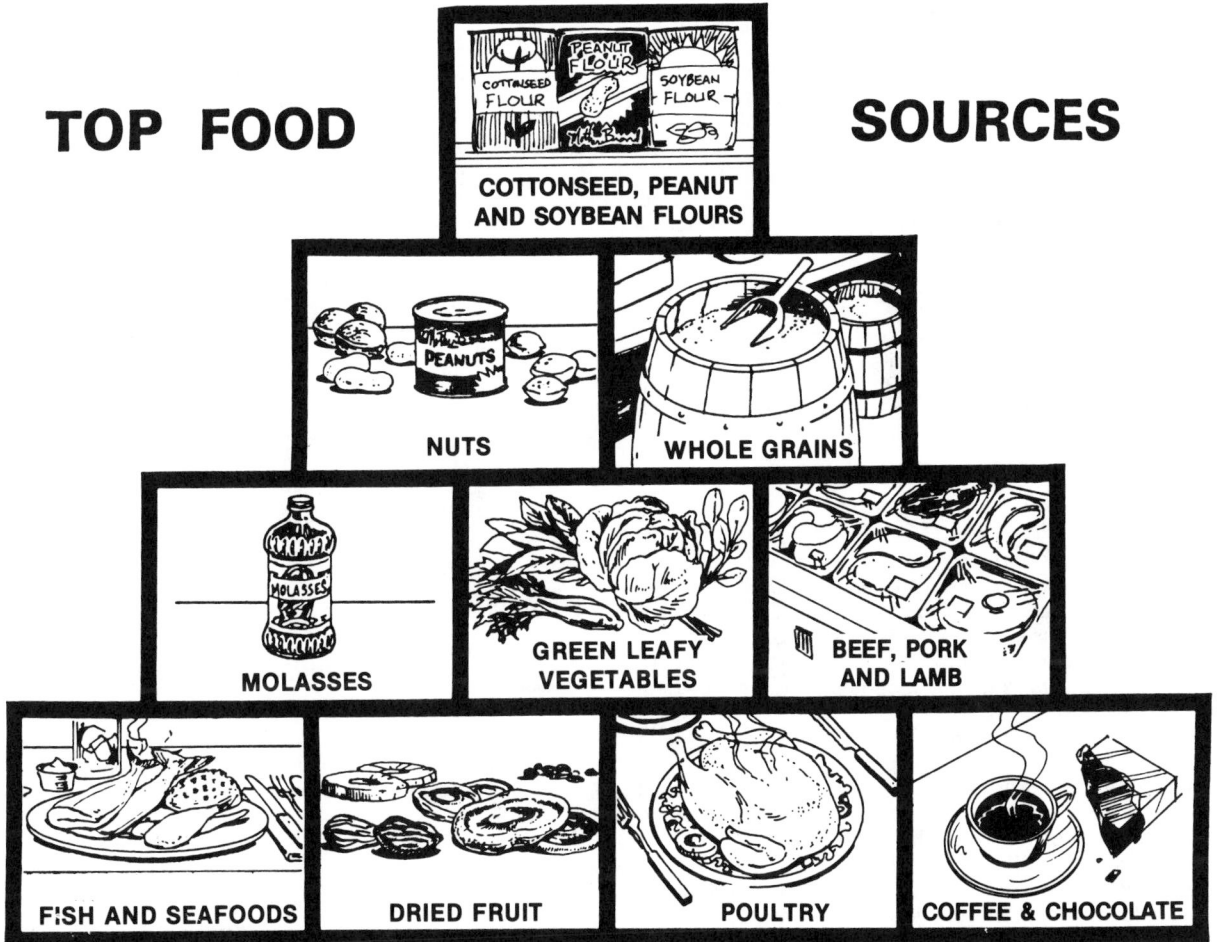

Fig. M-4.   Top food sources of magnesium.

Magnesium is an essential mineral that accounts for about 0.05% of the body's total weight, or about 20 to 30 g. Nearly 60% of this is located in the bones in the form of phosphates and carbonates, while 28% of it is found in the soft tissues and 2% in the body fluids. The highest concentration in the soft tissues is in the liver and muscles. The red blood cells also contain magnesium. Blood serum contains 1 to 3 mg of magnesium per 100 ml, most of which is bound to proteins; the rest is in the form of ions.

HISTORY. Centuries ago, the ancient Romans claimed that "magnesia alba" (white magnesium salts from the district of Magnesia in Greece, from which the element was eventually named) cured many ailments. But, it was not until 1808 that Sir Humphrey Davy, the British chemist, announced that he had isolated the element, magnesium.

In 1926, LeRoy, in France, using mice, first proved that magnesium is an essential nutrient for animals. Subsequently, McCollum and co-workers described several magnesium deficiency signs in rats and dogs, including magnesium tetany, a form of convulsions in which the nerves and muscles are affected. Indications that magnesium is required by man followed during the period 1933-1944.

ABSORPTION, METABOLISM, EXCRETION. From 30 to 50% of the average daily intake of magnesium is absorbed in the small intestine. Almost all of the magnesium in the feces represents unabsorbed dietary magnesium. Its absorption is interfered with by high intake of calcium, phosphate, oxalic acid (spinach, rhubarb), phytate (whole grain cereals), and poorly digested fats (long chain saturated fatty acids). Its absorption is enhanced by protein, lactose (milk sugar), vitamin D, growth hormone, and antibiotics.

Magnesium is generally reabsorbed in the kidneys, thus minimizing the loss of body reserves.

The main route of excretion of magnesium is the urine. Aldosterone, a hormone secreted by the adrenal gland, helps regulate the rate of magnesium excretion through the kidneys. Losses tend to increase with the consumption of alcohol or the use of diuretics.

FUNCTIONS OF MAGNESIUM.

Magnesium is involved in many functions. It is a constituent of bones and teeth; it is an essential element of cellular metabolism, often as an activator of enzymes involved in phosphorylated compounds and of the high energy phosphate transfer of ADP and ATP; and it is involved in activating certain peptidases in protein digestion. Magnesium relaxes nerve impulses and muscle contraction; functioning antagonistically to calcium which is stimulatory.

As the central component of chlorophyll, the green pigment of all higher plants, magnesium is essential for making glucose and oxygen from sunlight (energy source), water, and carbon dioxide by the process of photosynthesis. Magnesium is also a major mineral component of sea water (0.13%), from which life and chlorophyll originally evolved.

DEFICIENCY SYMPTOMS.

A deficiency of magnesium is characterized by (1) muscle spasms (tremor, twitching) and rapid heartbeat; (2) confusion, hallucinations, and disorientation; and (3) lack of appetite, listlessness, nausea, and vomiting.

Magnesium deficiency has been observed in alcoholics, in severe kidney disease, in acute diarrhea, and in kwashiorkor.

Some scientists have cautiously theorized a magnesium-cancer link. In support of this thinking, it is noteworthy that fewer cases of leukemia (a form of blood cancer characterized by abnormal increase of white blood cells) have been reported in Poland in areas where magnesium is plentiful in the soil and drinking water than in areas where it is scarce. At this time the magnesium-cancer link theory is without adequate proof, but it merits further research.

INTERRELATIONSHIPS.

When magnesium intake is extremely low, calcium is sometimes deposited in soft tissues forming calcified lesions.

An excess of magnesium upsets calcium and phosphorus metabolism. Also, with diets adequate in magnesium and other nutrients, increasing the calcium and/or phosphorus results in magnesium deficiency.

Magnesium activates many enzyme systems, particularly those concerned with transferring phosphate from ATP and ADP. Magnesium is also capable of inactivating certain enzymes, and is known to be a component of at least one enzyme.

Overuse of such substances as "milk of magnesia" (magnesium hydroxide, an antacid and laxative) or "Epsom salts" (magnesium sulfate, a laxative and tonic) may lead to deficiencies of other minerals, or even to toxicity.

RECOMMENDED DAILY ALLOWANCE OF MAGNESIUM.

The Food and Nutrition Board (FNB) of the National Research Council (NRC) recommended daily allowances of magnesium are given in Table M-2.

TABLE M-2
RECOMMENDED DAILY MAGNESIUM ALLOWANCES[1]

Group	Age	Weight		Height		Magnesium
	(yr)	(lb)	(kg)	(in.)	(cm)	(mg)
Infants	0–0.5	13	6	24	60	40
	0.5–1	20	9	28	71	60
Children	1–3	29	13	35	90	80
	4–6	44	20	44	112	120
	7–10	62	28	52	132	170
Males	11–14	99	45	62	157	270
	15–18	145	66	69	176	400
	19–24	160	72	70	177	350
	25–50	174	79	70	178	350
	51+	170	77	68	173	350
Females	11–14	101	46	62	157	280
	15–18	120	55	64	163	300
	19–24	128	58	65	164	280
	25–50	138	63	64	163	280
	51+	143	65	63	160	280
Pregnant	. . . .					320
Lactating	. . . .					355–340

[1]*Recommended Dietary Allowances*, 10th ed., 1989, NRC–National Academy of Sciences. p. 285.

Note that the daily magnesium allowances are as follows: For infants, 40 to 60 mg; for children, 80 to 170 mg; for adult males, 350 mg; for adult females, 280 mg; and for pregnant and lactating women, 320 to 355 mg.

• **Magnesium intake in average U.S. diet**—The U.S. Department of Agriculture reported that foods available for consumption in the United States in 1988 provided an average of 330 mg of magnesium per person per day, and that the leading sources were as follows: dairy products, 18.5%; flour and cereal products, 18.5%; meat, poultry, and fish, 15.4%; legumes, including dry beans and peas, nuts, soya flour, and grits, 12.7%; and vegetables, including tomatoes, 16.1%.

Surveys indicate that the magnesium content of the average American diet is about 120 mg per 1,000 Calories (kcal). Thus, a person consuming a varied diet of about 2,000 Calories (kcal) would get 240 mg of magnesium. However, a woman following diets limiting intake to 1,000 to 1,500 Calories (kcal) will likely have magnesium intakes below the recommended daily allowance.

TOXICITY.

Magnesium toxicity may occur when the kidneys are unable to get rid of a large overload; characterized by slowed breathing, coma, and sometimes death. It is noteworthy that magnesium salts taken by pregnant mothers may affect their newborn babies.

SOURCES OF MAGNESIUM.

Magnesium is relatively widespread in foods.

Human milk contains approximately 3 mg of magnesium per 100 g, while cow's milk contains about 13 mg/100 g. Processing grains causes them to lose most of their magnesium. Likewise, refined sugar, alcohol, fats, and oils do not contain magnesium. Excess cooking of foods in large amounts of water can cause losses.

Groupings by rank of common food sources of magnesium follow:

• **Rich sources**—Coffee (instant), cocoa powder, cottonseed flour, peanut flour, sesame seeds, soybean flour, spices, wheat bran, wheat germ.

• **Good sources**—Blackstrap molasses, nuts, peanut butter, whole grains (oats, barley, wheat, buckwheat), whole wheat flour, yeast.

• **Fair sources**—Avocados, bananas, beef and veal, breads, cheese, chicken, corn, cornmeal, dates, dehydrated fruit, fish and seafoods, lamb, liver, olives, pork, raspberries, rice, turkey, most green leafy vegetables.

• **Negligible sources**—Cabbage, egg plant, eggs, fats and oils, ice cream, lettuce, milk, most fruits, mushrooms, rhubarb, rutabagas, sausages and luncheon meats, sugar, tomatoes.

• **Supplemental sources**—Dolomite, magnesium gluconate, magnesium oxide, wheat germ.

For additional sources and more precise values of magnesium, see Food Composition Table F-36 of this book.

TOP MAGNESIUM SOURCES. The top magnesium sources are listed in Table M-3.

NOTE WELL: This table lists (1) the top sources without regard to the amount normally eaten (left column), and (2) the top food sources (right column); and the caloric (energy) content of each.

(Also see MINERAL[S], Table M-67.)

TABLE M-3
TOP MAGNESIUM SOURCES[1]

Top Sources[2]	Magnesium	Energy	Top Food Sources	Magnesium	Energy
	(mg/100 g)	(kcal/100 g)		(mg/100 g)	(kcal/100 g)
			Wheat bran	597	353
Coriander, leaf, dried	694	279	Brazil nuts, shelled	318	715
Cottonseed flour	650	356	Soybean flour, defatted	310	326
Wheat bran	597	353	Almonds, dried, shelled, whole	293	598
Dill weed, dried	451	253	Cashew nuts, unsalted	267	596
Celery seed	440	392	Molasses, blackstrap	258	230
Sage	428	315	Peanuts, roasted/skins, whole	175	582
Mustard, dried	422	580	Wheat-soy blend (WSB)/straight		
Basil	422	251	grade wheat flour	169	365
Cocoa powder	420	245	Wheat flour, whole		
Fennel seed	385	345	(from hard wheats)	150	361
Coffee, instant, dry	380	-	Oat flour	110	-
Savory	377	272	Beet greens, raw	106	24
Cumin seed	366	375	Spinach, frozen, chopped or leaf.	104	24
Wheat germ, toasted	364	391	Rye flour, medium or light	73	360
Peanut flour, defatted	360	371	Chard, Swiss, raw	65	25
Sesame seeds, dry,			Sugar, beet or cane, brown	62	373
decorticated	347	582	Figs, dried, uncooked	61	266
Tarragon	347	295	Turnip greens, raw	58	28
Marjoram, dried	346	271	Kingfish (southern, gulf, northern		
Poppy seed	320	533	whiting), cooked	56	255
Brazil nuts, shelled	318	715	Chickpeas, dry, cooked or canned.	54	179
			Apricots, dried, sulfured,		
			uncooked	50	236

[1]These listings are based on the data in Food Composition Table F-36. Some top or rich food sources may have been overlooked since some of the foods in Table F-36 lack values for magnesium.

Whenever possible, foods are on an "as used" basis, without regard to moisture content; hence, certain high-moisture foods may be disadvantaged when ranked on the basis of magnesium content per 100 g (approximately 3 1/2 oz) without regard to moisture content.

[2]Listed without regard to the amount normally eaten.

MAILLARD REACTION

Nonenzymatic browning that takes place upon heating or prolonged storage of food is caused by this reaction. The responsible chemical reaction occurs between a sugar and a free amino group (NH_2) of an amino acid. Once the reaction occurs the amino acid is no longer biologically available, thus reducing the nutritive value of the food. Most Maillard reactions take place with the essential amino acid lysine, since it has a free amino group not involved in a peptide bond. Dr. L. C. Maillard, who first described the reaction, died in 1936 without ever receiving recognition for the importance of his pioneering work.

(Also see LYSINE; and PRESERVATION.)

MALABSORPTION SYNDROME

This term is used to describe a number of symptoms and signs indicating a defect which limits or prevents absorption of one or more essential nutrient from the small intestine. Individuals suffering from a malabsorption syndrome display in varying degrees the following clinical manifestations: (1) diarrhea; (2) steatorrhea (fatty diarrhea) due to impaired fat absorption; (3) progressive weight loss and muscle wasting; (4) abdominal distention; and (5) evidence of vitamin and mineral deficiencies, such as macrocytic anemia due to inadequate folic acid and vitamin B-12 absorption, iron-deficiency anemia, hypocalcemic (low calcium) tetany, and inflammation of the tongue, mouth, and skin—glossitis stomatitis, and dermatitis, respectively. The laboratory findings characteristic of malabsorption consist of decreases in the blood concentrations of electrolytes, albumin, and carotene, and increases in fecal fat and nitrogen (protein).

Diagnosis of a malabsorption syndrome is based on the results of absorption tests such as xylose absorption, fat absorption balance study, the Schilling test for vitamin B-12 absorption, and the folic acid test. Also gastrointestinal x-ray studies, small intestine biopsy, pro-thrombin time, and serum levels of vitamin A are useful diagnostic tools.

Treatment is directed toward (1) eliminating, insofar as possible, the abnormality causing the malabsorption, (2) vitamin and mineral supplements, and (3) dietary modifications.

Dietary modification will differ due to the cause of the malabsorption syndrome. In general, the diet should be high in calories and protein, but some disorders require the elimination of certain carbohydrates, proteins, or amino acids. Persistent diarrhea may be dealt with by a soft or fiber-restricted diet. Furthermore, a modification of fat intake is beneficial; for example, the common practice of incorporating medium chain triglycerides (8- and 10-carbon chains) into the diet. Medium chain triglycerides substitution can reduce the steatorrhea and the losses of calcium, sodium, and potassium observed in many malabsorption syndromes.

Table M-4 outlines the causes and specific abnormalities of a variety of conditions which may create a malabsorption syndrome.

(Also see DIGESTION AND ABSORPTION; INBORN ERRORS OF METABOLISM; and MODIFIED DIETS.)

TABLE M-4
CLASSIFICATION OF MALABSORPTION SYNDROMES

Causes	Abnormality	Comments
Cardiovascular disorders (cardio-myopathies and blood vessel disorders) (Also see DIGESTION AND ABSORPTION; and HEART DISEASE.)	Constrictive pericarditis; congestive heart failure; insufficient blood supply to the intestine; inflammation of the blood vessels.	Excessive loss of protein into the intestine occurs in congestive heart failure, especially in constrictive pericarditis. Thus, excessive protein is lost in the feces. There is no clearance of absorbed nutrients away from the intestine due to the congestion in the veins or insufficient blood supply. Lymphatics in the intestine become dilated and their function impaired.
Endocrine gland disorders (Also see DIABETES MELLITUS; and ENDOCRINE GLANDS.)	Disorder of the pancreas.	In diabetes mellitus, steatorrhea (fatty diarrhea) may be due to (1) an accompanying deficiency of pancreatic enzymes and other secretions, (2) coexistent nontropical sprue, (3) abnormal numbers of bacteria in the small intestine, or (4) the nervous disorder, "diabetic diarrhea."
	Disorder of the parathyroid gland.	The cause of malabsorption in hypoparathyroidism (under secretion) is not clear. It is possible that the low blood calcium resulting from the under secretion of parathyroid hormone may lead to reduced motility of the intestine thereby allowing abnormal numbers of bacteria to occupy the intestine, alter the chemical nature of bile and utilize and/or bind vitamin B-12.
	Disorders of the adrenal gland cortex.	It is possible that the diarrhea, steatorrhea, and weight loss seen in adrenal insufficiency (Addison's disease) may in part be due to malabsorption.
	Thyroid gland disorders.	Hyperthyroidism (over secretion) produces malabsorption symptoms, which appear to be due to the rapid transit of food through the gastrointestinal tract.

(Continued)

TABLE M-4 (*Continued*)

Causes	Abnormality	Comments
Inadequate absorptive surface (Also see DIGESTION AND ABSORPTION.)	Surgical procedures such as massive intestinal resection or bypass and gastroileostomy.	Most nutrients are absorbed in the small intestine which is 12 to 15 ft (*4 to 5 m*) long. Any surgical procedure which alters the length or continuity of the small intestine produces symptoms of malabsorption. Loss of 50% of the small intestine poses only minor problems, while some individuals have survived with as little as 8 to 18 in. (*20 to 46 cm*) of small intestine. Attempts to increase absorption by the remaining intestine involve delaying transit time by (1) dietary modification, (2) drug therapy, and (3) other surgical measures.
Inadequate digestion (Also see ENDOCRINE GLANDS; DUMPING SYNDROME; and ZOLLINGER-ELLISON SYNDROME.)	Stomach removal (gastrectomy).	Following gastrectomy there is decreased release of the hormones secretin and cholecyslokinin-pancreozymin, decreased mixing of foods, and reduced passage time.
	Deficiency or inactivation of the enzyme pancreatic lipase.	Diseases which may be responsible are pancreatitis, pancreatic carcinoma, cystic fibrosis, and an ulcerogenic tumor of the pancreas (Zollinger-Ellison syndrome).
Lymphatic obstruction (Also see CHYLOMI-CRONS; DIGESTION and ABSORPTION; and LYMPH.) (Also see WHIPPLE'S DISEASE.)	Tumors of the lymph tissues and lymphangiectasia (dilation of the lymphatic vessels).	Both tumors and lymphangiectasia are associated with leakage of chylomicron fat and plasma proteins into the intestine. Also both are responsible for structural changes in the lining of the small intestine, the site of nutrient absorption.
	Whipple's disease (intestinal lipodystrophy).	There is evidence to suggest that the disease is caused by microorganisms; the disease does respond to antibiotics. Lymphatics are dilated and there is a loss of serum albumin and fat-soluble vitamins. However, malabsorption is caused by multiple defects.
Primary defects in the absorptive surface of the intestine (Also see BACTERIA IN FOOD; CANCER; DISEASES; GASTROENTERITIS; SCLERODERMA; and SPRUE.) (Also see ALLERGIES; CELIAC DISEASE; INBORN ERRORS OF METABOLISM; and SPRUE, NONTROPICAL.)	Inflamatory or infiltrative disorders of the small intestine.	Any of the following may produce some form of malabsorption: (1) regional enteritis; (2) amyloidosis; (3) scleroderma; (4) lymphoma; (5) radiation therapy for cancer of the uterus and vagina; (6) eosinophilic enteritis, red blood cell infiltration of the intestinal wall; (7) tropical sprue; (8) infectious gastroenteritis such as salmonellosis; (9) jejunitis; (10) mastocytosis; and (11) skin disorders such as psoriasis and eczema.
	Biochemical or genetic abnormalities.	The well-known gluten induced celiac disease and nontropical sprue belong to this group. Carbohydrate intolerances due to an enzyme deficiency; for example, lactase, also belong to this group. The hereditary deficiency of gamma globulin or B-lipoprotein in the blood creates a malabsorptive condition. Cystinuria and Hartnup disease are inborn errors in metabolism of amino acids which exhibit some malabsorption symptoms.
Protein-calorie malnutrition	Diarrhea, and malabsorption of sugars, starches, fats, and proteins.	One-fourth to one-half of medical and surgical patients hospitalized for longer than 2 weeks have been found to suffer from protein-calorie malnutrition, resulting from (1) nutritional deprivation, or (2) surgery, disease or other trauma. Inadequate energy and protein intake results in the body catabolizing its own protein tissue to provide energy and animo acids for synthesis of essential life-supporting proteins. Tissues with the most rapid turnover, including the intestinal mucosa and other visceral tissues, are utilized as a source of amino acids. This depletion of the gut results in a flattening of the intestinal villi and decreased levels of digestive enzymes, causing diarrhea and malabsorption. Repletion of nutritional status is essential for repair of the gut tissue and clinical improvement of diarrhea and malabsorption.[1]

Footnote at end of table

(*Continued*)

TABLE M-4 (*Continued*)

Causes	Abnormality	Comments
Reduced intestinal bile salt (Also see GALLSTONES.)	Hepatobiliary disease (liver and gallbladder disorders).	Diseases such as hepatitis, cirrhosis, and gallbladder diseases impair the synthesis or excretion of bile salts.
	Abnormal numbers of bacteria in the small intestine.	There is evidence of a vitamin B-12 deficiency due to binding and/or utilization of vitamin B-12 by bacteria. Also, bacteria are responsible for altering the chemical nature of bile making it ineffective. Problems occur in blind loop syndrome and diverticulosis, and other conditions which may hinder the passage of food through the small intestine.
(Also see BILE; GALLSTONES; and ILEITIS.)	Interrupted circulation of bile.	Surgical procedures involving the ileum, and ileitis are responsible for reducing the bile salt pool.
	Drug induced.	Drugs can impair emulsifying function of bile salts by chelating or precipitating bile salts; for example, neomycin, and cholestyramine.

[1]Coale, Margaret S. and John R. K. Robson, Dietary Management of Intractable Diarrhea in Malnourished Patients, *Journal of The American Dietetic Association*, Vol. 76, No. 5, May 1980, pp. 444-450.

MALAISE

A feeling of illness or depression.

MALARIA

Initially, there was some confusion over the cause-and-effect of this disease; hence, the name malaria which literally means "bad air." Swamps do produce bad air but, more importantly, they also produce *Anopheles* mosquitoes which carry the malaria parasites. In the cycle of this parasite man serves as an intermediate host, and the mosquito serves as a vector. Transmission of the disease requires at least two mosquito bites—one to pick up the malaria parasite, and another to infect the victim. Fig.M-5 illustrates the malaria cycle.

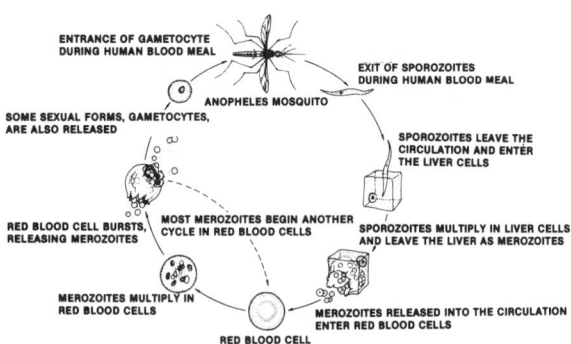

Fig. M-5.   The malaria cycle.

Ordinarily, man becomes infected with a species of *Plasmodium* when the female mosquito bites him to obtain a blood meal, though there have been cases of malaria transmission through transfusion blood, and contaminated needles and syringes of drug addicts. While biting, the mosquito injects saliva to prevent clotting, some digestive enzymes, and sporozoites of the malaria parasite. Once in the circulation of man, the sporozoites enter the liver cells within a short time. After about a week of growing and reproducing, they leave the liver as merozoites which enter the red blood cells. In the red blood cells the merozoites rapidly reproduce and eventually burst the infected red blood cell. This sets more merozoites free to infect other red blood cells, or to enter other tissues where they remain as a source for malarial relapses. The bursting of the red blood cells coincides with the characteristic malaria attacks of chills, fever, headache, sweating, and muscle pain leaving the patient exhausted.

While the asexual merozoites begin another cycle in the red blood cells, some sexual forms of the parasite—gametocytes—appear in the blood of the human host. These are transmitted back into another mosquito during another blood meal. In the gut of the new mosquito the male and female forms of the parasite—gametocytes—unite and form sporozoites which then migrate to the salivary gland where they will be discharged with the next blood meal. Thus, the cycle is completed.

There are four types of *Plasmodium* which are responsible for three distinct forms of malaria. Each form of malaria can be distinguished by the length of time between the recurrent malaria attacks.

• **Tertian malaria**—Merozoites are released every other day—every 48 hours. It is rarely fatal, and it can be caused by both *Plasmodium vivax* and *Plasmodium ovale*. However, infections of *Plasmodium ovale* tend to produce milder and shorter attacks.

• **Quartan malaria**—Attacks occur every fourth day, or 72 hours apart; hence, the name quartan. It is caused by *Plasmodium malariae.* Quartan is usually more disabling than tertian, but it responds well to treatment.

• **Falciparum malaria**—This is the most severe form, and it may be fatal if treatment is delayed or inadequate. It is caused by *Plasmodium falciparum.* Falciparum malaria block the capillaries to vital organs, and can prove fatal at any time during the course of the disease. In this form of malaria there is no characteristic length of time between attacks since the merozoites multiply in asynchronous cycles. The fever produced may be continuous or irregular.

It is not possible to prevent infection, but while residing in an area where there is a risk of contracting malaria, drugs can be taken that suppress the symptoms. Upon leaving the area proper, chemotherapy can "cure" a malaria infection. However, in "cured" malaria infections of particularly *Plasmodium malariae* relapses are known to occur years after the initial infection.

Prevention can only come about through public health programs that eliminate the *Anopheles* mosquito. Stagnant pools, swamps and marshes must be drained where possible, and insectides harmless to man should be used. In the United States during the mid-thirties the average yearly toll from malaria was 4 million cases. By the early 1950s, native malaria in this country was virtually eradicated. Worldwide prevention, however, may be a distant goal due to the emergence of insecticide-resistant mosquitoes, drug-resistant parasites, and a variety of administrative and socioeconomic problems. International travelers to areas where there is a risk of malaria—Central and South America, Africa, Southern Asia, and the Philippines—should consult a United States Public Health Official about precautions before arrival, during the visit, and after departure.

From a nutritional standpoint, malaria is important for two reasons. First, malaria survives in areas where the mosquito and the infected human population remain above a critical density for each. This situation often occurs in time of famine when people congregate, following which rains come producing breeding grounds for mosquitoes. Malaria then spreads rapidly among the weakened survivors of the famine. Second, malaria attacks, chronic malaria, or repeated infections of malaria are taxing on the nutritional reserves of the body. Good nutrition is essential to recovery. A high calorie, high protein, high fluid intake with vitamin supplementation is recommended.

(Also see MODIFIED DIETS.)

MALAY APPLE (POMERAC) *Eugenia malaccensis*

The fruit of an evergreen tree (of a family *Myrtaceae*) that is native to Malaysia and is now grown throughout the tropics. Malay apples are reddish-pink, oblong or pear-shaped fruit that are about 3 in. (*8 cm*) long. They have a white flesh that surrounds the single large seed. The rather bland fruit may be eaten fresh or made into jam or jelly.

Malay apples have a high water content (91%) and are low in calories (32 kcal per 100 g) and carbohydrates (8%). They are a fair source of vitamin C.

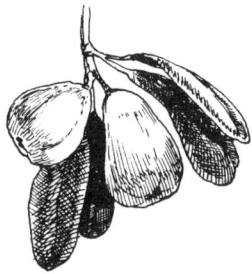

Fig. M-6. The Malay apple.

MALFORMATION

Any abnormal development in the physical and physiological makeup of the body.

MALIGNANT

Cancerous growth, as distinguished from a benign growth.
(Also see CANCER.)

MALNUTRITION

Contents | Page

This term refers to an impairment of health resulting from a failure of the diet, or from a failure of the physiologic processes of the body itself, to provide to the tissues the correct proportions of nutrients. Thus, malnutrition may involve nutrient deficiencies, excesses of nutrients such as carbohydrates, or a combination of deficiencies and excesses.
(Also see DISEASES.)

Disproportions or imbalances between the dietary supply and the tissue requirement for nutrients are responsible for severe deficiency diseases, like beriberi. Populations relying on dietary staples, such as commercially milled white rice, which is high in carbohydrates but low in the thiamin required for its metabolism, are very susceptible to beriberi. Other groups eating a similar diet may avoid the disease by using rice which has been parboiled prior to milling; parboiling rice drives the thiamin from the outside of the grain into the inner parts. As a result, less thiamin is lost when the outer layers of rice are removed during milling.

(Also see BERIBERI; and RICE, section headed "Nutritional Losses.")

Another example of a potential imbalance is the substitution of heat-processed polyunsaturated fats for saturated fats without the addition of vitamin E to the diet. The natural sources of these fats are plant seeds which usually contain ample amounts of vitamin E. But the vitamin E is easily destroyed in the extracted oils by exposure to heat, light, and oxygen. Although severe deficiencies of vitamin E are rare, marginal deficiencies may, over a long period, be responsible for cellular damage and premature senility. Both disorders may be caused by the peroxidation of polyunsaturated fatty acids, which is prevented by vitamin E.

(Also see VITAMIN E.)

Finally, there is evidence that high intake of dietary protein, such as 100 to 150 g/day, result in increased calcium excretion in the urine, thereby raising the requirement for dietary calcium to replace the extra loss from the body. Failure to provide the additional calcium in the diet may lead to the removal of calcium from bone, since the body maintains the level of the mineral in the blood by taking it from bone.

(Also see CALCIUM; and OSTEOPOROSIS.)

MALNUTRITION AROUND THE WORLD.

Many adverse physical conditions are brought about by prolonged periods of malnutrition, especially the absence of sufficient quantities of critical compounds in the diet. Rickets, scurvy, beriberi, pellagra, vitamin A deficiency (a major cause of blindness in many countries), anemia, iodine deficiency (which often leads to endemic goiter and cretinism), kwashiorkor, and marasmus are but a few of the many classical examples of nutritional deficiency diseases. When malnutrition begins at an early age and persists over a substantial period of time, a variety of defects may develop involving bone and body structures and mental condition, all of which may be irreversible. Unfortunately, in the developing countries, the basic problem is one of gross dietary inadequacies which may be compounded by specific vitamin or protein insufficiency.

The most malnutrition is found in the developing countries where 70% of the people in the world live, but where only 40% of the world's food is produced. Fig. M-7 shows the countries where the greatest deficits of protein and calories are found.

In Latin America, where protein-poor cereal grains are the imperfect staff of life, 82 out of every 1,000 children die before their first birthday; and another 12 die before they reach the age of 4. Even the survivors may envy the dead. Often brain damaged, they become the adults who are most in need of help and least able to help themselves.

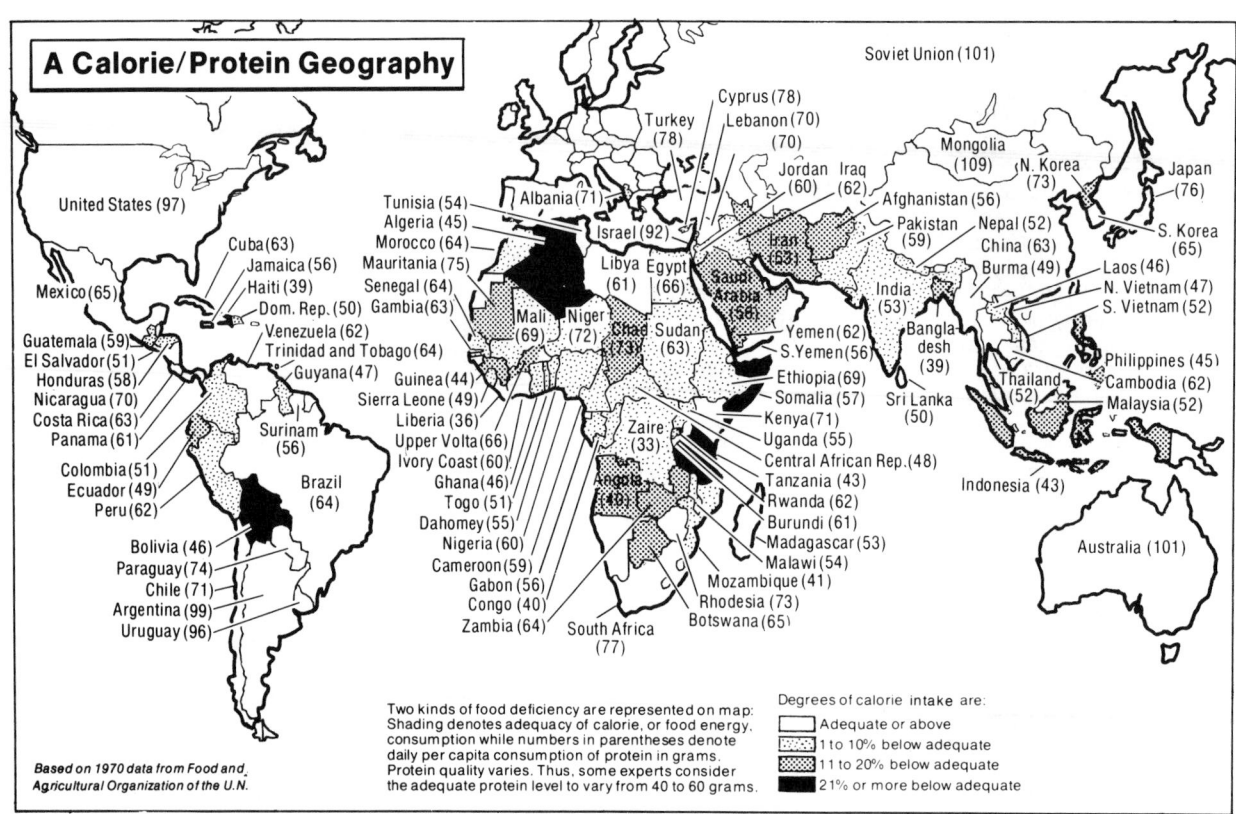

Fig. M-7. World geography of calories and proteins. (Courtesy, *The New York Times*)

In the Far East and Africa, 25 to 30% of the population is estimated to suffer from significant undernutrition. FAO estimates that (1) altogether in the developing world (exclusive of the Asian centrally planned economies for which insufficient information is available), malnutrition affects around 460 million people—that's nearly twice the population of the United States; and (2) one-half of the young children in the developing countries suffer in varying degrees from inadequate nutrition.[7]

According to the World Health Organization (WHO), 10 million children under the age of 5 are now chronically and severely malnourished, and 90 million more are moderately affected. While undernourished children may remain alive, they are extremely vulnerable to minor infectious diseases. WHO figures also show that of all the deaths in the poor countries, more than half occur among children under 5, and that the vast majority of all these deaths, perhaps as many as 75%, are due to malnutrition complicated by infection.

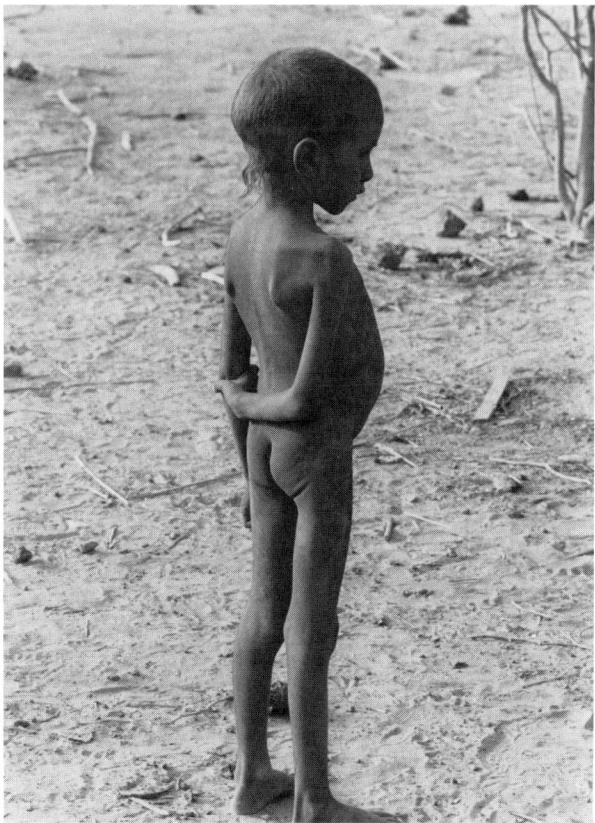

Fig. M-8. A malnourished youngster in the Sahel. Five years of drought caused human suffering and loss of cattle in the six countries along the southern edge of the Sahara. The Sahelian Zone includes Upper Volta, Mauritania, Niger, Senegal, Mali, and Chad. (Courtesy, Agency for International Development)

---

[7]*The World Food Situation and Prospects to 1985,* Foreign Ag. Econ. Report No. 98, Economic Research Service, USDA, p. 50.

CAUSES OF MALNUTRITION. Poor health due to malnourishment may be the result of one or more factors contributing to poor diets or reduced utilization of nutrients of the body. Some of the more important factors are outlined in Fig. M-9, and are discussed under the items which follow:

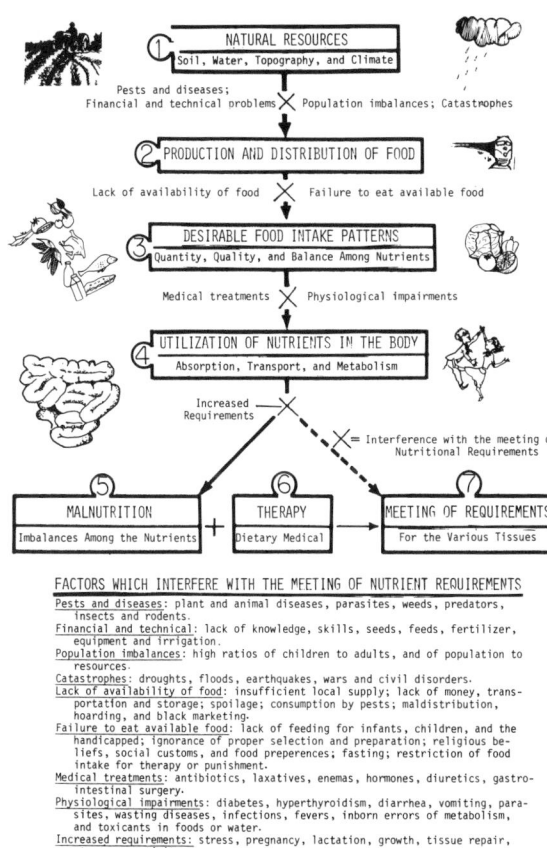

Fig. M-9. Causes of malnutrition.

- **Failure to cultivate arable land**—Although China has the smallest area of cultivated land per person of any nation in the world, she manages to feed her population by cultivating every inch of it. By contrast, central Africa cultivates less than 1/5 of its arable land, South America less than 1/6. However, some of the unused land could be brought under cultivation only with modern and costly technology.

- **Catastrophic events**—Droughts, floods, earthquakes, wars, and civil disorders may impede the process of agricultural development. For example, natural disasters and civil disorders have recently resulted in disruption of food production and distribution in Asia, Africa, and South America.

- **The population explosion**—Birthrates have continued to climb in many developing countries, partly because children who survive and reach adulthood may be a form of old age insurance for the parents.

• **Bad weather**—This has also been a major cause of malnutrition, since unexpected floods and droughts may disrupt the cycle of planting, growth, and harvesting of crops. Some of the high-yielding varieties of crops require a narrow range of soil, moisture, and temperature factors.

• **Inefficient food production**—About half of the world's potential for food production is not utilized. Improvements in the efficiency of agriculture require knowledge, skills, seeds, feeds, fertilizer, pesticides, farming equipment, irrigation, and health manpower. Developing areas frequently lack the funds and technical expertise to modernize readily their agricultural systems. Modest gains in production may be wiped out by field pests, diseases of plants and animals, predators, and storage pests—such as insects and rodents. Pests cause an estimated 30% annual loss in the worldwide production of crops, livestock, and forests.[8]

• **Reduced availability of grains**—These shortages force low-income people to resort to starchy plants, such as bananas, sweet potatoes, and cassava, for their staple foods. Nutritional problems are created by the low content of protein and other nutrients in these high-carbohydrate foods. They are particularly bad for the nutrition of infants and growing children, who require proportions of protein to energy (calories) similar to those in mixtures of grains and legumes in order to grow and remain in good health. Another reason for reliance on starchy roots, in tropical areas, is that grains do not store well under such conditions and are more susceptible to damage and destruction by insect pests and spoilage.

• **Lack of money**—Increasingly, this factor is becoming a cause of malnutrition due to the worldwide technical and socioeconomic changes spurred on by population growth, development of industry, and increased opportunities for trade. These developments result in higher costs of homes and land, and ultimately reduce the feasibility of obtaining food by hunting, fishing, gathering wild plants, and farming on small plots of land. The modernization of agriculture usually results in unemployment for some of the unskilled workers, who then move to urban areas to seek employment and food. Such developments around the world have been referred to as "the rural-to-urban malnutrition gradient." There is usually a modest reduction in malnutrition in the developing urban areas, compared to the rural areas, as a result of better opportunities for at least marginal employment which may cover the basic expenses of survival, low-cost health care, or various types of public and private assistance. In recent years, however, the ability to assist the unemployed and indigent has been sorely taxed in big cities, due to the large numbers seeking such assistance.

• **High food costs**—In developing countries and among the poor in all countries, expenditures for food may take 50% of private consumption expenditures; and cereals may account for as much as 50 to 70% of the cost of food. For these people, a doubling or tripling of the costs

of cereals during periods of scarcity, as happened in the early 1970s, is a major disaster.

The disparity that exists in the proportion of income spent for food from country to country is shown in Fig. M-10.

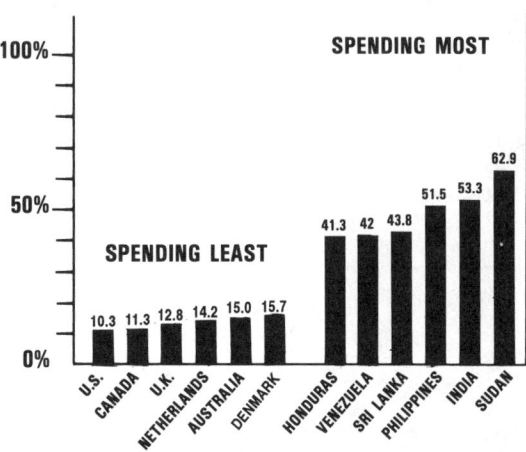

PERCENT OF INCOME SPENT ON FOOD

Fig. M-10. Proportion of income spent for food. As income rises, consumers spend a smaller proportion of their wages for food. Most countries are experiencing a decline in the amount of income spent for food due to greater efficiency in production, processing, and distribution. (Source: *Statistical Abstract of the United States 1991*, p. 843, and the USDA.)

• **Poor sanitation**—Foodborne and waterborne disease organisms are responsible for high incidences of gastrointestinal diseases in the developing countries. Also, infestation with parasites may greatly aggravate mild cases of deficiency diseases, such as the anemias.

• **Poor nutritional knowledge and practices**—Malnutrition is often present in areas other than "poverty pockets" and undeveloped regions, since persons having sufficient funds and availability of foods may have a poor diet due to personal reasons, such as religious beliefs, social customs, ignorance of proper selection and preparation of foods, and well-entrenched food habits. Americans, for example, consume per capita each year, refined, high-energy foods in the following amounts: sugar, 64.2 lb and corn sweeteners, 71.9 lb; fats, including butter, margarine and salad oils, 62.7 lb; white flour, 137.8 lb; and white rice, 16.1 lb.[9] An analysis of this data shows that 353 lb of food supplying mainly carbohydrates (and few other nutrients) provide approximately 598,187 Calories (kcal) per year or 1,638 Calories (kcal) per day. The 62.7 lb of separated fats (salad oil, butter, margarine, shortenings, etc.) provided 251,983 Calories (kcal) per year, or 690 Calories (kcal) per day. Thus, an average daily diet has most of its energy (about 2,000 Calories [kcal]) contributed by foods low in protein, vitamins, and minerals. These data are very alarming when one considers that the per capita figures are averages which include children (who eat less food than adults), and that the energy allowances per day for

---

[8]Ennis, Jr., W. B., W. M. Dowler, and W. Klassen, "Crop Production to Increase Food Supplies," *Science*, Vol. 188, No. 4188, May 9, 1975, p. 593.

[9]*Agricultural Statistics 1991*, USDA, p. 479, Table 672.

adult males and females are 2,700 Calories (kcal) and 2,000 Calories (kcal), respectively.[10]

• **Disorders which hamper the utilization of nutrients**— This refers to disorders which reduce the value of adequate diets. Uncontrolled diabetes, for example, is a condition where the victim literally starves on an adequate diet because the major nutrients do not enter the cells due to a lack of insulin. Other conditions responsible for hampering the utilization of nutrients are hyperthyroidism, hyperparathyroidism, diarrhea, vomiting, parasites, wasting diseases, infections, fevers, inborn errors of metabolism, and toxicants in food.

• **Iatrogenic malnutrition**—This refers to medical treatments which interfere with nutritional processes; among them, the administration of antibiotics, laxatives, enemas, hormones, anticonvulsants, diuretics, and gastrointestinal surgery, and the severe restriction of diet. For example, antibiotics may kill the microorganisms in the intestine which synthesize vitamins (such as vitamin K).

CONSEQUENCES OF MALNUTRITION. The
cost to the individual and to the society of illness, disability, and death from malnutrition far outweight the expense of adequate nutrition. Some of these consequences follow.

Impairment of Physical and Mental Development.
Physical development is determined by nutrition to such an extent that a high incidence of short stature in a population is now regarded as a sign that malnutrition exists in that population. The condition of nutritional dwarfing usually results fom protein-energy malnutrition; but impairment of growth may also result from deficiencies of vitamin A, B complex, C, and D, and from deficiencies of mineral elements such as iron, iodine, calcium, and phosphorus. Children may never catch up in growth if stunting occurs during a critical growth period. It is difficult to guess the ages of children in parts of the world where they may have a physical development like that of much younger children. Such malnutrition may pass undetected by the outside observer who is not aware of the ages of the children that he sees.

Development of the brain and nervous system may be hindered by severe malnutrition during fetal life and the first 2 years after birth. Some of the nutrients which are most needed for central nervous system activity are vitamin A, vitamin C, thiamin, riboflavin, niacin, pyridoxine, pantothenic acid, folic acid, and vitamin B-12. Mental functions derive not only from the physical structure of the brain, but from the interaction between children and other persons. Those who are frequently sick miss many school days and may drop out of school at a young age, thereby reducing their opportunities for escaping poverty and malnutrition and for receiving stimulation of intellectual growth.

Increased Susceptibility to Infectious Diseases.
Some forms of malnutrition reduce the response of the immune system to disease, while others slow the rate of recovery. Significantly greater numbers of children die in areas of malnutrition from diseases like measles, which are not usually fatal in healthier populations. There may be a reservoir of infection in poorly fed regions which makes more likely the exposure to contagious diseases. Fevers may be undetected, due to subnormal body temperatures resulting from malnutrition. Although protein deficiency is most likely to be the cause of reduced immunity, increased susceptibility to communicable diseases may also result from deficiencies of vitamin A, B complex, and C, and from iron.

Increased Susceptibility to Metabolic Disorders.
Nutritional imbalances cover a wide range of conditions ranging from starvation to obesity. It is ironic that both starvation, during early life, and obesity, later in life, may lead to increased tendencies toward the development of diabetes. Chronic low-protein intakes often lead to liver disorders. Kidney malfunction may be a response to stress induced by deficiencies of potassium, protein, and/or water; and increased stone formation may result from magnesium deficiency. Statistical studies have shown that there are higher incidences of bowel cancer in regions such as the United States where the fat content of diets is high.[11]

Chronic lack of dietary fiber is thought to contribute to a host of gastrointestinal problems plus diabetes and cancer. It also appears that there may be undiscovered relationships between nutrition and disease.

Reduced Work Capacity.
Slave owners in the Americas recognized that the productivity they received from their slaves improved in proportion to the quantity and quality of food issued to them. More precise observations were made during World War II on civilian workers and military personnel in order to learn how to obtain better performance. Energy from foods was found to be the first limiting factor for work performance, but protein, vitamin, and mineral deficiencies were accompanied by lack of initiative, reduced speed and coordination, and tendencies to become fatigued.

Increased per capita consumption of food energy in nine Latin American countries resulted in increased productivity which accounted for almost 5% of the average growth in national products. The contribution of diet almost equaled that of education. Mexico had the largest gain in productivity (10% of growth) which could be attributed to better nutrition.[12]

Another consequence of poor nutrition is reduced life expectancy and shortening of the working lifetime. Some very poorly fed populations have high ratios of infants and children to able-bodied adults workers, which results in lower per capita productivity of those populations.

---

[10]*Recommended Dietary Allowances*, 9th rev. ed., Food and Nutrition Board, NRC-National Academy of Sciences, Washington, D.C., 1980.

[11]Rose, D. P., "Update: Diet, Nutrition and Cancer," *The Professional Nutritionist*, Foremost Foods Company, San Francisco, Calif., Vol. 8, No. 4, Fall 1976, p. 1.

[12]Correa, H., and G. Cummins, "Contribution of Nutrition to Economic Growth," *American Journal of Clinical Nutrition*, Vol. 23, 1970, p. 560.

COMMON TYPES OF MALNUTRITION. About one billion cases of malnutrition around the world result mainly from lack of sufficient food.[13] However, hundreds of millions of people suffer from mild to severe nutritional deficiency diseases such as anemia, beriberi, blindness due to vitamin A deficiency (xerophthalmia), goiter, marasmus, pellagra, protein-energy malnutrition, rickets (children) or osteomalacia (adults), and scurvy.

Some of the more prevalent types of deficiencies are briefly described in the paragraphs which follow.

Protein-Energy Malnutrition. An insufficient intake of energy and/or protein needed to maintain the body functions—for activity, for growth, and for resistance to infectious diseases—may be manifested, in keeping with the severity of the deficiency, from the slight impairment of growth or thinness seen in mildly undernourished children to the gross alterations shown by persons suffering from kwashiorkor (protein deficiency) or marasmus (energy deficiency). There are many areas, particularly in the tropics and subtropics, where the inhabitants do not have enough food because of such factors as large populations, poor soils (heavy rainfall leaches out some minerals), and generally unfavorable climates for production of grains other than rice.

(Also see MALNUTRITION, PROTEIN-ENERGY; and STARVATION.)

Deficiencies of Minerals or Vitamins. The lack of sufficient quantities of critical vitamins or minerals may be the cause of many adverse conditions, even when the dietary amounts of protein and energy are adequate. Such deficiencies may result in disorders of specific organs and tissues, or of metabolic processes in general.

(Also see ANEMIA; BERIBERI; BLINDNESS DUE TO VITAMIN A DEFICIENCY; DEFICIENCY DISEASES; GOITER; PELLAGRA; RICKETS; and SCURVY.)

Disorders of Nutrient Utilization. Malnutrition may result even when the diet contains adequate amounts of all of the nutrients which are known to be required. In these cases, disease may be caused by a failure of the body to utilize fully certain nutrients, by accumulation of excess amounts of nutrients and/or their metabolites, or by diet-induced changes of the normal environment in and around tissues so that these areas develop increased vulnerability to pathogenic agents and stress factors. However, there may also be nonnutritional causes of some of these disorders, since it has been difficult to explain why a given diet results in disease for some, and fairly good health for others.

(Also see HEART DISEASE; DENTAL CARIES; DIABETES MELLITUS; INBORN ERRORS OF METABOLISM; MALABSORPTION SYNDROME; OBESITY; OSTEOPOROSIS.)

SIGNS OF MALNUTRITION. There are many signs which indicate moderate to severe malnutrition. Also, a number of laboratory tests are available for detection of tissue pathologies, metabolic imbalances, and deficiency diseases. It would be worthwhile, however, to be able to diagnose early stages of malnutrition, since prompt correction of dietary imbalances will, in the long run, be much less costly than later treatment of the more severe stages.

The incidence of malnutrition may be estimated for communities by examining hospital and autopsy records, and by interviewing the parents of deceased children. Also, some individual cases may be diagnosed by their features. Each of these types of assessment will be discussed under the items which follow.

Indicators of Malnutrition in Communities. Although cases of malnutrition may be found among all socioeconomic classes, one is most likely to find this condition in areas where there are serious problems concerning the following factors: the production and distribution of food, unemployment and low incomes, environmental sanitation, public health and other community services, and unusual food preferences.

A preliminary survey of the living conditions in a community might, therefore, save time and money in assessing the nutritional status of its residents. The following types of data might be collected in such a survey: (1) population from latest census; (2) total food consumption by the population (which may be roughly estimated from figures showing local production and shipments of food into the area); (3) foods and nutrients available per capita, which may be calculated from (1) and (2) and a food composition table; (4) morbidity and mortality statistics, plus estimates of school attendance and absenteeism in local industry; (5) infant feeding practices, such as breast feeding, use of formulas, baby foods, table foods, etc.; (6) food preferences and customs of the ethnic and religious groups in the community; (7) employment and income status; (8) water quality and sanitary facilities for disposal of garbage and human and animal waste; (9) food, health, and financial services provided by public and voluntary agencies; and (10) the professional training and number of workers in the service agencies. Personnel in these agencies may be requested to assist in such a survey, together with teachers, parents, and community leaders.

Analyses of the data should provide indications of the types of malnutrition and other health problems which are most likely to be present. Some examples of such analyses follow:

• **Nutrient consumption per capita**—The U.S. Department of Agriculture conducted a household food consumption survey which covered 14,500 persons.[14]

Part of the data was expressed as percentages of the Recommended Dietary Allowance (RDA) for each of the sex-age and income groups which were studied. Thus, it was shown that females 18 to 19 years of age, from low income families, consumed food which contained only 49% of the recommended daily allowance for calcium, and 57% of that for iron. Such dietary patterns might ultimately lead to increased incidences of osteoporosis and anemia for this group.

---

[13]McLaren, D. S., "Hunger/Malnutrition: Some Misconceptions," *The Professional Nutritionist*, Fall 1978, p. 13.

[14]*Dietary Levels of Households in the United States*, Ag. Res. Serv. Bull. No. 62–17, USDA.

• **Morbidity and mortality statistics**—A study in the state of Michigan showed that over half of a group of children under 5 years of age who died from measles had severe deficits in height and weight.[15]

It was suggested that the underlying cause of the unusual severity of these cases of measles was malnutrition.

Another study showed that Japanese men in Hawaii had higher rates of coronary heart disease than Japanese in Japan.[16]

The investigators suggested that the greater mortality in Hawaii compared to Japan might be explained by the greater variation in the caloric intake of the Hawaiians.

[15]Robson, J. R. K., and E. L. Jones, "Is the Child with Poor Growth Achievement More Likely to Die from Measles?," *Clinical Pediatrics,* Vol. 10, 1970, p. 270.

[16]Bassett, D. R., *et al.,* "Coronary Heart Disease in Hawaii: Dietary Intake, Depot Fat, 'Stress,' Smoking, and Energy Balance in Hawaiian and Japanese Men," *American Journal of Clinical Nutrition,* Vol. 22, 1969, p. 1483.

Signs of Malnutrition in Individuals. Assessment of the nutritional status of individuals by laboratory tests is expensive, so it is necessary to have some screening procedures for identifying persons who are most likely to suffer from malnutrition. Such screenings may include medical histories of individuals and their families; heights, weights, and other growth data for children; dietary histories; and observations of the face, tongue, mouth, eyes, skin, muscular and skeletal development, and weight in proportion to height.

Also, the following are valuable adjuncts in screening: measurements of hemoglobin in finger prick samples of blood, testing of urine with pretreated tapes for sugar and ketone bodies, and examination for the presence of sediment in the urine. In adolescents, the stage of sexual development in relation to age may be determined by physicians or nurses, since maturation may be delayed in malnutrition.

Criteria for the diagnosis of specific nutritional disorders are given in this book under the separate entries for each disease. Physical signs often associated with malnutrition are shown in Table M-5.

TABLE M-5
PHYSICAL SIGNS WHICH ARE OFTEN ASSOCIATED WITH MALNUTRITION[1]

Area of Body Examined	Normal Appearance	Common Signs of Malnutrition	Differential Diagnoses (other causes of clinical signs)
Appearance in general	Normal weight for age, sex, and height. Alert and emotionally stable. No areas of edema.	Significant overweight or underweight. Apathetic or hyperirritable. Loss or slowness of ankle or knee reflexes. Pitting edema.	Nonnutritional nervous or metabolic disorders. Endocrine diseases.
Eyes	Shiny and free from areas of abnormal pigmentation, opacity, vascularization, and dryness.	Paleness, dryness, redness, or pigmentation of membranes (conjunctiva). Foamy patches on conjunctiva (Bitot's spots). Dullness, softness, or vascularization of the cornea. Redness or fissures on eyelids.	Exposure to environmental or chemical irritants. Tissue changes accompanying aging.
Face	Skin is clear and uniform in color, free of all except minor blemishes. Free of swollen or lumpy areas.	Skin has lighter (depigmentation) and darker (over cheeks and under eyes) areas. Greasy scales around nose and lips. Swollen or lumpy areas.	Poor hygiene. Addison's disease (moonface).
Glands	No swollen areas on face or neck.	Swelling of parotids (enlarged "jowls") or thyroid (front of neck near its base).	Mumps. Inflammation, tumor, or hyperfunction of the thyroid.
Gums	Red, free from bleeding or swelling.	Receded. "Spongy" and bleeding. Swelling of the gingiva.	Medication. Periodontal disease. Poor oral hygiene.
Hair	Shiny, firmly attached to scalp (not easily plucked without pain to patient).	Dullness, may be brittle and easily plucked without pain. Sometimes lighter in color than normal (depigmentation may be bandlike when hair is held up to a source of light).	Endocrine disorders.

Footnotes at end of table

(Continued)

TABLE M-5 (Continued)

Area of Body Examined	Normal Appearance	Common Signs of Malnutrition	Differential Diagnoses (other causes of clinical signs)
Lips	Smooth, not chapped, cracked, or swollen.	Swollen, red, or cracked (cheilosis). Angular tissues and/or scars at the corners of the mouth.	Herpes (blisters). Exposure to strong sunshine, dry or cold climates.
Muscles	Muscles are firm and of normal size.	Wasting and flabbiness of muscle. Bleeding into muscle.	Wasting diseases. Trauma.
Nails	Firm, pink.	Spoon-shaped nails. Brittle and ridged nails.	Cardiopulmonary disease.
Organs, internal	Normal heart rate and rhythm. Normal blood pressure. Internal organs cannot be palpated (except the liver in children).	Racing heartbeat (over 100 beats per minute). Abnormal rhythm of heart. High blood pressure. Palpable enlargement of liver or spleen.	Rheumatic fever. Nonnutritional diseases of the heart, liver, spleen, and kidneys.
Skeleton	Bones have normal sizes and shapes.	Softening, swelling, or distorted shapes of bones and joints.	Nonnutritional connective tissue disorders.
Skin	Smooth, free of rashes, swellings, and discoloration.	Roughness (follicular hyperkeratosis), dryness, or flakiness. Irregular pigmentation, black and blue marks, "crazy pavement" lesions. Symmetrical, reddened lesions (like sunburn). Looseness of skin (lack of subcutaneous fat).	Secondary syphilis. Poor or improper hygiene (excessive washing with soap). Environmental irritants. Trauma. Anticoagulant therapy.
Teeth	Enamel is unbroken and unspotted. None or a few small cavities.	Caries. Mottled or darkened areas of enamel.	Developmental abnormalities. Stains from foods or cigarettes.
Tongue	Normal size of papillae (no atrophy or hypertrophy). Color is uniform and deep red. Sense of taste is without impairment.	Atrophy of papillae (the tongue is smooth) or hypertrophy of papillae. Irregularly shaped and distributed white patches. Swollen, scarlet, magenta (purple colored), or raw tongue.	Dietary irritants. Colors or dyes from food. Nonnutritional anemias. Antibiotics. Uremia. Malignancy.

¹Adapted by the authors from *American Journal of Public Health*, Vol. 63, November 1973 Supplement, p. 19, Table 1.

TREATMENT AND PREVENTION OF MALNUTRITION. The first step in the correction of a dietary imbalance is the use of a modified or supplemented diet, or when necessary, medical correction of a disorder which limits the utilization of nutrients.

(Also see MINERAL SUPPLEMENTS; MODIFIED DIETS; NUTRITIONAL SUPPLEMENTS; and VITAMIN SUPPLEMENTS.)

Sometimes it is necessary to administer nutrients by tube feeding to hospitalized patients who can't eat, or by injection to persons who require a supplement such as vitamin B-12, which is stored in the body and needs only to be supplied once a month.

Overtreatment of malnutrition by administration of excessive amounts of nutrients in a short period of time may be dangerous, since the victim usually has a reduced ability to detoxify and excrete excess materials. The treatment may, therefore, produce effects worse than the disease. All treatments require supervision by health professionals who are able to recognize the clinical signs of deterioration in the patient.

It may be more expeditious at the community, state, or national levels to enrich and fortify foods of low nutrient quality with amino acids, minerals, and vitamins, than to try to supply foods which naturally contain the optimal quantities of nutrients. this is particularly applicable to situations where foods, which are rich in the desired nutrients, are rejected by the population to be fed. For example, there is a high rejection rate for broccoli, carrots, and other vegetable sources of vitamin A in the U.S. School Lunch Program. Therefore, food technologists have proposed the development of a snack food, like a potato chip, which would contain spinach powder and be fortified with minerals and vitamins.

Prevention of malnutrition requires correction of the factors leading to a poor diet. This calls for education of the consumer; instituting new patterns of food selection, preparation, and consumption; and insuring that supplies of the appropriate foods are available.

(Also see ENRICHMENT [Fortification, Nutrification, Restoration].)

MALNUTRITION, PROTEIN-ENERGY

One of the most serious nutritional problems in the developing countries of the world is a group of disorders associated with inadequate or unbalanced intakes of protein and energy. It is often convenient to consider these disorders as various types of protein-energy malnutrition (PEM).

DIETARY ENERGY AND PROTEIN SUPPLIES AROUND THE WORLD. Although PEM may be found even in the developed countries, by far the greatest number of cases occur in the developing countries where food shortages limit the average consumption of energy and protein. Therefore, two rough indicators of the incidence of PEM are the per capita deficits in energy and in protein supplies of various countries. This means that there is the likelihood of there being a significant number of cases of PEM in countries where the per capita supplies of energy and/or protein fall below the recom-

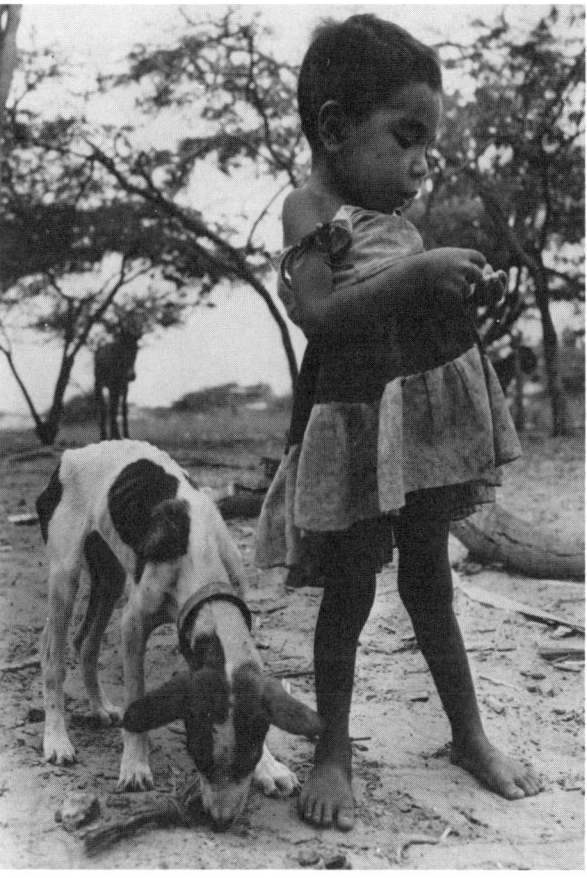

Fig. M-11. The world is rich, but not making good use of its riches. Too many people live in the shadow of chronic hunger and malnutrition. In this picture, the child with clear signs of malnutrition and poor development and the dog showing its ribs, indicate that they live little above the starvation level. (Courtesy, WHO, Geneva, Switzerland)

mended daily requirements defined by the Joint FAO/WHO Expert Committee on Energy and Protein Requirements.[17]

Information on energy and protein supplies is given in Tables M-6, M-7, and M-8. Table M-6 shows the ranking of countries in average available supplies of dietary energy in calories per capita, along with the percentage of requirements met by the available energy. Table M-7 shows the ranking of countries in average available supplies of protein in grams per capita. It is noteworthy that, of the 127 countries listed in these tables, 33 are classed as developed and 94 are developing. Table M-8 shows the per capita calories and proteins per day of countries in two groups: (1) developed countries, and (2) developing countries.

---

[17]Per capita requirements per day of 2,385 Calories (kcal) and 38.7 g of protein (as defined by the FAO/WHO Expert Committee in April 1971). From *Nutrition Newsletter*, Vol. 11, No. 4, FAO of the United Nations, October-December 1973, p. 4., Table 1.

TABLE M-6
WORLD DIETARY ENERGY SUPPLY[1]

Country	Dietary Energy Supply[2]	Percent-age of Require-ments[3]	Country	Dietary Energy Supply[2]	Percent-age of Require-ments[3]
	(Calories/ person/ day)	(%)		(Calories/ person/ day)	(%)
Ireland	3410	136	Paraguay	2740	119
			South Africa	2740	112
Belgium-Luxembourg	3380	128	Cuba	2700	117
United States	3330	126			
Netherlands	3320	123	Chile	2670	109
Austria	3310	126	Cyprus	2670	108
			Rhodesia	2660	111
Bulgaria	3290	126	Syrian Arab Rep.	2650	107
German Dem. Rep.	3290	126	Brazil	2620	110
Australia	3280	123	Costa Rica	2610	116
Hungary	3280	125	Spain	2600	106
Poland	3280	125			
U.S.S.R.	3280	131	Zambia	2590	112
Turkey	3250	129	Mexico	2580	111
Denmark	3240	120	Panama	2580	112
Germany, Fed. Rep.	3220	121	Libyan Arab Rep.	2570	109
France	3210	127	Thailand	2560	115
New Zealand	3200	121	Madagascar	2530	111
			Korea, Rep.	2520	107
Greece	3190	128	Japan	2510	107
Switzerland	3190	119	Egypt	2500	100
United Kingdom	3190	126			
Yugoslavia	3190	125	Gambia	2490	104
Italy	3180	126	Malaysia (West)	2460	110
Canada	3180	129	Nicaragua	2450	109
Czechoslovakia	3180	129	Surinam	2450	109
Romania	3140	118	Ivory Coast	2430	105
			Jordan	2430	99
Argentina	3060	115	Khmer Rep.	2430	98
Finland	3050	113	Venezuela	2430	98
			Cameroon	2410	104
Israel	2960	115			
Norway	2960	110	Albania	2390	99
Portugal	2900	118	Guiana	2390	105
			Mongolia	2380	106
Uruguay	2880	108	Trinidad and Tobago	2380	98
Malta	2820	114	Senegal	2370	100
Sweden	2810	104			

Footnotes at end of table

(Continued)

TABLE M-6 (*Continued*)
WORLD DIETARY ENERGY SUPPLY[1]

Country	Dietary Energy Supply[2]	Percentage of Requirements[3]	Country	Dietary Energy Supply[2]	Percentage of Requirements[3]
	(Calories/person/day)	(%)		(Calories/person/day)	(%)
Jamaica	2360	105	Guatemala	2130	97
Kenya	2360	102	Uganda	2130	91
Mauritius	2360	104	Dominican Rep.	2120	94
Vietnam Dem. Rep.	2350	114	Chad	2110	89
Togo	2330	101	Laos	2110	95
Ghana	2320	101			
Peru	2320	99	Nepal	2080	95
Vietnam, Rep. of	2320	107	Niger	2080	89
Iran	2300	96	India	2070	94
			Yemen, Dem. Rep.	2070	86
Lebanon	2280	92	Mali	2060	88
Sierra Leone	2280	99	Zaire	2060	93
Nigeria	2270	96	Mozambique	2050	88
Saudi Arabia	2270	94	Botswana	2040	87
Congo	2260	102	Burundi	2040	88
Dahomey	2260	98	Yemen Arab Rep.	2040	84
Tanzania	2260	98	Guinea	2020	88
Tunisia	2250	94	Ecuador	2010	88
Korea, Dem. Rep.	2240	89	Angola	2000	85
Gabon	2220	95			
Morocco	2220	92	Afghanistan	1970	81
Burma	2210	102	Mauritania	1970	85
Malawi	2210	95	Rwanda	1960	84
Central African Rep.	2200	98	Philippines	1940	86
Colombia	2200	95	El Salvador	1930	84
			Bolivia	1900	79
China	2170	91			
Liberia	2170	94	Bangladesh	1840	80
Sri Lanka	2170	98	Somalia	1830	79
Ethiopia	2160	93			
Iraq	2160	90	Indonesia	1790	83
Pakistan	2160	93	Algeria	1730	72
Sudan	2160	92	Haiti	1730	77
Honduras	2140	94	Upper Volta	1710	72

[1]Assessment of the *World Food Situation, present and future*, Item 8 of the Provisional Agenda, United Nations World Food Conference, Rome.
[2]Total food, including fish.
[3]Requirements may vary slightly from the overall world requirement of 2,385 Calories (kcal) per day due to differences in climate and estimated energy expenditures per capita.

TABLE M-7
WORLD DIETARY PROTEIN SUPPLY[1]

Country	Dietary Protein Supply[2]	Country	Dietary Protein Supply[2]	Country	Dietary Protein Supply[2]	Country	Dietary Protein Supply[2]
	(g/head/day)	(Continued from Col. 1)	(g/head/day)	(Continued from Col. 2)	(g/head/day)	(Continued from Col. 3)	(g/head/day)
Greece	113	Sweden	86	Cuba	63	Somalia	56
New Zealand	109	Portugal	85	Jamaica	63	Thailand	56
Australia	108	Spain	81	Lebanon	63	Togo	56
United States	106			Malawi	63	Khmer Rep.	55
Mongolia	106			Nigeria	63	Malaysia (West)	54
France	105	Japan	79	Sudan	63	Vietnam,	
Ireland	103	South Africa	78	Tanzania	63	Rep. of	53
Canada	101	Chile	77	Venezuela	63	El Salvador	52
Poland	101	Cyprus	76	Burundi	62	India	52
U.S.S.R	101	Rhodesia	76	Libyan Arab		Colombia	51
Argentina	100	Chad	75	Rep.	62	Sierra Leone	51
Bulgaria	100	Syrian Arab		Mexico	62	Burma	50
Hungary	100	Rep.	75	Morocco	62		
Italy	100	Albania	74	Saudi Arabia	62		
Uruguay	100	Niger	74	Panama	61	Central African	
		Korea, Dem.		Uganda	61	Rep.	49
Belgium-		Rep.	73	Yemen Arab		Ghana	49
Luxembourg	95	Paraguay	73	Rep.	61	Laos	49
Czechoslovakia	94	Ethiopia	72	China	60	Nepal	49
Yugoslavia	94	Nicaragua	71	Iran	60	Dominican	
Denmark	93			Iraq	60	Rep.	48
Finland	93	Egypt	69	Peru	60	Mauritius	48
Israel	93	Korea, Rep.	68			Sri Lanka	48
United		Mauritania	68	Guatemala	59	Ecuador	47
Kingdom	92	Zambia	68	Surinam	59	Philippines	47
Switzerland	91	Kenya	67	Upper Volta	59	Algeria	46
Turkey	91	Tunisia	67	Afghanistan	58	Bolivia	46
Austria	90	Costa Rica	66	Guiana	58	Guinea	45
Norway	90	Botswana	65	Madagascar	58	Congo	44
Romania	90	Brazil	65	Rwanda	58	Angola	42
		Jordan	65	Gabon	57	Mozambique	41
Germany, Fed.		Senegal	65	Yemen, Dem.		Bangladesh	40
Rep.	89	Cameroon	64	Rep.	57		
Malta	89	Gambia	64	Dahomey	56		
German Dem.		Mali	64	Honduras	56	Haiti	39
Rep.	87	Trinidad and		Ivory Coast	56	Liberia	39
Netherlands	87	Tobago	64	Pakistan	56	Indonesia	38
						Zaire	33

[1]Assessment of the World Food Situation, present and future, Item 8 of the Provisional Agenda, United Nations World Food Conference, Rome.
[2]Total food, including fish.

TABLE M-8
PER CAPITA CALORIES AND PROTEINS PER DAY
IN DEVELOPED COUNTRIES AND DEVELOPING COUNTRIES[1]

Year	Per Capita Calories/Day			Per Capita Protein/Day		
	World	Developed Countries	Developing Countries	World	Developed Countries	Developing Countries
	← — — — — — (kcal) — — — — — — — →			← — — — — — (g) — — — — — — — →		
1970	2,480	3,150	2,200	69.0	96.4	57.4
1985	2,610	3,220	2,400	72.6	100.0	63.3

[1]United Nations World Food Conference, Rome.

Additional facts pertinent to world per capita energy and protein supplies follow:

1. In general, countries that are low in calories are also low in protein supplies; and countries that are low in total protein are also low in animal protein (which generally has a higher biological value than protein from plant sources).

2. A total of 65 countries—over half of all countries—fail to meet the recommended daily requirement of 2,385 Calories (kcal) per person.

3. All but two of the 127 countries meet or exceed the recommended daily requirement of 38.7 g of protein per person. But it should be noted that, on a worldwide basis, much protein is diverted to meet dietary energy deficits; it is estimated that 11% of the energy comes from protein. Remember, too, that many of the countries that are low in total protein depend to a large extend on protein from plant sources which is required in greater amounts than animal protein.

4. The developed countries average over 3,150 Calories (kcal) per capita per day in their energy supplies (23% above requirement), whereas the developing countries average only 2,200 Calories (kcal) per capita per day (see Table M-8). Similarly, the protein supply is over 96 g per capita per day in the developed countries vs less than 58 g in the developing regions; and much of the latter is vegetable protein rather than animal protein, and is diverted in an attempt to meet the energy deficits (see Table M-8).

5. Despite an apparently adequate supply of energy and protein, a country may have a considerable number of people who fail to have their requirements met due to the unequal distribution of food between the different socioeconomic classes. There may also be disproportionate distributions of food within households, with the male head receiving well over his needs while the wife and children receive less than their needs.[18]

TYPES OF PROTEIN-ENERGY MALNUTRITION.

Depending upon the nature and extent of the deficiency, there is at one extreme *marasmus,* or severe deficiency of energy; and at the other, *kwashiorkor,* or deficiency of protein, in persons who have consumed marginal to adequate amounts of energy. In between are the combination disorders such as *marasmic kwashiorkor* and *nutritional dwarfing.* More than likely, deficiencies of certain vitamins and minerals accompany all of these disorders, except that the problems due to severe deficiencies of protein or energy overshadow the other problems. A discussion of the characteristics of each type of PEM follows.

---

[18]den Hartog, A. P., "Unequal Distribution of Food Within the Household," *Nutrition Newsletter,* Vol. 10, No. 4, FAO of the United Nations, October-December 1972, p. 8.

Kwashiorkor. Infants fed low-protein, starchy foods (such as bananas, yams, and cassava) after weaning may develop kwashiorkor. This imbalanced diet, which has a subnormal protein-to-calorie ratio for infants, prevents some of the adaptive mechanisms of the body from operating the way that they do in the case of starvation or marasmus.

In kwashiorkor there is less breakdown of protein and release of amino acids from muscle than in marasmus since provision of adequate energy in the diet reduces the adrenal cortical response to starvation and, consequently, the flow of amino acids from muscle to viscera. The release of amino acids from muscle is, therefore, not sufficient to meet the needs of the internal organs.

Particularly critical is the loss of tissue cells from the gastrointestinal lining which leads to various types of malabsorption. Also, the severe shortage of protein results in a reduction in synthesis of digestive enzymes, normally secreted from the pancreas or present in the intestinal wall. Thus, there is likely to be diarrhea which may cause excessive loss of water or dehydration, loss of mineral salts, and an electrolyte imbalance.

There may also be glucose intolerance, and, in some cases, elevated levels of plasma growth hormones, although the particular role of this hormone in malnutrition is not fully understood. Also, there may be reductions in the secretions of the thyroid gland which could lead to failure of the body to maintain its temperature.

Liver function is greatly reduced due to lack of protein for the synthesis of enzymes. Also, there is likely to be fat accumulation in the liver due to its inability to package fat with protein for transport in the blood. Low blood levels of albumin, along with anemia, result from the scarcity of amino acids for protein synthesis; and edema is a consequence of the depletion of plasma proteins and electrolytes.

The production of antibodies is likely to be greatly reduced and the victim, therefore, will be prone to infectious diseases. In chronic cases, there is likely to be delayed eruption of teeth, poor enamel with many caries, and pale gums and mucous membranes due to anemia.

Marasmus. Starvation in adults has a counterpart in children called marasmus. It is a severe deficiency of energy usually found in infants and young children who are not getting enough food or who have suffered from bouts of infection and diarrhea which have depleted body reserves. Marasmus in infants and children is more severe than starvation in adults, who can survive for a long period ((1 to 3 months) on their tissue stores of nutrients. An infant, or child, has very high requirements for nutrients in proportion to his size. His rate of metabolism is much higher than that of adults, and he has additional requirements for a rapid rate of growth.

Physiological adaptations in marasmus involve the breakdown of body tissues for energy which is stimulated by catabolic hormones, such as those from the adrenal cortex, and the reduction or cessation of protein synthesis and growth in many tissues. The specific effects of the adrenal cortical hormones are the breakdown of proteins to amino acids, and conversion of amino acids to glucose for use by the brain and nervous system.

Survival during extreme calorie deprivation is moderately enhanced by a large reduction in the utilization of nutrients for energy which is brought about by a diminished secretion of thyroid hormones and a reduced response of cells to insulin. Eventually, there may be dehydration and electrolyte imbalances due to depletion of sodium, potassium, magnesium, and chloride ions, which may in turn lead to disorders of the brain, heart, kidneys, and nerves. Therefore, these conditions can rapidly lead to death if not promptly corrected.

Marasmic Kwashiorkor.

This condition is found in many situations where children are fed diluted gruels after weaning. It is characterized by a combination of disorders which accompany both marasmus and kwashiorkor. Today, the tendency is to use the generalized term, protein-energy malnutrition, to describe this condition.

Nutritional Dwarfing or Growth Failure.

Nutritional dwarfing, or growth failure, while not always a severe handicap, is nonetheless an indicator of underlying protein-energy malnutrition, and may be the beginning of the development of marasmus or kwashiorkor.

Protein-Energy Malnutrition (PEM) in Adults.

These disorders may occur in adults under the following circumstances: chronic illness or alcoholism; unemployment or retirement—which means living on very limited resources; or hospitalized and maintained on intravenous glucose solutions without any other nutrients. The latter situation is particularly dangerous in the case of postsurgical patients who need extra amounts of protein for the healing of their tissues. These patients may show signs like those of kwashiorkor since calories are provided without protein.

SIGNS OF PROTEIN-ENERGY MALNUTRITION.

Every effort should be made to detect PEM in its early stages, since the cost of treating a severe case of this disorder in a hospital may easily be several times that of the treatment of a mild case on an outpatient basis.[19]

[19]Beghin, I. D., "Nutritional Rehabilitation Centers in Latin America: A Critical Assessment," *American Journal of Clinical Nutrition,* Vol. 23, 1970, p. 1412.

Indicators of Protein-Energy Malnutrition in Communities.

Even in the developed countries resources for health surveillance and follow-up care are limited. Therefore, it is necessary to identify communities where these services might yield maximum benefits. Regional health departments usually collect data which is helpful in locating areas where the needs for public health services are greatest. Statistics which suggest the possibility of finding PEM in a community are increased mortality and morbidity of preschool children, a high incidence of infectious diseases, and significant numbers of children who are below standard weights and heights for their ages. Unfortunately, it is not a common practice to obtain on a regular basis the heights and weights of preschool and school age children—not even in developed countries such as the United States.

Signs of Protein-Energy Malnutrition in Individuals.

The extreme forms of PEM (kwashiorkor and marasmus) are not often found in the developed countries, unless there are provocative factors such as parental neglect of children, untreated diseases such as those that affect the gastrointestinal tract, and improper infant feeding. For example, a case of kwashiorkor was identified by a foreign-trained physician in Bronx, New York.[20] The circumstances of the case follow: An attending physician in a clinic told the mother of a child suspected of having an allergy to cow's milk to feed her child soy milk and rice. The mother misunderstood the physician and fed her child only the rice, and the child became very ill. Another physician who was foreign trained, later saw the child in the hospital and recognized kwashiorkor (by the depigmented hair). Fortunately, the child was brought back to health. Thus, it is helpful for all health professionals to be able to recognize severe PEM. Some of the features of marasmus and kwashiorkor are given in Table M-9.

[20]Taitz, L. S., and L. Finberg, "Kwashiorkor in the Bronx," *American Journal of Diseases of Children,* Vol. 112, 1966, p. 76.

TABLE M-9
FEATURES OF MARASMUS AND KWASHIORKOR

Feature	Marasmus	Kwashiorkor
Albumin concentration in plasma[1]	Normal or slightly low	Markedly low
Anemia	Moderate	Moderate
Appetite	Normal to increased	Depressed

Footnote at end of table   *(Continued)*

TABLE M-9 *(Continued)*

Feature	Marasmus	Kwashiorkor
Dehydration............	Often	Sometimes
Edema[1]	Sometimes	Often on the legs and feet.
Electrolyte metabolism.	Near to normal	Potassium depletion
Endocrine function: Adrenal cortex (glucocorticoids)	Increased secretion	Normal to decreased secretion
Pancreas (insulin) ...	Normal to low secretion	Decreased secretion, impaired glucose tolerance.
Pituitary (growth hormone)..........	Increased secretion	Increased secretion
Thryoid	Decreased secretion	Decreased secretion
Essential/non-essential amino acids (blood)[1]	Normal ratio	Subnormal ratio
Gastrointestinal function	Atrophy of digestive tract	Decreased secretions, diarrhea.
Growth failure[1]	Severe	Moderate
Hair....................	Easily plucked	Depigmented in spots
Liver[1]	Atrophied	Fatty (may be palpated).
Mouth.................	Normal	Smooth tongue
Muscle wasting[1]	Noticeable	Masked by edema
Psychological	Alert (early stages)	Apathetic, miserable
Skin[1]	Dry and baggy	Depigmentation, rashes.
Weight (for age and height)[1]	Severely subnormal	Moderately subnormal

[1]Features which are commonly used to distinguish between marasmus and kwashiorkor.

It is also worthwhile to be able to distinguish between the types and degrees of PEM since in most cases the treatment should be directed towards correction of the causative factors and their resulting consequences. Distinguishing characteristics are discussed under the items which follow:

• **Kwashiorkor**—The specific features which distinguish this disorder from marasmus are (1) a significantly subnormal albumin concentration in plasma, (2) swollen parotid glands (just under and in front of the ears), (3) a depressed ratio of essential to nonessential amino acids in the blood plasma, (4) fatty liver (which often may be palpated), and (5) a moderate deficit in weight for height and age (the weight is usually 80% or more of normal).

Fig. M-12 shows a typical case of kwashiorkor.

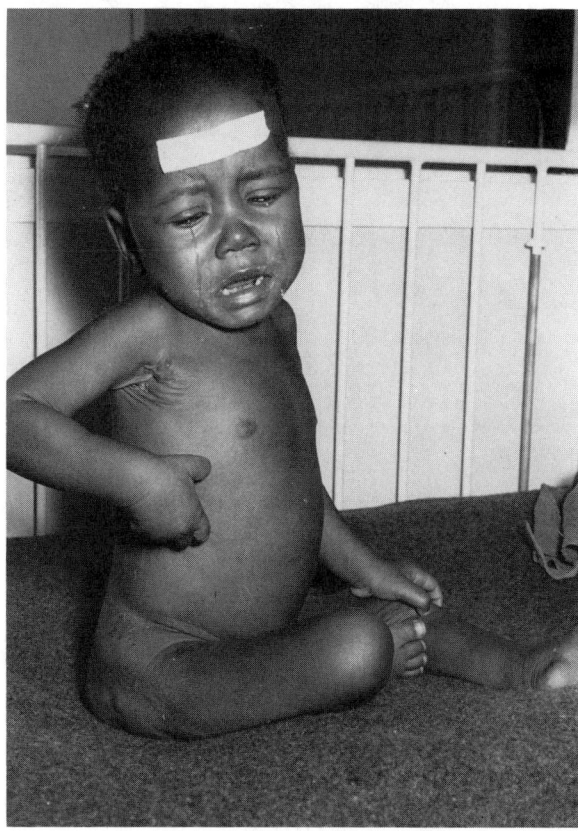

Fig. M-12.   An African boy suffering from kwashiorkor. Note the misery reflected in his expression and the characteristic signs of swollen parotid glands and distended abdomen, flabby thigh muscles, flaky and roughened skin (on his right thigh). (Courtesy, FAO, Rome, Italy)

• **Marasmus**—In contrast to kwashiorkor, this condition is distinguished by (1) severe growth failure where weight may be only 60 to 80% of normal, (2) noticeable muscle wasting, (3) dry and baggy skin (edema is not usually apparent), and (4) normal values for both the plasma albumin and the ratio of essential to nonessential amino acids.

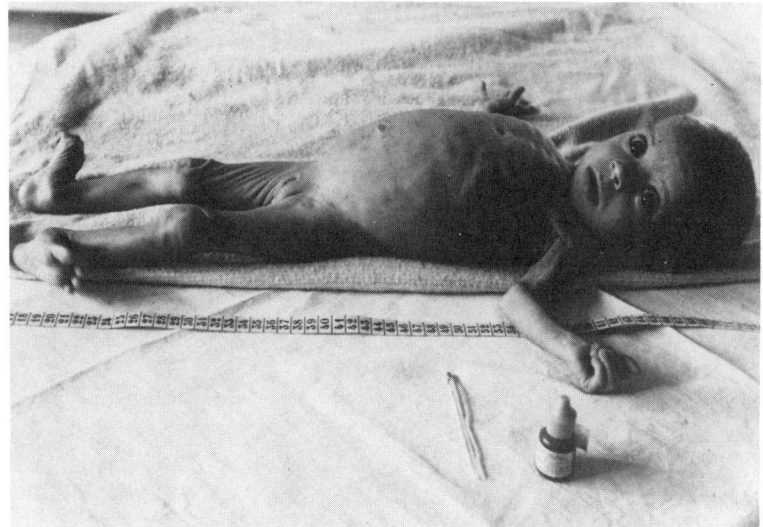 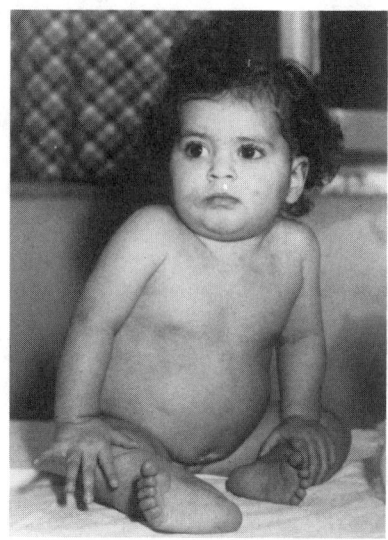

Fig. M-13. *Molok, a 4-month-old Iranian girl suffering from marasmus. Left*: When admitted to the demonstration foundling home in Teheran, she was 24 in. (*61 cm*) tall and weighed 7 lb (*3.2 kg*). *Right*: Following 10 months in the foundling home, Molok was 31 in. (*79 cm*) tall and weighed 16 lb (*7.3 kg*). She was restored to good health by a diet consisting of UNICEF milk powder, orange juice, green vegetables, potatoes, dried apricots, beef, liver, lentils, and bread. (Courtesy, FAO, Rome, Italy)

• **Marasmic kwashiorkor**—Patients who show features of both marasmus and kwashiorkor are usually given the general diagnosis of protein-energy malnutrition.

• **Nutritional dwarfing or growth failure**—One of the first effects of serious malnutrition in infants and children is growth retardation. Thus, it may often be possible to diagnose PEM in children who show none of the abnormal features other than growth deficits. New standard charts of growth curves are available for making comparisons.[21] These revised charts are now based on data from all contemporary U.S. children of the same age and sex, which is in contrast to the older standards based upon data from white, middle-class children living in Boston or Iowa 30 to 40 years ago.

Subnormal values for height and weight at a given age are considered to be those which are more than two standard deviations below the mean values (or below the curve representing the third percentile of values). Growth records should be kept over a period of time, since the child's placement on the chart for a single measurement is not as indicative of nutritional status as is the growth velocity, or increments of growth which occur between several measurements. For example, a child that was initially placed well up on a growth chart may subsequently experience protein-energy malnutrition and, as a result, drop down on the chart but still not fall below the curve representing the third percentile. When, however, the pattern of measurements is carefully examined, it can be seen that there has been a marked departure from the normal progress of growth.

• **Protein-energy malnutrition in adults**—Many of the signs observed in children suffering from PEM will be found in adult patients who have protein and/or energy deficiencies. However, in the case of adults, the ratio of weight to height has been found to be less sensitive than other indicators of PEM.[22] Better indicators of the severity of protein deficiency are serum albumin, triceps skinfold, and muscle circumference. These three measurements are distinctly subnormal in moderate to severe protein deficiencies.

[21]National Center for Health Statistics, *NCHS Growth Charts*, 1976, Health Resources Administration, Monthly Vital Statistics Report, Vol. 25, No. 3., June 1976 Supplement.

[22]Blackburn, G. L., and B. Bistrian, "Report from Boston," *Nutrition Today*, Vol. 9, No. 3, May/June 1974, p. 30.

TREATMENT AND PREVENTION OF PROTEIN-ENERGY MALNUTRITION.
Depending upon the severity of the disorder, the process of rehabilitation may require one or more levels of treatment. The main therapeutic levels follow.

Emergency Care of Severely Ill Patients.
The severely malnourished person has usually adapted over a period of weeks or even months to greatly reduced amounts of food and drink. Therefore, a great deal of care has to be exercised during rehabilitation in order to avoid overloading the patient's imbalanced physiologic functions. Death has frequently resulted from overzealous administration of food, fluids, and mineral salts. The priorities for rehabilitation follow:

• **Correction of dehydration of electrolyte imbalances**—Intravenous administrations of fluid may be harmful to a patient with impaired kidney function resulting from malnutrition. This therapy should be undertaken only when it is certain that there is dehydration (it is not usually present in the malnourished unless there has been diarrhea and/or vomiting). Signs of dehydration are dryness inside the mouth, and a rapid and weak pulse as a result of shrinkage of blood volume due to water loss, which, in turn, causes cardiac insufficiency. If there is no vomiting, oral administration of an electrolyte solution for rehydration is preferable to intravenous administration. Half-strength Darrow's solution with 2.5% dextrose is suitable for either mode of administration (32 ml of solution per pound of body weight over a period of 24 hours). This procedure should be stopped when the pulse slows to normal.

Repletion with magesium should *not* be undertaken until rehydration has been accomplished. Dangerously high levels of this element may accumulate when there is dehydration. Magnesium should not be given intravenously, because it may cause a dangerous drop in blood pressure. Instead, it should be given either orally (as magnesium hydroxide) or intramuscularly (as 50% solution of magnesium sulfate).

The malnourished patient usually has an excess of body sodium, so intravenous sodium bicarbonate should be given only when there is severe acidosis.

• **Feeding by nasogastric tube**—Acutely ill infants and children may be very irritable, making it difficult to feed them by spoon or bottle. Also, the feeding of large quantities of food in a short period of time may aggravate diarrhea. Therefore, some rehabilitation centers usually begin the refeeding procedure with administration of milk-oil formula[23] by nasogastric drip. The compositon of the formula is as follows (percent by weight): dried skim milk, 9.3%; vegetable oil (medium-chain triglycerides, a special dietetic fat derived from coconut oil, have also been used successfully in rehabilitation), 6.8%; magnesium hydroxide, 0.12%; potassium chloride, 0.4%; and water, 83.4%. One-half cup of this formula provides approximately 4 g of protein and 115 Calories (kcal). The formula is usually diluted at the beginning of rehabilitation and fed at a rate of 0.5, 1.0, or 1.5 g of protein per pound (*1.1, 2.2, or 2.3 g/kg*) of body weight per day. The lower concentrations are used in the case of diarrhea, but the amounts of magnesium and potassium salts should be proportionately increased. Following 1 to 3 days the nasogastric feeding may be replaced with bottle, spoon, or cup feeding of the full-strength mixture at the rate of 2 g protein/pound/day.

There may initially be a loss of weight due to correction of edema by protein repletion. The excess water in the tissues is gradually excreted. Once weight gain is steady, the dried skim milk may be replaced by dried whole milk, or by an equivalent quantity of evaporated or pasteurized milk, provided suitable sanitary storage facilities are available for these products.

Treatment of Protein Depletion in Hospital Patients (With Trauma, Infection, Burns, and After Surgery).
This has been most successfully accomplished by either (1) feeding meat, or (2) intravenous infusion of amino acids (compared to the lesser effect of intravenous glucose alone, or a combination of glucose and smaller amounts of amino acids).[24]

The rationale for not feeding patients who have had gastrointestinal surgery has been to prevent irritation or opening up of the surgical wounds. However, there are now available nutrient supplement powders which contain no indigestible residue, and which may be cautiously given to patients soon after surgery. These powders, generally called elemental diets, are marketed by several pharmaceutical companies.

Correction of Mild to Moderate Protein-Energy Malnutrition.
The rehabilitation procedure in developing countries usually consists of cautiously feeding nonfat dry milk (dietary fat is restricted at the start of treatment to avoid aggravation of diarrhea) reconstituted with boiled water (to avoid bacterial contamination) until other foods are tolerated. Supplements of vitamins and minerals are given along with the food to prevent or correct deficiencies. Vitamin A deficiency frequently accompanies kwashiorkor, but may not be noticed until the protein deficiency has been corrected. As soon as possible, part of the milk should be replaced with low-cost, nutritious foods which are readily available in the local community. Sometimes the milk may be mixed with foods of high-energy content, such as butter, banana, cassava, beans, and mixtures of grains.

Part of the rehabilitation procedure should involve teaching the patient (or the mothers in the cases of infants and children) the principles of selecting a diet containing the correct proportions of nutrients. This is not achieved easily where food supplies are scarce, or cultural practices limit the use of certain foods.

Prevention of Protein-Energy Malnutrition.
A high priority should be given to the identification of children who have been weaned early, or are being breast

[23]Robson, J. R. K., and C. de joya-Agregado, "The Operation and Function of Malward in the Philippines," *The Journal of Tropical Pediatrics and Environmental Child Health*, March 1973, p. 43, Table IV.

[24]"Protein Sparing Produced by Protein and Amino Acids," *Nutrition Reviews*, Vol. 34, 1976, p. 174.

fed by mothers who cannot produce adequate amounts of milk. They should be fed a supplemental formula. When feeding formulas under primitive or unsanitary conditions, every effort must be made to prevent contamination of the food given to the baby. Lack of proper preparation of formulas is the most common cause of diarrhea; spoilage of the milk formula is another.

The diets of infants after weaning should be carefully planned to include a high-quality protein source, since infants and children require suitable patterns of amino acids in their diets. This means that if grains are a major dietary staple, there should be supplementation with animal proteins—such as milk, eggs, fish, or if these are unavailable, with legumes such as soybeans or peanuts (which may be in the form of a powder). None of the commonly used grains—corn, rice, wheat, and barley—are adequate as the major source of protein for growing children, unless the grain preparations have been supplemented with lysine and/or other deficient amino acids.

Adults are not as likely to suffer from protein deficiencies as are children because (1) their requirements for protein, in proportion to their body size, are much less; and (2) they do not require high-quality proteins—for example, adults have been adequately nourished when wheat flour constituted the sole source of protein. Lysine is not required by adults at as high a level as it is for growing infants and children.

Many cultures believe that males require the most animal protein. So, they tend to feed women less meat than men, and to feed children largely on cereals. These priorities should be reversed by feeding young children the highest quality protein, including animal protein whenever possible; by giving women more meat than men, in order to offset menstrual losses of blood and iron; and, when necessary, by providing mainly vegetarian diets for men. However, some animal proteins, such as egg and milk, are needed by men in order to provide vitamin B-12.

RECENT DEVELOPMENTS IN THE TREATMENT AND PREVENTION OF PROTEIN-ENERGY MALNUTRITION.

A variety of new high-protein food products has been developed by large food concerns for distribution in developing countries. Many of these products are currently being test marketed in Latin American countries. For example, the protein quality of tortilla flour in Mexico has been enhanced by the mixing of soy flour with the traditional corn flour.

Another approach to meeting the protein needs of growing populations is the development of new, improved varieties of grains. Plant geneticists have recently produced high-lysine corn and both high-protein and high-yielding strains of wheat, rice, corn, barley, and sorghum; and they have crossed wheat and rye to obtain a nutritious new hybrid grain called *triticale*. Collectively, these developments, which are known as the "Green Revolution," have made these much-used cereals more nearly the staff of life for growing children.

(Also see DEFICIENCY DISEASES, Table D-1 Major Dietary Deficiency Diseases; ENRICHMENT [FORTIFICATION, NUTRIFICATION, RESTORATION]; GREEN REVOLUTION; HUNGER, WORLD; POPULATION, WORLD; PROTEIN; and WORLD FOOD.)

MALPIGHIA CHERRY (WEST INDIAN CHERRY) *Malpighia galbra*

The same as acerola, one of the world's richest natural sources of vitamin C.

(Also see ACEROLA; FRUITS, Table F-47 Fruits of the World—"Acerola.")

MALT

The term commonly applied to grains of barley which have been allowed to germinate under controlled conditions, then stripped of their sprouts and dried to prevent further sprouting or spoiling. However, the term malt may also refer to (1) the process of making malt; (2) germinated grains other than barley, such as wheat and rye; or (3) a water extract of the malted grain which may be either in the form of a dried powder or a concentrated syrup.

HISTORY OF MALTING.   The art of malting was probably discovered by accident when some stored barley became wet, started to sprout, then fermented. At some time man must have tasted the liquid which drained from the barmy barley. Hence, the practice of brewing most likely developed from attempts to produce intoxicating liquor from fermented barley. Apparently these discoveries were made by some of the earliest civilizations, for it is known that the Chaldeans and Egyptians brewed beer on a regular basis as early as 5000 B.C.

The ancient Egyptians became the first commercial malsters in 1300 B.C., when they produced malt for export by baking ground, malted barley into cakes which could be transported without spoilage. Beer was brewed from these malted cakes by soaking them in water until fermentation occurred.

Few technologies were so universally adopted throughout Europe and the Middle East as the practices of malting, fermenting, and brewing. The Greeks acquired these skills from the Egyptians around 700 B.C. About 300 years later, beer became a major beverage of the Roman legions when they learned about brewing from the Greeks. Shortly thereafter, all parts of the Roman Empire malted barley and brewed beer.

Although most of the malt which is produced today is used by brewers and distillers to make alcoholic beverages, some tasty, nonalcoholic foods are also made from malted grain.

PRODUCTION OF MALT AND ITS DERIVATIVES.   Fig. M-14 outlines the production of malt and some of its derivatives. A discussion of the procedure follows.

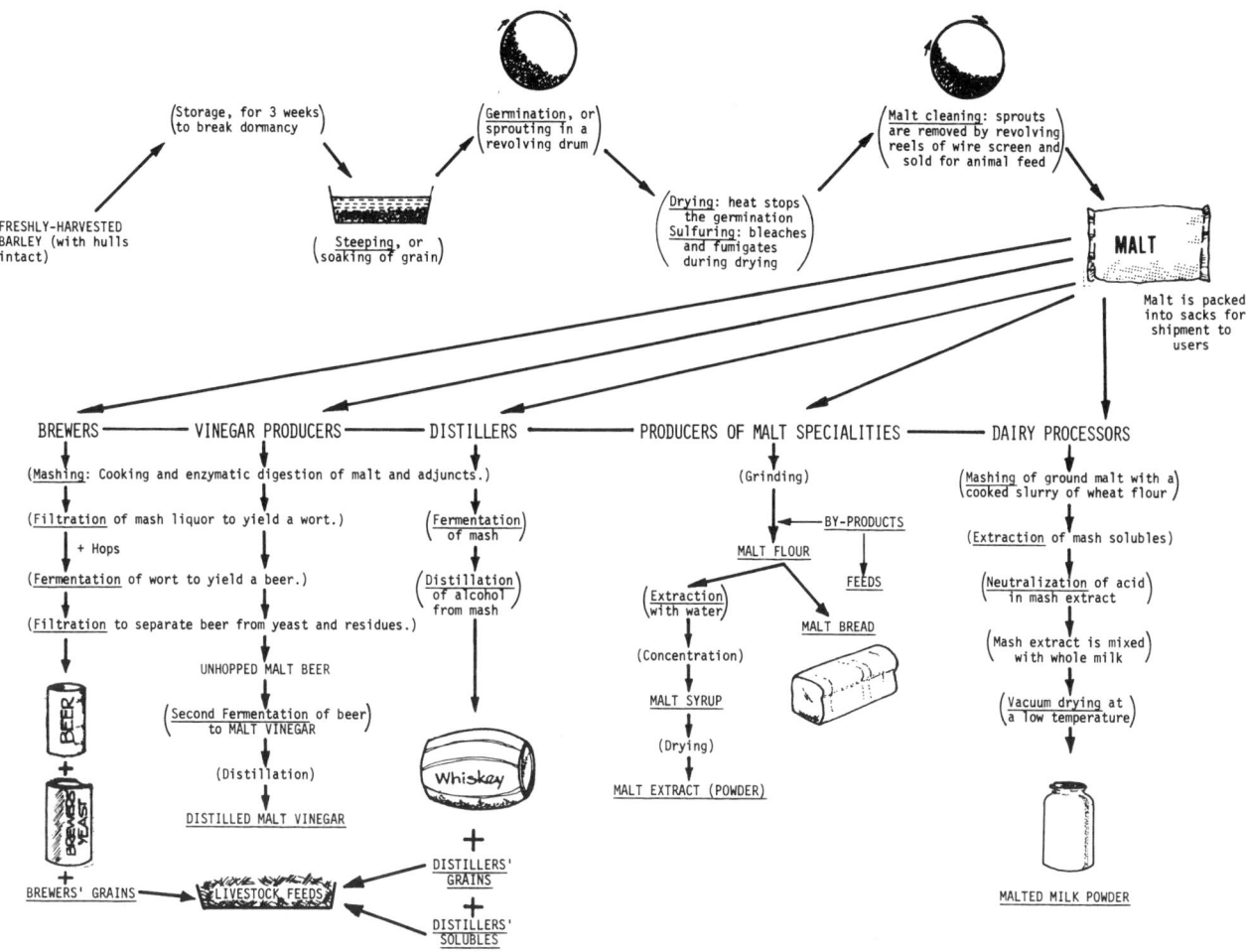

Fig. M-14.   Production of malt and some of its products.

Although malting is a simple process of germinating grains, careful scientific control of this process makes it possible to obtain from 97 to 99% germination of a batch of good barley.

Barley which is to be used to make malt has to be carefully selected for uniformity of protein content and kernel size, since it is important that all of the kernels germinate at the same rate. After grading, the barley has to be stored for at least 3 weeks in order to obtain the maximum rate of germination. (The dormancy of the seed is broken by either storage or careful heating of the grain to around 100°F, or [*38°C*].)

The first step of malting is the steeping or soaking of the grain in a tank of water at about 60°F (*16°C*) to bring the water content of the grain up to 42 to 46% moisture, which is required for germination. Then, the wetted grain is transferred to a revolving drum where the barley is turned and exposed to a stream of air during sprouting.

The malting of barley grains is characterized by a series of changes which are usually grouped together under the general term, *modification.* Some of the major aspects of modification follow:

1.   The development of enzyme activity in the aleurone layer results in a breakdown of part of the starch from the endosperm into maltose and other sugars, a splitting of cell-wall hemicelluloses (complex carbohydrates) into simple sugars, and a conversion of some of the insoluble proteins to more soluble fragments (peptides and peptones). A noticeable result of these enzyme actions or digestions is the tenderizing of the grain so it may be more easily crushed.

2.   Initiation of the growth of the embryonic roots (rootlets) is signaled by the appearance of "chits" or root sheaths which emerge through the seed coats of the grains. The growth and respiration of the rootlets and embryonic stems (plumules) consume part of the grain's supply of carbohydrates and proteins. Thus, there is a loss of from 6 to 12% of the dry matter from the original grain since the brewer cannot use the rootlets and plumules.

3.   The embryo in the sprouting grain secretes plant growth hormones called gibberellins which further stimulate the process of germination. Sometimes, growth

hormones obtained from outside sources, such as the mold *Gibberella fujikoroi,* may be added to the grain to hasten its germination.

Germination is stopped by slowly heating the malt up to about 170°F (*77°C*) after the rootlets have grown to about 1½ times the length of the grain or when the plumules are about ⅔ of the length of the grain. Usually the malt is dried to about 4% moisture content unless it is to be brewed immediately. After drying, the sprouts are removed and the malt is packed in cloth sacks for shipment or storage.

Malt produced by the processes described above retains most of its enzyme activity. Also, it contains maltose and other sugars which result from the breakdown of about 18% of the starch in the original grain. These properties lend themselves well to the production of the items which follow:

• **Beers**—These beverages are made by fermenting sugary solutions derived from the extraction of malted barley and other materials. First, *mashes* are prepared by cooking crushed grains of malt with or without other nonmalted grains such as wheat, corn, rice, or sorghum. (The nonmalted grains are called *adjuncts.*) During mashing, the enzymes from the malt liberate sugars, such as maltose, from the starches and other carbohydrates which are present in both the malted grains and the adjuncts. Then, the mash is filtered, and the sugary extract, or *wort,* is boiled with hops, followed by fermentation with yeast. The residue from extraction of the mash is called *brewers' grains.* Filtration, followed by clarification of the fermented wort yields beer. The *brewers' yeast* which is filtered out of the fermented liquor has usually grown to at least four times its original bulk, so some of it may be dried and packaged for uses other than brewing.

(Also see BEERS AND BREWING.)

• **Malt vinegar**—This product is made from an unhopped malt beer (produced from malt by a process very similar to that used to make regular beers) which is inoculated with acetic acid bacteria (*Acetobacter*) in a special tank or vat. The alcohol in the beer is converted by the bacteria to acetic acid, a major ingredient of all vinegars.

(Also see VINEGAR.)

• **Distilled malt vinegar**—This derivative of malt vinegar, which is produced by distillation, yields a colorless liquid containing only the volatile constituents of the original vinegar.

• **Whiskeys**—The production of these beverages involves the preparation of mashes like those used to make beer, except that the mashes are fermented without further clarification. Then, the alcohol resulting from fermentation is separated from the mash by distillation. Most of these distillates contain volatile substances, other than alcohol, which impart a fiery taste. Usually, the unwanted substances are removed by passage through absorbant charcoal (as in the case of vodka), or by storage and aging in special casks. The spent mash is called *distillers' slop or stillage.* Straining of the stillage yields (1) solids

(*distillers' grains*), and (2) a solution of various materials, called *distillers' solubles.*

(Also see DISTILLED LIQUORS.)

• **Malt flour**—This item is produced by grinding malt and sifting out the hulls.

(Also see FLOURS, Table F-26 Special Flours.)

• **Caramel malts**—These products are prepared by heating wetted malt at 150° to 170°F (*66° to 77°C*) for 1½ to 2 hours, then carefully increasing the temperature up to about 250°F (*121°C*) to produce caramelization (a process of browning sugar-rich materials).

• **Chocolate malts**—These items, which are similar in many ways to caramel malts, are made by roasting dry malt for about 2 hours at 420° to 450°F (*216° to 232°C*).

• **Malt extracts**—Extracts may be made of regular or special (such as caramel or chocolate) malts by grinding and mashing them (as in the production of beer), then concentrating the mash filtrates to *syrups,* or drying them (at low temperatures under vacuum) to powders.

• **Malt bread**—A tender bread with a sticky crumb is produced by the addition of small amounts of a diastatic malt product (usually malt flour, or malt syrup) to wheat flour doughs. The enzyme activity in the malt product converts some of the starch in the dough to sugar, and digests some of the protein.

• **Malted milk powder**—This product is made by combining whole milk with the filtrate from a mash made from barley malt and wheat flour, then vacuum drying the resulting mixture at a temperature below 140°F (*60°C*).

NUTRITIVE VALUES OF MALT PRODUCTS.
Table M-10 compares the nutrient content of the original barley grain, malt, and two of the products derived from it.

TABLE M-10
NUTRIENT COMPOSITION OF BARLEY AND MALT

	Unhulled Barley Grain	Dried Malt	Malt Extract, Dried[1]	Malted Milk Powder[1]
	← — —(per 100 g portion)- — — →			
Food energy . . kcal	274	368	367	410
Carbohydrates . g	66.6	77.4	89.2	72.9
Fat . . . . g	1.7	1.9	trace	8.3
Protein . . . . g	12.2	13.7	6.0	13.1
Fiber . . . . g	5.3	3.3	trace	.6
Calcium . . . . . . mg	40	60	48	266
Phosphorus . . . mg	330	460	294	380
Sodium . . . . mg	30	80	80	440
Magnesium . . . mg	140	180	140	93
Potassium . . . . mg	400	430	230	758
Iron . . . . mg	8	4	9	1
Niacin . . . . mg	8.5	5.7	9.8	.3
Riboflavin . . . . . mg	.2	.3	.4	.5
Thiamin . . . . mg	.4	.4	.4	.3

[1]Data from Food Composition Table F-36.

Table M-10 shows that malt contains higher levels of energy and protein, but less fiber, than the grain from which it was derived. In general, the grain is rendered more digestible by malting as a result of enzymatic activity generated in this process.

Malt extract is composed mainly of carbohydrates in the form of sugars, since much of the protein in malt is insoluble, and, therefore, is not extracted by water. Also, there is only a negligible content of fiber in the extract. Thus, the malt extract is not as complete a food as the malted grain.

Malted milk powder is the most nutritious of the products listed in Table M-10 since the whole milk used in its preparation contributes extra energy, fat, protein, calcium, phosphorus, sodium, and potassium. It may be mixed with milk and used as a nearly complete food for convalescents, except that supplemental vitamins, minerals, and fiber should be provided if it is the exclusive food for a long period of time.

Additional nutritional information may be found on malt and malt products in Food Composition Table F-36.

COMMERCIAL USES OF MALT AND ITS DERIVATIVES.

Although malt products are almost exclusively consumed by man in the form of beverages and foods, producers of these items recover and sell the by-products from their processes for use as ingredients in livestock feeds. A brief summary of some of the commercial uses of malt and its derivatives follows.

Beverages and Foods. The manufacturers of these products use malt because of (1) its enzymatic activity which helps to make foods more digestible, or more readily fermentable; (2) its content of sugars, such as maltose; and (3) its flavor. Examples of these applications follow:

• **Diastatic malts**—These products may be in the form of grains of malt, flours milled from malted grains, or malt extract in the form of dried powders or syrups. Although such malts are used mainly by brewers and distillers, they are also added by bakers to bread doughs at a level of around 2% in order to convert some of the starch in the flour to sugar for more rapid gas production (leavening) by yeast.

(Also see BEERS AND BREWING; BREADS AND BAKING; and DISTILLATION.)

• **Malt-flavored beverages and foods**—The distinctive flavor of malt is due in part to its constituents such as sugars, amino acids, and tannins; and in part to the products of the chemical reactions between these constituents which take place when the malted grain is heated. (Also see MALTOL.) Thus, malt or malt flavoring enhances the taste of such diverse products as breads, breakfast cereals, cakes, candies, crackers, coffee substitutes, dark beers, instant tea mixes, and nonalcoholic and carbonated beverages. Malted milk products are used for beverage powders, candies—such as malted milk balls, and infant foods.

• **Malt vinegars**—The undistilled vinegar has for a long time been used by the British more than any other vinegar. Americans have recently been introduced to the product as a seasoning for fish and chips. Distilled malt vinegar is used mainly in condiments, relishes, and sauces to which it contributes acidity.

Feeds. Even though malt has a higher nutritive value for feeding livestock than unmalted barley grain (see Table M-10), the higher cost of producing the malt makes such a use unprofitable. However, small amounts of diastatic malts are used to improve grains and silages. Also, the by-products which are not consumed by man make good ingredients for feeds. Details follow:

• **Diastatic malts**—Malts containing active enzymes (diastases, hemicellulases, and proteases) have been added experimentally in amounts of from 0.5 to 5.0% by weight to livestock feeds in order to break down complex carbohydrates and proteins. The results of these experiments were (1) more rapid fermentation of silage and therefore less spoilage, (2) more efficient utilization of feed for milk production by dairy cattle, and (3) better growth of chicks fed mixed barley and legume rations.

• **Malt hulls and malt sprouts**—These by-products are often sold as mixtures which are used at levels of some 8 to 16% in rations for ruminants and swine.

• **Other malt derivatives**—Miller's screenings (from the production of malt flour), brewers' grains, brewers' yeast, distillers' grains, and distillers' solubles are used with various other ingredients to make up rations for both nonruminants like chickens and hogs, and for ruminants such as sheep and cattle.

USING MALT EXTRACTS IN HOME RECIPES.

Diastatic malts are sold mainly by wholesalers to bakers, brewers, and distillers. Therefore, consumers are not likely to be able to purchase such products in retail stores.

Malt extracts are available in powdered and syrup form, but they are rather expensive since they are sold mainly in drug stores as laxatives and tonics. However, a slightly less expensive diastatic malt is sold by some health food stores.

An inexpensive, hop-flavored, nondiastatic malt syrup is sold in some supermarkets. This syrup might be used to flavor beverages where a bit of bitterness (from the hops) is desired. It would also make a good yeast food for bread baking because of its sugar content.

Although any of the whole cereal grains may be sprouted at home to make malts, care has to be taken to avoid excessive wetting of the grains which makes them susceptible to spoilage.

MALTASE

An enzyme which acts on maltose to produce glucose. Salivary amylase is present in saliva, and intestinal maltase is present in intestinal juice.

(Also see DIGESTION AND ABSORPTION.)

MALTHUS

In 1798, an English clergyman whose full name was Thomas Robert Malthus prophesied that world population grows faster than man's ability to increase food production. He stated, "The power of population is infinitely greater than the power in the earth to provide subsistence for man."

For 200 years, we proved Malthus wrong because, as the population increased, new land was brought under cultivation; and machinery, chemicals, new crops and varieties, and irrigation were added to step up the yields. Now, science has given us the miracle of better health and longer life; and world population is increasing at the rate of about 240,000 people a day, or 87.5 million per year; and it is predicted that world population will be 6.2 billion by the year 2000, and be doubled by the year 2045.

Despite an increase of 1.8 billion people in the world during the 25-year period 1961–63 to 1983–85, people as a whole were better fed than previously. On the average, the food available per capita rose from 2,320 Calories to 2,660 Calories. *But the exceptions were many!* In the low income countries as a group, apart from China and India, per capita food supplies in 1983–85 were no higher than 15 years earlier. More disturbing yet, over a billion people are seriously short of calories in their diets; ⅔ of these people lack good quality protein.

Seventy-five percent of the people in the world live in the developing countries where only 40% of the world's food is produced. Moreover, this is where most of the world's increase in population is occurring. Population growth in the developing countries averages 2.1% vs 0.6% in the developed countries. For every birth in the developed countries, there are three in the developing countries. The rapid population growth in the developing countries causes severe economic strains on food production, processing, and distribution.

To match population growth and feed people adequately, world food production needs to increase at an *average* rate of about 2.5% per year. This is feasible. Yet people in parts of the world will continue to starve to death, because of lack of food or lack of money. For them, a world average increase in food of 2.5% per year does nothing to satisfy their hunger pangs when they are far below the average.

(Also see HUNGER, WORLD; POPULATION, WORLD; and WORLD FOOD.)

MALTOL

This substance is used both for its own flavor and for enhancing the flavors of sweet, fruit-containing foods. It has a fragrant caramellike odor and a bittersweet taste. Chemically, the compound is known as 3-hydroxy-2 methyl-4H-pyran-4-one, with the structure shown in Fig. M-15.

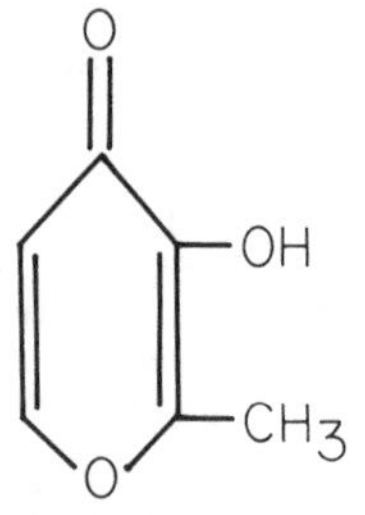

MALTOL
(3-hydroxy-2-methyl-4H-pyran-4-one)

Fig. M-15. Maltol. A food flavoring and a flavor enhancer.

FORMATION AND OCCURRENCE OF MALTOL. Chemists have demonstrated that maltol may be formed (1) by heating maltose at 375°F (*191°C*) for 1 hour (note the similarities of these conditions to those in baking), or (2) by heating mixtures of sugars, such as maltose and lactose, with amino acids, such as glycine (the latter procedure is known as nonenzymatic browning reaction of the Maillard type).

Maltol is found in roasted materials which have a moderate to high carbohydrate content, such as bread crusts, cocoa beans, cellulose, cereals, chicory, coffee beans, diastatic flour doughs (where some of the starch has been converted by enzyme action to maltose), malt products, soft woods, and soybeans. It is also found in heated products which contain moderate amounts of both sugars and amino acids, such as condensed and dried milks, dried whey, and soy sauce. Apparently heating is not always required for the production of maltol, since it also occurs in larch bark and the dry needles of cone-bearing evergreen trees.

USES OF MALTOL. When maltol flavor is desired in a food, it is often produced by careful attention to the conditions under which food is processed. For example, the roasting of cereal grains results in the production of maltol and other flavors which are similar to those in roasted cocoa and coffee. Thus, the distinctive flavors and aromas of many roasted foods are due to the different mixtures of the individual substances produced by the browning reactions.

The enhancement of fruit flavors in sweetened foods requires more precise control of the amounts of maltol in the food product than can be achieved by processing, since the flavor of maltol itself should not be evident in these foods. Thus, pure maltol is used in trace amounts ranging from 5 to 350 ppm (from about a teaspoon to 12 oz per ton of food) in products such as cakes, fruit drinks, gelatin desserts, ice cream, jams, soft drinks, and sweet rolls which have fruit flavors (strawberry, raspberry, pineapple, black cherry, and orange). Maltol also enhances the sensation of sweetness in sweet, fruit-containing foods, but it is less effective for this purpose than for enhancing fruit flavor.

ETHYL MALTOL. The strength of maltol as an enhancer of fruit flavors and as a sweetener is increased by a factor of from 4 to 6 when the methyl group (CH_3) in the molecule is replaced by an ethyl group (CH_2CH_3). Also, water solutions of ethyl maltol at room temperature are 9 times more volatile, and, therefore, more aromatic than those of maltol. The use of ethyl maltol as an additive in foods allows the sugar content to be reduced by 15%.

MALTOSE (MALT SUGAR)

A disaccharide with the formula $C_{12}H_{22}O_{11}$; obtained from the partial hydrolysis of starch; yields 2 molecules of glucose on further hydrolysis.

MAMEY SAPOTA *Calocarpum sapota; C. mammosum*

Fruit of a large, tall tree (of the family *Sapotaceae*) that is grown in the lowland of the West Indies and on the American mainland from Mexico to South America.

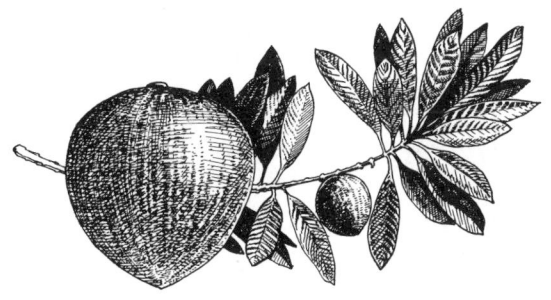

Fig. M-16.   The mamey sapota, a tropical fruit of the Americas.

Mamey sapotas are egg-shaped drupes, brown colored with reddish, sweet, spicy, nonacid flesh, and are from 3 to 6 in. (*7.5 to 15 cm*) long. The fruit is eaten fresh or made into jam. It is highly esteemed by the Indians in the rural areas.

Mamey sapotas are moderately high in calories (121 kcal per 100 g) and carbohydrates (31%). They are a fair to good source of iron and vitamin C.

MAMMEE APPLE (SANTO DOMINGO APRICOT) *Mammea americana*

The fruit of an evergreen tree (of the family *Guttiferae*) that is native to the West Indies, Central America, and South America.

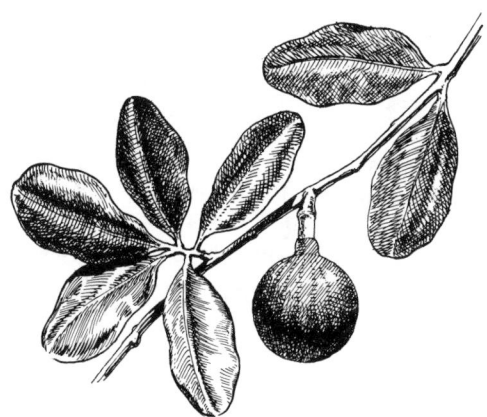

Fig. M-17.   The mammee apple.

The fruit is pear-shaped and from 3 to 6 in. (*7 to 14 cm*) in diameter with brown thick skin and an orange-colored flesh. It is eaten fresh, stewed and sweetened, or made into jam or jelly. Also, a liqueur is made from the flowers and a seasoning agent is made from the seeds of the fruit.

The fruit is fairly low in calories (59 kcal per 100 g) and carbohydrates (12%). It is a fair source of vitamin C.

MANATEE (MANATI; SEA COW)

A formerly common American herbivorous sea mammal of the West Indies and neighboring mainland coasts from Florida to Yucatan, now rare because of excessive killing. The manatee is about 10 ft long, nearly black, thick-skinned, and almost free from hair. The flesh of the manatee, which tastes something like pork, is much esteemed in the West Indies.

MANDARIN ORANGE (TANGERINE) *Citrus reticulata*

Contents   Page

The term "mandarin" refers to certain varieties of citrus fruits which resemble the sweet orange (*C. sinensis*), but which have loose skins that peel easily. (Many botanists classify all or most of the mandarins under the single species [*C. reticulata*], although some have assigned various varieties to other citrus species.) Certain types of mandarins are commonly called "tangerines," although the latter term is not an official botanical designation. Mandarin oranges, like the other citrus fruits, belong to the rue family (*Rutaceae*).

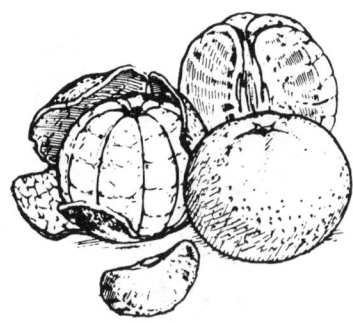

Fig. M-18.   The mandarin orange, a species of citrus fruit that has a loose, easily-peeled skin and a distinctive sweet flavor. Certain red-orange varieties are usually called tangerines.

TYPES OF MANDARIN ORANGES COMMONLY GROWN IN THE UNITED STATES.

The American tendency to call most types of mandarins "tangerines" is reflected in the naming of the major types of this fruit which are grown in the United States:

• **Tangerine**—Although this name may be given to all nonhybrid types of mandarins, it may also be reserved for those which have a deep orange or an orange-red color in the peel and the flesh of the fruit.

• **Tangelo**—This term designates the hybrids of the grapefruit and the tangerine. Usually, the fruits have the loose skin and sweetness of the latter parent, but they tend to have a distinctive flavor of their own.

• **Tangor**—Most lay people are unfamiliar with this name, which refers to hybrids of the tangerine and the sweet orange.

• **Temple orange**—This naturally occurring tangor was discovered in Jamaica. It is by far the most important hybrid of the mandarin.

ORIGIN AND HISTORY.

Mandarins are believed to have originated in Indochina and to have spread slowly northward and westward as migratory peoples took the fruits back to their native villages, where they planted the seeds. Many new varieties developed in the new environments as a result of (1) mutations, and (2) accidental or intentional crossbreeding (hybridization) with the local varieties. Some of the new varieties apparently originated in northeastern India, while others came from Indochina, China, and Japan. (It is often very difficult to trace the ancestry of mandarins because there are many new varieties.)

Although mandarin oranges were not introduced into Europe and the Americas until the 19th century, they were grown in China for about 3,000 years as evidenced by their description in the list of tribute articles sent to the Chinese ruler around 2200 B.C. One reason why mandarins were not brought westward from the Orient until recent times might be that their light, thin, loose skins made them much more susceptible to spoilage during the long, slow transport of ancient times than the citrus fruits which had thick, heavy peels.

The first mandarins grown in the Mediterranean region appear to have been those planted by the Arabs in various parts of North Africa. In the early part of the 19th century, several varieties of the fruit were introduced into Europe from the Orient and from north Africa. Around that time certain Europeans imported the fruit from Tangiers, Morocco and called it the tangerine. Shortly thereafter, several varieties of mandarin were introduced into Florida, where they were improved and crossbred with other citrus fruits.

Today, the mandarins and their hybrids are grown in most of the subtropical and tropical areas of the world.

PRODUCTION.   The annual world production of the major types of mandarins averages about 8.8 million metric tons.

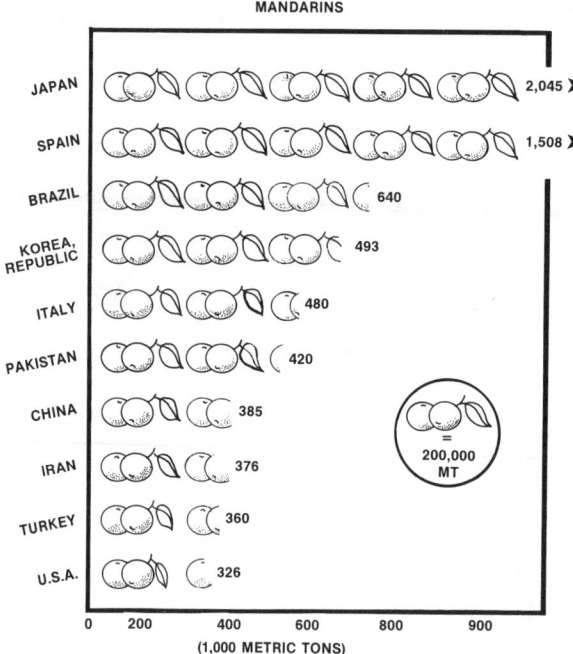

MANDARINS

JAPAN	2,045
SPAIN	1,508
BRAZIL	640
KOREA, REPUBLIC	493
ITALY	480
PAKISTAN	420
CHINA	385
IRAN	376
TURKEY	360
U.S.A.	326

= 200,000 MT

0   200   400   600   800   900
(1,000 METRIC TONS)

Fig. M-19. The leading mandarin-producing countries of the world. (Source: *FAO Production Yearbook*, 1991, FAO/UN, Rome, Italy, Vol. 44, pp. 163, 164, Table 71)

Most of the U.S. mandarin crop comes from Arizona which produces tangelos, Temple oranges, and tangerines. However, some of the tangerine crop is also produced in California, and Florida, as shown in Fig. M-20.

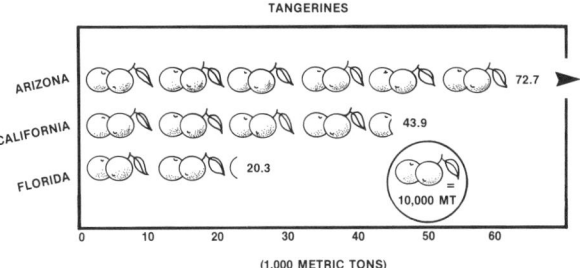

TANGERINES

ARIZONA .... 72.7 ▶
CALIFORNIA 43.9
FLORIDA 20.3
= 10,000 MT

0 10 20 30 40 50 60

(1,000 METRIC TONS)

Fig. M-20. The leading tangerine-producing states of the United States. (Source: *Agricultural Statistics*, 1991, USDA, p. 189, Table 278)

Mandarin orange trees are more cold resistant and heat resistant than the other citrus species. Hence, some varieties grow well as far north as Japan (dormant Satsuma mandarin trees have survived 15°F [-10°C] without severe injury), while others thrive near the Equator in Indonesia. However, the fruit is more readily damaged by frost than either the orange or the grapefruit, because mandarins have thinner, looser skins that confer little protection against low temperatures. Furthermore, the fruit is usually sweeter when grown in a hot, humid climate.

Details of citrus fruit growing are given elsewhere.

(Also see CITRUS FRUITS, section headed "Production.")

PROCESSING. A little over half of the U.S. crop of tangelos, tangerines, and Temple oranges is processed into single strength juices and frozen juice concentrates. Much of the fruit juice is blended into orange juice and frozen orange concentrates because the mandarins contribute a deep orange color. However, U.S. regulations limit the amount of mandarin juice in orange juice blends to 10%. Greater amounts impart off-flavors to the orange juice products.

Tangerines are not as likely to develop off-flavors during processing as tangelos and Temple oranges. Hence, some of the tangerine crop is made into single-strength tangerine juice and frozen tangerine juice concentrate. The latter product is by far the major one, because it is much more stable during storage.

Small amounts of mandarin orange segments are used in prepared citrus salads and gelatin desserts. It is noteworthy that almost all of the canned mandarin orange segments used in the United States are imported from the Orient.

More details regarding processed citrus products are given elsewhere.

(Also see CITRUS FRUITS, section headed "Processing.")

SELECTION. Fresh mandarin types of oranges are thin-skinned, and are usually oblate or decidely flattened at the ends. The skin is easily removed; there is little coarse fibrous substance between the skin and the flesh, and the segments of the fruit separate readily. The flavor is distinctive; the aroma is pungent and pleasant. Because of the looseness of the skin these oranges are likely to feel puffy; therefore, judgment as to quality should be based mainly on weight for size and deep yellow or orange color of the skin.

When present, decay is usually in the form of soft areas on the surface of the fruit that appear to be water-soaked. These areas may be covered by mold. In the early stages of decay, the skin in the affected area may be so soft that it breaks easily under pressure. Fruit with cut or punctured skins should be carefully examined for signs of spoilage.

Criteria for selecting processed citrus products are given elsewhere.

(Also see CITRUS FRUITS, section headed "Selection and Preparation.")

PREPARATION. Mandarin oranges are at their best when served fresh in appetizers, desserts, or toppings for frozen desserts and puddings. However, their juice and/or their peel may be used to flavor ice cream, ices, sauces, sherbets, and sauces.

NOTE: The light, loose skin on mandarins makes it necessary to use only light pressure when extracting the juice or grating the peel.)

CAUTION: Some people are allergic to one or more constituents of citrus peel. When such allergies are suspected, neither the peel nor products containing it should be consumed, and fruit juice should be extracted gently to avoid squeezing the oil and other substances from the peel into the juice. (It is noteworthy that some of the commercially prepared mandarin and sweet orange juice blends and drinks may contain peel and/or substances extracted from it, but that prepared citrus juice products for infants contain little or none of the peel constituents.)

Other suggestions for preparing citrus fruits and citrus products are given elsewhere.

(Also see CITRUS FRUITS, section headed "Selection and Preparation.")

NUTRITIONAL VALUE. The nutrient compositions of various types of mandarins and mandarin products are given in Food Composition Table F-36.

Some noteworthy observations regarding the nutrient composition of mandarins follow:

1. Fresh tangerines, fresh tangerine juice, and canned mandarin orange segments have similar nutritional values in that they are (a) moderately low in calories; (b) good sources of potassium and vitamin C; and (c) fair sources of vitamin A. Also, they all contain the vitaminlike bioflavonoids.

2. Frozen tangerine juice concentrate contains about 4 times the nutrient levels of the fresh, unconcentrated juice. Hence, the concentrate may make a significant nutritional contribution when it is added undiluted to drinks, sauces, and other preparations.

3. Canned tangerine juice has a nutritional value comparable to fresh juice, except that the canned product contains only two-thirds as much vitamin C.

4. Raw tangelos contain only half as much vitamin C as tangerines, but they supply about the same amount of potassium.

5. The peel of mandarin oranges and related citrus fruits contains citral, an aldehyde which antagonizes the effects of vitamin A. Hence, people should make certain that their dietary supply of the vitamin is adequate before consuming large amounts of peel from the various types of mandarin oranges.

(Also see FRUIT[S], Table F-47 Fruits of the World.)

MANGANESE (Mn)

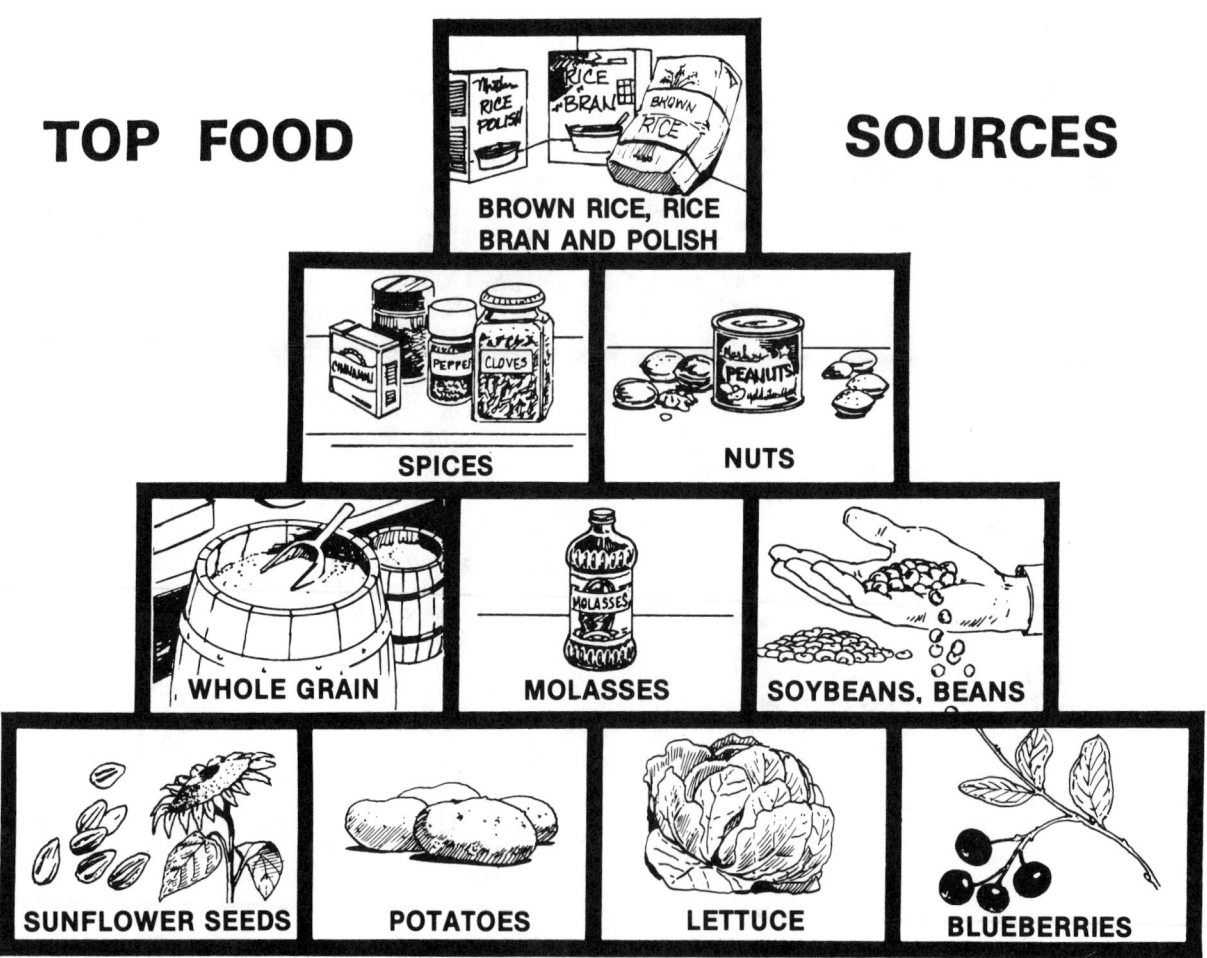

Fig. M-21.   Top food sources of manganese.

In industry, manganese is a metallic element used chiefly as an alloy in steel to give it toughness. In nutrition, it is an essential element for many animal species. Manganese is an activator of several enzyme systems involved in protein and energy metabolism and in the formation of mucopolysaccharides. The human body contains 12 to 20 mg of manganese. So, an essential function of the element must be assumed to exist in man.

HISTORY. Manganese was first recognized as an element in 1774 by the famous Swedish chemist Carl W. Scheele. It was isolated in the same year by his co-worker, Johann G. Ghan. The name *manganese* is a corrupted form of the Latin word for a form of magnetic stone, *magnesia.*

About 95% of the world's annual production of manganese is used by the steel industry. Also, manganese is essential for plant growth, and it is found in trace amounts in higher animals, where it activates many of the enzymes involved in metabolic processes.

In 1931, University of Wisconsin researchers reported that manganese was a dietary essential for growth of rats. Later, it was shown to be essential for poultry (a deficiency results in slipped tendon; see Fig. M-22), swine, guinea pigs, cattle, and other animals. Undoubtedly, manganese is an essential nutrient for man, even though the deficiency symptoms have never been determined with certainty.

ABSORPTION, METABOLISM, EXCRETION.
Manganese is rather poorly absorbed, primarily in the small intestine. In the average diet about 45% of the ingested manganese is absorbed, and 55% is excreted in the feces. Absorption can be depressed when excessive amounts of calcium, phosphorus, or iron are consumed.

Following absorption, manganese is loosely bound to a protein and transported as transmanganin. The bones, and to a lesser extent the liver, muscles, and skin, serve as storage sights.

Manganese is mainly eliminated from the body in the feces as a constituent of bile, but much of this is again reabsorbed, indicating an effective body conservation. Very little manganese is excreted in the urine.

The concentration of manganese in the various body tissues is quite stable under normal conditions, a phenomenon attributed to well controlled excretion rather than regulated absorption.

FUNCTIONS OF MANGANESE. Manganese is involved in the formation of bone and the growth of other connective tissues; in blood clotting; in insulin action; in cholesterol synthesis; and as an activator of various enzymes in the metabolism of carbohydrates, fats, proteins, and nucleic acids (DNA and RNA).

DEFICIENCY SYMPTOMS. Signs of deficiency in many animal species include poor reproductive performance, growth retardation, congenital malformations in the offspring, abnormal formation of bone and cartilage, and impaired glucose tolerance.

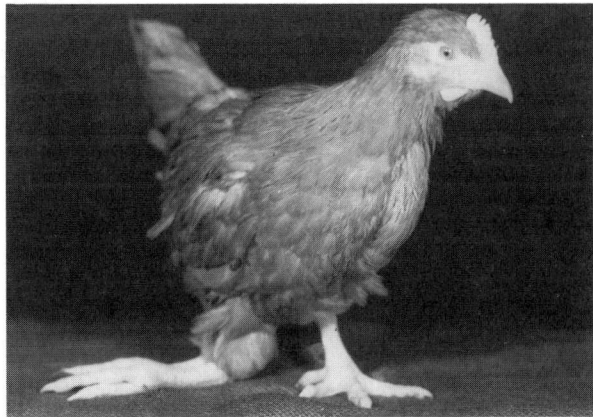

Fig. M-22. A bone disease known as perosis, or slipped tendon, in a chicken due to manganese deficiency. (Courtesy, Department of Poultry Science, Cornell University)

The only confirmed deficiency of manganese in man was in connection with a vitamin K deficiency, where administration of the vitamin did not correct the abnormality in blood clotting until supplemental manganese was provided.

Analyses of hair and blood samples for manganese content indicate that subclinical deficiencies of the mineral might aggravate such disorders as growth impairments, bone abnormalities, diabeticlike carbohydrate metabolism, lack of muscle coordination in the newborn, and abnormal metabolism of lipids (fatty acids, choline, and cholesterol).

In 1963, researchers at the University of California—Davis reported, in the *American Journal of Physiology*, on a study of convulsions in rats; they found that manganese levels helped determine the susceptibility to convulsions of rats subjected to electroshocks and a convulsive drug. In 1976, Yukio Tanaka, a clinical chemist at St. Mary's Hospital in Montreal, reported, before the American Chemical Society in Chicago, that about 30% of all children who have epileptic convulsions have low levels of manganese in their blood. These leads merit further study.

INTERRELATIONSHIPS. Manganese interacts with other nutrients. Excess calcium and phosphorus interfere with the absorption of manganese; the functions of manganese, copper, zinc, and iron may be interchangeable in certain enzyme systems; and manganese and vitamin K work together in the promotion of blood clotting.

RECOMMENDED DAILY ALLOWANCE OF MANGANESE. Extreme dietary habits can result in manganese intakes outside the limit suggested as safe, but the consumption of a varied diet, balanced with regard to bulk nutrients, can be relied on to furnish adequate and safe amounts.

Estimated safe and adequate intakes of manganese are given in Table M-11.

TABLE M–11
ESTIMATED SAFE AND ADEQUATE
DAILY DIETARY INTAKES OF MANGANESE[1]

Group	Age	Manganese
	(years)	(mg)
Infants	0–0.5	0.3–0.6
	0.5–1	0.6–1.0
Children and adolescents	1–3	1.0–1.5
	4–6	1.5–2.0
	7–10	2.0–3.0
	11+	2.0–5.0
Adults		2.0–5.0

[1]*Recommended Dietary Allowances,* 10th ed., 1989, NRC–National Academy of Sciences, pp. 230, 284.

• **Manganese intake in average U.S. diet**—In the United States, the normal daily intake of manganese varies from 2 to 9 mg/day in adults, depending on the composition of the diet.

TOXICITY. Toxicity in man as a consequence of dietary intake has not been observed. However, it has occurred in workers exposed to high concentrations of manganese dust in the air (such as in mining ores rich in manganese, and in the production of dry-cell batteries where manganese dioxide is used). The excess accumulates in the liver and central nervous system. The symptoms resemble those found in Parkinson's and Wilson's diseases.

SOURCES OF MANGANESE. The manganese content of plants is dependent on soil content. It is noteworthy, however, that plants grown on alkaline soils may be abnormally low in manganese.

Groupings by rank of common food sources of manganese follow:

• **Rich sources**—Rice (brown), rice bran and polish, spices, walnuts, wheat bran, wheat germ.

• **Good sources**—Blackstrap molasses, blueberries, lettuce, lima beans (dry), navy beans (dry), peanuts, potatoes, soybean flour, soybeans (dry), sunflower seeds, torula yeast, wheat flour, whole grains (barley, oats, sorghum, wheat).

• **Fair sources**—Brewers' yeast, liver, most fruits and vegetables, orange pekoe tea, white enriched bread.

• **Negligible sources**—Fats and oils, fish, eggs, meats, milk, poultry, sugar.

• **Supplemental sources**—Alfalfa leaf meal, dried kelp, manganese gluconate.

For additional sources and more precise values of manganese, see Table M-12 Some Food Sources of Manganese, which follows:

(Also see MINERAL[S], Table M-67.)

TABLE M-12
SOME FOOD SOURCES OF MANGANESE

Food	Manganese	Food	Manganese
	(mg/100 g)		(mg/100 g)
Rice bran	34.7	Barley, whole	
Cloves	30.3	grain	1.2
Rice polish	17.1	Wheat flour. .	1.0
Ginger	17.8	Lettuce	1.0
Walnuts	15.2	Potato, raw . . .	1.0
Wheat germ . . .	13.3	Blueberries,	
Wheat bran . . .	11.0	raw	1.0
Rice, whole		Spinach, raw. .	.8
grain	9.6	Beet, common	
Molasses,		red, raw	.7
blackstrap . .	4.3	Yeast,	
Wheat, whole		brewers'	.6
grain	3.7	Corn, whole	
Oats, whole		grain	.5
grain	3.7	Bananas, raw. .	.5
Alfalfa leaf		Carrot, raw . . .	.4
meal		Turnip, raw . . .	.4
(powder),		Cherries, raw. .	.4
dehydrated .	3.6	Green beans. .	.3
Soybean flour. .	3.2	Apple, raw	.3
Soybeans, dry. .	3.0	Bread, en-	
Peanuts	2.5	riched white. .	.3
Sunflower		Sweet potato. .	.3
seeds	2.3	Cabbage, raw. .	.3
Beans, navy,		Strawberries,	
dry	2.1	raw	.3
Beans, lima,		Liver	.2
dry	1.6	Orange pekoe	
Sorghum,		tea	.2
whole grain. .	1.6	Rutabaga, raw.	.1
Yeast, torula . .	1.3		

MANGO *Mangifera indica*

The mango is a tropical evergreen tree which produces the mango fruit—a slightly sour juicy oval fruit with a

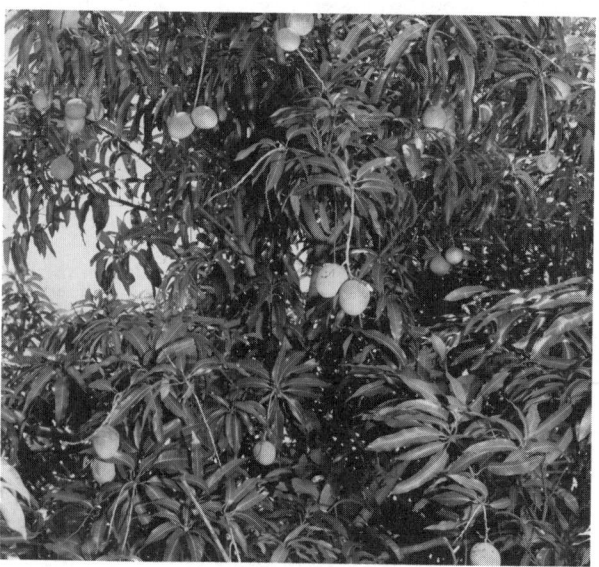

Fig. M-23. A fruiting mango tree. (Courtesy, USDA)

thick yellowish-red rind. Although not very popular in the United States, it is an important fruit crop of tropical countries—important enough to rank seventh among the top 20 fruits of the world. It is more important to the tropical countries than peaches and apples are to the countries in the temperate climates. Mangoes have a spicy flavor. Centuries of selection have produced mangoes free of fiber and offensive flavors.

ORIGIN AND HISTORY. Mangoes probably originated in an area from Burma to India, but they have been under cultivation for almost 6,000 years. The Indians probably took mangoes to the neighboring East Asian countries in the 5th or 4th century B.C., and the Persians transported them to the east African coast about the 10th century A.D. By the beginning of the 18th century, mangoes reached Brazil with the Portuguese colonists and then to the West Indies. In 1861, mangoes were successfully introduced into Florida. Today, they are grown in most tropical countries at lower altitudes.

PRODUCTION. India is by far the largest producer of mangoes. They have been an important item of the diet in India since ancient times, and they occupy an honored place in Hindu culture and ceremonies. Other leading mango-producing countries are shown in Fig. M-24.

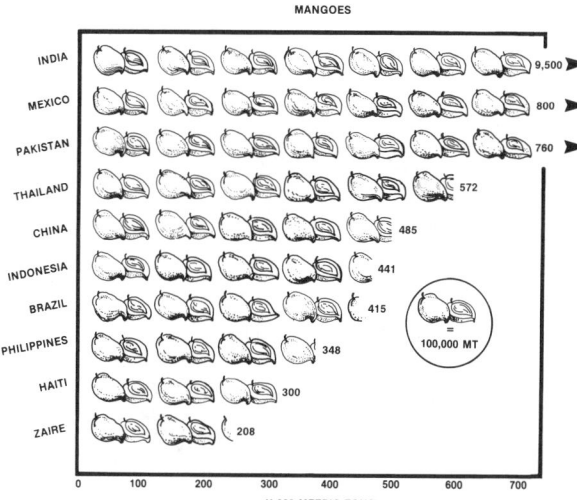

Fig. M-24. Leading mango-producing countries of the world. (Based on data from *FAO Production Yearbook*, 1990, FAO/UN, Rome, Italy, Vol. 44, pp. 167–168, Table 73)

Although the mango may be grown in California, Florida, and Hawaii, there are no production figures available. Florida and Hawaii grow some for commercial sale.

Propagation and Growing. Mature mango trees are 40 to 50 ft (*12.2 to 15.3 m*) tall with slender pointed leaves about 1 ft (*30 cm*) long. Mangoes may be grown from seeds, but the best varieties are clonal, propagated

by budding or by a type of grafting called inarching, on seedling stocks.

In the field, mangoes are spaced 30 to 35 ft (*9.2 to 10.7 m*) apart. By the tenth year following grafting or budding mango trees will produce 400 to 600 fruits, with further yield increases up to the twentieth year, and then declining after the fortieth year. Fruiting is best in humid climates that have a dry season. From 2 to 5 months are required for the fruit to mature.

Harvesting. When mangoes are to be consumed within the area of production, they are harvested when almost fully ripe. When picked for export purposes, mangoes are harvested at full size but before softening. If stored at 45° to 50°F (*7° to 10°C*), they keep as long as 1 month.

PROCESSING AND PREPARATION. Virtually all of the mango crop is marketed fresh. Ripe fruits are eaten raw as a dessert, fruit dish, or used in juice, jams, jellies or preserves. Small amounts are canned. Unripe mangoes are used in pickles and chutneys—a delicacy of India. Some are sun dried, and seasoned with turmeric to produce *amchur,* which may be ground and used in soups and chutneys.

NUTRITIONAL VALUE. Raw mangoes are about 82% water and contain 66 Calories (kcal) of energy per 100 g (about 3½ oz). Unripe fruits contain starch which changes to sugars during ripening. Furthermore, they are an excellent source of vitamin A and a fair source of vitamin C, containing 4800 IU/100 g and 35 mg/100 g, respectively. More complete information regarding the nutritional value of mangoes is presented in Food Composition Table F-36.

(Also see FRUIT[S], Table F-47 Fruits of the World.)

MANGO MELON *Cucumis melo*

This is a fairly uncommon variety (*Chito*) of muskmelon with fruit as small as lemons. The fruits are also called melon apples, orange melons, and vegetable oranges. They are used to make preserves.

MANGOSTEEN *Garcinia mangostana*

The fruit of a small, slow-growing evergreen tree (of the family *Guttiferae*) that is native to Malaysia. When ripe, the fruits have a brownish-purple color and are from 1½ to 3 in. (*4 to 7 cm*) in diameter.

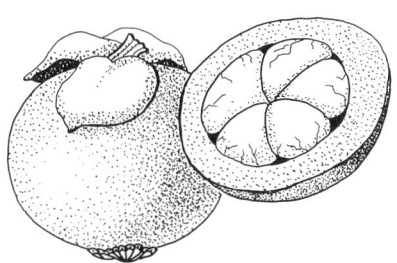

Fig. M-25. The mangosteen.

Mangosteens are usually eaten fresh, but they may be also cooked or made into a jam.

Mangosteen fruit is low to moderately high in calories (57 kcal per 100 g) and carbohydrates (15%). It is also high in fiber (5%), and is a fair to good source of potassium, and a poor source of vitamin C.

(Also see FRUIT[S], Table F-47 Fruits of the World.)

MANGROVE *Rhizophera mangle*

The fruit of a tree (of the family *Rhizophoraceae*) which grows along the Atlantic coast from South Carolina to the American tropics. Mangrove fruit is sweet and edible if it is picked before it starts to develop roots. It is one of the rare fruits that sprouts while on the tree.

MANNA

The food provided by God to the Israelites during their 40 years of wandering in the wilderness as they left Egypt for Canaan—the Promised Land. Manna fell from the sky every day except the Sabbath, for which an extra portion was gathered the previous day. (Exodus 16: Numbers 11)

Some historians say that manna was a gluey sugar from the tamarisk tree.

MANNITOL ($C_6H_{14}O_6$)

Mannitol is a sugar alcohol. The aldehyde group (C = O) of mannose is replaced by a hydroxyl group (OH). Mannitol tastes about 70% as sweet as sucrose—table sugar; hence, it is used as a sweetener in foods. As a sweetener, mannitol may be effective in preventing tooth decay, since oral bacteria are unable to form acid from mannitol. Furthermore, mannitol is slowly and incompletely absorbed from the intestine so it supplies only about one-half the calories of glucose. Much of the ingested mannitol appears unchanged in the urine. Since mannitol is absorbed slowly from the digestive tract, the ingestion of large amounts may cause an osmotic diarrhea. In some foods, mannitol serves as an anticaking or stabilizing-thickening agent. Natural sources of mannitol include pineapples, olives, asparagus, carrots, manna, seaweeds, and grasses.

In medicine, mannitol is used as a diuretic and to test kidney function.

(Also see ADDITIVES, Table A-3; CARBOHYDRATE[S]; and SWEETENING AGENTS.)

MANNOSE ($C_6H_{12}O_6$)

This is a hexose monosaccharide—a 6-carbon sugar. Mannose is not found free in foods, but it is derived from ivory nuts, orchid tubers, pine trees, yeast, molds, and bacteria. Although unimportant to human nutrition, it is a component of some glycoproteins and mucoproteins of the body. Its chemical structure is very similar to glucose.

(Also see CARBOHYDRATE[S]; and PROTEIN[S].)

MAPLE SYRUP

A product unique to North America, made by boiling the sap of the sugar maple (*Acer saccharum*). Collection of the sap commences in the spring of the year, when warm days begin to follow cool nights, causing the sap of the sugar maple to flow. During the winter, some of the starch that the tree made the previous summer and stored in its roots is converted to sugar, primarily sucrose, and carried in the first sap of the spring. Spring sap contains 4 to 10% sugar. Collected sap is boiled to concentrate the sugar and produce the characteristic flavor. Maple syrup is esteemed for its sweet taste and "maple" flavor. Interestingly, the maple flavor of the syrup, is not present in the sap, but develops during the boiling.

ORIGIN AND HISTORY. Years before the "White Man" arrived in North America, the northeast Indians tapped the maple trees by gashing the trunks with their tomahawks. As the sap flowed from the trees, it was collected in birch bark dishes. Then, by continually adding heated rocks to a hollowed-out cooking log, the Indians evaporated the sap down to a thick dark syrup. Upon arriving in the New World, the early settlers soon learned the art from the Indians, but they were able to improve upon the system by using iron drill bits to tap the trees and copper or iron kettles to boil the sap to syrup. During the 1700s and most of the 1800s maple syrup and maple sugar were important as foods, and as items of trade for other goods and services. However, by the late 1800s cane sugar became more available and less expensive, replacing maple sugar. Gradually, maple syrup has been replaced by blends of maple syrup and other syrups, which are less expensive.

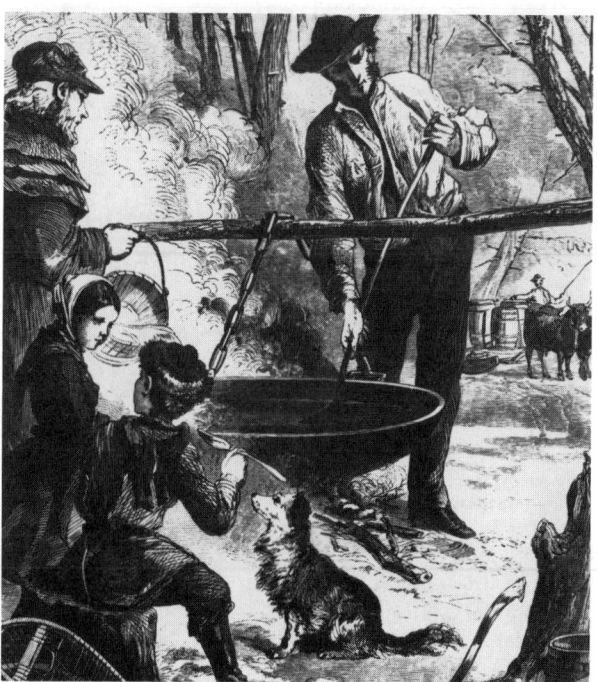

Fig. M-26. Making maple sugar in New England, during the 1800s. (Courtesy The Bettmann Archive, Inc., New York, N.Y.)

PRODUCTION. Nowadays, the methods of the Indians and early colonists have been refined, but the spring collection of maple sap and the production of maple syrup persists as an American tradition, and as a source of income, as shown in Fig. M-27.

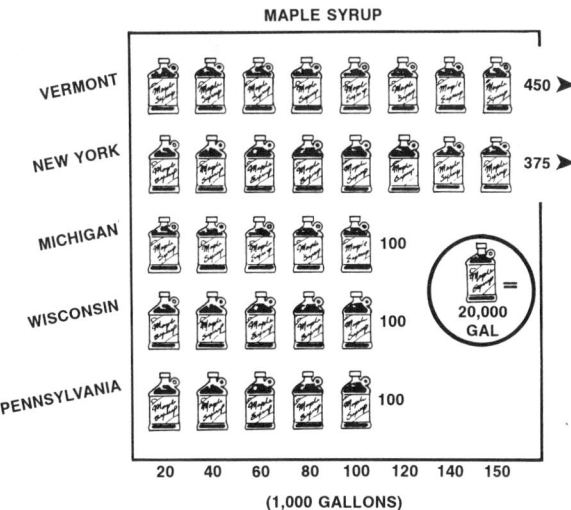

MAPLE SYRUP

VERMONT — 450 ▶

NEW YORK — 375 ▶

MICHIGAN — 100

WISCONSIN — 100

= 20,000 GAL

PENNSYLVANIA — 100

20   40   60   80   100   120   140   150
(1,000 GALLONS)

Fig. M-27. Maple syrup production in the United States. (Source of data: *Agricultural Statistics*, USDA)

Although the United States produces more than 2.6 million gallons of maple syrup yearly, this production is dwarfed by the Canadian province of Quebec which produces about 20 million gallons of maple syrup yearly. Maple syrup produced in the United States is for both home and commercial use.

Production of maple syrup begins with the spring tapping of maple trees. Although the sugar maple (*Acer saccharum*) is the major source of sap, the black maple (*Acer nigrum*) and the red maple (*Acer rubrum*) are also syrup sources. All of these types of maple trees are native to the eastern half of the North American continent. Their sap is harvested during a 4 to 6 week period before buds on the trees begin to open, usually between January and April.

Harvesting sap from the "sugar bush"—the stands of maple trees—is a rather picturesque operation in many locations. Holes are drilled into the tree about 2 to 3 in. (5 to 8 cm) deep and about 3 ft (1 m) above the ground. The number of holes depends on the size of the tree—larger trees may have four or more holes. Into each hole a metal spout is fitted and then a collection pail is hung below the spout.

Each day the accumulation of sap is collected from the pails, poured into a larger tank, and hauled by sled or wagon to the sugarhouse.

A more modern method of collecting the sap involves a system of plastic pipelines which transports the sap from the hole tapped into a tree to the sugarhouse. Regard-

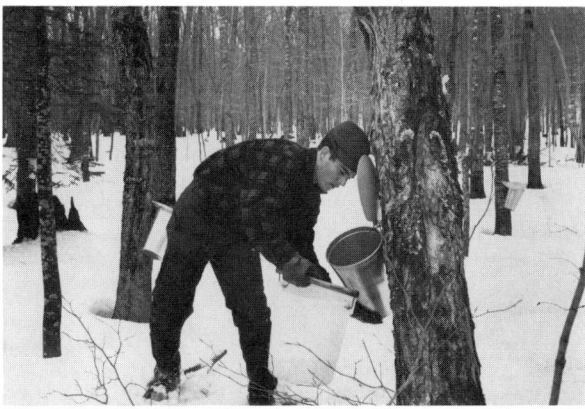

Fig. M-28. Collecting sap from a "sugar bush" in Quebec, Canada. (Courtesy, National Film Board of Canada, Ottawa, Ontario, Canada)

less of the method of collection, a good maple tree will yield 15 to 40 gal (*57 to 152 liter*) of sap in a season.

PROCESSING. Processing occurs in the sugarhouse. It is here that the sap is strained and then placed in shallow pans—evaporators—over wood, oil, or gas fires. As the sap boils, the water evaporates. When the sugar concentration reaches 66.5%, it is drawn off, filtered, and bottled as maple syrup. During the boiling and evaporation, the characteristic maple flavor and color develop. Depending on the sugar content of the sap, 30 to 50 gal (*115 to 190 liter*) of sap are required to make one gallon (*3.8 liter*) of maple syrup. Maple sugar is produced by further boiling and evaporation of most of the water. One gallon of syrup yields about 8 lb of sugar. An old-fashioned treat enjoyed by those making maple sugar is called Jack wax—a taffylike confection formed by pouring the hot syrup onto the snow. The process of forming maple sugar is referred to as sugaring off. Often sugaring off gatherings are held at which people sample the maple syrup and sugar.

NUTRITIONAL VALUE AND USES. During colonial times, maple syrup and sugar were important and abundant, but nowadays these products are rather a treat and a luxury. In 1990, a quart of maple syrup cost $10 to $12. Hence, true maple products contribute very little to our diets. Nevertheless, the composition of maple syrup is listed in the Food Composition Table F-36 of this book. Nutritionally, maple syrup is primarily a source of energy; 1 Tbsp (*15 ml*) of maple syrup contains about 50 Calories (kcal) of energy, along with some calcium and potassium.

No doubt, maple syrup is esteemed more for its flavor than its nutritional value. Maple syrup on pancakes, French toast, or ice cream, is a real treat. The flavor can also be enjoyed in glazed hams, glazed carrots, and baked beans—all made with maple syrup. A delicious hot toast spread can be made by boiling two cups of syrup in a pot to 230°F (110°C), placing the hot pan in ice water without stirring, cooling to tepid but pliant state, and then beating until creamy.

U.S. Grade A Light syrup has a subtle flavor, while Grade A Medium and Dark syrups have a more robust flavor for cooking; besides, they cost less.

(Also see SUGAR, section headed "Other Sources of Sugar.")

MARASMUS

From the Greek marasmos, meaning a dying away. A progressive wasting and emaciation.

This disease is due to chronic protein-calorie malnutrition. It is found in infants and young children in many areas of the world, particularly in the developing and over-populated countries, where protein-rich foods, especially those of animal origin, are practically unavailable to the poorer segments of the population. This is because (1) protein itself is deficient, and (2) total food consumption, and hence energy intake, is so inadequate that the protein eaten is not spared to function as an essential nutrient.

Physiological adaptations in marasmus involve the breakdown of body tissues for energy which is stimulated by catabolic hormones from the adrenal cortex. Moreover, there is a reduction or cessation of protein synthesis and growth in many tissues. Outward signs and symptoms include wasting of muscle, loss of subcutaneous fat, dry baggy skin, general appearance of old age, low body weight (often less than 60% of weight expected for age and height), large sunken eyes, diarrhea, subnormal body temperature, and malabsorption. Survival during marasmus is moderately enhanced by a large reduction in the utilization of nutrients for energy which is brought about by a diminished secretion of the thyroid hormones, and a reduced response of the cells to insulin. Eventually, there may be dehydration and electrolyte imbalances due to depletion of sodium, potassium, magnesium, and chloride ions, which may in turn lead to disorders of the brain, heart, kidneys, and nerves. These conditions can rapidly lead to death if not promptly corrected. Treatment of marasmus consists of feeding an easily digested diet, such as milk and oil, which supplies at least 1.0 g of protein and 50 to 60 kcal per lb of body weight (2.2 g of protein, 110 to 132 kcal per kg of body weight).

Also see DEFICIENCY DISEASES, Table D-1 Major Dietary Deficiency Diseases—"Marasmus"; and MALNUTRITION, PROTEIN-ENERGY.)

MARGARINE

This is an economical, nondairy product resembling butter in appearance, form, composition—and taste. Margarine contains about 80% fat as does butter, but the fat is generally entirely of plant origin—corn, soybean, safflower, and/or cottonseed, although a small amount of animal fat (not butterfat) is sometimes used by processors. Like many other products, margarine was developed in response to a need and an incentive.

ORIGIN AND HISTORY. Napoleon III, the ruler of France from 1852 to 1870, appealed to his people for an economical and nutritious butter substitute. Near the end of his rule, a chemist, Hippolyte Mege-Mouries, developed margarine, for which he was awarded a prize by the emperor. Mouries used oil obtained by pressing beef fat, oleo oil, salt, milk, and annatto for coloring. These ingredients were partially emulsified, then chilled rapidly with ice water to separate the solidified fatty granules from the excess water of the milk. This formed a solid emulsion which could be kneaded to the finished margarine. Even today, Mouries' method is the basis of margarine production. This first margarine had a pearly appearance and was called oleomargarine—a name derived from the oleo oil, and from the Greek word margaron, meaning pearl. In the United States, the name oleomargarine was required by law until 1952. Subsequently, the terms margarine and oleomargarine have been used interchangeably, but the term margarine is used most frequently.

While Napoleon appealed for the development of margarine and rewarded the inventor, the use of margarine in the United States was discouraged, and even penalized, almost as soon as it was introduced in the early 1870s. American dairymen protested, and in an effort to prevent immediate ruin to the butter market, Congress put a tax on margarine in 1886—forgetting the American ideal of free enterprise. By 1930, many states forbade the sale of yellow-colored margarine; furthermore, federal laws required restaurants which served margarine to post conspicuous notice indicating their substitution. Without doubt, government hurdles delayed change, but people still continued to buy margarine despite the restrictions. Finally, in 1950, criticism of the tax was so widespread that Congress ended it. Still, it took another 17 years before all states lifted the ban on the sale of yellow-colored margarine. Ironically, over the past 30 years, the per capita consumption of butter and margarine have switched positions. Today, Americans consume more margarine than butter, as Table M-13 shows. Most of the increased consumption of margarine can be explained by both the price difference between butter and margarine, and the nutritional comparison.

TABLE M-13
PER CAPITA CONSUMPTION OF BUTTER AND MARGARINE IN THE UNITED STATES SINCE 1950[1]

Year	Butter		Margarine	
	(lb)	(kg)	(lb)	(kg)
1950 . . .	10.7	4.9	6.1	2.8
1955 . . .	9.0	4.1	8.2	3.7
1960 . . .	7.5	3.4	9.4	4.3
1965 . . .	6.4	2.9	9.9	4.5
1970 . . .	5.3	2.4	11.0	5.0
1975 . . .	4.8	2.2	11.2	5.1
1980 . . .	4.5	2.0	11.4	5.2
1985 . . .	4.8	2.2	10.7	4.9
1990 . . .	4.3	2.0	10.9	5.0

[1]Data from Agricultural Statistics, USDA, 1965, p. 150, Table 220; 1980, p. 148, Table 208; and 1991, p. 139, Table 194.

PRODUCTION. Several types of plant oils may be used in the production of margarine. The most common is soybean oil, but corn, cottonseed, palm, peanut, and safflower oils may also be used by processors. Some of these oils may be hardened by hydrogenation. Also, some processors may employ a small amount of animal fat. Regardless of the oil source, the U.S. government stipulates that margarine must contain at least 80% fat.

Today, margarine is manufactured by first emulsifying —with the help of emulsifying agents—in water, milk, or a type of milk made from soybeans. Butterlike flavoring, salt, yellow coloring, preservatives, and vitamin A, and possibly other vitamins are added to the emulsion. In some processes beta-carotene is added for color as well as for supplying vitamin A. Next, this mixture is (1) agitated to distribute the water droplets uniformly; and (2) chilled, causing the oils to crystallize and solidify and trapping water droplets throughout, thus forming a mass with the desired semiplastic consistency. Nowadays, the whole process takes place in a completely closed, continuous churn—even shaping, wrapping, and packaging occurs as part of one continuous operation.

For consumer use, margarine is produced in the traditional hard sticks of 1-lb packages, as well as plastic tubs of soft margarine, liquid margarine in plastic squeeze bottles, or whipped with nitrogen gas. Whipped margarines have an increased volume and thus cut down on the amount used by calorie-conscious individuals. Also, a salt-free margarine is available for individuals on sodium restricted diets. In 1989, about 2.8 billion pounds of margarine were produced in the United States. Although most people consider margarine a household item, about 10 to 15% of the total production is used by the baking industry.

NUTRITIONAL VALUE. With the exception of the origin of the fat, the nutrient composition of margarine is very nearly the same as that of butter, as Table M-14 reveals.

TABLE M-14
COMPARISON OF THE NUTRIENT COMPOSITION
OF BUTTER AND MARGARINE[1]

Nutrient	Unit	Butter	Margarine
		◄ -(per 100 g)- - ►	
Food energy	kcal	717.0	718.7
Protein	g	0.9	0.9
Fats	g	81.1	80.5
Calcium	mg	24.0	29.9
Phosphorus	mg	23.0	22.9
Sodium	mg	826.0	943.4
Magnesium	mg	2.0	2.6
Potassium	mg	26.0	42.4
Iron	mg	0.2	—
Zinc	mg	0.1	—
Copper	mg	0.4	—
Vitamin A	IU	3058.0	3307.0[2]
Vitamin E	mg	1.6	15.0[3]
Thiamin	mcg	5.0	10.0
Riboflavin	mcg	34.0	37.0
Niacin	mcg	42.0	23.0
Vitamin B-6	mcg	3.0	9.0
Folic acid	mcg	3.0	1.2
Vitamin B-12	mcg	—	0.1

[1]Values from Food Composition Table F-36.
[2]Vitamin A must be added to yield a finished margarine with not less than 15,000 IU per pound (0.45 kg).
[3]Varies depending on the type of oil used.

The major difference between margarine and butter— the fat—is expanded in Table M-15.

TABLE M-15
COMPARISON OF THE FATS OF
BUTTER AND MARGARINE[1]

Fat	Butter	Margarine
	◄ — (g/100 g) - - ►	
Total fat	81.1	81.1
Animal fat	81.1	—
Plant fat	—	81.1
Saturated fat	50.5	14.8
Polyunsaturated fat	3.0	—
Oleic acid	20.4	41.4
Linoleic acid	1.8	22.2
Cholesterol	.2	.0

[1]Values from Table F-9, Fats and Fatty Acids in Selected Foods.

Table M-15 indicates a difference that has been exploited as a selling point—no cholesterol in margarine. Furthermore, margarine contains significant amounts of the essential fatty acid, linoleic acid.

Despite attempts to stymie the growth of the margarine industry, it has become a success and is established as a high-quality, wholesome, nutritious food, with worldwide acceptance.

(Also see ADDITIVES; FATS AND OTHER LIPIDS; MILK AND MILK PRODUCTS; and OILS, VEGETABLE.)

MARGARINE, KOSHER

Made only from vegetable fats, and fortified only with carotene (derived from vegetable sources.)

MARINADE

A mixture of liquids with herbs and spices which is used to steep meats and fish before cooking. By using pineapple juice, the marinade can be used to tenderize meats. The marinades containing oil and seasonings add oil and flavor to the fish or meat being cooked.

MARMITE

• A large metal or pottery soup kettle with a lid. Small individual ones are called *petite marmite.*

• Soup that is cooked in a marmite.

• A yeast product used for flavoring soups and meats; also as a spread or beverage.

MARRON

Chestnuts preserved in syrup flavored with vanilla.

MATE (BRAZILIAN TEA, PARAGUAY TEA, YERBA MATE)

This is a stimulating drink prepared from the dried leaves of mate or ilex plant (*Ilex paraguayensis*) of South America. It is prepared in much the same manner as tea. Boiling water is poured over mate leaves or powder and allowed to steep for about 10 minutes. Then the drink is strained and taken either hot or cold, with or without sugar. Mate is enjoyed throughout most of South America. It contains caffeine.

MATOKE *Musa paradisiaca* **var.** *sapientum*

The East African name for the local varieties of unripe bananas that are used mainly for cooking.
(Also see BANANA; and PLANTAINS.)

MATRIX

The ground work in which something is enclosed or embedded; for example, protein forms the bone matrix into which mineral salts are deposited.

MAY APPLE (INDIAN APPLE; MAYFLOWER) *Podophyllum peltatum*

The small, yellow fruit of a wild herb (of the *Podophyllaceae* family) which is native to eastern North America from southern Canada to the Gulf of Mexico.

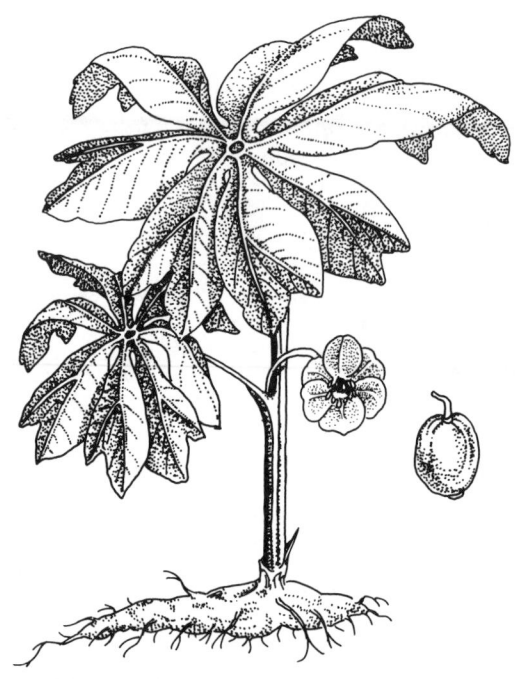

Fig. M-29. The may apple, a fruit that grows wild throughout the eastern United States and southeastern Canada.

It is good fresh or when made into fruit drinks, jam, jelly, marmalade, pies, and wine. It is noteworthy that the unripe fruit, leaves, and roots of the plant are poisonous.

MAYONNAISE

This is an oil-in-water type of semisolid emulsion with egg yolk acting as the emulsifying agent. It consists of vegetable oil, egg yolk or whole egg, vinegar, lemon and/or lime juice, with one or more of the following: salt, a sweetener, mustard, paprika or other spice, monosodium glutamate and other food seasonings. Vegetable oil comprises 65 to 80% of the composition. Thus, mayonnaise is high in calories. Each 3½ oz (*100 g*) contains 650 to 700 Calories (kcal). Vinegar and salt act as preservatives. A number of methods for manufacturing mayonnaise are available, but all of them make use of high-speed beating or dispersing equipment in some stage of the process. Manufacturers employ machines and systems which allow the semicontinuous and continuous production of mayonnaise. Mayonnaise may be packaged in glass or plastic wide-mouth jars, tubes, sachets, or individual portion cups. It is used on salads, fish, vegetables, other foods and in a variety of recipes.
(Also see OILS, VEGETABLE.)

MAYPOP *Passiflora incarnata*

The fruit of a wild species of passion fruit (family *Passifloraceae*) that grows in the southern United States. Maypop berries are yellow-colored, egg-shaped, and about 2 in. (*5 cm*) long. They may be eaten raw or made into jam, jelly, pies, and sauces.

The raw fruit is moderately high in calories (111 kcal per 100 g) and carbohydrates (21%). It is also high in fiber and a good source of iron.

MEAL

• A food ingredient having a particle size somewhat larger than flour.

• Mixtures of cereal foods, in which all of the ingredients are usually ground.
(Also see CEREAL GRAINS.)

MEAL PLANNING

Many factors enter into planning meals. Perhaps the most important one is nutritive value; but other things such as appearance, palatability, cost, and food preferences must be considered at the same time.

The procedure should begin by using the food groups as a pattern. Choose the entree from the protein group, then add the milk group, follow with the vegetable and the fruit, and finish up with the cereal group. It is quite simple if every meal is planned this way.

There are some well-known food combinations which have stood the test of time, thus when combining foods it is best not to try unorthodox combinations. The public has demanded that restaurant meals be well balanced; thus, when in doubt, their menus can be used as patterns.

Table M-16 Meal Planning Guide, can be used for the purpose of planning the day's meals. It gives the number of servings of each food group, for the different ages. Thus, one menu can take care of every age, merely by varying the number of servings from each food group.

TABLE M-16
MEAL PLANNING GUIDE

Food Group and Serving Size[1]			Servings Per Person Per Day											
			Infants under 1 yr	Children			Adolescent 12-19 yr		Adults (20-50 yr)				Persons Older than 50 Years	
Low-Energy Foods	Medium-Energy Foods	High-Energy Foods		1-3 yr	4-7 yr	8-11 yr	M	F	M	Non-Preg. F	Preg. F	Lac. F	M	F
MEATS, FISH OR SEAFOOD, EGGS, BEANS, PEAS, OR NUTS—each serving provides 12 to 20 g of protein			1/2	1	2	2	2	2	2	2	3	3	2	2
(50-150 kcal per serving) Cooked, lean meat such as beef, Canadian bacon, corned beef, ham, kidneys, lamb, liver, pork, or veal ......2 oz Cooked or canned fish such as cod, flounder, halibut, mackerel, perch, salmon, sardines, or tuna .....2 oz Canned crab .... 3 oz Eggs ......2 medium	*(200-300 kcal per serving)* Cooked brisket or shortribs of beef.........2 oz Salami ....2 oz Liverwurst or Polish sausage..3 oz Bologna .... 3½ oz Frankfurters .... 4 oz Cooked, dried beans or peas ......1 c	*(350-500 kcal per serving)* Sausage made from beef or pork.....2 oz Roasted nuts or seeds such as almonds, cashews, pecans, peanuts, sunflower seed kernels, or walnuts .... 3 oz Peanut butter .... 4 Tbsp												
MILK PRODUCTS—each serving provides 250 to 300 mg of calcium and 8 g of protein			1½-2	3	3	3	4	4	3	3	4	4	3	3
(about 100 kcal per serving) Skim or lowfat milk, buttermilk ....1 c Evaporated skim milk ....1/2 c Nonfat dry milk ......1/4 c Swiss cheese .... 1 oz	*(150-200 kcal per serving)* Whole milk or whole milk yogurt ....1 c Lowfat yogurt w/added dry milk, flavorings ....3/4 c Evaporated whole milk ....1/2 c American or cheddar cheese .... 1½ oz	*(300-500 kcal per serving)* Creamed cottage cheese ....2¼ c Ice cream ....1¾ c Light cream or sour cream ....3/4 c Sweetened, condensed whole milk ....1/3 c												
BREADS AND CEREALS—should be whole-grain or enriched. Each serving provides 70 kcal and 2 g of protein			2	3	4	4	6	6	4	4	6	6	4	4
Slice of bread, muffin, or biscuit .... 1 Hamburger bun ....1/2 Pancakes (4" dia) .... 2 Soda crackers .... 3 Ready-to-eat cereals....................1 oz Cooked cereal or cooked pasta ....3/4 c Flour .... 2½ Tbsp														

Footnote at end of table

(Continued)

TABLE M-16 (*Continued*)

Food Group and Serving Size[1]			Servings Per Person Per Day											
			Infants under 1 yr	Children			Adolescent		Adults (20-50 yr)				Persons Older than 50 Years	
Low-Energy Foods	Medium-Energy Foods	High-Energy Foods		1-3 yr	4-7 yr	8-11 yr	12-19 yr		M	Non-Preg. F	Preg. F	Lac. F	M	F
							M	F						
DARK-GREEN AND DEEP-YELLOW FRUITS AND VEGETABLES—each serving provides 3,000 or more IU of vitamin A			1/3	1/2	1/2	1/2	1	1	1	1	1½	1½	1	1
(less than 100 kcal per serving)	*(100-200 kcal per serving)*													
Raw or cooked item (or its unsweetened juice) such as apricots, beet greens, broccoli, carrots, chard, cherries, chickory, collards, cress, kale, mustard greens, peaches, peppers, pumpkin, squash, spinach, or turnip greens ....1/2 c Cantaloupe (6″ dia) 1/4	Sweet potatoes, cooked ....1/2 c													
CITRUS FRUITS OR THEIR EQUIVALENTS—each serving provides 30 or more mg of vitamin C and less than 100 kcal			1	1	1	1	1	1	1	1	2	2	1	1
Small orange, large tangerine or tomato........ 1 Canned pineapple, large slice ....1 Grapefruit ....1/2 Cantaloupe or honeydew melon (6″ dia) .....1/4 Juice from grapefruit, lemon, orange, pineapple, or tomato ....1/2 c														
OTHER FRUITS AND VEGETABLES—sources of carbohydrates, fiber, minerals, and vitamins			1/2	1	3	3	3	3	3	3	4	4	4	4
(less than 100 kcal per serving)	*(100-200 kcal per serving)*	*(200-350 kcal per serving)*												
Artichokes, asparagus, beans (snap), beets, blueberries, cabbage, cauliflower, celery, cucumbers, eggplant, grapes, lettuce, okra, onions, rutabagas, sauerkraut, turnips, or watermelon cubes ....1/2 c	Cooked corn (cut off cob), cooked dried legumes (beans, lentils, and peas), fresh figs, mashed potatoes ....1/2 c Avocado ....1 medium	Dried fruit (such as apricots, figs, peaches, prunes, raisins), french fried potatoes ....1/2 c												

Footnote at end of table

(Continued)

TABLE M-16 (*Continued*)

Food Group and Serving Size[1]			Servings Per Person Per Day											
			Infants under 1 yr	Children			Adolescent		Adults (20-50 yr)				Persons Older than 50 Years	
Low-Energy Foods	Medium-Energy Foods	High-Energy Foods		1-3 yr	4-7 yr	8-11 yr	12-19 yr		M	Non-Preg. F	Preg. F	Lac. F	M	F
							M	F						
ESSENTIAL FATS—each serving provides approximately 1 g of essential fatty acids and 40-70 kcal			1	1½	2	2½	3	2½	3	2	2½	2½	2½	2
Vegetable oil (corn, cottonseed, peanut, safflower, or soybean) ....1 tsp Margarine (contains liquid vegetable oil), mayonnaise, or peanut butter..............2 tsp French dressing .... 1 Tbsp Peanut .... 6 small (or 2 tsp)														
SUPPLEMENTAL SOURCES OF ENERGY— to bring the daily dietary energy up to the total allowance														
(less than 100 kcal per serving) Carbonated beverages or beer... 7 oz Gelatin dessert ....1/2 c Table wine .... 3 oz Gin, rum, vodka, whiskey .... 1 oz Crisp bacon .... 2 sl Butter, chicken fat, lard ....2 tsp Honey, molasses, sugar, syrup, tomato catsup .... 1 Tbsp Jam, jelly .... 2 Tbsp	*(150-300 kcal per serving)* Hot chocolate or cocoa ....1 c Dessert wine .... 4-7 oz Puddings ....1/2 c Cakes with frosting, pies ......1-3 oz piece Cookies .....3-5 small Candies .... 1-2 oz Ice cream cone ....1 medium scoop Eclair ....1 small Gin, rum, vodka, whiskey ....2-4 oz	*(350-500 kcal per serving)* Cheesecake, pie a la mode .... 1 3-oz pc Ice cream cone ...double dip													
ENERGY ALLOWANCES (kcal per person per day)			50/lb	1300	1800	2400	3000	2250	2700	2000	2300	2500	2400	1800

[1]To convert to metric, see WEIGHTS AND MEASURES.

Here is how to use Table M-16: Let us suppose that it is necessary to plan a daily meal pattern for a 25-year-old single, moderately active female, who is not overweight.

Step 1—Look down the column headed "Adults (20-50 years)" and subheaded "nonpregnant F." Note that the essential food groups and the number of servings are as follows:

Meat, Fish or Seafood, etc.—2

Milk Products—3
Breads and Cereals—4
Dark-Green Vegetables—1
Citrus Fruits—1
Other Fruits and Vegetables—2
Essential Fats—2
Optional items to make up a total of 2000 Calories (kcal).
(See next page for Steps 2 and 3)

Step 2—Select items from the essential groups. Take care to balance their distribution between the meals and snacks, but avoid exceeding the total allowance for energy—2000 Calories (kcal) per day. However, if the subject gains weight on 2000 Calories (kcal) per day, then it will be necessary to choose servings from the "Low-Energy Foods." On the other hand, if she wishes to gain weight, then choose servings from the "High-Energy Foods." Optional items may be added from the group "Supplemental Sources of Energy" in order to bring the total energy up to the amount allowed. However, it would be better to obtain the supplemental sources of energy from among the essential groups. A typical day's selection might be as follows:

MEAL	FOOD	AMOUNT	CALORIES
Breakfast	Grapefruit	½	100
	Poached egg	1	74
	Whole wheat toast	2 slices	109
	w/butter	2 tsp	70
	Coffee w/evapo-		
	rated milk	¼ c	50
	or Milk, 2%	1 c	122
Morning Snack	Yogurt, flavored	1 c	231
Lunch	Sandwich made w/		
	Cooked ham	2 oz	112
	Swiss cheese	½ oz	51
	Sliced tomato	4 slices	22
	Lettuce leaf		
	Mayonnaise	2 tsp	36
	Whole wheat		
	bread	2 slices	109
	Milk, nonfat	1 c	83
Dinner	Roast beef	3 oz	300
	Tomato catsup	1 Tbsp	16
	Baked potato	1	93
	Mixed vegetables	½ c	64
	Biscuits made w/		
	whole wheat		
	flour	2	204
	Butter	2 tsp	70
	Jam	1 Tbsp	54
Bedtime Snack	Apple	1	84
	Total		1932-2004

Step 3—After writing down the menu plan for the day, check the number of servings of each of the essential food groups and the total energy supplied as given in Table M-16.

Although Table M-16 is a useful guide in planning the day's diet, always remember the Golden Rule of Eating, which is—"The greater the variety of foods in the diet, the greater the chances of getting everything that the body requires."

(Also see FOOD GROUPS.)

MEAT(S)

Contents	Page

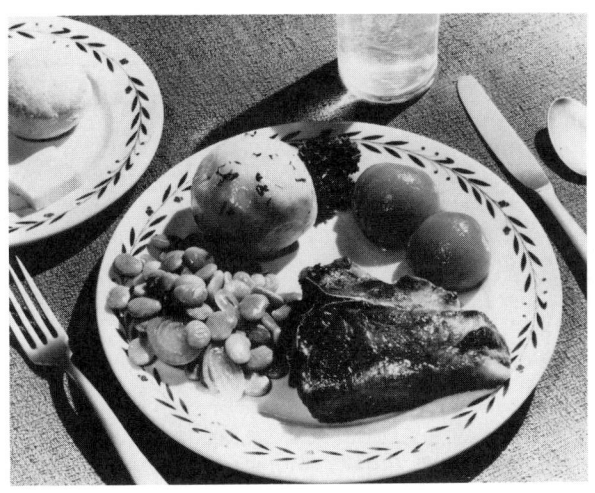

Fig. M-30. Meat on the table! People eat meat because it's good and good for them. (Courtesy, National Live Stock & Meat Board, Chicago, Ill.)

For centuries, animals have made a major contribution to human welfare as sources of food, pharmaceuticals, clothing, transportation, power, soil fertility, fuel, and pleasure. The most important of these is food—meat and other animal products. This section contains information on the value of animal foods to humans, with particular emphasis on the meat and meat by-product supply, along with their processing and utilization.

Meat is the edible flesh, organs, and glands of animals used for food. Meat by-products include all products, both edible and inedible, other than the carcass meat. In a broad sense, the term meat may include the flesh of poultry, fish and other seafoods, and game. In this section, however, the discussion of meat will largely be limited to red meat and to by-products therewith—to beef, lamb, and pork. Poultry, fish and seafoods, game, and milk and milk products will be treated in separate sections of this book.

That Americans enjoy eating meat is attested by the fact that, in 1990, the average American ate 112.3 lb of beef, veal, pork, and lamb. Of this total, beef accounted for 64 lb, pork for 46.3 lb, veal for 0.9 lb, and lamb for 1.1 lb.

Not only are meat and animal products good, but they are good for you. Foods from animals are the most nutritionally complete known. Today, they supply to the U.S. diet an average of 95% of the vitamin B-12, 79% of the calcium (mostly from milk and milk products), 55% of the riboflavin, 63% of the protein, 64% of the phosphorus, 51% of the vitamin B-6, 46% of the niacin, 36% of the vitamin A, 33% of the thiamin, 25% of the iron (in a readily absorbed form), and 34% of the magnesium. Additionally, animal proteins provide the nine essential amino acids in the proportions needed for humans; hence, they are *high quality* proteins.

Although this section is devoted primarily to the final product—meat, along with its processing—it must be remembered that this important food represents the culminatin of years of progressive breeding, the best in nutrition, vigilant sanitation and disease prevention, superior care and management, and modern marketing, processing, and distribution. Thus, the efficient availability of the highest quality meat is dependent upon the well-coordinated operation of the whole field of animal science. Much effort and years of progress have gone into the production of meat.

HISTORY OF MEAT. The use of meat by man antedates recorded history. Primitive man recognized that a meat-rich diet was far more concentrated than leaves, shoots, and fruits. Thus, the adoption of the meat-eating habit allowed him, if he was lucky in his kill, more time for other pursuits and skills, such as devising new tools and learning the beginnings of pictorial art.

Until less than 10,000 years ago, man obtained his food by hunting, scavenging, or gathering from the animal and vegetable kingdoms in his environment. It is probable that taming, and then domestication, of animals occurred without people being aware of what was happening. Certainly, gatherers and hunters—the people who first domesticated animals—could not forsee any use for them other than those they knew already—for meat and skins. Only later, after a change from a nomadic to a more settled life-style, were animals used for such things as milk, wool, motive power, war, sport, and prestige.

It is recorded that pork was used as a food in Egypt, probably at certain feasts, as early as 3400 B.C., and in China beginning in 2900 B.C. Old Testament Laws, written about 1100 B.C., dictated what meats were considered wholesome and sanitary. In I Corinthians, 15:39, written about 54 A.D., the Bible tells us—"All flesh is not the same flesh, but there is one kind of flesh of men, another flesh of beasts, another of fishes, and another of birds."

History of the Livestock and Meat Industry in the United States. Only the alpaca, bison (buffalo), deer, guinea pig, llama, and turkey were native to America at the time Columbus first landed in 1492. A chronology of the U.S. livestock and meat industry is given in Table M-17.

TABLE M-17
CHRONOLOGY OF THE U.S. LIVESTOCK AND MEAT INDUSTRY

Year	Event
1493	Christopher Columbus brought cattle, pigs, sheep, goats, and horses to the West Indies, on his second voyage.
1519	Cortez took cattle, sheep, and horses from Spain to Mexico.
1521	Ponce de Leon landed cattle, hogs, and sheep in what is now Florida.
1539	Hernando de Soto arrived in Tampa Bay (now Florida) with cattle, sheep, and horses.
1540	Coronado took cattle and sheep from Mexico into Arizona, and presumably into Texas, too.
1600	Spanish missionaries took Longhorn cattle with them for use in the Christian missions that they established among the Indians in the New World—missions that extended from the east coast of Mexico up the Rio Grande, thence across the mountains to the Pacific Coast.
1609	Colonists first brought cattle and sheep from England.
1610	Lord Delaware, who subsequently became the first Governor of the Virginia colony, arrived from England with oxen, cows, and goats for the Jamestown colony.
1641	John Pynchon founded the first meat packing plant in Springfield, Massachusetts; he packed salted pork in barrels for shipment to the West Indies, most of which was exchanged for sugar and rum.
1756	Brighton Market, near Boston, became the first public auction market and the slaughter center of the Northeast, although most slaughtering was still done on the farm.
1805	George and Felix Renick of the Scioto Valley of southern Ohio drove the first lot of fat steers across the Alleghenies to Baltimore.
1812	Samuel Wilson (1776-1854), an Army meat inspector and provisioner, became the symbol for mythical "Uncle Sam." The term "Uncle Sam," which originated as a derogatory nickname for the U.S. government during the war of 1812, was derived from the large initials "U.S." that Samuel Wilson stamped on barrels of salted beef which he had inspected. In the 1870s, Thomas Nast, a cartoonist, drew the figure commonly associated with Uncle Sam today. (A tall, slender figure with long white hair and beard, dressed in swallowtail coat decorated with stars, a pair of striped trousers, and a top hat with stars and stripes on it.) Uncle Sam changed from a character of derision to one of respectability in World Wars I and II. In 1961, Congress officially recognized Uncle Sam as the namesake of Samuel Wilson, a Troy, New York, Army meat inspector during the War of 1812.
1818	Elisha Mills established the first meat packing plant in Cincinnati. Other packing plants followed. By 1850, Cincinnati had become (1) the nation's main pork-packing center, and (2) known throughout the length and breadth of the land as "Porkopolis"; because it originated and perfected the system that packed 15 bushels of corn into a pig, packed that pig into a barrel, and sent it over the mountains and over the ocean to feed mankind.
1854	First railroad shipment of cattle was made by the Pennsylvania Railroad, using flat cars with slatted sides, but no roofs.
1866	Chisholm trail, the most famous of all trails, was laid out by Jesse Chisholm, a half-breed Cherokee Indian trader, who drove a wagon through Indian Territory (Oklahoma), to his trading post near Wichita, Kansas. When Abilene, Kansas became a railroad shipping center the next year, the cattle drovers followed Chisholm's wheel ruts and named the trail after him.
1875	G. H. Hammond, packer, after whom Hammond, Indiana was named, designed the first practical, though crude, refrigerated car.
1875	Gustave Swift, Chicago packer and founder of Swift & Company, perfected the refrigerated car.
1884	Congress established the Bureau of Animal Industry in the U.S. Department of Agriculture and gave the Secretary of Agriculture authority to enforce animal quarantine laws.
1906	Meat Inspection Act passed, providing for federal inspection of all meat intended for interstate and foreign commerce, including preslaughter inspection, postmortem inspection, and inspection at all stages of processing, livestock holding and meat packing, including inspection of meat packing equipment and facilities.
1906	L.L. Lewis of the Oklahoma Experiment Station described artificial insemination in horses, and in 1907 a calf was born in Oklahoma as a result of the dam being artificially inseminated; however, A. I. had been used in Europe much earlier.

(Continued)

TABLE M–17 (Continued)

Year	Event
1911	First shipment of livestock by motor truck to a public market was made, to the Indianapolis market.
1921	Packers and Stockyards Act passed by Congress, establishing the Packers and Stockyards Administration, to regulate livestock trading and related activities of packers and all others engaged in business at public stockyards.
1923	Federal grading of beef was started as a special service to U.S. Steamship Lines.
1925	Congress passed an act establishing a federal meat grading service.
1927	Federal meat grading of beef was initiated.
1949	Antibiotics were discovered as something new to be added to livestock feeds.
1954	Stilbestrol was approved by the Food and Drug Administration for use in cattle finishing rations; other hormones and hormonelike products followed.
1958	National Humane Slaughter Act set standards for slaughter methods; humane stunning methods for hogs and cattle improved.
1964	Congress enacted the Meat Import Law, to become effective January 1, 1965, providing for import quotas, based on a formula, for fresh, chilled, and frozen beef, veal, mutton (not lamb), and goat meat—including both carcass and boneless meat.
1967	Wholesome Meat Act extended meat inspection to products in intrastate commerce by a state-federal cooperative program.
1968	Wholesome Poultry Products Act passed, requiring inspection of poultry and poultry products by USDA, and extending poultry inspection to intrastate products.
1970	Dr. Norman Borlaug, an American agricultural scientist employed by the Rockefeller Foundation, and known as the *Father of the Green Revolution*, was awarded the Nobel Peace Prize for breeding new high-yielding, short-strawed varieties of wheat.
1977	Gene splicing, also known as recombinant DNA technique, ushered in a new era of genetic engineering, when scientists at the University of California-San Francisco reported a major breakthrough as a result of altering genes—turning ordinary bacteria into factories capable of producing insulin, a valuable hormone essential to the survival of diabetics.
1987	FDA approved an increase in the maximum allowance of selenium in complete feeds for cattle (beef and dairy), sheep, swine, chickens, turkeys, and ducks from 0.1 ppm to 0.3 ppm.
1990	Pollution control, sustainable agriculture, animal care and behavior, food safety, convenience foods, and human health came into vogue.

FROM WHENCE MEAT COMES. Animal agriculture is worldwide. Most of the livestock and poultry, along with 58% of the agricultural land, are found in Asia, Africa, and South America. Yet, North America, Europe, and Oceania, where scientific methods of production are most widely applied, produced 58% of the world's beef and veal, 62% of the milk, 41% of the lamb and mutton, 53% of the wool, 55% of the pork, 60% of the poultry meat, and 48% of the eggs.

Back of meat on the table are animals; and back of animals are vast expanses of pasture and range land, feed grains, and such by-product feeds as cull potatoes, beet by-products, and surplus fruit—all being utilized as feeds for cattle, hogs, and sheep. Back of all these is agriculture with assets of $834.6 billion in 1991, which ranks it as the nation's biggest single industry.

The business of agriculture is food. A total of $636.9 billion—representing 18.5% of the U.S. total disposable income of $3,450.1 billion—was spent for food in 1989. This vast sum went for the products and services of 2.2 million farms and ranches (1.4 million cattle farms and ranches, 329,833 hog farms, and 101,582 sheep farms), 42,081 feedlots; 676 marketing points; 6,753 meat packers and processors; 181,000 meat retailers; and more than 727,000 food service operators.

Consumers—all—need to know from whence their meat comes; they need to know that meat on the table is the ultimate objective in producing cattle, sheep, and swine. Consumers need to know that only farmers produce foods—that neither governments nor supermarkets produce foods; and they need to know that people do those things that are most profitable for them—and that farmers are people.

HOW MEAT REACHES THE TABLE

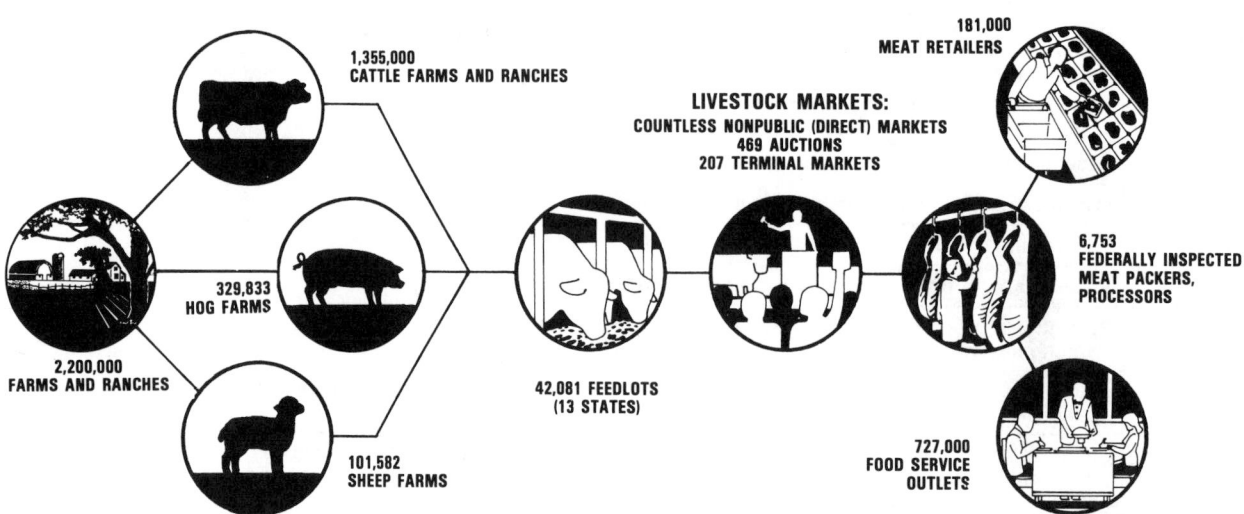

Fig. M-31. From whence meat comes. Back of meat on the table are 2,200,000 farms, of which 1,355,000 are cattle farms and ranches, 329,833 are hog farms, and 101,582 are sheep farms. All statistics are from the USDA, and for 1988, except number of cattle farms, number of hog farms, and number of sheep farms are from 1982 Agriculture Census.

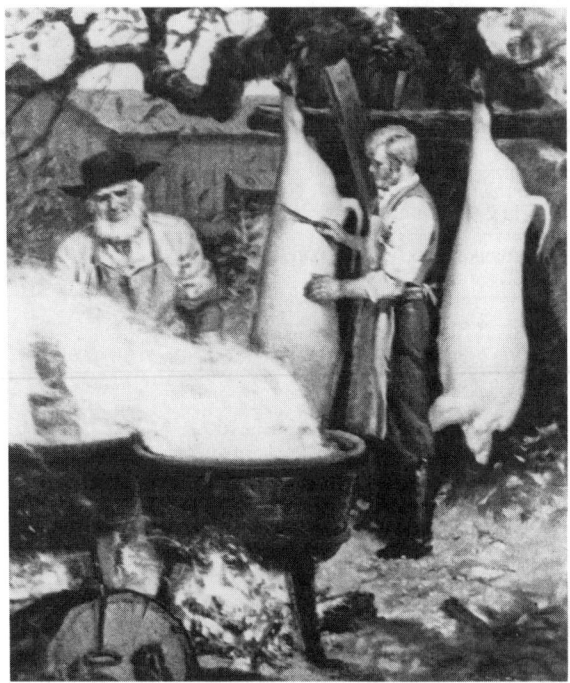

Fig. M-32. Old-time farm slaughter scene in the days before meat packing. When nearly all the people lived on the land—prior to the growth of cities and the rise of the town butcher—each family did its own slaughtering. (Courtesy, Swift and Company)

MEAT PACKING. *Meat packing is the business of slaughtering cattle, hogs, and sheep, and of preparing the meat for transportation and sale.* It is an important industry in many countries; the United States ranks first in meat packing. In 1986, 6,753 U.S. establishments slaughtered 37.6 million cattle, 3.5 million calves, 5.8 million sheep and lambs, and 80 million hogs; and produced 39.3 billion pounds of red meat. Also, the meat packing industry employed 143,000 people.

Today the name "packing" is a misnomer, for the barreled or pickled pork from whence the name originated is only a memory. But modern meat slaughtering and processing developed slowly, and the original name was so well established that there has been no attempt to rename the industry.

Packer Buying of Animals. In 1987, meat packers purchased their animals through the following channels:

Market Channel	Cattle	Calves	Sheep	Hogs
	(%)	(%)	(%)	(%)
Nonpublic markets ...	80.2	61.0	81.4	88.8
Auction markets ...	15.6	35.8	13.0	4.9
Terminal markets ...	4.2	3.2	5.5	6.3

Of course, these figures are continuing to shift, with terminal markets decreasing and direct buying and auctions increasing. Also, packers buy animals by other methods and channels, including carcass grade and weight basis, country commission firms, local markets and concentration yards, order buyers, local plants and retailers, cooperative shipping associations, cooperative selling associations, telephone auctions, telephone direct selling, teletype auctions, and selling on consignment (custom method).

Slaughtering and Processing. The slaughtering and dressing of animals is a "disassembly" operation—usually on-the-rail, whereas automobile manufacturing is an assembly line procedure.

Animals that are stressed before slaughter can result in marked changes in the appearance and value of carcasses and meat; so, slaughterers take great care to assure that stressful situations are avoided or minimized. Slaughtering is done under the surveillance of federal or state meat inspectors to assure that the carcass and edible by-products are wholesome and handled in a clean and sanitary manner. Though procedures vary among species, slaughtering and dressing usually include (1) rendering the animal unconscious, (2) bleeding, (3) removal of skin or hair, (4) removal of the abdominal viscera (stomach, intestines, liver, and reproductive organs), (5) detachment of the head and feet, and (6) removal of the thoracic cavity contents (trachea, lungs, heart, and esophagus). Minor variations in this procedure include the special requirements for ritualistic slaughter (e.g., Kosher slaughter) and for special age-species classes (e.g., hothouse lambs, roaster pigs, veal and calves with hide on). Carcasses are trimmed to remove bruises or surface contaminants, thoroughly washed to assure cleanliness, and rapidly chilled to 31° to 34°F (*0°-1°C*).

Today, new and innovative processing, tenderizing, curing, and sausage making generally follow standard slaughtering and dressing. The techniques and practices are presented under each of these headings.

MEAT PROCESSING. Meat is processed to convert it into forms that provide variety and convenience to consumers, to improve quality, to increase efficiency, and to save energy. Some new and innovative processing techniques follow:

• **Flaking, forming, restructuring**—Restructured steaks are made by (1) shaving (flaking) small sections from larger muscles, (2) compressing (forming) the flakes into the desired shape (usually a strip steak or a filet) in a cylindrical mold, and (3) cleaving the molded unit (log) into individual portions. The latest technology in restructuring makes use of an extrusion process, two hoppers (one filled with muscle, the other filled with fat), and a coextrusion manifold which produces a filet-shaped section of muscle that has a thin layer of fat attached to the outside surface—the result is a restructured steak that is a reasonable facsimile of the real thing.

The physical disruption of muscle associated with flaking should solve some, if not all, of the tenderness problems. The perfection of restructuring could make forage-fed beef an important source of red meat in the diet of America.

• **Massaging, tumbling, chunk-formed**—Meat massaging and tumbling are physical processes to which meat may be subjected for improving quality and accelerating meat product manufacture. Massaging is a rather gentle form of manipulation and mechanical agitation by use of a rotating drum and paddles or baffles, and is generally used on soft tissues. Tumbling is a more severe type of physical treatment, usually involving a drop of 3 ft (*1 m*) in the tumbler, which results in the transfer of kinetic energy into the muscle, disruption of muscle fibers, and abrasion of outer meat surfaces. Prior to, or during, tumbling, meat is usually injected or processed in cover cure (a mixture of flavorings, salt, and, sometimes, sodium nitrite). Tumbling improves and accelerates the distribution of cure in meat and increases the extraction of salt-soluble proteins; changes which make for a shorter curing process, assure the consumer of a more uniform product, and permit the use of muscle from any part of the animal to form products that resemble intact cuts.

Roast beef can be made by (1) tumbling chunks of meat with a small quantity of salt, (2) pressing and/or forming the chunks of meat into roast-size pieces, (3) cooking the chunked-form product, and (4) slicing into consumer portions. Such processing makes it possible to use lower quality beef.

• **Mechanical deboning**—Mechanical deboning is a process for salvaging most of the meat remaining on bones after conventional hand deboning. Following hand deboning, the bones and adhering meat are chopped in a grinder and then pressure-extruded through a screen or through slots of approximately 0.5 mm diameter to separate the bone from soft tissue. The resulting deboned meat is redder in color than regular ground meat because of its increased bone marrow content and the removal of much of the connective tissue.

Mechanically deboned meat has the estimated potential of adding one billion pounds of meat per year to the nation's food supply. Nutritionally, mechanically deboned meat (1) is rich in iron and calcium (up to 0.75% Ca)—nutrients often deficient in the U.S. diet, and (2) closely parallels hand-deboned meat in protein content and quality. Moreover, levels of fluoride and lead are not high enough to be of public health concern; and palatability and stability during frozen storage of ground beef products manufactured with mechanically deboned beef are equal to similar hand-boned products.

Mechanically deboned meat is suitable for use in sausages, bologna, and other similar products.

Despite the factors favorable to the use of mechanical deboning, prior to 1982 it had not been used extensively because of USDA labeling regulations which conveyed a negative connotation to consumers. In particular, the requirement that mechanically deboned meat carry a label indicating the percentage of powdered bone therein mitigated against sales. So, in 1982, the USDA eliminated this rule. Instead, mechanically deboned meat must now have a disclosure, either in the nutrition statement or somewhere else on the label showing the amount of calcium per serving.

It is noteworthy that mechanically deboned meat has been used by the U.S. fish and poultry industries for several years, and that mechanically deboned meat is approved for use in most countries.

• **Hot-boning**—This refers to the removal of soft tissue (muscle and fat) from the beef skeleton prior to chilling (usually 2 to 6 hours after slaughter). Because the meat industry is a very heavy user of energy, widespread adoption of hot-boning technology appears imminent; such processing makes it unnecessary to chill bones and undesired fat, thereby reducing energy requirements for chilling and for rendering, by a composite of 25 to 40%.

Presently, the main deterrents to the meat packing industry adopting hot-boning are: (1) toughening of muscle, which occurs if hot-boning is done too early postmortem; (2) the effect on the physical appearance of the cuts; and (3) federal grade standards make no provision for grading beef while it is "hot," with the result that block beef of the Prime, Choice, and Good grades cannot be graded as such.

MEAT TENDERIZING. Consumers want tenderness, as well as flavor, in the meat they buy. The common methods of tenderizing are:

• **Aging, Natural (low temperature)**—Following slaughter, dressed carcasses are rapidly chilled in a room at 32°F (0°C), at a relative humidity of about 85% in order to reduce moisture loss. The chilled side or cuts may be held for aging.

Aging is accomplished by holding the beef carcass or cuts for 1 to 6 weeks at a temperature of 38 to 40°F (3 to 4°C) and a relative humidity of 70 to 90%, with a gradual flow of air to provide a fresh atmosphere. These conditions permit selective enzymatic and bacterial action; the enzymes aid in the breakdown of various tissues, and the bacteria provide the nutlike flavor characteristic of aged beef. Today, very little beef is aged more than a week, because aging in carcass or wholesale cuts has become too costly in terms of shrinkage and cooler space.

Lamb carcasses are not aged.

(Also see subsequent section headed "Meat Packers and Retailers Court Consumers, • Aging.")

• **Vegetable enzymes and Pro-Ten**—Three enzymes of vegetable origin which dissolve or degrade collagen and elastin are:

1. *Papain,* secured from the tropical American tree, *Carica papaya* (Also see PAPAYA.)
2. *Bromelin,* secured from the juice of the pineapple (Also see PINEAPPLE.)
3. *Ficin,* secured from figs (Also see FIG.)

Swift and Company developed and patented the Pro-Ten process of tenderizing beef by injecting the standard proteolytic enzyme (papain) into the animal's jugular vein minutes (preferably, about 30 minutes) before slaughter. The tenderizing enzyme is carried to all parts of the body through the bloodstream and results in a significant increase in tenderness. Pro-Ten treated beef is sold as "Pro-ten beef."

A commercial tenderizer, known as Controlled Meat Tenderizer, consisting of hydrolyzed vegetable proteins, vegetable enzymes (papain, bromelin, and ficin), salt, monosodium glutamate, dextrose, propylene glycol, and other spices in a solution of water, is approved for use in government inspected plants.

The tenderizing action of enzymes does not occur until the meat is heated during cooking.

• **Mechanical tenderization (blade tenderization)**—Mechanical tenderizers, consisting of a machine that presses many sharp blades or needles through roasts and steaks, are being used by some segments of the meat trade. It is chiefly used on primal cuts (rib and loin) from lower quality grades and on the less tender cuts (chuck, round, shank) of higher grade carcasses. These machines have gained wide acceptance in the hotel, restaurant, and institutional trade in recent years. Research indicates that mechanical tenderization improves tenderness by 20 to 50%, without increasing cooking losses.

• **Electrical stimulation**—First observed in 1749 when Benjamin Franklin noted that meat from turkeys that had been electrically shocked was "uncommonly tender." Electrical stimulation has been adopted by the U.S. meat packing industry with unprecedented haste.

Electrical stimulation is a method of tenderizing meat with electricity. The passing of a current through the carcass causes the muscle fibers to loosen. Before rigor mortis sets in, the carcass is shocked until all the energy in the muscle that causes the fibers to contract is used up.

During the normal slaughter process, the carcass is cooled before being cut up. Rigor mortis pulls all the muscle fibers in the muscle into a bundle. Each fiber has smaller units within, that lengthen and shorten as the muscle works; when the carcass is cooled, these contract, also. This means that when a person is cutting and chewing on such a steak, he is chewing through a double thickness of fibers. By keeping them stretched out, there is less thickness; hence, less toughness.

The process, now used commercially, involves passing the just-killed carcass across a meta conductor. Research has shown that the optimum shock is 550 to 700 volts at 5 amps, and that 17 shocks are necessary to burn up all the energy left over in the muscle that would cause it to contract. The rest of the slaughter process remains the same, and there is no outward visual sign that the carcass has been shocked. Tests show that the tenderness is increased by 20 to 40%. Additional advantages of electrical stimulation include: (1) improved "set-up" of marbling, allowing grading at earlier time postmortem; (2) enhanced "aging" due to earlier release of the autolytic enzymes which increase meat tenderness during cooler storage; (3) reduced incidence of "heat-ring" in the ribeye; (4) brighter muscle color; (5) more desirable flavor; and (6) extended retail caselife. Packers view this processing technique as an easy means of assuring satisfactory palatability to their customers, and as a means of conserving energy (because less chilling time is required to increase grade, and less aging time is required to increase tenderness).

In the United States, Texas A&M University researchers have taken the lead in carcass tenderization by the electrical shock method. However, the process is not new; New Zealanders have been processing lamb through electrical stimulation for decades.

Electrical tenderizing is effective on beef, lamb, and goat carcasses, but not pork.

MEAT CURING. In this country, meat curing is largely confined to pork, primarily because of the keeping qualities and palatability of cured pork products. Considerable beef is corned or dried, and some lamb and veal are cured, but none of these is of such magnitude as cured pork.

Meat is cured with salt, sugar, and certain curing adjuncts (ascorbate, erythorbate, etc.); with sodium nitrite or sodium nitrate (the latter is used only in certain products); and with smoke. Each of the most common curing additives will be discussed:

• **Salt**—Sodium chloride is added to processed meats for preservative and palatability reasons. The addition of salt makes it possible to distribute certain perishable meats through what are often lengthy and complicated distribution systems. Also, in products such as wieners, bologna, and canned ham, fat solubilizes myosin, the major meat protein, and causes the meat particles to hold together; the meat can then be sliced without falling apart.

The amount of salt used in processed meat products could be reduced, but greater reliance would then have to be placed on refrigeration, and the margin of safety regarding product handling would be narrowed.

The salt added to certain meat products during processing does raise the sodium content sufficiently to make these products unsuited for persons who are on therapeutic, low-sodium diets.

(Also see SALT.)

• **Sodium nitrite (NaNO$_2$), sodium nitrate (NaNo$_3$), potassium nitrate or saltpeter (KNO$_3$)**—Nitrite and nitrate contribute to (1) the prevention of *Clostridium botulinum* spores in or on meat (*Clostridium botulinum* bacteria produce the botulin toxin that causes botulism, the most deadly form of food poisoning); (2) the development of the characteristic flavor and pink color of cured meats; (3) the prevention of "warmed-over flavor" in reheated products; and (4) the prevention of rancidity. Of all the effects of nitrite and nitrate, the antibotulinial effect is by far the most important. Nitrite is the essential ingredient for curing; the effectiveness of nitrate results from change of part of the nitrate to nitrite by reactions that occur during processing.

Nitrites may combine with certain nitrogen-containing substances and produce N-nitroso compounds, of which the most extensively studied have been the nitrosamines. Nitrosamines are sometimes found in very small amounts in meats cured with nitrite; for example, bacon cooked at high temperatures often contain detectable amounts of nitrosopyrrolidine (a specific kind of nitrosamine) as a result of the nitrite used in curing. Certain nitrosamines have been found to produce cancer when administered to test animals; hence, curing of meats with nitrite may create traces of carcinogens in at least some products under some circumstances.

No entirely satisfactory substitute is known for nitrite in meat curing. Two partial solutions are:

1. **A combination of nitrite and ascorbate.** For bacon curing, this consists of 120 parts of sodium nitrite and 550 parts of sodium ascorbate or sodium erythorbate per million parts of meat.

2. **A combination of sodium nitrite and potassium sorbate.** This consists of 40 ppm of sodium nitrite and 0.26% (2,600 ppm) of potassium sorbate.

NOTE WELL: If nitrite is not used to cure meat, the hazard of botulism will exist. Thus, discontinuance of nitrite use for meat curing could substitute one risk for another. Nevertheless, nitrite should be reduced in meat and other products to the extent that protection against botulism is not compromised, an extent yet to be determined.

• **Smoking**—Smoking produces the distinctive smoked-meat flavor which consumers demand in certain meats.

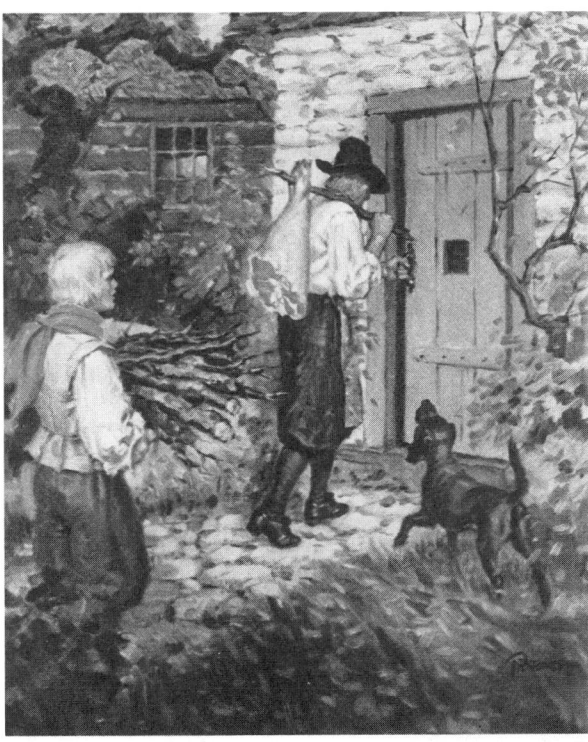

Fig. M-33. The Smoke House, in which meats were smoked in colonial days. This method of preserving meats is very old. Modern meat packers still smoke many of their products. (Courtesy, Swift and Company)

Wood smoke does contain known carcinogens. However, the situation is much like that with nitrite: carcinogens may be present in trace amounts, but there is no evidence that eating the meat products that have been smoked in the manner practiced in the United States influences the incidence of cancer. Many meat packers and processors now use either (1) "liquid smoke," made from natural wood smoke treated so as to remove certain components, or (2) a synthetic smoke made by mixing pure chemical compounds found in natural smoke; neither of which contains any carcinogens.

• **Phosphate (PO$_4$)**—Phosphate is added to increase the water-binding capacity of meat; its use increases yields up to 10%. Also, it enhances juiciness of the cooked product. Federal regulations restrict the amount of phosphates to: (1) not to exceed 0.5% in the finished product, and (2) not more than 5% in the pickle solution based on 10% pumping pickle. The addition of phosphate must be declared on the label.

SAUSAGE MAKING. *Sausage may be defined as minced meat, or a combination of meats, blended with various seasonings and spices and commonly stuffed into a casing or container.*

Although the origin of sausage is unknown, it was described as early as 900 B.C. Sausages were developed independently by people in several countries of Europe and Asia. National taste (flavor), climatic environment, and available seasoning ingredients largely determined the many varieties developed. The climate of southern Europe necessitated good-keeping qualities in sausages, so these people developed dry sausages. In the cooler climates of northern Europe, keeping qualities were less important than in the warmer southern climates; so, smoked and cooked sausages were developed in this area. Immigrants to America brought their sausage preferences and formulas with them; as a result, we have about 250 varieties of dried and smoked sausages in this country.

Each year, approximately 4.6 billion pounds (*2.1 billion kg*) of sausage are produced in the United States, which is about 11% of all meat consumed; making for an annual per capita consumption of 21 lb (*9.5 kg*) of sausage.

Sausage products provide a means of (1) storing meat for future use, (2) handling meat under adverse conditions, and (3) adding variety to meat products.

The flesh of any food animals, including fish, can be used in making sausage. In the United States, sausage is usually made from pork, beef, veal, and mutton. Trimmings are normally used as raw materials, rather than cuts, for which a ready market exists.

• **Classification of sausage**—Sausages may be classified as follows:

1. **Fresh sausage.** This sausage is made from chopped meats that are neither cured nor smoked. It may be sold in bulk, or stuffed into bags or casings. Examples are hamburger and fresh pork sausage.

2. **Uncooked smoked sausage.** This type of sausage is smoked, but not cooked. Smoked pork sausage is an example.

3. **Cooked smoked sausage.** This type of sausage is smoked lightly, then cooked. Frankfurters and bologna are examples.

4. **Dry sausage (summer sausage).** This sausage is made from pork or beef. Some dry sausage is cooked, but not smoked; other dry sausage is smoked and cooked. Dry sausage may be fermented with natural flora or with a starter culture. This sausage is often called *summer sausage* because of its superb keeping qualities. Dry salami is an example.

5. **Meat specialties.** This includes a great variety of products, consisting of chopped meats that are usually cooked or baked, rather than smoked. Examples are chili, souse, meat loaves, lunch meat, and minced ham.

Sausage may be further classified, based on variations in (1) ingredients and proportions of beef, pork, and/or veal, (2) fineness of chop or grind, (3) seasoning and spices, (4) smoking, (5) degree of cooking or drying, and (6) type of casing.

The most popular sausage in America is the frankfurter, or hot dog, or wiener.

Federal and State Meat Inspection. Most foods from animals are inspected by government officials to assure wholesomeness, proper labeling, and freedom from disease and adulteration. Federal inspection of animal products is the responsibility of the Food Safety and Quality Service of the U.S. Department of Agriculture. Imported meat and poultry are produced under USDA supervision in foreign countries where they originate, and samples are inspected by USDA upon arrival in the United States.

In 1906, the Meat Inspection Act was passed, providing for federal inspection of all meat intended for interstate and foreign commerce, including preslaughter inspection, postmortem inspection, and inspection at all stages of processing, livestock holding and meat packing, including inspection of meat packing equipment and facilities.

In 1967, the Wholesome Meat Act extended meat inspection to products in intrastate commerce by a state-federal cooperative program. The statute (1) requires that state standards be at least to the levels applied to meat sent across state lines; and (2) assures consumers that all meat sold in the United States is either inspected by the federal government or by an equal state program.

In 1968, the Wholesome Poultry Products Act was passed, requiring inspection of poultry and poultry products by the USDA and extending poultry inspection to intrastate products.

If meat passes federal inspection, an inspection stamp (Fig. M-34) is affixed to the wholesale cuts or package to assure the retailer and consumer that the products have been inspected. Products that do not pass inspection are denatured and rendered unusable for human consumption.

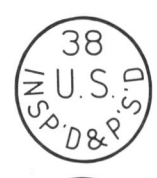

THIS IS THE STAMP USED ON MEAT CARCASSES. NOTE THAT IT ALSO BEARS THE OFFICIAL NUMBER ASSIGNED TO THE ESTABLISHMENT---IN THIS CASE NUMBER 38. THE STAMP IS USED ONLY ON THE MAJOR CUTS OF THE CARCASS; HENCE, IT MAY NOT APPEAR ON THE ROAST OR STEAK THE CONSUMER BUYS.

THIS MARK IS FOUND ON EVERY PREPACKAGED PROCESSED MEAT PRODUCT---SOUPS TO SPREADS--- THAT HAS BEEN FEDERALLY INSPECTED.

Fig. M-34.   Federal inspection marks used on animal products.

Federal Grades of Meats. *The grade of meat may be defined as a measure of its degree of excellence based on quality, or eating characteristics of the meat, and the* yield, or total proportion, of primal cuts. Naturally, the attributes upon which the grades are based vary between species. Nevertheless, it is intended that the specifications for each grade shall be sufficiently definite to make for uniform grades throughout the country and from season to season, and that on-hook grades shall be correlated with on-foot grades.

Federal grading of beef was first started as a special service to U.S. Steamship Lines in 1923; and on February 10, 1925, the 68th U.S. Congress passed an act setting up a federal meat grading service. But commercial meat grading was not inaugurated until 1927, at which time Prime and Choice grades of steer and heifer beef were stamped at Boston, New York City, Philadelphia, Washington, Chicago, Omaha, and Kansas City. A year later, the Good grade was added, and finally the service was broadened to include beef of all classes and grades.

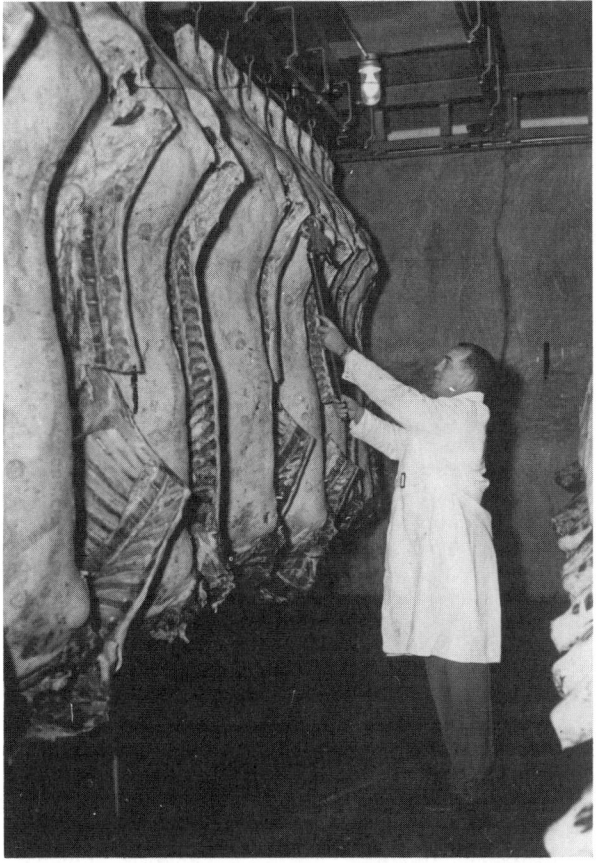

Fig. M-35.   Federal grader shown rolling (grading or stamping) beef with an edible vegetable dye. (Courtesy, *Livestock Breeder Journal*, Macon, Ga.)

At first, federal grading of meats was limited to beef, but it now includes mutton, lamb, calf, veal, and pork carcasses.

Government grading, unlike meat inspection, is not compulsory. Official graders are subject to the call of anyone who wishes their services, (packer, wholesaler, or retailer) with a charge per hour being made.

Consumers, especially the housewife who buys most of the meat, should know the federal grades of meats, because (1) in these days of self-service, prepackaged meats there is less opportunity to secure the counsel and advice of the meat cutter when making purchases, and (2) the average consumer is not the best judge of the quality of the various kinds of meats on display in the meat counter.

Federally graded meats are so stamped (with an edible vegetable dye) that the grade will appear on the retail cuts as well as on the carcass and wholesale cuts. These are summarized in Table M-18.

TABLE M-18
QUALITY GRADES OF MEATS BY CLASSES[1]

Beef[2]	Veal	Mutton and Lamb[2]	Pork
1. Prime[3]	1. Prime	1. Prime[4]	1. U.S. No. 1
2. Choice	2. Choice	2. Choice	2. U.S. No. 2
3. Select	3. Select	3. Select	3. U.S. No. 3
4. Standard	4. Standard	4. Utility	4. U.S. No. 4
5. Commercial	5. Utility	5. Cull[5]	5. U.S. Utility
6. Utility			
7. Cutter			
8. Canner			

[1]In rolling meat, the letters U.S. precede each federal grade name. This is important as only government-graded meat can be so marked. For convenience, however, the letters U.S. are not used in this table or in the discussion which follows.

[2]In addition to the quality grades given herein, there are the following yield grades of beef and lamb (and mutton) carcasses: Yield Grade 1, Yield Grade 2, Yield Grade 3, Yield Grade 4, and Yield Grade 5.

[3]Cow beef is not eligible for the Prime grade.

[4]Limited to lamb and yearling carcasses.

[5]Limited to mutton carcasses.

As would be expected, in order to make the top grade in the respective classes, the carcass or cut must possess a very high degree of the attributes upon which grades are based. The lower grades of meats are deficient in one or more of these grade-determining factors. Because each grade is determined on the basis of a composite evaluation of all factors, a carcass or cut may possess some characteristics that are common to another grade. It must also be recognized that all of the wholesale cuts produced from a carcass are not necessarily of the same grade as the carcass from which they are secured.

Until 1989, meat packers could choose to grade or not to grade beef. But, if they graded, they were required to grade for both quality and yield. In 1989, the law was changed, separating quality and yield grades of beef; and allowing packers to choose whether beef carcasses are graded for quality, for yield, or for both quality and yield. But packers could continue to choose between to grade or not to grade.

NOTE WELL: Federal grades of meats change from time to time, reflecting consumer preferences, technological developments in meat processing and marketing, and political expediency.

• **Proportion of U.S. meat federally graded**—In 1988, 93.6% of all lamb and mutton was quality graded, 56.4% of the beef was quality graded, but only negligible amounts of pork were quality graded.

TABLE M–19
U.S. BEEF GRADED IN 1983–1988[1]

	1983	1984	1985	1986	1987	1988
	(million pounds)					
Quality graded:						
Prime	472	363	456	400	383	380
Choice	11,152	10,829	11,875	12,053	11,463	11,598
Good/Select	423	430	386	344	266	579
Standard	13	12	11	6	3	2
Commercial	13	8	8	3	2	1
Utility	48	43	35	20	15	10
Cutter and Canner	1	1	4	1	1	1
Total	12,121	11,686	12,774	12,827	12,132	12,571
Yield Graded:						
Grade #1	275	406	461	507	448	456
Grade #2	4,221	4,923	5,195	5,360	5,048	5,052
Grade #3	6,672	5,767	6,387	6,286	5,989	6,275
Grade #4	856	550	667	621	593	717
Grade #5	97	40	63	53	53	71
Total	12,121	11,686	12,774	12,827	12,132	12,571
Total Commercial Beef Production	23,058	23,416	23,557	24,213	23,405	23,425

[1]Source: U.S. Department of Agriculture.

ADVANTAGES AND DISADVANTAGES OF FEDERAL MEAT GRADING.

Any system of evaluating products is certain to possess advantages and disadvantages—and meat grading is no exception.

• Some of the advantages of federal grading are—

1. Because the federal grade is applied by an independent agency, rather than an employee of the packinghouse, the average consumer is less likely to question it. Moreover, it reduces possible misunderstanding between buyers and sellers of meats.

2. The average consumer is not a good judge of the quality of the various kinds of meat that are on display. However, if the meat is correctly graded and labeled, the consumer is in a position to select the grade that meets his particular requirements.

3. Because there are fewer federal grades, the consumer is likely to become familiar with their significance more readily than with the more numerous packer brands.

4. Federal grading facilitates large-scale purchasing by federal, state, county, and city institutions and by hotels, restaurants, dining cars, and other large users of meats, chiefly because they can place large orders through one or several channels and obtain uniform products. Such large orders are usually on a contract basis, with grade specifications set forth.

5. The federal grades of meats correspond rather closely to the on-foot grades. They, therefore, provide a very important correlation for the benefit of producers. The payment of a premium for a quality product is a definite stimulation to improved breeding and feeding.

6. There is hardly any limit to the packer brands as established by different companies, whereas the federal grades are fairly comparable regardless of the area or ownership of the plant.

7. It is but natural that there should be less area or seasonal variation in appraisal of meat value or grades when a large overall agency is functioning than when

men are trained by many organizations, with only limited effort toward standardization between them.

8. Federal grading avoids any suspicion or temptation of upgrading, an alleged practice when demand for top grades exceeds the supply.

9. It makes meat market reports more intelligible.

10. The purchaser need not inspect carcasses or wholesale cuts to secure uniform products of merit to meet his requirements.

• Some of the disadvantages of federal grading are—

1. It ignores sex classes that are important. It would hardly be expected that a cow carcass grading U.S. Select would be comparable to a steer carcass of the same grade.

2. It does not provide sufficiently narrow classifications for a critical trade.

3. Many feel that packer brand names are more alluring to buyers than the rather unglamorous federal grades. Naturally, this feeling has been accentuated through advertising.

4. A meat packer's reputation is an individual proposition more than a collective one. It is argued, therefore, that he is more likely to uphold the reputation of his particular brand.

5. The national packers prefer advertising their brand names, claiming that to advertise federal grades places them in the position of helping the small packer, who does little or no advertising but who would greatly benefit therefrom.

Packer Brand Names. Practically all packers identify their higher grades of meats with alluring private brands so that the consumer as well as the retailer can recognize the quality of a particular cut.

A meat packer's reputation depends upon consistent standards of quality for all meats that carry his brand names. The brand names are also effectively used in advertising campaigns.

Kosher Meats.[25]

Meat for the Jewish trade—known as kosher meat—is slaughtered, washed, and salted according to ancient Biblical laws, called *Kashruth,* dating back to the days of Moses, more than 3,000 years ago. The Hebrew religion holds that God issued these instructions directly to Moses, who, in turn, transmitted them to the Jewish people while they were wandering in the wilderness near Mount Sinai.

The Hebrew word *kosher* means fit or proper, and this is the guiding principle in the handling of meats for the Jewish trade. Also, only those classes of animals considered clean—those that both chew the cud and have cloven hooves—are used. Thus, cattle, sheep, and goats—but not hogs—are koshered (Deuteronomy 14:4-5 and Leviticus 11:1-8).

Poultry is also koshered. Rabbinical law dictates that only cold water shall be used; hot or warm water cannot be used in defeathering or at any time in the processing of poultry products. Also, following picking and cleaning, kosher poultry must be washed, hung up to drip, hand-salted internally and externally, and rinsed; with constant inspection at all phases.

Both forequarters and hindquarters of kosher-slaughtered cattle, sheep and goats may be used by Orthodox Jews. However, the Jewish trade usually confines itself to the forequarters. The hindquarters (that portion of beef carcass below the twelfth rib) are generally sold as nonkosher for the following reasons:

1. The Sinew of Jacob ("the sinew that shrank," now known as the sciatic nerve), which is found in the hindquarters only, must be removed by reason of the Biblical story of Jacob's struggle with the Angel, in the course of which Jacob's thigh was injured and he was made to limp.

Actually, the sciatic nerve consists of two nerves; an inner long one located near the hip bone which spreads throughout the thigh, and an outer short one which lies near the flesh. Removal of the sinew (sciatic nerve) is very difficult.

The Biblical law of the sciatic nerve applies to cattle, sheep, and goats, but it does not apply to birds because they have no spoon-shaped hip (no hollow thigh).

2. The very considerable quantity of forbidden fat (Heleb) found in the hindquarters, especially around the loins, flanks, and kidneys, must be removed; and this is difficult and costly. Forbidden fat refers to fat (tallow) (a) that is not intermingled (marbled) with the flesh of the animal, but forms a separate solid layer; and (b) that is encrusted by a membrane which can be easily peeled off. The Biblical law of the forbidden fat applies to cattle,

sheep, and goats, but not birds and nondomesticated animals.

3. The blood vessels must be removed, because the consumption of blood is forbidden; and such removal is especially difficult in the hindquarters.

NOTE WELL: Forbidden fat and blood (the blood vessels) must be removed from both fore and hindquarters, but such removal is more difficult in the hindquarters than in the forequarters. However, the Sinew of Jacob (the sciatic nerve), which must also be removed, is found in the hindquarters only.

Because of the difficulties in processing, meat from the hindquarters is not eaten by Orthodox Jews in many countries, including England. However, the consumption of the hindquarters is permitted by the Rabbinic authorities where there is a special hardship involved in obtaining alternative supplies of meat; thus, in Israel the sinews are removed and the hindquarters are eaten.

Because the forequarters do not contain such choice cuts as the hinds, the kosher trade attempts to secure the best possible fores; thus, this trade is for high grade slaughter animals.

Kosher meat must be sold by the packer or the retailer within 72 hours after slaughter, or it must be washed (a treatment known as *begiss,* meaning to wash) and reinstated by a representative of the synagogue every subsequent 72 hours. At the expiration of 216 hours after the time of slaughter (after begissing three times), however, it is declared *trafeh,* meaning forbidden food, and is automatically rejected for kosher trade. It is then sold in the regular meat channels. Because of these regulations, kosher meat is moved out very soon after slaughter.

Kosher sausage and prepared meats are made from kosher meats which are soaked in water ½ hour, sprinkled with salt, allowed to stand for an hour, and washed thoroughly. This makes them kosher indefinitely.

The Jewish law also provides that before kosher meat is cooked, it must be soaked in water for ½ hour. After soaking, the meat is placed on a perforated board in order to drain off the excess moisture. It is then sprinkled liberally with salt. One hour later, it is thoroughly washed. Such meat is then considered to remain kosher as long as it is fresh and wholesome.

Meats and fowl are the only food items which require ritual slaughter, washing, and salting before they are rendered kosher.

• **Porging**—This is making a carcass commercially clean by drawing out and removing the sinews, the forbidden fat, and the blood vessels.

• **Porger**—A person whose business it is to do porging.

As would be expected, the volume of kosher meat is greatest in those Eastern Seaboard cities where the Jewish population is most concentrated. New York City alone uses about one-fourth of all the beef koshered in the United States.

While only about half of the total of more than six million U.S. Jewish population is orthodox, most members of the faith are heavy users of kosher meats.

---

[25]Authoritative information relative to kosher meats was secured from: (1) Grunfeld, Dayton Dr. I., *The Jewish Dietary Laws,* The Soncino Press, London/Jerusalem/New York, 1975; (2) a personal letter to M. E. Ensminger dated December 22, 1981, from Rabbi Menachem Genack, Rabbinic Coordinator, Union of Orthodox Jewish Congregations of America, New York, N.Y.; and (3) John Ensminger, Lawyer, New York, N.Y.

By-Products.

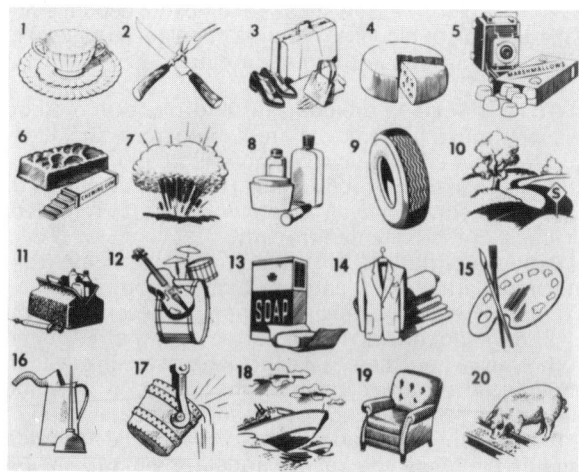

Fig. M-36. Some of the items for which by-products are used—items which contribute to the convenience, enjoyment, and health of people in all walks of life. (Courtesy, American Meat Institute, Washington, D.C.)

1. Bone for bone china
2. Horn and bone handles for carving sets
3. Hides and skins for leather goods
4. Rennet for cheese making
5. Gelatin for marshmallows, photographic film, printers' rollers
6. Stearin for making chewing gum and candies
7. Glycerin for explosives used in mining and blasting
8. Lanolin for cosmetics
9. Chemicals for tires that run cooler
10. Binders for asphalt paving
11. Medicines such as various hormones and glandular extracts, insulin, pepsin, epinephrine, ACTH, cortisone; and surgical sutures
12. Drumheads and violin strings
13. Animal fats for soap
14. Wool for clothing
15. Camel's hair (actually from cattle ears for artists' brushes
16. Cutting oils and other special industrial lubricants
17. Bone charcoal for high-grade steel, such as ball bearings
18. Special glues for marine plywoods, paper, matches, window shades
19. Curled hair for upholstery. Leather for covering fine furniture
20. High-protein livestock feeds

By-products include everything of value produced on the killing floor other than the dressed carcass; and they are classified as edible or inedible. The edible by-products include blood, brains, casings, fats, gelatin, hearts, kidneys, livers, oxtails, sweetbreads, tongues, and tripe. The inedible by-products include animal feeds, bone meal, bone products, brushes, cosmetics, feathers, fertilizer, glue, glycerin, hides and skins, lanolin, ligatures, lubricants, neat's foot oil, pluck (lungs, etc.), soap, and wool.

In addition to the edible (food) and nonfood (inedible) products, certain chemical substances useful as human drugs or pharmaceuticals are obtained as by-products. Among such drugs are ACTH, cholesterol, estrogen, epinephrine, heparin, insulin, rennet, thrombin, TSH, and thyroid extracts—all valuable pharmaceuticals which are routinely recovered from meat animals in the United States.

Newer Packing Developments.   Trends ahead in the meat packing industry include more prepackaging of retail meat items, along with recipes, detailed cooking instructions, chemical composition, and proportion of RDA provided per serving; portion control; precooked meat products; boneless beef; collecting and fractionating blood; refining tallow and edibles; recovery systems of inedible tallows and possibly other valuable items from waste water disposal; improved gelatin extraction and production; collagen extraction from hide trimmings; and more frozen beef, because it requires less energy to freeze at the point of origin.

KINDS OF MEAT.   The meat of cattle, hogs, sheep, and goats is known by several different names. These follow:

• **Beef**—This is the flesh of adult cattle. Good beef has white fat and bright cherry-red lean meat.

• **Veal**—This is the flesh of calves, usually 2 to 12 weeks old. Older calves are usually sold as "calves." Veal is pink in color and has a fine texture.

• **Mutton**—This is the flesh of mature sheep. It is darker colored and stronger flavored than lamb.

• **Lamb**—This is the flesh of young sheep. The meat of a sheep becomes mutton when the animal is about a year old. Lamb has a light-pink color and white fat, and a much milder flavor than mutton.

• **Pork**—This is the flesh of hogs. It is known as pork no matter how old the animal from which it comes. The eating quality of pork does not change much with the animal's age.

• **Chevon (goat meat)**—This is goat meat. The meat from young goats (kids) is delicious. Chevon from older goats is likely to possess a strong flavor.

• **Variety meat**—The various organs of animals are called variety meats. The heart, liver, brains, kidneys, tongue, cheek meat, tail, feet, sweetbreads (thymus and pancreatic glands), and tripe (pickled rumen of cattle and sheep) are sold over the counter as variety meats or fancy meats.

• **Game meat**—The flesh of wild animals or birds used as food.

MEAT PRESERVATION.   Methods of preserving meat were well established before the dawn of recorded history. Meat was dried by the aborigines; smoking and salting techniques were well established long before Homer's time (about 1000 B.C.); preparation and spicing of some kinds of sausages were common practices in Europe and in the Mediterranean countries before the time of the Caesars.

Fundamentally, meat preservation is a matter of controlling putrefactive bacterial action. Various methods of preserving meats have been practiced through the ages, the most common of which (listed alphabetically), are: (1) acidity, (2) air exclusion, (3) canning, (4) drying, (5) freeze-drying, (6) radiation, (7) refrigeration and freezing,

(8) salting, (9) dry sausage, (10) smoking, (11) spicing, and (12) sugar.

• **Acidity**—Commonly referred to as pickling or souring, an acid condition is unfavorable to bacteria. This method of preservation is used for pigs' feet, certain sausages, sauerkraut, pickles, and milk.

• **Air exclusion (vacuum packed)**—Vacuum packaging, or packaging with inert gas (e.g., N_2 or CO_2), are examples of the exclusion of air method. Elimination of oxygen from the package is the primary objective in vacuum and gas packaging. It extends the shelf life of fresh meats.

• **Canning**—*Canning is the temporary increasing of the heat content of a product that has been enclosed in an airtight container for the purpose of preventing the spoilage of the product being canned by the inactivation of particular organisms.* Two levels of heat may be applied in canning meat:

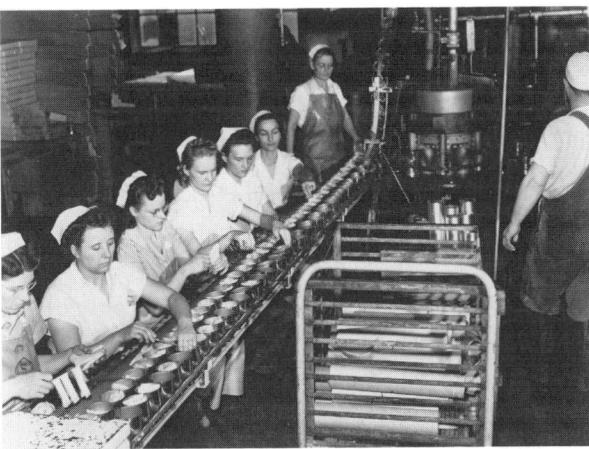

Fig. M-37. Canning meat, a method of meat preservation. (Courtesy, *Meat Magazine*)

1. **Pasteurization.** A low level of heat in the process of pasteurization, which is designed to kill all pathogenic organisms, but not all spoilage organisms. Since all spoilage organisms have not been destroyed, the product must still be stored under refrigeration. Most canned hams are pasteurized.

2. **Sterilization.** A high temperature in the process of sterilization. In this process, the canned meat is processed at a sufficiently high temperature and held there long enough to kill bacteria that cause spoilage, food poisoning, or infection. This calls for using a steam-pressure canner. By holding steam under pressure, one can get a temperature of 240°F (*115.5°C*) or more. Many luncheon meats are processed in this manner.

When canning, checking the sea level is important. More pressure in the canner is required at high altitudes than at low altitudes. A rule of thumb is: add 1 lb pressure for each 2,000 ft above sea level. Processing time depends on the container size.

Canning meat, as a method of meat preservation, was first initiated commercially in the United States by Arthur Libby in 1874.

• **Drying (beef jerky; dried beef; jerky; pemmican)**—The Spaniards who came to America following Columbus, found dried buffalo meat and dried venison in use by the Indians in southwestern United States, Mexico, Central America, and South America. Generally, the practice was to use only the tenderloin muscle and the eye muscle of the back from the hump to the rump. These muscles were cut in long, thin, flat strips and hung on poles, in trees, or in the tops of huts or tepees out of reach of dogs. The English adventurers called this dried meat "jerky."

The dried strips, which were very hard and inflexible, were powdered by beating them with stones or wooden mallets, then mixed with dried fruit and vegetables to form "pemmican."

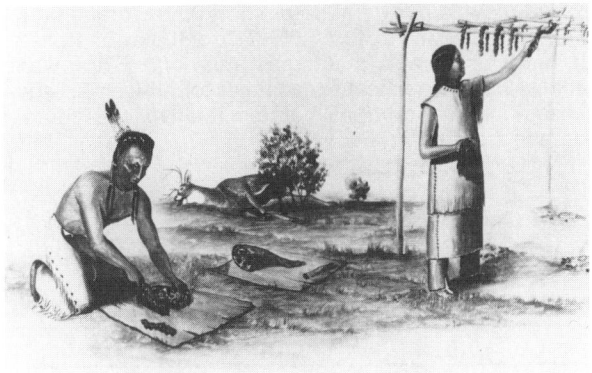

Fig. M-38. Indians drying and smoking venison. (Photo from a watercolor original by Ernest Smith. Owned by the Rochester Museum of Arts and Sciences)

Today, a limited amount of beef is cured and dried, in which form it is known as "beef jerky." It has a tough, chewy consistency and may be smoked, unsmoked, or air- or oven-dried.

• **Freeze-drying**—This process involves the dehydration of meat by the freeze-drying process, which consists of subjecting frozen pieces of meat to heat under vacuum. Products retain their shape and form and do not shrink as with other methods of dehydration. Freeze-dried meat and poultry have a moisture content of 2% or less and will not support the growth of most microbes.

• **Radiation**—This is the newest development in meat preservation. Nonionizing and ionizing radiation are capable of deactivating microorganisms.

Ultraviolet light is an example of nonionizing radiation; however, it does not sterilize beneath the surface.

Ionizing radiation, in the form of soft x rays or gamma rays, is capable of destroying organisms in canned, packaged, or exposed meat products without raising the temperature appreciably (hence, it is known as "cold sterilization"). Some researchers report that radiation may result in slight odor, flavor, and color changes. Also, it is noted that small doses of radiation do not completely inactivate all the proteolytic enzymes in meat, with the result that there is danger of these enzymes causing serious changes in the product during storage. However, much research is in progress; hence, these deficiencies may soon be overcome.

In 1981, the control of the Mediterranean fruit fly in California caused the Food and Drug Administration to ease the ban on treating food with gamma rays. However, each food processed by radiation requires FDA's approval. Also, labels on foods that have been irradiated must so indicate.

Consumer reaction to radiation of foods will be watched closely. It has great potential, provided people are not squeamish about the "dangers."

(Also see RADIATION PRESERVATION OF FOOD; and ULTRAVIOLET LIGHT.)

• **Refrigeration and freezing**—Meat is perishable, so proper care is essential to maintaining its keeping qualities.

Meat may be refrigerated for short-time storage, at a temperature of 36° to 40°F (2° - 4°C); or it may be frozen for longtime storage, at a temperature of 0°F or lower. Table M-20 gives recommended times for refrigerator and freezer storage. Additional pointers relative to refrigeration and freezing follow:

TABLE M-20
STORAGE TIME
FOR REFRIGERATED AND FROZEN MEATS[1]
(Maximum storage time recommendations for fresh, cooked, and processed meat)

Meat	Refrigerator	Freezer
	(36° to 40°F)[2]	(at 0°F or lower)
Beef (fresh)	2 to 4 days	6 to 12 months
Veal (fresh)	2 to 4 days	6 to 9 months
Pork (fresh)	2 to 4 days	3 to 6 months
Lamb (fresh)	2 to 4 days	6 to 9 months
Ground beef, veal and lamb	1 to 2 days	3 to 4 months
Ground pork	1 to 2 days	1 to 3 months
Variety meats	1 to 2 days	3 to 4 months
Luncheon meats	1 week	not recommended
Sausage, fresh pork	1 week	60 days
Sausage, smoked	3 to 7 days	—
Sausage, dry and semi-dry (unsliced)	2 to 3 weeks	—
Frankfurters............	4 to 5 days	1 month
Bacon..................	5 to 7 days	1 month
Smoked ham, whole....	1 week	60 days
Ham slices	3 to 4 days	60 days
Beef, corned	1 week	2 weeks
Leftover cooked meat ..	4 to 5 days	2 to 3 months
Frozen Combination Food		
Meat pies (cooked).....	—	3 months
Swiss steak (cooked)...	—	3 months
Stews (cooked)	—	3 to 4 months
Prepared meat dinners..	—	2 to 6 months

[1]*Lessons on Meat*, published by the National Live Stock and Meat Board, Chicago, Ill., p. 60.
[2]The range in time reflects recommendations for maximum storage time from several authorities. For top quality, fresh meats should be used in 2 or 3 days, ground meat and variety meats should be used in 24 hours.

1. **Storage of meat.** Fresh meat which is not to be refrozen should be stored in the coldest part of the refrigerator or, when available, in the compartment designed for meat storage. Additional guides for storage of meats follow:

a. **Fresh meat, prepackaged by the meat retailer (self-service).** It may be stored in the refrigerator in the original wrapping for not to exceed 2 days, or it may be frozen without rewrapping and stored in the freezer 1 to 2 weeks. For longer freezer storage, the original package should be overwrapped with special freezer material.

b. **Fresh meat, not prepackaged.** It should be removed from the market wrapping paper, wrapped loosely in waxed paper or aluminum foil, and refrigerated for not to exceed 2 days.

c. **Variety meats and ground or chopped meats.** They are more perishable than other meats; so, they should be cooked in 1 or 2 days if not frozen.

d. **Cured, cured and smoked meats, sausages, and ready-to-serve meats.** These should be left in their original wrapping and stored in the refrigerator.

e. **Canned hams, picnics and other perishable canned meats.** These should be stored in the refrigerator unless the directions on the can read to the contrary. These meats should not be frozen.

f. **Frozen meat.** Meat that is frozen at the time of purchase should be placed in the freezer soon after purchase unless it is to be defrosted for immediate cooking. The temperature of the freezer should not go above 0°F (-18°C). Packages should be dated as they are put into the freezer, and the storage time should be limited as recommended in Table M-20.

g. **Cooked meats.** Leftover cooked meats should be cooled within 1 to 2 hours after cooking, then covered or wrapped to prevent drying, and stored in the refrigerator. Meats cooked in liquid for future serving should be cooled uncovered for 1 to 2 hours, then covered and stored in the refrigerator.

2. **Freezing of meat.** Most meats may be frozen satisfactorily if properly wrapped, frozen quickly, and kept at 0°F or below. The following guides will help ensure good quality in frozen meats:

a. **Freeze meat while it is fresh and in top condition.** Properly done, freezing will maintain quality, but what comes out of the freezer will be no better than what goes in.

b. **Select proper wrapping material.** Choose a moisture-vapor-proof wrap so that air will be sealed out and moisture locked in. When air penetrates the package, moisture is drawn from the surface of the meat and the condition known as "freezer burn" develops. Several good feezer wraps are on the market.

c. **Prepare meat for freezing before wrapping.** Trim off excess fat and remove bones when practical; wrap in family-sized packages; place double thickness of freezer wrap between chops, patties, or individual pieces of meat, for easier separation during thawing.

d. **Label properly.** This should include the kind and cut of meat enclosed, the number of possible servings (including weight if convenient), and the date of packaging.

e. **Freeze immediately.** Start freezing immediately following wrapping and labeling.

f. **Keep freezer temperature 0°F (−18°C) or lower.** Higher temperatures and fluctuations above that temperature impair quality.

g. **Check freezer Table M-20 for maximum storage times.** Frozen meat will be of best quality if not held longer than indicated.

h. **Avoid refreezing if possible.** Refreezing results in loss of juices when rethawed, thereby affecting juiciness and flavor.

• **Salting**—Dry salting of meats has been practiced since the 5th century B.C., and possibly longer. However, it was not until the latter part of the 18th century that salt curing of meat was done on a scientific basis.

The presence of salt has an effect on osomotic pressure. In addition, the action of chloride on microorganisms is detrimental.

Currently, salt curing is limited to a few specialized products, such as hams and bacon. Although there is no specified salt content for products labeled "salt cured," most cured meats are acceptable at levels of 2.5 to 3% salt.

• **Dry sausages**—Dry sausages are often called summer sausages because of their keeping qualities. They can be held in a fairly cool room for a very long period of time. Dry salami is an example of a dry sausage.

• **Smoking**—This method of preserving meats is very old. The drying and smoking of meats was known to the Egyptians as well as to the ancient Sumerian civilization which preceded them. The advantage to this type of preservation lay in the fact that the smoke overcame objectionable flavors that developed if the drying did not proceed at a rapid rate. The favorite wood smoke in colonial America was produced by hickory or oak, although the Indians also used sage and various aromatic seeds and plants.

Smoking permits formaldehyde and phenolic compounds to accumulate on the surface of the meat. This, along with the surface drying, prevents microbial growth.

• **Spicing**—Many of the essential oils and other substances found in spices are effective bacteriostatic agents *provided* they are used at high levels. Mustard oil and allicin (allythiosulfinic allyl ester) in garlic are examples of effective bacteriostatic substances. Contrary to historical and popular belief, in the concentrations generally employed in flavoring agents, spices cannot be depended upon to have any preservative action. Rather, it appears that they gained early popularity as a means of masking undesirable flavors resulting from microbial spoilage and other causes.

• **Sugar**—A high concentration of sugar exerts a high osmotic pressure and causes water to be withdrawn from microorganisms. However, the sugar concentrations normally employed in meat curing are far short of those needed to contribute to any preservative action. Mincemeat, of which only a minor proportion is meat, is an example of a meat-containing food which is preserved by a combination of sugar, acetic acid, and spices.

MODERN MEAT MERCHANDIZING. Modern meat merchandizing involves the entire meat team—producers, promoters, packers, and retailers. The latter three are consumer oriented; hence, they will be detailed in the discussion that follows. Additionally, and most important, all members of the meat team should be cognizant of what the consumer wants.

Meat Promotion. Effective meat promotion—which should be conceived in a broad sense and embrace research, educational, and sales approaches—necessitates full knowledge of the nutritive qualities of the product. To this end, we need to recognize that (1) meat contains 15 to 20% high-quality protein, on a fresh basis; (2) meat is a rich source of energy, the energy value being dependent largely upon the amount of fat it contains; (3) meat is a rich source of several minerals, but it is especially good as a source of phosphorus and iron; (4) meat is one of the richest sources of the important B group of vitamins, especially thiamin, riboflavin, niacin, and vitamin B-12; and (5) meat is highly digestible, with about 97% of meat proteins and 95% of meat fats being digested. Thus, meat is one of the best foods with which to alleviate human malnutrition, a most important consideration in light of the estimation that 35 to 40% of the U.S. population is now failing to receive an adequate diet.

Also, it is noteworthy that the per capita consumption of red meat in five countries exceeds that of the United States; by rank, based on 1989 meat consumption, these are: (1) East Germany, 202.0 lb (*91.8 kg*); (2) Uruguay, 194.5 lb (*88.4 kg*); (3) Czechoslovakia, 188.8 lb (*85.8 kg*); (4) New Zealand, 176.0 lb (*80.0 kg*); and (5) Australia, 169.8 lb (*77.2 kg*). The United States ranked sixth, with a per capita consumption of 167.8 lb (*76.3 kg*).

Thus, based on (1) its nutritive qualities and (2) per capita consumption in those five countries exceeding us, it would appear that there is a place and a need for increased meat promotion, thereby increasing meat consumption and price.

• **Meat check-off**—Beef, lamb, and pork check-off programs are in operation. Each program is under different sponsorship.

Fabricated; Packaged Meat. With the advent of the refrigerator car, meat was shipped in exposed halves, quarters, or wholesale cuts, and divided into retail cuts in the back rooms of meat markets. But this traditional procedure leaves much to be desired from the standpoints of efficiency, sanitation, shrink, spoilage, and discoloration. To improve this situation, more and more packers are fabricating and packaging (boxing) meat in their plants, thereby freeing the back rooms of 200,000 supermarkets.

Today, modern packing plants are fabricating and packaging (boxing) meat. After chilling, the carcass is subjected to a disassembly process, in which it is fabricated or broken into counter-ready cuts; vacuum-sealed; moved into storage by an automated system; loaded into refrigerated trailers; and shipped to retailers across the nation.

The following benefits accrue from central fabricating, or cutting, of meats:

1.   Twenty-five percent of the weight of the carcass is removed at the packing plant. This results in a reduction in shipping costs because bones and trim do not have to be transported.

2.   Twenty to thirty percent of the carcass is bone and fat, which ends up as waste in the retail store. Where fabricating is done at the packing plant, trimmings, fats, and tallow are federally inspected and can be used as edible products; or they may be used as livestock feeds or for other purposes.

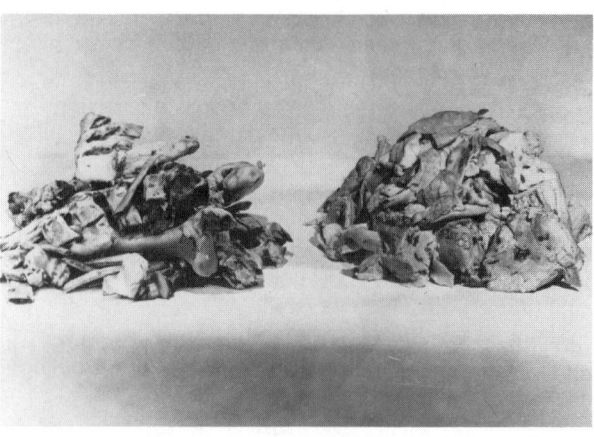

Fig. M-40. When beef is fabricated and boxed in the packing plant, fat and bone are removed from each carcass and remain at the plant. It's no longer necessary to ship unwanted fat and bone across the nation, pay freight charges, and receive only a token amount from the local renderer. (Courtesy, Iowa Beef Processors, Inc., Dakota City, Neb.)

3.   Processing equipment cost at the retail store level is usually high because of low volume and idle time. Hence, counter-ready cuts make for a saving in equipment cost at the retail store.

4.   Central fabricating permits a regulated aging process.

5.   Central fabricating aids in achieving uniformity of quality standards.

6.   Central fabricating improves merchandising through more uniformity of cuts, new cuts, more variety of cuts, matching cuts to area preferences, creating a more tenable situation for retail meat men who lack expertise and interest in cutting, and freeing the meat manager from butchering—thereby permitting him to devote his time to personal selling and customer relations.

Meat Packers and Retailers Court Consumers. There is much competition for the consumer's food dollar, both between and within different food industries. This is particularly true in the meat industry, as evidenced by modern packer technology and modern retailer meat counters and "meat specials"—all designed to attract customers.

Among the factors—some old, with new wrinkles added; others new—considered by packers and retailers in bringing meat to the consumer are the following:

• **Meat inspection stamp**—The primary purpose of Federal Meat Inspection is protection of the consumer by guaranteeing that all meat so inspected and passed is from healthy animals, slaughtered and passed under sanitary conditions; that the meat is entirely suitable for consumption when it leaves the processing establishment; and that no labels carrying misleading statements

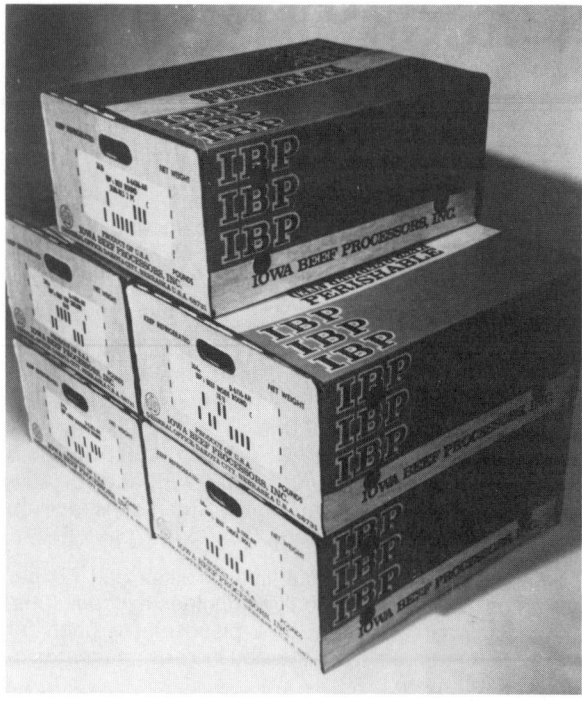

Fig. M-39.   Fabricated and boxed beef. Each cut is trimmed to rigid specifications, placed in a vacuum-sealed protective bag, and boxed for shipment. (Courtesy, Iowa Beef Processors, Inc., Dakota City, Neb.)

appear on it. Meat products which pass federal inspection standards are marked or stamped in abbreviated form, "U.S. Inspected and Passed." This stamp also bears the official number assigned to the establishment. The marking fluid used for this stamp is a vegetable coloring and is harmless; hence, it need not be trimmed from the meat.

(Also see earlier section headed "Federal and State Meat Inspection.")

• **Government grades and retailer and packer brand names**—The grades used on meat and meat products may include (a) the grade names of the U.S. Department of Agriculture, or (b) the brand and grade names of packers and retailers.

Both grade and brand names are applied to meat with a roller stamp which leaves its mark the full length of the carcass, or if cuts are being graded, the full length of the cuts. The vegetable-base marking fluid is similar to that used for the inspection stamp and is harmless.

Although the government meat grading program is administered by the U.S. Department of Agriculture, the cost of this service is born by those meat packers who use it.

Historically, government grade standards change from time to time reflecting changes in the industry.

(Also see earlier sections headed "Federal Grades of Meat" and "Packer Brand Names.")

• **Conformation, quality, and cutability of meat**—These are the primary factors which determine the value and general acceptability of the carcass.

1. **Conformation.** This refers to the general form, shape, or outline of the carcass. Superior conformation is characterized by thick backs with full loins and ribs; deep, plump rounds; thick shoulders; and short necks and shanks. Variations in conformation are related to the ratio of lean to bone.

2. **Quality.** This refers to those traits associated with the palatability of the lean—tenderness, juiciness, and flavor. Quality is evaluated on the basis of the following factors:
    a. **Maturity.** The age of the animal is indicated by (1) the ossification of the cartilages on the ends of the chine bone (the backbone), and (2) the texture and color of the lean. Increasing maturity is associated with decreasing tenderness.
    b. **Marbling.** This refers to flecks of fat within the lean. Marbling enhances palatability by increasing juiciness, flavor, and tenderness.
    c. **Color, firmness, and texture of the lean.** These traits also affect the quality of the meat. Bright colored, firm, fine textured lean is associated with high quality meat and has high consumer acceptability.

3. **Cutability.** This refers to the amount of usable meat in a carcass. High cutability carcasses combine a minimum of fat covering with very thick muscling. The USDA cutability grades are numered 1 to 5, with 1 having the highest cutability. The four factors which determine the cutability grade are:

a. The amount of external fat on the carcass
b. The amount of kidney, pelvic, and heart fat present on the carcass
c. The area of the ribeye muscle at the twelfth rib
d. The hot carcass weight

Although conformation, quality, and cutability are used in judging and grading beef, veal, pork, and lamb carcasses, the relative emphasis on the factors differs to some extent with each kind of meat. For example, veal shows practically no marbling within the lean and has a very thin outside covering of fat. Also, the firmness and distribution of fat varies with species and from grade to grade for each kind of meat. Lamb and mutton produce the hardest fat with the highest melting point, while pork fat is the softest with the lowest melting point.

• **Aging**—Usually, only ribs and loins of high quality beef, lamb, and mutton are aged. To be suitable for aging, meat must have a modest covering of fat to prevent discoloration of the lean and keep evaporation to a minimum. The three most widely used methods of aging are:

1. **Traditional aging.** This refers to holding meat at temperatures of 34 to 38°F (*1° to 3° C*) for 1 to 6 weeks. There is a difference of opinion as to the best cooler humidity; some prefer 70 to 75% so that the exposed surface of meat remains dry, others use humidities of 85 to 90% in order to develop a mold growth on the outside of the meat and reduce evaporation losses.

2. **Fast aging.** This refers to holding the meat at a temperature of about 70°F (*21°C*) for 2 days or less, at 85 to 90% humidity. Ultraviolet lights are used to reduce the microbial population in the aging room.

3. **Vacuum packaging.** This refers to the use of a moisture-vapor-proof film to protect the meat from the time it is fabricated until it reaches the consumer. Such packaging reduces weight loss and surface spoilage for 2 to 3 weeks.

In the normal process of moving fresh meat from packer to retailer to consumer to kitchen range, there is a time lapse of 6 to 10 days. This is long enough for considerable tenderizing to take place in vacuum packages.

(Also see earlier section headed "Meat Tenderizing.")

Qualities in Meat Desired by Consumers.
Consumers desire the following qualities in meats:
1. Palatability
2. Attractiveness; eye appeal
3. Moderate amount of fat
4. Tenderness
5. Small cuts
6. Ease of preparation
7. Repeatability

If these qualities are not met by meats, other products will. Recognition of this fact is important, for competition is keen for space on the shelves of a modern retail food outlet.

MEAT BUYING. Meat buying is important because, (1) meat prices change, (2) one-fourth of the disposable personal income spent on food goes for red meats, and (3) buying food for a family may be a more intricate affair than its prepartion at home. Hence, meat buying merits well informed buyers.

What Determines the Price of Meat?

During those periods when meat is high in price, especially the choicest cuts, there is a tendency on the part of the consumer to blame either or all of the following: (1) the farmer or rancher, (2) the packer, (3) the meat retailer, or (4) the government. Such criticisms, which often have a way of becoming quite vicious, are not justified. Actually, meat prices are determined by the laws of supply and demand; that is, the price of meat is largely dependent upon what the consumers as a group are able and willing to pay for the available supply.

• **The available supply of meat**—Because the vast majority of meats are marketed on a fresh basis rather than cured, and because meat is a perishable product, the supply of this food is dependent upon the number and weight of cattle, sheep, and hogs available for slaughter at a given time. In turn, the number of market animals is largely governed by the relative profitability of livestock enterprises in comparison with other agricultural pursuits. That is to say, farmers and ranchers—like any other good businessmen—generally do those things that are most profitable to them. Thus, a short supply of market animals at any given time usually reflects the unfavorable and unprofitable production factors that existed some months earlier and which caused curtailment of breeding and feeding operations.

Historically, when short meat supplies exist, meat prices rise, and the market price on slaughter animals usually advances, making livestock production profitable. But, unfortunately, livestock breeding and feeding operations cannot be turned on and off like a spigot. For example, a heifer cannot be bred until she is about 1½ years of age; the pregnancy period requires another 9 months; for various reasons only an average of 88 out of 100 cows bred in the United States conceive and give birth to young; and finally, the young are usually grown and fed until at least 1½ years of age before marketing. Thus, under the most favorable conditions, this production process, which is controlled by the laws of nature, requires about 4 years in which to produce a new generation of market cattle.

History also shows that if livestock prices remain high and feed abundant, the producer will step up his breeding and feeding operations as fast as he can within the limitations imposed by nature, only to discover when market time arrives that too many other producers have done likewise. Overproduction, disappointingly low prices, and curtailment in breeding and feeding operations are the result.

Nevertheless, the operations of livestock farmers and ranchers do respond to market prices, producing so-called cycles. Thus, the intervals of high production, or cycles, in cattle occur about every 10 years. In sheep, they occur about every 9 to 10 years; and in hogs—which are litter bearing, breed at an earlier age, have a shorter gestation period, and go to market at an earlier age—they occur every 4 years.

• **The demand for meat**—The demand for meat is primarily determined by buying power and competition from other products. Stated in simple terms, demand is determined by the spending money available and the competitive bidding of millions of housewives who are the chief home purchasers of meats. On a nationwide basis, a high buying power and great demand for meats exist when most people are employed and wages are high.

Also, it is generally recognized that in boom periods—periods of high personal income—meat purchases are affected in three ways: (1) More total meat is desired; (2) there is a greater demand for the choicest cuts; and (3) because of the increased money available and shorter working hours, there is a desire for more leisure time, which in turn increases the demand for those meat cuts that require a minimum of time in preparation (such as steaks, chops, and hamburger). Thus, during periods of high buying power, people not only want more meats, but they compete for the choicer and easier prepared cuts of meats—porterhouse and T-bone steaks, lamb and pork chops, hams, and hamburger (chiefly because of the ease of preparation of the latter).

Because of the operation of the old law of supply and demand, when the choicer and easier prepared cuts of meat are in increased demand, they advance proportionately more in price than the cheaper cuts. This results in a great spread in prices, with some meat cuts very much higher than others. While porterhouse steaks, or pork or lamb chops, may be selling for 4 or 5 times the cost per pound of the live animal, less desirable cuts may be priced at less than the cost per pound of the animal on foot. This is so because a market must be secured for all the cuts. (See Fig. M-41.)

But the novice may wonder why these choice cuts are so scarce, even though people are able and willing to pay a premium for them. The answer is simple. Nature does not make many choice cuts or top grades, regardless of price. Moreover, a hog is born with two hams only, a lamb with two hind legs; and only two loins (a right and a left one) can be obtained from each carcass upon slaughter. In addition, not all weight on foot can be cut into meat. For example, the average steer weighing 1,050 lb (477 kg) on foot will only yield 448.9 lb (204 kg) of retail cuts (the balance consists of hide, internal organs, etc.). Secondly, this 448.9 lb will cut out about 34.8 lb (15.8 kg) of porterhouse, T-bone, and top loin steaks. The balance of the cuts are equally wholesome and nutritious; and, although there are other steaks, many of the cuts are better adapted for use as roasts, stews, and soup

A STEER IS NOT ALL STEAK!

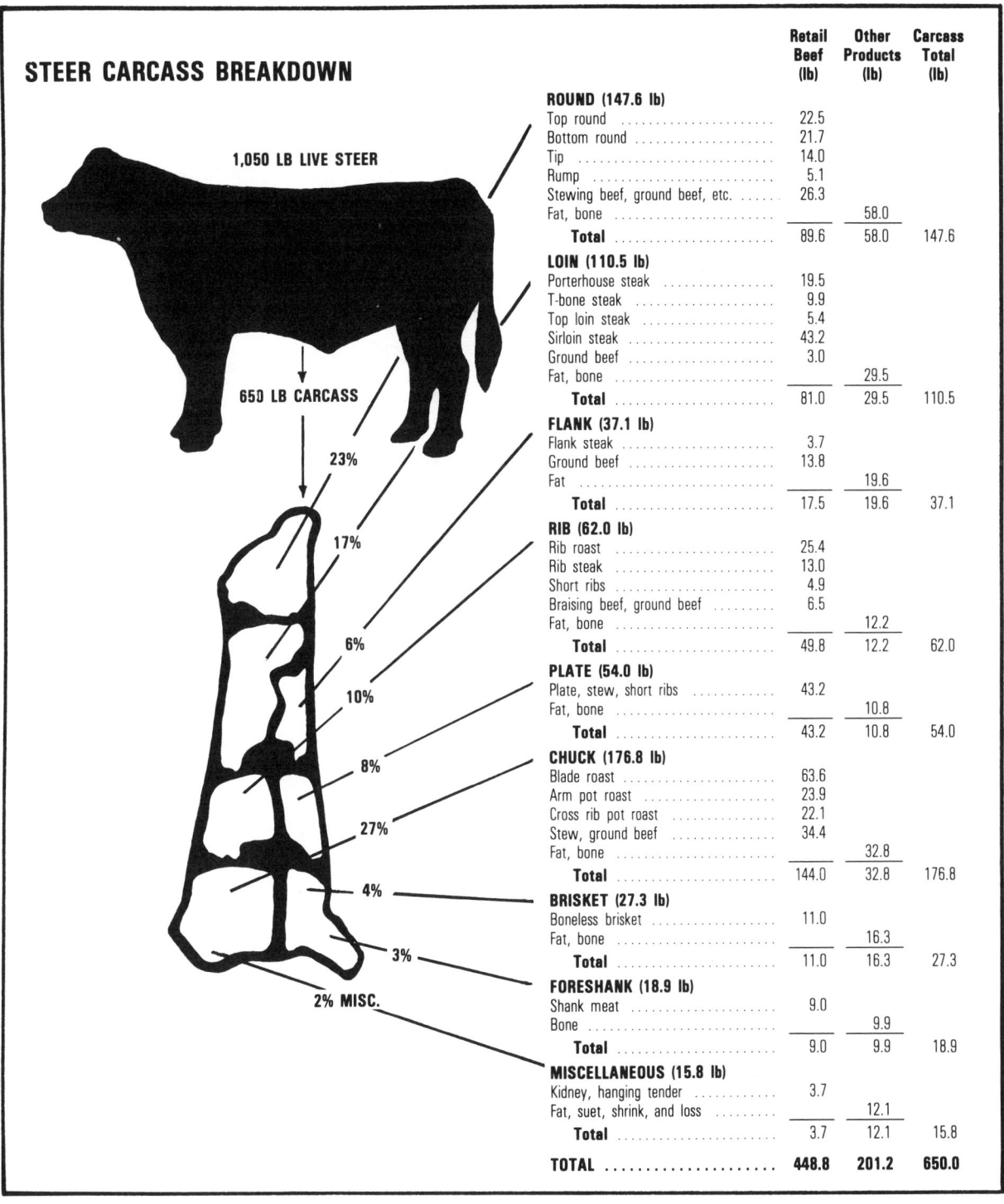

STEER CARCASS BREAKDOWN

1,050 LB LIVE STEER

650 LB CARCASS

23%

17%

6%

10%

8%

27%

4%

3%

2% MISC.

	Retail Beef (lb)	Other Products (lb)	Carcass Total (lb)
ROUND (147.6 lb)			
Top round	22.5		
Bottom round	21.7		
Tip	14.0		
Rump	5.1		
Stewing beef, ground beef, etc.	26.3		
Fat, bone		58.0	
Total	89.6	58.0	147.6
LOIN (110.5 lb)			
Porterhouse steak	19.5		
T-bone steak	9.9		
Top loin steak	5.4		
Sirloin steak	43.2		
Ground beef	3.0		
Fat, bone		29.5	
Total	81.0	29.5	110.5
FLANK (37.1 lb)			
Flank steak	3.7		
Ground beef	13.8		
Fat		19.6	
Total	17.5	19.6	37.1
RIB (62.0 lb)			
Rib roast	25.4		
Rib steak	13.0		
Short ribs	4.9		
Braising beef, ground beef	6.5		
Fat, bone		12.2	
Total	49.8	12.2	62.0
PLATE (54.0 lb)			
Plate, stew, short ribs	43.2		
Fat, bone		10.8	
Total	43.2	10.8	54.0
CHUCK (176.8 lb)			
Blade roast	63.6		
Arm pot roast	23.9		
Cross rib pot roast	22.1		
Stew, ground beef	34.4		
Fat, bone		32.8	
Total	144.0	32.8	176.8
BRISKET (27.3 lb)			
Boneless brisket	11.0		
Fat, bone		16.3	
Total	11.0	16.3	27.3
FORESHANK (18.9 lb)			
Shank meat	9.0		
Bone		9.9	
Total	9.0	9.9	18.9
MISCELLANEOUS (15.8 lb)			
Kidney, hanging tender	3.7		
Fat, suet, shrink, and loss		12.1	
Total	3.7	12.1	15.8
TOTAL	**448.8**	**201.2**	**650.0**

Fig. M-41. Cattle are not all beef, and beef is not all steak! This shows the approximate (a) percentage yield of carcass in relation to the weight of the animal on foot, and (b) the yield of different retail cuts. Note that a 1,050-lb live steer produces approximately a 650-lb carcass, and ends up with only 448.9 lb of retail beef. Note, too, the small amount of steaks. (Source: Adapted by the authors from *Meat Facts*, published by the American Meat Institute, Washington, D.C. Data derived from USDA and industry figures.)

bones. To make bad matters worse, not all cattle are of a quality suitable for the production of steaks. For example, the meat from most worn-out dairy animals and thin cattle of beef breeding is not sold over the block. Also, if the moneyed buyer insists on buying only the top grade of meat—namely, U.S. Prime or its equivalent—it must be remembered that only a small proportion of slaughter cattle produce carcasses of this top grade. To be sure, the lower grades are equally wholesome, but they are simply graded down because the carcass is somewhat deficient in conformation, finish, and/or quality.

Thus, when the national income is exceedingly high, there is a demand for the choicest but limited cuts of meat from the very top but limited grades. This is certain to make for high prices, for the supply of such cuts is limited, but the demand is great. Under these conditions, if prices do not move up to balance the supply with demand, there would be a marked shortage of the desired cuts at the retail counter.

Where the Consumer's Food Dollar Goes. In recognition of the importance of food to the nation's economy and the welfare of its people, it is important to know (1) what percentage of the disposable income is spent for food, and (2) where the consumer's food dollar goes—the proportion of it that goes to the farmer, and the proportion that goes to the middleman.

Table M-21 shows that the farmer's share of the retail price of food has decreased from 37% in 1980 to 30% in 1987. This means that the retailer's share has increased, reflecting increased wages and cost of retailing.

Fig. M-42 reveals that of each food dollar, the farmer's share ranged from 7¢ (for white bread) to 62¢ (for eggs). For choice beef, the farmer's share was 52¢ in 1987, the rest—48¢—went for processing and retailing. This means that about one-half of today's meat dollar goes for meat packing and meat retailing. Note, too, that the farmer's share of meat products has gone down and down, while the processing and retailing share has increased; reflecting increased wages and costs of meat processing and retailing.

The farmer's share of the retail price of eggs, meat products, poultry, and beef is relatively high because processing is relatively simple, and transportation costs are low due to the concentrated nature of the products. On the other hand, the farmer's share of bakery and cereal products is low due to the high processing and container costs, and their bulky nature and costly transportation.

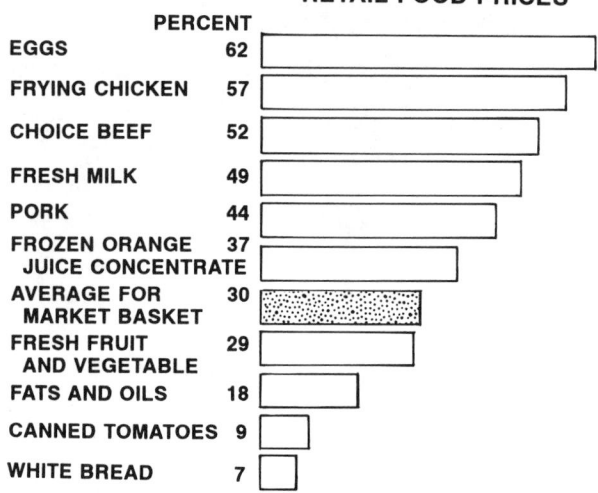

Fig. M-42. Farm share of retail food prices. (From: *1989 Handbook of Agricultural Charts,* Agricultural Handbook No. 684, USDA, p. 61)

Among the reasons why farm prices of foods fail to go up, thereby giving the farmer a greater share of the consumer's food dollar, are (1) rapid technological advances on the farm, making it possible for the farmer to stay in business despite small margins; (2) overproduction; and (3) the relative ease with which cost pressures within the marketing system can be passed backward rather than forward.

Over the years, processing and marketing costs have increased primarily because consumers have demanded, and gotten, more and more processing and packaging—more built-in services. For example, few consumers are interested in buying a live hog—or even a whole carcass. Instead, they want a pound of pork chops—all trimmed, packaged, and ready for cooking. Likewise, few housewives are interested in buying flour and baking bread. But consumers need to be reminded that, fine as these services are, they cost money—hence, they should be expected to pay for them. Without realizing it, American consumers have 1.3 million people working for them in food processing alone. These mysterious persons do not do any work in the kitchen; they're the 1.3 million people who work on the food from the time it leaves the farms and ranches until it reaches the nation's retail markets. They're the people who make it possible for the housewife to choose between quick-frozen, dry-frozen, quick-cooking, ready-to-heat, ready-

TABLE M–21
WHERE THE CONSUMER'S FOOD DOLLAR GOES AS SHOWN BY THE MARKET BASKET[1]

Year	Retail Price	Farm Value	Farm-to-Retail Spread	Farm Value Share of Retail Price
	◄— (Index, 82–84 = 100) —►			(%)
1980	88	97	83	37
1985	104	96	108	32
1987	112	97	119	30

[1]The market basket contains the average quantities of U.S. farm food products purchased annually per household. The farm value is the return to the farmer for the farm product equivalent of foods in the market basket. The spread between the retail cost and farm value represents charges for processing and marketing the product.

Source: *Food Cost Review, 1987,* USDA, ERS, Agricultural Economic Report No. 596, p. 10, Table 5, 1988.

to-eat, and many other conveniences. Hand in hand with this transition, and accentuating the demand for convenience foods, more women work outside the home; the proportion of the nation's labor force made up of women rose from 28% in 1947 to 44% in 1986. All this is fine, but it must be realized that the 1.3 million individuals engaged in processing foods must be paid, for they want to eat, too.

Income—Proportion Spent for Food; Food—Kinds Bought.

U.S. consumers are among the most favored people in the world in terms of food costs and the variety of food products available. In 1988, only 14.5% of the U.S. disposable income was spent for food; 18.8% of this was spent for red meats, with 9.5% of the red meat share spent for beef and 1.8% of it spent for pork (see Fig. M-43).

Food takes about ⅕ of the income in most other developed countries, and ½ or more of the income in most of the developing countries.

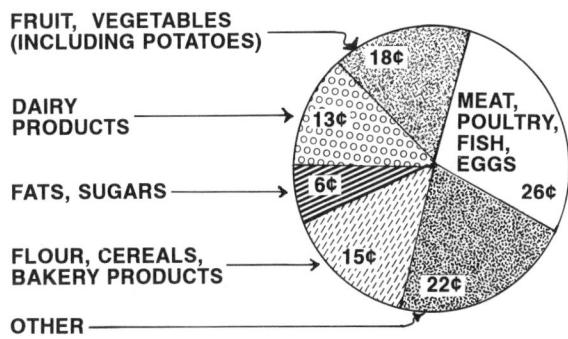

Fig. M-44. How the food dollar is spent. (From *Statistical Abstract of the United States 1991*, p. 448, Table 719)

(Also see INCOME, PROPORTION SPENT FOR FOOD.)

Selecting the Meat Market.

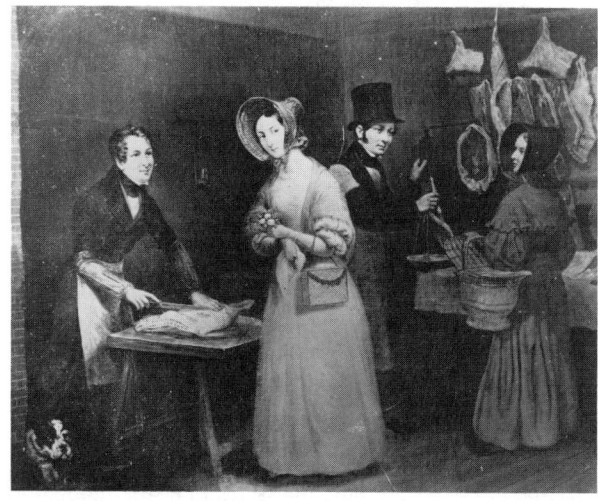

Fig. M-45. The way it used to be done. Early-day butcher shop, from a painting by W. S. Mount. There were neither wholesale cuts nor grades. (Courtesy, The Bettmann Archive)

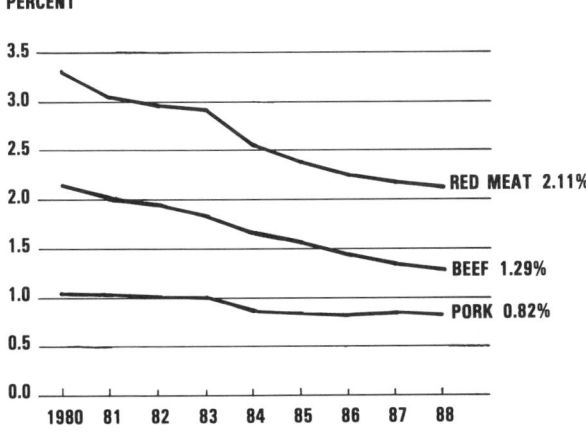

PERCENT OF INCOME SPENT FOR RED MEAT

PERCENT

RED MEAT 2.11%
BEEF 1.29%
PORK 0.82%

1980 81 82 83 84 85 86 87 88

Fig. M-43. Percent of U.S. disposable income spent for red meat and poultry 1980 to 1988. Red meat includes beef and pork only; poultry includes broilers and turkeys only; total meat includes beef, pork, broilers, and turkeys only. Note that the percent of income spent for red meat has declined, while percent of income spent for poultry meat has remained about the same. Since poultry meat consumption had increased markedly during this period, this indicates that poultry prices have decreased. (Source: USDA)

A further breakdown of how the food dollar is spent is given in Fig. M-44.

Today's family may need help in meat buying. Meat is available in many places, in both supermarkets and meat specialty stores. Also, there is a selection from different species; and meat comes in many forms—fresh, cured, cured and smoked, frozen, freeze-dried, canned, and ready-to-serve. Then, there is the matter of deciding on which of the popular cuts to buy and serve on different occasions. All this leads most consumers to shop around until they find a retailer who provides the quality of meat and customer services desired, then remain loyal to that food store.

Selecting the Cut of Meat.

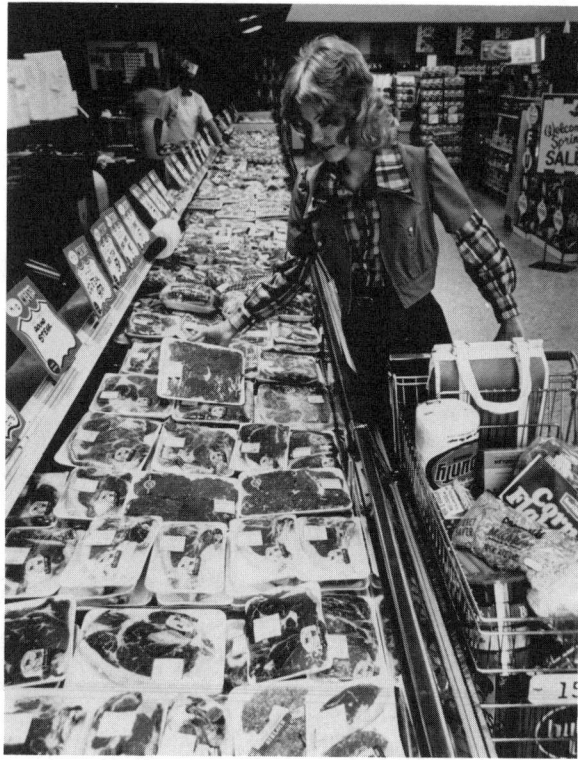

Fig. M-46. A modern meat market. (Courtesy, Iowa Beef Processors, Inc., Dakota City, Nebr.)

The open refrigerated cases in a modern supermarket or meat specialty store present a sea of appetizing meats and meat products. Generally, meats are displayed wrapped in polyvinyl chloride (PVC) film that is sealed, on an affixed label of which is stamped the net weight, total price, price per pound, and the name of the cut.

The arrangement for displaying meats is rather standard. They are segregated as to kind (beef, veal, pork, lamb, poultry) and type of cut (steak, roast, ground beef, etc.). Smoked meats have separate display space as do fish, liver and other specialty items. Usually a clerk behind the display cases adds a personal touch and furnishes a source of information.

As the consumer pushes the cart along the refrigerated cases, selection is based primarily on preference, satiety, and nutritional value, along with the following practical considerations:

1.   The kind of meat that is best for the use planned.

Skill in identifying cuts of meat and in cooking each of them properly is imperative.

2.   The best buy on the basis of cost per serving. Except for such items as chopped meat and stew, the price per pound includes bone and fat, which are not eaten. Sometimes cuts like spareribs seem relatively inexpensive, but the amount of edible meat is small.

(Also see BEEF AND VEAL, section headed "Beef Cuts and How to Cook Them"; PORK, section headed "Pork Cuts and How to Cook Them"; and LAMB AND MUTTON, section headed "Lamb Cuts and How to Cook Them.")

Watching for Specials. Most meat retailers feature a good many meat specials. Experienced homemakers watch for these announcements and take advantage of them. When a home freezer is available, it may be possible to effect additional savings by buying extra large amounts of meat during special sales, then storing them.

Deciding How Much to Buy. Each meat shopper needs to be able to estimate how much meat, fish, or poultry to buy. Consideration should be given to the appetites and preferences of the members of the family. For example, active men and teen-agers generally have hearty appetites, and one child may like pork chops while another prefers hamburgers.

Besides allowing for individual preference, this type of planning is beneficial because it helps to eliminate problems with leftovers which may go to waste.

Two to three ounces of cooked lean meat is considered by nutritionists to be one standard size serving, but most American families serve portions larger than 3 oz since meat is one of the most popular foods.

Depending on the kind of cut, a pound of meat will provide the following number of 3-oz servings:

Bony meat	1 to 2 servings per pound
Moderate bone .	2 to 3 servings per pound
Little bone	3 to 4 servings per pound
No bone	4 to 5 servings per pound

Other factors that should be considered in determining how much meat to buy are:

1.   **Time available for preparation.** This often determines whether to select one of the larger cuts suitable for roasting, braising, or cooking in liquid, or to select smaller cuts.

2.   **It may be practical to buy a particular cut for more than one meal.** Sometimes it may be best to buy and cook a larger cut of meat, and to serve it either the same way or in different ways for more than one meal. At other times, it may be advantageous to buy a large cut of meat and ask the retailer to divide it into smaller cuts. For example, a pot-roast might be cut into two portions; one portion for a one-meal pot-roast or Swiss steak, and the second for stew.

3.   **Storage facilities.** Available storage facilities have a bearing on the amount of meat to purchase. Where a freezer is available, larger quantities of fresh meats may be stored. Pantry or other storage space help to determine the quantity of canned meats that may be kept on hand.

MEAT COOKING[26]—Every grade and cut of meat can be made tender and palatable provided it is cooked by the proper method. Also, it is important that meat be cooked at low temperature, usually between 300° and 350°F (*149 and 177°C*). At this temperature, it cooks slowly; and, as a result, it is juicier, shrinks less, and is better flavored than when cooked at high temperatures.

The method used in meat cookery depends on the nature of the cut to which it is applied. A summary of each type of meat cookery follows.

• **Roasting**—Roasting is dry-heat cooking. It is recommended for preparing large tender cuts of beef, veal, pork, and lamb. The following steps should be followed for best results:

1. Season with salt and pepper, if desired.

2. Place meat, fat side up, on rack in open shallow roasting pan.

3. Insert a meat thermometer so that the bulb is in the center of the largest muscle.

4. Do not add water or cover.

5. Roast in a slow oven—300° to 350°F (*149 to 177°C*).

6. Roast to the desired degree of doneness.

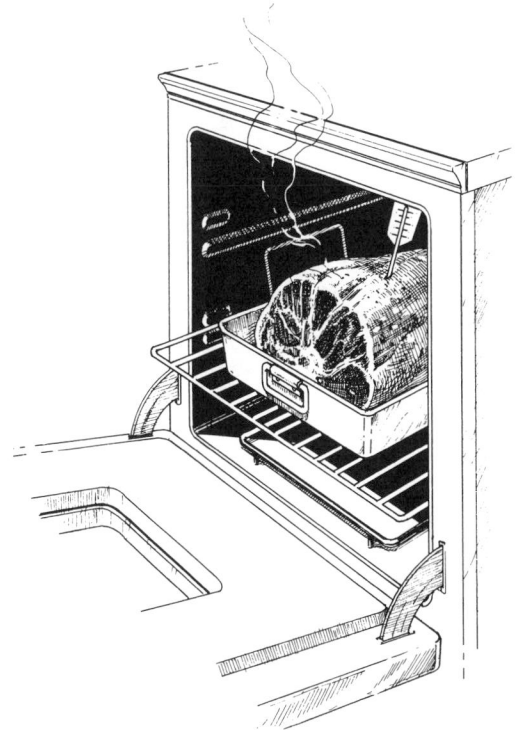

Fig. M-47. Roasting, suitable for large tender cuts of beef, veal, pork, and lamb.

---

[26]In the preparation of this section the authors adapted materials from *Lessons on Meat,* published by the National Live Stock and Meat Board, 4444 N. Michigan Avenue, Chicago, Ill.; with the permission of Mr. John L. Huston, President.

• **Broiling**—Broiling is dry-heat cooking. It is used to prepare the more tender cuts—those that contain little connective tissue; it is suitable for beef steaks, lamb chops, pork chops, sliced ham, bacon, and ground beef or lamb. Steaks and chops should be at least ¾ in. (*19 mm*) thick, and ham should be at least ½ in. (*13 mm*) thick. For best results, the following steps should be followed:

1. Set the oven regulator for broiling.

2. Place the meat on the rack of the broiler pan, 2 to 5 in. (*5 to 13 cm*) from the heat.

3. Broil until top side is brown. (Lightly browned for cured and smoked pork.)

4. Season the top side with salt and pepper, if desired.

5. Turn and brown the other side.

6. Season if desired, and serve at once.

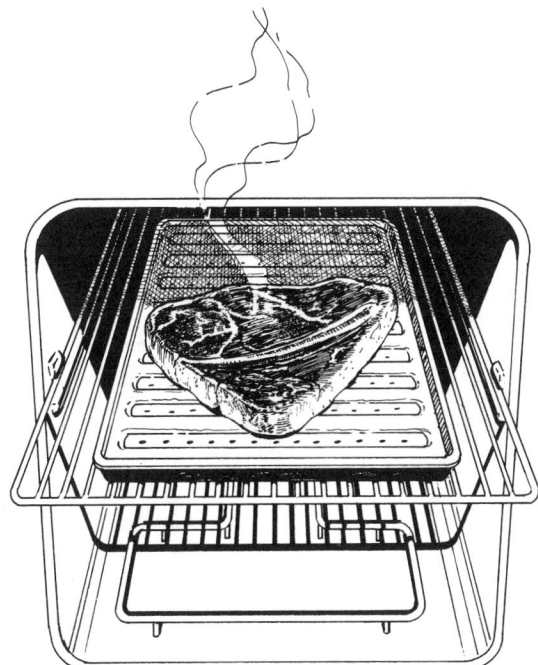

Fig. M-48. Broiling, suitable for tender beef steaks, lamb chops, pork chops, sliced ham, bacon, and ground beef or lamb.

• **Panbroiling**—Panbroiling is dry-heat cooking. It is suitable for tender cuts when cut to a thickness of 1 in. (*2.5 cm.*) or less. It is also a convenient method for a small steak or a few chops. For best results, these steps should be followed:

1. Place meat in a heavy frying pan or a griddle.

2. Do not add fat or water.

3. Cook slowly, turning occasionally.

4. Pour off or remove fat as it accumulates.

5.   Brown meat on both sides.

6.   Do not overcook. Season if desired, and serve at once.

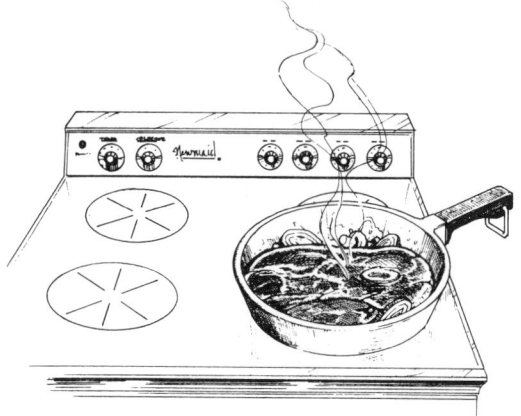

Fig. M-49.   Panbroiling, suitable for tender cuts when cut 1 in., or less, thick.

• **Panfrying**—When a small amount of fat is added before cooking, or allowed to accumulate during cooking, the method is called panfrying. This is suitable for preparing comparatively thin pieces of tender meat, or those pieces made tender by pounding, scoring, cubing, or grinding, or for preparing leftover meat. Follow these steps for panfrying:

1.   Brown meat on both sides in a small amount of fat.
2.   Season with salt and pepper, if desired.
3.   Do not cover the meat.
4.   Cook at moderate temperature, turning occasionally, until done.
5.   Remove from pan and serve at once.

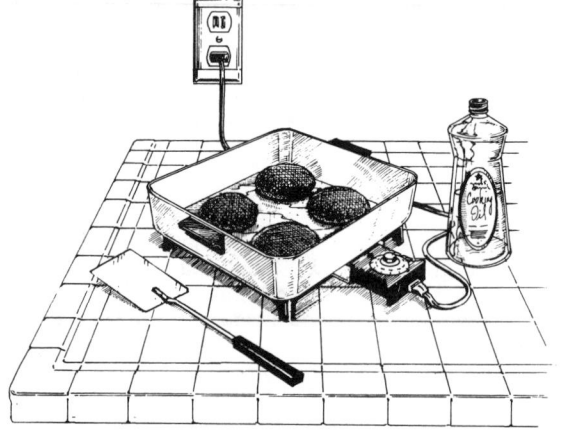

Fig. M-50.   Panfrying, suitable for comparatively thin pieces of tender meat.

• **Deep-fat frying**—When meat is cooked immersed in fat, it is called deep-fat frying. This method of cooking is sometimes used for preparing brains, sweetbreads, liver, croquettes, and leftover meat. Usually the meat is coated with eggs and crumbs or a batter, or dredged with flour or cornmeal. For best results, follow these steps:

1.   Use a deep kettle and a wire frying basket.

2.   Heat fat to frying temperature.

3.   Place meat in frying basket.

4.   Brown meat and cook it through.

5.   When done, drain fat from meat into kettle and remove meat from basket.

6.   Strain fat through cloth; then cool.

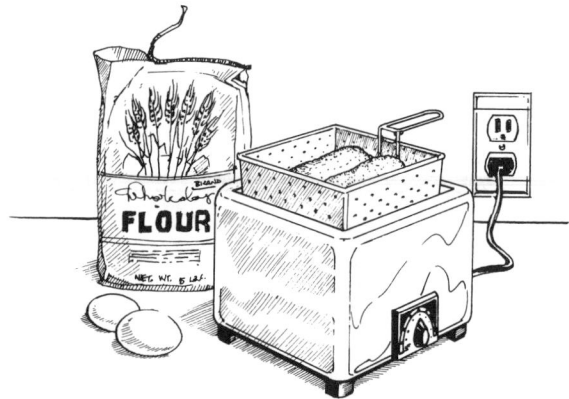

Fig. M-51.   Deep-fat frying, suitable for cooking brains, sweetbreads, liver, croquettes, and leftover meat.

• **Braising**—Braising is suitable for less tender cuts of meat, although some tender cuts are usually best if braised, including pork steaks and cutlets; veal chops, steaks and cutlets; and pork liver. For best results in braising, follow these steps:

1.   Brown meat slowly on all sides in heavy utensil.

2.   Season with salt, pepper, herbs and spices, if desired.

3.   Add a small amount of liquid, if necessary.

4.   Cover tightly.

5. Cook at low temperature until tender.

6. Make sauce or gravy from the liquid in the pan, if desired.

6. Add vegetable to the meat just long enough before serving to be cooked.

7. When done, remove meat and vegetable to a pan, platter or casserole and keep hot.

8. If desired, thicken the cooking liquid with flour for gravy.

9. Serve the hot gravy (or thickened liquid) over the meat and vegetable or serve separately in a sauce boat.

10. Meat pies may be made from the stew; a meat pie is merely a stew with a top on it. (The top may be made of pastry, biscuits or biscuit dough, mashed potatoes, or cereal.)

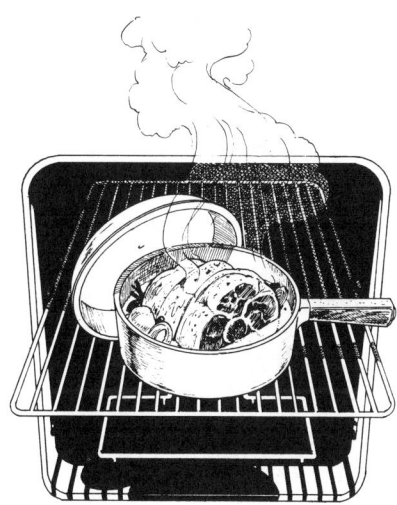

Fig. M-52. Braising, suitable for less tender cuts of meat.

• **Cooking in liquid**—Large less tender cuts and stews are prepared by cooking in liquid, although, for variety, a few of the tender cuts may also be cooked in liquid. This method is usually used when making meat soups. Follow these cookery steps.

Large cuts:
1. Brown meat on all sides, if desired.
2. Cover the meat with water or stock.
3. Season with salt, pepper, herbs, spices and vegetables, if desired. (Cured or smoked meat and corned beef do not require salt.)
4. Cover kettle and simmer (do not boil) until tender.
5. If the meat is to be served cold, let it cool and then chill in the stock in which it was cooked.
6. When vegetables are to be cooked with the meat, as in "boiled" dinners, add them whole or in pieces, just long enough to cook them before the meat is tender.

Stews:
1. Cut meat in uniform pieces, usually 1- to 2-in. (2.5 to 5.1 cm) cubes.
2. If a brown stew is desired, brown meat cubes on all sides.
3. Add just enough water, vegetable juices or other liquid to cover the meat.
4. Season with salt, pepper, herbs and spices, if desired.
5. Cover kettle and simmer (do not boil) until meat is tender.

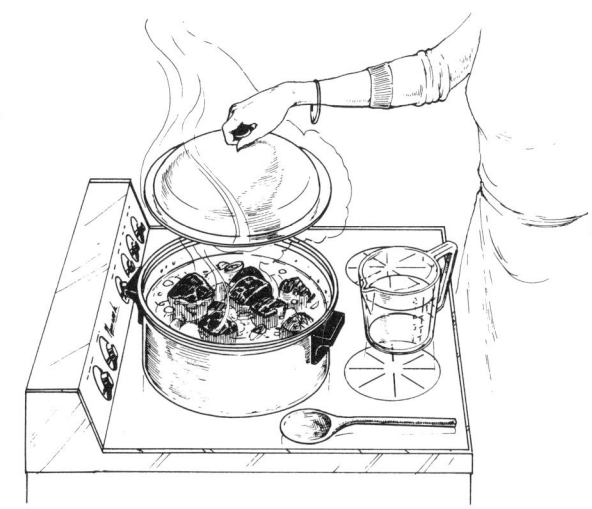

Fig. M-53. Cooking in liquid, suitable for large less tender cuts and stews.

• **Cooking variety meats**—Variety meats include liver, brains, heart, kidneys, sweetbreads, tongue, tripe, and others. Like the other retail cuts, there is a pronounced similarity among the variety meats from beef, veal, pork, and lamb; with the size of the variety meat consistent with the size of the animal from which it came, in most cases. The recommended methods of cookery for the more common variety meats follow:

Liver: The membrane should be peeled or trimmed from liver before cooking. Beef and pork liver are frequently braised or fried and are sometimes ground for loaves and patties. Veal, lamb and baby beef liver are usually broiled, panbroiled, or panfried.

Brains: Brains are soft in consistency, very tender, and have a delicate flavor. They should be washed before cooking, and the membrane should be removed before or after cooking. If they are not to be used immediately after purchase, they should be precooked. Brains may be broiled, fried, braised, or cooked in liquid.

Heart: This is a less tender variety meat. Therefore, braising and cooking in liquid are the preferred cookery methods.

Kidneys: Veal and lamb kidneys are often attached to chops (as veal chops and English lamb chops), although both varieties are sold separately. Before cooking, remove membrane and hard parts. If desired, kidneys may be sliced or cut in pieces. Lamb kidneys are usually split or left whole. Beef kidney is less tender than other kidneys and should be cooked in liquid or braised.

Sweetbreads (thymus glands): Veal and young beef furnish nearly all of the sweetbreads on the market; as the animals mature, the thymus gland disappears. Sweetbreads may be broiled, fried, braised, or cooked in liquid.

The same procedure for precooking and preparation recommended for brains should be followed in preparing sweetbreads.

Tongue: Tongue may be purchased fresh, pickled, corned, smoked, or canned. Tongue is a less tender cut; hence, it needs long, slow cooking in liquid. After cooking, the skin is removed and the tongue may be (1) molded and weighted, then cut crosswise and served cold, or (2) reheated (whole or sliced), in a spicy sauce.

Tripe: Tripe may be purchased fresh, partially cooked, fully cooked, pickled, or canned. It is a less tender cut; hence, it requires long, slow cooking in liquid. Tripe is precooked in salted water; 1 tsp salt for each quart of water.

• **Cooking sausage—**

Fresh sausage or uncooked smoked sausage: This type of sausage may be cooked by one of the following methods:

1. **Panfried.** Place links or patties in cold frying-pan; add 2 to 4 tsp (*10 to 20 ml*) water; cover tightly and cook slowly 5 to 8 minutes—depending on size and thickness; remove cover and brown slowly; cook until well done.

2. **Cooked in oven.** Arrange sausage in single layer in shallow baking pan; bake in a hot oven (400°F, or *204°C*) 20 to 30 minutes, or until well done; turn to brown evenly; pour off drippings as they accumulate.

Frankfurters or other cooked smoked sausage links: This type of sausage does not require cooking, but may be heated by one of the following methods:

1. **Simmered.** Drop frankfurters or sausage into boiling water; cover and let water simmer (not boil) until heated through, about 5 to 10 minutes, depending on size.

2. **Panbroiled (or griddle-broiled).** Melt a small amount of fat (1 to 2 Tbsp, or *15 to 30 ml*) in a heavy frying pan or on a griddle and brown meat by turning slowly with tongs. Do not pierce with fork.

3. **Broiled.** Brush each frankfurter or sausage with butter, margarine or other fat, if desired; broil about 3 in. (*8 cm*) from the heat; turn to brown evenly, using tongs.

• **Cooking frozen meat—**Frozen meat may be cooked satisfactorily by defrosting prior to cooking or during cooking. Commercially frozen products should be prepared according to package directions.

The following pointers are pertinent to cooking frozen meat:

1. **When defrosting meat before cooking.** The most desirable method of defrosting is in the refrigerator, and in the original wrapping. Defrosting in water is recommended only if the meat is to be cooked in liquid; e.g.,

meat stews. Following defrosting, the meat should be cooked in the same way as other fresh meat. See Table M-22 for timetable for defrosting frozen meat in the refrigerator.

TABLE M-22
TIMETABLE FOR DEFROSTING FROZEN MEAT[1]

Cut of Meat	In Refrigerator (36° to 40°F)
Large roast	4 to 7 hr per lb
Small roast	3 to 5 hr per lb
1-in. steak	12 to 14 hr

[1]To convert to metric, see WEIGHTS AND MEASURES.

2. **When cooking meat from the frozen state.** This requires additional time; frozen roasts require approximately a third to a half again as long for cooking as roasts which have been defrosted. The additional time for cooking steaks and chops varies according to the surface area and the thickness of the meat, as well as the broiling temperature used when broiling meats.

3. **When broiling thick frozen steaks, chops, and ground meat patties.** These must be farther from the heat than defrosted ones in order that the meat will be cooked to the degree of doneness without becoming too brown on the outside.

4. **When panbroiling frozen steaks and chops.** A hot frying pan should be used so that the meat browns before defrosting on the surface. The heat should be reduced after browning and the meat turned occasionally so it will cook through without becoming too brown.

• **Cooking meat outdoors—**In recent years, cooking outdoors has become increasingly popular.

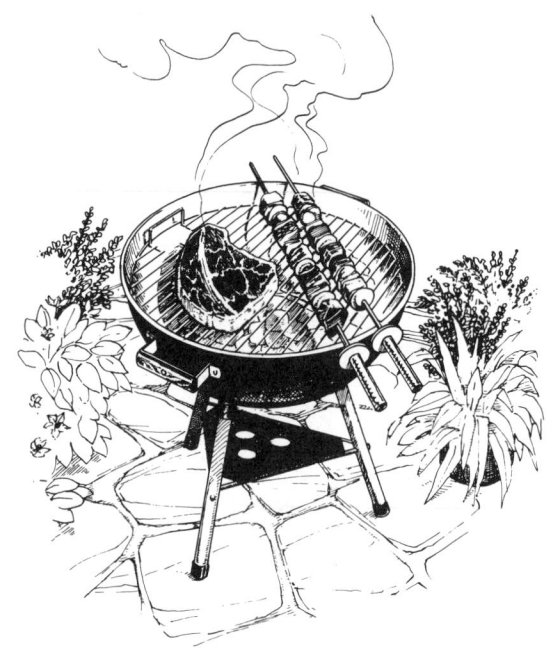

Fig. M-54. Cooking meat over the coals is popular.

Selecting the cut: Practically any cut of meat that is suitable for broiling, panbroiling (or griddle-broiling), panfrying, or roasting may be successfully cooked over the coals if the appropriate equipment is on hand and the recommended procedure is followed. The following factors will help determine the type of cut to choose:

1.   **The equipment.**   A shielded or covered rotisserie is needed for cooking roasts. All cuts normally roasted may be cooked outdoors.

For cooking on the grill, good choices are tender steaks, chops, meat patties, pork or lamb ribs, sliced, cured and smoked meat, frankfurters or other types of sausage; for the skewer or rotisserie basket, selected tender cubes.

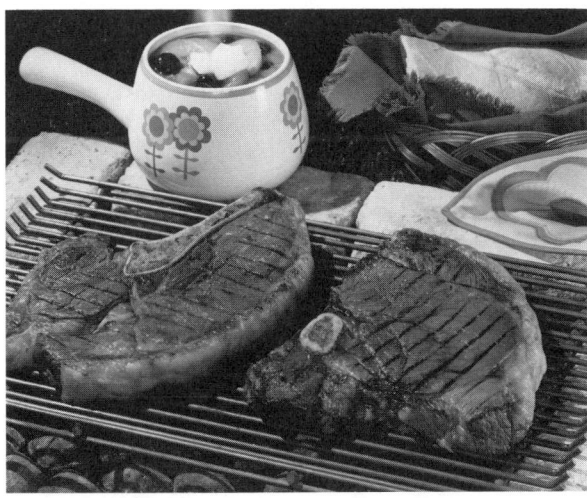

Fig. M-55.   Cooking beef sirloin steaks on the grill. (Courtesy, National Live Stock and Meat Board, Chicago, Ill.)

2.   **The number to be served.**   Generous servings of meat should be planned for the outdoor menu. For bone-in cuts, ¾ to 1 lb *(0.34 to 0.45 kg)* should be allowed. For boneless cuts, ⅓ to ¾ lb *(0.15 to 0.34 kg)* should be planned, depending on the type of meat.

3.   **The time available for preparation.**   Allow 3½ to 5 hr for a large boneless rib roast; 1 to 1½ hr for spareribs; 8 to 10 minutes for frankfurters; and 15 to 20 minutes per side for a 2-in. *(5 cm)* steak cooked medium rare.

Starting the fire and arranging the charcoal: Successful outdoor cooking requires great skill in starting the fire and arranging the charcoal. Instruction in these arts can best be learned by observing and working with a person who has expertise in outdoor cookery, rather than by reading a set of instructions.

Cooking reminders:

1.   Low to moderate temperatures for cooking meat apply when cooking on a rotisserie or grill just as when roasting or broiling in the kitchen range.

2.   The cooking time required will depend on the kind, size and shape of the meat cut; the temperature of the meat when cooking begins; the equipment used; the heat maintained during cooking; and the degree of doneness desired.

3.   A meat thermometer is the most accurate guide to the doneness of roasts.

4.   Basting of meat may be done, if desired, during the entire cooking time or during the last half hour, depending upon the basting ingredients.

Tips for the rotisserie: For even cooking and easy turning of the rotisserie rod, these tips should be observed:

1.   **For roasts.**   Insert rod lengthwise through center of roast, then fasten meat securely so that it turns only with the rod.

2.   **For ribs.**   Weave rod in and out of ribs forming accordianlike folds. Tighten screws with pliers.

3.   **Kabobs.**   This is meat, or meat and vegetables, or meat and fruit pieces alternated on a skewer and cooked on the grill.

• **Microwave cooking**—In electronic or microwave cooking, food is cooked by the heat generated in the food itself.

The primary advantage of microwave cooking is speed.

There are still some problems with microwave cooking, especially with regard to the cookery of basic meat cuts. For example, electronically cooked roasts have a higher shrinkage; microwaves frequently do not penetrate a roast uniformly, with the result that there may be variations in doneness of meat; the amount of food electronically cooked greatly affects cooking time; and foods cooked solely by microwave do not brown.

Although emphasizing that there had been no reported cases of illness resulting from pork cooked in a microwave oven, in 1981 the USDA issued a warning that pork cooked in a microwave oven should be at a temperature of 170°F *(77°C)* "*throughout* to destroy any microorganisms that might be present." This caution was taken because preliminary unpublished studies brought to the department's attention indicated that, "under certain circumstances, trichinal and food poisoning bacteria may not be destroyed by microwave cooking."
(Also see TRICHINOSIS.)

MEAT CARVING.

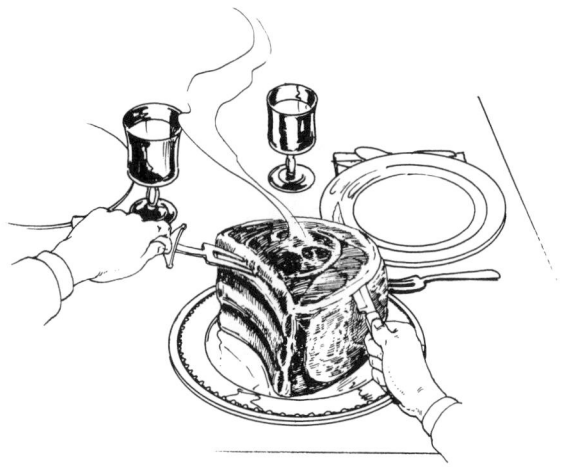

Fig. M-56.   Carving a "standing rib roast." The roast is placed on the platter with the small cut surface up and the rib side to your left. With the guard up, insert the fork firmly between the two top ribs. From the fat outside edge, slice across the grain toward the ribs. Make the slices an eighths to three-eighths of an inch thick.

Carving is the art of cutting up meat, poultry, or game to serve at the table. In royal households, the *ecuyer tranchant* was usually a nobleman who always carried out his duties with his sword at his side. The art of skillful carving was considered essential by our forefathers and was taught to well-born young men as an indispensable part of good education.

Carving should be a proud accomplishment rather than drudgery. To master carving for the best presentation and maximum yield, the following simple rules should be observed:

1.   **Have proper tools.**   Most carving needs can be met with a standard carving set and a steak set.

The standard carving set consists of a knife, fork, and steel. The knife has an 8- to 9-in. *(20 to 23 cm)* blade. There is a guard on the fork for protecting the hand when cutting toward the fork. With this set, all-around carving of roasts and fowl can be done.

The steak set consists of a knife with a 6- or 7-in. *(15 or 18 cm)* blade and matching fork which may or may not have a guard. This set is used to carve all steaks and is a convenient size for small roasts and small fowl.

2.   **Use sharp knife.**   Always use a sharp carving knife (and never sharpen it at the table).

3.   **Stand up if you prefer.**   It is perfectly proper for the carver to stand if he prefers to do so. (Standing may make carving easier for those with oversize waistlines.)

4.   **Know bone structure.**   The carver should know something about anatomy; otherwise, the bones will get in his way.

5.   **Know direction of muscle fiber and cut across the grain.**   Except for steaks, meat should always be cut across the grain to avoid long meat fibers giving a stringy texture to the slices.

6.   **Have a plan.**   Start with a plan, cut with a plan, and make neat slices.

7.   **Have ample platter or carving board.**   The carving platter or board should be of ample size; large enough to accommodate slices. (It is embarrasing to serve cuts from the tablecloth or the lap.)

8.   **Have elbow room.**   The carver must have plenty of elbow room.

9.   **Use fork to hold cut.**   The fork should be used for its intended purpose—to hold the cut; and not to dull the knife.

10.   **Cut large and even slices.**   The slices should be as large and even as possible.

11.   **Be at ease.**   The carver should always appear at ease. If the carver is nervous, the guests will be nervous, too.

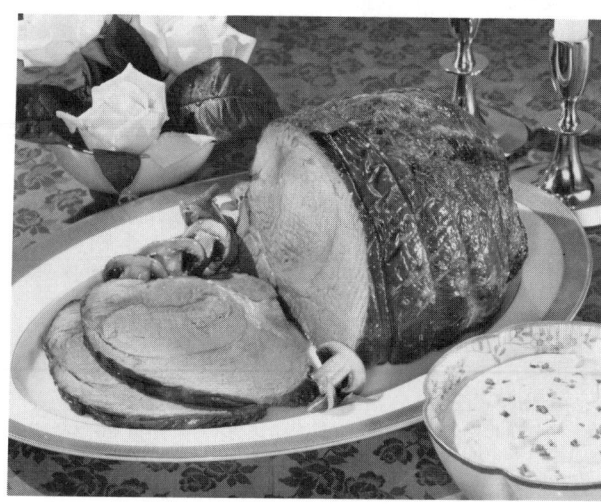

Fig. M-57.   Properly carved roast of beef. (Courtesy, National Live Stock & Meat Board, Chicago, Ill.

U.S. MEAT PRODUCTION.

U.S. MEAT PRODUCTION.   U.S. production of red meat (total and by kinds) is shown in Table M-23. This reveals that (1) beef accounts for approximately 60% of all U.S. meat production, and (2) veal and lamb-mutton production account for a very small proportion of the total red meat production.

TABLE M–23
U.S. PRODUCTION OF MEAT[1]

Year	All Meats (excluding lard)		Beef		U.S. Meat Prod.	Veal		U.S. Meat Prod.	Lamb and Mutton		U.S. Meat Prod.	Pork (excluding lard)		U.S. Meat Prod.
	(million)													
	(lb)	(kg)	(lb)	(kg)	(%)	(lb)	(kg)	(%)	(lb)	(kg)	(%)	(lb)	(kg)	(%)
1970	36,220	16,429	21,652	9,821	60	588	267	1.6	551	250	1.5	13,429	6,091	37
1975	36,760	16,674	23,974	10,874	65	873	396	2.4	410	186	1.1	11,503	5,218	31
1980	38,977	17,717	21,644	9,838	56	400	182	1.0	318	145	0.8	16,615	7,552	43
1985	39,404	17,910	23,728	10,785	60	514	234	1.0	357	162	0.9	14,805	6,730	38
1990	38,785	17,630	22,743	10,338	59	327	149	0.8	362	165	0.9	15,353	6,979	40

[1]From *Agricultural Statistics* 1980, p. 344; and 1991, p. 287.

U.S. PER CAPITA MEAT CONSUMPTION.
Although comprising only 5.0% of the world's population, the people of the United States consume 10.5% of the total world production of meat. The amount of meat consumed in this country varies from year to year (see Fig. M-58). In 1990, the average per capita red meat consumption was 163.2 lb, with distribution by types of meat as shown in Table M-24.

TABLE M–24
U.S. PER CAPITA CONSUMPTION OF MEAT, BY KINDS, 1990[1]

Type of Meat	Annual per Capita Consumption (carcass weight basis)	
	(lb)	(kg)
Beef	96.1	43.7
Veal	1.3	0.6
Lamb and mutton . .	1.7	0.8
Pork	64.1	29.1
Total meat	163.2	74.2

[1]Carcass weight equivalent or dressed weight. (From: USDA)

For the most part, meat consumption in this country is on a domestic basis, with only limited amounts being either imported or exported. Although cured meats furnish somewhat of a reserve supply—with more meats going into cure during times of meat surpluses—meat consumption generally is up when livestock production is high. Also, when good crops are produced and feed prices are favorable, market animals are fed to heavier weights. On the other hand, when feed-livestock ratios are unfavorable, breeding operations are curtailed, and animals are marketed at lighter weights. But during the latter periods, numbers are liquidated, thus tending to keep the meat supply fairly stable.

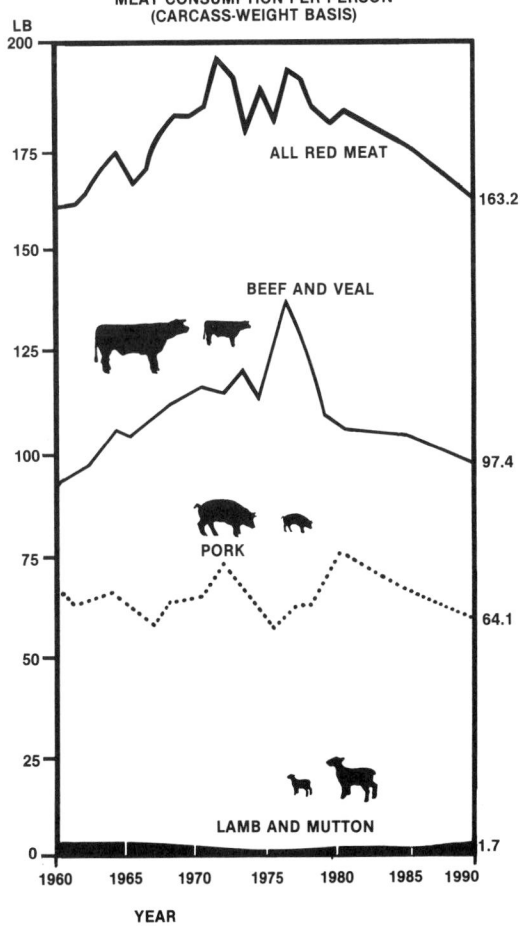

Fig. M-58. Per capita meat consumption in the United States, by kind of meat. As noted, the amount of meat consumed in this country varies from year to year. In recent years, the average American has consumed more beef than any other kind of meat. (Based on USDA figures)

EATING HABIT TRENDS. Figs. M-59 thru M-63 clearly point up the following U.S. trends in eating habits in per capita consumption of meat and other foods by groups:

• The consumption of crop products is increasing, while the consumption of animal products is decreasing.

• Consumption of poultry and fish is on the increase; consumption of eggs continues to decrease; consumption of meat and dairy products has leveled off.

• Consumption of fruits stays about the same, vegetables show a slight increase, and cereal products continue to rise.

• Total consumption of sugars and sweeteners is rising again after a flat period during the 1970s. The consumption of sugar has dropped because it has been replaced by corn sweeteners, which are used primarily in soft drinks.

• Consumption of coffee, tea, and cocoa has declined rather sharply.

• Consumption of vegetable oils has increased, while consumption of animal fats has fallen.

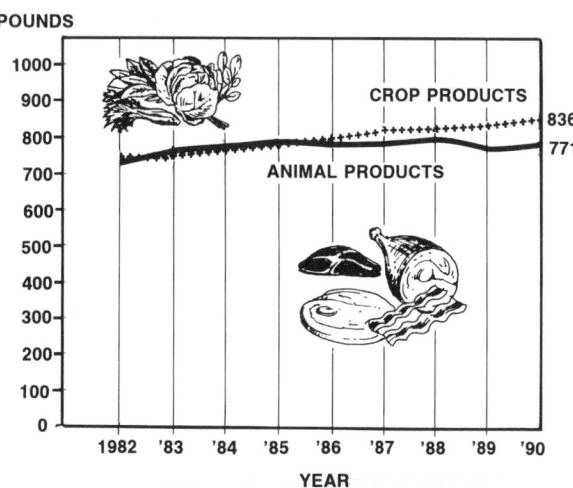

Fig. M-59. Per capita consumption of animal products vs crop products. (*Agricultural Statistics*, 1991, USDA, p. 479, Table 672)

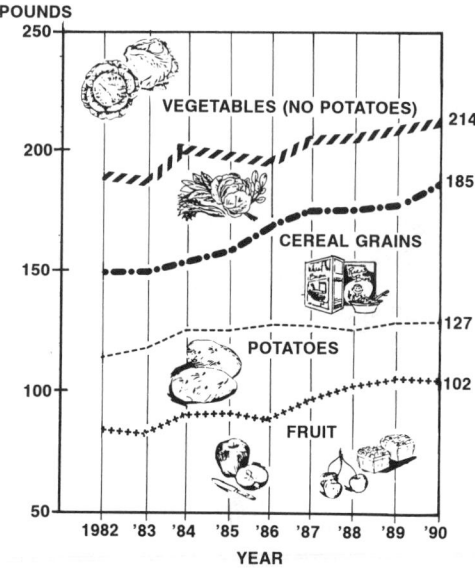

Fig. M-61. Per capita consumption of cereal grains, fruits, vegetables, and potatoes. (*Agricultural Statistics*, 1991, USDA, p. 479, Table 672)

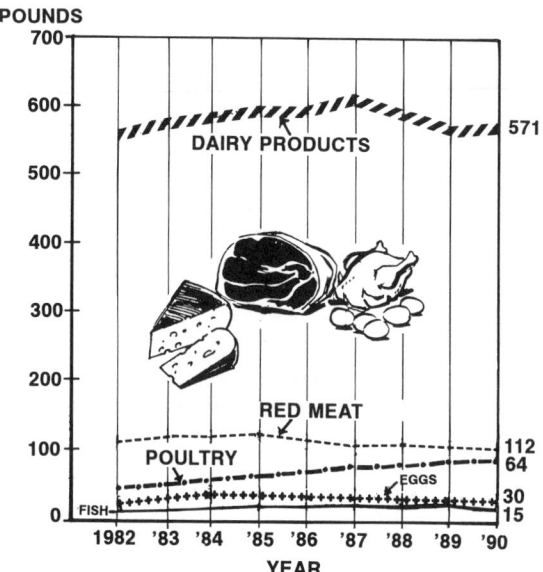

Fig. M-60. Per capita consumption of red meat, fish, poultry, eggs, and dairy products. (*Agricultural Statistics*, 1991, USDA, p. 479, Table 672)

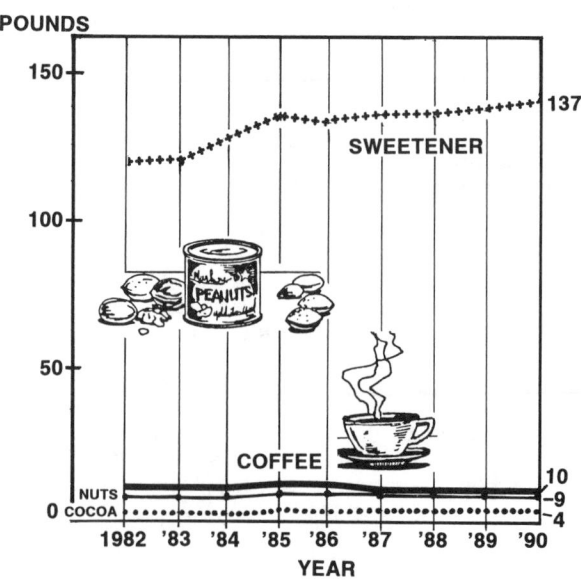

Fig. M-62. Per capita consumption of sweeteners (sugar, corn, and honey), coffee, cocoa, and nuts. (*Agricultural Statistics*, 1991, USDA, p. 479, Table 672)

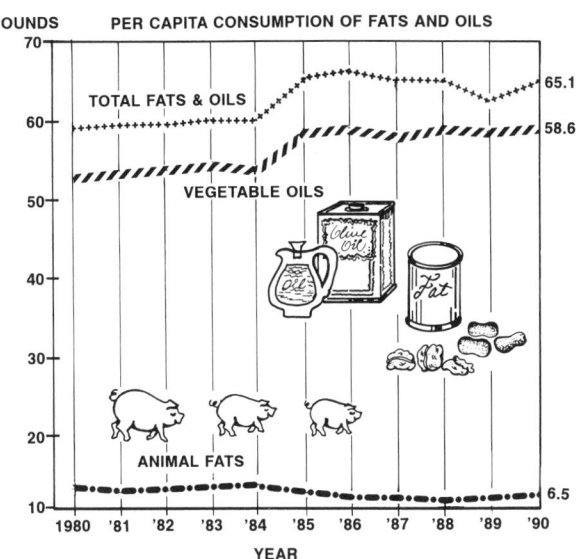

Fig. M-63. Consumption of animal fats vs vegetable oils. (*Agricultural Statistics*, 1991, USDA, p. 139, Table 194)

The selection of food is based on taste preference, relative prices, dietary guidelines issued by government agencies and scientific groups, and myths.

U.S. MEAT IMPORTS AND EXPORTS. Stockmen are prone to ask why the United States, which produces nearly one-fourth of the world's meat, buys meat from abroad. Conversely, consumers sometimes wonder why we export meat. Occasionally, there is justification for such fears. Table M-25 gives a comparison of U.S. meat imports and production for 1990.

TABLE M–25
U.S. PRODUCTION OF MEAT
COMPARED WITH U.S. IMPORTS

Kind of Meat	Production		Imports		Imports as Percent of Production
	◄――― (million) ―――►				(%)
	(lb)	*(kg)*	(lb)	*(kg)*	
Beef and veal	23,070	*10,486*	2,356	*1,071*	10.2
Pork	15,354	*6,979*	898	*408*	5.8
Lamb and mutton ..	363	*165*	59	*27*	16.3
Total	38,787	*17,630*	3,313	*1,506*	8.5

The column on the right shows imports as a percent of production. As shown, lamb imports were equivalent to

16.3% of U.S. production, beef imports were equivalent to 10.2% of U.S. production, pork imports were negligible, and total meat imports were equivalent to only 8.5% of our production.

Figs. M-64 and M-65 show a breakdown by kinds of meat imports and exports.

U.S. Imports of red meat

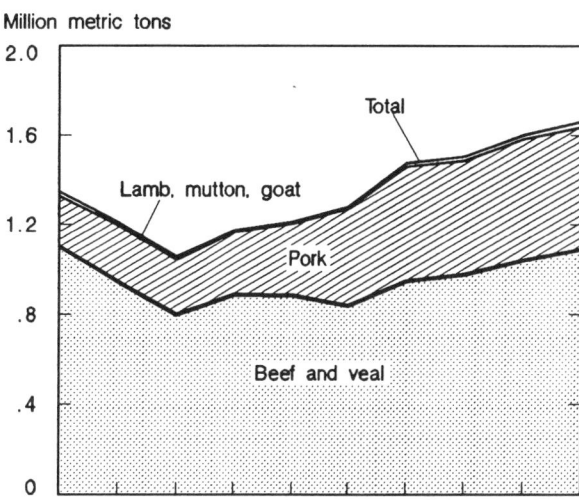

Fig. M-64. U.S. imports of red meats. Note the dominant position of beef and veal. (*1989 Agricultural Chartbook*, USDA, p. 87, Chart 189)

U.S. exports of livestock products

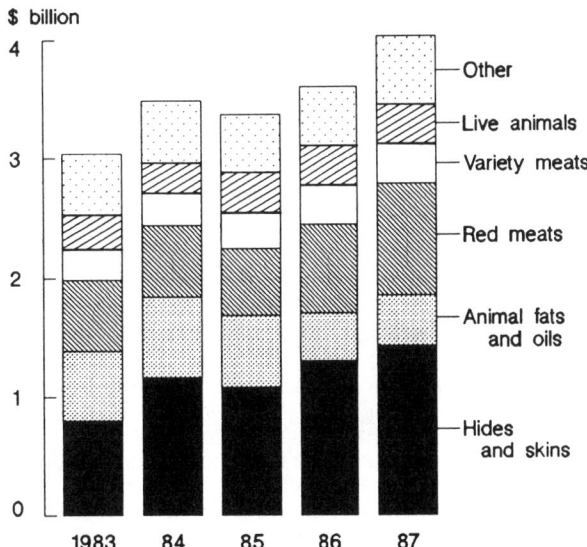

Fig. M-65. U.S. exports of meat, livestock products, and live animals. Note that lard, tallow, hides, and skins are the chief exports. (*1989 Agricultural Chartbook*, USDA, p. 87, Chart 188)

Table M-26 reveals that the United States imports more meat than it exports, but that total meat imports actually constitute a very small percentage of the available U.S. supply.

TABLE M–26
U.S. MEAT EXPORTS AND IMPORTS[1]

Year	Beef and Veal		Pork		Lamb and Mutton		All Meat	
	Exports	Imports	Exports	Imports	Exports	Imports	Exports	Imports
	(million lb)							
1986	526	2,156	86	1,122	2	41	614	3,319
1987	604	2,293	109	1,195	1	44	721	3,532
1988	681	2,407	195	1,136	1	51	887	3,594
1989	1,023	2,179	262	896	2	63	1,287	3,138
1990	1,006	2,356	239	898	3	59	1,248	3,313

[1]Carcass weight equivalent of all meat. (Data from *Agricultural Statistics 1991*, USDA, p. 295, Table 451)

The quality of meat and animals imported from abroad depends to a substantial degree on (1) level of U.S. meat production, (2) consumer buying power, (3) livestock prices, (4) quotas and tariffs, and (5) the need for manufacturing-type beef (the kind that is boned and used in making hamburgers, franks, sausages, and bologna). When animal prices are high, more meat is imported. Actually, there may some virtue in *judiciously* increasing imports of meat and animals during times of scarcity and high prices, as an alternative to pricing meat out of the market.

Because of restrictions designed to prevent the introduction of foot-and-mouth disease, neither fresh nor salted refrigerated beef can be imported to the United States from South America; beef importations from these countries must be canned or fully cured (i.e., corned beef).

Our meat imports came from many countries, but our chief sources, in order of importance in 1990, were:

• **Beef and veal**—from Australia, New Zealand, Canada, Guatemala, Costa Rica, Dominican Republic, and Honduras.

• **Lamb and mutton**—from Australia and New Zealand.

• **Pork**—from Canada, Denmark, Poland, Yugoslavia, and Hungary.

• **Total meat** (beef and veal, lamb and mutton, and pork)—from Australia, Canada, New Zealand, Denmark, Argentina, and Poland.

The quantity of meat and animals exported from this country is dependent upon (1) the volume of meat and the number of animals produced in the United States, (2) the volume of meat and the number of animals produced abroad, and (3) the relative vigor of international trade, especially as affected by buying power and trade restrictions.

Our export of animal products consists largely of those by-products which are surplus in the United States. As shown in Fig. M-65, hides and skins lead, with red meats next in importance, followed by animal fats and oils, variety meats, live animals, and other livestock products such as wool and mohair. The major markets for each of these products are: *Lard*—Mexico, Canada, Belize, and Haiti. *Tallow*—Mexico, Republic of Korea, Turkey, Venezuela, Algeria, and Spain. *Hides and skins*—Korea, Japan, Taiwan, and Mexico.

The United States exports more cattle than any other class of animal, followed, in order, by sheep and hogs.

• **Meat Import Law (Public Law 88–482)**—Because of cheaper labor (and often cheaper feed supplies), farmers in the surplus meat producing countries can produce meat at a lower cost than the American producer. Transportation distances and costs are not prohibitive in obtaining meat from these countries. For these reasons, only protective walls—tariffs, quotas, and embargo legislation enacted by the U.S. Government—can stand in the way of increased meat competition from foreign sources.

But the question of regulating the supply of meat, like regulating any other commodity, raises extremely complex issues and makes for conflicts of interest between producers and consumers.

The U.S. Congress enacted the Meat Import Law (Public Law 88–482) in August 1964, which became effective January 1, 1965. This law provides for import quotas, based on a formula, for fresh, chilled, and frozen beef, veal, mutton (not lamb), and goat meat—including both carcass and boneless meat. It does not include lamb or canned meats. The law is for the purpose of limiting annual imports of the specified meats to a level comparable to the designated base period of 1959–1963, with an adjustment, or "growth factor," based on changes in domestic production relative to the base period.

The base quota was established as the average annual quantity imported during the base period (1959–1963), which was 725,400,000 lb, or 4.6% of domestic production during those years.

It appears that voluntary agreements will be the chief means of controlling future imports. But the fact that a law exists may have considerable psychological effect on negotiations.

WORLD MEAT PRODUCTION AND CON-SUMPTION. In general, meat production and consumption are highest in those countries which have extensive grasslands, temperate climates, well-developed livestock industries, and sparse populations. In many of the older and more densely populated regions of the world, insufficient grain is produced to support the human population even when consumed directly. This lessens the possibility of keeping animals, except for consuming forages and other humanly inedible feeds. Certainly, when it is a choice between the luxury of meat and animal by-products or starvation, people will elect to accept a lower standard of living and go on a grain diet. In addition to the available meat supply, food habits and religious restrictions affect the kind and amount of meat produced and consumed.

Table M-27 shows the beef and veal; pork; mutton, lamb, and goat meat; and total red meat production in the ten leading red meat producing countries of the world in 1990. Note the favored position of beef. In 1990, the United States produced 10.4 million metric tons of beef, or about 22% of the world production of beef.

TABLE M–27
MEAT PRODUCTION, BY TYPES OF RED MEATS, IN TEN LEADING COUNTRIES OF THE WORLD[1,2]

Country (leading countries, by rank, of all meats)	Beef and Veal	Pork	Mutton, Lamb, and Goat Meat	Total Red Meat Production
	(1,000 metric tons)	(1,000 metric tons)	(1,000 metric tons)	(1,000 metric tons)
China	1,250	22,700	1,090	25,040
U.S.A.	10,464	6,964	165	17,593
U.S.S.R.	8,700	6,800	1,000	16,500
Germany	2,121	3,811	50	5,982
Brazil	4,180	1,050	0	5,230
France	1,710	1,870	160	3,740
Argentina	2,650	0	100	2,750
Australia	1,695	305	666	2,666
Mexico	1,790	792	76	2,658
Poland	799	1,814	28	2,641
World Total	47,739	64,325	6,413	118,477

[1]*Agricultural Statistics 1991*, USDA, p. 288, Table 443.
[2]Carcass weight basis; excludes offals.

Table M-28 shows the per capita consumption, by species, of the leading red meat-eating (beef and pork) countries of the world.

As shown in Table M-28, in 1990 the United States, with a per capita consumption of 97.2 lb (*44.2 kg*), ranked third in consumption of beef and veal, edging out

TABLE M–28
LEADING RED MEAT-EATING COUNTRIES OF THE WORLD[1]

Country	Beef and Veal Quantity[2]	Beef and Veal Rank	Country	Pork Quantity	Pork Rank
	(lb)			(lb)	
Argentina	143.3	1	Hungary	168.7	1
Uruguay	127.0	2	Denmark	147.7	2
U.S.A.	97.2	3	Czechoslovakia	130.3	3
Australia	88.9	4	Austria	116.0	4
Canada	86.2	5	Germany	115.8	5
New Zealand	79.6	6	Belgium-Luxembourg	105.0	6
U.S.S.R.	67.7	7	Poland	103.2	7
Czechoslovakia	65.7	8	Bulgaria	103.0	8
France	63.7	9	Spain	100.5	9
Italy	58.9	10	Netherlands	99.0	10
Switzerland	55.6	11	Hong Kong	94.2	11
Greece	54.5	12	Switzerland	90.2	12
Panama	51.8	13	China: Taiwan	85.8	13
Germany	50.3	14	France	82.2	14
Colombia	49.6	15	U.S.A.	63.9	15

[1]*Statistical Abstract of the United States 1991*, U.S. Dept. of Commerce, p. 843, Table 1452.
[2]Pounds per capita. To convert to kilograms divide by 2.2.

the Australians who averaged 88.9 lb (*40.4 kg*). But the United States was exceeded in per capita red meat consumption by Argentina, with 143.3 lb (*65.1 kg*); and Uruguay, with 127 lb (*57.7 kg*).

In per capita pork consumption, the five leading countries in 1990 were: Hungary, 168.7 lb (*76.7 kg*); Denmark, 147.7 lb (*67 kg*); Czechoslovakia, 130.3 lb (*59 kg*); Austria, 116 lb (*52.7 kg*); and Belgium-Luxembourg, 105 lb (*47.7 kg*). The United States ranked twenty-fourth in per capita pork consumption.

Fig. M-66 shows the total per capita consumption of all red meat of selected countries in 1989.

The per capita red meat consumption of the leading meat-eating countries changes from time to time. Thus, from 1965 to 1968, New Zealand was the world's largest per capita consumer of red meat, followed closely by Australia. In 1969, Australia took the lead. In 1989, the leading countries in red meat consumption by rank were: East Germany, Uruguay, Czechoslovakia, New Zealand, Australia, and the United States (see Fig. M-66).

WORLD'S RED MEAT EATERS

PER CAPITA CONSUMPTION

Country	Pounds
EAST GERMANY	202.0 LB
URUGUAY	194.5 LB
CZECHOSLOVAKIA	188.8 LB
NEW ZEALAND	176.0 LB
AUSTRALIA	169.6 LB
UNITED STATES	167.6 LB
HUNGARY	166.1 LB
CANADA	159.1 LB
ARGENTINA	155.1 LB
SWITZERLAND	150.7 LB

POUNDS 0   50   100   150   200   250

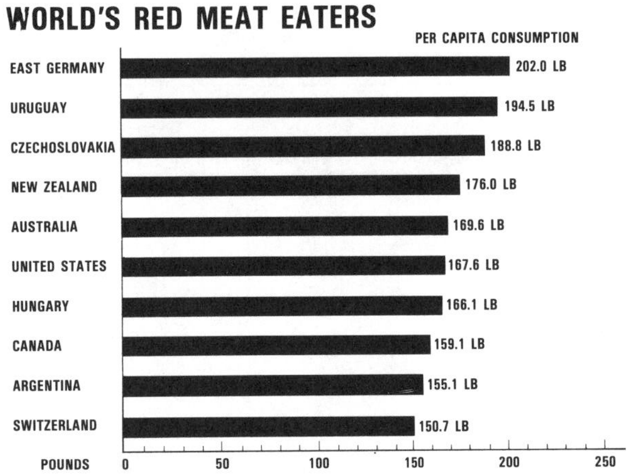

Fig. M-66. Total per capita consumption of all red meat—beef, veal, pork, mutton, lamb, and goat meat—in selected countries in 1989. (Source: *World Livestock Situation,* USDA, FAS, Nov. 1989)

NUTRITIVE COMPOSITION OF MEATS. Meat is far more than just a very tempting and delicious food. From a nutritional standpoint, it contains the essentials of an adequate diet. This is important, for how we live and how long we live are determined in large part by our diet.

Meat is an excellent source of high-quality protein, of certain minerals, especially iron, and of the B-complex vitamins. It supplies nutrients which contribute significantly to the dietary balance of meals, and it is easily digested.

Table M-29 shows the contribution (1) of red meat (beef, pork, and lamb) and (2) of meat, poultry, and fish combined, to meeting the recommended daily nutrient allowance (RDA) of the various nutrients.

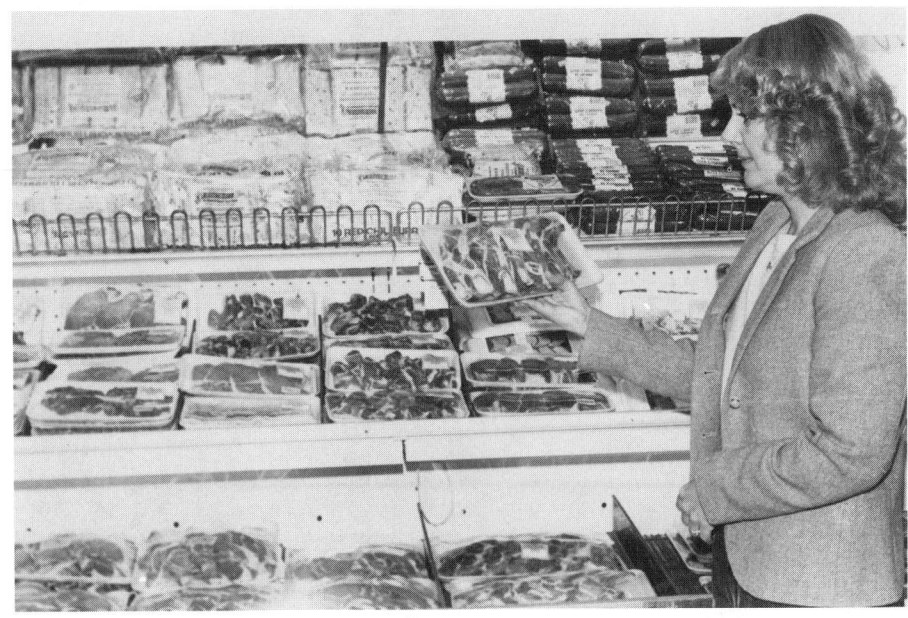

Fig. M-66a. In most areas of the world, the meat consumer has a wide choice of cuts from which to select. In addition, there are a myriad of processed meats and meat dishes. (Photo by A. H. Ensminger)

TABLE M–29
CONTRIBUTIONS OF MEAT TO THE RECOMMENDED NUTRIENT ALLOWANCES IN THE UNITED STATES[1]

Nutrient	United States Recommended Daily Allowances (RDA)[2]	Contribution from Meat-Poultry-Fish, Combined	
		Total Amount/Day[3]	RDA[4]
			(%)
Energy	2,900 kcal	676.8 kcal	23.3
Carbohydrate	Not established	0.4 g	—
Fat	Not established	53.3 g	—
Protein	63 g	45.5 g	72.2
Calcium	800 mg	34.7 mg	4.3
Phosphorus	800 mg	450 mg	56.2
Magnesium	350 mg	50.8 mg	14.5
Copper	1.5–3 mg	0.30 mg	13.2
Iron[5]	10 mg	3.78 mg	37.8
Zinc	15 mg	5.99 mg	40
Vitamin A[6]	1,000 R.E.	336 R.E.	33.6
Folate	200 mcg	27.8 mcg	13.9
Niacin	19 mg	11.6 mg	61.3
Riboflavin	1.7 mg	0.53 mg	31.3
Thiamin	1.5 mg	0.55 mg	36.7
Vitamin B-6	2.0 mg	0.89 mg	44.6
Vitamin B-12	2.0 mcg	6.93 mcg	346.3
Vitamin C	60 mg	2.6 mg	4.3

[1]From: Agricultural Statistics 1991, USDA, pp. 474–478.

[2]National Research Council (1989 for adult male 25-50 years of age).

[3]USDA (1988).

[4]Calculated as follows: % RDA = Avg $\dfrac{\text{daily per capita intake}}{\text{RDA}}$

[5]RDA value used for iron based on adult male, whereas, adult premenopausal female has an RDA of 15 mg/day.

[6]Vitamin A is given in terms of retinol equivalents (R.E.), one R.E. = 3.3 IU of vitamin A activity, which was assumed to be the predominant form in meat, poultry, and fish.

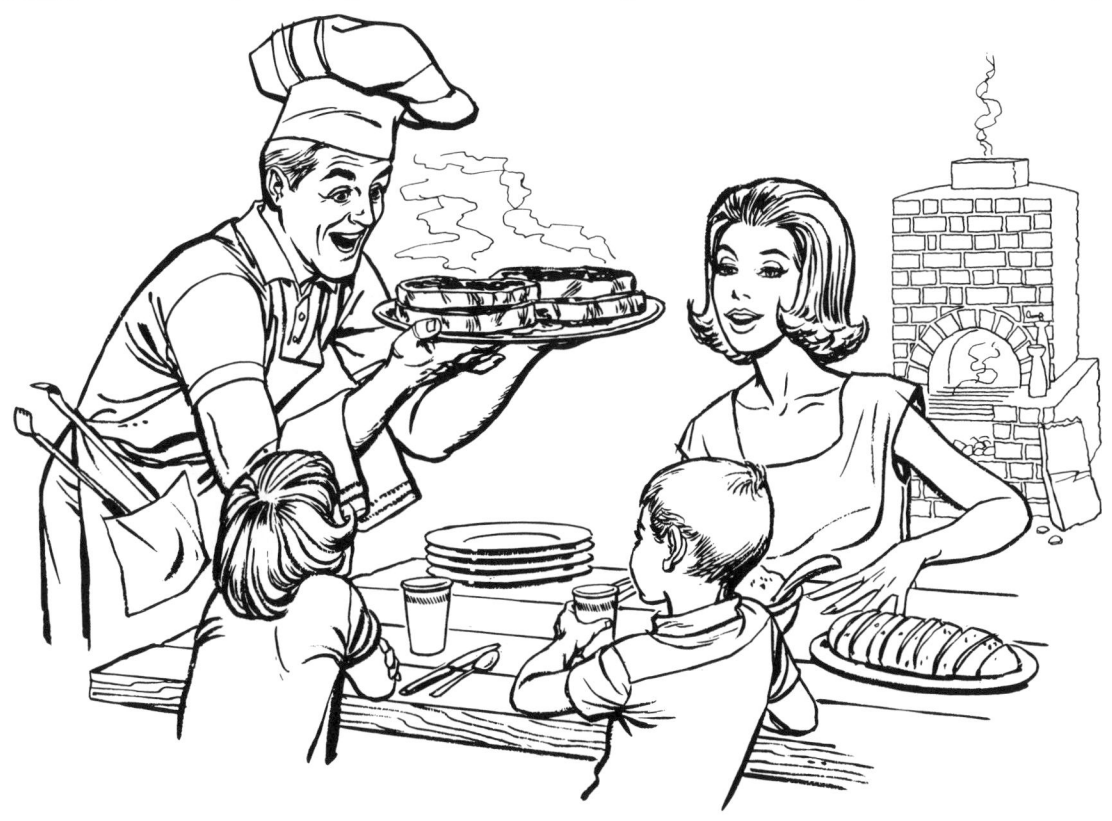

Although the RDAs are believed to be more than adequate to meet the requirements of most consumers, it is recognized that individuals vary greatly in their requirements—by as much as twofold. So, Table M-30 presents data showing the contribution (1) of red meat and (2) of meat, poultry, and fish combined, toward the total dietary intake of each of the nutrients.

TABLE M–30
CONTRIBUTIONS OF MEAT TO THE
DIETARY INTAKE IN THE UNITED STATES[1,2]

Nutrition	Average Per Capita Consumption Per Day	Total Consumption Contributed by Meat-Poultry-Fish Combined
		(%)
Energy	3,600 kcal	18.8
Carbohydrate ..	425 g	0.1
Fat	168 g	31.7
Protein	105 g	43.3
Calcium	890 mg	3.9
Phosphorus ...	1,540 mg	29.2
Magnesium	339 mg	15.4
Copper	1.7 mg	17.5
Iron	17.1 mg	22.1
Zinc	12.7 mg	47.2
Vitamin A (R.E.)	1,630 mcg	20.6
Folate	284 mcg	9.8
Niacin	26 mg	44.8
Riboflavin	2.4 mg	22.2
Thiamin	2.2 mg	25.0
Vitamin B-6	2.2 mg	40.5
Vitamin B-12 ...	9.1 mcg	76.1
Vitamin C	118 mg	2.2

[1]Agricultural Statistics 1991, USDA, pp. 474–479.

[2]The average yearly per capita consumption (carcass basis) amounted to 112.3 lb of red meat, 63.8 lb of poultry, and 15.4 lb of fish that was consumed in 1990.

It should be noted that the values given in both Tables M-29 and M-30 are calculations based on food disappearance data and may not accurately reflect actual consumption; and that there is considerable variation in the composition of meat from animal to animal and cut to cut.

The nutritive qualities of meats are detailed in the sections that follow.

Energy.[27]   The energy value of meat is largely dependent upon the amount of fat that it contains. Thus, fatback and other fat meats once provided much of the food energy of lumberjacks and other men of brawn, some of whom consumed up to 9,000 Calories (kcal) per day. But machines replaced muscles; and with the transition, animals were slenderized and leaner meats were produced.

Today, meat-poultry-fish combined supply 25.1% of the RDA for energy (Table M-29). But of the total energy intake, meat-poultry-fish combined supply only 18.8% of the total energy intake (Table M-30). Thus, meat is not a major contributor to excess energy intake. Nevertheless, it should be pointed out that the values given are averages, and that anyone greatly exceeding the average could be adding to the caloric burden unless other sources of energy are controlled.

(Also see CALORIE [ENERGY] EXPENDITURE; and ENERGY UTILIZATION BY THE BODY.)

Carbohydrate.   Although the carbohydrates provide a major source of energy for man, they are found only in very limited amounts in meats and other animal products.

About half the carbohydrate is distributed through the muscles and in the bloodstream; the other half is stored in the liver in the form of glycogen (animal starch), where it constitutes 3 to 7% of the weight of that organ. Yet, most animal products contain little, if any, carbohydrate, for the reason that when an animal is slaughtered, the glycogen stored in the liver and muscles is rapidly broken down to lactic acid and pyruvic acid. Oysters and scallops contain some glycogen, but the amount is not significant to the diet. Milk, which contains the carbohydrate lactose or milk sugar, is the only animal food of importance as a carbohydrate source.

Only 0.4 g of carbohydrate comes from red meat daily, with most of it derived from the glycogen and reducing tissues naturally present in the tissues (Table M-29). Neither meat nor meat-poultry-fish make any significant contribution to total carbohydrate consumption; in each case they account for only 0.1% (Table M-30). A small amount of carbohydrate in the diet also comes from sugars and other carbohydrates added to sausages. The low level of carbohydrate in meat helps to keep its caloric contribution to a minimum. On the other hand, there is evidence that complex carbohydrates, i.e., fiber, con-

[27]Although the National Research Council nutrient allowances recognize that energy requirements vary depending upon sex, age, and physical activity, in Table M-29 adult males 25 to 50 years of age were chosen, so the data needs to be adapted when applied to other groups. The range in energy needs is given, but the values used for the calculations are based on the average of 2,700 Calories (kcal).

tribute to bowel movement and the elimination of toxic substances from the digestive tract. Thus, it is recommended that fruit and vegetables be included in the diet to provide fiber.

(Also see CARBOHYDRATE[S].)

Fats. Energy is supplied by animal fats, which are highly digestible. Fats also supply needed fatty acids, transport fat-soluble vitamins (A, D, E, K), provide protection and insulation to the human body, and add palatability to lean meat. Highly unsaturated fats are soft and oily (as in soft pork). Generally, animal fats contain higher levels of saturated fat than vegetable oils.

The amount and composition of fats in the animal body are highly variable, depending upon the species, diet, and maturity. The species differences in the composition of fats are particularly noticeable between ruminants and nonruminants; ruminants (through rumen microorganisms) may alter the composition of the dietary fats, whereas nonruminants tend to deposit lipids in the form found in the diet. Australian researchers have developed a procedure for protecting dietary fats from the action of the rumen organisms by encapsulation of the fat, thus permitting alteration of the characteristic fatty acid composition in both meat and milk.

The fats of the diet serve as a source of the essential fatty acids—arachidonic, linoleic, and linolenic acid, but only linoleic acid is required preformed in the diet. Although meats provide fat, the vegetable oils are generally richer sources of the essential fatty acids than animal fats; hence, no deficiency of fatty acids is likely to develop on a meatless diet unless there is impaired lipid absorption.

There is no RDA for fat consumption since there is seldom a deficiency. Rather, the main problem from fat consumption is its contribution to obesity.

Meat-poultry-fish combined contribute 53.3 g of fat per capita per day (Table M-29) and account for 31.7% of the total consumption (Table M-30).

(Also see FATS AND OTHER LIPIDS.)

Protein. The need for protein in the diet is actually a need for amino acids, of which nine are essential for humans. (Ten are essential for animals; they require arginine, which is not required by humans.) But all proteins are not created equal! Some proteins of certain foods are low or completely devoid of certain essential amino acids. Hence, meeting the protein requirement demands quality as well as quantity. It is noteworthy that all the essential amino acids are present in muscle meats, heart, liver, and kidney. However, there is considerable variation in the protein content of meat, depending on the degree of fatness and the water content; the total protein content of animal bodies ranges from about 10% in very fat, mature animals to 20% in thin, young animals.

Because animal proteins are in short supply in the developing countries, it has been estimated that 20 to 30% of the children in these countries suffer severe protein-calorie malnutrition, and that it may contribute to as much as 50% of the mortality for this group. Kwashiorkor and marasmus are common manifestations of protein and protein-calorie deficiencies in infants and children. Also, the ability of the human body to produce antibodies (substances that attack specific foreign bodies) is dependent upon an adequate supply of amino acids in the diet. (The antibody molecule is actually a molecule of globulin—a class of protein.)

Table M-29 shows that the RDA for protein for the 25 to 50-year-old man is 63 g, with meat-poultry-fish supplying 72.2% of this amount. Table M-30 shows that meat-poultry-fish supply 43.3% of the total protein intake.

In spite of the high level of high-quality protein in the average American diet, there is evidence that some protein deficiencies occur in young children shortly after weaning. In these cases, it appears that protein intake is low either due to their economic status or a strict vegetarian diet. Regardless of the reason for the deficiency, inclusion of small amounts of meat or other animal protein would alleviate all signs of protein deficiency.

(Also see PROTEIN[S].)

Minerals. Meat is a rich source of several minerals, but it is an especially rich source of phosphorus and iron.

In the discussion that follows, minerals are divided into macrominerals or microminerals, based on the relative amount needed in the diet.

(Also see MINERAL[S].)

MACROMINERALS. The macrominerals, or major minerals, are those that are needed in greatest abundance.

• **Calcium**—Meat is a poor source of calcium. Table M-29 shows that meat-poultry-fish combined provide only 4.3% of the RDA. Table M-30 shows that meat-poultry-fish combined provide 3.9% of the calcium intake.

It is noteworthy that mechanically deboned meat contains up to 0.75% calcium, and that it can make a considerable contribution to the calcium of the diet of man.

(Also see CALCIUM.)

• **Phosphorus**—Although meat is a poor source of calcium, it is usually a good source of phosphorus. Meat-

Meat Is A Good Source of Phosphorus

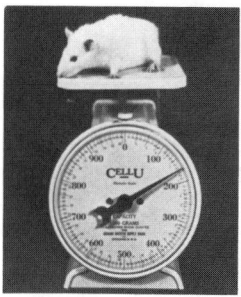
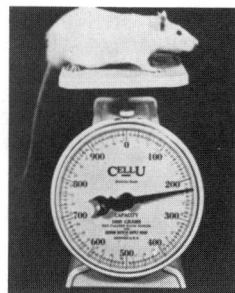

Low phosphorus diet
(no meat)
Wt. 168 grams

Same diet plus meat
Wt. 225 grams

Fig. M-67. This shows that meat is a rich source of phosphorus. Minerals are necessary in order to build and maintain the body skeleton and tissues and regulate body functions. Although meat is a good source of several minerals, it is especially rich as a source of phosphorus and iron. (Courtesy, National Live Stock and Meat Board and Rush Medical College)

poultry-fish combined contribute 56.2% of the RDA (Table M-29). Meat-poultry-fish combined provide 29.2% of the phosphorus intake (Table M-30).

(Also see PHOSPHORUS.)

• **Sodium**—Most of the sodium in the diet is in the form of salt (sodium chloride—NaCl). Deficiencies of sodium are rare because nearly all foods contain some sodium. However, excess dietary salt over a long period of time is believed to lead to high blood pressure in susceptible people. Also, excess salt may cause edema. So, a prudent diet should limit excess salt intake; this would call for limiting the intake of cured meats.

(Also see SODIUM.)

• **Chlorine**—Chlorine is provided by table salt (sodium chloride—NaCl) and by the foods that contain salt. Persons suffering from diseases of the heart, kidney, or liver, whose sodium intake is severely restricted by deleting table salt and such salty foods as cured meats, may need an alternative source of chloride; a number of chloride-containing salt substitutes are available for this purpose.

(Also see CHLORINE.)

• **Magnesium**—Meat, poultry, and fish are low in magnesium; they supply only 14.5% of the RDA of this mineral (Table M-29). Most of the magnesium in meat is found in the muscle and liver.

(Also see MAGNESIUM.)

• **Potassium**—Potassium is the third most abundant element in the body, after calcium and phosphorus; and it is present in twice the concentration of sodium.

Potassium is widely distributed in foods. Meat, poultry, fish, many fruits, whole grains, and vegetables are good sources. (Although meat, poultry, and fish are good sources of potassium, these items may be restricted when dietary sodium is restricted.)

(Also see POTASSIUM.)

• **Sulfur**—Meeting the sulfur needs of the body seems to be primarily a matter of providing sulfur for the sulfur-containing amino acids: methionine, cystine, and cysteine.

Inorganic sulfur is poorly utilized by man. Thus, meat, poultry, and fish, which are good sources of sulfur, serve an important function in supplying the body with its sulfur requirements.

(Also see SULFUR.)

MICROMINERALS. The microminerals, or trace or minor minerals, are those that are needed in least amounts.

• **Chromium**—Chromium, which has a number of important functions in the human body, is widely distributed in animal tissues and in animal products. In the section on Chromium, Table C-30, of this book, the chromium content of the following foods of animal origin, in mcg/100 g is reported: dried liver, 170; egg, 52; cheese, 51; fresh liver, 50; and beef, 32.

(Also see CHROMIUM.)

• **Cobalt**—This mineral, which is an integral part of vitamin B-12—an essential factor in the formation of red blood cells, must be ingested in the form of vitamin B-12 in order to be of value to man; hence, a table showing the cobalt content of human foods serves no useful purpose. The organ meats (liver, kidney) are excellent sources of vitamin B-12 (hence, of cobalt). The vitamin B-12 content, in mcg/100 g, of some rich animal food sources follows: beef liver, 111; clams, 98; lamb kidneys, 63; turkey liver, 48; and calf kidney, 25.

(Also see COBALT.)

• **Copper**—Organ meats (liver, kidney, brains) and shell fish are rich sources of copper. Table M-29 shows that meat-poultry-fish combined supply 13.2% of the RDA of copper.

(Also see COPPER.)

• **Fluorine**—Fluorine, which is necessary for sound bones and teeth, is widely, but unevenly, distributed in nature. Seafoods and tea are the richest dietary sources.

Because fluorine tends to concentrate in the bones and teeth and is toxic if used in excess, there has been some concern about fluorine levels in deboned meat. Yet, there seems to be little basis for such apprehension unless the bones come from animals suffering from fluorosis.

(Also see FLUORINE.)

• **Iodine**—Most of the iodine need of humans is met by iodized salt. Saltwater fish and most shellfish are rich sources of iodine. Dairy products and eggs may be good sources if the producing animals have access to iodine-enriched rations. Red meats and poultry are poor sources of iodine.

(Also see IODINE.)

• **Iron**—Liver is an excellent source of easily assimilated iron and is prescribed in the diet of anemia sufferers. Muscle meat, poultry, and fish are good sources of iron, but they contain less than half as much iron as liver.

There are two forms of food iron—heme (organic) and nonheme (inorganic). Of the two, heme is absorbed from food more efficiently than inorganic iron and is independent of vitamin C or iron binding chelating agents. Although the proportion of heme iron in animal tissue varies, it amounts to about 1/3 of the total iron in all animal tissues—including meat, liver, poultry, and fish. The remaining 2/3 of the iron in animal tissues and all the iron of vegetable products are treated as nonheme iron.

Meat also enhances the absorption of iron, as does vitamin C; it improves iron absorption by supplying what is referred to as the "meat factor." It has been demonstrated that beef, veal, lamb, pork, liver, chicken, and fish all increase iron absorption by two to fourfold, while milk, cheese, and egg do not increase iron absorption.

The data in Table M-29 are calculated using an RDA of 10 mg of iron, which is the level recommended for an adult man.

As shown in Table M-29, meat-poultry-fish combined provide 37.8% of the RDA. Table M-30 shows that the total intake of iron in the diet is 17.1 mg/day; and that meat-poultry-fish combined provide 22.1% of the total intake.

But there are four situations in life in which the RDA is higher than the RDA of 10 mg for adult men (according to *Recommended Dietary Allowances, NRC–National Academy of Sciences*, 1989, p. 201: (1) in infancy; (2) during rapid growth and adolescence; (3) during the female reproductive period; and (4) in pregnancy. So, for females age 11 to 50, NRC recommends an RDA of 15 mg of iron, *plus* 30 mg of supplemental iron daily during pregnancy, and dropping to 15 mg daily during lactation. During these four stages in life, the iron status could be greatly improved by including meat, poultry, and fish in the diet on a regular basis.

(Also see IRON.)

• **Manganese**—Only a trace of manganese is found in muscle meat. Liver is a fair source.

(Also see MANGANESE.)

• **Molybdenum**—The organ meats (liver, kidney) are a good source of molybdenum.

(Also see MOLYBDENUM.)

• **Selenium**—Meat, poultry, and fish all contain small amounts of selenium, but liver and kidney are the best sources. The selenium content of animal products depends upon the content of the element in livestock feeds; for example, the Ohio Station reported that the addition of 0.1 ppm selenium to the animal's diet increased the selenium content of beef liver by 72%.[28]

Fortunately, foods eaten in the United States are generally varied in nature and origin; so, there does not appear to be any deficiency of selenium in man. However, a deficiency of selenium has been reported in a localized area in China where only locally produced foods are consumed.

(Also see SELENIUM.)

• **Silicon**—Meat, poultry, and fish all contribute silicon to the diet in appreciable quantities. However, the best sources of silicon are the fibrous parts of whole grains, followed by various organ meats (liver, kidney, brain), and connective tissues.

Because of the abundance of silicon in all but the most highly refined foods, it is of little concern in the human diet.

(Also see SILICON.)

• **Zinc**—Meat, poultry, fish, eggs, and dairy products are good sources of zinc. The animal proteins are generally much better sources of dietary zinc than plants because the phytate present in many plant sources complexes the zinc and makes it unavailable.

Table M-29 shows that meat-poultry-fish combined supply 40% of the recommended zinc allowance.

Since meat, poultry, fish, eggs, and dairy products are good sources of zinc, they should be included regularly in the diet. This recommendation is further reinforced by the fact that zinc deficiency is virtually unknown on a diet containing animal products.

(Also see ZINC.)

Vitamins. Many phenomena of vitamin nutrition are related to solubility—vitamins are soluble in either fat or water. This is a convenient way in which to discuss vitamins in meats; hence, they are grouped and treated as fat-soluble vitamins or water-soluble vitamins.

Data showing the contribution of meat-poultry-fish combined is presented in Table M-29. Total consumption data and the proportion of the total contributed by meat-poultry-fish combined are summarized in Table M-30.

(Also see VITAMINS.)

---

[28]Moxon, A. L. and D. L. Palmquist, "Selenium Content of Foods Grown or Sold in Ohio," *Ohio Report*, Ohio State University, Columbus, Ohio, January-February 1980, pp. 13-14, Table 1.

FAT-SOLUBLE VITAMINS. The fat-soluble vitamins are stored in appreciable quantities in the animal body, whereas the water-soluble vitamins are not. Any of the fat-soluble vitamins can be stored wherever fat is deposited; and the greater the intake of the vitamin, the greater the storage. It follows that most meats, poultry, and fish are good sources of the fat-soluble vitamins.

• **Vitamin A**—Both vitamin A and the carotenes are found in the animal body associated with fats (lipids).

Cod and other fish liver oils are extremely high in vitamin A, sufficiently so that they are used as supplemental sources. Livers of all kinds are rich food sources of vitamin A, exceeding raw carrots.

The values given in Table M-29 were calculated on the assumption that most of the vitamin A activity in meat, poultry, and fish is present as vitamin A, although it is recognized that some carotene is present. As indicated in Table M-29, meat-poultry, fish combined provide 33.6% of the RDA. Table M-30 shows that meat-poultry-fish combined contribute 20.6% of the average daily per capita consumption of vitamin A (retinol).

(Also see VITAMIN A.)

• **Vitamin D**—Fish liver oils (from cod, halibut, or swordfish) are very high in vitamin D, sufficiently so that they are used as supplemental sources. Fatty fish and fish roe are rich food sources, while liver, egg yolk, cream, butter, and cheese are fair sources. Muscle meats and unfortified milk are negligible sources.

(Also see VITAMIN D.)

• **Vitamin E**—Meat and animal products are good to fair sources of vitamin E (the tocopherols); plant materials are much richer sources, especially vegetable oils, some grains, nuts, and green leafy vegetables.

The amount of vitamin E in animal tissues and products is influenced by the dietary consumption of tocopherols by the animal. Good animal sources are: beef and organ meats, butter, eggs, and seafoods. Cheese and chicken are fair sources.

(Also see VITAMIN E.)

• **Vitamin K**—Certain animal foods are good to fair sources of vitamin K, although they are far outranked by green tea, turnip greens, and broccoli. Beef liver is a rich source of vitamin K; bacon, cheese, butter, and pork liver are good sources; and beef fat, ham, eggs, pork tenderloin, ground beef, and chicken liver are fair sources.

(Also see VITAMIN K.)

WATER-SOLUBLE VITAMINS. The water-soluble vitamins are not stored in the animal body to any appreciable extent.

• **Biotin**—Biotin is widely distributed in foods of animal origin, with liver and kidney being rich sources, followed by eggs, sardines and salmon, cheese, chicken, oysters, and pork.

(Also see BIOTIN.)

• **Choline**—All animal tissues contain some choline, although it is more abundant in fatty than in lean tissues. Rich sources are: eggs, liver, and dried buttermilk.

(Also see CHOLINE.)

• **Folacin (folic acid)**—Folacin is widely distributed in animal foods, with liver and kidney being particularly rich sources. Eggs and fish are good sources, while cheese, cod, and halibut are fair sources. Chicken, milk, and most muscle meats are poor sources of folacin.

(Also see FOLACIN [FOLIC ACID].)

• **Niacin (nicotinic acid; nicotinamide)**—Generally speaking, niacin is found in animal tissue as nicotinamide. Animal foods are excellent dietary sources, with the richest sources being liver, kidney, lean meats, poultry, fish, and rabbit. Although low in niacin content, milk, cheese, and eggs are good sources because (1) of their tryptophan content (which may yield niacin), and (2) of their niacin being in available form.

The role of niacin-rich animal foods in eliminating pellagra, which was once a serious scourge in the United States, is generally recognized.

As shown in Table M-29, meat-poultry-fish combined contribute 61.3% of the RDA of niacin.

As shown in Table M-30, meat-poultry-fish provide 44.8% of the total dietary intake of niacin.

(Also see NIACIN.)

• **Pantothenic acid (vitamin B-3)**—Pantothenic acid is widely distributed in animal foods, with organ meats (liver, kidney, and heart) being particularly rich sources. Salmon, blue cheese, eggs, and lobster are good sources, while lean muscle and chicken are only fair sources.

(Also see PANTOTHENIC ACID.)

• **Riboflavin**—The organ meats (liver, kidney, heart) are rich sources of riboflavin; lean meat (beef, pork, lamb), cheese, eggs, and bacon are good sources; while chicken and fish are only fair sources.

Meat-poultry-fish combined supply 31.3% of the RDA of riboflavin (Table M-29). Meat-poultry-fish combined supply 22.2% of the per capita daily consumption of riboflavin (Table M-30).

(Also see RIBOFLAVIN.)

• **Thiamin (vitamin B-1)**—Some thiamin is found in a large variety of animal products, but it is abundant in few.

MEAT IS A GOOD SOURCE OF THIAMIN (VITAMIN B-1)

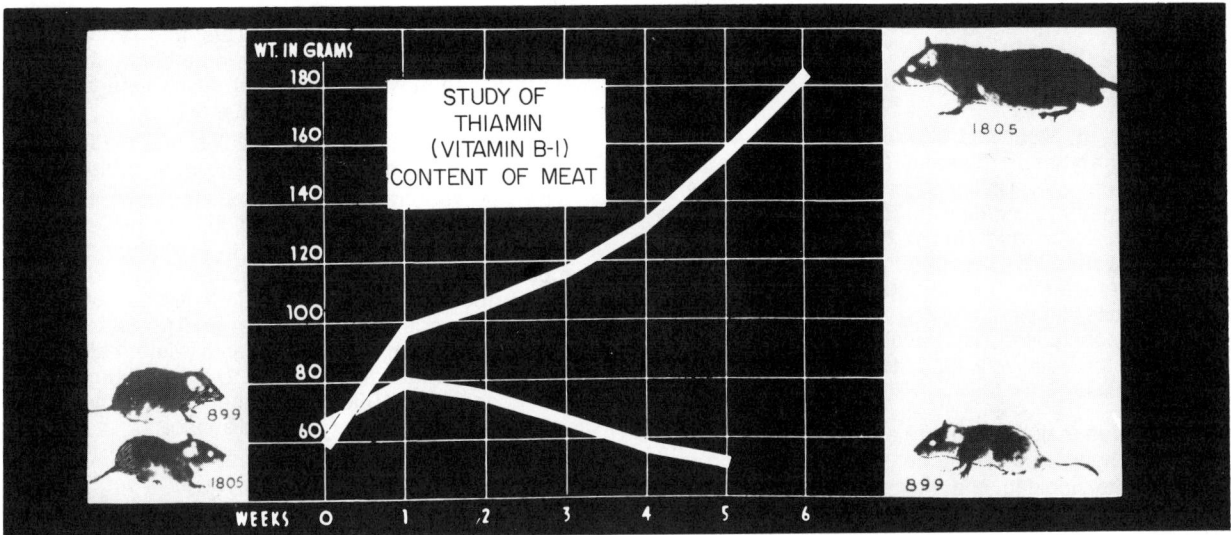

RAT NO. 899 RECEIVED ADEQUATE DIET EXCEPT FOR THIAMIN
RAT NO. 1805 RECEIVED SAME DIET + 2% DRIED PORK HAM WHICH IS RICH IN THIAMIN

Fig. M-68. Meat is a good source of thiamin (vitamin B-1). (Studies by the University of Wisconsin; supported by the National Live Stock and Meat Board)

Lean pork (fresh and cured) is a rich source; kidney is a good source; while egg yolk, poultry, beef liver, luncheon meat, and fish are only fair sources. The thiamin content of pork can be greatly altered by the thiamin level of the feed. Curing of meat causes only small losses.

Meat-poultry-fish combined contribute 36.7% of the RDA of thiamin (Table M-29). Meat-poultry-fish combined contribute approximately 25% of the total thiamin intake (Table M-30).

(Also see THIAMIN.)

• **Vitamin B-6 (pyridoxine; pyridoxal; pyridoxamine)**—In animal tissues, vitamin B-6 occurs mainly as pyridoxal and pyridoxamine. Vitamin B-6 is widely distributed in foods of animal origin. Liver, kidney, lean meat, and poultry are good sources; eggs are a fair source; and fat, cheese, and milk are negligible sources.

Meat-poultry-fish combined supply 44.6% of the RDA (Table M-29). Meat-poultry-fish combined contribute 40.5% of the total vitamin B-6 intake (Table M-30).

(Also see VITAMIN B-6.)

• **Vitamin B-12 (cobalamins)**—Vitamin B-12 is found in all foods of animal origin. Plants cannot manufacture vitamin B-12; hence, except for trace amounts absorbed from the soil (because of soil bacteria, soil is a good source of B-12) by the growing plant, very little is found in plant foods.

Liver and other organ meats—kidney, heart—are rich sources of vitamin B-12; muscle meats, fish, shellfish, eggs, and cheese are good sources; and milk, poultry, and yogurt are fair sources.

Meat-poultry-fish combined provide 346.3% of the RDA of the vitamin B-12 (Table M-29). This means that most meat eaters have an abundance of dietary vitamin B-12. Table M-30 shows that meat-poultry-fish contribute 76.1% of the average per capita consumption of vitamin B-12 per day. Thus, there is a great excess of vitamin B-12 in the average diet.

(Also see VITAMIN B-12.)

• **Vitamin C (ascorbic acid)**—Vitamin C is found only in small amounts in animal tissues, with the largest amounts being localized in the adrenal glands. Vitamin C is added to cured meats at a level of 550 ppm to reduce nitrosamine formation.

Table M-29 shows that meat-poultry-fish combined contribute only 4.3% of the RDA of vitamin C. Table M-30 shows that meat-poultry-fish combined provide only 2.2% of the total intake of vitamin C.

(Also see VITAMIN C.)

Summary. The unique contributions of meat, poultry, and fish to the nutritional needs of man have been presented in this section. In summary form, the major nutritive contribution of foods of animal origin are:

1. They are an excellent source of protein, from the standpoint of both quantity and quality; they supply all the essential amino acids.

2. They are rich sources of phosphorus, iron, copper, and zinc.

3. They are the major dietary source of vitamin B-12 and vitamin B-6, and they supply appreciable amounts of vitamin A, biotin, niacin, pantothenic acid, riboflavin, and thiamin.

MEAT FACTS AND MYTHS. Much has been spoken and written linking the consumption of meat to certain health related problems in humans, including heart disease, cancer, high blood pressure (hypertension), and harmful residues. A summary of four incorrect statements, along with the correct facts, follows:

• **Fact or Myth: Meat fats cause coronary heart disease**—Coronary heart disease (CHD) is the leading cause of death in the United States, accounting for one-third of all deaths, according to *The Surgeon General's Report on Nutrition and Health* (1988, p. 4, Table 2). The major form of CHD results from atherosclerosis, a condition characterized by fatty deposits in the coronary arteries. These deposits are rich in cholesterol, a complex fatlike substance. Also, in general, serum cholesterol levels are relatively high among individuals with atherosclerosis.

Fact: Three major factors are associated with the risk of coronary heart disease; namely, elevated blood pressure, cigarette smoking, and elevated serum cholesterol. A serum cholesterol level in excess of 280 mg/dl is considered a major risk for heart disease. The concentration of cholesterol in the blood is strongly affected by the degree of saturation of the dietary fat.

Professional groups suggest that many people would benefit (1) if the amount of fat in the diet were reduced from the present level of 37% to less than 30% of the total calories; (2) if the amount of dietary cholesterol were restricted to less than 300 mg per day; (3) if polyunsaturated fats were substituted for some of the saturated fat in the diet so that the distribution among polyunsaturated, monounsaturated, and saturated fatty acids would be about equal; (4) if saturated fat were limited to 10% of the total caloric intake; and (5) if caloric intake were adjusted to maintain desired body weight.

The major dietary sources of fat in the American diet are meat, poultry, fish, dairy products, and fats and oils. Animal products tend to be higher in both total and saturated fats than most plant sources. Also, dietary cholesterol is found only in foods of animal origin.

The intake and types of fatty acids that made up an average American diet in 1956 is shown in Table M-31.

Since the 1956 report by the U.S. Department of Agriculture (Table M-31), health and dietary professionals have urged the American people to (1) reduce the consumption of total fat, especially saturated fat and cholesterol; (2) increase the intake of fruits, vegetables, and whole grain products and cereals; and (3) increase the consumption of fish, poultry prepared without skin, lean meats, and low-fat dairy products. Dietary changes have been made since 1956, but further improvements will lessen the risk of coronary heart disease.

(Also see HEART DISEASE.)

• **Fact or Myth: Meat causes bowel cancer**—This question has been prompted by the following reports: (1) that the age-adjusted incidence of colon cancer has been found to increase with the per capita consumption of meat in countries; (2) that, in a study done in Hawaii, the incidence of colon cancer in persons of Japanese ancestry was found to be greater among those who ate Western-style meals, especially those who ate beef; and (3) that an examination of (a) international food consumption patterns, and (b) food consumption survey data from the United States showed that a higher incidence of colon cancer occurred in areas with greater beef consumption.

TABLE M–31
AVERAGE CONSUMPTION, IN GRAMS PER PERSON PER DAY, OF FATTY ACIDS FROM FOODS THAT MADE UP AN AVERAGE AMERICAN DIET AS REPORTED BY THE U.S. DEPARTMENT OF AGRICULTURE IN 1956[1]

Commodity	Total Saturated Acids	Oleic Acid	Other Monounsaturated Acids	Linoleic Acid	Other Polyunsaturated Acids
Dairy products (milk, cheese, butter)	28.2	7.5	3.0	0.8	0.4
Fats, oils	10.0	18.9	0.4	9.5	0.4
Flour, cereal products	0.7	1.5	—	2.2	0.2
Bakery products, purchased	2.7	3.7	—	2.4	0.3
Meats, poultry, eggs	14.1	17.0	0.8	3.8	0.6
Sugar, sweets	1.1	1.0	—	0.4	—
Potatoes	0.4	0.3	—	0.3	0.2
Fruits, vegetables	0.3	0.6	—	0.4	0.1
Miscellaneous foods	0.9	2.2	—	0.7	—
Totals	58.4	52.7	4.2	20.5	2.2
% of Total	42.3	38.2	3.0	14.9	1.6

[1]From: *Diet and Health,* Council for Agricultural Science and Technology, Report No. 111, March 1987, p. 25. Obtained from a 1956 report from the U.S. Department of Agriculture. The per capita fat consumption represented 96.4% of the fat consumed.

Fact: A direct cause-effect relationship between diet and cancer has not been established. Such studies as the three cited provide valuable leads for researchers who are trying to determine the cause of a certain disease such as colon cancer, but they do not establish the cause. The reason is that the factor measured and found associated with the incidence of colon cancer or other condition is not the only difference among the population groups studied, and the factor measured in the study may be only associated in some way with the real cause.

Rather than incriminating meat as the cause of cancer, the above studies raise the following questions:

1. In countries with high per capita meat consumption, the consumption of plant products and fiber tends to be low (for meat is devoid of fiber). It is conceivable that a low intake of fiber might cause colon cancer, but this hypothesis is without proof.

2. In the case of the Japanese, eating more beef wasn't the only change. They changed their life-styles, too; and they also ate less of some Japanese foods which could have been functioning as suppressants.

3. In the countries where meat consumption is high, some plausible associations of colon cancer with meat intake meriting further study are:

    a. That the higher incidence of colon cancer may be due to higher fat consumption, part of which is derived from meat.

    b. That the way in which the meat is prepared may be a causative factor.

(Also see CANCER.)

• **Fact or Myth: Meat causes high blood pressure (hypertension)**— Some have implicated meat as a cause of high blood pressure.

Fact: There is no evidence that meat per se has any major effect on high blood pressure. However, consumption of cured meat containing large amounts of salt should be minimized as should the amount of salt used as a condiment on meat and other foods. Other dietary factors that contribute to high blood pressure include obesity and excessive intake of alcohol.

(Also see HIGH BLOOD PRESSURE [HYPERTENSION].)

• **Fact or Myth: Meat contains harmful residues**—Do meats contain harmful toxic metals, pesticides, insecticides, animal drugs and additives?

Fact: If one pushed the argument of how safe is "safe" far enough, it would be necessary to forbid breast feeding as a source of food, because, from time to time, human milk has been found to contain DDT, antibiotics, thiobromine, caffeine, nicotine, and selenium.

Here are the facts relative to toxic metals, pesticides, insecticides, and animal drugs and additives in meats:

1. All metals are present in at least trace amounts in soil and water. It follows that they are also present in small amounts in plants and animals. But samplings of meat and poultry have not shown any toxic levels of these metals; hence, the normal intake of these metals in meats does not present any known hazard.

2. More than 1,000 drugs and additives are approved by the Food and Drug Administration (FDA) for use by livestock and poultry producers. They include products that fight disease, pesticides and insecticides to control pests and insects, protect animals from infection, and make for higher and more efficient production of meat, milk, and eggs. Some of these drugs and additives can leave potentially harmful residues. For this reason, the FDA requires drug withdrawal times on some of them, in order to protect consumers from residues. Additionally, federal agencies (USDA and/or FDA), as well as certain state and local regulatory groups, conduct continuous surveillance, sampling programs, and analyses of meats and other food products on their content of drugs and additives.

(Also see FOOD MYTHS AND MISINFORMATION; and POISONS.)

MEAT SUBSTITUTES (Meat Analogs). *An analog is something that is similar to some other thing. A meat analog is an engineered or fabricated protein food product.* For the most part, meat substitutes are either vegetable proteins or single-cell proteins. Among the factors favoring meat substitutes are: economy, convenience, dietary restrictions, religious preferences, and functionality.

In the American diet and economy, meat and poultry will continue to be important. Worldwide, the opportunities for meat substitutes are encouraging, due to doubling of the global population soon after the year 2000 and a shortage of meat in the developing countries.

Vegetable Meat Substitutes. Soybean protein is the most commonly used meat substitute at this time, but a wide range of other vegetable proteins are potential sources, including cottonseed, peanuts, safflower, and sunflower.

Soybeans have long been used by Asian cultures as a substitute for meat. Soy protein is commonly produced and marketed in three forms:

1. Flour or soy grits—40 to 60% protein.
2. Soy protein concentrate—not less than 70% protein.
3. Soybean protein isolates—not less than 90% protein.

Further processing of the basic forms—flours and grits, concentrates, and isolates—is now practiced to give soybean proteins a texture that resembles specific types of meat; these items range from extenders to be used with ground meats to complete meat analogs.

Two basic types of textured soybean protein products are now available:

1. *Extruded*, made by cooking soybean flour and other ingredients and forcing the mixture through small holes into a chamber of lower temperature and pressure. Granules of these expanded materials are available in both colored and uncolored and flavored and unflavored forms.

For the most part, extruded soy is used in combination with meat, as a ground meat extender.

2. *Spun*, made by spinning the fibers and then flavoring, coloring, and forming them in shapes which resemble pieces of meat, poultry, and fish.

Generally, spun soy is used as meat analogs; as baconlike bits, simulated sausages, simulated ham chunks, simulated chicken chunks, and simulated bacon slices.

Single-Cell Protein (SCP). *Single-cell protein (SCP) is protein obtained from single-cell organisms, such as yeast, bacteria, and algae, that have been grown on specially prepared growth media.* Production of this type of protein can be attained through the fermentation of petroleum derivatives or organic waste or through the culturing of photosynthetic organisms in special illuminated ponds.

Of course, yeast and bacteria have been used for centuries in the baking, brewing, and distilling industries, in making cheese and other fermented foods, and in the storage and preservation of foods. Dried brewers' yeast, a residue from the brewing industry, and torula yeast, resulting from the fermentation of wood residue and other cellulose sources, have been marketed as animal feeds for years.

A wide variety of materials can be used as substrates for the growth of these organisms. Current research deals with the use of industrial by-products which otherwise would have little or no economic value. By-products from the chemical, wood and paper, and food industries have shown considerable promise as sources of nutrients for single-cell organisms; among them, (1) crude and refined petroleum products, (2) methane, (3) alcohols, (4) sulfite waste liquor, (5) starch, (6) molasses, and (7) cellulose.

The potential of single-cell protein as a high-protein source for both man and livestock is enormous, but many obstacles must be overcome before it becomes widely used. It has been calculated that a single-cell protein fermenter covering .386 square mile (*1 km²*) could yield enough protein to supply 10% of the world's needs. To put this potential in a different perspective, a 1,000-lb steer will produce about 1 lb (*0.45 kg*) of protein per day. One thousand pounds of rapidly growing soybeans will produce 80 lb of protein per day. One thousand pounds of single-cell organisms might well produce up to 50 tons of protein per day. There is a limited amount of single-cell protein on the market in the form of brewers' yeast and torula yeast, but these products are generally too expensive to use as a major protein supplement; besides, they lack appetite appeal.

• **Types of single-cell protein**—Single-cell protein can be produced by nonphotosynthetic and photosynthetic organisms. Of the nonphotosynthetic organisms, yeasts are the most popular sources, but bacteria and fungi are also currently being investigated as potential sources. The photosynthetic organisms—algae—are grown in ponds that are illuminated and fortified with simple salts such as carbonates, nitrates, and phosphates.

• **Current problems associated with single-cell protein**—Although single-cell protein appears to be an excellent alternative source to the protein foods currently used, several problems must be overcome before it becomes a widely used foodstuff; among them, palatability, digestibility, nucleic acid content, toxins, protein quality, and economics.

(Also see SINGLE-CELL PROTEIN; SOYBEANS; and VEGETARIAN DIETS.)

MEAT ANALOGS

Food material usually prepared from vegetable protein to resemble specific meats in texture, color, and flavor.
(Also see SOYBEANS; and VEGETARIAN DIET.)

MEAT EXTRACT

This is a boiled down and concentrated extract of beef, veal, poultry, or game. Meat extracts should be regarded as condiments which impart the same flavor as the meat stock from which they were obtained.

MEAT FACTOR

A factor in meat which enhances the absorption of iron in the body. It has been demonstrated that beef, veal, pork, liver, chicken, and fish all increase iron absorption by two- to fourfold, while milk, cheese, and egg do not increase iron absorption.

MECHANICALLY EXTRACTED

A method of extracting the fat content from oilseeds by the application of heat and mechanical pressure. The hydraulic and expeller processes are both methods of mechanical extraction.
(Also see OILS, VEGETABLE.)

MEDICINAL PLANTS

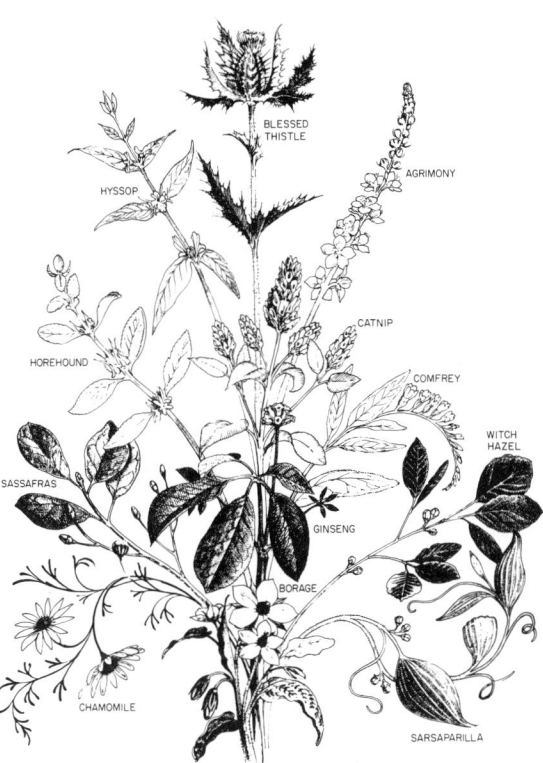

Fig. M-69. A bouquet of familiar medicinal herbs.

HISTORY. Almost every civilization has a history of medicinal plants. Perhaps, one of the oldest civilizations to record their use of plants for medicine is China. Books describing the use of plants as medicine are sometimes called herbals, and one of the earliest known herbals was supposedly written by the Chinese emperor Shen-Nung about 2700 B.C. About the time of the Chin and Han dynasties (202 B.C. to 220 A.D.), the first Chinese book on pharmacology was written. In it, 365 medicinal substances were recorded, with notes on the collection and preparation of the drugs. During the Tang dynasty, the government established a pharmacological institute which was called the Herbary. A total of 850 medicinal plants were grown on its 50 acres of fertile land. The cultivation, collection, and preparation of drugs were taught as basic subjects in this institute. In his *Magnum Opus*, Li Shih-chen (1518 to 1593 A.D.), the pharmacologist, recorded 1,892 drugs. In China today there is an attempt to mesh traditional Chinese medical practices with Western medical practices. Chinese traditional medical prescriptions are the roots, stems, bark, leaves, flowers, and fruits of shrubs and trees. A small part comes from birds, animals, insects, fish, and minerals. About 70% of the prescriptions made out in the hospitals and in the rural areas are for herbal medicine.

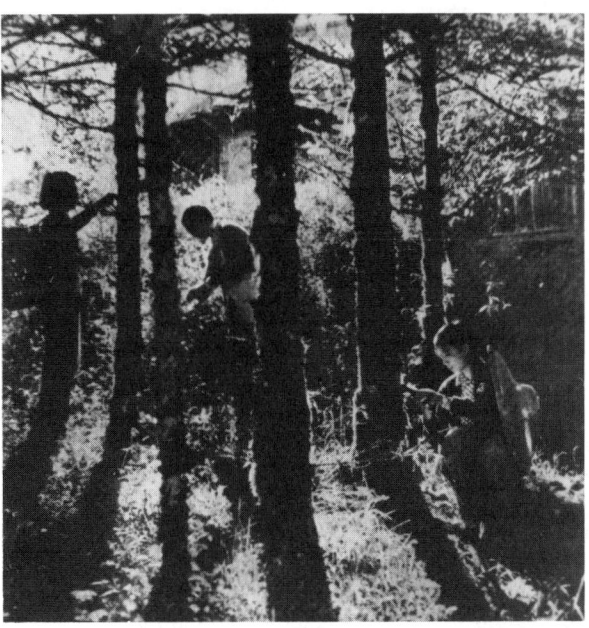

Fig. M-70. Gathering medicinal herbs on Omei Mountains in Szechwan Province, China.

Through the ages various plants have been tried as medicine to see which ones helped cure certain ailments of mankind. Thus, by trial and error, men came to use thousands of plants as remedies for their ills. For example, many American Indian tribes used willow bark to treat pain, but how the Indians came to choose willow bark is not known. Willow bark contains salicin, a forerunner of aspirin. While not all plants actually cured or relieved ailments, many did. Prescribing and dispensing medicinal plants, was the pharmaceutical industry of the past. Then, as science advanced, those plants which demonstrated positive effects on certain ailments were extracted, chemically analyzed, and their active chemicals were discovered. Thus, some traditional medicinal plants became stepping stones for the development of modern day drugs as active chemicals were isolated from plants, or were synthesized in laboratories. Although drugs used in medicine today are composed of specific chemicals extracted or derived from plants or synthesized by other methods, the direct use of plants for medicine still survives. There are endless books available describing the medicinal plants, their combinations, and conditions which they prevent, relieve, or cure. Sometimes it is called folk medicine, or herbal medicine. Indeed, whole businesses have grown up around the uses of herbs or medicinal plants. This article deals specifically with plants used directly for medicinal purposes.

In India, the oldest sacred writings of the Hindus, the four Vedas, refer to many healing plants.

Ancient Egyptian doctors practiced a combination of herbal medicine and faith healing. Carvings on tomb and temple walls indicate that people used plants for medicine around 3000 B.C., while a document written about 1500 B.C. described more than 800 remedies.

Hippocrates, the Father of Medicine, and other Greeks probably copied some of their plant lore from the Egyptians. About 370 B.C., Theophrastus, a pupil of Plato, wrote *An Enquiry Into Plants*, which contained a section on the medicinal properties of plants.

Dioscorides, a Greek surgeon in the Roman army, recorded the combined Egyptian, Greek, and Roman knowledge on the properties of plants. Much of the work of Dioscorides remained the basis of European medical practice for nearly 1500 years.

During the Middle Ages, Moslem pharmacists prepared herbal medicines for the disease-plagued Europeans. Men paid fantastic prices for these remedies since the Arabs controlled the drug and spice trade.

With the invention of printing, all knowledge became more widespread, and some of the first works printed following the *Bible* were books dealing with medicinal plants. In 1471, *De Agricultura* by Peter Crescentius, was published, containing complete, woodcut illustrated references to the useful and medicinal plants of southern Europe. More and more publications followed, and in 1597 *Gerard's Herbal* was published in England. Therefore, explorers of the New World must have been well versed in medicinal plants.

In the New World, Spanish explorers found the Incas and Aztecs using medicinal plants. The British and French explorers found the American Indians using still other plant remedies. As these plants were brought back to Europe, they were added to the European medicine chest and studied.

As the New World was settled, the herbal knowledge of the English soon meshed with that of the Indians who depended upon their medicine men. Benjamin Rush, a Philadelphia physician, investigated and wrote about the Indian cures. Soon, other compilers began to publish guides to Indian medicines during the early 1800s.

In the late 18th century and early 19th century, medicinal plants were primarily available to those who collected them in the wild. However, members of the Church of the United Society of Believers—the Shakers—were the first to mass produce herbs. By 1857, a Shaker settlement in New Lebanon, New York produced tons of medicinal plants which were shipped to every state and to England and Australia.

Gradually, as curiosity increased, scientists studied these medicinal plants handed down through the ages. They sought to discover the chemicals responsible for the healing properties of medicinal plants.

PLANT REMEDIES TO MODERN MEDICINE.

As scientists studied the medicinal plants, they isolated the active chemicals, which could then be put into liquids or pills. Furthermore, once the active chemicals were discovered, the hope was that these chemicals could be synthesized in the laboratory, thus eliminating the need for collecting and extracting tons of plants to meet medicinal needs. Discovery of some active chemicals did lead to their laboratory synthesis, while some drugs still must come from plants. Examples of some important chemicals derived from plants include (1) the pain killer morphine from the opium poppy, (2) the tranquilizer reser-pine from the snakeroot plant (rauwolfia), (3) the anesthetic cocaine from the coca plant, (4) the muscle relaxant and deadly poison curare from the curare vine, (5) the first malaria treatment, quinine from the bark of the cinchona tree, (6) the heart stimulant digitalis from the foxglove plant, and (7) the pupil-dilating drug atropine from the deadly nightshade. Thus, many medicinal plants handed down through the ages possess a chemical reason for their action. Other medicinal plants have been handed down through the ages, but without any specific reason for their success. No doubt other important drugs will be discovered in plants as the search continues with more sophisticated techniques. Drug companies and government agencies are screening and testing thousands of plants yearly in an effort to find new and more effective cures for the ailments of mankind.

LANGUAGE OF PLANT REMEDIES.

Along with the knowledge of the use of medicinal plants, a particular language has resulted which describes the method of use and the ailments for which plant remedies are employed. Some of the more important words commonly used follow:

• **Alteratives**—These are medicines that produce a gradual change for the better, and restore normal body function.

• **Anodyne**—Agents which relieve pain are called anodynes.

• **Astringent**—Substances which contract tissues and check the discharge of blood or mucus are termed astringents.

• **Carminative**—This is a substance that acts to reduce flatulence (gas).

• **Cathartics**—These are plant substances which relieve constipation by stimulating the secretions of the intestines.

• **Decoctions**—Decoctions are medicines made by simmering plant parts in water.

• **Demulcents**—These plant medicines are soothing to the intestinal tract and usually are of an oily or mucilaginous nature.

• **Diaphoretic**—This type of substance has the ability to produce sweating.

• **Emollients**—These act similar to demulcents but their soothing action is for the skin rather than the intestines.

• **Emmenagogues**—Plant remedies with this action are said to promote menstrual discharge.

• **Expectorants**—These are remedies which aid the patient in bringing up and spitting out excessive secretions of phlegm (mucus) from the lungs and windpipe.

• **Febrifuges**—These are the same as antipyretics—agents which help dissipate a fever.

• **Infusion**—This term applies to soaking of plant parts in water to extract their virtues. Infusions provide a quick and simple method for removing the medicinal principle from dried plant parts.

• **Nervines**—These substances are said to calm, soothe, and relax tensions caused by nervous excitement, strain, or fatigue.

• **Ointments and linaments**—The major difference between these is largely their consistency. An ointment is a semisolid in a fatty material, while a linament is a liquid or semiliquid preparation in a base of alcohol or oil.

• **Stimulants**—These are plant medicines which temporarily increase mental or physical activity.

• **Stomachics**—Plants with this property stimulate stomach secretions.

• **Tincture**—This refers to a solution of plant substances in alcohol. Tinctures contain those oils, resins, or waxes not soluble in water.

• **Tonic**—A tonic is said to be an agent which restores and invigorates the system and stimulates the appetite.

• **Vulneraries**—This word is often found in old herbals. It refers to medicines useful in healing wounds.

Table M-32 groups some of the medicinal plants according to the language of herbal medicine.

TABLE M-32
SOME MEDICINAL PLANTS GROUPED ACCORDING TO THEIR REPORTED EFFECTS AND USES

Alterative	Anodyne	Appetite Stimulation	Astringent	Calmative
agrimony	birch bark	alfalfa	agrimony	catnip
black cohosh root	hops	anise	bayberry	chamomile
blue flag root	white willow bark	chamomile	blackberry	fennel seeds
burdock root	wintergreen	celery	valerian	linden flowers
dandelion		dandelion	witch hazel	
echinacea		ginseng		
ginseng		juniper		
goldenseal		mint		
red clover flowers		parsley		
sarsaparilla root		rosemary		
sassafras root		sweet cicely		
		Virginia snakeroot		
		winter savory		
		wormwood		

Carminative	Cathartic	Demulcent	Diaphoretic	Diuretic
anise seed	barberry	borage	angelica root	alfalfa
capsicum	buckthorn bark	comfrey	borage	angelica
cardamom	chicory	marshmallow	catnip	bearberry leaves
catnip	colcynth		chamomile	buchu leaves
cumin	dandelion		ginger root	celery
fennel seed	senna		hyssop	chicory
ginger root			pennyroyal	cleaver's herb
goldenrod			sassafras	corn silk
lovage root			senega root	dandelion
nutmeg			serpentaria root	elecampane root
peppermint				goldenrod
spearmint				horehound
valerian root				horse tail grass
				juniper berries
				parsley root
				wild carrot

Expectorant	Febrifuge	Nervine	Stimulant	Tonic
acacia	angelica	catnip	angelica	barberry root
angelica	balm	chamomile	bayberry leaves	and bark
colt's foot	birch bark	hops	capsicum fruit	cascarilla bark
garlic	borage	linden flower	cardamom	celery seed
horehound	dandelion	passion flower	mayweed	dandelion root
licorice root	eucalyptus	skullcap	Paraguay tea	gentian root
senega root	lobelia	valerian root	sarsaparilla root	ginseng
	meadowsweet	yarrow	tansy	goldenseal
	pennyroyal		vervain	hops
	senna		wintergreen	mugwort
	willow bark			wormwood

COMMON MEDICINAL PLANTS AND THEIR REPORTED USES. Herbal medicine still lives in this day and age of antibiotics, antibodies, vaccines, and synthetic chemicals. In fact, there seems to have been a revitalization of herbal medicine with numerous new books printed on the subject and reprints of old books on the subject with increased sales of herbs, and mixtures of herbs to cure, relieve, or prevent almost every ailment. In Table M-33 which follows, some of the most common medicinal plants and their reported uses are described.

NOTE WELL: As part of the search for new and better drugs, thousands of plants are collected worldwide, and the information contained in old medical texts, herbals, and world folklore is also collected. This table is presented for informational purposes only, and perhaps to stimulate interest and research. No claim is made as to the efficacy of these medicinal plants.

TABLE M-33
SOME COMMON MEDICINAL PLANTS

Common and Scientific Name	Description	Production	Part(s) of Plant Used	Reported Uses
Agrimony *Agrimonia gryposepala*	Small yellow flowers on a long spike; leaves hairy and at least 5 in. (*13 cm*) long, narrow and pointed; leaf edges toothed; a perennial.	Needs good soil and sunshine; grows in New England and Middle Atlantic states.	Whole plant including roots.	A tonic, alterative, diuretic, and astringent; infusions from the leaves for sore throats; treatment of kidney and bladder stones; root for jaundice.
Aletris root (white-tube stargrass) *Aletris farinosa*	Grasslike leaves in a flat rosette around a spike-like stem; white to yellow tubular flowers along stem.	Moist locations in woods, meadows or bogs; New England to Michigan and Wisconsin; south to Florida and west to Texas.	Leaves; roots.	Poultice of leaves for sore breast; liquid from boiled roots for stomach pains, tonic, sedative, and diuretic.
Alfalfa *Medicago sativa*	Very leafy plant growing 1 to 2 ft (*30 to 61 cm*) high; small green leaves; bluish-purple flowers; deep roots.	A legume cultivated widely in the United States.	Leaves	Powdered and mixed with cider vinegar as a tonic; infusions for a tasty drink; leaves may also be used green.
Aloe vera *Aloe barbadensis*	A succulent plant with leathery sword-shaped leaves, 6 to 24 in. (*15 to 61 cm*) long.	A semidesert plant which grows in Mexico and Hawaii; temperature must remain above 50° F (*10° C*); can be a house plant.	Mucilaginous juice of the leaves.	Effective on small cuts and sunburn; speeds healing; manufactured product for variety of cosmetic purposes.
Angelica *Angelica atropurpurea*	Shrub growing to 8 ft (*2.4 m*) high; stem purplish with 3 toothed leaflets at tip of each leaf stem; white or greenish flowers in clusters at end of each stalk.	Grows in rich low soil near streams and swamps and in gardens; from New England west to Ohio, Indiana, Illinois, and Wisconsin; south to Delaware, Maryland, West Virginia, and Kentucky.	Roots; seeds.	Small amounts of dried root or seeds for relief of flatulence; roots for the induction of vomiting and perspiration; roots for treatment of toothache, bronchitis, rheumatism, gout, and fever; and to increase menstrual flow.
Anise (Anise seed) *Pimpinella anisum*	Annual plant, 1 to 2 ft (*30 to 61 cm*) high; belongs to carrot family; small white flowers on long hairy stalk; lower leaves egg-shaped; upper leaves feathery.	Grown all over the world; grows wild in countries around the Mediterranean; much is imported to United States.	Seed	As a hot tea to relieve flatulence or for colic.

(Continued)

TABLE M-33 *(Continued)*

Common and Scientific Name	Description	Production	Part(s) of Plant Used	Reported Uses
Asafetida *Ferula* sp	A coarse plant growing to 7 ft (*2.1 m*) high with numerous stem leaves; pale green-yellow flowers; flowers and seeds borne in clusters on stalks; large fleshy root; tenacious odor.	Indigenous to Afghanistan, but some species grow in other Asiatic countries.	Gummy resin from the root.	As an antispasmodic; to ward off colds and flu by wearing in a bag around the neck.
Barberry *Berberis vulgaris*	Perennial shrub growing to 8 ft (*2.4 m*) high; leaves are small and green on top and gray below; flowers yellow; the fruit scarlet to purple; inner wood yellow.	Grows along thickets and fence rows wild in New England, Delaware, and Pennsylvania, west to Minnesota, Iowa, and Missouri; introduced from Europe.	Stem bark; root bark; fruit.	Berries for drink to reduce fever; drink made from root bark steeped in beer for jaundice and hemorrhage; bark used to treat dysentery and indigestion; mashed roots for sore throats.
Bayberry (Southern wax myrtle) *Myrica cerifera*	Perennial shrub growing to 30 ft (*9.2 m*) high; waxy branchlets; narrow evergreen leaves tapering at both ends; yellowish flowers; fruits are grayish berries.	Grows in coastal regions from New Jersey, Delaware and Maryland to Florida, Alabama, Mississippi, and Arkansas.	Root bark; leaves and stems.	Decoction of root bark to treat uterine hemorrhage, jaundice, dysentery, and cankers; leaves and stems boiled and used to treat fevers, decoction of boiled leaves for intestinal worms.
Bearberry *Arctostaphylos uva-ursi*	Creeping evergreen shrub with stems up to 6 in. (*15 cm*) high; reddish bark; bright green leaves, 1 in. (*3 cm*) long; white flowers with red markings, in clusters; smooth red fruits.	Grows in well-drained soils at higher altitudes; from Oregon, Washington, and California, to Colorado and New Mexico.	Leaves	As a diuretic; also boiled infusions used as a drink to treat sprains, stomach pains, and urinary problems; poison oak inflammations treated with leaf decoction by pioneers.
Blackberry (brambleberry, dewberry, raspberry) *Rubus*	Shrubby or viny thorny perennial; numerous species; large white flowers; red or black fruit.	Grows wild or in gardens throughout the United States; wild in old fields, waste areas, forest borders, and pastures.	Roots; root bark, leaves; fruit.	Infusion made from roots used to dry up runny noses; infusion from root bark to treat dysentery; fruit used to treat dysentery in children; leaves also used in similar manner.
Black cohosh *Cimicifuga racemosa*	Perennial shrub growing to 9 ft (*2.7 m*) or more in height; leaf has 2 to 5 leaflets; plant topped with spike of slender candlelike, white or yellowish flowers; rhizome gnarled and twisted.	Grows throughout eastern United States; commercial supply from Blue Ridge Mountains.	Rhizomes and roots.	Infusion and decoctions used to treat sore throat, rheumatism, kidney trouble, general malaise; also used for "women's ailments" and malaria.

(Continued)

TABLE M-33 *(Continued)*

Common and Scientific Name	Description	Production	Part(s) of Plant Used	Reported Uses
Black Walnut *Juglans nigra*	A tree growing up to 120 ft (*36.6 m*) high; leaflets alternate 12 to 23 per stem, finely toothed and about 3 to 3 1/2 in. (*8 to 9 cm*) long; nut occurs singly or in clusters with fleshy, aromatic husk.	Native to a large section of the rich woods of eastern and midwestern United States.	Bark; nut husk; leaves.	Inner bark used as mild laxative; husk of nut used for treating intestinal worms, ulcers, syphilis, and fungus infections; leaf infusion for bedbugs.
Blessed thistle *Cnicus benedictus*	Annual plant growing to 2 ft (*61 cm*) high; spiny tooth, lobed leaves; many flowered yellow heads.	Grows along roadsides and in waste places in eastern and parts of southwestern United States.	Leaves and flowering tops in full bloom; seeds.	Infusions from leaves and tops for cancer treatment, to induce sweating, as a diuretic, to reduce fever, and for inflammations of the respiratory system; infusion of tops as Indian contraceptive; seeds induce vomiting.
Boneset *Eupatorium perfoliatum*	Perennial bush growing to 5 ft (*1.5 m*) in height; heavy stems with leaves opposite; purplish to white flowers borne in flat heads.	Commonly found in wet areas such as swamps, rich woods, marshes, and pastures; grows from Canada to Florida and west to Texas and Nebraska.	Leaves; flowering tops.	Infusion made from leaves used for laxative, and treatment of coughs and chest illnesses—a cold remedy; Negro slaves and Indians used it to treat malaria.
Borage *Borago officinalis*	Entire plant not over 1 ft (*30 cm*) high; nodding heads of starlike flowers grow from clusters of hairy obovate leaves.	Introduced in United States from Europe; occasionally grows in waste areas in northern states; cultivated widely in gardens.	Leaves	Most often used as an infusion to increase sweating, as a diuretic, or to soothe intestinal tract; can be applied to swellings and inflamed areas for relief.
Buchu *Rutaceae*	Low shrubs with angular branches and small leaves growing in opposition; flowers from white to pink.	Grown in rich soil in warm climate of South Africa.	Dried leaves.	Prepared as tincture or infusion; used for genito-urinary diseases, indigestion, edema, and early stages of diabetes.
Buckthorn *Rhamnus purshiana*	Deciduous tree growing to 25 ft (*7.6 m*) high; leaves 2 to 6 in. (*5 to 15 cm*) long; flowers small greenish yellow; fruit globular and black, about 1/4 in. (*6 mm*) across.	Grows usually with conifers along canyon walls, rich bottom lands and mountain ridges in western United States.	Bark; fruit.	Bark used as a laxative and tonic; fruit (berries) used as a laxative.
Burdock *Arctium minus*	Biennial or perennial growing 5 to 8 ft (*1.5 to 2.4 m*) high; large leaves resembling rhubarb; tube-shaped white and pink to purple flowers in heads, brown bristled burrs contain seeds.	Grows in wastelands, fields, and pastures throughout the United States.	Root	Infusion of roots for coughs, asthma, and to stimulate menstruation; tincture of root for rheumatism and stomachache.

(Continued)

TABLE M-33 (Continued)

Common and Scientific Name	Description	Production	Part(s) of Plant Used	Reported Uses
Calamus (Sweet flag) *Acorus calamus*	Perennial growing 3 to 5 ft (1.0 to 1.5 m) high; long narrow leaves with sharp edges; aromatic leaves; flower stalk 2 to 3 in. (3 to 8 cm) long and clublike; greenish-yellow flowers.	Grows in swamps, edges of streams and ponds from New England west to Oregon and Montana, and from Texas east to Florida and north.	Rhizomes	Root chewed to clear phlegm (mucous) and ease stomach gas; infusions to treat stomach distress; considered useful as tonic and stimulant.
Catnip *Nepeta cataria*	Perennial growing to 3 ft (1 m) in height; stem downy and whitish; leaves heart-shaped, opposite coarsely toothed and 2 to 3 in. (3 to 8 cm) long; tubular whitish with purplish marked flowers in compact spikes.	Grows wild along fences, roadsides, waste places, and streams in Virginia, Tennessee, West Virginia, Georgia, New England, Illinois, Indiana, Ohio, New Mexico, Colorado, Arizona, Utah, and California; readily cultivated in gardens.	Entire plant.	Infusions for treating colds, nervous disorders, stomach ailments, infant colic, and hives; smoke relieves respiratory ailments; poultice to reduce swellings.
Celery *Apium graveolens*	A biennial producing flower stalk second year; terminal leaflet at end of stem; fruit brown and round.	Cultivated in California, Florida, Michigan, New York, and Washington.	Seeds	As an infusion to relieve rheumatism and flatulence (gas); to act as a diuretic; to act as a tonic and stimulant; oil from seeds used similarly.
Chamomile *Anthemis nobilis*	Low growing, pleasantly strong-scented, downy and matlike perennial; daisylike flowers with white petals and yellow center.	Cultivated in gardens; some wild growing which escaped from gardens.	Leaves and flowers.	Powdered and mixed with boiling water to stimulate stomach, to remedy nervousness in women, and stimulate menstrual flow, also a tonic; flowers for poultice to relieve pain; Chamomile tea known as soothing, sedative, completely harmless.
Chaparral *Croton corynbulosus*	Shrubby perennial plant of the Spurge family.	Grows in dry rocky areas from Texas west.	Flowering tips.	Infusions act as laxative; some claims as cancer treatment.
Chickweed *Stellaria media*	Annual growing 12 to 15 in. (30 to 38 cm) high; stems matted to somewhat upright; upper leaves vary but lower leaves ovate; white, small individual flowers.	Grows in shaded areas, meadows, wasteland, cultivated land, thickets, gardens, and damp woods in Virginia to South Carolina and southeast.	Entire plant in full bloom.	Poultice made to treat sores, ulcers, infections, and hemorrhoids.
Chicory *Cichorium intybus*	Easily confused with its close relative the dandelion; in bloom bears blue or soft pink blooms not resembling dandelion.	Introduced from Europe, now common wild plant in United States; some grown in gardens.	Roots; leaves.	No great medicinal value; some mention of diuretic, laxative, and tonic use; mainly added to give coffee distinctive flavor.

(Continued)

TABLE M-33 *(Continued)*

Common and Scientific Name	Description	Production	Part(s) of Plant Used	Reported Uses
Cinnamon *Cinnamomum zeylanicum*	An evergreen bush or tree growing to 30 ft *(9 m)* high.	A native plant of Sri Lanka, India, and Malaysia; tree kept pruned to a shrub; bark of lower branches peeled and dried.	Bark	Treatment for flatulence, diarrhea, vomiting, and nausea.
Cleaver's herb (Catchweed bedstraw) *Galium aparine*	Annual plant; weak reclining bristled stem with hairy joints; leaves in whorls of 8; white flowers in broad, flat cluster; bristled fruit.	Grows in rich woods, thickets, seashores, waste areas, and shady areas from Canada to Florida and west to Texas.	Entire plant during flowering.	To increase urine formation; to stimulate appetite; to reduce fever; to remedy vitamin C deficiency; also used to remove freckles.
Cloves *Syzygium aromaticum*	Dried flower bud of a tropical tree which is a 30-ft *(9 m)* high red flowered evergreen.	Tree native to Molucca, but widely cultivated in tropics; flower bud picked before flower opens and dried.	Flower bud.	To promote salivation and gastric secretion; to relieve pain in stomach and intestines; applied externally to relieve rheumatism, lumbago, toothache, muscle cramps, and neuralgia; clove oil used, too; infusions with clove powder relieves nausea and vomiting.
Colt's foot (Canada wild ginger) *Asarum canadense*	Low growing stemless perennial; heart-shaped leaves; flowers near root and brown and bell-shaped.	Found in moist woods from Maine to Georgia and west to Ohio.	Roots; leaves.	Infusion of root to relieve flatulence; powdered root to relieve flatulence; induce sweating, and to relieve aching head and eyes; leaves substitute for ginger.
Comfrey *Symphytum officinale*	A perennial which reaches about 2 ft *(61 cm)* in height; leaves are large and broad at base but lancelike at terminal; fine hair on leaves; tail-shaped head of white to purple flowers at terminal.	Prefers a moist environment; a European plant now naturalized in the United States.	Roots; leaves.	Numerous uses including treatments for pneumonia, coughs, diarrhea, calcium deficiency, colds, sores, ulcers, arthritis, gallstones, tonsils, cuts and wounds, headaches, hemorrhoids, gout, burns, kidney stones, anemia, and tuberculosis; used as a poultice, infusion, powder, or in capsule form.
Dandelion *Taraxacum officinale*	Biennial or perennial growing 2 to 12 in. *(5 to 30 cm)* high; leaves deeply serrated forming a basal rosette in spring; yellow flower but turns to gray upon maturing.	Weed throughout the United States; the bane of lawns.	Flowers; roots; green leaves.	Root uses include diuretic, laxative, tonic and to stimulate appetite; infusion from flower for heart troubles; paste of green leaves and bread dough for bruises.

(Continued)

TABLE M-33 *(Continued)*

Common and Scientific Name	Description	Production	Part(s) of Plant Used	Reported Uses
Echinecea (Purple echinacea) *Echinacea purpurea*	Perennial from 2 to 5 ft (0.6 to 1.5 m) high; alternate lance-shaped leaves; leaf margins toothed; top leaves lack stems; purple to white flower.	Grows wild on road banks, prairies, and dry, open woods in Ohio to Iowa, south to Oklahoma, Georgia, and Alabama.	Roots	Treatment of ulcers and boils, syphilis, snakebites, skin diseases, and blood poisoning; used as powder and in capsules.
Eucalyptus *Eucalyptus globulus*	Tall, fragrant tree growing up to 300 ft (92 m) high; reddish-brown stringy bark.	Native to Australia but grown in other semitropical and warm temperate regions.	Leaves and oil distilled from leaves.	Antiseptic value; inhaled freely for sore throat; asthma relief; local application to ulcers; used on open wounds.
Eyebright (Indian tobacco) *Lobelia inflata*	Branching annual growing to 3 ft (1 m) high with leaves 1 to 3 in. (3 to 8 cm) long; small violet to pinkish-white flowers in axils of leaves; seed capsules at base of flower containing many tiny brown seeds.	Roadside weed of eastern United States, west to Kansas.	Entire plant in full bloom or when seeds are formed.	Treatment of whooping cough, asthma, epilepsy, pneumonia, hysteria, and convulsion; alkaloid extracted for use in antismoking preparations.
Fenugreek *Trigonella foenum-graceum*	Annual plant similar to clover in size.	Native to the Mediterranean region and northern India; widely cultivated; easily grown in home gardens.	Seed	Poultice for wounds; gargle for sore throat.
Flax (Linseed) *Linum usitatissimum*	Herbaceous annual; slender upright plant with narrow leaves and blue flowers; grows to about 2 ft (61cm) high.	Originated in Mediterranean region; cultivated widely for fiber and oil.	Seed	Ground flaxseed mixed with boiling water for poultice on burns, boils, carbuncles, and sores; internally as a laxative.
Garlic *Allium sativum*	Annual plant growing to 12 in. (30 cm) high; long, linear, narrow leaves; bulb composed of several bulblets.	Throughout the United States under cultivation; some wild.	Entire plant when in bloom; bulbs.	Fresh poultice of the mashed plant for treating snake bite, hornet stings, and scorpion stings; eaten to expel worms, treat colds, coughs, hoarseness, and asthma; bulb expressed against the gum for toothache.
Gentian (Sampson's snakeroot) *Gentiana villosa*	Perennial with stems growing 8 to 10 in. (20 to 25 cm) high; opposite ovate, lance-shaped leaves; pale blue flowers.	Grows wild in swampy areas Florida west to Louisiana, north to New Jersey, Pennsylvania, Ohio, and Indiana.	Rhizomes and roots.	Treatment of indigestion, gout, and rheumatism; induction of vomiting; aid to digestion; a tonic.
Ginger *Zingiber officinale*	Perennial plant; forms irregular shaped rhizomes at shallow depth.	Native to southeastern Asia; now grown all over tropics.	Rhizome	An expectorant; treatment of flatulence, colds, and sore throats.

(Continued)

TABLE M-33 *(Continued)*

Common and Scientific Name	Description	Production	Part(s) of Plant Used	Reported Uses
Ginseng *Panax quinquefolia*	Hollow stems solid at nodes; leaves alternate; root often resembles shape of a man; small, inconspicuous flowers; vivid, shiny, scarlet berries.	Grows in eastern Asia, Korea, China, and Japan; some grown in United States.	Root	As a tonic and stimulant; treatment of convulsions, dizziness, vomiting, colds, fevers, headaches, and rheumatism; commonly believed to be an aphrodisiac.
Goldenrod *Solidago odora*	Grows 18 to 36 in. *(46 to 91 cm)* high with narrow leaves scented like anise; inconspicuous head with 6 to 8 flowers.	Grows throughout the United States.	Leaves	Infusions from dried leaves as aromatic stimulant, a carminative and a diuretic.
Goldenseal *Hydrastis canadensis*	Perennial growing to about 1 ft *(30 cm)* high; one stem with 5 to 7 lobed leaves near top; several single leafstalks topped with petalless flowers; raspberrylike fruit but inedible.	Grows in rich, shady woods of southeastern and midwestern United States; grown under cultivation in Washington.	Roots; leaves, and stalks.	Root infusion as an appetite stimulant and tonic; root powder for open cuts and wounds; chewing root for mouth sores; leaf infusion for liver and stomach ailments.
Guarana *Paullinia cupana*	Climbing shrub of the soapberry family; yellow flowers; pear-shaped fruit; seed in 3-sided, 3-celled capsules.	Grows in South America particularly Brazil and Uruguay.	Seeds	Stimulant, seeds high in caffeine.
Hawthorn *Crataegus oxycantha*	Hardy shrub or tree depending upon growth conditions; small, berry fruit; cup-shaped flowers with 5 parts; thorny stems.	Originally grown throughout England as hedges; also grows wild; some introduced in the United States.	Berry	Tonic for heart ailments such as angina pectoris, valve defects, rapid and feeble heart beat, and hypertrophied heart; reverses arteriosclerosis.
Hop *Humulus lupulus*	Twining, perennial growing 20 ft *(6 m)* or more; 3 smooth-lobed leaves 4 to 5 in. *(10 to 13 cm)* long; membranous, conelike fruit.	Grows throughout the United States; often a cultivated crop.	Fruit (hops).	Straight hops or powder used; hot poultice of hops for boils and inflammations; treatment of fever, worms, rheumatism; as a diuretic; as a sedative.
Horehound (White horehound) *Marrubium vulgare*	Shrub growing to 3 ft *(1 m)* in height; fuzzy ovate-round leaves which are whitish above and gray below; foliage aromatic when crushed.	Grows wild throughout most of United States in pastures, old fields, and waste places, except in arid southwest.	Leaves and small stems; bark.	Decoctions to treat coughs, colds, asthma, and hoarseness; other uses include treatments for diarrhea, menstrual irregularity, and kidney ailments.
Huckleberry (Sparkleberry) *Vaccinium arboreum*	Shrub or tree growing to 25 ft *(7.6 m)* high; leathery, shiny, thick leaves; white flowers; black berries; other species.	Grows wild in woods, clearings, sandy and dry woods in Virginia, Georgia, Florida, Mississippi, Indiana, Illinois, Missouri, Texas, and Oklahoma.	Leaves, root bark, and berries.	Decoctions of leaves and root bark to treat sore throat and diarrhea; drink from berry for treating chronic dysentery.

(Continued)

TABLE M-33   *(Continued)*

Common and Scientific Name	Description	Production	Part(s) of Plant Used	Reported Uses
Hyssop *Hyssopus officinalis*	Hardy, fragrant, bushy plants belonging to the mint family; stem woody; leaves hairy, pointed and about 1/2 in. (20 mm) long; blue flowers in tufts.	Grows in various parts of Europe including the Middle East; some grown in United States.	Leaves	Infusions for colds, coughs, tuberculosis, and asthma; an aromatic stimulant; healing agent for cuts and bruises.
Juniper (Common juniper) *Juniperus communis*	Small evergreen shrub growing 12 to 30 ft (3.7 to 9.2 m) high; bark of trunk reddish-brown and tends to shred; needles straight and at right angles to branchlets; dark, purple, fleshy berrylike fruit.	Widely distributed from New Mexico to Dakotas and east; dry areas.	Fruit (berries).	Used as a diuretic, to induce menstruation, to relieve gas, and to treat snake bites and intestinal worms.
Lemon balm *Melissa officinalis*	Persistent perennial growing to 1 ft (30 cm) high; light green, serrated leaves; lemon smell and taste to crushed leaves.	Wild in much of the United States, grown in gardens.	Leaves	Infusion used as a carminative; diaphoretic or febrifuge.
Licorice (Wild licorice) *Glycyrrhiza lepidota*	Erect perennial growing to 3 ft (1 m) high; pale yellow to white flowers at end of flower stalks; brown seed pods resemble cockleburrs.	Grows wild on prairies, lake shores, railroad-right-of-ways throughout much of the United States.	Root *Caution:* Licorice raises the blood pressure of some people dangerously high, due to the retention of sodium.	Root extract to help bring out phlegm (mucus); treatment of stomach ulcers, rheumatism and arthritis; root decoctions for inducing menstrual flow, treating fevers, and expulsion of afterbirth.
Marshmallow *Althaea officinalis*	Stems erect and 3 to 4 ft (0.9 to 1.2 m) high with only a few lateral branches; roundish, ovate-cordate leaves 2 to 3 in. (5 to 8 cm) long and irregularly toothed at margin; cup-shaped, pale colored flowers.	Introduced into United States from Europe; now found on banks of tidal rivers and brackish streams; grew wild in salt marches, damp meadows, by ditches, by the sea, and on banks of tidal rivers from Denmark south.	Root	Primarily a demulcent and emollient; used in cough remedies; good poultice made from crushed roots.
Motherwort *Leonurus cardiaca*	Perennial growing 5 to 6 ft (1.5 to 1.8 m) high; lobed, dented leaves, 5 in. (13 cm) long; very fuzzy white to pink flowers.	Grows wild in pastures, waste places, and roadsides from northeastern states west to Montana and Texas, south to North Carolina and Tennessee.	Entire plant above ground.	Used as a stimulant, tonic, and diuretic; Europeans used for asthma and heart palpitation; usually taken as an infusion.

(Continued)

TABLE M-33   *(Continued)*

Common and Scientific Name	Description	Production	Part(s) of Plant Used	Reported Uses
Mullien (Aaron's rod) *Verbascum thapsus*	At base a rosette of woody, lance-shaped, oblong leaves with a diameter of up to 2 ft (61 cm); yellow flowers along a clublike spike arising from the rosette to a height of up to 7 ft (2.1 m).	Grows wild throughout the United States in dry fields, meadows, pastures, rocky or gravelly banks, burned areas, etc.	Leaves; roots; flowers.	Infusions of leaves to treat colds and dysentery; dried leaves and flowers serve as a demulcent and emollient; leaves smoked for asthma relief; boiled roots for croup; oil from flowers for earache; local applications of leaves for hemorrhoids, inflammations, and sunburn.
Nutmeg *Muristica fragrans*	Evergreen tree growing to about 25 ft (7.6 m) high; grayish-brown, smooth bark; fruit resembles yellow plum, the seed of which is known as nutmeg.	Native to Spice Islands of Indonesia; now cultivated in other tropical areas.	Seed	For the treatment of nausea and vomiting; grated and mixed with lard for hermorrhoid ointment.
Papaya *Carica papaya*	Small tree seldom above 20 ft (6.1 m) high; soft, spongy wood; leaves as large as 2 ft (61 cm) in diameter and deeply cut into 7 lobes; fruit oblong and dingy green-yellow.	Originated in South American tropics; now cultivated in tropical climates.	Leaves	Dressing for wounds, and aid to digestion; contains proteolytic enzyme, papain, used as a meat tenderizer.
Parsley *Petroselinum crispum*	Biennial which is usually grown as an annual; finely divided, often curled, fragrant leaves.	Originated in the Mediterranean area; now grown worldwide.	Leaves; seeds; roots.	As a diuretic with aromatic and stimulating properties.
Passion flower (Maypop passion-flower) *Passiflora incarnata*	Perennial vine growing to 30 ft (9.2 m) in length; alternate leaves composed of 3 to 5 finely toothed lobes; showy, vivid, purple, flesh-colored flowers; smooth, yellow ovate fruit 2 to 3 in. (5 to 8 cm) long.	Grows wild in West Indies and southern United States; cultivated in many areas.	Flowering and fruiting tops.	Crushed parts for poultice to treat bruises and injuries; other uses include treatment of nervousness, insomnia, fevers, and asthma.
Peppermint *Mentha piperita*	Perennial growing to about 3 1/2 ft (1m) high; dark, green, toothed leaves; purplish flowers in spike-like groups.	Originated in temperate regions of the Old World where most is still grown; grows in shady damp areas in many areas of the United States; grown in gardens.	Flowering tops; leaves.	Infusions for relief of flatulence, nausea, headache, and heartburn; fresh leaves rubbed into skin to relieve local pain; extracted oil contains medicinal properties.
Plantain *Plantago* sp	Low perennial with broad leaves; flowers on erect spikes.	Grows wild throughout the United States in poor soils, fields, lawns, and edges of woods.	Leaves; seeds; root.	Infusion of leaves for a tonic; seeds for laxative; soaking seeds provides sticky gum for lotions; fresh, crushed leaves to reduce swelling of bruised body parts; fresh, boiled roots applied to sore nipples.

(Continued)

TABLE M-33   (Continued)

Common and Scientific Name	Description	Production	Part(s) of Plant Used	Reported Uses
Pleurisy root (Butterfly milkweed) *Asclepias tuberosa*	Leafy perennial growing to 3 ft (*1 m*) high; alternate leaves which are 2 to 6 in. (*5 to 15 cm*) long and narrow; bright orange flowers in a cluster; root spindle-shaped with knotty crown.	Grows in sandy, dry soils; pastures, roadsides, and gardens; south to Florida and west to Texas and Arizona.	Root	Small doses of dried root as a diaphoretic, diuretic, expectorant, and alterative; ground roots fresh or dried for poultice to treat sores.
Queensdelight *Stillingia sylvatica*	Perennial growing to 3 ft (*1 m*) high; contains milky juice; leathery, fleshy, stemless leaves; yellow flowers.	Grows wild in dry woods, sandy soils and old fields; Virginia to Florida, Kansas, and Texas, north to Oklahoma.	Root	Treatment of infectious diseases; as an alterative.
Red clover *Trifolium pratense*	Biennial or perennial legume less than 2 ft (*61 cm*) high; 3 oval-shaped leaflets form leaf; flowers globe-shaped and rose to purple colored.	Throughout United States; some wild, some cultivated.	Entire plant in full bloom.	Infusions to treat whooping cough; component of salves for sores and ulcers; flowers as sedative; to relieve gastric distress and improve the appetite.
Rosemary *Rosmarinus officinalis*	Low-growing perennial evergreen shrub; leaves about 1 in. (*3 cm*) long and dark green on top and paler below; flowers small and pale blue.	Native to Mediterranean region; now cultivated in most of Europe and the Americas.	Leaves	Used as a tonic, astringent, diaphoretic, stimulant, carminative, and nervine.
Saffron (Safflower) *Carthamus tinctorius*	Annual with alternate spring leaves; grows to 3 ft (*1 m*) in height; orange-yellow flowers; white, shiny seeds.	Wild in Afghanistan; cultivated in the United States primarily in California.	Flowers; seeds; entire plant in bloom.	Paste of flowers and water applied to boils; flowers soaked in water to make a drink to reduce fever; as a laxative; to induce perspiration; to stimulate menstrual flow; to dry up skin symptoms of measles.
Sage (Garden sage) *Salvia officinalis*	Fuzzy perennial belonging to the mint family; leaves with toothed edges; terminal spikes bearing blue or white flowers in whorls.	Originated in the Mediterranean area where it grows wild and is cultivated; grown throughout the United States, some wild.	Leaves	Treatment for wounds and cuts, sores, coughs, colds, and sore throat; infusions used as a laxative and to relieve flatulence; major use for treatment of dyspepsia.
Sarsaparilla *Smilax* sp	Climbing evergreen shrub with prickly stems; leaves round to oblong; small, globular berry for fruit.	Grown in tropical areas of Central and South America and in Japan and China.	Root	Primarily an alterative regarded as an aphrodisiac; for colds and fevers; to relieve flatulence; best used as an infusion.

(Continued)

TABLE M-33 *(Continued)*

Common and Scientific Name	Description	Production	Part(s) of Plant Used	Reported Uses
Sassafras *Sassafras albidum*	Tree growing to 40 ft (*12.2 m*) high; leaves may be 3-lobed, 2-lobed, mitten-shaped, or unlobed; yellowish-green flowers in clusters; pea-sized, 1-seeded berries in fall.	Originated in New World; grows in New England, New York, Ohio, Illinois, and Michigan, south to Florida and Texas; grows along roadsides, in woods, along fences, and in fields.	Root bark.	Sassafras was formerly used for medical purposes. But the use of the roots was banned by the FDA because of their carcinogenic qualities.
Saw palmetto *Serenoa serrulata*	Low-growing fan palm; whitish bloom covers saw-toothed, green leaves; flowers in branching clusters; fruit varies in size and shape.	Grows in warm, swampy, low areas near the coast.	Fruit (berries).	To improve digestion; to treat respiratory infections; as a tonic and as a sedative.
Senna (Wild senna) *Cassia marilandica*	Perennial growing to 6 ft (*1.8 m*) in height; alternate leaves with leaflets in pairs of 5 to 10; bright yellow flowers.	Grows along roadsides and in thickets from Pennsylvania to Kansas and Iowa, south to Texas and Florida.	Leaves	Infusions primarily employed as a laxative.
Skullcap *Scutellaria lateriflora*	Perennial growing 1 to 2 ft (*30 to 61 cm*) high; toothed, lance-shaped leaves; blue or whitish flowers.	Native to most sections of the United States; prefers moist woods, damp areas, meadows, and swampy areas.	Entire plant in bloom.	Powdered plant primarily a nervine.
Spearmint *Mentha spicata*	Perennial resembling other mints; grows to 3 ft (*1 m*) in height; pink or white flowers borne in long spikes.	Throughout the United States in damp places; cultivated in Michigan, Indiana, and California.	Above ground parts.	Primarily a carminative; administered as an infusion though extracted oils.
Tansy *Tanacetum vulgare*	Perennial growing to 3 ft (*1 m*) in height; pungent fernlike foliage with tops of composite heads of buttonlike flowers.	Grown or escaped into the wild in much of the United States.	Leaves and flowering tops.	Infusions used as stomachic, emmenagogue, or to expel intestinal worms; extracted oil induced abortion often with fatal results; poultice for sprains and bruises.

(Continued)

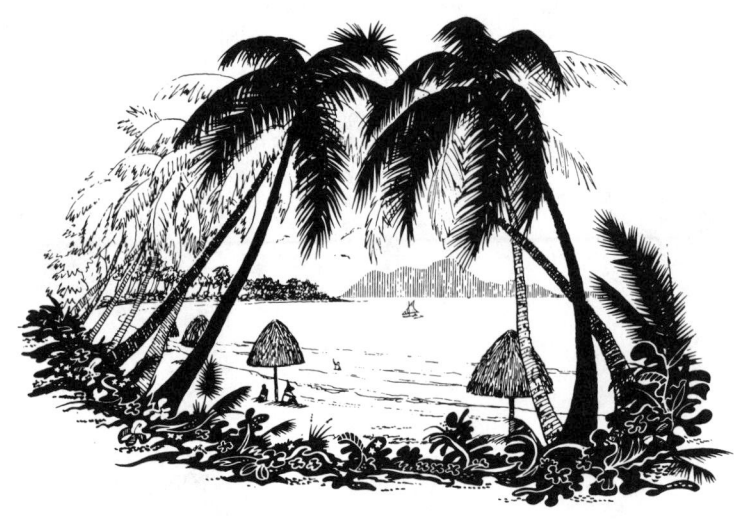

TABLE M-33 *(Continued)*

Common and Scientific Name	Description	Production	Part(s) of Plant Used	Reported Uses
Valerian *Valeriana officinalis*	Coarse perennial growing to 5 ft (*1.5 m*) high; fragrant, pinkish-white flowers opposite pinnate leaves.	Native to Europe and Northern Asia; cultivated in the United States.	Root	As a calmative and as a carminative.
Witch hazel *Hamamelis virginiana*	Crooked tree or shrub 8 to 15 ft (*2.4 to 4.6 m*) in height; smooth, brown bark; roundish to oval leaves; yellow, thread-like flowers; fruits in clusters along the stem eject shiny, black seeds.	Found in damp woods of North America from Nova Scotia to Florida and west to Minnesota and Texas.	Leaves; bark and twigs.	Twigs, leaves, and bark basis for witch hazel extract which is included in many lotions for bruises, sprains, and shaving; bark sometimes applied to tumors and skin inflammations; some preparations for treating hemmorrhoids.
Yerba santa *Eriodictyon californicum*	Evergreen shrub with lance-shaped leaves.	Part of flora of the west coast of the United States.	Leaves	As an expectorant; recommended for asthma and hay fever.

WORDS OF CAUTION. Herbal medicine, folk medicine, or whatever it is called is back in vogue. It is appealing because most remedies are handy, inexpensive, and "natural." Moreover, folk medicine gives people the feeling that they are taking care of themselves. With this return to folk medicine, there are numerous purveyors; hence, people should be wary. Many generalized and meaningless claims are employed to describe the action of certain plant remedies. For example, such claims include the following: purify the blood; strengthen the glands; establish a normal balance; strengthen the nerves; balance the female organism; encourage rejuvenation; and ease nerve pain. These claims could describe any number of symptoms or cures—or none at all. Moreover, some plant remedies are still recommended on the basis of the "doctrine of signatures," which held that plant remedies could be identified by their resemblance to the afflicted part of the body. Names like liverwort and heartsease recall this belief.

As long as herbal medicine is not poisonous and does not replace traditional, professional medicine in serious ailments, no harm is likely. However, the individual subscribing to herbal medicine should be certain of the identity of the plants used since some are poisonous and others may have serious side effects. Overall, herbal medicine is safe, fun, and some of it probably even helps ease minor ailments.

(Also see POISONOUS PLANTS; and WILD EDIBLE PLANTS.)

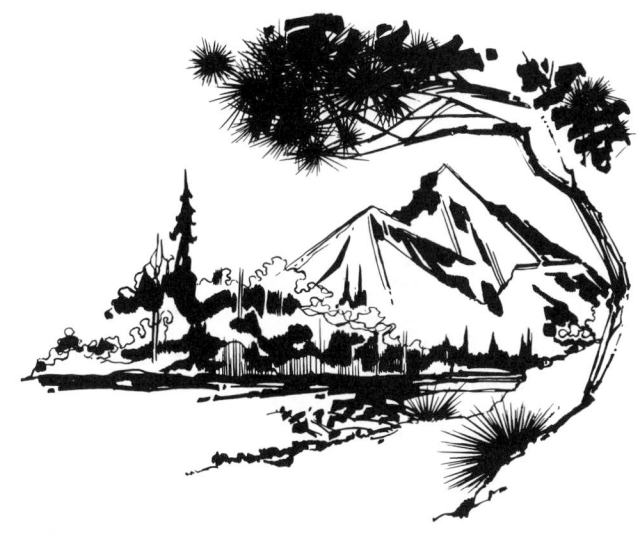

MEDIUM CHAIN TRIGLYCERIDES (MCT)

This is a special dietary product made from coconut oil by (1) steam and pressure hydrolysis of the oil into free fatty acids and glycerol, (2) separation of the resulting hydrolysate into medium-chain and long-chain fatty acids, and (3) recombination of the medium-chain fatty acids with glycerol to form MCT oil. It is composed of about ¾ caprylic acid, a saturated fatty acid containing 8 carbon atoms; and about ¼ capric acid, a saturated fatty acid containing 10 carbon atoms. The special nutritive values of this product are as follows:

1. It is much more readily digested, absorbed, and metabolized than either animal fats or vegetable oils which contain mainly long-chain triglycerides. The enzyme, pancreatic lipase, can easily break down MCT. Hence, MCT oil is valuable in the dietary treatment of fatty diarrhea and other digestive disorders in which the absorption of fat is impaired—malabsorption.

2. Medium-chain triglycerides, unlike other saturated fats, do *not* contribute to a rise in blood cholesterol. Therefore, they are used to treat some forms of hyperlipoproteinemia.

At the present time, MCT oil is used almost exclusively for special dietary formulations in the United States, but it is also available in various nonmedical consumer products in Europe.

(Also see HYPERLIPOPROTEINEMIAS; and MALABSORPTION SYNDROME.)

MEGADOSE

A very large dose; for example, taking 20 to 100 times the recommended allowance of vitamin C.

MEGAJOULE (MJ)

A metric unit of energy, equivalent to 240 kcal.

MEGALOBLAST

A large embryonic type of red blood cell with a large nucleus; present in the blood in cases of pernicious anemia, vitamin B-12 deficiency, and/or folacin deficiency.

MELANIN

Any of the various dark brown or black pigments of the skin, hair, and certain other tissues; derived from tyrosine metabolism.

MELBA TOAST

This is very thin bread which is toasted or baked until crisp and well browned. Thus, rusks, croutons, and Melba toast all have one thing in common—all of them are made from bread which is baked until dry and crisp.

MELON(S)

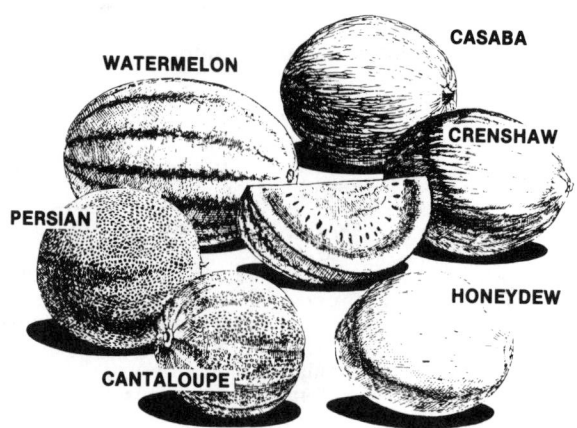

Fig. M-71. Common melons—all sizes, shapes, colors, and flavors.

The term *melon* is applied to the fruit of several closely related plants of the cucurbit family (*Cucurbitaceae*)—a family whose members include cucumbers, pumpkins, squashes, watermelons, and gourds.

Melons grow on plants that are either climbing or trailing vines with round, pointed or folded leaves, and small, yellow flowers. Melons are oblong to round. The surface of the melon is a skin called a rind which may be smooth, wrinkled, warty, netted, or ridged, and colored tan and yellow to light or dark green. The edible flesh—the pulp—may be green, white, yellow, pink, or red.

Melons include the summer melons, muskmelons, or cantaloupes; the winter melons, casaba, honeydew, crenshaw, and Persian melon; and watermelons. Brief descriptions of these melons follow:

• **Cantaloupe**—This is a variety of muskmelon, sometimes it is even called muskmelon. The netted-rind of the cantaloupe is yellow-green while the pulp is orange. Cantaloupes range in size from 4 to 7 in. (*10 to 17.5 cm*) in diameter. Although there are several varieties of cantaloupes which are grown in different climatic regions of the United States, California is by far the largest producer of the fruit. Usually, cantaloupes require about 3 months or so to reach maturity. Most of the crop is sold fresh, but some is canned or frozen in the form of melon balls.

• **Casaba**—The casaba is a golden-yellow, wrinkled-rind, round variety of muskmelon which has a white-colored flesh. Casabas range from 6 to 8 in. (*15 to 20 cm*) in diameter. This fruit requires a hot, dry climate and reaches maturity in about 3½ months. Most of the U.S. production is grown on irrigated fields in the southwestern and western states. All of the crop is marketed fresh right after harvesting or after a brief period of storage.

• **Honeydew**—This variety of melon has a white, smooth rind and light-green pulp. It is about 7 in. (*17.5 cm*) in diameter and 8 in. (*20 cm*) long. Honeydew melons grow best in hot, dry climates and require about 4 months to reach maturity. They are called winter melons because they ripen late in the season and are marketed during the winter. Most of the U.S. production comes from irrigated fields in the southwestern and western states. They are usually used fresh and as canned or frozen melon balls packed in syrup.

• **Crenshaw**—Crenshaw melons are oblong, with a yellow-tan, smooth rind. Their pulp is salmon-orange in color. Crenshaws are usually about 6 in. *(15 cm)* in diameter and about 7 in. *(17.5 cm)* long. These melons require a hot, dry climate and reach maturity in about 4 months. Most of the U.S. production is grown in irrigated fields in the southwestern and western states. All of this crop is marketed fresh.

• **Persian**—These melons are round with a dark green netted, rind and orange pulp. There are small Persian melons that are 4 to 5 in. *(10 to 12.5 cm)* in diameter and large types that are 7 to 10 in. *(17.5 to 25 cm)* in diameter. Persian melons require a hot, dry climate and reach maturity in about 4 months. Most of the U.S. crop is grown in the southwestern states.

• **Watermelon**—All the melons listed above belong to the genus and species *Cucumis melo*, but the scientific name for watermelon is *Citrullus vulgaris*. Depending upon the variety, watermelons weigh 5 to 85 lb *(2.3 to 38.3 kg)* and vary in shape from round to oval to oblong-cylindrical. The rind may be very light to very dark-green with stripes or mottling, while the pulp is red, pink, orange, yellow, or white. Watermelons are grown in tropical, semitropical, and temperate climates. In the United States commercial watermelon production occurs primarily in the southern states.

Nutritionally, melons are all quite similar containing only about 30 Calories (kcal) per 100 g and being good sources of potassium, vitamin C, and vitamin A when the flesh is deep orange. Melons are all about 90% water. More complete information regarding the nutritional value of melons is in Food Composition Table F-36.

(Also see CANTALOUPE; FRUIT[S], Table F-47 Fruits of the World; and WATERMELON.)

MELON PEAR (PEPINO) *Solanum Muricatum*

The yellow and purple streaked fruit of a shrub (of the family *Solanaceae*) that is native to Peru, but is now grown in various parts of the American tropics. It is between 4 and 6 in. *(10 and 15 cm)* long, and has an aromatic pulp that is used to make drinks, jams, and jellies.

The pulp of the fruit is high in water content (92%) and low in calories (32 kcal per 100 g) and carbohydrates (6%). It is a good source of vitamin C.

MENARCHE

The initiation of menstruation.

MENIERE'S SYNDROME

Most common in the fifth decade of life, Meniere's syndrome denotes symptoms resulting from a disturbance of the inner ear due to fluid accumulation. The disease, whose symptoms were first collectively described by Prosper Meniere in 1861, is characterized by the sensation of whirling around in space—vertigo—fluctuating incidents of deafness, high pitch ringing or buzzing in the ear, nausea, vomiting and headache. Many inner ear disorders can be traced to a variety of causes. However, the cause of Meniere's syndrome is difficult to pinpoint and it is rarely traceable to a disease or infection. Treatment, therefore, may proceed on a trial-and-error basis. Bed rest is an effective treatment since the sufferer can usually find a position in which vertigo is minimal. Other forms of treatment consist of diuretics and low salt diets to relieve the fluid accumulation in the inner ear and the use of sedatives and tranquilizers. A preparation such as Dramamine may be given to relieve the vertigo. Should the condition become so annoying that normal activities are impossible, then surgery is often the only cure.

Some sufferers of Meniere's syndrome report obtaining relief from taking niacin (both oral and injections simultaneously) and other B-complex vitamins, and from adding yogurt or buttermilk to the diet. Also, a diet low in (1) saturated fats, (2) carbohydrates (especially sugar), and (3) salt has been found to be helpful.

(Also see MODIFIED DIETS.)

MENTAL DEVELOPMENT

Mental development is a complex, on-going process influenced by a multitude of factors. Furthermore, it is difficult to assess and compare due to various social, racial, and ethnic backgrounds. In general, mental development may be defined as the increased ability to function. It involves motor skills, social traits, behavioral traits and learning skills. Normal mental development is evidenced by the gradual development of certain skills— roll over, sit, creep, walk, coordination of eyes and hands, formation of words, formation of whole thoughts, and ability to relate to people. The overall desired outcome of mental development is the attainment of an individual's full genetic potential.

In humans, it is difficult to say whether nutrition *per se* contributes to mental development since the conditions of malnutrition and deprived social and environmental conditions coexist. However some animal models have been designed to separate the effects of nutrition and environment on mental development. Therefore, animal models and observations of human populations combine to form the following salient points in regards to nutrition and mental development:

1. The brain and spinal cord continue rapid growth during infancy.
2. Malnutrition during the early life of animals and humans alters the number of brain cells, brain cell size and/or other biochemical parameters depending upon the time of onset and the duration of the malnutrition.
3. Malnourished animals demonstrate impaired learning abilities.

4. Teachers have observed that hungry, undernourished children are apathetic and lethargic.

5. Children suffering from kwashiorkor are apathetic, listless, withdrawn and seldom resist examination or wander off when left alone.

6. Children who recover from marasmus have a reduced head circumference—brain size—even after five years of rehabilitation.

7. Numerous studies suggest that infants subjected to acute malnutrition during the first years of life develop irreversible gaps in mental development, and thus never attain their full genetic potential.

Nevertheless, no amount of food can compensate for the emotional and social deprivation, resulting primarily from the lack of fulfilling infant-parent interaction.

(Also see MALNUTRITION; and STARVATION.)

MENTAL ILLNESS

This is a catchall term referring to any alteration in the normal function of the mind, ranging from periods of brief depression to severe, long lasting, disabling personality disorders. Rather broadly, mental illnesses can be classified as (1) neuroses, (2) psychophysiologic disorders, (3) personality disorders, (4) psychoses, and (5) transient situational disturbances. It can be characterized by lack of control over emotions and actions plus anxiety and even the stimulation of various physical disorders; for example, a peptic ulcer. Mental illness may be inherited and/or induced by environmental factors—chemical, bacterial, viral, nutritional, psychological, and social. Indeed there are probably as many or more forms of mental illness as there are physical illnesses. It should also be noted that no sharp line exists between mental health and mental illness because every human is unique. What is normal or abnormal may be merely a matter of degree and the manner in which a person's behavior is interpreted by family, friends, and physicians. However, it is well documented that there are certain nutritional disorders which cause some modifications in normal nervous system function—mental illness. The following examples demonstrate that nutritional states modify nervous system function:

1. **Vitamins and minerals.** Dietary deficiencies of thiamin, riboflavin, niacin, pantothenic acid, vitamin B-6, and vitamin B-12 will modify sensory functions, motor ability and personality. Deficiencies of minerals such as sodium and magnesium, and toxic intakes of minerals such as lead and mercury, produce mild to severe forms of mental disorders—hyperactivity, learning difficulties, hallucinations, confusion, and giddiness.

(Also see MINERAL[S]; and VITAMIN[S].)

2. **Hypoglycemia.** When hypoglycemia (low blood sugar) develops over a short period of time, the symptoms include rapid pulse, trembling, hunger, and a slight amount of mental confusion. However, hypoglycemia which has developed over many hours—meal skipping—is characterized by headache, depression, blurred vision, incoherent speech, and considerable mental confusion.

(Also see HYPOGLYCEMIA.)

3. **Starvation.** Short periods of starvation—4 days of water only—in healthy individuals decreases coordination and ability to concentrate. Semistarvation over long periods of time, such as existed in World War II concentration camps, decreased the ability to concentrate, lessened interests, decreased the ability of sustained mental effort, and created irritability, apathy, and sullenness.

(Also see STARVATION.)

4. **Beriberi.** Beriberi is a disease due to thiamin deficiency. Behavioral changes which have been noted include mental depression, loss of interest, diminution of the sense of humor, loss of ability to concentrate, and loss of patience with others. Rapid reversal of these symptoms depends upon restoration of thiamin to the diet.

(Also see BERIBERI.)

5. **Alcoholism.** Alcoholics make up about 10% of the first admissions to psychiatric wards. They possess some of the same symptoms noted in thiamin deficiency, and indeed respond to thiamin therapy. Often Korsakoff's syndrome—confusion, confabulation, fear, impaired learning, delirium—is associated with alcoholism. Vitamin therapy helps to restore the individual's attentiveness, alertness, and responsiveness.

(Also see ALCOHOLISM.)

One other aspect of mental illness is that of providing nutrition for the mentally ill. Of course, every case is different, but some of the feeding problems encountered are: (1) fears and suspicions about food; (2) lost interest in food; (3) overeating; or (4) refusal to eat. Appealing, well-planned meals with added verbal encouragement and assurance will help.

(Also see ANOREXIA NERVOSA; DEFICIENCY DISEASES; INBORN ERRORS OF METABOLISM; MENTAL DEVELOPMENT; MENTAL RETARDATION; and STRESS.)

MENTAL RETARDATION

Various degrees of mental retardation occur, but all are characterized by faulty development or set-back in the mental processes which impairs an individual's ability to cope with and adapt to the demands of society. In the United States, there are about 6 million mentally retarded individuals. It is generally recognized that there are three classes of mental retardation: (1) high grade or educable; (2) middle grade or trainable; and (3) low grade. A physical injury to the brain; some childhood diseases; an infection such as rubella, syphilis or meningitis during pregnancy; a genetic defect such as Down's syndrome; and inborn errors of metabolism such as phenylketonuria and galactosemia without dietary adjustments can all cause mental retardation. Nutritionally, a low iodine intake by the mother during pregnancy may result in cretinism in the baby, and alcohol consumption during pregnancy may contribute to varying degrees of mental retardation in the infant. A poor diet by the mother during pregnancy, and/or a poor diet by the infant may contribute to abnormal mental development. In fact, a large number of cases of mild mental retardation, which are educable, are not related to any known physical or organic cause. In these cases, genetic, environmental, nutritional, or psychological factors, or a combination of factors, may be the cause. Depending upon the degree, a mentally retarded person can present some obvious feeding problems. Feeding may be messy and slow, and thus require frequent small feedings in an effort to provide adequate food. Like any normal person, mentally retarded individuals have food likes and dislikes, and, despite their mental differences, their nutritional requirements are like those of a normal individual.

(Also see ALCOHOLISM; INBORN ERRORS OF METABOLISM; IODINE; and MENTAL DEVELOPMENT.)

MERCURY (Hg)

The element mercury is discharged into air and water from industrial operations and is used in herbicide and fungicide treatments. Although known cases of mercury poisoning have been limited, there is widespread concern over environmental pollution by this element.

(Also see MINERAL[S], section on "Contamination of Drinking Water, Foods, or Air With Toxic Minerals"; and POISONS.)

MESOMORPH

A type of body build according to one system of classification.

(Also see BODY TYPES.)

METABOLIC POOL

The nutrients available at any given time for the metabolic activities of the body; e.g., the amino acid pool, the calcium pool.

METABOLIC RATE

Essentially all of the energy released from foods becomes heat. Therefore, the metabolic rate is a measure of the rate of heat production by the body. It is expressed in Calories (Kcal) and can be determined by direct calorimetry which measures the heat given off by a person engaged in various activities. However, indirect calorimetry is more frequently used. This method determines the heat produced by measuring the oxygen consumed, since it is known that on the average for each liter of oxygen burned by the metabolic fires of the body 4.825 Calories (kcal) of energy are released. When a normal person is in a quiet resting state the metabolic rate is about 60 to 80 Calories (kcal) per hour. However, a variety of factors influence the metabolic rate. Many of these factors are interrelated and some are more important than others:

• **Exercise**—Perhaps, muscular activity is the most powerful stimulus for increasing the metabolic rate. Short bursts of strenuous exercise can increase the metabolic rate to 40 times that of the resting state.

• **Recent ingestion of food**—Following a meal the metabolic rate rises. This increase is dependent upon the type of food eaten. Carbohydrates and fats elevate the metabolic rate 4 to 15%, whereas proteins increase the rate 30 to 60%. This phenomenon is known as the specific dynamic action of foods (SDA).

• **Environmental temperature**—Increases or decreases in the environmental temperature increase the metabolic rate.

• **Body surface area**—Body surface area is a function of height and weight. A person weighing 200 lb (*91 kg*) has about 30% more surface area than a person weighing 100 lb (*45 kg*), when both are the same height. Hence, the larger person's metabolic rate is about 30% greater, not twice as great as is the weight.

• **Sex**—Females have a slightly lower metabolic rate than males throughout life.

• **Age**—Metabolic rate gradually declines with age.

• **Emotional state**—Various emotional states—fear, anger, rage—stimulate the release of epinephrine and norepinephrine which can increase the metabolic rate 100% on a short term basis.

• **State of nutrition**—During prolonged undernutrition the body adapts by decreasing the metabolic rate by as much as 50%.

• **Body temperature**—For every one degree increase in body temperature during a fever, the metabolic rate increases 7%.

• **Thyroid hormones**—On a long term basis, increased secretion of the thyroid hormones, thyroxine and triiodothyronine, can raise the metabolic rate by as much as 100%. Conversely, undersecretion can cause the rate to fall to 50% below normal.

• **Pregnancy and lactation**—The metabolic rate rises during pregnancy and lactation.

(Also see CALORIC [ENERGY] EXPENDITURE; CALORIMETRY: and METABOLISM.)

METABOLIC REACTIONS

The chemical changes that occur in the body; some are synthetic (the formation of new compounds), others are degradative (the breaking down of compounds).

METABOLIC WATER

Water formed within the cells of the body during the combustion (breakdown) of nutrients for the release of energy. On the average 13 ml of metabolic water are formed for every 100 kcal of metabolizable energy in the typical diet of a human. It contributes to the daily intake of water, and must be accounted for in the maintenance of water balance. Table M-34 illustrates the oxygen requirement and the production of carbon dioxide, water and energy for carbohydrates, proteins, and fats.

(Also see METABOLISM; and WATER BALANCE.)

TABLE M-34
OXYGEN REQUIREMENTS AND CARBON DIOXIDE, WATER, AND ENERGY PRODUCTION FOR THE BREAKDOWN OF EACH 100 GRAMS OF CARBOHYDRATE, PROTEIN, AND FAT

Nutrient	Oxygen Consumed	Carbon Dioxide Produced	Water Produced	Energy Released
	(liter)	(liter)	(ml)	(kcal)
Carbohydrate	82.9	82.9	60	410
Protein	96.6	78.2	40	410
Fat	201.9	142.7	110	930

METABOLISM

Contents   Page

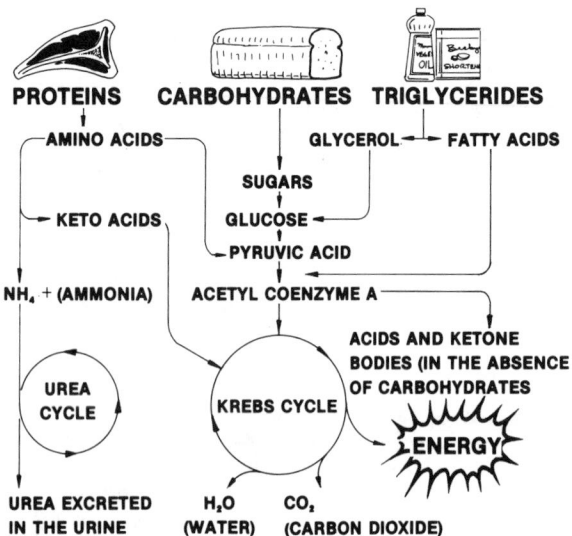

Fig. M-72. Metabolism of foods for the production of energy—the number one need.

Beefsteak, lettuce, tomatoes, and beans never get to the cells and tissues of our bodies, including our brains. But the nutrient chemicals—more than 40 of them, including amino acids, minerals, vitamins—do reach the body cells and tissues and are essential to their life. These are the ABCs of modern nutrition.

Once foods are eaten and digested, the nutrients are absorbed into the blood and distributed to the cells of the body. Still more chemical changes are required before the nutrients can be put to work in the body, by transforming them into energy or structural material. Thus, nutrients—carbohydrates, fats, proteins, minerals, vitamins, and water—are subjected to various chemical reactions. These chemical reactions occur on the cellular and subcellular level. The sum of all of these chemical reactions is termed metabolism. It has two phases: (1) catabolism, and (2) anabolism:

1. **Catabolism.** Catabolism is the oxidation—burning—of nutrients, liberating energy which is used to fulfill the body's immediate demands. When reactions liberate energy they are termed *exergonic reactions*.

2. **Anabolism.** Anabolism is the process by which nutrient molecules are used as building blocks for the synthesis of complex molecules. Anabolic reactions are endergonic—they require the input of energy into the system.

Basic to understanding the process of metabolism, is the realization that all of the reactions are catalyzed by enzymes—protein molecules which speed up biochemical reactions without being used up in the reactions. Furthermore, most all of the biochemical reactions of the metabolic processes are reversible. This is an important concept.

Life is a conquest for energy. Energy is required for practically all life processes—for the action of the heart, maintenance of blood pressure and muscle tone, transmission of nerve impulses, ion transport across membranes, reabsorption in the kidneys, protein and fat synthesis, the secretion of milk, and muscular contraction. A deficiency of energy is manifested by slow or stunted growth, body tissue losses, and/or weakness.

The diet contains carbohydrates, fats, and proteins. Although each of these has specific functions in maintaining a normal body, all of them can be used to provide the number one requirement—energy. Hence, the following discussion of their metabolism centers first, on their catabolism, and second, on their anabolism. Although they are not used for energy, minerals, vitamins, and water are essential to the metabolic processes.

In many ways, metabolism is similar to a factory. Like any manufacturing process, there are waste products with which to be dealt. Since the waste products of metabolism are toxic to the body at high levels, the body has developed reliable means for the removal of these wastes. Also, like any manufacturing process, there must be controls. Various factors control the rate and the direction of metabolism—anabolism or catabolism. Occasionally, a faulty piece of equipment hinders a manufacturing process. The body, too, can inherit faulty equipment for performing the metabolic processes.

CELLS—FUNCTIONAL UNITS.

Every living thing is composed of cells and cell products. In an organism as complex as a human—with trillions of cells—the proper function of the body processes is dependent upon each individual cell carrying out its proper metabolic processes for the organ or tissue in which it is located. Just as the body has organs, the cells of the body contain organelles (little organs) which are involved in the metabolic processes:

• **Cell membrane**—This membrane, which surrounds the cell like skin on the body, (1) gives shape to the cell, (2) contains the cytoplasm, and (3) serves to control the passage of substances into and out of the cells.

• **Nucleus**—The nucleus contains the DNA, the genetic material with coded information which directs the formation of protein molecules—primarily enzymes, necessary for the cell to perform its metabolic role.

• **Endoplasmic reticulum**—There are two types of endoplasmic reticulum: rough and smooth. Rough endoplasmic reticulum is the site of protein synthesis, while the smooth endoplasmic reticulum is involved in lipid synthesis and detoxification. Structurally, the endoplasmic reticulum is a complex series of tubules in the cytoplasm continuous with the cell membrane. The rough type is due to the attachment of ribosomes—the actual sites of protein synthesis.

• **Golgi complex**—This is another series of tubules usually located near the nucleus. Its function is believed to be that of "packaging" proteins, such as enzymes and hormones, secreted by the cell. Also, lysosomes are formed by the golgi complex.

• **Mitochondria**—These are sausage-shaped structures that are the power generating units of the cell. The mitochondria contain enzymes which release much of the energy contained in nutrients. Cells which have high energy requirements have the most mitochondria.

• **Lysosomes**—These large and somewhat irregular-shaped structures are packages of enzymes capable of destroying most of the cellular components if they are released. Lysosomes are the "digestive system" of the cell. Large molecules, engulfed particles, and old cells can be broken down by the enzymes within the lysosomes.

A typical cell with the structures involved in metabolic processes is shown in Fig. M-73.

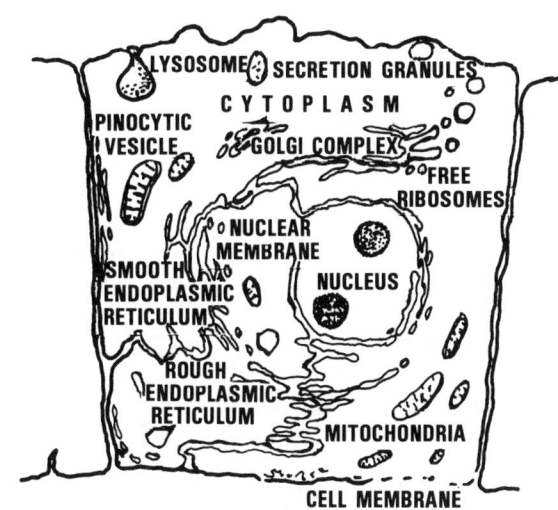

Fig. M-73. A typical cell showing some of the structural components most cells have in common, though cells of the body are variable in structure and function.

NUTRIENTS FOR METABOLISM.

From the standpoint of supplying the normal energy needs, carbohydrates are by far the most important, with fats second, and proteins third. Carbohydrates are usually more abundant and cheaper, and most of them are easily digested and absorbed. Moreover, excess carbohydrates can be transformed into body fat or into amino acids for protein synthesis.

Carbohydrates. The carbohydrates are organic compounds composed of carbon (C), hydrogen (H), and oxygen (O). They are formed in the plant by photosynthesis as follows: $6CO_2 + 6H_2O$ + energy from sun = $C_6H_{12}O_6$ (glucose) + $6O_2$. Carbohydrates form the woody framework of plants as well as the chief reserve food stored in seeds, roots, and tubers. As far as man is concerned, starch and sugars, primarily 6-carbon sugars, are the carbohydrates available for his use. Starch is composed of long chains of glucose which the digestive processes split into individual glucose molecules. Fructose (fruit sugar), glucose (grape sugar), sucrose (table sugar), and lactose (milk sugar) are the important dietary sugars. Other carbohydrates such as cellulose, hemicellulose, and pectin are not digestible; hence, they are unavailable for the metabolic processes. Sometimes these carbohydrates are called fiber or roughage. Ultimately, after being digested and absorbed, carbohydrates are converted to glucose.

No appreciable amount of carbohydrate is found in the body at any one time, but the blood supply of glucose is held rather constant at about 70 to 100 mg/100 ml. However, this small quantity of glucose in the blood, which is constantly replenished by changing the glycogen of the liver back to glucose, serves as the chief source of fuel with which to maintain the body temperature and to furnish the energy needed for all body processes. Maintenance of the blood glucose level is so important that at times amino acids and part of the fat molecule (glycerol) may be used to make glucose. The storage of glycogen (so-called animal starch) in the liver amounts to 3 to 7% of the weight of that organ. Glycogen is also stored in the muscles, but the latter is not available to raise blood glucose.

(Also see CARBOHYDRATE[S]; FIBER; HYPOGLYCEMIA; and STARCH.)

CATABOLISM. The primary use for carbohydrates is to produce energy. In the presence of oxygen, glucose will produce a maximum of 686 kcal/mole (*180.2 g*), as seen in the following equation:

$$C_6H_{12}O_6 + 6 O_2 \rightarrow 6 CO_2 + 6 H_2O + 686 \text{ kcal/mole (heat)}$$

The above reaction is a combustion or burning reaction. Hence, the expression of "burning off calories" can be understood.

No physiological system can approach 100% efficiency in the production of energy from the catabolism of a nutrient. Likewise, the body cannot produce 686 kcal from one mole (*180.2 g*) of glucose. Nevertheless, a great deal of energy is produced from the catabolism of glucose by a series of enzymatic reactions which permit the orderly transfer of energy from glucose to energy-rich compounds:

• **ATP—energy currency**—For metabolism to permit the orderly transfer of energy from foods to processes requiring energy, there must be a common carrier of energy—something cells can use to exchange goods for services. The energy currency—the primary mechanism by which energy is captured and stored—is a compound called adenosine triphosphate, often abbreviated ATP. Just as pennies are small units of a dollar, ATP is a small unit of energy.

ATP is a compound formed from the purine adenine, the 5-carbon sugar ribose, and three phosphate molecules as shown in Fig. M-74. Two of the phosphates are joined by high energy bonds.

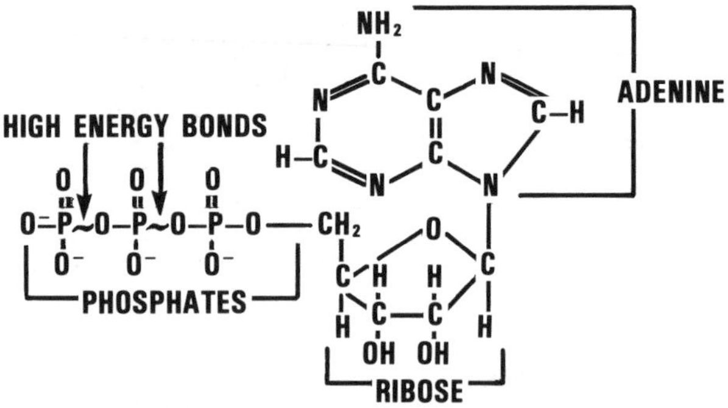

storage compound for the energy produced in the catabolism of various nutrients. When energy is required for body functions, ATP is broken down to ADP by releasing one phosphate and 8 kcal/mole of energy.

Releasing all of the energy contained in carbohydrates (fats and proteins, too) in one step would result in lost and wasted heat energy. Instead, energy is released in steps. The body utilizes a series of biological oxidations to form ATP. Oxidation refers to the loss of electrons (or hydrogen) by a compound. Conversely, reduction refers to the acceptance of electrons (or hydrogen) by a compound. Chemical energy is released as the lost electrons flow down energy gradients of an elevated state to the next lower hydrogen (electron) acceptor or carrier. Several coenzymes act as hydrogen (H^+) acceptors, many of which involve vitamins; for example, niacin and riboflavin. Compounds such as nicotinamide adenine dinucleotide (NAD^+), nicotinamide adenine dinucleotide phosphate ($NADP^+$), and flavin adenine dinucleotide (FAD) can accept and transfer hydrogen (or electrons) through a cytochrome system known as the electron transport system. Cytochromes are pigmented proteins similar to hemoglobin. In the electron transport system, electrons cascade from one intermediate carrier molecule—cytochrome—to the next lower in line, like water over the small waterfall. For every two electrons that tumble down the cytochrome system enough energy is released to form three ATP molecules by adding a high energy phosphate to ADP. The ultimate hydrogen acceptor in the system is oxygen; hence, water (H_2O) is formed. This is metabolic water. Production of ATP through this system is known as oxidative phosphorylation. Oxygen is required. It should be noted that when oxidation is initiated and NAD^+ carries the hydrogen ($NADH + H^+$) there is a net production of three ATP molecules. Only two ATPs are yielded, however, when hydrogen is transferred by FAD ($FADH_2$).

Fig. M-75 illustrates the cytochrome system, and the formation of ATP as hydrogen drops to different energy levels.

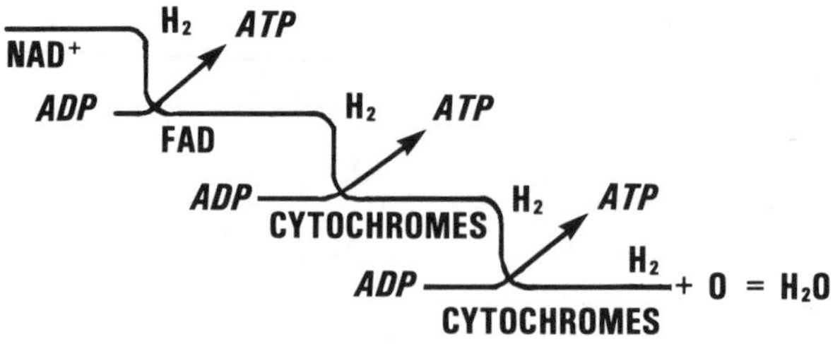

Fig. M-74.   Structure of adenosine triphosphate.

Fig. M-75.   The formation of adenosine triphosphate (ATP) from adenosine diphosphate as hydrogen tumbles down a chain of hydrogen carriers—the electron transport system. NAD^+ stands for nicotinamide adenine dinucleotide, and FAD stands for flavin adenine dinucleotide—both hydrogen carriers similar to the cytochromes.

When ATP is formed from ADP (adenosine diphosphate) by the addition of another phosphate, 8 kcal/mole must be put into the system—like a deposit in a bank account. The ATP then acts as a high-energy

• **Glycolysis**—Before glucose can be used by the cells it must first enter from the blood. Entry into the cells depends upon the hormone insulin from the pancreas.

Without insulin, glucose stays in the blood and creates the condition known as diabetes mellitus. Once inside the cell, the initial steps in the catabolism of glucose begin with a process called glycolysis—meaning glucose destruction. This pathway of chemical changes is referred to as the Embden-Meyerhof or glycolytic pathway. It is a series of reactions that are oxygen independent—no free or molecular oxygen needs to be involved; hence, these reactions are said to be anaerobic. The first reaction of glucose is that of providing activation energy—energy to get glucose "over a hump" before proceeding "downhill." This is accomplished by a reaction in which ATP donates a high energy phosphate yielding a new compound called glucose-6-phosphate.

Next, glucose atoms are slightly rearranged to yield fructose-6-phosphate. Then another phosphate is added by a donation from ATP. The compound is now called fructose-1, 6-phosphate. Another enzyme splits this 6-carbon compound into two 3-carbon compounds each containing a phosphate. One compound is glyceraldehyde-3-phosphate and the other is dihydroxyacetone phosphate. Dihydroxyacetone phosphate can be converted to glyceraldehyde-3-phosphate which receives another phosphate after two hydrogen atoms are removed via NADH + H$^+$. When oxygen is present (aerobic), this hydrogen enters the electron transport system and yields three ATP. Next, the compound with two phosphates—1, 3, diphosphoglyceric acid—loses a phosphate thus forming ATP from ADP and converting the compound to 3-phosphoglyceric acid. Eventually, the other phosphate is lost to convert ADP to another ATP and pyruvic acid is formed. Since each glucose provides two 3-carbon compounds for glycolysis, the net gain in ATP to this point is two ATP. Two ATP were used to add phosphate to the 6-carbon compounds while two were gained for each 3-carbon compound converted to pyruvic acid.

Lactic acid is produced only under anaerobic conditions such as exercise, when oxygen cannot be delivered fast enough by the blood. Since the conversion of pyruvic acid to lactic acid requires the input of two hydrogen atoms, the NADH + H$^+$ generated earlier in glycolysis can be reconverted to NAD$^+$ thus allowing glycolysis to continue. Normally, NADH + H$^+$ would go to the electron transport system, but this requires oxygen. Lactic acid is a dead end. In order for the body to use it, it must be reconverted to pyruvic acid, and in some cases glucose.

The whole scheme of glycolysis is presented in Fig. M-76.
The following items are important features of glycolysis:

1. Two ATP are netted for each glucose.
2. The system allows for the anaerobic breakdown of glucose.
3. It provides a system whereby energy from glucose stored as glycogen can be made readily available in muscle even when oxygen is in short supply during exercise.
4. Intermediates for the synthesis of other nutrients, such as glycerol and amino acids, are provided.

5. In the step whereby glyceraldehyde-3-phosphate is converted to 1, 3-diphosphoglyceric acid, 2 moles of NADH + H$^+$ are produced which can subsequently be oxidized in the electron transport system under aerobic conditions to produce 6 additional ATP.

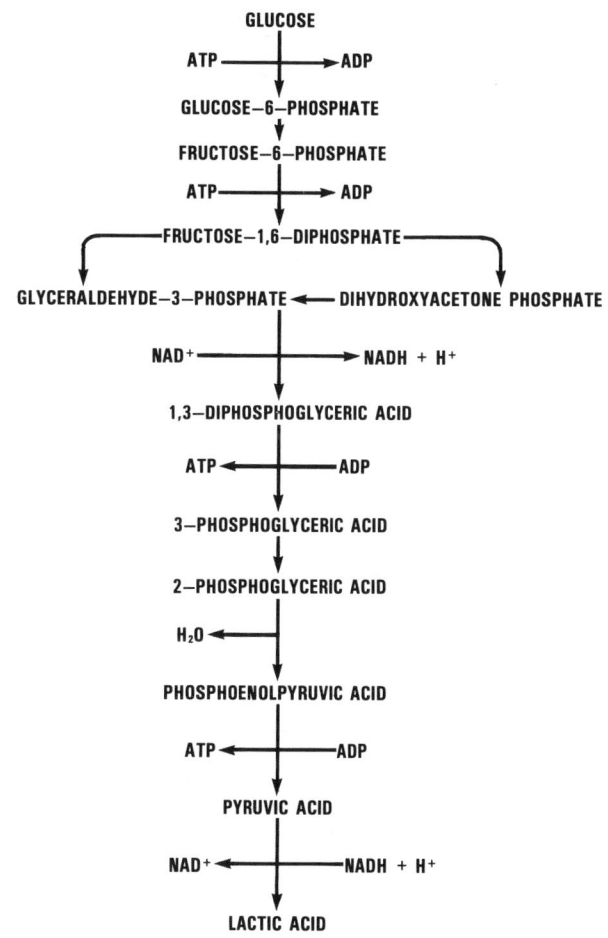

Fig. M-76. Glycolytic or Embden-Meyerhof pathway.

Through more chemical reactions, more energy can be derived from glucose which has reached the point of pyruvic acid. These additional reactions take place in a cellular structure appropriately called the powerhouse of the cell. These are the mitochondria.

• **Mitochondria**—These are watermelon-shaped microscopic structures within the cells of the body. The number and distribution of mitochondria within a cell depends upon the energy requirement of the cell. Those cells with large energy requirements possess a large number of mitochondria. The mitochondria contain the electron transport system. Moreover, they contain the enzymes necessary for the further metabolism of pyruvic acid, and other chemical transformations. It is their unique internal structure of cristae—a series of baffles—that allows for very efficient production of ATP.

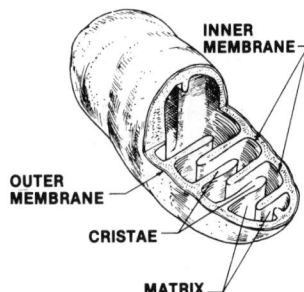

Fig. M-77.   Microscopic view of a mitochondrion—powerhouse of the cell.

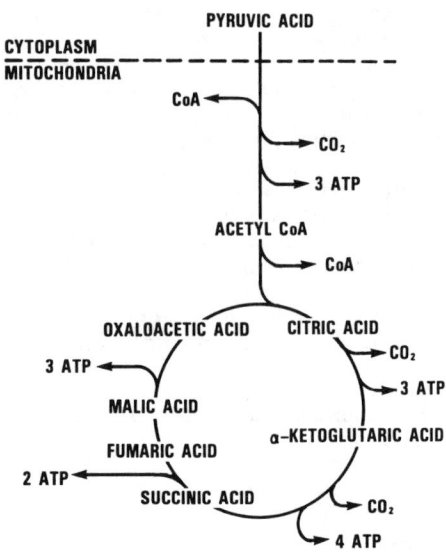

Fig. M-78.   The Krebs cycle.

Pyruvic acid enters the mitochondria of the cell and begins another series of reactions variously referred to as the Krebs cycle, the tricarboxylic acid (TCA) cycle, or the citric acid cycle. First, pyruvic acid is converted to acetyl coenzyme A (acetyl CoA) by a loss of a carbon atom as carbon dioxide (CO_2) and two hydrogen atoms. This conversion yields 3 ATP, since the hydrogen atoms enter the electron transport system via NADH + H$^+$. Acetyl CoA is then condensed with oxaloacetic acid to form citric acid, thus initiating the Krebs cycle. As the cycle progresses, more electrons (hydrogens) are transferred to different coenzymes, which, in turn, enter the electron transport chain producing ATP. One complete turn of the cycle (1) produces 12 ATP and the loss of two carbons as carbon dioxides (CO_2) from citrate, and (2) the restoration of oxaloacetic acid; completing the cycle. Since 2 pyruvic acid molecules can be formed from 1 glucose molecule, 24 ATP are produced via the Krebs cycle. Thus, 38 ATP are produced from 1 molecule of glucose: 8 from glycolysis, 6 in the conversion of pyruvic acid to acetyl CoA, and 24 from the Krebs cycle. Each pass of the 2-carbon acetyl CoA through the Krebs cycle results in the formation of CO_2 (carbon dioxide) and H_2O (water), the end products of catabolism.

Fig. M-78 illustrates the simplified version of the Krebs cycle, named after the scientist who discovered it.

• **Energy efficiency**—One ATP molecule will yield about 8 Calories (kcal). Since 38 ATP are derived from the complete oxidation of glucose, 304 Calories (kcal) of energy are formed (38 × 8 = 304). Under ideal conditions, the oxidation of glucose yields 686 Calories (kcal). Hence, the human body is 44% efficient in converting glucose to energy (304 ÷ 686 × 100 = 44). Diesel engines have a maximum efficiency of about 40%, while many gasoline engines only convert about 25% of their fuel energy into work. The human body burns its fuel quite efficiently.

• **Hexosemonophosphate pathway**—Not all glucose enters the glycolytic pathway. A small amount continually enters another pathway known as the pentose shunt or hexosemonophosphate (HMP) pathway. The functions of this pathway are twofold: (1) to provide some energy in the form of NADPH, another hydrogen carrier, which will function in the formation of fatty acids; and (2) to provide the 5-carbon sugar ribose for use in the nucleic acid DNA and RNA, or nucleotide coenzymes such as ATP. Products of this pathway eventually reenter the glycolytic pathway.

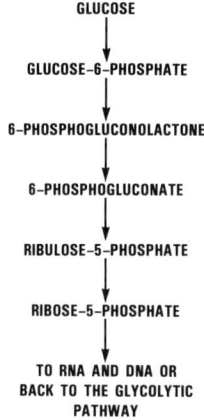

Fig. M-79.   The pentose shunt or hexosemonophosphate pathway.

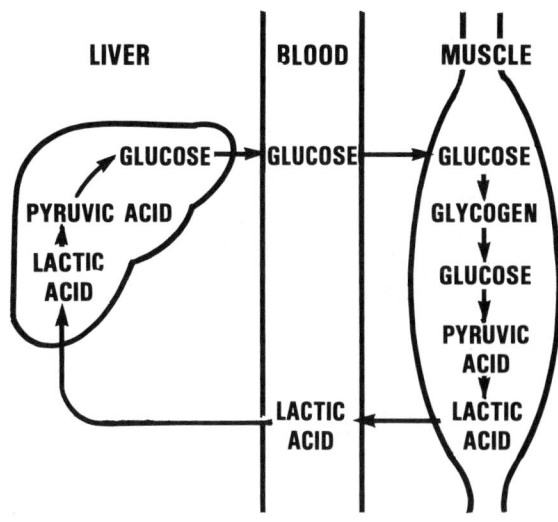

Fig. M-80.   The lactic acid or Cori cycle.

ANABOLISM. Two processes involved in carbohydrate metabolism may be considered anabolic in that they require energy: (1) storage of glucose as glycogen; and (2) the formation of glucose from noncarbohydrate sources, or gluconeogenesis.

• **Glycogen**—Upon absorption into the bloodstream, glucose travels to the liver where it is incorporated into glycogen. Glycogen is composed of numerous glucose molecules which are all chemically joined. Starch in plants is also composed of numerous glucose molecules joined together; hence, glycogen is sometimes referred to as animal starch. Each time a glucose molecule is linked with the glycogen already in the liver, two high-energy phosphate bonds are required. Then, as glucose is needed to maintain the blood glucose levels, glycogen is broken down to release glucose.

Some glycogen is manufactured and stored in the muscles. However, glucose derived from this glycogen is available only for use by the muscle and not the general circulation. Lactic acid may leave the muscle and be reconverted to glucose in the liver and released into the blood. This process requires six ATP for each glucose molecule, and is referred to as the lactic acid cycle or Cori cycle. A husband and wife team, Carl and Gerty Cori, described it; and they were jointly awarded the Nobel Prize in 1947.

• **Gluconeogenesis**—Gluconeogenesis is the formation of glucose from nutrients other than carbohydrates. This pathway is extremely important when there is an insufficiency of dietary carbohydrates. The liver is the main site for gluconeogenesis. Amino acids are the primary precursors in gluconeogenesis. However, amino acids must first have their amino group (NH_2) removed by a process called deamination, following which the remaining carbon skeleton can enter the Krebs cycle and, essentially, be worked backwards through glycolysis to glucose. All of the amino acids except leucine are glycogenic—capable of forming glucose. Production of glucose by this means is possible since most reactions catalyzed by enzymes are reversible. There is, however, one exception. Pyruvic acid in the mitochondria of cells cannot be directly converted to phosphoenolpyruvic acid. Rather, it is transformed into oxaloacetic acid and malic acid. Malic acid is then able to cross the mitochondrial membrane into the cytoplasm where it is reconverted to oxaloacetic acid. Oxaloacetic acid is then converted to phosphoenolpyruvic acid due to the presence of a specific enzyme in the cytoplasm. Once this is accomplished, the process closely resembles the reverse of the glycolytic pathway. (See Figs. M-76 and M-78.) The whole process requires an expenditure of energy.

Table M-35 indicates where each amino acid fits into the metabolic scheme following deamination.

TABLE M-35
GLUCONEOGENESIS FROM AMINO ACIDS

Amino Acid	Compounds Formed Following Deamination	Metabolic Fate[1]
Alanine	Pyruvic acid	Glycogenic
Arginine	Alpha-ketoglutaric acid	Glycogenic
Aspartate	Fumaric acid	Glycogenic
Cysteine	Pyruvic acid	Glycogenic
Glutamate	Alpha-ketoglutaric acid	Glycogenic
Glycine	Pyruvic acid	Glycogenic
Histidine	Alpha-ketoglutaric acid, beta-ketoglutaric acid	Glycogenic
Proline	Alpha-ketoglutaric acid	Glycogenic
Hydroxy-proline	Alpha-ketoglutaric acid	Glycogenic
Methionine	Succinyl CoA	Glycogenic
Serine	Pyruvic acid	Glycogenic
Threonine	Succinyl CoA	Glycogenic
Valine	Succinyl CoA	Glycogenic
Isoleucine	Acetyl CoA, succinyl CoA	Glycogenic and ketogenic
Lysine	Alpha-ketoglutaric acid, acetyl CoA, acetoacetyl CoA	Glycogenic and ketogenic
Phenylalanine	Fumaric acid, acetyl CoA	Glycogenic and ketogenic
Tryptophan	Succinyl CoA, acetyl CoA	Glycogenic and ketogenic
Leucine	Acetyl CoA, acetoacetic acid	Ketogenic

[1]Glycogenic forms glucose while ketogenic forms ketone bodies—acetoacetic acid, beta-hydroxybutyric acid, and acetone.

Fats. Fats are compounds composed of carbon, hydrogen, and oxygen—much like carbohydrates. However, because of the larger portion of carbon and hydrogen in their makeup, fats provide about 2.25 times as much energy as do the carbohydrates—more hydrogen atoms for the electron transport system. Dietary fats are primarily compounds composed of three fatty acid molecules linked to one glycerol molecule—a combination called triglycerides.

(Also see FATS AND OTHER LIPIDS.)

CATABOLISM. When fats are hydrolyzed (water added), glycerol and fatty acids are released and subsequently catabolized separately. Glycerol is converted to glycerol-3-phosphate, then to dihydroxyacetone phosphate. Dihydroxyacetone phosphate can be readily converted to 3-phosphoglyceraldehyde which enters the last part of the glycolytic pathway and eventually enters into the Krebs cycle (See Fig. M-78). Thus, it yields an amount of energy similar to that of one-half of the glucose molecule passing through glycolysis and the Krebs cycle.

The catabolism of fatty acids occurs in the mitochondria through a systematic process called beta-oxidation, whereby 2-carbon fragments are successively chopped

from the fatty acid molecule to form acetyl CoA which then enters the Krebs cycle (see Fig. M-78). The term lipolysis indicates mobilization of fats and their oxidation. Carnitine, a vitaminlike substance, facilitates the transport of fatty acids across the mitochondrial membrane. The first step in the beta-oxidation of a fatty acid is the addition of coenzyme A (CoA) to the end of the molecule. This requires energy, but not nearly as much energy as is subsequently generated. For example, the 16-carbon fatty acid palmitic acid can be oxidized seven times. Each time a 2-carbon fragment—acetyl CoA—is released from a fatty acid, 5 ATP are formed. However, 1 ATP is consumed in activating the fatty acid with CoA. Then, each acetyl CoA enters the Krebs cycle and produces 12 ATP. The energy balance sheet is as follows:

$$\begin{array}{llr}
 & & \text{ATP} \\
\text{Palmitic acid} & \longrightarrow \text{Palmitoyl CoA} \ldots\ldots\ldots & -1 \\
\text{Palmitoyl CoA} & \longrightarrow 8 \text{ Acetyl CoA } (7 \times 5 \text{ ATP}) & 35 \\
8 \text{ Acetyl CoA} & \longrightarrow H_2O + 18 \, CO_2 \, (8 \times 12 \text{ ATP}) & \underline{96} \\
& \text{Net} \ldots\ldots\ldots\ldots\ldots\ldots\ldots\ldots\ldots\ldots\ldots & 130
\end{array}$$

Each mole of ATP contains about 8 Calories (kcal). Therefore, 1 mole of palmitic acid yields 1,040 Calories (kcal), which demonstrates that fats are high-energy compounds. Comparing this value to that obtained by burning fat in a laboratory bomb calorimeter, the efficiency of the biological burning of palmitic acid is about 42%—not bad for any machine.

Fig. M-81 summarizes beta-oxidation. Of course, the long-chain fatty acids yield more ATP than do the short-chain fatty acids.

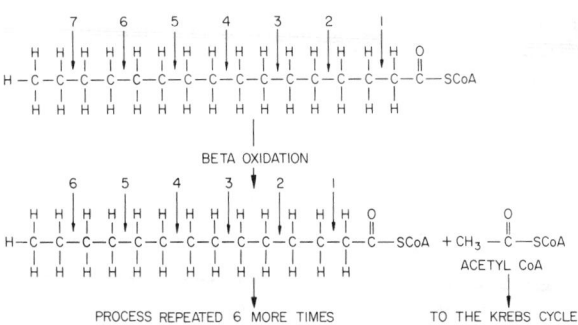

Fig. M-81. The combination of the fatty acid palmitic acid and CoA (palmitoyl CoA) with the subsequent removal of acetyl CoA. The numbered arrows indicate the number of beta-oxidations possible.

Acetyl CoA is a common point—a crossroad— for many of the biochemical reactions of the body. It can be used for building other substances including (1) new fatty acids and cholesterol, (2) the formation of the ketone body, acetoacetic acid, and (3) the nerve transmitter substance, acetylcholine. It is formed during the catabolism of fatty acids, glucose, and amino acids; hence, excesses of these nutrients can be stored as fat. As already pointed out, acetyl CoA can enter the Krebs cycle. However, entry into this cycle is dependent upon continued availability of carbohydrates.

• **Ketosis**—Pyruvate, a product of carbohydrate catabolism, is needed to produce oxaloacetic acid. Oxaloacetic acid must then condense with acetyl CoA in order to produce citric acid. If there is insufficient oxaloacetic acid in the cell to keep the Krebs cycle functioning efficiently, the acetyl CoA is converted to acetoacetic acid, beta-hydroxybutyric acid, and acetone. These ketone bodies accumulate in the blood; and if the condition goes unchecked, acidosis will occur, often resulting in coma and death. Ketosis can be a complication of diabetes mellitus and starvation.

(Also see DIABETES MELLITUS; and STARVATION.)

ANABOLISM. Saturated fatty acids and mono-unsaturated fatty acids are rapidly and abundantly formed from acetyl CoA. Hence, any nutrient capable of yielding acetyl CoA during the metabolic processes can potentially contribute to fatty acid synthesis—a process called lipogenesis. While a limited amount of fat synthesis occurs in the mitochondria of the cell, most synthesis takes place outside the mitochondria via enzymes in the cytoplasm when supplemented with energy (ATP), carbon dioxide (CO_2), hydrogen, and the mineral magnesium (Mn^+). The 2-carbon compound, acetyl CoA, is the primary building block. It is first carboxylated (organic acid group COOH added) to form malonyl CoA, and then it is transferred to a carrier protein—acyl-carrier protein (ACP). Malonyl-ACP then combines with acetyl CoA via acetyl ACP to form acetoacetyl-ACP which then has hydrogen added by NADPH generated in the pentose shunt to convert to butyryl-ACP. More and more acetyl CoA and hydrogen are added to this molecule until the chain is 16 carbons long—palmitic acid. All fatty acids formed as described above are then transported back into the mitochondria where three fatty acids are joined—esterified—with one glycerol molecule, thus forming triglycerides. The glycerol is derived from the glycolytic pathway. Fatty acids may also be elongated in the mitochondria.

Acetyl CoA, may also be used to synthesize cholesterol in many tissues, but the liver is the major site of synthesis.

(Also see CHOLESTEROL; and FATS AND OTHER LIPIDS.)

Proteins. Proteins are complex organic compounds made up chiefly of amino acids, which are present in characteristic proportions for each specific protein. This nutrient always contains carbon, hydrogen, oxygen, and nitrogen; and, in addition, it usually contains sulfur and frequently phosphorus. Proteins are essential in all plant and animal life as components of the active protoplasm of each living cell. The need for protein in the diet is actually a need for its constituents—the amino acids. For more than a century, the amino acids have been studied and recognized as important nutrients.

The dietary proteins are broken down into amino acids during digestion. They are then absorbed and distributed by the bloodstream to the body cells, which rebuild these amino acids into body proteins. Although the primary use of amino acids in the body is synthesis, amino acids can be catabolized as a source of energy.

CATABOLISM. Amino acids from the proteins are the primary sources of carbon skeletons utilized in gluconeogenesis—a process previously explained. In order that amino acids may enter energy metabolic pathways, they must first have their amino (NH_2) group removed—a process called oxidative deamination. This forms ammonia and a carbon skeleton that can be used for energy.

Following deamination, the carbon skeletons, depending upon their structure, can enter the Krebs cycle as pyruvic acid, alpha-ketoglutaric acid, succinic acid, fumaric acid, or oxaloacetic acid and be completely oxidized to carbon dioxide and water yielding the production of ATP (See Table M-35). Transamination—the transfer of an amino group (NH_2) to synthesize new amino acids—also forms carbon skeletons which can enter the Krebs cycle.

Most deaminated amino acids can be used to synthesize glucose by working backwards through glycolysis. This process is called gluconeogenesis, and amino acids capable of this are called gluconeogenic or glycogenic. Alanine is an important gluconeogenic amino acid. Alanine is formed in the muscles by transamination. When it is deaminated in the liver, it becomes pyruvic acid which the liver converts to glucose. Leucine is the only amino acid incapable of gluconeogenesis.

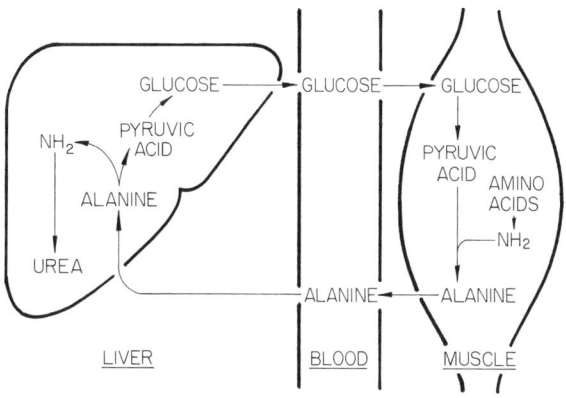

Fig. M-82.   The alanine cycle.

• **Urea**—The fate of the amino group (NH_2) split off from amino acids, presents a special metabolic problem. Fortunately, the body has developed the urea cycle for handling this substance. Most of the NH_2 is converted to urea in the liver for excretion by the kidneys. To facilitate elimination, 1 mole of ammonia (NH_3) combines with 1 mole of carbon dioxide (CO_2), another metabolic waste product. Phosphate is then added to this compound to produce carbamyl phosphate. Carbamyl phosphate then combines with ornithine to form citrulline—an intermediate in the urea cycle. The amino acid, aspartic acid, contributes another amino group (NH_2), and citrulline is then converted to the amino acid arginine.

Urea splits off from arginine forming ornithine, and the cycle is completed. The kidneys remove urea from the blood and excrete it in the urine.

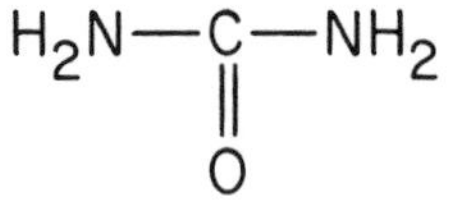

$$H_2N - \overset{\displaystyle \underset{\parallel}{C}}{\underset{O}{}} - NH_2$$

Fig. M-83.   The structure of urea—the means of eliminating amino groups from amino acids.

(Also see UREA CYCLE.)

ANABOLISM. The various amino acids are systematically joined together to form peptides and proteins. The amino portion (NH_2) of one amino acid will combine with the carboxyl (COOH) portion of another amino acid releasing water (H_2O) and forming a peptide linkage—like railroad cars joining to form a train. When numerous of these junctions occur, the resulting molecule is called a protein. The proteins of the body are the primary constituents of many structural and protective tissues—bones, ligaments, hair, fingernails, skin, organs, and muscles. Perhaps, most importantly enzymes are proteins, and they are responsible for most all of the catabolic and anabolic reactions.

Protein synthesis is not a random process whereby a number of amino acids are joined together; rather, it is a detailed predetermined procedure. Within the cell, DNA contains the coded information concerning the amino acid sequences of the various proteins to be synthesized in the cell. When DNA is decoded, amino acids are linked to form a specific protein which has its own particular physiological function.

Protein synthesis involves a series of reactions which are specific for *each* protein. A four step outline of this procedure follows:

1.   Messenger RNA (ribonucleic acid) transcribes the sequence "message" from DNA to form a template (a pattern or guide) for protein synthesis. The sequences of the nucleotides in the DNA are the keys to the sequence pattern forming this template. This is possible because the nucleotides always pair off in the following manner: adenine (A) and thymine (T); adenine (A) and uracil (U); and guanine (G) and cytosine (C). Triplets of the purine (adenine and guanine) and pyrimidine (cytosine, thymine, and uracil) bases in the DNA form "codons" which correspond to specific amino acids and are signals which control protein synthesis. For example, the codon AGG (adenine, guanine, and guanine) signals the incorporation of arginine.

2.   A specific transfer RNA (tRNA) combines with each respective amino acid to form an aminoacyl complex. This reaction requires the expenditure of energy. There is at least one specific tRNA for most of the 22 amino acids.

3.   The initiation of protein synthesis occurs when the ribosome of the rough endoplasmic reticulum (site of protein synthesis) recognizes a codon specific for initiation. This first amino acid will be the amino (NH_2) terminal end of the protein. This amino acid is formulated to prevent the amino group of the amino acid from being incor-

porated in a peptide bond. Upon completion of the protein, the N-formyl group is cleaved from the protein.

4.   Once synthesis has been initiated, the protein is elongated through a series of successive additions of amino acids as determined by the messenger RNA template. Each new amino acid is linked to the next by the formation of a peptide bond. Eventually the procedure will be terminated when a codon specific for terminating protein synthesis is reached. Thereupon, the protein splits off from the ribosomes.

Fig. M-84 graphically demonstrates the complete process of protein synthesis.

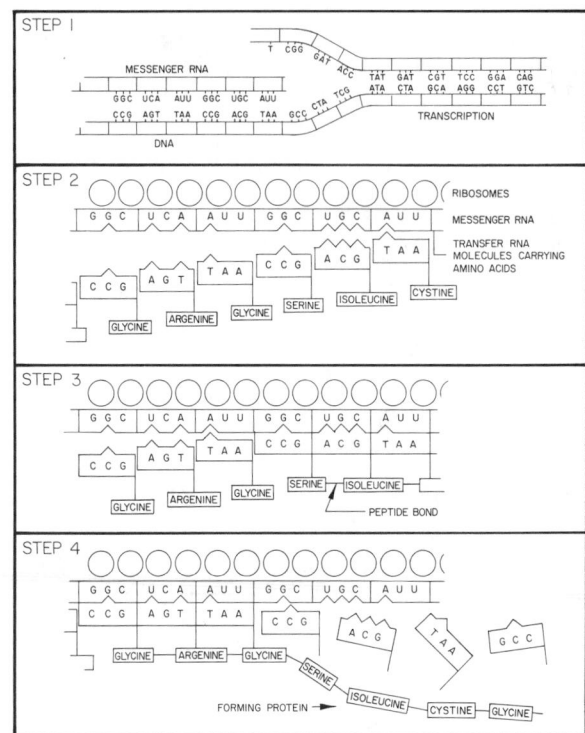

Fig. M-84.   Four steps of protein synthesis directed by the coded master plans contained in DNA.

Each sequence of amino acids is a different protein. Hence, different proteins are able to accomplish different functions in the body. With 22 amino acids, the different arrangements possible are endless, yielding a variety of proteins. For example, egg albumin, a small protein, contains approximately 288 amino acids. Thus, if one assumes that there are about 20 different amino acids in the albumin molecule, then mathematical calculations show that the possible arrangements of this number of amino acids are in excess of 10^{300}. (For comparison, one million is equal to 10^6.)

Since the DNA of each cell carries the master plan for forming proteins, genetic mutations often are manifested by disorders in protein metabolism. Many metabolic defects—inborn errors of metabolism—are the result of a missing or modified enzyme or other protein. The misplacement or omission of just one amino acid in a protein molecule can result in a nonfunctional protein.

Therefore, when proteins are formed three requirements must be met: (1) the proper amino acids, (2) the proper number of amino acids, and (3) the proper order of the amino acid in the chain forming the protein. Meeting these requirements allows the formation of proteins which are very specific and which gives tissues their unique form, function and character.

(Also see INBORN ERRORS OF METABOLISM; and NUCLEIC ACIDS.)

Minerals And Vitamins. The metabolism of minerals and vitamins does not produce energy. However, minerals and vitamins are involved in many of the reactions in the body which comprise metabolism. The following table indicates some of the areas where minerals and vitamins are directly involved in metabolism. More information may be gained about minerals and vitamins under their separate entries.

(Also see MINERAL[S]; and VITAMIN[S].)

TABLE M-36
MINERAL AND VITAMIN
FUNCTIONS IN METABOLISM

Mineral or Vitamin	Function
Minerals:	
Calcium	Cell wall permeability; enzyme activation; hormone secretion.
Phosphorus	Energy utilization (ATP formation); amino acid metabolism; protein formation; enzyme systems; formation of some fats (phospholipids).
Sodium	Acid-base balance of the body; absorption of sugars.
Chlorine	Acid-base balance; stomach acid; enzyme activation.
Magnesium	Enzyme activation.
Potassium	Acid-base balance; enzyme reactions; nutrient transfer.
Sulfur	Component of the vitamin biotin and thiamin; component of coenzyme A (CoA).
Chromium	Component of the Glucose Transfer Factor; enzyme activation; stimulation of fatty acid synthesis.
Copper	Constituent of several enzyme systems.
Iodine	Constituent of thyroid hormones which act to regulate metabolism.
Iron	Component of cytochromes; component of hemoglobin which brings oxygen to the tissues.
Manganese	Enzyme activator.
Molybdenum	Component of enzyme systems.
Selenium	Enzyme component.

(Continued)

TABLE M-36 *(Continued)*

Mineral or Vitamin	Function
Zinc	Component of enzyme systems.
Vitamins:	
A	Synthesis of protein, some hormones, and glycogen.
D	Regulates calcium and phosphorus.
E	Regulator of DNA synthesis, and coenzyme Q, a hydrogen carrier.
Biotin	Coenzyme in decarboxylation (removal of carbon dioxide) and carboxylation (addition of carbon dioxide) reactions of carbohydrate, fat, and protein metabolism; for example, pyruvic acid to oxaloacetic acid, and acetyl CoA to malonyl CoA; formation of purines; formation of urea; deamination of amino acids.
Choline	Transport and metabolism of fats; source of methyl groups (CH_3).
Folacin	Formation of coenzymes for synthesis of DNA and RNA; amino acid synthesis.
Niacin	Constituent of the two coenzymes nicotinamide adenine dinucleotide (NAD) and nicotinamide adenine dinucleotide phosphate (NADP) which transport hydrogen during energy formation.
Pantothenic acid . . .	Form part of coenzyme A (CoA) and the acyl carrier protein (ACP).
Riboflavin	Forms coenzymes like flavin adenine dinucleotide (FAD) which is responsible for transport of hydrogen ions.
Thiamin	A coenzyme in energy metabolism via decarboxylation of pyruvic acid and formation of acetyl CoA.
Vitamin B-6	As a coenzyme for: transamination, decarboxylation, deamination, transsulfuration, absorption of amino acids, conversion of glycogen to glucose, and fatty acid conversions.
Vitamin B-12	Coenzyme in protein synthesis.
Vitamin C	Makes iron available for hemoglobin synthesis, metabolism of the amino acids tyrosine and tryptophan.

Water. Water is a vital nutrient. It is the solvent wherein the metabolic reactions of the body take place. Also, as a solvent, water carries (1) the nutrients which are subjected to cellular metabolism, and (2) the waste products of metabolism. Also, it serves to disperse the heat generated by the metabolic reactions. In many of the metabolic reactions water is either added or subtracted. Subtracted water is termed metabolic water. The addition of water is termed hydrolysis.

(Also see WATER; and WATER AND ELECTROLYTES.)

EXCRETION. Products not used and products formed during metabolism must be continually removed from the body. The three major routes of removal are: (1) feces, (2) urine, and (3) lungs. The feces serve to remove materials that cannot be digested or absorbed. Urea, produced from the metabolism of amino acids is excreted by the kidneys into the urine, along with excess water, mineral salts, and some other compounds formed during metabolism. Carbon dioxide produced during metabolism is excreted from the body via the lungs. For every 2,100 Calories (kcal), about 327 liters of carbon dioxide are produced in the body.

FACTORS CONTROLLING METABOLISM. The rate at which the body utilizes nutrients, and the direction of metabolism—anabolism or catabolism, are controlled by a variety of factors, but primarily the nervous system and endocrine systems. Many of these factors are interrelated and some are more important than others. Generally, metabolism is discussed in terms of energy, since energy to drive the machinery of the body is the first concern. The metabolic rate is the rate at which the body uses energy—calories—packaged in ATP. Some factors affecting metabolism follow:

• **Exercise**—Perhaps, muscular activity is the most powerful stimulus for increasing the metabolic rate. Short bursts of strenuous exercise can increase the metabolic rate to 40 times that of the resting state.

• **Recent ingestion of food**—Following a meal, the metabolic rate rises. This increase is dependent upon the type of food eaten. Carbohydrates and fats elevate the metabolic rate 4 to 15%, whereas proteins increase the rate 30 to 60%. This phenomenon is known as the specific dynamic action of foods (SDA).

• **Environmental temperature**—Increases or decreases in the environmental temperature increase the metabolic rate.

• **Body surface area**—Body surface area is a function of height and weight. A person weighing 200 lb (91 kg) has about 30% more surface area than a person weighing 100 lb (45.5 kg), when both are the same height. Hence, the larger person's metabolic rate is about 30% greater, not twice as great as is the weight.

• **Sex**—Females have a slightly lower metabolic rate than males throughout life.

• **Pregnancy and lactation**—The metabolic rate rises during pregnancy and lactation.

• **Age**—Metabolic rate gradually declines with age. During growth, energy is needed for the anabolic processes.

• **Emotional state**—Various emotional states—fear, anger, shock—stimulate the release of the hormones epinephrine and norepinephrine which can increase the metabolic rate 100% on a short term basis.

• **State of nutrition**—During prolonged undernutrition the body adapts by decreasing the metabolic rate by as much as 50%.

• **Body temperature**—For every one degree increase in body temperature during a fever, the metabolic rate increases 7%.

• **Hormones**—Many of the above changes in metabolism are ultimately due to some hormonal change. Most of the hormones direct the metabolic processes. The storage and release of glucose is hormone mediated. Protein synthesis is hormone mediated, as is the release of fatty acids from fats. The thyroid hormones can, on a long term basis, raise the metabolic rate 100%. Conversely, undersecretion can cause the metabolic rate to fall 50% below normal. Other hormones control water and minerals, and still others control the digestive processes.

(Also see CALORIC [ENERGY] EXPENDITURE; ENDOCRINE GLANDS; and ENERGY UTILIZATION BY THE BODY.)

INBORN ERRORS OF METABOLISM. At times the metabolism of the nutrients cannot proceed normally due to some defect in the genetic information that exists at birth or shortly thereafter. These defects can affect the metabolism of carbohydrates, proteins, and fats; hence, they are referred to as inborn errors of metabolism. Often they are due to production of a nonfunctional enzyme or complete lack of an enzyme involved in the metabolic scheme. Since enzymes are protein, their production relies upon correct genetic information. Many of these inborn errors have serious consequences, but fortunately most are rare. Familiar examples of errors in carbohydrate metabolism include lactose intolerance and galactosemia. Familiar examples of errors in protein metabolism include albinism, maple syrup urine disease, and phenylketonuria. The hyperlipoproteinemias are familiar examples of inborn errors of fat metabolism.

(Also see INBORN ERRORS OF METABOLISM.)

SUMMARY. Although metabolism is discussed in parts—pathways, nutrients, and cycles—it is an interrelated, continuous process—the sum of all chemical changes in the body. While some organs have more important roles, metabolic processes occur in every cell of the body—from those in the big toe to brain cells. Energy production in the form of ATP is the first concern of metabolism, and water (H_2O), carbon dioxide (CO_2), and urea are the major waste products of metabolism. Fig. M-85 presents a simplified overview of metabolism showing the major interrelationships, the waste product formation, and the production of ATP for work—mechanical work, transport work, or biosynthetic (anabolic) work.

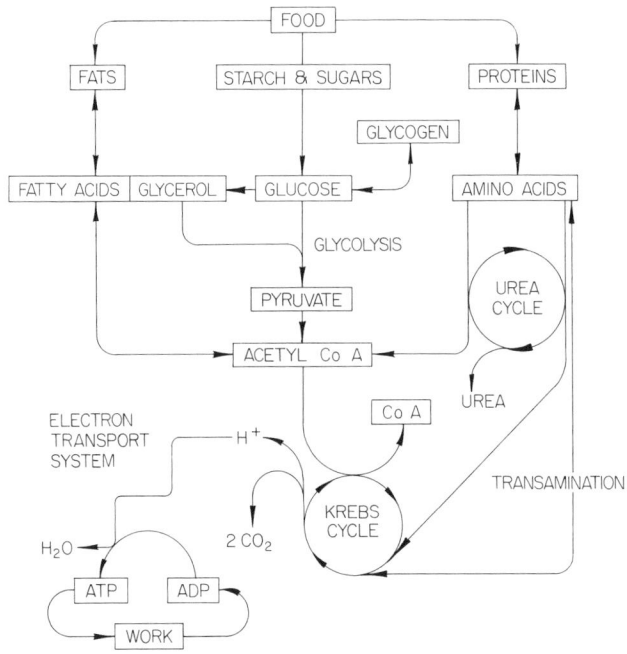

Fig. M-85. A simplified summary of metabolism.

METABOLITE

Any substance produced by metabolism or by a metabolic process.

METALLOENZYME

An enzyme of which a metal (ion) is an integral part of its active structure. Examples: carbonic anhydrase (zinc) and cytochromes (iron, copper).

METHIONINE

An essential amino acid which contains sulfur. Furthermore, methionine participates in a biochemical reaction in the body called transmethylation by donating a methyl group (CH_3).
(Also see AMINO ACID[S].)

METHYL ALCOHOL (WOOD ALCOHOL; CH_3OH METHANOL)

The simplest of the alcohols, but it is highly toxic when ingested. As little as 20 ml may cause (1) permanent blindness as a result of the formaldehyde formed by the metabolism of the methyl alcohol damaging the retina of the eye, or (2) death due to severe acidosis. Poisoning due to methyl alcohol is almost always a case of ingestion as a substitute for ethyl alcohol—the alcohol of liquors. Rather ironically, part of the treatment for methyl alcohol poisoning consists of administering ethyl alcohol. Aside from its adverse effects when ingested, methyl alcohol is an important industrial chemical utilized for numerous processes and products.

METHYLATED SPIRITS

Ethyl alcohol to which methyl alcohol has been added to render it unfit for consumption as a beverage. Often called denatured alcohol. The added methyl alcohol makes it highly poisonous.
(Also see METHYL ALCOHOL.)

MEULENGRACHT DIET

A diet for peptic ulcer patients first introduced by the Danish Physician Meulengracht in 1935. It is more liberal than the *Sippy Diet*, which was initiated in 1915 by the American Physician, Bertram Sippy. The Sippy Diet holds rather rigidly to a program of milk and cream feeding with slow additions of single soft food items over a prolonged period of time. To begin with, the Meulengracht Diet consists of milk, eggs, pureed fruits and vegetables, custard, ice cream, gelatin, plain pudding, crackers, bread and butter. Then, after 2 days, ground or minced meats and broiled, baked or creamed fish are included. Taboo foods are coffee, tea, cocoa, soft drinks, alcoholic beverages, spices, nuts and pastries.
(Also see MODIFIED DIETS; and ULCERS, PEPTIC.)

MEVALONIC ACID ($C_6H_{12}O_4$)

In the human body, mevalonic acid occurs as a precursor in the manufacture of cholesterol. In bacterial cultures, mevalonic acid can replace acetate as a growth promoting factor for *Lactobacillus acidophilus*, a bacterium producing lactic acid.

MEXICAN STRAWBERRY

The two most common meanings of this term follow:

• A variety of abundantly-bearing strawberry (fruit of the family *Rosaceae*) that once grew wild in the mountainous area north of Mexico City. It is noteworthy that a very large crop of the fruit is currently produced in this area, which includes the states Guanajuanto and Michoacan. Irapuato City in Guanajuanto is sometimes called the strawberry capital of the world.

• A southwestern cowboy expression for the kidney bean (a vegetable of the family *Leguminosae*.)

MICELLAR BILE-FAT COMPLEX

A micelle is a particle formed by an aggregate of molecules—a microscopic unit of protoplasm. In the micellar bile-fat complex, the particle is formed by the combination of bile salts with fat substances (fatty acids and glycerides) to facilitate the absorption of fat across the intestinal mucosa.

MICELLE

A microscopic particle of lipids and bile salts.

MICROCYTE

A small red blood cell.

MICROGRAM

A metric measure of weight which is equal to one millionth of a gram or one thousandth of a milligram. One ounce of a substance weighs over 28 million micrograms.

MICRONUTRIENTS

These are nutrients that are present in the body, and required by the body in minute quantities, ranging from millionths of a gram (microgram) to thousandths of a gram (milligram). Examples are vitamin B-12, pantothenic acid, chromium, cobalt, copper, fluorine, iodine, iron, manganese, molybdenum, selenium, silicon, and zinc. Their minuteness in no way diminishes their importance to human nutrition—many are known to be absolutely essential.

(Also see MINERAL[S]; TRACE ELEMENTS; and VITAMIN[S].)

MICROVILLI

Minute (visible only through an electron microscope) surface projections that cover the edge of each intestinal villus, called the brush border. The microvilli add a tremendous surface area for absorption.

MICROWAVE COOKING

Although microwave cooking has been available since the 1950s, it took 20 years for the microwave oven to become a common item on the market.

The magnetron tube is a vacuum tube which can convert electricity into electromagnetic energy radiation. In microwave cooking, food is cooked by the heat generated in the food itself.

The frequencies for microwave heating come under the rules of the Federal Communications Commission, which has designated four frequencies—915, 2450, 5800, and 22,125 mc/sec. The majority of the microwave ovens on the market today use 2450 megacycles.

It requires skill and experience to use the microwave oven successfully. Although it cooks foods in ½ to ⅓ the time of an electric oven, there are the following problems:

1. The microwave oven does not brown the food.
2. Frequently, microwaves do not penetrate a roast uniformly, with the result that there may be variations in doneness of meat. Thus, unless pork cooked in a microwave oven is subjected to a temperature of 170°F (77°C) *throughout* to destroy any organisms that might be present, *Trichinella spiralis* (the parasite that causes trichinosis) and food poisoning bacteria may not be destroyed.

(Also see FOOD—BUYING, PREPARING, COOKING, AND SERVING, section headed "Methods and Media of Cooking"; and MEAT[S], section headed "Meat Cooking".)

MIDDLINGS

A by-product of flour milling comprising several grades of granular particles containing different proportions of endosperm, bran, and germ, each of which contains different percentages of crude fiber.

(Also see CEREAL GRAINS; and FLOURS.)

MILK-ALKALI SYNDROME

A condition usually associated with sufferers of peptic ulcers wherein the sufferer consumes large amounts of milk and a readily absorbed alkali over a period of years resulting in hypercalcemia—high levels of calcium in the blood. Symptoms consist of vomiting, gastrointestinal bleeding, and increased blood pressure. Furthermore, kidney stones are common and calcium may be deposited in other soft tissues. The use of nonabsorbable antacids in peptic ulcer therapy seems to have lessened the prevalence of the milk-alkali syndrome.

(Also see ANTACIDS; CALCIUM; and HYPERCALCEMIA.)

MILK AND MILK PRODUCTS

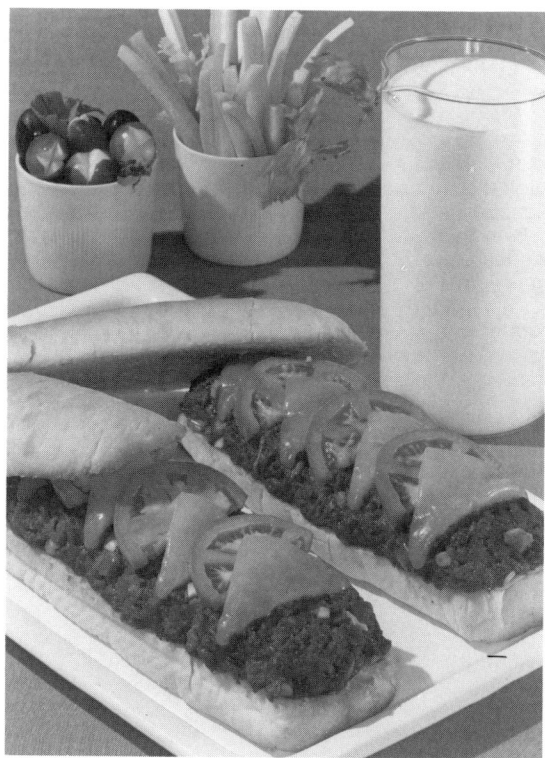

Fig. M-86.   Milk and cheeseburger; nutritious, economical, and easy to prepare. (Courtesy, United Dairy Industry Association, Rosemont, Ill.)

Milk is the fluid normally secreted by female mammals for the nourishment of their young.

Milk products include a diverse group of foods made from milk, including butter, cheese, dried nonfat milk, condensed and evaporated milk, yogurt, etc.

In different parts of the world, milk from various species of animals is used for food. In the United States, however, the cow furnishes virtually all the available market milk. Therefore, unless otherwise stated, the terms "milk" and "milk products" as used in this section refer to cow's milk.

MILK FROM VARIOUS SPECIES. Most of the world's milk is produced by cows. However, 8.6%—slightly less than one-twelfth—of the global milk supply comes from buffaloes, goats, and sheep. Yet, in 16 Asian countries for which data are available, only 51.5% of the milk is from cows, while water buffaloes, goats, and sheep produce 11.1, 15.2, and 22.2%, respectively. Mares are also used for producing milk for human consumption in different parts of the world.

A comparison of milks from various species, including humans, is given in Table M-37.

TABLE M-37
COMPOSITION OF MILKS FROM DIFFERENT SPECIES[1]
(Amount in 100 g edible portion. Dashes denote lack of reliable data for a constituent believed to be present in measurable amounts.)

Nutrient	Species				
	Cow	Human	Buffalo	Goat	Sheep
Water .... (g)	87.99	87.50	83.39	87.03	80.70
Food energy .... (kcal)	61	70	97	69	108
.... (kj)	257	291	404	288	451
Carbohydrate, total .... (g)	4.66	6.89	5.18	4.45	5.36
Fat .... (g)	3.34	4.38	6.89	4.14	7.00
Protein (N x 6.38) ...... (g)	3.29	1.03	3.75	3.56	5.98
Fiber .... (g)	0	0	0	0	0
Ash .... (g)	.72	.20	.79	.82	.96
Macrominerals					
Calcium .... (mg)	119	32	169	134	193
Phosphorus .... (mg)	93	14	117	111	158
Sodium............. (mg)	49	17	52	50	44
Magnesium.......... (mg)	13	3	31	14	18
Potassium .... (mg)	152	51	178	204	136
Microminerals					
Iron .... (mg)	.05	.03	.12	.05	.10
Zinc .... (mg)	.38	.17	.22	.30	—
Fat-soluble vitamins					
Vitamin A .... (RE)	31	64	53	56	42
.... (IU)	126	241	178	185	147
Water-soluble vitamins					
Folacin .... (mcg)	5	5	6	1	—
Niacin .... (mg)	.084	.177	.091	.277	.417
Pantothenic acid .... (mg)	.314	.223	.192	.310	.407
Riboflavin .... (mg)	.162	.036	.135	.138	.355
Thiamin .... (mg)	.038	.014	.052	.048	.065
Vitamin B-6 .... (mg)	.042	.011	.023	.046	—
Vitamin B-12 .... (mcg)	.357	.045	.363	.065	.711
Vitamin C (ascorbic acid) .... (mg)	.94	5.00	2.25	1.29	4.16
Cholesterol .... (mg)	14	14	19	11	—

[1]*Newer Knowledge of Milk and Other Fluid Dairy Products,* National Dairy Council, Rosemont, Ill., 1979, p. 44, Table D.

Goat Milk.

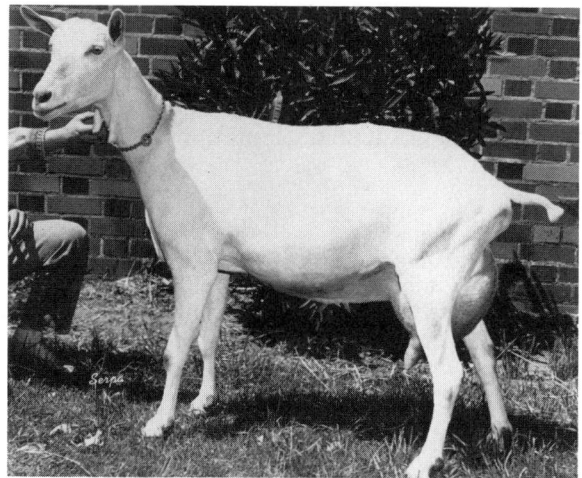

Fig. M-87. Saanen doe, Laurelwood Acres Merna, owned by Laurelwood Acres, Ripon, Calif. (Courtesy, *Dairy Goat Journal*)

Goats have played an important role in supplying milk for man since prehistoric times, and they still do so in many areas. Approximately 400 million goats, including milk, mohair and meat goats, exist throughout the world, most of them in India, China, Turkey, Ethiopia, Iran, and Brazil. Although goats supply less than 3% of the worldwide milk supply for man, it is believed that more people consume goat milk than cow's milk, even though the per capita consumption may be small. This is because the highly populated countries of Asia and Africa have 70% of the world's goats.

Dairy goats commonly produce 3 to 4 qt (*2.9 to 3.8 liter*) of milk (6 to 8 lb) daily, although some yield 20 lb (*9.1 kg*) or more daily at the peak of lactation. Goat milk resembles cow's milk in composition (see section headed "Milk From Various Species," Table M-37). However, the fat globules of goat milk are smaller and tend to remain suspended (little cream rises to the top); hence, homogenization is unnecessary. Also, goat milk is whiter in color than cow's milk, because the goat is essentially 100% efficient in converting carotene to vitamin A; it follows that butter made from goat milk is white, also. Goat milk produced under sanitary conditions is sweet, tasty, and free of off-flavors. Goat milk should be produced, handled, and processed much like cow's milk. The most important dairy goat products are milk and cheese, although goat milk can be manufactured into all the products made from cow's milk.

Since the time of Hippocrates, physicians have recommended goat milk for infants and invalids because it is easily digested. Also, those allergic to cow milk can usually drink goat milk without ill effects; and goat milk is widely used by persons afflicted with stomach ulcers.

MILK FROM COW TO TABLE. Fig. M-88 illustrates how milk gets from the cow to the table.

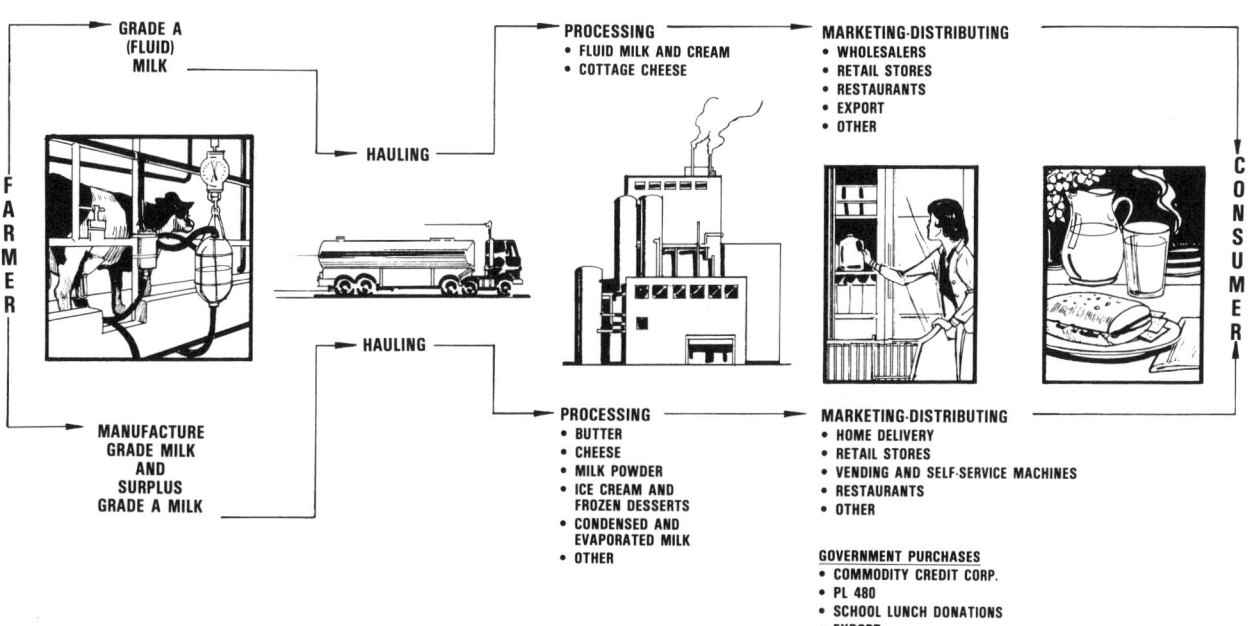

Fig. M-88. Steps and channels for getting milk from cows to table.

In summary form, the stages in getting milk from the cow to the table follow:

1. Milk is secreted by the mammary glands of a cow, beginning with the birth of a calf and continuing for about 305 days.

2. Milk is removed through the teats, generally by machine milking, although hand milking is still done.

3. Milk is cooled, usually in bulk tanks, to at least 50°F (preferably 40°F) as soon after milking as possible in order to inhibit bacterial growth.

4. Insulated trucks usually pick up milk from dairy farms daily and transport it to processing plants.

5. Processors (a) process and package fluid milk, or (b) manufacture milk into various products.

6. Milk and milk products are distributed through wholesale and retail channels to consumers.

NUTRIENTS OF MILK.[29]

Hippocrates, often referred to as the father of medicine, described milk in his

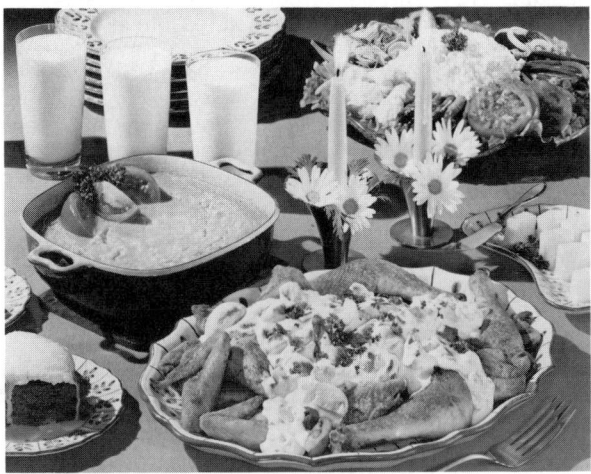

Fig. M-89. Milk is good and good for you; it's the most nearly perfect food. (Courtesy, American Dairy Association, Chicago, Ill.)

---

[29]In the preparation of this section, the authors adapted material from the following publications by the National Dairy Council: *Newer Knowledge of Milk and Other Fluid Dairy Products*, and *Dairy Council Digest*, Vol. 48, No. 5; published by National Dairy Council, Rosemont, Ill.

writings as "the most nearly perfect food." Indeed, this must be so, for the newborn mammal relies almost totally on its mother's milk for food. Its digestive tract is largely undeveloped, and its food must be nutritionally complete and easily digested and absorbed. The body of the newborn mammal grows rapidly and must cope with a great deal of stress. If milk were anything less than complete, survival of young would be difficult.

Although fluid whole milk is a liquid food (88% water), it contains an average of 12% total solids (total solids includes all the constituents of milk except water) and 8.6% solids-not-fat (includes carbohydrate, protein, minerals, and water-soluble vitamins).

More than 100 components have been identified in milk. Two glasses (1 pt) of whole milk provides approximately 23 g of carbohydrate (total), 16.3 g of fat, 16 g of protein, 3.5 g of minerals, plus fat-soluble and water-soluble vitamins. But the composition of milk varies in response to physiological factors (inherited or genetic) and environmental factors. Variations in composition occur among breeds, between milkings, and between milk taken from different sections of the udder. Also, the composition of milk is affected by the feed, the environmental temperature, the season, and the age of the cow.

Milk plays an important role in the diet of the average American, as is shown in Table M-38 and Fig. M-90. The major nutrients provided by dairy products in the American diet are food energy (9.6%), fat (11.7%), protein (19.5%), calcium (75.1%), phosphorus (34.3%), vitamin A (15.8%), and riboflavin (32.6%).

The major components of milk—carbohydrate, fat, and protein—possess a wide range of nutritional and functional properties which lend themselves to application in a variety of food formulations. Milk is also a valuable source of certain minerals and vitamins.

TABLE M–38
FOOD NUTRIENTS:
U.S. PERCENTAGE OF TOTAL CONTRIBUTED BY LIVESTOCK AND POULTRY PRODUCTS, 1988[1]

	Food Energy	Carbo-hydrates	Fat	Pro-tein	Cal-cium	Phos-phorus	Mag-nesium	Iron	Vita-min A Value	Nia-cin	Ribo-flavin	Thia-min	Vita-min B-6	Vita-min B-12
	◄——————————————————————— (%) ———————————————————————►													
Dairy products, excluding butter	9.6	5.3	11.7	19.5	75.1	34.3	18.5	2.4	15.8	1.6	32.6	7.5	10.2	18.5
Meat, fish, and poultry	18.8	0.1	31.7	43.3	3.9	29.2	15.4	22.1	20.6	44.8	22.2	25.0	40.5	76.1
Eggs	1.4	0.1	2.0	4.0	1.9	3.9	1.0	2.9	4.0	0.1	7.2	0.9	2.2	3.7
Total	29.8	5.5	45.4	66.8	80.9	67.4	34.9	27.4	40.4	46.5	62.0	33.4	52.9	98.3

[1]*Agricultural Statistics 1991*, p. 478.

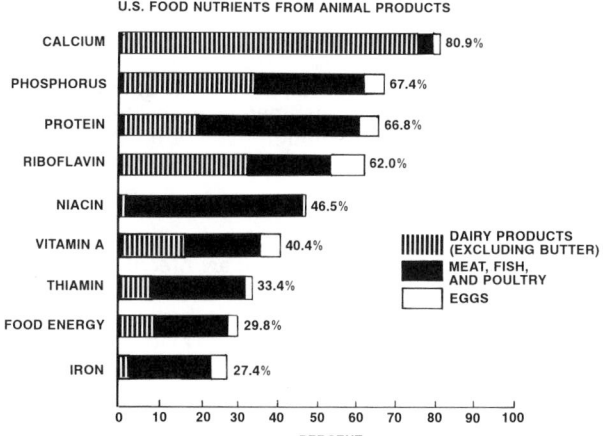

U.S. FOOD NUTRIENTS FROM ANIMAL PRODUCTS

CALCIUM 80.9%
PHOSPHORUS 67.4%
PROTEIN 66.8%
RIBOFLAVIN 62.0%
NIACIN 46.5%
VITAMIN A 40.4%
THIAMIN 33.4%
FOOD ENERGY 29.8%
IRON 27.4%

DAIRY PRODUCTS (EXCLUDING BUTTER)
MEAT, FISH, AND POULTRY
EGGS

PERCENT

Fig. M-90. Percentage of food nutrients contributed by animal products of the total supply in the U.S.

Carbohydrates In Milk. Lactose is, by far, the most abundant sugar in milk, constituting about 4.9% of cow's milk and 7.0% of human milk. This disaccharide, consisting of glucose and galactose, is only one-sixth as sweet as sucrose (table sugar) and is less soluble in water. In the small intestine, lactose is cleaved to form its constituent monosaccharides. Glucose is readily absorbed, while galactose is slowly absorbed, thereby serving as a growth promotant for intestinal bacteria that synthesize the vitamins biotin, folacin, and riboflavin in the intestine. Lactose is also converted to lactic acid by intestinal bacteria. When lactic acid is produced in the intestines, growth of pathogenic bacteria is inhibited.

Lactose has been shown to facilitate the absorption of calcium. Also, there are reports that lactose enhances the absorption of barium, magnesium, phosphorus, radium, strontium, and zinc.

Glucose and galactose are the products of lactose hydrolysis by the enzyme lactase. Some individuals are unable to metabolize lactose because of reduced lactase levels, a condition termed lactose intolerance. Preparations of the enzyme lactase are now being marketed for commercial or consumer addition to milk. The resulting milk is sweeter tasting because the majority of the lactose is hydrolyzed to glucose and galactose.

Lactose has many food uses; among them, the following: as an anticaking ingredient in dry mixtures such as nondairy coffee whiteners; as a flavor enhancer in dusting powders to flavor potato chips, barbecue sauces, salad dressings, pie fillings, and puddings; in candies and confectionery products; and in the bakery industry.

(Also see subsequent section headed "Lactose Intolerance.")

Milk Fat. Milk fat, sometimes called butterfat, contributes about 48% of the calories of whole milk. Fat also gives milk its flavor.

Milk fat is highly emulsified, which facilitates its diges-

tion. Since fats must be liquid or emulsified at body temperature to be digested and absorbed, and since milk fat has a melting point lower than body temperature, it is efficiently utilized—particularly by the young and the elderly.

Fat is the most variable constituent of milk, the amount being affected primarily by such factors as breed of cow and environmental temperature (a given cow will produce higher fat milk in cool weather than in hot weather). Minor factors affecting the amount of milk fat include the type and amount of feed and the stage of lactation. Feed also influences the fatty acid composition of the fat produced; for example, cows consuming succulent feed or pasture produce much more oleic acid than cows receiving dry roughage.

Milk fat consists of 12.5% glycerol and 87.5% fatty acids, by weight. The fatty acids combine with glycerol in units of three fatty acid molecules per glycerol molecule to form triglycerides which make up 95 to 96% of the total milk fat.

Milk fat contains a greater number of different fatty acids than any other food fat; approximately 500 different fatty acids and fatty acid derivatives have been identified in milk. Milk fat contains a relatively high proportion of short-chain fatty acids. These short-chain fatty acids (which are virtually absent in most vegetable oils) are water-soluble, are absorbed through the intestinal wall without being resynthesized to glycerides, and are transported in the portal vein directly to the liver where they are immediately converted to forms utilizable for energy. For this reason, they serve as a quick source of energy, which may be important—especially early in life.

Generally, the fatty acids are approximately 66% saturated (devoid of double bonds between the carbon atoms), 30% monounsaturated, and 4% polyunsaturated. The saturated fatty acids present in largest amounts in milk fat are myristic, palmitic, and stearic. The chief unsaturated (double-bond linkage between the carbon atoms) fatty acids are oleic, linoleic, and linolenic. Arachidonic acid, which has four double bonds, is present in trace amounts. Arachidonic acid and its precursor, linoleic acid, are essential fatty acids—they are not synthesized in the human body, or they are not synthesized fast enough; consequently, they must be supplied in the diet.

Milk fat is available in the food industry as conventional butter, anhydrous milk fat, or anhydrous butter oil.

Besides butter, fluid whole milk, cheeses, and ice cream are the main dairy foods in which milk fat is consumed in the United States. Milk fat is also used in the candy industry, in the baking industry, and, in the form of butter, in soups and sauces for frozen and canned vegetables.

Cholesterol is the principal sterol in milk. An 8-oz (1 cup, or *240 ml*) serving of whole fluid milk (3.34% fat) contains 33 mg of cholesterol, whereas a similar serving of fluid skim milk (0.1% fat) contains 4 mg of cholesterol. In order to limit the consumption of cholesterol to 300 mg per day, as is recommended by most health professionals, low-fat dairy products may be used.

Protein in Milk. Fluid whole milk contains an average of 3.3% protein, mainly casein and whey proteins. Protein accounts for about 38% of the total solids-not-fat content of milk and for about 22% of the calories of whole milk. Dairy products (excluding butter) contributed 19.5% of the total protein in the U.S. diet in 1990.

The proteins of milk are of very high quality, having a biological value of 85 as compared to 50 to 65 for the cereal proteins. They contain, in varying amounts, all of the amino acids required by man. Except for the sulfur-containing amino acids (methionine and cystine), 1 pt (*470 ml*) of milk supplies the recommended daily allowance of all the essential amino acids. Additionally, the protein to calorie ratio is very favorable in milk, assuring that the consumer is not ingesting "empty" calories.

It is also noteworthy that milk is rich in the amino acid tryptophan, a precursor of niacin; hence, milk is an excellent source of niacin equivalents. (One niacin equivalent is defined as 1 mg of niacin or 60 mg of tryptophan.) It is noteworthy, too, that the immunoglobulins in milk are a heterogeneous group of antibody proteins that serve as a source of passive immunity for the newborn, and that colostrum contains large quantities of globulins. A discusion of milk proteins follows:

• **Casein**—Comprising about 82% of the total protein content, casein is found only in milk, in which it is the principal protein. It gives milk its white color. Casein alone has a somewhat lower biological value than the whey proteins because of the limited quantity of the sulfur-containing amino acids. Commercial casein is made by either of two techniques: (1) precipitation by acid, or (2) coagulation by rennin. This procedure is followed by washing and drying the casein curd to a granular powder. The caseins and caseinates (sodium caseinate and calcium caseinate) are concentrated forms of proteins which have exceptional water-binding, fat-emulsifying and whipping capabilities.

Casein has been utilized as the main source of protein in the manufacture of meat analogs and as a protein supplement in some meat products. Also, it has found application in baked goods and as an ingredient of coffee whitener and whipped toppings.

Sodium caseinates are used in the meat industry as water-binding agents, as well as in the preparation of toppings, cream substitutes, and numerous desserts as whip-imparting agents.

Calcium caseinate, while significantly less soluble than the sodium salt, is used in various specialized dietary foods where low sodium intake is essential.

• **Whey protein**—A by-product of cheese and casein manufacture, whey is the liquid that remains after the removal of casein and fat from milk.

Like casein, whey protein is a complex mixture of a large number of protein fractions, with beta-lactoglobulin and alpha-lactalbumin being the principal ones of commercial interest. The whey proteins have a relative surplus of the sulfur-containing amino acids.

Recent advances have made the production of undenatured whey protein concentrates (WPC) a commercial reality. Among the uses made of WPC in food products are: in the fortification of acid fruit drinks and carbonated beverages; in cake flour; in dessert topping; and

as a binder in the production of textured vegetable protein products. Also, the excellent binding, emulsifying, and gelling properties of WPC have been utilized in the formulation of meat products, soups, and sauces. In addition to the contributions that whey proteins make toward improved organoleptic characteristics in other foods, their nutritional contributions should not be underestimated.

• **Co-precipitates**—As the name implies, co-precipitates contain the total milk proteins that are precipitated from fresh milk. They are unique in that they contain both caseins and whey proteins, thus making them of high nutritional value. The low content of lactose also makes these co-precipitates useful in formulations where the use of dry milk powder may be unacceptable. Co-precipitates have found uses in baking, in dessert and confectionery products, and in meat analogs.

Minerals In Milk. Minerals are generally classified as macrominerals or microminerals, according to the amounts needed in the diet. These two groupings will be used in the discussion that follows:

• **Macrominerals**—Minerals that are needed at levels of 100 mg or more daily are generaly classified as macrominerals.

1. **Calcium.** Of all the foods commonly eaten in the American diet, milk is one of the best and most commonly consumed sources of calcium. Dairy products (exclusive of butter) contributed 75.1% of the total calcium in the U.S. diet in 1990.

It is difficult to meet the RDA for calcium without including milk or milk products in the diet. Two 8-oz glasses (1 pt or *480 ml*) of milk daily will provide about 73% of the adult RDA for calcium. An additional allowance of 400 mg of calcium per day (a total of 1.2 g) during pregnancy and lactation will provide for the needs of the mother, the growing fetus, and the infant; a quart (*950 ml*) of milk will meet approximately 97% of this calcium allowance. For children 1 to 10 years of age, 800 mg of calcium daily are recommended, an allowance which is amply met by three 8-oz glasses of milk. During periods of rapid growth in preadolescence and puberty, 1.2 g of calcium per day are recommended, an amount supplied by 1 qt of milk.

2. **Phosphorus.** Dairy products (exclusive of butter) contributed 34.3% of the total phosphorus in the U.S. diet in 1990.

The RDA for phosphorus is the same as that for calcium after 1 year of age, thus two glasses (*480 ml*) of milk will supply the same percentage of the RDA for phosphorus as that for calcium.

3. **Magnesium.** Dairy products (exclusive of butter) contributed 18.5% of the total magnesium in the U.S. diet in 1990.

The RDA for magnesium is about 350 and 280 mg for adult males and females, respectively. Milk contains about 13 mg per 100 g; so, two 8-oz glasses (1 pt) furnish about 19% of the magnesium RDA for the adult male and 20.5% for the adult female.

• **Microminerals**—These are the minerals which are needed at levels of a few milligrams daily. Of the 103 known microminerals, 17 exhibit biological function in man and animals. The contribution which milk makes to the essential trace element intake is greatest with respect to zinc and possibly iodine.

The microminerals in milk are derived from the cow's feedstuffs, water, and environment. The concentrations are highly variable due to stage of lactation, season, milk yield, amount of the trace element in the cow's diet, handling of the milk following pasteurization, and storage conditions.

1. **Iodine.** Iodine is present in milk, but in variable amounts. As sea water is rich in iodine, milk from coastal agricultural areas contains more iodine than milk from inland areas. The iodine content of milk is highly dependent upon the composition of the animal's feed; it can be increased by as much as 200 times by adding iodine to the feed or by giving iodized salt blocks. Whole milk normally contains 13 to 37 mcg iodine per 100 g. So, two 8-oz glasses (*480 ml*) of milk supply about 25 to 69% of the iodine RDA for an adult man, 25 to 50 years of age.

2. **Iron.** Milk is a poor source of iron. The iron content of milk ranges from 10 to 90 mcg per 100 g. Feeding supplemental iron to cows does not increase the iron content of milk. However, milk is a very satisfactory food for iron fortification.

Two 8-oz glasses (1 pt) of milk provide about 1% of the iron recommended for women of childbearing age.

3. **Zinc.** This mineral occurs in many foods, including milk. The zinc content of milk varies from 0.3 to 0.6 mg per 100 g of milk, with an average of 0.38 mg. It may be slightly increased by feeding zinc supplement to the cow. About 88% of zinc in milk is associated with casein; thus, the level of zinc in milk is mostly related to the milk protein content. It follows that the zinc content of lowfat and skim milk is virtually identical to that of whole milk.

Two 8-oz glasses (1 pt) of milk provide about 14% of the zinc RDA for adults.

(Also see MINERAL[S].)

Vitamins in Milk. For convenience, the vitamins in milk are grouped and discussed as fat-soluble vitamins and water-soluble vitamins in the discussion that follows:

• **Fat-soluble vitamins**—Vitamins A, D, E, and K are associated with the fat component of milk. Their quantities in milk, with the exception of vitamin K are dependent upon the dietary intake of the cow.

1. Vitamin A and its precursors, the carotenoids (principally beta-carotene), are present in high, but variable, quantities in milk. The carotenoids, which give milk its characteristic creamy color, constitute from 11 to 50% of the total vitamin A activity of milk. The carotenoid intake of the cow varies seasonally, generally being highest when the animals are on pasture.

One hundred grams of whole milk contain about 126 IU of vitamin A (31 RE); so, 1 qt (*960 ml*), of whole milk will supply about 30% of the vitamin A recommended dietary allowance (RDA) of 5,000 IU (1,000 RE) for the adult male.

2. **Vitamin D.** Vitamin D (ergocalciferol and cholecalciferol), the ricket-preventing vitamin, is present in low concentrations in unfortified milk. However, approximately 98% of the fluid milk marketed in the United States is fortified with vitamin D to obtain standardized amounts of 400 IU (10 mcg cholecalciferol) per quart, the recommended intake for most persons.

The addition of vitamin D to fluid whole milk—thereby resulting in a widely used food providing calcium, phosphorus, and vitamin D—has been credited with the virtual eradication of rickets among children in the United States. The vitamin D fortification of milk to provide a concentration of 400 IU per quart has been endorsed by the Food and Nutrition Board, National Research Council/National Academy of Sciences; the American Academy of Pediatrics; and the American Medical Association.

3. **Vitamin E.** Vitamin E (principally alpha-tocopherol) is present in low concentrations in milk.

4. **Vitamin K.** Vitamin K is found only in trace amounts in milk. Also, there is some indication that part of the vitamin K of milk is destroyed by pasteurization.

• **Water-soluble vitamins**—All of the vitamins known to be essential for man have been detected in milk. The water-soluble vitamins are in the nonfat portion. The content of water-soluble vitamins in milk is relatively constant and not easily influenced by the vitamin content of the cow's ration.

1. **Biotin.** Milk is a fairly good source of biotin, generally providing about 3 mcg per 100 g. Two glasses of milk would provide between 7 and 23% of the average daily dietary intake of this vitamin. Less than 10% of biotin is destroyed by pasteurization.

2. **Folate (folic acid).** According to recent analyses, milk contains an average of 5 mcg of folate per 100 g. Two glasses (*480 ml*), of milk would supply about 12% of the 200 mcg RDA. Folate of milk is decreased by heat, but this can be minimized by excluding oxygen.

3. **Niacin.** The average niacin content of milk is only 0.08 mg per 100 g; so, two glasses of milk make little contribution (2 to 3%) to the 15 mg niacin RDA for adults. Nevertheless, milk and milk products are among the most effective pellagra-preventive foods because of (a) the complete availability of niacin in milk; and (b) the presence of the amino acid tryptophan (about 46 mg tryptophan per 100 g milk) in milk protein, which can be used for the synthesis of niacin in the body. (A dietary intake of 60 mg tryptophan is equivalent to 1 mg niacin.) Thus, the niacin value of milk is considerably greater than is reflected by its niacin concentration. Also, it is noteworthy that pasteurization does not destroy the niacin content of milk.

4. **Pantothenic acid (vitamin B-3).** Milk is a good source of pantothenic acid; it averages abut 0.31 mg of pantothenic acid per 100 g. Pasteurization does not destroy the pantothenic acid in milk.

5. **Riboflavin (vitamin B-2).** Milk is an important source of this vitamin; dairy products (excluding butter) contributed 32.6% of the total riboflavin in the U.S. diet in 1990. The average riboflavin content of fluid whole milk is about 0.16 mg per 100 g. Two glasses (*480 ml*) of milk would supply between 45 and 60% of the 1.3 to 1.7 mg RDA for adults. Although riboflavin is not sensitive to heat, it can be destroyed by exposure to light. Riboflavin losses due to light can be minimized by protecting milk from exposure to strong light through utilizing opaque containers, transporting milk in special trucks, and storing milk in darkened refrigerators.

6. **Thiamin (vitamin B-1).** Significant quantities of this vitamin are found in milk—an average of 0.04 mg per 100 g. Since the RDA for thiamin is between 1.1 and 1.5 mg for the adult, two glasses of milk per day would supply about 13 to 18% of the RDA. Pasteurization results in the loss of about 10% of the thiamin.

7. **Vitamin B-6 (pyridoxine, pyridoxal, pyridoxamine).** An average of about 0.04 mg of vitamin B-6 are found in 100 g of milk; but there is considerable variation in the content of this vitamin in milk. Two glasses of milk furnish about 10% of the 2 mg RDA for adults. Pasteurization does not affect the vitamin B-6 content of milk.

8. **Vitamin B-12.** Milk is a good source of vitamin B-12; it contributed 18.5% of the total vitamin B-12 in the U.S. diet in 1990. Milk averages about 0.36 mcg of vitamin B-12 per 100 g. Two glasses of milk would furnish about 88% of the 2 mcg RDA for most adults. Pasteurization causes only minor destruction of the vitamin B-12 in milk.

9. **Vitamin C (ascorbic acid).** Fresh raw milk contains a small amount of ascorbic acid (about 0.94 mg per 100 g of milk), but processing and exposure to light and heat reduce the amount.

10. **Other vitamins.** Milk also contains choline, myoinositol, and para-aminobenzoic acid, the quantitative requirements of which have not been established.

(Also see VITAMIN[S].)

MILK AS A FOOD.[30]

Milk is often referred to as "the most nearly perfect food." It is consumed as a liquid and in the form of such products as butter, cheese, ice cream, and numerous other foods. Milk contains all the nutrients (food elements) needed for growth and good health.

The milk food group makes important contributions to the diet. Milk and milk products are the leading source of calcium and a good source of phosphorus. Also, they provide high-quality protein, the fat-soluble vitamins—A, D (when fortified), E, and K, and all the water-soluble vitamins. Lowfat or skim-milk products fortified with vitamins A and D have essentially the same nutrients as whole milk products, but with fewer calories.

No food has a wider acceptability or offers a greater variety of uses than milk. It is the first food of newborn babies, whether they are breast-fed or bottle-fed; and milk and milk products are important throughout life. For this reason, milk and dairy foods comprise a separate group in The Four Food Groups.

The sections that follow deal primarily with the role of milk in meeting the nutrient needs of various age groups.

(Also see FOOD GROUPS.)

Milk for Pregnant and Lactating Women.

The recommended nutrient allowances (RDA) during pregnancy and lactation are given in the section on Nutrients: Requirements, Allowances, Functions, Sources, Table N-6.

---

[30]In the preparation of this section, the authors adapted material from the following publication by the National Dairy Council: *Newer Knowledge of Milk and Other Fluid Dairy Products*, National Dairy Council, Rosemont, Ill.

Milk has an important role during pregnancy and lactation. The extent to which milk would supply the RDA for nutrients during pregnancy and lactation is shown in Table M-39.

NOTE WELL: Table M-39 calls for 4 cups (*950 ml*) of 2% milk during both pregnancy and lactation.

TABLE M–39
THE EXTENT TO WHICH SUGGESTED QUANTITIES OF MILK SUPPLY THE RDA FOR VARIOUS NUTRIENTS FOR WOMEN 25 TO 50 YEARS OF AGE[1]

Nutrient	Percentage of RDA		
	Amount in Adulthood 2 cups	Amount in Pregnancy 4 cups	Amount in Lactation 4 cups
	◄——— (%) ———►		
Energy	11	19.5	18.1
Protein	32	54	50
Macrominerals			
Calcium	74	99	99
Phosphorus	58	77	77
Magnesium	24	43	39
Microminerals			
Iron	1.6	1.6	3.2
Zinc	15.8	25	20
Fat-soluble vitamins			
Vitamin A (RE)	37.5	75	46
Vitamin D[2]	100	100	100
Water-soluble vitamins			
Folate	13.6	12.2	17.4
Niacin	2.8	4.9	4.2
Riboflavin	61.5	100	88.9
Thiamin	18.2	26.7	25
Vitamin B-6	13.8	20	21
Vitamin B-12	89.0	162	137
Vitamin C (ascorbic acid)	7.7	13	10

[1]Calculated from: *Recommended Dietary Allowances*, 1989, National Research Council and Table F-36, Food Composition Table, p. 942, using 2% milk.

[2]Milk fortified with 400 IU vitamin D per quart. One cup equals about 240 ml.

Further information in support of including milk in the diet of pregnant and lactating women follows:

• **Protein**—Growth of the fetus and the production of breast milk require additional protein. The National Research Council (NRC), National Academy of Sciences, recommends an additional 10 g of protein per day during pregnancy. Thus, a pregnant female 25 to 50 years of age whose nonpregnant allowance is 50 g/day would have a total protein allowance of 60 g/day.

The NRC recommends the addition of 15 g of protein daily to the allowance during lactation. So, a lactating female 25 to 50 years of age whose normal allowance is 50 g/day would have a total protein allowance of 65 g/day.

In addition to providing added quantity of protein during pregnancy and lactation, it is noteworthy that the proteins of milk are of high biological value due to the excellent assortment of amino acids.

• **Calcium, phosphorus, and vitamin D**—Calcium is one of the most important nutrients in the diet of pregnant and lactating women. During the last trimester of pregnancy, calcium is deposited in the fetus at the rate of 200 to 300 mg daily. Also, phosphorus and vitamin D are important. As shown in Table M-39, milk is an excellent way in which to provide added calcium, phosphorus, and vitamin D during the critical periods of pregnancy and lactation.

• **Vitamins**—The allowances of most of the vitamins are increased during pregnancy and lactation. Four cups (*950 ml*) of milk daily during these critical periods will contribute significantly to the increased vitamin allowances except for ascorbic acid.

(Also see PREGNANCY AND LACTATION NUTRITION.)

Milk for Infants. Human milk of high quality is regarded as the best source of nourishment of the infant. The curd formed is exceedingly fine and flaky, thus aiding digestion. Also, it is important that newborn babies receive colostrum, the secretion of the mammary glands, for the first 2 to 4 days following birth. Colostrum contains more protein, minerals, and vitamin A than regular milk, but less carbohydrate and fat. Also, and most important, it is a rich source of bacteria and viral antibodies which may provide the infant with resistance to infections by organisms that enter the body through the gastrointestinal tract. Iron supplements can be prescribed if the infant's body stores are insufficient. Vitamin D and fluoride can also be supplied by supplements. The sanitary quality of the milk can be assured by the personal hygiene of the nursing mother.

A comparison between the nutrient content of human and cow's milk is given under the heading "Milk of Different Species," Table M-37. As noted, human milk is lower in protein (1.0% in human milk vs 3.3% in cow's milk), and the protein of human milk contains a higher ratio of whey proteins to casein, whereas casein is the predominant protein of cow's milk. Also, human milk is higher in carbohydrate (7.0% carbohydrate in human milk vs 4.8% in cow's milk); lower in ash (0.20% in human milk vs 0.72% in cow's milk); and, with the exception of ascorbic acid, vitamin B-12, and vitamin A, the vitamins are present in smaller quantities in human milk than in cow's milk. Considering both preformed niacin and the amino acid tryptophan, cow's milk contains almost twice the niacin equivalent of human milk.

For infant feeding, cow's milk should be modified so that it more closely meets the nutrient and physical requirements of infants. Its high casein content is responsible for forming the large, tough curd, which is difficult to digest, compared with the curd from human milk. However, when cow's milk is heated, homogenized, or acidified to prevent curd formation, the protein is utilized as efficiently as that of human milk. The types of formulas most commonly used are evaporated milk and commercially prepared formulas. Evaporated milk is heated, homogenized, concentrated whole cow's milk available in 13-oz cans. It is reconstituted with water. Carbohydrate (corn syrup or another carbohydrate source) is added to maintain a relatively constant proportion of the total calories being provided by carbohydrate. Evaporated milk is fortified with vitamin D, but iron and ascorbic acid may need to be added. The latter is usually provided from 2 weeks of age by supplements, fortified infant fruit juices, or orange juice.

The transition to solid foods is a gradual process, as is the transition from human milk or formula to fresh fluid milk. It is recommended that whole milk rather than skim or lowfat milk be fed to children under 2 years of age.

Even after other foods are introduced, milk will supply over half the calories and many essential nutrients in the infant diet. It should continue to play an essential role in nourishing the infant throughout childhood.

(Also see INFANT DIET AND NUTRITION.)

Milk for Children and Adolescents.

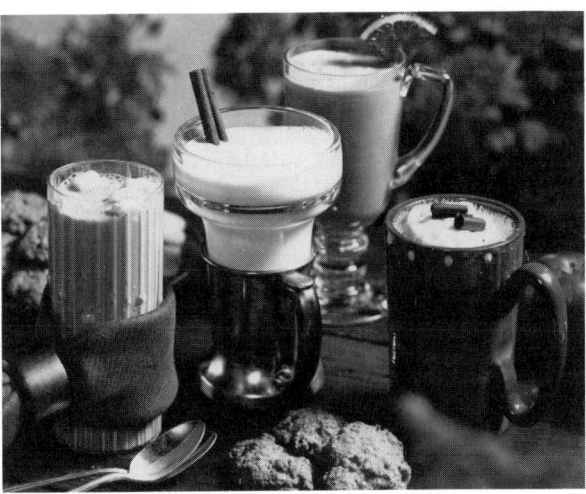

Fig. M-91. Zippy milk drinks. Children and adolescents should come to know that milk is a "fun drink" and good for them. (Courtesy, American Dairy Association, Chicago, Ill.)

As used herein, the "child and adolescent" stage covers the period from weaning to the completion of physical growth, although some people continue to grow in height up to age 30. A further breakdown into the child and adolescent stages is sometimes made; with the childhood stage covering the period from weaning to pubescence, and the adolescence period extending from the end of pubescence to the completion of physical growth—between 16 and 18 years of age in girls, and around 18 to 21 in boys.

During the preschool period, there is a slowing of the growth rate and a lessening of the appetite. Nevertheless, the bones and teeth continue to develop throughout the preschool years, requiring a basic supply of protein, calcium, phosphorus, and vitamin D. Abundant quantities of protein, vitamins, and minerals are also needed for soft tissue growth, which is rapid at this time, and for the development and maintenance of the blood supply.

A daily intake of 2 cups (*480 ml*) of milk, or even less, is not uncommon just before or during the second year of life. Some compensation for reduced milk intake at this stage in life may be made by offering milk puddings, cheese, yogurt, or ice cream. Three glasses (*720 ml*) of milk daily, incorporated with the meat, eggs, fruits, vegetables, cereals, bread and butter will usually supply the nutrients needed. Vitamin D can be obtained from vitamin D fortified milk and from exposure to sunlight which enables the body to synthesize it.

By 6 years of age, the appetite and rate of growth increase. Three cups (*720 ml*) of milk daily, along with generous amounts of other wholesome foods, will supply the nutrient needs for the average child. Three cups of milk will supply the calcium RDA (800 mg daily) for children 1 to 10 years of age; and 3 cups of vitamin D milk will also provide 75% of the 10 mcg of vitamin D recommended for proper calcification of bones and teeth.

The increased nutritional requirements of the adolescent are conditioned primarily by the growth spurt associated with pubescence (period of sexual development, ending with the capacity for sexual reproduction). The pubescent growth spurt is characterized by an increase in body size, a rate of increase which is matched or exceeded only by the developing fetus and the infant during the first year of life. This growth spurt occurs earlier and less extensively in girls than in boys.

At least 1 qt (*950 ml*) of milk daily, or its equivalent in cheese, yogurt, ice cream, or other milk products, is recommended for this period of growth. This amount of milk or its equivalent in other milk products will provide all the calcium and 55% of the protein recommended for teenagers. One quart of vitamin D milk also supplies the vitamin D recommended, generous amounts of vitamin A and riboflavin—which are important for growth and skin health, along with significant amounts of all major nutrients except iron and ascorbic acid.

(Also see CHILDHOOD AND ADOLESCENT NUTRITION.)

Milk for Adults. A nutritionally adequate diet for adults is of paramount importance, particularly with increased life expectancy.

The concept that dietary calcium is no longer required after bony structures are fully formed is erroneous. The RDA calls for 800 mg calcium daily for adults. Two glasses (*480 ml*) of milk provide almost 75% of this amount. Some individuals may adapt to lower calcium intakes. However, moderate deficiencies of calcium over a long time may cause decreased bone density, predisposing to osteoporosis and possibly periodontal disease (through loss of alveolar bone).

Two glasses (1 pt) of milk also provide the adult with about 30% of the protein RDA, generous amounts of vitamin A and riboflavin, and smaller but significant amounts of all major nutrients except iron and ascorbic acid. In view of these contributions, the caloric yield of two glasses of whole milk, 300 calories, or 2% milk, 244 calories, is indeed moderate.

(Also see ADULT NUTRITION.)

Milk for the Elderly. The fundamental nutrient needs of the healthy older adult are the same as those of the younger adult. However, the gradual decline in the basal metabolic rate as the body ages, and the decrease in physical activity that usually occurs, reduce caloric requirements. Men and women over 51 years of age need 300 to 200 fewer calories per day, respectively, than they did between 25 and 50 years of age. However, their needs for the other essential nutrients, such as calcium and protein, are unchanged. So, the caloric intake must not be reduced at the expense of essential nutrients. Requirements for protein and calcium may even be increased, depending upon previous nutriture and general health. Digestion, absorption, and even utilization of nutrients may be less efficient. Hence, it is wise to supply all nutrients in recommended amounts.

Milk is an important food for the elderly as it furnishes a generous supply of nutrients in relation to calories. That is, milk has high nutrient density. Moreover, if mastication becomes difficult, as it may with dentures, milk alone or in combination with eggs may be the major source of high-quality protein in the diet. Also, milkfat is sometimes more readily digested than other fats.

With aging, there is increased prevalence of the disabling symptoms of osteoporosis, a problem of bone demineralization. Since osteoporosis involves the loss of bone matrix and minerals, a diet generous in protein, calcium, vitamin D, and fluoride has been recommended. Thus, milk, due to its content of calcium and other nutrients, is an important food for this segment of the population. Furthermore, for the elderly, milk is an efficient source of nutrients readily tolerated by a sometimes weakened digestive system.

(Also see GERONTOLOGY AND GERIATRIC NUTRITION.)

Milk for Therapy. Therapeutic diets are fundamentally adaptations of the regular diet, planned to maintain or restore good nutrition in the individual under treatment. Recovery in many illnesses may be hastened by fulfilling all nutritional requirements. For this reason, therapeutic diets should meet or exceed the RDA for a normal individual, except when less than normal nutrient requirements are indicated, as in caloric or sodium restrictions. In planning hospital diets, daily milk intake for adults is frequently increased from 2 to 3 cups (*480 to 720 ml*) because milk provides many essential nutrients in a form easily consumed.

In an analysis of specific therapeutic diets frequently used, milk (whole, lowfat, or skim) is found to be incorporated either in generous or in specified amounts in all the therapeutic diets except in clear-fluid diets, very low-residue and protein-free diets, galactose-free and low phenylalanine diets, and in the dumping syndrome (a complication associated with gastric resection which limits the stomach's capacity as a reservoir so that ingested material enters the intestine in larger quantities and more rapidly; symptoms such as abdominal fullness, distention, weakness, and sweating ensue.)

Specific therapeutic diets are the province of the medical and dietetic professions. However, the wide use of milk in therapeutic diets in addition to clinical evidence attests to milk's value as a food and to its unique physical adaptability to the nourishment of humans with abnormal as well as normal capacity to ingest food.

HEALTH ASPECTS OF MILK CONSUMPTION.

Numerous advantages, along with some disadvantages, should be considered when incorporating milk in a nutrition program.

Health Benefits from Milk. The health, strength and vitality of people is dependent upon their getting an adequate supply of the right nutrients and foods. Milk, the most nearly perfect food, contributes richly to these needs. It bridges the gap all the way from the dependent fetus to independent old age.

The health imparting qualities of milk are indicated by the fact that daily consumption of a quart (*950 ml*) of cow's milk furnishes an average adult approximately all the fat, calcium, phosphorus, and riboflavin; ½ the protein; ⅓ of the vitamin A, ascorbic acid, and thiamin; ¼ of the calories; and, with the exception of iron, copper, manganese, and magnesium, all the minerals needed daily. These and other nutritional and health benefits of milk are detailed under two earlier headings of this section entitled "Nutrients of Milk" and "Milk as a Food"; hence, the reader is referred thereto.

Additional health benefits of milk are evidenced by its contribution to longevity, tranquilizing effect, ulcer therapy, symbolic meaning, and, perhaps, lessening stomach cancer; each of which is discussed in a separate section that follows.

LONGEVITY. As shown in Table M-40, most of the countries with high life expectancies, produce considerable quantities of milk on a per capita basis.

TABLE M-40
PER CAPITA MILK PRODUCTION OF COUNTRIES WITH HIGHEST LIFE EXPECTANCY AT BIRTH

Longevity Rank	Country	Life Expectancy[1]	Per Capita Milk Production[2]	
		(years)	(lb)	(kg)
1	Japan	79.3	146	66
2	Switzerland	78.9	1,269	577
3	Spain	78.2	343	156
4	Italy	78.0	413	188
5	Sweden	77.7	895	407
6	Greece	77.6	141	64
7	Netherlands	77.6	1,650	750
8	France	77.6	1,033	470
9	Canada	77.3	656	298
10	Austria	77.1	958	435
11	Belgium	76.9	816	371
12	Australia	76.6	838	381
13	United Kingdom	76.3	575	261
14	Denmark	75.7	2,018	917
15	**United States**	**75.6**	**593**	**270**
16	Germany	75.5	952	433
17	Cuba	75.5	N/A	N/A
18	Portugal	74.4	315	143

[1]*Statistical Abstract of the United States 1991*, U.S. Dept. of Commerce, p. 834, Table 1436.

[2]*Milk Facts 1991*, Milk Industry Foundation, p. 32.

TRANQUILIZING EFFECT. Soon after consumption of milk, a general mild tranquilizing effect can be felt. While the exact cause of this effect has not been determined, some researchers feel that it may be due to the high concentration of calcium in milk.

ULCER THERAPY. Formerly, milk was commonly used in duodenal ulcer therapy. While milk does relieve duodenal ulcer pain, the acid neutralizing effect is slight; its buffering action may be overweighed by its ability to stimulate acid production. So, the use of milk therapy has been greatly reduced in recent years, owing to more knowledge of its side effects and allergic reactions. Nevertheless, the controversy regarding the use of milk in ulcer therapy continues. There are those who still advocate the regular use of milk, primarily during the active stage of duodenal ulcer. Whether or not milk is included, duodenal ulcer therapy generally calls for a bland diet of soft creamy foods, eaten frequently and in small quantities and supplemented with vitamins to compensate for lacking nutrients.

SYMBOLIC MEANING. Milk is imbued with more physiologic meaning than any other food. To many persons, it symbolizes security and comfort, especially if the individual's early relationships with the mother were happy; it conjures up the recollection of an infant held lovingly in its mother's arms. Such a person away from home, or ill, relishes milk as symbolic of the comfort and security of home.

On the other hand, milk may be refused because it imparts a feeling of dependence to an individual, which he does not want to admit. This type of person is prone to remark that he does not "want to be treated like a baby."

LESSENING STOMACH CANCER. Several studies have shown that populations consuming small amounts of milk have a higher incidence of stomach cancer than populations that consume large amounts of milk. Since this trend is largely based on statistical surveys of populations, and not physiological experiments, it cannot be accepted as conclusive.

Health Problems from Milk. Several metabolic disorders are found in certain individuals when milk is introduced into the diet; among them, milk allergy, lactose intolerance, milk intolerance, galactose disease, milk anemia, or following gastric surgery.

MILK ALLERGY (MILK SENSITIVITY). Cow's milk is probably the most common food allergen in the United States, estimates of the incidence of which range from 0.3 to 3%. It tends to run in families; and an infant who has an allergy to milk may also be allergic to other foods, such as eggs.

The common symptoms of milk allergy are colic, spitting up the feeding, irritability, loose stools, respiratory problems, and/or allergic skin reactions—usually eczema. Other signs may include asthma, headache, tension, fatigue, and possibly hyperactivity. More serious problems, such as shock (cardiovascular collapse), may rarely occur. In some infants, the incidence of hypochromic anemia has been attributed to sensitivity to milk. Following the ingestion of milk by these sensitive infants, some blood is lost from the gastrointestinal tract.

The blood loss may go unnoticed until the anemia becomes apparent months later. In other cases, the infants may have a sufficiently high intake of other iron-rich foods so that the anemic tendency is counteracted. The symptoms may occur as early as 2 to 4 weeks of age, or they may appear later. In a susceptible breast-fed baby, the symptoms will begin soon after the cow's milk feeding starts.

Where allergy to cow's milk exists, the following dietary alternatives are suggested:

1. Substitute goat's milk.
2. Change the form of the milk; that is, try boiled, powdered, acidulated, or evaporated milk.
3. Eliminate cow's milk and milk products from the diet, and substitute formulas in which the protein is derived from meat or soybeans.
(Also see ALLERGIES.)

LACTOSE INTOLERANCE.   During digestion, nature ordained that lactose (milk sugar) be hydrolyzed (split) into its component monosaccharides, glucose and galactose, by the enzyme lactase. Sometimes this physiological process does not occur, and lactose intolerance results.

Lactose intolerance is the malabsorption of the milk sugar lactose due to a decrease in, or absence of, the enzyme lactase, which results in characteristic clinical symptoms (abdominal pain, diarrhea, bloating, flatulence). Three types of lactose intolerance are known:

1. Congenital lactose intolerance (often regarded as an inborn error of metabolism), a relatively rare condition, caused by an absence of lactase from birth.
2. Secondary lactose intolerance caused by damage by viruses, bacteria, allergens, etc. to the outer cell layer of the intestinal epithelium, possibly the brush border or the glycocalyx which surrounds the cell membrane, where the enzyme is confined.
3. Primary lactose intolerance due to an apparently normal developmental decrease in lactase activity.

The latter type—primary lactose intolerance—involving a normal decrease in the enzyme lactase after early childhood, is the most common type; hence, the discussion that follows pertains primarily thereto.

Normally, the enzyme lactase reaches maximum activity soon after birth, and its activity remains high throughout infancy (the suckling period). But, by late childhood, it decreases to a very low level in all but the Caucasian race.

Because of low intestinal lactase activity in a high proportion of non-Caucasian adults, their consumption of appreciable quantities of lactose can create considerable problems. In such cases, only a portion of the lactose is hydrolyzed; the excess passes down into the lower regions of the gastrointestinal tract, where it undergoes bacterial fermentation. As a consequence, large quantities of fluids are drawn into the lumen of the gut due to the osmotic effect of the uncleaved lactose molecule and its fermented by-products. A reaction follows, generally characterized by abdominal bloating, gaseousness, cramps, flatulence, and watery diarrhea. Initial symptoms are usually observed 30 to 90 minutes after the administration of the disaccharide; diarrhea usually occurs within 2 hours; and the symptoms disappear within 2 to 6 hours after the intake of lactose.

Lactose intolerance is of practical concern in developing countries, as well as in school lunch programs, where milk is commonly used in attempts to correct or avoid serious nutritional problems.

This metabolic disorder interests the anthropologist as well as the physiologist because certain populations throughout the world show extremely high rates of lactose intolerance. Less than 15% of Scandinavians and those of Western and Northern European extraction exhibit this affliction, while 60 to 80% of Greek Cypriots, American Indians, Arabs, Ashkenazi Jews, Mexican-Americans, and American Negroes, and 90% of African Bantus and Orientals have been reported to be lactose intolerant. An estimated 30 to 50 million Americans are lactose intolerant. In general, populations in which dairying is traditional seem to tolerate lactose, whereas people from nondairying parts of the world do not; and the inability to utilize lactose in the latter groups persist in successive generations in spite of migration. The question posed by anthropologists is whether the intolerance to lactose evolved due to the inadequate consumption of milk over a period of generations or whether the low consumption of milk was a result of low gut lactase activity originally. That is, did these people once have the ability to digest lactose and eventually lose it, or have they always had this lactase insufficiency?

Fortunately, many people having lactose intolerance can digest most cheeses and other fermented dairy products, such as yogurt. Fortunately, too, lactase is now on the market. By adding it to milk, lactose is changed into two simple sugars, glucose and galactose. The resulting milk is four times sweeter than regular milk, but is otherwise unchanged. Another alternative is lactose-reduced low fat milk currently available in many supermarkets that contains 70% less lactose than milk.

MILK INTOLERANCE.   Milk intolerance is not the same as lactose intolerance. Rather, it refers to the development of significant symptoms similar to those described for lactose intolerance following the consumption of usual amounts of milk or milk-containing products. However, many persons with lactose intolerance (lactase deficiency) can consume milk in 1-cup quantities at meals without discomfort, and others can tolerate smaller quantities.

Suitable alternatives for milk-intolerant individuals should provide the same nutrients as does milk. Lactose hydrolyzed milk has been shown to be a suitable alternative in most cases. In addition, other dairy foods such as cheese and other fermented dairy products are well tolerated by the truly milk-intolerant individual.

On the basis of present evidence, it would appear inappropriate to discourage supplemental milk feeding programs targeted at children on the basis of primary lactose intolerance. Also, the use of milk should not be discouraged in feeding malnourished children—except when they have severe diarrhea.

GALACTOSE DISEASE (GALACTOSEMIA).   Galactose disease, an inborn error of carbohydrate metabolism, inherited as an autosomal recessive trait, is caused by insufficient levels of the enzyme galactose-1-phosphate uridyl transferase, sometimes abbreviated P-

Gal-transferase, which is needed in the liver for the conversion of galactose to glucose. Galactose is derived from the hydrolysis of lactose (milk sugar) in the intestine. (The enzyme lactase splits lactose into glucose and galactose.)

Where this genetic defect exists, galactose disease becomes apparent within a few days after birth by such symptoms as loss of appetite, vomiting, occasional diarrhea, drowsiness, jaundice, puffiness of the face, edema of the lower extremities, and weight loss. The spleen and liver enlarge. Mental retardation becomes evident very early in the course of the disease, and cataracts develop within the first year.

Dietary treatment consists of early diagnosis and the complete exclusion from the diet of milk, the only food that supplies lactose, along with all foods that contain milk. As a rule, the substitution of a nonmilk formula (usually a meat-base or a soy-base formula, supplemented with calcium gluconate or chloride, iron, and vitamins) leads to rapid improvement. All the symptoms disappear except the mental retardation which has already occurred and is not reversible.

Complete elimination of galactose is necessary for the young child, but breads and other prepared foods containing milk are usually permitted when the child enters school. Milk must be permanently excluded from the diet, however.

(Also see INBORN ERRORS OF METABOLISM.)

MILK ANEMIA. *Milk anemia is the condition that results when infants and children drink milk over an extended period without iron supplementation by an iron salt or an iron-rich food(s).*

During growth, the demand for positive iron balance is imperative. At birth, a newborn infant has about 3 to 6 months' supply of iron, which was stored in the liver during fetal development. Since milk does not supply iron, supplementary iron-rich foods must be provided to prevent the classic milk anemia of young children fed cow's milk only after 6 months of age.

Iron is also needed for continued growth during the toddler stage (1 to 3 years). Sometimes excess milk intake during this period, a habit carried over from infancy, may exclude some solid foods from the diet. As a result, the child may be lacking iron and develop a milk anemia.

AFTER GASTRIC SURGERY. The patient whose gastric or duodenal ulcer does not respond to medical treatment is the most common candidate for gastric surgery.

Immediately after gastric surgery, milk may or may not be included in the small frequent feedings, for the reason that the contents of the stomach may pass into the small intestine before it is in proper solution and cause distention of the jejunum. When this happens, the patient experiences nausea, cramps, diarrhea, light-headedness, and extreme weakness. This occurs 15 to 30 minutes after meals and is known as the "dumping syndrome."

Also, some, but not all, individuals develop lactose intolerance following gastric surgery; therefore, some physicians regularly exclude milk after such surgery. However, other physicians exclude milk only after the patient has experienced distention and diarrhea that are relieved by the exclusion of milk.

Milk Myths. Some myths and misconceptions related to health concerns appear to have acted as barriers to milk consumption; among them, the following:

Milk is toxic to nonwhite people.
Milk causes coronary heart disease.
Milk causes cancer.
Milk causes iron deficiency anemia.
Milk causes urinary calculi.
Milk causes acne.

• **Myth: Milk is toxic to nonwhite people**—This myth had its beginning with lactose intolerance; and it received widespread attention when studies revealed that 70% of the black population but only 6 to 12% of the white population in the United States had low lactase (the lactose-splitting enzyme) levels in their digestive tract.

Fact: While a person may be lactose intolerant, he is not necessarily milk intolerant.

Experimental studies involving (1) American Indian adults and children, and (2) young black and white children reinforce the recommendations of the Protein Advisory Group of the United Nations, the Food and Nutrition Board, and the American Academy of Pediatrics that existing milk programs for young children should not and need not be limited because of lactose intolerance.

Symptoms of lactose intolerance often have been attributed to milk allergy, which is a totally different medical condition. Milk allergy affects from 0.3 to 7.0% under 2 years of age, after which it is generally outgrown.

• **Myth: Milk causes coronary heart disease**—Intake of excessive amounts of fats, saturated fats, and cholesterol, which generally are found in milk and other animal foods, has been associated with a rise in blood serum cholesterol. In turn, dietary cholesterol, along with other substances, becomes deposited in the artery wall resulting in atherosclerosis and finally heart attack (blockage of the coronary artery which delivers blood to the heart muscle). Also, the American Heart Association has continually recommended that the entire U.S. population modify its diet as a measure of general insurance against heart disease. The dietary recommendations include, among others, a reduction in intake of fats, saturated fats, and cholesterol, with an increase of polyunsaturated fatty acids.

Fact: The per capita consumption of dairy products has been declining since 1960, despite an increase in the sales of yogurt, low-fat milk, and cheese. The decline has been attributed primarily to concern about blood cholesterol levels, along with lack of understanding of the nutritive value of milk.

Those who question that milk causes coronary heart disease cite the following supporting evidence:

1. Indication that milk may have a lowering effect on serum cholesterol was found in studies of the Masai, a nomadic tribe inhabiting parts of southern Kenya and

northern Tanzania. These people live almost exclusively on milk, averaging approximately 4 qt daily, supplemented occasionally by blood and meat. Yet, it was found that serum cholesterol among Masai averaged 135 mg per 100 ml, whereas normal values in other populations range from 190 to 250 mg per 100 ml.[31]

2.   Pennsylvania State University ascertained that rats fed milk developed lower serum cholesterol and had reduced liver production of cholesterol.[32]

3.   In a 10-year study, initiated in 1980, with the results reported in 1991, involving 4,200 middle-aged men in Britain, conducted by researchers at Llandough Hospital and funded by the U.K. Medical Research Council, it was found (a) that men who drank a pint of milk a day were nearly 10 times less likely to suffer heart attacks than those drinking no milk at all, and (b) that heart attacks in middle-aged butter-eaters occurred at half the rate of margarine-eaters.

Also, heart disease is seen by most health authorities as being due to multiple causes, including hypertension, cigarette smoking, and elevated serum cholesterol level.

Despite all the superior nutritional qualities of milk, it is important that consumers be aware of, and heed, the following recommendations of most professional health groups in order to lessen coronary heart disease: (1) lower the fat in the diet from the present 37% to less than 30% of the total calories, (2) restrict the intake of cholesterol to less than 300 mg per day, and (3) limit saturated fat to 10% of the calorie intake. To help reduce consumption of total fat, saturated fat, and cholesterol, consumers should consider low-fat dietary products. Thus, it is noteworthy that an 8-oz glass of whole milk contains 33 mg of cholesterol, whereas the same amount of skim milk contains only 4 mg of cholesterol.

• **Myth: Milk causes cancer**—Some people say that milk causes cancer. So, they recommend avoiding butter, drinking only skim milk, and eating only low fat cheeses.

Fact: There is substantial, but not conclusive evidence that dietary fat increases the risk of cancers of the breast, colon, rectum, endometrium, and prostate. Both animal and international epidemiologic data suggest that a decrease in fat consumption from the current 37% of total caloric intake to less than 30% of the total calories may reduce the risks of certain cancers. To help reduce the consumption of total fat, consumers should consider low-fat dairy products.

• **Myth: Milk causes iron deficiency anemia**—Another health concern adversely affecting milk consumption is iron deficiency anemia, considered the most prevalent nutritional disorder among infants and children in the United States.

Fact: The alleged relationship of milk to iron deficiency anemia may be explained in two ways:

1.   When fed during the first 6 months of life, milk may cause gastrointestinal blood loss in some infants.

2.   Excess consumption of milk precludes or limits consumption of iron-rich foods.

Of course, the first contention can be alleviated by either breast feeding or using a formula which does not contain cow's milk. The second argument relative to excessive consumption of milk would apply to any food eaten to excess. Physicians and nutritionists do not recommend that milk be consumed to the exclusion of other foods.

• **Myth: Milk causes urinary calculi (kidney stones)**—Since approximately 95% of renal calculi contain calcium and phosphorus, and since milk and other dairy foods are rich in calcium and phosphorus, they have been implicated as causing urinary calculi.

Fact: There is no evidence that the formation of urinary calculi is caused by foods rich in calcium and phosphorus. Moreover, there is no evidence of a higher incidence of kidney stones in parts of the world where there is higher consumption of dairy products than in areas where consumption of dairy products is low.

• **Myth: Milk causes acne**—Claims have been made by some people that milk contributes to the development of acne, based on the supposition that milk contains sufficient concentrations of sex hormones known to produce acne. Male hormones (androgens) and perhaps progestigens are known to stimulate the sebaceous glands, an initial step in the onset of acne. Secondly, progesterone and androgens have been shown to occur in bovine tissue.

Fact: Studies of the acne-producing hormone content of milk show that milk could not be the cause of acne.

HISTORY AND DEVELOPMENT OF THE DAIRY INDUSTRY.

Long before recorded history, the first food provided for mankind was from women's mammary glands. In remote times, when nature failed to bless the newborn

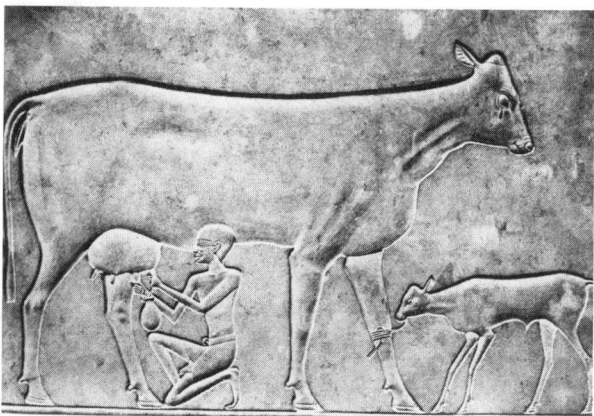

Fig. M-92.   Dairy scene from ancient Egypt, from bas-relief found in the tomb of Princess Kewitt. Note man milking cow while calf is fastened to left foreleg. (Courtesy, The Bettmann Archive, Inc., New York, N.Y.)

[31]McCarthy, R. D. and G. A. Porter, "Milk Has Lowering Effect On Blood Serum Cholesterol," The Pennsylvania State University, *Science In Agriculture,* Vol. XXV, No. 4, Summer 1978, p. 3.

[32]*Ibid.*

child with a lactating mother, the baby either suckled another mother, or an animal, or died.

In due time, man found that milk was good—and good for him—with the result that he began domesticating milk-producing animals. However, under natural conditions, wild animals produce only enough milk for their offspring. So, man began selecting them for higher production for his own use. For the most part, this included the cow, the buffalo, and the goat—although the ewe, the mare, the sow, and other mammals have been used for producing milk for human consumption in different parts of the world. The importance of the cow in milk production is attested to by her well-earned designation as "the foster mother of the human race."

As the cow population expanded throughout the world and as milk production became a specialized phase of agriculture, methods were developed for concentrating and preserving milk foods for future use, barter, and/or international trade. Dairying progressed from an art to a science—drawing upon genetics, chemistry, physics, bacteriology, heat, refrigeration, engineering, business, and other branches of knowledge, in order to improve dairy commodities, create new ones, and profitably distribute them in both domestic and world commerce.

Hand in hand with improvements and expansion in production and processing, recognition of the nutritional importance of milk and milk products increased. Following World War II, milk and milk foods were established as one of the groups of foods contributing the essentials of an adequate diet—first as one division of the Seven Food Groups, and later in the Four Food Groups.

WORLD DAIRY PRODUCTION. Table M-41 shows the ten leading milk cow producing countries of the world, ranked by cow numbers. As noted, the U.S.S.R. has a commanding lead. Table M-41 also shows the proficiency of cows in the principal countries of the world. It is noteworthy that the United States ranks third in average milk production per cow, being outproduced by both Israel and Japan.

TABLE M–41
TEN LEADING COUNTRIES IN
(1) MILK COWS ON FARMS, AND
(2) MILK PRODUCTION PER COW, 1990[1]

Country	No. Milk Cows on Farms	Country	Average Milk Production Per Cow	
	(1,000 head)		(lb)	(kg)
U.S.S.R.	41,734	Israel	20,299	9,227
India	30,000	Japan	16,667	7,526
Brazil	14,800	U.S.A.	14,612	6,642
U.S.A.	10,127	Sweden . . .	13,690	6,223
Germany	6,801	Denmark . .	13,548	6,158
Mexico	6,410	Netherlands .	13,259	6,027
France	5,489	Norway . . .	12,294	5,588
Poland	4,900	Finland . . .	12,267	5,576
United Kingdom	3,224	Canada . . .	12,162	5,528
Italy	2,931	Switzerland .	10,875	4,943

[1]*Agricultural Statistics 1991*, USDA, p. 309.
[2]Israel average milk production per cow is from *Hoard's Dairyman*, April 10, 1992.

Some countries produce more dairy products than they can use, whereas others are importers. New Zealand accounts for about one-third of the total world dairy exports. The United Kingdom is an especially heavy importer of butter, cheese, and condensed milk.

Among the factors that determine the present development of the dairy industry in different countries are the character and preferences of the people; the adaptation of the country to dairying—dairying is not adaptable to areas that are excessively hot or cold, or where soils are poor; the relative size of urban and rural population; and the extent and effectiveness of dairy research and education.

Role of Dairy Cow in Feeding a Hungry World. As the ghost of hunger stalks the world before the year 2000 A.D., the focus will be on animals, including the dairy cow.

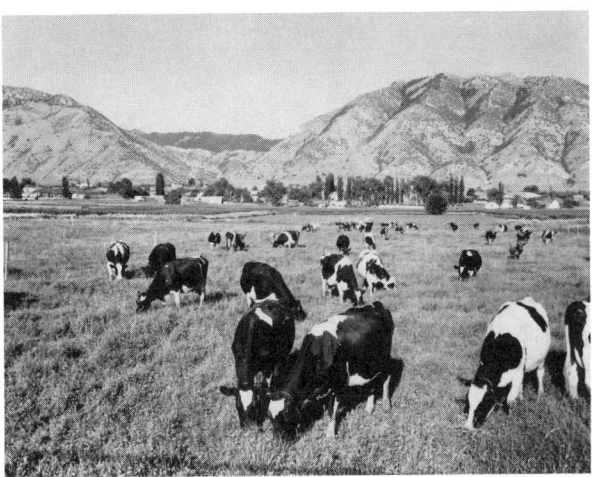

Fig. M-93. Cows convert the photosynthetic energy derived from solar energy and stored in grass into milk for humans. (Courtesy, Union Pacific Railroad, Omaha, Nebr.)

Based on FAO estimates, only about 11% of the land area of the world is utilized as permanent crop land, another 25% is used for permanent pasture and meadow, and about 31% is covered with forests. About 32% is not available for agricultural production.

Some pasture land may be shifted to crop land by making major investments in reclamation and irrigation projects. But the high costs involved and climatic limitations will restrict the conversion of grassland to crop use.

Shipping cereal grains to the food deficit areas has received much attention. In the short run, shipping grain is the logical way to deal with floods, drought, and similar emergency problems. Over the long run, however, food security can best be assured by improving the ability of each area of the world to feed itself.

What then, will the role of the dairy cow be in feeding a hungry world?

It is generally agreed that, in order to maximize world food production, the emphasis must be on animals which are able to convert materials nonedible to humans into high-quality essential nutrients.

Ruminant animals, such as the cow, possess a unique digestive system which is able to convert inedible plant materials to human food in the form of milk and meat.

About 60 to 65% of the feed nutrients used for milk production comes from forages and fibrous feeds. Also, by-products from the processing and refining of food crops for human consumption can be utilized to supplement forages and reduce need for feed grains.

Basically, the feed to food efficiency—the proportion of a specific plant nutrient recovered in the animal product—has been used to express the biological efficiency of conversion of crop nutrients to human foods. Estimates of the efficiency of conversion of energy and protein by various classes of livestock are presented in Table M-42.

TABLE M–42
FEED TO FOOD EFFICIENCY RATING BY SPECIES OF ANIMALS

Class	Efficiency of Conversion	
	Energy or Calories	Protein
	(%)	(%)
Nonruminants:		
Broiler	8.1	52.4
Fish	14.5	47.6
Turkey	5.3	31.7
Hen (layers)	8.3	25.9
Swine	5.3	24.4
Ruminants:		
Dairy cow	17.2	37.0
Beef steer	2.9	9.4
Lamb	2.3	6.0

Note that the dairy cow is the most efficient of the species listed in converting feed energy to food energy. Note, too, that the dairy cow is third only to broilers and fish in the efficiency of conversion of feed protein to food protein.

In the United States and other temperate zone countries, milk has been an important part of the national diets, providing a large amount of high-quality protein, calcium, phosphorus, and riboflavin, and a moderate amount of vitamin A and energy or calories.

In the last 30 years, as new knowledge of genetics and inheritance, feeding and management of dairy cows was applied, feed efficiency in U.S. milk production increased about 54%. Therefore, the total feed used for milk production was reduced.

Under adverse conditions of animal production, efficiencies of conversion of feed by animals are not obtained. This is evidenced by the fact that the developing countries maintain about 60% of the world's livestock but produce only 20 to 30% of the world's livestock products. In those countries where the milk supply is very limited, the average diet tends to be low in protein, calcium, and riboflavin. These nutrient deficiencies are especially critical with recently weaned children. Thus, expansion and improvement in dairy production are needed in the developing countries, so that more milk will be available.

In summary, the future role of the dairy cow in world production appears favorable because:

1. Much of the world's land is not suited to crop production; instead, its highest and best use is, and will remain, for grazing.

2. The dairy cow efficiently converts pasture and other roughages, feed crop by-products, nonprotein nitrogen, and feed grains to a high-quality human food.

3. The dairy cow converts the chemical energy in plants (produced by photosynthesis and utilizing solar energy) into a form (milk) available to man.

4. High-quality milk protein effectively balances the amino acid patterns of plant proteins.

5. Milk is a critical source of nutrients for most infants and children.

6. Dairying favorably affects land use by using forage crops, preventing soil erosion, and returning animal manure to the land to maintain fertility.

U.S. PRODUCTION OF MILK. The United States ranks fourth in number of milk cows and third in production per cow, among the leading dairy countries of the world (see Table M-41).

The process of getting milk to the consumer involves the coordinated efforts of many people, from production through marketing. This process can be broken down into three primary divisions or stages: (1) producing and assembling, (2) processing, and (3) marketing and distributing milk and dairy products.

Leading Dairy States. Milk is produced in every state of the Union. However, the greatest concentration of dairy cows is found in those areas with the densest human populations. This is as one would expect from the standpoint of the demand for, and the marketing of, fresh milk—a highly perishable product.

Table M-43 lists the ten leading states in dairy cattle numbers by rank. Human population centers, which provide a large market for milk, have been a major factor in determining the intensity of dairying. Also land, climate, and feed exert a considerable influence. Wisconsin is, by far, the leading dairy state in the United States, having the most milk cows on farms and the highest total production of milk. Some states have a well-managed dairy industry; but because of their small size, they do not have a large total dairy cattle population. Therefore, proficiency of dairy herd management is best indicated by average production per cow. Additionally, several states have highly intensified dairy farms due to the limitation of arable land and the cost of irrigation. They must have high-producing cows in order to meet high overhead. New Mexico leads the United States in milk production per cow, with an average in excess of 18,552 lb (*8,433 kg*).

TABLE M–43
TEN LEADING STATES IN (1) MILK COWS ON FARMS,
(2) MILK PRODUCTION PER COW, AND (3) TOTAL MILK PRODUCTION, 1989[1]

Ranking	State	No. Milk Cows on Farms	State	Milk Production Per Cow		State	Total Milk Production	
		(thousands)		(lb)	(kg)		(mil lb)	(mil kg)
1	Wisconsin	1,739	New Mexico	18,552	8,419	Wisconsin	24,000	10.909
2	California	1,104	Washington	18,209	8,277	California	19,420	8,827
3	New York	776	California	17,591	7,996	New York	11,071	5,032
4	Minnesota	734	Colorado	16,803	7,638	Minnesota	10,108	4,595
5	Pennsylvania	698	Arizona	16,758	7,617	Pennsylvania	9,998	4,545
6	Ohio	349	Oregon	15,884	7,220	Texas	5,170	2,350
7	Michigan	345	Idaho	15,608	7,095	Michigan	5,152	2,342
8	Iowa	309	Connecticut	15,412	7,005	Ohio	4,535	2,061
9	Missouri	228	Utah	15,395	6,998	Iowa	4,202	1,910
10	Washington	225	Michigan	14,933	6,788	Washington	4,097	1,862

[1]*Agricultural Statistics 1991*, USDA, p. 306.

Milk Cow Production as Related to Human Population. The average annual production per cow in the United States has steadily increased from 3,138 lb (1,423 kg) in 1920 to 14,612 lb (6,642 kg) per cow in 1990; simultaneously, cow numbers have declined while the human population has increased (see Table M-44 and Fig. M-94). This increase in average production per cow can be attributed to recent progress in improved breeding, feeding, disease control, and management. With this increased production, efficiency has increased, also.

TABLE M–44
U.S. MILK PRODUCTION PER COW, MILK COW NUMBERS, AND HUMAN POPULATION

Year	Milk Production Per Cow[1]		Number of Milk Cows[2]	Human Population[3]	Ratio of Milk Cows to Humans
	(lb)	(kg)			(Cows:Humans)
1920	3,138	1,423	21,455,000	105,710,620	1:4.9
1930	4,508	2,045	23,032,000	122,775,046	1:5.5
1940	4,625	2,098	24,940,000	131,699,275	1:5.6
1950	5,314	2,410	23,853,000	150,697,361	1:6.6
1960	7,002	3,176	19,527,000	180,684,000	1:9.3
1970	9,385	4,257	12,483,000	202,711,000	1:16.2
1980	11,875[4]	5,398	10,815,000	221,700,000	1:20.5
1990	14,612	6,642	10,127,000	250,000,000	1:24.7

[1]*Agricultural Statistics*, USDA.
[2]*Livestock and Meat Statistics*, USDA.
[3]*Statistical Abstract of the United States*, 1949, and *The World Almanac and Book of Facts*, 1966, 1970, 1977, and 1991.
[4]*1981 Dairy Producer Highlights*, National Milk Producers Federation, p. 6.

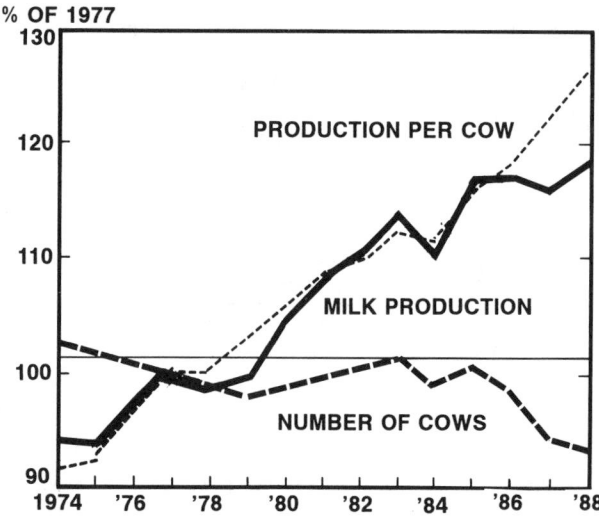

Fig. M-94. Although cow numbers have gone down, milk production has increased due to higher production per cow. (Courtesy, USDA. From: *1989 Handbook of Agricultural Charts*, p. 89, Chart 198)

The cows which were in record-keeping dairy herd improvement associations and which obviously were the more efficient ones, produced an average of 18,031 lb (*8,196 kg*) of milk and 662 lb (*301 kg*) of butterfat in 1990.

Dairy Producers. It is impossible to describe the "average" American dairy farm, for the dairyman can choose to tailor his operation in an infinite number of ways. Herd size, breeds, milking equipment, frequency of milking, and intensity of production all enter into the makeup of the dairy farm.

In general, however, dairy operations can be classified in the following manner:

1. **Grade or mixed herds.** These herds may consist of a mixture of registered and unregistered cows and may range in size from about 20 to 5,000, or more, lactating cows. Production is the sole determinant of whether a cow is kept or culled and is the primary basis for providing income for the dairy operator. If a cow becomes a health problem or fails to meet the production standards set by the operator, she is generally sent to slaughter.

2. **Registered herds.** The operator of a registered dairy herd is interested in two aspects of dairying: (a) production, and (b) improvement of genetic potential. Through careful record keeping and well-planned breeding programs, the registered dairy herd operator provides the industry with top bulls and heifers. Thus,

premium prices are paid for young stock from a registered herd, thereby supplementing the income received from milk production.

3. **Dairy herds as sideline.** In many areas which are not conducive to large, intensified dairy production, farmers maintain a small dairy herd for supplemental income. In addition to the dairy cows kept on the farm, the farm operator may grow cash crops or raise other livestock.

4. **Part-time dairying.** Many part-time farmers keep a few milk cows in addition to holding a full-time job off the farm.

5. **Dairy beef.** When prices are favorable, dairy steers are fed for beef or young dairy bulls are raised for early slaughter as veal calves. With the increasing consumer demand for leaner beef, more and more dairy steers have gone into the feedlot for finishing. In addition, many virgin heifers are bred to beef bulls so that the resulting calves will be smaller and pose fewer calving problems. Thus, a good market for crossbred dairy-beef calves is available.

Through the years, dairy farms have become larger and more specialized. Separating cream, making butter, processing market milk, growing and mixing concentrates, and keeping bulls have largely disappeared fom the average dairy farm; and this trend will continue. Dairymen tend to buy more of their feed and replacements, instead of investing in more land. A few produce part or all of their forage requirements. Some have specialized heifer-raising operations.

Most dairy farms in the major dairy areas—especially the Lake States, Corn Belt, and Northeast—continue to be operated as family enterprises. However, as dairy farms become multiple units, operating agreements—such as father-son agreements—become more important. Through a partnership, or by incorporating, it is possible (1) to assure continuity of the enterprise by transfer of ownership from one generation to the next without excessively heavy tax penalty, and (2) to arrange for the necessary capital for a prospective dairyman who cannot finance his own operation.

A limited number of dairy farms are owned and operated by milk-processing plants, or are under corporations, or in cow pools and cooperatives.

The trends in the U.S. dairy industry are as follows:

1. **Dairy farms declining; herd size increasing.** The number of farms reporting dairy cows has declined sharply and will, in all likelihood, continue to decline in the future. But herd size has increased. As shown in Table M-45, from 1950 to 1989, 3,443,000 dairy farms went out of business, while, during this same period, average herd size increased more than eight fold—from 5.8 cows to 49.0 cows.

TABLE M–45
TOTAL NUMBER OF FARMS WITH
MILK COWS AND AVERAGE HERD SIZE[1,2]

Census of	Farms Reporting Milk Cows	
	Total	Average Herd Size
	(1,000)	(number)
1900	4,514	3.8
1910	5,141	3.3
1920	4,461	4.4
1930	4,453	4.6
1940	4,644	5.2
1950	3,648	5.8
1960	1,792	9.2
1970	568	19.7
1989	205	49.0

[1]Data through 1975 from *1978 Dairy Producers Highlights*, National Milk Producers Federation, p. 2.

[2]Data for 1989 from *Dairy Background for 1990 Farm Legislation*, USDA, ERS, Commodity Economics Division, p. 4, Table 1. In 1989, commercial dairy farms (farms with 10 or more milk cows) were estimated at around 160,000 with an average of around 65 cows per farm.

2. **Cow numbers decreasing.** During the period 1950 to 1990, the numbers of milk cows in the United States declined from 23,853,000 to 10,127,000 (see Table M-44).

3. **Production per cow increasing.** From 1950 to 1990, production per cow increased from 5,314 to 14,612 lb. Table M-44 shows this trend well.

4. **Confinement systems increasing.** Confinement systems away from pasture have increased. In such an operation, the entire ration may be mixed together and distributed in a bunk by a self-unloading truck to cows separated into corrals according to level of production.

MILKING AND HANDLING MILK. Milk is secreted by the mammary glands of mammals. In the United States, cows furnish virtually all market milk.

Lactation begins at freshening, when a calf is born, and usually lasts 305 days. Milk is removed through the teats (the elongated nipples). Milking is carried out by either of two methods: (1) hand milking, or (2) machine milking.

The composition of milk depends mainly on the breed of cows. The flavor and quality of milk vary according to how the cows are cared for, what they are fed, and how the milk is handled. Milk must be kept cool and clean from the moment it comes from the cows.

Milk possesses two characteristics which make it ideal for the development of bacteria: (1) It is a well-balanced food in which bacteria thrive; and (2) the temperature, as it comes from the cow, is ideal for bacterial growth. For these reasons, milk must be cooled to at least 50°F (preferably 40°F, or *4°C*) as soon as possible in order to inhibit bacterial growth.

Milk may be handled by either of two systems: the can system, or the bulk system. Today, the trend is to more and more bulk tanks, with the milk piped directly from

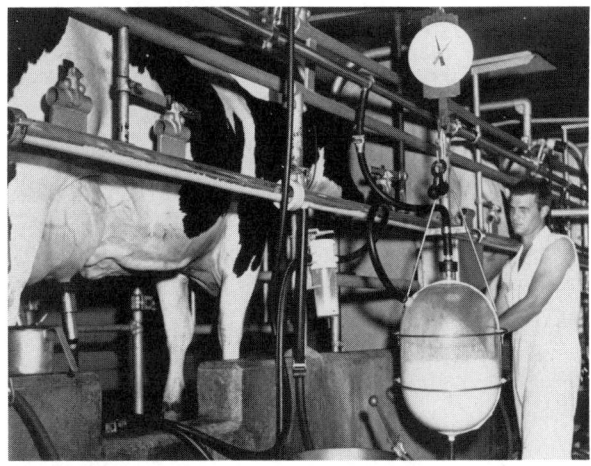

Fig. M-95. Cow being machine milked in a milking parlor. Note that the milk is weighed, then piped directly into a refrigerated storage tank; without exposure of the milk—all very sanitary. (Courtesy, Holstein-Friesian Assn. of America, Brattleboro, Vt.)

milking machines into refrigerated storage tanks. Almost all fluid milk is now delivered to processors in bulk tanks, and the conversion to bulk tanks has been substantial with manufacturing milk.

Insulated trucks usually pick up milk from dairy farms daily and transport it to processing plants.

Quality milk can be produced only when dairymen pay special attention to a number of factors; among them, herd health, clean cows, care of the milking equipment, cooling and storage of milk, and proper transportation of milk to market.

HAULING MILK. Ownership of milk changes at the farm when milk becomes commingled with other milk in the truck tank. However, producers pay all or part of the cost of hauling to most processors.

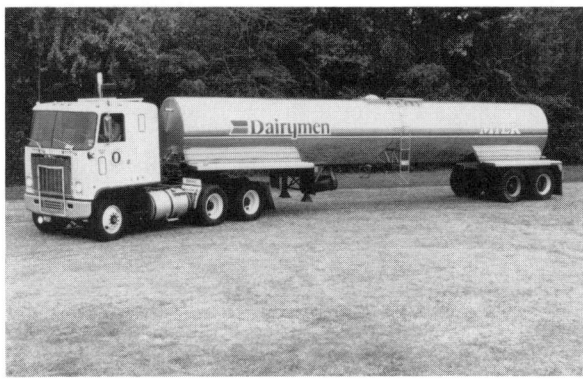

Fig. M-96. The bulk, system of handling milk. This over-the-road transport is capable of moving 6,000 gal (*22,800 liter*) of milk. The insulated stainless steel tank holds milk within a few degrees of its original temperature. (Courtesy, Dairymen, Inc., Lexington, Ky.)

Practically all milk is now (1) placed in mechanically cooled bulk tanks on farms, and (2) transported to processing plants in bulk tank trucks with capacities ranging from 15,000 to 50,000 lb (*6,803 to 22,676 kg*).

Because ownership changes at loading, this places responsibility on the truck operator to evaluate odor, flavor, and appearance of the milk, and to measure and sample the milk accurately and properly.

The basis for truck costs for hauling milk vary. Some costs are computed on a flat-rate basis per cwt of milk. Others pay according to the distance traveled. Still others use a formula based on (1) distance by all-weather roads, (2) density of producers on the route, (3) volume—with discount per cwt if over 2,500 lb, and (4) minimum charge per stop.

DAIRY FARM INCOME.   Table M-46 shows the importance of the U.S. dairy industry. As noted, cash farm income from dairy projects totaled almost $20 billion in 1990.

TABLE M–46
U.S. DAIRY FARM DATA[1]

Milk cows on farms (not including heifers not fresh) . . . .(no.)		10,127,000
Farm milk production . . . . (lb)		148,284,000,000
(kg)		67,538,000,000
Average production per cow . . . (lb)		14,642
(kg)		6,655
Cash farm income from milk and cream . . . . ($)		19,952,300,000

[1]*1991 Milk Facts*, Milk Industry Foundation, pp. 22, 23.

Table M-47 shows the importance of dairy products as compared to the other sources of farm and ranch income. Dairy products rank second only to cattle and calves in percent of livestock receipts. The importance of dairy cattle as a source of farm revenue is further magnified when one considers that the income from the sale of cows, heifers, and calves from dairy herds amounted to about $3.1 billion in 1990—a figure that is included in the total income from the sale of cattle and calves.

TABLE M–47
U.S. FARM INCOME BY COMMODITY[1]

Commodity	Income	Percent of Commodity Group	Percent of Total Income
	(million $)	(%)	(%)
Livestock & poultry:			
Cattle and calves .	39,748	44.4	23.4
Dairy products . . .	20,199	22.5	11.9
Hogs	11,516	12.8	6.8
Broilers	8,366	9.3	4.9
Eggs	4,044	4.5	2.4
Turkeys	2,383	2.7	1.4
Sheep and lamb . .	412	0.5	0.2
Misc. livestock and poultry[2]	2,954	3.3	1.7
Total	89,623	100	
Crops:			
Feed crops	19,116	23.8	11.2
Oil bearing crops .	12,403	15.4	7.3
Vegetables[3]	11,533	14.4	6.8
Fruits and tree nuts	9,306	11.6	5.5
Food grains	7,876	9.8	4.6
Cotton (lint and seed)	5,234	6.5	3.1
Tobacco	2,736	3.4	1.6
Other crops[4]	12,160	15.1	7.2
Total	80,364	100	
Total livestock & crops	169,987		100

[1]*Agricultural Statistics 1991*, p. 389, Table 570.
[2]Wool, horses and mules, mohair, honey, beeswax, bees, goats, rabbits, and fur animals. Also, farm chickens, ducks, geese, guineas, pigeons, quail, pheasants, and turkey hatching eggs.
[3]Includes melons.
[4]Sugar crops, floriculture and ornamentals, forest products, mushrooms, legume and grass seeds, hops, mint, broomcorn, popcorn, hemp fiber and seed, and flax fiber.

PROCESSING MILK.[33]   Upon arrival at the processing plant, trained laboratory technicians make many tests to ensure the quality and purity of milk, including temperature, flavor, odor, and appearance. They reject milk that does not meet the required high standards for quality.

---

[33]In the preparation of this section, the authors adapted material from *Newer Knowledge of Milk and Other Fluid Dairy Products,* National Dairy Council, Rosemont, Ill.

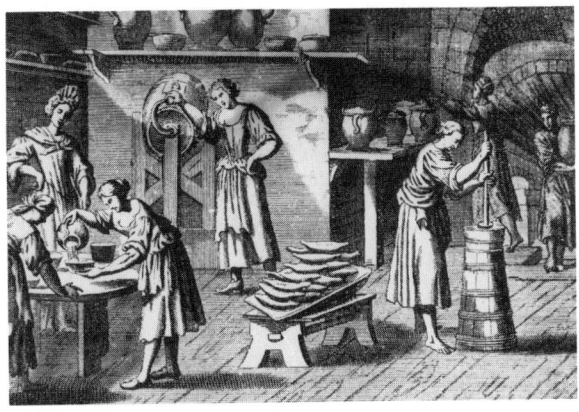

Fig. M-97. Seventeenth century dairy manufacturing plant. Note (1) division of labor among women workers; and (2) buttermaking, using two different types of churns: a barrellike churn with paddles inside (elevated in back of room and to the left), and a churn with a stirring stick called a *dasher* (right). (Courtesy, The Bettmann Archive, New York, N.Y.)

Also milk is tested to determine its fat content; and different batches may be blended, in a process called standardization, to adjust the fat content.

Today, most milk is homogenized, pasteurized, and fortified (at least with vitamin D), the details of which follow:

• **Homogenization**—Most whole milk is homogenized to prevent formation of a cream layer. Homogenization is accomplished by passing hot milk under high pressure through a narrow constriction with a specially designed pump. In the process, fat globules are reduced in size so that they are no longer acted upon by force of gravity and remain evenly dispersed throughout the milk. The keeping quality and nutritive value of homogenized and nonhomogenized milk are similar. The main *advantages* of homogenizing are: (1) no separation of the cream—the product retains uniform consistency; and (2) a softer curd forms in the stomach, which aids digestion. The main *disadvantages*: (1) The protein is more readily coagulated by heat or acid so that care must be taken to avoid curdling; and (2) increased susceptibility of off-flavor induced by sun or fluorescent light.

• **Pasteurization**—*Pasteurization is the heating of raw milk in properly approved and operated equipment at a sufficiently high temperature for a specified length of time to destroy pathogenic bacteria.* Pasteurization is required by law for all Grade A fluid milk and milk products moved in interstate commerce for retail sale. This process was developed by and named after Louis Pasteur, the French scientist who in the early 1860s demonstrated that wine and beer could be preserved by heating above 135°F (*57.2°C*).

In addition to extending the shelf life of milk, pasteurization destroys pathogens that might be conveyed from infected cows to man.

Various time-temperature relationships are utilized in the pasteurization process. The first three that follow are most commonly used by milk processors. The fourth—sterilized or aseptic—milk is a relatively new development.

1. **Low temperature pasteurization.** Milk is heated to a minimum of 145°F (*63°C*) for at least 30 minutes.

2. **High temperature pasteurization.** Milk is heated to a minimum of 160.7°F (*71.5°C*) for at least 15 seconds, following which it is immediately cooled.

(Also see PASTEURIZATION.)

3. **Ultrapasteurization.** Milk is heated to 191.3°F (*88.5°C*) for 1 second. This method is common in Europe and is widely used for cream and eggnog in the United States.

4. **Sterilized milk (aseptic milk).** This refers to ultrapasteurized milk products which are packaged aseptically. They can be stored at room temperature for several weeks.

• **Fortification**—Fortified milks are those that contain added minerals, vitamins, and/or milk solids-not-fat. Details follow:

1. **Fortification with vitamin D.** 400 IU of vitamin D per quart (*950 ml*) are added to most milk and low fat milk. This has been common practice for many years. It has contributed significantly to a reduction in the incidence of rickets in infants. Milk provides the necessary calcium and phosphorus, but vitamin D must also be present for normal calcification of bones and teeth.

2. **Fortification of skim milk with vitamin A.** 2,000 to 4,000 IU of vitamin A per quart may be added to skim milk in most states, in addition to vitamin D.

3. **Multivitamin-mineral milk.** In addition to vitamins A and D, multivitamin-mineral milk typically has the following vitamins and minerals added per quart: thiamin (1 mg), riboflavin (2 mg), niacin (10 mg), iron (10 mg), and iodine (0.1 mg).

4. **Protein fortified low fat and skim milks.** Federal standards for low fat and skim milks provide for a protein fortified product containing a minimum of 10% milk-

derived nonfat solids, with the stipulation that the product must be labeled "protein fortified" or "fortified with protein." Fortification of milk with nonfat solids is desirable for two reasons: (1) The flavor of most milk is improved, and (2) the nutritive value is increased.

NOTE WELL: The Food and Drug Administration requires that fortified foods or foods that are labeled or advertised with a claim to their nutrition be labeled to show content, in terms of percent Recommended Daily Allowance, of protein, vitamin A, vitamin C, thiamin, riboflavin, niacin, calcium, and iron. Also, serving size and quantities per serving must be stated for calories, fat, protein, and carbohydrate.

State laws vary relative to fortification. In those states permitting such fortification, the levels are regulated by law.

Dairy Processing Plants.

Dairy plants process fluid milk and/or manufacture dairy products from milk. Some of them produce several kinds of milk and milk products, others specialize—for example, they make cheese only, or they may condense and evaporate milk.

Fluid milk processors are located in and near population centers, where most fluid milk is consumed. The Great Lakes and Midwest regions of the United States are the primary centers for manufacturing grade milk. Thus, with the exception of ice cream production, the processing of manufactured dairy products—butter, nonfat dry milk, cheese, evaporated and condensed milk, and other products of minor importance—is concentrated near these areas of production. Other major production areas—California, New York, and Pennsylvania—produce substantial quantities of manufactured dairy products from excess Grade A milk.

In recent years, the number of milk manufacturing plants has decreased, while the output per plant has increased. This can be attributed to the advances in food technology and processing that have made the manufacturing of dairy products more efficient.

In 1987, there were a total of 1,933 U.S. dairy plants manufacturing one or more dairy products.

PACKAGING MILK.

The evolution of milk packaging in the United States can be traced from milk can to pitcher and bottle, bottle to paper, paper to plastic, and plastic to sterilized container.

Milk packaging and distribution in this country began as a home delivery service, with metal cans hauled in a horse-drawn wagon; and with the milkman alerting his early-morning customers with the familiar call, "Mulluk, Mulluk, Mulluk." With one hand clutched to the lid of the can and the other to the quart measure, the deliveryman

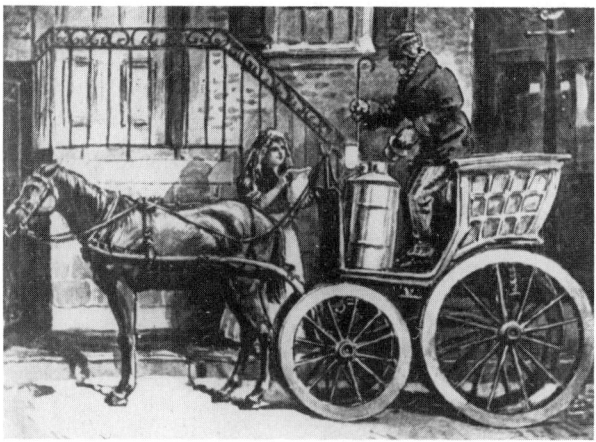

Fig. M-98.   How it used to be done. Milkman transferring milk from can into customer's own pitcher, using a quart measure. (Courtesy, The Bettmann Archive, Inc., New York, N.Y.)

poured the amount of milk the customer wanted into her own pitcher. Stirrers, the forerunners of homogenization, were used to mix the milk and avoid one customer getting mostly cream while others received skim milk. Pasteurization was not used until the end of the 19th century, so shelf life was never very long.

In 1878, the first glass milk container was patented—a jar that featured a metal device with a rubber gasket and thumbscrew on top to hold down the glass cover.

In 1884, Harvey D. Thatcher, a small town druggist, designed a milk bottle, which became the first container to gain nationwide popularity.

Glass bottles dominated milk packaging during the first half of the 1900s. But they were expensive because of breakage, washing, and lost bottles. Besides, when exposed to light, vitamin D was destroyed.

In 1907, *Scientific American* reported on a plain paper cylinder for milk, thereby ushering in the era of paper containers. War time restrictions in the early 1940s slowed the use of paper, but following the war paper containers increased rapidly. By 1952, nearly 40%, and by 1967 approximately 70%, of the packaged fluid milk in this country was in waxed or plastic-coated paper containers.

The latest development is presterilized containers. Known as aseptic packaging, these sterile containers are used to package milk processed by ultrahigh temperature—temperature ranging from 275° to 300°F (*135° to 148.8°C*) from 2 to 8 seconds, followed by rapid cooling. With this packaging, milk can be stored for several weeks without refrigeration.

Table M-48 portrays the changes in fluid milk packaging since 1975, both in type and size of containers. Note the shift to paper and plastic and to larger containers.

TABLE M–48
TYPE OF CONTAINER AND SIZE OF CONTAINER
(FEDERAL ORDER MARKETS)[1]

	1975[2]	1980	1985	1990
Number of markets[3] ...	56	47	NA	42
	◄——————— (%) ———————►			
Type of container:				
Glass	3	1	—[4]	—[4]
Paper	67	45	34	32
Plastic	30	54	66	68
Metal cans	—[4]	—[4]	—[4]	—[4]
Total	100	100	100	100
Size of container:				
Gallon	42	54	60	62
Half-gallon	34	25	22	21
Quart	7	5	5	4
Pint	2	1	2	2
Half-pint	11	11	9	9
Other	1	1	—[4]	—[4]
Bulk:[4]				
5 to 10 qt	—[4]	—[4]	2	2
Over 10 qt	3	3	—	—
Total	100	100	100	100

[1]*1991 Milk Facts*, Milk Industry Foundation, p. 19.

[2]Estimated by Milk Industry Foundation.

[3]Markets for which complete data were available include the New York-New Jersey market. Data for 1988.

[4]Less than 0.5%.

Kinds And Uses Of Milk And Milk Products.
Table M-49 shows the quantity of milk going into different uses, and Fig. M-99 shows the relative importance of each use.

TABLE M–49
HOW THE U.S. MILK SUPPLY IS USED[1]

Product	Milk Equivalent	
	(mil lb)	(*mil kg*)
Fluid milk and cream sales (25.8 billion quart)	55,370	*25,168*
Cheese	47,368	*21,531*
Creamery butter	25,043	*11,383*
Frozen dairy products[2]	12,307	*5,594*
Used on farms where produced	2,048	*931*
Evaporated and condensed milk ...	1,926	*875*
Other uses	4,413	*2,006*

[1]*1991 Milk Facts*, Milk Industry Foundation, Washington, D.C., p. 29.

[2]Plus 2,014 mil lb of milk equivalent in other manufactured dairy products used in production of frozen dairy products.

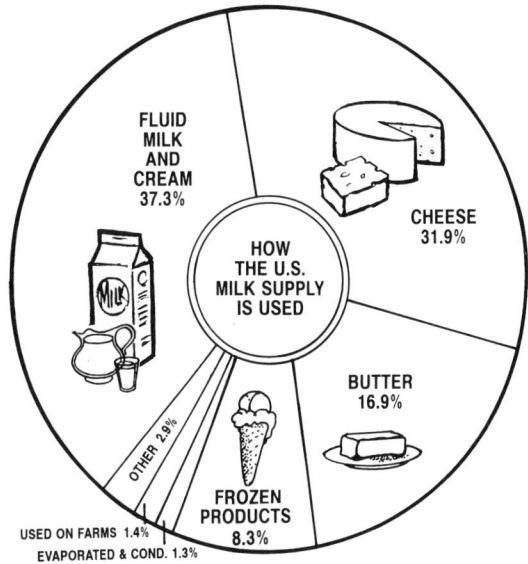

Fig. M-99. The uses of milk, in percentages. (From *1991 Milk Facts*, Milk Industry Foundation, p. 28)

Milk is processed for subsequent marketing in a number of ways, ranging from fluid milk to cheese. In 1990, 37.3% of the milk marketed by dairy farmers was consumed in fluid form. Fluid milk is retailed as pasteurized milk, homogenized milk, fortified milk (vitamin D), skim milk, or flavored milk. In 1990, 62.7% of the milk marketed by dairy farmers went into manufactured dairy products. Of the milk used for manufactured dairy products in 1990, 31.9% was used for making cheese (excluding creamed cottage cheese) and 16.9% was used for making butter. It is noteworthy that, today, more milk is used for the manufacture of cheese than for butter.

Standards of composition for milk and milk products in the United States have generally been established by state and local governments. Also, federal standards of identity have been promulgated for several of the products that are shipped in interstate commerce.

Each of the branches of the dairy processing segment and each of the products will be listed and described briefly in the sections that follow.

FLUID MILK. This type of processing requires only a minimum of product alteration. Milk is usually homogenized, pasteurized, and fortified with vitamin D. The common forms of fluid milk follow:

• **Whole milk**—*Raw whole milk is defined as the lacteal secretion, practically free from colostrum, obtained by milking one or more cows.* Federal regulations require that whole milk as marketed contain not less than 3.25% milkfat and not less than 8.25% milk solids-not-fat. (Solids-not-fat include carbohydrate, protein, minerals, and water-soluble vitamins, whereas the total solids of milk includes all the constituents of milk except water.)

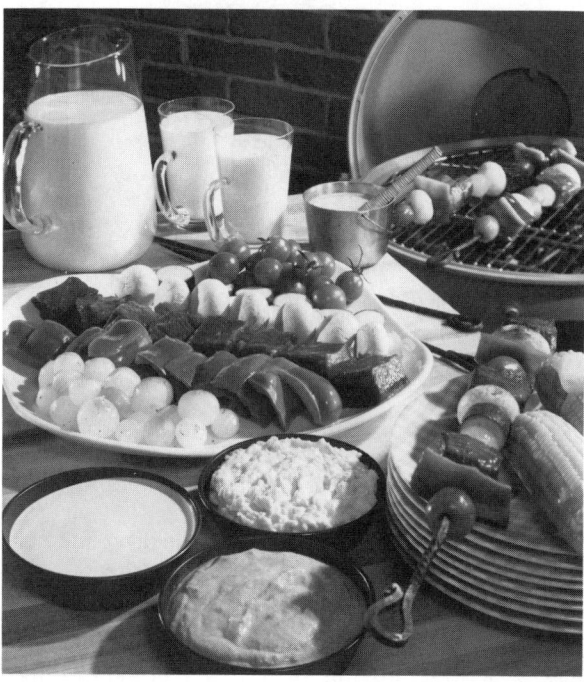

Fig. M-100. Fluid milk can be used in many form and in may ways. This shows milk served with kabobs in outdoor cooking. (Courtesy, United Dairy Industry Association, Rosemont, Ill.)

Various state standards provide that milkfat minimums may vary from 3.0 to 3.8% and solids-not-fat minimums from 8.0 to 8.7%. At the milk plant, the milk from different farms is pooled and "standardized" by removing excess milkfat or by adding cream, concentrated milk, dry whole milk, skim milk, concentrated skim milk, or nonfat dry milk to meet or exceed the minimum legal standards.

Whole fluid milk shipped in interstate commerce is usually pasteurized or ultrapasteurized; it must be pasteurized or ultrapasteurized before being sold for beverage use. Where milk is ultrapasteurized, it must be so indicated on the label.

The addition of vitamin A and/or vitamin D to fresh fluid milk is optional. If added, vitamin A must be present at a level not less than 2,000 IU per quart (*950 ml*) and vitamin D must be present at a level of 400 IU per quart. These amounts must be stated on the label. Milk is an excellent food for vitamin D fortification as it contains the proportion of calcium and phosphorus desirable for normal calcification of bones and teeth. Either vitamin D_2 or D_3 can be added to milk. Although vitamin D fortification of milk is optional, estimates indicate that approximately 98% of all homogenized milk contains vitamin D.

• **Lowfat milk**—Lowfat milk is milk from which sufficient milkfat has been removed to produce a food having one of the following milkfat contents: 0.5, 1.0, 1.5, or 2.0%; along with not less than 8.25% milk solids-not-fat.

In 1987, for the first time ever, low-fat fluid milk consumption in the United States exceeded whole fluid milk consumption.

The addition of vitamin A to low fat milk to a level of 2,000 IU per quart is mandatory. The addition of vitamin D is optional, but if added it must be present at a level of 400 IU per quart. If nonfat milk solids are added to reach the 10% solids-not-fat level, the product must be labeled "protein fortified" or "fortified with protein."

• **Skim or nonfat milk**—This is milk from which as much fat as possible has been removed. But the milk solids-not-fat must be a minimum of 8.25%. The provisions for the additions of vitamins A and D and nonfat milk solids to skim or nonfat milk are identical to those described for lowfat milk.

• **Chocolate milk; other flavored milks**—Chocolate whole, lowfat, and skim milk are flavored with a chocolate syrup, cocoa, or a chocolate powder to give a final chocolate solids concentration of 1 to 1.5%. Additionally, a nutritive sweetener (about 5 to 7% sucrose) is added. Chocolate lowfat and skim milk must contain not less than 2,000 IU of vitamin A per quart. If vitamin D is added, it must be present in not less than 400 IU per quart.

Numerous other flavorings may also be added to milk; among them, strawberry, cherry, raspberry, pineapple, apple, orange, and banana. But chocolate is the most popular flavoring of milk.

EVAPORATED AND CONDENSED MILK. The introduction of condensed milk in 1853 (patented in 1856) made available dairy products that expanded markets at home and abroad and significantly enhanced growth of the U.S. dairy industry. Today, candy manufacturers, bakers, and ice cream processors are large users of concentrated milk.

The primary products within this cateogry are evaporated and concentrated (condensed) milk packed in cans for consumer use, and concentrated whole and skim milk shipped in bulk.

• **Evaporated milk**—Evaporated milk is made by preheating to stabilize proteins, concentrating in vacuum pans at 122° to 131°F (*50° to 55°C*) to remove about 60% of the water, homogenizing (which is mandatory), standardizing to the required percentage of components, adding vitamins (vitamin D must be added to provide 400 IU per reconstituted quart), canning, and stabilizing (sealed in the container, then heat treated [240° to 245°F, or *115.5° to 118.5°C,* for 15 minutes] to sterilize).

Federal standards require that the milkfat and total milk solids content of evaporated milk be not less than 7.5 and 25.5%, respectively. Evaporated skim milk is concentrated, fortified skim milk containing not less than 20% milk solids.

In recent years, per capita consumption of evaporated milk has declined, but bulk shipments of unsweetened concentrated milk to food and ice cream processors have increased.

• **Concentrated or condensed milk**—This is similar to evaporated milk because it is made by the partial removal of water from fluid milk; hence, the milkfat and total milk solids must not be less than 7.5 and 25.5%, respectively. Unlike evaporated milk, however, concentrated milk is usually not subjected to further heat treatment to prevent spoilage. The product is perishable and spoilage may occur rapidly at temperatures above 44.6°F (7°C).

• **Sweetened condensed milk**—This product is made by the removal of approximately 60% of the water from whole milk and the addition of a suitable sweetener such as sucrose. The amount of the sweetener (40 to 45% of the condensed milk) used is sufficient to prevent spoilage. Federal standards of identity require that sweetened condensed milk contain not less than 8.5% of milkfat and not less than 28% of total milk solids.

DRY MILK. Perishability and bulk of fluid milk have been a major drawback to transporting milk over long distances. However, the development of the dry milk industry made it possible to export milk abroad. Also, dry milk may be transported over relatively long distances domestically (1) to consumers who desire a less costly source of milk, and (2) to processors of other dairy products in areas where milk for manufacturing may not be readily available. The leading states producing dry milk are California, Wisconsin, and Minnesota. A discussion of each of the common dry milks follows:

• **Nonfat dry milk**—This product is prepared by removing water from pasteurized skim milk. Federal standards of identity require that it contain not more than 5% by weight of moisture and not more than 1.5% by weight of milkfat unless indicated. Except for small losses of ascorbic acid, thiamin, vitamin B-12, and biotin, the processing has no appreciable effect on the nutritive value of the milk. Due to its low moisture content, it can be kept for long periods.

• **Nonfat dry milk fortified with vitamins A and D**—This

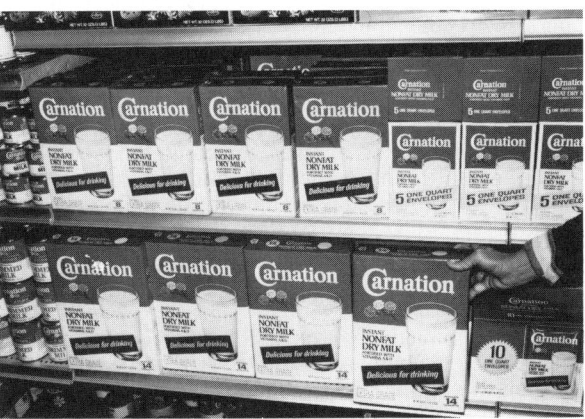

Fig. M-101. Nonfat dry milk fortified with vitamins A & D, displayed on a supermarket shelf. (Courtesy, Carnation Company, Los Angeles, Calif.)

product is similar to nonfat dry milk except that it contains 2,000 IU of vitamin A and 400 IU of vitamin D per quart (950 ml) when reconstituted according to label directions. Almost all nonfat dry milk sold retail is fortified with vitamins A and D.

• **Dry whole milk**—This product is made from pasteurized whole milk from which water has been removed. Except for losses in ascorbic acid (20% for spray dried), vitamin B-6 (30% for spray dried), and thiamin (10% for spray dried, and 20% for roller dried), the processing has no appreciable effect on the nutritive value of the product. The major deterioration of dry whole milk is oxidative changes in the fat. Stability of the product can be increased by special packaging, such as gas-pack (removal of air and replacement with inert gas such as nitrogen) or vacuum-pack containers.

CULTURED MILK AND OTHER PRODUCTS. Cultured milks are fluid products that result from the souring of milk or its products by bacteria that produce lactic acid, whereas acidified milks are obtained by the addition of food-grade acids to produce an acidity of not less than 0.20%, expressed as lactic acid. The word *cultured* is used because pure bacterial cultures are employed in commercial manufacture. It is proper also to use the words *fermented* or *sour* because lactic acid, which imparts sourness,is produced by fermentaton of milk sugar (lactose). Kefir, koumiss, acidophilus milk, cultured buttermilk, sour cream, and yogurt are examples of lactic acid fermentations.

Sales of cultured products are increasing as consumers recognize their nutritional value and appreciate their flavors. Cultured products are also a practical means of introducing large numbers of particular organisms into the intestinal tract.

The body, flavor, and aroma developed in the finished product vary with the type of culture and milk, the concentration of milk solids-not-fat, the fermentation process, and the temperature. The vitamin concentration may be altered; the variation of specific vitamins depends on both the types of culture and the length of ripening. A discussion of each of the common cultured milk products follows:

• **Kefir and koumiss**—These are the two major types of cultured milks which have been subject to both acid and alcoholic fermentation.

Kefir, made from the milk of mares, goats, or cows, is popular in countries of southwestern Asia.

Koumiss, made from unheated mare's milk, is the typical fermented milk of the U.S.S.R. and western Asia.

• **Acidophilus milk**—Pasteurized milk, usually lowfat or skim, cultured with *Lactobacillus acidophilus* and incubated at 100.4°F (38°C) for at least 18 hours until a soft curd forms, is called acidophilus milk.

Today, there is increasing demand for health foods; and, frequently, acidophilus milk is promoted as such a food. Although much research is still needed, *L. acidophilus* is believed to be a normal bacterial component of the gut microflora that helps to maintain the balance of microorganisms in the intestinal tract. Cultures of products containing *L. acidophilus* are sometimes used to regenerate intestinal flora after antibiotic treatment or other conditions that upset the microfloral balance in the gut.

• **Cultured buttermilk; Bulgarian buttermilk**—The fluid remaining after churning cream to make butter is called buttermilk. Today, this product is used primarily by the baking industry; and most buttermilk for beverage purposes is a cultured product. Most of the cultured buttermilk marketed in the United States is made from fresh pasteurized skim or lowfat milk with added nonfat dry milk solids, cultured with *Streptococcus lactis*. However, cultured buttermilk can also be made from fluid whole milk, concentrated fluid forms, or reconstituted nonfat dry milk.

Bulgarian buttermilk is made with *Lactobacillus bulgaricus*.

• **Sour cream or cultured sour cream**—Pasteurized, homogenized cream cultured with *Streptococcus lactis* at 71.6°F (22°C) until the acidity is at least 0.5%, calculated as lactic acid, results in an acid gel product known as cultured sour cream. Federal standards of identity specify that cultured sour cream contain not less than 18% milkfat. If nutritive sweeteners or bulky flavoring ingredients are added, the product must not contain less than 14.4% milkfat.

Cultured sour cream is a uniformly textured, smooth product that is widely used for flavoring.

• **Acidified sour cream**—This product results from the souring of pasteurized cream with safe and suitable acidifiers, with or without the addition of lactic acid producing bacteria. Federal standards of identity call for not less than 18% milkfat and a titratable acidity of not less than 0.5% calculated as lactic acid. In the event nutritive sweeteners or bulky flavoring ingredients are added, the product may not contain less than 14.4% milkfat.

• **Sour half-and-half or cultured half-and-half**—The federal standards of identity state that this is the product of pasteurized half-and-half containing not less than 10.5% and not more than 18% milkfat and containing lactic acid producing bacteria.

• **Acidified sour half-and-half**—This product results from the souring of half-and-half with safe and suitable acidifiers, with or without the addition of lactic acid producing bacteria.

• **Sour cream dressing and sour half-and-half dressing**—The word dressing denotes a product in which other dairy ingredients such as butter have been substituted for cream and/or milk. Sour cream dressing is similar to sour cream and contains not less than 18% milkfat or not less than 14.4% milkfat if nutritive sweeteners or bulky ingredients are added. Sour half-and-half dressing is made in semblance of sour half-and-half and contains not less than 10.5% milkfat or not less than 8.4% if nutritive sweeteners or bulky ingredients are added.

• **Yogurt**—This product can be manufactured from fresh whole milk, lowfat milk, or skim milk. In the united States, yogurt usually is made from a mixture of fresh, partially skimmed milk and nonfat dry milk; and fermentation is generally accomplished by a one-to-one mixed culture of *Lactobacillus bulgaricus and Streptococcus thermophilus*, in a symbiotic relationship, with each microorganism metabolizing milk products which are subsequently used by the other.

The milk is pasteurized, homogenized, inoculated, incubated at 107.6° to 114.8°F (*42° to 46°C*) until the desired stage of acidity and flavor is reached, and chilled to 44.6°F (*7°C*) or lower to halt further fermentation. The usual milkfat levels of current products are: yogurt, at least 3.25% milkfat; lowfat yogurt, 0.5 to 2% milkfat; and nonfat yogurt, less than 0.5%. Milk solids-not-fat range from 9 to 16%, the higher amount reflecting the addition of solids. Today, three main types of yogurt are produced:

1. Flavored, containing no fruit.
2. Flavored, containing fruit.
3. Unflavored yogurt.

The rise in popularity of yogurt in the United States in recent years has been phenomenal. This increased consumption is largely attributed to development of fruit-flavored yogurts and the promotion of low-calorie, but highly nutritional, yogurts as diet foods.

• **Eggnog**—Eggnog is a mixture of milk, cream, sugar, milk soids, eggs, stabilizers, and spices that is pasteurized, homogenized, cooled, and packaged. Eggnog may refer to a product with 6.0 to 8.0% milkfat, 1.0% egg yolk solids, and 0.5% stabilizer. Also, eggnog-flavored milk is available; it contains a minimum milkfat level of 3.25%, minimum egg yolk solids of 0.5%, and a maximum stabilizer level of 0.5%.

SPECIALTY MILKS. Several specialty milks are on the market, including certified milk, low sodium milk, imitation milk, and filled milk. A discussion of each of these follows:

• **Certified milk**—The first certified milk was produced in 1893, in Essex County, New Jersey, before dairy sanitation had achieved the excellence that now exists in producing Grade A milk. Certified milk refers to raw or pasteurized milk produced and handled by dairies that operate according to the rules and sanitary regulations stated in the book *Methods and Standards for the Production of Certified Milk* issued and revised periodically by the American Association of Medical Milk Commissioners, Inc. Today, the quality of Grade A milk is so high that it has largely replaced certified milk—and at a lower cost, so certified milk is produced in only a few localities. The production of certified milk, conducted under the auspices of a Medical Milk Commission, involves the veterinary examination of cows, the sanitary inspection of the dairy farm and equipment, and the medical examination of employees who handle the milk.

• **Low sodium milk**—Ninety-five percent or more of the sodium that occurs naturally in milk can be removed by ion-exchange. Thus, the sodium content of whole milk generally can be reduced from a normal amount of about 49 mg to about 2.5 mg per 100 g of milk. Fresh whole milk is passed through an ion-exchange resin to replace the sodium in milk with potassium, following which the milk is pasteurized and homogenized.

Low sodium milk permits the inclusion of milk and milk-containing foods that might otherwise be limited in therapeutic diets because of their sodium content.

• **Imitation milk**—Imitation milks purport to substitute for and resemble milk. These products usually contain water, corn syrup solids, sugar, vegetable fat (coconut, soybean, cottonseed), and protein from soybean, fish, sodium caseinate, or other sources. Although imitation fluid milks do not contain dairy products as such, they may contain derivatives of milk such as casein, salts of casein, milk proteins other than casein, whey, and lactose. Sometimes vitamins A and/or D are added. Ingredient composition, and hence nutrient composition, vary widely. The American Academy of Pediatrics considers imitation milk products inappropriate for feeding infants and young children.

• **Filled milk**—These are milk products (milk, lowfat milk, half-and-half or cream, whether or not condensed, evaporated, concentrated, powdered, dried, or desiccated) from which all or part of the milkfat has been removed and to which any fat or oil other than milkfat has been added. The American Academy of Pediatrics does not recommend the use of filled milks for feeding infants and small children.

CREAM.   Cream is the liquid milk product, high in fat, separated from milk, which may have been adjusted by the addition of milk, concentrated milk, dry whole milk, skim milk, concentrated skim milk, or nonfat dry milk. Federal standards of identity require that cream contain not less than 18% milkfat. The several cream products on the market are:

• **Half-and-half**—This is a mixture of milk and cream containing not less than 10.5% nor more than 18% milkfat. It is pasteurized or ultrapasteurized, and it may be homogenized.

• **Light cream (coffee cream, table cream)**—This product contains not less than 18% nor more than 30% milkfat. it is pasteurized or ultrapasteurized, and it may be homogenized.

• **Light whipping cream (whipping cream)**—This cream contains not less than 30% nor more than 36% milkfat. It is pasteurized, or ultrapasteurized, and it may be homogenized.

• **Heavy cream (heavy whipping cream)**—This cream contains not less than 36% milkfat. It is pasteurized or ultrapasteurized, and it may be homogenized.

ICE CREAM AND FROZEN DESSERTS.

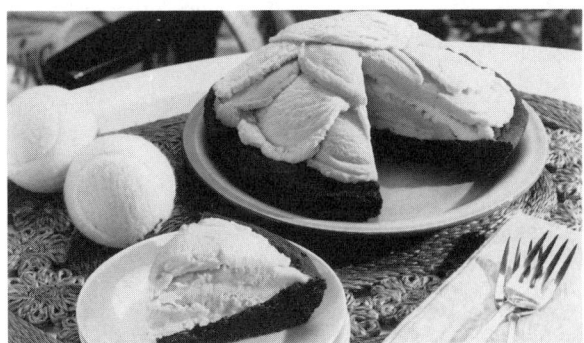

Fig. M-102.   Brownie baked as a pie shell and an a la mode topping of vanilla ice cream and orange sherbet—a frozen dessert. (Courtesy, United Dairy Industry Assn., Rosemont, Ill.)

The following excerpts from the pages of history tell how ice cream and frozen desserts started:

• In the 4th century B.C., Alexander the Great was reputed to be fond of iced beverages.

• In 62 A.D., the Roman Emperor, Nero, sent fleets of slaves to the mountains of the Apennines to fetch snow and ice which were then flavored with nectar, fruit pulp, and honey.

• In the 13th century, Marco Polo, bard and adventurer, brought with him to Europe from the Far East recipes for water ices—said to have been used in Asia for thousands of years.

• In 1812, at the second inaugural ball, Dolley Madison created a sensation when she served ice cream as a dessert at the White House.

• In 1904, the first ice cream cone was made and sold at the St. Louis World's Fair.

Today, the ice cream manufacturing industry is one of the largest in the realm of dairy processing. U.S. production of frozen dairy products increased from 936 million gallons (*3.5 billion liter*) in 1960 to 1.3 billion gallons (*4.9 billion liter*) in 1988 (see Table M-50).

TABLE M–50
FROZEN DAIRY PRODUCTS AND FROZEN PRODUCTS
CONTAINING SUBSTITUTES FOR BUTTERFAT, PRODUCTION[1]

Year	Ice Cream		Milk Sherbets		Ice Milk		Frozen Products Made from Fats, Oils Other Than Butterfat		Total[2]	
	◄——————————————————————— (in mil gal or liter) ———————————————————————►									
	(gal)	(liter)	(gal)	(liter)	(gal)	(liter)	(gal)	(liter)	(gal)	(liter)
1970	762	*2,884*	49	*185*	287	*1,086*	52	*197*	1,156	*4,376*
1975	833	*3,157*	48	*182*	295	*1,118*	30	*114*	1,217	*4,612*
1980	830	*3,146*	45	*171*	292	*1,107*	13	*49*	1,181	*4,476*
1985	901	*3,415*	48	*182*	301	*1,141*	9	*34*	1,259	*4,772*
1988	882	*3,343*	52	*197*	354	*1,342*	10	*38*	1,298	*4,919*

[1]*1989 Dairy Producer Highlights,* National Milk Producers Federation, p. 16.
[2]Includes other frozen dairy products through 1975.

Several products are classified under the category of frozen desserts. Some of these follow:

1. **Ice cream**. Of all the frozen dairy desserts, ice cream contains the most milk solids (about 16 to 24%). It consists primarily of milk fat, nonfat milk solids, sugar, flavoring, and stabilizers.

2. **Custards and French ice cream**. These products closely resemble ice cream except they must contain at least 1.4% egg yolk solids, additionally.

3. **Ice milk**. Ice milk contains less fat and less total solids than ice cream; hence, it contains fewer calories It must contain at least 2%, but not more than 7%, milkfat.

4. **Mellorine**. Mellorine is essentially the same product as ice cream except that vegetable fat is used in place of milkfat.

5. **Sherbet**. Sherbet is a sweet, tart-flavored frozen dairy product that is low in total milk solids (about 3 to 5%). It can be made either by mixing water with ice cream or by manufacturing from the raw ingredients. Since its melting point is lower than ice cream, it is softer than ice cream when the two products are stored at the same temperature.

BUTTER. Butter is made from cream. As marketed, it contains about 80 to 82% butterfat, 14 to 16% water, 0 to 4% salt, and 0.1 to 1.0% curd. *Sweet cream butter* is made from pasteurized sweet cream to which no starter has been added. *Ripened cream butter* is made by starter ripened cream. *Sweet butter* contains no salt. *Unsalted butter* is butter to which no salt has been added. *Salted butter* is butter to which salt has been added.

Butter is classed as Grade AA, A, B, or C based on flavor, body, color, and salt (see Table M-51). Butter which

does not meet the standards of Grade C cannot carry a USDA label.

Butter is sometimes referred to as the "balance wheel" of the dairy industry. This designation comes from the fact that milk is not used for butter until all other demands have been met, with the result that butter manufacture increases or decreases as necessary to balance out total milk production with utilization. The wholesale price received for butter (as well as the wholesale price for cheese and nonfat dry milk) is based on the price support of the Commodity Credit Corporation (CCC). The CCC is the governmental agency that purchases excesses of butter to help establish market price floors. If shortages occur, the CCC may sell butter supplies to enhance commercial availability, provided, according to the present regulations, the selling price is not less than 110% of the CCC purchase price.

Table M-52 shows the per capita consumption of butter and margarine for selected years from 1910 to 1990. Per capita consumption of margarine surpassed butter in 1957. In 1990, the per capita consumption of butter was 4.4 lb, as compared to 10.9 lb of margarine. The controversy about cholesterol and heart disease are the primary reasons for the decrease in both margarine and butter consumption.

TABLE M-51
GRADES OF BUTTER

Grade	Numerical Rating	Description
AA ...	93	Pleasing flavor; smooth texture with good spreadability; well blended; and completely dissolved salt in a desirable amount (1-2%).
A ...	92	Distinct feed and cooked flavor; slight intensity of bitter, acid flat, or storage flavors.
B ...	90	Generally manufactured from sour cream. May be used for table use. Off-flavors allowed: 1. Slight intensity—malty, neutralizer, rancid, sweet, scorched, unclean, weed, musty, whey. 2. Definite intensity—bitter, acid, storage, old cream. 3. Pronounced intensity—feed.
C ...	89	Low quality. Off-flavors allowed: 1. Slight intensity—barny, onion, garlic, sour, yeasty. 2. Definite intensity—malty, musty, rancid, neutralizer, storage, unclean, whey, weed.

TABLE M-52
PER CAPITA CONSUMPTION
OF BUTTER AND MARGARINE[1]

Year	Per Capita Consumption			
	Butter		Margarine	
	(lb)	(kg)	(lb)	(kg)
1910	18.3	8.3	1.6	0.7
1920	14.9	6.8	3.4	1.5
1930	17.6	8.0	2.6	1.2
1940	17.0	7.7	2.4	1.1
1950	10.7	4.9	6.1	2.8
1960	7.5	3.4	9.4	4.3
1970	5.3	2.4	11.0	5.0
1980	4.5	2.0	11.4	5.2
1990	4.4	2.0	10.9	4.5

[1]*Dairy Statistics Through 1960*, Stat. Bull No. 303, Supp. for 1963–64, Economic Research Service, USDA; *National Food Situation*, Economic Research Service, USDA, February 1966; *Agricultural Statistics 1980*, USDA, p. 148 and *1991*, p. 479.

State and federal laws and regulations prevent additives to or changes in butter. Nevertheless, experiments are being conducted on low butterfat spreads. Besides their appeal to homemakers, these products would be better able to compete with oleomargarine.

Production of butter in the United States in 1990 totaled 1.3 billion pounds (*592 million kg*). Wisconsin, the leading state, accounted for 25% of the total. California produced 21%, followed by Minnesota with 9%.

CHEESE. *Cheese may be defined as the fresh or matured product obtained by draining after coagulation of milk, cream, skimmed or partly skimmed milk, buttermilk, or a combination of some or all of these products.*

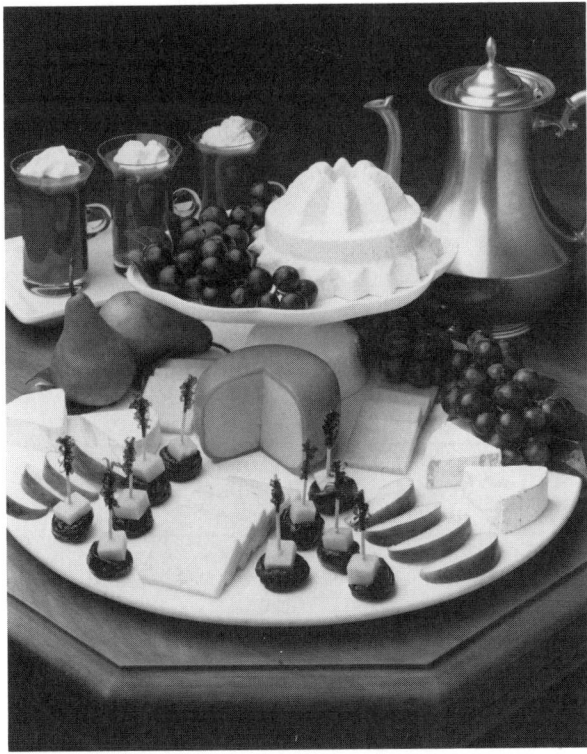

Fig. M-103. Assorted cheeses for dessert. (Courtesy, United Dairy Assn., Rosemont, Ill.)

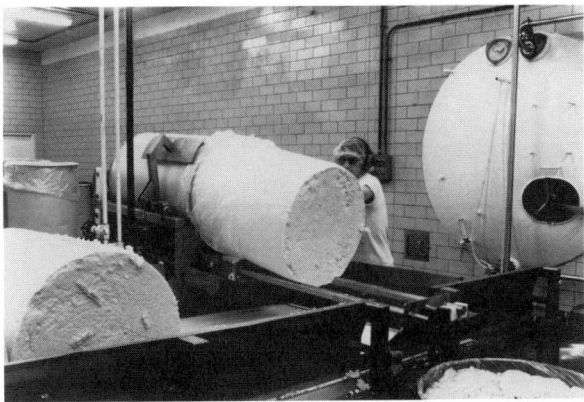

Fig. M-104. Cheddar cheese, which accounts for more than 40% of the U.S. total cheese production. This shows a 500-lb (*227 kg*) cheddar cheese being removed from a barrel and moved onto a conveyor. (Courtesy, Borden Inc., Columbus, Ohio)

According to legend, cheese was discovered several thousand years before Christ by an Arabian traveler who, starting on a trip across the desert, placed milk in a pouch made of a sheep's stomach and tied it to his camel saddle. During the journey, the combined action of the sun's heat and the enzymes in the lining of the pouch-stomach changed the milk into curds of cheese and liquid whey. From that time forward, cheese became a popular food.

Cheese graced the banquet tables of Roman emperors and served as part of the rations of their conquering armies, just as it serves armies around the world in our present day.

Cheese is manufactured by: (1) exposing milk to specific bacterial fermentation, and/or (2) treating with enzymes; to coagulate some of the protein. The first step in cheese making is to separate the casein and milk solids from the water in milk. The coagulated milk is then cut into small pieces and the water separated from the solids by a series of drainings and pressings. The characteristic flavor of the cheese is created by bacteria growth and subsequent acid production in the cheese during the cheese-making process and also by the bacteria and mold development during a period of curing.

Milk can be, and is, processed into many different varieties of cheese. In fact, there are over 2,000 different named cheeses. Some are made from whole milk, others from milk that has had part of the fat removed, and still others from skim milk. (The most important variety produced from skim milk is cottage cheese.) In 1990, American types of cheese accounted for 50% of the U.S. total cheese production, of which 96% was American Cheddar and 2.2% was other American types (Colby, washed curd, stirred curd, Monterey). Other important types of cheese are Italian (mostly soft varieties), Swiss, Muenster, cream, blue, and Neufchatel.

Fig. M-105 shows the kinds of cheese produced in 1990, exclusive of cottage cheese.

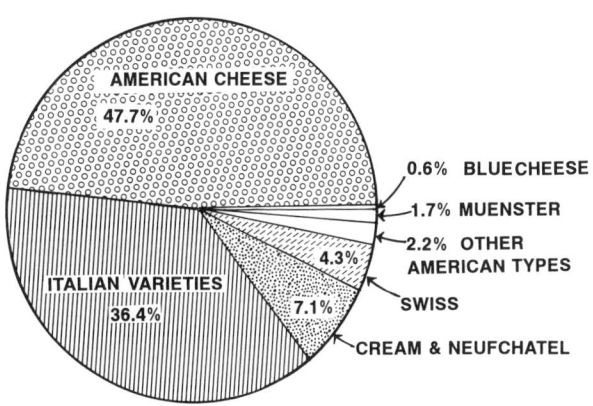

Fig. M-105. Relative importance of kinds of cheeses produced in the United States. (Source: USDA)

Table M-53 shows the per capita consumption of selected cheese varieties, 1950 to 1988. Table M-54 gives the origin, characteristics and mode of serving the commonly used varieties of natural cheeses.

TABLE M–53
PER CAPITA CONSUMPTION OF SELECTED CHEESE VARIETIES[1]

Year	American	Italian Types[2]	Swiss[3]	Cream and Neufchatel	Muenster	Blue-Cheese[4]	Edam and Gouda
				◄——————— (lb)[5] ———————►			
1950	5.5	0.54	0.70	0.46		0.08	0.04
1960	5.4	1.0	0.76	0.60	0.13	0.11	0.06
1970	7.1	2.09	0.90	0.63	0.17	0.14	0.11
1980	9.7	4.4	1.3	1.0	0.31	0.17	0.13
1988	11.4	8.1	1.3	1.5	0.34	0.17	0.19

[1]*1991 Dairy Producer Highlights*, National Milk Producers Federation, p. 18
[2]Includes Romano, Pecorino, Reggiano, Parmesano, Provolone, and Provelette.
[3]Includes Gruyere and Emmenthaler.
[4]Includes Gorgonzola.
[5]One lb equals 0.45 kg.

TABLE M-54
NAME, ORIGIN, CHARACTERISTICS,
AND MODE OF SERVING THE COMMONLY USED VARIETIES OF CHEESE[1]

Name	Origin	Consistency and Texture	Color and Shape	Flavor	Basic Ingredient	Normal Ripening Period	Mode of Serving
Cheddar	England	Hard; smooth, firm body, can be crumbly.	Nearly white to orange; varied shapes and styles.	Mild to sharp.	Cow's milk, whole.	60 days minimum; 3 to 6 months usually; 12 or longer for sharp flavor.	As such; in sandwiches, cooked foods.
Colby	United States	Hard, but softer and more open in texture than Cheddar.	White to light yellow orange; cylindrical.	Mild to mellow.	Cow's milk, whole.	1 to 3 months.	As such; in sandwiches, cooked foods.
Cream	United States	Soft; smooth, buttery.	White; foil-wrapped in rectangular portions.	Mild, slightly acid; flavoring may be added.	Cream and whole cow's milk.	Unripened	As such; in salads, in sandwiches, on crackers.
Edam	Holland	Semisoft to hard; firm crumbly body; small eyes.	Creamy yellow with natural or red paraffin coat, flattened ball or loaf shape, about 4 lb.	Mild, sometimes salty.	Cow's milk, lowfat.	2 months or longer.	As such; on crackers; with fresh fruit.
Gouda	Holland	Hard, but softer than Cheddar; more open mealy body like edam, small eyes.	Creamy yellow with or without red wax coat, oval or flattened sphere of about 10 to 12 lb.	Mild, nutlike, similar to edam.	Cow's milk, lowfat but more milk-fat than edam.	2 to 6 months.	As such; on crackers, with fresh fruit; in cooked dishes.

Footnote at end of table

(Continued)

TABLE M-54 *(Continued)*

Name	Origin	Consistency and Texture	Color and Shape	Flavor	Basic Ingredient	Normal Ripening Period	Mode of Serving
Monterey Jack	United States	Semisoft (whole milk), hard (lowfat or skim milk); smooth texture with small openings throughout.	Creamy, white; round or rectangular.	Mild to mellow.	Cow's milk, whole, lowfat or skim.	3 to 6 weeks for table use; 6 months minimum for grating.	As such; in sandwiches, grating cheese if made from lowfat or skim milk.
Mozzarella	Italy	Semisoft; plastic.	Creamy white, rectangular and spherical, may be molded into various shapes.	Mild, delicate.	Cow's milk, whole or lowfat; may be acidified with vinegar.	From unripened to 2 months.	Generally used in cooking, pizza; as such.
Muenster	Germany	Semisoft; smooth, waxy body, numerous small mechanical openings.	Yellow, tan, or white surface, creamy white interior; cylindrical and flat or loaf shaped, small wheels and blocks.	Mild to mellow, between brick and limburger.	Cow's milk, whole.	2 to 8 weeks.	As such; in sandwiches.
Neufchatel	France	Soft; smooth; creamy.	White; foil-wrapped in rectangular retail portions.	Mild	Cow's milk, whole or skim, or a mixture of milk and cream.	3 to 4 weeks or unripened.	As such; in sandwiches, dips, salads.
Parmesan	Italy	Very hard (grating), hard brittle rind.	Light yellow with brown or black coating; cylindrical.	Sharp; piquant.	Cow's milk, lowfat.	10 months minimum.	As such; as grated cheese on salads and soups.
Provolone	Italy	Hard; stringy texture, cuts without crumbling, plastic.	Light golden-yellow to golden-brown, shiny surface bound with cord, yellow-white interior. Made in various shapes (pear, sausage, salami) and sizes.	Bland acid flavor to sharp and piquant, usually smoked.	Cow's milk, whole.	6 to 14 months.	As such (dessert) after it has ripened for 6 to 9 months; grating cheese when aged.

Footnote at end of table

(Continued)

TABLE M-54 (*Continued*)

Name	Origin	Consistency and Texture	Color and Shape	Flavor	Basic Ingredient	Normal Ripening Period	Mode of Serving
Ricotta	Italy	Soft, moist and grainy, or dry.	White; packaged fresh in paper, plastic, or metal containers, or dry for grating.	Bland but semisweet.	Whey and whole or skim milk or whole and lowfat milk.	Unripened	As such; in cooked foods; as seasoning (grated) when dried.
Romano	Italy	Very hard, granular interior, hard brittle rind.	Round with flat sides, various sizes.	Sharp, piquant if aged.	Cow's (usually lowfat), goat's milk or mixtures of these.	5 months minimum; usually 5 to 8 months for table cheese; 12 months minimum for grating cheese.	As such; grated and used as a seasoning.
Swiss	Switzerland	Hard; smooth with large gas holes or eyes.	Pale yellow, shiny; rindless rectangular blocks and large wheels with rind.	Mild, sweet, nutty.	Cow's milk, lowfat.	2 months minimum; 2 to 9 months usually.	As such; in sandwiches; with salads; fondue.

[1]From *Newer Knowledge of Cheese and Other Cheese Products*, National Dairy Council, Rosemont, Ill., pp. 14 and 15.

Cheeses are generally classified as to hardness. Hardness is largely a function of moisture content with the very hard cheeses containing as little as 30% moisture while the soft cheeses may contain up to 80% moisture.

The USDA has recommended that cheeses be graded as AA, A, B, and C, with AA being the highest quality cheese. Cheeses failing to Grade C are termed undergrade. The bulk of American cheese is graded as U.S. Extra, U.S. Standard, and U.S. Commercial. Grading is based primarily on flavor, texture, and body, but other factors, such as color and appearance, are often considered.

In 1990, the leading states, by rank, in the production of cheese, excluding cottage cheese, were: Wisconsin, 32%; California, 12%; Minnesota, 11%; and New York, 8%.

Cheese consumption has risen steadily over the years. Table M-53 shows the per capita consumption of selected cheese varieties. In 1990, the U.S. per capita consumption of all cheeses totaled 24.7 lb (*11 kg*).

Although less than 1% of the cheese marketed is traded on the Wisconsin Cheese Exchange, the exchange prices are generally considered to be a good basis for establishing prices for buyers and sellers of American-type or Swiss cheeses. Depending on the needs of the buyer, premiums are often paid for cheese having desirable age, moisture, fat, or flavor.

In cheese making, changes in the composition of the original milk occur at two stages: (1) at the separation of the curd from the whey, and (2) during ripening. The removal of whey, concentrates in the curd (cheese) many of the nutrients of milk. The degree of concentration depends largely on the type of cheese being manufactured, on the type of milk (whole or skimmed) initially used, and on the manner of coagulation. Almost all of the water-insoluble and some water-soluble components are retained in the curd resulting in approximately an eight to tenfold increase in protein, fat (when whole or partially skimmed milk is used), calcium, phosphorus, and vitamin A over those in milk. Most of the water-soluble components, on the other hand, are retained by the whey. As a result, lactose, soluble proteins, and water-soluble salts are not all concentrated and thus may be relatively lower in cheese than in the original milk.

Ripening involves intentional exposure to controlled temperature for long or short periods of time—depending on the type of cheese—to allow bacteria and enzymes to transform the fresh curd into a cheese of a specific flavor, texture, and appearance. The extent of these changes, which inevitably affect nutrient content of the product, depends largely on the microorganisms introduced as a starter culture prior to ripening and/or present initially.

Hard cheese, such as Cheddar, is one of the most concentrated of common foods; 100 g (about 3.5 oz) supplies about 36% of the protein, 80% of the calcium, and 34% of the fat in the recommended daily allowances. Cheese is also a good source of some minerals and vitamins.

Cheese is a high-protein food, and the protein (principally casein) is partially digested. It is rich in the essential amino acids, calcium, phosphorus, certain other minerals, and vitamins, and has a high caloric value. Only a trace of the lactose present in milk remains in the cheese.

Cottage cheese (as made from skim milk) is low in fat and high in protein, but has only about one-eighth of the calcium content of American (Cheddar) cheese. Cream cheese differs from other soft cheeses in having more fat and less protein.

One ounce (*about 28 g*) of Cheddar-type cheese provides about the same nutritive value as a glass of milk. It is a particularly good food for children.

• **Processed cheese**—This product is formed by grinding, heating, and mixing hard-type cheeses. This type of cheese serves as an outlet to salvage defective cheeses as well as provide a uniform, widely marketable product.

• **Nutritive value of cheeses**—The composition and nutritive value of a number of varieties of cheeses is given in Food Composition Table F-36, in the section on "Milk and Products."

CASEINATES (COFFEE WHITENERS; WHIPPED TOPPINGS).

Caseinates are salts of casein. They are classified as food chemicals derived from milk and are commonly used in (1) nondairy coffee whiteners (coffee whiteners are made from sodium caseinate) and (2) whipped toppings.

To produce caseinates, enough alkali, commonly calcium hydroxide or sodium hydroxide, is added to acid coagulated casein to reach a pH of 6.7. The resulting suspension is pasteurized and spray dried.

WHEY.

Whey is the watery part of milk separated from the curd. Whey is available as dried whey, condensed whey, dried whey solubles, condensed whey solubles, dried hydrolyzed whey, condensed hydrolyzed whey, condensed whey product, dried whey product, and condensed cultured whey.

Whey provides food processors with an inexpensive product that can be used as a source of lactose, milk solids, milk proteins, or total solids. Additionally, whey, which is relatively high in digestibility and nutritive value, is commonly used as a livestock feed.

MARKETING AND DISTRIBUTING MILK.

Marketing milk is that all-important end of the line; it's that which give point and purpose to all that has gone before.

Satisfactory milk marketing requires one basic ingredient—quality milk; and this begins with production on the farm.

The difference in price between Grade A milk and the lower grades is substantial. But it goes beyond this; quality influences consumer demand.

Buyers, health departments, and consumers share a common interest in the quality of milk marketed as fresh milk or used in manufacturing. In recent years, there has arisen a great interest by people pertaining to the quality of the food they eat. Food must be wholesome and free from contamination lest it be deemed unsafe or unfit for consumption.

In our present system, the vast majority of the marketing of milk and dairy products is handled by specialists, usually under a myriad of complex regulations and controls. Both successful milk producers and enlightened consumers should be familiar with milk markets, regulations and controls, and pricing systems, along with the factors affecting them.

Milk Supply. In 1990, a total of 148 billion pounds (*67 billion kilograms*) of milk were marketed by U.S. dairy farmers for $20 billion delivered to plants. Of this amount, 37.3% was consumed in fluid form and 62.7% was processed into manufactured dairy products.

Fluid milk is retailed as pasteurized milk, homogenized milk, fortified milk (usually vitamin D), skim milk, and flavored milk. Of the milk used for manufacturing in 1990, 31.9% was used for making cheese (exclusive of creamed cottage cheese) and 16.9% was used for making butter.

Future milk supply will depend primarily on the profitability of dairy enterprises, for, like all other businesses, dairies are owned by people—and all people like to make a profit. In turn, profitability is determined by milk prices and cost of production. Also, dairy farmers will consider alternative farm and off-farm opportunities.

SEASONALITY OF MILK PRODUCTION. Milk production is seasonal in nature, and the economic principles of supply and demand dictate that prices decline when milk availability increases. Fig. M-106 shows that milk production peaks in May and reaches its yearly low in November.

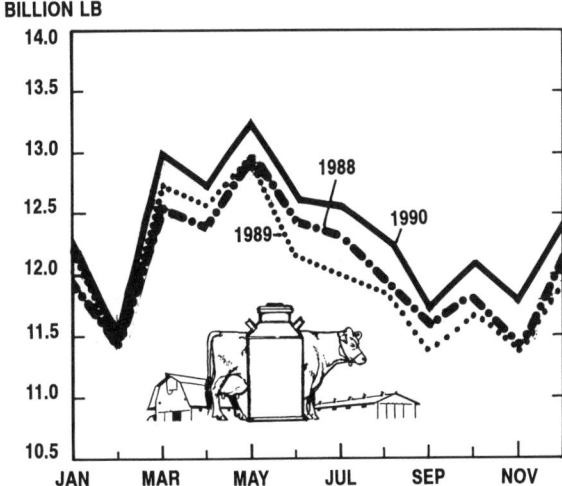

U.S. MILK PRODUCTION BY MONTHS

Fig. M-106. U.S. milk production by months. (From: *Dairy Situation and Outlook Report*, USDA, ERS, DS-429, April 1991, p. 61)

Milk Demand. There have been dramatic changes in the per capita consumption of milk and manufactured dairy products in recent years. Fig. M-107 clearly shows these changes.

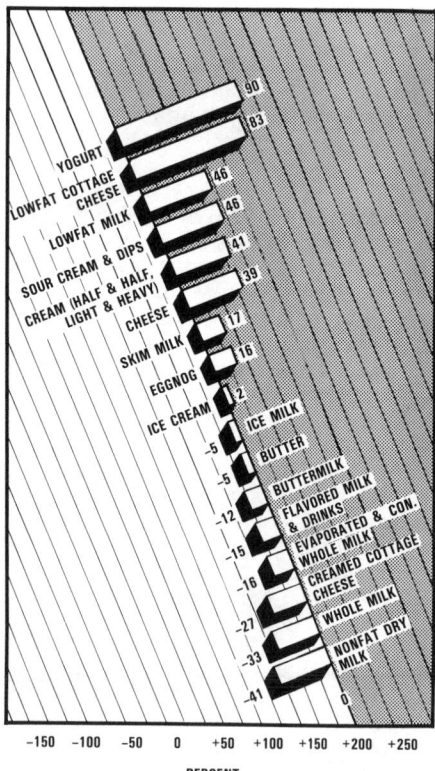

PERCENT CHANGE IN PER CAPITA SALES
1977–87

Fig. M-107. Change in U.S. per capita consumption of milk and dairy products 1977 to 1987, based on sales. Bars to the left of the vertical line represent decreases; bars to the right represent increases. (Source: *1988 Milk Facts,* Milk Industry Foundation, Washington, D.C., p. 16)

Because of increasing consumer infatuation with weight watching, low calorie diets, and cholesterol levels, it appears that present trends will continue. It is noteworthy that declines in per capita consumption were registered in the following products: ice milk, butter, buttermilk, flavored milk and drinks, evaporated and condensed whole milk, creamed cottage cheese, whole milk, and nonfat dry milk. It is noteworthy, too, that yogurt and low fat cottage cheese led the increases. Increases in yogurt reflect the rising interest in health foods, whereas increased consumption of low fat cottage cheese reflects weight watching.

Contrary to popular opinion, the United States ranks low among nations in per capita consumption of dairy products (see Table M-55). As shown, of the 18 major countries in per capita consumption of fluid milk, the United States ranks fifteenth in per capita consumption of fluid milk, last in consumption of butter, seventh in consumption of cheese, and twelfth in consumption of dry milk.

TABLE M–55
PER CAPITA CONSUMPTION
OF DAIRY PRODUCTS BY COUNTRIES[1]

Country	Consumption			
	Fluid Milk[2]	Butter[3]	Cheese[4]	Nonfat Dry Milk[5]
	◄—————— (pounds per capita)[6] ——————►			
Norway	513	7.3	28.4	N.A.[7]
Ireland	394	10.1	13.2	6.8
Poland	338	18.3	7.3	7.3
Finland	336	15.4	25.4	7.9
Sweden	318	12.1	32.6	6.2
New Zealand ...	308	34.8	20.1	19.4
Netherlands ...	302	8.8	32.4	25.1
Austria	293	11.2	18.7	2.9
Romania	284	5.3	9.3	N.A.[7]
Denmark	269	21.4	31.8	6.0
United Kingdom	267	7.7	18.5	2.6
Spain	239	1.3	9.0	1.5
Canada	237	7.1	22.5	4.0
Switzerland	234	13.5	32.0	9.7
U.S.A.	229	4.4	24.7	2.6
Australia	227	7.1	18.3	5.5
Czechoslovakia	204	21.2	19.8	N.A.[7]
Hungary	188	6.8	8.4	N.A.[7]

[1]From: *1991 Milk Facts,* Milk Industry Foundation, p. 32.
[2]Whole milk equivalent (fat solids basis) of fluid milk and cream.
[3]Includes anhydrous milkfat, butter oil and ghee.
[4]Cured cheese only.
[5]Includes both human and animal use.
[6]One lb equals 0.45 kg.
[7]N.A. Not available. (Source: USDA).

FACTORS INFLUENCING DEMAND. The demand for milk and milk products depends on a number of factors, chief of which are those which follow:

● **Price**—An increase in price of milk and manufactured dairy products does result in lowered consumption; however, the consumption of fluid milk is less affected than the consumption of manufactured products. Thus, a 10% increase in price may lower fluid milk consumption by 1.4% compared to lowering butter consumption by 7.3% (in the latter case, margarine is likely to be substituted for butter). Decrease in consumer purchases, or the substitution of another food item that costs less results in increased dairy surpluses followed by lower farm prices.

● **Availability and price of substitute products**—Imitation milk and filled milk are substitute products, prepared from ingredients that make it possible for them to sell for less than milk. (See earlier section on "Specialty Milks.") Consumption of price-attractive imitation and filled milks may increase in the future because of their improved product stability and taste, increased promotion, retail price increases in milk, and recent court rulings.

Among other substitute products presently on the market, or developed, are the following:

1. **Mellorine.** This is a vegetable fat ice cream. Until July 1, 1975, federal standards of identity required that it be labeled "imitation ice cream." Now that the more appealing name *mellorine* may be used, mellorine sales are increasing and adversely affecting sales of ice cream and milk fat.

2. **Imitation and filled cheese.** Today, several companies are developing different imitation and filled cheese variations. Imitation cheese, like imitation milk, contains vegetable fat, rather than milk fat, and protein from soybeans and other sources than milk. Filled cheese contains vegetable oil (coconut, soybean, cottonseed, or corn oil) in place of milk fat. Some of these substitutes for processed cheese taste like the real thing.

These products have aroused considerable apprehension on the part of established cheese producers, ever mindful of what margarine has done to butter consumption in this country.

• **Consumer income**—Milk consumption increases with income. Conversely, lower per capita income, unemployment, and inflation encourage the purchase of lower-priced substitutes.

• **Population growth**—The more people, the more milk drinkers. Thus, population growth within itself, even if per capita consumption remains the same, makes for increased demand for milk.

• **Changes in consumer preference**—Shifts in consumer preferences, affect consumer demand for food products, and milk is no exception. (See the previous section on "Milk Demand.")

• **Age and sex**—Both the proportion of people drinking milk and the per capita consumption decrease with age. Ninety-five percent of children under 6 years of age of both sexes consume an average of 1.5 pints (*920 ml*) of milk daily. During the teenage stage, boys continue to consume an average of 1.5 pints daily, but girls drink only 0.95 of a pint. Average daily consumption of people over 35 years of age is less than 0.5 of a pint. So, convincing teenage girls and adult males and females that continuation of their earlier milk drinking habits would be nutritionally advantageous would immensely increase milk consumption.

• **Carbonated beverages**—An increase in the consumption of carbonated beverages normally results in decreased consumption of fluid milk. One-third of the children and one-half of the teenagers drink carbonated beverages regularly at mealtime and between meals. Convincing children and teenagers that milk is a "fun drink" and "better for them" would increase sales.

• **Type and size of container**—Glass bottles have been largely replaced by paper and plastic containers, with 32 and 68%, respectively, of 1990 Federal Order milk packaged in these containers. In 1990, 83% of the Federal Order milk was packaged in gallon and half-gallon containers. Only 4% of Federal Order milk was still packaged in quart containers.

The availability of larger sized paper and plastic containers has increased sales of fluid milk because of greater consumer convenience associated with these containers.

(Also see earlier section on "Packaging Milk," Table M-48 Type of Container and Size of Container.)

• **Promotion of milk and dairy products**—Nutritional merit of milk alone will not assure its optimal acceptance and use. A joint effort by all segments of the dairy industry is needed to educate the public concerning the values and qualities of milk and milk products, with this effort amplified and extended through promotion and advertising.

Dairy promotion assessments on farm milk were first authorized in Federal Milk Order markets in 1971. Under the terms of the law, an agency can be organized within a Federal order by producers and producers' associations to administer the program using money paid by dairymen (usually 5¢ per cwt) for their milk sold (mandatory checkoff). However, individual dairymen may request and receive refunds of money deducted from their payments if they do not wish to participate.

The primary organization that receives funds deducted in either mandatory or voluntary checkoff programs is the United Dairy Industry Association (UDIA).

Milk Price Supports. Chaotic conditions in milk marketing, resulting from the breakdown of private controls and the serious economic plight of farmers during the depression years of the 1930s, brought requests from organized producers and distributors for government control. Out of this evolved the Agricultural Act of 1949, which assures consumers of an adequate milk supply at reasonable prices. Although this Act has been amended several times since, it still provides the authority for the milk price support program. In 1981, federal legislation departed from the parity concept for the first time and parity has not been used as a basis of establishing dairy price supports since then. The Food Security Act of 1985 set the support price of milk from 1986 to 1990. On January 1, 1990, the support price was $10.10 per cwt.

The minimum price for raw milk is established indirectly by the support prices of the federal government, but not every transaction is supported. Processors compete for supplies of manufacturing milk through price competition. Normally, it is only when there is a surplus of manufacturing milk that the federal government must provide price support through the purchase of butter, nonfat dry milk, and/or cheese.

In carrying out milk price supports, the U.S. Department of Agriculture, through the Commodity Credit Corporation (CCC), offers to buy on the open market at announced prices carlots of butter, cheese, and nonfat dry milk which meet certain CCC specifications, including federal grade standards.

MILK PARITY. *Parity may be defined as a yardstick for measuring the relationship between the prices farmers receive for the products they sell and the prices they pay for the things they buy, including interest, taxes, and farm wage rates.* The term parity comes from the Latin word *paritas*, meaning equal.

The price of a farm commodity may be said to be at parity when a given unit has the same purchasing power that it had in the base period. Thus, if a dairyman received parity price per hundredweight for milk, he should be able to take the money and buy as much with it as he could back in 1910 to 1914, the base period. If the price of things farmers buy for their production program doubles, the parity price of farm commodities also doubles, to keep in line or equal parity.

In 1981, the U.S. Congress departed from the parity concept as a basis of establishing support prices for dairy products, and parity hasn't been used since. For the time being, parity is gone but not forgotten.

COMMODITY CREDIT CORPORATION (CCC).
In order to provide price supports for manufactured dairy products, the Commodity Credit Corporation (CCC) purchases butter, Cheddar cheese, and nonfat dry milk for the various programs of the USDA; with these purchases made on the open market at prices that, with average yields and processing-marketing costs for these products, enable dairy plants to pay farmers the support price. By providing an outlet for excess quantities of these three major dairy products, market prices of all manufactured dairy products are maintained, because of competition among plants for milk supplies.

Table M-56 shows the CCC purchase prices for dairy products for 1951 to 1989. Beginning in 1956 and continuing to 1973, there was a steady increase in the price of butter, Cheddar cheese, and nonfat dry milk. However, butter prices declined sharply in 1973 and 1974, then rose rapidly thereafter. Likewise, the price of Cheddar cheese and nonfat milk has risen rapidly since 1973.

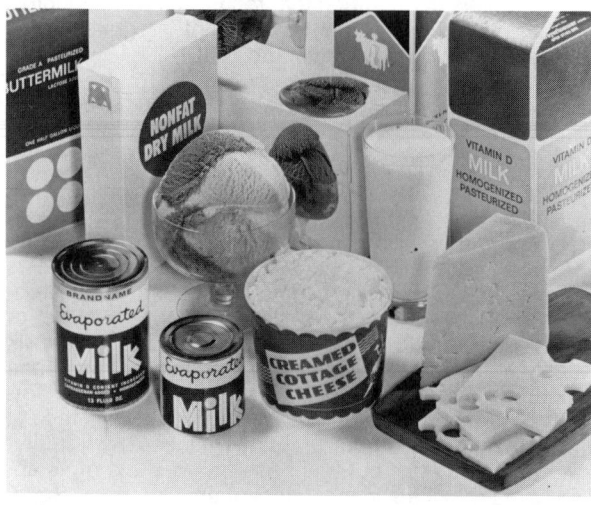

Fig. M-107 a. Milk and milk products. The retail price of milk and milk products is determined by the support price of milk, processing cost, marketing costs, and supply and demand. (Courtesy, USDA)

TABLE M–56
CCC PURCHASE PRICES FOR DAIRY PRODUCTS[1]

Effective Date[2]	Support Price at National Standard Fat Test	Butter — Grade A New York	Cheddar Cheese — Grade A or Higher	Cheddar Cheese — Barrels, Extra Grade	Nonfat Dry Milk, Extra Grade Spray
		(¢ per lb)			
1951	3.60	66.00	36.00	—	15.0
1956	3.15	58.25	34.00	—	16.0
1961	3.40	61.25	36.10	—	15.9
1966	3.50	61.75	39.30	—	16.6
1971	4.93	68.75	54.75	—	31.7
1976	8.13	87.75	90.50	—	62.4
1981	13.49	152.00	139.50	136.50	94.0
1985	12.10	143.25	128.75	124.50	84.8
1989	11.10	132.00	120.25	116.25	79.0

[1]*1989 Dairy Producer Highlights*, National Milk Producers Federation, p. 32.

[2]Price established as of April of the respective year.

Table M-57 shows how the dairy products purchased by the CCC were utilized in 1987 and 1988. All of the butter and cheese purchased by the CCC were used for domestic distribution. However, substantial quantities of the nonfat dry milk purchased by the CCC were shipped for foreign distribution. Foreign utilization of nonfat dry milk constituted 41 and 30% of the CCC dairy products for the years 1987 and 1988, respectively.

TABLE M–57
UTILIZATION OF CCC DAIRY PRODUCTS[1]

	Butter				Cheese				Nonfat Dry Milk			
	1987		1988		1987		1988		1987		1988	
	←					(million)						→
	(lb)	*(kg)*	(lb)	*(kg)*	(lb)	*(kg)*	(lb)	*(kg)*	(lb)	*(kg)*	(lb)	*(kg)*
Domestic:												
Commercial domestic sales	0.1	*0.05*	0.1	*0.05*	21.9	*10.0*	0.3	*0.1*	71.9	*32.8*	1.1	*0.5*
Transfers ..	35.7	*16.2*	44.8	*20.4*	19.3	*8.8*	27.4	*12.5*	392.1	*178.3*	135.5	*61.6*
Domestic donations	165.7	*75.3*	182.5	*83.0*	639.6	*290.7*	340.8	*154.9*	149.0	*67.8*	103.2	*46.9*
Total domestic	201.5	*91.55*	227.4	*103.45*	680.8	*309.5*	368.5	*167.5*	613.0	*278.9*	239.8	*109.0*
Foreign:												
Donations Title II, PL-480 Section 416	49.6	*22.5*	0.0	*0.0*	16.7	*7.6*	0.0	*0.0*	422.6	*192.1*	102.2	*46.5*
Total	251.1	*114.05*	227.4	*103.45*	697.5	*317.1*	368.5	*167.5*	1,035.6	*471.0*	342.0	*155.5*

[1]*1989 Dairy Producer Highlights*, National Milk Producers Federation, p. 34.

• **Storage of CCC-owned dairy commodities**—On September 30, 1989, the Commodity Credit Corporation reported that, as of that date,—

1. The CCC inventories consisted of approximately 407.6 million pounds (*185.3 mil kg*) of butter, 48.9 million pounds (*22.2 mil kg*) of cheese, and 32 million pounds (*14.5 mil kg*) of nonfat dry milk.
2. Nearly three-fourths of the dairy products in storage were less than 1 year old.
3. The Government's value for the above inventory was over $658 million.
4. Relatively small quantities of these products are lost due to spoilage while in storage, although some loss in quality or product deterioration can occur.
5. Only the nonfat dry milk is sold on a restricted basis (not to be used for human consumption).

Federal Milk Marketing Orders. Federal Milk Marketing Orders are established and administered by the Secretary of Agriculture under acts of Congress passed in 1933 and 1937. They are legal instruments, and they are very complex. However, stated in simple terms, they are designed to stabilize the marketing of fluid milk and to assist farmers in negotiating with distrib-

utors for the sale of their milk.

Federal Milk Orders (1) regulate only Grade A farm milk prices—they do not regulate Grade B milk prices, and (2) establish minimum, not maximum, farm milk prices. Prices paid to farmers are controlled, but there is no direct control of retail prices.

Federal orders are not concerned with sanitary regulations. These are administered by state and local health authorities.

In 1988, there were 42 different federal milk market orders, each with a market administrator and provision for setting minimum farm prices and regulating transactions between farmers and milk dealers in their area.

Milk handlers are the only entities actually regulated under a Federal Milk Order. Handlers include fluid milk processors who distribute milk to consumers and retailers, and also persons who sell milk to other milk dealers for fluid distribution. (Handlers may be individuals, partnerships, corporations, or cooperatives.) In 1988, there were 796 handlers.

Prices in other Grade A markets are influenced by prices established under federal orders or state control programs. Additionally, dairy support programs directly affect the prices of both manufacturing grade milk marketed by farmers and the milk farmers sell as farm-separated cream.

Table M-58 shows the scope of the federal milk marketing order program from 1960 to 1988. It is noteworthy that, in 1988, slightly more than two-thirds of all milk marketed in the country and almost 80% of the Grade A milk were covered by federal orders. Gross value of this milk was $12 billion.

TABLE M–58
SCOPE OF FEDERAL MILK MARKET ORDER PROGRAM[1]

Year	Milk Sold to Plants and Dealers				Receipts Federal Order Markets			Class 1 Sales in Federal Order Markets			Price per 100 Lb 3.5% Milk		Number of Federal Order Markets[2]
	Total		Fluid Use		Quantity		Milk Sold to Plants and Dealers	Quantity		U.S. Total Fluid Use	Class 1	Blend	
	(billion)						(%)	(billion)		(%)	($)	($)	
	(lb)	(kg)	(lb)	(kg)	(lb)	(kg)		(lb)	(kg)				
1960	103.9	47.1	50.9	23.1	44.8	20.3	43.1	28.8	13.1	56.6	4.88	4.47	80
1970	111.0	49.9	50.3	22.8	65.1	29.5	59.6	40.1	18.2	79.7	6.74	5.95	62
1980	124.5	56.6	50.9	23.1	84.0	38.1	67.5	41.0	18.6	80.6	13.77	12.86	47
1988	142.1	64.6	54.5	24.8	100.1	45.5	70.4	43.1	19.6	79.1	13.42	12.14	42

[1] *1989 Dairy Producer Highlights,* National Milk Producers Federation, p. 20.
[2] At end of year.

Methods of Pricing and Paying for Milk. Economists refer to the different systems of paying for milk as *price plans.* These plans, which in actual practice generally involve two or more plants—for example, pricing based on (1) class, (2) grade, and (3) base surplus—are:

1. **Flat price plan.** This was the common method up to World War I. The milk producer was paid a uniform price for all milk sold, regardless of quality or the use made of it.

2. **Use classification plan.** Most marketing orders established two use classes—Class I and Class II.

Class I milk generally includes milk used in fluid form such as whole fluid milk, or milk for creamed drinks which must be made from milk approved by local health authorities. Generally speaking, Class I prices are 10 to 15% higher than Class II prices.

Class II milk usually includes milk in excess of fluid needs, which is used to make manufactured dairy products—primarily butter, nonfat dry milk, and cheese.

On some markets, a further division is made, primarily for milk going into cottage cheese, with the result that there are three classes of milk—Class I, Class II, and Class III.

3. **Blend prices.** When dealers buy according to classification prices, they may pay producers a blend price. The blend is an average of class prices weighted by the volume of milk in each class, usually quoted at a specific point and for a specific test of milk.

4. **Quality grade plan.** Frequently, the terms Grade A and Grade B (Grade B is usually called *Manufacturing Grade Milk*) are encountered in milk marketing. Although there may be some local variations in their use, Grade A usually refers to milk produced under conditions which make it acceptable for fluid use in a given market. Grade B often refers to milk produced under conditions which do not make it acceptable for fluid milk use—it is manufacturing milk.

The production of Grade A milk relative to that of Grade B milk has been increasing in recent years. In 1987, U.S. farmers marketed 139,058 million pounds of milk, of which 123,768 million pounds, or 89%, was Grade A, and 15,290 million pounds, or 11%, was Grade B.

5. **Base surplus plan.** The base surplus plan (or base rating plant) is designed to encourage that a uniform supply of milk be available. It compensates the producers who maintain a high fall production, when more milk is needed. The base period is established during the lowest production months, usually over a period of 3 to 6 months. Then, a producer's base is established by the average amount of milk delivered during the base period. The producer's base may be modified from time to time.

6. **Butterfat test price plan.** The butterfat test of milk affects the price. The common practice is to establish a price for 100 lb of milk of a specified butterfat test. Usually 3.5% butterfat is the basis for pricing, although several markets have established their base as high as 4% butterfat. Then, a price differential (per point or 0.1%) is set up for milk testing above or below this amount.

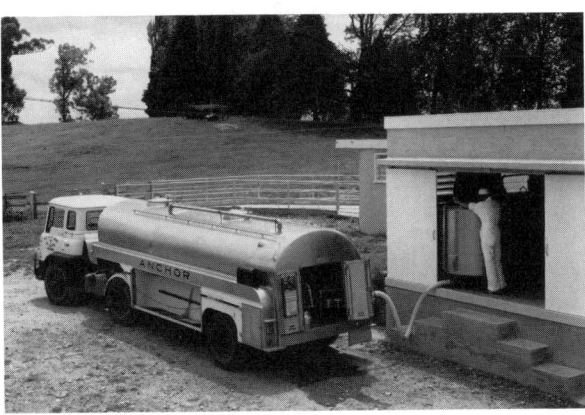

Fig. M-107 b. Transferring milk from a cooled bulk tank in the milk room to a cooled bulk tank truck for transporting to the processing plant.

supplies milk to a distributor on a per gallon or per quart basis. Since average milk weighs 2.15 lb to the quart and 8.6 lb to the gallon, 100 lb of milk would be equivalent to 46.5 qt or 11.6 gal. Thus, one can easily compute the possible returns from selling milk by different methods.

10. **Special milks.** Certain milks are sold under special labels. Among them are:

a. **Certified milk.** This is milk that is produced under special sanitary conditions prescribed by the American Association of Medical Commissioners. It is sold at a higher price than ordinary milk.

b. **Golden Guernsey milk.** Golden Guernsey milk is produced by owners of purebred Guernsey herds who comply with the regulations of the American Guernsey Cattle Association. Such milk is sold under the trade name *Golden Guernsey,* at a premium price.

c. **All-Jersey milk.** This is produced by registered Jersey herds whose owners comply with the regulations of the American Jersey Cattle Club. It is sold at a premium price under the trademark *All Jersey.*

7. **Solids-not-fat price plan.** Today, the emphasis on the food value of milk is shifting from fat content to the other solids, especially protein. This is feasible because tests for solids-not-fat have been devised, and these are proving practical for field use. It is anticipated that this system of pricing milk will expand in the future.

On the average, whole milk contains about 2¼ lb of solids-not-fat for each pound of milk fat. Thus, milk testing 4% butterfat contains approximately 9 lb of solids-not-fat, to a total of 13 lb of solids per hundredweight.

8. **Component pricing plans.** Although various component pricing plans being formulated or adopted are not uniform, they continue to give price credit for butterfat in farm milk; in addition, they give credit for solids-not-fat, including protein. Some also involve end product pricing in which farm milk prices are based on the yield and market value of cheese and other dairy products that can be manufactured from the milk. Most also either (a) establish a maximum somatic cell count at which component premiums will be paid, or (b) pay a premium of 6 to 12¢ per hundredweight of milk for minimum somatic cell counts.

On the average, farm milk contains about 3.7% butterfat and 8.55% solids-not-fat, including 3.2% protein. A one point (0.1%) change in milk fat test is normally associated with a 0.4 point (0.04%) change in solids-not-fat. However, considerable variation in this average relationship does occur. Component pricing takes into consideration the value of variations in solids-not-fat as well as fat; thus, its advocates feel that it would correct an inequity to dairy farmers under current butterfat differential pricing.

In 1988, the Federal Milk Marketing Administrator reported that 48% of all federal order milk was eligible for multiple component pricing (MCP), meaning that if the milk meets the minimum component, quality, and/or other requirements established by producers, cooperatives, or plants, payment may be based upon two or more components. If we include the non-federal order milk eligible for MCP, then approximately 60% of U.S. milk production is eligible for MCP. More and more component pricing will be implemented.

9. **Gallon or quart plan.** Occasionally, a producer

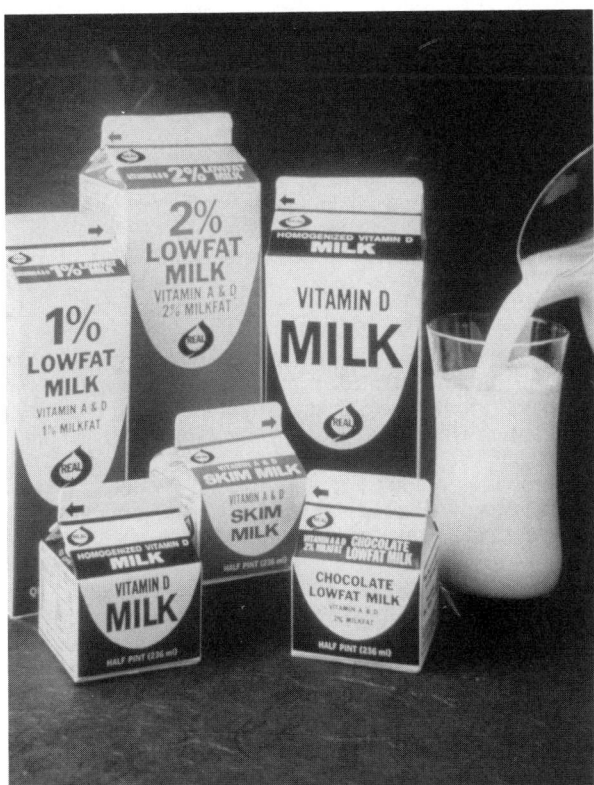

Fig. M-107 c. Choice of milks. (Courtesy, American Dairy Assn., Rosemont, Ill.)

State Milk Controls. Several of the states have milk control programs that also include some authority over milk prices.

In setting minimum farm prices, state control agencies often operate in a manner similar to Federal Milk Orders. They price only Grade A milk. State orders price milk only within the particular state whereas Federal Orders can cover several states. Federal Milk Orders establish only farm milk prices, while State Orders establish prices at various stages along the way—farm, wholesale, retail, as well as regulating trade practices.

Some states set maximum prices at either wholesale or retail, or at both levels. Others set both minimum and maximum wholesale and retail milk prices. Still others require a minimum markup by retailers, while others require that milk prices be reported to the state. Most states specify Class I prices in their Orders.

All state control agencies have authority to require distributors to be licensed and to inspect and investigate operations of milk dealers and audit their records.

Among the unfair trade practices prohibited or controlled by the State Orders are: (1) free service or equipment; (2) discounts or rebates to some, but not all; (3) sales below cost; and (4) price discrimination.

Also state programs generally include advertising, merchandizing, research, and education. A few states appropriate funds for promotion, but most assess producers for most or all of their operational costs.

Cooperatives.
An individual dairyman has little influence on the price for which his product is to be sold. Thus, cooperatives developed. These are organizations run by members who pool their resources as collective bargaining groups. These cooperative associations are of two general types:

1. Bargaining associations which do not handle any milk, but make all business arrangements.
2. Associations which process and distribute milk or assemble it for fluid use.

Today, more than 75% of the total deliveries of milk to plants and dealers in the United States is handled by cooperatives.

In the last decade, a large number of small cooperatives have merged together to form regional organizations that offer a more powerful position for bargaining and more efficient use of marketing channels.

Cooperatives allow the dairyman of a given area to integrate the various aspects of marketing. Procurement, assembling, marketing, and routing of milk are all handled by the cooperative. Thus, the member of a cooperative is assured of a market for his milk.

Other Regulatory Programs.
Because of the essential nature of milk, plus the fact that it is easily contaminated and a favorable medium for bacterial growth, it is inevitable that numerous regulatory programs have evolved around it—federal, state, and local—some having been designed to control prices and assure a reasonably uniform flow of milk, and others for sanitary reasons.

SANITARY REGULATIONS.
The sanitation of milk and dairy products is assured by the enforcement of sanitary regulations by federal, state, and local authorities.

All major cities and states have sanitary regulations governing the production, transportation, processing, and delivery of milk. Unfortunately, from area to area, there are a bewildering number of different regulations, with the result that milk going to more than one city market is often subjected to duplication and confusion in inspection. Also, sanitary and health regulations have sometimes been used as barriers to keep milk out of a certain area for competitive reasons.

In 1923, the U.S. Public Health Service (USPHS) established an Office of Milk Investigations; and, in 1924, the USPHS published its first Grade A pasteurized milk ordinance. Subsequently, this regulation has been revised several times.

Producers are issued permits allowing them to ship Grade A milk. The permit is revoked if either the bacteria count of raw milk exceeds 100,000 per milliliter or the cooling temperature exceeds 40°F in three of the last five samples.

The standard plate count of Grade A pasteurized milk may not exceed 20,000 per milliliter nor the coliform count 10 per milliliter in three of the last five samples or the processor's permit will be revoked.

A sample must be taken from each bulk tank at each farm every time the milk is collected.

The Food and Drug Administration (FDA) is charged with inspecting dairy products and processing plants for contamination and adulteration.

STANDARDS AND GRADES.
Milk standards are established on the state and local levels and are patterned after the Pasteurized Milk Ordinance (PMO) formulated by the Food and Drug Administration (FDA). Essentially, the PMO is a set of recommendations for voluntary adoption by state and local regulatory agencies. Legal responsibility for the provision of quality milk rests mostly with state and local governments whose requirements are in some instances more stringent than the guidelines of the PMO.

The common grades are Grade A, manufacturing grade, or reject. In some areas, Grades A, B, and C are used.

Details relative to *Grade A Milk* and *Manufacture Grade Milk* follow, with a separate section devoted to each. For more specific regulations concerning the grading of milk in any particular area, the reader is advised to contact his local dairy extension agent.

Grade A Milk.
Grade A milk is milk that meets certain quality standards and is produced, processed, and handled in a stipulated manner in approved facilities and equipment.

Grade A milk is produced and processed in accordance with the quality standards of the Pasteurized Milk Ordinance (PMO) formulated (and revised from time to time) by the Food and Drug Administration (FDA) for voluntary adoption by state and local milk regulatory agencies and the dairy industry. Federal specifications for the procurement of Grade A milk and milk products are based on the PMO, as are sanitary regulations for Grade A milk and milk products entering interstate commerce.

The Pasteurized Milk Ordinance is a very effective instrument for protecting milk quality. Strict compliance therewith is imposed so that the milk will be of high uniform quality. The sanitary dairy practices outlined by the PMO include:

1. Inspection and sanitary control of farms and milk plants.
2. Examination and testing of herds for the elimination of bovine diseases related to public health.

3. Regular instruction on desirable sanitary practices for persons engaged in production, processing, and distribution of milk.

4. Proper pasteurizatin or ultrapasteurization of milk.

5. Laboratory examination of milk.

6. Monitoring of milk supplies by federal, state, and local health officials to protect against unintentional chemical, physical, and microbiological adulterants.

Most rigid control is placed on the production and processing of Grade A market milk which is sold to consumers in its fluid state. Grade A pasteurized milk is obtained from dairy farms that conform with the sanitary requirements of the PMO or its equivalent as enforced by state or local authorities. The milk must be obtained from cows tested and found free of disease and disease-producing organisms. The raw milk is cooled immediately to the specified legal temperature and maintained at no higher temperature from the completion of milking until processing at a dairy plant that also conforms with state and local sanitation requirements.

At the processing plant, the milk is analyzed to be sure it contains not more than a specified bacterial count and is pasteurized according to the specified time-temperature relationships. Public health authorities advocate pasteurization since it is the only practical commercial process that destroys all disease-producing organisms that may be present in fluid milk. After processing, the milk is cooled again to the specified legal temperature and maintained at no higher temperature until sold. Today, practically all fluid market milk sold to consumers is Grade A pasteurized milk.

In order to become a producer of Grade A milk, the milking and milk storage facilities of the dairy must first pass the careful inspection of the state inspector. If approved by the inspector, the dairy is granted a permit for the shipment of Grade A Milk. Once a permit is issued, the dairy operation is periodically inspected by a local health department official to ensure that adequate sanitation practices are maintained. The permit may be revoked if the bacteria count is too high, if the cooling temperature exceeds 40°F, and/or if the producer is found in repeated violation of other requirements of the ordinance.

Manufacture Grade Milk. As with Grade A Milk, each state adopts and enforces its own regulations for the production, processing, and handling of Manufacture Grade Milk, which is produced for, and processed into, ice cream, cheeses, etc. There is much less uniformity in the regulations governing Manufacture Grade Milk than in Grade A Milk, and the standards are not so high (although the trend is higher and more rigid).

Dairy farms producing Manufacture Grade Milk must also conform to the sanitary requirements of state and local authorities, and the milk must come from cows tested and found free of disease and disease-producing organisms.

Processing plants manufacturing dairy products are subjected to general sanitation requirements similar to those for plants processing Grade A Milk. Additionally, there are supplemental and specific requirements for plants that process dry milk products, butter, cheeses, and evaporated, condensed, or sterilized milk products.

Market Distribution of Fluid Milk. Once milk is processed, it must be marketed rather rapidly because of its highly perishable nature. When a consumer has a bad experience with milk, it is difficult to get him or her back into the habit of drinking milk. Hence, it is imperative that fluid milk be of high quality and possess desirable taste and packaging.

Milk is distributed in a number of ways: (1) home delivery, (2) retail stores, and (3) vending machines and self-service. Table M-59 portrays the changes in fluid milk sales since 1970 in distribution methods. As shown, the distribution of fluid milk through wholesale channels increased, while home delivery decreased.

TABLE M–59
PERCENT OF FLUID MILK
SOLD BY DISTRIBUTION METHOD
(FEDERAL ORDER MARKETS)[1]

	1970	1975	1980	1985	1990
Number of markets[2]	—	56	47	44	42
	←		(%)		→
Distribution method:					
Wholesale	83	93	97	99	99
Home Delivered ...	17	7	3	1	1
Total	100	100	100	100	100

[1]*1991 Milk Facts*, Milk Industry Foundation, p. 19.

[2]Markets for which complete data were available include the New York-New Jersey market, starting in 1969.

HOME DELIVERY. Throughout the first half of the 20th century, home delivery was the primary means of distributing milk. In fact, home delivery constituted one-fourth of all milk distributed from federal milk orders as late as 1966. However, in recent years retail sales have shifted from home delivery to retail stores. In 1990, only 1% of U.S. milk was home delivered.

RETAIL STORES. Today, the vast majority of milk is sold in retail stores. This is largely due to (1) the increased mobility of the public through the use of cars; (2) new technology in processing that increases the storage life of milk; (3) the widespread use of efficient refrigerators; (4) the increase in the methods of packaging milk (plastic and paper containers); (5) the increase in the number of supermarkets that offer low-priced milk; (6) the sales of milk by the retailer through the use of dairy industry personnel rather than wholesale middlemen; and (7) increased costs involved with home deliveries.

Many stores today offer only milk brands that are processed by their own plants. Through this sales practice, the stores are able to reduce marketing costs, gain a better control of inventory, and predict sales volume more closely.

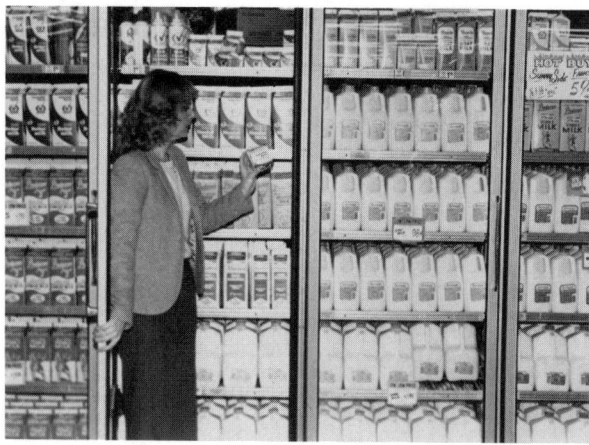

Fig. M-108. Milk and milk products in a modern retail store. (Photo by A. H. Ensminger)

Other retail stores sell their own brand of milk at a lower price than the regional or national brands, but continue to offer the competitive brands so as to provide customers a wider choice. Through the use of private brands, the store has considerably more control over pricing and merchandising than with outside brands.

A third type of retail outlet is the milk store operated by a large dairy, integrated from production through processing and marketing. As dairy operations become larger and more integrated in the future, the number of these specialty markets will likely increase.

VENDING AND SELF-SERVICE MACHINES. In areas where people congregate, vending machines containing milk can be effectively utilized. Little labor is involved, and the customer has ready access to the product.

Dairy Imports and Exports. In order to protect the dairy industry from depressed prices caused by other countries dumping dairy products onto American markets, import quotas have been established. A number of dairy products, including several types of cheeses, butter, malted milk, butter oil, and dried milk are covered by specific import quotas. Although not formally restricted, certain other dairy products may be limited by agreement between the United States and the exporting country. Total imports on a milk equivalent basis have been very small. In 1988, imports of dairy products amounted to 2.4 million pounds (*1.1 mil kg*) (see Table M-60) when total milk production was more than 148 billion pounds (*67 bil kg*). Hence, imports of dairy products were equivalent to only 0.002% of the total U.S. market milk

As long as domestic prices are above world prices and world supplies are ample, exporting countries will look to the United States as a possible market. The four countries exporting the largest amount of dairy products are Italy, New Zealand, Denmark, and The Netherlands. As a result, import pressure will persist; yet, it is expected that imports of many commodities will continue to be limited by quotas.

TABLE M-60
SUMMARY OF DAIRY PRODUCT IMPORTS FOR SELECTED YEARS[1]

Year	Imports		Cheese Imports			Imports Other than Cheese		
	Total Imports	Total Import Quotas	Total	Within Quota	Outside Quota	Total	Within Quota	Outside Quota
	(thousand metric tons)							
1984	1,233	1,005	1,095	878	217	138	138	0
1985	1,250	1,005	1,079	856	222	171	171	0
1986	1,230	1,005	1,059	845	214	162	162	0
1987	1,121	1,005	945	731	214	176	176	0
1988	1,077	1,005	900	702	198	NA	NA	0

[1]*1989 Dairy Producer Highlights*, National Milk Producers Federation, p. 38.

As with imports, exports of dairy products by the United States are rather small. They fluctuate from year to year, but never amount to more than about 1% of the total milk supply. Table M-61 shows the exports of dairy products in 1988, 1989, and 1990.

TABLE M–61
EXPORTS OF DAIRY PRODUCTS[1]

Product	1988	1989	1990
	← (metric tons) →		
Butter	6,804	27,142	52,449
Cheese	13,602	10,111	11,885
Evaporated milk ...	1,010	11,323	1,180
Condensed milk ...	2,467	2,455	2,753
Dry whole milk	8,394	39,976	5,113
Nonfat dry milk	218,356	117,120	7,722

[1]*Agricultural Statistics 1991*, USDA, p. 334, Table 497.

In recent years, exports of butter, condensed milk, dried milk, and evaporated milk have exceeded imports, whereas imports of casein and cheese have exceeded exports.

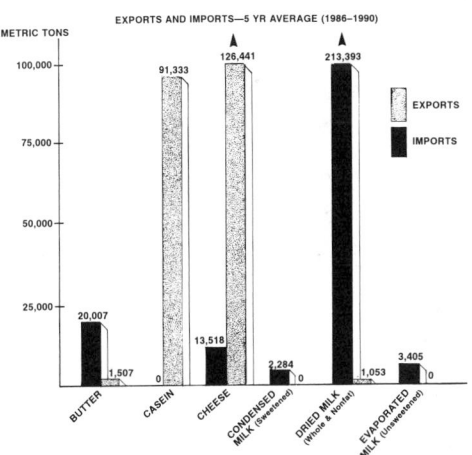

Fig. M-109. Dairy exports and imports, 5-year average (1986–1990.) (From *Agricultural Statistics*, 1991, USDA, pp. 329 and 334, Tables 492 and 497)

Exports of dairy products will continue to be influenced by the availability of surplus products, the demand for dairy products abroad, and foreign policy. A more active role in meeting food deficiencies in the less developed countries of the world could increase total demand for dairy products and demand for export products.

•**Public Law 480**—The United States established a program called "Food for Peace" with the passage of the Agricultural Trade Development and Assistance Act of 1954 (Public Law 480). Title I sales of dairy products involve the tailoring of purchase agreements with other countries; and Title II donations provide a mechanism for distributing free food to help improve the nutrition of the people in developing countries.

MILK FACTS. Some pertinent milk facts are contained in the sections that follow.

Per Capita Consumption of Milk and Milk Products. Milk is an important constituent of the American diet in terms of per capita consumption (Table M-62).

In 1990, the total milk equivalent consumption of all dairy products was 570.6 lb (*259.4 kg*), a 13% decline from 1960. But the growth in human population offset per capita decline, with the result that total consumption increased. From Table M-62, several trends are apparent: Americans have become weight conscious in recent years leading to a decreased per capita consumption of fluid whole milk and cream and an increased per capita consumption of low-fat milk. Per capita fluid whole milk consumption declined 67% from the period of 1960 to 1990, while per capita low-fat milk consumption increased 313%. Of the manufactured dairy products, per capita consumption of butter declined 41%, and evaporated milk 42%, in the period 1960 to 1990. Per capita total cheese consumption increased 34% in this same period. Per capita consumption of ice cream declined due to the increased popularity of frozen yogurt.

TABLE M–62
DAIRY PRODUCTS: U.S. PER CAPITA CIVILIAN CONSUMPTION,

	Fluid Milk Products										Manufactured					
Year	Fluid Whole Milk		Cream		Low-fat Milk		Total Product		Whole Milk Equiv. of Butterfat		Butter		Total Cheese		Cottage Cheese	
	(lb)	(kg)	(lb)	(kg)	(lb)	(kg)	(lb)	(kg)	(lb)	(kg)	(lb)	(kg)	(lb)	(kg)	(lb)	(kg)
1960	276	125	9.1	4.1	23.8	10.8	309	140	309	140	7.5	3.4	8.3	3.8	4.8	2.2
1965	264	120	7.6	3.4	34.0	15.4	306	139	294	133	6.4	2.9	9.6	4.4	4.7	2.1
1970	229	104	5.6	2.5	57.5	26.1	292	132	260	118	5.3	2.4	11.5	5.2	5.1	2.3
1975	195	88	5.9	2.7	84.7	38.4	286	130	244	111	4.8	2.2	14.5	6.6	4.7	2.1
1980	148	67	5.7	2.6	97.8	44.5	251	114	231	105	4.1	1.9	17.1	7.8	4.6	2.1
1985	120	55	6.0	2.7	107.0	48.6	239	109	186	85	4.9	2.2	22.6	10.3	4.1	1.9
1988	100	45	6.0	2.7	132.0	60.0	238	108	184	84	4.4	2.0	23.6	10.7	3.8	1.7

[1]*1989 Dairy Producer Highlights*, National Milk Producers Federation, p. 17.

Milk a Good Buy. Although the per capita consumption of milk has declined in recent years (see Fig. M-110), it still remains one of the best food buys. In fact, the real price of milk as shown by minutes of work required to buy ½ gal of milk has been declining (see Table M-63). In 1950, it took the average worker 15.8 minutes to earn enough money to buy ½ gal (*1.9 liter*) of milk. In 1990, this figure was only 7.9 minutes.

TABLE M–63
THE REAL PRICE OF MILK[1]

Year	Average Hourly Wages of Production Workers	Average Retail Price of ½ Gal of Milk[2]	Minutes of Work Required to Buy ½ Gal of Milk
	($)	($)	(minutes)
1950		0.39	15.8
1955		0.44	13.8
1960	2.03[3]	0.49	12.8
1965	2.57	0.47	10.9
1970	3.64	0.57	10.3
1975	5.21	0.79	9.8
1980	6.66	1.05	8.7
1985	8.57	1.13	7.1
1990	9.66	1.27	7.9

[1]*1981 Milk Facts*, Milk Industry Foundation, pp. 5 and 7; and *Statistical Abstract of the United States 1991*, Dept. of Commerce, p. 488, Table 785.

[2]*1981 Dairy Producer Highlights*, National Milk Producers Federation, p. 23.

[3]*1981 Milk Facts*, p. 5, 1958 data.

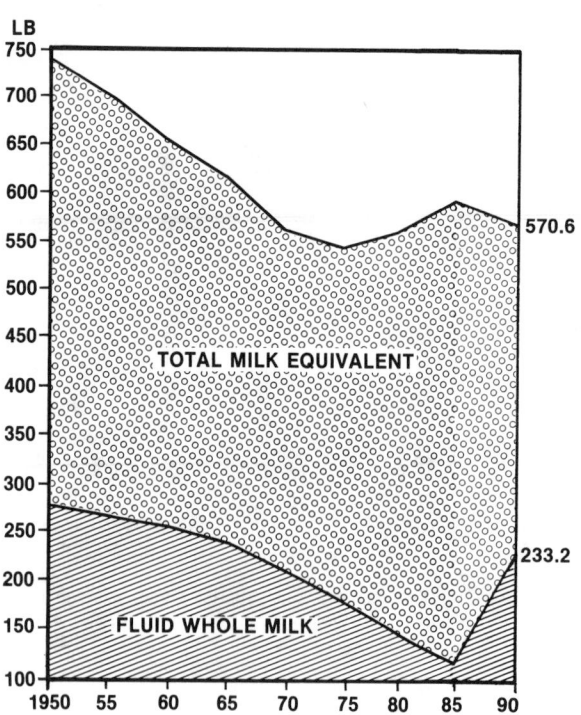

PER CAPITA CONSUMPTION OF MILK IN THE U.S.

Fig. M-110. Per capita consumption of milk in the U.S.A.

SELECTED YEARS 1960–88[1]

Milk Products

Ice Cream		Evap. & Cond. Milk		Nonfat Dry Milk		Yogurt		All Milk Equiv- alent	
(lb)	(kg)	(lb)	(kg)	(lb)	(kg)	(lb)	(kg)	(lb)	(kg)
18.3	8.3	13.7	6.2	6.2	2.8	0.3	0.1	653	296
18.5	8.4	10.7	4.9	5.6	2.5	0.3	0.1	620	281
17.7	8.0	7.1	3.2	5.4	2.4	0.9	0.4	561	254
18.6	8.4	5.3	2.4	3.3	1.5	2.1	1.0	546	248
17.6	8.0	7.2	3.3	3.0	1.3	2.5	1.1	554	252
18.0	8.2	7.9	3.6	2.2	1.0	4.1	1.9	593	270
17.8	8.1	7.9	3.6	2.7	1.2	4.7	2.1	585	266

Care Of Milk In The Home.[34]   The consumer also has responsibility for protecting the quality of milk. Proper handling of dairy products and open dating are designed to assure consumers of dairy products with a good shelf life, which is the length of time after processing that the product will retain its quality.

Open dating is the sometimes mandatory, often voluntary, inclusion of a date on milk containers to indicate when they should be withdrawn from retail sale. It is used by industry to reflect the age of individual packages. It does not indicate the shelf life of products. Generally, depending upon storage conditions and care in the home, a product will remain fresh and usable for a few days beyond this "pull date," or "sell-by-date." Regulation of open dating varies among states and municipalities.

Dairy products are highly perishable, therefore, it is recommended that consumers observe the following practices to preserve quality:

1.   Use proper containers to protect milk from exposure to sunlight, bright daylight, and strong fluorescent light to prevent the development of off-flavor and a reduction in riboflavin, ascorbic acid, and vitamin B-6 content.
2.   Store milk at refrigerated temperatures 44.6°F (7°C) or below as soon as possible after purchase.
3.   Keep milk containers closed to prevent absorption of other food flavors in the refrigerator. An absorbed flavor alters the taste, but the milk is still safe.
4.   Use milk in the order purchased.
5.   Serve milk cold.
6.   Return milk container to the refrigerator immediately to prevent bacterial growth. Temperatures

above 44.6°F (7°C) for fluid and cultured milk products for even a few minutes reduces shelf life. Never return unused milk to the original container.
7.   Keep canned milk in a cool, dry place. Once opened it should be transferred to a clean opaque container and refrigerated.
8.   Store dry milk in a cool, dry place and reseal the container after opening. Humidity causes dry milk to lump and may affect flavor and color changes. If such changes occur, the milk should not be consumed. Once reconstituted, dry milk should be treated like any other fluid milk: covered and stored in the refrigerator.

Guidelines on the storage life of various milk products at specific temperatures are shown in Table M-64. In this table, storage life refers to the approximate length of time after processing, not after purchasing, that the product will retain its quality.

TABLE M-64
APPROXIMATE STORAGE LIFE OF
MILK PRODUCTS AT SPECIFIC TEMPERATURES
(Storage life refers to the length of time after processing—not after purchasing— that the product will retain its quality.)

Product	Approximate Storage Life at Specific Temperatures	(°F)	(°C)
Fresh fluid milk (whole, lowfat, skim, chocolate, and unfermented acidophilus............	8 to 20 days below	39.2	4
Sterilized whole milk ..	4 months at	69.8	21
	12 months at	39.2	4
Frozen whole milk	12 months at	-2.2	-23
Evaporated milk	1 month at	89.6	32
	12 to 24 months at	69.8	21
	24 months at	39.2	4
Concentrated milk	2 or more weeks at	34.7	1.5
Concentrated frozen milk.	6 months at	-6.8	-26
Sweetened condensed milk	3 months at	89.6	32
	9 to 24 months at	69.8	21
	15 months at	39.2	4
Nonfat dry milk, extra grade.................. (in moisture-proof pack)	6 months at	89.6	32
	16 to 24 months at	69.8	21
	24 months at	39.2	4
Dry whole milk, extra grade.................. (gas pack: maximum oxygen 2%)	6 months at	89.6	32
	12 months at	69.8	21
	24 months at	39.2	4
Buttermilk	2 to 3 weeks at	39.2	4
Sour cream	3 to 4 weeks at	39.2	4
Yogurt	3 to 6 weeks at	39.2	4
Eggnog.................	1 to 2 weeks at	39.2	4
Ultrapasteurized cream ..	6 to 8 weeks at	39.2	4

[34]This section and Table M-64 were adapted by the authors from *Newer Knowledge of Milk and Other Fluid Dairy Products,* National Dairy Council, Rosemont, Ill.)

Three to five days may elapse between processing and purchasing, so the shelf life from the point of purchasing would be correspondingly less.

Various dairy products such as fluid and concentrated milk may be preserved by freezing. Milk has a lower freezing point than water due to dissolved constituents such as lactose and salts. The average freezing point of milk is 31°F (*-0.54°C*).

A very low temperature is needed to freeze milk completely. About 75% of the milk will freeze at 14°F (*-10°C*). A temperature below 7.6°F (*-18°C*) is recommended for frozen storage.

Milk can be frozen and thawed in the refrigerator; however, it is not recommended. The quality of milk is impaired by freezing due to protein destabilization and settling of some milk solids. A watery wheylike liquid may collect on the top and curd particles may also appear. Mixing returns the product to its normal dispersion and subsequent separation does not occur. However, thawed milk may be susceptible to the development of an oxidized flavor. The homogenization of milk overcomes the problem of demulsification of fat, a result of freezing milk.

Cream can be frozen, as evidenced by the successful use of frozen cream by the ice cream industry for several decades. However, particles of fat are evident when frozen cream is thawed. Homogenization of high-fat products such as cream has little effect in preventing demulsification of fat which occurs during freezing. The addition of sugar and very rapid freezing tend to retard the fat coalescence. Generally, the home freezing of cream produces an unsatisfactory product. Similarly, sour cream does not freeze well, although some dishes prepared with sour cream can be frozen without adverse effects.

Freezing buttermilk is not advocated due to the separation of the watery portion from the solids. If inadvertently frozen, buttermilk can be thawed in the refrigerator, gently mixed and used in cooked products.

Freezing *per se* of milk, cream, and other dairy products does not influence their nutritional properties. However, ascorbic acid and thiamin levels in dairy products may decrease during frozen storage.

OUTLOOK. Per capita consumption of milk and most dairy products appears to have reached a somewhat stable stage. The most important factors affecting the future demand for dairy products will continue to be changes in population, income, consumer preferences, and new products.

It is expected that per capita consumption of various dairy products will follow the trend of recent years; products high in fat will decline in per capita consumption, while those low in fat will increase. The proportion of milk consumed in fluid form will decrease; per capita consumption of butter and evaporated milk will likely decline still further; and low-fat fluid milk, cheese, ice cream and similar frozen desserts, cultured milk products (yogurt, cultured buttermilk, cultured sour cream, and acidophilus milk), and caseinates will likely increase in per capita consumption.

Without doubt, new low-fat dairy products and non-dairy substitutes will replace some of the consumption of similar products higher in fat; and the use of man-made milk will increase.

The trend toward a single grade of milk—Grade A—will continue; and the standards for Grade B will continue to be raised, so that they approach Grade A.

The dairy farm handling of manufacturing milk in cans will almost completely disappear, with manufacturing milk handled like fluid milk—in bulk tanks.

MILK CHOCOLATE

Chocolate is made by (1) first roasting and grinding fermented cacao beans (cocoa beans), and (2) then adding cocoa butter (fat), sugar, and various flavors. In 1876, M. D. Peter of Switzerland put milk into chocolate, producing a new flavor and a new product—milk chocolate. Today's milk chocolate contains 15 to 20% milk solids, and is still a favorite. Milk chocolate is lighter in color and milder in taste than regular sweet chocolate.

(Also see COCOA AND CHOCOLATE; and MILK AND MILK PRODUCTS, section headed "Fluid Milk.")

MILK, FERMENTED

Milk is fermented with selected bacteria, which convert some of the milk sugar, lactose, into lactic acid. In selected cases, some alcohol is formed additionally.

(Also see MILK AND MILK PRODUCTS, section headed "Cultured Milk and Other Products.")

MILK FREEZING POINT TEST

This test serves as an indicator of adulteration, especially the addition of water. Most milk samples freeze within the range of 31.01° to 31.05°F (*-0.530° to -0.550°C*). The addition of 1% of water to milk will raise the freezing point slightly more than 0.011°F (*0.006°C*). Thermistor cryoscopes are sensitive to changes in temperature of 0.002°F (*0.001°C*).

MILK, FROZEN OR FRESH FROZEN

This is milk that has been pasteurized, treated with an ultrasonic vibrator at 5 million cycles per second for 5 minutes, then frozen to 10°F (*-12.2°C*). It will keep for a year; when thawed, it is indistinguishable from the original milk.

MILK SHAKE

Milk and a flavored syrup sometimes with added ice cream either shaken up and down with a hand shaker or blended in an electric mixer.

MILK, TURBIDITY TEST

This is a test to distinguish sterilized milk from pasteurized milk. During sterilization, all the albumin is precipitated. So, in the test the filtrate from an ammonium sulfate precipitation should remain clear on heating, indicating that no albumin was present in solution and the milk had therefore been sterilized.

MILLET *Panicum miliaceum*

Millet provides the major part of the diet of millions of poor people living on the poor, dry lands of India, Africa, China, Russia, and elsewhere. Also, millet is now sold in many U.S. health food stores. The forage, and sometimes a small part of the grain, is fed to animals.

ORIGIN AND HISTORY. Although millet has been grown in Asia and North Africa since prehistoric times, little is known of its origin. It probably came from Eastern and Central Asia. Millet was important in Europe during the Middle Ages, before corn and potatoes were known there. But it is of minor importance in Europe today.

WORLD AND U.S. PRODUCTION. The annual production of millet totals 30 million metric tons, grown on some 94 million acres (*38 million hectares*), more than 87% of which is produced in Asia and Africa. India alone produces 39% of the world's millet, followed by China and Nigeria, each produces 13% of the global total.

Millet has never been of major agricultural importance in the United States. It is grown primarily as a substitute or emergency crop in the Great Plains and southeastern states.

THE MILLET PLANT. Millet is a rapid-growing, warm weather cereal grass of the family, *Gramineae*, genus *Panicum* and species *miliaceum*, whose small grains are used primarily for human food. The plant normally grows to 1 to 4 ft (*30 to 122 cm*) tall, although pearl millet may grow to a height of 10 ft (*3.1 m*) or more. The plants have long, narrow-bladed leaves, with variable seed heads. The heads of pearl and foxtail millets are long, compacted and cylindrical. Proso seed is in a loose, open panicle. The finger millet head has several short fingers with seed on each. Except for bulrush millet, all millet seeds remain enclosed in hulls after threshing.

MILLET CULTURE. In much of the world, millet is grown by primitive methods; the crop is cut by hand with sickles and threshed by treading and winnowing.

In the United States, the growing of millet is mechanized. It is seeded by broadcasting or drilling, much like wheat, barley, or oats. In order to lessen shattering

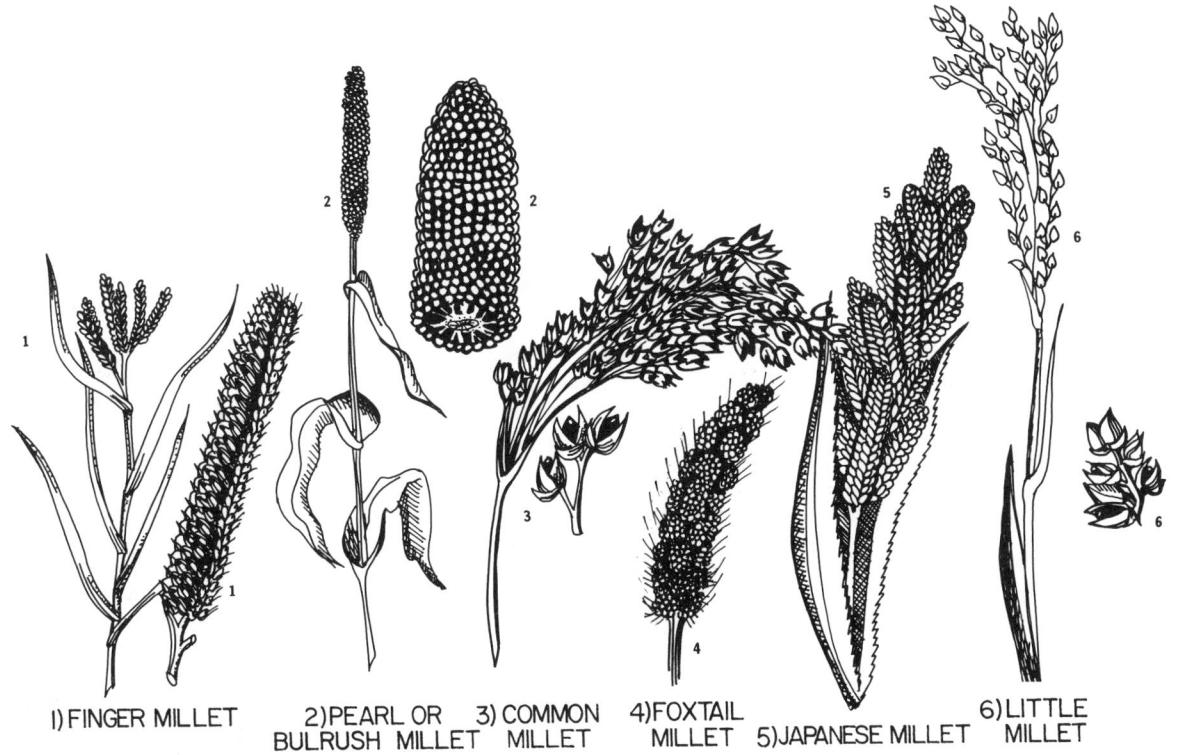

1) FINGER MILLET 2) PEARL OR 3) COMMON 4) FOXTAIL 6) LITTLE
BULRUSH MILLET MILLET MILLET 5) JAPANESE MILLET MILLET

Fig. M-111. Heads of major millet species of the world.

losses, the seed is usually not harvested by direct combining; instead, it is cut, windrowed, allowed to dry, then threshed by a combine equipped with a pickup attachment. When intended for hay, it is harvested much like any other hay crop.

KINDS OF MILLET.

Millets differ widely botanically. The major millet species of the world are:

1. **Common millet** (*Panicum miliaceum*), **also known as Proso, Indian, Broomcorn, and Hog millet.** It has been cultivated since prehistoric times. In Ezekiel 4:9, there is reference to its use for making bread. Today, common millet is widely grown as a food crop for man and livestock in the U.S.S.R., China, Japan, India, Southern Europe, and parts of North America.

2. **Finger millet** (*Eleusine coracana*). It is appropriately named because the ear consists of about five spikes which radiate like fingers, sometimes in a curving manner, from a central point. Finger millet probably originated in India. It is an important food crop of India, Ceylon, and Africa. It has the best storage properties of all the millets.

3. **Foxtail millet** (*Setaria italica*). Foxtail millet originated in Asia. It was a sacred plant in China as early as 2700 B.C., and it was known to the Swiss Lake Dwellers of the stone age. Introduced in the United States in 1849, it is the most common millet species of this country. In the U.S., it is grown for hay, silage, and pasture. In the Soviet Union, it is used for brewing beer. In Britain, it is best known as a bird seed. Throughout the subtropical and warm temperate countries, it is a human food.

4. **Japanese millet** (*Echinochloa frumentacea*). It is widely cultivated in warm regions, for use as food or forage. In Japan and Korea, the grain is ground into meal and made into a porridge. In America, it is primarily a forage crop for animals.

5. **Little millet** (*Panicum miliare*). It is chiefly grown in India. Its main virtues are its capacity to produce a moderate yield on very poor soils and to withstand both drought and water logging better than most crops.

6. **Pearl millet or Bulrush millet** (*Pennisetum typhoideum*). It probably originated in Africa, where it provides a very important food supply. It is also an important food crop in some of the driest areas of India and Pakistan.

Sorghum is not considered a millet, although it is sometimes erroneously referred to as such.

MILLING MILLET.

Little millet is processed commercially. In those parts of Africa and India where millet is the staple diet, the whole grain is stored as such. Then the requirements for flour or meal are prepared daily. In hot climates, the storage of meal is not practiced because of the rapidity with which the undegerminated meal becomes rancid. Most millet is either hand ground with a rubbing stone or in a stone or wooden mortar and pestle, or ground in a small burrstone or hammer mill.

As with other cereal grains, the nutritive value of millet depends on the milling method and refinement. One reason for the higher nutritive value of millet diets than predominantly wheat, rice, or corn diets is that millet products are generally less refined.

NUTRITIONAL VALUE OF MILLET.

Food Composition Table F-36 provides nutritional information regarding millet.

Some salient points concerning the nutritional value of millet follow:

1. Millet is high in starch—about 70%; hence, it serves as an energy food.

2. Like other grains, millet is low or lacking in calcium, vitamins A, D, C, and B-12.

3. The protein content varies greatly among various types, ranging from 5 to 20%, with an average of 10 to 12%. Millet is generally superior to wheat, rice, and corn in protein quality. However, it is low in the essential amino acid lysine; so, when it is used for human food, the quality of the protein should be improved by the inclusion of animal products and fish in the diet. Generally speaking, the higher the protein content of millet, the lower the lysine:protein ratio (mg/g protein) tends to become.

Table M-65 compares the essential amino acid content of millet to that of cow's milk—a high-quality protein—showing that it contains less than one-half of the lysine, phenylalanine, and tyrosine necessary.

(Also see PROTEIN[S].)

TABLE M–65
PROFILE OF ESSENTIAL AMINO ACIDS IN MILLET COMPARED TO COW'S MILK—A HIGH-QUALITY PROTEIN

Amino Acid	Millet	Cow's Milk[1]
	← (mg/g protein) →	
Histidine	19	27
Isoleucine	40	47
Leucine	102	95
Lysine	20	78
Methionine and cystine	25	33
Phenylalanine and tyrosine	49	102
Threonine	36	44
Tryptophan	14	14
Valine	51	64

[1]*Recommended Dietary Allowances*, 10th ed., 1991, National Academy of Sciences, p. 67, Table 6–5.

MILLET PRODUCTS AND USES.

In Asia and Africa, millet is grown as a seed crop for food. In Europe and the United States, it is grown primarily for forage.

Globally, about 85% of the millet crop is used for food. Millions of the poor in India, Africa, China, and parts of the U.S.S.R. depend on millet for 70% or more of their food calories.

Millet grain does not contain any gluten; hence, it is unsuited for making leavened breads. Millet meal and flour are used primarily for making flat breads and griddle-type cakes, and in boiled gruels. Ground millet is used in puddings, steamed meals, and deep-fried doughs, and is mixed with pulses (peas, beans, and lentils), vegetables, milk, cheese, or dates. Whole grains are eaten with soups and stews, or they're popped, roasted, sprouted, or malted. Millet is also consumed in the form of a porridge made from dry parched grain, or cooked with sugar, peanuts, or other foods to make desserts. In the U.S.S.R., the porridge made by cooking dehulled grains, either whole or cracked, is called kaska.

In North America, a limited acreage of millet is produced for forage; and some proso and foxtail millets are grown for grain for stock feed and bird seed. Millet compares favorably with other cereals as livestock and poultry feed, except for horses; neither millet hay nor seed should be fed to horses at high levels over an ex-tended period. The seeds are hard, so they should be ground or crushed for cattle and hogs; but whole seed may be fed to poultry.

Table M-66 presents, in summary form, the use of millet (1) in fortified foods, based on millet, for developing countries, and (2) in fermented beverage.

(Also see CEREAL GRAINS, Table C-18 Cereal Grains of the World; and FLOURS, Table F-26 Special Flours.)

TABLE M-66
MILLET PRODUCTS AND USES

Product	Description	Uses	Comments
FORTIFIED FOOD, BASED ON MILLET, FOR DEVELOPING COUNTRIES			
Aliment de Sevrage	Mixture of millet flour, peanut flour, skim milk powder, sugar, calcium, and vitamins A and D. It contains 20% protein.	High-protein infant food.	Only the Senegal version of this food contains millet. The Algerian version contains wheat.
FERMENTED BEVERAGES			
Millet beers	Brewed beverages made from finger millet, with or without corn (maize) and sorghum.	Alcoholic beverages.	The beers are made by (1) sprouting millet by immersion in a stream, (2) drying and grinding the sprouted grain, (3) preparing a yeasty mixture from part of the sprouted grain by exposure to wild yeasts in the air, or on the surface of the brewing vessel, (4) mixing the freshly prepared yeast with a batch of sprouted grain, and pouring the mixture into gourds where fermentation occurs, (5) diluting the crude beer paste with hot water, and (6) allowing sediment to settle out prior to drinking.

MILLIEQUIVALENT (mEq)

An expression of concentration of a substance per liter of solution calculated by dividing the concentration in mg percent by the molecular weight.

MILLIGRAM

Metric unit of weight equal to 1/1,000 gram.

MINCE

To mince is to chop very finely. Sometimes the food is put through a food grinder to get it as fine as desired.

In England, mince refers to ground beef or hamburger. Therefore, in England, rather than going for a hamburger, you would go for a mince; and the sign would read: "McDonald's Minces."

MINCEMEAT

A special mixture used in pies, coffee cakes, and cookies. It is made with raisins, citron, apple, sugar and spices and usually contains some cooked beef and suet, which has been put through the food chopper along with the apple. The whole mixture is then simmered together. It can be used immediately, packed in sterilized jars, or put in the freezer.

MINERAL(S)

In nutrition, the term *mineral* denotes certain chemical elements which are found in the ash that remains after a food or a body tissue is burned. Some of these elements are essential to the proper functioning of the body—hence, they must be regularly supplied by the diet. Other elements are not known to be essential, yet they may get into the body by various means. The essential minerals are often called "inorganic" nutrients so that they may be distinguished from the "organic" or carbon-containing nutrients such as carbohydrates, fats, proteins, and vitamins.

Each of the essential elements is considered to be either a macromineral or a micromineral, depending upon the quantity which is required in the diet.

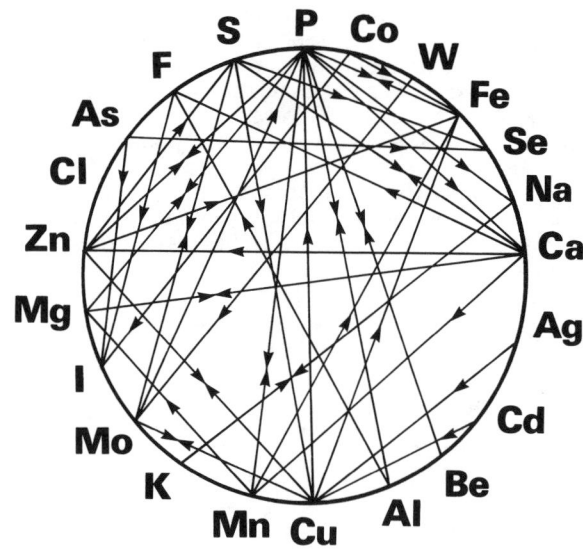

Fig. M-112.   Mineral interaction chart, showing the interrelationship of minerals. The importance of such relationships is evidenced by the following relationships:

1.   A great excess of dietary calcium and/or phosphorus interferes with the absorption of both minerals, and increases the excretion of the lesser mineral.

2.   Excess magnesium upsets calcium metabolism.

3.   Excess zinc interferes with copper metabolism.

4.   Copper is required for the proper utilization of iron, but excess copper can markedly depress iron absorption.

And there are others! The maze of connecting lines in this figure shows the relation of each mineral to other minerals.

• **Macrominerals**—These elements—which include calcium, phosphorus, sodium, chlorine, magnesium, potassium, and sulfur—are required in amounts ranging from a few tenths of a gram to one or more grams per day.

• **Microminerals**—These elements are also known as *trace* elements because they are required in minute quantities, ranging from millionths of a gram (micrograms) to thousandths of a gram (milligram) per day. As of this writing, the trace elements known to be essential for humans are chromium, cobalt, copper, fluorine, iodine, iron, manganese, molybdenum, selenium, silicon, and zinc. It seems likely that arsenic, vanadium, tin, and nickel may soon be added to this list.

Fig. M-113 shows by means of bar graphs the amounts of essential macrominerals and microminerals which are present in the adult body.

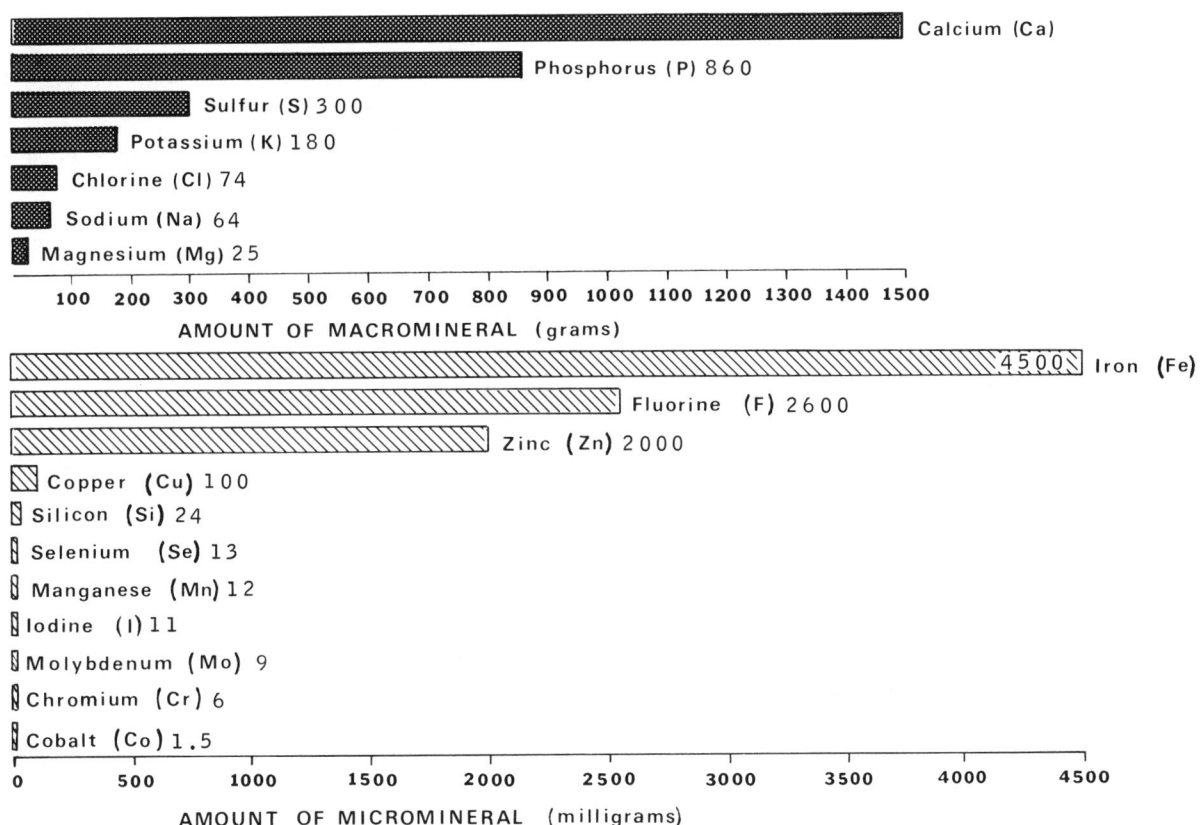

Fig. M-113. Amounts of essential minerals in the adult human body. *Top*: Macrominerals (amounts in grams). *Bottom*: Microminerals (amounts in milligrams). (The data used to construct the graphs are from Scrimshaw, N. S., and V. R. Young, "The Requirements of Human Nutrition," *Scientific American*, Vol. 235, 1976, p. 64.)

HISTORICAL BACKGROUND. It is noteworthy that certain ancient peoples recognized and treated mineral deficiencies, although they did not understand the bases of their treatments. For example, a Chinese document dated about 3000 B.C. described goiter and recommended that the afflicted people eat seaweed and burnt sponge, which are good sources of the trace element iodine. Another deficiency disease, anemia, was treated in ancient Greece (around the time of Hippocrates, or about 4th century, B.C.) by giving the patient iron-containing water in which heated swords had been quenched. However, the effects of such treatments were often unpredictable, because there were no means of identifying or measuring the quantity of the active ingredients in the various medicinal substances.

The breakthroughs in our understanding of the functions of minerals in the body did not come for many centuries because laboratories for research were not developed until the Renaissance; although the medieval alchemists appear to have invented some of the techniques and tools of chemistry in their futile efforts to change base metals into gold. Furthermore, all of the elements which are essential for human life are so highly reactive that they are usually found in chemical combination with other elements, except when they are present in minute amounts as charged particles (ions) in the blood. Hence, it was an important breakthrough when the German chemist Brand reported in 1669 that he had identified the highly combustible and toxic phosphorus as a constituent of a compound in human urine.

It is noteworthy that the great French chemist Lavoisier, who is credited with being the founder of the science of nutrition, predicted in 1799 that such elements as sodium and potassium would soon be discovered because he believed that they were present in certain mineral compounds which were then known as "earths." Sure enough, within a few years the British chemist Davy discovered not only sodium and potassium, but also calcium, sulfur, magnesium, and chlorine. Davy's discoveries were so highly regarded by the French Academy that in 1806 they awarded him their new Volta medal, even though France and England were at war when the award was presented.

The pace of progress quickened as the noted Swedish chemist Berzelius added to our knowledge of minerals by (1) reporting his analysis of the calcium and phosphorus content of bone in 1801, and (2) concluding in 1838 that the iron in hemoglobin made it possible for the blood to absorb much oxygen. Similar contributions were made by the Frech chemist Boussingault, who (1) noted in 1822 that South American villagers who used salt containing iodine were protected from goiter which affected those who used plain salt; and (2) showed by means of animal feeding trials the necessity of providing dietary calcium and iron. Calcium studies were also conducted by Chossat, a physician in Switzerland, who won a prize in 1840 for his demonstration that the addition of calcium carbonate to a diet of wheat and water improved bone growth in pigeons.

From the mid-19th century to the present, most of the great advances in our knowledge of minerals had to do with the roles of the trace elements. However, these advances were hard won and slow in coming, because of such difficulties as those which dogged the French chemist Chatin from 1850 to 1876. Chatin conducted analyses for iodine on soil and water samples from various regions where cretinism and goiter were prevalent; and he tried to convince his contemporaries that these diseases were due to lack of iodine. He met with little success because (1) his critics claimed that his analytical procedures were not sufficiently sensitive to detect minute traces of iodine; and (2) the overzealous use of iodine against the cautions of various scientists had given the mineral a bad name, because excessively large doses did more harm than good. Almost another half century elapsed before the value of iodine became widely accepted; thanks to (1) the discovery by the German biochemist Baumann in 1895 that the thyroid gland contained iodine, and (2) the demonstrations by the American medical scientist Marine and his co-workers between 1907 and 1918 that the administration of minute amounts of iodine prevented goiter in animals and in school children.

It is noteworthy that by the end of the 19th century only about one-third of the minerals now accepted as essential were known to be required in the diet. This state of affairs existed in spite of the many nutritional investigations which were conducted during that century because the need for vitamins had not yet been discovered. Hence, it was difficult to differentiate between the deficiency diseases due to lack of minerals and those due to lack of vitamins.

The first two decades of the 20th century were marked by a flurry of discoveries concerning the roles of various vitamins. Then, various minerals were found to be required by animals and man, as indicated by the dates of the discoveries which follow: phosphorus, 1918; copper, 1925; magnesium, manganese, and molybdenum, 1931; zinc, 1934; and cobalt, 1935. However, there was often uncertainty as to the metabolic roles of various minerals, even though they were known to be essential. For example, it was not until 1948 that it was established that cobalt functions as a component of vitamin B-12. Hence, the two decades between the 1930s and the 1950s were marked by feverish activity aimed at learning how each of the newly discovered essential elements acted in the body.

The most recent chapter in this story began when Schwarz, a medical scientist who had emigrated to the United States from Germany, and his co-workers discovered the essentiality of selenium in 1957, and of chromium in 1959. They then developed isolation equipment for shielding their animals and their ultrapure diets from contamination by minute amounts of elements in the environment. Their painstaking work paid off because in 1972 they were able to show that fluorine and silicon were also essential. It is ironic that only a short time ago each of these four trace elements was considered to be only an unwanted toxic contaminant of foods, water, and air. However, it might be worthwhile for the enthusiastic user of food supplements to take heed of the fact that fairly small excesses of certain essential trace elements are toxic. Hence, much work remains to be done in the areas of (1) testing whether other elements might be essential, (2) defining the limits of safe and toxic doses for those already known, and (3) determining how the various elements interact with each other in the human body.

MINERAL TABLE. The general functions of minerals are as follows:

1. Give rigidity and strength to the skeletal structure.

2. Serve as constituents of the organic compounds, such as protein and lipid, which make up the muscles, organs, blood cells, and other soft tissues of the body.

3. Activate enzyme systems.

4. Control fluid balance—osmotic pressure and excretion.

5. Regulate acid-base balance.

6. Exert characteristic effects on the irritability of muscles and nerves.

7. Act together with hormones, vitamins, and other metabolic regulators.

In addition to the general functions in which several minerals may be involved, each essential mineral has at least one specific role. It is noteworthy that those which are present in large amounts, like calcium and phosphorus, are likely to have multiple and diverse roles. However, trace elements that are present at barely detectable levels, such as chromium and cobalt, appear to have highly specific functions centered around the organic molecules to which they are bound.

A summary of individual mineral functions, deficiency

and toxicity symptoms, recommended daily allowance, and sources is given in Table M-67, Mineral Table, which follows. (Calcium, phosphorus, sodium, and chlorine are listed in this order, and first, under macrominerals, then the rest of the minerals are listed alphabetically under their respective categories—as macromineral or micromineral.)

Additionally, a separate and more complete presentation relative to each mineral appears alphabetically in the encyclopedia under its respective name.

TABLE M-67
MINERAL TABLE

Functions	Deficiencies and Toxicity Symptoms	Recommended Daily Allowance			Sources	Comments
		Age	Years	Mineral		
MACROMINERALS: **Calcium (Ca)** The primary function of calcium is to build the bones and teeth, and to maintain the bones. Other functions are: 1. Blood clotting. 2. Muscle contraction and relaxation, especially the heartbeat. 3. Nerve transmission. 4. Cell wall permeability. 5. Enzyme activation. 6. Secretion of a number of hormones and hormone-releasing factors. (Also see CALCIUM.)	**Deficiency symptoms**—The most dramatic deficiency symptoms are manifested in the bones and teeth of the young, evidenced in— 1. Stunting of growth. 2. Poor quality bones and teeth. 3. Malformation of bones—rickets. The clinical manifestations of calcium related diseases are— 1. Rickets in children. 2. Osteomalacia, the adult counterpart of rickets. 3. Osteoporosis, a condition of too little bone, resulting when bone resorption exceeds bone formation. 4. Hypercalcemia, characterized by high serum calcium. 5. Tetany, characterized by muscle spasms and muscle pain. 6. Kidney stones. **Toxicity**—Normally, the small intestine prevents excess calcium from being absorbed. However, a breakdown of this control may raise the level of calcium in the blood and lead to calcification of the kidneys and other internal organs. High calcium intake may cause excess secretion of calcitonin and such bone abnormalities as osteopetrosis (dense bone). High calcium intakes have also been reported to cause kidney stones.	Infants Children Males Females Pregnant Lactating	0–0.5 0.5–1.0 1–3 4–6 7–10 11–14 15–18 19–24 25–50 51+ 11–14 15–18 19–24 25–50 51+	*Calcium*[1] (mg) 400 600 800 800 800 1,200 1,200 1,200 800 800 1,200 1,200 1,200 800 800 1,200 1,200	**Rich sources**— Cheeses, wheat-soy flour, black-strap molasses. **Good sources**— Almonds, Brazil nuts, caviar, cottonseed flour, dried figs, fish with soft edible bones, green leafy vegetables, hazel nuts, ice cream, milk, oysters, sour cream, soybean flour, yogurt.	Calcium is the most abundant mineral in the body. It makes up about 2.0% of the body weight, or about 40% of the total mineral present; 99% of it is in the bones and teeth. Normally, only 20 to 30% of the calcium in the average diet is absorbed from the intestinal tract and taken into the bloodstream. But growing children and pregnant-lactating women utilize calcium most efficiently— they absorb 40% or more of the calcium in their diets. Calcium is involved in a number of relationships, which are detailed in the Calcium section of this book. Generally, nutritionists recommend a calcium-phosphorus ratio of 1.5:1 in infancy, decreasing to 1:1 at 1 year of age and remaining at 1:1 throughout the rest of life; although they consider ratios between 2:1 and 1:2 as satisfactory.

[1]*Recommended Dietary Allowances*, 10th ed., NRC–National Academy of Sciences, 1989, p. 285.

Fair sources— Beans, bread, broccoli, cabbage, clams, cottage cheese, crab, dehydrated apricots, dehydrated peaches, eggs, legumes, lettuce, lobster, okra, olives, oranges, parsnips, peanut butter, prunes, raisins, rhubarb, spinach, Swiss chard, turnips, wheat germ. **Negligible sources**— Asparagus, beef, beets, Brussels sprouts, carrots, cauliflower, corn and cornmeal and other grains and cereals, cucumbers, fats and oils, juice, kohlrabi, most fish, most fresh fruits, mushrooms, peas, pickles, popcorn, pork, potatoes, poultry, pumpkin, radishes, roe, squash, sugar, tomatoes. **Supplemental sources**— Bone meal, calcium carbonate, calcium gluconate, calcium lactate, dicalcium phosphate, dolomite, kelp. If calcium is taken as a pill, it should be in the form of some soluble salt, such as calcium lactate.

(Continued)

TABLE M-67 (Continued)

Functions	Deficiencies and Toxicity Symptoms	Recommended Daily Allowance			Sources	Comments
		Age	Years	Mineral		

Phosphorus (P)

Functions	Deficiencies and Toxicity Symptoms	Age	Years	Phosphorus[1] (mg)	Sources	Comments
Essential for bone formation and maintenance. Important in the development of teeth. Essential for normal milk secretion. Important in building muscle tissue. As a component of nucleic acids (RNA and DNA), which are important in genetic transmission and control of cellular metabolism.	**Deficiency symptoms**—General weakness, loss of appetite, muscle weakness, bone pain, demineralization of bone, and loss of calcium. Severe and prolonged deficiencies of phosphorus may be manifested by rickets, osteomalacia, and other phosphorus related diseases. **Toxicity**—There is no known phosphorus toxicity *per se*. However, excess phosphate consumption may cause hypocalcemia (a deficiency of calcium in the blood).	Infants	0–0.5	400	**Rich sources**—Cocoa powder, cottonseed flour, fish flour, peanut flour, pumpkin and squash seeds, rice bran, rice polish, soybean flour, sunflower seeds, wheat bran. **Good sources**—Beef, cheeses, fish and seafood, lamb, liver, nuts, peanut butter, pork, poultry, whole grain flours.	Phosphorus comprises about 1/4 the total mineral matter in the body. Eighty percent of the phosphorus is in the bones and teeth in inorganic combination with calcium. Normally, 70% of the ingested phosphorus is absorbed. Generally, nutritionists recommend a calcium-phosphorus ratio of 1.5:1 in infancy, decreasing to 1:1 at 1 year of age, and remaining at 1:1 throughout the rest of life; although they consider ratios between 2:1 and 1:2 as satisfactory.
			0.5–1.0	600		
		Children	1–3	800		
			4–6	800		
			7–10	800		
		Males	11–14	1,200		
			15–18	1,200		
			19–24	1,200		
			25–50	800		
			51+	800		
		Females	11–14	1,200		
			15–18	1,200		
			19–24	1,200		
			25–50	800		
			51+	800		
		Pregnant		1,200		
		Lactating		1,200		

[1]*Recommended Dietary Allowances*, 10th ed., NRC–National Academy of Sciences, 1989, p. 285.

Maintenance of osmotic and acid-base balance.
Important in many metabolic functions, especially—
1. Energy utilization.
2. Phospholipid formation.
3. Amino acid metabolism; protein formation.
4. Enzyme systems.

(Also see PHOSPHORUS.)

Fair sources—Breads and cereals, cottage cheese, dehydrated fruits, eggs, ice cream, kidneys, milk, molasses, most vegetables, mushrooms, sausages and luncheon meats, white flour, yogurt.
Negligible sources—Fats and oils, juices and beverages, raw and canned fruits, some vegetables (lettuce, celery, carrots, tomatoes), sugar.
Supplemental sources—Ammonium phosphate, bone meal, calcium phosphate, dicalcium phosphate, lecithin, monosodium phosphate, wheat germ (toasted), yeast (brewers', torula).

Sodium (Na)

Functions	Deficiencies and Toxicity Symptoms	Age	Years	Sodium[1] (mg)	Sources	Comments
Helps to maintain the balance of water, acids, and bases in the fluid outside the cells. As a constituent of pancreatic juice, bile, sweat, and tears. Associated with muscle contraction and nerve functions. Plays a specific role in the absorption of carbohydrates. (Also see SODIUM.)	**Deficiency symptoms**—Reduced growth, loss of appetite, loss of body weight due to loss of water, reduced milk production of lactating mothers, muscle cramps, nausea, diarrhea, and headache. Excess perspiration and salt depletion may be accompanied by heat exhaustion. **Toxicity**—Salt may be toxic when (1) a high intake is accompanied by a restriction of water, (2) when the body is adapted to a chronic low salt diet, or (3) when it is fed to infants or others whose kidneys cannot excrete the excess in the urine.	Infants	0–0.5	120	Generally speaking, the need is for low sodium diets, which calls for avoiding high sodium foods. Groupings of common food sources of sodium in descending order follow: **Rich sources**—Anchovy paste, bacon, bologna, bran cereal, butter and margarine, Canadian bacon, corned	Most of the salt in the diet is in the form of sodium chloride (NaCl). Excess dietary salt, over a long period of time, is believed to lead to high blood pressure in susceptible people. Also, excess sodium may cause edema, evidenced by swelling of such areas as the legs and face. The simplest way to reduce sodium intake is to
			0.5–1.0	200		
		Children and adolescents	1	225		
			2–5	300		
			6–9	400		
			10–18	500		
		Adults	18+	500		

[1]*Note well:* The sodium values are "Estimated Minimum Requirements," from *Recommended Dietary Allowances*, 10th ed., NRC–National Academy of Sciences, 1989, p. 253, Table 11–1.

(Continued)

TABLE M-67 (*Continued*)

Functions	Deficiencies and Toxicity Symptoms	Recommended Daily Allowance			Sources	Comments
		Age	Years	Mineral		

Sodium (Na) (*Continued*)

| | | | | | beef, cornflakes cereal, cucumber | eliminate the use of table salt. Deficiencies of sodium may occur from strict vegetarian diets without salt, or when there has been heavy, prolonged sweating, diarrhea, vomiting, or adrenal cortical insufficiency. In such cases, extra salt should be taken. |

pickles, cured ham, dehydrated cod, dried squid, frankfurters, green olives, luncheon meats, oat cereal, parmesan cheese, pasteurized process cheese, potato chips, pretzels, sausages, seaweed, shrimp, smoked herring, soda crackers, soy sauce, tomato catsup, wheat flakes cereal.

Good sources—Breads and cookies, canned vegetables, cheeses, condensed soups, many prepared foods and mixes, peanut butter, pickled foods, salad dressings, seafoods.

Fair sources—Beef, desserts and sweets, eggs, lamb, milk, pork, poultry, salt-loving vegetables (spinach, beets, chard, celery, carrots), some fish (cod, haddock, salmon, tuna) depending upon preparation, veal, yogurt.

Negligible sources—Lard, legumes, most fresh fruits and vegetables, rye flour, shortening, soybean flour, sugar, vegetable oils, wheat bran, wheat flour.

Supplemental sources—Salt (sodium chloride), baking soda, monosodium glutamate (MSG), sodium-containing baking powder.

Functions	Deficiencies and Toxicity Symptoms	Age	Years	*Chlorine*[1] (mg)	Sources	Comments
Chlorine (Cl) Plays a major role in the regulation of osmotic pressure, water balance, and acid-base balance. Required for the production of hydrochloric acid of the stomach; this acid is necessary for the proper absorption of vitamin B-12 and iron, for the activation of the enzyme that breaks down starch, and for suppressing the growth of microorganisms that enter the stomach with food and drink. (Also see CHLORINE OR CHLORIDE.)	**Deficiency symptoms**— Severe deficiencies may result in alkalosis (an excess of alkali in the blood), characterized by slow and shallow breathing, listlessness, muscle cramps, loss of appetite, and, occasionally, by convulsions. Deficiencies of chloride may develop from prolonged and severe vomiting, diarrhea, pumping of the stomach, injudicious use of diuretic drugs, or strict vegetarian diets without salt. **Toxicity**—An excess of chlorine ions is unlikely when the kidneys are functioning properly.	Infants	0–0.5 0.5–1.0	180 300	Table salt (sodium chloride) and foods that contain salt. Persons whose sodium intake is severely restricted (owing to diseases of the heart, kidney, or liver) may need an alternative source of chloride; a number of chloride-containing salt substitutes are available for this purpose.	Chlorine is an essential mineral, with a special function in forming the hydrochloric acid (HCl) present in the gastric juice.
		Children and adolescents	1 2–5 6–9 10–18	350 500 600 750		
		Adults	18+	750		

[1]*Note well:* The chloride values are "Estimated Minimum Requirements," from *Recommended Dietary Allowances,* 10th ed., NRC–National Academy of Sciences, 1989, p. 253, Table 11–1.

(Continued)

TABLE M-67 (*Continued*)

Functions	Deficiencies and Toxicity Symptoms	Recommended Daily Allowance			Sources	Comments
		Age	Years	Mineral		

Magnesium (Mg)

Functions	Deficiencies and Toxicity Symptoms	Age	Years	*Magnesium*[1] (mg)	Sources	Comments
Magnesium (Mg) Constituent of bones and teeth. Essential element of cellular metabolism, often as an activator of enzymes involved in phosphorylated compounds and of high energy phosphate transfer of ADP and ATP. Involved in activating certain peptidases in protein digestion. Relaxes nerve impulses, functioning antagonistically to calcium which is stimulatory. (Also see MAGNESIUM.)	**Deficiency symptoms**—A deficiency of magnesium is characterized by (1) muscle spasms (tremor, twitching) and rapid heartbeat; (2) confusion, hallucinations, and disorientation; and (3) lack of appetite, listlessness, nausea, and vomiting. **Toxicity**—Magnesium toxicity is characterized by slowed breathing, coma, and sometimes death.	Infants	0–0.5 / 0.5–1.0	40 / 60	Groupings by rank of common food sources of magnesium follow: **Rich sources**— Coffee (instant), cocoa powder, cottonseed flour, peanut flour, sesame seeds, soybean flour, spices, wheat bran, wheat germ. **Good sources**— Blackstrap molasses, nuts, peanut butter, whole grains (oats, barley,	Overuse of such substances as "milk of magnesia" (magnesium hydroxide, an antacid and laxative) or "Epsom salts" (magnesium sulfate, a laxative and tonic) may lead to deficiencies of other minerals, or even to toxicity.
		Children	1–3 / 4–6 / 7–10	80 / 120 / 170		
		Males	11–14 / 15–18 / 19–24 / 25–50 / 51+	270 / 400 / 350 / 350 / 350		
		Females	11–14 / 15–18 / 19–24 / 25–50 / 51+	280 / 300 / 280 / 280 / 280		
		Pregnant		320		
		Lactating		355		

[1]*Recommended Dietary Allowances,* 10th ed., NRC–National Academy of Sciences, 1989, p. 285

wheat, buckwheat), whole wheat flour, yeast.
Fair sources—Avocados, bananas, beef and veal, breads, cheese, chicken, corn, cornmeal, dates, dehydrated fruit, fish and seafoods, lamb, liver, olives, pork, raspberries, rice, turkey, most green leafy vegetables.
Negligible sources—Cabbage, egg plant, eggs, fats and oils, ice cream, lettuce, milk, most fruits, mushrooms, rhubarb, rutabagas, sausages and luncheon meats, sugar, tomatoes.
Supplemental sources—Dolomite, magnesium gluconate, magnesium oxide, wheat germ.

Potassium (K)

Functions	Deficiencies and Toxicity Symptoms	Age	Years	*Potassium*[1] (mg)	Sources	Comments
Potassium (K) Involved in the maintenance of proper acid-base balance and the transfer of nutrients in and out of individual cells. Relaxes the heart muscle—action opposite to that of calcium, which is stimulatory. Required for the secretion of insulin by the pancreas, in enzyme reactions involving the phosphorylation of creatine, in carbohydrate metabolism, in protein synthesis. (Also see POTASSIUM.)	**Deficiency symptoms**— Potassium deficiency may cause rapid and irregular heartbeats, and abnormal electrocardiograms; muscle weakness, irritability, and occasionally paralysis; and nausea, vomiting, diarrhea, and swollen abdomen. Extreme and prolonged deficiency of potassium may cause hypokalemia, culminating in the heart muscles stopping. **Toxicity**—Acute toxicity from potassium (known as hyperpotassemia or hyperkalemia) will result from sudden increases of potassium to levels of about 18 g per day for an adult, provided the kidneys are not functioning properly and there is not an immediate and sharply increased loss of potassium from the body. The condition may prove fatal due to cardiac arrest.	Infants	0–0.5 / 0.5–1.0	500 / 700	**Rich sources**— Dehydrated fruits, molasses, potato flour, rice bran, seaweed, soybean flour, spices, sunflower seeds, wheat bran. **Good sources**— Avocado, beef, dates, guavas, most raw vegetables, nectarine, nuts, pork, poultry, sardines, veal. **Fair sources**— Breads, cereals, cheeses, cooked or canned vegetables, eggs, fruit juices, milk, raw,	Potassium is the third most abundant element in the body, after calcium and phosphorus; and it is present in twice the concentration of sodium. Sources of potassium other than foods, such as potassium chloride, should be taken only on the advice of a physician or nutritionist.
		Children and adolescents	1 / 2–5 / 6–9 / 10–18	1,000 / 1,400 / 1,600 / 2,000		
		Adults	18+	2,000		

[1]*Note well:* The potassium values are "Estimated Minimum Requirements," from *Recommended Dietary Allowances,* 10th ed., NRC–National Academy of Sciences, 1989, p. 253, Table 11–1.

cooked, or canned fruits, shellfish, whole wheat flour, wine, yogurt.
Negligible sources—Cooked rice, cornmeal, fats and oils, honey, olives, sugar.
Supplemental sources—Potassium gluconate, potassium chloride, seaweed, yeast (brewers', torula), wheat germ.

(Continued)

TABLE M-67 (Continued)

Functions	Deficiencies and Toxicity Symptoms	Recommended Daily Allowance			Sources	Comments
		Age	Years	Mineral		

Sulfur (S)

Functions	Deficiencies and Toxicity Symptoms	Recommended Daily Allowance	Sources	Comments
As a component of the sulfur-containing amino acids methionine, cystine, and cysteine. As a component of biotin, sulfur is important in fat metabolism. As a component of thiamin and insulin, it is important in carbohydrate metabolism. As a component of coenzyme A, it is important in energy metabolism.	**Deficiency symptoms—** Primarily retarded growth, because of sulfur's association with protein synthesis. **Toxicity—**Except in rare, inborn errors of metabolism where the utilization of the sulfur-containing amino acids is abnormal, excess organic sulfur intake is essentially nonexistent. However, inorganic sulfur can be dangerous if ingested in large amounts.	There are no recommended allowances for sulfur because it is assumed that the sulfur requirements are met when the methionine and cystine intakes are adequate.	For the most part, the sulfur needs of the body are met from organic complexes, notably the amino acids of proteins, rather than from inorganic sources. Good food sources are: cheese, grains and grain products, eggs, fish, legumes, meat, nuts, and poultry.	Sulfur is found in every cell in the body and is essential for life itself. Approximately 10% of the mineral content of the body is sulfur.

As a component of certain complex carbohydrates, it is important in various connective tissues.
As a component of insulin and glutathione, it regulates energy metabolism.
As a converter of toxic substances to nontoxic forms, it rids the body (via excretion) of such toxic substances as phenols and cresols.

(Also see SULFUR.)

MICROMINERALS OR TRACE ELEMENTS:
Chromium (Cr)

Functions	Deficiencies and Toxicity Symptoms	Age	Years	Chromium[1,2] (mcg)	Sources	Comments
Component of the Glucose Tolerance Factor (GTF), which enhances the effect of insulin. Activator of certain enzymes, most of which are involved in the production of energy from carbohydrates, fats, and proteins. Stabilizer of nucleic acids (DNA and RNA). Stimulation of synthesis of fatty acids and cholesterol in the liver.	**Deficiency symptoms—** Impaired glucose tolerance, which may be accompanied by high blood sugar and the spilling of sugar in the urine; seen especially in older persons, in maturity-onset diabetes, and in infants with protein-calorie malnutrition. Disturbance in lipid and protein metabolism. (Also see DIABETES.) **Toxicity—**Chromium is seldom toxic because (1) only small amounts are present in most foods, (2) the body utilizes it poorly, and (3) there is a wide margin of safety between helpful and harmful doses. *Note well:* Excesses of inorganic chromium are much more toxic than similar amounts of GTF-chromium.	Infants Children and adolescents Adults	0–.5 .5–1.0 1–3 4–6 7–10 11+	10–40 20–60 20–80 30–120 50–200 50–200 50–200	Groupings by rank of some common food sources of chromium follow: **Rich sources—** Blackstrap molasses, cheese, eggs, liver. **Good sources—** Apple peel, banana, beef, beer, bread, brown sugar, butter or margarine,	Further studies are needed to determine chromium's role in metabolism and its nutritional significance. Chromium levels in the body decline with aging. Hence, it is suspected that some of the cases of adult-onset diabetes are due to lack of GTF-chromium.

[1]*Note well:* The chromium values are "Estimated Minimum Requirements," from *Recommended Dietary Allowances*, 10th ed., NRC–National Academy of Sciences, 1989, p. 284.

(Also see CHROMIUM.)

chicken, cornflakes, cornmeal, flour, oysters, potatoes, vegetable oils, wheat bran, whole wheat.
Fair sources—Carrots, green beans, oranges, spinach, strawberries.
Negligible sources—Milk, most fruits and vegetables, sugar.
Supplemental sources—Brewers' yeast, dried liver.
Note well: The content and/or availability of chromium in foods may be affected by the following:
1. The chromium content of the soil.
2. The processing of grain.
3. The refining of molasses.
4. The type of cooking utensil.
5. Fermentation.
6. The alcohol-extractable fraction.

(Also see GLUCOSE TOLERANCE FACTOR.)

TABLE M-67 (Continued)

Functions	Deficiencies and Toxicity Symptoms	Recommended Daily Allowance			Sources	Comments
		Age	Years	Mineral		

Cobalt (Co)

Functions	Deficiencies and Toxicity Symptoms	Recommended Daily Allowance	Sources	Comments
The only known function of cobalt is that of an integral part of vitamin B-12, an essential factor in the formation of red blood cells. (Also see COBALT; and VITAMIN B-12.)	A cobalt deficiency as such has never been produced in humans. The signs and symptoms that are sometimes attributed to cobalt deficiency are actually due to lack of vitamin B-12, characterized by pernicious anemia, poor growth, and occasionally neurological disorders. (Also see ANEMIA, PERNICIOUS.)	There is no known human requirement for cobalt, except for that contained in vitamin B-12. the cobalt content of human foods serves no useful purpose. Instead, the need is for rich sources of vitamin B-12—liver, kidneys, fish, poultry, eggs, and tempeh.	Cobalt is present in many foods. However, the element must be ingested in the form of vitamin B-12 in order to be of value to man; hence, a table showing	Cobalt is an essential constituent of vitamin B-12 and must be ingested in the form of the vitamin molecule inasmuch as humans synthesize little of the vitamin. (A small amount of vitamin B-12 is synthesized in the human colon by *E. coli*, but absorption is very limited.)

Copper (Cu)

Functions	Deficiencies and Toxicity Symptoms	Age	Years	Copper[1] (mg)	Sources	Comments
Facilitating the absorption of iron from the intestinal tract and releasing it from storage in the liver and the reticuloendothelial system. Essential for the formation of hemoglobin, although it is not a part of hemoglobin as such. Constituent of several enzyme systems. Development and maintenance of the vascular and skeletal structures (blood vessels, tendons, bones). Structure and functioning of the central nervous system. Required for normal pigmentation of the hair. Component of important copper-containing proteins. Reproduction (fertility). (Also see COPPER.)	**Deficiency symptoms**—Deficiency is most apt to occur in malnourished children and in premature infants fed exclusively on modified cow's milk and in infants breast fed for an extended period of time. Deficiency leads to a variety of abnormalities, including anemia, skeletal defects, demyelination and degeneration of the nervous system, defects in pigmentation and structure of the hair, reproductive failure, and pronounced cardiovascular lesions. **Toxicity**—Copper is relatively nontoxic to monogastric species, including man. The recommended copper intake for adults is in the range of 2 to 3 mg/day. Daily intakes of more than 20 to 30 mg over extended periods would be expected to be unsafe.	Infants Children and adolescents Adults	0–0.5 0.5–1.0 1–3 4–6 7–10 11+	0.4–0.6 0.6–0.7 0.7–1.0 1.0–1.5 1.0–2.0 1.5–2.5 1.5–3.0	Groupings by rank of common food sources of copper follow: **Rich sources**—Black pepper, blackstrap molasses, Brazil nuts, cocoa, liver, oysters (raw). **Good sources**—Lobster, nuts and seeds, olives (green),	Most cases of copper poisoning result from drinking water or beverages that have been stored in copper tanks and/or pass through copper pipes. Dietary excesses of calcium, iron, cadmium, zinc, lead, silver, and molybdenum plus sulfur reduce the utilization of copper.

[1]*Note well:* The copper values are "Estimated Minimum Requirements," from *Recommended Dietary Allowances*, 10th ed., NRC–National Academy of Sciences, 1989, p. 284.

soybean flour, wheat bran, wheat germ (toasted).
Fair sources—Avocado, banana, beans, beef, breads and cereals, butter, Cheddar cheese, coconut, dried fruits, eggs, fish, granola, green vegetables (turnip greens, collards, spinach), lamb, peanut butter, pork, poultry, turnip, yams.
Negligible sources—Fats and oils, milk, and most milk products (ice cream, cottage cheese), other fruits and vegetables, sugar.
Supplemental sources—Alfalfa leaf meal, brewers' yeast, copper carbonate, copper sulfate.
Note well: Copper sulfate or copper carbonate should only be taken on the advice of a physician or nutritionist.

(Continued)

TABLE M-67 (*Continued*)

Functions	Deficiencies and Toxicity Symptoms	Recommended Daily Allowance			Sources	Comments
		Age	Years	Mineral		
Fluorine (F) Constitutes .02 to .05% of the bones and teeth. Necessary for sound bones and teeth. Assists in the prevention of dental caries. (Also see FLUORINE.)	**Deficiency symptoms—** Excess dental caries. Also, there is indication that a deficiency of fluorine results in more osteoporosis in the aged. However, excesses of fluorine are of more concern than deficiencies. **Toxicity—**Deformed teeth and bones, and softening, mottling, and irregular wear of the teeth.			*Fluorine*[1] (mg)	Fluorine is found in many foods, but seafoods and dry tea are the richest food sources. A few rich sources follow: *Source Fluorine (F)* (ppm) Dried seaweed 326.0 Tea 32.0 Mackerel 19.0 Sardines 11.0 Salmon 6.8 Shrimp 4.5 Fluoridation of water supplies to bring the concentration of fluoride to 1 ppm.	Large amounts of dietary calcium, aluminum, and fat will lower the absorption of fluorine. Fluoridation of water supplies (1 ppm) is the simplest and most effective method of providing added protection against dental caries.
		Infants	0–.5 .5–1.0	.1–.5 .2–1.0		
		Children and adolescents	1–3 4–6 7–10 11+	.5–1.5 1.0–2.5 1.5–2.5 1.5–2.5		
		Adults		1.5–4.0		
	[1]*Note well:* The fluoride values are "Estimated Minimum Requirements," from *Recommended Dietary Allowances*, 10th ed., NRC–National Academy of Sciences, 1989, p. 284.					
Iodine (I) The sole function of iodine is making the iodine-containing hormones secreted by the thyroid gland, which regulate the rate of oxidation within the cells; and in so doing influence physical and mental growth, the functioning of the nervous and muscle tissues, circulatory activity, and the metabolism of all nutrients. (Also see IODINE.)	**Deficiency symptoms—** Iodine deficiency is characterized by goiter (an enlargement of the thyroid gland at the base of the neck), coarse hair, obesity, and high blood cholesterol. Iodine-deficient mothers may give birth to infants with a type of dwarfism known as cretinism, a disorder characterized by malfunctioning of the thyroid gland, goiter, mental retardation, and stunted growth. A similar disorder of the thyroid gland, known as myxedema, may develop in adults. **Toxicity—**Long-term intake of large excesses of iodine may disturb the utilization of iodine by the thyroid gland and result in goiter. (Also see ENDOCRINE GLANDS: and GOITER.)			*Iodine*[1] (mcg)	Among natural foods the best sources of iodine are kelp, seafoods, and vegetables grown on iodine-rich soils. Dairy products and eggs may be good sources if the producing animals have access to iodine-enriched rations. Most cereal grains, legumes, roots, and fruits have low iodine content. Of the various methods for assuring an adequate iodine intake, iodized salt has thus far proved to be most successful, and therefore the most widely adopted method. In the U.S. iodination is on a voluntary basis, nevertheless	The enlargement of the thyroid gland (goiter) is nature's way of attempting to make sufficient thyroxine under conditions where a deficiency exists. Certain foods (especially plants of the cabbage family) contain goitrogens, which interfere with the use of thyroxine and may produce goiter. Fortunately, goitrogenic action is prevented by cooking. For intakes of iodine, man is dependent upon food, soil, and water. The iodine content of food varies widely, depending chiefly on (1) the iodine content of the soil, (2) the iodine content of the animal feeds (to which iodized salt is routinely added in most
		Infants	0–0.5 0.5–1.0	40 50		
		Children	1–3 4–6 7–10	70 90 120		
		Males	11–14 15–18 19–24 25–50 51+	150 150 150 150 150		
		Females	11–14 15–18 19–24 25–50 51+	150 150 150 150 150		
		Pregnant		175		
		Lactating		200		
	[1]*Recommended Dietary Allowances*, 10th ed., NRC–National Academy of Sciences, 1989, p. 285.					

(*Continued*)

TABLE M-67 (*Continued*)

Functions	Deficiencies and Toxicity Symptoms	Recommended Daily Allowance			Sources	Comments
		Age	Years	Mineral		
Iodine (I) (*Continued*)					slightly more than half of the table salt consumed is iodized. Stabilized iodized salt contains 0.01% potassium iodide (0.0076% I), or 76 mcg of iodine per gram. Iodine may also be provided in bread. But the practice of using iodates in bread making appears to be on the decline.	countries), and (3) the use of iodized salt in food processing operations. Iodine in drinking and cooking water varies widely in different regions; in some areas, such as near oceans, it is high enough to meet the daily requirement.

Functions	Deficiencies and Toxicity Symptoms	Age	Years	*Iron*[1] (mg)	Sources	Comments
Iron (Fe) Iron (heme) conbines with protein (globin) to make hemoglobin, the iron-containing compound in red blood cells; so, iron is involved in transporting oxygen. Iron is also a component of enzymes which are involved in energy metabolism. (Also see IRON.)	**Deficiency symptoms**—Iron-deficiency (nutritional) anemia, the symptoms of which are: paleness of skin and mucous membranes, fatigue, dizziness, sensitivity to cold, shortness of breath, rapid heartbeats, and tingling of the fingers and toes. **Toxicity**—Approximately 2,000 cases of iron poisoning occur each year in the U.S., mainly in young children who ingest the medical iron supplements of their parents. The lethal dose of ferrous sulfate for a 2-year-old is about 3 g; for an adult it's between 200 and 250 mg/kg of body weight. (Also see ANEMIA.)	Infants Children Males Females Pregnant[2] Lactating	0–0.5 0.5–1.0 1–3 4–6 7–10 11–14 15–18 19–24 25–50 51+ 11–14 15–18 19–24 25–50 51+	6 10 10 10 10 12 12 10 10 10 15 15 15 15 10 30 15	Groupings by rank of common sources of iron follow: **Rich sources**— Beef kidneys, blackstrap molasses, caviar, chicken giblets, cocoa powder, fish flour, liver, orange pekoe tea, oysters, potato flour, rice polish, soybean flour, spices, sunflower seed flour, wheat bran, wheat germ, wheat-soy blend flour. **Good sources**— Beef, brown sugar, clams, dried fruits, egg yolk, heart, light or medium molasses, lima beans (cooked), nuts, pork, pork and lamb kidneys. **Fair sources**— Asparagus, beans, chicken, dandelion	About 70% of the iron is present in the hemoglobin, the pigment of the red blood cells. The other 30% is present as a reserve store in the liver, spleen, and bone marrow. An excess of iron in the diet can tie up phosphorus in an insoluble iron-phosphate complex, thereby creating a deficiency of phosphorus. Babies are not born with sufficient iron to meet their needs beyond 6 months. Milk and milk products are poor sources of iron. About 20% of the iron in the average U.S. diet comes from fortified products. Ferrous sulfate is the supplemental iron source of choice.

[1]*Recommended Dietary Allowances*, 10th ed., NRC–National Academy of Sciences, 1989, p. 285.

[2]The increased requirement during pregnancy cannot be met by the iron content of habitual American diets nor by the existing iron stores of many women; therefore, the use of 30 to 60 mg of supplemental iron is recommended. Iron needs during lactation are not substantially different from those of nonpregnant women, but continued supplementation of the mother for 2 to 3 months after parturition is advisable in order to replenish stores depleted by pregnancy.

greens, enriched bread, enriched cereals, enriched cornmeal, enriched flour, enriched rice, fish, lamb, lentils, mustard greens, peanuts, peas, sausages and luncheon meats, spinach, Swiss chard, turkey, turnip greens, whole eggs.

Negligible sources—Cheese, fats and oils, fresh and canned fruits, fruit juices and beverages, ice cream, milk, most fresh and canned vegetables, sour cream, sugar, yogurt.

Supplemental sources—Dried liver, ferrous gluconate, ferrous succinate, ferrous sulfate, iron fumarate, iron peptonate, seaweed, yeast.

TABLE M-67 (*Continued*)

Functions	Deficiencies and Toxicity Symptoms	Recommended Daily Allowance			Sources	Comments
		Age	Years	Mineral		
Manganese (Mn) Formation of bone and the growth of other connective tissues. Blood clotting. Insulin action. Cholesterol synthesis. Activator of various enzymes in the metabolism of carbohydrates, fats, proteins, and nucleic acids, (DNA and RNA). (Also see MANGANESE.)	**Deficiency symptoms**—The only confirmed deficiency of manganese in man was in connection with a vitamin K deficiency, where administration of the vitamin did not correct the abnormality in blood clotting until supplemental manganese was provided. Analysis of hair and blood samples for manganese content indicate that sub-clinical deficiencies of the mineral might aggravate such disorders as growth impairments, bone abnormalities, diabeticlike carbohydrate metabolism, lack of muscle coordination of the newborn and abnormal metabolism of lipids (fatty acids, choline, and cholesterol). **Toxicity**—Toxicity in man as a consequence of dietary intake has not been observed. However, it has occurred in workers (miners, and others) exposed to high concentrations of manganese dust in the air. The symptoms resemble those found in Parkinson's and Wilson's diseases.	Infants Children and adolescents Adults	0–0.5 0.5–1.0 1–3 4–6 7–10 11+	*Manganese*[1] (mg) 0.3–0.6 0.6–1.0 1.0–1.5 1.5–2.0 2.0–3.0 2.0–5.0 2.0–5.0	Groupings by rank of common food sources of manganese follow: **Rich sources—** Rice (brown), rice bran and polish, spices, walnuts, wheat bran, wheat germ. **Good sources—** Blackstrap molasses, blueberries, lettuce, lima beans (dry), navy beans (dry), peanuts, potatoes, soybean flour, soybeans (dry), sunflower seeds, torula yeast, wheat flour, whole grains (barley, oats, sorghum, wheat). **Fair sources**—Brewers' yeast, liver, most fruits and vegetables, orange pekoe tea, white enriched bread. **Negligible sources**—Fats and oils, eggs, fish, meats, milk, poultry, sugar. **Supplemental sources**—Alfalfa leaf meal, dried kelp, manganese gluconate.	In average diets, only about 45% of the ingested magnesium is absorbed. The manganese content of plants is dependent on soil content. It is noteworthy, however, that plants grown on alkaline soils may be abnormally low in manganese.

[1]*Note well:* The manganese values are "Estimated Minimum Requirements," from *Recommended Dietary Allowances*, 10th ed., NRC–National Academy of Sciences, 1989, p. 284.

Functions	Deficiencies and Toxicity Symptoms	Recommended Daily Allowance			Sources	Comments
		Age	Years	Mineral		
Molybdenum (Mo) As a component of three different enzyme systems which are involved in the metabolism of carbohydrates, fats, proteins, sulfur-containing amino acids, nucleic acids (DNA and RNA), and iron. As a component of the enamel of teeth, where it appears to prevent or reduce the incidence of dental caries, although this function has not yet been proven conclusively. (Also see MOLYBDENUM.)	**Deficiency symptoms—** Naturally occurring deficiency in man is not known, *unless* utilization of the mineral is interfered with by excesses of copper and/or sulfate. Molybdenum-deficient animals are especially susceptible to the toxic effects of bisulfite, characterized by breathing difficulties and neurological disorders.	Infants Children and adolescents Adults	0–0.5 0.5–1.0 1–3 4–6 7–10 11+	*Molybdenum*[1] (mcg) 15–30 20–40 25–50 30–75 50–150 75–250 75–250	The concentration of molybdenum in food varies considerably, depending on the soil in which it is grown. Most of the dietary molybdenum intake is derived from organ meats, whole grains, leafy vegetables, legumes, and yeast.	The utilization of molybdenum is reduced by excess copper, sulfate, and tungsten. In cattle, a relationship exists between molybdenum, copper, and sulfur. Excess molybdenum will cause copper deficiency. However, when the sulfate content of the diet is increased, the symptoms of toxicity are avoided inasmuch as the excretion of molybdenum is increased.

[1]*Note well:* The molybdenum values are "Estimated Minimum Requirements," from *Recommended Dietary Allowances*, 10th ed., NRC–National Academy of Sciences, 1989, p. 284.

Severe molybdenum toxicity in animals (molybdenosis), particularly cattle, occurs throughout the world wherever pastures are grown on high-molybdenum soils. The symptoms include diarrhea, loss of weight, decreased production, fading of hair color, and other symptoms of copper deficiency.
Toxicity—In the USSR, molybdenum toxicity in man is reported to have caused a high incidence of goutlike syndrome associated with elevated blood levels of molybdenum, uric acid, and xanthine oxidase.

TABLE M-67 (*Continued*)

Functions	Deficiencies and Toxicity Symptoms	Recommended Daily Allowance			Sources	Comments
		Age	Years	Mineral		
Selenium (Se) Component of the enzyme glutathione peroxidase, the metabolic role of which is to protect against oxidation of polyunsaturated fatty acids and resultant tissue damage. Protecting tissues from certain poisonous substances, such as arsenic, cadmium, and mercury. Interrelation with vitamin E—they spare each other, and with the sulfur-containing amino acids. (Also see SELENIUM.)	**Deficiency symptoms**— There are no clear-cut deficiencies of selenium, because this mineral is so closely related to vitamin E that it is difficult to distinguish deficiency due to selenium alone. The selenium content of the blood, hair, and fingernails may be used as rough indicators of the selenium content of the rest of the body. **Toxicity**—Poisonous effects of selenium are manifested by (1) abnormalities of the hair, nails, and skin; (2) garlic odor on the breath; (3) intensification of selenium toxicity by arsenic or mercury; (4) higher than normal rates of dental caries.			*Selenium*[1] (mcg)	The selenium content of plant and animal products is affected by the selenium content of the soil and animal feed, respectively. Nevertheless, such data are useful as they show which foods are likely to be good sources of the mineral. Groupings by rank of some common food sources of selenium follow:	The high selenium areas are in the Great Plains and the Rocky Mountain States—especially in parts of the Dakotas and Wyoming. The functions of selenium are closely related to those of vitamin E and the sulfur-containing amino acids. Selenium-rich supplements should be taken only on the advice of a physician or dietitian.
		Infants	0.0–0.5	10		
			0.5–1.0	15		
		Children	1–3	20		
			4–6	20		
			7–10	30		
		Males	11–14	40		
			15–18	50		
			19–24	70		
			25–50	70		
			51+	70		
		Females	11–14	45		
			15–18	50		
			19–24	55		
			25–50	55		
			51+	55		
		Pregnant		65		
		Lactating		75		

[1]*Note well:* The selenium values are "Estimated Minimum Requirements," from *Recommended Dietary Allowances*, 10th ed., NRC–National Academy of Sciences, 1989, p. 285.

Rich sources—Brazil nuts, butter, fish flour, lobster, smelt.
Good sources—Beer, blackstrap molasses, cider vinegar, clams, crab, eggs, lamb, mushrooms, oysters, pork kidneys, spices (garlic, cinnamon, chili powder, nutmeg), Swiss chard, turnips, wheat bran, whole grains (wheat, barley, rye, oats).
Fair sources—Cabbage, carrots, cheese, corn, grape juice, most nuts, orange juice, whole milk.
Negligible sources—Fruits and sugar.
Supplemental sources—Wheat germ, yeast (brewers' and torula).
Note well: Many drug stores and health food stores now carry special types of yeast which were grown on media rich in selenium; hence, they contain much greater amounts of this mineral than ordinary yeast. Tablets made from high-selenium yeast are also available.

Functions	Deficiencies and Toxicity Symptoms	Recommended Daily Allowance	Sources	Comments
Silicon (Sl) Necessary for normal growth and skeletal development of the chick and the rat. These findings suggest that it may also have essential functions in man. (Also see SILICON.)	**Deficiency symptoms**— Deficiencies in chicks and rats are characterized by growth retardation and skeletal alterations and deformities, especially of the skull. Deficiencies of silicon have not been produced in man. **Toxicity**—Silicon does not appear to be toxic in the levels usually found in foods.	A human requirement for silicon has not been established. The silicon intake in the average U.S. diet has been estimated at approximately 1 g per day.	The best sources of silicon are the fibrous parts of whole grains, followed by various organ meats (liver, lungs, kidneys, and brain) and connective tissues. Much of the silicon in whole grains is lost when they are milled into highly refined products.	A common nondietary form of silicon toxicity is a fibrosis of the lungs known as silicosis, due to inhalation of airborne silicon oxide dust.

TABLE M-67 (*Continued*)

Functions	Deficiencies and Toxicity Symptoms	Recommended Daily Allowance			Sources	Comments
		Age	Years	Mineral		
				Zinc[1] (mg)		
Zinc (Zn) Needed for normal skin, bones, and hair. As a component of several different enzyme systems which are involved in digestion and respiration. Required for the transfer of carbon dioxide in red blood cells; for proper calcification of bones; for the synthesis and metabolism of proteins and nucleic acids; for the development and functioning of reproductive organs; for wound and burn healing; for the functioning of insulin; and for normal taste acuity. (Also see ZINC.)	**Deficiency symptoms**—Loss of appetite, stunted growth in children, skin changes, small sex glands in boys, loss of taste sensitivity, lightened pigment in hair, white spots on the fingernails, and delayed healing of wounds. In the Middle East, pronounced zinc deficiency in man has resulted in hypogonadism and dwarfism. In pregnant animals, experimental zinc deficiency has resulted in malformation and behavioral disturbances in offspring. **Toxicity**—Ingestion of excess soluble salts may cause nausea, vomiting, purging.	Infants	0–0.5	5	Groupings by rank of common food sources of zinc follows: **Rich sources**— Beef, liver, oysters, spices, wheat bran. **Good sources**— Cheddar cheese, crab, granola, lamb, peanut butter, peanuts, popcorn, pork, poultry. **Fair sources**— Beans, clams, eggs, fish, sausages and luncheon meats,	The biological availability of zinc in different foods varies widely; meats and seafoods are much better sources of available zinc than vegetables. Zinc availability is adversely affected by phytates (found in whole grains and beans), high calcium, oxalates (in rhubarb and spinach), high fiber, copper (from drinking water conveyed in copper piping), and EDTA (an additive used in certain canned foods).
			0.5–1.0	5		
		Children	1–3	10		
			4–6	10		
			7–10	10		
		Males	11–14	15		
			15–18	15		
			19–24	15		
			25–50	15		
			51+	15		
		Females	11–14	12		
			15–18	12		
			19–24	12		
			25–50	12		
			51+	12		
		Pregnant		15		
		Lactating		19		

[1]*Recommended Dietary Allowances*, 10th ed., NRC–National Academy of Sciences, 1989, p. 284.

turnip greens, wheat cereals, whole grain products (wheat, rye, oats, rice, barley). **Negligible sources**—Beverages, fats and oils, fruits and vegetables, milk, sugar, white bread. **Supplemental sources**—Wheat germ, yeast (torula), zinc carbonate, zinc gluconate, zinc sulfate. (Zinc carbonate or zinc sulfate are commonly used where zinc supplementation is necessary.)

CAUSES OF MINERAL DEFICIENCIES AND/OR TOXICITIES.

Recently, there has been much speculation as to whether many people in the United States might have subclinical deficiencies of certain minerals. It has also been speculated that mild, but chronic, toxicities, due to excesses of certain nutrients, might contribute to the development of such disorders as atherosclerosis, diabetes, heart failure, high blood pressure, and kidney stones. In light of these concerns, one often wonders if our distant ancestors were also prone to similar diet-related problems. Hence, it is worth reviewing briefly certain aspects of man's early existence in order to compare dietary factors of the past with those of the present.

Our knowledge of prehistoric diets has been derived mainly from archaeological studies of charred food remains and dried fecal material found in caves and at the sites of ancient camps. Also, there have been many studies of the aborigines who are still engaged in stone age practices in such parts of the world as Africa, Australia, New Guinea, and the Philippines. These lines of research have established that man's practice of agriculture on a regular basis has been limited to only the last 10,000 years or so of the more than 2 million years that humans have lived on the earth.[35] During the long preagricultural period, people obtained a much greater variety of foods from hunting, fishing, and gathering than their agricultural descendants did from the cultivation

[35]Robson, J. R. K., "Foods from the Past; Lessons for the Future," *The Professional Nutritionist*, Vol. 8, Spring 1976, p. 13.

of plants and the domestication of animals.

Other primitive practices which provided people with essential minerals were (1) the use of salt obtained by evaporating sea water, and (2) seasoning foods with ashes from burnt plant materials.[36]

Therefore, it seems that mineral needs might have been met better in prehistoric times than in the more recent agricultural societies. However, certain other practices and conditions became established with the rise of the great civilizations, and these, too, might be responsible for the development of mineral deficiencies and/or toxicities.

Agricultural Practices Which May Be Harmful.
Plants use the energy of the sun, gases from the air, and water and minerals from the soil, to make the various substances which are essential for their life processes and for those of animals and man. Hence, the mineral composition of the soil is one of the major factors affecting the nutritive composition of the foods we eat. Agricultural practices affect the utilization of soil minerals by plants in ways which may, in turn, affect animals and people that eat the plants. However, the reader should note that the discussions which follow are not intended to be condemnations of certain practices; rather, they are designed to point out some pitfalls of carrying them to extremes. Consider:

• **Application of sewage sludge to soils**—Although it is a good idea to apply organic wastes to the soil in order to improve its chemical and physical characteristics, sewage sludge may contain such toxic elements as cadmium, lead, and mercury—particularly when the sludge comes from highly industrialized areas.

• **Close grazing of seleniferous ranges**—This practice forces the grazing animals to eat plants which may contain extremely high levels of selenium. Some of these plants would not be eaten under conditions of light or moderate grazing because the animals prefer grains and various grasses which are much lower in selenium content.

• **Depletion of soil minerals by intensive single cropping**—Growing the same crop on the same area year after year may deplete the soil of certain minerals because they are removed more rapidly than they are replaced by the commonly used fertilizers.

(Also see DEFICIENCY DISEASES, section headed "Eating Patterns Which Lead to Dietary Deficiencies.")

• **Excessive use of copper-containing sprays**—Plants are sprayed with copper compounds in order to prevent certain fungus diseases. However, overspraying may cause the buildup of toxic levels of copper in the plants and/or the soil, which may interfere with the utilization of other minerals.

• **Feeding livestock unsupplemented feeds and forages which have been grown on mineral-deficient soils**—It is well known that products obtained from animals given such feedstuffs are likely to reflect the mineral deficiencies of the soils on which the feeds and/or forages were grown.

• **Overfertilization of soils with certain minerals**—The overapplication of such minerals as nitrogen, potash, potassium, lime, and sulfur to soils may (1) kill soil microorganisms which convert minerals to forms which are readily picked up by plants, and (2) change the chemical composition of the soil so that certain minerals form insoluble compounds which are not available to plants.

Contamination of Drinking Water, Foods, or Air with Toxic Minerals.
Toxic chemical elements—which include some of the essential trace minerals—may get into foods or drinking water from the environment, piping, commercial processing equipment, packaging, or utensils used in the home. In certain cases, such contamination might even be beneficial, if it results in the ingestion of essential minerals which are not supplied in adequate amounts by the foods or the drinking water. However, the margins between beneficial or harmless amounts and toxic levels are rather narrow for certain elements. Furthermore, excesses of certain elements may produce deficiencies of others that they counteract. Hence, it is important to consider how potentially toxic elements get into water, foods, or air so that appropriate measures might be taken to control the amounts which are ingested or inhaled. Consider:

• **Aluminum**—It is not certain whether it is safe to cook such highly acid foods as rhubarb and tomatoes in aluminum pots and pans, because aluminum is dissolved by acid solutions. Abnormally large intakes of aluminum have irritated the digestive tract. Also, unusual conditions have sometimes permitted the absorption of sufficient aluminum from antacids to cause brain damage.[37] Even if the amounts of aluminum leached from aluminum utensils by acid foods are not toxic, there is the possibility that insoluble complexes might be formed between the aluminum and some of the trace minerals, so that the absorption of these nutrients is blocked.

(Also see ANTACIDS; and POISONS, Table P-11 Some Potentially Poisonous [Toxic] Substances.)

• **Arsenic**—Although the public has long thought arsenic to be synonymous with poison, it may be less toxic than the essential trace element selenium, which it counteracts within the body. Also, recent studies on rats suggested that arsenic may be essential. Furthermore, organic arsenic compounds, such as the arsonic acids, are used as growth stimulants for poultry and swine.

---

[36]Townsend, P. K., S-C. Liao, and J. E. Konlande, "Nutritive Contributions of Sago Ash Used as a Native Salt in Papua, New Guinea," *Ecology of Food and Nutrition*, Vol. 1, 1973, p. 1.

[37]"Possible Aluminum Intoxication," *Nutrition Reviews*, Vol. 34, 1976, pp. 166-167.

Minute amounts of arsenic are widely distributed in the common foods, in quantities that are more likely to be beneficial than toxic. However, poisoning may result from foods contaminated with excessive amounts of arsenic-containing sprays used as insecticides and weed killers. Acute arsenic toxicity is characterized by weakness and digestive disorders such as burning of the mouth and throat, nausea, vomiting, abdominal pains and diarrhea, whereas chronic poisoning may result in goiter and deaf mutism.

(Also see POISONS, Table P-11 Some Potentially Poisonous [Toxic] Substances.)

• **Cadmium**—In the early 1970s there were many cases of cadmium toxicity in the Jinzu River basin near Toyama, Japan, which is about 160 miles northwest of Tokyo. The disease that resulted was known as itai-itai, or "ouch-ouch" disease, because of the pains the victims had in their bones. Eventually, the poisonings were traced to the chronic consumption of rice and soybeans containing about 3 ppm (parts per million) of cadmium, a nonessential trace mineral which came from the wastes of nearby mines and smelters. Therefore, it is noteworthy that cadmium levels of around 1 ppm have been found in soybeans grown in soil fertilized by sewage sludge, and that oysters taken from waters contaminated by industrial wastes contained about 3 ppm of cadmium.

Other sources of potential environmental contamination by cadmium are cigarette smoke, electroplating processes, paint pigments, the cadmium-nickel type of automobile storage battery, certain phosphate fertilizers, and some of the older types of galvanized water tanks.

While severe cadmium toxicity like that which occurred near Toyama has not been found elsewhere, it is suspected that mild to moderate types of chronic cadmium toxicity may cause disorders of the kidneys leading to high blood pressure. However, the milder forms of cadmium poisoning may be counteracted by such essential minerals as calcium, copper, iron, manganese, selenium, and zinc. Therefore, a few scientists believe that high ratios of cadmium to zinc in the diet and in the various tissues of the body are better indicators of potential cadmium toxicities than the dietary and tissue levels of this toxicant alone.

• **Chlorine**—This element may be ingested as essential chloride ions from inorganic salts, or as toxic organic compounds such as chlorinated hydrocarbons, which may cause liver damage, or even cancer.[38] The toxic chlorine compounds are formed when lake or river water containing nonchlorinated hydrocarbons is chlorinated prior to its use as drinking water. Chlorinated hydrocarbons have been found to be present at various levels in many of the drinking water supplies in the United States, but information is lacking as to the levels which pose either short-term or long-term hazards.

(Also see CHLORINE OR CHLORIDE.)

• **Copper**—Several groups of scientists have recently warned about the possibility of copper poisoning by acid and/or soft drinking water which has been conveyed through copper piping. The blue stains on the surface of sinks where the water drips from the faucet are an indication that drinking water may contain too much copper. About twice as much copper may be present in hot tap water as in cold tap water. Infants are particularly susceptible to the toxic effects of copper in tap water because (1) their water needs are high relative to their size, so they ingest more water in proportion to their body weights than adults; and (2) their diets are usually limited in variety, which means that they may not receive much of the other mineral elements which counteract the effects of copper.

Acute copper toxicity is characterized by headache, dizziness, metalic taste, excessive salivation, nausea, vomiting, stomachache, diarrhea, and weakness. If the disease is allowed to get worse, there may also be racing of the heart, high blood pressure, jaundice, hemolytic anemia, dark-pigmented urine, kidney disorders, or even death. Chronic copper toxicity is more subtle in that its effects may appear to be caused by other factors. For example, it has been suggested that excess copper in the body might sometimes be a contributory factor to iron-deficienciy anemia, mental illness following childbirth (postpartum psychosis), certain types of schizophrenia, and maybe, heart attacks.

In view of the disorders associated with copper toxicity, it is heartening to note that many of these conditions may be counteracted by increasing the dietary levels of iron, molybdenum, sulfur, zinc, and vitamin C. However, in cases of severe poisoning, it is necessary to administer special metal-binding (chelating) agents which draw copper out of the body.

(Also see POISONS, Table P-11 Some Potentially Poisonous [Toxic] Substances.)

• **Fluorine**—This essential element, like chlorine, is beneficial when it is provided in ionic form (inorganic fluorides) at levels up to 1 ppm in drinking water. The major benefit obtained from such fluoridated water is the increased resistance to tooth decay which occurs when it is consumed by children whose teeth are developing. Higher levels of fluoride (3 to 10 ppm), such as may occur in certain naturally fluoridated waters, may cause mottling of the teeth in some of the children who drink it, although this does not occur if the initial exposure to excessive fluoride takes place after the teeth are fully developed. Furthermore, growing children appear to have greater resistance than adults to the other toxic effects of fluoride, like the development of brittleness in bones and the inhibition of certain enzymes, because growing bones apparently take up fairly large amounts of fluoride without harm.

It is suspected that fluoride deposits in the bones may help to prevent the demineralization (osteoporosis) which often occurs with aging, although various investigators have obtained contradictory results. The answer to this dilemma might be that extra vitamin D is needed to promote the incorporation of calcium and fluoride into the bones of older adults, since administration of the vitamin apparently minimized the development of brittleness due

[38]Ibrahim, M.A., and R. F. Christman, "Drinking Water and Carcinogenesis: The Dilemmas," *American Journal of Public Health,* Vol. 67, 1977, p. 719.

to fluoride treatment.[39] Fluoridated water, or treatment with fluoride, may be hazardous to people with various types of kidney diseases, because they may not be able to excrete excesses of the mineral. Furthermore, susceptibility to fluoride toxicity is increased by deficiencies of calcium, vitamin C, and protein.[40]

In addition to fluoridated water, some other sources of significant amounts of fluoride are (1) the environments around aluminum refining plants; and (2) the consumption of tea, crude sea salt, bone meal, or fish (particularly, fish bones). However, the effects of excess fluoride may be reduced somewhat by diets rich in calcium and magnesium.

(Also see POISONS, Table P-11 Some Potentially Poisonous [Toxic] Substances.)

• **Iodine**—Only the radioactive isotope of this element—Iodine 131—is likely to be an environmental hazard, because it emits dangerous radiation. It is formed during the explosions of nuclear weapons; and it may get into foods.

When the contaminated foods are eaten, the radioactive iodine is utilized by the body as if it were normal, nonradioactive iodine. Most of it is picked up by the thyroid gland, which may be injured by the radioactivity that is emitted.

(Also see RADIOACTIVE FALLOUT.)

• **Iron**—The worldwide concern over iron-deficiency anemia has often obscured the fact that exceses of dietary iron might sometimes lead to such disorders as toxic accumulations of the mineral in the liver, spleen, pancreas, heart muscle, and kidneys. This overloading of the body with iron, called hemochromatosis, is most likely to occur in adult males who consume liberal amounts of alcohol. Females are less likely to have such an accumulation of iron because they regularly lose significant amounts of the mineral during their menstrual flow, or as a result of pregnancy and childbirth.

Moderate excesses of iron, which do not have direct toxic effects, may produce nutritional deficiencies by interfering with the absorption of copper, manganese, and zinc, and by destroying vitamins C and E.

Some of the sources of iron which may lead to overaccumulation of the mineral in the body are (1) acid foods which have been cooked in iron pots, (2) certain ciders and wines, and (3) occasionally, drinking water. Fortunately, diets containing abundant quantities of phosphorus, copper, manganese, and zinc tend to protect against excesses of iron, because these minerals interfere with its absorption.

• **Lead**—Apparently, lead poisoning had dogged man for a longer time than most people might suspect, because toxic levels of this nonessential mineral were found in the disinterred bones of ancient Romans. In fact, the use

of lead for household utensils and wine containers by the Romans is suspected of having been responsible for widespread lead poisoning which, it is conjectured, may have led to weakness and infertility, and the eventual decline of the empire.

Today, there is great concern over acute lead poisoning in young children (ages 1 to 6) who live in urban slums where they may eat chips of lead-containing paints, peeled off from painted wood. The effects of such poisoning may be anemia, hyperactivity, learning difficulties, mental retardation, or even death.[41] There is also concern for older children and adults who might develop chronic lead poisoning from (1) exposure to such sources of toxic mineral as automobile exhaust fumes, cigarette smoke, fumes from lead smelters, or smoke from coal fires; or (2) consumption of beer held in lead-containing pewter mugs, fruits from orchards sprayed with lead arsenate, fruits and vegetables grown near heavily traveled highways.

Children and pregnant women appear to be most susceptible to lead poisoning because (1) they are likely to have deficiencies of calcium and iron, minerals which protect against lead toxicity; (2) rapidly growing children absorb more lead and excrete less of this metal than other people, and (3) there is a rapid transfer of lead from the blood of pregnant women, through the placenta, to the fetus.

(Also see POISONS, Table P-11 Some Potentially Poisonous [Toxic] Substances.)

• **Mercury**—This nonessential and toxic mineral element was known in ancient times as "quicksilver," because of its shiny appearance and existence as a slippery liquid at room temperature. Its inorganic compounds, such as calomel (mercurous chloride), have long been used to treat a variety of ailments, ranging from constipation to syphilis. Also, it is common knowledge that mercury fumes may be responsible for the mental deterioration encountered by some workers in the felt hat industry (often called "mad hatters"). Yet, widespread concern over environmental pollution by the mineral did not develop until the late 1950s when an epidemic of mercury poisonings occurred in Japan.

The mercury poisonings in Japan—which were characterized by losses of balance, hearing, speech, and vision; and by mental disorders—came to be known as "Minamata Disease," because they first occurred in people who lived around Minamata Bay, about 50 miles (80 km) southeast of Nagasaki. However, another rash of poisonings occurred around the Agano River in Nugata, a region about 150 miles (240 km) north of Tokyo. Eventually, investigators identified more than 700 cases of mercury toxicity at Minamata, and more than 500 cases at Nugata.[42] The poisonings were traced to the consumption of large amounts of fish and shellfish which con-

[39]Jowsey, J., et al., "Effect of Combined Therapy with Sodium Fluoride, Vitamin D, and Calcium in Osteoporosis," *American Journal of Medicine,* Vol. 53, 1972, p. 43.

[40]"Skeletal Fluorosis and Dietary Calcium, Vitamin C, and Protein," *Nutrition Reviews,* Vol. 32, 1974, p. 13.

[41]King, B. G., A. F. Schaplowsky, and E. B. McCabe, "Occupational Health and Child Lead Poisoning: Mutual Interest and Special Problems," *American Journal of Public Health,* Vol. 62, 1972, pp. 1056-1058.

[42]*An Assessment of Mercury in the Environment,* National Academy of Sciences, 1978, p. 90.

tained methylmercury, an organic compound of the element that is much more toxic than its inorganic compounds. It appears that the chain of events which led to the buildup of methylmercury in the fish was as follows:

1. Certain industries discharged their inorganic mercury wastes into Minamata Bay and the Agano River.

2. The bay and the river contained abundant amounts of microscopic organisms which converted inorganic mercury into methylmercury. It also appears likely that the profuse growth of these organisms was promoted by the dumping of organic wastes into these waters.

3. The minute organisms which methylated and stored the mercury were eaten by larger forms of life, which in turn stored the methylmercury. Hence, the poisonous compound eventually became concentrated in the bodies of fish and shellfish.

Fig. M-114 depicts some of the ways by which mercury from mineral deposits may get into the foods eaten by man.

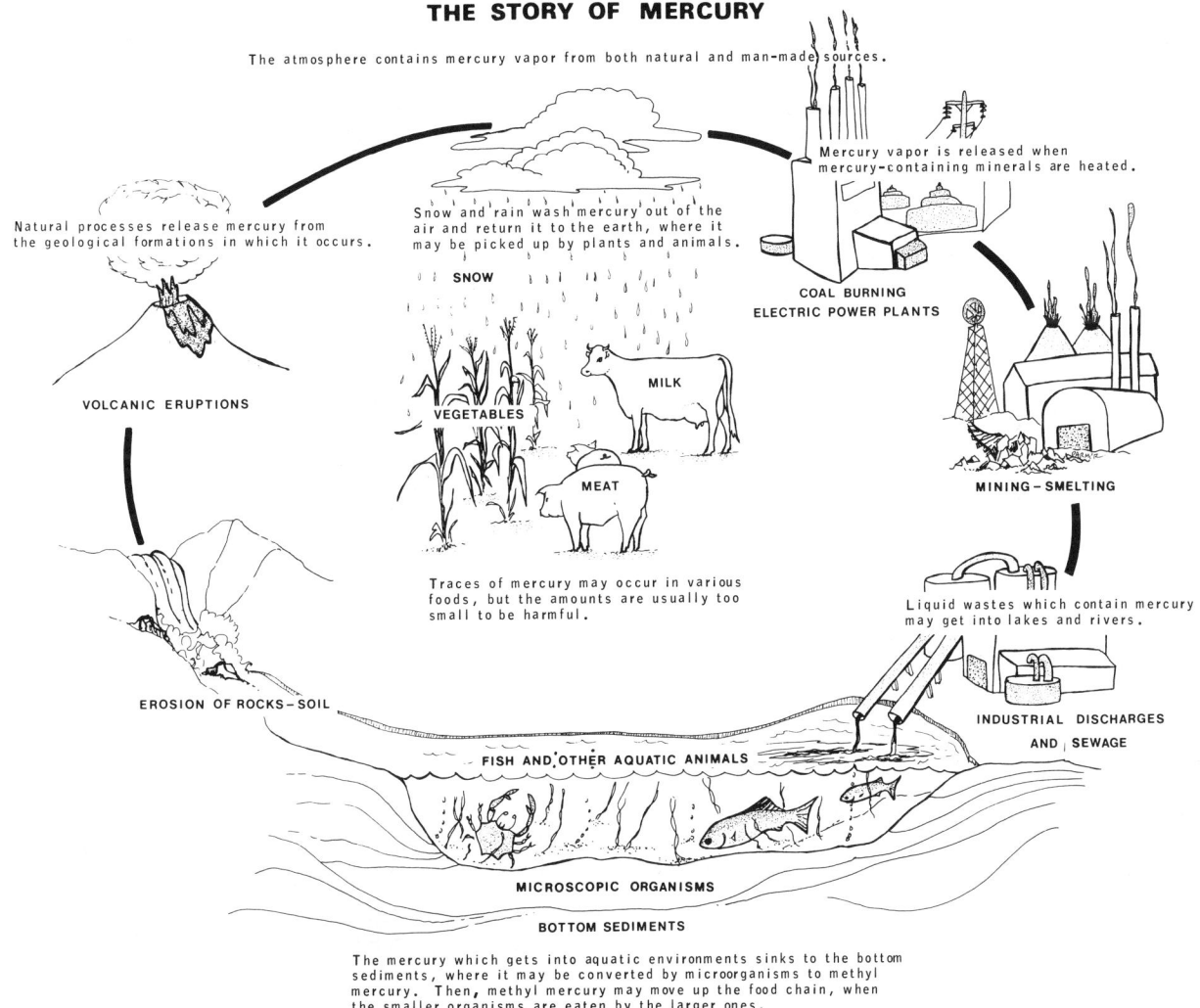

Fig. M-114. Natural and man-made pollution of the environment by mercury.

Another recent outbreak of mercury poisonings occurred in Iraq, where more than 6,000 people were hospitalized after eating bread baked from wheat seed that had been treated with a methylmercury fungicide.[43]

The poisonous seed grain had not been intended for human consumption; rather, it had been sent to Iraq for planting. Such fungicide-treated seed does not produce poisonous plants, because the methylmercury is detoxified in the soil.

Around the world, investigations were triggered by the

[43]*Ibid*, p. 91.

reports of mercury poisonings. Only a few people were found to have unmistakable signs of mercury toxicity, even though some had abnormally high levels of the metal in their tissues. Recently, it has been found that the essential trace mineral selenium sometimes protects people against the toxic effects of mercury. Hence, a food which contains both mercury and selenium may not be as dangerous as one which contains mercury alone. Furthermore, the selenium in one food might also provide some protection against mercury in other foods.[44]

(Also see POISONS, Table P-11 Some Potentially Poisonous [Toxic] Substances.)

• **Selenium**—Although it is suspected that people living in areas with high levels of selenium in the soil may occasionally suffer from such effects of selenium toxicity as dental caries and dermatitis, poisoned livestock commonly develop severe deformities; or they may even die from eating excessive amounts of this essential mineral. It is not that people are immune to severe poisoning from selenium; rather, the grains eaten by people are relatively low in selenium compared to the forage plants eaten by grazing animals. Furthermore, high selenium soils alone will not yield wheat containing abnormally large amounts of the mineral unless it is in a form which is readily available to the growing wheat. Usually, this requires that "selenium converter plants," such as *Astragulus racemosus,* be present to convert soil selenium to a form which is absorbable by wheat.

Fig. M-115 shows how various natural processes cause the foods produced in certain areas to be rich in selenium.

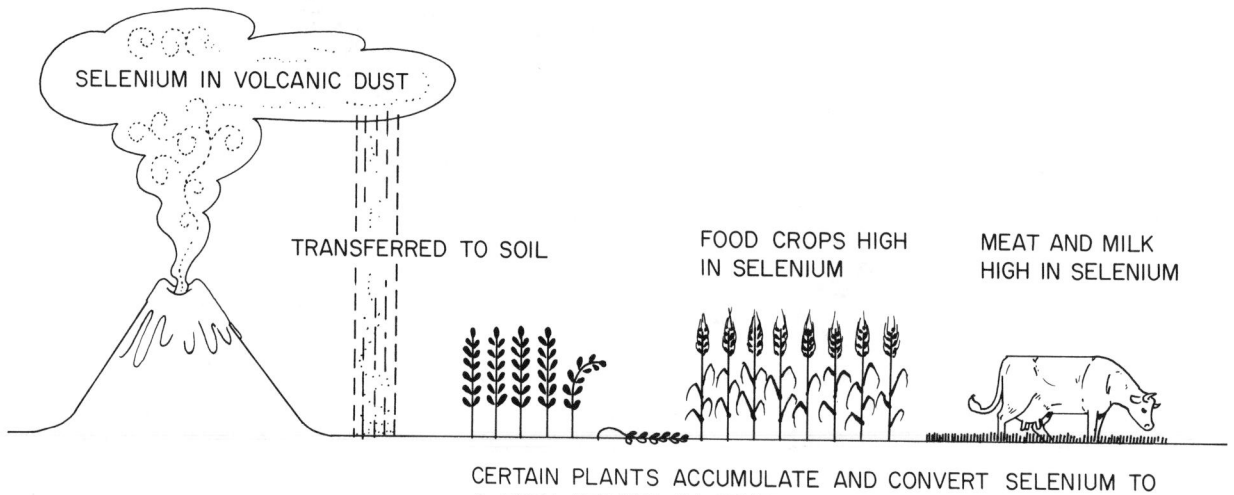

CERTAIN PLANTS ACCUMULATE AND CONVERT SELENIUM TO A FORM UTILIZED BY OTHER PLANTS

Fig. M-115.   The selenium chain. Natural factors which are responsible for the high levels of selenium that are found in certain foods.

In the event that conditions in high-selenium areas should be conducive to the poisoning of people, it is noteworthy that selenium toxicity may be counteracted by arsenic and copper, which are less toxic.

(Also see SELENIUM.)

• **Strontium**—This nonessential element, which is normally nontoxic, has an artificial radioactive isotope—strontium 90—that is produced in man-made nuclear reactions, such as those occurring during the explosion of nuclear weapons or during the generation of nuclear energy. Strontium 90 is toxic because it is absorbed by the body and deposited in the bones, where it continuously emits radiation which may cause such disorders as bone cancer and leukemia.

Strontium is chemically similar to calcium, and is likely to be mixed with this element in foods such as milk, vegetables, and cereals. Hence, it follows that the foods which are most frequently fed to infants and young children are those most likely to be contaminated with radioactive strontium. However, diets high in noncontaminated calcium tend to reduce the absorption of strontium 90.

In the long run, the best protection against the buildup of radioactive strontium in the environment is the cessation of nuclear weapons tests conducted in the atmosphere.

(Also see RADIOACTIVE FALLOUT.)

• **Zinc**—It is not likely that people will receive toxic excesses of zinc from eating ordinary, unsupplemented diets unless some of the foods were stored in zinc-coated (galvanized) containers, because most of the common foods contain only small fractions of the levels of zinc which may be ingested safely. However, zinc toxicity due to contamination of food by galvanized containers or

[44]"Mercury Toxicity Reduced by Selenium," *Nutrition Reviews,* Vol. 31, 1973, p. 25.

similar means may be accompanied by nausea, vomiting, stomachache, diarrhea, and fever.

Dietary and Medical Treatments. Various types of therapies may eventually lead to deficiencies or toxic excesses of certain essential minerals because they alter the ways in which the body absorbs, utilizes, retains, or excretes these nutrients. Often, countermeasures may be used to offset the undesirable effects of treatments, while retaining the desirable effects. Hence, the typical treatments and effects which follow are noteworthy:

• **Blood transfusions**—Sometimes, blood is given regularly, and over a period of time, to people with various diseases characterized by short-lived red cells. The danger of this practice is that it may lead to the overaccumulation of iron, since each pint of blood contains over 200 mg of the mineral, most of which is likely to be retained within the body.

• **Dialysis of patients with kidney failure**—Dialysis procedures, which are used to remove wastes from the blood of people whose kidney function is impaired, also remove essential minerals. Although certain procedures are designed to prevent the withdrawal of such major minerals as calcium, magnesium, potassium, and sodium, there is still the likelihood that various bloodborne trace elements will be reduced to deficient levels.

• **Dietary modifications**—Restriction or elimination of certain foods in order to produce diets which are low in carbohydrates, fats, or protein may lead to mineral deficiencies, unless great care is taken to provide other sources of the deleted elements. For example, it was found that some typical hospital diets tended to be deficient in copper, iron, magnesium, and manganese.[45]

Even more likely to lead to mineral deficiencies are the "crash diets" which cause rapid loss of weight primarily through loss of water, because there also may be excessive losses of minerals in the urine.

• **Intravenous administration of glucose and/or other nutrients**—Long-term maintenance of hospitalized patients on intravenous solutions may accentuate the effects of mild to moderate deficiencies of chromium, manganese, and zinc, because (1) each of these essential trace elements is involved, somehow, in the actions of insulin, and (2) increases in blood sugar add to the workload of the insulin-secreting system. Also, it is noteworthy that the solutions commonly used for total parenteral nutrition may or may not contain manganese and zinc, and that most do not contain chromium.

• **Pumping the stomach**—Normally, the minerals which are abundantly present in the digestive juices secreted by the stomach are almost totally absorbed in the intestine so that only negligible amounts of these essential substances are lost in the stool. However, the pumping of gastric fluid from the stomach results in the removal of large quantities of chloride and potassium ions, so that deficiencies of these elements may result, unless measures are taken to replace them.

• **Tube feeding**—When concentrated liquid formulas are fed too rapidly to sick people by stomach tube, there may be diarrhea, dehydration, and losses of both the minerals which are present in the formulas and those which are secreted in the digestive juices. The causes of these undesirable effects are (1) reductions in the secretion of the digestive juices which would normally dilute the formula, due to the illness and the unnatural means of feeding; and (2) the drawing of water from the intestinal wall by the formula, so that a strong laxative effect is produced.

Drugs Which May Affect the Utilization of Minerals by the Body. Certain commonly used drugs affect the utilization of both essential and nonessential minerals by the body. Furthermore, many of these medicines may be used to treat chronic conditions over long periods of time. Therefore, brief descriptions of the effects of some of the most frequently used drugs are presented, so that appropriate measures may be taken to prevent mineral deficiencies or toxicities:

• **Antacids**—The nonabsorbable types of these compounds, such as aluminum hydroxide, may form insoluble complexes in the intestine, which reduce the absorption of phosphate, fluoride, and other essential minerals. Furthermore, it recently became apparent that certain patients with kidney diseases who had been put on diets low in phosphate and who were given regular dialysis treatments absorbed considerable amounts of aluminum from antacids, because they developed toxic deposits of the metal in the brain and the bones.[46]

On the other hand, excessive consumption of antacids which yields such absorbable ions as calcium, magnesium, sodium, and bicarbonate may lead to toxic excesses of these ions in the body.

(Also see ANTACIDS.)

• **Antibiotics**—The tetracycline types of these drugs may form insoluble, unabsorbable complexes with such essential minerals as calcium, iron, and magnesium.

• **Anticonvulsants**—Epileptic patients given these drugs for the prevention of seizures have sometimes developed softening and distortion of their bones which may lead to rickets in children, or to softening of the bones (osteomalacia) in adults.[47] Apparently, the drugs produce their harmful effects on the bones by provoking increased rates of destruction of vitamin D and its active metabolites, so that the absorption and utilization of dietary calcium is reduced. Sometimes, their effects have been overcome by providing extra vitamin D and/or additional exposure to sunlight.

[45]Gormican, A., "Inorganic Elements in Foods Used in Hospital Menus," *Journal of the American Dietetic Association*, Vol. 56, 1970, p. 403.

[46]Alfrey, A. C., *et al.*, "The Dialysis Encephalopathy Sydrome," *The New England Journal of Medicine*, Vol.294, 1976, p. 184.

[47]"Anticonvulsant Drugs and Calcium Metabolism," *Nutrition Reviews*, Vol. 33, 1975, pp. 221-222.

• **Blood-cholesterol-lowering agents**—It is suspected that the types of these drugs which bind with cholesterol and bile salts in the intestine may similarly tie up calcium and other minerals so that their absorption is reduced.

• **Diuretics ("water pills")**—Usually, these drugs are given to people with water accumulation in their tissues and/or high blood pressure. Some of them may promote excessive urinary losses of potassium and other essential minerals.

• **Hormones**—Although the administration of adrenocorticotropic hormone (ACTH) and cortisone has often provided great relief for those who suffer from allergies and from inflammatory diseases like arthritis, the long-term use of these hormones has sometimes caused loss of bone minerals to the extent that weakening of the bones (osteoporosis) and/or collapse of the spine have occurred.

• **Laxatives**—Habitual use of these drugs may result in mineral deficiencies because they reduce the intestinal absorption of (1) dietary minerals, and (2) minerals secreted in the various digestive juices.

• **Mineral supplements**—The consumption of excessive amounts of certain minerals in the form of pills or tonics may lead to the deficiencies of other minerals, because there are diverse interactions between the various essential elements. For example, high intakes of iron may interfere with the absorption of copper, phosphorus, and zinc.

• **Oral contraceptives (birth control pills)**—The full details are still uncertain, but it appears that these drugs alter the metabolic processes which involve calcium, magnesium, and phosphorus.

Food Additives. Many natural and synthetic substances are added to foods to improve their color, odor, texture, and taste. The U.S. Food and Drug Administration has established strict regulations governing food additives so that there is little likelihood of any direct toxic effects resulting from the proper use of such ingredients. However, some of these substances affect the utilization of certain minerals. Such effects may not be important to people who eat a little of everything, but they may be responsible in part for mineral deficiencies or toxicities in people whose diets are narrowly limited by choice, economic circumstances, or other factors. Therefore, some effects of various food additives on mineral metabolism follow:

• **Aluminum compounds**—The amounts of aluminum that most people consume in the form of food additives—mainly present in such items as baking powder, pickles, and processed cheeses—are probably less than that ingested by people who regularly take aluminum-containing antacids. For example, 3½ oz (*100 g*) of one brand of processed American cheese was found to contain 70 mg of aluminum,[48] which is about the amount present in a single tablet of a commonly used antacid. Nevertheless, even small amounts of aluminum may form nonabsorbable complexes with essential trace elements such as iron.

• **Bran**—This product of flour milling is sometimes added to breads and cereals to increase their fiber content. However, it is rich in phytates, phosphorus compounds that bind many of the essential minerals so that they are not readily absorbed. It is noteworthy that the leavening of breads with yeast overcomes much of the effects of phytates.[49]

• **Chelating agents**—These additives are used to bind metallic mineral elements like copper, iron, and zinc, because the unbound forms of the minerals may promote the deterioration and/or discoloration of foods.[50]

The effects of added chelating agents may be beneficial, unfavorable, or uncertain with respect to mineral nutrition, because (1) foods may contain naturally occurring chelating agents which interact with the food additives; (2) some agents interfere with mineral absorption, while others enhance it; (3) sometimes, agents which enhance the absorption of metals also increase their urinary excretion; and (4) the overall mineral content of the diet often determines which of the various metals will be bound to the chelating agent(s), and which will remain free.

• **Gums**—These water-soluble mucilaginous materials may be added to a wide variety of processed foods to produce clarification (by binding with clouding agents), gelling, stabilization (prevention of the separation of various components), and thickening. Many of the gums used in foods are neither digested nor absorbed by man; hence, they may tie up essential minerals so that they are poorly absorbed. For example, sodium alginate—a seaweed derivative which is sometimes added to beers, cheeses, ice creams, salad dressings, sausages, whipped toppings, and wines—forms insoluble, nonabsorbble complexes with iron and copper.

• **Iodates**—Some nutritionists have expressed concern lest the use of these compounds as dough conditioners in the baking industry may lead to excessive consumption of iodine. Hence, it is noteworthy that the iodate fortification of bread for the prevention of goiter in Tasmania was accompanied by an increased incidence of iodine-induced overactivity of the thyroid gland (hyperthyroidism) in goiter-prone people.[51]

• **Iron**—In 1970, the American Bakers Association and the Millers' National Federation asked the U.S. Food and Drug Administration to triple the amount of iron permitted in the enrichment of flour and bread because there was

[48]Gormican, A., "Inorganic Elements in Foods Used in Hosptial Menus," *Journal of the American Dietetic Association*, Vol. 56, 1970, p. 399, Table 1.

[49]"Zinc Availability in Leavened and Unleavened Bread," *Nutrition Reviews,* Vol. 33, 1975, pp. 18-19.

[50]Furia, T. E., "Sequestrants in Foods," *Handbook of Food Additives*, 2nd ed., edited by T. E. Furia, CRC Press, Cleveland, Ohio, 1972, pp. 278-287.

[51]"Iodine Fortification and Thyrotoxicosis," *Nutrition Reviews*, Vol. 28, 1970, pp. 212-213.

widespread concern over iron-deficiency anemia in women and children.[52] However, it was strongly opposed by some of the leading blood specialists on the grounds that it might lead to toxic accumulations of iron in the tissues of susceptible people.

Finally, in late 1977, the FDA decided that there were too many unresolved questions regarding the safety of adding the proposed levels of iron to breads and flour, so they rejected the proposal by the bakers and the millers.

There is no evidence that the current amounts of iron which are added to foods pose any hazards.

• **Phosphates**—It has been estimated that the widespread use of phosphates as food additives may make the calcium to phosphorus ratio in the American diet as low as 1:4. This mineral imbalance may lead to poor absorption and utilization of dietary calcium, and perhaps even to certain bone disorders.

Sometimes, these effects may be prevented by extra dietary vitamin D, or by exposure to sunlight. However, newborn infants, whose kidneys do not excrete excess phosphate as well as those of older infants and children, may develop high blood levels of phosphate and have seizures when they are fed evaporated milk containing phosphate additives.[53] The seizures are attributed to the fact that cow's milk contains almost four times the calcium and over six times the phosphorus present in human breast milk.[54] Furthermore, extra phosphate is often added to evaporated milk to lengthen its shelf life. Hence, newborn babies fed evaporated milk (diluted with an equal volume of water) may receive between seven and eight times the phosphorus they would get from the same amount of human breast milk. An elevation of the blood level of phosphate causes a corresponding drop in the level of ionized calcium. The direct cause of the milk-induced seizures is the lack of sufficient ionized calcium in the blood.

Fortunately, such seizures have become much less of a problem in the United States, because (1) the use of commercial infant formulas which contain much less phosphate have essentially replaced the use of evaporated milk for feeding newborn infants; and (2) pediatricians generally advise mothers who neither breast feed nor use commercial formulas to either dilute fresh cow's milk, or use extra water in diluting evaporated milk.

Another problem which may result from high levels of dietary phosphate is the formation of nonabsorbable complexes with essential trace elements such as iron.

• **Sodium compounds**—It is suspected that high intakes of sodium may be one of the factors which lead to the development of high blood pressure in susceptible peo-

ple. Natural, unprocessed foods contain only small amounts of sodium compared to most commercially processed foods. Furthermore, in addition to being present in foods in the form of common salt (sodium chloride), sodium may also be present in such additives as sodium bicarbonate, monosodium glutamate, and various types of phosphates. Therefore, the consumer who is on a low-sodium diet must read carefully the labels of food products because items which are low in salt may contain liberal amounts of other sodium compounds.

(Also see SODIUM.)

Food Processing. The development of food processing has enabled man to modify such undesirable qualities of natural foods as bulkiness, toughness, susceptibility to spoilage, and in some cases, even toxicity. However, certain processes may detract from the mineral values of foods, while others may enhance them. The favorable effects are given in the section of this article headed, "Production and Preparation of Foods so as to Maximize Their Mineral Values." The details which follow cover some of the detrimental effects:

• **Canning fruits and vegetables**—Some of the minerals in canned fruits and vegetables escape into the packing fluid, which may be discarded. The amount of mineral loss depends upon such factors as the type of processing, degree of acidity of the packing medium, and the length of storage.

• **Cheese making**—During this process, milk is clotted by either acid or rennet (an enzyme-containing substance derived from animal stomachs) so that it separates into cheese and whey. Usually, much more calcium and phosphorus are lost in the whey from acid-clotted items like cottage cheese than from the rennet-clotted cheeses like Cheddar and Swiss.

• **Milling grains**—The greater part of the mineral content of grains is lost during milling because these elements are usually concentrated in the outer layers of the seed. Hence, such by-products of milling as bran, hominy feed, and rice polishings are excellent sources of many essential minerals. Usually, these by-products are fed to livestock, although they are sometimes added to special breads and cereals.

• **Refining sugar**—Most of the minerals that are present in raw sugar made from either sugarcane or sugar beets are (1) removed as the sugar is refined, and (2) end up in the crude molasses, which is a by-product. Cane molasses may be marketed for human consumption as dark molasses, or "blackstrap" molasses, but because beet molasses is bitter, it is sold as a feed ingredient.

Metabolic Disorders Which May Alter Mineral Metabolism. Various disorders of metabolism may interfere with the ways in which the body normally absorbs, utilizes, and excretes essential minerals, so that deficiencies and/or toxicities may result. Sometimes, the disorders produce conditions so precarious that the maintenance of the proper blood levels of sodium, potassium, calcium, and magnesium may become a matter of life or death. Brief descriptions of some of these medical problems are given so that the reader may realize

[52]"Anatomy of a Decision," *Nutrition Today,* Vol. 13, January/February 1978, pp. 6-7.

[53]Filer, L., Jr., "Excessive Intakes and Imbalance of Vitamins and Minerals," *Nutrients in Proposed Foods: Vitamins-Minerals,* (Papers from a symposium sponsored by the American Medical Association), Publishing Sciences Group, Inc., Acton, Mass., 1974, p. 27.

[54]Robson, *et al., Malnutrition: Its Causation and Control,* Gordon and Breach, Science Publishers, Inc., 1972, Vol. 1, p. 125, Table 12.

the importance of consulting a doctor before taking mineral supplements or making drastic dietary changes, since people differ widely in their susceptibility to these metabolic disorders. Metabolic disorders which may alter mineral metabolism follow:

• **Acidosis**—This condition is characterized by an excess of acid in the blood which may result from such diverse causes as diabetes; diarrhea; diets which are high in fat and protein, but low in carbohydrates; fever; kidney diseases; lung diseases; severe stress; starvation; or trauma. If prolonged, acidosis may lead to (1) excessive urinary loss of calcium and demineralization of the bones; (2) depletion of water, sodium, and potassium; and (3) retention of excessive amounts of phosphate and sulfate ions. The blood levels of potassium may be normal, even when the cells are low in the mineral. Hence, the feeding of injured, sick, or starved people must be done cautiously so as not to aggravate the imbalances in the body's mineral salts.
(Also see ACID-BASE BALANCE.)

• **Addison's disease**—Victims of this disorder have abnormally low secretions of adrenal cortical hormones, so they are unable to retain sufficient amounts of sodium and water in their bodies to counter such stresses as dehydration and low sodium diets. However, they may retain excessive amounts of potassium in their blood, which may cause cardiac arrest.
(Also see ADDISON'S DISEASE; and ENDOCRINE GLANDS.)

• **Alkalosis**—The main causes of alkalosis, which is an excess of alkali in the blood, are: (1) the consumption of large amounts of such absorbable antacids as sodium bicarbonate, (2) the loss of large amounts of stomach acid through vomiting, (3) the depletion of the body's supply of chloride ions through vomiting or diarrhea, and (4) excessively deep breathing—due to nervousness or overdoses of aspirin—which eliminates too much carbon dioxide. Alkalosis may be accompanied by the development of a potassium deficiency, due to an excessive loss of the mineral in the urine; and a reduction in the blood level of calcium ions, so that muscle spasms may occur.
(Also see ACID-BASE BALANCE.)

• **Congestive heart failure**—Abnormalities such as the accumulation of fluid in the tissues, and an overtaxing of the heart muscle, make the patient with heart failure extra susceptible to the toxic effects of imbalances between the blood and tissue levels of such ions as sodium, potassium, calcium, and magnesium. Extra magnesium and potassium may be given to prevent irregular heartbeats when digitalis is used as a medication. However, too much potassium may cause cardiac arrest, if the kidneys are not able to excrete excesses of this mineral in the urine.
(Also see HEART DISEASE.)

• **Cushing's syndrome**—This disorder is characterized by oversecretion of adrenal cortical hormones which cause the breakdown and loss of protein from the bones and muscles. Potassium is lost along with muscle protein, and the bone minerals—mainly calcium and phosphorus-are lost when the protein structure of bone breaks down. People with Cushing's syndrome often have an accumulation of salt and water in their tissues, a condition which gives rise to a rounded body "moon-face," and high blood pressure.
(Also see CUSHING'S SYNDROME; and ENDOCRINE GLANDS.)

• **Diabetes**—Uncontrolled diabetes is frequently accompanied by acidosis and ketosis—conditions characterized by excesses of acid and ketones in the blood—which may lead to depletion of bone calcium and of muscle potassium. It is noteworthy that the treatment of diabetes with insulin results in the rapid uptake of bloodborne potassium by the tissues. Hence, there may be a dangerous drop in the blood level of this mineral, unless extra amounts are given.
(Also see DIABETES MELLITUS.)

• **Goiter**—People with goiter may be overly susceptible to the toxic effects of excess iodine because their thyroid glands have become extra efficient in the utilization of this mineral. Therefore, they may develop oversecretion of thyroid hormones (hyperthyroidism) when given extra iodine. This toxic condition may sometimes be accompanied by the loss of calcium from the bones, and of potassium from the muscles.
(Also see ENDOCRINE GLANDS; GOITER; and IODINE.)

• **Hemolytic anemia**—Several types of anemias are characterized by an overly rapid breakdown of red blood cells, which may be caused by genetic, nutritional, and/or toxic factors. Administration of extra iron or blood transfusions to people with these disorders may be dangerous because the iron which is released during the destruction of red cells may accumulate in various tissues where it may cause damage.
(Also see ANEMIA.)

• **High blood pressure**—Sometimes, this condition results from a failure of the kidneys to excrete excess sodium, which promotes the accumulation of water in the body. Certain people appear to be overly susceptible to the effects of only moderate excesses of dietary sodium, so they should restrict their salt intake in order to avoid high blood pressure.
(Also see HIGH BLOOD PRESSURE.)

• **Ketosis**—The most common causes of this condition —which is characterized by an excess of ketones in the blood—are (1) diabetes; (2) diets high in fat and protein, but low in carbohydrate; (3) fevers; and (4) starvation. A mild ketosis in normally healthy people is usually not dangerous, unless it occurs regularly over a long period of time. Then, it may lead to such problems as (1) excessive urinary loss of sodium and water; (2) acidosis which provokes the loss of calcium from bone, and potassium from muscle; and (3) the accumulation of uric acid (a waste product of protein metabolism) in the blood, and sometimes in the soft tissues where it causes damage and pain (the latter disorder is commonly called gout). Uric acid buildup is usually treated with alkalizers to prevent the formation of kidney stones. However, the alkalizers may cause other alterations in mineral metabolism.

It is noteworthy that two men who lived for 1 year on a ketogenic diet consisting only of beef, veal, lamb, pork, and chicken lost about 300 mg of calcium from their bodies each day.[55]

(Also see DIABETES MELLITUS; MODIFIED DIETS; and STARVATION.)

• **Kidney diseases**—These disorders are usually accompanied by excessive loss of certain minerals in the urine and/or excessive retention of others, depending upon the parts of the kidney which are diseased. Kidney function may also be impaired whenever the blood supply to the organs is reduced, such as occurs in heart failure and shock. Furthermore, certain kidney diseases impair the metabolism of vitamin D, so that the utilization of calcium and phosphorus may be greatly reduced.

(Also see KETOSIS; and KIDNEY DISEASES.)

• **Lack of stomach acid**—Older people may have a deficiency of stomach acid. This may contribute to mineral malnutrition because acid is needed to offset the alkalinity of bile and pancreatic juice which tends to reduce the absorption of certain minerals.

• **Oversecretion of parathyroid hormone (PTH)**—This condition may be due to (1) a tumorous growth of the parathyroid glands, or (2) enlargement of the glands due to prolonged stimulation by a chronically low blood level of calcium ions. The hormone raises the blood calcium by causing its withdrawal from the bones. Hence, the chronic oversecretion of PTH may lead to such troubles as demineralization of bones, excessive excretion of phosphorus so that muscle weaknesses result, and deposition of calcium in tissues such as the kidneys.

(Also see CALCIUM; ENDOCRINE GLANDS: and PHOSPHORUS.)

• **Rickets**—This disease of infancy and childhood, which is usually due to a deficiency of vitamin D, is characterized by poor utilization of dietary calcium and phosphorus for the mineralization of bones. A similar condition, which may occur in adults, is called "softening of the bones" or osteomalacia.

(Also see CALCIUM; PHOSPHORUS; RICKETS; and VITAMIN D.)

• **Starvation**—The extreme deprivation of food is increasingly being used as a means to achieve a rapid loss in body weight, even though there may be such harmful effects as severe depletion of water, sodium, and potassium. These effects have often led to serious disorders of the heart, and even death—in cases of both voluntary and involuntary starvation. Furthermore, there

may be abnormal shifts of mineral salts and water between the tissues and the blood, so it may be difficult to decide how to rehabilitate starved people without aggravating their water and salt imbalances.

(Also see STARVATION.)

• **Vitamin D poisoning**—Overdoses of this vitamin may raise the blood calcium so high that the mineral forms harmful deposits in many of the soft tissues in the body. If this toxicity is prolonged, there may be demineralization of the bones since the high blood calcium is maintained at the expense of the bones. A similar, but milder type of poisoning may result from the overexposure of fair-skinned people to sunlight or other forms of ultraviolet light, such as sun lamps.

(Also see VITAMIN D.)

Mineral Composition of the Soil. There has been continuing controversy over how the mineral composition of the soil might affect the nutrient levels of the plants grown on it. The U.S. Food and Drug Administration has long maintained that (1) mineral deficiencies in soils may lead to reduced yields of plants rather than to plants containing subnormal levels of minerals; and (2) most people eat a wide variety of foods from different areas of the United States, so that variations in the mineral contents of foods tend to average out. On the other hand, certain proponents of organic farming may go so far as to assert that various human nutritional deficiencies may be due to the consumption of products grown on mineral-deficient soils. It is difficult to evaluate the information presented in support of each side of the controversy, because comparisons have often been made between different nutrients in different crops which have been grown on different soils.

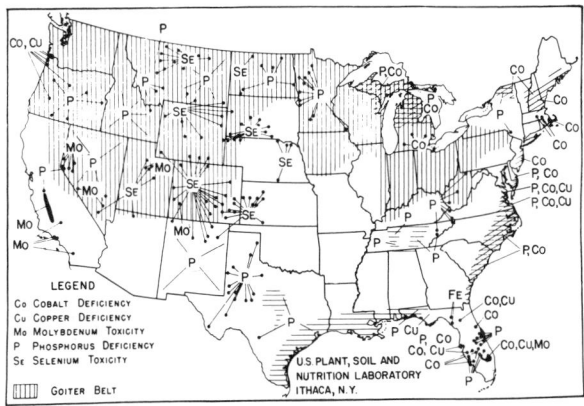

Fig. M-116. Known areas in the U.S. where mineral nutritional diseases of animals occur. The dots indicate approximate locations where troubles occur. The lines not terminating in dots indicate a generalized area or areas where specific locations have not been reported.

People need to be aware of any soil mineral deficiencies or of certain minerals that may cause toxicities because there is a direct and most important relationship between soil minerals and plant composition. (Courtesy, USDA)

[55]Randall, H. T., "Water, Electrolytes, and Acid-Base Balance," *Modern Nutrition in Health and Disease*, 5th ed., edited by R. S. Goodhart and M. E. Shils, Lea & Febiger, Philadelphia, Pa., 1973, p. 360.

Present research, together with practical observation, points to the fact that the mere evaluation of crop yields in terms of tons of forage or bushels of grain produced per acre is not enough. Neither does a standard food analysis (a proximate analysis) tell the whole story. Rather, there is a direct and most important relationship between the fertility of the soil and the composition of the plant.

The land surface of the earth is covered with many kinds of soil. Some of them naturally contain an abundant supply of most of the elements needed by both plants and animals. Other soils may have an abundant supply of most required elements and yet be deficient in one or more essential. For example, southwestern United States is known as a phosphorus-deficient area; northwestern United States and the Great Lakes region are iodine-deficient areas, and southeastern United States is a cobalt-deficient area.

At every step in the chain from soils to man, the essential mineral elements interact with other elements, and these interactions may profoundly affect the availability of essential elements or the amount of the essential element required for normal growth or metabolic function. For example, a high level of sulfate in the soil may depress the uptake of selenium by plants, and cause the people that eat the plants to suffer from selenium deficiency. The availability of zinc may be depressed if the diet is high in calcium. These and other interactions must be considered in assessing whether a given soil will supply plants with needed nutrients, and, in turn, whether plants will supply the people that consume them with needed nutrients.

Thus, the transfer of essential nutrient elements from soils to plants, thence to man, is a complicated process.

Some of the pathways and relationships of soil elements pertinent to human nutrition follow:

1. **Cobalt (Co).** Cobalt moves from the soil into plants. When plants are eaten by grazing cattle and sheep, the cobalt is combined with other materials in the digestive tract to form vitamin B-12, which then enriches the meat and milk from these animals. Areas of low-cobalt soils in the United States occur in the New England states and along the South Atlantic Coastal Plain.

Adding cobalt to soils, either as cobalt sulfate or as cobaltized superphosphate, can be used to increase the level of cobalt in plants and to prevent cobalt deficiency in cattle and sheep.

2. **Copper (Cu).** Copper is required by plants, animals, and man. In some parts of Australia, livestock production was impossible until copper fertilizers were used on pastures.

3. **Fluorine (F).** Low levels of fluorides have beneficial effects on teeth and bone structure. But excessive levels of certain fluorine compounds—from fumes and dust emitted from industrial plants, and from high levels of fluoride in water—are very toxic.

Where increased fluoride intake is desirable to prevent dental caries, carefully controlled direct additions to the drinking water are more promising than adding fluorides to soils that produce food crops.

4. **Iodine (I).** The relationship between the iodine levels of the soil and the incidence of iodine deficiency (goiter) in man is well known. Iodine is not required by plants. Nevertheless, if iodine is present in the soil, it is taken up by most plants and moves on into man's diet in forms that are effective in preventing goiter. However, there are important differences among plant species, and even among varieties of the same species, in their tendency to take up iodine from the soil.

Many of the iodine-deficient areas of the world have been identified and mapped. Thus, northwestern United States and the Great Lakes region are well-known iodine deficient areas.

The use of iodized salt is such an effective and low-cost way of supplying this element to people that there is little need to include iodine in fertilizers.

5. **Iron (Fe).** Iron deficiency is a serious problem in crop production in certain areas, and some nutritionists consider iron-deficiency anemia to be the most frequently observed mineral deficiency in people. Nevertheless, iron fertilization of soils is not likely to be effective in decreasing the incidence of iron deficiency in people. Actually, most soils contain plenty of iron; however, it may not be soluble. Some soils that are red from iron compounds contain too little available iron for normal plant growth.

6. **Magnesium (Mg).** The level of magnesium in plants is affected by soil content, plant species, and the presence of potassium. The leguminous plants (beans and peas) usually contain more magnesium than corn and other nonleguminous plants. Also, a very high level of available potassium in the soil interferes with the uptake of magnesium by plants; hence, magnesium deficiency in plants is often found on soils that are very high in available potassium.

7. **Manganese (Mn).** Manganese is required by plants, animals, and man. The uptake of manganese in food plants is more dependent on the acidity or alkalinity of the soil than on the amount of manganese used in fertilizers.

8. **Phosphorus (P).** When phosphorus is added to soils deficient in available forms of this element, increased crop yields usually follow. Sometimes the phosphorus concentration in the crop is increased, but this is not always the case.

Washington State University produced alfalfa hay on soils containing two different levels of phosphorus, then fed it to rabbits. The rabbits in the low-phosphorus group made slower growth, required more matings per conception, and had more fragile bones than the high-phosphorus group. There is reason to believe that soil nutrients affect animals and man similarly—in growth, conception, and soundness of bone; but more experimental work on this subject is needed.

(Also see PHOSPHORUS, section headed "Phosphorus Related Diseases.")

9. **Potassium (K).** Potassium is required by most plants and animals. Most soils contain an abundance of total potassium, but the level of available, or soluble, forms of potassium is frequently inadequate. The role of potassium fertilizers is to increase crop yields rather than to improve the nutritional quality of the crop produced.

10. **Selenium (Se).** Selenium is not required by plants, but it is required in very small amounts by animals and man. But the dividing line between requirement and selenium toxicity is very narrow, and excess selenium

produces toxicity.

In large areas of the United States, the soils contain little available selenium. Crops produced in these areas are low in selenium, and selenium deficiency in livestock is a serious problem. On the other hand, the soils in some areas of the Great Plains and Rocky Mountain states are rich in readily available selenium, with the result that the plants produced thereon are so high in selenium that they are poisonous to the animals that eat them.

In 1957, selenium was found to be essential in preventing liver degeneration of laboratory rats. Subsequent studies revealed that selenium compounds, either added to the diet or injected, would prevent certain diseases of lambs, calves, and chicks. Further, it was shown that diets high in vitamin E necessitated less selenium. In selenium-deficient areas of the United States, farmers and ranchers frequently inject young calves and lambs with small amounts of selenium to protect them from white muscle disease. Also, selenium is now being added to certain commercial livestock and poultry feeds. However, swine fed grains grown on selenium-rich soil which contain organic compounds of the mineral have more selenium in their muscle meat than similar swine fed equal amounts of selenium in the form of an inorganic compound added to their feed.[56]

(Also see SELENIUM.)

11. **Zinc (Zn).** Zinc was one of the first trace elements known to be essential for plants, animals, and man. The zinc content of grains and legumes may be raised by zinc fertilization of the soils upon which they are grown.

12. **Chlorine (C1)** is required by plants, animals, and man, but deficiencies of this element under practical conditions are relatively rare. The addition of salt (sodium chloride) to human diets has been a common practice for centuries. Salt accomplishes two things: (1) It improves flavor; and (2) it ensures an adequate intake of chlorine.

13. **Chromium (Cr)** is one of the most recent elements to be added to those required by animals and man. It appears that certain compounds of chromium activate insulin during sugar metabolism. Chromium is not required by plants.

14. **Silicon (S)** is an essential element for both plants and animals. However, it is one of the most abundant elements of the earth's crust and a major component of most soils.

15. **Sodium (Na)** is required by all animals. Adding salt to animal and human diets is the oldest known dietary supplementation practice.

16. **Sulfur (S)** is an important component of most proteins and an essential element of all living organisms. This element may be supplied by decaying organic matter or by inorganic salts called sulfates. However, cabbages which were grown on sand beds containing high levels of sulfate were goitrogenic (that is, they contained something that interfered with the utilization of iodine by the thyroid gland), whereas cabbages grown on similar beds which were low in sulfate had no goitrogenic activity.[57] The most goitrogenic plants contained the most sulfur.

Naturally Occurring Mineral Antagonists in Foods. Although there has been much recent praise of the virtues of natural, unprocessed foods, certain naturally occurring substances present in foods may interfere with the absorption and utilization of minerals by the body. Sometimes, these interfering substances or antagonists may contribute to the development of mineral deficiencies, when diets are barely adequate with respect to these nutrients. Hence, it is important to identify the most common types of naturally occurring mineral antagonists, such as—

• **Fiber**—Plant foods that contain large amounts of indigestible carbohydrate (fiber) tend to stimulate more rapid movements of the intestine, so that the absorption of minerals and other nutrients may be reduced. Another way in which fiber may reduce mineral absorption is by enveloping certain mineral elements so that they pass into the stool with the indigestible matter.

• **Goitrogens**—Certain plants contain substances called goitrogens, which interfere with the utilization of iodine by the thyroid gland, so that the gland becomes enlarged. An enlarged thyroid gland is called a goiter. The most common food sources of goitrogens are Brussels sprouts, cabbage, kohlrabi, rutabaga, and turnip. Even the milk of cows which have been fed substantial amounts of these plants may be goitrogenic. Also, it is noteworthy that soybeans contain a goitrogen, which may be rendered less toxic by heating.[58]

(Also see DEFICIENCY DISEASES, section headed "Major Dietary Deficiency Diseases"; and GOITER.)

• **Interacting minerals**—Excesses of various essential or nonessential minerals may reduce the absorption and/or the activity in the body of other minerals. Such interferences are most likely to happen when large excesses of special mineral supplements are taken. However, they may occur to a lesser degree when (1) the diet lacks variety, and disproportionate amounts of phosphate are obtained from foods like fish, meats, nuts, and poultry; and (2) most of the foods have been produced in a particular area where the environment is heavily contaminated with such toxic elements as arsenic, cadmium, copper, lead, mercury, and selenium.

(Also see Table M-67 for additional details on mineral interrelationships.)

• **Naturally occurring chelating agents**—Many naturally occurring substances in foods—such as amino acids and other organic acids like citric, oxalic, salicylic, and tartaric—may bind with (chelate) metallic mineral elements in the digestive tract. The effects of such chelating agents may be either beneficial or detrimen-

[56]Ullrey, D. E., "The Selenium-Deficiency Problem in Animal Agriculture," *Trace Element Metabolism in Animals-2*, edited by W. G. Hoekstra, *et al.*, University Park Press, Baltimore, Md., 1974, p.61.

[57]Wills, J. H., Jr., "Goitrogens in Foods," *Toxicants Occurring Naturally in Foods*, National Academy of Sciences, 1966, p. 5.

[58]*Ibid.*, p. 8.

tal, depending upon whether mineral absorption is enhanced or reduced. Also, the effects of chelating agents may be counteracted by dietary excesses of metal which are chemically similar, because such metals may compete for binding to the chelator. Therefore, it is not known at the present time whether these agents may have significant effects on mineral nutrition when ordinary, mixed diets are consumed.

• **Oxalates**—Nutritionists have long been concerned about whether oxalates, which are present in such foods as rhubarb and spinach, might bind with sufficient amounts of calcium and/or iron so as to produce deficiencies of these minerals. However, experiments have shown that such effects are not likely to occur in man unless (1) the mineral intake is marginal and (2) unusually large amounts of these foods are eaten, along with other sources of oxalates like almonds, beet greens, cashew nuts, cocoa, and tea.[59]

• **Phytates**—These poorly utilized compounds of phosphorus—which are present in the outer layers of grains—bind with such minerals as calcium, iron, and zinc and interfere with their absorption. Hence, mineral deficiencies may occur in people whose diets are composed mainly of whole grain breads. For example, diets based upon these breads were found to be the cause of combined zinc and protein deficiencies which led to stunting of growth and impaired sexual development of males in rural Iran.[60]

The interference of phytates with calcium absorption may be counteracted by supplemental vitamin D and/or exposure of the skin to ultraviolet light from the sun, or from an artificial source such as a sun lamp.[61]

Overconsumption of Alcohol.
Alcoholics may suffer from deficiencies of minerals such as magnesium, potassium, and zinc, provoked in part by erratic eating habits and in part by an increased urinary loss of these minerals due to the effects of alcohol.

Alcoholism may also increase the toxicity of certain dietary minerals by causing alterations in the ways in which the body absorbs, utilizes, and excretes these substances. For example, iron deposits in organs such as the liver, pancreas, and spleen may sometimes result from the enhancement of iron absorption by alcohol. Similarly, a moderate to heavy consumption of alcohol appears to have contributed to the cobalt poisoning of certain beer drinkers, because the amounts of cobalt ingested by these people were less than the doses of the mineral which have been used medicinally without such ill effects.[62]

Poor Food Choices.
Although a wide variety of foods rich in minerals is available in most supermarkets, people may eat only a few of them for reasons such as (1) lack of money to buy certain items, (2) dependence upon eating most meals away from home, (3) dislike of many types of nutritious foods, and (4) lack of knowledge of and/or the facilities for the preparation of various items. Even the consumption of a wide variety of foods may not guarantee the achievement of adequate mineral nutrition if most of the foods selected are high in fats and carbohydrates, but low in minerals.

Procedures Used in the Preparation of Meals.
The preparation of meals may involve procedures which result in the loss of essential minerals. These losses may be great enough to make the difference between adequate and inadequate mineral nutrition. Hence, the food preparation procedures that follow are noteworthy:

1. The thawing of frozen fish, meat, and poultry results in the loss of some of the juices, but data on their mineral content are scarce. Usually, the amount of fluid which is lost increases as the amount of cut surface increases. Thus, small cubes of beef for stewing will have greater losses than large pieces of meat. It may not always be safe to save the thaw juices from the food, because there may be considerable bacterial growth in the fluids during the period of thawing.

2. Large amounts of peelings and trimmings may be removed from fruits and vegetables during meal preparation. Often, the material which is removed and discarded may be richer in certain minerals than the part which is retained for eating. For example, the outer green leaves of cabbage may contain from 1.5 to 3 times as much iron as the inner bleached leaves.

3. Soaking vegetables in water prior to cooking tends to leach out some of the water-soluble minerals.

4. Cooking fruits and vegetables in lots of water, then throwing away the cooking water, is a sure way to lose plenty of minerals. For example, the boiling of cabbage led to the following losses of minerals: calcium, 72%; magnesium, 76%; phosphorus, 60%; and iron, 67%.[63] Boiling results in much greater losses of minerals than pressure cooking, baking, frying, steaming, or roasting. The greater the amount of cut surface, the greater the mineral losses. Hence, French cut green beans are subject to greater losses during cooking than cross cut beans.

Stress and Trauma.
Many types of stresses and traumas (the term used for sudden shocks, injuries, or wounds to the body) may alter various aspects of mineral metabolism. The reactions of the body to various types of stresses and traumas are similar because (1) such stresses as the deprivation of food or water, extremes of heat or cold, or emotional upsets may damage the body tissues in ways which are similar to the effects of

[59]Fassett, D. W., "Oxalates," *Toxicants Occurring Naturally in Foods*, National Academy of Sciences, 1966, pp. 259-264.

[60]Prasad, A. S., "Nutritional Aspects of Zinc," *Dietetic Currents*, Vol. 4, September/October 1977, p. 27.

[61]"Phytates and Rickets," *Nutrition Reviews*, Vol. 31, 1973, pp. 238-239.

[62]"Synergism of Cobalt and Ethanol," *Nutrition Reviews*, Vol. 29, 1971, pp. 43-45.

[63]Lachance, P. A., "Effects of Food Preparation Procedures on Nutrient Retention with Emphasis upon Food Service Practices," *Nutritional Evaluation of Food Processing*, 2nd ed., edited by R. S. Harris and E. Karmas, The Avi Publishing Company, Inc., Westport, Conn., 1975, p. 476.

trauma; and (2) most traumas provoke substantial increases in the secretion of stress hormones by the pituitary and adrenal glands. The prolonged secretion of abnormally high levels of stress hormones may lead to excessive losses of potassium, phosphorus, calcium, magnesium, and zinc in the urine. Usually, such conditions are accompanied by greater than normal retention of sodium and water, so that fluid sometimes accumulates in tissues and the blood pressure may be raised.

Bad burns produce effects somewhat different from those due to other stresses and traumas because substantial amounts of body fluid and mineral salts may be lost. Hence, burn patients are often very thirsty and drink large amounts of water, which can be dangerous because there may be excessive dilution of the body fluids and the salts which remain. A severe deficiency of sodium might occur under such conditions. Therefore, considerable care must be taken to replenish the body with the proper mixture of mineral salts and water. It is noteworthy that attempts to replace the large losses of calcium and phosphorus rapidly have sometimes led to kidney stones, because the body was unable to use all of the minerals which were provided, so the excesses were filtered through the kidneys.

Another factor which causes increased mineral loss in the urine after an injury is the confinement of the patient to a bed and/or wheel chair. It seems that a certain amount of physical activity is required for the maintenance of optimal bone mineralization.

DIAGNOSIS OF MINERAL DEFICIENCIES.
There are various degrees of mineral deficiencies, ranging from a mild depletion of the body's stores of the mineral(s), to severe clinical disorders which may result in disability or even death. Hence, it may be possible to improve health and increase longevity if mineral malnutrition is detected early by means such as those which follow:

Dietary Histories. Dietary patterns which might lead to mineral deficiencies may sometimes be discovered by (1) asking people to list the types and amounts of food that they usually eat; (2) calculating their mineral intakes with the help of food composition tables (see Food Composition Table F-36); and (3) comparing their mineral intakes with the mineral allowances which have been set by the Food and Nutrition Board of the National Research Council. These dietary histories may also reveal the presence of conditions that are known to interfere with the absorption and/or the utilization of certain minerals.

Table M-67, Mineral Table, gives the mineral allowances recommended by the Food and Nutrition Board, National Academy of Sciences. However, official allowances are given for only six essential elements, while estimated safe and adequate ranges of intakes are given for nine others, because limited data is available for establishing precisely defined intakes of the latter minerals.

The Recommended Daily Allowances in Table M-67, Mineral Table, may be used for purposes of comparing the official mineral allowances with the actual mineral intakes of people who may be eating inadequate diets. However, a person who consumes a diet which lacks sufficient amounts of certain minerals may *not* necessarily have deficiencies of these minerals because (1) individual needs for minerals vary widely; (2) other dietary and non-dietary factors affect the ways in which minerals are utilized; and (3) there may be stores of the minerals in that individual's body, which may be used to offset inadequacies of the diet. Nevertheless, the chances are that a markedly inadequate diet will eventually lead to nutritional deficiencies.

Calculating individual mineral intakes for large groups of people is an expensive and time-consuming procedure. Hence, a practical shortcut is to try to identify the most likely candidates for mineral deficiencies by scanning individual patterns of food selection. Some guidelines for identifying diets which may lead to certain mineral deficiencies follow:

1. **Calcium deficiency** may result from diets containing only small amounts of dairy products and/or green, leafy vegetables.
2. **Phosphorus deficiency** is likely only when the diet is low in protein foods.
3. **Iodine deficiency** usually occurs in areas where the soil is low in the mineral, unless iodized salt is used or there are such unsuspected sources of dietary iodine as (a) breads containing iodates as additives or (b) milk from cows which have been fed supplemental iodine, and/or which have had their udders washed with disinfectant solutions that contain iodine compounds.
4. **Iron deficiency** may often be due to lack of sufficient meat in the diet, because the forms of iron which are present in blood and muscle are utilized about three times as well as those in cereals, legumes, and vegetables; and about twice as well as those in fish.
5. **Magnesium deficiency** is not thought to be common in the United States, except among people whose diets consist mainly of highly milled grains and cereal products, and which are lacking in whole grains, leafy green vegetables, nuts, legumes, fish, and meats.
6. **Zinc deficiency** may occur in a mild form when the diet lacks meat, poultry, or fish.

Signs and Symptoms of Mineral Deficiencies.
Only a few clinical signs, such as a goiter which may result from an iodine deficiency, are specific indicators of certain mineral deficiencies. Other signs, like stunted growth, may be due to deficiencies of one or more minerals, vitamins, carbohydrates, fats, and/or proteins. (See Table M-67, Mineral Table, for a more complete coverage of the symptoms associated with various mineral deficiencies.) Hence, it is not wise to rely upon signs and symptoms for the early diagnosis of mineral deficiencies. Some other types of diagnostic measures are discussed in the next section.

Laboratory Tests for Mineral Deficiencies.
Tests for iron-deficiency anemia are widely used all over the world; but most of the tests for other mineral deficiencies are limited mainly to research studies, because

there is a lack of information regarding normal values for such groups as infants, children, adults, and pregnant or nursing mothers. Nevertheless, a growing number of commercial laboratories offer analyses of hair and/or urine directly to customers. These laboratories may also sell mineral and vitamin supplements to the people who use their services.

It is not wise for lay people to attempt to interpret laboratory tests for mineral deficiencies without the aid of a doctor, because many factors other than the diet may raise or lower the levels of minerals in the body liquids and the tissues. Therefore, some of the better-known types of diagnostic tests are covered briefly, so that the reader may be knowledgable when discussing them with his or her physician. These follow:

• **Blood levels of various minerals**—Mild to moderate deficiencies of minerals may not be detected by analysis of the blood, because in mild deficiencies blood levels of essential elements are maintained at the expense of tissue supplies. Hence, subnormal blood values are likely to mean that the mineral reserves have been depleted. Unfortunately, there are only a few convenient procedures for measuring minerals in the tissues.

• **Bone marrow biopsies**—This procedure involves the sampling (by means of a needle) of a small amount of bone marrow for its iron content. It gives an indication of the amount of iron which is stored in the skeleton. However, it is used mainly in research studies.

• **Hair levels of minerals**—Hair is one of the last tissues of the body to be nourished and one of the first to show the effects of poor nutrition. Hence, there is much current interest in the use of hair as a test medium for various mineral deficiencies and/or toxicities. New analytical methods are now available for the rapid analysis of hair for more than a dozen minerals, so certain laboratories offer this service to the public. Some of the merits and demerits of these tests follow:

1. Abnormally high amounts of arsenic, lead, and mercury in hair usually indicate internal poisoning by these toxic elements.

2. Subnormal levels of such trace elements as chromium, manganese, and zinc are usually correlated with deficiencies of these essential minerals.

3. Sometimes, the minerals in hair originate from environmental contamination—from hair dyes, shampoos, and swimming pool water, rather than from the diet.

4. Standards for the mineral content of hair should take into consideration the color of the hair because certain minerals are constituents of hair pigments. For example, blonde hair has lower ratios of zinc to copper than dark shades of hair.[64] Also, red hair contains more iron than other colors, because iron is present in the red

pigment.[65] Also, age and sex can affect hair analyses.

Many of the laboratories that analyze hair recommend supplements to correct deficiencies. It's no small coincidence, of course, that they just happen to sell the supplement that they are recommending.

(Also see HAIR ANALYSIS.)

• **Urinalysis**—Mineral deficiencies are likely to result in reductions in the amounts of the elements which are excreted in the urine, as the body attempts to conserve its dwindling supply of these essential nutrients. The trouble with urinalysis as a test for mineral nutrition status is that other factors, such as dehydration or stress, may raise or lower the rate of urinary excretion of minerals; hence, the effects of nutritional status alone cannot be readily measured.

• **X rays of bone**—X rays are used to diagnose demineralization of bones—which is usually due to deficiencies of calcium, phosphorus, and/or vitamin D—and the deposition of lead in the bones whch occurs in lead poisoning.

Often, tests such as those described are used in conjunction with tests of other metabolic functions, because the metabolic activities of certain minerals are not always correlated with the levels of the elements which are present in body fluids and tissues. For example, hair may be analyzed for its chromium content in order to determine whether a diabeticlike response to a glucose tolerance test is due to a lack of chromium in the form of the glucose tolerance factor (GTF).

More details on the detection of specific mineral deficiencies will be found in the articles dealing with each of the individual minerals.

PREVENTION AND TREATMENT OF MINERAL DEFICIENCIES AND/OR TOXICITIES.
The prevention and treatment of the various mineral deficiencies require the cautious use of mineral-rich foods or special supplements because (1) there is a narrow range between the safe levels and the toxic levels of such trace elements as iron, copper, fluorine, and selenium; (2) excesses of certain minerals are likely to reduce the absorption and utilization of others; and (3) large excesses of most minerals—except for potassium, sodium, and chloride—are not well absorbed, but are excreted in the stool. Therefore, lay persons should *not* dose themselves with "shotgun" amounts of mineral supplements; rather, they should limit themselves to more prudent measures, such as those which follow:

Selection of Foods Rich in Essential Minerals.
Foods which comprise the most vital tissues of plants and animals are likely to be the richest in essential minerals, because mineral elements participate in the important life functions of these organisms. Hence, the

---

[64]Eads, E. A., and C. E. Lambdin, "A Survey of Trace Metals in Human Hair," *Environmental Research*, Vol. 6, 1973, p. 251.

[65]Schwartz, I. L., "Extrarenal Regulation with Special Reference to the Sweat Glands," *Mineral Metabolism*, edited by C. L. Comar and F. Bronner, Academic Press, Inc., New York, N.Y., Vol. 1, Part A, 1960, p. 374.

animal products highest in mineral content are blood, bones, milk, and the vital organs, whereas leaves and seeds contain the highest levels of minerals found in the plant foods. Therefore, a mineral-rich diet may be assured by including a wide variety of such foods as dairy products; fish and other seafoods; meats and poultry (hearts, kidneys, and livers are much richer in minerals than the muscle meats); beans and peas; molasses; nuts; herbs; spices; tea; raw, unpeeled vegetables; and whole grain breads and cereal products.

Generally, foods which are only minimally refined contain the most minerals, because these elements are often present in the parts which are removed during processing. However, certain types of food processing may favorably alter the forms of the minerals present in foods so that these nutrients are better absorbed and utilized by the body. For example, yeast fermentation during the leavening of whole grain bread doughs is known to increase the availability of zinc and other minerals.

Production and Preparation of Foods to Maximize Their Mineral Values.

Sometimes, animals and plants which have been produced "naturally"—with a minimum of interference from man—are not as nutritious as they might be. Correction of certain soil deficiencies and problems may enhance the mineral value of plants, and, likewise, the supplementation of natural animal feeds may improve the nutritive value of meat, milk, and eggs. Also, the procedures used in processing foods and in preparing meals may contribute to better mineral nutrition. Therefore, it is worth noting how the mineral values of various foods may be maximized through careful attention to certain details of food production and preparation.

BENEFICIAL PRACTICES IN AGRICULTURAL PRODUCTION.

The profitable production of both animal and plant foods depends partly on the minerals which are provided by the farmers as supplements to the feedstuffs for livestock and as fertilizers for the soil. Although large excesses of certain elements will interfere with the utilization of other elements, it seems that small excesses—beyond the minimal amounts required for good production—may raise the levels of minerals present in the food products. However, this concept is highly controversial, so some of the evidence favoring liberal mineral supplementation for animals and plants follow:

1. Feeding livestock extra amounts of certain minerals like copper, iodine, manganese, selenium, and zinc tends to raise the levels of these elements in meat (including poultry) and eggs. But the amounts of mineral supplements which are required are considerably greater than the gains in mineral content of products achieved; hence, the method is inefficient.

2. Practices which encourage the growth of certain soil microorganisms may also enhance the uptake of minerals by plants because the microorganisms convert insoluble mineral compounds to more soluble forms, which are more readily utilized by plants. The growth of beneficial microorganisms in the soil is favored by (a) organic matter, which may be added as compost or manure; (b) the proper balance between acidity and alkalinity; and (c) minerals which are required by the microorganisms for growth and reproduction.

3. The improvement of mineral-depleted soils by balanced mineral fertilization has often resulted in both better overall crop yields and higher levels of certain minerals in individual plants. However, there are limits of the extent to which the mineral composition of plants may be improved by fertilization, because the utilization of minerals by plants is controlled mainly by genetic factors.

FOOD PROCESSING PROCEDURES WHICH RAISE THE MINERAL VALUES OF FOODS.

It is well known that certain types of food processing are detrimental to nutritive values. On the other hand, mention is seldom made of the types of food processing which either raise the level(s) of one or more minerals, or which alter foods in ways that make their minerals more available. Details follow:

1. The preparation of purees by homogenizing vegetables in water makes the iron in these items more available, because it breaks down the fibrous cell walls which enclose minerals and other nutrients.

2. Yeast fermentation which occurs during the leavening of whole grain breads breaks down the phytates (poorly utilized phosphorus compounds in the bran of the wheat grain) that interfere with mineral absorption.[66] Hence, there is better utilization of the minerals in such breads when yeast is used instead of baking powder.

3. The production of undistilled alcoholic beverages (beers and wines) from grains, grapes, and other plant materials appears to render minerals like iron more available for absorption. Alcoholic iron tonics have long been used to treat anemia. Also, alcoholic fermentation by yeast may convert the inorganic chromium which is present in various fermentable materials to the glucose tolerance factor (GTF)—an organically complexed form of chromium that augments the effects of insulin. (GTF has been found in beer and in yeast which has been grown on chromium-containing nutrient broths. Hence, it seems likely that yeast might similarly convert the chromium that is abundantly present in grape juice into GTF.)

(Also see BEERS AND BREWING; GLUCOSE TOLERANCE FACTOR; and WINE.)

4. Cheese making may raise or lower the amount of calcium in 100-Calorie (kcal) portions of the product compared to the original milk because variable amounts of calcium, phosphorus, protein, and lactose are lost in the whey, depending upon whether the milk is clotted with

---

[66]"Zinc Availability in Leavened and Unleavened Bread," *Nutrition Reviews*, Vol. 33, 1975, pp. 18-19.

rennet, or with acid alone. Table M-68 shows how the contents of calories, calcium, and phosphorus vary between milk and several types of popular cheeses.

TABLE M-68
SELECTED COMPONENTS OF MILK
AND FOUR TYPES OF CHEESES[1]

Component	Milk[2]	Cheddar Cheese	Swiss Cheese	Cottage Cheese
Calories .. (kcal/100 g)	62	402	372	90
Calcium ... (mg/100 g)	119	718	961	68
Phosphorus .... (mg/100 g)	89	510	605	150
Calcium in 100 kcal portion of food ....(mg)	192	179	258	76
Calcium to phosphorus ratio	1.33:1	1.41:1	1.59:1	.45:1
Amount of product needed to supply 800 mg calcium .... (oz)	23.7	3.9	2.9	41.5
.... (g)	672	111	83	1,176
Amount of energy which must be consumed to obtain 800 mg calcium ... (kcal)	417	446	309	1,058

[1]The food composition data were obtained from Food Composition Table F-36 of this book.
[2]Milk which contains 3.5% fat.

Dieters seeking to cut down their caloric intake while obtaining most of their calcium requirements from dairy products can use a few ounces of Swiss and/or Cheddar cheeses instead of cupfuls of whole milk or cottage cheese. However, each unit of calcium from Cheddar or Swiss cheese costs about 50% more than an equivalent amount from fresh whole milk.

5.   The extraction of fat from soybean products prior to production of flour may raise the ratio of the mineral content (as represented by ash content) to the caloric content by more than 60%. This means that the consumer gets more minerals, but fewer calories, when defatted soybean products are selected.

6.   Ascorbic acid (vitamin C) is a beneficial food additive because it converts oxidized iron to the reduced form, which is better absorbed. Also, the addition of sulfites (substances used to prevent discoloration and/or microbial growth) to foods may indirectly promote better utilizatin of iron, because these additives preserve ascorbic acid against oxidation.

7.   The use of limewater (calcium hydroxide solution) in the production of tortillas (flat, thin cakes made of corn meal) adds about 100 mg of calcium per 100 g of product.

8.   Heat treatment of soybeans improves the utilization of copper, iron, manganese, and zinc from this food because it inactivates a metal-binding constituent.

MEAL PREPARATION PRACTICES WHICH CONSERVE ESSENTIAL MINERALS.
It may not have been too important for prehistoric man to minimize the loss of mineral nutrients during cooking because the lack of laborsaving devices made it necessary to eat large amounts of food so as to provide for great expenditures of energy. Today, people expend much less energy and eat considerably less food; so, it is now necessary to use better methods of meal preparation. Some guidelines for conserving minerals follow:

1.   Soaking spinach and rhubarb in water removes some of the oxalic acid from these items so that dietary minerals are better utilized. Oxalic acid forms insoluble, unabsorbable compounds with calcium, iron, and other minerals.

2.   Cleaning fruits and vegetables with a stiff brush is preferable to peeling them, because the outer layers of many items are much richer in minerals than the inner parts. Hence, the mineral losses due to peeling may be disproportionately high for the amount of material that is removed.

3.   It is better to purchase smaller amounts of fresh, leafy vegetables more frequently than to store large amounts in the refrigerator for long periods of time, because cutting down on storage time minimizes wilting and the need to discard the wilted outer leaves, which are the richest in minerals.

4.   The loss of minerals during pressure cooking or steam cooking of vegetables is significantly less than that during boiling. Other ways of cooking which conserve minerals are baking and microwave heating. When other conditions are the same, mineral losses may also be minimized by cooking vegetables in large pieces rather than small pieces, and by keeping the cooking time as short as possible.

5.   There are considerable amounts of minerals in the packing fluids used in most canned foods, so the fluids should be saved and used whenever feasible.

6.   The thawing of frozen foods results in losses of minerals with the juices which escape during thawing. Freezing food ruptures cell walls so that the cell contents escape readily during thawing. Although the thaw juices might be used in meal preparation, it may be dangerous to do so if there has been considerable time for the growth of microorganisms during thawing. Hence, it may be desirable to cook frozen foods without preliminary thawing so that the juices which escape may be used safely.

Microwave heating may be preferable to other ways of cooking unthawed frozen foods because when food is penetrated by the microwaves cooking proceeds uniformly throughout, whereas in other ways of cooking the heat acts mainly on the outside of the food, which may become overcooked, while the interior is undercooked.

ENRICHMENT AND FORTIFICATION OF FOODS WITH MINERALS.
Extra minerals may be added to foods so as to (1) to restore those lost during processing (such restoration is called *enrichment*), or (2) to make certain popular foods are richer in various nutrients than is natural for these items (this process is called *fortification*). For example, the level at which iron is added to white flour and other refined cereal products constitutes enrichment or restoration of the iron lost during milling, whereas the addition of iron to milk-based infant formulas is fortification, because milk is normally low in iron.

From such early beginnings as the iodine fortification of salt in the 1920s, and the enrichment of flour and bread with iron and vitamins in the 1930s, the addition of essential minerals has been extended to both traditional foods and new items which have been recently concocted by food technologists. Therefore, it is important to be knowledgeable relative to the following items that may be enriched or fortified with minerals:

• **Breakfast cereals**—Many of these items are made from highly milled grains, so they are often fortified with vitamins and iron, and sometimes with calcium. However, milling removes large amounts of other minerals like magnesium, chromium, manganese, copper, zinc, selenium, and molybdenum, which are not usually added during enrichment or fortification, unless the manufacturer does so indirectly by adding wheat germ, bran, or rice polish to his products. (The by-products of milling removed from the whole grains are rich sources of the minerals.) Hence, the consumer receives better overall mineral nutrition with whole grain cereals than with those made from refined grains which have been enriched or fortified with one or two minerals.

• **Complete diet formulas**—There are various types of powders and liquids, which usually contain skim milk or other sources of protein, that are fortified with minerals and vitamins so that they may be taken instead of regular meals. Nevertheless, they are not likely to contain adequate amounts of such newly discovered trace minerals as chromium, selenium, and silicon, because these elements are not usually added to the products. Hence, the formulas are best used as replacements for only one or two meals per day, so that the missing minerals may be obtained from regular foods.

• **Flour, grains, and bakery goods**—Usually, iron is the only mineral used to enrich these products when they are made from milled grains. It may be wise to avoid these items and select whole wheat or bran breads and muffins, and brown rice, unless the rest of the diet makes up for the mineral deficiencies in the highly refined products.

• **Imitation foods or analogs**—High prices for such staple foods as fruit juices, milk, ice cream, butter, meats, and poultry, along with the concern over the cholesterol and fat content of certain of these foods, have stimulated the development of imitation products or analogs. These products are made from lower-cost materials, like soybean derivatives, and they are usually fortified with minerals, vitamins, and amino acids so as to be nutritionally equivalent to the items which they are designed to replace in the diet.

Analogs are generally wholesome and nutritious for most healthy people. However, those who are prone to heart disorders and/or high blood pressure should note that (1) some of the soybean-based imitations of meats and poultry contain much more sodium than the authentic animal products, and (2) artificial fruitlike drinks may contain little or none of the potassium present in real fruit juices, which are often prescribed as sources of the mineral for therapeutic diets. Hence, there is a need for more extensive nutritional labeling on the packages of imitation foods.

• **Infant cereals**—These products generally provide better mineral nutrition than the breakfast cereals designed for older children and adults, because they are often fortified with calcium, iron, copper, and other minerals. Of course, whole grain cereals are also good, but the fiber they contain may have too much of a laxative effect on infants.

• **Infant formulas**—The manufacturers of these products have usually designed them to be nutritionally equivalent to human breast milk, perhaps with the following notable exceptions:

1. The calcium and phosphorus levels in the formulas may be considerably higher than those in human milk, but they are usually somewhat lower than those in fresh or evaporated cow's milk. Newborn infants may have seizures if they are fed excessive amounts of phosphorus. Hence, the formulas are safer than either undiluted, fresh cows' milk or evaporated milk diluted with only an equal volume of water.

2. The iron levels may be unusually high in certain formulas, because it is believed that the very low levels of this mineral in both human and cow's milk may sometimes be responsible for the development of anemia in infants and children.

• **Instant breakfast powders**—These powders, which are usually designed to be mixed with a glass of milk, are fortified with minerals and vitamins so as to supply at least one-fourth of the daily nutrient requirement for an adult. Probably they supply better balanced mineral nutrition than most people regularly receive from ordinary types of breakfast foods. However, they may not be suitable for people prone to constipation, unless the low fiber content of the formulas is offset by eating pulpy fruits or drinking unstrained juices.

• **Milk**—Minerals are not usually added to ordinary cow's milk, but vitamin D is usually added, so that the calcium and phosphorus which are present in the milk will be well utilized.

• **"Nutrified" cakes, cookies, and food bars**—The new term *nutrification,* which is derived from the words nutrient and fortification, was coined by food scientists to denote the providing of nutrients through fabricated, fortified foods such as snack cakes, cookies, food bars, and "chips" laced with minerals, vitamins, and amino acids. However, some of these products are too high in fats and/or sugars to be used by sedentary adults, who might easily eat too much of these concentrated sources of calories.

• **Salt**—Slightly more than half of the salt sold at the retail level is fortified with iodine for the purpose of preventing iodine-deficiency goiter.

Special Dietary Products. The use of special foods and mineral supplements may be justified when it appears that the diet is deficient in certain essential elements. Ordinary diets may not suffice to meet mineral needs under circumstances such as (1) pregnancy; (2) breast feeding of infants; (3) illnesses which depress the appetite; (4) types of malnutrition that require rapid restoration of the body's supply of certain minerals (*these conditions require the attention of physicians who are proficient in nutritional therapy*); (5) sharp restrictions in caloric intake in order to achieve rapid reduction in body weight; or (6) shortages of wholesome, nutritious foods.

The authors do *not* wish to suggest that any of the conditions just mentioned are to be treated with special dietary products; rather, they wish to point out that certain products may be used to fill the gaps in mineral nutrition which may result from inadequate diets. Furthermore, the nutritional assessment of diets and the selection of products to provide minerals may be hazardous for a lay person to undertake without the assistance of a doctor or a dietitian. Unfortunately, this type of assistance is not always readily available. Hence, some practical guidelines are presented with the hope that they may help to counteract the current tendency for many people to select nutritional products on the basis of questionable advertising claims.

SPECIALTY FOODS AND HIGHLY POTENT NUTRITIONAL SUPPLEMENTS.   It is fortunate that most consumers are not able to purchase pure mineral salts and to mix them into their foods, because without special measuring equipment and experience in preparing such mixtures, it is very easy to add toxic excesses of trace elements like iodine and selenium to foods. However, even some of the products that are sold by health food stores may have undesirable, or even toxic effects, because they are very rich in certain minerals. The potentially hazardous products may be considered as "highly potent nutritional supplements," in order to distinguish them from the less potent specialty foods, which are usually safe in the amounts consumed. Table M-69 shows the approximate amounts of these minerals that are provided by various specialty foods and nutritional supplements.

TABLE M–69
AMOUNTS OF SELECTED MINERALS IN SOME SPECIALTY FOODS AND NUTRITIONAL SUPPLEMENTS[1]

Product	Macrominerals					Microminerals					
	Calcium (Ca)	Phosphorus (P)	Potassium (K)	Sodium (Na)	Magnesium (Mg)	Iron (Fe)	Zinc (Zn)	Copper (Cu)	Selenium (Se)	Iodine (I)	Chromium (Cr)
	(mg/100 g)	(mg/100 g)	(mg/100 g)	(mg/100 g)	(mg/100 g)	(mg/100 g)	(mg/100 g)	(mg/100 g)	(mcg/100 g)	(mcg/100 g)	(mcg/100 g)
SPECIALTY FOOD:											
Alfalfa (leaf) powder	1,640	230	2,070	60	350	36.0	1.6	1.0	28	—	—
Almonds, dried	234	504	773	4	293	4.7	3.1	1.2	—	—	—
Bran	119	1,276	1,121	9	598	11.0	10.4	1.3	63	6	40
Flaxseeds	271	462	1,460	30	400	9.0	—	—	—	—	—
Nonfat milk, dried, powder	1,308	1,016	1,794	532	144	.3	4.1	.5	—	—	12
Peanuts, roasted w/skins	72	407	701	5	175	2.2	3.0	.3	—	—	—
Rice polishings	69	1,106	714	100	650	16.1	2.6	.7	—	7	—
Sesame seeds	131	776	407	40	347	7.8	10.3	1.6	—	—	—
Soybean flour (low fat)	263	634	1,859	1	289	9.1	2.0	1.6	—	—	—
Sunflower seeds ...	120	837	920	30	38	7.1	4.6	1.8	—	—	—
Wheat germ, toasted	47	1,084	947	2	365	8.9	15.4	1.3	111	—	25
NUTRITIONAL SUPPLEMENT:											
Blackstrap molasses	684	84	2,927	96	209	16.1	2.2	6.0	—	158	115
Bone meal	29,820	12,490	180	5,530	320	85.0	12.6	1.1	—	—	—
Brewers' yeast.....	210	1,753	1,894	121	231	17.3	3.9	3.3	125	—	118
Dolomite..........	22,080	40	360	—	9,870	76.0	—	—	—	—	—
Kelp	1,904	240	5,273	3,007	213	89.6	3.5	.6	43	62,400	Trace
Liver, dried, powder	40	830	930	450	—	20.0	—	9.0	180	—	170
Torula yeast.......	424	1,713	2,046	15	165	19.3	1.9	1.4	132	—	—

[1]A dash indicates a lack of authoritative data, *not* that the mineral is absent.

It may be seen from Table M-69 that it is safer to use specialty foods as sources of minerals than it is to use highly potent nutritional supplements because the former contain considerably lower levels of minerals than the latter, so the chance of receiving dangerous excesses of any of the elements is much less. For example, 3½ oz (*100 g*) of wheat germ contain about half of the daily allowance for copper, whereas an equal amount of liver powder contains seven times as much of the mineral. Furthermore, the contents of protein, vitamins, and other nutrients in the different products vary considerably. Hence, it is desirable to use a variety of these items, rather than a single one, to meet specific mineral needs. Some guidelines for using the various products follow.

Specialty Foods. The following items are good to excellent sources of energy, minerals, protein, and vitamins; so, they may be used by themselves as foods, or they may be mixed with other items:

• **Alfalfa (leaf) powder or tablets**—Because of its grasslike taste, alfalfa powder should be mixed with other foods like baked goods (not more than a tablespoon per cup of flour), thick vegetable soups, or "green sauces" for pasta. It is noteworthy that the flavor of alfalfa blends well with mint or spices. Alfalfa is also available in the form of tablets that contain no other ingredient. Tablets avoid flavor problems because they may be swallowed whole. Alfalfa powder is an excellent source of calcium, iron, and magnesium.

• **Almonds, dried**—Although these nuts cost about twice as much as peanuts, they may be worth the price because (1) they are tasty without salt, and (2) their mineral content is higher than peanuts (three times the calcium, one and one-half times the magnesium, and two times the iron). Many people eat them plain, but they are also good in toppings, coatings (such as fish almondine), or in pastries and other desserts. Almonds, like other nuts, are also good sources or protein, polyunsaturated fats, and vitamins. Also, they are easy to carry while backpacking or on other pleasure trips, or when on business trips.

• **Bran**—This product has about nine times the overall mineral content of white flour. It may be (1) used alone as a cereal (a little goes a long way, because it soaks up liquid and is, therefore, very filling); (2) mixed with other cereals; (3) used as a breading for baked, broiled, or fried foods; or (4) mixed with chopped fish, meat, and poultry as a filler which aids in the retention of their juices. However, bran may have a laxative effect on some people, varying according to the amount eaten and individual susceptibilities. So, it should be added cautiously to the diet, in small amounts, until the level of tolerance is known. Also, plenty of liquid should be taken with bran, or it may cause irritation in the digestive tract. Bran is an excellent source of many of the essential minerals.

• **Flaxseeds**—These seeds, when ground, have long been used as the basis of various "natural" laxative preparations. They contain a mucilaginous material which thickens the porridge that is formed when they are cooked in water with other grains. Their bland taste makes it convenient to add them to various cereal products, where their ample supply of calcium, iron, and magnesium adds to the mineral values.

• **Nonfat milk powder**—This product, when mixed with water, yields a drink which is equal in mineral value to whole milk, but which is lower in calories. However, even greater mineral nutrition may be promoted by adding the dry powder to various foods, to which it contributes calcium and magnesium. For example, it blends well with the other ingredients in items such as cooked cereals, doughs, fudge-type candies, puddings, coffee, cocoa, and tea. Furthermore, milk sugar—lactose, which is abundantly present in nonfat milk powder, appears to promote the absorption of calcium and other essential elements.

• **Peanuts**—Peanuts and peanut butter are often used as meat substitutes, because of their protein content. However, they contain much more calcium, chromium, copper, magnesium, and calories than do muscle meats. Like almonds, they may be eaten alone, or in various combinations with other foods.

• **Rice polishings**—This product, like wheat bran, contains the minerals removed from whole grains (brown rice) during milling. It is an excellent source of iron, magnesium, and the vitamin B complex. The bland taste makes it a good additive for fortifying baked items, breading, and breakfast cereals.

• **Sesame seeds**—These seeds are often sprinkled over breads, cookies, crackers, and rolls. Like peanuts, they outstrip muscle meats in their content of several minerals and calories. Sesame seed butter (which resembles peanut butter) is sold in many health food stores.

• **Soy flour**—Usually soybeans have had most of their fat removed by crushing and extraction prior to being ground into flour. Hence, soy flour contains more minerals, but fewer calories, than most nuts and seeds. It is a good source of calcium and magnesium, as well as protein and certain vitamins. However, the use of this product is limited by (1) the beany flavor; and (2) its content of certain carbohydrates, which ferment in the digestive tract to form gas. Some ways of overcoming these disadvantages are: (1) adding soy flour to highly spiced foods like gingerbread cookies and ground sausage meat, so that the beany taste is disguised; and (2) using small amounts of soy flour at first, until the limit of one's tolerance to the gas-producing effects is determined.

• **Sunflower seeds**—Although many Americans formerly considered this chewy product to be best suited for feeding birds, it is now sold as a snack food. The seeds keep very well without refrigeration, because of their protective outer covering. Their content of copper and iron, along with protein and vitamins, makes them a much better snack item than popcorn, potato chips, and sweets. Some health food stores carry sunflower seed butter and sunflower seed meal; but these items sometimes have a bitter taste, which may be due to rancidity that develops when the seed is crushed and the oil exposed to the air.

• **Wheat germ**—This by-product of wheat milling has about the same overall mineral content as bran, but it is better digested and it provides more protein, calories, and vitamins. Also, it ranks close behind the vegetable oils as a source of vitamin E. It may be used alone as a breakfast cereal, or it may be added to various cereal products.
(Also see BREAKFAST CEREALS; and WHEAT.)

Highly Potent Nutritional Supplements. The following products should be used with caution so as to avoid overdoses of certain minerals or other potentially harmful substances:

- **Blackstrap molasses**—About two heaping tablespoons (40 g total) per day of this thick, sugary fluid will furnish liberal amounts of calcium, magnesium, chromium, copper, iodine, iron, and zinc. However, many people may find its licoricelike taste too strong for their liking when they attempt to take it alone, like a tonic. Also, it may be a strong laxative for some people. Hence, it might be mixed cautiously into other foods where its flavor may be either diluted or masked by other strong flavors. For example, it may be added to items like (1) a glass of milk, because the addition of 1 teaspoon (5 ml) of molasses per 1 or 2 teaspoons of carob powder makes a drink that is more nutritious than chocolate milk; (2) spice cakes or gingerbread cookies, which may also contain added soy flour; or (3) pumpernickel or other dark breads leavened with yeast, because the yeast may convert the inorganic chromium from the molasses into the glucose tolerance factor, an organic form of the mineral, which acts along with insulin in promoting the metabolism of carbohydrates.

(Also see MOLASSES, section headed "Food.")

- **Bone meal powder or tablets**—A little of this item goes a long way. A teaspoon of the powder provides over 1,000 mg of calcium, which appears to be more than enough for people other than pregnant or nursing mothers. Tablets may be more convenient than powder for most people, who usually lack scales for accurately measuring small quantities of powder. However, if the powder is to be mixed into such items as cereals, doughs, gravies, and sauces—*not* more than ¼ teaspoon per person per serving should be used. Careful trials should be conducted on a small scale, before adding the powder to recipes, because bone meal imparts a slightly gritty texture to foods.

- **Brewers' yeast powder or tablets**—This special product has long been used to prevent or treat malnutrition by providing extra protein and the vitamin B complex. However, it is also one of the richest sources of both chromium and selenium—minerals that are likely to be supplied inadequately by ordinary diets. Furthermore, the chromium is present in an organic form (glucose tolerance factor) which is much more beneficial to the body than the inorganic forms of the mineral.

Brewers' yeast is also rich in nucleic acids, which are substances that may cause certain susceptible people to develop high blood levels of uric acid (hyperuricemia) and/or gout. These disorders tend to run in certain families, so it may be wise to inquire whether any close relatives have had these disorders, before taking this supplement on a regular basis.

A suitable daily portion of the dried yeast—for people who are *not* prone to either hyperuricemia or gout—is 1 or 2 tablespoons (15 or 30 ml). It may be mixed in vegetable drinks like tomato juice, cooked cereals, flavored instant breakfast drinks, gravies, meat loaves, or various sauces. If there is a choice of product, one that is "debittered" should be selected. Tablets are also available for those who prefer a more convenient form of the product.

- **Dolomite tablets**—Usually, each tablet supplies about 130 mg of calcium, and about 60 mg of magnesium. Four such tablets daily should be an adequate supplement for most people, except for pregnant or nursing mothers, who may need as many as six tablets to fill the gap between intake and recommended allowances of these minerals. However, excesses of calcium and magnesium may interfere with the utilization of other essential minerals.

- **Kelp tablets**—Just about every brand of these tablets contains an amount of iodine equal to the U.S. RDAs for adults (150 mcg per day) in each tablet. It is not wise to exceed this amount because people who have tendencies to develop goiter are extra susceptible to iodine toxicity. Those who have suffered from dietary iodine deficiency may have thyroid glands which have adapted to low intakes of the mineral by becoming very efficient in the production of thyroid hormones. Thus, their glands may overproduce these hormones when the dietary level of iodine is raised.

CAUTION: Due to its high content of iodine, it is very easy to get an overdose of iodine from only small amounts of kelp powder.

(Also see ENDOCRINE GLANDS; and GOITER.)

- **Liver, dried, powder**—This excellent source of chromium, copper, iron, and selenium may also be rich in cholesterol and fat, unless it has been defatted. Also, the defatted types of liver powder have a more pleasant taste. However, this supplement should *not* be used by people who might have tendencies to develop high blood levels of uric acid or gout because it is rich in nucleic acids, which are converted into uric acid in the body.

Two teaspoons (10 ml) of liver powder per day provide plenty of extra minerals for most people, when it is used on a regular basis. It may be added to gravies, meat loaves, or various sauces, provided sufficient seasonings are used to disguise the liver flavor.

MINERAL SUPPLEMENTS. Sometimes, it may be more convenient and economical to provide supplementary minerals in pill form than to attempt to meet all of one's mineral needs through ordinary foods and/or specialty products. However, mineral pills or tablets have certain disadvantages in that (1) people may neglect to take their pills regularly; and (2) small pills which contain large amounts of certain minerals may lead to overdosage by people who are impatient to obtain the expected beneficial effects, and to poisoning of small children who might be tempted to sample the pills. Nevertheless, there are circumstances under which it is necessary to take mineral pills in order to prevent nutritional deficiencies. Hence, some suggestions for using these products follow:

1. Whenever feasible, consult with a doctor or a dietitian before attempting to correct dietary inadequacies by means of special supplements.

2. Buy mineral pills which are labeled in accordance with the U.S. RDAs proposed by the Food and Drug Administration.

3. Use mineral supplements according to the directions on their labels.

4. Keep all types of pills out of the reach of infants and children.

5. Report any unusual signs or symptoms, such as changes in bowel habits, to a physician.

(Also see NUTRIENTS: REQUIREMENTS, ALLOWANCES, FUNCTIONS, SOURCES; NUTRITIONAL SUPPLEMENTS; and U.S. RECOMMENDED DAILY ALLOWANCES.)

MINERALOCORTICOIDS

A term describing the hormones secreted from the adrenal cortex which control the metabolism of the minerals sodium (Na) and potassium (K). The major mineralocorticoid is aldosterone.
(Also see ENDOCRINE GLANDS; and HORMONES.)

MINERAL OIL

A mixture of liquid hydrocarbons obtained from petroleum. It is practically tasteless and odorless, and has no caloric value. In the past, mineral oil has enjoyed widespread use as a laxative due to its lubricating properties. It is not, however, the laxative of choice since it has three disadvantages: (1) it may lead to lipid pneumonia if inhaled; (2) it leaks (drips) from the rectum and may cause embarrassment; and (3) it interferes with the absorption of the fat-soluble vitamins A, D, E, and K.
(Also see CONSTIPATION; and LAXATIVE.)

MINERAL SALTS

The term includes all inorganic salts of such elements as sodium, calcium, magnesium, copper etc. As a general rule salts are formed by the chemical reaction of an acid and a base. By far, the most common mineral salt is sodium chloride (NaC1) or table salt.
(Also see MINERAL[S]; and SALT.)

MINERAL SUPPLEMENTS

Rich sources of one or more of the inorganic elements needed to perform certain essential body functions.
(Also see MINERAL[S].)

MINERAL WATERS

Based on some of their descriptions one would think mineral waters possessed some mystical power to improve health. Actually, mineral waters come from natural springs and contain small amounts of sodium chloride, sodium carbonate, sodium bicarbonate, salts of calcium and magnesium, and occasionally iron or hydrogen sulphide. Each mineral spring is said to have its own special properties. Many are naturally impregnated with carbon dioxide. Some are bottled and sold worldwide. They make refreshing drinks. However, the main health benefit derived from drinking them may be that they limit the intake of other less desirable beverages such as soda pop. Actually, all drinking water contains minerals. More important than mineral content, drinking water should be free of disease causing microorganisms, and free of toxic substances like lead, mercury, cadmium, nitrates, and other industrial chemicals or wastes.
(Also see WATER.)

MINERS' CRAMPS (HEAT CRAMPS)

Muscle cramps which usually occur after strenuous exercise and excessive sweating. They are common to athletes, individuals in the tropics, and miners working in hot pits. Muscles of the arms and legs exhibit painful spasms due to the loss of salt from the body. Examination of the blood reveals that there is an increased concentration of the red blood cells and decreased concentration of the sodium and chloride. Prevention and treatment consists of consuming more salt (sodium chloride).
(Also see SODIUM.)

MINIMUM DAILY REQUIREMENTS (MDR)

Guidelines used for many years in the labeling of vitamins, mineral supplements, breakfast cereals, and some special foods; now obsolete. They have now been replaced by the United States Recommended Daily Allowances (U.S. RDA) to express daily nutrient needs. The U.S. RDAs are set higher than the MDRs, and they are based on the Recommended Dietary Allowances established by the Food and Nutrition Board of the National Academy of Sciences-National Research Council (NAS/NRC). Unlike the MDRs which represented the minimum amount of a nutrient needed to maintain health, the U.S. RDAs are said to include a generous amount above the minimum.
(Also see NUTRIENTS: REQUIREMENTS, ALLOWANCES, FUNCTIONS, SOURCES; and U.S. RECOMMENDED DAILY ALLOWANCES.)

MIRACLEBERRY *Richardello dulcifica; Synsepalum dulcifium*

A tropical berry that is native to Africa and contains a substance that makes sour foods such as vinegar taste sweet. The substance, which is a glycoprotein, has been isolated and given the name miraculin (after the name of the berry).

MISCIBLE

Capable of being mixed easily with other substances.

MITOCHONDRIA

Minute spheres, rods, or filaments in the cytoplasm. Mitochondria are the sites of numerous biochemical reactions including amino acid and fatty acid catabolism, the oxidative reactions of the Krebs cycle, respiratory electron transport, and oxidative phosphorylation. As a result of these reactions, mitochondria are the major producers of the high energy compound adenosine triphosphate (ATP) in aerobically grown cells.

MODIFIED DIETS

This term refers to modifications of the ordinary American diet which are made for the purpose of providing nourishment when the consumption of a normal diet is inadvisable. (Strictly speaking, the term diet alone refers to whatever pattern of foods is consumed regularly, whether it conforms to a normal pattern or not.)

There is widespread current interest in various types of modified diets because many people are interested in increasing their productive years while minimizing the amounts spent on medical care. Also, an ever increasing number of nutritional supplements and special dietary products are marketed each year.

HISTORY. During most of human history, food patterns for most people have been based mainly upon whatever edible items could be obtained readily from nearby fields, forests, oceans, rivers, and streams, although some prehistoric peoples traveled long distances while hunting and gathering their foods. However, it appears that each of the preagricultural societies had some type of lore that attributed curative powers to certain special animal foods and druglike preparations from plants. For example, it was widely believed that eating the eyes of animals was the proper treatment for disorders of vision. (This idea was confirmed as valid in the 20th century, when it was found that eyes and other rich sources of vitamin A helped to cure visual problems due to deficiencies of this nutrient.)

The rise of agriculture made it possible for large numbers of people to dwell together in complex societies, but it also brought new health and nutritional problems because (1) infectious diseases spread rapidly through densely populated regions, and (2) the need to provide for large populations resulted in fewer types of foods being produced and consumed. The latter condition increased the likelihood of nutritional deficiencies because there were no means of identifying specific deficiencies and the nutrients that prevented them until a more scientific approach to nutrition was initiated by the great French chemist Antoine Lavoisier in the latter part of the 18th century. Nevertheless, the actual practice of dietetics began much earlier.

Dietetic concepts in the ancient civilizations of Babylon, China, Egypt, and India were based on various combinations of religious beliefs, superstitions, taboos, and trial-and-error observations. Even the last-named basis of judgment was clouded frequently by illness due to a contagious disease, contaminated water, or spoiled food. (The longstanding bias of some Greek and Roman physicians against the eating of fruit is believed to have been due to the fact that fruits were usually abundant in warm weather when diarrheal diseases were rampant because the conditions favored the rapid growth of microorganisms.) Another common type of prescientific concept was that (1) all matter was constituted of varying proportions of the elements air, earth, fire, and water (the Hindus believed that there were three elements, whereas the Chinese postulated five); and (2) the characteristic temperament of the patient (choleric, melancholic, phlegmatic, or sanguine) was due to the excess of one of the elements. Hence, it was considered desirable for an ill person to eat foods which counteracted the excess rather than those which augmented it. For example, a person with a fiery (choleric) temperament was usually told to eat only "cool" foods. In this case, coolness or hotness of foods referred to attributes other than temperature, which were deduced by rather convoluted reasoning. It is noteworthy, that beliefs in cool and hot foods are still held by many poorly educated groups of people around the world.

Two major developments which contributed to the beginnings of modern dietetics in the 18th century were (1) the experiments on metabolism by Lavoisier whose career was literally cut short by the guillotine, and (2) founding of voluntary hospitals in England by private philanthropy. (The latter development helped to fill the gap created by the closing of the many hospitals operated by Catholic religious orders that occurred during the Reformation.) At first, the diet which was given to all patients was based mainly on beef, beer, and bread. Later, the diet was modified for (1) convalescent patients who were given "half diets" consisting of smaller quantities of meat that were augmented with light puddings, soups, broths, and vegetables; and (2) febrile patients who were fed "low diets" of gruels, milk, porridges, puddings, and small portions of cheese and/or meat. Use of these diets and variations of them persisted until the 20th century, because the nutritional science of the 19th century was dominated by the belief that adequate amounts of carbohydrates, fats, proteins, and minerals were all that were required to maintain good health. The need to prevent scurvy and other nutritional deficiencies by the provision of fruits and vegetables was not common knowledge until the latter part of the 19th century. Also, these items spoiled readily.

The major factors which accelerated the growth of modern dietetics in the first few decades of the 20th century were (1) the discoveries of the requirements for certain amino acids, trace minerals, and vitamins; (2) the founding of the American Dietetic Association in 1917 (this organization has contributed greatly to the stan-dardization of the education and training of dietitians and the types of diets used for treating various disorders); and (3) the widespread recognition of the need for dietary modification in the treatment of certain conditions. (The designation "dietitian" originated in 1899 at the meeting of the National Home Economics Association at Lake Placid, New York.) It is noteworthy that the dramatic recoveries of some critically ill patients which resulted from the appropriate diet therapy led to a certain amount of unscrupulous promotion of nutritional supplements. These abuses inspired leading dietitians, doctors, and public health professionals to conduct vigorous educational campaigns against food faddism and nutritional hucksterism. The campaigns also emphasized that balancing diets with respect to all of the essential nutrients was much more important than relying on unusual dietary modifications or large quantities of a few minerals and vitamins to bring about the desired improvement of health.

Today, there are many types of modified diets that are used regularly in the treatment of a wide variety of abnormal conditions. However, there is a need for more accurate record keeping and monitoring of the patient's daily food intake so that the efficacy of these modifications may be judged with more certainty.

COMMON TYPES OF DIETARY MODIFICATIONS.
Two of the most important principles of dietary modification are (1) only necessary changes should be made in order to minimize the difficulty the patient will have in following the dietary prescription, and (2) every effort should be made to ensure that a modified diet is an adequate source of all essential nutrients, or if this is not feasible, appropriate nutritional supplementation should be recommended. The most common dietary modifications are given in Table M-70.

NOTE: This table lists only diets comprised of common beverages and foods that are taken orally because special formulas that may be administered by oral or other means are covered in the articles ELEMENTAL DIETS; INTRAVENOUS (PARENTERAL) NUTRITION, SUPPLEMENTARY; LIQUID DIETS; and TOTAL PARENTERAL (INTRAVENOUS) NUTRITION.

TABLE M-70
MODIFIED DIETS

Diet	Composition		Uses	Comments
	Foods Included	**Foods Excluded**		
General diet	The regular diet consumed by most Americans.	None	Patients who do not require any dietary modifications.	This is also called the house or full hospital diet and varies somewhat from one institution to another.
I. *Modifications in texture and consistency*				
General diet, pureed	Same as general diet.	None	Toothless patients.	
General diet, liquid (Also see LIQUID DIETS.)	Finely homogenized and strained fish, meat, or poultry (visible fat should be removed before homogenization).	All other forms of fish, meat, or poultry.	For patients who are unable to chew and/or swallow foods due to circumstances such as surgery on the face, oral cavity, neck, or throat; fractures of the jaw; esophageal strictures; partial paralysis; or unconsciousness. As nutritional supplements for people who find it difficult to eat sufficient amounts of ordinary foods. By athletes prior to, and/or during sporting events because liquids leave the stomach more rapidly than solid foods. Weight reduction, when a low-calorie liquid diet is used at one or more daily meals in place of solid foods which contain more calories.	The daily allotment is usually divided into 6 feedings. Milk, milk drinks, and strained fruit or vegetable juices may be served between meals. Underweight patients may need supplemental feedings (commonly called "nourishments") that are rich in calories from foods such as melted butter or margarine (added to hot liquids), or honey, sugar, or syrups (added to fruit juices). Liquid diets are usually deficient in certain nutrients. Hence, the doctor or dietitian may recommend certain mineral and vitamin supplements if the diet is to be used for more than a week or so.
	Any type or kind of milk or cream.	None		
	Strained cottage cheese.	All other forms of cheese.		
	Eggs in cooked foods such as puddings and soft custards.	All other forms of eggs.		
	Strained fruit juices, pureed and strained fruits.	Berries with small seeds.		
	Strained vegetable juices, pureed and strained mild flavored vegetables such as asparagus, beans (green and wax), beets, carrots, peas, potatoes, spinach, squash, sweet potatoes, and tomatoes.	Strong flavored vegetables.		
	Cereal gruels made from enriched refined cooked cereals.	All prepared or dry cereals, and whole grain cooked cereals. All forms of bread.		
	Moderate amounts of butter, margarine, oil, or cream.	All other forms of fat.		
	Cream or broth-type soups made with pureed vegetables; strained fish, meats, or poultry; broth, bouillon, or consomme.	Highly seasoned soups or those containing pieces of vegetables, meats, or poultry.		
	Sugar, honey, syrups, jelly, and plain sugar candy.	Jams and marmalades.		
	Plain ice cream, sherbets, ices, puddings, junket preparations, soft custard, tapioca, and plain dessert gels.	Desserts that contain nuts, fruit, coconut, or other solids.		

(Continued)

TABLE M-70 *(Continued)*

Diet	Composition		Uses	Comments
	Foods Included	**Foods Excluded**		
General diet, liquid *(Continued)*	Carbonated beverages, cocoa, coffee, tea, and coffee substitutes.	All other beverages.		
	Salt, mild spices, and vanilla and other mild flavorings in moderate amounts.	All other types of condiments, flavorings, seasonings, and spices.		
Soft diet	Fresh, canned, or frozen fish; beef, lamb, liver, lean roast pork or ham, crisp bacon; or poultry meat. (These items should be cooked by baking, broiling, pan-broiling or roasting.)	Fried or deep fat fried fish, meats, or poultry; fish, meats or poultry with small bones, gristle, or skin; fatty pork or ham, franks, corned beef; spiced or smoked items.	An intermediate diet that is given after a full liquid diet, and before a regular diet. Patients who are bedridden and likely to suffer from gas and other digestive problems when coarser foods are consumed. When difficulties in chewing and/or swallowing are present.	The compositions of soft diets vary somewhat between different hospitals. This diet may not furnish enough iron for women unless there is a liberal use of meats, enriched breads, and strained legumes. (The latter may be made into dips, soups, or spreads for bread.) Soft diets can be used for long periods of time, but they should not be used longer than necessary or the patient may lose his or her tolerance for coarser foods.
	Any type or kind of milk or cream.	None		
	Cottage and other mild-flavored varieties of cheeses.	Sharp or strong-flavored cheeses.		
	Eggs that are baked, hard or soft cooked, poached, or scrambled without fat (cooked in a nonstick fry pan).	Fried eggs or scrambled eggs cooked in fat.		
	All fruit juices; cooked and canned apples (without skin), applesauce, apricots, cherries, peaches, pears, plums, and prunes; and raw ripe banana, grapefruit and orange sections, ripe peeled peaches, and ripe peeled pears.	All fruits with small seeds or tough skins, unless these parts are removed completely. Dates, figs, and raisins.		
	All vegetable juices; cooked and canned asparagus, beets, carrots, eggplant, green beans, peas, pumpkin, spinach, squash, and tomatoes; corn and lima or navy beans that have been passed through a sieve; and raw lettuce.	Cooked broccoli, Brussels sprouts, cabbage, cauliflower, corn, cucumbers, kale, onions, parsnips, and whole lima or navy beans. All raw vegetables except lettuce.		
	Day old or toasted white bread; salted, soda or graham crackers; refined cereals such as cornmeal, cream of wheat, oatmeal, or rice; dry cereals such as cornflakes.	All whole grain breads and cereals except oatmeal. Hot breads.		
	Sweet or white potatoes (without skins); macaroni, noodles, or spaghetti made with white flour; and white rice.	Spicy dressings or sauces on potatoes, pasta, or rice.		

(Continued)

TABLE M-70 *(Continued)*

Diet	Foods Included	Foods Excluded	Uses	Comments
	Composition			
Soft diet *(Continued)*	Butter or margarine, cooking oils, cream, crisp bacon, mild-flavored salad dressings.	Fried foods and gravies.		
	Canned or homemade broths or soups made from items in this column.	Spicy soups or those containing large amounts of fat.		
	Sugar, syrups, honey, and clear jellies in moderation.	Jams and preserves which contain nuts, seeds, or skins.		
	Cakes (angel food, mild chocolate, plain white, sponge, yellow); cookies; custards; fruit whips; gelatin desserts with allowed fruits; ice cream or sherbet without fruit pulp or nuts; and puddings (bread, butterscotch, chocolate, rice, tapioca, vanilla).	Pastries; pies; excessively sweet desserts; or those containing dates, fruits with small seeds, or raisins.		
	Carbonated beverages, coffee, coffee substitutes, and tea in moderation.	Alcoholic beverages, unless ordered by the doctor.		
	Salt, lemon juice, vanilla, cocoa, cinnamon, allspice and ripe olives.	Spicy or fibrous condiments.		
Soft diet, pureed	Same foods as in the soft diet.	Same foods as in the soft diet.	Patients who have considerable difficulty in chewing and/or swallowing.	All solid foods are chopped fine, strained, or blended.
Bland diet	All of the foods in the soft diet, except the excluded items listed in the next column.	Those excluded from the soft diet *plus* chocolate, cocoa, coffee, decaffeinated coffee, cola beverages, tea; tomatoes, tomato juice, and citrus juices; and excessively fatty foods.	In some cases of chronic digestive disorders such as esophagitis, hiatus hernia, ulcers, colitis, diverticulitis, etc.	There is now some doubt as to whether the traditional types of bland diets promote healing any faster than regular diets which are free of strong irritants such as mustard and pepper. Pureed vegetables may also be used to make bland dressings and sauces. A vitamin C supplement is advisable.

(Continued)

TABLE M-70 (*Continued*)

Diet	Composition		Uses	Comments
	Foods Included	**Foods Excluded**		
Bland diet, low fiber	All of the foods listed for the soft diet, except the excluded items listed in the next column.	Those excluded from the soft diet *plus* chocolate, coffee, decaffeinated coffee, cola beverages, tea; all fruit juices and fruits; all vegetables other than those pureed, strained, and prepared in cream soups; excessively fatty foods; and all spices other than salt.	In some cases of chronic digestive disorders such as esophagitis, hiatus hernia, ulcers, colitis, diverticulitis, etc.	The foods are usually distributed between 6 small meals per day. Additional feedings of milk and/or cream may be given between meals. A vitamin C supplement should be given. There is no reason for continuing this diet after the acute inflammatory stage of the disorder has subsided.
Milk and cream diet	A 1:1 mixture of whole milk and cream; or "coffee cream" with 12.5% butterfat; or if calories are to be reduced, only whole milk or skim milk.	All others	Acute stages of gastrointestinal disorders such as high gastric acidity, gastritis, ulcers, etc.	Generally, about 4 oz (*120 ml*) of the mixture are given every hour to keep some food in the stomach at all times. Mineral and vitamin supplements are needed.
Clear liquid diet (Also see LIQUID DIETS.)	Fat-free broth, bouillon, carbonated beverages, coffee, decaffeinated coffee, flavored gelatin, honey, popsicles, strained fruit juices, sugar, syrups (clear), and tea.	All others	Zero residue feeding used for (1) preparation for a barium enema and/or bowel surgery, (2) after surgery, (3) diarrhea, and (4) very weakened patients.	Supplies only a few calories (from the sugars in the allowed items) and some electrolytes (mainly sodium, chloride, and potassium).
Tea and fat-free broth diet	Tea and fat-free broth (the doctor may allow the use of sugar).	All others	First feeding after surgery on the digestive tract.	Provides mainly water and little in the way of nutrients.

(Continued)

TABLE M-70 (*Continued*)

Diet	Composition		Uses	Comments
	Foods Included	**Foods Excluded**		
II. Modifications of caloric content				
High-calorie diet (Also see UNDER-WEIGHT.)	The regular American diet, with an emphasis on eating greater-than-usual quantities of carbohydrate-rich items (breads, desserts, pasta products, and sweets); fat-rich items (bacon, butter, cream, marga-rine, mayonnaise, oils, peanut butter, salad dressings, and sour cream); and protein-rich items (cheeses, cus-tards, eggs, eggnogs, fish, meats, poultry, and undiluted evaporated milk).	None, but low calorie foods should be replaced in part by calorie-rich foods.	Providing the energy needs of (1) hypermetabolic patients (in cancer, hyperthy-roidism, severe burns, and trauma), (2) underweight peo-ple, (3) victims of malnutrition and malabsorption syndromes, and (4) very active people such as athletes, explor-ers, laborers, min-ers, and soldiers.	Many of the people who have high energy needs also have high protein require-ments. Hence, extra protein sources should be given. The metabolic sta-tus of the patient should be con-sidered in deter-mining whether the extra calories should be sup-plied as carbohy-drates, fats, and/or proteins.
Low-calorie diet (Also see OBESITY.)	Low-calorie items that are rich in protein, fiber, minerals, and vitamins, such as eggs, fish, lean meats, poultry, lowfat cheeses and milk prod-ucts, low-carbohydrate fruits and vegetables, and whole grain and bran types of breads and cereals. (The last named group of foods is not much lower in calo-ries than those made from refined flour, but it contains very filling items that reduce the desire to overeat.)	Those which supply mainly calories, but little else in the way of nu-trients (alcoholic and carbonated beverages, cakes, cookies, des-serts, highly refined fatty, starchy, and sugary foods, and many of the common snack foods).	Weight reduction for overweight peo-ple. (Loss of weight may also help to correct other undesirable conditions such as high blood pressure, an impaired utiliza-tion of sugars, and elevations in the blood levels of cholesterol and triglycerides.)	Drastic restrictions in dietary calories may lead to great reductions in cer-tain energy-rich foods that are good sources of minerals and vitamins. There-fore, nutritional supplements may be needed in these cases. Vigorous exercise may offset some of the need for dietary re-strictions. People attempting to lose consider-able weight should be exam-ined by a doctor before going on a very low calorie diet.

(Continued)

TABLE M-70 *(Continued)*

Diet	Composition		Uses	Comments
	Foods Included	**Foods Excluded**		
III. Modifications in the intakes of specific nutrients				
Carbohydrate restricted diet (Also see DUMPING SYNDROME; HYPO— GLYCEMIA; and OBESITY.)	All types of cheeses, eggs, fish, meats, and poultry; milk products without added sweetener; nuts; and peanut butter.	Sweetened milk products.	Treatment of the dumping syndrome in patients who have had all or part of their stomach removed. Correction of elevated blood levels of triglycerides when used with concurrent restrictions of alcohol, cholesterol, and saturated fats. Stabilization of the blood sugar in people with a tendency to low blood sugar (hypoglycemia). Weight reduction of patients who are obese due to an over secretion of insulin in response to dietary sugars. Management of some types of juvenile diabetes in which it is difficult to adjust the dosages of insulin, or in the control of adult onset diabetes.	Some patients may also require the restriction of all milk products after they have had stomach surgery. This diet is high in cholesterol, saturated fats, and fats in general and should not be used without further modification for patients with high blood levels of lipids (hyperlipoproteinemias). The high protein content of this diet may be dangerous for people with certain kidney disorders. (Also see the ketogenic diet which is outlined in this table.)
	Unsweetened fruit juices and fruits (limited to 3 exchanges per day).	Sweetened fruit juices and fruits.		
	Low-carbohydrate vegetables (limited to 2 exchanges per day).	Vegetables prepared with sweetener.		
	Unsweetened breads, cereals, pasta, and starchy vegetables (limited to 5 exchanges per day).	Breads and cereals with sugar, dates, or raisins (includes granola types).		
	Bacon, butter or margarine, cream (unsweetened), fats, French dressing, mayonnaise, shortenings, and vegetable oils.	Sweetened imitation cream toppings.		
	Soups made with allowed foods (starchy items limited as above).	Gravies thickened with cornstarch or flour.		
	Custards, gelatin desserts, and junket puddings made without a natural sweetener (an artificial sweetener may be used).	All desserts made with natural sweeteners.		
	Artificially sweetened carbonated beverages, coffee, herb teas, and tea (only artificial sweetener may be used in coffee and teas).	Alcoholic beverages, naturally sweetened carbonated beverages, sweetened coffee, imitation coffee creams, and sweetened iced tea.		
	Unsweetened condiments and spices.	Honey, jams, jellies, marmalade, molasses, sugar, and syrups.		

(Continued)

TABLE M-70 *(Continued)*

Diet	Composition		Uses	Comments
	Foods Included	**Foods Excluded**		
Carbohydrate, fiber, and fluid restricted diet	All of the foods listed for the soft diet, except the excluded items listed in the next column. Fluid intake should be restricted to 4 to 8 oz (120 to 240 ml) taken at each of 6 small meals per day. (The patient may be allowed to sip water or suck on cracked ice between meals.) Strained fruit juices should be diluted 1:1 with water. Only unsweetened cooked or canned fruits are allowed. The only allowed desserts are gelatin or baked custard made without added sugar (artificial sweeteners may be used).	Those excluded from the soft diet *plus* dried fruits, sweetened cooked or canned fruits, sweet potatoes, graham crackers, all types of sweetened desserts, all forms of sugar and sweets, all foods preserved with sugar or salt, and salt that is added at the table. (Some salt may be used in cooking.)	After gastrointestinal surgery when it is necessary to reduce the volume of fluids and foods in the stomach and intestines.	The amounts of food fluid served at each of the 6 daily meals should be increased cautiously in accordance with the patient's tolerance for food. Most nutrient requirements will be met if a variety of the allowed foods are consumed, and adequate amounts of food are eaten. However, a vitamin C supplement should be provided to compensate for the small amount of fruits.
Fat restricted diet (Also see HYPERLIPO-PROTEIN-EMIAS.)	Canned fish (water pack), fresh or frozen fish (skinless and unbreaded), lean meats, and poultry prepared by baking, or broiling (the pieces may be wrapped in foil to retain the juices), panbroiling (in a nonstick frying pan without added fat), and roasting.	Fish canned in oil, fresh or frozen salmon, fish cakes and frozen fish sticks, bacon, ham, pork, duck, goose, sandwich meats and sausages, canned and frozen meat dishes.	Patients who show signs of an impairment in the clearing of blood-borne fats such as chylomicrons and triglycerides from the blood within a normal period after a fat-containing meal. The major signs of this condition (Type I Hyper-lipoproteinemia) are (1) a creamy upper layer that forms on a sample of blood plasma left overnight in a refrigerator, (2) abdominal pain after the consumption of fat, and (3) visible deposits of fat under the skin (eruptive xanthomas). Other uses are in disorders of the biliary tract and/or the pancreas in which dietary fats are digested poorly and likely to cause a fatty	This diet imposes a drastic restriction on the dietary fats which form chylomicrons. However, the fat-soluble vitamins (vitamins A, D, E, and K) are absorbed and transported in the blood along with these fats. Hence, deficiencies of these vitamins may result from the diet unless supplements containing water-soluble forms of the vitamins are provided. Sometimes, patients are allowed to use specially prepared fats called medium chain triglycerides (MCT) because they do not accumulate in the blood.
	Evaporated skim milk, fat-free buttermilk, nonfat dry milk, and skim milk.	Chocolate milk, cultured buttermilk, whole milk, and yogurt.		
	Fat-free cottage cheese, pot cheese, and other skim-milk cheeses.	All other cheeses.		
	Medium to hard cooked, poached, or scrambled egg (in a nonstick pan without added fat). Limit of 1 whole egg per day, but whites are not limited.	Eggs cooked with added fat or in omelets or souffles with fatty foods.		
	All fruits and their juices, except avocado and coconut.	Avocado and coconut.		
	All canned, fresh, or frozen vegetables prepared without a cream sauce, an oil, a fat, or a fatty food (such as a rich cheese).	Creamed vegetables or those prepared with a fat or an oil.		

TABLE M-70 (*Continued*)

Diet	Composition		Uses	Comments
	Foods Included	**Foods Excluded**		
Fat restricted diet (*Continued*)	Breads and other baked goods made with little or no fat.	All other breads and baked goods.	diarrhea (steatorrhea).	
	All cooked and dry cereals (served with skim milk).	None		
	Baked, boiled, or mashed (with skim milk) potatoes served without any fat; hominy (corn), pasta, or rice without a fatty sauce; and unbuttered popcorn.	Escalloped, creamed or fried potatoes; potato chips, ovenbrowned potatoes; buttered popcorn; and egg noodles.		
	Lowfat desserts such as cake (angel food), cookies (arrowroot, ladyfingers, and vanilla wafers), crackers (graham), fruit whips made with egg whites or gelatin, gelatin desserts, meringues, puddings (cornstarch, junket, rice, and tapioca) made with skim milk and egg whites, and water ices.	All cakes, cookies, ice cream, pastries, puddings, and other desserts made with eggs, egg yolks, fats, and whole milk.		
	Hard candy, fondant, jelly beans, honey, jams, and other lowfat sweets.	Candy made with fats or nuts, chocolate candy or chocolate syrup.		
	Carbonated beverages, coffee, grain beverages, and tea.	Alcoholic beverages, chocolate drinks.		
	Condiments, pickles, spices, white sauce made with skim milk.	Fat-containing gravies and sauces.		
Cholesterol and saturated fat restricted diet (Also see HEART DISEASE; and HYPER—LIPOPRO—TEINEMIAS.)	A modified regular diet that emphasizes foods containing little or no cholesterol and/or saturated fat (typical items are breads, cereals, egg whites, fish, fruits, lean muscle meats, legumes [beans and peas], lowfat cheeses [such as cottage], margarines made from liquid vegetable oils other than coconut, nonfat milk products, oils, peanut butter [nonhydrogenated], poultry breast meats, salad dressings made from vegetable oils, and vegetables). Also, it is usually recommended that polyunsaturated vegetable oil products replace most of the elim-	The foods that follow are *not* excluded, but should be eaten only in limited amounts: bacon, brains, butter, coconut oil, cream, creamy or fatty cheeses, chicken fat, egg yolks, kidneys, lard, liver, margarines made from animal fats, mayonnaise, meat fats, rich ice creams, sandwich meats and sausages, shellfish, sour cream, and whole milk products.	To prevent or treat certain hyper-lipoproteinemias (high blood levels of cholesterol and/or triglycerides) in patients who (1) have a family history of early cardiovascular and/or cerebrovascular diseases (tendencies to have heart attacks and/or strokes), (2) are overweight and have high blood fats, or (3) have an abnormally rapid clotting of the blood.	The replacement of dietary saturated fats with polyunsaturated vegetable oils is considered by some doctors to be potentially hazardous because it may (1) increase the risk of cancer, (2) aggravate gallbladder disease, and (3) produce a deficiency of vitamin E, unless supplements of the latter are taken. It is not certain whether this diet is of any benefit to people other

(*Continued*)

TABLE M-70 (*Continued*)

Diet	Composition		Uses	Comments
	Foods Included	**Foods Excluded**	**Uses**	**Comments**
Cholesterol and saturated fat restricted diet (*Continued*)	inated saturated fats.			than those who tend to accumulate fats in the blood. Hyperlipemic patients should be given a glucose tolerance test before being put on this diet (to rule out the possibility that their condition is induced by dietary carbohydrates).
High fiber diet (Also see FIBER.)	A modification of the diet consumed by most Americans, with an emphasis on consuming greater-than-usual amounts of milk products, fruits, vegetables, whole-grain and bran-type breads and cereals, and nuts.	None, but some or all of the highly refined carbohydrate foods should be replaced by their unrefined equivalents.	Stimulation of larger, more frequent bowel movements in order to correct or prevent chronic constipation and its consequences (diverticulitis, hemorrhoids and narrowing of the colon diameter).	Dietary fiber should be increased gradually for people accustomed to low fiber diets in order to prevent flatulence and looseness of the bowels. Should *not* be used when the bowel is inflamed.
Fiber-restricted diet	All of the foods for the soft diet, except the excluded items listed in the next column. Milk intake should be restricted to 2 cups per day.	Those excluded from the soft diet *plus* all fruit and vegetable products other than strained fruit and vegetable juices and cooked white potatoes without skin; popcorn and potato chips, and prune juice (even when strained it has a laxative effect).	When gastrointestinal passages such as the esophagus or the intestines are narrowed by strictures and there is danger of blockage. Severe inflammation of the bowel in diverticulitis, infectious enterocolitis, or ulcerative colitis. As an intermediate diet that is used after a full liquid diet, and before a soft or a regular diet.	A low fiber diet should not be used any longer than necessary because it produces small infrequent stools. This condition may encourage (1) excessive constriction of the colon, (2) narrowing of its diameter, (3) herniation of the colonic muscles and the production of pouches (diverticula), and (4) general aggravation of bowel problems.

(*Continued*)

TABLE M-70 (*Continued*)

| Diet | Composition | | Uses | Comments |
	Foods Included	Foods Excluded		
Nonfiber, milk-free diet	All of the foods listed for the soft diet, except for the excluded items listed in the next column.	Those excluded from the soft diet *plus* all milk products and cheeses, all fruit products other than strained fruit juices, all vegetable products other than strained tomato juice, potatoes, and all spices and condiments other than salt.	After intestinal surgery or trauma, when it is necessary to reduce bowel movements to a minimum.	This diet is usually given for only a few days until healing occurs because small, infrequent stools may result in (1) excessive constriction of the colon, (2) narrowing of its diameter, and (3) general aggravation of bowel problems. A calcium supplement should be given.
High protein, high calorie diet	The normal American dietary pattern supplemented by extra servings of protein-rich foods such as cheeses, eggs, fish, meats, milk products, peanut butter, poultry, and special proprietary formulas when necessary.	None, although certain filling low protein foods such as fruits and vegetables may be replaced in part by high protein foods.	Patients recovering from burns, cancer therapy, injuries, hepatitis, malnutrition, surgery, and ulcerative colitis and/or other inflammatory conditions of the gastrointestinal tract, and underweight.	High protein diets often increase the urinary losses of calcium so that a calcium supplement may be advisable. Should not be used when protein metabolism or nitrogen excretion is impaired.
Controlled protein, potassium, sodium, and water diet	A daily food pattern that provides 30 g of protein and about 800 mg each of potassium and sodium follows: 1 1/2 oz (*28 g*) of unsalted eggs, fish, liver or muscle meat, or poultry.	Brains; kidneys; salted eggs, fish, meats, or poultry; sandwich meats; and sausages.	To provide as much nourishment as possible to patients with advanced kidney disease while preventing the accumulation in the body of excessive amounts of nitrogenous wastes and mineral salts. However, patients who are being treated regularly with hemodialysis or peritoneal dialysis may usually be given more liberal diets.	This type of diet should not be used until it is absolutely necessary, because if given prematurely, the patient may tire of it by the time it is needed the most. The diet may not supply sufficient calories for all patients and may need to be supplemented with intravenous feeding. Also, a mineral and vitamin supplement is required when a patient is given the diet for more
	1/2 cup (*120 ml*) of unsalted cottage cheese or 1/2 oz (*14 g*) of unsalted American cheese.	All other forms of cheese and milk products.		
	1/2 cup (*120 ml*) of a canned, fresh, or frozen noncitrus-type of fruit.	Citrus fruits and dried fruits.		
	1 cup (*240 ml*) of cranberry juice or reconstituted frozen lemonade or limeade.	All other fruit juices.		

(*Continued*)

TABLE M-70   *(Continued)*

Diet	Composition		Uses	Comments
	Foods Included	**Foods Excluded**		
Controlled protein potassium, sodium, and water diet *(Continued)*	1 cup *(240 ml)* of salt-free or unsalted cooked or raw cabbage, canned carrots, canned green beans, canned peas, canned wax beans, fresh cucumber or lettuce.	All vegetables prepared with salt, and all others not listed.		than a few days.
	3 slices of enriched white bread or 5 saltine crackers.	All other breads and baked goods.		
	1/2 cup *(120 ml)* of cooked cream of wheat, farina, or hominy grits served without milk.	All other cereals.		
	1 cup *(240 ml)* of cooked enriched pasta or enriched white rice that has been prepared without salt.	All forms of sweet and white potatoes, potato chips, and brown rice.		
	3 tsp *(15 ml)* of butter, cream cheese, marga-rine, mayonnaise, or salad dressing; and unrestricted amounts of corn oil.	Cream gravies and all other fatty foods.		
	No types of soups. 1 tsp *(5 ml)* of jam or jelly; moderate amounts of gum drops, hard candy, marshmallows, and sugar syrup (colorless-type).	All types of soups. All other types of sugars and sweets.		
	Moderate amounts of a homemade gelatin des-sert prepared with sugar and artificial flavoring; dietetic gelatin; or lime ice.	Commercial gelatin des-serts and all other types of desserts.		
	2 cups *(480 ml)* of ginger ale, or root beer.	All other beverages.		
	Unlimited amounts of cin-namon, mace, nutmeg, peppermint extract, vanilla, vinegar, and white pepper.	All other condiments, fla-vorings, herbs, and spices.		
Purine restricted diet	Cheeses; eggs; fishes and meats, except for those listed in the next column as excluded; and sea-foods.	Brains, kidneys, liver, and sweetbreads; broths, extracts, gravies, sau-ces, and soups made from meats; fried meats; and anchovies, caviar, roe, and sardines.	Patients with high blood levels of uric acid (hyperu-ricemia), gout, and gouty arth-ritis.	A high fat diet may aggravate hyper-uricemia. Hence, the amounts of dietary fats should be mod-erately restricted.

(Continued)

TABLE M-70   (*Continued*)

Diet	Composition		Uses	Comments
	Foods Included	**Foods Excluded**		
Purine restricted diet (*Continued*)	All milk products, except that high fat products should be used in moderation.	None		The blood level of uric acid is also raised by the heavy consumption of alcoholic beverages and fasting. Vegetarian diets that are rich in microbically-fermented products, seeds, and yeast or yeast derivatives may furnish more purines (uric-acid forming substances) per calorie than diets which contain fish, meats, and poultry.
	All fruits and fruit juices.	None		
	Vegetables and vegetable juices as desired, except that cooked dried beans and peas should be limited to 1/2 cup (*120 ml*) per day.	None		
	Most breads and cereals.	Wheat germ.		
	Most forms of sweet and white potatoes; and all pasta and rice products.	Fried potatoes and potato chips.		
	All types of fats, when used in moderation.	None		
	Desserts that contain only small to moderate amounts of fats, such as custards made with skim milk, gelatin desserts, lowfat cakes, cookies, ice cream, and puddings.	High fat items such as rich cakes, cookies, ice cream, mince meat, pastries, and whipped cream or imitation whipped toppings.		
	Carbonated beverages and cereal beverages (coffee substitutes).	Alcoholic beverages, chocolate, cocoa, coffee, and tea.		
	Condiments, herbs, nuts, olives, peanut butter, pickles, popcorn, relishes, salt, spices, vinegar, and white sauce.	Fatty broths, extracts, gravies, sauces, and soups; and yeast.		
Ketogenic diet	This diet is very low in carbohydrates, high in fat content and contains moderate amounts of protein. It is characterized by (1) the use of large and carefully calculated amounts of bacon, butter, cheese, cream, eggs, fish, meats, and poultry; (2) minimal amounts of low carbohydrate fruits and vegetables; and (3) exclusion of foods of moderate to high carbohydrate contents (such as those listed in the next column).	Beverages that contain sugar, breads and cereals, desserts other than small amounts of fruits with plenty of whipped cream, fruits and vegetables of moderate to high carbohydrate contents, milk products other than butter and cream, and all forms of sweets.	Prevention of seizures in epileptic children by inducing and maintaining a state of ketosis (the presence of ketone bodies in the blood and urine). Sometimes, this type of diet is used by doctors to induce a rapid loss of body weight in patients who find it difficult to reduce by other means. (The weight loss is largely made up of lost fluid.)	Some patients on this diet are prone to abdominal cramps, nausea, and vomiting. Small, frequent feedings are tolerated better than a few large meals per day. A special fat preparation called medium chain triglycerides is often given to patients on these diets.

(Continued)

TABLE M-70 *(Continued)*

Diet	Composition		Uses	Comments
	Foods Included	**Foods Excluded**		
Gluten-free diet	All types of cheeses, eggs, fish, meats, and poultry that are *not* breaded creamed, extended, or served with a gravy made from barley, oats, rye, or wheat; sandwich meats and sausages if labeled as "pure meat."	Cheese, egg, fish, meat or poultry mixtures such as chili, croquettes, meat loaf, and canned products that are likely to contain flour.	The life-long diet of patients who have an intolerance to foods that contain the cereal protein gluten.	Sometimes, adults who had no previous history of gluten sensitivity have developed this condition after surgery on the digestive tract. (It has been suggested that any condition which allows incompletely digested gluten-containing proteins to be absorbed may lead to the development of a sensitivity.)
	Milk products that are not likely to contain cereal ingredients.	Chocolate and malted milk products that contain cereals or flours.		
	All fruit juices and fruits.	None		
	All vegetable juices, vegetables, except those listed in the next column as excluded.	Items prepared with bread, bread crumbs, or wheat flour.		
	Baked goods, breads and cereals made from corn, potato, rice, soybean, and/or tapioca flours or meals only.	Products containing barley, oat, rye, or wheat flour or meal.		
	Sweet or white potatoes other than those prepared by breading or flouring.	Macaroni, noodles, and spaghetti.		
	All types of fat, except those listed in the next column as excluded.	All commercial salad dressings except pure mayonnaise.		
	Clear broths, consomme, and soups that contain no barley, oats, rye, or wheat; and cream soups that are thickened only with cornstarch or potato flour.	All canned soups other than clear broth; and all creamed soups that are thickened with the excluded grain products.		
	Gluten-free desserts such as custards, fruit products made without flour, gelatin desserts, homemade ice cream, ices and sherbets, and junket, rice and other puddings thickened only with cornstarch, potato flour or tapioca.	Cakes, cookies, ice cream containing a stabilizer made from wheat, ice cream cones, commercial baking mixes other than those labeled "gluten-free," and commercial puddings.		
	Corn syrup, honey, jams and jellies, molasses, and brown and white sugars.	Commercial candies that contain the excluded grain products.		

(Continued)

TABLE M-70   (*Continued*)

Diet	Composition		Uses	Comments
	Foods Included	**Foods Excluded**		
Lactose-free diet	All types of eggs, fish, meats, nuts, and poultry without added lactose or milk.	Creamed or breaded preparations, sandwich meats and sausages unless labelled "all meat," and omelets and souffles made with cheeses or milk.	For people who cannot digest milk sugar (lactose) and suffer from unpleasant symptoms when lactose-containing foods are consumed. In many cases the intolerance is congenital or hereditary, but it may also occur spontaneously in people who showed no prior indications of the condition. Usually, acquired lactose intolerance occurs as a result of injury to the intestinal lining in celiac disease (gluten intolerance), gastrointestinal milk protein allergy, irritable bowel syndrome, kwashiorkor, malnutrition, regional enteritis (Crohn's disease), ulcerative colitis, viral enteritis; and after some types of gastrointestinal surgery.	It is believed that a large percentage of the world's people may have mild to severe symptoms of lactose intolerance (abdominal cramps, diarrhea, distention, gas, and malabsorption of nutrients) after the consumption of fairly small amounts of milk (as little as 1/4 cup or *60 ml*). However, some types of fermented milks contain little or no unfermented lactose and do not produce the symptoms. (Many of the brands of yogurt sold in the U.S. contain added nonfermented skim milk solids.) Patients should be taught to scrutinize food labels for the presence of butter, casein, cheese, cream, lactose, milk, or whey. A commercial enzyme preparation that digests lactose in milk to harmless products is now available.
	Nondairy creamers and similar lactose-free substitutes for milk.	All forms of milks, cheeses, ice creams, malted milks, etc.		
	All fruits and vegetables and their juices that have been prepared without cheeses, cream sauces, lactose, or other milk products.	Fruit and vegetable products prepared with lactose or a milk product (such as breaded, buttered, or creamed items, corn curls, frozen french fries and instant potatoes.)		
	Breads, cereals, and pasta made without lactose or milk.	Breads and other baked goods made from prepared mixes that contain lactose or milk products, cereals and pasta made from milk.		
	Dressings, margarines, and shortenings made without any milk products; bacon; meat fats; nut butters that are lactose-free; oils, and certain brands of nondairy creamers and whipped toppings that contain no milk derivatives.	Dressings, margarines, certain nondairy creamers, peanut butter, and whipped toppings made with butter, cheese, cream lactose, or other milk products.		
	Broths, consomme, cream soups, and soups without milk products.	Items containing lactose or milk.		
	Candies, cakes, cookies, pies, and puddings made without milk.	Dessert items that contain milk.		
	Alcoholic and carbonated beverages, coffee, milk substitutes, tea.	Hot chocolate and some types of cocoa.		
	Condiments, jams, jellies, marmalades, spices, and sweeteners.	Artificial sweeteners that contain lactose.		
Calcium restricted diet	Most common foods, except those that are rich in calcium and are listed in the excluded list in the next column. However, meats are limited to 6 oz (*170 g*) per day, eggs to 1 per day, nonexcluded vegetables to 1 cup (*240 ml*) per day, and potatoes (prepared without milk) to 1 cup (*240 ml*) per day.	All milk products (except butter); canned mackerel, salmon, sardines; shellfish; foods that contain milk; baking powders and products made from them; green leafy vegetables; and molasses.	When the blood calcium of a patient is excessively high, and in certain tests of calcium metabolism. (Usually, only a few days of dietary calcium restriction will bring the blood calcium down to normal.)	This diet is *no longer* used to prevent the formation of calcium-containing kidney stones because keeping the urine acid (by feeding cranberry juice or other means) works better.

(Continued)

TABLE M-70   *(Continued)*

Diet	Composition		Uses	Comments
	Foods Included	**Foods Excluded**		
Phosphorus restricted diet	3 oz (*85 g*) of cod, crab, flounder, haddock, lobster, and oysters; beef, bologna, corned beef, frankfurters, ham, heart, pork, tongue; and chicken and duck.	Other fish and shellfish; bacon, brains, lamb, liver, turkey, and veal.	In hyperphosphatemia (excessively high blood levels of phosphate that occurs in hyperparathyroidism) and certain kidney diseases. Sometimes, a diet that is low in both phosphorus and calcium is given to prevent or treat calcium phosphate kidney stones.	When a rapid reduction in blood phosphate is essential to the patient's health, the diet is used in conjunction with the oral dosage of aluminum hydroxide antacids that bind with phosphate and prevent its absorption.
	1/2 cup (*120 ml*) of heavy cream (35% butterfat).	All other milk products.		
	No cheeses	All cheeses		
	No eggs	All forms of eggs		
	3 cups (*720 ml*) of any canned, fresh, or frozen fruit or juice other than those listed as excluded in the next column.	Avocado, banana, blackberries; and all dried fruits.		
	1 1/2 cups (*360 ml*) beets (roots are permitted, but not the leaves), cabbage, carrots, chicory, cucumbers, green beans, green peppers, lettuce, sauerkraut, spinach, squash, and tomatoes.	All dried beans and peas, and beet greens, broccoli, Brussels sprouts, and corn.		
	5 slices of enriched white bread or the equivalent in crackers made from enriched white flour.	Breads made from rye, or whole or cracked wheat, and all items made with baking powder.		
	1/2 cup (*120 ml*) of a dry or a cooked cereal made from refined grain.	All cereals made from whole or cracked (but not fully refined) grains.		
	1/2 cup (*120 ml*) of sweet or white potato; pasta made from refined white flour, and white rice.	No milk products except the cream allowance may be used in dressings or sauces.		
	8 tsp (*120 ml*) of butter, margarine.	All other types of fats and salad dressings.		
	3 tsp (*15 g*) of white sugar, or 3 Tbsp (*45 ml*) of honey, jam, or jelly; and/or hard candy, drops, fondant, and mints as desired.	Candies that contain chocolate, cream or milk, dried fruits, or nuts; and all other desserts.		
	Unlimited coffee and tea. Unlimited olives and pickles.	All other beverages. All other condiments and snacks.		

(Continued)

TABLE M-70 (*Continued*)

Diet	Composition		Uses	Comments
	Foods Included	**Foods Excluded**		
High potassium diet	A regular diet that emphasizes the consumption of potassium-rich foods such as those which follow: milk, citrus fruits and juices, apricots, bananas, cantaloupe, dates, figs, prunes, raisins, cooked dry beans and peas, green leafy vegetables, tomatoes and tomato juice, whole-grain and bran-type breads and cereals, nuts, catsup, chocolate, cocoa, herbs, spices, and sauces.	None. However, it would be wise to substitute the high potassium foods in each food group (such as fruits and vegetables) for the low-potassium items in each group.	Patients who have become potassium depleted as a result of diarrhea, malnutrition, stresses, surgery, and treatment with certain diuretics.	When there is only mild to moderate potassium depletion it is generally safer to supply it in foods than as pure potassium salts which may cause gastrointestinal irritation. Potassium containing salt substitutes should be used cautiously, and only after a doctor has authorized their use.
Sodium restricted diet	The plan for a moderately restricted diet (800 to 1,000 mg of sodium per day) follows: 10 oz (*284 g*) of unsalted canned, fresh, or frozen fish, meats, or poultry; except the types listed as excluded in the next column. (Liver may be served only once every 2 weeks.)	All types of fish; cured meats such as bacon and ham; and poultry that contains added salt. (Also see Sodium, Table S-14.)	Patients with (1) fluid and sodium retention that is associated with congestive heart failure, liver disease such as cirrhosis, and certain types of kidney diseases; and (2) high blood pressure (hypertension).	Careful adherence to a moderately low salt diet may reduce or eliminate the need for some people to take diuretics and other medications. Many low salt foods are now available in health food stores, large supermarkets, and pharmacies. (A pharmacist can prepare a low sodium baking powder if a commercial product is not available.)
	3 cups (*720 ml*) of skim milk, unsalted buttermilk, and/or whole milk; or the equivalent in evaporated or nonfat dry milk.	Condensed milk, cultured buttermilk, and yogurt; all milk drinks containing chocolate syrup, ice cream, or a malt product.		
	1 oz (*28 g*) of unsalted American cheese, unsalted cottage cheese, or unsalted cream cheese.	All other cheeses.		
	2 eggs boiled, poached, scrambled, or fried in unsalted butter.	None		
	1 1/2 cups (*360 ml*) of canned, fresh, or frozen fruit juice(s) and fruits, one of which should be citrus.	Candied fruits, dried figs, or raisins; tomato juice; all fruit drinks, juices, and other products to which sodium coloring, flavoring, or preservatives have been added.		

(Continued)

TABLE M-70 *(Continued)*

Diet	Composition		Uses	Comments
	Foods Included	**Foods Excluded**		
Sodium restricted diet *(Continued)*	1 1/2 cups (*360 ml*) of salt-free canned, fresh, and frozen vegetables except those listed as excluded in the next column; dried lima beans, lentils, soybeans, and split peas, prepared without salt, salted pork, or a salty sauce.	Canned vegetables and vegetable juices that contain added salt; and frozen vegetables processed with salt.		
	6 slices of unsalted yeast bread, quick breads made with low sodium baking powder, and unsalted crackers. (Salt-containing yeast bread may be permitted, but not salt sticks.)	Products prepared with salt and/or baking powder or baking soda that contains sodium.		
	1/2 cup (*120 ml*) of an unsalted, slow-cooking cereal such as barley, buckwheat groats (kasha), cornmeal, and hominy grits; unsalted dry cereals such as puffed rice and puffed wheat and some brands of shredded wheat (unsalted corn flakes are available in some health food stores).	Quick-cooking and enriched hot cereals; and dry cereals that contain salt.		
	1 cup (*240 ml*) of pasta, potatoes, and/or rice cooked without salt.	Potato chips and prepared potato products.		
	6 tsp (*30 ml*) of unsalted butter, cream, margarine, and homemade salt-free mayonnaise and salad dressings (commercial salt-free products are sold in some health food stores); cooking oils, salt-free shortenings and gravies.	Bacon, pork fat, salted butter and mayonnaise and salad dressings unless labeled "salt-free".		

(Continued)

TABLE M-70 *(Continued)*

Diet	Composition		Uses	Comments
	Foods Included	**Foods Excluded**		
Sodium restricted diet *(Continued)*	1 cup (*240 ml*) of unsalted broth, consomme, cream soup (made with part of the day's allowances for butter and milk), and other soups made from allowed foods listed in this column.	All canned, dehydrated, and frozen broths, bouillon cubes, consomme, extracts and soups that contain salt.		
	Moderate amounts of hard candy, honey, jams and jellies made without sodium benzoate, maple syrup, and brown and white types of sugar.	Chocolate syrups, commercial soft candies or syrups, molasses, and artificial sweeteners that contain sodium.		
	1/2 cup (*120 ml*) of unsalted desserts such as custards (made with part of the day's allowances for eggs and milk), fruit ices, gelatin desserts made with fresh fruit juices, ice cream and sherbets (commercial types must be deducted from the day's milk allowance), and salt-free puddings (cornstarch, rice, and tapioca).	All commercial cakes, cookies, gelatin desserts, chocolate junket desserts, pies, and puddings unless labeled "salt free"; and all other desserts made with baking powder, soda, or salt.		
	Unlimited cocoa (milk deducted from day's allowance), coffee, decaffeinated coffee, fruit drinks without sodium benzoate or an artificial sweetener. Limit of 1 cup of carbonated drink.	Commercial chocolate drinks, diet soft drinks, ginger ale, and instant cocoa.		
	All seasonings, spices, and unsalted condiments except those excluded; unsalted nuts and popcorn; and low sodium catsup.	Salted condiments, seasonings, snacks, and spices; celery seed and dried celery leaves.		

Use of Exchange Lists in Planning Diets.
Table M-70 shows that many types of modified diets are based upon the selection of certain allowed foods and the exclusion of others. However, it is often necessary also to control the composition of diets quantitatively in regard to the levels of protein, carbohydrates, fats, and calories. In the early days of prescribing diets for diabetics this was done by stipulating the weights of the foods that were allowed. The preparation of

meals for these patients was a tedious task for homemakers, who had to control their recipes carefully and weigh each portion of food that was served. This laborious task was simplified greatly in 1950, when the food exchange lists prepared by a joint committee of the American Dietetic Association, American Diabetes Association, and the U.S. Public Health Service were published. A revised version of this system is outlined in Table M-71.

TABLE M-71
FOOD EXCHANGE LISTS GROUPED ACCORDING TO CALORIC CONTENT AND SIZE OF PORTION[1]

Name and Description of Exchange	Low-Calorie Items	Medium-Calorie Items	High-Calorie Items
Meat and protein-rich meat substitutes 1 oz (28 g) of cooked fish, meat, or poultry; or the protein equivalent in cheese, eggs, cooked dried beans or peas, peanut butter, or a vegetable protein product.	*Lean meats and other protein-rich foods:* 1 exchange furnishes about 7 g of protein, 3 g of fat, and 55 kcal Baby beef, chipped beef, chuck, flank steak, tenderloin, plate ribs, plate skirt steak, round (bottom, top), all cuts rump, spare ribs, tripe ....1 oz (28g) Leg, rib, sirloin, loin, shank, shoulder of lamb ....1 oz (28g) Leg (whole rump, center shank) of pork, smoked ham (center slices) ....1 oz (28g) Leg, loin, rib, shank, shoulder, cutlets of veal...................1 oz (28 g) Meat without skin of chicken, turkey, Cornish hen, guinea hen, pheasant ....1 oz (28 g) Any fresh or frozen fish ....1 oz (28 g) Canned crab, lobster, mackerel, salmon and tuna ....1 oz (28 g) Clams, oysters, scallops, shrimp ....5 or 1 oz (28 g) Sardines, drained ....3 Cheeses containing less than 5% fat...........................1 oz (28 g) Cottage cheese, dry and 2% fat ....1/4 c (60 ml) Cooked dried peas and beans (omit 1 bread exchange) .. 1/2 c (120 ml)	*Medium fat meats and other protein-rich foods:* 1 exchange furnishes about 7 g of protein, 5 g of fat and 75 kcal (*omit 1/2 fat exchange*)[2] Canned beef, corned beef, ground (15% fat), ground round, rib eye ......1 oz (28 g) Loin of pork (all cuts), tenderloin, picnic, shoulder arm, shoulder blade (Boston butt), Canadian bacon, boiled ham, loin, picnic ham, shoulder............1 oz (28 g) Liver, heart, kidney, sweetbreads ....1 oz (28 g) Cheese (farmer's, mozzarella, Neufchatel, ricotta)...............1 oz (28 g) Cheese, Parmesan ......3 Tbsp (45 ml) Egg...................1 Peanut butter (omit 2 fat exchanges) .... 2 Tbsp (30 ml)	*High fat meats and other protein-rich foods:* 1 exchange furnishes about 7 g of protein, 8 g of fat and 100 kcal (*omit 1 fat exchange*)[2] Brisket of beef, corned beef (brisket), ground beef (more than 20% fat), ground chuck, hamburger, rib roasts, club and rib steaks................1 oz (28 g) Breast of lamb ....1 oz (28 g) Ground pork loin (back ribs), spare ribs, country-style ham, deviled ham.........1 oz (28 g) Breast of veal ....1 oz (28 g) Capon, duck, goose ....1 oz (28 g) Cheddar cheese and similar types ....1 oz (28 g) Cold cuts—4½" (113 mm) diameter x 1/8" (3 mm) thick ....1 slice Frankfurter 1

Footnotes at end of table

(Continued)

TABLE M-71 (*Continued*)

Name and Description of Exchange	Low-Calorie Items	Medium-Calorie Items	High-Calorie Items
Milk and milk products 1 cup (*240 ml*) or the equivalent in evaporated or nonfat dry milk.	*Nonfat items:* 1 exchange furnishes about 8 g of protein, 12 g of carbohydrate, a trace of fat and 80 kcal Fluid nonfat or skim milk.......................1 c (*240 ml*) Buttermilk made from skim milk.......................1 c (*240 ml*) Plain (unflavored) yogurt made with skim milk.................1 c (*240 ml*) Canned evaporated skim milk .... 1/2 c (*120 ml*) Nonfat dry (powdered skim) milk...........................1/3 c (*80 ml*)	*Lowfat items:* 1 exchange furnishes about 8 g of protein, 12 g of carbo-hydrate, 5 g of fat, and 125 kcal (*omit 1 fat exchange*) Low fat (2% fat) fluid milk ....1 c (*240 ml*)	*Medium fat items:* 1 exchange furnishes about 8 g of protein, 12 g of carbohydrate, 8.5 g of fat, and 160 kcal (*omit 2 fat exchanges*) Buttermilk made from whole milk ....1 c (*240 ml*) Canned evaporated whole milk ...... 1/2 c (*120 ml*) Fluid whole milk ....1 c (*240 ml*) Yogurt made from whole milk ....1 c (*240 ml*)
Fruits and fruit juices Each of the desig-nated portions furnishes 10 g of carbohydrate and 40 kcal.	*Large portions:* 4½ to 7 oz.................. (130 to 200 g) Cantaloupe, 6" (*152 mm*) diameter...................... 1/4 Grapefruit, small............ 1/2 Honeydew melon 7" (*178 mm*) diameter.................... 1/8 Raspberries .... 2/3 c (*160 ml*) Strawberries .... 3/4 c (*180 ml*) Watermelon ....1 c (*240 ml*)	*Medium portions:* 2¼ to 4½ oz (*65 to 129 g*) Apple juice or apple cider ....1/3 c (*80 ml*) Apple, 2" (*51 mm*) diameter ....1 Applesauce, unsweetened .... 1/2 c (*120 ml*) Apricots, fresh, medium ....2 Apricot nectar .....1/3 c (*80 ml*) Blackberries...... 1/2 c (*120 ml*) Blueberries....... 1/2 c (*120 ml*) Fruit cocktail..... 1/2 c (*120 ml*) Grapefruit juice .... 1/2 c (*120 ml*) Grapes............. 12 Mango, small .... 1/2 Nectarine, small ....1 Orange, small.......1 Orange-apricot nectar ....1/3 c (*80 ml*) Orange juice ..... 1/2 c (*120 ml*) Papaya, medium .... 1/3 Peach, medium .....1 Peach nectar.......1/3 c (*80 ml*) Pear, small ....1 Pear nectar.........1/3 c (*80 ml*) Pineapple .... 1/2 c (*120 ml*) Pineapple juice ....1/3 c (*80 ml*) Plums, medium.....2 Tangerine, medium 1	*Small portions:* 1/2 to 2¼ oz (*15 to 64 g*) Apricots, dried ....4 halves Banana, small........ 1/2 Dates....................2 Fig, dried, small ....1 Fig, fresh, large ....1 Grape juice.........1/4 c (*60 ml*) Prunes, dried, medium ....2 Prune juice ....1/4 c (*60 ml*) Raisins........... 2 Tbsp (*30 ml*)

Footnotes at end of table

(Continued)

TABLE M-71 (*Continued*)

Name and Description of Exchange	Low-Calorie Items	Medium-Calorie Items	High-Calorie Items

Vegetables and vegetable juices
 	
(The caloric contents of these items are dependent upon the carbohydrate contents. Hence, the low-calorie items are also low-carbohydrate items, and vice versa.)
	Free items to be used as desired when consumed raw: (If cooked, 1 c [240 ml] may be used without counting it, but the second cup of the cooked item should be counted as furnishing 2 g of protein, 5 g of carbohydrates, and 25 kcal)
	
	Celery
	Chicory
	Chinese cabbage
	Cucumbers
	Endive
	Escarole
	Lettuce
	Watercress
		Counted items: Each 1/2 c of the cooked or raw items (or their corresponding juices) that follow are to be counted as furnishing 2 g of protein, 5 g of carbohydrates, and 25 kcal
		
		Asparagus
		Bean sprouts
		Beets
		Broccoli
		Brussels sprouts
		Cabbage
		Carrots
		Cauliflower
		Eggplant
		Green pepper
		Greens:
		  Beet
		  Chard
		  Collard
		  Dandelion
		  Kale
		
		Greens:
		  Mustard
		  Spinach
		  Turnip
		Mushrooms
		Okra
		Onions
		Radishes
		Rhubarb
		Rutabaga
		Sauerkraut
		String beans, green or wax
		Summer squash
		Tomatoes
		Tomato juice
		Turnips
		Vegetable juice cocktail
		Zucchini
			Starchy vegetables:
			1 exchange furnishes 2 g of protein, 15 g of carbohydrates, and 70 kcal
			
			Baked beans, no pork (canned) ....1/4 c (60 ml)
			Cooked dried beans, lentils, peas
			.... 1/2 c (120 ml)
			Corn kernels, regular or cream-style
			..................1/3 c (80 ml)
			Lima beans....... 1/2 c (120 ml)
			Parsnips .... 2/3 c (160 ml)
			Peas, green (canned or frozen)
			.... 1/2 c (120 ml)
			Potato, white, small
			1
			Pumpkin.......... 3/4 c (180 ml)
			Winter squash, acorn or butternut ... 1/2 c (120 ml)
			Yam or sweet potato
			..................1/4 c (60 ml)

Breads and cereals	*Low-fat items:* 1 exchange furnishes 2 g of protein, 15 g of carbohydrate, and 70 kcal Bread (French, Italian, pumpernickel, raisin, rye, white, whole wheat) .... 1 slice Bread crumbs, dry .... 3 Tbsp (45 ml) English muffin, small .... 1/2 Frankfurter roll .... 1/2 Hamburger bun .... 1/2 Pancake 5" (127 mm) diameter .... 1 Roll, plain, small 1	*Medium-fat items:* 1 exchange furnishes 2 g of protein, 15 g of carbohydrate, 5 g of fat, and 115 kcal (omit 1 fat exchange) Biscuit, 2" (51 mm) diameter ....1 Corn muffin, 2" (51 mm) diameter..................1 Crackers, round butter-type ....5 Muffin, plain, small ....1 Potatoes, french fried 2 to 3½" (51 to 89 mm) long 8	*High-fat items:* 1 exchange furnishes 2 g of protein, 15 g of carbohydrate, 10 g of fat, and 160 kcal (omit 2 fat exchanges) Corn or potato chips ....15 Ice cream......... 1/2 c (120 ml)

Footnotes at end of table

(Continued)

TABLE M-71 (*Continued*)

Name and Description of Exchange	Low-Calorie Items	Medium-Calorie Items	High-Calorie Items

Breads and cereals (*Continued*)	Tortilla 6" (*152 mm*) diameter 1
	Waffle 5" (*127 mm*) square 1
	Cooked cereals.............. 1/2 c (*120 ml*)
	Ready-to-eat cereals:
	  Bran flakes.................. 1/2 c (*120 ml*)
	  Others (unsweetened) .... 3/4 c (*180 ml*)
	  Puffed grains ....1 c (*240 ml*)
	Pastas, cooked .... 1/2 c (*120 ml*)
	Flour .... 2½ Tbsp (*38 ml*)
	Wheat germ ....1/4 c (*60 ml*)
	Crackers:
	  Arrowroot.............................3
	  Graham 2½" (*64 mm*) square 2
	  Matzoh 4" x 6" (*102 x 152 mm*) 1/2
	  Oyster 20
	  Pretzels 3⅛" (*80 mm*) long x ⅛" (*3 mm*) diameter 25
	  Rye wafers 2" (*51 mm*) x 3½" (*89 mm*) 3
	  Saltines...............................6
	  Soda 2½" (*64 mm*) square 4
	Sponge cake, plain, 1½" (*38 mm*) cube........................1
	Vanilla wafers 5		

Fats
 	
Each of the designated portions furnishes 5 g of fat and 45 kcal.
	Least concentrated sources:
	  2 to 3 Tbsp (*30 to 45 g*)
	
	Avocado 4" (*102 mm*) diameter 1/8
	Cream, light, sweet or sour .... 2 Tbsp (*30 ml*)
	Half and half .... 3 Tbsp (*45 ml*)
	Olives, green, medium 3
		Intermediate sources:
		  1 to 2 Tbsp (*15 to 30 g*)
		
		Cream, heavy ... 1 Tbsp (*15 ml*)
		Cream cheese .... 1 Tbsp (*15 ml*)
		French dressing .... 1 Tbsp (*15 ml*)
			Most concentrated sources:
			  1 to 3 tsp (*5 to 15 g*)
			
			Bacon, crisp .... 1 strip
			Butter, lard, margarine, mayonnaise, meat fat (melted), oil, shortening .... 1 tsp (*5 ml*)
			Nuts, shelled, small 6
			Salad dressing, mayonnaise type .... 2 tsp (*10 ml*)

¹Adapted by the authors from *Exchange Lists for Meal Planning*, The American Dietetic Association and the American Diabetes Association, in cooperation with the National Institute of Arthritis, Metabolism and Digestive Diseases and the National Heart, Blood and Lung Institute, Public Health Service, U.S. Dept. HEW, 1976.
²Most diets are based upon the use of lean meats and nonfat milk products. Hence, the use of items richer in fat must be compensated for by the deduction of fat exchanges from the total allowed.

The use of the food exchange lists presented in Table M-71 is illustrated by the sample calculations shown in Table M-72 and the typical menu in Table M-73.

TABLE M-72
CALCULATION OF FOOD EXCHANGES FOR A PRESCRIBED DIET

Prescription: 1,800 kcal   20% protein (*90 g*), 45% carbohydrate (*202 g*), 35% fat (*70 g*)

Exchange	No. of Exchanges	Protein, g	Carbohydrate, g	Fat, g		Calories (kcal)
Meat, lean	3	(x 7) = 21	—	(x 3) = 9		(x 55) = 165
Meat, medium fat	3	(x 7) = 21	—	(x 5) = 15		(x 75) = 225
Running subtotal		(42)		(24)		(390)
Milk, lowfat	2	(x 8) = 16	(x 12) = 24	(x 5) = 10		(x 125) = 250
Milk, medium fat	1	(x 8) = 8	(x 12) = 12	(x 8.5) = 8.5		(x 160) = 160
Running subtotal		(66)	(36)	(42.5)		(800)
Fruit	3	—	(x 10) = 30	—		(x 40) = 120
Running subtotal		(66)	(66)	(42.5)		(920)
Vegetables, free items	unlimited	—	—	—		—
Vegetables, counted	2	(x 2) = 4	(x 5) = 10	—		(x 25) = 50
Vegetables, starchy	2	(x 2) = 4	(x 15) = 30	—		(x 70) = 140
Running subtotal		(74)	(106)	(42.5)		(1,110)
Bread, lowfat	3	(x 2) = 6	(x 15) = 45	—		(x 70) = 210
Bread, medium fat	2	(x 2) = 4	(x 15) = 30	(x 5) = 10		(x 115) = 230
Bread, high fat	1	(x 2) = 2	(x 15) = 15	(x 10) = 10		(x 160) = 160
Running subtotal		(86)	(196)	(62.5)		(1,710)
Fats	2	—	—	(x 5) = 10		(x 45) = 90
Total x calorie factor		86 x 4	196 x 4	72.5 x 9		1,800
Calories		344	+ 784	+ 652.5 =		1,781

The bases of the calculations shown in Table M-72 and the typical daily menu in Table M-73 are as follows:

1.   A 48-year-old businessman who is 6 ft, 2 in. (*188 cm*) tall is of medium build, and weighs 198 lb (*90 kg*) has been diagnosed recently as an adult onset diabetic who does not require insulin injections but would benefit from a reduction of his body weight to one that is more desirable for his age, height, and condition.

2.   The ideal weight of the patient is 176 lb, or *80 kg* (from a standard life insurance table) and the caloric intake for a sedentary person at that weight should be 176 lb x 13 Calories (kcal) per pound (*28.6 kcal/kg*), or 2,288 kcal per day. (This allowance may be rounded to 2,300 kcal per day.)

3.   It is decided that the weight reduction of the patient should be gradual (about 1 lb per week). Hence, his dietary prescription is for 1,800 kcal per day, distributed as follows: 20% from proteins, 45% from carbohydrates, and 35% from fats. (A caloric deficit of 500 kcal per day equals a weekly deficit of 3,500 kcal, or the amount needed to lose 1 lb [*0.45 kg*] of body weight.) The daily allowances (in grams) of proteins, carbohydrates, and fats are determined by dividing the caloric factors for nutrients (proteins, 4 kcal/g; carbohydrates, 4 kcal/g; and fats, 9 kcal/g) into the kcal contributed by each nutrient.

$$\text{Proteins} = \frac{1,800 \text{ kcal x } 20\%}{4 \text{ kcal/g}} = 90 \text{ g}$$

$$\text{Carbohydrates} = \frac{1,800 \text{ kcal x } 45\%}{4 \text{ kcal/g}} = 202 \text{ g}$$

$$\text{Fats} = \frac{1,800 \text{ kcal x } 35\%}{9 \text{ kcal/g}} = 70 \text{ g}$$

4.   The allowed food exchanges are worked out by (1) considering the meat and milk items to have the highest

A TYPICAL DAILY 1800-CALORIE MENU THAT WAS PLANNED FROM FOOD EXCHANGE LISTS[1]

Type of Food Exchange	No. of Exchanges	Typical Foods in Designated Exchange	Type of Food Exchange	No. of Exchanges	Typical Foods in Designated Exchange
Breakfast:					extra fat exchanges may be allowed.
Meat, medium fat.	1	An egg, a 1 oz-slice of boiled ham, Canadian bacon, or 1 lamb kidney (cooked without fat, unless 1 of the allowed fat exchanges is used).	Fat.............	1	Dressing for salad or vegetable, or spread for bread.
			Unrestricted items	—	Coffee, cereal beverage, dietetic soft drink, herb tea, etc. (See Breakfast).
Milk, lowfat (2%)..	1	Taken as a beverage, in coffee or tea, and/or on cereal.			
Fruit	1	Glass (4 oz, or *120 ml*) of fruit juice, or a serving of a fruit.	**Midafternoon:**		
			Unrestricted items	—	Coffee, cereal beverage, dietetic soft drink, herb tea, etc. (See Breakfast).
Bread, lowfat	2	Bread and/or cereal.			
Unrestricted items	—	Coffee, cereal beverage (coffee substitute), dietetic (artificially sweetened) soft drink, herb tea, or tea without a natural sweetener (unless 1/3 bread exchange is deducted for each tsp of sweetener used during the day).	Bread, if *not* used at breakfast or lunch	1 to 2	Bread, cake, cookies, or crackers.
			Milk, if not used as allowed at another meal...	—	(See the note next to milk under Midmorning.)
Midmorning:			**Supper:**		
Unrestricted items	—	Coffee, cereal beverage, dietetic soft drink, herb tea, etc. (See Breakfast).	Meat, lean	3	Fish, meat, poultry, or a meat substitute.
			Fruit	1	Glass (4 oz, or *120 ml*) of fruit juice, or a serving of a fruit.
Bread, if *not* used at breakfast ...	1	Bread, cake, cookies, or crackers.	Vegetable, free ..	—	Celery, cucumber, lettuce, etc. as desired.
Milk, if *not* used at breakfast ...	1	Part of the allowed medium fat milk exchange (whole or evaporated milk) may be used in the unrestricted beverage.	Vegetable, counted.......	1	Beets, carrots, green pepper, mushrooms, onions, tomatoes, etc.
			Vegetable, starchy	1	Baked beans (without pork), cooked dried beans or peas, corn, green peas, sweet or white potato.
Lunch:			Bread, lowfat	1	Bread, roll, tortilla, etc.
Meat, medium fat.	2	2 slices (2 oz, or *56 g*) of broiled or roasted (not fried) meat.	Bread, high fat...	1	Items such as 1 serving of ice cream or potato chips (If low or medium-fat bread is used instead, an extra fat exchange may be allowed).
Fruit	1	Glass (4 oz, or *120 ml*) of fruit juice, or a serving of a fruit.			
Vegetable, free ..	—	Celery, cucumber, lettuce, etc. as desired.	Fat.............	1	Dressing for salad or vegetable, or spread for bread.
Vegetable, counted.......	1	Beets, carrots, green pepper, mushrooms, onions, tomatoes, etc.	Unrestricted items	—	Coffee, cereal beverage, dietetic soft drink, herb tea, etc. (See Breakfast).
Vegetable, starchy	1	Baked beans (without pork), cooked dried beans or peas, corn, green peas, sweet or white potato.	**Bedtime:**		
Bread, medium fat	2	Allowance is intended to cover items such as a small serving of french fried potatoes, biscuits, or corn muffins. If 1 or more lowfat items are used instead, 1 or more	Milk, lowfat (2%)..	1	
			Bread, if the exchanges allowed at meals during the day are not all used	1 to 3	Bread, cake, cereal, cookies, or crackers.

[1]See Table D-72 and the accompanying text for the calculations used to determine the numbers of allowed food exchanges.

priorities, and (2) keeping a running count of the dietary content of proteins, carbohydrates, fats, and calories as the various exchanges are added to the diet. This calculation is simplified by the tabular format of Table M-72 in which the values shown in parentheses represent the nutrient values of the exchanges listed in the column on the left margin. The values shown after the equal signs were obtained by multiplying the nutrient values for the exchanges by the number of exchanges selected. It is noteworthy that the patient was allowed some medium fat exchanges for meat, milk, and bread products because he has to eat his lunch in a fast food restaurant.

5.   After the bread exchanges were added to the diet, the running subtotal showed that only two separate fat exchanges could be added. Then, a check of the dietary totals of proteins, carbohydrates, fats, and calories showed that they were reasonably close to those in the dietary prescription.

6.   The menu shows how the allowed exchanges may be used in meals. Although it may not always be possible to adhere perfectly to the plan, lapses on certain days should be noted carefully in terms of the allowances that were exceeded and they should be compensated for in the days that follow the deviations. For example, extra fat taken on one day should be compensated for by an equivalent deduction the next day, such as the substitution of a lowfat exchange for an allowed medium fat exchange.

Special Dietetic Foods.   Many types of special dietary products are now available for people who must limit their consumption of substances present in ordinary foods. For example, there are artificially sweetened jams, jellies, salad dressings, sauces, and soft drinks. (The term "dietetic" does not always mean that the product contains an artificial sweetener. Rather, it may mean that considerably less than the normal amounts of natural sweetener were used in the recipe. It may also be used to designate lowfat varieties of items such as salad dressings. Also, both dry and liquid forms of low-cholesterol egg products are sold in most supermarkets. However, it is best for anyone who has been placed on a modified diet to consult his or her doctor or dietitian before using any special dietetic foods because use of the new product may result in a significant alteration in the nutritional value of the prescribed diet.

SUMMARY.   The proper types of modified diets may be very useful in the treatment of people with various disorders or undesirable conditions such as overweight or underweight. Nevertheless, the combined expertise of a doctor and a dietitian are usually needed to determine the dietary patterns most suitable for individual patients.

MOIETY

Any equal part.

MOISTURE

A term used to indicate the water contained in foods—expressed as a percentage.

MOISTURE-FREE (M-F, oven-dry, 100% dry matter)

This refers to any substance that has been dried in an oven at 221°F (105°C) until all the moisture has been removed.

(Also see ANALYSIS OF FOODS.)

MOLASSES

Molasses is the thick brownish syrup by-product of the manufacture of cane or beet sugar from which part of the crystallizable sugar has been removed. However, molasses is also the by-product of several other industries. Citrus molasses is produced from the juice of citrus wastes. Wood molasses is a by-product of the manufacture of paper, fiberboard, and pure cellulose from wood; it is an extract from the more soluble carbohydrates and minerals of the wood material. Starch molasses, Hydrol, is a by-product of the manufacture of dextrose (glucose) from starch derived from corn or grain sorghums in which the starch is hydrolyzed by use of enzymes and/or acid. Cane molasses is, by far, the most extensively used type of molasses. The different types of molasses are available in both liquid and dehydrated forms.

Molasses still contains sugar, which forms the basis of determining its quality. The sugar content is expressed as *Brix*. Brix is determined by measuring the specific gravity of molasses. After the specific gravity has been obtained, the value is applied to a conversion table from which the level of sucrose (or degrees Brix) can be determined. As sugar content increases, degrees Brix likewise increases. Since molasses also contains lipids, protein, inorganic salts, waxes, gums, and other material, the Brix classification can often be misleading, because each of these contaminants has an influence on the specific gravity of the solution. However, degrees Brix does give a relatively accurate indication of the sugar content of molasses and is, therefore, a good means of determining quality.

PRODUCTION.   As early as 1900, sugar planters in Louisiana fed cane molasses in long, open troughs to mules, cows, and hogs. Feeding was a sticky, messy business, and there were swarms of flies. Even so, molasses was fed simply because it had to be disposed of, and the animals liked it. It couldn't be sold for the price of the barrel container, and there was still the matter of freight charges. Now, molasses production (including cane, beet, starch, and citrus molasses) amounts to about 638 million gallons (*2,414 million liter*) annually in the United States. In addition, more than 900,000 metric tons are imported annually; the majority of this, however, is not for human consumption. In the United States, Louisiana is the center of molasses production.

Molasses may be made by the open kettle method or by the vacuum pan method. In the open kettle method, the cane juice is boiled in a large open pan. Large sugar factories generally use the vacuum pan method, in which large, covered vacuum pans are used.

USES. Only a small portion of the molasses available in the United States is consumed by humans. Some molasses is used in industries for the production of yeast and organic fermentation chemicals. But the major utilization of molasses in the United States is in animal feeds, as blackstrap molasses—the molasses left after several boilings.

Food. As a food, molasses is not as popular as it once was. Consumption declined from 1945 to 1970, then stabilized. (See Fig. M-117.)

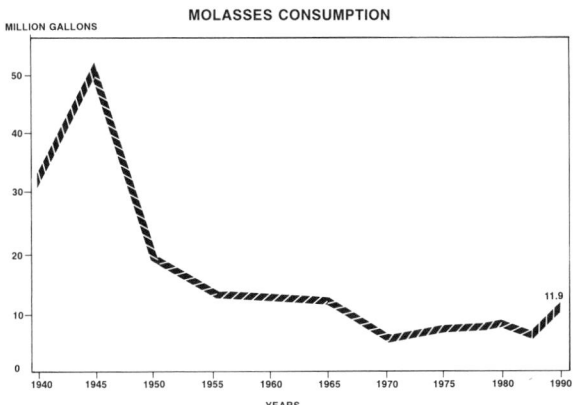

Fig. M-117. Consumption of edible molasses in the United States since 1940. (Source of data: *Agricultural Statistics*, 1951–1991, USDA)

The baking industry is the largest consumer of edible molasses. It imparts a pleasant flavor to breads, cakes, and cookies. Additionally, molasses serves as a humectant—helping to maintain the freshness of baked goods, and enhances the flavor of chocolate in baked goods or drinks.

In home cooking, molasses is employed for the same purposes as in the baking industry. Also, molasses is often incorporated in baked beans, and in glazes for sweet potatoes and meats such as hams. The flavor of toffees and caramel may be rounded out with molasses. Some table syrups contain molasses, and some individuals sweeten foods with molasses, while others mix a spoonful or two with hot water for a hot beverage. Many recipes have been developed which take advantage of the pleasant flavor and smell of molasses.

Generally, molasses is eaten in such small amounts it does not make an important contribution to the diet. However, the nutritional value of molasses is indicated in Table M-74.

TABLE M-74
NUTRITIONAL VALUE OF CANE MOLASSES[1]

Nutrient[2]	Unit	Molasses		
		Light	Medium	Blackstrap
		◄ — —(Per 100 g) — — ►		
Food energy	kcal	270.0	250.0	230.0
Protein	g	2.4	2.4	2.4
Carbohydrates ...	g	65.0	60.0	55.0
Calcium	mg	165.0	290.0	684.0
Phosphorus	mg	45.0	69.0	84.0
Sodium	mg	15.0	37.0	96.0
Magnesium	mg	209.3	81.0	209.3
Potassium........	mg	917.0	1063.0	2927.0
Iron	mg	4.3	6.0	16.1
Zinc..............	mg	.4	.4	.4
Copper	mg	.6	.6	.6
Thiamin	mg	.1	.1	.1
Riboflavin	mg	.1	.1	.2
Niacin............	mg	.2	1.2	2.0
Pantothenic acid.	mg	.4	.4	.4
Pyridoxine	mg	.2	.2	.2
Folic acid	mcg	13.0	9.5	9.5
Biotin	mcg	9.0	9.0	9.0

[1]Values from Food Composition Table F-36.
[2]Nutrients not listed are not present.

Table M-74 indicates that (1) molasses is a good source of some minerals—especially calcium, magnesium, potassium, and iron; (2) molasses is a concentrated energy source; (3) blackstrap contains several of the minerals at higher levels than light or medium molasses; and (4) vitamins are present only in low levels, or nonexistent.

NOTE WELL: Dark molasses (blackstrap molasses) is a fair, but variable and unreliable, source of iron. Today, there is less iron in molasses that is processed in stainless steel or aluminum vessels than in molasses processed in old-fashioned iron vats and pipes. Besides, molasses is generally eaten infrequently and/or in small servings. Some opinions to the contrary, molasses has no miraculous curative properties; rather, it should be eaten for reason of taste.

The alcoholic fermentation and distillation of molasses yields rum, which in a crude form was a drink of early sailors trading with the sugarcane growing West Indies. Also, molasses from the West Indies was imported to New England where it became rum in colonial days. Through the Molasses Act of the British Parliament in 1733, an attempt was made, by high taxes, to discourage the American colonies from trading with the parts of the West Indies not under British rule. The Molasses Act further provoked the pre-Revolutionary unrest in colonial America.

Rum still is produced from the fermentation of molasses. After distillation, it is aged from 5 to 7 years. Rum gets its color from the oaken cask in which it is aged and from caramel added before aging. Some light rums are rapidly fermented with cultured yeast and aged from 1 to 4 years.

(Also see ALCOHOLIC BEVERAGES.)

Industry. Molasses provides carbohydrates, minerals, and some vitamins for the culture of yeast. Cane and beet molasses are employed for the commercial production of baker's and brewers' yeast. The culture of yeast for food—human food or animal feed—may utilize beet, cane, starch, citrus, or wood molasses as a carbohydrate source. Furthermore, the fermentation of molasses provides a source of industrial alcohol (ethyl alcohol) and other important industrial organic chemicals.

(Also see SINGLE-CELL PROTEIN.)

Animal Feeds. Molasses (including cane, beet, citrus, wood, and starch molasses) is an extremely palatable and excellent source of energy for animals, particularly cattle. It (1) adds energy, (2) reduces dustiness, (3) serves as a binder, (4) provides minerals, (5) serves as an appetizer, (6) stimulates rumen microbial activity, and (7) provides unidentified factors. In cattle feeds, molasses is restricted to the level of 10 to 15% of the ration.

Including imports, about 600 million gallons (*2,280 million liter*) of all types of molasses are available each year for feed and industrial purposes. Human consumption of molasses is minor when compared to this amount.

(Also see CARBOHYDRATE[S]; and SUGAR.)

MOLD INHIBITORS

Substances such as sodium and calcium propionate which are added to foods to prevent the growth of mold. Often, substances with this action are referred to as antimicrobials.

(Also see ADDITIVES.)

MOLDS (FUNGI)

Fungi which are distinguished by the formation of mycelium (a network of filaments or threads), or by spore masses.

(Also see POISONS, Table P-11 Some Potentially Poisonous [Toxic] Substances—Mycotoxins; and SPOILAGE OF FOOD.)

MOLECULE

A chemical combination of two or more atoms.

MOLYBDENUM (Mo)

Although the essential role of molybdenum in plants is well known, the essentiality of this element in man is less well established. Evidence that molybdenum is an essential trace element is based on the facts that it is part of the molecular structure of two enzymes, xanthine oxidase (involved in the oxidation of xanthine to uric acid) and aldehyde oxidase (involved in the oxidation of aldehydes to carboxylic acids), and that diets low in molybdenum adversely affect growth in small animals. There is no evidence, however, that a low molybdenum intake produces deficiency signs and symptoms in man.

The adult human body contains only about 9 mg of molybdenum.

HISTORY. In 1778, Karl Scheele of Sweden recognized molybdenite as a distinct ore of a new element. Then, in 1782, P. J. Hjelm obtained the metal by reducing the oxide with carbon and called it molybdenum. The name molybdenum is derived from the Greek *molybdos*, meaning lead.

Molybdenum was long known as essential for the growth of all higher plants. Then, in 1953 it was found in the essential enzyme, xanthine dehydrogenase.

ABSORPTION, METABOLISM, EXCRETION. Molybdenum is readily absorbed as molybdate in the small intestine, although some absorption occurs throughout the intestinal tract. There is little retention of this element except in the liver, adrenals, kidneys, and bones. Molybdenum is excreted rapidly in the urine, and in limited amounts via the bile and feces.

FUNCTIONS OF MOLYBDENUM. Molybdenum is a component of three different enzyme systems which are involved in the metabolism of carbohydrates, fats, proteins, sulfur-containing amino acids, nucleic acids (DNA and RNA), and iron. Also, it is found in the enamel of teeth, where it appears to prevent or reduce the incidence of dental caries, although this function has not yet been proven conclusively.

DEFICIENCY SYMPTOMS. Naturally occurring deficiency of molybdenum in human subjects is not known, *unless* utilization of the mineral is interfered with by excesses of copper and/or sulfate.

Molybdenum-deficient animals are especially susceptible to the toxic effects of bisulfite, which is both a food additive and a product of the metabolism of sulfur-containing amino acids. Bisulfite toxicity is characterized by breathing difficulties and neurological disorders.

INTERRELATIONSHIPS. The utilization of molybdenum is reduced by excess copper, sulfate, and tungsten (an environmental contaminant). Also, even a moderate excess of molybdenum causes significant urinary loss of copper; and toxicity due to excess copper is counteracted by molybdenum.

In cattle, an interesting relationship has been observed between molybdenum, copper, and sulfur. Molybdenum competes with copper for some of the main metabolic sites, with the result that an excess of molybdenum will cause copper deficiency. However, when the sulfate content of the diet is increased, the symptoms of toxicity are avoided inasmuch as the excretion of molybdenum is increased.

RECOMMENDED DAILY ALLOWANCE OF MOLYBDENUM. Man's requirement for molybdenum is so low that it is easily furnished by the diet.

The Food and Nutrition Board of the National Research Council (FNB-NRC) recommends that the molybdenum intake of an adult be within the range of 0.15 to 0.5 mg/day, with a maximum habitual intake not to exceed 0.5 mg per day.

Estimated safe and adequate intakes of molybdenum are given in Table M-75.

**TABLE M–75
ESTIMATED SAFE AND ADEQUATE
DAILY DIETARY INTAKES OF MOLYBDENUM[1]**

Group	Age	Molybdenum
	(years)	(mcg)
Infants	0.0–0.5	15–30
	0.5–1.0	20–40
Children and adolescents . .	1–3	25–50
	4–6	30–75
	7–10	50–150
	11+	75–250
Adults		75–250

[1]*Recommended Dietary Allowances*, 10th ed., 1989, NRC–National Academy of Sciences, p. 284.

• **Molybdenum intake in average U.S. diet**—The daily intake from a mixed diet in the United States has been estimated at between 0.1 and 0.46 mg.

TOXICITY. The greatest concern about molybdenum is its toxicity. Adverse effects of high molybdenum concentrations in the environment have been reported in the human population living in a province of the U.S.S.R.[67] According to the U.S.S.R. report, an excessive dietary intake of 10 to 15 mg/day of molybdenum caused a high incidence of a goutlike syndrome associated with elevated blood levels of molybdenum, uric acid, and xanthine oxidase.

[67]Kovalskiy, V. V., and G. A. Yarovaya, Molybdenum-infiltrated Biogeochemical Provinces, *Agrokhimiya*, Vol. 8, 1966, pp. 68-91.

Severe molybdenum toxicity in animals (molybdenosis), particularly cattle, occurs throughout the world wherever pastures are grown on high-molybdenum soils. The symptoms include diarrhea, loss of weight, decreased production, fading of hair color, and other symptoms of a copper deficiency.

Potentially toxic levels of molybdenum are contained in some soils and herbage in parts of Florida, California, and Manitoba.

SOURCES OF MOLYBDENUM. The concentration of molybdenum in food varies considerably, depending on the soil in which it was grown. Most of the dietary molybdenum intake is derived from organ meats, whole grains, wheat germ, legumes, leafy vegetables, and yeast. Table M-76 gives the molybdenum content of some common foods. The molybdenum requirement should be met by most diets. Supplements of additional molybdenum are not recommended.

(Also see MINERAL[S], Table M-67.)

**TABLE M-76
MOLYBDENUM CONTENT
OF SOME COMMON FOODS**

Food	Molybdenum
	(mg/100 g)
Lima beans, dry	.323
Wheat germ	.210
Liver	.150
Green beans	.067
Eggs	.050
Whole wheat flour	.048
Poultry	.040
White flours	.025
Spinach	.025
Cabbage	.017
Potato	.016
Cantaloupe	.016
Apricot	.011
Carrot	.010
Banana	.003
Milk	.003
Lettuce	.002
Celery	.002

MONOGLYCERIDE

An ester of glycerol with one fatty acid.
(Also see ADDITIVES, Table A-3.)

MONOPHAGIA

The habit of eating, or the desire to eat, only one type of food.
(Also see APPETITE.)

MONOSACCHARIDE

Any one of several simple, nonhydrolyzable sugars. Glucose, fructose, galactose, arabinose, xylose, and ribose are examples.

(Also see CARBOHYDRATE[S]; and SUGARS.)

MONOUNSATURATED

Having one double bond, as in a fatty acid; e.g., oleic acid.

MONOVALENT

Having a valence (the power of an atom to combine with another atom) of one. Example: sodium ($Na+$) has a valence of one; it combines with chloride (Cl-) to form sodium chloride ($NaCl$).

MORBIDITY

A state of sickness.

MORTADELLA

A dry or semidry sausage made of chopped pork and pork fat; seasoned with red pepper and garlic; stuffed in large casings; and cooked and smoked.

MOTILITY

The power of spontaneous movement.

MUCIN

A glycoprotein secreted by the secretory cells of the digestive tract. It functions to (1) facilitate the smooth movement of food through the digestive tract, and (2) provide a protective coating to the gastric and duodenal mucosa against the corrosive action of hydrochloric acid.

(Also see DIGESTION AND ABSORPTION; and ULCERS, PEPTIC.)

MUCOPOLYSACCHARIDE (GLYCOSAMINO -GLYCAN)

A group of polysaccharides which contains hexosamine (as glucosamine), which may or may not be combined with protein, and which, dispersed in water, form many of the mucins—thick gelatinous material that cements cells together and lubricates joints and bursas.

MUCOPROTEIN

Substances containing a polypeptid chain and disaccharides, found in mucous secretions of the digestive glands.

MUCOSA (MUCOUS MEMBRANE)

A membrane rich in mucous glands which lines the gastrointestinal, respiratory, and genitourinary tracts.

MUCOUS MEMBRANE

A membrane lining the cavities and canals of the body, kept moist by mucus.

(Also see BODY TISSUES.)

MUCUS

A slimy liquid secreted by the mucous glands and membranes.

MULTIPLE SCLEROSIS (MS)

A strange and baffling disease of the nervous system of unknown origin whose victims are between the ages of 20 and 40. Some evidence suggests that it is caused by a slow-acting virus to which the body's immune system does not respond. Nerve tracts of the brain and spinal cord develop areas of faulty nerve transmission due to the development of areas of demyelination—loss of myelin, the insulation of nerves—which is thought to be the result of some alteration in lipid metabolism. These areas occur at random and may come and go. Symptoms signaling the onset of multiple sclerosis may be so minor that they are overlooked; for example, blurred or double vision. Once the initial symptoms disappear they may never recur, and a period of months or years may pass before other symptoms appear such as weakness of certain muscles, unusual tiring of a limb, minor interference with walking, muscle stiffness, dizziness, loss of bladder control and disturbances in the senses of touch, pain, and heat. Each symptom may appear and then disappear only to be followed by another. The disease continues to progress, and eventually the victim becomes crippled and even bedridden. However, the progression and remission of multiple sclerosis is different for every victim. Maintenance of good physical health, resistance to infection, and good mental health play a role in the severity of the symptoms. To this end a nutritionally adequate and appealing diet simply prepared is recommended. As the disease progresses, a pureed or liquefied diet may be necessary since victims have difficulty swallowing.

(Also see MODIFIED DIETS.)

MUNG BEAN (GOLDEN GRAM; GREEN GRAM) *Phaseolus aureus*

Americans usually consume this legume in the form of bean sprouts. Mung bean seeds grow in hairy pods and are generally utilized when fully mature. Fig. M-118 shows part of a mung bean plant.

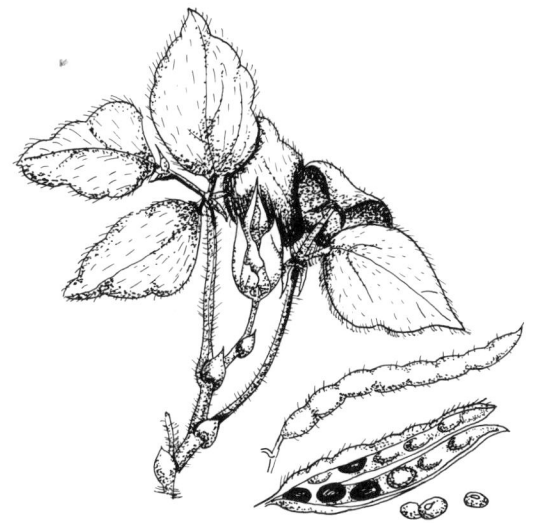

Fig. M-118. Mung bean.

ORIGIN AND HISTORY. This crop has been cultivated in India for thousands of years. It was brought to China and southeast Asia centuries ago. In recent times it has been introduced into Africa, the United States, and the West Indies.

PRODUCTION. Much of the world's mung bean crop is grown in India and Pakistan, but small amounts are also produced in subtropical and tropical regions of Africa, the Americas, and Asia, because the crop does well when the temperature ranges between 68°F (*20°C*) and 113°F (*45°C*). The number of beans produced per plant can be increased dramatically by inoculation of the seeds with *Rhizobium* (a family of nitrogen-fixing species of bacteria). A series of experiments showed that yields were increased by 50%, or more, in plants grown from inoculated seeds compared to those grown from uninoculated seeds. The pods are sometimes harvested green and used as a fresh vegetable in India, but elsewhere they are usually picked only when the beans are fully mature.

PROCESSING. The beans are dried, debranned, and ground into flour in India and Pakistan, whereas in China and the United States they are usually allowed to sprout for about 4 days. Certain American producers of Chinese foods either can the sprouts (1) alone in water, or (2) mixed with other Chinese vegetables such as water chestnuts.

SELECTION AND PREPARATION. Usually, the dried bean seeds are sold only in (1) stores that cater to customers of Chinese descent, and (2) health or natural food stores. However, the canned sprouts are available in most large supermarkets. Sprouts may be prepared from the dry beans by (1) soaking in water overnight, (2) draining the water and placing the soaked beans in a container in the dark for 4 to 7 days, and (3) keeping the beans moist while draining off the old water two or more times daily. (Allowing the seeds to stand for too long in the old water may bring about spoilage before sprouting.) A pound (*0.45 kg*) of dry beans yields from 6 to 8 lb (*2.7 to 3.6 kg*) of sprouts.

Sprouts may be added to salads without further preparation, or they may be stir-fried briefly with other items such as celery, cheese, eggs, fish, green peppers, legumes, meat, onions, poultry, and/or water chestnuts. (Most of these items should be cut into small pieces prior to stir frying.) Also, the sprouts may be used in quiches and in homemade chop suey or chow mein. Some people make sandwiches with whole wheat bread, sprouts, sliced cheese, lettuce, and Tamari sauce.

NUTRITIONAL VALUE. The nutrient composition of mung bean sprouts is given in Food Composition Table F-36.

The high water content (about 90%) makes mung bean sprouts low in solids, calories, and most other nutrients. Also, the sprouts supply about 11 g of protein per 100 Calories (kcal). However, their bulkiness makes it necessary to eat from 5 to 6 cups (about *680 g*) to obtain the protein in 3 oz (*85 g*) of meat. Furthermore, the protein in mung beans is quite deficient in the sulfur amino acids methionine and cystine. In China, this deficiency is corrected in part by eating the beans or their sprouts with cereal products such as rice, or with small amounts of eggs, fish, meat, or poultry. (The other protein sources balance the amino acid deficiencies in the legume.) People who have ravenous appetites and an enormous capacity for food might do well to eat lots of mung bean sprouts, which are very filling but not very fattening.

(Also see BEAN[S], Table B-10 Beans of the World; LEGUMES, Table L-2 Legumes of the World; and VEGETABLE[S], Table V-6 Vegetables of the World.)

MUSCLES

All physical functions of the body involve muscular contractions, which, in turn, require nutrients derived from the diet. Muscles conduct nervous impulses, contract in response to nervous impulses, and modify their activity according to the degree they are stretched. In the body, there are three types of muscles:

1. **Skeletal muscles.** These are attached to the 206 bones that make up the skeleton. Their coordinated contraction and relaxation results in the movement of body parts. Skeletal muscles are voluntarily controlled. They are also classified as striated muscles due to their microscopic appearance.

2. **Smooth muscles.** Most of the internal organs of the body contain smooth muscles. They are responsible for contractions of such organs as the intestines, blood vessels and uterus. For the most part, smooth muscles are involuntarily controlled.

3. **Cardiac muscle.** Obviously, it is found only in the heart. Continually contracting and relaxing with a built in rhythmicity until death, it pumps about 8,000 gallons (*30,400 liter*) of blood through 12,000 miles (*19,200 km*) of blood vessels each day.

Muscular contraction is a complicated process involving the actin and myosin filaments of the cell; requiring chemical energy and oxygen. It forms heat and a force capable of performing work.

(Also see ENERGY UTILIZATION OF THE BODY; METABOLISM; and MUSCULAR WORK.)

MUSCOVADO

Unrefined raw sugar obtained from the juice of sugarcane by evaporation and drawing off the molasses.

MUSCULAR DYSTROPHY (MD)

Any of the hereditary diseases of the skeletal muscles characterized by a progressive shrinking or wasting of the muscles. At the onset only certain muscles seem affected, but ultimately all muscles become involved. The exact cause is not known. The most common form of muscular dystrophy occurs almost entirely in males since its inheritance is sex linked—passed from mother to son on the X chromosome. There is no effective treatment. Physical therapy may delay the progression of the disease. Dietary adjustments due to limited mobility and feeding difficulties are necessary as the disease advances.

(Also see DISEASES; and MODIFIED DIETS.)

MUSCULAR WORK

Energy is the ability to do work. Mechanical work is accomplished when a force acts to move an object some distance. Muscles require chemical energy derived from the diet to contract and produce a force capable of performing work. Contraction of the heart produces a force which propels the blood through the blood vessels. Contracting limb muscles are capable of exerting a force to move an object from the floor to a table. Contracting limb muscles work to move the body—exercise. The amount of energy required is in direct relation to the intensity of the muscular work.

(Also see CALORIC [ENERGY] EXPENDITURE.)

MUSH

This is a dish made by boiling cornmeal in water, which is eaten as a hot cereal; or it can be put into a mold until cold, then sliced and fried in a little butter.

MUSHROOMS, CULTIVATED *Basidiomycetes, Ascomycetes*

Contents   Page

These much esteemed foods are the fleshy, fruiting bodies of higher fungi that grow in soil rich in organic matter, or on living trees or dead wood. From a strict botanical point of view, the term mushroom designates certain club fungi (*Basidiomycetes*). However, many people extend the term to cover cup fungi (*Ascomycetes*) such as truffles.

This article deals only with cultivated mushrooms. Edible and poisonous wild mushrooms are covered elsewhere.

(Also see POISONOUS PLANTS; and WILD EDIBLE PLANTS.)

MAJOR TYPES. There are about 38,000 known species of mushrooms. Of course, it is impossible in this article to list or describe all the kinds of mushrooms. However, brief descriptions of the five most commonly cultivated mushrooms follow.

• **Common Cultivated Mushroom** (*Agaricus bisporus*)— This is the type that is best known to Americans. It is light colored and very mild flavored.

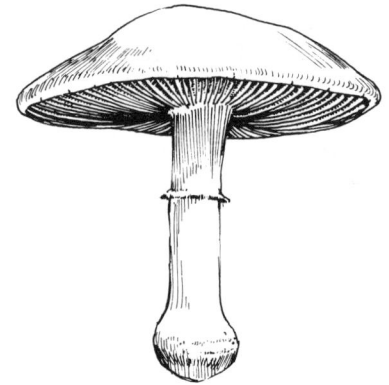

Fig. M-119. The Common Cultivated Mushroom (*Agaricus bisporus*).

• **Oyster Mushroom** (*Pleurotus ostreatus*)—The color and shape of this type are like those of an oyster. It is grown mainly in the Orient and in Europe. The canned oyster mushrooms sold in the United States are usually imported from Taiwan.

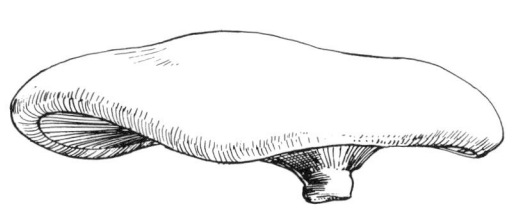

Fig. M-120. The Oyster Mushroom (*Pleurotus ostreatus*).

• **Padi Straw Mushroom** (*Volvariella volvaceae*)—Most of this crop is produced in the Orient, where it is grown on rice (paddy) straw. These mushrooms are usually sold in the dried form.

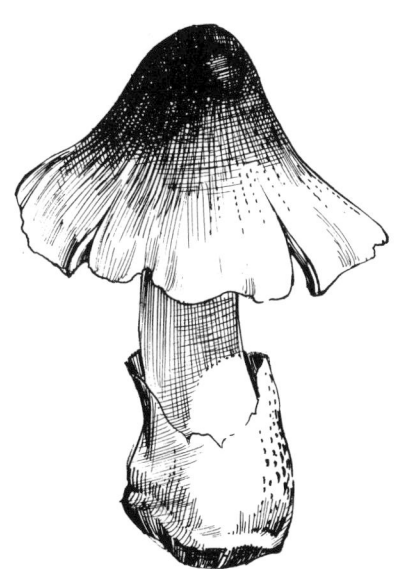

Fig. M-121. The Padi Straw Mushroom (*Volvariella volvaceae*).

• **Shiitake** (*Lentinus edodes*)—This type is grown mainly in China and Japan, and is exported in canned, dried, and pickled forms.

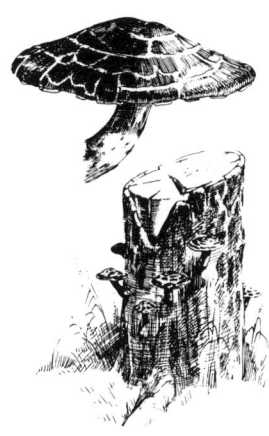

Fig. M-122. Shiitake (*Lentinus edodes*), a mushroom which grows on hardwood logs.

• **Truffles** (*Tuber melanosporum; Tuber magnatum*)—These are by far the most sought after and expensive of the mushrooms. Actually, they are cup fungi (*Ascomycetes*), rather than mushrooms, and they grow underground in association with the roots of oak and beech trees. Most of the world's supply of this delicacy is produced in France and Italy. Terfezios are fungi that resemble truffles closely and are found mainly in the desert areas of North Africa and the Middle East.

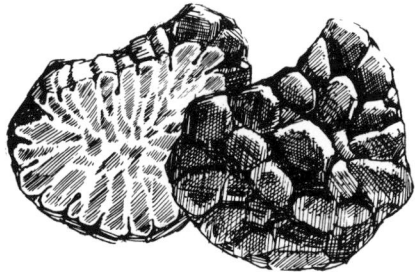

Fig. M-123. Truffles (*Tuber melanosporum*), a gourmet fungus that is highly esteemed for its fragrant aroma.

ORIGIN AND HISTORY. Wild Mushrooms and other edible fungi were consumed by primitive peoples long before the dawn of agriculture. Many centuries elapsed, and a wide variety of green plants were grown around the world before even a few of the many species of edible mushrooms were cultivated on a regular basis. Mushroom cultivation was not developed as early as the growing of other plants because the edible fleshy fungi grow only under special conditions that are often difficult to arrange.

One of the consequences of man's long dependence on wild mushrooms was the possibility of poisoning by toxic species that were difficult to distinguish from edible ones. History records that certain Roman emperors, a couple of European kings, and even a pope died from mushroom poisoning. Furthermore, it is suspected that the notorious poisoner Lucretia Borgia (1480-1519) utilized poisonous mushrooms to dispatch at least one of her victims. Even in modern times there have been outbreaks of mushroom poisonings, such as the one which occurred in the New York City area in 1911. This outbreak involved immigrants from southern Europe who collected and ate some wild mushrooms which they had thought were edible ones they had long used in their homeland.
The cultivation of edible species of mushrooms in various parts of the world was a noteworthy achievement because it vanquished the specter of poisoning and provided wholesome food that might be produced in abundance on small areas of land.

Man's servant, the horse, played an important role in the cultivation of the Common Cultivated Mushroom because it was noted that this type grew in abundance on horse manure. The first people to cultivate these mushrooms appear to have been the French, since the cultural methods were first described in their agricultural writings of the early 18th century. By the end of that century, there was a large-scale production of the fungi in underground caverns around Paris. About the same time Kennett Square, Pennsylvania (in the southeastern part of the state near the border with Delaware) became the American center of mushroom growing because it was the site where the horses, used to draw the Philadelphia streetcars, were stabled. Even today horse manure is a major ingredient of the medium used to produce this fungi.
The Oyster Mushroom was recently brought into commercial production in Taiwan, where many of the producers have large families that supply the required labor at a low cost.
Padi Straw Mushrooms were first cultivated in southeastern China by rice farmers who probably observed the wild species growing on the straw remaining in the fields after the rice harvest. Now this type of mushroom is grown throughout the warm regions of the Orient.
Shiitake has been used as a food in China and Japan for about 2,000 years. However, it is not certain when it was first cultivated.
Truffles (or a closely-related species of *Ascomycetes*) are described in ancient Babylonian and Roman writings, but the conditions which favored their growth were not understood very well until 1810, when a Frenchman found them growing under some young oak trees he had

planted. In the following year, it became known that Napolean had fathered his only son after eating truffles, thereby giving rise to the claim that truffles impart virility. After that, the demand for the fungi increased and many groves of oaks were established. To this day, the virility myth still persists in France and Italy. So, truffles are one of the most expensive foods because of (1) the demand for them as gourmet items, and (2) the limited supply.
Plant scientists are currently conducting research on the commercial production of other edible mushrooms such as the Ear Fungi (*Auricularea polytricha*), Fairy Ring Mushrooms (*Marasmius oreades*), and certain types of morels (*Morchella* spp.).

PRODUCTION. Statistics on the world production of cultivated mushrooms are not readily available. The U.S. production averages about 700 million pounds (*318,000 metric tons*) each year. Another 110 million pounds (*50,000 metric tons*) of canned mushrooms are imported by the United States primarily from the following countries (listed in descending order of tonnage imported in 1990): Taiwan, Hong Kong, Indonesia, China, Spain, and India. Furthermore, the U.S. per capita consumption continues to increase more rapidly than the U.S. production.

Mushrooms, like other fungi, lack the green pigment chlorophyll which is needed for the production of organic nutrients by photosynthesis. Hence they will grow only on media that are rich in organic matter. Mushroom growth is characterized by (1) a vegetative phase during which a network of threadlike filaments called a mycelium spreads throughout the medium, and (2) a fruiting (reproductive) phase when certain areas of the mycelium develop swellings that enlarge and emerge from the medium as fleshy fruiting bodies. The biological function of the fruiting bodies is the release of spores contained in the mushroom caps, thereby achieving the propagation of the species. The main parts of a typical cultivated mushroom are shown in Fig. M-124.

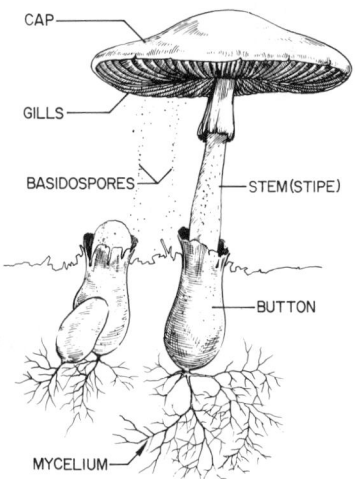

Fig. M-124. The major stages of mushroom growth.

Details regarding the production of the major types of cultivated mushrooms follow:

Common Cultivated Mushroom.
Each stage of production is carefully controlled to ensure that there will be an optimal yield of a high-quality product.

Spores from carefully selected mushrooms are germinated, then grown to produce mycelia in sterile cultures containing millet or rye grain, water, and nutrients. Sometimes the culture medium is prepared from chopped tobacco stems, humus or peat, and inorganic salts.

Beds of compost are prepared by fermenting a mixture of horse manure and various extenders (straw, deep litter poultry manure, cottonseed meal, and/or brewers' grains) until it resembles humus. The fermented compost is placed in mushroom-growing trays and is allowed to ferment again until it reaches the pasteurization temperature of 140°F (60°C), after which it is cooled down to the spawning temperature.

The prepared mycelia (spawn) are introduced into the trays of compost and allowed to grow for about 4 weeks. Then, the trays are cased (covered with a shallow layer of a mildly alkaline loam) and watered every other day. Casing usually induces the emergence of mushrooms within a week or two. The emergence of the buttons from the compost is called a "break."

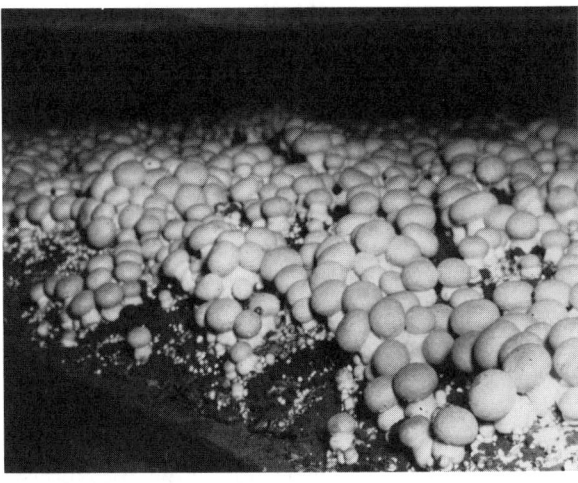

Fig. M-125. A good "break" of mushrooms. (Courtesy, USDA)

Mushrooms are usually harvested at the button stage because they are more perishable when they are allowed to reach greater maturity. Repeated harvests may be obtained for 3 to 7 months until the nutrients in the compost are depleted. Then, new beds have to be prepared.

In the United States, the average yield of mushrooms is about 3 lb (1.4 kg) per square foot of growing bed, whereas in Great Britain it ranges from 3.5 to 4 lb (1.6 to 1.8 kg) per square foot. Hence, the yields produced on small areas of land may be very high, provided that (1)

multiple crops (the total amount produced on a prepared bed constitutes a single crop) are produced each year, and (2) the trays are stacked in tiers. For example, five crops per year from tiers of five trays each, and a yield of 3 lb per square foot would produce 75 lb of mushrooms per square foot of space in the mushroom house. However, some space has to be allotted for the various other functions that are essential to mushroom production.

Oyster Mushroom and Shiitake.
These two different types are covered together because (1) both grow on deciduous hardwood trees, and (2) the methods of production are quite similar.

The logs used for growing the mushrooms are cut from the trunks of small trees, and from the branches of larger trees. Mycelium-containing material for inoculating the logs is produced from cultures grown on sterilized sawdust or autoclaved pegs or wedges of wood.

Preparation of the logs for inoculation consists of soaking in water and drilling holes to receive the cultured mycelia. After inoculation the logs are propped up at a slight angle to the ground in a "laying yard" where they are left for 5 to 8 months and watered periodically to prevent them from drying out.

The emergence of mushrooms is induced by standing the logs upright against supports in a "raising yard" and keeping them damp. Two crops of mushrooms per year are produced, and the same logs may be used for 3 to 6 years before they become unsuitable for profitable production.

Padi Straw Mushroom.
This type is usually grown on rice straw, although the straw by-products from the production of other cereal grains may also be used.

The straw is prepared by tying it into bundles and immersing the bundles in water for 1 to 2 days. Then, the water-soaked bundles are laid horizontally in layers on soil bases that are built up to about 1 ft (30 cm) above the ground. Each layer is wetted down with a preparation made from distillery waste. The masses of straw are allowed to ferment for a few days until the internal temperature reaches about 147°F (64°C) and a sticky material is exuded.

After preparation by fermentation, the straw bundles are removed from the soil bases, untied, and rebundled. Then, they are replaced on the bases as before, but this time the layers are interspersed with pieces of mycelia-rich straw cut from exhausted old beds. The newly prepared beds are kept moist, but not wet, by watering judiciously at regular intervals. The mushrooms usually appear after 2 to 4 weeks. Repeated "breaks" will occur about every 10 days until the beds are exhausted.

Truffles.
The best varieties of these fungi grow in the Perigord region of France and in the Piedmont area of Italy. Furthermore, they are most likely to be found growing in association with the roots of certain species of oak trees. Hence, truffle growers usually adhere to a procedure similar to that which follows:

The acorns used to grow the oak trees are collected in the fall after they have lain for a while on ground permeated with truffle mycelia. They are stored in moist sand over the winter and planted in the spring. Poor, chalky soil favors the development of the oak root-truffle association. Also, a heavy clay-type soil makes the oak roots grow horizontally near the surface of the soil, where the truffles may be harvested readily. The trees are pruned regularly to stimulate the growth of young roots, which apparently encourages the production of truffles.

Usually, specially trained dogs and pigs are used to hunt truffles. They can smell a truffle from a distance and will run quickly to the spot and dig it out. However, experienced truffle hunters know about where to dig for the fungi after taking note of the locations of oak trees, appearance of the soil, and the type of ground cover.

(Also see TRUFFLE.)

PROCESSING. Fresh mushrooms spoil readily. Hence, those that are not likely to be used fresh within a short time after harvesting are processed in various ways as follows:

• **Common Cultivated Mushroom**—The most common forms of processing consist of (1) canning (in brine, marinated in oil and various seasonings, pickled, or as an ingredient of gravies, sauces, and soups); and (2) freezing (in combination with other foods in hors d'oeuvres, pizzas, or mixtures of vegetables). However, this species does not dry well. The dried mushrooms imported from Europe are usually wild *Boletus edulis,* which is commonly called boletus or ceps.

• **Oyster Mushrooms**—This type is usually canned and imported from Taiwan.

• **Padi Straw Mushrooms**—Canned or dried forms are usually imported from Hong Kong, Taiwan, and other parts of the Orient.

• **Shiitake**—This item is usually canned, dried, or pickled and is imported from the Orient, although small amounts are produced in California.

• **Truffles**—Processing may result in the loss of much of the aroma for which the most desirable varieties are noted. Nevertheless, they are available canned, dried, and powdered—unless a dedicated gourmet is willing to pay the cost of having the fresh fungi shipped by air from France or Italy. It is noteworthy that some brands of canned truffles are made from the less expensive, more mildly aromatic varieties.

SELECTION AND PREPARATION. Best quality fresh mushrooms are clean, fresh in appearance, white to creamy-white in color, and free from open caps, pitting, discoloration, wilting, or other injury. For most purposes, sizes ranging from ¾ in. to 3 in. in diameter are usually preferred. If mushroom caps are partially open, the "gills" (fluted formation between cap and stem) should be light in color. Brown or black gills indicate overage mushrooms which should be avoided.

Much of the characteristic flavor is lost when mushrooms are canned. Therefore, some suggestions for preparing fresh mushrooms follow:

1. Mushrooms lose their flavor if soaked in water. Hence, they should be rinsed quickly and blotted dry.

2. A little lemon juice prevents fresh mushrooms from darkening when they are cut or bruised.

3. Just a touch of garlic brings out the mushroom flavor.

4. Fresh, clean mushroom caps may be used raw in salads.

5. The stems of fresh mushrooms are a little chewy for serving raw, but they are good in cooked dishes.

6. Cook mushrooms briefly to retain their flavor and texture.

7. A tasty way of serving fresh mushrooms is on toast after sauteeing them briefly in melted butter or margarine that contains various seasonings.

8. Large caps may be stuffed with chopped cheese or cooked ingredients such as fish, meat, poultry, or seafood, and then baked or broiled briefly.

Canned Oyster Mushrooms generally cost less and have a more pronounced flavor than canned Common Cultivated Mushrooms.

Dried mushrooms should be rehydrated by soaking in water *before* cooking in order to keep the cooking time to a minimum.

All forms of mushrooms mix well with most other foods in dishes such as appetizers, baked breads and similar items, casseroles, Chinese stir-fried dishes, gravies, hors d'oeuvres, omelets, pates, pizzas, relish trays, salads, sauces, soups, stuffings, and vegetable combinations.

Canned condensed cream of mushroom soup is a very versatile convenience food that may save the cook considerable time in the preparation of casseroles, sauces, soups, and stews because it mixes well with other foods such as eggs, fish, meat, pasta products, poultry, seafood, and vegetables. However, most brands of the canned soup are quite salty. Hence, it would be wise not to use any additional salt in the dishes that contain substantial amounts of the condensed soup.

NUTRITIONAL VALUE. The nutrient compositions of various forms of mushrooms are given in Food Composition Table F-36.

Some noteworthy observations regarding the nutrient composition of mushrooms follow:

1. Mushrooms are high in water content (90%) and low in calories (28 to 35 kcal per 100 g). They contain about 20% more protein than potatoes, but they furnish less than half as many calories. Furthermore, they are very low in calcium, vitamin A, and vitamin C; moderately low in thiamin and riboflavin; and a good source of phosphorus, potassium, and niacin. However, many of the nutrients that are lacking in mushrooms may be provided by green leafy vegetables and milk products, which go well with the fungi.

2. Cream of mushroom soup is most nutritious when it is prepared with milk. For example, a 1-cup serving (*245 g*) of the soup (made by mixing the canned condensed soup with an equal volume of milk) furnishes about 7 g of protein, the amount provided by a cup of canned beans

and pork in tomato sauce. Furthermore, the mushroom soup provides two-thirds of the calcium content of a cup of milk.

3.   All types of mushrooms are rich sources of nucleic acids, which are generally thought to be produced in adequate amounts within the body. Nevertheless, certain doctors and nutritionists believe that it may be beneficial to consume foods containing these substances in the event that the body's production fails to meet its needs. For example, some of the undesirable physiological changes that occur with aging might be due to (1) a gradual depletion of the nucleic acids present in various cells, and/or (2) a failure of the genetic and reproductive material of cells (mainly DNA and RNA, which are composed of nucleic acids) to repair itself when damaged by certain environmental and dietary factors.

CAUTION: People who have gout and/or high blood levels of uric acid are usually advised to avoid eating mushrooms and other foods that are rich in nucleic acids.

(Also see GOUT; and NUCLEIC ACIDS.)

FUTURE PROSPECTS. Agricultural and nutritional researchers are beginning to explore the possibility that various species of mushrooms might serve as supplemental protein sources for the undernourished peoples of the developing countries. A major reason for this interest is that certain types of mushroom culture produce more protein per unit of land area than most of our other forms of food production. However, this means of protein production might seem impractical to many Americans who are familiar with the rather high prices charged for mushrooms in the United States. Therefore, it is noteworthy that the current high costs of mushrooms in the developed countries of the world are due mainly to the costs of the labor and the specialized facilities that are needed to produce the fleshy fruiting bodies which are practically the only form of these fungi that are now consumed. However, there are a couple of approaches which might bring these costs down.

First, labor costs in the developing countries are much lower than those in the developed countries. Hence, the major difficulties that are involved in setting up mushroom cultivation in developing countries are (1) establishing the specialized production facilities, and (2) developing the technical skills that are needed to produce optimal yields of a fully wholesome product. Low labor costs are the main reason why the countries of the Orient are claiming an ever-increasing share of the U.S. market for mushrooms.

A more radical approach to mushroom growing is the production of mycelia without attempting to induce the formation of the fleshy fruiting bodies. The mycelia may be grown in nutrient solutions, then harvested and processed by canning, drying, or freezing. It is not expected that the mycelia will be consumed in the same ways as ordinary cultivated mushrooms, but that they may be added to meat dishes, sauces, and soups. It is noteworthy that the mycelia of Common Cultivated Mushrooms are 38% higher in protein (on a dried basis) than the fruiting bodies of these fungi. Furthermore, mycelia can be produced at a much lower cost than the fleshy fruiting bodies.

(Also see VEGETABLE[S], Table V-6 Vegetables of the World.)

MUSKRAT *Ondatra zibethicus*

A small rodent found throughout the United States and Canada, and in parts of Europe, living in the holes in the banks of ponds and streams or in dome-shaped houses of rushes and mud. The muskrat is about the size of a small cat, has a long tail and webbed hind feet, is brown in color and possesses small glands that give off a musky odor. Muskrat fur is sold as "Hudson seal." Muskrat meat is tasty and is sold as "marsh rabbit."

MUSTARD GREENS (INDIAN MUSTARD)
Brassica juncea

Indian mustard is one of several plants bearing the name mustard, all of which belong to the mustard family (*Cruciferae*). This plant may be grown either for its green leaves, which are used as a vegetable, or for its seeds, which are ground and used to make the seasoning called mustard. Unfortunately, it is not practical to obtain both products from the same crop because the leaves are suitable for harvesting at an earlier stage of growth than the seeds. This article deals with the production and utilization of the plant for its green leaves. The condiment, called mustard, is prepared from the seeds of Indian mustard and several other species. Hence, the production of mustard seasoning is covered in a separate article entitled Mustard Seed.

Fig. M-126 shows the curled leaves of a popular variety of mustard greens.

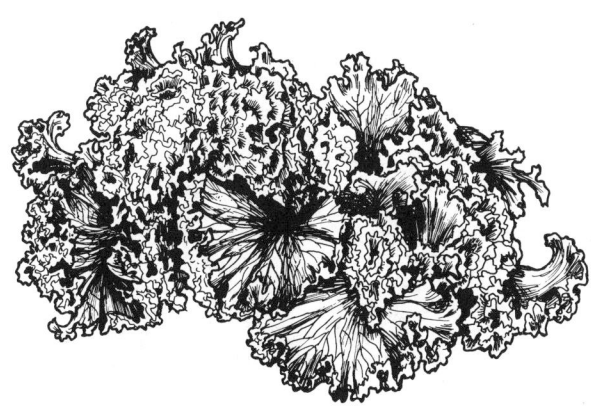

Fig. M-126.   Mustard greens, a nutritious leafy vegetable.

ORIGIN AND HISTORY. Most mustard species were native to Europe and western Asia.

It is not certain how this vegetable came to be cultivated for its "greens" in the southeastern United States, nor is there much information regarding the breeding of the plant for succulent leaves. Perhaps, little or no effort has been made in this direction, since the raw vegetable has a very distinct mustard flavor. This may be the reason why the popularity of the fresh vegetable has declined somewhat, in favor of other "greens" such as collards, kale, and spinach.

PRODUCTION. Statistics for the total U.S. production of mustard greens are not readily available, but the American Frozen Food Institute reported that an average of 12.2 million pounds (*5.5 thousand metric tons*) are frozen each year.[68]

Indian mustard goes to seed rapidly when the weather gets warm. Hence, for harvesting in the spring, it is planted as early in the year as possible, and for harvesting in the fall, it is planted in the summer. Mustard requires a fertile soil with plenty of organic matter. These requirements are usually met by various combinations of (1) inorganic fertilizers supplying nitrogen, phosphorus, and potassium, (2) green manure, and/or (3) animal manure.

PROCESSING. The annual production of frozen mustard greens has fluctuated from year to year, but the total in 1990 was about the same as in 1969. By contrast, during this same period, the production of all frozen vegetables increased by about 65%.

SELECTION AND PREPARATION. High quality mustard greens are fresh, young, tender, and green. Leaves which show insect injury, coarse stems, dryness or yellowing, excessive dirt, or poor development, are usually lacking in quality and may cause excessive waste.

Mustard greens are almost always cooked before eating. Steaming is better than boiling because the latter procedure extracts water-soluble minerals and vitamins, which are lost if the cooking water is discarded. Mustard greens may also be cooked by (1) sauteeing the leaves with or without bacon, onions, and/or pork; or (2) adding the leaves to casseroles, omelets, or soups. Plain cooked greens may be dressed up with a cheese sauce, hollandaise dressing, or a white sauce. Sliced, hard cooked eggs also go well with the cooked greens.

CAUTION: Mustard greens and other vegetables of the mustard family (*Cruciferae*) contain small amounts of substances called goitrogens that interfere with the utilization of iodine by the thyroid gland. Hence, people who eat very large amounts of these vegetables when on an iodine-deficient diet may develop an enlargement of the thyroid, commonly called a goiter. The best insurance against this potentially harmful effect is the consumption of ample amounts of dietary iodine, which is abundantly present in iodized salt, ocean fish, seafood, and edible seaweeds.

---

[68]*Agricultural Statistics 1980*, USDA, p. 200, Table 285.

NUTRITIONAL VALUE. The nutrient composition of mustard greens is given in the Food Composition Table F-36.

Some noteworthy observations regarding the nutrient composition of mustard greens follow:

1. Mustard greens contain over 90% water and furnish only about 30 Calories (kcal) per cup (*240 ml*).

2. A 1-cup serving of the vegetable supplies about two-thirds as much calcium as a cup of milk. Furthermore, the calcium content is four times the phosphorus content. Hence, mustard greens complement cereals, eggs, fish, legumes, meats, poultry, and seafood, which provide much less calcium than phosphorus.

3. Mustard greens are an excellent source of iron, potassium, vitamin A, and vitamin C. One cup of the cooked greens supplies as much vitamin C as an orange.

(Also see MUSTARD SEED; and VEGETABLE[S], Table V-6 Vegetables of the World.)

MUSTARD SEED *Sinapis alba; Brassica* **spp**

Mustard, which is made from the seeds of certain plants of the mustard family (*Cruciferae*), is the leading spice in worldwide usage. The four species of mustard seeds used for this purpose are: (1) white mustard (*Sinapis alba*), (2) brown mustard (*Brassica juncea*), (3) black mustard (*Brassica nigra*), and (4) Ethiopian mustard (*Brassica carinata*). It is noteworthy that brown mustard, which is also called Indian mustard, may also be grown for its green leaves rather than for its seeds.

Fig. M-127 shows a typical mustard plant.

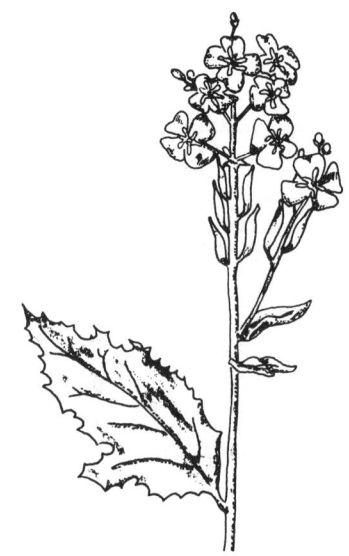

Fig. M-127. A flowering mustard plant. The plants of the mustard family are called *Cruciferae*, because the four petals of each flower form a cross.

ORIGIN AND HISTORY. The four different species which yield the spice-bearing seed originated in different parts of Eurasia. It is believed that (1) white mustard came from the eastern Mediterranean, (2) brown mustard originated along the western foothills of the Himalayas, (3) black mustard came from somewhere between Asia Minor and Iran, and (4) Ethiopean mustard resulted from a crossing (hybridization) between black mustard and a cabbagelike plant.

Brown mustard appears to have been used for about 5,000 years, since it is mentioned in ancient Sanskrit writings. The mustard seed is also mentioned in the New Testament (Matthew 13:31), a parable in which Christ compared the kingdom of heaven to a grain of mustard seed. Also, various writers of ancient Greece and Rome described the use of this seasoning. It appears that the Romans made a paste from ground mustard seed mixed with must (the unfermented juice pressed from grapes). The name mustard appears to have been derived from the Latin words *must* and *ardens,* meaning burning (hot).

PRODUCTION. Accurate statistics on the production of mustard seed are not readily available, although it has been reported that the worldwide demand exceeds 400 million pounds (*182,000 metric tons*) per year.[69]

In the United States, mustard seed production is confined to California, the Dakotas, Montana (probably the leading state), Oregon, and Washington.

The planting of mustard in the spring is timed so that the seed pods may be harvested in dry weather. It is necessary to harvest the seeds before they are fully ripe; otherwise the pods may burst open and scatter their seeds.

PROCESSING. Mustard seed is usually marketed as a dry powder, or as a preparation with a pastelike consistency. Both of these forms are made by grinding the dry seed into a powder, then removing the seed hulls by milling, screening, and sifting. The dried mustard powder has no pungent odor because the "hot" components are present in a chemically inactive form. However, wetting the powder brings about an enzymatic action which liberates the pungent components.

Most prepared mustard is made by mixing the dried mustard powder with salt, vinegar, and other spices. Also, mustard is utilized in other products such as mayonnaise, salad dressings, and pickles.

SELECTION AND PREPARATION. Mustard powder, which is available in most supermarkets, may be added directly to casseroles (such as baked beans and

pork), soups, stews, and other mixed dishes. However, it should be used cautiously, since the enzymatic action which releases the pungent components from the wetted powder requires a bit of time in which to develop the maximum flavor intensity. It is noteworthy that mixing the powder with very hot water, or with moderately strong acid such as lemon juice or vinegar, stabilizes the flavor intensity by stopping the enzyme action.

Prepared mustard may be used to spice up deviled eggs, fish, meats, and poultry. It also enhances the flavor of dressings and sauces.

NUTRITIONAL VALUE. Mustard seed is rich in nutrients (469 kcal per 100 g, 25% protein, and 29% fat), but it is not likely to contribute much to the diet, nutritionally, because the acrid components limit the amounts which may be consumed safely. (Mustard oil blisters the skin.) Nevertheless, the small amounts normally used are helpful in enhancing the taste of food and in stimulating the appetite. The nutrient composition of mustard powder is given in Food Composition Table F-36.

(Also see MUSTARD GREENS.)

MUTAGENS

Any of a number of chemical compounds capable of inducing mutations (gene changes) in DNA and in living cells. The alkyl mustards, as well as dimethyl sulfate, diethyl sulfate, and ethylmethane sulfonate, comprise a group of alkylating agents, reacting with the nitrogen atoms of quanine (a purine base), a constituent of both RNA and DNA. This reaction affects the quanine molecule in such a way as ultimately to induce a mutation in DNA. Nitrous oxide can deaminate (remove the amino group from) both quanine and cytosine (a pyrimidine base).

Caffeine appears to be a weak mutagen in some nonmammalian systems. But its significance as a mutagen in humans is unknown. It is noteworthy, however, that studies of the caffeine intake of pregnant women have shown no association between caffeine and birth defects.

(Also see NUCLEIC ACIDS.)

MYASTHENIA GRAVIS

An autoimmune disease—failure of the body's immune system to recognize self—in which the body forms antibodies against its own muscle cell membranes. The antibodies attack the muscle cell membranes and destroy their responsiveness to nerve impulses. Nerve impulses fail to reach the muscle and contraction fails. Muscles unable to contract are paralyzed.

The cause of the disease is not known, but it is associated with an enlarged thymus. Myasthenia gravis is characterized by various groups of muscles which become easily fatigued and weakened. Respiratory, neck,

---

[69]Clarke, R. J., and J. W. Drummond, "Spices, Hot Beverages and Tobacco," *Chemical Technology: An Encyclopedic Treatment,* Vol. VII, edited by L. W. Codd, *et al.,* Barnes & Noble Books, New York, N.Y., 1975, p. 646.

tongue, trunk and shoulder muscles are affected. Some drugs are capable of improving muscular fuctions. Due to the muscles involved, there are some feeding difficulties as swallowing, and coughing; and grasping abilities are impaired.

MYCOTOXINS

Poisonous substances produced by some yeasts and molds. Some mycotoxins are capable of causing liver cancer or cirrhosis. It is important to know that mycotoxins remain in food long after the organisms that produced them have died. Fortunately, not all yeasts and molds produce mycotoxins.

(Also see POISONS, Table P-11 Some Potentially Poisonous [Toxic] Substances—"Ergot," and "Mycotoxins.")

MYELIN

The white, fatlike substance which forms a sheath around certain nerve fibers.

MYO-

Prefix meaning muscle.

MYOCARDIAL INFARCTION

A disorder of the heart occurring when the coronary artery or one of its branches is obstructed (occluded). Tissue may be damaged if there are areas of the heart muscle which do not receive sufficient blood. These damaged areas are called *infarcts,* and the *coronary occlusion* is simply called a *coronary.* Usually, a myocardial infarction is accompanied by severe pain which does not subside upon resting. The victim's skin turns pale, cold and sweaty. The pulse is weak and breathing is labored. Sudden death may occur. A few people may have "silent" attacks in which there is no noticeable pain. The presence of infarcts may often be confirmed by an electrocardiogram or by elevations in the blood levels of enzymes which leak out of the damaged heart muscle.

(Also see HEART DISEASES.)

MYOCARDIUM

The heart muscle.

MYOFIBRILS

The hundreds of small contractile units found in each muscle fiber. Myofibrils are composed of the muscle protein filaments, myosin and actin.

MYOGEN

A muscle protein, an albumin, that is found in the cytoplasm of the muscle cell. It is not a protein of the actin and myosin filaments.

MYOGLOBIN

A protein similar to hemoglobin in structure and function, found only in the muscles. Myoglobin receives oxygen from the blood and stores it for use by the muscle cells. It is responsible for the red color of meat.

(Also see HEMOGLOBIN.)

MYOSIN

One of two muscle cell proteins which play an important role in the contraction and elasticity of muscles. The other protein is actin.

(Also see MUSCLES.)

MYSORE FLOUR

This flour was developed in India and used for large-scale feeding trials as a partial substitute for cereals. It is a mixture of 75% tapioca flour and 25% peanut flour.

MYXEDEMA

A disease due to undersecretion of the thyroid hormones, thyroxine and triiodothyronine, in the adult. Doctors say it is the one disease that "can be diagnosed over the phone" as the voice is husky and slow, and memory is poor. In addition, persons suffering from myxedema, usually females between 40 and 60 years of age, are lethargic, susceptible to chills, overweight, lack muscle tone, have coarse skin and hair, and poor circulation. It is named after the fluid accumulation appearing in the face and other areas of the body.

Treatment consists of the administration of thyroid gland extract under the direction of a physician.

(Also see ENDOCRINE GLANDS; and GOITER, section headed "Myxedema.")

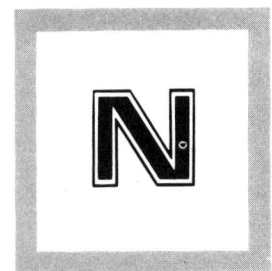

NAILS (FINGERNAILS)

Nails may be a sign of good health or of poor health. In good health, the nails are firm and pink. In poor health, the nails are rigid and brittle. In chronic iron deficiency anemia, the nails may be spoon-shaped (*koilonychia*). Severe protein deficiency may result in transverse white bands in the nails, occurring symmetrically on both hands. In other forms of malnutrition, the nails may be brittle, thickened, or lined on the surface either transversely or longitudinally; but these changes may also be seen in well-nourished people.

(Also see DEFICIENCY DISEASES, Table D-2 Minor Dietary Deficiency Disorders; and HEALTH, Sections headed "Signs of Good Health" and "Signs of Ill Health.")

NAPHTHOQUINONE

A derivative of quinone. Some of these derivatives have vitamin K activity.

NARANJILLA *Solanum quitoense*

The fruit of a very large herbaceous plant (of the family *Solanaceae*) that is 6 to 10 ft (*2 to 3 m*) tall and a native of the northern Andes.

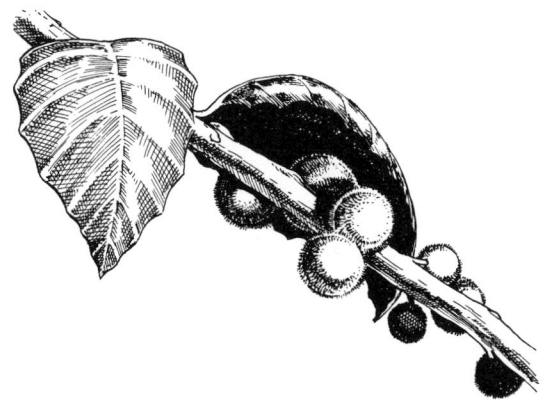

Fig. N-1. Naranjilla fruits.

Naranjilla fruits are orange-colored, fuzzy tomatolike fruits that have a sour green pulp. They are used mainly to make jam, jelly, juice, and pies.

The pulp of the fruit has a high water (92%) and a low content of calories (28 kcal per 100 g) and carbohydrates (7%). It is a good source of vitamin C.

NATAL PLUM *Carissa grandiflora*

Fruit of a shrub (of the family *Apocynaceae*) that is native to South Africa. Natal plums are pear-shaped and are up to 2 in. (*5 cm*) long. They have a reddish skin and reddish pulp with a white milky latex. The ripe fruits are used for making jellies and sauces. They may also be eaten fresh or stewed.

Natal plums are moderately high in calories (68 kcal per 10 g) and carbohydrates (16%). They are a good source of iron and ascorbic acid.

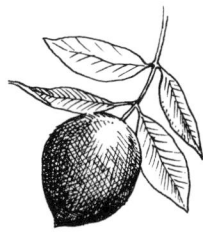

Fig. N-2. The natal plum.

NATIONAL FLOUR

Presently, this is the name given to 85% extraction wheat flour in the United Kingdom.

NATIONAL RESEARCH COUNCIL (NRC)

A division of the National Academy of Sciences established in 1916 to promote the effective utilization of scientific and technical resources. Periodically, this private, nonprofit organiation of scientists publishes bulletins giving nutrient requirements and allowances for man and domestic animals, copies of which are available on a charge basis through the National Academy of Sciences, National Research Council, 2101 Constitution Avenue, N.W., Washington, D.C. 20418.

NATURAL FOODS

Natural foods are those that are grown naturally and subjected to little or no processing. But there is no official definition of a natural food. The Food and Drug Administration's policy on food labeling only prohibits a manufacturer from calling an entire food natural if it contains artificial colors or flavors or any synthetic ingredients.

Natural food enthusiasts stress nature and the return to a more primitive way of life. Some of these advocates go so far as to suggest that something valuable has been removed from the traditional foods sold in the supermarket; that they are counterfeit, prefabricated, worthless, or devitalized. It is inferred that processing destroys the nutritive value of the food. Such notions have created doubts in the minds of some Americans about the integrity, purity, and nutritive content of the nation's food supply. It is true that modern food refining removes some valuable nutrients from such foods as white flour and wild rice. However, these foods, and many other processed foods, are enriched with minerals and vitamins to make them nutritious.

Usually, natural foods are grown with organic fertilizer and without chemical sprays in a garden, on a tree, or a farm, and just washed, possibly hulled and cracked, or cut before eating raw or cooked. And they contain no chemical additives, such as preservatives, emulsifiers, and antioxidants. Such foods include fresh fruits and vegetables, nuts, seeds, and stone-ground cereals. Honey, brown sugar, and fertile eggs are other foods which natural food enthusiasts consider to have superior power over their actual nutritive content.

The back-to-nature movement popularized granola, a "natural" food that had been around for years. Granola is a heavy, chewy, dry cereal made from such "healthy" ingredients as whole grains, nuts, seeds, raisins, and honey, and often (though not always) without chemical preservatives. The granola labels proclaim "all natural." To its credit, granola does contain more protein, fiber, vitamins, and minerals than most popular cereals. However, its nutritious aspects may be offset by lots of fats (especially highly saturated coconut oil), and sugars (after all, honey is sugar, natural or not), and calories—four to six times as many calories as the same volume of more traditional cereals.

Some natural food advocates use raw milk, despite the hazard of brucellosis (undulant fever) and tuberculosis—disease-producing organisms that are destroyed by pasteurization. Others consider fish, chicken, and animal flesh as natural foods so long as the animals are grown without the use of commercial feeds, hormones, and antibiotics. Still, others imagine that natural vitamins are superior to synthetic vitamins; despite the fact that a vitamin is a vitamin whatever its source, and that a vitamin has a chemical formula and functions in a certain manner in the body whether it is natural or synthetic.

But the natural food movement has made for nutritional awareness and interest. In this respect, it has succeeded where mothers have failed. Many young people are now eating vegetables and a greater variety of other foods. Also, they are turning away from highly refined foods like candy, soft drinks, and other "empty calories."

(Also see FOOD MYTHS AND MISINFORMATION; HEALTH FOODS; and ORGANICALLY GROWN FOODS.)

NAUSEA

Sickness at the stomach associated with an urge to vomit.

NEAT'S-FOOT OIL

A pale yellow fatty oil made by boiling the feet and shinbones of cattle, used chiefly as a leather dressing and fine lubricant.

NECROSIS

Death of a part of the cells making up a living tissue.

NECTAR

The two major nutritional meanings of this term are as follows:

• A syrupy liquid produced by special glands of flowers that is collected by bees and converted by them into honey. The unique flavors of the honeys derived from the different nectars are due mainly to the essential oils and other aromatic substances produced by the flowers.
(Also see HONEY.)

• A pulpy fruit drink made from various combinations of ingredients such as water, fruit puree, fruit pulp, fruit juice, sweetener(s), citric acid, and vitamin C. The minimum amounts of fruit ingredient for each of the types of nectar are specified in the Standards Of Identity which have been established by the FDA. Some of the fruit nectars sold in the United States are apricot, guava, mango, papaya, peach, and pear.
(Also see the articles on the individual fruits for details regarding the various nectars.)

NECTARINE

A fuzzless (smooth-skinned) variety of peach that is otherwise almost identical to the peach.

However, nectarines are more susceptible to disease when grown in hot, humid climates such as those of the major peach-growing areas of southeastern United States. Hence, most of the U.S. nectarine production comes from the Pacific Coast.
(Also see PEACH AND NECTARINE.)

NEONATE

A newborn baby.

NEOPLASM (TUMOR)

A new and abnormal growth—a tumor, which serves no physiological purpose.

NEPHRITIS

Inflammation of the kidneys.
(Also see DISEASES.)

NEPHRON

The structural and functional unit of the kidneys consisting of a tuft of capillaries known as the glomerulus attached to the renal tubule. Urine is formed by filtration of blood in the glomerulus and by the selective reabsorption and secretion of solutes by cells that comprise the walls of the renal tubules. There are aproximately 1 million nephrons in each kidney.
(Also see GLOMERULONEPHRITIS [Nephritis].)

NEPHROSCLEROSIS

Hardening and narrowing of the arteries of the kidneys, a condition usually associated with high blood pressure and arteriosclerosis. Nephrosclerosis causes degeneration of the renal tubules, and fibrosis of the glomeruli, the points where filtration occurs. Its incidence increases with age but it often produces no outward symptoms. It may, however, account for the decrease in kidney reserve noted in the elderly. During its late stages some sodium and protein restrictions may be necessary.

NEPHROSIS

A degenerative kidney disease occurring without signs of inflammation. It may occur as a consequence of acute glomerulonephritis, lupus erythematosus, an allergic reaction, diabetes mellitus, or mercury poisoning. In children it appears for no apparent reason. Clinically, the patient exhibits massive losses of protein in the urine—proteinuria; low blood protein—hypoproteinemia; and water in the tissues of the body—edema. Treatment consists of replacing protein losses with a high protein diet, and controlling the edema with a restricted sodium intake. Possibly diuretics or steroids may also be involved in the treatment. Successful therapy is a long term process. Full recovery seldom requires less than 2 years.
(Also see DIABETES MELLITUS; MODIFIED DIETS; GLOMERULONEPHRITIS; and LUPUS ERYTHEMATOSUS.)

NEROLI OIL

This is a fragrant essential oil obtained from certain flowers, especially the sour orange, which is used chiefly in perfumes, but which is also used in flavoring foods.
(Also see SEVILLE ORANGE.)

NERVOUS SYSTEM

The entire nerve apparatus of the body consisting of the brain and spinal cord, nerves, ganglia, and parts of the receptor organs that receive and interpret stimuli and transmit impulses to the effector organs.

NERVOUS SYSTEM DISORDERS

These may encompass everything from numbness in a limb to quadraplegia to mental illness, which in itself includes a multitude of disorders. Nutritional factors which may cause or contribute to some nervous system disorders include:

• **Energy**—About 1/5 of the basal metabolic rate is due to the brain. Thus, the brain requires a continuous and adequate supply of glucose and oxygen. Any interruptions in this supply can result in irreversible damage. Low blood sugar, hypoglycemia, is manifest by altered mental states. Hypothyroid conditions alter the utilization of energy, and can have profound effects on the function of the nervous system.
(Also see GOITER; and HYPOGLYCEMIA.)

• **Protein**—Severe protein restriction during pregnancy or during infancy can alter brain development. Inborn errors in the metabolism of amino acids which result in high blood levels of certain amino acids can cause mental retardation.

(Also see INBORN ERRORS OF METABOLISM; MALNUTRITION; PROTEIN[S]; and PROTEIN AS ENERGY SOURCE.)

• **Lipid**—Lipid metabolism seems correlated with the development of atherosclerosis. If blood vessels in the brain become occluded, a stroke may result. Also, in multiple sclerosis, which is a nervous system disorder, there is an alteration in the metabolism of lipids and some suggestion that the disease may be treated with the essential fatty acid linoleic acid.

(Also see FATS AND OTHER LIPIDS.)

• **Vitamins**—Deficiencies of the vitamin B complex may induce a variety of nervous system disorders; for example, poor memory, depression, irritability, lack of interest, hallucination, weakness, forgetfulness, and vision impairment. The Wernicke-Korsakoff syndrome indicates a whole list of nervous system disorders due mainly to a thiamin deficiency.

(Also see DEFICIENCY DISEASES; VITAMIN[S]; and VITAMIN B-COMPLEX.)

• **Minerals**—Lead and mercury poisoning can disrupt mental function causing hyperactivity, learning difficulties, weakness, and mental retardation. On the other hand, deficiencies of minerals like sodium, magnesium, and potassium can produce some symptoms which can be termed nervous system disorders—giddiness, confusion, and irritability. A high salt (sodium) intake seems related to high blood pressure, and, in turn, high blood pressure may predispose a person to a stroke.

(Also see BLOOD PRESSURE; MINERAL[S]; and POISONS.)

• **Toxins**—A variety of toxins, both man-made and naturally occurring, can find their way into the food supply, or be ingested by accident. Many toxins have detrimental effects on the nervous system; for example, pesticides, ergot, mycotoxins, polybrominated biphenyls (PBBs), polychlorinated biphenyls (PCBs), neurotoxins, hallucinogens, and cholinesterase inhibitors.

(Also see POISONOUS PLANTS; and POISONS.)

The above discussion is by no means a complete review of the role of nutrition in nervous disorders. Rather, it provides some indications of the variety of interrelationships that exist between the two. Hopefully, awareness of the relationships between the two will continue to increase.

Nutrition and nervous system disorders are further related since nervous disorders often require special dietary adjustments, and may present some feeding difficulties.

(Also see MODIFIED DIETS; MENTAL DEVELOPMENT; and MENTAL ILLNESS.)

NEURITIC

Of, relating to, or affected by neuritis.

NEURITIS

Inflammation of the peripheral nerves—the nerves which link the brain and spinal cord with the muscles, skin, organs, and other parts of the body.

NEUROPATHY

Disease of the nervous system, especially when involving degenerative changes.

NEUTROPENIA

The presence of neutrophile cells (white blood cells which do not stain readily) in abnormally small number in the peripheral bloodstream.

NEW PROCESS

Pertains to the extraction of oil from seeds. Same as solvent process.

(Also see OILS, VEGETABLE; and FATS AND OTHER LIPIDS.)

NIACIN (NICOTINIC ACID; NICOTINAMIDE)[1]

[1]Niacin has, along the way, been known as vitamin P-P, pellagra-preventive vitamin, vitamin G, vitamin B-3, vitamin B-4, and vitamin B-5.

NIACIN

IT'S ESSENTIAL FOR HUMANS TOO!

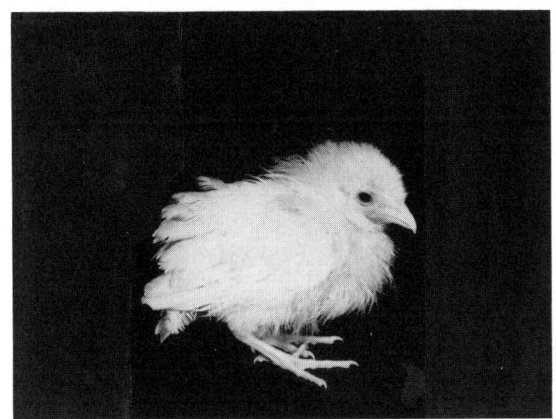 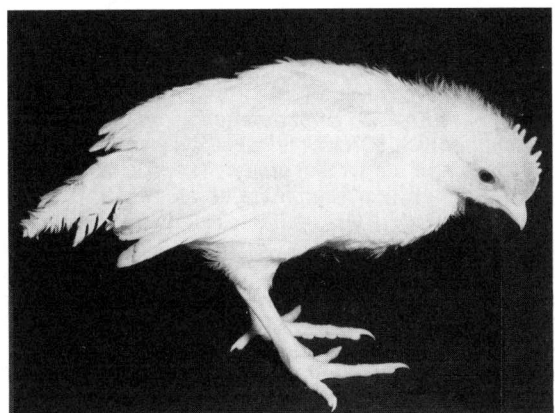

NIACIN MADE THE DIFFERENCE! <u>LEFT</u>: CHICK ON NIACIN-DEFICIENT DIET. NOTE POOR GROWTH AND ABNORMAL FEATHERING. <u>RIGHT</u>: CHICK THAT RECEIVED PLENTY OF NIACIN. (COURTESY, UNIVERSITY OF WISCONSIN)

TOP FOOD SOURCES

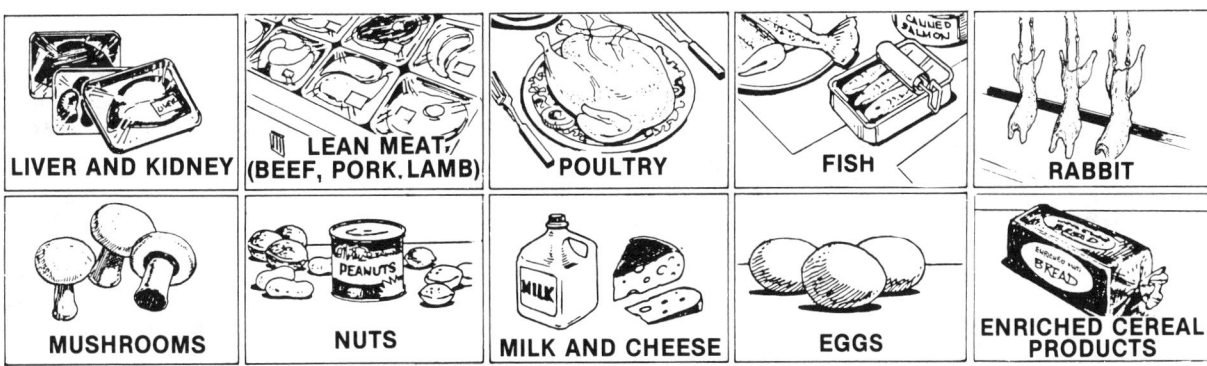

LIVER AND KIDNEY | LEAN MEAT (BEEF, PORK, LAMB) | POULTRY | FISH | RABBIT

MUSHROOMS | NUTS | MILK AND CHEESE | EGGS | ENRICHED CEREAL PRODUCTS

Fig. N-3. Niacin made the difference! *Left*: Chick on niacin-deficient diet. Note poor growth and abnormal feathering. *Right*: Chick that received plenty of niacin. (Courtesy, H. R. Bird, Department of Poultry Science, University of Wisconsin) Note, too, ten top food sources of niacin.

Niacin, a member of the B complex, is a collective term which includes nicotinic acid and nicotinamide, both natural forms of the vitamin with equal niacin activity. In the body, they are active as nicotinamide adenine dinucleotide (NAD) and nicotinamide adenine dinucleotide phosphate (NADP) and serve as coenzymes, often in partnership with thiamin and riboflavin coenzymes, to produce energy within the cells, precisely when needed and in the amount necessary.

The discovery of the role of niacin as a vitamin of the B group was the result of man's age-old struggle against pellagra. The disease was first described by the physi-

cian Gaspar Casal in Spain in 1730, soon after the introduction of corn (maize) into Europe; and it was given the name pellagra (*pelle,* for skin; and *agra,* for sour) by physician Francesco Frapoli in Italy in 1771.

Pellagra spread with the spread and cultivation of corn. In the 19th century, it was common in almost all of the European and African countries bordering on the Mediterranean sea; and it later spread to other African countries. Pellagra had long been present in both North and South America, but it reached epidemic proportions in southern United States after the Civil War, which left poverty in its wake, as a result of which many of the poor subsisted almost entirely on corn. Outbreaks of the disease were so widespread and severe that most physicians considered the cause to be either an infectious agent or a toxic substance present in spoiled corn.

HISTORY. Nicotinic acid was first discovered and named in 1867, when Huber, a German chemist, prepared it from the nicotine of tobacco. But for the next 70 years it remained idle on the chemist's shelves because no one thought of it, even remotely, as a cure for pellagra. In the meantime, thousands of people died from the disease.

Subsequent to 1867, nicotinic acid was "rediscovered" many times as a compound present in foods and tissues. In 1912, Funk, in England, isolated nicotinic acid from rice polishings while attempting to isolate the antiberiberi vitamin; and, that same year, Suzuki, in Japan, isolated nicotinic acid from rice bran. But both researchers lost interest in the acid when they found it ineffective in curing beriberi.

In the early 1900s, pellagra reached epidemic proportions in southern United States, where the diet was based primarily on corn, which is extremely low in both available niacin and in tryptophan. In 1915, 10,000 people died of the disease; and, in 1917-18, there were 200,000 cases of pellagra in this country.

In 1914, the U.S. Public Health Service dispatched a team under the direction of Dr. Joseph Goldberger, a physician-researcher, to study the cause of, and hopefully find a cure for, pellagra. In a series of studies initiated in 1914 and continuing throughout the 1920s, Goldberger proved that the disease was caused by a dietary deficiency, and not an infection or toxin. A chronological summary of Dr. Goldberger's classical clinical nutrition studies follows:

In 1914, Dr. Goldberger observed an orphanage. On his first visit to the Baptist Orphanage in Jackson, Mississippi, to study the problem, Goldberger proved to be a very observant person. He noted that 68 of the 211 children suffered from pellagra, but that none of the employees in the institution had ever contracted the disease. This caused him to doubt the prevailing theory that pellagra was a communicable disease. Shrewdly, Goldberger traced the absence of pellagra among the better-fed employees to the presence of meat and milk on their tables, and of at least some of the pellagra-free orphans to their pilfering milk and meat from the orphanage's limited supply.

As a result of these observations, Dr. Goldberger improved the orphan's diets through the addition of milk, eggs, and meat. Within a few weeks, all children suffering from pellagra recovered and no new cases developed. This convinced him that he was on the right track.

In 1915, Dr. Goldberger used prisoners as subjects. In order to confirm that pellagra results from deficiencies in the diet, Goldberger enlisted the cooperation of 12 volunteers (all men) in the Mississippi State Penitentiary in a classic experiment designed to study the effect of subsisting on a diet similar to that consumed in areas where pellagra was a problem; and Governor Brewer of Mississippi agreed to grant unconditional pardons to those prisoners who participated in the study for a period not to exceed 6 months. Five of the inmates on the study developed pellagra, which was cured by the addition of yeast to the diet.

In 1916, Goldberger experimented on himself and his friends. Despite the evidence of the well designed studies cited above, most medical practitioners refused to reject the long-held belief that pellagra was infectious. So, in an heroic and crucial experiment, Dr. Goldberger and his faithful disciple, Dr. G. A. Wheeler, made themselves the first subjects of a series of experiments designed to prove that pellagra could not be contagious. On April 25, 1916, both of them swabbed their throats with secretions obtained from the nose and naso-pharynx of pellagra patients, but they did not contract the disease. Further experiments continued into June of that year. During this period seven separate groups, involving 21 men and one woman, swallowed in capsule a nauseating concoction made up of blood, feces, and urine of pellagra patients. Dr. Goldberger's wife, Mary Farrar, begged to join them, but the men wouldn't consent to her swallowing the capsule; instead, she was given by hypodermic needle in the abdomen an injection of the blood of a woman dying of pellagra. Although some of the volunteers reported feeling a bit squeamish (as who wouldn't?), none developed pellagra.

In 1925, Goldberger and Tanner classified common foods on the basis of their effectiveness in preventing or curing human pellagra. They studied the effects of supplementing a pellagra-producing diet with certain foods. From these results, (1) they concluded that there is a specific dietary factor of unknown nature present in certain foods, which is involved in preventing and curing pellagra; and (2) they rated foods on their content of this factor as follows: *abundant,* yeast; *good,* lean meat and milk; *fair,* peas and beans (and other vegetables).

In 1926, Goldberger and Wheeler showed that pellagra in man and blacktongue in dogs were similar. Goldberger and his associates observed that in towns where many people suffered from pellagra, a large percentage of the dogs had blacktongue, thereby noting the similarity between pellagra in man and blacktongue in dogs. Further, they confirmed that dogs with blacktongue could be cured by yeast. Goldberger and Wheeler designated this preventive and curative factor, present in certain foods, as P-P (pellagra-preventive); others designated it vitamin G for Goldberger.

In 1935, von Euler, Albers, and Schlenck studied the preparation of cozymase, the coenzyme which is necessary for the alcoholic fermentation of glucose by apozymase, shown later to be diphosphopyridine nucleotide (DPN). On hydrolysis, cozymase yielded nicotinic acid. This was the first evidence that nicotinic acid (in the form of its amide) formed a part of the structure of an enzyme, and placed it among the organic compounds of great importance in biological chemistry.

In 1936, two German scientists, Warburg and Christian, showed that nicotinamide was an essential component of the hydrogen transport system in the form of nicotinamide adenine dinucleotide (NAD).

In 1937, Dr. Conrad Elvehjem, and co-workers, at the University of Wisconsin, discovered that niacin (as either nicotinic acid or nicotinic acid amide, which he isolated from liver) cured blacktongue in dogs, a condition recognized as similar to pellaga in man. Shortly thereafter, several investigators found that niacin was effective in the prevention and treatment of pellagra in humans. Soon, the vitamin became recognized as a dietary essential for man, monkeys, pigs, chickens, and other species.

In 1945, Willard Krehl and his associates at the University of Wisconsin finally solved another mystery in the story of pellagra prevention when they discovered that tryptophan is a precursor of niacin, thereby explaining two things: (1) why milk, which is low in niacin but high in tryptophan, will prevent or cure pellagra; and (2) why, in earlier concepts, protein deficiency was often related to pellagra—for without protein, there could be no tryptophan (the precursor of niacin). Corn is low in tryptophan whereas meat contains both tryptophan and niacin.

In 1971, the name *niacin* was adopted by the American Institute of Nutrition and international agencies for all forms of the vitamin.

It is noteworthy that recent findings indicate that most persons suffering from pellagra have multiple deficiencies—that certain symptoms formerly associated with the disease are not relieved until thiamin and riboflavin are supplied along with niacin.

Today, pellagra is rare in the United States. Even in Latin America and Mexico, where many people eat large amounts of corn, pellagra is seldom seen. This is because of their common practice of soaking the corn in lime, which makes the niacin present in the corn in the bound form (niacytin) more available to the body. This probably explains why Mexicans who eat tortillas are relatively free of pellagra. In making tortillas, the pre-Columbian civilizations of Mexico (Aztec, Mayan, Toltec) devised a procedure to treat corn flour with lime water (alkali) before cooking in order to improve the plastic properties of the dough; and, presumably unbeknown to them, the lime water treatment also freed the niacin from the niacytin and made it fully available to the body tissues.

Africa is the only continent in which pellagra is still a public health problem.

CHEMISTRY, METABOLISM, PROPERTIES.
The chemistry, metabolism, and properties of nicotinic acid and nicotinamide follow:

• **Chemistry**—The structure of nicotinic acid and nicotinamide are shown in Fig. N-4.

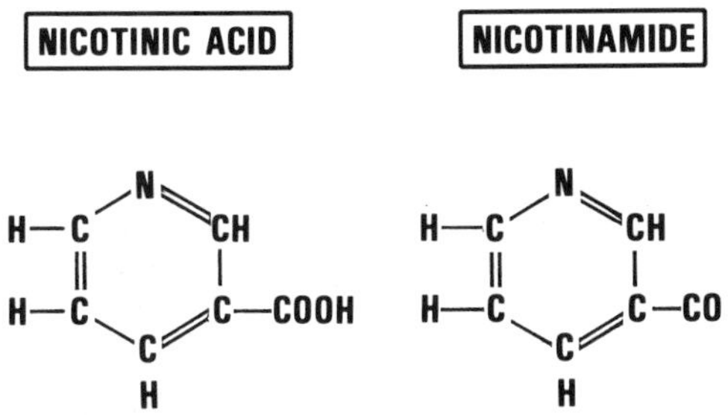

Fig. N-4. The formulas of nicotinic acid and nicotinamide reveal that the compounds are derivatives of pyridine.

• **Metabolism**—Niacin is readily absorbed from the small intestine into the portal blood circulation and taken to the liver. There it is converted to the coenzyme nicotinamide adenine dinucleotide (NAD). Also, some NAD is synthesized in the liver from tryptophan. NAD formed in the liver is broken down, releasing nicotinamide, which is excreted into the general circulation. This nicotinamide and the niacin that was not metabolized in the liver are carried in the blood to other body tissues, where they are utilized for the synthesis of niacin-containing coenzymes.

Niacin is found in the body tissues largely as part of two important coenzymes, nicotinamide adenine dinucleotide (NAD) and nicotinamide adenine dinucleotide phosphate (NADP); together, NAD and NADP are known as the pyridine nucleotides. The structure of NAD is given in Fig. N-5.

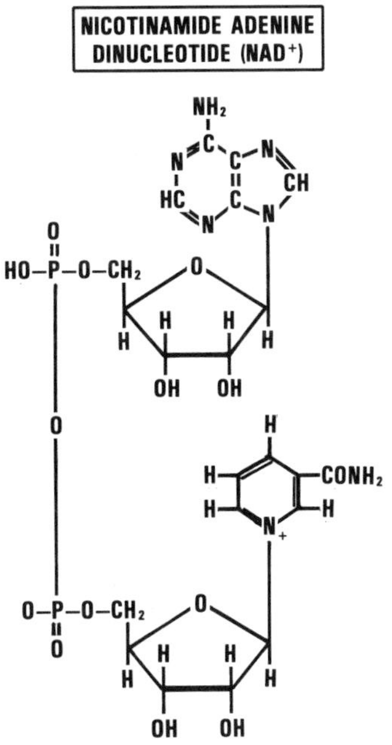

Fig. N-5. Structure of NAD.

NAD is composed of nicotinamide, adenine, two molecules of ribose, and two molecules of phosphate. NADP is similar in structure except it contains three phosphate groups.

Little niacin is stored in the body. Most of the excess is methylated and excreted in the urine, principally as N-methylnicotinamide and N-methyl pyridine (in about equal quantities). Also, small amounts of nicotinic acid and niacinamide are excreted in the urine. With a low niacin intake, there is a low level of metabolite excretion in any form.

• **Properties**—Nicotinic acid appears as colorless nee-dlelike crystals with a bitter taste, whereas nicotinamide is a white powder when crystallized. Both are soluble in water (with the amide being more soluble than the acid form) and are not destroyed by acid, alkali, light, oxidation, or heat.

Nicotinic acid is easily converted to nicotinamide in the body. In large amounts, nicotinic acid acts as a mild vasodilator (as a mild dilator of blood vessels), causing flushing of the face, increased skin temperature, and dizziness. Since nicotinamide does not cause these unpleasant reactions, its use is preferred in therapeutic preparations.

MEASUREMENT/ASSAY. Niacin in foods and niacin requirements are expressed in milligrams of the pure chemical substance.

Chemical and microbiological methods for niacin assay are now generally used rather than animal assays.

The biological vitamin activity of new compounds can be assayed by the curative dog test (blacktongue disease) or by growth test with chicks and rats.

FUNCTIONS. The principal role of niacin is as a constituent of two important hydrogen-transferring coenzymes in the body: nicotinamide adenine dinucleotide (NAD) and nicotinamide adenine dinucleotide phosphate (NADP). These coenzymes function in many important enzyme systems that are necessary for cell respiration. They are involved in the release of energy from carbohydrates, fats, and protein. Along with the thiamin- and riboflavin-containing coenzymes, they serve as hydrogen acceptors and donors in a series of oxidation-reduction reactions that bring about the release of energy (see Fig. N-6).

$$NAD^+ + 2H^+ \rightleftharpoons NADH + H$$

Fig. N-6. Hydrogen acceptor function of nicotinamide containing coenzymes. R = adenine dinucleotide (= NAD): = adenine dinucleotide phosphate (= NADP).

Also, NAD and NADP are involved in the synthesis of fatty acids, protein, and DNA. For many of these processes to proceed normally, other B-complex vitamins, including vitamin B-6, pantothenic acid, and biotin, are required. .

Niacin also has other functions. It is thought to have a specific effect on growth. Also, there are reports that nicotinic acid (but not nicotinamide) reduces the levels of cholesterol; and that niacin in large doses is slightly beneficial in protecting to some degree against recurrent nonfatal myocardial infarction. However, because of possible undesirable effects, ingestion of large amounts (therapeutic doses) of niacin should be under the direction of a physician.

DEFICIENCY SYMPTOMS. In man, a deficiency of niacin results in pellagra, which generations of medical students have remembered as the disease of the three "Ds"—dermatitis, diarrhea, and dementia (insanity).

The typical features of pellagra are: dermatitis, particularly of areas of skin which are exposed to light or injury; inflammation of mucous membranes including the entire gastrointestinal tract, which results in a red, swollen, sore tongue and mouth, diarrhea, and rectal irritation; and psychic changes, such as irritability, anxiety, depression, and, in advanced cases, delirium, hallucinations, confusion, disorientation, and stupor.

Dogs develop a characteristic black tongue and lesions in the mouth, along with a skin rash, bloody diarrhea, and wasting; followed by eventual death.

(Aslo see PELLAGRA.)

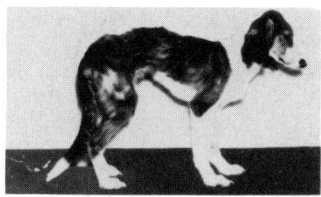
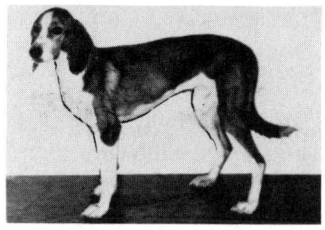

Fig. N-7. Niacin made the difference! *Top*: A dog that had been fed a diet extremely low in niacin. *Bottom*: The same dog after having been fed meat—a good source of niacin—for only 2 weeks. (Studies by Dr. C. A. Elvehjem; courtesy, University of Wisconsin)

RECOMMENDED DAILY ALLOWANCE OF NIACIN. Estimation of niacin requirements are complicated (1) by the fact that some tryptophan is converted to niacin in man, (2) by the paucity of people of different ages receiving diets varying in niacin and tryptophan content, and (3) by the possible unavailablity of niacin in some foods (such as corn).

The Food and Nutrition Board (FNB) of the National Research Council (NRC) recommended daily allowances of niacin are given in Table N-1. Allowances for niacin are commonly related (1) to energy expenditure, based on the essential role of niacin in energy formation—the involvement of the coenzymes NAD and NADP in the functions of respiratory enzymes; and (2) to protein intake, because (a) a diet that furnishes the recommended allowances of protein usually also provides enough niacin through the conversion of tryptophan to niacin, and (b) protein-rich foods are generally, except for milk, rich in preformed niacin. Hence, Table N-1 gives niacin equivalent allowances in relation to both calories and protein.

In Table N-1, the recommended dietary allowances for niacin have been presented as niacin equivalents (NE), recognizing that the contribution from tryptophan may be variable and unpredictable but may represent a substantial portion of the niacin activity of the diet. In estimating the amount of niacin available from foods, the average value of 60 mg of tryptophan should be considered equivalent to 1 mg of niacin.

As with the other B-complex vitamins, the niacin requirements are increased whenever metabolism is accelerated as by fever or by the stress of injury or surgery.

TABLE N-1
RECOMMENDED DAILY NIACIN ALLOWANCES[1]

Group	Age	Weight		Height		Calories	Protein	Niacin
	(yr)	(lb)	(kg)	(in.)	(cm)		(g)	(mg NE)[2]
Infants	0.0–0.5	13	6	24	60	650	13	5
	0.5–1.0	20	9	28	71	850	14	6
Children	1–3	29	13	35	90	1,300	16	9
	4–6	44	20	44	112	1,800	24	12
	7–10	62	28	52	132	2,000	28	13
Males	11–14	99	45	62	157	2,500	45	17
	15–18	145	66	69	176	3,000	59	20
	19–24	160	72	70	177	2,900	58	19
	25–50	174	79	70	176	2,900	63	19
	51+	170	77	68	173	2,400	63	15
Females	11–14	101	46	62	157	2,200	46	15
	15–18	120	55	64	163	2,200	44	15
	19–24	128	58	65	164	2,200	46	15
	25–50	138	63	64	163	2,200	50	15
	51+	143	65	63	160	1,900	50	13
Pregnant						+300	60	17
Lactating						+500	65	20

[1]Recommended Dietary Allowances, 10th ed., 1989, NRC-National Academy of Sciences, p. 285. Calorie values from p. 33, Table 3–5 of the same report.
[2]On the average, 1 mg of niacin is derived from each 60 mg of dietary tryptophan.

Additional pertinent information relative to Table N-1 follows:

• **Recommended allowance for infants, children, and adolescents**—Human milk contains approximately 0.17 mg of niacin and 22 mg of tryptophan per 100 ml or 70 Calories (kcal). Milk from a well-nourished mother appears to be adequate to meet the niacin needs of the infant. Therefore, the niacin allowance recommended for infants up to 6 months of age is 7.7 niacin equivalents per 1,000 Calories (kcal), about two-thirds of which will ordinarily come from tryptophan. The niacin allowance for children over 6 months of age and for adolescents is 7.1 niacin equivalents per 1,000 Calories (kcal).

• **Recommended allowance for adults**—The allowance recommended for adults, expressed as niacin equivalents, is 6.6 niacin equivalents per 1,000 Calories (kcal) and not less than 13 niacin equivalents at caloric intakes

of less than 2,000 Calories (kcal). This amount provides an allowance for the differences in the contributions from tryptophan and the availability of niacin in diets.

• **Recommended allowances for pregnancy and lactation**—The recommended allowance provides an increase of 2 niacin equivalents daily during pregnancy, based on the recommended increase in energy intake of 300 Calories (kcal) daily.

With a recommended increase of 500 Calories (kcal) to support lactation, an additional intake of 3.3 niacin equivalents would be indicated; hence, a total additional intake of 5 niacin equivalents per day is recommended during lactation.

• **Pharmacological intakes of niacin**—Niacin in large doses has been found to be slightly beneficial in protecting to some degree against recurrent nonfatal myocardial infarction. However, ingestion of large amounts of nicotinic acid (3 g or more daily), but not of the amide, may produce vascular dilation, or ''flushing,'' along with other harmful side affects. So, it is recommended that great care and caution be exercised if this vitamin is to be used for the treatment of individuals with coronary heart disease. Mega doses of niacin should be taken under the supervision of a physician.

• **Niacin intake in average U.S. diet**—Average diets in the United States for women ages 19 to 50 supply 700 mg of tryptophan daily, and for men 19 to 50, 1,100 mg. The corresponding values for preformed niacin are 16 and 24 mg, respectively. Thus, the calculated intakes of total NEs are 27 mg for women and 41 mg for men. Proteins of animal origin (milk, eggs, and meat) contain approximately 1.4% tryptophan; most vegetable proteins contain about 1% tryptophan; whereas corn products contain only 0.6%. Some foodstuffs, such as corn, contain niacin-containing compounds from which the niacin may not be completely available. It has been estimated that the enrichment of cereal products adds about 20% more niacin to the food supply than would be provided if these products were not enriched.

The U.S. Department of Agriculture reported that, in 1979, there were sufficient available food sources in the United States to provide an average consumption of 26.7 mg of niacin per person per day; with 45% of the total contributed by meat, poultry, and fish, and 27.4% contributed by flour and cereal products.

TOXICITY. Only large doses of niacin, sometimes given to an individual with a mental illness, are known to be toxic. However, the ingestion of large amounts of nicotinic acid (2 to 3 g per day) may result in vascular dilation, or "flushing" of the skin, itching, liver damage, elevated blood glucose, elevated blood enzymes, and/or peptic ulcer. So, high doses which are sometimes prescribed for cardiovascular diseases and other clinical symptoms, should only be taken on the advice of a physician.

NIACIN LOSSES DURING PROCESSING, COOKING, AND STORAGE. Niacin is the most stable of the B-complex vitamins. It can withstand reasonable periods of heating, cooking, and storage with little loss.

Canning, dehydration, or freezing result in little destruction of the vitamin.

Because niacin is water-soluble, some of it may be lost in cooking, but in a mixed diet usually such losses do not amount to more than 15 to 25% Using a small amount of cooking water will minimize this loss.

Storage results in little loss. In a study of the niacin content of potatoes stored for 6 months at 40°F (4.4°C), only small losses of niacin were observed.

SOURCES OF NIACIN. Generally speaking, niacin is found in animal tissues as nicotinamide and in plant tissues as nicotinic acid; both forms of which are of equal niacin activity and commercially available. For pharmaceutical use, nicotinamide is usually used; for food nutrification (fortification), nicotinic acid is usually used.

As is true of other B vitamins, the niacin content of foods varies widely. A grouping and ranking of foods on the basis of normal niacin content follows:

• **Rich sources**—The best niacin sources are liver, kidney, lean meats, poultry, fish, rabbit, corn flakes (enriched), nuts, peanut butter.

• **Good sources**—Milk, cheese, and eggs, although low in niacin content, are good antipellagra foods (1) because of their high tryptophan content, and (2) because their niacin is in available form. Also, enriched cereal flours and products are good sources of niacin.

• **Negligible sources**—Cereals (corn, wheat, oats, rice, and rye) as a group tend to be low in niacin. Moreover, approximately 80 to 90% of their niacin is in the seed coats, which are removed in the milling process; and the niacin may be present in bound form (i.e., niacytin) and unavailable. Whole grains, enriched cereal flours and other products, and "converted" rice contains considerable niacin. Fruits and vegetables (other than mushrooms and legumes) are variable, but generally poor sources. Also, butter and white sugar are insignificant sources.

• **Supplemental sources**—Synthetic nicotinamide and nicotinic acid; yeast.

NOTE WELL: Most foods that are rich in animal protein are also rich in tryptophan.

Food Composition Table F-36 gives the niacin content of foods. Proteins and Amino Acids in Selected Foods, Table P-37, gives the tryptophan content on a limited number of foods. In the absence of information on the tryptophan content of foods, the following thumb rules for estimating tryptophan content may be used: Proteins of animal origin (milk, eggs, and meat) contain about 1.4% tryptophan, those of vegetable origin about 1.0%, and corn products about 0.6%. An average mixed diet in the United States provides about 1% of protein as tryptophan. Thus, a diet supplying 60 g of protein contains about 600 mg of tryptophan, which will yield about 10 mg of niacin (on the average, 1 mg of niacin is derived from each 60 mg of dietary tryptophan).

Niacin may be present in foods in a "bound" form (i.e., niacytin in corn) which is not absorbable. This is particularly true of corn, wheat, oats, rice, and rye. Yet, pellagra occurs less frequently than one might expect in Mexico, where corn consumption is high. Born of centuries of experience, it is the custom in Mexico to treat corn with limewater before making tortillas, thereby liberating the nicotinic acid. Likewise, the Hopi Indians of Arizona roast sweetcorn in hot ashes, another traditional practice that liberates the nicotinic acid. But the ways of food preparation in Africa do not have this effect.

Coffee is a good source of niacin (a dark roast provides about 3 mg of niacin per cup). In certain areas of the world where the diet of the people is low in niacin and tryptophan, their high consumption of coffee may explain their low incidence of pellagra.

EXAMPLE OF CALCULATING NIACIN EQUIVALENTS

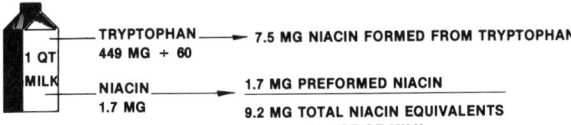

Fig. N-8. How to calculate the niacin equivalents in a quart of milk. A quart of milk containing 449 mg of tryptophan will form 7.5 mg of niacin (449 ÷ 60) from tryptophan. So, this is added to the 1.7 mg of niacin found as such in the milk, bringing the total niacin equivalents of milk to 9.2.

When considering sources of niacin, it should be noted that niacin can be, and is, synthesized by the intestinal flora. However, the amount produced is only of minor importance in the human. By contrast, as with thiamin and riboflavin, ruminants (cattle, sheep, etc.) have no dietary requirements for niacin because of bacterial synthesis in the rumen.

Niacin was one of the original vitamins, along with thiamin and riboflavin, first added to white flour in the United States in 1941; and later to other processed cereal products. Nicotinic acid is the form usually added to foods.

As with most other vitamins, the most inexpensive source of niacin is the synthetic source. Nicotinamide (niacinamide), the form usually taken as a vitamin supplement, is available in most food stores and pharmacies at a very reasonable cost.

TOP FOOD SOURCES OF NIACIN. The top food sources of niacin are listed in Table N-2.

NOTE WELL: This table lists (1) the top sources without regard to the amount normally eaten (left column), and (2) the top food sources (right column); and the caloric (energy) content of each food.

As noted in the preceding section entitled "Sources of Niacin," in estimating the total amount of niacin supplied in the diet, the tryptophan content of the foods should be considered, also.

(Also see VITAMIN[S], Table V-9.)

TABLE N-2
TOP SOURCES OF NIACIN AND THEIR CALORIC AND PROTEIN CONTENT[1]

Top Sources[2]	Niacin (mg/100 g)	Energy (kcal/100 g)	Protein (g/100 g)	Top Food Sources	Niacin (mg/100 g)	Energy (kcal/100 g)	Protein (g/100 g)
Yeast, torula	44	277	39				
Brewers' yeast, tablet form	40	--	--	Peanuts, roasted and salted	17	570	26
Yeast, brewers', debittered	38	283	39	Liver, beef or calf, fried	17	242	28
Yeast, baker's, dry (active)	37	282	37	Chicken, broiler/fryer, breast meat w/ skin, fried, flour coated	14	203	33
Coffee, instant, dry	31	--	15				
Rice, bran	30	276	13	Tuna, canned in water, solid/- liquid, salt or no salt	13	123	28
Rice, polished	28	265	12	Corn flakes, w/added nutrients	12	380	8
Peanut flour, defatted	28	371	48	Rabbit, domesticated, flesh only stewed	11	216	29
Sunflower seed flour, partially defatted	27	339	45	Turkey, all classes, light meat, cooked, roasted	11	176	33
Liver, lamb, broiled	25	261	32	Salmon, broiled or baked	10	182	27
Liver, hog, fried in margarine	22	241	30	Mackerel, cooked	8	230	23
Wheat bran	21	353	16	Peaches, dehydrated, sulfured, uncooked	8	340	5
Cereal bran/sugar and malt extract	18	240	13	Pork, fresh, loin, lean	7	300	25
Peanuts, roasted and salted	17	570	26	Lamb leg or loin, separable lean, roasted	6	245	25
Liver, beef or calf, fried	17	242	28	Beef[3]	6	350	25
Paprika, domestic	15	289	15	Nuts, mixed, dry roasted	5	590	22
Peanut butter	15	594	25	Wheat flour, all-purpose, enriched	5	365	10
Liver, turkey, simmered	14	174	28	Wheat flour, whole (from hard wheats)	4	361	13
Cereal bran/sugar and defatted wheat germ	14	238	11	Mushrooms (*Agaricus campestris*), raw	4	28	2
Chicken, broiler/fryer, breast meat w/skin, fried in flour	14	203	33	Cornmeal, degermed, enriched	4	362	8
				Rice, white, enriched, raw	4	363	7
				Bread, white, enriched	3	270	9

[1]These listings are based on the data in Food Composition Table F-36. Some top or rich sources may have been overlooked since some of the foods in Table F-36 lack values for niacin.

Whenever possible, foods are on an "as used" basis, without regard to moisture content; hence, certain high-moisture foods may be disadvantaged when ranked on the basis of niacin content per 100 g (approximately 3 1/2 oz) without regard to moisture content.

[2]Listed without regard to the amount normally eaten.

[3]Includes a variety of lean cuts including lean ground hamburger.

NIACINAMIDE

The biologically active form of niacin occurring in the tissues.

NIACIN EQUIVALENT (NE)

Because tryptophan is a precursor of niacin and thus an additional source, dietary requirements for niacin are usually given in terms of total niacin or niacin equivalents. Niacin equivalent is the total niacin available from the diet including (1) preformed niacin, plus (2) niacin derived from the metabolism of tryptophan (60 mg tryptophan = I mg niacin).

(Also see NIACIN.)

NICKEL (Ni)

This element, first discovered in 1751 by Cronstedt and named nickel after "Old Nick," a demon, is the same nickel that the U.S. five-cent piece is named after.

In 1970, F.H. Nielsen, of the U.S. Department of Agriculture, reported that chickens deficient in nickel (Ni) developed slightly enlarged hocks, thickened legs, bright orange leg color (instead of pale yellow-brown), a dermatitis, and a less friable liver; deficiency symptoms which were corrected by adding nickel at a level of 3 to 5 mg per kg of diet. Subsequently, deficiencies have also been reported in rats, pigs, and goats, and nickel has been found in a serum protein (called nickeloplasmin) in rabbits and humans.

NICOTINAMIDE

The amide of nicotinic acid. It has niacin (one of the B vitamins) activity as a constituent of two coenzymes.
(Also see NIACIN; and VITAMIN[S].)

NICOTINAMIDE ADENINE DINUCLEO-TIDE (NAD)

A coenzyme formed by the chemical combination of nicotinamide, adenine, ribose and phosphate. Its formation requires the vitamin niacin. In the body it is employed as a hydrogen (electron) acceptor during the oxidation (breakdown) of foods to form energy.

(Also see METABOLISM; and NIACIN.)

NICOTINAMIDE ADENINE DINUCLEO-TIDE PHOSPHATE (NADP)

A coenzyme of niacin with three high-energy phosphate bonds which facilitates oxidation within the cells.

NICOTINIC ACID

Another name for niacin.
(Also see NIACIN; and VITAMIN[S].)

NIGHT BLINDNESS

A minor dietary deficiency disorder due to the deficiency of vitamin A. Characteristically, an abnormally long time is required for adaptation from vision in a strong light to vision in a dim light or darkness. It is one of the earliest signs of a vitamin A deficiency.

(Also see BLINDNESS DUE TO VITAMIN A DEFICIENCY; DEFICIENCY DISEASES, Table D-2 Minor Dietary Deficiency Disorders; and VITAMIN A.)

NISIN

A naturally-occurring antibiotic, sometimes found in milk. Many countries use nisin as a food preservative. However, the direct addition of antibiotic to food is not permitted in the United States.
(Also see ANTIBIOTICS.)

NITRATES AND NITRITES

Nitrate refers to the chemical union of one nitrogen (N) and three oxygen (O) atoms, or NO_3, while nitrite refers to the chemical union of one nitrogen (N) and two oxygen (O) atoms, or NO_2. These terms are frequently used by the news media and others when referring to four specific chemicals contained in foods.

CHEMISTRY. Of prime concern are sodium nitrate (Chile saltpeter), potassium nitrate (saltpeter), sodium nitrite, and potassium nitrite.

• **Sodium nitrate ($NaNO_3$)**—A colorless, odorless, but somewhat bitter tasting, chemical which can be in the form of crystals or powder. It occurs as a mineral in Chile; hence, the name Chile saltpeter. Sodium nitrate is very soluble in water; 1 g dissolves in 1.1 ml of water.

• **Potassium nitrate (KNO₃)**—A colorless, white compound, which occurs in either powder or crystal form. It tastes slightly salty and pungent, and can be used as a diuretic. Potassium nitrate is soluble in water, but not as soluble as sodium nitrate—only 1 g per 2.8 ml.

• **Sodium nitrite (NaNO₂)**—A white or slightly yellow chemical existing as granules, rods, or powder. In the air, it oxidizes very slowly to nitrate. It is very soluble in water; 1 g dissolves in 1.5 ml of water.

• **Potassium nitrite (KNO₂)**—A white or slightly yellow compound existing in the form of granules or rods which pick up moisture from the air and become liquid upon exposure to the air.

Both sodium and potassium nitrite are unstable when exposed to heat, while the nitrates are stable to heat but can be reduced to nitrites by bacteria.

OCCURRENCE AND EXPOSURE.
Nitrates and nitrites are common chemicals in our environment whether they come from "natural" or "unnatural" sources.

Naturally Occurring. Most green vegetables contain nitrates. The level of nitrates in vegetables depends on (1) species, (2) variety, (3) plant part, (4) stage of plant maturity, (5) soil condition such as deficiencies of potassium, phosphorus, and calcium or excesses of soil nitrogen, and (6) environmental factors such as drought, high temperature, time of day, and shade. Regardless of the variation of nitrate content in plants, vegetables are the major source of nitrate ingestion as Table N-3 shows.

Those vegetables which are most apt to contain high levels of nitrates include beets, spinach, radishes, and lettuce. Despite the shift from manure to chemical fertilizers over the years, the overall average concentration of nitrate in plants has remained unchanged. Other natural sources of nitrate are negligible.

Nitrite occurrence in foods is minimal. Interestingly, a naturally occurring source of nitrites appears to be the saliva. Table N-3 demonstrates that more nitrite is derived from the bacterial action on nitrate in the mouth than from any other source. However, this source is directly dependent upon the amount of nitrate ingested. Bacteria in the intestine probably produce another 80 to 130 mg of nitrite daily.

Food Additives. Both nitrates and nitrites are used as food additives, mainly in meat and meat products, according to the guidelines presented in Table N-4. Their use in meat has been the subject of much publicity, though their use to cure meat is lost in antiquity. The role of nitrates in meats is not clear, though it is believed that they provide a reservoir source of nitrite since microorganisms convert nitrate to nitrite. It is the nitrite which decomposes to nitric oxide, NO, and reacts with heme pigments to form nitrosomyoglobin giving meats their red color. Furthermore, taste panel studies on bacon, ham, hot dogs, and other products have demonstrated that a definite preference is shown for the taste of those products containing nitrites. In addition, nitrites retard rancidity, but more importantly, nitrites inhibit microbial growth, especially *Clostridium botulinum*. Hence, cured meats provide a source of ingested nitrates and nitrites. However, as a source of nitrate, cured meats are minor compared to vegetables. The major dietary source of nitrites is cured meats, but this is small when compared to that produced by the bacteria in the mouth and swallowed with saliva. Currently, there is no other protection from botulism as effective as nitrites. So, for those wishing to eliminate nitrites, possible carcinogens, there is a Catch 22—eliminate the nitrites and increase botulism poisoning, a proven danger.

Note: Since 1990, 90% of the cured meat samples have contained less than 50 ppm nitrate; only 0.1% have contained more than 200 ppm.

TABLE N-3
ESTIMATED AVERAGE DAILY INGESTION OF NITRATE AND NITRITE PER PERSON IN THE UNITED STATES[1]

Source	Nitrate (NO₃₋)	Nitrite (NO₂₋)
	(mg)	(mg)
Vegetables	86.1	.20
Cured meats	9.4	2.38
Bread	2.0	.02
Fruits, juices	1.4	.00
Water	.7	.00
Milk and products . . .	.2	.00
Total	99.8	2.60
Saliva[2]	30.0	8.62

[1]*Nitrates: An Environmental Assessment*, 1978, National Academy of Sciences, p. 437, Table 9.1.

[2]Not included in the total since the amount of nitrite produced by bacteria in the mouth depends directly upon the amount of nitrate ingested.

TABLE N-4
FEDERAL NITRATE AND NITRITE ALLOWANCES IN MEAT

Meat Preparation	Level Allowed	
	Sodium or Potassium Nitrate	Sodium or Potassium Nitrite
Finished product ..	200 ppm or 91 mg/lb (maximum)	200 ppm or 91 mg/lb (maximum)
Dry cure	3.5 oz/100 lb or 991 mg/lb	1.0 oz/100 lb or 283 mg/lb
Chopped meat	2.75 oz/100 lb or 778 mg/lb	0.25 oz/100 lb or 71 mg/lb

Other Sources. Aside from very unusual circumstances other sources of exposure to nitrates and nitrites are relatively minor. (See Table N-3.) Nitrate concentrations in groundwater used for drinking range from several hundred micrograms per liter (1.06 qt) to a few milligrams per liter. Nitrates are generally higher in groundwater than surface water since plants remove nitrates from surface water. Surveys of public water supplies have shown that nitrate concentrations above 10 mg/liter, a standard for nitrate in drinking water recom-

mended by the U.S. Public Health Service, are extremely rare in the United States. Furthermore, high levels of nitrate are more likely to occur in well water in regions where conditions favor the accumulation of nitrates in groundwater. Some private wells on small farms contain several hundred mg/liter of nitrate.

Strategies to reduce the nitrate content of water are frustrated by the complexity of the nitrogen cycle which makes determining the source of the nitrate difficult. As Fig. N-9 illustrates, nitrogen, nitrates, and other nitrogen compounds are everywhere.

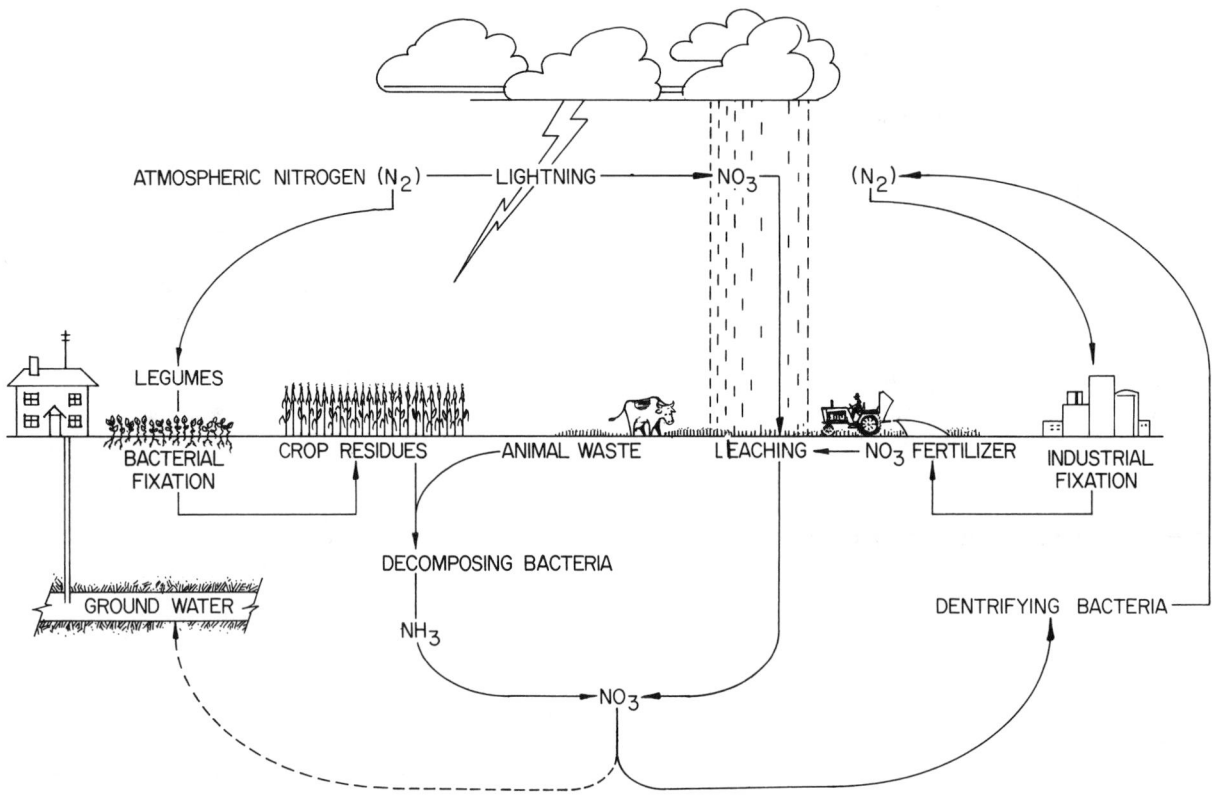

Fig. N-9.   The nitrogen cycle emphasizing activities that affect fluxes of nitrogen.

Very little is known about the contribution of airborne nitrates and nitrites to human exposure. Some evidence shows an increase in nitrites due to pollution, while most nitrates occur in the atmosphere as the result of normal

processes of the nitrogen cycle. Although both nitrates and nitrites are present in the atmosphere, there is no definite indication that these pose a health hazard.

DANGERS OF NITRATES AND NITRITES.
Possibly these chemicals may present a hazard to man through two routes. First, under certain circumstances nitrates and nitrites can be directly toxic. Second, nitrates and nitrites contribute to the formation of cancer causing nitrosamine.

Toxicity. Our knowledge of the toxic effects of nitrates and nitrites is derived from its long use in medicine, accidental ingestion, and ingestion by animals. Overall, poisoning by nitrates is uncommon. An accidental ingestion of 8 to 15 g causes severe gastroenteritis, blood in the urine and stool, weakness, collapse, and possibly death. Fortunately, nitrate is rapidly excreted from the adult body in the urine, and the formation of methemoglobin generally is not part of the toxic action of nitrates.

Nitrites are more toxic than nitrates; and nitrate can be reduced to nitrite by the rumen bacteria of cattle and sheep, resulting in nitrite poisoning from plants or water high in nitrates. Upon absorption into the bloodstream, nitrite reacts with the red oxygen-transporting pigment, hemoglobin, to form a chocolate brown pigment, methemoglobin, that cannot carry oxygen. Death occurs when about three-fourths of the oxygen-carrying hemoglobin is converted to methemoglobin. Adults have been poisoned by overdoses of drugs such as amyl nitrite which is used to relax involuntary muscles, particularly those in the blood vessels. However, during the first 3 to 6 months of life, an infant's stomach pH is high—between 5 and 7—thus, it does not inhibit the growth of nitrate-reducing bacteria which are later confined to the intestine. Hence, infants can reduce nitrate to nitrite in their stomach. In older children and in adults, the nitrate is absorbed in the stomach before reaching the nitrate-reducing bacteria in the intestine. Despite this unique condition of the infant's stomach, only rarely has methemoglobinemia resulted from eating nitrate-containing vegetables or cured meats. Almost all cases of nitrate-induced methemoglobinemia in the United States have resulted from the ingestion of infant formula made with water from a private well containing an extremely high nitrate level. Overall, it is comforting to note that several hundred million pounds of beets and spinach—nitrate-containing vegetables—are eaten yearly without injury.

The Cancer Question. Without doubt, the greatest concern of people is the involvement of nitrates and nitrites in directly causing cancer, or in indirectly pro-ducing compounds known as nitrosamines. Since nitrosamines are definitely accepted as carcinogens in test animals, a majority of the furor around nitrates and nitrites stems from this fact.

CONVERSION TO NITROSAMINES. The conversion of nitrate to nitrite to nitrous acid and then combining with secondary amines (NH) to form nitrosamines in the body (as shown in Fig. N-10) is potentially possible, but it has not been clearly demonstrated. However, what really started the whole nitrate and nitrite issue was the discovery that nitrite-containing bacon when fried at very high temperatures of 350° to 400°F (*177 to 204°C*) or higher, yielded some nitrosamines. There is a whole family of nitrosamines; and their carcinogenic activity, in a variety of animals, varies from harmless to very carcinogenic.

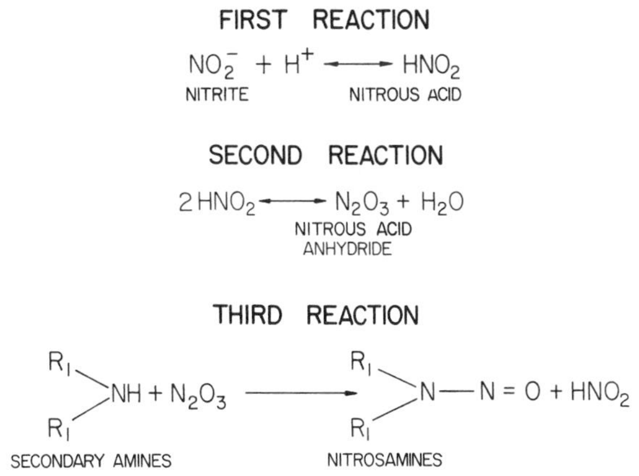

FIRST REACTION

$$NO_2^- + H^+ \longrightarrow HNO_2$$
NITRITE   NITROUS ACID

SECOND REACTION

$$2\,HNO_2 \longrightarrow N_2O_3 + H_2O$$
NITROUS ACID ANHYDRIDE

THIRD REACTION

$$\begin{array}{c} R_1 \\ \diagdown \\ R_1 \end{array} NH + N_2O_3 \longrightarrow \begin{array}{c} R_1 \\ \diagdown \\ R_1 \end{array} N-N=O + HNO_2$$
SECONDARY AMINES   NITROSAMINES

Fig. N-10. Reactions occurring in the formation of nitrosamines from nitrites in water solutions. In the third reaction, R_1 and R_2 represent carbon chains of various lengths.

CARCINOGENIC ACTIVITY OF NITROSAMINES. It cannot be stated that any human cancer has been positively attributed to nitrosamines. However, some nitrosamines have caused cancer in every laboratory animal species tested. Four of the more carcinogenic nitrosamines are indicated by name and chemical structure in Table N-5.

TABLE N-5
THE NAME, STRUCTURE, AND CARCINOGENIC ACTIVITY OF SELECTED NITROSAMINES

Name	Structure	Carcino-genicity[1]	Cancer Types in Experimental Animals	Possible Routes of Human Exposure[2]
N-nitrosodiethylamine or diethylnitrosamine (DEN)	CH_3—CH_2 $\backslash$ N—NO / CH_3—CH_2	3.20	Esophagus; larynx; liver; lung; nasal cavities; stomach; trachea.	New car interiors; whiskey; iron foundry.
N-nitrosopyrrolidine (NPYR)	H_2C—CH_2 / H_2C CH_2 $\backslash$ N / NO	2.64	Liver; lung; trachea; nasal cavities; testes.	Cooked nitrite cured bacon; sausage; cured meat.
N-nitrosodimethylamine or dimethylnitrosamine (DMN)	CH_3 $\backslash$ N—NO / CH_3	2.27	Kidney; liver; lung; nasal cavity.	Leather tannery; smoked fish; rubber tire plant; canned fish; new car interiors; cooked bacon; beer; herbicides; fish meal; iron foundry; frankfurters; powdered milk.
Nitrosomorphololine (NMOR)	O / \ H_2C CH_2 H_2C CH_2 \ / N NO	1.95	Esophagus; kidney; liver; lung; nasal cavities; ovary; testes.	Leather tannery; rubber tire plant; new car interiors.

[1]Defined as the logarithm of one divided by D_{50}, where D_{50} is the molar dose required to induce tumors in 50% of the test animals.
[2]Too few food samples have been analyzed to comment on the frequency of nitrosamine contamination in the human food supply. Furthermore, when samples are analyzed, only a fraction of the samples are positive for nitrosamines.

Experimental animals such as mice, rats, hamsters, pigs, dogs, monkeys, and fish all have demonstrated cancer formation in various organs from exposure to certain nitrosamines. The most common organ affected by all nitrosamines is the liver. Still, it is not known how humans respond to nitrosamines, nor is the hazardous level of exposure known.

EXPOSURE TO NITROSAMINES. When nitrosamines are mentioned, foods are the first items which come to mind. However, as Table N-5 shows there are numerous other sources of nitrosamines. Furthermore, people are exposed to some other nitrosamines not listed in Table N-5; namely, cosmetics, lotions, and shampoos containing N-nitrosodiethanolamine (NDELA), which is carcinogenic in the rat. Other preformed nitrosamines have been found in tobacco and tobacco smoke. Hence, human exposure can result from breathing or eating preformed nitrosamines, or by applying them to the skin. Foods are not the only source of nitrosamines.

THE FDA AND THE DELANEY CLAUSE. To ban or not to ban the use of nitrates and nitrites in foods is the question. In the summer of 1978, this "fire" received more fuel when a study conducted for the FDA by Dr. Paul Newberne of Massachusetts Institute of Technology (MIT) reported that nitrite alone fed to rats increased the incidence of cancers of the lymphatic system. Immediately, and before the study was properly reviewed, the USDA and the FDA announced they would soon ban nitrites. Tempers flared and pork producers lost money due to the implication of bacon containing a cancer-causing substance. The MIT study has now been reviewed by an independent group, and the research has been shown to be in error. For the time being, the FDA and USDA have backed down from their earlier stand to ban nitrite; they now say that the evidence is insufficient to initiate any action to remove nitrite from foods. However, it is noteworthy that the U.S. Supreme Court has cleared the way for the USDA to approve no-nitrate labels in processed meats, should they wish to do so.

In February 1981, the Supreme Court announced that it would not hear an appeal from the Eighth Ciruit Court of Appeals, thereby signaling that the National Pork Producers Council (NPPC) had lost its lengthy court battle against the U.S. Department of Agriculture, on the no-nitrite label which it was promulgating. The NPPC argument: Botulism or cancer; which is the greatest threat? Apparently this paves the way for the USDA to approve labels for "no nitrite, look alike" processed meats. At this writing, industry observers aren't sure what the ruling will mean. The USDA may review the whole case and decide to drop the no-nitrite label effort. Even if the USDA does go ahead with the labeling, meat industry representatives aren't really certain how much no-nitrite product will go on the market.

On an individual basis, after carefully considering the issue, it is the old question of benefit versus risk. The risk of botulism in cured meats in the absence of nitrite is both real and dangerous, while the risk of cancer from low levels of nitrosamines and/or nitrites remains uncertain. Furthermore, no acceptable alternative is as effective as nitrite in preventing botulism, and foods represent only one source of exposure to nitrosamines. Nevertheless, nitrite should be reduced in all products to the extent protection against botulism is not compromised, an extent yet to be determined.

(Also see ADDITIVES; BACTERIA IN FOOD; CANCER; DELANEY CLAUSE; and MEAT[S].)

NITROGEN (N)

A chemical element essential to life. All plant and animal tissues contain nitrogen. Animals and humans get it from protein foods; plants get it from the soil; and some bacteria get it directly from the air. Nitrogen forms about 80% of the air.

(Also see METABOLISM; and PROTEIN[S].)

NITROGEN BALANCE

The nitrogen in the food intake minus the nitrogen in the feces, minus the nitrogen in the urine is the nitrogen balance. Normal adults are in nitrogen balance—intake equals output. Nitrogen is obtained from the proteins we eat.

• **Positive nitrogen balance**—When nitrogen intake exceeds nitrogen output a positive nitrogen balance exists. Such a condition is present in the following physiological states: pregnancy, lactation, recovery from a severe illness, growth, and following the administration of an anabolic steroid such as testosterone. A positive nitrogen balance indicates that new tissue is being built.

• **Negative nitrogen balance**—This occurs when nitrogen intake is less than output. Starvation, diabetes mellitus, fever, surgery, burns or shock can all result in a negative nitrogen balance. This is an undesirable state since body protein is being broken down faster than it is being built up.

(Also see METABOLISM; PROTEIN[S]; and BIOLOGICAL VALUE OF PROTEINS.)

NITROGEN DEFICIT

The term used to describe the condition when more nitrogen is being lost from the body in the urine and feces than is being consumed in the diet, a negative nitrogen balance.

(Also see NITROGEN BALANCE.)

NITROGEN EQUILIBRIUM

A term sometimes used in place of nitrogen balance. (Also see NITROGEN BALANCE.)

NITROGEN-FREE EXTRACT (NFE)

It consists principally of sugars, starches, pentoses, and nonnitrogenous organic acids in any given food. The percentage is determined by subtracting the sum of the percentages of moisture, crude protein, crude fat, crude fiber, and ash from 100. This fraction represents a catch-all for the organic compounds for which there is no specific analysis when performing a proximate food analysis.

(Also see ANALYSIS OF FOODS.)

NITROGEN, METABOLIC

That nitrogen which is lost in the urine and feces due to the metabolic processes of the body and not due to that derived from the diet. Metabolic nitrogen consists of digestive enzymes, cells from the lining of the gastrointestinal tract and bacteria.

(Also see NITROGEN BALANCE.)

NITROSAMINES

A whole family of chemical compounds formed when chemicals containing nitrogen dioxide (NO_2)—so called nitrites—react with amine (NH_2) groups of other chemicals. Many nitrosamines are potent carcinogens when tested in animals. Because there are numerous chemicals capable of reacting with nitrite, nitrosamines have been found in the air, water, tobacco smoke, cured meats, cosmetics, pesticides, tanneries, alcoholic beverages, and tire manufacturing plants. It is even possible that they are formed in our body, though this process is not clearly demonstrated. Thus, human exposure may result from several routes. However, very few data are available to make estimates of levels of exposure by each route. Some epidemiological studies have associated increased incidence of human cancer with the presence of nitrosamines in the diet. Direct evidence that nitrosamines are carcinogenic for humans is lacking.

(Also see CANCER; and NITRATES AND NITRITES, section headed "Conversion to Nitrosamines.")

NITROSOMYOGLOBIN

The chemical responsible for the red color of cured meat. It is formed by the decomposition of nitrites to nitric oxide (NO) which reacts with the myoglobin of the muscle.

(Also see MEATS, section headed "Meat Curing"; MYOGLOBIN; and NITRATES AND NITRITES.)

NITROUS OXIDE (N₂O)

To most people it is better known as laughing gas, an inhalation anesthetic and analgesic. However, in the food industry it is approved by the FDA as a propellant and aerating agent in certain sprayed foods canned under pressure such as whipped cream or sprayed vegetable fats.

(Also see ADDITIVES.)

NOCTURIA

Excessive urination at night.

NOGGIN

• A small cup or mug of ¼ pt, (*120 ml*) usually for liquor.

• A person's head.

NONESSENTIAL AMINO ACID

Any one of several amino acids that are required by animals but which can be synthesized in adequate amounts by an animal in its tissues from other amino acids.

(Also see AMINO ACID[S].)

NONESTERIFIED FATTY ACIDS (NEFA)

Those fatty acids which are freed from triglycerides, and released into the blood. Often they are called free fatty acids (FFA).

(Also see FATS AND OTHER LIPIDS; FREE FATTY ACIDS; and TRIGLYCERIDES.)

NONFAT DRY MILK (NDM)

The product obtained by removing water from pasteurized skim milk.

(Also see MILK AND MILK PRODUCTS.)

NONHEME

Iron that is not a part of the hemoglobin molecule; a designation for iron in foods of plant origin.

(Also see IRON, section headed "Absorption, Metabolism, Excretion.")

NONPAREILS

Another name for colored sugar crystals used in decorating candies, cakes, or cookies.

NONPROTEIN NITROGEN (NPN)

Nitrogen which comes from other than a protein source but which under certain circumstances may be used by man in the building of body protein. NPN sources include compounds like urea and salts of ammonia. Persons on low protein diets make better use of NPN than those fed adequate or high levels of protein.

(Also see UREA.)

NONVEGAN

A nonvegetarian; a person who includes animal proteins in the diet.

NORDIHYDROGUAIARETIC ACID (NDGA)

An antioxidant used in fats and oils. At one time, it was on the GRAS list of approved substances, but the FDA now prohibits its use.

(Also see ADDITIVES.)

NOURISH

To furnish or sustain with food or other substances necessary for life and growth.

NUCLEIC ACIDS

Nucleic acids were so named because they were originally isolated from cell nuclei. They are the carriers and mediators of genetic information, of which there are two types: *deoxyribonucleic acid (DNA)* and *ribonucleic acid (RNA)*. The two types of nucleic acids, DNA and RNA, differ in that DNA has one less oxygen molecule (carbon atom number 2) in its component sugar ribose, and is a double strand.

Every cell of the body contains the same amount of DNA with the exception of the sperm and egg cells. It is the DNA of the chromosomes in the nuclei of cells that carries the coded master plans for all of the inherited characteristics—size, shape, and orderly development from conception to birth to death. DNA is different for each species, and even for each individual within a species. These differences consist of minor rearrangements of sequences among the nitrogenous bases, which constitute a code containing all the information on the heritable characteristics of cells, tissues, organs, and individuals.

The messages carried by DNA are put into action in the cells by the other nucleic acid, RNA. To do this, DNA serves as a template (as the pattern or guide) for the formation of RNA. The genetic message is coded by the sequence of purine and pyrimidine bases attached to the "backbone"of the DNA structure—a long chain of the sugar deoxyribose and phosphoric acid. Purine bases in DNA include adenine and guanine, while pyrimidine bases include cytosine and thymine. One molecule of DNA may contain 500 million bases. The "backbone" of RNA is also a sugar, the sugar ribose, plus phosphoric acid. However, in RNA the pyrimidine base thymine is replaced by uracil, another pyrimidine. RNA molecules are considerably smaller than DNA, containing from less than a hundred to hundreds of bases—not millions.

(Also see METABOLISM, section headed "Proteins.")

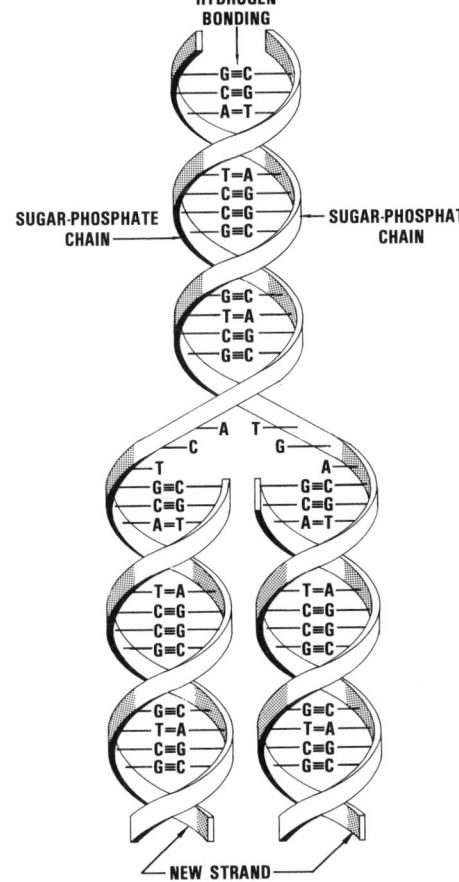

Fig. N-11. The spiral structure of deoxyribonucleic acid, or DNA—the basic building block of life on earth. It's a double helix (a double spiral structure), with the sugar (deoxyribose)-phosphate (phosphoric acid) "backbone" represented by the two spiral ribbons. Connecting the "backbone" are four nitrogenous bases (a base is the nonacid part of a salt): adenine (A) paired with thymine (T), and guanine (G) paired with cytosine (C); with the parallel spiral ribbons held together by hydrogen bonding between these base pairs. Adenine and guanine are purines, while thymine and cytosine are pyrimidines.

HISTORY. The study of nucleic acids began in the 1860s with the Austrian monk, Gregor Mendel, experimenting with garden peas. He showed that heredity could be understood in terms of simple mathematical ratios. Although Mendel was not able to explain how hereditary characteristics are transmitted to offspring, he was observing nucleic acids in action. An explanation of Mendel's work was not available until 1916, when Thomas Hunt Morgan and his group at Columbia University, using the fruit fly, demonstrated that genes on the chromosomes carried hereditary information from parent to offspring. In 1933, Morgan won a Nobel Prize for his work. Before 1950, George W. Beadle and Edward L. Tatum demonstrated that genes were long-chain polymers in which proteins are linked with nucleic acids. They received a Nobel Prize in 1958. Next, Alfred E. Mirsky and V. G. Allfrey of the Rockefeller Institute showed that DNA was necessary for the manufacture of RNA in the cell and for the buildup of proteins in the nucleus. Then, Erwin Chargoff noted the important relationship between the bases—adenine and thymine occur in equal amounts, as do cytosine and guanine. Armed with this information and the x-ray diffraction studies of Maurice Wilkins of King's College in London, James Watson, an American biochemist, and Francis Crick, an English physical chemist, set out to determine the actual structure of DNA.

Working together, they explored many possible structures, out of which they finally concluded that DNA was composed of two polynucleotide chains joined by bonds between the bases and wrapped around each other in the form of a double helix. In 1962, those three scientists—Wilkins, Watson, and Crick—shared the Nobel Prize for physiology and medicine for their work. But the story did not end! Building upon the present knowledge and understanding of the nucleic acids DNA and RNA, scientists are making such ideas as genetic engineering and cloning into realities. Thus, mankind is coming closer and closer to understanding the very essence of life—DNA.

SYNTHESIS.   Each time a cell divides, a new DNA is made, while within most cells RNA is continually being synthesized and broken down into its components. When the purines and pyrimidines are combined with the sugars ribose or deoxyribose, the resultant compound is referred to as a *nucleoside. Nucleotides* are nucleosides that are esterified (acid and alcohol combination) with phosphoric acid. When a series of nucleotides are joined together, nucleic acids are formed. The secret of the code is a process called base pairing.

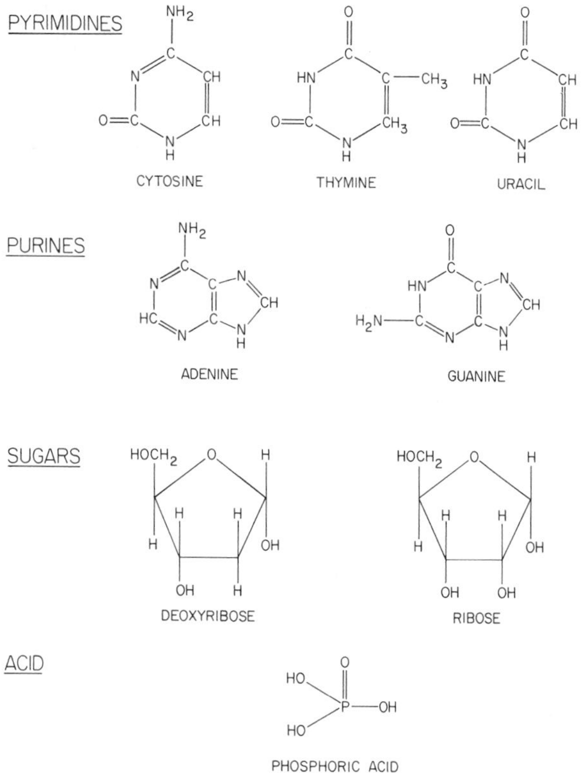

Fig. N-12.   Components of nucleic acids.

During the formation of new DNA or RNA, the same bases always pair off—guanine with cytosine, adenine with thymine, and adenine with uracil in RNA. This ensures that the code is duplicated time and time again. During synthesis, the double helix splits, pulling the base pairs apart. New bases line up with the proper partner and form another sugar-phosphoric acid "backbone" (see Fig. N-11).

Purines, pyrimidines, ribose, and deoxyribose may be synthesized in the body from other compounds, or they may be recycled. Phosphorus, for the formation of phosphoric acid, is a required dietary mineral, and it is employed in a variety of other compounds besides DNA and RNA.

DIGESTION, ABSORPTION, AND METABOLISM.   The enzymes from the pancreas, called nucleases, split the nucleic acids into nucleotides. Then the nucleotides are split into nucleosides and phosphoric acid by other enzymes in the intestine. Finally, the nucleosides are split into their (1) constituent sugars (deoxyribose or ribose, (2) purine bases (adenine and guanine), and (3) pyrimidine bases (cytosine, thymine, and uracil). These bases are then absorbed into the blood via active transport. The sugars are absorbed slowly, and, as far as is known, there is no specific transport mechanism.

Once in the body, the purine and pyrimidine bases may be reused. They are not only used for DNA and RNA but also as components of a variety of coenzymes. If not used, pyrimidines are catabolized to beta-alanine, beta-aminoisobutyric acid, carbon dioxide (CO_2), and ammonia (NH_3), while the purines are converted to uric acid. Ammonia, uric acid, and beta-aminoisobutyric acid are excreted in the urine.

Ribose can be metabolized via the pentose shunt or hexosemonophosphate pathway—the same metabolic pathway that produces ribose.

(Also see METABOLISM.)

FUNCTIONS.   DNA is the component of the chromosomes that carries the blueprint for a species—the heritable characteristics of each cell in the body and its descendants. It functions in the egg and sperm cells to pass the blueprint along from parent to offspring. Messages are relayed from DNA in the nucleus of cells to the cytoplasm by RNA, whereupon the sequences of amino acids in protein synthesis are dictated by the order of the purine and pyrimidine bases transcribed from the DNA. Each cell of the body contains a full genetic blueprint, but only small parts of the genetic message are normally transcribed by RNA for cells to fulfill their role in whatever tissue they are located.

REQUIRED INTAKE.   There is no required level of intake of nucleic acids per se. A nutritious, well-balanced diet provides the precursors necessary for the synthesis of the purines, pyrimidines, and ribose sugar in the body. The only direct requirement is for the mineral phosphorus. Since it is a component of DNA and RNA, it is in every cell of the body. Children and adults require 800 to 1,200 mg daily.

• **Aging**—While there is little doubt that aging involves changes in the body's DNA and RNA, there is some doubt that increasing the dietary intake of DNA and/or RNA will prolong life, prevent aging, or rejuvenate the aged as some promoters claim. Any possible benefits to accrue from supplemental nucleic acid await further research.

Currently, the Committee on Dietary Allowances and the Food and Nutrition Board recognize nucleotides and nucleic acids as substances known to be growth factors for lower forms of life, but for which no dietary requirement for higher humans or animals is known.

(Also see PHOSPHORUS.)

SOURCES. Since DNA and RNA are components of all cells, any food in which the cells are concentrated is a rich source of nucleic acids. Organ meats such as liver, kidneys and pancreas are rich sources. Since these meats are rich sources of nucleic acids, it follows that they are rich sources of purines; hence, sufferers of gout are advised to avoid them. Other meats, poultry, and fish, the embryo or germ of grains and legumes, and the growing parts of young plants are good sources of nucleic acids. Butter and other fats, cheese, eggs, fruits, milk, nuts, starch, sugar, and vegetables are low in nucleic acids.

(Also see ARTHRITIS, section headed "Gout [Gouty Arthritis].")

GENETIC ENGINEERING. The recent development of gene-splicing (also known as recombinant DNA) ushered in a new era of genetic engineering—with all its promise and possible peril. The scientific community is bitterly divided about the unknown risks of "tinkering with life." Proponents of research in DNA are convinced that it can help point the way to new scientific horizons—of understanding and perhaps curing cancer and such inherited diseases as diabetes and hemophilia; of a vastly improved knowledge of the genetics of all plants and animals, including eventually humans. The outcome being the potential of creating new or improved animals and plants, and correcting errors in human genetics. On May 23, 1977, scientists at the University of California-San Francisco reported a major breakthrough as a result of altering genes—turning ordinary bacteria into factories capable of producing insulin, a valuable hormone previously extracted at slaughter from pigs, sheep, and cattle, so essential to the survival of 1.8 million diabetics.

The feat opened the door to further genetic engineering or splicing. Already, this genetic wizardry has been used in transplanting into bacteria (and recently into yeast cells) genes responsible for many critical biochemicals in addition to insulin; among them, the following:

• **Endorphin**—A recently discovered group of polypeptides that influence nerve transmission, referred to as the brain's own opiate (because they bind to those receptors which bind opiates [morphine, naloxone, etc.]) and thus mimic some of the pharmacological properties of morphine. Now beta-endorphin—which may prove effective in the treatment of schizophrenia, depression, and pain—can be available in abundance for tests because bacteria can be used to mass produce it.

• **Somatotropin**—This is the human growth hormone, used to treat dwarfism in children. To date, the hormone has been rare and expensive because the only source has been the pituitary gland taken from cadavers; and about 50 pituitaries are needed to produce enough hormone to treat one child for a year.

• **Interferon**—A protein produced by the body as part of its response to viral infection, which may have anticancer potential. Currently, researchers produce interferon for about $100 per gram; and it is being used experimentally to treat a few cancer patients at a cost of $30,000 a year per patient.

• **Vaccines**—Safer and more effective vaccines are coming. Already, a vaccine against foot-and-mouth disease, one of the world's most serious animal diseases, has been developed by recombinant DNA technology, or cloning.

Also, the advocates of DNA research argue, recombinant DNA techniques are of enormous help to scientists in mapping the positions of genes and learning their fundamental nature. They also point out that man has been intervening in the natural order for centuries—by breeding animals and hybrid plants, and more recently by the use of antibiotics. On the other hand, the opponents of tinkering with DNA raise the specter (1) of reengineered creatures proving dangerous, and ravaging the earth, and (2) of moral responsibility in removing nature's "evolutionaly barrier" between species that do not mate.

Genetic manipulation to create new forms of life make biologists custodians of a great power. Despite different schools of thought, scare headlines, and political hearings, molecular biologists will continue recombinant DNA studies, with reasonable restraints, and work ceaselessly away at making the world a better place in which to live. (See Fig. N-13.)

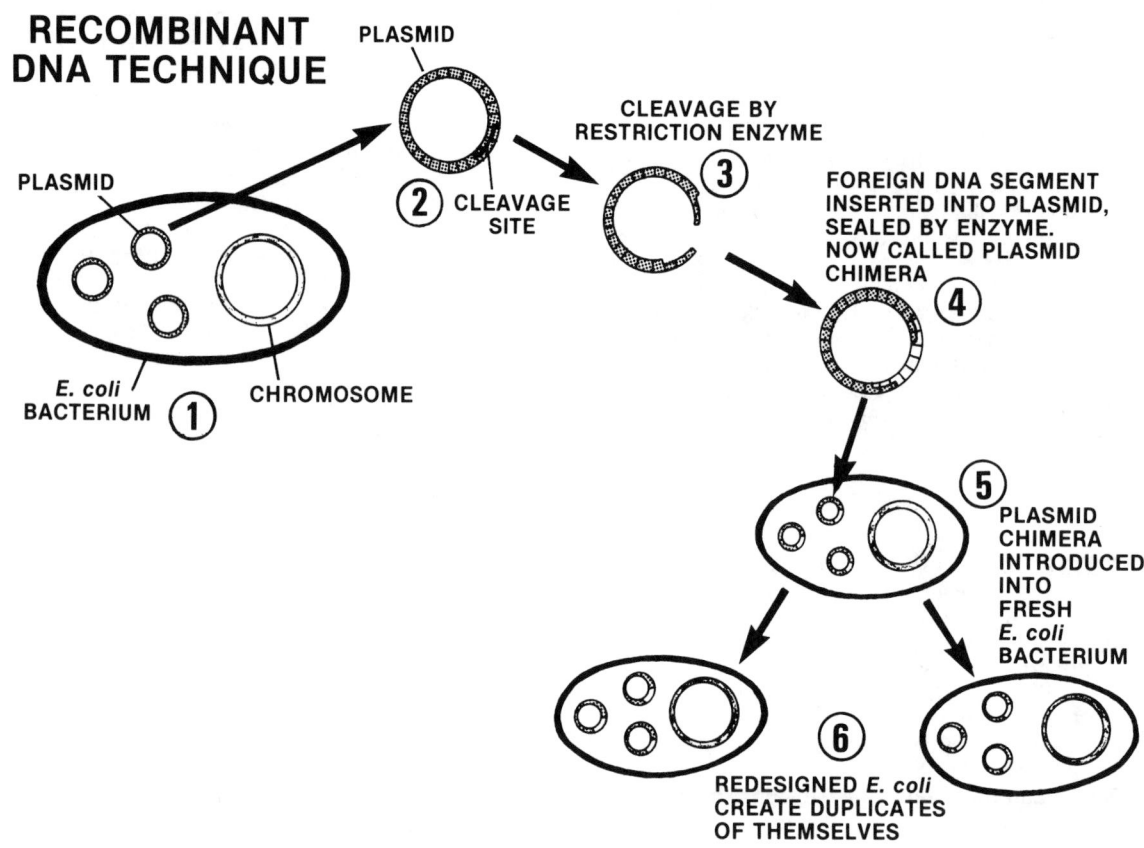

Fig. N-13. Redesigning *E. coli*, common bacteria of animal and human intestines. The steps:

1. The scientist places the bacterium in a test tube with a detergent. This dissolves the microbe's outer membrane, causing its DNA strands to spill out.

2. The plasmids (the closed loops), which are genetic particles found in bacteria, are separated from the chromosomal DNA in a centrifuge.

3. The plasmids are placed in a solution with a chemical catalyst called a restriction enzyme, which cuts through the plasmids' DNA strips at specific points.

4. The opened plasmid loops are then mixed in a solution with genes—also removed by the use of restriction enzymes—from the DNA of a plant, animal, bacterium, or virus. In the solution is another enzyme called a DNA ligase, which cements the foreign gene into place in the opening of the plasmids. These new loops of DNA are called plasmid chimeras because, like the chimera—the mythical lion-goat-serpent after which they are named—they contain the components of more than one organism.

5. The chimeras are placed in a cold solution of calcium chloride containing normal *E. coli* bacteria. Then the solution is suddenly heated, at which time the membranes of the *E. coli* become permeable, allowing the plasmid chimeras to pass through and become a part of the microbe's new genetic structure.

6. When the redesigned *E. coli* reproduce, they create duplicates of themselves, new plasmids—and DNA sequences—and all.

NUCLEOLUS

The nucleus usually contains a distinct body—the *nucleolus*, which is rich in RNA.

NUCLEOPROTEIN

A compound of one or more proteins and nucleic acid found in the nuclei of cells; found in large amounts in glandular tissue.

NUCLEOTIDES

Hydrolytic products of nucleic acid; they contain a sugar-phosphate component and a purine or pyrimidine base.

NUCLEUS

That part of the cell that contains the chromosomes; it's the control center of the cell, for both chemical reactions and reproduction; it contains large quantities of DNA.

NUTRIENT ENEMA

Another term for the discontinued practice of rectal feeding.

(Also see RECTAL FEEDING.)

NUTRIENTS: REQUIREMENTS, ALLOW-ANCES, FUNCTIONS, SOURCES

Nutrients are the chemical substances found in food that can be used, and are necessary for the maintenance, growth, and health of people. There are more than 40 nutrients, including minerals, vitamins, and the amino acids from protein. Specific amounts of the nutrients are required, but their intake in the diet is expressed as allowances. Each nutrient from the various food sources reaches the cells of the body where it performs essential functions.

• **Requirements**—Nutrient requirements are the amount of nutrients necessary to meet an individual's minimum needs, without margins of safety, for maintenance, growth, pregnancy, and lactation. To meet nutrient requirements, individuals must receive sufficient food to furnish the necessary quantity of energy, protein, minerals, and vitamins. However, good nutrition is more than just meeting minimal needs.

• **Allowances**—To ensure good nutrition, allowances for the daily intake of nutrients are determined. These allowances provide reasonable margins of safety because of variations in such things as food composition, environment, stress, and individuality. Moreover, the nutritive needs vary according to age, sex, pregnancy, and lactation. Allowances must be determined; otherwise, imbalances may result, excesses may cause toxicity and needless expense, or deficiency diseases may develop. Recommended daily allowances of nutrients for humans are based on the *Recommended Dietary Allowances* compiled by the Committee on Dietary Allowances and the Food and Nutrition Board, National Research Council. These allowances are arrived at by (1) determining the nutrient intake in apparently normal healthy people, (2) biochemical studies, (3) examining clinical cases of nutrient deficiencies, (4) nutrient balance studies, (5) some human experimentation using diets low or deficient in nutrients, and (6) animal experiments. The most recent edition of the *Recommended Dietary Allowances* is the tenth revised edition, 1989, published by the National Research Council, National Academy of Sciences.

• **Functions**—Nutrients perform a variety of specific functions in the body, from providing energy, to becoming tissue components, to acting as cofactors in enzymatic reactions. Altogether, the functions of these nutrients ensure good health as reflected in the general appearance, weight, posture, muscles, nerves, digestive system, heart, lungs, skin, hair, teeth, eyes, nails, and skeleton.

• **Sources**—However, nutrients are more than just chemicals. They are the components of foods, but nutrient distribution in foods is not equal. Some foods may contain virtually no nutrients, while others are good sources of several nutrients. Since there are thousands of foods from which to select, knowledge of foods providing good nutrition becomes very important.

Table N-6 provides summary information relative to the recommended daily allowance of each nutrient, its function in the body, and some of the best foods for obtaining the nutrient. More information about specific nutrients and their food sources may be obtained from individual articles on each nutrient. Also, Food Composition Table F-36 of this book lists complete nutrient composition data for a large number of foods.

Nutrient	Recommended Daily Dietary Allowances By Age Group																
	Infants		Children			Males					Females						
Years	0–0.5	0.5–1	1–3	4–6	7–10	11–14	15–18	19–24	25–50	50+	11–14	15–18	19–24	25–50	50+	Pregnant	Lactating
Calories																	
REE ...... kcal	320	500	740	950	1130	1440	1760	1780	1800	1530	1310	1370	1350	1380	1280	+300	+300
Energy allowance																	
.... kcal/kg	108	98	102	90	70	55	45	40	37	30	47	40	38	36	30		
Total ...... kcal	650	850	1300	1800	2000	2500	3000	2900	2900	2300	2200	2200	2200	2200	1900	2500	2700
Protein ...... g	13	14	16	24	28	45	59	58	63	63	46	44	46	50	50	60	65
Macrominerals																	
Calcium ....mg	400	600	800	800	800	1200	1200	1200	800	800	1200	1200	1200	800	800	1200	1200
Phosphorus mg	300	500	800	800	800	1200	1200	1200	800	800	1200	1200	1200	800	800	1200	1200
Sodium[2] ....mg	120	200	225	300	400	500	500	500	500	500	500	500	500	500	500	500	500
Chloride ....mg	180	300	350	500	600	750	750	750	750	750	750	750	750	750	750	750	750
Magnesium mg	40	60	80	120	170	270	400	350	350	350	280	300	280	280	280	320	355
Potassium ..mg	500	700	1000	1400	1600	2000	2000	2000	2000	2000	2000	2000	2000	2000	2000	2000	2000

Footnotes at end of table.

SOURCES[1]

Nutrient	Major Function(s) in the Body	Best Food Source
Calories		
Carbohydrates	Supply food energy; in certain cases, fiber and bulk.	Bread and cereal products made from whole grains, starchy vegetables, fruits, and sugars.
Fats	Provide food energy and the essential fatty acid; carrier of fat-soluble vitamins; body structure; and regulatory functions.	Vegetable oils, butter, whole milk and cream, margarine, lard, shortening, salad and cooking oils, nuts, and meat fat.
Protein	Formation of new tissues; maintenance, regulatory functions; and provide energy.	Meat, fish, poultry, eggs, cheese, dried beans, soybeans, peas, lentils, nuts, and milk.
Macrominerals Calcium	Builds and maintains bones and teeth; blood clotting, muscle contraction and relaxation, cell wall permeability; enzyme activation; and nerve transmission.	Milk and milk products, most nuts, dried figs, fish with soft edible bones, and green leafy vegetables.
Phosphorus	Bone formation and maintenance, development of teeth, building muscles, genetic transmission and control of cellular metabolism, maintenance of osmotic and acid-base balance, and important in many metabolic functions.	Milk and milk products, rice bran, rice polish, wheat bran, sunflower seeds, beef, lamb, pork, poultry, liver, fish and seafoods, nuts, and whole grains.
Sodium	Helps maintain balance of water, acids, and bases in fluids outside of cells; a constituent of pancreatic juice, bile, sweat, and tears; associated with muscle contraction and nerve functions; involved in absorption of carbohydrates.	Table salt, and most fresh or processed foods other than fresh fruits and vegetables. *Note well:* Generally, the need is for low-sodium diets, which calls for avoiding high-sodium foods.
Chlorine	Helps regulate osmotic pressure, water balance and acid-base balance; necessary for stomach acid formation and vitamin B-12 and iron absorption.	Table salt and foods containing table salt.
Magnesium	Constituent of bones and teeth; essential element of cellular metabolism; involved in protein metabolism; relaxes nerve impulses.	Nuts, sesame seeds, spices, wheat bran, wheat germ, whole grains, and molasses.
Potassium	Involved in acid-base balance and transfer of nutrients in and out of individual cells; relaxes heart muscle; required for secretion of insulin phosphorylation of creatin, carbohydrate metabolism, and protein synthesis.	Fruits, molasses, rice bran, sunflower seeds, wheat bran, beef, most raw vegetables, nuts, pork, poultry, and sardines.

(Continued)

TABLE

| Nutrient | Recommended Daily Dietary Allowances By Age Group | | | | | | | | | | | | | | | | |
| | Infants | | Children | | | Males | | | | | Females | | | | | | |
Years	0–0.5	0.5–1	1–3	4–6	7–10	11–14	15–18	19–24	25–50	50+	11–14	15–18	19–24	25–50	50+	Preg-nant	Lacta-ting
Microminerals																	
Chromium[2] mcg	10–40	20–60	20–80	30–120	50–200	50–200	50–200	50–200	50–200	50–200	50–200	50–200	50–200	50–200	50–200	50–200	50–200
Copper[2] . . . . mg	.4–.6	.6–.7	.7–1.0	1.0–1.5	1.0–2.0	1.5–2.5	1.5–2.5	1.5–3.0	1.5–3.0	1.5–3.0	1.5–2.5	1.5–2.5	1.5–3.0	1.5–3.0	1.5–3.0	1.5–3.0	1.5–3.0
Fluoride[2] . . . . mg	.1–.5	.2–1.0	.5–1.5	1.0–2.5	1.5–2.5	1.5–2.5	1.5–2.5	1.5–4.0	1.5–4.0	1.5–4.0	1.5–2.5	1.5–2.5	1.5–4.0	1.5–4.0	1.5–4.0	1.5–4.0	1.5–4.0
Iodine . . . . . mcg	40	50	70	90	120	150	150	150	150	150	150	150	150	150	150	175	200
Iron . . . . mg	6	10	10	10	12	12	10	10	10	15	15	15	15	15	10	30[3]	15[3]
Manganese[2] mg	.3–.6	.6–1	1–1.5	1.5–2	2–3	2–5	2–5	2–5	2–5	2–5	2–5	2–5	2–5	2–5	2–5	2–5	2–5
Molybdenum[2] . . . . mcg	15–30	20–40	25–50	30–75	50–150	75–250	75–250	75–250	75–250	75–250	75–250	75–250	75–250	75–250	75–250	75–250	75–250
Selenium . . mcg	10	15	20	20	30	40	50	70	70	70	45	50	55	55	55	65	75
Zinc . . . . mg	5	5	10	10	10	15	15	15	15	15	12	12	12	12	12	15	19
Fat-soluble vitamins																	
Vitamin A . . . . . . mcg RE	375	375	400	500	700	1000	1000	1000	1000	1000	800	800	800	800	800	1300	1200
Vitamin D . . mcg	7.5	10	10	10	10	10	10	10	5	5	10	10	10	5	5	10	10
Vitamin E . . mg alpha TE	3	4	6	7	7	10	10	10	10	10	8	8	8	8	8	10	12
Vitamin K . . mcg	5	10	15	20	30	45	65	70	80	80	45	55	60	65	65	65	65

Footnotes at end of table.

N-6 *(Continued)*

Nutrient	Major Function(s) in the Body	Best Food Source
Microminerals Chromium[2]	Component of the Glucose Tolerance Factor (GTF) which enhances the effect of insulin; enzyme activator; stabilizer of nucleic acids.	Apple peel, banana, beef, beer, blackstrap molasses, bread, brown sugar, butter or margarine, cheese, eggs, flour and whole wheat, liver, oysters, and potatoes.
Copper[2]	Facilitates iron absorption and release from storage; necessary for hemoglobin formation; hair pigmentation; component of important proteins.	Black pepper, blackstrap molasses, cocoa, green olives, liver, nuts and seeds, oysters, soybean flour, and wheat bran and germ.
Fluoride[2]	Necessary for sound bones and teeth.	Dry tea, fluoridated water, and seafoods.
Iodine	Essential component of hormones secreted by the thyroid gland.	Iodized table salt, kelp, seafoods, and vegetables grown on iodine-rich soils.
Iron	Iron (heme) combines with protein (globin) to make hemoglobin for red blood cells. Also, iron is a component of enzymes which are involved in energy metabolism.	Organ meats (liver, kidney, heart) blackstrap molasses, oysters, rice polish, wheat bran, beef, brown sugar, egg yolk, lima beans, nuts, pork, and iron-fortified products.
Manganese[2]	Formation of bone and growth of connective tissues; blood clotting; insulin action; enzyme activation.	Brown rice, legumes, rice bran and polish, spices, and whole grains.
Molybdenum[2]	Component of enzymes which metabolize carbohydrates, fats, proteins, and nucleic acids; component of tooth enamel.	Leafy vegetables, legumes, organ meats (liver, kidney, heart), whole grains, and yeast.
Selenium	Component of the enzyme glutathione peroxidase; interrelated with vitamin E as an antioxidant.	Beer, blackstrap molasses, Brazil nuts, butter, clams, crab, egg, lamb, lobster, mushrooms, oysters, smelt, Swiss chard, turnips, and whole grains.
Zinc	Needed for normal skin, bones, and hair; component of many enzymes of energy metabolism and of protein synthesis.	Beef, lamb, liver, oysters, peanuts, pork, poultry, spices, and wheat bran.
Fat-soluble vitamins Vitamin A	Necessary for vision in dim light, the growth and repair of certain tissues, and resistance to infection.	Dark-green leafy vegetables, yellow vegetables, yellow fruits, crab, halibut, oysters, salmon, swordfish, butter, cheese, egg yolk, margarine (fortified), and whole milk.
Vitamin D	Essential for the absorption and utilization of calcium in the building of strong bones and teeth.	Fatty fish, liver, egg yolk, cream, butter, cheese, milk fortified with vitamin D. Exposure of the skin to sunlight results in the conversion of provitamin D (converted in the body to vitamin D).
Vitamin E	Serves along with selenium as an antioxidant; protects fatty acids from oxidative destruction.	Wheat germ, salad and cooking oils, margarine, nuts, sunflower seed kernels, beef and organ meats, butter, eggs, green leafy vegetables, oatmeal, and seafoods.
Vitamin K	Necessary for the clotting of the blood.	Green leafy vegetables, green tea, beef liver. Produced by microorganisms in the intestine.

(Continued)

TABLE

Nutrient	Recommended Daily Dietary Allowances By Age Group																
	Infants		Children			Males					Females						
Years	0–0.5	0.5–1	1–3	4–6	7–10	11–14	15–18	19–24	25–50	50+	11–14	15–18	19–24	25–50	50+	Pregnant	Lactating
Water-soluble vitamins																	
Biotin[2] . . . . . mcg	10	15	20	25	30	30–100	30–100	30–100	30–100	30–100	30–100	30–100	30–100	30–100	30–100	30–100	30–100
Folate . . . . . mcg	25	35	50	75	100	150	200	200	200	200	150	180	180	180	180	400	280
Niacin . . . mg NE	5	6	9	12	13	17	20	19	19	15	15	15	15	15	13	17	20
Pantothenic acid[2] . . . . mg	2	3	3	3–4	4–5	4–7	4–7	4–7	4–7	4–7	4–7	4–7	4–7	4–7	4–7	4–7	4–7
Riboflavin (vitamin B-2) . . . . mg	.4	.5	.8	1.0	1.2	1.5	1.8	1.7	1.7	1.4	1.3	1.3	1.3	1.3	1.2	1.6	1.8
Thiamin (vitamin B-1) . . . . mg	.3	.4	.7	.9	1.0	1.3	1.5	1.5	1.5	1.2	1.1	1.1	1.1	1.1	1.0	1.5	1.6
Vitamin B-6 (pyridoxine) mg	.3	.6	1.0	1.1	1.4	1.7	2.0	2.0	2.0	2.0	1.4	1.5	1.6	1.6	1.6	2.2	2.1
Vitamin B-12 (cobalamins) . . . . mcg	.3	.5	.7	1.0	1.4	2	2	2	2	2	2	2	2	2	2	2.2	2.6
Vitamin C (ascorbic acid) . . . . mg	30	35	40	45	45	50	60	60	60	60	50	60	60	60	60	70	95

[1]Compiled from *Recommended Dietary Allowances*, 10th ed., National Academy of Sciences, 1989.

[2]These figures are given in the form of ranges of recommended intakes, since there is insufficient information to determine allowances.

[3]The increased requirement during pregnancy cannot be met by the iron content of habitual American diets nor by the existing iron stores of many women; therefore the use of 30–60 mg of supplemental iron is recommended. Iron needs during lactation are not substantially different from those of nonpregnant women, but continued supplementation of the mother for 2 to 3 months after parturition (birth) is advisable in order to replenish stores depleted by pregnancy.

N-6 *(Continued)*

Nutrient	Major Function(s) in the Body	Best Food Source
Water-soluble vitamins Biotin[2]	Essential for the metabolism of carbohydrates, fats, and proteins.	Cheese (processed), kidney, liver, most vegetables, eggs, nuts, sardines, salmon, and wheat bran. Also, considerable biotin is synthesized by the microorganisms in the digestive tract.
Folate	Important in metabolism, in cell division and reproduction, and in the formation of heme—the iron-containing protein in hemoglobin.	Liver and kidneys, beans, beets, eggs, fish, green leafy vegetables, nuts, oranges, and whole wheat products.
Niacin	Constituent of coenzymes that function in cell respiration and in the release of energy from carbohydrates, fats, and protein; involved in synthesis of fatty acids, protein, and DNA.	Liver, kidney, lean meats, poultry, fish, rabbit, cornflakes (enriched), nuts, milk, cheese, and eggs.
Pantothenic acid[2]	Functions as part of two enzymes important in metabolism, nerve impulses, hemoglobin synthesis, synthesis of steroids, maintenance of normal blood sugar, and formation of antibodies.	Organ meats (liver, kidney, heart), wheat bran, rice bran, rice polish, nuts, salmon, eggs, brown rice, and sunflower seeds.
Riboflavin (vitamin B-2)	Essential for metabolism of amino acids, fatty acids, and carbohydrates, accompanied by release of energy; and necessary for formation of niacin from the amino acid tryptophan.	Organ meats (liver, kidney, heart), cheese, eggs, lean meat (beef, pork, lamb), enriched breads, turnip greens, wheat bran, and bacon.
Thiamin (vitamin B-1)	Energy metabolism—without thiamin there could be no energy; needed for conversion of glucose to fats, healthy nerves, normal appetite, muscle tone, and good mental attitude.	Rice bran, wheat germ, rice polish, lean pork, sunflower seeds, nuts, wheat bran, kidney, enriched breads, rye bread, whole wheat bread, and soybean sprouts.
Vitamin B-6 (pyridoxine)	In its coenzyme forms, involved in a number of physiologic functions, particularly (1) protein metabolism, (2) carbohydrate and fat metabolism, and (3) central nervous system disturbances.	Rice polish, rice bran, wheat bran, sunflower seeds, bananas, corn, fish, kidney, liver, lean meat, nuts, poultry, brown rice, and whole grains.
Vitamin B-12 (cobalamins)	Needed for red blood cell production, healthy nerves, and metabolism.	Organ meats, muscle meats, fish, shellfish, egg, cheese. Most plant foods contain little or none of this vitamin.
Vitamin C (ascorbic acid)	Formation and maintenance of collagen; involved in metabolism of amino acids tyrosine and tryptophan, absorption and movement of iron, metabolism of fats and lipids and cholesterol control; and makes for sound teeth and bones, and strong capillary walls and blood vessels.	Citrus fruits, guavas, peppers (green or hot), green leafy vegetables, cantaloupe, papaya, strawberries, and tomatoes.

NUTRITION

Nutrition can be defined as the science of food and its nutrients and their relation to health.

NUTRITIONAL DEFICIENCY DISEASES

Those disorders in normal structure and function of the body resulting from dietary shortages of one or more essential nutrients. They may be prevented or cured by the administration of the missing nutrient(s), except when there is irreparable damage to vital tissues of the body.
(Also see DEFICIENCY DISEASES.)

NUTRITIONAL STATUS

An evaluation or assessment of how well the needs of the body for essential nutrients are being met.

NUTRITIONAL SUPPLEMENTS

A nutritional supplement is any food(s) or nutrient(s), or a mixture of both, used to improve the nutritional value of the diet. Usually, a nutritional supplement consists of minerals, vitamins, and unidentified factor source(s), although it may include protein, one or more amino acids, and other substances.

Clearly, the above definition states that a nutritional supplement is "used to improve." It follows that if the diet is complete and balanced, and not in need of improvement, no supplementation is necessary. Certainly, nutritional supplementation is unnecessary for anyone who always eats a balanced diet consisting of such foods as fresh fruit, fresh vegetables, an animal protein (meat, milk, and/or eggs), whole grain breads and cereals, unroasted nuts, and honey—all produced on unleached, mineral-rich soils; the type of good eating that grandmother served up. But how many people eat such foods regularly today? Also, and most important, there is a wide difference between (1) the amount of a nutrient(s) required to prevent deficiency symptoms, and (2) the amount required for buoyant good health.

The rule, therefore, is: If you eat *enough* of *proper* foods *regularly*, you'll get your full complement of needed nutrients. But for many people throughout the world these three key words—*enough, proper, and regularly*—are the catch. In the first place, many folks don't know what constitutes a good diet. Worse yet, altogether too many people neglect or ignore the rules even if they know them. In either case, the net result is always the same. We shortchange ourselves on the amounts of certain nutrients, especially on some needed minerals and vitamins. As a result, more and more doctors and nutritionists are recommending judicious nutritional supplementation.

Undoubtedly, the use of nutritional supplements far exceeds the need for them in many cases. Also, the potency of preparations on the market varies widely, and the number of nutrients present differs from one product to another. Further, the consumer may be unable to interpret the label information in terms of his own requirements. Moreover, the supplemental nutritional program will and should vary according to needs. With these facts fully understood, the following nutritional supplemental program presently used by the two senior authors of this encyclopedia, Dr. and Mrs. M. E. Ensminger, for whom work is fun and fun is work—is presented with the admonition that it be used for guide purposes only as each person confers with his or her physician or other competent nutrient advisor to develop a similar program for his or her own use.

(Also see VITAMIN[S], section headed "Vitamin Supplementation of the Diet.")

	Each of 3 meals (pills)	or	Per Day (pills)
Alfalfa tablets	3		9
Brewers' yeast tablets	3		9
Liverall tablets	3		9
High selenium brewers' yeast . .	1		3
or selenium tablets			300 mcg
Vitamin A (10,000 IU) and D (400 IU)	—		1
Vitamin B complex (50 mg of B-1, B-2, B-6)	—		1
Vitamin B-6 (25 mg)	1		3
Vitamin E (400 IU)	—		1
Kelp (according to directions) . . .	—		1
Vitamin C (500 mg) with bioflavonoids and rutin	—		2
Minerals—amino acid chelated multimineral formula (2 tablets contain 750 mg Ca, 375 mg Mg)	1		3
Lecithin-19 grains (1,200 mg) . .	1		3
Wheat germ (untreated)	—		1–3 tsp

NUTRITION EDUCATION

Nutrition education is concerned with (1) imparting sound knowledge of how food selection influences the health and well being of the individual, and (2) motivating the individual to use that information in daily living. Nutrition is, amongst other things, a behavioral science. It follows that nutrition education needs to be a practical program with a positive approach based on nutrition science and food composition, along with an understanding of human behavior. Additionally, cognizance should be taken that American consumers want freedom of choice in what they believe and in what they consume. This challenges nutrition educators to present scientifically based nutrition information in such a way that its authenticity is recognized and acted upon.

More people in the United States are malnourished because of nutritional ignorance and misinformation than because of poverty. The explanation is simple: In human folly, facts have never stood in the way of myths and misinformation. Faddism is costly, too. Americans spend more than $10 billion each year on magic to lose weight—more than is spent on research to discover the major causes of diseases that kill. Only a massive program of nutrition education can hope to have any overall effect in raising the quality of diets.

In the developing countries of the world where population growth is resulting in hunger and malnutrition, food production is the first requisite. Nutrition education has little effect where people have neither the food nor the money with which to buy food to quiet their hunger pangs.

NUTRITION EDUCATORS. All consumers, regardless of age, lifestyle, and cultural and socio-economic background, need nutrition education. To reach everyone will require the enormous team approach of the following:
1. Government agencies
2. Educational institutions
3. Professional organizations
4. Voluntary agencies
5. Food industries

Each of the above agencies or groups has its own special resources, facilities, programs, and opportunities to contribute to a national nutrition education program. Pertinent information about each of them follows:

Government Agencies. The golden rule is that "those who have the gold make the rules." It follows that government programs have the greatest impact of any agency or group on foods and nutrition.

The two government agencies having most to do with foods and nutrition issues are the U.S. Department of Agriculture (USDA), and the U.S. Department of Health and Human Services—notably two of its agencies, the Food and Drug Administration (FDA) and The National Institute of Health (NIH).

The USDA is involved in massive food and nutrition programs, such as the School Lunch Program, the School Breakfast Program, and the Special Milk Progam—all for children; the special supplemental food program for Women, Infants, and Children (WIC); and the Food Stamp

Programs. These food programs cost more than $21.7 billion in 1990. Additionally, through its Cooperative Extension Programs, the USDA has a vast network of home economists who reach a large segment of the consuming public and have a tradition of success in consumer education programs.

The FDA is charged with protecting the safety of the food supply. Through its dietary guidelines for a variety of food products, and through its regulation of "standards of identity," the FDA can also influence the food supply in very significant ways. More recently, the FDA has become involved in nutrition education efforts through its nutrition labeling program, as a consequence of which more and more foods appearing on supermarket shelves are nutritionally labeled. This program, which represents the first effort in this country to provide nutrition information for consumers, should be augmented with adequate education efforts.

The National Institute of Health supports nutrition and health research.

A host of other government agencies have an impact, in one way or another, upon the nation's food and nutrition. The Federal Trade Commission regulates food advertising and the application of anti-trust laws. The Office of Education supports educational research.

Also, Congress has become interested and involved in food and nutrition issues. Thus, there are more and more hearings dealing with nutrition topics. The dietary goals prepared by the Senate Select Committee on Nutrition and Human Needs indicate the tremendous impact which Congress can have on nutrition programs of this country.

All of the above comments indicate that the government recognizes that foods and nutrition are clearly linked to health and, as an important factor in the maintenance of health, demand government attention.

(Also see FOOD STAMP PROGRAM; GOVERNMENT FOOD PROGRAMS; HOME ECONOMISTS; SCHOOL LUNCH PROGRAM; U.S. DEPARTMENT OF AGRICULTURE; and U.S. DEPARTMENT OF HEALTH AND HUMAN SERVICES.)

Educational Institutions. Teachers (including physical education teachers and coaches, science teachers, and home economics teachers), doctors, nurses, dietitions, and social workers must receive adequate training in nutrition if they are to be competent educators in the area of health protection. Only through adequate training of these key personnel can sound nutrition education be imparted to students, patients, clients, and parents.

There is need for expanded nutrition instruction in higher education. For example, the professional preparation of most elementary school teachers does not include a single course in nutrition. It is noteworthy, however, that several American universities do have excellent postgraduate courses in nutrition.

In medical schools, some nutrition is taught as part of the undergraduate courses in biochemistry, physiology, pharmacology, pathology, internal medicine, pediatrics, obstetrics, surgery, and dentistry. However, there is a scientific core to nutrition which is unlikely to be covered except in one or more basic courses in nutrition. This includes such topics as the assessment of nutritional status, interactions of nutrients with one another and with diseases, recommended intakes of nutrients, food composition, food technology, world food problems, and psychological and sociological aspects of food habits. The final report of the 1969 White House Conference on Food, Nutrition and Health stressed the urgent need to take positive steps to incorporate nutrition in the medical curriculum.

Nurses should also have a sound elementary knowledge of nutrition and dietetics because of their responsibility in feeding patients.

Professional Organizations.

Professional organizations engaged in human nutrition work need to be active in nutrition education. A number of these organizations are listed in the last section of this article, under the heading "Nutrition Education Sources."

Voluntary Agencies.

Nutrition programs at the community level are greatly augmented by voluntary agencies; among them, parent-teachers associations, church organizations, the Salvation Army, children's camps, and day nurseries. Voluntary agencies are supported by private funds, such as the United Fund, foundations, and other means.

Food Industries.

Government alone cannot meet the need for nutrition education, nor can a single agency, organization, institution or group accomplish what is needed. The demands are too great.

Some early leaders of our basic food industries perceived that their success depended both on quality of production and on consumers who were well informed about the nutritive value of their products and how to use them. Thus, in the 1920s, organizations came into being which were concerned with production, processing, distribution and household use of specific foodstuffs—organizations that were variously named councils, boards, institutes, or foundations. They were primarily concerned with kinds of food, rather than brand names. Earliest among these organizations were the National Live Stock and Meat Board and the National Dairy Council. Other food industries followed in the ensuing years. The Nutrition Foundation, an organization of many industries, was formed in 1941 and "dedicated to the advancement of nutrition knowledge and its effective application in improving the health and welfare of mankind."

(Also see FOOD INDUSTRY.)

NUTRITION EDUCATION CHANNELS.

The solution lies in instituting and/or enlarging nutrition education programs through the following channels:

1. Elementary and secondary schools.
2. Doctors, nurses, dietitians, teachers, and social workers.
3. News media and community programs.
4. Food Industries.
5. Regulatory controls.
6. Food Assistance.
7. Source information.

Pertinent information about the role of each of the above channels follows.

Nutrition Education In Elementary And Secondary Schools.

Nutrition education must become an integral part of the curriculum in elementary and secondary schools.

Food habits are dependent on attitudes, prejudices, and taboos acquired early in life. It follows that schools afford the single best opportunity to help the child establish attitudes and practices concerning food selection which will lead him to a more healthful, productive life. Nutrition education must begin in the Kindergarten and continue through the twelfth grade if it is to achieve maximum effectiveness. It is the primary responsibility of the elementary teacher, along with the teachers of home economics, health, and physical education. Also, the school physician, nurse, and dentist may have opportunities to note defects in health that suggest the need for improved nutrition. And the classroom instruction can find application in the meals provided through school food services, with the school dietitians serving as teachers and as consultants to teachers.

Nutrition Education By Doctors, Nurses, Dietitians, Teachers, and Social Workers.

More can be done in medical care settings such as hospitals and clinics. Even though education about proper nutrition is often provided to patients suffering from health problems such as diabetes and kidney disease, it is uneven in quality. And although pediatricians, obstetricians, and health workers often include some sort of nutrition education as part of their care of infants, mothers, and pregnant women, rarely do they take advantage of this opportunity to build nutritional knowledge and positive attitudes for future decision-making.

Nutrition Education Through News Media and Community Programs.

Nutrition education must continue throughout the individual's life in order to accommodate for developments in nutrition science and for changing economic circumstances, health requirements, and new food products being developed for the nation's markets. To reach the millions of people will require greatly expanded use of the news media—newspapers, radio, and television—and the involvement of governmental and private agencies, universities, and food industries.

But nutrition news as reported by the mass media is often misleading. Both the public and the mass media need to challenge the credentials of "self-styled experts," people who base their information on emotion and hearsay rather than on training ad experience. To rectify this situation, a spokesman for the American Medical Association has recommended that professional and scientific organizations help the media, and thus the public, to determine the validity of proposed releases of information in the field of nutrition.

To reach the citizenry, nutrition education at the community level needs to be carried out in health centers, maternal and child-care centers, day-care centers, programs for the elderly, Head Start and Get Set programs, youth organizations, and women's clubs. Public health nutritionists, dietitians, nurses, home economists, and social workers have direct rolls to fulfill in implementing many of the community programs required for the improvement of nutrition.

Nutrition Education Through Food Industries. A number of food industries have proud records of accomplishment in nutrition education.

Some food industry organizations have the professional personnel and resources to create and distribute imaginative, reliable publications and visual materials for educational programs at all levels, especially for schools. Also, in comparison with traditional government and educational agencies, food industry nutrition education programs have the advantage of being flexible enough to adjust rapidly to changing educational needs, and the capacity to develop special programs for the interest of groups such as teenagers, the elderly, and the handicapped.

Nutrition Education Through Regulatory Controls. We need to enforce regulatory controls, so that food advertising claims conform to scientific facts.

The Food and Drug Administration has the responsibility of policing the veracity of labels and the safety of the products sold to the public. And the Federal Trade Commission regulates food advertising and the application of anti-trust laws.

(Also see FOOD MYTHS AND MISINFORMATION; and GOVERNMENT FOOD PROGRAMS.)

Nutrition Education Through Food Assistance. Education efforts must be augmented by direct food assistance to segments of the population which find it difficult to meet basic nutritional needs. Many of the elderly, for example, are the victims of inflation and fixed incomes.

A number of federal food distribution and supplemental food programs have been established to provide poor people with better diets; among them, the School Lunch Program, the Food Stamp Program, and the special supplemental program for Women, Infants, and Children. Nutritional education programs are needed to assist people in using these food programs properly and effectively.

(Also see FOOD STAMP PROGRAMS; GOVERNMENT FOOD PROGRAMS; and SCHOOL LUNCH PROGRAMS.)

Nutrition Education Sources. Sound nutrition information should be disseminated through good books and the news media.

All consumers, and all those who counsel with them—doctors, dentists, nutritionists, health experts, and others in allied fields—should have a book shelf on which good nutrition books are readily available (see section on Books).

Today's superstar M.D. will be tomorrow's mediocre M.D. without a continuing effort to keep abreast of medical progress. There are several ways to do this, but reading good books is one of the best. Look at the books in your doctor's office. Are they new editions, or are they dusty with disuse and tattered with age?

Sound nutrition information should also involve the news media—newspapers, radio, and television. Food advertising, particularly on the television, has a powerful influence on food choices. Many foods are promoted for their convenience and ease of preparation or for their taste, rather than for nutritional value. Although convenience and good taste are important considerations, a balanced presentation should also consider nutritional value.

Recommended sources of information about foods and nutrition follow:

• **Books**—Good books are listed in this encyclopedia under BOOKS.

• **County Agricultural Extension (Farm Advisor)**—Information can be secured from these centers in each county.

• **State Universities**—A list of available bulletins and circulars, including information regarding foods and nutrition, can be obtained by writing to (1) the Foods and Nutrition Department, or (2) the Agricultural and Home Economics Extension Service at each State University.

• **U.S. Department of Agriculture, Washington, D.C. 20250**—The following USDA services can be contacted for information:
  Agricultural Research Service
  Consumer and Marketing Service
  Cooperative State Research Service
  Economic Research Service
  Federal Extension Service
  Foreign Agricultural Service
  International Agricultural Development Service
  Office of Communication

• **U.S. Department of Health and Human Services, F St. between 18th & 19th Streets N.W., Washington D.C. 20006**—
  Administration on Aging
  Children's Bureau
  Food and Drug Administration, 5600 Fishers Lane, Rockville, MD 20857
  Maternal and Child Health Services
  Office of Education
  Public Health Service
    National Institutes of Health, Bethesda, MD 20205

● **U.S. Department of State—**

Agency for International Development, U.S.A.I.D. Administration, 2401 E. St. N.W., Washington, DC 20523

● **Professional Societies and Voluntary Health Associations—**

American Academy of Pediatrics, P.O. Box 1034, Evanston, IL, 60204

American Council on Science and Health, 1995 Broadway, New York, NY 10023

American Dental Association, 211 E. Chicago Ave., Chicago, IL 60611

American Diabetes Association, 2 Park Ave., New York, NY 10016

American Dietetic Association, 430 North Michigan Ave., Chicago, IL 60611

American Heart Association, 7320 Greenville Ave., Dallas, TX 75231

American Home Economics Association, 2010 Massachusetts Ave. N.W., Washington, DC 20036

American Institute of Nutrition, 9650 Rockville Pike, Bethesda, MD 20814

American Medical Association, Council on Foods and Nutrition, 535 N. Dearborn St., Chicago, IL 60610

Council for Agricultural Science and Technology (CAST), 137 Lynn Ave., Ames, IA 50010–7197

Institute of Food Technologists, Suite 2120, 221 North LaSalle St., Chicago, IL 60601

National Academy of Sciences, National Research Council, 2101 Constitution Ave., Washington, DC 20418

Nutrition Today Society, 703 Giddings Ave., P.O. Box 1829, Annapolis, MD 21404

Society for Nutrition Education, 1736 Franklin St., Oakland, CA 94612

● **Foundations—**

Ford Foundation, 320 East 43rd St., New York, NY 10017–4801

Kellogg Foundation, 400 North Ave., Battle Creek, MI 49017–3398

Medical Education and Research Foundation, 1100 Waterway Blvd., Indianapolis, IN 46202

Vitamin Information Bureau, 612 N. Michigan Ave., Chicago, IL 60611

The Nutrition Foundation, 489 Fifth Ave., New York, NY 10017

Rockefeller Foundation, 1133 Avenue of the Americas, New York, NY 10036

● **Industry-Sponsored Groups—**

American Meat Institute (AMI), 1700 N. Moore St., Suite 1600, Arlington, VA 22209–1995

Cereal Institute, 1111 Plaza Drive, Schaumburg, IL 60195

National Dairy Council, 6300 North River Road, Rosemont, IL 60018

National Livestock and Meat Board, 444 North Michigan Ave., Chicago, IL 60611

● **International Organizations—**

Food and Agriculture Organization (FAO) of the United Nations, Via delle Terme di Caracalla, 00100 Rome, Italy

League for International Food Education, 1126 Sixteenth St., N.W., Washington, DC 20036

United Nations Children's Fund (UNICEF), 331 East 38th St., New York, NY 10016

United Nations Scientific and Cultural Organization (UNESCO), 7, Place de Fontenoy, 75700 Paris, France

World Health Organization (WHO, Geneva, Switzerland), WHO Publication Centre, 49 Sheridan Ave., Albany, NY 12210

SUMMARY. Food choices are determined primarily by availability, personal and family likes and dislikes, marketing and advertising, and disposable income. There is need that the person who buys and prepares the food should give greater consideration to nutritional need.

Without sacrificing soundness and accuracy in the least, we need to emulate the purveyors of myths and misinformation when it comes to communicating effectively. Through whatever channel—books, news media, lecturers, schools, seminars, counselors—the chosen words and terms should always convey the intended meaning and concept. But a big word should not be used if it can be avoided. Choose words that are clear, specific, and simple, and that come alive. As an illustration, consider the words used by one of the masters of the English language, Sir Winston Churchill. During World War II, Churchill could never have rallied the British people to defend their country if he had called on them for "hemorrhage, perspiration, and lachrymation." Instead, he used the immortal words, "blood, sweat, and tears"—words that continue to live in history.

NUTRITION REVIEWS

This journal is published by the International Life Sciences Institute (formerly known as the Nutrition Foundation, Inc., which was formed in 1941 by the food and allied industries). The Institute's goal is to make essential contributions to the advancement of nutrition knowledge and its effective application, and thus serve the health and welfare of the public. *Nutrition Reviews* contains abstracts of current scientific literature in nutrition. Also, throughout the years, the Institute has published semi-popular brochures on current topics in nutrition.

NUTRITIONIST

An individual who is trained in and able to apply a knowledge of foods and their relationship to growth, maintenance and health. A nutritionist may apply his or her training and knowledge in clinics, consultation, medicine, public health, research, and teaching.

(Also see DIETITIAN and DIETETICS.)

NUTRITIVE RATIO (NR)

The ratio of digestible protein to other digestible nutrients in a food. It is the sum of the digestible protein, fat, and carbohydrate divided by the digestible protein.

NUTS

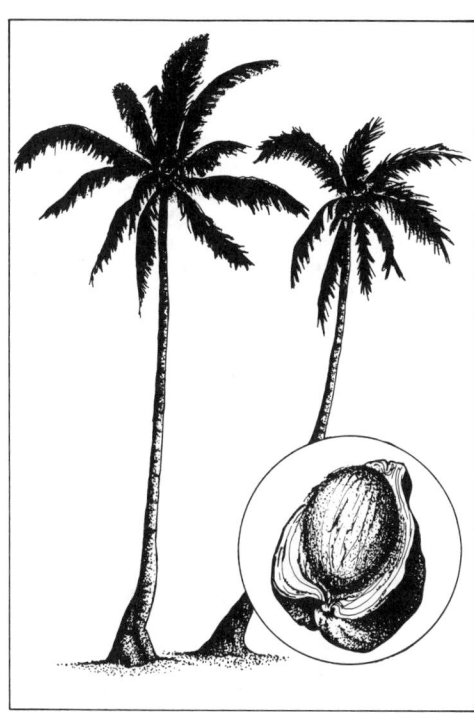

Fig. N-14. Coconut palm, the world's leading nut tree.

This name is commonly given to the shell-encased seeds of nonleguminous trees, although various other seeds commonly called nuts may not grow on trees, and may even be legumes. (The peanut is the seed from a leguminous plant.) Mankind has long depended upon nuts for food, as have various species of wild animals and birds. Now, some of these seeds are being utilized around the world as protein supplements to cereal diets, especially where animal protein foods are scarce. Fig. N-14 shows a coconut tree, which provides a major part of the world's nut crop.

History. Archaeological evidence shows that between 20,000 B.C. and 10,000 B.C. various nomadic peoples around the world began to form permanent settlements in certain areas where wild animals and plants were abundant. However, the numbers of large wild game species dwindled as the human populations grew. As a result, the settlers in the temperate regions came to depend upon small game and wild grains, legumes, and acorns and other nuts to meet the greater part of their food requirements. It is noteworthy that many types of acorns contained toxic levels of tannins (bitter tasting substances which are also present in tea leaves and in many fruits), which the primitive peoples removed by soaking in water. In the tropical parts of the world the coconut became a staple food. These trees grow wild on many tropical beaches because the nuts float readily and retain their viability even after crossing an ocean.

Shortly after 10,000 B.C., some of the settled peoples began to cultivate the plants they favored. By Biblical times, almonds, pistachio nuts and walnuts were grown in southwestern Asia; and Brazil nuts, cashew nuts, and peanuts were grown in South America. The early agricultural societies experimented with various ways of processing nuts, which eventually resulted in the production of such items as "milks," oils, and nut powders. For example, the North American Indians made milks from hickory nuts and pecans; the southeastern Asians made milk from coconuts; and the Middle Eastern peoples made milks from almonds and walnuts. Similarly, oils were obtained from almonds, coconuts, and walnuts. Finally, the use of almond and pistachio nut powders in a variety of dishes appears to have been passed by the Persians to the Arabs, who in turn spread the practice westward throughout the Mediterranean, and eastward to India.

The first Spanish explorers to reach the Americas found peanuts growing on some of the Carribean islands, to which they had apparently been brought by earlier migrations of South American Indians. These nuts were taken to Africa, where they soon became an important crop. It is ironic that peanuts were once thought to have originated in Africa, because the slaves had carried them to the Americas. This erroneous belief was corrected when the nuts were found in the ruins of an ancient settlement in Peru. South America also gave the world Brazil nuts and cashew nuts.

The peanuts brought to the southeastern United States by the African slaves were soon grown extensively in the semitropical region. However, there was not much of a market for them as food (they had long been given to livestock) until 1890, when a St. Louis physician prepared peanut butter for his aged, toothless patients. A crude peanut butter had been prepared hundreds of years previously by South American Indians. About the same time, Dr. J. H. Kellogg promoted peanut butter as a food for the vegetarian patients at the Battle Creek Sanitarium in Michigan. Finally, the subsequent research of G. W. Carver at the newly founded Tuskegee Institute in Alabama resulted in hundreds of new food and nonfood uses for peanuts, which by then had become an important crop in the southern states.

At the present time, food technologists are striving to perfect modern day counterparts of the nut products prepared by ancient peoples. Also, scientists have invented some new products such as defatted nut flours and nut protein concentrates. Hence, there is little doubt that various types of nuts will continue to be important foods for people, providing that the trees which yield these valuable fruits are maintained and replaced when necessary.

PRODUCTION AND PROCESSING. World nut production is small compared to grain, oilseed, and legume production.

Fig. N-15 presents the yearly production data for the most important nut crops of the world.

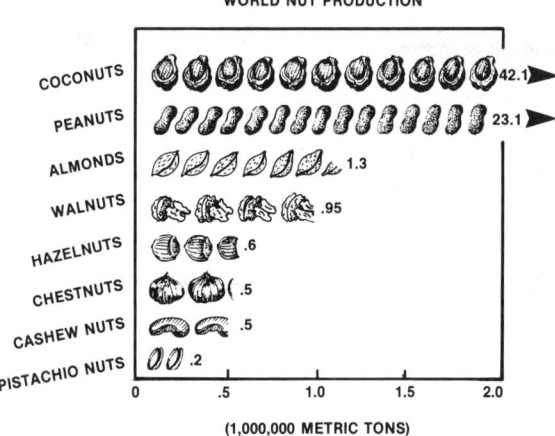

Fig. N-15. The world production of the leading nut crops. (Source: *FAO Production Yearbook*, 1990, FAO/UN, Rome, Italy, Vol. 44)

Fig. N-15 shows that coconuts and peanuts are by far the most important nut crops. Together, they account for about 94% of the world nut production. This situation prevails because coconut and peanut oils are among the leading ingredients of margarines and shortenings.

The production of nuts in the United States represents only a small fraction of the world production of these crops (except in the case of almonds, where the United States contributes almost one-third of the world's production). Fig. N-16 shows the tonnages of each of the four most important nut crops in the United States.

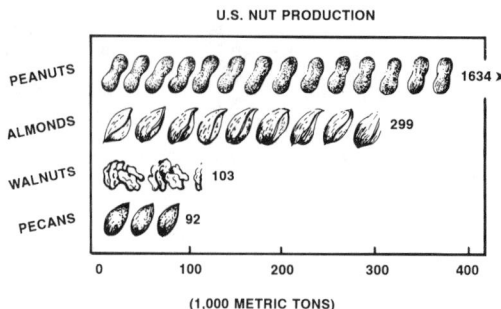

Fig. N-16. The U.S. production of nut crops. (Source: *Agricultural Statistics*, 1991, USDA, pp. 370-371, Table 548)

Fig. N-16 shows that the peanut crop accounts for most (about 77%) of the nut production in the United States. It is noteworthy that the per capita consumption of peanuts in the United States is the highest in the world.

Nuts are still gathered from wild trees in many parts of the world. However, the recent growth in demand for nuts together with the rapid loss of stands of wild trees to other land uses has now made it profitable to utilize more intensive and scientific methods of production. In California, for example, nut trees are planted in large orchards where they are pruned, sprayed, and watered regularly, and even provided with resident bees for pollenation. Usually, beekeepers are invited to place their hives in the orchards.

Many species are propagated by vegetative methods, such as the grafting of slips onto sturdy and disease resistant rootstock, which may sometimes be that of a different variety, or even of a different species. Almond slips may be budded onto almond, peach, or plum rootstocks.

Nuts are often harvested in the United States by mechanical tree shakers or by merely allowing them to fall when ripe. Then, they are gathered from the ground by hand, by sweeping or by vacuum machines.

Peanuts are harvested with a special digger-shaker, windrower. Then, the pods are dried. Fig. N-17 shows the loading of dried peanuts for shipment.

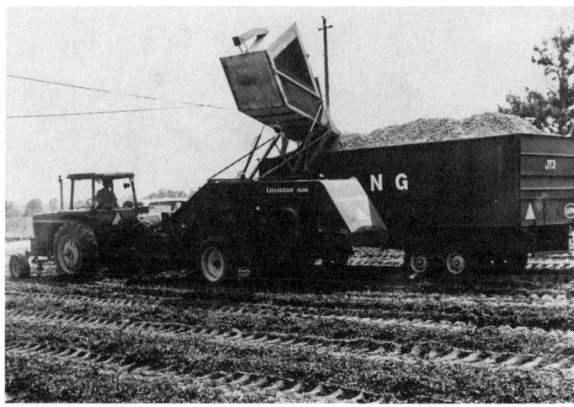

Fig. N-17. Newly harvested peanuts being loaded for shipment to a processing plant. (Courtesy, National Peanut Council, Washington, D.C.)

Shelling may also be done mechanically. Certain types of nut meats are often roasted and salted, while others are packed without further processing. The most common types of packaging are plastic bags, glass jars, and metal cans. However, some nuts are still sold unpacked or loose from bins or cannisters. Other details of the production and processing of certain types of nuts are given in Table N-8.

NUTRITIVE VALUES. Nuts, like grains and legumes, are seeds that contain abundant quantities of the nutrients needed by the embryonic plant until it is sufficiently developed to provide for itself. Fortunately, the nutritive needs of all living cells are quite similar. Hence, the cells of the human body may benefit greatly from the nutrients stored in nuts. The Food Composition Table F-36 gives the nutrient composition of some of the commonly used nuts and nut products.

A few salient points concerning the nutritive value of nuts follow:

1. Most nuts contain about 500 or more Calories (kcal) per 100 g portion (140 or more kcal per oz) due to their high fat content. This explains why energy-rich "trail mixes" contain lots of nuts; hikers need concentrated sources of calories and proteins.

2. The protein content of nuts is about the same as that of legumes (close to 20%, on the average), except that the protein-to-calorie ratio for most nuts (about 4 g of protein per 100 kcal) is only two-thirds of that for legumes.

3. Defatted products, such as almond meal and peanut flour, are much better sources of protein (they contain 40% or more) and substantially lower in calories than nondefatted products.

4. Nuts contain only one-quarter to one-third as much carbohydrate as grains and legumes. Hence, nuts may be useful for low-carbohydrate diets.

5. Almonds, Brazil nuts, and filberts are moderately good sources of calcium (100 g furnish from 1/5 to 1/4 of the Recommended Dietary Allowance [RDA] for adults). Almost all nuts furnish at least 1/3 of the RDA for phosphorus, and are fair to good sources of iron.

6. Nuts are also good sources of the B-complex vitamins, as indicated by the values for thiamin, riboflavin, and niacin. However, roasting destroys much of the thiamin. Nuts also furnish biotin, pantothenic acid, vitamin B-6, and vitamin E.

7. Nuts are good sources of (a) magnesium, a macromineral that activates enzymes and aids functioning of nerves and muscles, (b) zinc, a component of various enzymes, and (c) copper, the mineral that functions in enzyme actions, hair growth and pigmentation, connective tissue development, and red blood cell formation.

Details regarding some of the nutritive values not indicated in Food Composition Table F-36 are discussed in the sections that follow.

Fatty Acid Content. The fats in all of the common edible nuts, with the exception of coconuts, contain 77% or more of unsaturated fatty acids. Coconut fat contains over 90% saturated fatty acids. Table N-7 lists the un-

saturated and polyunsaturated fatty acid content, as well as the content of the essential fatty acid linoleic acid in some common nuts.

TABLE N-7
FATTY ACID CONTENT OF SOME COMMON NUTS[1]

Nut	Saturated Fatty Acids	Polyunsaturated Fatty Acids	Linoleic Acid
	←------ (g/100 g) ------→		
Almond............	4.3	10.5	9.9
Brazil nut..........	17.4	25.7	25.4
Cashew............	9.2	7.7	7.3
Coconut..........	31.2	.8	.7
Filbert (hazelnut) ..	4.6	6.9	6.6
Hickory nut........	6.0	12.7	12.0
Peanut	8.6	13.3	13.3
Pecan	6.1	18.3	17.0
Pistachio	7.4	7.3	6.8
Walnut, black......	5.1	40.9	36.8
Walnut, English	6.9	42.0	34.9

[1]Data from Table F-9, Fats and Fatty Acids in Selected Foods.

All of the nuts in Table N-7, except almonds, cashews, coconuts, filberts, and pistachios contain liberal amounts of linoleic acid—the essential polyunsaturated fatty acid. One ounce (*28 g*) of peanuts, Brazil nuts, or English walnuts provides about 4, 7, and 10 g of linoleic acid, respectively. Therefore, it may be better to rely on nuts rather than vegetable oils to supply the essential fatty acid linoleic acid because the nuts also furnish protein, minerals, and certain vitamins that are not supplied by the oils. Shelled nuts, like vegetable oils, should be kept refrigerated to prevent them from becoming rancid.
(Also see FATS AND OTHER LIPIDS.)

Protein Quantity and Quality. Like legumes, nuts contain about twice as much protein as the common cereal grains and have amino acid patterns that generally complement those of the cereals. However, nuts contain less of the amino acid lysine than legumes. Hence, the age-old practice of combining nut milks with cooked cereals made a lot of sense when animal protein was scarce. The American version of these complementary protein mixtures is peanut butter sandwiches, which children should eat with milk to offset the mild deficiency of lysine in the sandwich.
(Also see PROTEIN[S], section headed "Sources.")

Minerals and Vitamins. In addition to the minerals listed in Food Composition Table F-36, nuts are also good sources of (1) chromium, a micromineral which renders insulin more effective in promoting the passage of nutrients into cells; (2) manganese, an element required for growth of bones and other connective tissues, insulin action, blood clotting, and enzyme actions in many aspects of metabolism; and (3) selenium, which is present in an enzyme that detoxifies dangerous peroxides formed during metabolism. In general, nuts contain from

1 to 7 times the amounts of these minerals present in the other types of fresh, minimally processed natural foods.[2]

Nuts also supply choline, a vitaminlike factor required for the transport of fats from the liver. Normally, the body synthesizes choline, but sometimes the amounts may be insufficient to meet its needs.

In general, the nutritive values of nuts are sufficient to enable people to live healthfully on them (provided that 12 to 16 oz [*340 to 454 g*] are consumed daily), plus some fruits and/or vegetables to supply the missing vitamin A and vitamin C. However, the prices of nuts have recently become so high that it is now more economical to eat dietary combinations of animal foods, cereals, and legumes instead of nuts. Also, the other foods are lower in calories. Therefore, it seems that with the exception of a few undeveloped areas blessed with an abundance of wild nut trees, most people of modest means will have to settle for using nuts as occasional snacks and garnishes for dishes based mainly upon other foods.

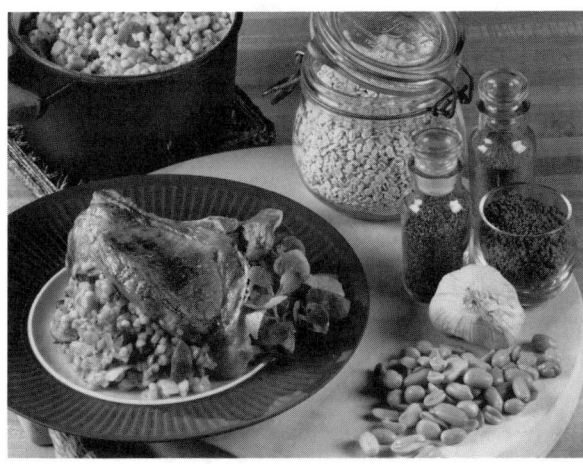

Fig. N-18. Peanut-barley stuffing for meat dishes. (Courtesy, National Peanut Council, Washington, D.C.)

NUTS OF THE WORLD.   Each type of nut tree (or vine in the case of peanuts) originated in an area with a particular climate and certain soil condition. Also, the growing conditions, harvesting, and processing for the

market may vary for each species, as may the most important food uses. Fig. N-18 shows a typical use of nuts.

Finally, nutritive values vary over a spectrum ranging from fair to excellent with regard to the major nutrients. Information on these aspects is given in summary form in Table N-8.

---

[2]Schroeder, H. A., "Losses of vitamins and trace minerals resulting from processing and preservation of foods," *The American Journal of Clinical Nutrition*, Vol. 24, 1971, p. 570, Table 7.

TABLE N–8
NUTS OF THE WORLD

Popular Name; Scientific Name; Origin and History	Importance; Principle Areas; Growing Conditions	Processing; Preparing; Uses	Nutritive Value[1]

Almond
Source: The seed of the almond fruit.
Scientific Name of the Almond Tree:
  Family: *Rosaceae*
  Genus: *Prunus*
  Species: *P. amygdalus*
Origin and History: Believed to have originated in Persia and to have been introduced into Arabia by Persian conquerors. Arabs in turn took the tree west to Spain and east to India. (Also see ALMONDS.)
	Importance: The fourth leading nut crop in the world, and the second leading one in the U.S. An estimated 1.3 million metric tons are produced worldwide each year.
	Principal Areas: U.S.A., Italy, and Spain.
	Growing Conditions: Almonds need a dry, semi-tropical, frostfree climate like that in the Mediterranean region. Thrive under high summer temperatures and withstand moderate droughts. Cross-pollination is essential for the bearing of fruit, so different varieties must be planted in close proximity. Also, bees are often kept in the orchards to insure pollination.
		Processing: Harvesting is done by hand in the Mediterranean, but in California shaking machines are used to bring down the nuts so that they may be gathered by mechanical sweepers. Then, they are mechanically cracked and cleaned, after which they are sorted into grades. Some nuts are blanched, while others are roasted and salted.
		Preparing: Shelled almonds may be roasted, blanched, ground into meal, or made into paste. Sometimes the oil is extracted.
		Uses: Snacks, ingredient of baked goods, breading for fried foods, casseroles, confections, desserts, ice cream, mixed nuts, salads, and toppings.
			Almonds are an excellent source of calories, essential polyunsaturated fatty acids, magnesium, and phosphorus; and a good source of protein, calcium, iron, and vitamin B complex. It is noteworthy that the roasting of almonds destroys about 80% of the thiamin content.
			A 3½ oz (*100 g*) portion of almonds supplies 598 kcal (170 kcal per oz).

TABLE N–8 *(Continued)*

Popular Name; Scientific Name; Origin and History	Importance; Principle Areas; Growing Conditions	Processing; Preparing; Uses	Nutritive Value[1]
Brazil Nut **Source:** The seed of the Brazil nut tree. **Scientific Name of the Brazil Nut Tree:** Family: *Lecythidaceae* Genus: *Bertholletia* Species: *B. excelsa* **Origin and History:** Originated in the Amazon valley in Bolivia and Brazil, the only region where it now grows.	**Importance:** An important native food in the areas around where it is grown. Also, from 30,000 to 40,000 metric tons are exported annually to the U.S.A. and Europe. **Principal Areas:** The Amazon valley in Bolivia and Brazil. **Growing Conditions:** Grows wild in the forests of the Amazon valley.	**Processing:** The nut-bearing fruits are allowed to fall to the ground when ripe. Then, the tough fruit capsules are cracked open and 15 to 30 nuts are removed. The hard shells may be either removed or left on the nuts prior to shipping and marketing. **Preparing:** No treatment is required for the shelled nuts. Sometimes, the kernels are crushed and oil is extracted. **Uses:** Snacks, ingredient of baked goods, confections, and nut mixtures. The oil may be used in salads.	Brazil nuts are similar in nutritive value to almonds, except that they furnish more calories, essential fatty acids, phosphorus, and thiamin. Also, they contain less calcium, iron, magnesium, riboflavin, and niacin. The shelled nuts should be refrigerated or at least kept under cool conditions because their high oil content makes them very susceptible to rancidity. A 3½ oz *(100 g)* portion of Brazil nuts furnishes 627 kcal (178 kcal per oz).
Cashew Nut **Source:** The seed adhering to the cashew apple. **Scientific Name of the Cashew Tree:** Family: *Anacardiaceae* Genus: *Anacardium* Species: *A. occidentale* **Origin and History:** Native to coastal areas of northeastern Brazil. Introduced into India and Africa by the Portuguese.	**Importance:** The fifth leading nut crop in the world. An estimated 478,832 metric tons are produced annually. **Principal Areas:** India, Brazil, Nigeria, Mozambique, and Tanzania. **Growing Conditions:** Dry, tropical climate. Well adapted to poor soils and sandy soils.	**Processing:** Nuts are allowed to fall to the ground. The shell around the nuts contains a caustic oil that blisters the hands. Hence, the shell oil is often extracted with solvents or by roasting or steaming after the nuts have been dried in the sun, cleaned, moistened, and allowed to stand in heaps. Then, the nuts are cracked and the kernel removed, after which the adhering skin is removed from the kernel. **Preparing:** Cashew nut kernels are usually consumed raw or after roasting and salting. **Uses:** Nut kernels are used as snacks, and as ingredients of baked goods and confections. Shell oil is used as a food and as a flavoring.	Cashew nuts are similar in nutritive value to almonds, except that they contain more phosphorus and thiamin. Also, they contain a little less energy (calories), protein, phosphorus, and iron; and much less essential fatty acids, calcium, riboflavin, and niacin. Oleic acid accounts for about 90% of the unsaturated fatty acids, and linoleic only 10%. Hence, cashew nuts are less likely to grow rancid than some of the other nuts which are much richer in linoleic acid. A 3½ oz *(100 g)* portion of cashew nuts contains 561 kcal (160 kcal per oz).

Footnote at end of table

(Continued)

TABLE N–8 *(Continued)*

Popular Name; Scientific Name; Origin and History	Importance; Principle Areas; Growing Conditions	Processing; Preparing; Uses	Nutritive Value[1]
Chestnut **Source:** The seed of the chestnut tree. **Scientific Name of the Chestnut tree:** Family: *Fagaceae* Genus: *Castanea* Species: *C. crenata* (Japanese), *C. dentala* (N. American), *C. mollissima* (Chinese), *C. sativa* (European) **Origin and History:** Native to southern Europe and Asia Minor. Taken to other areas by the Romans.	**Importance:** The sixth leading nut crop in the world. An estimated 488,161 metric tons are produced annually. **Principal Areas:** China, South Korea, Italy, Japan, and Spain. **Growing Conditions:** Mild, temperate climate with few frosty nights. Does best on well drained soils. The North American chestnut is the hardiest of the varieties, but it was practically wiped out by chestnut blight. Hence, hybrids of the American and Oriental chestnuts are now being grown.	**Processing:** The fallen burrs are gathered and the chestnuts removed. After roasting, the nuts may be left whole or ground into a flour. **Preparing:** Roasting, boiling, making into puree, grinding into a flour, preserving with sugar or syrup. **Uses:** Snacks; ingredient of confections, desserts, fritters, porridges, soups, stews, and stuffings.	Dried chestnuts differ greatly from all the other nuts in that they contain considerably more carbohydrate (3 to 4 times as much), and only fractions of the protein (about ⅓) and fat (about ¹⁄₁₅) content. Also, they furnish little more than ½ the calories of other nuts. The overall nutrient composition of chestnuts is quite close to that of dry cereal products made from corn or rice. A 3½ oz *(100 g)* portion of dried chestnuts contains 377 kcal (107 kcal per oz).
Coconut **Source:** The nut (fruit) of the coconut palm tree. **Scientific Name of the Coconut Palm:** Family: *Palmae* Genus: *Cocos* Species: *C. nucifera* **Origin and History:** Originated in Southeast Asia and on the islands of Melanesia in the Pacific Ocean. Widely distributed by water (coconuts float) and man to all parts of the tropical and subtropical world. (Also see COCONUT.)	**Importance:** Coconuts are by far the most extensively grown and used nuts in the world; an estimated over 42 million metric tons of nuts are produced annually. **Principal Areas:** The tropical sea coastal areas of the Old World. The leading coconut-producing countries of the world are: Indonesia, Philippines, India, Sri Lanka, and Malaysia. **Growing Conditions:** The trees thrive best in tropical countries, near the coast, and on rich, sandy soil. Salt water is tolerated, provided the water table fluctuates so as to give the roots aeration.	**Processing:** To make copra, the husks are removed and the coconuts are split open and dried in the sun, by smoking, or in tunnels or ovens. Most of the world production of oil is extracted by continuous screw pressed, sometimes followed by solvent extraction. In some areas, hydraulic cage and box presses continue to be used. **Preparing:** Crude coconut oil is refined and deodorized to remove free fatty acids and flavors. About 70% of the desiccated or shredded coconut is sold directly to bakery and confectionery manufacturers without further processing. The other 30% is further processed to produce (1) white sweetened coconut, by adding powdered sugar, propylene glycol, salt, and moisture; (2) toasted coconut, by adding powdered sugar, dextrose, and salt, then belt-conveying through toasting ovens; or (3) creamed coconut, by grinding, aerating chilling, and whipping desiccated coconut to a smooth consistency.	Nutritionally, coconuts and their products are characterized as follows: 1. The fresh nut contains about 50% water and 30 to 40% oil. 2. Coconut oil has the highest percentage of saturated fatty acids of all common food oils. This imparts long stability. Also when fed to milk cows, it produces hard butter, and when fed to hogs, it produces firm pork. 3. Coconut meal or copra meal contains about 21.2% crude protein. It is deficient in the amino acids lysine and methionine.

Footnote at end of table

(Continued)

TABLE N–8 *(Continued)*

Popular Name; Scientific Name; Origin and History	Importance; Principle Areas; Growing Conditions	Processing; Preparing; Uses	Nutritive Value[1]
Coconut *(Continued)*		**Uses:** The coconut palm is one of the most useful trees. Its most common food uses are: for consumption of the meat and sugary interior liquid of green or mature nuts; for use of the oil for confections, bakery goods, deep frying, and candies; for use of shredded coconut as a topping agent, bulking agent, nutmeat, or flavoring; for making toddy, a beverage which is consumed either fresh or fermented, from the unopened flower stalks (toddy is sometimes distilled to produce a spirit called arrack); and for palm cabbage, a salad made from buds cut from the top of the tree.	
Hazelnuts (Filberts) **Source:** The seed of the hazel or filbert tree. **Scientific Names of the Hazel and Filbert:** Family: *Betulaceae* Genus: *Corylus* Species: *C. maxima* (Filbert) *C. avellana* (Hazel) **Origin and History:** Various species are native to Europe, Asia, and North America.	**Importance:** The seventh leading nut crop in the world. Over 561,000 metric tons are produced annually. **Principal Areas:** Turkey, Italy, and Spain. In the U.S.A., most commercial growing of filberts is in Oregon, Washington, and California. **Growing Conditions:** Moist, temperate climate. The filbert tree is usually larger and more hardy than the hazel tree.	**Processing:** Fallen nuts are gathered by hand or by mechanical sweepers. After shelling, the nuts may be dried and/or the oil extracted. **Preparing:** No treatment is required for the shelled nuts. **Uses:** Snacks; ingredients of chocolates and other confections, and desserts. Filbert oil is used in the manufacture of cosmetics and perfumes.	Filberts are similar in nutritive value to almonds, except that they furnish more calories, fat, and thiamin; but less protein (only ⅔ as much), calcium, phosphorus, iron, and niacin. A 3½ oz (*100 g*) portion of filberts supplies 634 kcal (180 kcal per oz).

Footnote at end of table

(Continued)

TABLE N–8 *(Continued)*

Popular Name; Scientific Name; Origin and History	Importance; Principle Areas; Growing Conditions	Processing; Preparing; Uses	Nutritive Value[1]
Macadamia Nut **Source:** The seed of the macadamia tree. **Scientific Name of the Macadamia Tree:** Family: *Proteaceae* Genus: *Macadamia* Species: *M. ternifolia* **Origin and History:** Native to Australia. Brought to Hawaii, where it has prospered.	**Importance:** One of the leading orchard crops of the Hawaiian Islands, but does not contribute significantly to world nut production. **Principal Areas:** Australia and Hawaii. **Growing Conditions:** Moist semitropical climate. Does best on well-drained soils.	**Processing:** Fallen nuts are gathered and the outer husk is removed by a special machine. The unshelled nuts can be stored safely in a dry environment. Shelling is done by a cracking machine after the nuts have been air dried to a low moisture content. The shelled nuts are fried in deep fat, then salted and packaged. **Preparing:** No treatment is needed for packaged nuts. **Uses:** Snacks; ingredients of cakes, candy, and ice cream.	Macadamia nuts are very high in fat (72%), but low in protein (8%), calcium, phosphorus, iron, and the vitamin B complex. A 3½ oz (*100 g*) portion furnishes 691 kcal (196 kcal per oz).
Peanut **Source:** The seed of the peanut plant. **Scientific Name of the Peanut Plant:** Genus: *Arachis* Species: *A. bypogaea* **Origin and History:** Originated somewhere between Brazil and Bolivia. Spanish and Portuguese traders took peanuts to Africa. Later, African slaves brought them to the U.S.A. (Also see PEANUTS.)	**Importance:** The second leading nut crop in the world, and by far the leading one in the U.S.A. An estimated 23.1 million metric tons are produced worldwide each year. **Principal Areas:** India, Africa (Mauritius), China, Cyprus, and U.S.A. **Growing Conditions:** Tropical or subtropical climate. Needs a frost-free growing period of 4 to 5 months and adequate amounts of both sunshine and rainfall. Grows best on light, well-drained sandy soils.	**Processing:** The mature pods and seeds are dug and lifted from the ground by a digger-shaker-windrower. After drying in windrows the pods are cleaned, graded, and shelled. Oil is extracted from some of the crop by hot pressing and/or solvent extraction; and the residue from the extraction made into a flour or a meal. The rest of the crop is (1) left raw, (2) roasted and salted, or (3) made into peanut butter. **Preparing:** Raw peanuts may be boiled or roasted. **Uses:** Snack, peanut butter, salted peanuts, mixed nuts, baked goods, confections, salads, desserts, and meat analogs.	Peanuts are the highest in protein (26%) among the leading nuts. Compared to almonds, they are richer in essential fatty acids and the vitamin B complex, but lower in calcium and iron. However, roasting destroys about ⅔ of the thiamin. A 3½ oz (*100 g*) portion of roasted peanuts furnishes 582 kcal (165 kcal per oz).

Footnote at end of table

(Continued)

TABLE N–8 (Continued)

Popular Name; Scientific Name; Origin and History	Importance; Principle Areas; Growing Conditions	Processing; Preparing; Uses	Nutritive Value[1]
Pecan **Source:** The seed of the pecan tree. **Scientific Name of the Pecan Tree:** Family: *Juglandaceae* Genus: *Carya* Species: *C. illinoensis* **Origin and History:** Native to the river valleys of the south central U.S.A. and adjoining parts of Mexico. (Also see PECAN[S].) 	**Importance:** The fourth leading nut crop in the U.S.A. (after peanuts and almonds) with an average annual production of over 90,000 metric tons. **Principal Areas:** Southern U.S.A. **Growing Conditions:** Temperate or subtropical climate with long, warm summers. Best yield of nuts is obtained when coldest winter month averages less than 60°F (*18°C*).	**Processing:** The mature nuts may be knocked from the trees with long poles, or just allowed to fall. After gathering, the unshelled nuts are dried prior to cracking or storage under controlled temperature and humidity. Cracking is done by machine. **Preparing:** No further treatment is required for shelled nuts. **Uses:** Snack, baked goods, confections, casseroles, desserts, ice cream, pecan pie, puddings, souffles, and stuffing.	Pecans contain about the same amount of fat (71%) as macadamia nuts, along with similar levels of other nutrients, except that they contain 2½ times the thiamin. A 3½ oz (*100 g*) portion of pecans contains 739 kcal (211 kcal per oz).
Pine Nuts (Pinon Nuts) **Source:** The seeds of various species of pine trees. **Scientific Names of the Nut-bearing Pine Trees:** Family: *Pinaceae* Genus: *Pinus* Species: *P. cembra* (Swiss stone pine), *P. cembroides* (Mexican nut pine), *P. edulis* (pinon pine of southwestern U.S.A.), and *P. pinea* (stone pine of the Mediterranean) **Origin and History:** Trees are native to the areas noted under Species. 	**Importance:** Little of the crop enters the nut trade. The annual production in northern Mexico and southwestern U.S.A. averages 3,000 or more metric tons. **Principal Areas:** Northern Mexico, southwestern U.S.A, Europe, and Asia. **Growing Conditions:** Varies according to species. Generally, the nut-bearing species grow wild in the temperate zones of the Northern Hemisphere. The nut pines of North America are adapted to an arid climate.	**Processing:** Most harvesting consists of picking the cones from the tree before the cone scales separate. Then, the cones are dried to free the nuts. Machines are used to shell the nuts. (American Indians gathered fallen nuts and cracked them with hand tools.) Some species require roasting to remove a turpentine flavor. **Preparing:** No further treatment is required for commercially processed nuts, but unprocessed items may require roasting. **Uses:** Snacks; ingredient of baked goods, confections, desserts, and vegetarian dishes.	The European types (generally called pignolias) are very rich in protein (31%), but lower in fat (47%) and carbohydrates (12%) than the American types (pinon nuts) which contain 13% protein, 60% fat, and 20% carbohydrates. Compared to almonds, pinon nuts are richer in phosphorus, iron, and the vitamin B complex, but lower in calcium. A 3½ oz (*100 g*) portion of pignolia nuts supplies 552 kcal (157 kcal per oz), whereas the same amount of pinon nuts furnishes 653 kcal (180 kcal per oz). All types of pine nuts contain fats that are highly susceptible to rancidity. Hence, they should be stored in a refrigerator.

Footnote at end of table

(Continued)

TABLE N–8 *(Continued)*

Popular Name; Scientific Name; Origin and History	Importance; Principle Areas; Growing Conditions	Processing; Preparing; Uses	Nutrtive Value[1]
Pistachio Nut **Source:** The seed of the pistachio tree. **Scientific Name of the Pistachio Tree:** Family: *Anacardiaceae* Genus: *Pistacia* Species: *P. vera* **Origin and History:** Native to western Asia. Has now been introduced to the central valley of California.	**Importance:** The eighth leading nut crop in the world. An estimated 220,490 metric tons are produced annually. **Principal Areas:** Iran, U.S.A., Turkey, Syria. **Growing Conditions:** Temperate to subtropical climate. Requires well-drained soils, and thrives on sandy loams. Tolerates drought well, and often grows wild on dry wastelands.	**Processing:** The nuts are harvested by picking the clusters or by beating them from the trees onto cloths. They may be husked immediately or after drying in the sun followed by soaking in water. Some of the nuts are roasted and salted in brine while in the shell, while others are cracked and the shells removed. **Preparing:** None required. **Uses:** Snacks; ingredient of confections, desserts, and ice cream.	Pistachio nuts are very similar in nutritional value to almonds, except that they are richer in iron and thiamin, and lower in calcium and niacin. A 3½ oz (*100 g*) portion contains 594 kcal (168 kcal per oz).
Walnut, Black, English, and White **Source:** The seeds of black walnut, English (Persian) walnut, and white walnut (butternut) trees. **Scientific Names of Walnut Trees:** Family: *Juglandaceae* Genus: *Juglans* Species: *J. cinerea* (white walnut or butternut), *J. nigra* (black walnut), *J. regia* (English or Persian walnut) **Origin and History:** The black and white walnuts are native to North America, whereas the English walnut originated in Persia. (Also see WALNUT[S].)	**Importance:** The fourth leading nut crop in the world, and the third in the U.S.A. An estimated 946,626 metric tons are produced worldwide each year. The English walnut accounts for most of the walnut crop. **Principal Areas:** U.S.A., China, Turkey, U.S.S.R., Romania, and Yugoslavia. **Growing Conditions:** Temperate to subtropical climate. Well-drained soils are required. Extremes of temperature reduce the yields of nuts, although a moderately cold winter is needed to break the dormancy of the trees.	**Processing:** Nuts are harvested by hand in many areas of the world. However, in California, English walnuts are mechanically shaken from the trees onto the ground, where they are gathered by a sweeping machine. After hulling, washing, and drying, the unshelled nuts are graded and bleached for sale. Some nuts are mechanically shelled. It is difficult to remove the hulls of black walnuts, so they are usually allowed to rot away. The nutmeats are sold in broken pieces because it is difficult to remove the whole nuts from the shell. **Preparing:** None required. **Uses:** Snacks; ingredient of baked goods, confections, desserts, ice cream.	Black walnuts are very similar in nutritional value to almonds, whereas English walnuts are higher in fat and thiamin, but lower in protein, phosphorus, and iron. Also, both types of walnuts contain much less calcium than almonds. Walnuts are the richest sources of essential polyunsaturated fatty acids, among the leading nuts. Hence, they should be kept refrigerated to prevent rancidity. A 3½ oz (*100 g*) portion of black walnuts supplies 628 kcal (178 kcal per oz), whereas the same amount of English walnuts supplies 651 kcal (185 kcal per oz).

[1]Additional details on the nutritive values are given in the Food Composition Table F-36, Table P-37, Proteins and Amino Acids In Selected Foods, and Table F-9, Fats and Fatty Acids in Selected Foods.

Additional details are given for the different types of nuts in the individual articles bearing their popular names.

NYCTALOPIA

The medical term for night blindness.
(Also see NIGHT BLINDNESS.)

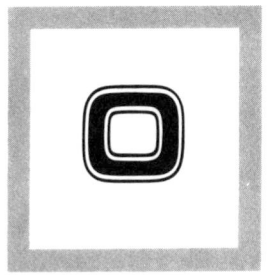

OATS *Avena sativa*

Oats are grown in most temperate countries of the world for grain, straw, and/or pasture. In general, they are a cool-season crop which require a moist climate.

ORIGIN AND HISTORY. Oats are believed to have developed from wild stocks that first grew in Asia. For many years, the common wild oat was considered to be the ancestor of oats, but a recent theory, supported by considerable evidence, postulates that wild red oats are the ancestor of all the oats with 42 chromosomes (21 pairs). Different kinds of oats were likely taken from various parts of Asia to Europe. As a cultivated crop, oats were substantially later in origin than wheat. Not until about 2,000 years ago, at the beginning of the Christian era, are references to oats as a cultivated crop found in the literature. Early use of oats appears to have been medicinal, rather than as a food crop. Cultivation of oats was extensive in Europe prior to the discovery of America. In the 1200s, it was known as pilcorn in England. Oats were introduced into North America in 1602, for plantings made on the Elizabeth Islands off the coast of Massachusetts.
(Also see CEREAL GRAINS.)

WORLD AND U.S. PRODUCTION. In 1990, 44 million metric tons of oats were produced in the world, almost exclusively in temperate North America and

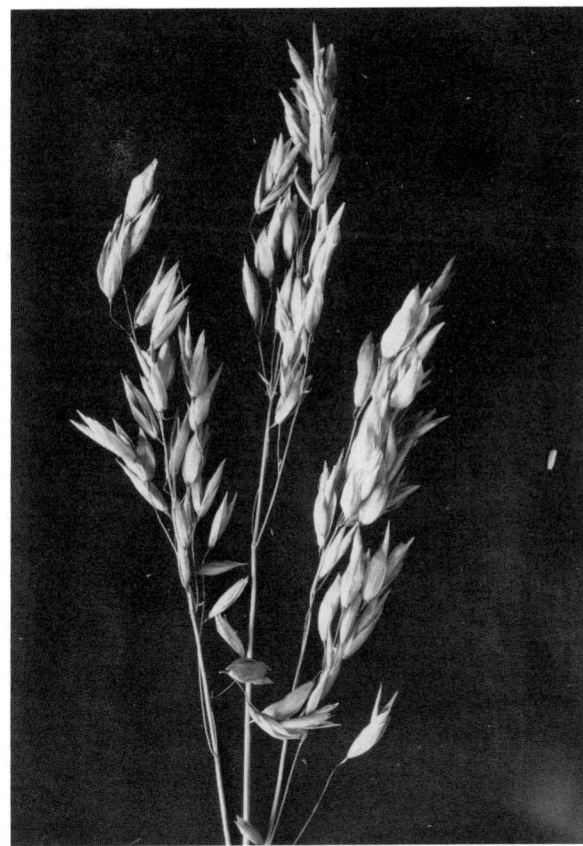

Fig. O-1. Oat panicles with many branches and spikelets. Note the loose-fitting hulls surrounding the grain, which are inedible by humans and must be removed when oats are processed for food. (Photo by J. C. Allen & Sons, West Lafayette, Ind.)

Europe. Oats rank sixth among the cereal grains, but account for only 2.2% of the total cereal grain produced globally. The ten leading oat-producing countries of the world by rank are: The Soviet Union, United States,

Canada, Germany, Poland, Finland, Sweden, Australia, France, and Argentina (see Fig. O-2).

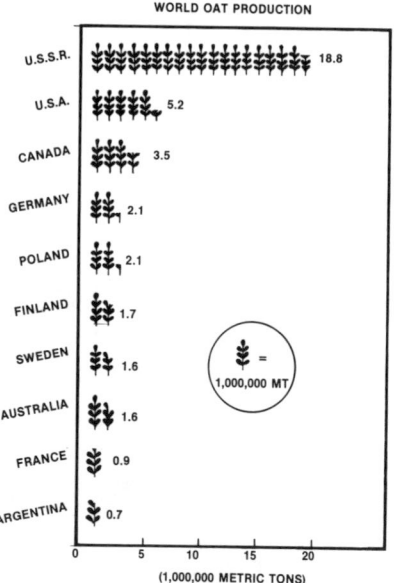

Fig. O-2.   Leading oat-producing countries. (From: *FAO Production Yearbook*, 1990, FAO/UN, Rome, Italy, Vol. 44, p. 82)

Oats rank fifth as a cereal crop, in bushels produced, in the United States, being exceeded only by corn, wheat, grain sorghum, and barley. The ten leading oat-producing states, by rank, in 1991 were: South Dakota, Minnesota, Wisconsin, Iowa, North Dakota, Ohio, Pennsylvania, Nebraska, Michigan, and Illinois (see Fig. O-3).

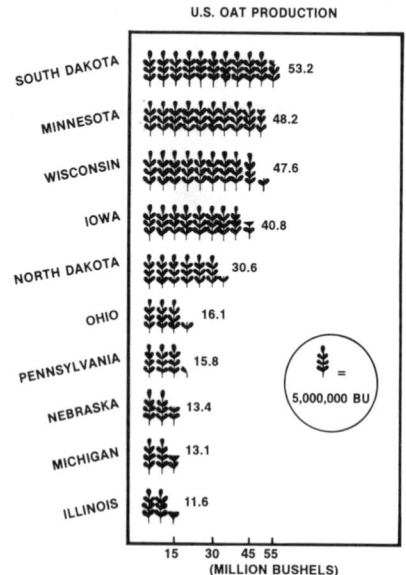

Fig. O-3.   Leading U.S. oat-producing states. (Source: *Agricultural Statistics*, 1991, USDA, p. 41, Table 51)

The U.S. average yield per harvested acre is about 60.1 bu *(2.1 MT/ha)*, compared to the world average yield of 55.6 bu per acre *(2 MT/ha)*. However, in the Netherlands, Ireland, Switzerland, United Kingdom, and New Zealand, yields are double or more than double those of the United States or the world average.

THE OAT PLANT *Avena sativa.*   Oats belong to the grass family, *Gramineae.* Most cultivated oats have been developed from the genus *Avena*, species *A. sativa.*

The oat plant forms a crown at the soil surface from which the fibrous root system penetrates the soil. The leaves are thin, narrow, and long. The stalk (culm) usually grows 2 to 5 ft *(61 to 152 cm)* tall and terminates in the panicle. Each panicle usually bears 10 to 75 spikelets on its numerous branches. The oat kernel, called the groat, is protected by a covering of hulls—the lemma and palea, which are not removed by threshing. At maturity, the lemma may be white, yellow, gray, brown, red, or black, depending on the variety. The oat kernel, or groat, is the part remaining after removal of the palea and lemma. It is spindle shaped—up to ½ in. *(13 mm)* in length and 1/8 in. *(3 mm)* or less in width; and it includes the seed coat layers of cells, the starch endosperm, and the embryo.

OAT CULTURE.   In the Corn Belt, oats usually follow one of the row crops—corn, sorghum, or soybeans. It may be used as a companion or nurse crop for forage seeding; for example, oats and alfalfa may be planted simultaneously, with the oats harvested for grain the first year and alfalfa harvested for hay in subsequent years. Spring oats are drilled or broadcast in March or April, at the rate of 2 to 3 bu per acre *(74 to 111 kg/ha)* in a seedbed prepared by discing or plowing. Winter oats are seeded in October or November. When ripe, oats are harvested with a combine, either direct or after being windrowed to dry. For safe storage, the grain should not contain more than 13% moisture. Straw is either baled and used as bedding or worked into the soil for humus.

FEDERAL GRADES OF OATS.   The Official United States Standards For Grain, established by the U.S. Department of Agriculture, divide oats into the following five color classes: white oats, red oats, gray oats, black oats, and mixed oats. Then, within each class, there are five grades: U.S. No. 1, U.S. No. 2, U.S. No. 3, U.S. No. 4, and U.S. Sample grade. The grades are determined by test weight per bushel, sound cultivated oats, heat-damaged kernels, foreign material, and wild oats.

KINDS OF OATS.   Three broad groupings based on chromosome number—14, 28, or 42—are recognized in the general botanical classification of oats. But only those having 42 chromosomes will be considered here. The species represented in this group are:

Common oats
Common wild oats
Cultivated red oats
Large naked oats (hull-less oats)
Side oats
Wild red oats

Common oats, and to a lesser extent cultivated red oats, comprise most of the acreage in the United States. Side oats and large seeded naked or hull-less oats are of only minor importance in oat production. The common wild oat is a particularly troublesome weed in many states.

Like wheat, oats are broadly classified into spring or winter types, depending upon the season of planting. It is noteworthy that the world collection of oats, maintained by the U.S. Department of Agriculture, contains more than 14,000 lines of 42-chromosome types.

PROCESSING OATS.

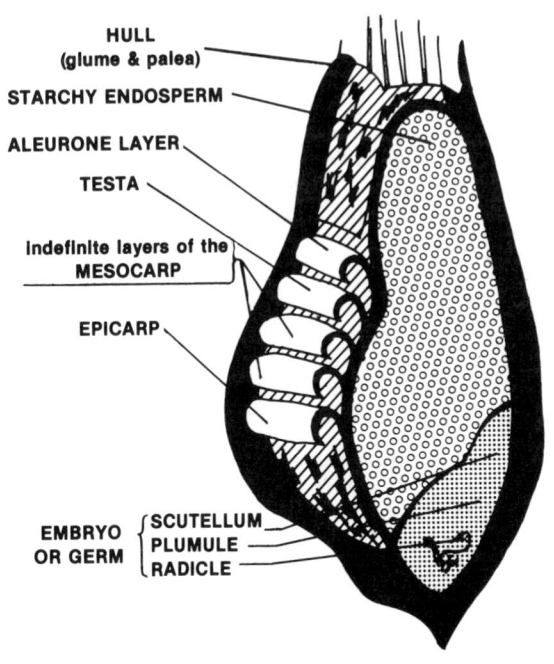

HULL
(glume & palea)

STARCHY ENDOSPERM

ALEURONE LAYER

TESTA

Indefinite layers of the
MESOCARP

EPICARP

EMBRYO   SCUTELLUM
OR GERM   PLUMULE
          RADICLE

Fig. O-4.   Covered kernel (caropsis) of oats.

Only about 15% of the U.S. oat crop is processed for food.

The oat kernel has a fibrous hull, which is inedible by humans. So, the goal in milling oats is to obtain the maximum yield of clean, uniform, sound, whole oat kernels which are free from hulls, floury material, extraneous matter, and undesirable flavors. The hulls range from 21 to 43%, with an average of 25%.

The milling of oats involves the following steps:

1. **Cleaning.** Foreign material and oats not suitable for milling are first removed.

2. **Drying and roasting.** The grain is subjected to heat and the moisture is reduced to somewhere between 7 and 8½%. This process develops flavor, improves keeping quality, and facilitates the subsequent separation of the hull from the groats.

3. **Cooling.** After drying, the oats are cooled by air circulation.

4. **Hulling.** The hulling machine separates the groat kernel from the surrounding hull. The following products are obtained from the hullers: hulls, groats, broken groats and meal, flour, and unhulled oats. These materials are separated by air aspiration and screening. The choicest, plumpest groats are used to make package-grade rolled oats, while the less choice groats make either bulk or feed rolled oats. The broken kernels are used as livestock feed.

5. **Cutting.** The purpose of cutting is to convert groats to uniform granules.

6. **Flaking.** The granules are flaked between rolls to produce a quick-cooking breakfast cereal.

NUTRITIONAL VALUE OF OATS. The nutrient composition of oats and oat products are given in Food Composition Table F-36.

A few salient points regarding the nutritional value of oats follow:

1. Oat cereals are palatable, rich in carbohydrates (starch), a good source of thiamin and vitamin E, but deficient in minerals, especially calcium.

2. Oat groats contain more protein than wheat. The protein is not of the glutenin type; hence, oat flour is not suitable as the sole flour for breads. However, it may be used for cakes, biscuits, and breakfast foods.

3. Oats lack protein quantity and quality. While dry oatmeal is about 14% protein, cooked oatmeal is only about 2% protein. Moreover, it is deficient in the essential amino acid lysine as shown in Table O-1.

4. The oat grain very closely resembles a kernel of wheat in structure. Unlike wheat, however, the nutritious bran and germ are not removed in the normal processing because oats are not refined. The most important nutritional advantage of oats is the soluble fiber which helps to lower the cholesterol in the blood. Oat bran is a major source of this fiber.

When oats are processed, the hull is removed, leaving the whole grain. After further processing, the whole grain oat will become rolled, steelcut, or instant oats. The outer covering of the whole grain oat is bran. In the production of oat bran, however, the bran plus 3 to 4 layers of cells called aleurone layers are included in the final product.

(Also see CEREAL GRAINS and PROTEIN[S].)

TABLE O-1
PROFILE OF ESSENTIAL AMINO ACIDS IN OATMEAL COMPARED TO MILK— A HIGH-QUALITY PROTEIN

Amino Acid	Oatmeal (dry)	Cow's Milk[1]
	← (mg/g protein) →	
Histidine	18	27
Isoleucine	52	47
Leucine	75	95
Lysine	37	78
Methionine and cystine	36	33
Phenylalanine and tyrosine	90	102
Threonine	33	44
Tryptophan	13	14
Valine	60	64

[1]*Recommended Dietary Allowances*, 10th ed., 1989, NRC-National Academy of Sciences, p. 67, Table 6–5.

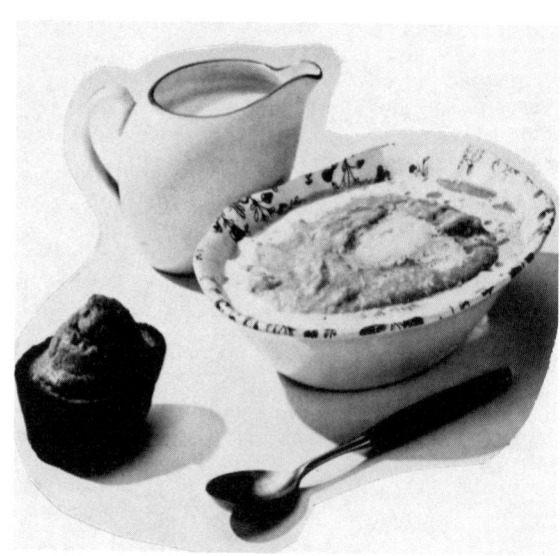

Fig. O-5. Many a schoolchild has been raised on a breakfast of hot oatmeal porridge. (Courtesy, Elam's, Broadview, Ill.)

OAT PRODUCTS AND USES. The products from the milling of oats are: oat hulls, oat groats, steel-cut oats, oatmeal, rolled oats, oat flakes, oat flour, and the feed by-products.

Eighty-five percent of the oats grown in the United States are used as livestock feed; hence, they enter the human diet primarily as meat, milk, and eggs.

Table O-2 presents in summary form the story of oat products and uses.

(Also see BREAKFAST CEREAL[S]; and CEREAL GRAINS, Table C-18 Cultural Characteristics of Selected Grains; FLOURS, Table F-26 Special Flours.)

TABLE O-2
OAT PRODUCTS AND USES

Product	Description	Uses	Comments
HUMAN FOODS			
Oat flakes	The product made from the whole groats through (1) by-passing the cutting system, and (2) subjecting the whole kernel to steaming and flaking to a slightly greater thickness than regular rolled oats.	Porridge	This product is sometimes referred to as "old fashioned" or "5-minute" oat flakes.
Oat flour	The product produced by grinding and screening the oat flakes from the rolls.	As an antioxidant, as a constituent of baby foods, and in soaps and cosmetic preparations.	The antioxidant property of oat flour is due to the presence of caffeic acid derivatives which act as strong antioxidants. This explains why properly processed oatmeal is extremely stable and can be maintained in good quality in closed containers for many years.
Oatmeal	Uniform granules of a mealy texture, with a minimum of fine granules and flour.	Porridge	The decline in the consumption of oatmeal porridge is attributable to the greater convenience and speed of ready-cooked breakfast cereal. Oatmeal is made by subjecting groats to cutters, which convert them to uniform granules.

(Continued)

TABLE O-2 (*Continued*)

Product	Description	Uses	Comments
HUMAN FOODS (*Continued*)			
Rolled oats	The product resulting from rolling the groats after treating them with live steam, then passing the flakes through separators to remove all the fine material.	Breakfast foods, cookies, and breads. Granola (homemade or commercially prepared), eaten either— 1. As a ready-to-eat breakfast cereal; or 2. As a snack.	Rolled oats and oatmeal contain about 1,850 calories (kcal) per lb (4,079 calories [kcal] per kg); hence, they are an excellent food for the winter diet. Granola is a mixture of rolled oats, honey, vegetable oil, chopped nuts, shredded coconut, sunflower seeds, raisins, chopped dates, cinnamon, vanilla, and/or other ingredients. The raw granola is usually heated in an oven until crisp and slightly browned.
LIVESTOCK FEEDS			
Whole oats	Whole oats with hulls.	Used for all farm animals. Their use for poultry is generally limited to pullet developer feeds and as a scratch feed for hens.	Oats are superior to other cereals as a feed for horses and are excellent for breeding animals and young stock. Their value as feed for these classes of livestock is due to their bulkiness and fairly high-protein content. Because of their bulkiness, they are also one of the safest feeds to use in starting finishing cattle and sheep on feed. For most animals, ground oats have considerably higher feeding value than whole oats. The high-fiber content of oats limits their use in the rations of monogastric animals.
Chipped oat product	The product obtained in the manufacture of chipped oats, consisting of the material broken from the ends of the hulls, empty hulls, light immature oats, and dust. It must not contain an excessive amount of oat hulls.	Used chiefly as an ingredient in mixed feeds.	
Feeding oatmeal	This product, which is obtained in the manufacture of rolled groats or rolled oats, consists of broken oat groats, oat groat chips, and the floury portions of the oat groats, with only such quantity of finely ground oat hulls as is unavoidable in normal milling. It must not contain more than 4% crude fiber.	Chick mashes and pig starters.	

(Continued)

TABLE O-2 (*Continued*)

Product	Description	Uses	Comments
		LIVESTOCK FEEDS (*Continued*)	
Oat groats	Cleaned oats with the hulls removed.	Sometimes oat groats are ground and used in pig starters or in mashes for chicks.	
Oat hulls	The outer covering of oats, obtained in the milling of table cereals or in the groating of oats.	Oat hulls may be used as a low-grade roughage for ruminants; as deep litter for chickens.	
Oat mill by-product	The by-product obtained in the manufacture of oat groats, consisting of oat hulls and particles of the groat. It must not contain more than 22% crude fiber.	Oats mill by-product is a low-protein roughage.	
Oat forages: **Oat hay**	The entire oat plant cut and cured for hay.	Chiefly as a feed for horses.	Oat hay should be cut in the soft dough stage.
Oat pasture	Young oat plants.	For temporary and supplemental pastures for cattle, sheep, and swine.	
Oat plants, young	Young oat plants before they begin to joint, cut and dehydrated.	Consumed by both livestock (chiefly poultry) and people as a rich source of the "grass juice factor."	
Oat silage	The entire oat plant cut and cured for silage.	Fed to beef cattle, dairy cattle, and sheep.	Cut in the soft dough stage.
Oat straw	The stalk that remains following threshing.	Roughage for cattle and horses. Bedding for animals.	Oat straw is more nutritious and palatable than wheat straw.
		OTHER USES	
Oat hulls	The outer covering of oats, obtained in the milling of table cereals or in the groating of oats.	Furfural, which is used as a solvent and in the manufacture of plastics and nylon.	

OATCAKES

These are thin, flat cakes made by mixing oatmeal with either water, milk, or sour milk, then cooked on a griddle.

OATMEAL

(See OATS.)

OBESE

Overweight due to a surplus of body fat.
(Also see OBESITY.)

OBESITY

Contents   Page

This term means an excess of body fat beyond that needed for optimal maintenance of body functions. Obesity is *not* synonymous with overweight because (1) a person may have an optimal body weight, yet have an excess of fat and less than the normal amount of lean (non-fat) tissue; or (2) some overweight people may have above average amounts of bone and muscle, but only normal amounts of body fat.

Some of our leading medical people consider obesity to be the most widespread nutritional disorder in the United States.[1] An estimated 100 million Americans are obese. In 1990, Americans spent an estimated $33 billion on diets and diet-related products. Statistics gathered by life insurance companies show that obese people are more likely to develop degenerative diseases and die early. However, these statistics have limited value when applied to the U.S. population at large because (1) they are based upon the characteristics of people who purchased life insurance policies; (2) the distinction between obesity and overweight is not made, since no measurements of fatness, other than body weight, are made; (3) the high sickness and death rates of overweight people who have diseases that are aggravated by the gaining of weight, such as diabetes, heart disease, high blood fats, and high blood pressure, tend to distort the overall rates for overweight people who have none of these disorders, because unhealthy people are not considered separately from healthy people; and (4) the ranges of desirable weights for small, medium, and large frames were established arbitrarily, with no attempts to define criteria for assigning people to the appropriate categories.

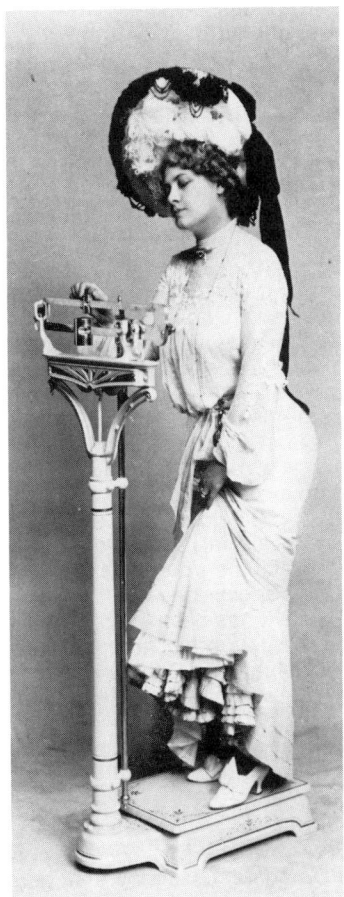

Fig. O-6. Down through the ages, people have been concerned with their weight. (Courtesy, The Bettmann Archive, Inc.)

---

[1]Sebrel, W. H., Jr., "Changing Concept of Malnutrition," *The American Journal of Clinical Nutrition*, Vol. 20, 1967, p. 653.

In spite of the great uncertainty as to what constitutes the "ideal" weight for any particular person, the attainment of such a weight has long been promoted as a goal for those who wish to remain in good health. Some doctors devote their entire medical practice to the treatment of obesity. Also, great amounts of money are now being made by manufacturers of such items as dietetic foods, exercise devices, jogging attire, liquid and powdered formulas for losing weight, "rainbow" pills (mixtures of drugs for losing weight), and special suits which cause loss of weight by inducing a heavy loss of water as sweat. Therefore, both the obese and the nonobese may be interested in the discussions that follow.

TYPES OF OBESITY.   Although all fat people may look alike to the untrained observer, there seems to be considerable variation in the physiological characteristics of obese people, judging from the many recent reports on this subject. Studies of the development of obesity in both animals and man have shown that there are two major types of obesity: early-onset and late-onset.[2] Descriptions follow:

• **Early-onset obesity**—This type is characterized by an abnormally large number of fat cells because it originates in childhood while the cells in the fatty tisues are still dividing. Early-onset obesity is often accompanied by extra nonfat tissue because the dietary, hereditary, and hormonal factors which spur the proliferation of fat cells also stimuate extra growth of bone and muscle.

For example, it is well known that females who have been obese since childhood tend to have heavier upper arms, larger rib cages, and earlier onset of puberty than those who were leaner during their periods of growth. Although obese children may often be taller than lean children of the same age, adult heights are about the same for the lean and obese because the obese usually stop growing at an earlier age. Obesity in boys and girls is different from "baby" fat which tends to disappear during periods of rapid growth.

Childhood obesity is a subject of great concern among health professionals, particularly those whose experiences have shown that most efforts to correct this condition, once it has been established, are doomed to failure. One reason for this difficulty in obtaining permanent loss of weight is that there is often a combination of both excessive numbers of fat cells and greatly enlarged fat cells. While the size of these cells may be reduced, there is no way to reduce the numbers of extra cells, short of surgical removal of fatty tissues.

• **Late-onset obesity**—This type, in contrast to early-onset type, is characterized by enlargement of normal numbers of fat cells because it usually begins after the division of cells in the tissues has ceased. Sometimes, adult obesity may be distinguished from that which began in childhood because the former is characterized by proportionately greater deposits of excess fat on the trunk of the body than on the arms and legs. Those who first became obese in adulthood are usually more successful in achieving long-term control of their body weight.

CAUSES OF OBESITY.   There are many different opinions as to the cause(s) of obesity. The simplest concept is that it is almost always due to a combination of overeating and underactivity. Hence, there tends to be an attitude of moral superiority in some people who flaunt their leanness at those who are obese. However, there may be many other reasons for obesity and leanness. Some of the current ideas on this subject follow:

Fattening Aided Survival of Early Man.   In preagricultural times man depended upon the hunting and gathering of foods. When, for various reasons, the food supply in the local area became exhausted, it was often necessary to travel long distances to another place where food was more plentiful. Each pound of body fat sustained a person for a day or two when no food was available. Hence, people who had a tendency to fatten easily were more likely to survive than those lacking this tendency. Even today, lack of sufficient calories is a major cause of disability and death of malnourished people in some of the developing countries.

Hereditary and Acquired Traits.   Each newborn baby has unique features which are determined mainly by heredity. However, the eventual development of the baby into a fat or lean adult depends upon a combination of both hereditary and environmental factors. It is noteworthy that the ancient Greek physicians in the time of Hippocrates attempted to take into consideration the characteristics of their patients by classifying them according to both (1) their body builds; and (2) their predominant temperament, with the latter classed as either choleric, melancholic, phlegmatic, or sanguineous. Even today, some well-known anthropologists, physicians, and psychologists believe that tendencies toward fatness or leanness may depend somewhat upon body build and other traits. Explanations follow.

BODY BUILDS (Somatotypes).   Dr. Sheldon, an American physical anthropologist, and his co-workers have described the temperaments they observed to be associated with each of three types of physique: ectomorph, mesomorph, and endomorph.[3] These types are shown in Fig. O-7.

---

[2]Winick, M., "Childhood Obesity," *Nutrition Today*, Vol. 9, May/June 1974, p. 6.

[3]Sheldon, W. H., and S. S. Stevens, *The Varieties of Temperament*, Harper and Row, New York, N.Y., 1942.

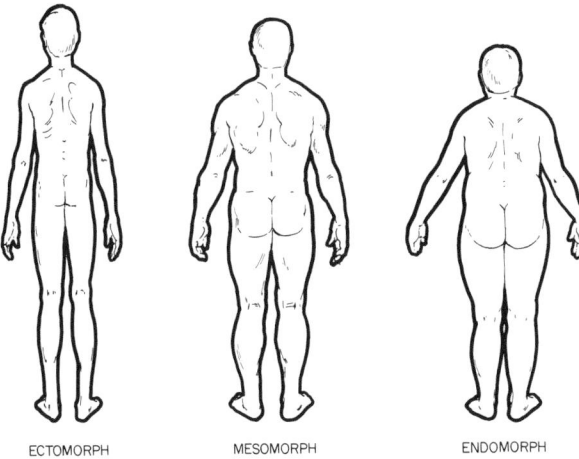

ECTOMORPH   MESOMORPH   ENDOMORPH

Fig. O-7. Sheldon's three extreme types of body build.

Details follow:

• **Ectomorph**—This type of physique is tall and slender with long arms and legs, but the trunk is short compared to the rest of the body. The personality of the person who has such a physique is closest to the introvert type, which was first described by the Swiss psychiatrist Jung.[4] Most of the introvert's drive originates from within, so he or she works well alone, and with minimal supervision. Ectomorphs are often characterized by other people as ambitious and persevering, but also as somewhat inhibited and tense. Statistics which have been compiled by life insurance companies show that people with this physique live the longest. Hence, the tables of ideal weights for various heights tend to be closer to those of ectomorphs than to those of endomorphs or mesomorphs.

• **Mesomorph**—This body build has traditionally been viewed as the epitome of masculinity, although some women may also have this physique yet be truly feminine in every respect. It is characterized by an athletic build with good proportions between the arms, legs, and trunk. Usually, the chest is more prominent than the abdomen. Mesomorphs are rarely extreme extroverts or extreme introverts, but they are energetic and perform well in such team sports as football and hockey. Although life insurance statistics suggest that mesomorphs do not usually live as long as ectomorphs in sedentary, urban societies, it might be possible for people with this body build to live longer than expected by regularly engaging in strenuous physical activities. For example, a study of San Francisco longshoremen showed that those who

consistently performed the heaviest work in loading cargo had only about ½ the death rate and ⅓ the sudden death rate as those who did lighter loading work.[5]

• **Endomorph**—People with this body build usually have large abdomens, long trunks, but short arms and legs. They are closest in personality to the extrovert type described by Jung.[6] In contrast to the introvert, the extrovert's drive depends mainly upon stimulation by such external factors as good food, interaction with other people, and a comfortable environment. Others often see endomorphs as good natured, pleasure loving, talkative, and on the lazy side. Extroverts sometimes have difficulty working alone. Many endomorphs may appear to be obese, but this designation may often be made without taking into consideration their marked differences in body build from the ectomorphic physique.

Readers should not conclude that the characteristics associated with various physiques are immutable, inherited tendencies which predetermine certain aspects of an individual's life from birth to death; rather, they should be viewed as fairly stable patterns which at a given time are resistant to change. For example, it may require starvation to bring the weight of an endomorph down to that of an ectomorph. Also, nutrition in infancy and childhood apparently has a major role in the development of the adult physique since it is well known that protein-energy deficiencies early in life are much more limiting to the growth of limbs than to the growth of the trunk. Thus, it seems that nature protects females against problems in childbearing since the length of the trunk and the width of the pelvis are important for success in this regard. It may be readily observed that, in any gathering of women, there will be fairly great variations in standing height, but much smaller variations in sitting height.

Many psychologists have found fault with attempts to relate personality traits to such constitutional factors as body build. They maintain that when behavior fits certain stereotypes, it is because society tends to reinforce the traits that it expects of (1) males vs females; and (2) people who are either lean, muscular, or obese. On the other hand, evidence is beginning to accumulate concerning a third set of factors which appear to be related to both behavior and physical characteristics; namely, inherited or acquired differences in metabolism, which are discussed in the sections that follow.

DIFFERENCES IN THE UTILIZATION OF FOOD ENERGY. It has long been known that energy production by the body is stepped up after a meal has been consumed. The extra energy is usually lost from the body in the form of heat. *Hence, this effect of eating food is called thermogenesis (heat production) or specific dynamic action (SDA).* Thermogenesis is taken into con-

[4]Jung, C. G., *Psychological Types*, translated by H. G. Brynes, Harcourt Brace, New York, N.Y., 1923.

[5]Paffenbarger, R. S., Jr., and W. E. Hale, "Work Activity and Coronary Heart Mortality," *New England Journal of Medicine*, Vol. 292, 1975, p. 545.

[6]Jung, C. G., *Psychological Types*, translated by H. G. Brynes, Harcourt Brace, New York, N.Y., 1923.

sideration in caloric allowances since they are usually increased by 10% after the energy costs of (1) basal metabolism, and (2) the daily activities have been estimated. However, the amount of extra heat production after meals varies considerably for different people, depending upon circumstances such as those which follow:

• **Degree of fatness or leanness**—Certain obese patients had lower metabolic rates after eating, whereas thin patients had a rise in heat production in response to the test meal.[7] These results suggest there may be great differences in the efficiency with which various people utilize food energy, and that the obese may be able to maintain their body weights on below average caloric intakes.

• **Level of physical activity**—Subjects who exercised before and after a high calorie breakfast lost twice as much heat after eating as those who did not exercise.[8]

Hence, exercising before and after meals may result in a greater expenditure of calories than performance of the same amount of exercise at other times.

• **Prior level of dietary calories**—People who have long tried to lose weight by dieting sometimes find it difficult, if not impossible, to maintain a steady pattern of weight loss after having had some initial success in this regard. A study showed that about one-third of a group of women who had participated in weight control groups for 6 months or more could not lose weight on a diet containing 1,350 Calories (kcal).[9] Generally, the women who failed to lose weight had subnormal basal metabolic rates and low total energy expenditures. It was suspected that the low basal metabolism was an adaptation to the long use of low calorie diets.

• **Cellular metabolism**—Not all fat people are guilty of gluttony and sloth. On this point increasing physiological evidence agrees with the anguished testimony of overweight men and women. By and large, obese people do not eat more than thin people. As for sloth, it is noteworthy that physical activity accounts for only about 20% of most adults' energy expenditure. Why, then, do some people gain weight on a diet that allows others to remain slim, even at the same level of physical activity? It is not that the metabolic engine runs steadily at a lower energy cost in fat people than in thin people; it does not. Rather, it is because people with a tendency to obesity apparently are deficient in a particular cellular mechanism that in other people switches on automatically to burn off excess calories.

On being overfed, most people do not gain weight in proportion to the amount of overfeeding; they dispose of the extra energy by generating heat—through nonshivering thermogenesis (the production of heat in the body by oxidation). However, diet-induced thermogenesis is significantly reduced in obese and formerly obese individuals. This diminished thermogenesis may be due to a metabolic defect in brown fat, a particular tissue long known to be associated with heat production in young animals, and found mainly in the chest, upper back, and near the kidneys of adult animals. Brown fat is brown because it has more iron containing cytochrome molecules than white fat. The cytochromes are components of the membrane of the mitochondria; the cells of brown fat are packed with these organelles which carry out cellular respiration by oxidizing nutrient molecules. In the mitochondria of brown-fat cells, a proton leak bypasses the coupling of oxidation with adenosine triphosphate (ATP) production. As a result, the mitochondria, oxidizing local stores of fat, generate heat instead of ATP.

Although more experimental work is needed, it does seem clear that there is diminished capacity in many obese people for thermogenesis induced by dietary fat. The defect seems to be associated with brown fat. It could be that the amount of tissue is inadequate, or that there is a difference in the proton-leakage pathway, or that there is a failure at some stage of the switching-on process.

Of course, not all fat people suffer from a metabolic defect; many people do eat too much. However, because of the possibility of a metabolic defect, a physician should not too readily condemn his fat patients for lack of willpower while he, unwittingly, enjoys a physiological system that allows him to stabilize his own weight with effortless ease.

HORMONAL INFLUENCES ON METABOLISM.

The knowledge of the effects of the various hormones is at best a science in its infancy, since most of the major discoveries in this field have been made in the 20th century. When the early breakthroughs were first publicized, many doctors had high hopes of being able to treat obesity and other disorders with specific hormones which might produce immediate results like those seen in diabetics given insulin. The failure of these expectations to materialize led some doctors to abandon their interest in endocrinology. However, Dr. Bieler, a physician with a lifelong practice of medicine in California, has often classified his patients according to traits that he associates with the activity of various endocrine glands.[10] He believes that a careful scrutiny of a patient's features (body build, distribution and type of hair, facial characteristics, head shape and size, skin, and trunk) will usually reveal which of three endocrine glands is most active: the adrenals, the pituitary, or the thyroid. Greater activity of a particular gland may not necessarily indicate excessive secretion; rather, it may mean that the other glands are not fully active. Descriptions of Dr. Bieler's endocrine types follow:

---

[7]Robson, J. R. K., *et al.*, "Metabolic Response to Food," *The Lancet*, December 24 & 31, 1977, p. 1367.

[8]Miller, D. S., P. Mumford, and M. J. Stock, "Gluttony: 2. Thermogenesis in Overeating Man," *The American Journal of Clinical Nutrition*, Vol. 20, 1967, pp. 1228-1229.

[9]Miller, D. S., and S. Parsonage, "Resistance to Slimming: Adaptation or Illusion?," *The Lancet*, April 5, 1975, p. 773.

[10]Bieler, H. G., *Food is Your Best Medicine*, Random House, New York, N.Y., 1965, p. 83.

• **Adrenal**—This type is close in characteristics to the mesomorph which was described by Sheldon. However, Bieler adds additional physiological characteristics such as ease of childbirth in women, excellent digestive functions, immunity to infections, and steady nerves. Greater than normal secretion of the adrenals might confer abundant physical energy and drive, traits that are highly revered around the world. Nevertheless, other doctors believe that overactivity of the adrenal glands may also lead to the early development of coronary heart disease, particularly when the "physical" types of men and women spend most of their waking hours engaged in predominantly sedentary activities. Their good appetites and remarkable digestions may lead to obesity unless time is allotted for sufficient exercise, while frustration of their physical drives may lead to stress-induced disorders.

• **Pituitary**—A dominant pituitary gland often leads to tallness (due to abundant secretion of growth hormone), a large skull, and long fingers. Dr. Bieler considers this type to be highly creative and intellectual, but he admits that the information on this subject is limited. It would seem that pituitary types might be either lean or obese, since oversecretion of adrenocorticotrophic hormone (ACTH) from this gland may lead to Cushing's syndrome and its characteristic obesity.

• **Thyroid**—The body build of this type is very close to the ectomorphic type, and is characterized by slenderness. A high level of thyroid activity results in the rapid utilization of nutrients for calories. People in this group tend to be nervous, and are prone to becoming irritated with co-workers, family members, and friends. Although thyroid deficiency leads to obesity, most obese people have normal thyroid function since their obesity usually has other causes.

These generalizations should not be considered as hard and fast criteria for classifying the lean and the obese because most people have combinations of the features described under each of the endocrine types.

HORMONAL ABNORMALITIES IN THE OBESE. It is well known that patterns of endocrine secretion may be altered by such factors as the climate, diet, emotions, and the amount of body fat. For example, the development of obesity often results in increases in the secretion of insulin from the pancreas and of steroid hormones from the adrenal cortex; and by a decreased rate of secretion of growth hormones from the pituitary.[11] However, this does not mean that such abnormalities are the causes of obesity, since they often disappear when the body weight is reduced to normal. Nevertheless, once the abnormalities are established, they may make it difficult to lose weight.
Details of these abnormalities follow:

• **Adrenal cortical hormones**—The reason for oversecretion of these hormones in obesity is not known, except in the specific case of the uncommon disorder known as Cushing's syndrome which is accompanied by a peculiar type of obesity caused by large excesses of these hormones. Whatever the cause, an important effect of such hormonal excess is the development of resistance to the effects of insulin by tissues, a situation leading to elevated blood levels of insulin (hyperinsulinism) because the pancreas is overstimulated by the prolongation of high blood sugar levels after meals. This abnormality may bring on the clinical signs of diabetes in people who have a tendency to develop the adult-onset form of this disease.
(Also see DIABETES MELLITUS.)

• **Growth hormone**—Although it is suspected that oversecretion of this pituitary hormone may promote the development of obesity in growing children, secretion of the hormone is subnormal once obesity is established.[12] Reduction of obesity may be more difficult when growth hormone secretion is subnormal because this hormone promotes the release of fatty acids from stored fat during fasting, an action which helps to whittle down deposits of fat.

• **Insulin**—Oversecretion of this hormone by the pancreas helps to perpetuate obesity by (1) promoting the synthesis and storage of fat; and (2) causing the blood sugar to drop to low levels between meals, a condition which may lead to excessive appetite and overeating.

Thus, it seems that while some people may have inborn tendencies to fatness or leanness, others may somehow have become obese, then found it difficult to change their status because they developed hormonal abnormalities which made it difficult to lose weight. Although it might be convenient to assume that there are people who are destined to become obese because of subtle, hard-to-detect differences in their physiological or psychological traits, this concept leaves some unanswered questions. For example, it is well known (1) that the ancestors of many obese people were much leaner, and (2) that their relatives who are living under different circumstances may also be much leaner. Hence, it seems that there may be various external factors which promote obesity. These factors are discussed in the next section.

External Factors Which May Spur the Development of Obesity. Many of the lean people who believe that they have stronger character traits than the obese may not owe their success in staying lean to their own efforts; rather, they may owe them to complex physiological processes which regulate their appetites.

[11]Albrink, M. J., "Overnutrition and the Fat Cell," *Duncan's Diseases of Metabolism*, 7th ed., edited by P. K. Bondy and L. E. Rosenberg, W. B. Saunders Co., Philadelphia, Pa., 1974, pp. 428-429.

[12]Cheek, D. B., and J. J. White, "Obesity in Adolescents: Role of Hormones and Nutrition," *Proceedings of the Ninth International Congress of Nutrition (Mexico, 1972)*, edited by A. Chavez, S. Karger, Basel, Switzerland, 1975, p. 291.

There is evidence for both the short-term and the long-term regulation of food intake in species of animals which are similar to man in their physiology.[13] Details of appetite regulation are given elsewhere in this book.

(Also see APPETITE.)

Animal experiments have also shown that under various circumstances, appetite control may be interfered with, or bypassed, so that the animals will eat sufficient food for fattening to occur. For example, it is well known that confining livestock in pens speeds up their gains in weight. Likewise, other procedures, such as changing the composition of rations and/or administering hormones, helps the farmer to fatten his animals. Therefore, it is reasonable to expect that similar factors may spur the development of human obesity. Discussions of these factors follow:

• **Birth-control pills (oral contraceptives)**—These agents may provoke elevated blood levels of insulin,[14] a condition which is known to favor the development of obesity.

• **Climate**—It is well known that natives of tropical regions have basal metabolic rates that are, on the average, about 10% lower than those of people who live in cooler regions. Also, it is uncomfortable for many people to engage in strenuous physical activity when the weather is hot and humid. On the other hand, extremely cold weather may keep all but a few people indoors where their activities are usually sedentary. Also, it is noteworthy that people who live, work, and play in cold environments may expend extra energy to maintain their body temperatures.[15] Yet, the effect of cold environments on obese people is greatly diminished because their extra body fat acts as a layer of insulation which slows heat loss.

• **Cultural factors**—Until recently, obesity was considered to be very desirable by various peoples. For example, in certain parts of Africa women are still being fattened up prior to marriage, and a man's worth may be partly based upon the total weight of his wives. It is easy to understand how obesity came to be regarded as a sign of affluence by certain cultures, particularly when they had experienced many periods of deprivation. Even the practice of fattening children had considerable merit, because fat babies were most likely to survive the frequent bouts of infectious disease and diarrhea which were common before modern sanitary measures were established. Therefore, people who still adhere to the dietary patterns of their ancestors may become obese since such patterns were based upon much harsher ways of life.

• **Eating in response to external cues**—Many people are literally conditioned to eat, whether they require food or not, in response to such cues as the sight and smell of food, social gatherings, or while viewing movies or television. Hence, these people are likely to overeat and become obese if they are regularly exposed to these cues. A tendency to overindulge in eating desserts and sweets when lonely or depressed may be established in childhood by parents and relatives who use these foods as rewards or tokens of affection.

• **Emotional stresses**—Dr. Bruch, a psychiatrist on the faculty of Baylor College of Medicine in Texas who has long studied the psychiatric problems of obese children and adults, believes that for some people overeating and obesity may stem from chronic emotional disturbances.[16] For example, parents who impose the amounts and types of food that they think should be eaten may make it difficult for their children to learn how to recognize and satisfy their own hunger. Their children may develop tendencies to eat as a reaction to emotional stresses, or in response to such external cues as the presence of food. Needless to say, this inappropriate eating may lead to obesity. Emotional stresses in the obese may be further aggravated by condemnatory attitudes of other people. The sad irony of this situation is that the endomorphic, extroverted person, who is so dependent upon the stimulation derived from social interaction, may become isolated from others and develop severe depression.

• **Excessive dietary carbohydrates**—This nutrient, particularly when it is in a form which is rapidly digested and readily absorbed, is the strongest stimulator of the secretion of insulin, the hormone that promotes the synthesis and storage of fat. The most readily utilized forms of carbohydrates occur in such highly refined foods as table sugar and white flour, so it has often been suggested that overconsumption of foods containing these ingredients may be a major cause of obesity.

• **Excessive dietary fats**—It may seem strange that modern man worries about eating too much fat when it is considered that the earliest primitive societies depended on hunting animals and gathering plants for survival, which sometimes resulted in the eating of large quantities of meat and fat from the animals they killed. However, modern man lives in a different environment in which (1) the energy expenditures of most people are small compared to those of their distant ancestors; (2) it is now possible to have three meals a day, year in and year out, while in the past there were frequent periods of food deprivation due to scarcity; and (3) there are now available concentrated sources of fat such as butter, cream, margarine, and vegetable oils, which may be eaten separately or combined with cereals, fruits, and vegetables. Although it is said that dietary fat has a high satiety value (it may trigger an intestinal response which generates a satiety signal), its low bulk may allow some people to consume excessive calories before feeling satisfied. The filling of the small intestine seems to be

[13]Van Itallie, T. B., N. S. Smith, and D. Quartermain, "Short-Term and Long-Term Components in the Regulation of Food Intake: Evidence for a Modulatory Role of Carbohydrate Status," *American Journal of Clinical Nutrition*, Vol. 30, 1977, p. 742.

[14]Spellacy, W. N., K. L. Carlson, and S. A. Birk, "Carbohydrate Metabolic Studies after Six Cycles of Combined Type Oral Contraceptive Tablets. Measurement of Plasma Insulin and Blood Glucose Levels," *Diabetes*, Vol. 16, 1967, p. 590.

[15]Danowski, T. S., *Sustained Weight Control*, F. A. Davis Co., Philadelphia, Pa., 1973, p. 125.

[16]Bruch, H., "Psychological Implications of Obesity," *Nutrition News*, Vol. 35, 1972, p. 9.

one of the other factors which produce satiety. Furthermore, there is evidence that high-fat diets may impair the utilization of carbohydrates,[17] an effect which is undesirable because it might lead to adult-onset diabetes.

• **Excessive dietary proteins**—The test feeding of meals high in both proteins and carbohydrates provoked a marked increase in the secretion of insulin by adult males,[18] a situation which is well known to accelerate the laying down of fat. However, test feedings consisting only of lean meat were potent stimulators of the copious secretion of the growth hormone, mentioned earlier in this article as an agent favoring the development of obesity in growing children. These findings suggest the need for investigations of the long-term effects of eating excess protein.

• **Fatigue**—It is not a good idea to eat when one is excessively tired, unless the tiredness is due to lack of food and/or low blood sugar, because (1) it may lead to a habit of eating when tired; (2) the feeling of satiety may be dulled due to the fatigue, so one might overeat; and (3) the combination of fatigue and a meal might induce sleepiness so that physical activity is greatly reduced after eating. Therefore, it is a very bad practice to eat the bulk of the day's food at a late dinner after most of the day's activities are over.

• **Lack of exercise**—Research studies of both animals and humans by Dr. J. Mayer (an internationally known nutritionist, formerly at Harvard, now President of Tufts University) showed that at low levels of physical activity control of appetite falters so that there is usually consumption of excess energy and a gaining of weight.[19] He found that workers who had sedentary jobs ate more than those whose positions required more physical activity.

• **Lack of fiber**—It may be that there is a minimum requirement for bulk in the diet so that distention of the small intestine may make its contribution to feelings of satiety. Diets in the developed countries are usually low in fiber because (1) comparatively small amounts of food are eaten since energy expenditures are low, and (2) the food which is eaten is either naturally low in fiber (for example, meats) or there has been removal of fiber during processing.
(Also see FIBER.)

• **Meal patterns**—Recent research has shown that the eating of two or three large meals per day is more likely to result in excessive fattening than five or six smaller meals, even when the amounts and types of foods eaten are the same for the two different meal patterns.[20] A particularly bad practice is the skimping on food at breakfast and lunch so that more food may be eaten at supper, because the food deprivation during most of the day stimulates the body's fattening processes.

• **Nutritional deficiencies**—Metabolic and nervous abnormalities may result from deficiencies of minerals and vitamins, so it seems reasonable to suspect that these nutritonal deficiencies may lead to derangements in appetite control. Depraved appetites are often noted in malnourished livestock.

Disturbances in the utilization of carbohydrates may be produced by deficiencies of the nutrients chromium, iodine, magnesium, manganese, potassium, pyridoxine (vitamin B-6), and zinc. The utilization of carbohydrates somehow affects the functioning of the satiety center in the brain, which is a factor in the regulation of food intake. Hence, the advice to eat a wide variety of foods may not be helpful in avoiding obesity, since restrictions on calorie consumption mean that great care must be taken so as to obtain all of the required nutrients from the limited amounts of food which may be eaten.

• **Overfeeding of infants and children**—Many bottle-fed babies are literally force fed, particularly when mothers enlarge the holes in the rubber nipples, then prop up the bottle so that the milk runs down the throats of their babies. Another practice is holding the infant and spooning in as much baby food as will be tolerated. A recent study of infant feeding practices by a team at the Gerber Research Center in Michigan showed that mothers fed their children only slight excesses of calories, but great excesses of protein.[21] The effects of so much extra protein on children are not known, but it seems reasonable to suspect that it might force rapid growth, and perhaps contribute to obesity, because high-protein meals may overstimulate the secretion of both growth hormone and insulin.

As indicated in the earlier section headed "Early-onset obesity," it is extremely difficult to correct obesity which developed during childhood.

• **Overseasoning of food**—Heavy use of the seasoning agents catsup, garlic, onions, mustard, pepper, and sugar may make food highly palatable, increase the flow of digestive juices, and generally promote overeating. For example, it is difficult to imagine anyone but a very hungry person continuously overeating unseasoned cereal grains, lean meats, and vegetables. Another consequence of the overseasoning is the irritation of the tongue, esophagus, stomach, intestines, and anus (where the irritation may result in hemorrhoids).

• **Pregnancy**—Many women gain weight after each pregnancy. There is no general agreement as to why this occurs, although it may be for the same reason that fat-

[17]Anderson, J. W., and R. H. Herman, "Effects of Carbohydrate Restriction on Glucose Tolerance of Normal Men and Reactive Hypoglycemia Patients," *American Journal of Clinical Nutrition*, Vol. 28, 1975, p. 748.

[18]Pallotta, J. A., and P. J. Kennedy, "Response of Plasma Insulin and Growth Hormone to Carbohydrate and Protein Feeding," *Metabolism*, Vol. 17, 1968, p. 901.

[19]Mayer, J., "Why People Get Hungry," *Nutrition Today*, Vol. 1, June 1966, p. 2.

[20]Leveille, G. A., and D. R. Romsos, "Meal Eating and Obesity," *Nutrition Today*, Vol. 9, November/December 1974, p. 4.

[21]Purvis, G. A., "What Nutrients Do Our Infants Really Get?," *Nutrition Today*, Vol. 8, September/October 1973, p. 28.

tening occurs in the users of birth control pills (excessive secretion of insulin due to resistance of tissues to insulin). There is need for studies relative to the energy requirements during pregnancy and lactation, since the allowances used by nutritionists are at best only educated guesses.

• **Prenatal and early postnatal influences**—Many recent research reports have suggested that, if not genetic, the tendency towards lifelong obesity begins in a child at some time between the latter part of pregnancy and the end of the first year after birth.[22] For example, studies at age 19 of the boys born to mothers who were pregnant during the Dutch Famine of World War II (October 1944 to May 1945) showed that there was a higher incidence of obesity among those whose mothers were deprived of food early in pregnancy than among those whose mothers suffered deprivation later in pregnancy. Although the lower birth weights of the latter group might partly account for their lower incidence of obesity, it is noteworthy that another group of boys, who had equally low birth weights, but whose mothers had been starved in mid-pregnancy, had a higher incidence of obesity.

It seems likely that the diets and/or the hormonal patterns of pregnant mothers may affect the hormonal secretions of their offspring, since animal studies have shown that maternal overfeeding near the end of pregnancy resulted in oversecretion of insulin by the newborn.[23]

• **Rapid eating**—It has often been noted that many obese people appear to eat their food more rapidly than the nonobese. Hence, some doctors have instructed their patients who are trying to lose weight to eat slowly and to pause frequently between mouthfuls of food. Perhaps there is a delay in the operation of the various satiety mechanisms which allows rapid eaters to consume more than is required.

• **Sexual and other frustrations**—From time to time there are reports of studies which show that more obese than lean people complain of sexual frustration. There is usually a tendency to conclude from these reports that obesity may be caused or perpetuated by overeating in response to sexual and/or other types of frustrations. These generalizations are hard to verify because (1) the sex drive in humans is partly due to innate biological factors and partly due to cultural factors; (2) various ethnic, religious, and social groups may have different expectations concerning sex; and (3) people responding to questioning may find it easier to attribute feelings of general dissatisfaction with their circumstances to sexual frustration rather than attempt to look deeper into the root causes of their feelings. At any rate, the belief that various frustrations lead to overeating merits further investigation.

• **Social customs**—Eating is often an important part of baptisms, bar mitzvahs or confirmations, business luncheons, funerals, professional meetings, and weddings. Usually, each person is served much more food than they should eat; and in small, intimate gatherings it may be difficult for some to refuse what is offered when it is very appealing. While these infrequent binges may seem to be unimportant, it may be difficult for some people to regain control of their eating.

• **Types of food**—Overeating is more likely to occur when the forms and types of food are high in calories, low in fiber, and do not require much chewing. For example, mashed potatoes and gravy, soft puddings, tender meat which is highly marbled with fat, and white bread and butter are easy to eat compared to boiled potatoes, raw carrot sticks and celery, less tender cuts of lean meat, and unbuttered whole wheat bread.

People trying to lose weight have long been instructed to chew their food well, but the faithful following of such advice requires that much of the food eaten consists of items which cannot be comfortably swallowed without thorough chewing.

DISORDERS WHICH ARE OFTEN AGGRAVATED BY OBESITY.

Statistics from the Metropolitan Life Insurance Company show that obese people (those who are more than 20% overweight) have significantly higher death rates than the nonobese from such conditions as appendicitis, cancers of the gallbladder and liver, cirrhosis of the liver, diabetes, gallstones, heart disease, hernia and intestinal obstruction, kidney disease, stroke, and toxemia of pregnancy.[24] They are also more likely to die in automobile accidents. However, they have significantly lower rates of death by suicide.

The statistical associations between obesity and various medical problems do not necessarily mean that the former is always the cause of the latter. For example, a tendency towards diabetes may make some people more susceptible to obesity and other problems, whereas similar problems may be absent in others who are obese. Furthermore, it is important to distinguish between those problems which are directly aggravated by obesity and those which are only indirectly affected, because the choice of the most effective treatment for a disorder depends upon identification of the primary causative factor. Therefore, the effects of obesity on the disorders which follow are noteworthy:

• **Angina pectoris**—This term refers to a sharp pain in the chest and shoulder which regularly accompanies physical exertion, and which sometimes precedes a heart attack. It is due to an insufficient flow of blood to the heart muscle, which may often be the result of advanced atherosclerosis. Data collected in the well-known Framingham study showed that the risk of this condition

[22]"Influence of Intrauterine Nutritional Status on the Development of Obesity in Later Life," *Nutrition Reviews*, Vol. 35, 1977, p. 100.

[23]Butterfield, W. J. H., "Obesity—a Problem in a Changing World," *Nutritional Problems in a Changing World*, edited by D. Hollingsworth and M. Russell, Applied Science Publishers, Ltd., Essex, England, 1973, p. 13.

[24]Mayer, J., "Obesity," *Modern Nutriton in Health and Disease*, 5th ed., edited by R. S. Goodhart and M. E. Shils, Lea & Febiger, Philadelphia, Pa., 1973, p. 635, Table 22-4.

for obese males was about twice as great as that for nonobese males.[25] This study was conducted on over 5,000 men and women, aged 30 to 62, in Framingham, Massachusetts, which is about 20 miles (*32 km*) southwest of Boston.

(Also see HEART DISEASE.)

• **Breathing difficulties**—The weight of extra fat on the chest wall makes breathing more difficult in the grossly obese. It is noteworthy that obese infants and children have more respiratory problems than their nonobese counterparts.

• **Coronary heart disease**—This term is synonymous with *ischemic heart disease,* which means that there is an abnormal and dangerous reduction in the flow of blood through the coronary arteries to the heart muscle, a condition which is often due to atherosclerosis. It includes (1) myocardial infarction, which is death of part of the heart muscle due to lack of blood; (2) angina pectoris (which was discussed earlier in this section); and (3) sudden and unexpected death (to be discussed later in this section). The Framingham data suggest that the obese are much more likely than the nonobese to experience angina pectoris and sudden death, but that there is about an equal chance of the obese and nonobese suffering from myocardial infarction.

(Also see HEART DISEASE.)

• **Diabetes**—The life insurance statistics, which were mentioned earlier in this section, show that the obese are 3 to 4 times as likely to die from diabetes and/or its complications as are the nonobese. Perhaps the high death rate of the obese is due to the fact that when the cells of fatty tissues become engorged with fat, they develop a resistance to the effects of insulin, a condition which may greatly aggravate a diabetic tendency.

(Also see DIABETES MELLITUS.)

• **Easy fatigability**—Exercise is often difficult for the obese because of (1) the extra weight which has to be put into motion, and (2) the slower breathing which results in a subnormal oxygen content of arterial blood.[26] A considerable amount of extra effort must be expended by the obese to overcome these difficulties; hence, they may tire easily. Another cause of fatigue is low blood sugar, a frequent consequence of the excessive secretion of insulin which is often found in the obese.

• **Enlargement of the heart**—This condition may be first noticed when an obese person has either a chest x ray, or an electrocardiogram. It usually occurs on the left side of the heart (left ventricular hypertrophy) and is believed to result from the extra load on the heart which has been imposed by the obesity. However, it has also been found

in athletes who regularly participate in grueling events such as 6-day bicycle races. Excessive enlargement may dangerously weaken the heart muscle.

• **Excessive numbers of red blood cells and abnormal clotting of the blood**—The production of extra red cells is provoked by tissue shortages of oxygen, a situation which may occur when obese people have difficulty in breathing. An excessive number of red blood cells (polycythemia) is often accompanied by a thickening of the blood (increased resistance to flow) and a more rapid clotting.

• **Gallstones**—It is not known why gallstones and inflammation of the gallbladder occur more often in people characterized by the four f's (fair, fat, female, and forty). Some medical people believe that high-energy, high-fat diets may also spur the development of this condition.

(Also see GALLSTONES.)

• **Gout**—This disorder is a form of arthritis in which there are crystalline deposits of uric acid in such joints as the one in the middle of the big toe. The condition is usually accompanied by elevated blood levels of urates (salts of uric acid), which may sometimes be caused by crash diets low in carbohydrates, but high in fats and proteins. No one knows why highly successful, middle-aged, obese men have this disorder more often than other groups of people, although it appears to run in certain families.

(Also see GOUT.)

• **Hernia**—Large deposits of abdominal fat are often accompanied by weaknesses of the abdominal muscles. Hence very obese people are more prone to navel hernias. Also, the extra fat may crowd the stomach so that it pokes up through the opening in the diaphragm, producing the condition known as hiatus hernia.

• **High blood pressure**—Data from the Framingham study show that the risk of developing high blood pressure (systolic pressure 160 or over, or diastolic pressure 95 or over) was almost double for obese men and women compared to those with normal weight.

• **High levels of fats in the blood (hyperlipoproteinemias)**—Here again, the Framingham data showed that blood cholesterol changed in the same direction as changes in body weight. However the declines in blood triglycerides which accompany weight loss are usually much more dramatic than the changes in blood cholesterol. It seems that high blood triglycerides are often due to the insulin resistance which accompanies obesity.[27]

(Also see HYPERLIPOPROTEINEMIAS.)

• **Increased sweating and susceptibility to heat exhaustion**—An extra layer of body fat acts as insulation which slows the loss of heat from the body. Hence, keeping an obese body cool requires more sweating than

[25]Kannel, W. B., "The Disease of Living," *Nutrition Today,* Vol. 6, No. 3, May/June 1971, pp.2-11.

[26]Holley, H. S., *et al.,* "Regional Distribution of Pulmonary Ventilation and Perfusion in Obesity," *The Journal of Clinical Investigation,* Vol. 46, 1967, p. 475.

[27]Davidson, P. C., and M. J. Albrink, "Insulin Resistance in Hyperglyceridemia," *Metabolism,* Vol. 14, 1965, p. 1059.

is required for a lean body under similar conditions. A recent research study showed that when both obese and nonobese women were required to walk rapidly in a hot environment, the heavier ladies were under a greater heat stress as shown by the more pronounced increases in their body temperatures.[28]

• **Infertility in men**—Human sperm cells rapidly lose their vitality in warm environments, but their storage in the scrotum usually protects them against excessive heat. However, the scrotum in obese males may be surrounded by layers of fat on the thighs which block the loss of heat. Also, it is believed that the regular taking of excessively hot baths may similarly lower the fertility of some men.

• **Kidney disease**—Although insurance statistics show that obese policyholders have about twice the death rate from kidney diseases as the nonobese, these data do not necessarily prove that obesity is a direct cause of various kidney diseases. Rather, it may be that the higher rate of kidney disease in heavy people may stem from obesity-related disorders such as diabetes, gout (deposits of uric acid may damage the kidneys), and high blood pressure.

(Also see KIDNEY DISEASES.)

• **Low blood sugar (hypoglycemia)**—Many obese people have an abnormal condition in which high blood sugar coexists with high blood levels of insulin. Normally, a high level of insulin might be expected to cause a rapid drop in the blood sugar. However, in some people the abnormality may persist for only an hour or so after meals, after which there may be a drop in the blood sugar to an abnormally low level. Symptoms of low blood sugar may usually be relieved by eating some food, an act likely to help perpetuate overeating and obesity unless the diet is carefully planned.

• **Osteoarthritis**—This condition, unlike rheumatoid arthritis, is due mainly to the wear and tear on the joints which bear most of the weight of the body. Hence, it occurs mainly in the hips and knees and is aggravated by obesity.

• **Skin problems**—These problems are most common in heavy people because (1) they sweat more (moist skin is more susceptible to irritation and injury), and (2) folds of skin and fat rub together and sometimes cause chafing in sensitive areas.

• **Sleepiness**—Drowsiness may occur when the oxygen content of the blood is subnormal. It was mentioned earlier that many of the obese have shallow breathing because it requires extra effort for them to breathe hard enough to meet their oxygen needs. This tendency may lead to excessive inactivity and increased obesity.

• **Stroke**—The Framingham data suggested that obesity only slightly increased the risk of stroke, since this disorder appeared to be much more closely associated with abnormalities of heart function (as shown by an electrocardiogram) and with high blood pressure.[29]

• **Sudden-unexpected death**—Sixty percent of those who die from coronary heart disease in the United States die suddenly and unexpectedly.[30] Although the Framingham data showed that the risk to middle-aged males of sudden death due to a heart attack was about three times as great for the obese as for the nonobese, a more detailed analysis of this data shows that the male and female diabetics among the obese made a disproportionately high contribution to these statistics because they had more than four times the death rate of nonobese, nondiabetics.[31] When the data for diabetics were excluded, it appeared that the risk of sudden death for nondiabetic, obese males and females is about one and a half times as great as that for nondiabetic, nonobese people. It is not surprising that diabetes greatly increases this risk since many of the complications of the disease render a person more susceptible to ventricular fibrillation, a condition where the individual heart muscle fibers no longer beat in unison, and sudden death often occurs.

• **Surgical dangers**—Although precise statistics are not available, it is well known that obesity may greatly increase the risk of dire consequences from surgery. Some of the reasons for this increased risk are (1) it is difficult to judge the correct amount of anesthetic for an obese person, (2) there are more likely to be hidden abnormalities like diabetes in the obese, and (3) breathing difficulties may make it dangerous to use inhalation anesthetics.

• **Toxemia**—It is not known why obese women are more susceptible to toxemia of pregnancy, although the disorder is related to high blood pressure, a condition which is more likely to occur in obesity.

• **Troubles with the feet and legs**—As in the case of asteoarthritis, the extra weight in obesity puts greater stress on the lower limbs. Obese women seem to have more trouble with ulceration of varicose veins, but the obesity is not likely to be the cause of varicosities.

WAYS OF DETECTING BORDERLINE OBESITY.

The standard practice of doctors and life insurance companies has been to consider their clients to be obese when their body weight is greater than their ideal weight

---

[28]Bar-Or, O., H. M. Lundegren, and E. R. Buskirk, "Heat Tolerance of Exercising Obese and Lean Women," *Journal of Applied Physiology*, Vol. 26, 1969, p. 403.

[29]Kannel, W. B., G. Pearson, and P. M. McNamara, "Obesity as a Force of Morbidity and Mortality," *Adolescent Nutrition and Growth*, F. P. Heald, editor, Appleton-Century-Crofts, New York, N.Y., 1969, p. 62.

[30]Kuller, L. "Sudden Death in Atherosclerotic Heart Disease. The Case for Preventive Medicine," *American Journal of Cardiology*, Vol. 24, 1969, p. 617.

[31]Kannel, W. B., G. Pearson, and P. M. McNamara, "Obesity as a Force of Morbidity and Mortality," *Adolescent Nutrition and Growth*, F. P. Heald, editor, Appleton-Century-Crofts, New York, N.Y., 1969, p. 60.

(for their height and body build) by some arbitrary figure—commonly 20%. This arbitrary figure may be an unsatisfactory boundary between normal weight and obesity when (1) it is too low, as in the cases of people who have heavy bones and muscles; or (2) it is too high, as in the case of people with abnormally slender bones and muscles. Nevertheless, it is not wise to wait until someone is grossly obese before taking corrective measures, since the difficulty in achieving weight reduction increases with the degree of obesity. Therefore, it is worth noting the diagnostic standards which follow.

Formulas for Estimating Desirable Body Weights. Doctors and dietitians commonly estimate desirable weights for (1) adult males by allowing 106 lb for the first 5 ft of height and 6 lb for each additional inch of height over 5 ft, and (2) adult females by allowing 100 lb for the first 5 ft of height and 5 lb for each additional inch. According to the formula for males, a man who is 6 ft 2 in. tall has a desirable weight of 106 lb + 14 × 6 lb (for each inch of height over 5 ft) = 190 lb.

Height-Weight Tables. The first of these tables to be published in the United States was compiled from data on people who purchased life insurance policies between 1885 and 1908. There were two such tables, one for men and one for women, which listed the average weights found for people of various heights and ages. However, as the number of people purchasing life insurance policies increased over the years, these tables were found to have their limitations in that (1) the data were based mainly on sedentary, prosperous people who were not typical of the rest of the population; (2) the average weights for older people were heavier than those for younger people, although the weight gained in adulthood tends to be mostly fat, which is likely to be more of a detriment than a benefit to health; and (3) no provision had been made for differences in body builds.

The limitations of the earlier tables led the Metropolitan Life Insurance Company to introduce new ones in 1943. These new tables had no classification of weight by age since their weights were based mainly on those found in young adults. Also, a range of weights was substituted for single values of average weights, and each height category had weight ranges for small, medium, and large body builds. However, no details were given as to the means for distinguishing between the various body builds. A major limitation of these new tables was that even though the average weights of younger people were used as standards, there was no certainty that these weights were associated with longevity.

Finally, representatives from 26 life insurance companies in the United States and Canada pooled and analyzed their data on body weight and mortality which had been compiled from the records of several million policyholders over a period of 20 years. The data in this study were published in 1959.[32] Shortly thereafter, the Metropolitan Life Insurance Company issued new,

revised tables of desirable weights, which were those found to be associated with the greatest longevity. These tables, like the ones which preceded them, give a range of weights for each of the three categories of build. It should be noted that the values for heights and weights which are presented in these tables represent those obtained from people wearing shoes and their usual indoor clothing. This means that the heights have been obtained from men wearing shoes with 1-in. heels, and from women wearing 2-in. heels; and that the total extra weight for clothing in the men was about 8 lb, while in women it was about 5 lb. Here again, it is necessary for the examiner to decide on a person's body build, since no directions are given for making such determinations. Even if body build were to be determined more precisely, there would still be considerable variation of the relative proportions of fat and lean tissues within each body build.

Therefore, desirable weights obtained from the life insurance tables, or from the formula given in the preceding section, give at best only rough indications of the most desirable body characteristics.

An Index of Slenderness (Ponderal Index). This derived quantity represents an attempt to express relative leanness as a function of height and weight. It is obtained through the use of the following formula:

$$\text{Ponderal Index (PI)} = \frac{\text{Height (in.)}}{\sqrt[3]{\text{Weight (lb)}}}$$

This quantity may also be calculated using metric units. However, the values so obtained cannot be compared with those obtained using English units because the ratios of the height to weight units differ between the two systems of measurement. The ponderal index has the applications that follow:

PREDICTION OF THE EFFECTS OF BODY WEIGHT ON HEALTH. The higher the ponderal index, the greater the leanness and the lower the risk of cardiovascular disease since values under 12.0 are associated with higher rates of this type of disorder.[33] People who have ponderal indexes of 13 or more have very low risk for cardiovascular disease because they are more slender than average. The major limitations of the use of the ponderal index for evaluating adult body weights are (1) it is distorted on the low side for people who are very short of stature, so it tends to overestimate the risks due to weight in these people; and (2) it is distorted on the high side for very tall people, so it underestimates the risks due to weight in these people. For example, a short man (5 ft 1 in.) with a heavy build whose weight (126 lb)

[32]*Build and Blood Pressure Study*, 1959, Society of Actuaries, Chicago, Ill., 1959.

[33]Seltzer, C. C., "Some Re-evaluations of the build and Blood Pressure Study, 1959, as Related to Ponderal Index, Somatotype and Mortality," *New England Journal of Medicine*, Vol. 274, 1966, p. 254.

is right in the middle of the range of desirable weights given in the Metropolitan Life Insurance Tables has a ponderal index of 12.2, which suggests that he is close to the high-risk category. On the other hand, a tall, heavy-built man (6 ft 3 in.) whose weight (193 lb) is also right in the middle of the range of desirable weights has a ponderal index of 13.0, which suggests that he is a low risk. Hence, in these cases the ponderal indexes are not in line with the weight categories in the life insurance tables, which are backed up by considerably more data than the ponderal index.

ESTIMATION OF TRENDS TOWARDS FATNESS OR LEANNESS IN GROWING CHILDREN.

In this application, a ponderal index which increases with growth in height supposedly indicates a thinning out; while an index which decreases with growth indicates fattening. Although there has been little use of the ponderal index for this purpose, it has been suggested that a value of less than 12.4 might indicate obesity in adolescent girls.[34]

Pinch Tests for Hidden Fat.

Skinfold measurements are more precise versions of the long used "pinch" tests for obesity. In a pinch test, one selects an area of the body where fat is likely to be deposited and grasps a double fold of skin between his thumb and forefinger. Excessive fat is present when the thickness of the double fat is an inch (2.5 cm) or more. Special calipers are available for accurately measuring skinfold thicknesses. The use of these calipers is shown in Fig. O-8.

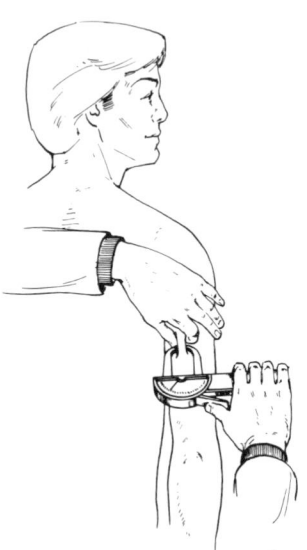

Fig. O-8.   The use of skinfold calipers.

Fig. O-8 shows a skinfold measurement being made on the triceps at a point on the back of the arm which is midway between the shoulder and the elbow. Other sites where skinfold measurements are often taken are (1) the subscapular region, which is just below the bottom of the shoulder blade; (2) the skin over the midpoint of the biceps; (3) the lower abdominal region, halfway between navel and the groin; and (4) the skin just above the top of the hip bone.

It is easiest to obtain the thickness of the skinfold over the triceps, because it may usually be measured without the removal of indoor clothing. Hence, it has been proposed that abnormally high values of this measurement be considered as indicative of obesity.[35] However, the thickness of the subscapular skinfold has been found to be more closely correlated with elevated blood fats.[36] (It is a good indicator of fatness on the trunk of the body.) Finally, it may not be advisable to base standards for skinfolds on pooled data which have been gathered from different ethnic groups, because there is evidence suggesting that there might be considerable differences in the distribution of body fat in people from such diverse groups.[37]

Weighing People Under Water.

Anyone observing obese people swimming can hardly fail to notice that their bodies float higher in the water than those of nonobese people. The reason for the greater buoyancy in the obese is that a given volume of fatty tissue weighs only about 90% as much as an equal volume of lean tissue. While it appears obvious that differences in the body fat content of people might be detected by immersing them in water, it took an unusual set of circumstances to generate interest in this procedure.

During World War II, a group of young men who were professional football players were rejected from service in the U.S. Navy because of overweight. However, the fact that they were well muscled and did not appear to be obese attracted the attention of the naval surgeon, Behnke, who with the help of his associates, studied the body compositions of these men and others.[38] Body densities were determined by weighing them (1) in air, and (2) while immersed in water. Calculations based upon these data showed that the athletes had unusually small amounts of fat in their bodies, and that their extra weights were due to lean tissue made up of bone, muscle, and water. Some of the athletes had as little as 4%

[34]Canning, H., and J. Mayer, "Obesity—Its Possible Effect on College Acceptance," *The New England Journal of Medicine*, Vol. 275, 1966, p. 1172.

[35]Seltzer, C. C., and J. Mayer, "Simple Criterion of Obesity," *Postgraduate Medicine*, Vol. 38, 1965, p. A101.

[36]Albrink M. J., and J. W. Meigs, "The Relationship between Serum Triglycerides and Skinfold Thickness in Obese Subjects," *Annals of the New York Academy of Sciences*, Vol. 131, 1965, p. 673.

[37]Robson, J. R. K., M. Bazin, and R. Soderstrom, "Ethnic Differences in Skinfold Thickness," *The American Journal of Clinical Nutrition*, Vol. 24, 1971, p. 864.

[38]Welham, W. C., and A. R. Behnke, Jr., "The Specific Gravity of Healthy men; Body Weight ÷ Volume and Other Physical Characteristics of Exceptional Athletes and of Naval Personnel," *Journal of the American Medical Association*, Vol. 118, 1942, p. 498.

body fat, whereas the average amount found in young, adult men is about 25%.[39] Although measurement of body density is generally limited to research studies, it is a useful tool for evaluating other more convenient measurements such as skinfold thicknesses.

Detection of Early Signs of Obesity in Children.
Much might be done to prevent hard-to-manage obesity in adults if more efforts were made to detect and treat the early stages of fattening in children. However, children tend to grow at variable rates so many doctors are reluctant to advise dietary restriction for heavier than average children for fear of slowing their rates of growth.

One means of detecting fattening in children is to pay close attention to the long-term pattern of growth in each child, rather than attempting to make a judgment on the basis of one-time measurements of height and weight. The pattern of growth is determined by plotting the monthly values of a child's height and weight on a standard growth chart. The standard charts usually have curved lines corresponding to growth rates for the 97th, 90th, 75th, 50th, 25th, 10th, and 3rd percentiles of the population of children. There are separate charts for boys and girls.

For example, an infant, who at the age of 6 months had a height and weight corresponding to the 75th percentile of the population, would usually be judged to be growing at a normal rate, because the statistical range of normal values extends from the 3rd to the 97th percentiles. However, if the same infant had from birth up to age 5 months followed the curves for the 25th percentile of heights and weights, then there would be reason to suspect that the child's growth might have been excessively rapid between 5 and 6 months of age, because of the progression from the 25th to the 75th percentiles in a month. This finding should lead the doctor or other examiner to question the parent as to the feeding of the infant, since overfeeding may force rapid growth and ultimately produce an obesity that is difficult to correct. Likewise, a body weight which is disproportionately high (for example, in the 75th percentile) for height (which might be in the 25th percentile) should lead an examiner to suspect excessive fattening.

TREATMENT OF OBESITY.
While the prospects of developing any of the deadly disorders associated with obesity are enough to make anyone shudder, there are rarely good reasons for crash dieting, since extremely rapid rates of weight loss are metabolically equivalent to the eating of extraordinary quantities of dietary fat. Hence, the cure may be worse than the disease. Furthermore, many other metabolic abnormalities may accompany drastic changes in body weight. Therefore, it is worth noting the principles of weight control that follow.

Principles of Weight Reduction.
It is often said that all a person has to do to lose weight is to eat fewer calories than is needed to meet his or her requirements. While this statement may be true over a long period of time, short-term changes in body weight often appear to defy these scientific principles. For example, a very lean person who skips supper one night might lose as much as 2 lb (0.9 kg) while a very obese person may go without food for two whole days and yet lose no weight. Furthermore, even very obese people might lose as much as 2 lb (0.9 kg) per day, when their daily diet is restricted to 400 Calories (kcal) from fat or protein alone, or from mixtures of these nutrients. The secret behind such seemingly contradictory observations is that weight losses may be due not only to loss of fat, but also to losses of variable amounts of water and protein from the lean tissues of the body. Explanations follow:

- **Different types of weight loss**—The major objective of losing weight should be to get rid of excess fat, but people often go on crash diets, take drugs, or engage in other activities that cause abnormal losses of lean tissue, which is composed of protein and water. Since more than 60% of the body is water, it stands to reason that measures which provoke loss of body water may produce immediate and drastic losses of weight, whereas loss of fat may proceed much more slowly because each pound (454 g) of body fat will supply the caloric needs of a starved adult female for 2 days.

- **How loss of body fat is provoked by shortages of calories**—Right after a meal, the dietary sources of calories (carbohydrates, fats, and proteins) are first used to meet the immediate needs of the body; then what remains is stored as fat. Between meals, there is a gradual, but steady, release of fats from tissue stores because the body's needs for calories are continuous, even during the hours of sleeping. The metabolism of fats for calories results in the production of chemical energy (which is used for such purposes as muscle contraction), heat energy, carbon dioxide, and water. A net loss of body fat usually occurs when energy utilization outstrips energy intake, a condition which is called a calorie deficit. Generally, there will be a loss of a pound of body weight, which is mainly fat, when there is a deficit of 3,500 Calories (kcal). However, the loss of body fat does not necessarily mean that there will be a loss of weight because the 1.12 lb (0.51 kg) of water which is derived from the metabolism of each pound of fat is not always excreted promptly.

- **Reasons why it may be difficult for some obese people to lose weight**—A sharp restriction of calories sometimes fails to result in a loss of weight because (1) the fatty tissues may not release fats when calories are needed, due to a shortage of growth hormone which often accompanies obesity, (2) some people retain the water from the metabolism of their body fat, or (3) there may be a more efficient utilization of energy (less escapes in the form of heat) by some people.[40]

---

[39]Mayer, J., *Human Nutrition*, published by Charles C. Thomas, Springfield, Ill., 1972, p. 324.

[40]Bray, G. A., "Effect of Diet and Triiodothyronine on the Activity of sn-Glycerol-3-Phosphate Dehydrogenase and the Metabolism of Glucose and Pyruvate by Adipose Tissue of Obese Patients," *Journal of Clinical Investigation*, Vol. 48, 1969, p. 1413.

• **Differences between the nutrients metabolized and those supplied in the diet**—There is a tendency to identify the composition of the metabolic mixture which is used for energy by the body with the nutrient composition of the diet. However, the two mixtures may be quite different because (1) the fat content of the mixture of nutrients which is metabolized by the body may be much higher than that in the diet, particularly when the diet is low in calories and large amounts of body fat must be utilized; (2) even on low-carbohydrate diets, the metabolism of carbohydrates may be greater than expected when there is a large-scale conversion in the body of proteins to carbohydrates, which occurs under various conditions of stress; (3) lean people who are deprived of dietary calories may be forced to derive them from the destructive metabolism of their body proteins. Therefore, special tests of metabolic functions may be needed in order to determine correctly the proportions of carbohydrate, fat, and protein which are utilized for energy by the body.

• **The effects of skipping meals on very lean people**— Fat stores may be minimal in some very lean people who may therefore have unusually large losses of weight when deprived of food. For example, a daily deficit of 500 Calories (kcal) will usually produce a weight loss of about 1 lb (0.45 kg) per week in people who have ample body fat, but the same energy deficit may cause the loss of as many as 8 lb, (3.6 kg) more, in lean people who must utilize their body protein for calories. (One pound of body protein is equivalent to 1,800 Calories [kcal], but each pound of protein is associated with an additional 3 lb [1.4 kg] of water which is usually lost from the body when the protein is metabolized for energy.)

• **How low-carbohydrate diets promote rapid loss of weight**—These diets produce their effects by means of a carbohydrate deficiency which (1) greatly slows the production and storage of fat, but accelerates the rate of fat release from the tissues into the blood; (2) impedes the complete metabolism of fats for energy, so that there is a production of ketones which reduce the appetite; (3) may cause the breakdown and conversion of tissue protein to carbohydrates for maintenance of the blood sugar; and (4) promotes an increased loss of water and various mineral salts in the urine. Low-carbohydrate diets may also produce metabolic adaptations in the body which lead to rapid gains in weight whenever one resumes the eating of normal amounts of carbohydrates. Most of these diets are high in fats and proteins from such foods as cheeses, eggs, and meats, but they contain only small amounts of the carbohydrate-rich fruits, grains, and vegetables.

Hence, mineral and vitamin supplements may be required in order to make up for missing nutrients which would normally be provided by the latter foods.

• **Protein-sparing fasts, the latest dietary concept for weight reduction**—Complete abstinence from food during fasting or starvation results in a rapid loss of weight due to the destructive metabolism of both fatty and lean tissues for energy. While the swift loss of body fat may often be desirable, the loss of substantial amounts of protein from the lean tissues might result in a weakening of the body, and perhaps some damage to vital organs. Hence, an ideal diet seems to be one which produces a rapid loss of fat while sparing the body's essential proteins.

The concept of protein-sparing is not new, it has merely been revised recently by medical researchers in Boston who were seeking means of preventing protein loss in hospital patients whose diets had to be restricted after surgery.[41] They found that (1) obese volunteers who were fed only 12 oz (340 g) of lean meat, fish, or poultry per day lost little of their body's protein while losing weight, whereas similar volunteers who were starved lost considerable amounts of protein; and (2) the intravenous injection of an amino acid solution in amounts equivalent to the protein fed to the obese volunteers almost completely halted the losses of body protein in surgical patients who were not given any food.

The reports of protein-sparing by these medical researchers inspired the promotion of various "predigested" liquid protein diets for weight reduction. Many of these diet formulas consist of water solutions of acid-digested proteins from such cartilaginous items as beef tendon, cowhide, or pork skin—to which various flavorings and supplementary amino acids, minerals, and vitamins may be added. However, there does not seem to be any advantage to the feeding of digested proteins to normal, healthy people. (The main medical use of predigested protein formulas is in the feeding of people with digestive problems.)

NOTE: The Food and Drug Administration (FDA) of the U.S. Department of Health, Education, and Welfare announced on November 10, 1977 that it intended to ask the manufacturers of predigested liquid protein diets to state on their labels that *these products should not be used without medical supervision*. This announcement came after it was learned that about a dozen or more obese women who used these diets died from various heart disorders.

Although the frequent occurrence of nonrhythmic heartbeats in the stricken dieters suggested that the cause of the heart problems was potassium deficiency, it is noteworthy that three liquid protein dieters in California were similarly afflicted, although each of them took potassium supplements with their diets.[42] Unfortunately, there is often a tendency to overlook the fact that magnesium is required for the "pumping" of potassium from the blood into the cells of the heart muscle.[43] Hence, potassium supplements may not be fully effective when magnesium is lacking.

[41]"Protein-Sparing Produced by Proteins and Amino Acids," *Nutrition Reviews*, Vol. 34, 1976, p. 174.

[42]Bishop, J. E., "Deaths of 2 Liquid Protein Dieters Tied to Unusual Heart Rhythm Abnormalities," *The Wall Street Journal*, December 1, 1977, p. 8.

[43]Seelig, M. S., and H. A. Heggtveit, "Magnesium Interrelationships in Ischemic Heart Disease: A Review," *The American Journal of Clinical Nutrition*, Vol. 27, 1974, p. 59.

Another cause of the heart problems might have been lack of vitamin E, since nonrhythmic heartbeats also occurred in the case of a woman who died after 30 weeks of total starvation.[44] An autopsy showed that her heart muscle contained brown pigment, a characteristic sign of vitamin E deficiency. Also found was the wasting of the heart muscle fibers which commonly occurs when large amounts of body protein are metabolized for energy.

Finally, there is a lack of information concerning the long-term effect of these diets because the Boston studies of protein sparing lasted for only a few weeks. It is noteworthy that the FDA announced on December 7, 1977, that tests of three well-known brands of liquid protein showed that the protein quality of these formulas was extremely poor because they failed to support the growth of laboratory rats. Hence, people who use these formulas as their sole source of dietary protein might have excessive breakdown of their tissue proteins as their bodies attempt to make good the deficiencies of the liquid diets.

• **Dangers of diets based upon imbalances between the major nutrients**—The greatest danger of imbalanced diets is their potential for inducing abnormalities in such vital processes as acid-alkali (base) balance; excretion of wastes; fluid distribution in the blood and various tissues; metabolism of carbohydrates, fats, and proteins; and the patterns of hormonal secretion. For example, low-carbohydrate diets produce, in addition to the effects mentioned earlier, high blood levels of uric acid and ketones. These are conditions which may aggravate or precipitate such metabolic disorders as electrolyte imbalances, gout, or ketoacidosis.

• **Fiber and water; substances that fill, but do not fatten** —Many people who are trying to lose weight search for tasty, low-calorie foods which are filling but not fattening. Most of our traditional, well-liked foods are high in calories—a habit inherited from bygone days when almost everyone expended much more energy in physical activity. The demand for low-calorie items has led to the fortification of cereal products with such high-fiber items as bran and refined forms of cellulose, substances which add bulk to the diet because (1) they are only minimally digested, and (2) they absorb and hold water in the digestive tract. People who are avoiding cereals because of their carbohydrate content may obtain plenty of fiber and water from low-calorie vegetables such as artichokes, asparagus, beet greens, broccoli, cabbage, carrots, cauliflower, celery, chicory, cucumbers, eggplant, green peppers, kale, lettuce, mustard greens, okra, sauerkraut, snapbeans, and turnip greens. These vegetables provide fewer calories when served raw because cooking increases the availability of the small amounts of carbohydrates which are present.

(Also see CARBOHYDRATE[S], UNAVAILABLE; and FIBER.)

44Holden, E. M., "Fragmentation of Cardiac Myofibrils After Therapeutic Starvation," *The Lancelot*, Vol. ii, 1969, p. 55.

Planning Diets and Selecting Foods. Anyone with a tendency to become obese needs to plan a balanced diet which provides the required nutrients, but which does not contain excess calories. It is easy to do such planning when one follows the procedures used by dietitians and others with expertise in planning such meals. Simplified versions of these procedures follow.

MODIFIED DIETS. This term is now used instead of the older designation of "special diets" because nutritionists want to advance the idea that one should start with a basic diet which is suitable for most people, then modify it so as to achieve whatever composition may be desired. The modifications which are usually made for low-calorie diets involve reduction in the number of items high in carbohydrates and fats, but retention of those which are good sources of proteins, minerals, and vitamins. For example, it might be desirable to avoid candy, cookies, cakes, ice cream, butter or margarine, and table sugar, and to substitute in their place, whole grain breads, fruits, vegetables, and salad oils. Also, the leaner cuts of meat such as round steak might be used in place of short ribs, porterhouse steak, and luncheon meats (which tend to have higher fat contents).

However, such dietary modifications may not in themselves be sufficient to produce loss of weight, because excessive quantities of the low-calorie foods may be eaten. Therefore, it is often necessary to calculate caloric requirements so that the dietary calorie content may be low enough to produce the appropriate caloric deficit. Descriptions of such calculations follow:

• **Estimating requirements for calories**—The equation for this calculation is: Calories (kcal) in modified diet equal caloric requirement minus caloric deficit for weight loss.

Most people require 15 Calories (kcal) or less per pound of desirable weight. (Desirable weights may be estimated by the means described in the section headed "Ways of Detecting Borderline Obesity.")

The caloric deficit is 500 Calories (kcal) per day to lose 1 lb (0.45 kg) per week, or 1,000 Calories (kcal) to lose 2 lb. People who wish to lose weight more rapidly should only do so under a doctor's supervision.

• **Selecting foods to make up a diet**—It is not wise to select foods solely on the basis of their calorie contents (a practice that is sometimes called "counting calories") because it may lead to dietary deficiencies. Instead, one should select items from each of the various food groups so as to obtain a nutritionally balanced diet. Even then, the diet may not furnish all of the required nutrients unless special effort is made to select foods which are good sources of these nutrients, such as dairy products, eggs, fish, fresh or frozen fruits and vegetables, meats, and whole grain cereal products. However, the amounts of these highly nutritious items must be limited in order to keep the energy content of the diet low enough for weight loss to occur. Hence, it is best to use the exchange system for planning diets. Table O-3 gives some typical diets planned by this system.

TABLE O-3
TYPICAL MENUS FOR VARIOUS TYPES OF LOW-ENERGY DIETS

Types of Food Exchanges[1] (used for each meal or snack)	Number of Exchanges Per Meal (based upon daily energy requirements)					
	Low Carbohydrate Diet		Low-Fat Diet		High Carbohydrate Very Low-Fat Diet	
	1,200 kcal per day	1,500 kcal per day	1,200 kcal per day	1,500 kcal per day	1,200 kcal per day	1,500 kcal per day
Breakfast:						
Bread (or biscuits, cereals, crackers, muffins, pancakes, waffles, etc.)	1	1	1	1	1	2
Fat (bacon, butter, coffee lightener, margarine, mayonnaise, etc.)[2]	1	1	1	1	0	1
Fruit (or its equivalent in juice)	1	1	1	1	1	1
Lean meat (or low-fat cheese, fish, fowl, etc.)	1	1	1	1	0	0
Milk, nonfat[2]	0	0	0	0	1	1
Optional beverage: bouillon (fat free), clear broth, club soda, coffee, herb tea, tea, water	◀————— Any amount, but limit sweetener[3] —————▶					
Mid-morning snack:						
Bread	0	0	1	1	1	1
Fat	0	1	0	0	0	0
Milk, nonfat	1	1	1	1	0	0
Optional beverage (see Breakfast)	◀————— Any amount, but limit sweetener[3] —————▶					
Lunch:						
Bread	1	1	1	2	2	3
Fat	2	2	0	2	0	1
Fruit (or juice)	0	0	0	1	1	1
Meat, lean (see Breakfast)	3	3	3	3	2	2
Optional beverage (see Breakfast)	◀————— Any amount, but limit sweetener[3] —————▶					
Raw vegetable, or salad without dressing	1	1	1	1	1	1
Mid-afternoon snack:						
Bread	0	0	1	1	0	1
Fat	0	1	0	0	0	0
Milk, nonfat	1	1	1	1	1	1
Optional beverage (see Breakfast)	◀————— Any amount, but limit sweetener[3] —————▶					
Supper:						
Bread	1	1	1	2	2	2
Fat	3	3	1	2	0	1
Fruit	0	1	0	0	1	1
Meat, lean (see Breakfast)	3	4	3	3	3	3
Optional beverage (see Breakfast)	◀————— Any amount, but limit sweetener[3] —————▶					
Nonstarchy vegetable, cooked	1	1	1	1	1	1
Raw vegetable, or salad without dressing	1	1	1	1	1	1
Late evening snack:						
Bread	0	1	0	0	1	1
Fat	0	1	0	0	1	0
Fruit (or juice)	0	0	1	1	0	0
Milk, nonfat	1	1	1	1	1	1

[1]Exchanges are portions of food which have been grouped together because they contain similar proportions of carbohydrates, fats, proteins, and calories. Portion sizes have been calculated so that the exchanges within each group may be substituted for one another because their nutritive values are approximately equal. (Also see MODIFIED DIETS, section headed "Use of Exchange Lists in Planning Diets.")

[2]The distribution of fat at meals may have to be adjusted if the foods chosen from among the other groups of exchanges contain more or less fat than the amount which is typical for each of the groups. For example, two fat exchanges should be deducted from the amounts allowed each time that whole milk is used instead of the nonfat type, or one fat exchange deducted to compensate for the use of 2% milk or plain yogurt in lieu of nonfat milk. Similarly, one fat exchange should be deducted for each exchange of high-fat meat used instead of lean meat, or ½ fat exchange deducted for each exchange of medium-fat meat. Also, many doctors recommend that, wherever possible, the items used as fat exchanges be chosen from such sources of polyunsaturated fats as salad oils and soft margarines because ample amounts of saturated fats are provided by the meat exchanges.

[3]These fluids contain few calories, so they may be taken as desired. However, the use of sugar and other sweeteners should be limited because 4 tsp (*20 ml*) of sugar furnish about the same amount of carbohydrates as one bread exchange, 1¾ fruit exchanges, one nonfat milk exchange, or three exchanges from the cooked vegetables.

Table O-3 gives typical menus for diets which are (1) low in carbohydrates (thought to be useful for abnormally high levels of blood triglycerides), (2) moderately low in fat content (the basis of the most commonly used standard diets), and (3) high in carbohydrates and very low in fats (this type of diet may be helpful in preventing heart disease). However, it was noted earlier that when the dietary energy deficit is great enough to bring about the metabolism of large amounts of body fat, the mixture of nutrients metabolized by the body will have a much higher fat content than the diet. Hence, even low-fat diets may make it necessary for the body to burn considerable amounts of fat, which is mostly saturated because it is derived mainly from the fatty tissues. Therefore, one should avoid crash diets which result in the loss of more than 2 lb per week because the metabolic consequences of such programs are uncertain.

The procedure for using the table follows:

1.   Determine your desirable body weight by either referring to a standard height-weight table, or by using the appropriate formula given in the section headed "Formulas for Estimating Desirable Body Weights."

2.   Calculate your caloric requirement for maintenance of weight by multiplying your ideal body weight by 15.

3.   Choose a dietary calorie level by deducting a caloric deficit of either 500 Calories (kcal) (to lose 1 lb [0.45 kg] per week) or 1,000 Calories (kcal) (to lose 2 lb per week) from your caloric requirement calculated in step 2. Do not select a diet which furnishes less than 1,000 Calories (kcal) per day without consulting a physician.

4.   Set up a daily menu by selecting exchanges from the food groups listed in Table O-3.

(Also see MODIFIED DIETS, section headed "Use of Exchange Lists in Planning Diets.")

EXAMPLE: An adult female who is 5 ft 4 in. (163 cm) tall and has a medium body build, weighs 140 lb (63 kg). She would like to get her weight down to normal as soon as possible. Her ideal body weight is 120 lb (54 kg) and her energy requirement for maintenance of this weight is 1,800 Calories (kcal) per day. It is not advisable for her to try and lose more than 1 lb (0.45 kg) per week because diets containing less than 1,200 Calories (kcal) per day are neither nutritious nor satisfying. Hence, it might take her about 17 weeks to reach her ideal weight if she sticks to her diet. (Her weight loss might be accelerated by extra activity.) Some typical meals and snacks for a 1,200 Calorie (kcal) low-fat diet are given in the column on the right. Generally, such low-fat, high-carbohydrate diets are more filling than low-carbohydrate, high-fat diets because the former contain more high-fiber foods like bread (if whole grain varieties are used) and fruits, while the latter are based upon foods where the calories are concentrated in a small amount of bulk.

(Also see FIBER.)

Meal	Menu		Calorie (kcal)
Breakfast ...	Ready-to-eat cereal	¾ c......	70
	with nonfat milk	¾ c......	60
	and sliced fresh	1 whole	
	peaches	peach ..	40
	Coffee	1 c......	0
	Evaporated skim		
	milk	2 Tbsp ...	20
	Sugar..........	½ tsp	9
Mid-morning Snack	Graham crackers .	two 2½ in. square ...	70
	Tea with lemon ..	1 c......	0
Lunch	Sandwich made with whole-rye		
	bread..........	2 slices ..	140
	boiled ham	2 slices ..	110
	lettuce, tomato, and mustard...	no limit ..	0
	Clear, fat-free hot		
	broth	1 c......	0
	Apple..........	one 2 in. diameter	40
Mid-afternoon snack	Nonfat milk	1 c......	80
Supper	Tossed salad made with chicory, chopped green peppers, mushroom slices, oregano (dried), and vinegar	no limit ..	0
	Flank steak	three 1 oz slices ...	165
	Horseradish sauce	2 tsp	0
	Mashed potato without butter or margarine	½ c......	70
	Carrots, cooked..	½ c......	25
	Cantaloupe......	¼ of 6 in. diameter fruit.....	40
	Whole-wheat bread..........	1 slice ...	70
	Mint tea	1 c......	0
Late-evening snack	Tortilla..........	one 6 in. diameter	70
	Low-fat yogurt, plain	1 c......	125

Total food energy 1,204

SUGGESTIONS FOR PREPARING MEALS AT HOME. A good deal of study and planning is necessary in order for weight reduction to be achieved through dieting. One must learn (1) which foods are low in energy, yet are nutritious; (2) how to estimate correct portion sizes for various types of foods; and (3) ways of combining separate items in such dishes as casseroles, desserts, soups, and stews. Then, the necessary food ingredients must be purchased and kept available for meal preparation. In short, safe and successful weight reduction may require the expenditure of extra effort, money, and time. Suggestions for easing the task follow.

Selecting Low-Energy Foods. Within each major food group there are certain foods which are more filling, but less fattening than others. In general, these items contain smaller amounts of carbohydrates and fats, but greater quantities of fiber and/or water. Descriptions of such items follow:

• **Beverages, alcoholic**—It does not make much sense for a person who is trying to lose weight to spend much of a limited calorie allowance on these items. For example, 1 oz (*30 ml*) of hard liquor (gin, rum, vodka, or whiskey), 2 oz of dessert wine (these wines are fortified with extra alcohol), 3½ oz table wine (unfortified), or 7 oz beer, each provide about 80 Calories (kcal), or approximately the amount in 2 cups of fresh strawberries.

• **Beverages, nonalcoholic**—The items which are so low in calories that they may be taken without limit are coffee, fat-free bouillons or broths, herb teas, teas, and unsweetened, carbonated beverages (club sodas). Each cup of a sweetened, carbonated beverage has about the same amount of calories (80 Calories [kcal]) as the alcoholic items listed in the preceding paragraph. Therefore, mixing the two types of high-calorie drinks makes no more sense for a dieter than does drinking either type alone.
(Also see BEVERAGES.)

• **Breads and cereal products**—The low-calorie items are the breads, breakfast cereals, crackers, and macaroni products (pastas) which contain little added fat or sugar, while the high-calorie items are biscuits, cakes, cookies, donuts, muffins, pies, stuffing (usually contains meat drippings), and waffles.
(Also see BREADS AND BAKING; and CEREAL GRAINS.)

• **Cheeses**—Although there are great variations in caloric values within this group, generally the lowest priced items are lowest in calories, because prices increase along with the amounts of fat and solids. The lowest priced items are creamed cottage cheese (4% fat, 78% water, and about 60 Calories [kcal] per 2 oz [*57 g*] serving) and "imitation" processed cheese spread (3% fat, 62% water, and 48 Calories [kcal] per ounce). (Federal regulations require that products which resemble, but differ in composition from those which have official standards of identity, be labeled "imitation.") However, uncreamed, or dry curd cottage cheese contains no fat and the same amount of water as the creamed variety, yet costs more and is not always available. Cream cheese and American Cheddar cheese, which are usually the highest priced items, contain about ⅓ water, ⅓ fat, and over 100 Calories (kcal) per ounce.

• **Egg products**—A whole egg, which weighs about 1¾ oz (*50 g*), yields about 80 Calories (kcal). However, the protein is divided almost equally between the yolk and the white, but the yolk contains 6 to 7 times as many calories (due to its high-fat content). Hence, dieters might do well to eat the whites and save the yolks for others. There are now available several different brands of egg substitutes where egg whites have been mixed with vegetable oils, yellow food coloring, vegetable gums, emulsifying agents, and other ingredients so that they resemble beaten eggs. Such products are about 20% lower in calories than whole eggs.
(Also see EGG[S].)

• **Fatty foods**—The energy yields of these items are almost entirely due to their fat contents. Hence, dietitians group them under fat exchanges. One of these exchanges contains 45 Calories (kcal), which is furnished by 1 tsp (*5 ml*) each of such foods as butter, cooking oil, lard, margarine, mayonnaise, and shortening; one strip of bacon; five small olives; ten whole peanuts; 1 Tbsp (*15 ml*) of cream cheese, French dressing, or heavy cream; or 1 oz (*28 g*) of light cream, or sour cream. It is noteworthy that "imitation" or whipped margarines may contain extra water and/or air and fewer calories than regular margarines.
(Also see FATS AND OTHER LIPIDS.)

• **Fish and seafood**—Almost all of these items are considerably lower in energy and fat than most meats, but about equal to meats in protein content. For example, flounder contains only about one-half as many calories as an equal weight of rib roast.
(Also see FISH AND SEAFOOD[S].)

• **Frozen desserts**—These items are like cake and cookies because their calories are derived mainly from fats and sugars. However, there is wide variation in their caloric values. For example, a 2-oz (*57 g*) scoop of various items yields calories as follows: vanilla ice milk, 46; soft serve frozen custard, 56; regular vanilla ice cream or orange sherbet, 67; rich vanilla ice cream, 87; and French style soft serve, 94.[45]

• **Fruits and fruit drinks**—These items are made up of fruit pulp, sugar (which supplies most of the calories), and water. The standard fruit exchange contains 40 Calories (kcal), the amount furnished by about (1) ¼ cup (*60 ml*) of grape juice or prune juice; (2) ½ cup of unsweetened items such as applesauce, blackberries, blueberries, grapefruit juice, orange juice, pineapple, and raspberries; (3) ¾ cup of strawberries or papaya; or (4) 1 cup of cataloupe or watermelon. There are now many mixed fruit drinks in the supermarkets. However, their caloric contents are variable because the amounts of added sugar vary. Therefore, a good practice for dieters

---

[45]"Composition and Nutritive Value of Dairy Foods," *Dairy Council Digest*, Vol. 47, September/October 1976, p. 28.

is to buy pure fruit juices, then dilute them 50/50 with water and a little lemon juice.

(Also see FRUIT[S].)

• **Gelatin desserts**—These items are more filling, but less fattening than cakes, cookies, frozen desserts, or pies. Hence, a dieter may take larger portions of dessert gels than of the other items. For example, a 4 oz (*113 g*) serving of a gelatin dessert is equivalent in energy value (105 Calories [kcal]) to 3 oz of fruit sherbet, 1½ oz of vamilla ice cream, or 1 oz of devil's food cake.

(Also see GELATIN.)

• **Jams and jellies**—Federal standards of identity require that such products have specified compositions with respect to fruit, sugar, and water. Therefore, each teaspoon of these items contains about 14 Calories (kcal) from sugar. (A fruit exchange equals 40 Calories [kcal], or about 3 tsp [*15 ml*] of jam or jelly; while a bread exchange contains 70 Calories [kcal], the equivalent of 5 tsp of these spreads.) However, there are now available so-called "imitation" jams and jellies, which contain more water, less sugar, and only about half as many calories as the standard products.

(Also see JELLY.)

• **Meats (beef, lamb, pork, and veal)**—Although the standard lean meat exchange contains 55 Calories (kcal) per ounce (*28 g*), the medium-fat cuts contain 78 Calories (kcal) per ounce, and the high-fat cuts contain 100 Calories (kcal) per ounce. The latter group contains country-style ham, porterhouse steak, prime ribs of beef, rib lamb chops, and spareribs. It is noteworthy that the leanest cuts come from the most-exercised muscles like the shoulder (chuck cuts) and the hindquarters (round cuts) of the younger animals; while the fattest cuts come from the loin and ribs of the older animals.

The luncheon meats, which are processed, ground meat formed into loaf or sausage shapes, range in caloric values from 40 Calories (kcal) per ounce for chicken and turkey products to about 135 Calories (kcal) per ounce for such high-fat items as capicola, cervelet, dry salami, and pork sausage. The various meat products obtained from poultry will be discussed separately.

(Also see MEAT[S].)

• **Milk products**—Generally speaking, the items made from skim milk have only about half of the energy content of those made from whole milk. However, there are also items made from various low-fat milks which usually contain about 1 to 2% fat, compared to over 3% fat in whole milk. In addition, items such as chocolate milk, fruit-flavored yogurt, and sweetened condensed milk may contain added sugars. These products may be too high in calories for use in energy-restricted diets. Caloric values (kcal per cup [*240 ml*]) for some typical products are as follows: skim or nonfat milk, 80; low-fat (1%) milk, 103; low-fat (2%) milk, 125; plain, unflavored yogurt made from whole milk, or whole milk (3.5% fat), 170; and chocolate milk made with whole milk, 213.

(Also see MILK AND MILK PRODUCTS.)

• **Nuts**—Although nutritious (because they contain minerals, polyunsaturated fats, protein, vitamins, and fiber), these foods may be the downfall of dieters because they are so high in calories that a handful or two may contain the caloric value of a small meal. For example, almonds, cashew nuts, dried coconut, peanut butter, peanuts, pumpkin seeds, sunflower seeds, and walnuts contain from 160 Calories (kcal) to 170 Calories (kcal) per ounce (*28 g*), while pecans contain about 200 Calories (kcal) per ounce. Hence, dieters should *not* consume more than an ounce or two of these foods per day. Even then, they would do well to choose the low-calorie varieties of breads, meats, and milk products. Nutlike foods which contain about two-thirds as much energy (110 Calories [kcal] to 120 Calories [kcal] per ounce) as nuts are roasted chickpeas (garbanzos) and soybeans. The latter items, if roasted without additional fat, contain about 1 to 2 tsp (*5 to 10 ml*) of fat per ounce.

• **Poultry**—Chicken and turkey are usually good items for dieters because the broiled or roasted meat with the skin removed contains about 40 Calories (kcal) to 50 Calories (kcal) per ounce (*28 g*). However, the skin and its underlying fat add so many calories to cooked pieces of poultry that these pieces may yield from 60 Calories (kcal) to 65 Calories (kcal) per ounce. Because fried, breaded chicken parts are so high in fat, dieters should peel off and discard the fried coating and skin when they eat this type of food. Soup chickens (old hens and roosters) are up to 50% higher in fat than broilers.

(Also see POULTRY.)

• **Purees**—Watery, blended foods are generally thought of as being mainly suitable for babies, convalescent patients, and invalids. Only a few people appreciate the fact that purees may have many functions in meals because they are convenient forms of foods for inclusion in various recipes, or they may be eaten alone. Their caloric values depend upon (1) the original ingredients, and (2) the amounts of water used in preparing these mixtures. For example, some of the commercial baby foods have caloric values (kcal/ounce [*28 g*]) like those that follow: applesauce with pineapple, but without added sugar, 13; beef, 34; beets, 11; carrots, 8; chicken, 36; creamed spinach, 12; green beans, 6; lamb, 35; liver, 28; peas, 15; squash, 7; and sweet potatoes, 12. If baby food meats are used in diets for weight control, it should be noted that 2 oz of each of these purees are approximately equivalent to 1 oz of cooked, lean meat. Ideas for the incorporation of purees in recipes are given in the next section, which deals with the preparation and serving of foods.

(Also see BABY FOODS.)

• **Raw vegetables which may be eaten as desired**—Although each of these items contains a few calories in the form of carbohydrates, the amounts are so small that for all practical purposes they need not be measured. The most common of these vegetables are artichokes, asparagus, beet greens, broccoli, Brussels sprouts, cabbage, cauliflower, celery, chard, chicory, collards, cucumbers, dandelion greens, eggplant, endive, green peppers, kale, lettuce, mushrooms, mustard greens, okra, parsley, radishes, sauerkraut, spinach, string beans, summer squash, tomatoes, watercress, and wax beans.

However, cooking makes available more of the carbohydrates in these items, so the first cup (240 ml) of cooked vegetable may be taken "free" (without counting), but the second such cup should be counted as furnishing 25 Calories (kcal).

• **Relishes**—These appetizers, which consist of various raw vegetables with or without dressing and/or sweetener, vary widely in their energy content from such items as chopped sour pickles (only 3 Calories [kcal] per ounce [28 g]) to cranberry-orange relish (51 Calories [kcal] per ounce). The items lowest in calories are made from the "free" vegetables listed in the preceding paragraph, with only herbs and/or a little lemon juice or vinegar used for seasoning, but with no added dressings, oils, sauces, or sweeteners. Relishes may be great bonuses to dieters since they (1) are filling; (2) may be substituted (when finely chopped) for such high-calorie items as gravies, salad dressings, sauces, and spreads for bread; and (3) are often good sources of vitamin C and other essential nutrients.

(Also see RELISH, CHUTNEY, AND PICCALILLY.)

• **Salad dressings**—Too often a person trying to lose weight will conscientiously eat plenty of salads, but then greatly exceed the caloric allowances of his or her diet by using excessive amounts of dressings. These items range in their caloric values from vinegar at 4 Calories (kcal) per ounce (30 ml) up to pure salad oil at over 250 Calories (kcal) per ounce (1 oz = 2 Tbsp). The most commonly used dressings (blue or roquefort, French, Italian, mayonnaise type, Russian, and thousand island) range in calorie values from 110 Calories (kcal) to 160 Calories (kcal) per ounce because they contain from 2 tsp to 3½ tsp of oil per ounce. It is noteworthy that many people fail to distinguish between the mayonnaise type of salad dressing (124 Calories [kcal] per ounce) and mayonnaise itself (206 Calories [kcal] per ounce), which has almost twice the fat content of the dressing.

There are now available in the supermarkets various types of dietetic dressings, which are low in fat, and are stabilized and thickened by such additives as emulsifying agents and vegetable gums.

• **Sauces**—Many of the famous restaurant chefs owe their reputations to their special sauces. Although low-calorie sauces are easy to prepare, some cooks use excessive fats and sugars. Hence, the dieter must beware, for the energy content of the most popular sauces vary from 11 Calories (kcal) per ounce (30 ml) for prepared horseradish to 152 Calories (kcal) per ounce for tartar sauce (a mixture which is predominantly mayonnaise plus chopped onion, pickles, olives, and capers). Often, dietitians wil allow their patients to use without counting calories moderate amounts (1 tsp to 3 tsp) of such products as barbecue sauce, horseradish, prepared mustard, soy sauce, Tabasco sauce, and Worcestershire sauce. However, these items often are very salty, which is not good for people prone to obesity and high blood pressure, conditions where there may be excessive retention of fluid.

(Also see SAUCES.)

• **Snack items**—Unfortunately, the most popular items in this category are high in carbohydrates and/or fats, but low in proteins, minerals, and vitamins. Plain, unbuttered, unsweetened snacks like popcorn, pretzels, and soda crackers contain around 115 Calories (kcal) per ounce (28 g), while the richer items like chocolate candy, potato chips, and puffed corn snacks contain over 150 Calories (kcal) per ounce, which is close to that for the various types of nuts.

(Also see SNACK FOODS.)

• **Soups**—A high water content makes these foods desirable for dieters. Certain items, like beef broth, bouillon, and consomme, are so low in calories that they may be taken as desired, while other types range from 20 to 100 Calories (kcal) per 7-oz (210 ml) bowl. However, soups containing substantial quantities of beans, fats, meats, peas, and starch thickeners may have even higher values.

(Also see SOUPS.)

• **Spices**—Most of these products may be taken as desired, since they contain few calories. However, consumers should read the labels carefully when purchasing spices, because in some cases the major ingredient (listed first) may be salt.

(Also see SPICES.)

• **Starchy vegetables**—These foods are usually grouped under the bread exchanges because most of their calories are contributed by carbohydrates. They may be furher divided into three categories, with the following portions equivalent in caloric content (70 Calories [kcal]) to one slice of bread:
1.   One-half cup (120 ml) each of cooked corn, cowpeas, green peas, Irish potatoes (baked or boiled), or mixed vegetables (carrots, corn, lima beans, peas, and snap beans)
2.   One-third cup each of most types of cooked dry beans, lentils, mature peas, or rice
3.   One-fourth cup each of cooked mature lima beans, scalloped or au gratin potatoes, or sweet potatoes.

(Also see VEGETABLE[S].)

• **Sweeteners**—Saccharin, a nonnutritive sweetener, has long been used in special dietary foods and beverages. In 1981, aspartame, a low calorie artificial sweetener, was approved for human consumption by the FDA. However, most of the sweetening agents used in foods are carbohydrates which contain from 15 to 20 Calories (kcal) per teaspoon (5 ml). Many food processors add four or more types of sugar to such products as cakes, cookies, and various snack items, so the consumer should know the various names for these ingredients. Some of the most commonly used sweetening agents are: corn syrup, corn sweeteners, dextrins, dextrose, fructose, glucose, honey, invert sugar, lactose, levulose, malto-dextrins, maltose, molasses, sorbitol, sucrose, and sugar. It makes sense to choose products which contain the fewest sweeteners.

(Also see SWEETENING AGENTS.)

• **Vegetables which contain small amounts of carbohydrates**—These vegetables, unlike those which may be eaten as desired when raw, contain about 25 Calories (kcal) per ½ cup (120 ml) serving. This includes bean sprouts, beets, carrots, onions, pumpkin, rutabagas, turnips, and winter squash. One cup of such vegetables equals a slice of bread in energy value.

(Also see VEGETABLE[S].)

Preparing Dietetic Dishes. First of all, a good cook needs the proper tools for preparing low-energy recipes. Some special utensils which may be helpful are a blender, crock pot, food chopper, grater, measuring cups, plastic knives, pressure cooker, scale for weighing portions, a sprouter for seeds, strainers, Teflon-coated skillet, and a wire rack for use in an electric broiler or oven.

Some suggestions for modifying standard recipes follow:

• **Better uses of breads and cereals**—People become obese from eating these items when they have been over-processed, overshortened (too much fat), and over-sweetened. Therefore, it makes sense to (1) add bran and wheat germ to homemade breads and to breakfast cereals so that these products are made more filling and nutritious, (2) use salad dressings instead of butter and margarines as spreads because the former have more flavor and may be spread thinner than the latter, and (3) use brown rice and other whole grains whenever possible.

A dietetic rice pudding may be made by cooking rice, raisins, cinnamon, and nutmeg powder with the appropriate amount of water (2½ cups [600 ml] of water per cup of rice and raisins) for 10 minutes (at least 15 minutes for brown rice) in a pressure cooker. The rice is more tender when the counterweight is kept over the steam vent until the cooker has cooled to room temperature.Then, evaporated skim milk may be added to taste, and the pudding chilled in individual cups or dishes in a refrigerator. Sweetness may be increased by increasing the proportion of raisins to rice.

Leftover breads are excellent extenders for high-protein foods. For example, expensive parmesan cheese may be stretched by mixing it with finely ground, dry bread crumbs. Similarly, bread may be soaked in evaporated skim milk and mixed with chopped meat to make meatballs and patties.

• **Dietetic dairy products**—Evaporated skim milk has a smooth, creamy texture even though it contains only traces of butterfat. Its smoothness is due to the vegetable gum that it contains, which ties up some of the water that is present. Similarly, low-fat yogurt is thicker than might be expected because it contains extra nonft milk solids which were added after the lactic acid fermentation, plus, in some brands, such other additives as gelatin and/or vegetable gums. Although these products are made by commercial dairies, the homemaker may readily prepare equally desirable items from low-fat milk products. Details follow.

When mixed with a small amount of ice water, nonfat milk powder may be whipped to a creamy consistency. The directions on the package usually suggest mixing 1 part of milk powder with about 3 parts of water. However, only ⅓ to ½ as much water should be used when a thicker, creamier product is desired. Evaporated skim milk may also be chilled and whipped (without any additional water) to a similar consistency. The resulting "dietetic whipped cream" may be flavored with dietetic gelatin dessert powders, pureed fruits, or vanilla extract. These whips stand up better when small amounts of a gelatin or vegetable gelling agent are added.

Nonfat types of buttermilk or yogurt may be used in recipes in place of sour cream, except that ⅓ cup (80 ml) of water or other fluid should be omitted for each cup of the nonfat products. Uncreamed cottage cheese can be blended with skim milk, then seasoned for a mock sour cream dressing.

• **Flavorful fruit items**—Fruit and juice items made from apples, apricots, grapes, peaches, pears, and prunes are usually sufficiently sweet so that extra sugar is not needed. For example, one package of unflavored gelatin may be dissolved with gentle heating in 1½ cups (360 ml) of juice from these fruits and the resulting mixture may then be allowed to gel in a refrigerator. Other such fruits as pieces of grapes, oranges, peaches, and pineapple might be added to these mixtures before chilling.

• **Frying without fat**—Foods may be fried without added fat in skillets coated with Teflon or another type of nonstick coating. There is now available a spray-on coating which comes in pressurized cans.

• **Greasless, low-starch, gravies and sauces**—Meat drippings may be chilled in the refrigerator so that the fat solidifies and is easily removed. The remaining meat juice may then be thickened with vegetable purees made from beets, carrots, spinach, tomatoes, or turnips. Vegetable baby foods are convenient forms of such purees. However, the gravy or sauce may have to be boiled to evaporate some of the water.

• **High-protein, low-calorie entrees**—Selection of low-fat entrees allows a dieter to have more breads and other starchy items. Therefore, suggestions for such main course foods follow.

Use dry curd cottage cheese (35 Calories [kcal] per ounce [28 g]) instead of creamed cottage cheese (62 Calories [kcal] per ounce). The dry curd may be moistened with low-fat buttermilk, skim milk, or yogurt. When this type of cottage cheese is unavailable, it may be prepared from the creamed type by placing the latter in a strainer over a clean glass or jar and rinsing off the cream with nonfat milk. The rinsings should be saved for others who do not have to watch their diets so closely.

The leaner, tougher cuts of meat (beef heart, chuck, and round) should be cooked at low temperatures (250°F [121°C] or less). Many people are using crock pots for cooking stews made with such cuts. Chopped beef heart is especially good in such dishes as chili and meat sauce for spaghetti.

The fat may be easily removed from stews which have been chilled in a refrigerator.

Marbled, tender cuts (loin and ribs) might be cooked on a rack so that the fat drips off. They also contain less fat when well done. It might also be a good idea to broil frankfurters (split in half lengthwise) and luncheon meats similarly, so as to remove some of the fat they contain.

Cheese omelets may be made from egg whites beaten with dry curd cottage cheese (35 Calories [kcal] per ounce) or small cubes of imitation process cheese spread (48 Calories [kcal] per ounce) plus diced peppers and tomatoes. Then, the omelet may be cooked without added fat in a Teflon-coated skillet.

Pour off and save the oil from unhomogenized peanut butter for salads. If the partially defatted peanut butter is too dry, moisten it by mixing in such fruit items as applesauce, fruit purees, and prune juice. Seasonings like allspice, cinnamon, and nutmeg may please some tastes. Open-face peanut butter sandwiches are also good when lightly toasted under a broiler.

• **Special salad dressings**—Many of the popular dressings are high in fat, so it makes good sense to dilute them with pickle juice, tomato juice, and/or vegetable purees. Another type of dressing may be prepared by blending cottage cheese, buttermilk and/or yogurt, with beets or parsley (for color), plus herbs and spices.

• **Super sandwiches**—The amount of bread which is eaten in a "hero" or "submarine" sandwich may be reduced by removing bread from the center thereof, thereby making more room for such items as lettuce, mushrooms, onions, peppers, tomatoes, cheese, fish, meats, and/or poultry breast meat. The pieces of bread which are removed may be saved for extending meatballs or patties, or for toasting and use as croutons.

Try a sandwich made with pumpernickel or whole grain bread spread with yogurt and filled with apricot halves, canned peach halves, or carrot and raisin salad. The latter items also go well with chunky style peanut butter which might first be partially defatted and moistened as described under "High-protein, low-caloric entrees."

• **Sweetening with less sugar**—One way to decrease the amount of sugar needed in a recipe is to cut down on the amounts of the bitter or sour ingredients like baking powder (use yeast instead), lemon juice (use orange), or citrus peel (replace with citrus pulp). Carob powder is a good substitute for chocolate or cocoa because it contains less fat and is sweeter. Pure vanilla extract (not the imitation type) also gives a sensation of sweetness so that less sugar need be used when the amount of this rather expensive ingredient is increased. However, the reduced sugar intake justifies the increased cost.

• **Variety in vegetable dishes**—Many of the immigrants who came to the United States brought with them such high-energy vegetable dishes as string beans cooked with garlic and oil, beans or greens with fatback pork, or tossed salads literally doused with blue cheese dressing. Although most vegetables by themselves contain only low to moderate amounts of calories, many people do not like the tastes of such plain items. Therefore, suggestions for improvement follow.

The butter, gravy, margarine, or sour cream which is often used on baked, boiled, or mashed potatoes may be replaced by such low-calorie items as dietetic salad dressings; fat-free bouillon, broth, or consomme; such spices as celery powder, chili powder, chives, garlic powder, horseradish, onion powder, oregano, paprika, parsley, pepper, poppy seeds; and/or plain, unflavored low-fat yogurt.

A meal in a salad bowl might contain liberal amounts of raw, "free" vegetables, chopped pieces of cheese, egg, fish, meat, poultry, or seafood; plus croutons made from dry or toasted whole grain bread. A dressing may be made according to the suggestions given earlier, but it would be wise *not* to have more than 1 teaspoon (5 ml) of oil per serving.

Sprouts from such seeds as alfalfa, mung beans, oats, soybeans, and wheat are lower in energy, but higher in certain vitamins, than the original seeds. They make excellent ingredients for relishes, salads, and soups. A sprouter may be used, or the seeds may be placed between moist paper towels until they sprout.

Low-energy tubers such as Jerusalem artichokes and salsify (oyster plant) may be substituted for potatoes or other starchy vegetables.

Less dressing, fat, or sauce need be used for cooked vegetables when they are either cooked with no water remaining, or are drained well after cooking. Save the cooking water and use it for other dishes, such as soups, so as to benefit from the minerals and vitamins it contains.

A nutlike snack may be prepared by slicing fresh mushrooms and toasting them until brown under a broiler.

Raw vegetables may be chopped or sliced, soaked in leftover pickle juice, then mixed to make tasty relishes.

EATING AWAY FROM HOME. Too many people who are frequently away from home may put on fat because they eat whatever is served to them. However, dieters should have a preplanned strategy for coping with the pitfalls of eating away from home. Suggestions follow:

Lunches Brought from Home. It seems obvious that with careful planning it is possible to both stick to a diet and to save money by bringing food from home for lunches, picnics, and short automobile trips. However, there is also the hazard of poisoning due to food spoilage if such highly perishable items as dairy products and fresh fish are kept in a warm place. So-called "salad sandwiches" containing chopped cheese, eggs, meat, or poultry mixed with mayonnaise do not keep well either. An important principle in this regard is that foods which are alkaline or neutral tend to spoil more rapidly than those which are acid (such as fermented milk products like cheeses and yogurt, fruits and their juices, and vinegary salad dressings). Therefore, catsup, horseradish, mustard, pickles, pickle relishes, and acid tomato sauces (they should taste slightly sour) are good ingredients for sandwiches containing cheese and/or *cooked* meats or poultry. Rare roast beef spoils much more rapidly than when it is well done. Other lunch items follow:

• **Breads**—Almost all types of biscuits, breads, crackers, muffins, and rolls keep well at room temperature when they are not too moist. However, whole grain types or those containing bran are more filling and nutritious.

• **Cooked meats and similar items**—Well-cooked meats, such as chops, meatballs, pieces of steak, sausages, slices from roasts, and whole pieces of poultry, keep reasonably well for about a day at room temperature if they are on the dry side. It also might be wise to broil luncheon meats which are to be kept without refrigeration.

CAUTION: In spite of a well-done appearance on the outside, meats which were frozen before cooking may still be almost raw on the inside. It may be necessary to break or cut open the item to inspect the inside. People who like canned fish might leave it in the closed can until lunchtime.

• **Fresh vegetables**—The following low-energy raw vegetables are fairly resistant to spoilage: carrots, celery, lettuce, and radishes. Ripe tomatoes are very susceptible to mold growth which may sometimes be tasted before it may be seen.

• **Fruits**—Whole apples, apricots, oranges, peaches, and plums keep for a day, or more, at room temperature if they are firm and not too ripe.

• **Ingredients for drinks**—Nonperishable ingredients which may be mixed with water to make drinks are carob powder, canned juices, evaporated milk in cans, herb teas, instant coffee or tea, nonfat dry milk powder, powders for various diet drinks, and purees (fruits and vegetables) for babies which come in glass jars.

(Also see BABY FOODS.)

• **Miscellaneous items**—Nuts and seeds keep well, but they are high in calories. Roasted chickpeas (garbanzos) and soybeans contain about two-thirds as many calories.

Eating in Restaurants.   Although the staff in the better restaurants will usually make every effort to accommodate diners who are on diets, dieters must also be prepared to cope with a lot less flexibility in such places as fast food establishments where the foods and the cooking systems are designed for rapid turnover. Some suggestions follow:

Buffets usually have some nutritious, low-calorie items, but they may tempt the diner to overeat other items so as to obtain a bargain. Good rules for such situations are: (1) concentrate on the fruit and vegetables, (2) select only *one* serving each of a meat and a starchy dish, (3) forego fatty or other high-calorie sauces, and (4) omit desserts.

Cafeterias usually charge for each item, a practice which may discourage overeating unless one chooses a "special" which includes one or more fattening foods. Avoid places where most of the fish and meat items are either breaded and fried in deep fat, or are floating in rich sauces; instead, choose those featuring fresh salads, broiled fish, and roast meats. However, when necessary,

the diner might peel off and discard fried coatings or ask the servers to let most of the sauce drain back into the serving pan.

Coffee shops usually feature cakes, doughnuts, french fries, grilled sandwiches, hamburgers, and pies; but have only limited selections of other foods. Nevertheless, a dieter can usually order a cheese, lettuce, and tomato sandwich on toast, but he should make sure that the toast is prepared in a toaster, not fried on a greasy grill.

Delicatessen items, except for coleslaw and other salads, are usually high in carbohydrates and fats. Those who dine in "deli's" should stick to plain meat items like chicken, roast beef, or turkey, and avoid ordering fatty items like liverwurst, pastrami, and salami.

Eating establishments with blackened, greasy grills or fryers bubbling with smoking fat should not be patronized, since toxic substances are formed in over-heated fats. (Research studies on animals suggest that chronic consumption of such fats might lead to tumors.) Furthermore, a dieter should steer clear of foods cooked by these methods, even when fresh fats are used.

French and Italian dishes like casseroles, lasagna, and pasta with various sauces are traps for the dieter because these items are usually high in fats and starches. However, *small* side dishes of these foods may be eaten if the rest of the meal is low in calories.

Hamburger or hot dog lunches aren't bad if the diner enriches the sandwich with plenty of lettuce, onions, relish, sauerkraut, or tomato, and avoids ordering french fries. Chili and crackers are fine when eaten alone, but not when combined with a hamburger or a hot dog.

Ice cream parlors, pancake houses, and pizza parlors serve items that are usually very fattening. Hence, dieters might well avoid such places, except those in which they may order fruits or salads.

Oriental dishes, like those containing meat, rice, and vegetables, are often complete meals in themselves, so the diner should not order extra fattening items like barbecued spareribs, egg or shrimp rolls (which have usually been fried in deep fat), or dessert.

Seafood is a good choice for people who want to lose weight because clams, crabs, fish, lobsters, oysters, and shrimp are low in energy, but high in protein. However, these foods should be baked, boiled, broiled, or raw, and not used in such rich forms as au gratin, chowders, or deep fried. Seafood salad platters are usually filling, but not so fattening.

Steak dinners usually provide about twice as many calories as a dieter should eat at a single meal. The person who orders such a meal may cut down on his or her caloric intake by (1) having the steak cooked well done; (2) cutting all visible fat from the cooked meat; (3) eating only about 3 oz (*85 g*) of the steak and taking the rest home for another meal; (4) using only a *small* amount of oil and/or vinegar on the salad, and avoiding such dressings as blue cheese; (5) passing up butter, margarine, or sour cream for the baked potato, instead, using the juice from the meat and the dressing which drains to the bottom of the salad; and (6) omitting the dessert.

Tacos and similar Mexican foods that have bean or meat fillings may contain liberal amounts of fat. However, there is considerable variation in the amounts and types of ingredients in such fillings. Therefore, it is better to have only small portions of such foods as accompaniments to other items, rather than to have larger portions as main courses for meals.

Changing Eating Behavior.

This method of combating obesity, which is sometimes called "behavior mod" (mod is short for modification), differs from "crash" dieting in that it seeks permanent modification of the behavior that led to the obesity. Many people regain weight they lost by crash dieting because they failed to change their eating habits. However, before a person starts on such a program, it is a good idea to try and identify each of the factors which might be cues for his or her overeating. For example, some people habitually may eat, whether hungry or not, at such times and places as: (1) while engaged in such activities as conversation, reading, or watching television; or (2) in response to such emotions as anger, anxiety, boredom, excitement, frustration, happiness, or loneliness.[46] Hence, it might be necessary for a compulsive eater to keep a detailed diary for a week or so, noting both the circumstances (time, place, emotions, etc.) that prompt eating, and the amounts and types of foods which are eaten. Suggestions for coping with various situations follow.

ORGANIZING AGAINST IMPULSIVE EATING.

Some do's and don'ts to prevent impulsive eating are:

1. Prepare a list before shopping for food. Plan to get items which require some type of preparation, but avoid buying ready-to-eat snack items other than low-energy fruits and vegetables.

2. Do not shop when hungry, or take small children to food stores when it can be avoided. Tell older children that you will not take them unless they promise not to pester you to buy snacks or sweets.

3. As soon as possible, after returning home from shopping, divide fish, meats, and similar items into individual portions before putting them into the freezer. This should be done so as to make it unnecessary to thaw and/or cook more food than is necessary for a single meal. However, large roasts might be handled by cooking them, cutting off just what is needed for a single meal, then promptly storing the remainder so as to prevent nibbling. At this time, it might also be wise to wash and package fresh fruits and vegetables so that they are in convenient forms for use at every meal.

EATING BEHAVIOR AT HOME.

Some do's and don'ts in changing eating behavior at home are:

1. Establish specific times and places for eating, then eat *only* under those circumstances. For example, this might mean that when one is home, eating is done only in the dining room at 7:30 a.m., 6:30 p.m., and 10:00 p.m.; and *never* while working in the kitchen or when people unexpectedly drop in between meals. Visitors may be served food, but a dieter should learn to avoid eating just because others are doing so if the time is not in accordance with the new behavior pattern which is being established.

[46]Leon, G. R., "A Behavioral Approach to Obesity," *The American Journal of Clinical Nutrition*, Vol. 30, 1977, p. 785.

2. When eating, concentrate only on that activity. It might be necessary to ask other members of the family to cooperate by refraining from starting intense discussions at meals. One way to emphasize the importance of eating without distractions is to establish a regular etiquette for each meal and snack by using place settings and saying grace.

3. Do *not* put platters and bowls of food on the dining table so that diners may readily refill their plates; rather, put out only the servings of food needed for those present. It is rarely necessary to prepare more than one serving of foods per person, other than salads, since underweight members of the family would probably be better off eating extra food between meals; instead of eating more food at meals. However, the athletes or laborers in the family might go into the kitchen and serve themselves extra food, if such is absolutely necessary.

4. Put individual servings of all of the courses on the dining table before sitting down to eat. That way, everyone may see the total meal and thereby find it easier to avoid overeating the items which are normally served early in the meal. Using small dishes helps to emphasize the size of food portions.

5. Slow down your rate of eating by (a) breaking or cutting off only one small bite of food at a time, (b) chewing each bite of food thoroughly, and (c) swallowing each chewed bite before taking another. Development of a habit of chewing rather than bolting food may require the eating of such foods as dry breads, tough meats, and fibrous fruits and vegetables—all items which cannot be comfortably swallowed without thorough chewing.

6. The pace of eating may also be slowed by serving foods that require more time to eat like (a) fish or meat containing bones, (b) nuts with shells, and (c) fruits with rinds and seeds. Also, according to the rules of etiquette, one should *not* bring to the mouth a large piece of food, then chew off pieces; rather, he should use fingers (in the case of breads) or utensils to remove one bite size piece at a time.

7. When everyone has eaten, the leftovers should immediately be removed from the dining table and stored. Do *not* provide opportunities for nibbling after meals have been completed.

8. Allow sufficient time for meals and snacks each day so that food never has to be eaten on the run.

EATING BEHAVIOR AWAY FROM HOME.

Some do's and don'ts in changing eating behavior away from home are:

1. Try to avoid conducting business or talking about work while eating, since emotionally disturbing discussions may (a) stimulate the flow of extra stomach acid and intensify movements of the digestive tract, two conditions which may increase the urge to eat more; (b) distract from the enjoyment of food so that the meal is completed without the usual satisfaction; and (c) provoke compulsive eating by susceptible people. There are very few people who cannot comfortably eat a moderate-sized meal in 30 minutes or less. Expenditure of this amount of time just for eating and small talk might in the long run prove to be a good investment, since a friendly relationship might be established at the meal so that unnecessary argumentation might be avoided when discussing

business *after* the meal.

2. Planning in advance for uncertain eating conditions while traveling. For example, find out whether or not food will be served on an airline flight, so that one does not eat both before and during the flight. Not all airline terminals have shops where nutritious, low-calorie snacks may be purchased. Some of those near large cities have various types of restaurants which serve a variety of salads, main dishes, and other items suitable for dieters. However, there are often long waits for service at the better restaurants, so at least an extra hour should be allowed for eating at airline terminals.

3. Learn to be firm when coaxed by dining companions to have more food or drink. One may be gracious to hosts by praising them for their hospitality, rather than by trying to eat every morsel which is served. The old notion that guests should be filled almost to bursting is now considered passe.

USING IMAGES TO MODIFY BEHAVIOR. Although it has long been thought to be a waste of time for a person to daydream, it has recently been found that people may be taught to imagine scenes which help them to develop desirable eating habits.[47] Mental images may be used in a negative way to keep from eating on impulse, or in a positive way to reward (reinforce) good behavior. It is noteworthy that Saint Ignatius of Loyola, a 16th-century Spanish priest who founded the Jesuit order, recommended in his classic *Spiritual Exercises* that people should attempt to improve their behavior by imagining vivid scenes of heaven and hell.

For example, a person tempted to eat a piece of candy might imagine that he or she is out on a vast, sun-baked dessert with only a little water, where eating anything so sweet would cause a burning thirst. On the other hand, a reward for picking a vegetable dish might be the visualization of a walk through a multicolored garden where a mild breeze is rippling the leaves of fruit-laden plants. A brief daydream might also be used as a temporary escape from an emotionally charged situation which regularly leads to compulsive eating.

PARTICIPATION IN WEIGHT CONTROL GROUPS.
It may be difficult for highly extroverted obese people to persist in dieting when the required sacrifices depend entirely upon their own initiative. Therefore, they might consider joining a dieting group which meets weekly to share experiences in the battle against the bulges. These groups differ in that (1) a few are affiliated with teaching hospitals whose doctors and dietitians provide guidance to members, (2) others operate as private, profit-making organizations which have paid nutrition consultants, and (3) still others are private, nonprofit clubs where there may be some voluntary participation by medical and/or nutrition professionals. It is desirable for weight control groups to have persons trained in food and nutrition as consultants because many members would benefit from professional evaluations of the new dietary concepts and

the various dietetic foods which are promoted through the mass media. For example, one of the better known profit-making groups recently hired a prominent nutritionist who promptly updated their dietary plans to incorporate the latest ideas in the field.[48]

Before joining a weight control group, a prospective member should obtain a thorough medical examination so as to rule out the possibility that a metabolic problem might be accompanying or contributing to his or her obesity. Then, the obese person might make certain that overeating is not a response to one or more emotional problems which are not related to foods. If the latter is the case, it might be necessary for the dieter to find some other means for coping with this situation. Finally, the prospective member should investigate the club to determine (1) whether the diet(s) recommended might be considered both safe and suitable by his or her doctor, and (2) if the techniques used by the group to modify behavior are compatible with the personality of the dieter. For example, some people might find it annoying to be chided, or even ridiculed, for dietary indiscretions, while others might find such tactics to be just what is needed to give a boost to their will power. However, certain members may so value the esteem of the group that a day or so prior to meetings they may resort to such drastic measures as depriving themselves of fluids and food, or taking enemas or strong laxatives. Hence, these groups might do well to advise against such practices.

People may find out about weight control groups in their local community by asking their doctor.

Drugs Which Affect Appetite and Metabolism.
Certain types of drugs, taken alone or in combination with others, may help to speed loss of weight when they (1) reduce appetite (these are called anorexic agents), (2) promote loss of water through urination (diuretics), and (3) increase the proportion of food energy lost as heat (thyroid hormones). In addition to these types of substances, other drugs might be used to counteract some of the undesirable side effects of those which promote the loss of weight.

NOTE: Each of the drugs which follow may have harmful side effects. Hence, their use in the treatment of obesity should be done only under the close supervision of a physician. It would be much better to attempt to reduce the body weight by dieting and exercise, and to use drugs only as a last resort. Some reducing drugs follow:

• **Anorexic agents**—These drugs are appetite suppresants which might be used as *part* of the treatment for obesity, augmenting the other part of the treatment consisting of a nutritious, calorie-restricted diet. There is widespread misuse of these substances as stimulants. Hence, they are also known as "bennies," "pep pills," and "uppers." People taking this type of drug may also need to take "downers," or sleeping pills (barbiturates) in order to be able to go to sleep. There are now available nonamphetamine appetite depressants which do not have such stimulatory effects on the nerves.

[47]Stern, F., "Weight Control Through Imagery Training," *Nutrition News*, Vol. 39, 1976, p. 13.

[48]"Tops, Weight Watchers, and Other Groups," *Rating the Diets*, by T. Berland and the editors of *Consumer Guide*, Publications International, Ltd., Skokie, Ill., 1974, Chapter 17.

• **Atropine**—This antispasmodic drug slows excessive activity of the digestive tract, a condition sometimes resulting from the use of amphetamines. Hence, the two types of drugs may be combined in an antiobesity formulation.

• **Barbiturates**—These drugs, also known as "downers," depress the activity of the central nervous system. Hence they may be combined with amphetamines.

• **Digitalis**—This substance slows the heart rate, so it may be used in combination with thyroid hormones, which speed up the heart rate. *The combination of these two types of drugs is considered to be both dangerous and unwarranted in the treatment of obesity.*[49]

• **Diuretics**—These agents increase the amounts of water lost from the body through urination. Some of the diuretic drugs also cause marked losses of potassium in the urine, a situation which might result in increased susceptibility of the heart muscle to the toxic effects of digitalis. Patients treated for congestive heart failure with combinations of these drugs are usually warned to obtain sufficient dietary potassium to compensate for urinary losses.

• **Hormones**—Thyroid hormones are often used to treat obesity because they increase the amount of food energy lost as heat so that the total energy metabolism of the body must be increased in order to meet the needs of the body tissues. However, the hormones may also cause palpitations of the heart. Therefore, many doctors believe that the use of these agents should be limited to people who have thyroid deficiencies.

The much-heralded HCG (human chorionic gonadotropin), a hormone found in the urine of women who have recently become pregnant, has been promoted for weight reduction, but recent studies have shown it to be ineffective for this purpose.[50]

• **Laxatives**—Drugs such as atropine and diuretics may make some people constipated, so laxatives may sometimes be added to such mixed medications. Some misinformed people also use excessive amounts of laxatives to cause weight loss which results in an increased loss of nutrients and water in the stool.

• **Rainbow pills**—These are multicolored pills which often contain mixtures of such drugs as amphetamines, barbiturates, digitalis, diuretics, laxatives, and thyroid hormones. It appears that rainbow pills were responsible for the deaths of six women, and illness in two others; according to an investigation in Oregon.[51] The dead women had no abnormal characteristics other than accumulation of excessive fluid in the lungs, a condition which often accompanies congestive heart failure, whereas those who survived showed signs of potassium deficiency. Dr. Henry, Chief Medical Examiner for the Oregon State Board of Health, reasoned that (1) none of the victims consumed sufficient potassium because the amphetamines depressed their appetites, (2) loss of potassium from the body was accelerated by the diuretic and the laxative, and (3) depletion of potassium from the heart muscle rendered it more susceptible to the toxic effects of digitalis.

Exercise.   Although most people would not be able to exercise vigorously enough to lose weight by this method alone, more and more programs for weight control and physical fitness emphasize the need for frequent and brief periods of strenuous activity, e.g., bicycling, jogging, tennis, or swimming, all of which result in deep breathing and a speeding of the heart rate. These activities should be engaged in for at least 4 hours a week, and if possible, at least 1 hour every day. However, some people may be in such poor physical condition that they would be risking excessive strain on their hearts, joints, and muscles if they were suddenly to begin such exercises. Therefore anyone who wishes to start an exercise program should first obtain a thorough physical examination, then ask his or her physician how much should be done. People unaccustomed to exercise might begin with walking at a moderate pace for an extra 30 minutes to 1 hour each day.

It is noteworthy that regular participation in vigorous activity might slow weight loss because the building up of muscles involves both protein and water. However, one might determine whether or not fat is being lost by periodically taking measurements of the skinfold thickness at various sites on the body.

Many of the dangerous tendencies which may accompany obesity might be reduced or eliminated by regular exercise, even when the rate of weight loss may be very slow. Therefore, some health benefits of exercise follow:

• **Appetite reduction**—It was mentioned earlier in this article that appetite decreases when sedentary people take up moderate physical activity. Hence, a good time for jogging or similar exercise would be after work, and just before supper.

• **Clearing of fats from the blood**—Many studies have shown that blood triglycerides often drop sharply when a person undertakes a daily program of exercise. This improvement in the levels of blood fats may occur even when the energy expended is compensated for by eating extra food.[52] There may also be gradual, but significant, declines in blood cholesterol.

[49]"No End to the Rainbow," *Nutrition Today*, Vol. 3, June 1968, p. 24.

[50]Stein, M. R., *et al.*, "Ineffectiveness of Human Chorionic Gonadotropin in Weight Reduction: A Double-Blind Study," *The American Journal of Clinical Nutrition*, Vol. 29, 1976, p. 940.

[51]Henry, R. C., "The Fatal Interaction," *Nutrition Today*, Vol. 3, March 1968, p. 18.

[52]Gyntelberg, F., *et al.*, "Plasma Triglyceride Lowering by Exercise Despite Increased Food Intake in Patients with Type IV Hyperlipoproteinemia," *The American Journal of Clinical Nutrition*, Vol. 30, 1977, p. 716.

• **Extra energy expenditure and loss of weight**—About the most weight which may be lost through extra exercise is 1 lb per week, when an additional 500 Calories (kcal) are expended each day, and no extra food is taken. However, it is not difficult at all to expend an extra 250 Calories (kcal) per day by jogging for half an hour, which will result in the loss of 13 lb (*5.9 kg*) over 6 months. Extra exercise might also help to rid the body of excess weight due to the buildup of water.

• **Firming up of muscles and improvement in appearance**—Men and women who lose weight without exercise may retain a protruding pot-belly or drooping breasts because flabby muscles allow these tissues to sag. Although most experts state that one cannot preferentially reduce certain fatty spots in the body without equally reducing all such deposits, the firming up of adjacent muscles helps to prevent unsightly sagging of flesh.

• **Improved tolerance for heat stress**—It was recently found that the tolerance of men for heat stress was improved when they underwent a 6-week training period where they engaged in such vigorous activities as basketball, handball, jogging, and running for 1 hour per day, 5 times a week.[53]

• **Increased flow of blood to vital organs and tissues**—Exercise speeds the heart rate and the flow of blood around the body. However, if the flow of blood in the muscles is greatly increased, as in strenuous exercise, there is likely to be a decreased flow to the visceral organs. Hence, it is *not* wise to do such exercises right after meals, since it may result in digestive problems.

• **Lowering of blood pressure**—Two conditions which may contribute to a drop in blood pressure during exercise are (1) the opening up of small blood vessels in the muscles, and (2) a similar dilation of blood vessels in the skin as part of the body's means of dissipating heat.

• **Lowering of elevated blood sugar**—It is well known that exercise lowers blood sugar, even in diabetics, since there appears to be an insulinlike effect of strenuous activity. Hence, diabetics who are required to take injections of insulin may often lower the dosage of this hormone when they take extra exercise.

• **Opening up of "emergency" blood vessels in the heart muscle**—Regular exercise may be one of the best forms of insurance against dying of a heart attack, since moderate working of the heart muscle causes enlargement of the branches of the coronary artery. Hence, if there is an obstruction to the flow of blood in one part of this system, the chances for survival are greatly enhanced when one has a highly functional system of alternative blood vessels for supplying the heart muscle.

• **Prevention of varicose veins**—Frequent exercising of the legs during the day helps to force the blood in the veins back up to the heart. It is believed that the enlargement of the leg veins is at least partly due to the pooling of blood in them when insufficient exercise is taken.

• **Reduction in the loss of calcium from bones**—Among the other benefits which accrue to older people from exercise is a dramatic decrease in the loss of calcium from their bones, which is considerable when people take little exercises.[54]
(Also see OSTEOPOROSIS.)

• **Relaxation of tensions**—Getting out and exercising may help compulsive eaters since it helps to dissipate some of the tension which may build up from emotional stresses. Remember, that man's physiology is oriented towards "fight or flight" when confronted by various threats.

• **Slowing of the resting heart rate**—One of the signs that a person has achieved a high level of physical fitness is the slowing of his or her heart rate to as low as 60 beats per minute. A slower resting heart rate means that the organ has more time to rest between each beat.

• **Thinning of the blood**—Some obese, middle-aged men have excessive numbers of red blood cells (polycythemia) which increases the thickness (viscosity) of their blood along with its tendency to clot. It is believed that one cause of this condition may be a lack of oxygen in certain tissues, a condition which stimulates the production of extra red cells by the bone marrow. However, it has been found that vigorous exercise may cause a drop in the red cell count.[55] The lowering of the blood sugar by exercise might also help to prevent thickening of the blood since excess sugar produces excess glycoproteins, substances which contribute resistance to the flow of blood in the small blood vessels.
(Also see DIABETES MELLITUS.)

Surgery and Other Drastic Measures.   When all else fails to produce the desired loss in weight, drastic surgical measures may be taken. For example, one type of operation removes deposits of fat and some of the excess skin from the abdomen. Then, the wound is sewn together at the edges.
Another type of surgery is the removal of part of the small intestine so that the absorption of nutrients is greatly reduced. However, this operation may be followed by liver disorders, kidney stones, and other problems, and even death.[56] Hence, many doctors do not recommend it unless the risks of obesity are greater than those of the surgery.

[53]Gisolfi, C., and S. Robinson, "Relations between Physical Training, Acclimatization, and Heat Tolerance," *Journal of Applied Physiology*, Vol. 26, 1969, p. 530.

[54]Sidney, K. H., R. J. Shephard, and J. E. Harrison, "Endurance Training and Body Composition of the Elderly," *The American Journal of Clinical Nutrition*, Vol. 30, 1977, p. 326.

[55]Yoshimura, H., "Anemia during Physical Training (Sports Anemia)," *Nutrition Reviews*, Vol. 28, 1970, p. 251.

[56]Bray, G. A., and J. R. Benfield, "Intestinal Bypass for Obesity: A Summary and Perspective," *The American Journal of Clinical Nutrition*, Vol. 30, 1977, p. 121.

Finally, a few people have had their jaws wired shut so that they might drink fluids, but could not take any solid foods. Dramatic losses of weight have occurred, but there has been no news as to whether these losses were sustained after the wires were removed.

SUMMARY. This important subject warrants a summary. No matter what the reason may be for obesity, it is not to be desired and should be avoided or treated promptly if it develops. The two most important points are:

1. Total caloric consumption must be reduced, and a new permanent pattern of eating established—otherwise, the weight will be regained eventually.
2. Exercise should be increased on a daily basis.

OBESITY DRUGS

Generally, this refers to anorexic agents—those drugs which suppress the appetite. Originally, amphetamines were used for this purpose but now a number of other drugs are available; among them, diuretics, hormones, barbiturates, and atropine, used alone or in combination. Drugs may be used as *part* of the treatment for obesity, with the other part of the treatment consisting of a nutritious calorie-restricted diet. But they should only be used as a last resort, and then only under the close supervision of a doctor.

(Also see MODIFIED DIETS; and OBESITY.)

OCTACOSANOL ($C_{28}H_{58}O$)

This substance, which exists in nature as a constituent of many plant oils and waxes, including the oil of raw wheat germ, is reputed to be important in physical fitness. Based on a long series of human experiments on physical fitness conducted by Dr. Thomas Kirk Cureton of the University of Illionis Physical Fitness Institute, it appears that octacosanol is one of the factors responsible for the beneficial effects of unrefined, unheated wheat germ oil. Vitamin E alone was not effective.

Dr. Cureton's subjects were tested for pulse rates, breath-holding ability, basal metabolism, heart action, reaction time, agility, bicycling, strength and many other physical activities. Improvements were noted in stamina, speed, reflexes, agility, and heart action.

Octacosanol, which has been concentrated from wheat germ oil, will be listed on any product that contains it.

NOTE WELL; More experimental work is needed relative to the importance of octacosanol as part of a nutritional program for persons engaged in strenuous activities where agility, speed, and endurance are important. Also, persons eating plenty of whole grain cereals, unheated seeds and nuts, and other foods rich in this substance, do not need supplemental sources of octacosanol.

OFFAL

Formerly, the term offal, which literally means "off fall," included all parts of the animal that fell off during slaughtering. As our knowledge of nutrition improved, the edible portions—liver, tongue, sweetbread, heart, kidney, brain, tripe, and oxtail—were upgraded and classed as *variety meats*. Hand in hand with this transition, the hide, wool, and tallow became known as by-products. Thus, in a modern packing plant, only the entrails and inedible trimmings are referred to as offal.

OIL

Although fats and oils have the same general structure and chemical properties, they have different physical characteristics. The melting points of oils are such that they are liquid at ordinary room temperatures.

(Also see OILS, VEGETABLE.)

OIL CROPS

The main oil crops are soybeans, cottonseed, peanuts, and flaxseed. Sunflower, safflower, castor bean, and corn are also used for making oil.

OIL PALM *Elaeis guineensis*

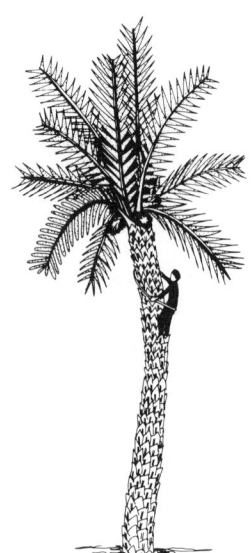

Fig. O-9.   Oil palm of West Africa, showing climber ascending tree to harvest the fruit.

The oil palm is one of the world's most important sources of edible and soapmaking oil. It yields more per acre than can be obtained from any other vegetable oil; hence, its importance is not likely to decline.

ORIGIN AND HISTORY. The oil palm is indigenous to tropical West Africa, where it grows wild in great numbers. A large proportion of the commercial palm oil comes from the fruits collected from wild palm groves. But plantations have also been established in the Congo, in Tanzania, along the Ivory Coast, and in Malaysia and Indonesia.

PRODUCTION. The oil palm thrives only where the rainfall is fairly high, but it will do rather well on poor soils.

For plantation purposes, seedlings are raised in a nursery, then transplanted to the field when 12 to 18 months old. Bearing begins at 5 years, reaches a maximum at 10 years, and the trees live to 50 years of age. A tree may produce 2 to 6 bunches of fruit per year, with each bunch containing up to 200 fruits. Harvesting from trees, which may be 30 to 60 ft (9 to 18 m) high, is usually done by a climber who places a rope around the trunk of the tree and behind his buttocks.

In 1990, the world production of palm oil totaled 11,084,344 metric tons, and the world production of palm kernels totaled 3,468,186 metric tons. That year, the leading palm oil producing countries, by rank, were: Malaysia, Indonesia, Nigeria, Colombia, and Thailand.

PROCESSING. In order to understand the processing of oil palm, it is necessary to know something about the fruit. Each individual fruit is between 1 in. and 2 in. (2.5 and 5.1 cm) in length and ¾ to 1 in. (1.5 to 2.5 cm) in diameter, and weighs from 3 to 25 g. Beneath the outer skin of the fruit is a layer of fibrous pulp, called the pericarp, which contains 30 to 70% oil and yields the palm oil proper of commerce. Inside this is the seed, consisting of a hard, black outer shell (which is useless except for fuel) and an inner kernel which contains approximately 50% by weight of palm kernel oil, suitable for making margarine.

The primitive method of processing, which is still used by many small African farmers, consists of leaving the bunches of fruit to ferment for a few days (usually in holes in the ground); stripping off the fruits, then boiling and pounding them; and skimming off the oil from the surface of the water. The shells of the nuts are broken between two stones or in a hand-operated cracking machine. The kernels are usually sold for export, with their oil extracted by the importing country.

But modern oil processing factories are gradually replacing the primitive method, and recovering a larger percentage of oil from the fruits than can be secured by hand processing. The trend is toward steam distillation, followed by centrifuging and even hydraulic expression. In industrialized nations, the kernels are either expressed or solvent-treated.

The amount and proportion of the two oils (palm oil and palm kernel oil) produced also varies according to the variety of oil palm.

PREPARING. Although liquid when first extracted, palm oil sets about as thick as butter at normal temperatures. It has a yellowish color due to the carotene pigment, and a pleasant aroma.

NUTRITIONAL VALUE. Palm oils vary; in some cases resembling kernel oil, and in others olive oil. But they are always a rich source of vitamin A; they contain from 37,300 to 128,700 mcg of beta-carotene equivalent per 100 g. All kernel oils are very similar—they're high in lauric acid and high in saturation. Food Composition Table F-36 lists the nutrient composition of palm oil and palm kernel oil.

USES. Perhaps half of the oil produced in Africa is used locally as food in all kinds of cookery; the rest is exported.

When exported, palm oil is used chiefly for soapmaking and industrial purposes; but with suitable treatment it may also be used in margarine. Palm kernel oil, which is white or pale yellow, is largely used for margarine. Following extraction, the oilcake is used as a protein supplement for livestock.

As with many other palms, wine may be prepared from the oil palm by tapping and fermenting the sugary sap, which contains a useful content of B vitamins.

OILSEED

Seeds from which oil is extracted for commercial use are termed oilseeds, including castor bean, cottonseed, flaxseed, peanut, safflower, sesame, soybean, and sunflower.

(Also see OILS, VEGETABLE, Table O-6.)

OILS, VEGETABLE

These products are obtained from the seeds and fruits of various plants. Many of their characteristics are similar to those of animal fats, which is fortunate because the per capita supply of the latter is ever dwindling as the human population grows larger. In fact, the past century has been marked by a continual effort to modify vegetable oils so that they may serve as replacements for butter, cream, and lard. Recently, there has been considerable controversy regarding the possible roles of the various fatty foods in the prevention or provocation of such disorders as atherosclerosis, cancer, heart disease, and obesity. Apparently, there are no simple answers to these questions, since dietitians, doctors, and nutritionists disagree on the relative merits and demerits of the different products. Therefore, some noteworthy background material on the vegetable oils is presented in the sections that follow.

HISTORY.

The first fats produced by primitive peoples were those rendered from animal carcasses. Later, butter was obtained by churning the milk from domesticated animals. However, certain areas of the world became too densely populated to support a large population of wild or domesticated animals, and so the people in these places came to depend upon plants as sources of fats and oils.

It appears that olives may have been cultivated in various places around the eastern end of the Mediterranean Sea for at least 6,000 years. Similarly, the sesame plant has been grown for thousands of years in the tropical belt extending from Africa to India. Other sources of oil, such as coconut palm and the oil palm, have long grown wild in the tropics, where people gathered the nuts and extracted the oil. These oils (olive, sesame, coconut, and palm) keep better without refrigeration than most of the other vegetable oils. Hence, the stable oils have long been shipped to various parts of the world. Other, more perishable oils, such as safflower, were not articles of worldwide commerce until recently, when certain technological developments made it possible to reduce the potential for spoilage, or breakdown during frying.

Attempts to produce semisolid cooking fats from vegetable oils led to the blending of these oils with tallow. The products of the blending were acceptable as crude substitutes for lard, but not for butter. This type of imitation lard was produced in the United States during the latter part of the 18th century. However, the most significant breakthrough in the production of a butter substitute occurred in 1869, when Napoleon III offered a prize for its development. This inducement led the French chemist Mege-Mouries to (1) separate tallow into two fractions, one hard, and the other soft like butter; (2) mix the butterlike fraction with skim milk to form an imitation cream; and (3) churn the "cream" to produce the first margarine. Shortly thereafter, some margarines were extended with coconut oil, palm oil, whale oil, and other liquid oils, but the amounts used had to be limited in order to avoid making the margarine too soft. The first practical process for the hardening (hydrogenation) of vegetable oils was developed by the English chemist Normann early in the 20th century.

At first, the production of margarine in the United States was mainly the province of the meat packing industry. After hydrogenation was perfected, soap companies and other concerns became involved in the production of vegetable oil margarines. At about the same time, the production of hydrogenated shortenings (vegetable oil substitutes for lard) came onto the market. Since then, the demand for vegetable oils has grown steadily, because hardened oils keep much better than

unhardened oils and are less likely to break down during frying. Lately, the use of hardened fats in margarines has abated somewhat, due to the promotion of polyunsaturated fats as a preventive measure against atherosclerosis and heart disease.

PRODUCTION AND PROCESSING.

The utilization of the major fat and oil products in the United States is shown in Fig. O-10.

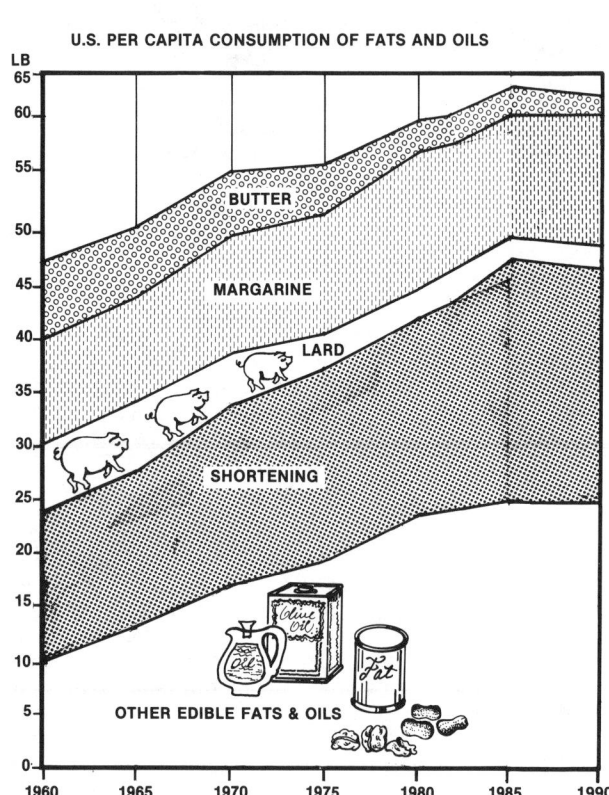

Fig. O-10. Per capita consumption trends of fats and oils in the United States between the years 1960 and 1990. (Source: *Statistical Abstract of the United States 1980*, p. 131, No. 211; and *Agricultural Statistics, 1991*, p. 135, Table 190)

It may be seen from Fig. O-10 that the per capita consumption of both butter and lard has declined significantly in recent years, whereas the consumption of vegetable oil products has risen sharply. The categories of margarine, shortening, and other edible fats and oils represent mainly items made from vegetable oils.

At the present time, vegetable oils contribute the major share of the world production of fats and oils. Fig. O-11 shows the contribution to world production of each of the important fats and oils.

WORLD PRODUCTION OF FATS & OILS

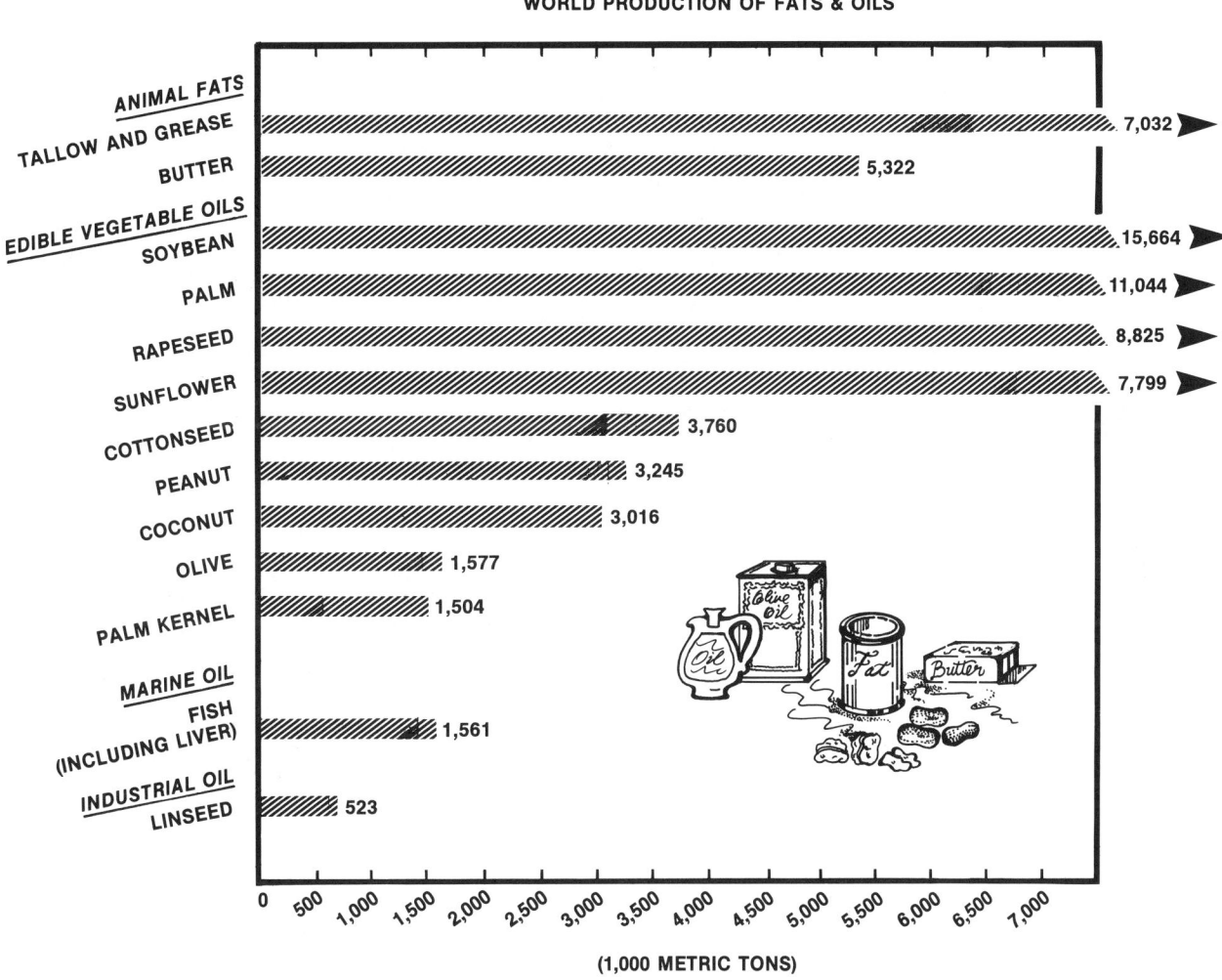

Fig. O-11. World production of fats and oils. (Source: *Agricultural Statistics 1991,* USDA, p. 135, Table 190)

Descriptions of the processes used in the production of vegetable oils and related products follow.

Extraction of Oils.

Vegetable oils are enclosed within the cells of seeds or fruits. Hence, the plant tissues must be broken so that the oil may be extracted. Various processes have been developed to insure the maximum yield of oil because this product has generally brought considerably more profit than the extracted plant residue. Details of the more commonly used processes are noteworthy:

• **Cracking, crushing, flaking, or grinding of the oil-bearing tissue**—Depending upon the nature of the plant material, one or more of these processes are used to prepare the oil source for extraction; sometimes, the broken pieces are also cooked prior to extraction.

• **Pressing**—Various devices, ranging from small hand-operated presses to large mechanically driven expellers, are used to squeeze the oil from the pretreated pulverized plant tissue.

• **Solvent extraction**—Often, the residues from pressing are further treated with solvents such as ethylene dichloride or hexane to remove the remaining oil. Then, the oil and solvent mixture is heated to drive off the solvent.

Refining.

Different processes may be used to refine each of the various oils, because the undesired constituents vary in each case:

• **Agitation with caustic soda**—The freshly extracted oil is stirred with alkali and heated in order to convert any free fatty acids to soaps. Then, centrifugation is used to remove the soaps, gums, sludge, and other undesirable materials. All traces of alkali are then removed by one or more washings with water, followed by centrifugation.

• **Bleaching (Decolorization)**—After alkali treatment, colored materials are removed from the oil by (1) the addition of fine particles of filtering clay and activated charcoal, and (2) passage of the mixture through a filter press to remove the colored materials absorbed into the clay and charcoal.

• **Deodorization**—Odoriferous materials are removed by the passage of steam through the heated oil in a vacuum chamber.

• **Winterization**—Certain oils contain fats which solidify (crystalize) at refrigerator temperatures and cause cloudiness. These harmless, but esthetically undesirable, components are removed by chilling the oil and filtering.

Hardening (Hydrogenation).

This process is used to reduce the polyunsaturation of certain oils in order to (1) make them more solid at room temperature (for use in margarines and shortenings), and (2) increase their stability against deterioration when stored for long periods or when heated. It consists of (1) adding a trace amount of a nickel catalyst to the oil; (2) heating, and passing hydrogen gas through the oil in a converter kept under a vacuum; and (3) rebleaching, and removing the catalyst from the hydrogenated oil by filtration.

CHEMICAL COMPOSITION AND OTHER CHARACTERISTICS.

Both vegetable oils and animal fats are comprised mainly of mixtures of triglycerides, which are chemical compounds containing three molecules of fatty acids combined with one molecule of glycerol. Triglycerides differ from one another because their fatty acid content varies, while the glycerol in each triglyceride remains the same. Hence, the chemical and physical characteristics of vegetable oils depend ultimately on the types and amounts of chemically-combined fatty acids that they contain.

Fatty Acid Composition.

Fatty acids are made up of hydrocarbon chains that contain an organic acid (COOH) grouping at one end. The backbone of the chain consists of carbon atoms connected by either single (saturated) or double (unsaturated) linkages (valence bonds). Saturated linkages are more stable than unsaturated linkages because the latter have the ability to combine readily with oxygen or other substances. Furthermore, fatty acids which contain two or more unsaturated bonds per molecule (polyunsaturated fatty acids or PUFA) are prone to rancidity (oxidative deterioration).

Another variable factor in the makeup of fatty acid molecules is the number of carbon atoms. Fatty acids are designated as having (1) short chains when the number of carbon atoms is 6 or less, (2) medium chains when there are 8 or 10 carbon atoms, and (3) long chains when the number of carbon atoms is 12 or more.

The properties of the various fatty acids depend mainly upon the combination of (1) the number of unsaturated bonds present, and (2) the length of the carbon chain.

TABLE O-4
CHEMISTRY OF FATTY ACIDS COMMONLY PRESENT IN VEGETABLE OILS

Name	Structure	Chain Length	Melting Point	
		(no. C atoms)	(°F)	(°C)
Saturated:				
Caproic	$CH_3 (CH_2)_4COOH$	6	18	*− 8*
Caprylic	$CH_3 (CH_2)_6COOH$	8	62	*16*
Capric	$CH_3 (CH_2)_8COOH$	10	88	*31*
Lauric	$CH_3 (CH_2)_{10}COOH$	12	112	*44*
Myristic	$CH_3 (CH_2)_{12}COOH$	14	129	*54*
Palmitic	$CH_3 (CH_2)_{14}COOH$	16	146	*63*
Stearic	$CH_3 (CH_2)_{16}COOH$	18	157	*70*
Arachidic	$CH_3 (CH_2)_{18}COOH$	20	170	*76*
Lignoceric	$CH_3 (CH_2)_{22}COOH$	24	187	*86*
Monounsaturated:				
Palmitoleic	$CH_3 (CH_2)_5CH = {}^1CH(CH_2)_7COOH$	16	31	*− 1*
Oleic	$CH_3 (CH_2)_7CH = CH(CH_2)_7COOH$	18	56	*13*
Polyunsaturated:				
Linoleic	$CH_3 (CH_2)_4CH = CHCH_2CH = CH(CH_2)_7COOH$	18	23	*− 5*
Linolenic	$CH_3CH_2CH = CHCH_2CH = CHCH_2CH = CH(CH_2)_7COOH$	18	12	*− 11*
Arachidonic	$CH_3 (CH_2)_4CH = CHCH_2CH = CHCH_2CH = CHCH_2CH = CH(CH_2)_3COOH$	20	− 57	*− 50*

[1]The symbol = indicates a double valence (unsaturated) bond between adjacent carbon atoms.

Table O-4 shows how these chemical characteristics affect melting points. Melting points of fats are very important in nutrition, because fats that remain solid in the digestive tract are utilized poorly.

It may be noted from Table O-4 that there is a steady rise in melting points as the chain lengths of fatty acids increase. However, for a given chain length, the melting points decrease as the degree of unsaturation increases. The latter principle is exemplified in the fatty acids with 18 carbon atoms by the high melting point for stearic acid (157°F, or *69°C*), which is saturated; compared to those for monounsaturated oleic acid (56°F, or *13°C*) and polyunsaturated linolenic acid (12°F, or *-11°C*).

Although it is not shown in Table O-5, it is noteworthy that melting points of fats containing both low- and high-melting fatty acids are intermediate between the two extremes.

The relative amounts of saturated, monounsaturated, and polyunsaturated fats present in each of the commonly used vegetable oils are given in Table O-5.

TABLE O-5
FATTY ACID CONTENT OF 1-TBSP PORTIONS
OF SELECTED VEGETABLE OILS[1]

Oil	Total Fat	Satu-rated	Mono-unsat-urated	Poly-unsat-urated	Other Minor Fats
	(g)	(g)	(g)	(g)	(g)
Coconut	13.6	11.8	0.8	0.2	0.8
Corn	13.6	1.7	3.3	8.0	0.6
Cottonseed	13.6	3.5	2.4	7.1	0.6
Olive	13.6	1.8	9.9	1.1	0.7
Peanut	13.6	2.3	6.2	4.3	0.7
Safflower	13.6	1.2	1.6	10.1	0.7
Sesame	13.6	1.9	5.4	5.7	0.6
Soybean	13.6	2.0	3.2	7.9	0.5
Sunflower, commercial	13.6	1.4	2.7	8.9	0.6
Sunflower, southern	13.6	1.4	6.2	5.5	0.5

[1]*Composition of Foods*, Ag. Hdbk. No. 8–4, USDA, 1979.

Chemical and Physical properties. The wide variety of ways in which vegetable oils are utilized makes it necessary to have expeditious means for determing certain characteristics of these products. It is too expensive and time consuming for many commercial users of vegetable oils to assess the chemical and physical properties by the more comprehensive methods used in research studies. Some of the commonly conducted tests follow:

• **Iodine Value**—This test measures the degree of unsaturation of a fat. The higher the number, the greater the unsaturation. For example, the highly saturated coconut oil has an iodine value of only 9, whereas the highly unsaturated soybean oil has a value of 134. Susceptibility to oxidative rancidity increases, and the melting point decreases with the iodine value. It is noteworthy that this test is used to assess the amount of hydrogenation applied to vegetable oils. The value is usually given in the purchasing specifications for these products.

• **Saponification Value**—The name of this test is derived from the reaction (saponification) in which fats react with alkalis to form soaps, because the higher the value, the better the soap making potential. What is actually measured is the average length of the carbon chains in the fatty acids which constitute the fat. A high saponification value signifies a low melting point and a short chain length, and vice versa. For example, the value for coconut oil ranges between 250 and 264, because this product is rich in the fatty acids which contain 12 or fewer carbon atoms per molecule. On the other hand, the value for rapeseed oil ranges between 170 and 180, due to the high content of long-chain fatty acids.

• **Melting Point**—This is an important value for food processors because (1) consumers expect certain items to be solid at ordinary room temperatures, and others to be liquid; and (2) most shortenings should be at least semisolid at room temperature because flakiness of pastry depends upon the production of layers of solid fat. In common language, an item is called a fat if solid under ordinary conditions, or an oil if liquid. Ordinary conditions usually imply a temperature between 64°F (18°C) and 75°F (24°C). Products with a suitable melting point may be obtained by mixing high-melting items with low-melting ones.

NUTRITIVE VALUES.

The nutrient compositions of the common vegetable oils are given in Food Composition Table F-36, and their fatty acid contents are given in Table F-39, Fats and Fatty Acids In Selected Foods.

Vegetable oils, like other highly edible fats, furnish about 9.3 Calories (kcal) per gram. Hence, 1 Tbsp (13.6 g) furnishes about 127 Calories (kcal). However, the most valuable nutritional assets of these products are the content of polyunsaturated fats and vitamin E. Nevertheless, the merits of the former may have been exaggerated somewhat over the past 3 decades, as exemplified by the growing doubts as to whether polyunsaturated fatty acids are efficacious in the prevention of heart disease. Also, the consumption of large amounts of vegetable oils might under certain conditions be hazardous to health. Therefore, some of the basic principles that bear on these and other controversial issues are noteworthy.

Essential Fatty Acids. The polyunsaturated fatty acid, linoleic acid, is required in the diet because it cannot be synthesized in the body. Linoleic appears to be needed in amounts of about 7.5 g per day.

Corn, cottonseed, safflower, soybean, and sunflower oils are excellent sources of linoleic acid, which comprises about one-half of the fatty acid content of these oils. Hence, about 1 Tbsp per day of any of them will provide the requirement for adults.

NOTE: The polyunsaturated fatty acid content of each of the oils listed in Table O-5 is mainly linoleic acid.

The essential fatty acids serve important functions in cell membranes, and as raw materials for the synthesis of hormonelike agents called prostaglandins. Deficiencies of these fatty acids result in skin disorders, reproductive difficulties, loss of hair, and perhaps even an increased susceptibility to high blood pressure. It is suspected that certain prostaglandins, that are synthesized from the essential fatty acids, help to control blood pressure.

(Also see FATS AND OTHER LIPIDS, section headed "Essential Fatty Acids.")

Polyunsaturated vs. Saturated Fats. Most vegetable oils, with the exception of cocoa butter, coconut oil, and the palm oils, are more unsaturated (they have higher iodine numbers) than most fats from land animals. Marine animals and fish may also be rich in unsaturated fats. Also, vegetable oils are free of cholesterol, which is suspected of contributing to the development of atherosclerosis and heart disease, when excessive amounts of the sterol are consumed by susceptible people over long periods of time. Furthermore, the substitution of substantial amounts of vegetable oils for saturated animal fats such as butter, cream, lard, and meat drippings has sometimes led to (1) a modest (up to 20%) drop in blood cholesterol, and (2) a reduction in the tendency of the blood to form clots.[57] However, arachidonic acid, a polyunsaturated fatty acid found mainly in peanut oil, promotes clotting.[58]

The effects of polyunsaturated fatty acids on the heart muscle are uncertain, since it has been found that the lifetime feeding of corn, cottonseed, or soybean oils produced more heart lesions in rats than beef fat, butter, chicken fat, or lard.[59]

[57]Iacono, J. M., "The Influence of Dietary Fats on Hypercoagulation and Thrombosis," *Diet and Atherosclerosis*, edited by C. Sirtori *et al*., Plenum Press, New York, N.Y., 1975, p. 191.

[58]"Dietary Essential Fatty Acids, Prostaglandin Formation and Platelet Aggregation," *Nutrition Reviews*, Vol. 34, 1976, p. 243.

[59]Kaunitz, H., and R. E. Johnson, "Influence of Dietary Fats on Disease and Longevity," *Proceedings of the Ninth International Congress of Nutrition (Mexico, 1972)*, Vol. 1, edited by A. Chavez, *et al*., published by S. Karger, Basel, Switzerland, 1975, p. 369, Table III.

Some of the other findings which call into question the wisdom of consuming large amounts of polyunsaturated vegetable oils have been summarized in a recent review.[60] They are as follows:

1. The drop in blood cholesterol may be due mainly to a shifting of the sterol from the blood to the tissues.

2. Polyunsaturated fats cause an increase in the amount of cholesterol secreted in the bile, a condition that sometimes leads to the formation of cholesterol gallstones.

3. Extra vitamin E is required to prevent the formation of toxic peroxides when the dietary level of polyunsaturated fats is raised. However, diets containing ample amounts of the essential trace mineral selenium (which is a part of the enzyme that breaks down the peroxides) may also help to offset this danger.

Medium-Chain Triglycerides (MCT Oil) This special dietary product is made from coconut oil by (1) steam and pressure hydrolysis of the oil into free fatty acids and glycerol, (2) fractionation of the resulting hydrolysate into medium-chain and long-chain fatty acids, and (3) recombination of the medium-chain fatty acids with glycerol to form MCT oil, which is made up of about ¾ caprylic acid (a saturated fatty acid containing 8 carbon atoms) and about ¼ capric acid (a saturated fatty acid containing 10 carbon atoms). The special nutritive values of this product are as follows:

1. It is much more readily digested, absorbed, and metabolized than either animal fats or vegetable oils which contain mainly long-chain triglycerides. Hence, MCT oil is valuable in the dietary treatment of fatty diarrhea and other digestive disorders in which the absorption of fat is impaired.

2. Medium-chain triglycerides, unlike other saturated fats, do *not* contribute to a rise in blood cholesterol.

At the present time, MCT oil is used almost exclusively for special dietary formulations in the United States, but it is also available in various nonmedical consumer products in Europe.

Vitamin E and Other Beneficial Substances. Vegetable oils and the seeds from which they are derived are the best food sources of vitamin E. For example, the amounts supplied by some typical oils (mg of vitamin E per 100 g [about 3½ oz] of oil) are as follows: wheat germ, 115; safflower, 34; cottonseed, 32; peanut, 19; corn, 12; and soybean, 7.[61] It is noteworthy that these figures apply only to the amounts of alpha-tocopherol, which is the official standard for vitamin E activity. However, most vegetable oils also contain substantial quantities of related compounds (nonalpha-tocopherols) that have a reduced vitamin activity, but which, nevertheless, contribute to the total vitamin E value. Hence, some nutritionists have suggested that allowances also be made for the contributions of the other tocopherols.

Vegetable oils also contain plant sterols (phytosterols) that resemble cholesterol in structure, but which help to lower blood cholesterol by (1) interfering with its absorption, and (2) possibly accelerating its removal from the body.[62] It is noteworthy that vegetable oils which are very similar in fatty acid composition lower blood cholesterol by markedly different amounts. However, the anticholesterolemic effects of the oils are often in direct proportion to their content of plant sterols. For example, wheat germ oil, which contains approximately 5% phytosterols, has been shown to produce a much greater lowering of blood cholesterol than the other vegetable oils, which contain from 0.4% to about 1.0% phytosterols.[63] The higher plant sterol content of corn oil (about 1.0%) might also be the reason why this product is much more anticholesterolemic than soybean oil, which contains only about 0.4% phytosterols.

Antinutritional and/or Toxic Factors. Under certain conditions, small amounts of potentially harmful substances may be formed from polyunsaturated fatty acids. These substances present hazards only when large amounts of the affected oil products are consumed. This is *not* to suggest that these products be avoided, but rather that they should be used judiciously, while keeping in mind the possible consequences of misuse. Consider:

• **Peroxides**—The highly polyunsaturated fatty acids that are abundantly present in corn, cottonseed, safflower, soybean, and sunflower oils may be oxidized to toxic peroxides when exposed to air, heat, light, and metals such as copper and iron. Also, the long reuse of frying fats that have been overheated repeatedly is likely to result in the production of peroxides and other toxic substances.

Peroxides destroy vitamin E and help to speed the breakdown of polyunsaturated fatty acids in cell membranes. It is even suspected that these chemical reactions are responsible for some of the degenerative changes in the aging process because, upon autopsy, the brains of some senile people have been found to contain oxidized fats from cell membranes.

Some of the means by which the formation of peroxides in oils may be minimized are: (1) the addition of trace amounts of antioxidants; (2) storage of the oils in tightly capped, dark brown bottles in a refrigerator; (3) careful heating during frying so that smoking does not occur (a thermometer may be helpful to inexperienced cooks); and (4) straining of the oil after frying to remove food particles, because they increase the tendency of the oil to smoke.

[60]"The Biological Effects of Polyunsaturated Fatty Acids," *Dairy Council Digest*, Vol. 46, 1975, p. 31.

[61]Slover, H. T., *et al.*, "Vitamin E in Foods: Determination of Tocols and Tocotrienols," *Journal of the American Oil Chemists' Society*, Vol. 46, 1969, p. 420, Table VII.

[62]Konlande, J. E., and H. Fisher, "Evidence for a Nonabsorptive Antihypercholestrolemic Action of Phytosterols in the Chicken," *The Journal of Nutrition*, Vol. 98, 1969, p. 435.

[63]Alfin-Slater, R. B., 1961, "Factors Affecting Essential Fatty Acid Utilization," *Drugs Affecting Lipid Metabolism*, edited by S. Garattini, and R. Paoletti, Elsevier Publishing Company, Amsterdam, Netherlands, 1961.

TABLE O–6
VEGETABLE OILS

Oil; Source; Scientific Name; Origin and History	Importance; Principal Areas; Growing Conditions	Processing; Preparation; Uses	Nutritional Value[1]
Coconut Oil **Source:** The nut (fruit) of the coconut palm tree, one of the world's most important crop trees. **Scientific Name of Coconut Palm:** Family: *Palmae* Genus: *Cocos* Species: *C. nucifera* **Origin and History:** Originated in Southeast Asia on the islands of Melanesia in the Pacific Ocean. Widely distributed by water (coconuts float) and man to all parts of the tropical and subtropical world. (Also see COCONUT.)	**Importance:** The world production of coconuts averages over 42 million metric tons, and the production of coconut oil over 9.6 million metric tons. **Principal Areas:** Tropical, sea coastal areas of the Old World. In 1990, the seven leading coconut-producing countries of the world, by rank, were: Indonesia, Philippines, India, Sri Lanka, Thailand, Malaysia, and Mexico. **Growing Conditions:** The trees grow wild on the coasts of all tropical countries. They thrive best on rich, sandy soil near the coast. Most of the coconuts of commerce today come from natural groves of seedling trees, harvested and processed in a crude, laborious fashion.	**Processing:** Most coconut oil is obtained from copra by pressing in mechanical screw presses, sometimes followed by solvent extraction. In some areas, hydraulic cage and box presses are still used. **Preparation:** Crude coconut oil is refined and deodorized to remove free fatty acids and flavors. **Uses:** Because of the high percentage of lauric acid (45%), a saturated fatty acid, confectioners and bakers use coconut oil in coatings and fillings for baked goods and candy which may stand for a relatively long time between manufacture and consumption. Major uses of coconut oil are in shortening and oleomargarine, deep fat frying, detergents, laundry, and toilet soaps. Minor uses are in filled milk, imitation milk, prepared flours and cake mixes; lotions, rubbing creams, and in pressurized toppings. Recently, coconut oil has served as the raw material for producing medium chain triglycerides, which are very useful in the treatment of certain digestive disorders.	The fatty acids of coconut oil are: 		%	 	Lauric	44	 	Myristic	18	 	Palmitic	11	 	Oleic	7	 	Caprylic	6	 	Capric	6	 	Stearic	6	 	Linoleic	2	 Coconut oil has the highest percentage of saturated fatty acids of all common food oils; 86% vs 11% for corn oil. Hence, it is very stable, either alone or in products. Iodine value: 9 (This indicates the degree of unsaturation; it is the number of grams of iodine absorbed by 100 cm of fat. The higher the iodine value the greater the degree of unsaturation.) The high content of lauric, caprylic, and capric acids is a nutritional asset because these fatty acids are very useful in the dietary treatment of certain digestive disorders. However, the high degree of saturation of coconut oil may raise the blood cholesterol in some people, even though the oil itself contains no cholesterol.

Footnote at end of table

(Continued)

TABLE O–6 *(Continued)*

Oil; Source; Scientific Name; Origin and History	Importance; Principal Areas; Growing Conditions	Processing; Preparation; Uses	Nutritional Value[1]
Corn Oil **Scientific Name:** Family: *Gramineae,* the grass family Genus: *Zea* Species: *Z. mays* **Origin and History:** Corn is indigenous to North America. Fossilized pollens estimated to be 80,000 years old, have been found in soil profiles near Mexico City; and ears of corn about the size of strawberries, estimated to be 3,000 years old, have been discovered in Mexico. Archaeological discoveries almost as ancient as those in Mexico have been found in South America, so, it may have been domesticated simultaneously in two different areas. (Also see CORN.)	**Importance:** Corn is the leading cereal grain in the United States. Corn has always been important in North America. It accounts for 48% of the total world production of 475 million metric tons; the United States alone produces 43% of the world total. World production of corn oil averages 520,000 metric tons. **Principal Areas:** Although corn is grown throughout the United States, the greatest production is in the area of the Midwest called the Corn Belt, consisting of the seven states of Illinois, Indiana, Iowa, Kansas, Missouri, Nebraska, and Ohio. In 1980, 66% of the corn grown for grain was produced in the Corn Belt, and more than ⅓ of it was produced in Illinois and Iowa. **Growing Conditions:** Corn does best in areas with ample moisture, fertile soil, and warm nights. It is grown primarily in the north central states, but it has expanded over a wider area with the development of new hybrids. The growing of corn requires a high level of technology, including selecting hybrids adapted to the area, using adequate fertilizer of the right kind, planting enough seed to establish a good, uniform stand, applying effective weed control, and using specialized machinery to carry out the necessary operations from planting to harvesting and storing effectively, on time, and with a minimum of labor.	**Processing:** Each year, about 6% of the U.S. corn crop is milled. Corn is wet milled for the production of starch, sweeteners, and oil; and corn is dry milled for the production of grits, flakes, meal, oil, and feeds. **Preparation:** Corn oil is further refined before using for food. **Uses:** Corn oil is used for salad dressings and cooking oil; and in such products as margarine and shortening. It is also used in paints, varnishes, soaps, glycerine, and linoleum.	Corn oil is rich in essential fatty acid and contains moderate amounts of vitamin E. The chief fatty acids of corn oil are: % Linoleic 54 Oleic 29 Palmitic 13 Stearic 4 Iodine value: 127

Footnote at end of table

A 1917 government poster promoting wholesome and nutritious foods from corn. (Courtesy, The Bettmann Archive, Inc., New York, NY)

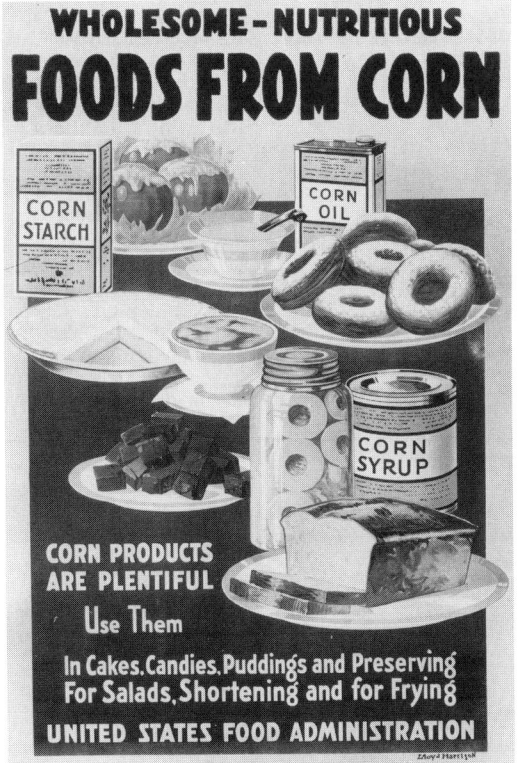

TABLE O–6 *(Continued)*

Oil; Source; Scientific Name; Origin and History	Importance; Principal Areas; Growing Conditions	Processing; Preparation; Uses	Nutritional Value[1]
Cottonseed Oil **Source:** Derived from the seed of the cotton plant. **Scientific Name:** Family: *Malvaceae* Genus: *Gossypium* Species: There are about 20 species, of which the following four are cultivated: *G. hirsutum,* American upland cotton; *G. barbadense,* Egyptian and Sea Island cottons; *G. herbaceum* and *G. arboreum,* the Asiatic cottons. **Origin and History:** Cotton has been grown for fiber for centuries. The Aztec Indians of Mexico grew cotton for textile purposes nearly 8,000 years ago. A record of cotton textiles, dating back about 5,000 years, was found in the Indus River Valley in what is now Pakistan. Excavations in Peru have uncovered cotton cloth identified as 4,500 years old. Cotton fabrics have also been found in the Pueblo ruins in Arizona and in the ruins of some of the early civilizations of Egypt. Although the ancient peoples used cotton for clothing, cottonseed was once largely wasted; hence, little or no oil was produced until the 19th century. (Also see COTTONSEED.)	**Importance:** Today, cottonseed oil is one of the most important food oils. It is the second most widely consumed vegetable oil in the United States. A ton of seed yields an average of 336 lb *(152 kg)* of oil. The United States and the U.S.S.R. are the leading cotton-producing countries of the world, with the ranking of the two countries shifting back and forth according to the growing conditions during the year. Production figures are in bales, with a net weight per bale of about 480 lb *(218 kg).* The world total production is approximately 86.7 million bales; and the world total cottonseed oil production is approximately 3.8 million metric tons. **Principal Areas:** The ten leading cotton-producing countries, by rank, are: China, U.S.A., U.S.S.R., India, Pakistan, Brazil, Turkey, Egypt, Australia, and Argentina. The U.S.A., China, and the U.S.S.R. accounted for 56% of the world total. The seven leading U.S. cotton producing states in total bales produced, by rank, are: Texas, California, Mississippi, Louisiana, Arkansas, Arizona, and Tennessee. **Growing Conditions:** Cotton requires a warm to hot climate with about 180 frost-free days during the growing season. It thrives best in fertile, well-drained soil that gets adequate moisture during the growing season. U.S. cotton production is highly mechanized. However, in many parts of the world, cotton is still grown and harvested in a relatively unmechanized fashion.	**Processing:** The oil is removed by three methods. The methods, along with the proportion of the U.S. cottonseed production processed by each, follows: screwpressing, 40%; prepress solvent extraction, 28%; and direct solvent extraction, 32%. **Preparation:** The crude oil extracted from the seed is usually subjected to the following processes: (1) refined, (2) bleached, (3) deodorized, and (4) winterized. **Uses:** The principal use of cottonseed oil in the United States is in salad and cooking oils. It is also used in shortening, margarine, and mellorine—a frozen dessert that is comparable to ice cream in appearance and nutritive value. Cottonseed oil is also used in emulsifiers, pharmaceuticals, insecticides and fungicides, cosmetics, rubber, plastics, and finishes for leather, paper, and textiles.	Two major technological breakthroughs have largely eliminated gossypol as a barrier to cottonseed oil in food: (1) the separation of the pigment glands in processing; and (2) glandless cottonseed. Cottonseed oil is classified as a polyunsaturated vegetable oil. Linoleic acid, its principal fatty acid, comprises about 47 to 50% of the total fatty acids. Its unique crystalline properties result from the presence of about 26% palmitic acid. Its good flavor is generally attributed to the absence of linolenic acid. Cottonseed oil is a preferred human food oil because of its flavor stability. Iodine value: 109

Footnote at end of table

(Continued)

TABLE O–6 *(Continued)*

Oil; Source; Scientific Name; Origin and History	Importance; Principal Areas; Growing Conditions	Processing; Preparation; Uses	Nutritional Value[1]

Olive Oil
Source: Derived from the olive, a fruit tree.
Scientific Name of the Olive Tree:
    Family: *Oleaceae*
    Genus: *Olea*
    Species: *O. europae*
Origin and History: It is not known when wild olives were first brought under domestication. Records point to Attica, the Greek peninsula, as the seat of the first cultivation.
(Also see OLIVE.)
	Importance: In the United States, olive oil is a sideline. The major portion of the fruit is processed for eating. There are about 13.5 million acres (*5.5 million ha*) of olive trees in the world; and over 1.7 million metric tons of olive oil are produced.
	Principal Areas: Seventy-five percent of the world's olive oil is produced in Spain, Greece, and Italy. There are about 32,000 acres (*12,598 ha*) of olive trees in central and southern California.
	Growing Conditions: Olives are adapted to hot, semiarid regions, and are tolerant of alkaline soils. Irrigation is usually required.
		Processing: Olives are processed by crushing between stone or steel rollers. Then the crushed pulp is pressed, after which the oil is separated from the liquor.
		Preparation: Olive oil of good quality is ready to use following extracting, without refining.
		Uses: Olive oil is used chiefly in salad dressings and as a cooking oil. It is also used in soaps, perfumes, and medicines.
			Olive oil is one of the most digestible of the edible oils. The fatty acid content of olive oil is:
			
			    %
			Oleic 75
			Palmitic 13
			Linoleic 9
			Stearic 2
			Palmitoleic 1
			
			Iodine value: 84
			A medium size olive averages about 3.8 Calories (kcal). Olives are a good source of calcium, iron, and vitamin A.

Palm Oil
Source: Derived from the oil palm tree.
Scientific Name of Oil Palm:
    Family: *Palmae*
    Genus: *Elaeis*
    Species: *E. guineensis*
Origin and History: The oil palm is indigenous to tropical West Africa, where it grows wild in great numbers.
(Also see OIL PALM.)
	Importance: Palm oil is one of the world's most important edible and soap-making oils. Moreover, the yield per acre is higher than can be obtained by any other vegetable oil.
	The world production of palm oil totals over 11 million metric tons, plus approximately 3 million metric tons of palm kernels.
	Principal Areas: The five leading palm oil producing countries of the world, by rank, are: Malaysia, Nigeria, Indonesia, Colombia, and Thailand.
	Growing Conditions: The oil palm thrives only where the rainfall is fairly high, but it will do rather well on poor soils.
		Processing: The traditional method of processing by African farmers consists of (1) fermenting the fruits, followed by boiling, pounding, and skimming off the oil; and (2) cracking the nuts and exporting the kernels for processing. Modern factories process by steam distillation, followed by centrifuging or hydraulic expression. In industrialized nations, the kernels are either expressed or are solvent extracted. Correctly speaking, the fruits yield palm oil and the kernels yield palm kernel oil. But usually both are referred to as palm oil.
		Preparation: Palm oil of good quality is ready for certain uses following extracting without refining. Although it is liquid when first extracted, it sets about as thick as butter at normal temperature.
		Uses: An estimated half of the palm oil produced in Africa is used locally as food in all kinds of cookery. The rest is exported. When exported, palm oil is used chiefly for soap-making and industrial purposes. But, with suitable treatment, it may also be used in margarine. Palm kernel oil, which is white or pale yellow, is largely used for margarine.
			Palm oils vary; in some cases, they resemble kernel oil, and in others olive oil.
			The fatty acid profile of palm oil is:
			
			    %
			Palmitic 48
			Oleic 38
			Linoleic 9
			Stearic 4
			Myristic 1
			
			The fatty acid profile of palm kernel oil is:
			
			    %
			Lauric 51
			Myristic 17
			Oleic 13
			Palmitic 8
			Capric 4
			Caprylic 3
			Stearic 2
			Linoleic 2
			
			Iodine value of palm oil: 51
			Iodine value of palm kernel oil: 16

Footnote at end of table

TABLE O–6 *(Continued)*

Oil; Source; Scientific Name; Origin and History	Importance; Principal Areas; Growing Conditions	Processing; Preparation; Uses	Nutritional Value[1]
Peanut Oil **Source:** Derived from the peanut; a member of the pea family. **Scientific Name:** Family: *Leguminosae* Genus: *Arachis* Species: *A. hypogaea* **Origin and History:** Peanuts (also called *groundnuts*) originated in South America. The South American Indians were growing peanuts at least 1,000 years ago. Early North American settlers grew peanuts, but no one knows whether peanuts were cultivated in North America before the settlers arrived. Peanuts did not become an important commercial crop in the United States until after 1917. (Also see PEANUTS.)	**Importance:** Peanuts, which contain 47 to 50% oil, are an important crop, especially in the warm regions of the world. World production totals: (1) peanuts in the shell, over 23 million metric tons; (2) peanut oil, 3.76 million metric tons. About ⅔ of the world's peanut crop is crushed for oil. Peanuts supply about 8% of the world's edible oil production, and almost 70% of the oilseed crops of India. **Principal Areas:** More than 80% of the global production is in Asia and Africa. The ten leading peanut-producing countries of the world, by rank, are: India, China, U.S.A., Nigeria, Indonesia, Senegal, Brazil, Zaire, Myanmar, and Argentina. The leading peanut-growing states of the United States, by rank, are: Georgia, Texas, North Carolina, Alabama, Virginia, Oklahoma, and Florida. **Growing Conditions:** Peanuts are an annual legume, adapted to warm climates. They need much sunshine, warm temperature, moderate rainfall, and a frost-free growing period of 4 to 5 months. They thrive best in light, well-drained, sandy soil. Loose soil is important so that the pegs can penetrate the ground easily.	**Processing:** The oil from peanuts is extracted by one of three methods: (1) hydraulic extraction, (2) expeller extraction, or (3) solvent extraction. **Preparation:** Following extracting, peanut oil is refined. The major portion of the characteristic peanut aroma and flavor is retained in the oil. **Uses:** In the United States, only a small proportion of the crop is processed for oil and protein concentrate. But in the rest of the world, peanuts are primarily processed for their separate constituents—oil and protein. Peanut oil is used primarily for food purposes: for frying foods, in salad oils, dressings, and margarine, and along with other vegetable shortenings. Also, peanut oil is used in soaps, face powders, shaving creams, shampoos, paints, as machinery oil, and in making nitroglycerin.	Peanut oil contains the following fatty acids: % Oleic 61 Linoleic 22 Palmitic 6 Stearic 5 Behenic 3 Arachidic 2 Lignoceric 1 Iodine value: 101 The major portion of the characteristic peanut aroma and flavor is imparted by the oil.

Footnote at end of table

(Continued)

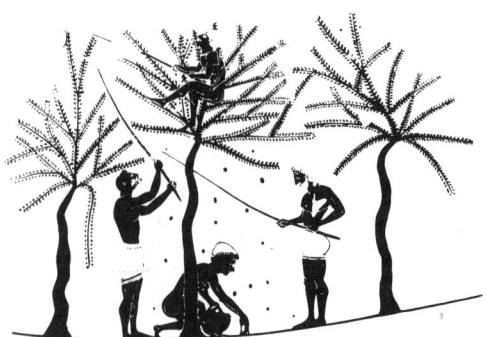

Romans gathering olives. From a vase of the 6th century B.C. (Courtesy, the Bettmann Archive, Inc., New York, NY)

TABLE O–6 *(Continued)*

Oil; Source; Scientific Name; Origin and History	Importance; Principal Areas; Growing Conditions	Processing; Preparation; Uses	Nutritional Value[1]
Rapeseed Oil **Source:** Derived from the rape plant, a member of the mustard family. **Scientific Name:** Family: *Cruciferae* Genus: *Brassica* Species: *B. napus* and *B. camtestris* **Origin and History:** The primary types of rape come from Asia, the Mediterranean, and western Europe. It has a long history, with earliest reference to it made in Indian Sanskrit writings of 2000 to 1500 B.C. (Also see RAPE.)	**Importance:** Rape oil is the only oil derived from an oilseed crop grown successfully in all parts of the world. World production of rapeseed totals approximately 24.5 million metric tons, and world production of rapeseed oil totals over 8.8 million metric tons. **Principal Areas:** The leading producing nations, by rank, are: China, India, Canada, Germany, France, U.K., and Poland. U.S. production of rapeseed and rapeseed oil is insignificant. **Growing Conditions:** Rape is a cool climate oilseed. But it does well in such subtropical areas as northern India, Japan, and Mexico, where it is grown as a cool season or winter crop. It grows well on a wide variety of soils.	**Processing:** The processing of rapeseed to obtain oil is similar to that of other oilseeds. There are three methods: (1) mechanical pressing, (2) straight solvent, or (3) pre-press solvent-extraction. The latter is the method of choice. **Preparation:** The crude oil must still be refined. **Uses:** The primary use of rapeseed oil is for human food. Its relatively low linolenic acid content permits it to compete with other vegetable oils in shortenings, margarine, salad oils, and frying oils. Oils which are almost free of erucic acid will open up new uses of rapeseed oil.	In the past, rapeseed oil was high (it contained 40 to 45%) in the long-chain fatty acid erucic acid. Since nutritional studies indicate that this substance, along with glucosinolates which the meal formerly contained, can be detrimental to human and animal health if consumed in substantial quantities, plant breeders were stimulated to make genetic changes in the composition of rapeseed—to lower or eliminate erucic acid and glucosinolate. This change has proceeded at different rates in different countries, but is now nearly complete in Canada—one of the leading rapeseed producers of the world. Oil made from the new varieties of rape is almost free of the long-chain fatty acid, erucic acid, while the oleic acid content is significantly higher. Except for the presence of linolenic acid, the composition of the new oil greatly resembles olive oil. Canada renamed the changed plant; it is called *canola.*
Safflower Oil **Source:** Safflower, a relative of the thistle. **Scientific Name:** Family: *Compositae* Genus: *Carthamus* Species: *C. tinctorius* **Origin and History:** Safflower is native to Southeastern Asia, but it has long been cultivated in India, Egypt, China, and North Africa. It was taken to Mexico by the early Spanish explorers. (Also see SAFFLOWER.)	**Importance:** The importance of safflower oil stems from its unique fatty acid composition, which places it highest in polyunsaturates and lowest in saturates of all commercial fats and oils. World safflower seed production averages approximately 922,000 metric tons. **Principal Areas:** India is far in the lead in safflower oil production, followed by Mexico, then the U.S.A. **Growing Conditions:** Climatically, the safflower is adapted to a dry climate and is salt-tolerant.	**Processing:** In the U.S.A., extraction of the oil is largely by the continuous screw-press solvent-extraction method. **Preparation:** The oil must be refined. Due to the susceptibility of safflower oil to oxidation, care is taken to exclude air during storage, transport, and packaging. **Uses:** Safflower oil is used principally in the production of margarine, salad oils, mayonnaise, shortening, and other food products. The oil is also used as a drying agent in paints and varnishes.	Safflower oil is (1) extolled as a preventative of cholesterol build-up in the blood, and (2) recommended in the diets of persons suffering from heart disease and hypertension. The value of polyunsaturated fatty acids for such treatments, however, remains a matter of controversy. Safflower oil averages about 6.6% saturated acids and 93.4% unsaturated acids, with the latter consisting of 77.0% linoleic acid and 16.4% oleic acid. Linolenic acid is absent.

Footnote at end of table

(Continued)

TABLE O–6 *(Continued)*

Oil; Source; Scientific Name; Origin and History	Importance; Principal Areas; Growing Conditions	Processing; Preparation; Uses	Nutritional Value[1]
Sesame Oil **Source:** Derived from the sesame plant, an annual herb. **Scientific Name:** Family: *Pedaliaceae* Genus: *Sesamum* Species: *S. indicum* **Origin and History:** Sesame has been grown in tropical countries for edible oils since time immemorial. It appears to be the oldest crop grown for edible oil. In 1298, Marco Polo observed the Persians using sesame oil for cooking, body massage, medicinal purposes, illumination, cosmetics, and lubricating primitive machinery. (Also see SESAME.)	**Importance:** The world production of sesame seed now exceeds 2 million metric tons. **Principal Areas:** Production of sesame is limited to countries where labor is plentiful and inexpensive, and will so remain until and unless nonshattering varieties with satisfactory yields and/or improved mechanical harvesting techniques are developed. The seven leading nations, by rank, are: India, China, Myanmar, Mexico, Nigeria, Sudan, and Somalia. Sudan is the largest exporter of seed. **Growing Conditions:** Most sesame is produced in tropical areas that are not agriculturally mechanized, and where harvesting is usually done by hand—by flailing pods with a stick.	**Processing:** In those areas where sesame is primarily processed for its oil content, the seed is not dehulled; rather, the entire seed is crushed. There is a U.S. patented process for extraction of oil from crushed sesame seed with hot calcium hydroxide solution. **Preparation:** Sesame oil is a natural salad oil requiring little or no winterization and is one of the few vegetable oils that can be used without refining. These are factors of increasing importance as energy costs escalate. **Uses:** Sesame oil is popular because of its pleasant, mild taste and remarkable stability—it is the most stable naturally occurring liquid vegetable oil. Sesame oil is much sought because of the presence of a natural antioxidant, sesamol, and because of its high content of unsaturated fatty acids, 40% oleic and 44% linoleic. The oil is used as a substitute for olive oil—primarily as a salad and cooking oil and for margarine and soap. Also, a significant quantity of oil is used by the cosmetic industry for softening and soothing purposes and by the pharmaceutical industry as a carrier for medicines.	Due to the presence of natural antioxidants in the crude oil, sesame oil is the most stable naturally occurring liquid vegetable oil. It will keep for several years without turning rancid. The fatty acid composition of sesame oil is: % Linoleic 44 Oleic 40 Palmitic 9 Stearic 5 Linolenic 2 Sesame oil is classified as polyunsaturated. Iodine value: 114

Footnote at end of table

(Continued)

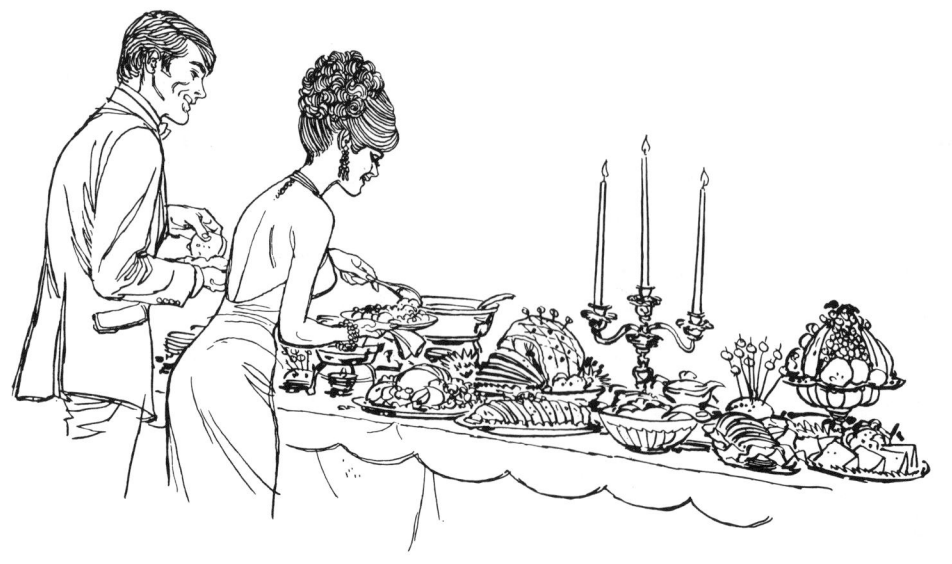

TABLE O–6 *(Continued)*

Oil; Source; Scientific Name; Origin and History	Importance; Principal Areas; Growing Conditions	Processing; Preparation; Uses	Nutritional Value[1]

Sorghum Oil
Source: Derived from the grain of the sorghum plant.
Scientific Name:
  Family: *Gramineae*
  Genus: *Sorghum*
  Species: *S. bicolor*
Origin and History: Sorghum has been cultivated in Africa and Asia for 4,000 years. Under the name "chicken corn," sorghum was introduced along the southern Atlantic coast of the United States in colonial times.
(Also see SORGHUM.)
 	
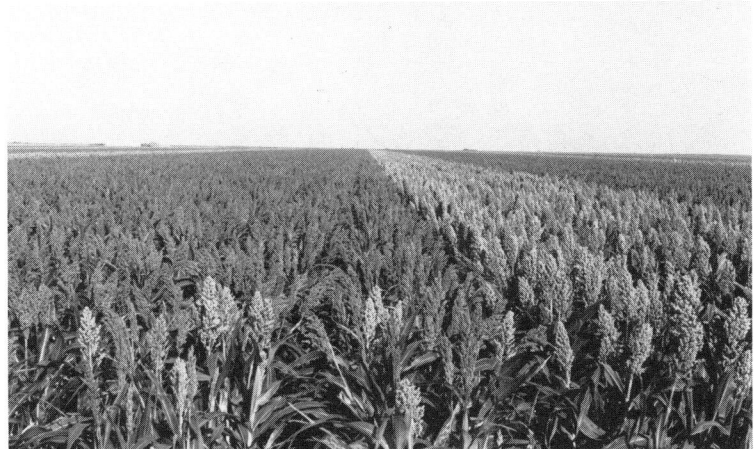
	Importance: Sorghum is the staple food in parts of Asia and Africa. In the United States, where it is used primarily as an animal feed, it is the third ranking cereal crop in acreage harvested, being exceeded only by corn and wheat.
	Sorghum is the fifth ranking cereal food crop of the world, being exceeded by wheat, rice, corn, and barley. The world sorghum crop totals over 58 million metric tons.
	Principal Areas: The ten leading producing countries of the world, by rank, are: U.S.A., India, Mexico, China, Nigeria, Argentina, Sudan, Australia, Ethiopia, and Burkina Faso.
	In the United States, which produced 25% of the world's sorghum grain in 1990, the Sorghum Belt is in the Southern Great Plains.
	Growing Conditions: Sorghum is a tropical or subtropical plant, grown mainly in hot, dry regions where corn, rice, and wheat cannot be produced successfully. Although well adapted to semiarid conditions, sorghum makes efficient use of irrigation.
		Processing: As with corn, sorghum may be either dry milled or wet milled. However, most sorghum is dry milled, simply because it is easier to accomplish.
		Sorghum oil is extracted from the germ of the grain.
		Preparation: For food use, sorghum oil must be refined, much like corn oil.
		Uses: Cooking oil; and in such products as margarine and shortenings.
			The oil of sorghum is important nutritionally, and it influences flavor and acceptability of sorghum products.
			The fatty acid composition of sorghum germ oil is similar to corn oil.
			(See CORN OIL.)
			The ether extract of sorghum bran is composed mainly of long-chain alcohols and esters with some long-chain hydrocarbons.

Footnote at end of table

(Continued)

A field of grain sorghum, headed out. Sorghum oil, which is similar to corn oil, is extracted from the germ of the grain. (Courtesy, Funk Seeds International, Bloomington, Ill.)

TABLE O–6 (Continued)

Oil; Source; Scientific Name; Origin and History	Importance; Principal Areas; Growing Conditions	Processing; Preparation; Uses	Nutritional Value[1]
Soybean Oil **Source:** Soybean oil is derived from seeds produced by soybean plants. **Scientific Name:** Family: *Leguminosae* Genus: *Glycine* Species: *G. max* **Origin and History:** The soybean plant is native to eastern Asia. It was among the first crops grown by man. Soybeans emerged as a cultivated crop in China in the 11th century B.C. (Also see SOYBEANS.)	**Importance:** Soybean oil is the leading vegetable oil for human food in the United States. In the Far East, soybean oil is consumed extensively as a food. World production of soybeans now totals about 108 million metric tons, and world production of soybean oil is approximately 15.7 million metric tons. **Principal Areas:** The eight leading soybean producing countries, by rank, are: U.S.A., Brazil, China, Argentina, India, Paraguay, Indonesia, and Italy. The United States produces over 52 million metric tons of soybeans, about 49% of the world total. Most of the soybeans in the United States are produced in the Corn Belt and in southern and southeastern United States. **Growing Conditions:** Soybeans produce maximum yields in soils where residual fertility has been maintained at a high level and the pH is between 6.0 and 6.5. Because soybeans are legumes, they can obtain part of their nitrogen enrichment from the air through the action of certain nodule-forming bacteria living in the roots of the plant, provided the seed is inoculated. In the United States, soybeans are usually planted in rows in a well prepared seedbed, in May or early June. Most soybeans are harvested by means of a combine, which threshes as it reaps.	**Processing:** There are three basic processing methods of obtaining oil from soybeans: solvent extraction, hydraulic extraction, or expeller extraction. Today, almost all of the oil is extracted by the solvent process. **Preparation:** About 93% of soybean oil is used for food. To be suitable for human consumption, the extracted crude oil must undergo further processing, which is generally referred to as refining. **Uses:** Soybean oil is widely used throughout the world for human consumption as margarine, salad and cooking oils, and shortening. Also, soybean oil is used in paints, varnishes, enamels, soaps, linoleum, pharmaceuticals, cosmetics, core oil, synthetic rubber, and printing ink.	The fatty acid profile of soybean oil follows: % Linoleic 54 Oleic 24 Palmitic 12 Linolenic 8 Stearic 2 Soybean oil is low in saturated fat and free of cholesterol. Iodine value: 134

Footnote at end of table

(Continued)

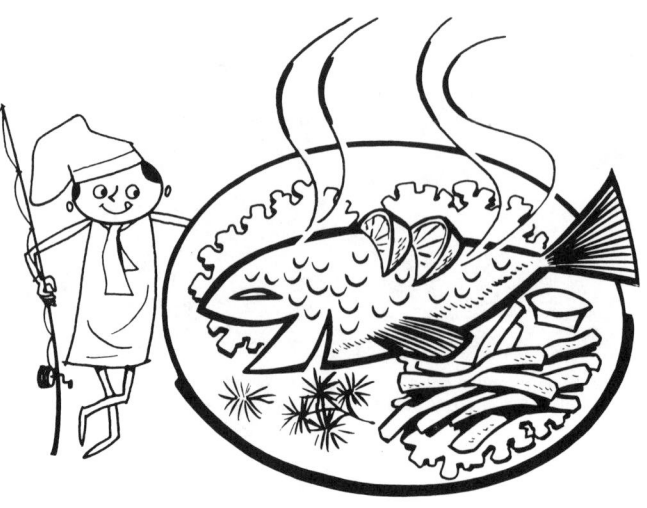

TABLE O–6 *(Continued)*

Oil; Source; Scientific Name; Origin and History	Importance; Principal Areas; Growing Conditions	Processing; Preparation; Uses	Nutritional Value[1]
Sunflower Oil **Source:** Sunflowers **Scientific Name:** Family: *Compositeae* Genus: *Helianthus* Species: *H. annuus* **Origin and History:** The sunflower was first domesticated in the United States, although there is evidence that this honor should be shared with Peru and Mexico. (Also see SUNFLOWERS.) 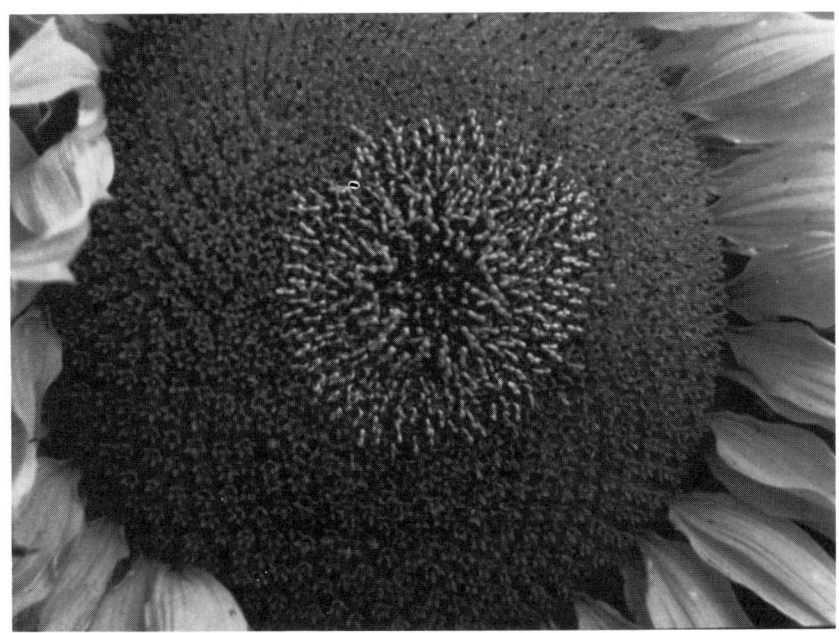	**Importance:** Today, sunflower oil holds undisputed claim to third place among vegetable oils. World sunflower seed production is approximately 22 million metric tons, and world sunflower oil production totals 7.8 million metric tons. Twenty-nine percent of the world sunflower seed is produced in the U.S.S.R. Eighty percent of the vegetable oil produced in the Soviet Union comes from sunflowers. **Principal Areas:** The ten leading sunflower-producing countries, by rank, are: U.S.S.R., Argentina, France, China, Spain, U.S.A., Turkey, Hungary, South Africa, and Romania. U.S. sunflower production is centered in North and South Dakotas, Minnesota, and Texas. **Growing Conditions:** Sunflowers are drought resistant except for the 3-week interval during flower and seed development. They demand proper management, and they yield poorly when the management practices are not good. Sunflowers are adapted to most of the climates and cultivated soils of the United States.	**Processing:** The separation of the oil from the seed may be achieved (1) by direct solvent-extraction, (2) by pre-press solvent-extraction, or (3) by mechanical means (screwpressing). In the United States, sunflower oil is processed primarily by the prepress solvent-extraction method; and only small quantities of seed are dehulled prior to extraction. **Preparation:** Crude sunflower oil is stored in tanks following extraction until further processing. After refining, it has an attractive color and a pleasant, faintly nutty flavor. **Uses:** Cooking oil, salad oil, shortening, margarine, or for frying foods, making potato chips, producing a modified butter with improved low temperature spreadability, and blending with other vegetable oils.	The fatty acid composition of sunflower oil makes it desirable as an edible oil. It follows: $\quad\quad\quad$ % Linoleic $\quad$ 66 Oleic $\quad\quad$ 21 Palmitic $\quad$ 8 Stearic $\quad\;$ 5 As noted, sunflower oil is relatively low in the saturated fatty acids, palmitic and stearic. The high linoleic acid content and the high ratio of polyunsaturated to saturated fatty acid prompts some nutritionists to believe that sunflower oil might be useful in the prevention and treatment of high blood cholesterol and heart disease. Iodine value: 134

[1]Food Composition Table F-36 and Table F-9, Fats and Fatty Acids in Selected Foods contain additional information.

A close-up view of a sunflower head in full bloom. (Courtesy, National Sunflower Assn., Bismark, N.D.)

OKRA (GUMBO) *Hibiscus esculentus; Abelmoschus esculentus*

This plant bears edible seed-filled pods. Although the vegetable itself is sometimes called "gumbo," this name is more often given to the soups and stews in which it is an important ingredient. Okra is a member of the Mallow family (*Malvaceae*), which includes cotton and various other plants grown for fiber, flowers, and/or food. Fig. O-12 shows a typical okra plant.

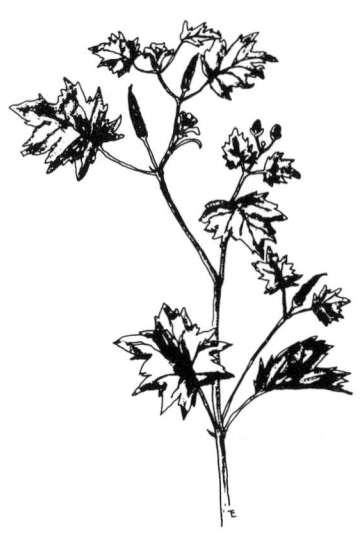

Fig. O-12.   Okra, a plant that furnishes the pods used in gumbo soups and other Creole dishes which characterize the French cuisine of New Orleans. (Courtesy, USDA)

ORIGIN AND HISTORY.   Okra is believed to be native to Africa, where it was first cultivated. However, wild species have also been found in India, which suggests that the wild ancestor(s) of the plant was widely distributed throughout the Old World. Some historians suspect that okra was taken from Africa to Spain by the invading Moors of the 8th century. The vegetable was introduced into the tropical areas of the Americas shortly after the discovery of these lands by Columbus. Although okra was once grown as far north as Philadelphia, almost all of the commercial crop is now produced in the southern United States, where the climate favors a rapid rate of growth.

PRODUCTION.   This vegetable is grown throughout the subtropical and tropical areas of the world, including the southern United States. However, statistics on the world and U.S. production are not readily available, though the USDA reports that each year more than 12 million pounds of okra are shipped within the United States, and more than 65 million pounds are frozen.

Okra seeds require warm soil for germination. Therefore, it is noteworthy that this plant has about the same planting, fertilization, and watering schedule as corn.

The pods should be harvested when they are 3 or 4 days old because (1) after that they become more fibrous and tough, and (2) harvesting the pods before they reach maturity stimulates the plant to bear more.

PROCESSING.   A large part of the crop is frozen, while much of the remainder is canned alone or in various soups. In some parts of Europe and Asia the young pods are dried for export. Also, the gummy extract from the pods is used to make an extender for blood plasma.

SELECTION AND PREPARATION.   Young, tender, fresh, clean pods of small to medium size (2 to 4 in. [5 to 10 cm] in length) are usually of good quality. Such pods snap easily when broken and are easily punctured. Dull, dry-appearing pods indicate excessive age and are usually hard, woody, and fibrous, with hard seeds. Also, pods that are not fresh may be shriveled, discolored, and lacking in flavor. Depending on variety, okra pods may be green or whitish-green, varying somewhat in size and ridging.

Young okra pods require only brief cooking (not more than 5 minutes). Usually, they are cut crosswise, and prepared by (1) boiling or steaming, then served with butter, margarine, or a sauce; (2) dipping in egg, dredging in cornmeal, and frying; or (3) cooking in soups and stews to which they contribute flavorful bite-sized pieces of vegetable, and a thickening effect (due to the mucilaginous substance they contain). Also, okra and stewed tomatoes are commonly served as a vegetable dish. Finally, the Creole cuisine of New Orleans includes various "gumbos," or okra-containing stews of vegetables, seasonings, and crabs, fish, meat, and/or poultry.

CAUTION: Okra may become discolored if it is cooked in a utensil made from brass, copper, or iron. However, the discoloration is not harmful; it is only unsightly. Nevertheless, it would be best to use aluminum, stainless steel, or enamel-coated utensils for cooking okra.

NUTRITIONAL VALUE.   The nutrient compositions of various forms of okra are given in Food Composition Table F-36.

Some noteworthy observations regarding the nutrient composition of okra follow:

1.   Okra is low in calories (only about 30 to 40 kcal per 100 g), but it is a fair to good source of calcium, potassium, vitamin A, and vitamin C. Also, it supplies about 7 g of protein per 100 Calories (kcal). However, about 10½ oz (*300 g*) would have to be eaten to supply these amounts of calories and protein. Therefore, okra is a good food for hearty eaters, since it is filling, but not fattening.

2.   The mucilaginous material from cooked okra is very soothing to irritations of the digestive tract. Hence,

ulcer patients may be fed the extracted "goo" without the seeds and fibrous matter of the vegetable.

(Also see VEGETABLE[S], Table V-6 Vegetables of the World.)

OLD PROCESS

Pertains to the extraction of oil from seeds. Same as hydraulic process.

(Also see OILS, VEGETABLE)

OLEIC ACID

An 18-carbon unsaturated fatty acid (one double bond) which reacts with glycerol to form olein.

(Also see FATS AND OTHER LIPIDS.)

OLEOMARGARINE

A nondairy butter substitute made of not less than 80% vegetable and/or animal fat. The first butter substitute was made by a French chemist, H. Mege-Mouries, in response to an appeal by Napoleon III. Mouries used oil obtained by pressing beef fat (oleo oil), to produce a pearly appearing product. His product was and still is called oleomargarine—a name derived from the oleo oil, and from the Greek word *margarites*, meaning pearly. The words margarine and oleomargarine are used interchangeably.

(Also see MARGARINE.)

OLFACTORY

Pertaining to the sense of smell.

OLIGOSACCHARIDE

A complex carbohydrate which contains 2 to 10 molecules of monosaccharides combined through glycoside bonds.

OLIGURIA

Scanty urination.

OLIVE *Olea europaea*

Legend has it that Athena (Greek goddess of war) and Poseidon (Greek god of the sea) once disputed the allegiance of a small settlement on a rock in eastern Greece. A jury of gods agreed to decide in favor of the one who could most benefit the primitive inhabitants. Poseidon struck a salt spring from the rock. Athena turned and pointed to an olive tree, the very first one, which she had caused to grow from the soil. With great discernment, the gods ruled in favor of Athena, with her gifts of agriculture.

ORIGIN AND HISTORY. The olive is one of the oldest known fruit crops; man grew olive trees even before recorded history. It is not known when the wild olive was first brought under cultivation. But records point to the limestone hills of Attica, the Greek peninsula, as the seat of its first cultivation. The olive is frequently mentioned in the Bible. The Spanish brought the olive to California in 1769; in the early Franciscan missions, the fruit was pressed for oil and used in the diet and burned in lamps.

PRODUCTION. There are about 13.5 million acres (*5.5 million ha*) of olive trees in the world. Each year, about 9 million metric tons of olives and 1.6 million metric tons of olive oil are produced. The countries bordering the Mediterranean Sea grow most of the world's olives; Italy and Spain produce 50% of the olives and 54% of the olive oil. Olives are also grown in Greece, Turkey, Syria, Morocco, Tunisia, Portugal, and the U.S.A. In Spain, trees yield about one-third ton per acre; in California, yields are higher.

There are about 32,000 acres (*12,598 ha*) of olive trees in central and southern California. The United States produces an average of about 110,000 tons of olives. In this country, over 90% of the fruit is processed for table eating; only blemished and small fruit are processed for oil.

The olive tree is adapted to a hot, dry climate; and it does well on many different soils. For bearing fruit, it must have water (usually irrigation), along with good drainage. Trees come into production at 5 years of age, but are not in full production until 15 to 20 years old; and they are long lived. Some of the trees brought to the United States by the Spaniards are still bearing fruit.

For the production of high quality table olives, the fruit is picked by hand. But harvesting for the oil industry has been mechanized, either by knocking the fruit from the tree with slender poles, or by use of shakers.

PROCESSING. Olives were one of the first crops that man learned to adapt to his needs by developing special techniques for making the fruit edible and for extraction of the oil.

The methods of processing olives for the table vary widely. However, the three major commercial methods, known after the countries of their origin, are: (1) the Spanish method, in which unripe yellowish-green olives are fermented; (2) the American method, in which half-

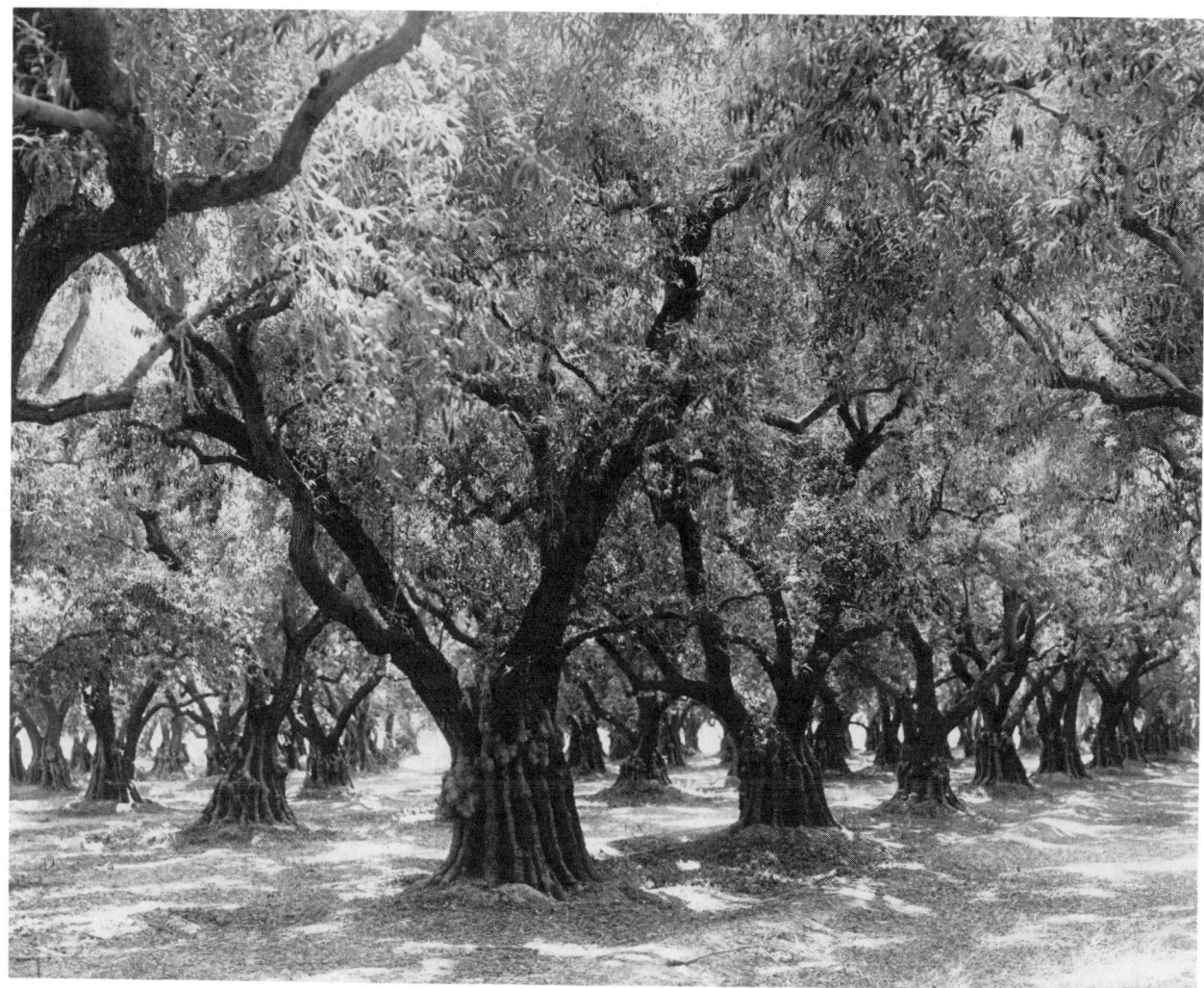

Fig. O-13.   Olive grove. (Courtesy, California Olive Industry, Fresno, Calif.)

ripe, reddish fruit is used; and (3) the Greek method, in which the fully ripe, dark purple fruit is preserved. Additionally, there are numerous local methods of processing, including pitting, stuffing, chopping, and spicing. In most processing methods, a weak solution of lye is applied for the purpose of neutralizing the bitter principle; the lye penetrates the olives and hydrolyzes the bitter phenolic glycoside, oleuropeen. The lye-treated olives are immediately rinsed and soaked in water with frequent changes in order to remove the lye. The washed olives are then placed in fermentation tanks and barrels and covered with brine. (See Fig. O-14.)

The use of lye is not permitted in Greece; instead, they rely on brine (salt solution) to lessen and mask the bitterness.

Olive oil is produced by mechanical extraction of the ground fruit. Traditionally, this involves three steps: (1) crushing the fruit, (2) pressing (usually 2 to 4 times) the paste, and (3) separating the oil from the liquor. After the second pressing, the cake is usually solvent-extracted. Unlike most other vegetable oils, olive oil prepared from properly matured, harvested, and stored fruit is consumed without any refining treatment, thereby alleviating the need for added energy.

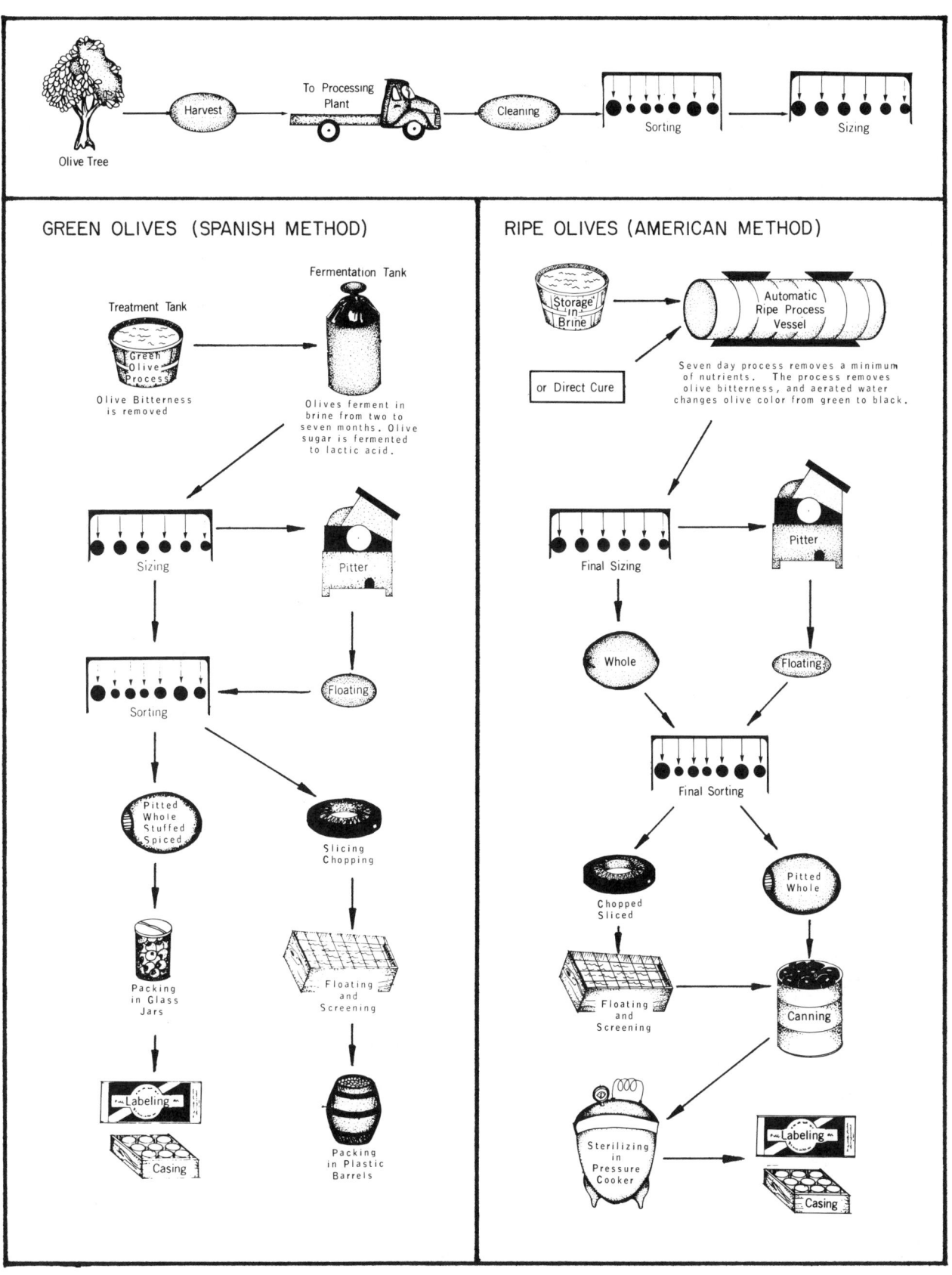

Fig. O-14. Olive process flow chart; from harvesting through processing by either (1) Spanish method—green fermented, or (2) American method—ripe olives. (Adapted from flow chart provided by Lindsay Olive Growers, Lindsay, Calif.)

PREPARING. Most table olives are prepared commercially in ready-to-serve form, using one of the following methods:

1. **Canned or bottled green fermented olives (Spanish method).** This refers to green olives that are fermented, then put in jars or barrels. Increasingly, green olives are being pitted and the pit cavity stuffed with either pimentos, onions, almonds, anchovies, or other edibles.

2. **Canned ripe olives (American method).** The production of canned ripe olives is centered in California. The olives are picked when straw yellow to cherry red in color. In the curing process, the olives darken progressively due to the oxidation of the phenolic substances in a basic environment. The cured olives are packed in enamel-lined cans, covered with salt solution, sealed, and sterilized. More and more canned ripe olives are being pitted and stuffed.

A combination of the American and Spanish methods, known as green-ripe olives, is also used in California. In it, greener, less-mature fruit is used than for the method described above.

3. **Black, naturally ripe olives (Greek method).** Olives to be prepared by this method are kept on the trees until they are fully matured and completely dark. The fruit is brined, with frequent change of water in order to hasten the destruction of the bitter principle. Pretreatment with lye solution before brining, such as is used in the Spanish method, will hasten debittering and fermentation.

In addition to the above three major commercial procedures, a large number of different techniques for preparing olives for table use exist. Olives are often pitted, stuffed, chopped, and spiced, and put in fancy packs.

Olive oil of good quality needs no refining.

NUTRITIONAL VALUE. The nutrient compositions of olives and olive oil are given in Food Composition Table F-36.

A few salient points regarding the nutritional value of olives follow:

1. At full maturity, the fruit meat (mesocarp) contains 15 to 35% oil. The pit, which accounts for 15 to 30% of the weight of the fruit, contains about 5% oil. The characteristic bitter glycoside, oleuropein, present in fresh olives, is concentrated close to the peel (exocarp).

2. Olive oil consists chiefly of glycerides formed by a mixture of unsaturated and saturated fatty acids. Unsaturation is due primarily to oleic acid (67% to 83%). It has a saponification number of 187 to 191 (vs 87 to 93 for corn) and an iodine number of 78 to 90 (vs 105 to 125 for corn). (The larger the saponification number, the smaller the average chain length; and the higher the iodine number, the greater the degree of unsaturation.)

3. Olives are low in calories, with variation according to size and oil content. On a per olive basis, they average about as follows:

Olive Size	Calories/Olive
Medium	3.84
Large	4.50
Extra Large	5.31

4. Olives contain fair amounts of iron and calcium and some vitamin A.

USES. Increasingly, table olives are becoming luxury products in countries with high standards of living.

The oil is highly esteemed by the gourmet. It is used chiefly in salad dressings, as a cooking oil, and for canning sardines. The oil is also used for medicinal purposes in the pharmaceutical industry, and for cosmetic and toilet preparations. In some countries, olive oil is prescribed for burning in sanctuary lamps and for anointing.

The press residue remaining after extracting the oil from the olives may be used (1) for livestock feed (after removal of the pieces of pits), (2) for fuel or fertilizer, or (3) for the production of charcoal.

(Also see OILS, VEGETABLE, TABLE O-6; and VEGETABLE[S], Table V-6 Vegetables of the World.)

OLIVE OIL

Oil extracted from olives that are crushed into a pulp and then pressed. Olive oil is ready for use following extraction. It is one of the most digestible of the edible oils. Its chief uses are salad dressings and cooking oil.

(Also see OLIVE; and OILS, VEGETABLE, Table O-6 Vegetable Oils—"Olive Oil.")

-OLOGY

Suffix meaning science of, or study of.

OMOPHAGIA

The practice of eating foods, particularly flesh, raw. The primitive diet of Eskimos consisted of raw meat and fish.

ONION *Allium cepa,* **variety** *cepa*

The underground bulb of this plant is one of the leading vegetable crops of the world. It is distinguished by its pungency when raw and the appetizing flavor it imparts when cooked with various other foods. The odor is due to an oil, which readily forms a vapor and escapes into the air when onions are peeled or cut. It affects nerves in the nose connected with the eyes, and makes tears flow.

The onion, like the other related vegetables (*Allium* genus), has long been classified as a member of the Lily family (*Liliaceae*), but now some botanists place the onion and its close relatives in a new family called the *Alliaceae*. The common onion is classified as the variety *cepa* to distinguish it from other varieties of onions such as the shallot, which is the *aggregatum* variety. Fig. O-15 shows a typical onion bulb.

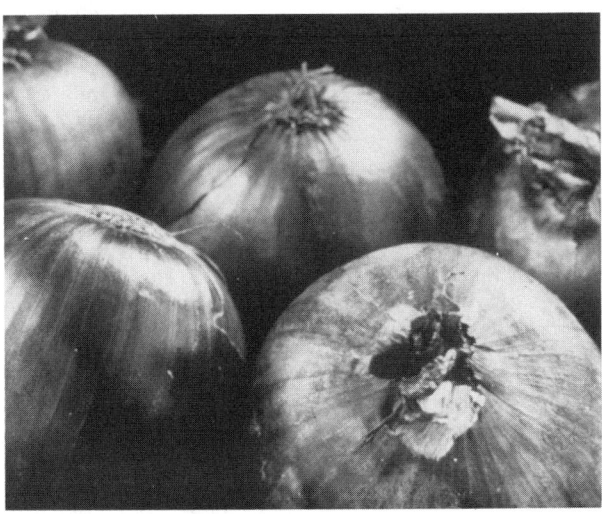

Fig. O-15. Onions, a leading vegetable crop of the world. (Courtesy, USDA)

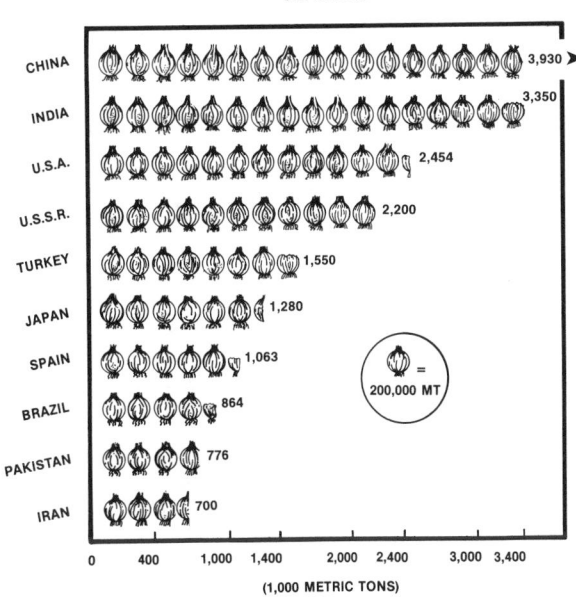

Fig. O-16. The leading onion-producing countries of the world. (Based upon data from *FAO Production Yearbook*, 1990, FAO/UN, Rome, Italy, Vol. 44, p. 141, Table 58)

ORIGIN AND HISTORY.

Onions originated in the central part of Asia which extends eastward from Iran to Pakistan, and northward into the southern part of the Soviet Union. It seems likely that prehistoric man gathered and cooked wild onions along with various other bulbs, roots, and tubers long before the first crops were planted. Some time after the dawn of agriculture in the Middle East, onions were grown in ancient Chaldea and ancient Egypt. They were used as early as 5,000 years ago in the First Egyptian Dynasty. Onions were represented on ancient Egyptian monuments, and one variety cultivated in Egypt was accorded divine honors.

Ancient Greek and Roman literature attests to the popularity of onions in those times. However, they did not seem to be spicy enough to suit the upper-class Romans, who often dressed them with asafetida (a pungent resin). During the Middle Ages, onions were consumed throughout all of Europe. Peasants in China also used this vegetable in many dishes and developed certain unique varieties of the plant. The widespread production of onions in the Old World made it possible for many of the poor to add some much needed flavor to their otherwise bland diet. Later, the New World benefitted similarly when the crop, which was planted by Columbus in the West Indies, was brought to many parts of this new land.

The status of onions rose significantly after the popularization of French onion soup by Stanislaus I, the former king of Poland who had close ties to France. (His daughter was married to King Louis XV.) Recently, it was found that the allicin present in the bulbs inhibits the growth of certain bacteria.

PRODUCTION.

About 30 million metric tons of dry onions are produced worldwide each year. Fig. O-16 shows the amounts contributed by the ten top producers

The annual production of onions in the United States is over 2.4 million metric tons. Fig. O-17 shows the amounts produced in the leading states.

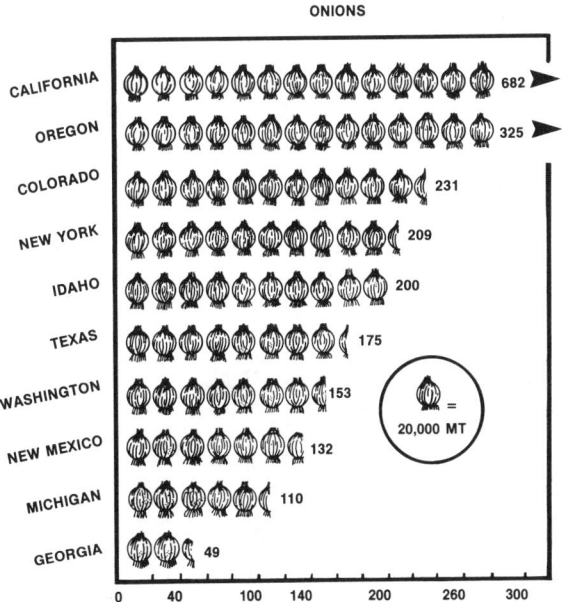

Fig. O-17. The ten top onion-producing states. (Based on data from *Agricultural Statistics*, 1991, USDA, p. 157, Table 222)

Onions are propagated by planting either seeds or small bulbs (sets). Fig. O-18 shows onion plants that were grown for their seeds. Sets are produced by sowing onion

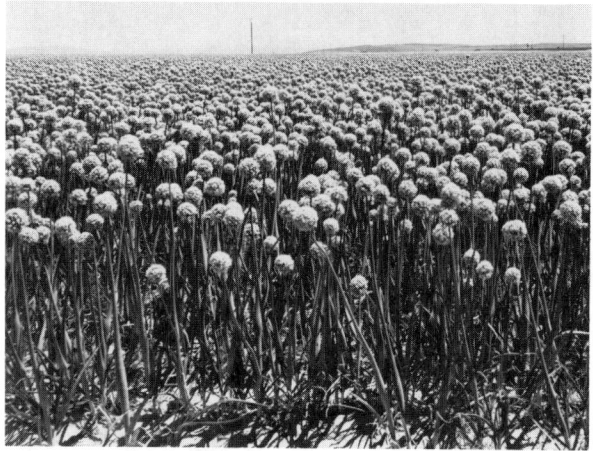

Fig. O-18.   Flowering onion plants. The seeds produced by these plants will be used to plant the next crop of onion bulbs. (Courtesy, Union Pacific Railroad Company, Omaha, Nebr.)

seed very thickly so that the plants grow very close together and produce only small bulbs. Bulbs for planting usually range from ¼- to 1-in. (0.6 to 2.5 cm) in diameter. Planting should be done as early as possible (in cold climates as soon as the danger of a hard frost has passed) so that there will be an adequate development of foliage before the formation of bulbs occurs. Foliage grows best in cool weather, and the bulbs thrive in warm weather. Each onion variety will begin to form bulbs at a particular time in the growing season, regardless of when planting was done, but the plants with the most foliage will produce the largest bulbs.

Most of the U.S. crop is planted in well-drained organic (muck) soils which have been well pulverized. Clay soils usually require the addition of humus to make them loose enough for onion growing. Whenever feasible, the crop is irrigated in areas where there is insufficient rainfall, although it is grown without irrigation (dry-land production) in certain parts of Texas.

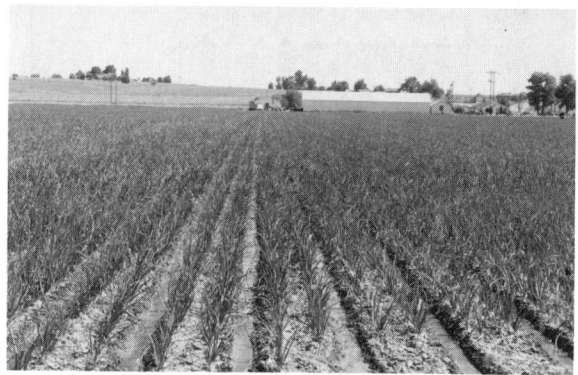

Fig. O-19.   An irrigated field of onions. (Courtesy, Union Pacific Railroad Company, Omaha, Nebr.)

Young onion plants usually require careful cultivation and weeding until they are well established. Cultivation should not be deeper than an inch or so, because onion roots lie close to the surface of the soil. Sometimes, chemical weed killers are applied to the soil, but this practice may be inadvisable when chemical-sensitive crops are to be planted after the onions.

Onion bulbs may be harvested for use as (1) green onions, when the bulbs are immature and range from ¼ to 1 in. (0.6 to 2.5 cm) in diameter; or (2) mature (dry) onions, when the top of the plant has started to turn yellow and wither. The average yield of onions in the United States is 38,200 lb per acre (42,888 kg/ha). Yields as high as 47,500 lb (53,200 kg/ha) are obtained in Idaho and Oregon.

Fresh green onions do not keep well, so they must be used or processed within a short time after harvesting. Mature onions are often dried in the field if the weather permits. After drying, the tops are cut from the bulbs. It is noteworthy that the most pungent varieties of dry onions keep the best in storage because the pungency is due to a component that acts as a preservative. Fig. O-20 shows dry onions ready for marketing.

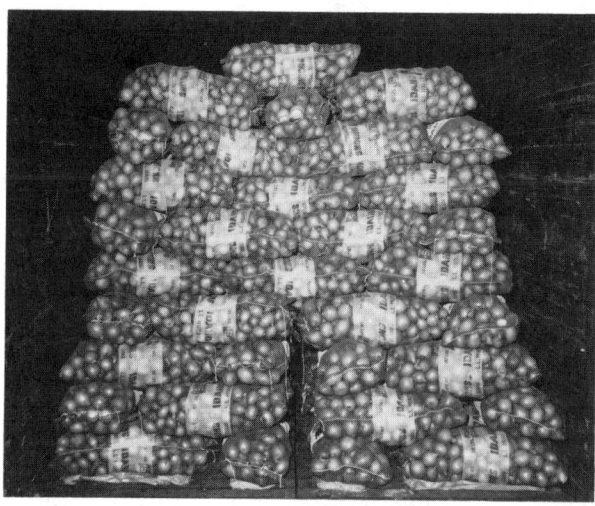

Fig. O-20.   Dry onions packed in 50-lb (23 kg) bags. (Courtesy, Union Pacific Railroad Company, Omaha, Nebr.)

PROCESSING. The length of time that unprocessed onions may be stored without spoilage varies from a few days to as long as several months, depending upon the variety, stage of maturity, and degree of pungency. Furthermore, the producers of items such as condiments, prepared ethnic foods (Chinese, Italian, and Mexican dishes, mainly), sauces, and soups often find it more convenient to incorporate preprocessed onions in their products than to process raw onions in their own plants. Therefore, the most common means of processing are noteworthy:

• **Canning**—White-skinned onions, which are the most desirable ones for canning, are processed by removal of the papery skin, blanching, packing into cans, acidifying, and processing in a boiling water bath. Onions are also canned in prepared soups that require only heating.

• **Dehydration**—This procedure involves (1) burning off the onion skin and pieces of adhering roots, (2) washing with a high pressure stream of water to remove the charred pieces of skin, (3) slicing the deskinned onions thinly, (4) drying the slices with hot air, and (5) packaging the dehyrated pieces. Sometimes, dehydrated onion pieces are ground finely to make onion powder and onion salt.

• **Freezing**—Onions are commonly frozen in forms such as chopped raw onions, French fried onion rings, prepared soups, and TV dinners.

• **Pickling**—Small, immature onion bulbs are pickled by soaking in several changes of a salt solution (brine), boiling in fresh brine, and packing in a well-seasoned mixture of vinegar and sugar. Pickled onions are quite popular as an appetizer, and in certain cocktails.

SELECTION AND PREPARATION.
Professional chefs select types of onions according to how they will be utilized, since there are notable differences in flavor, pungency, and quality among the varieties commonly available in the United States. Hence, some guidelines for selecting and utilizing the various kinds of onions follow:

Dry Onions. Most people expect to be able to store mature onions in their refrigerator for considerable periods of time. However, some of the mild varieties may spoil rapidly, therefore, the discussions which follow are noteworthy.

TYPES. Two general classes of dry onions grown in the United States are found in retail markets: the mild flavored types, either large and elongated, or flat; and the usually stronger flavored types, generally globe shaped and medium in size. The former are *Spanish* or *Bermuda* types, and the latter are known as *globe* or *late crop* types.

The Bermuda type is flat in shape, sweet and mild, and usually may be found in markets from March to June in either yellow, white, or red varieties. The Spanish or Valencia type is a large, somewhat elongated, mild, sweet onion which may be either light-yellowish, brown, or white in color. They are available in most markets from August through April.

Globe or other late crop onion types are mostly somewhat globular in shape, with yellow, white, red, or brown skins, depending on variety. These onions usually keep extremely well under proper storage conditions and are marketed throughout the year.

Boiler is a term used to designate small-size onions.

JUDGING QUALITY. Bright, clean, hard, well-shaped, mature onions with dry skins are usually of good quality. Onions in which the seedstem has developed are undesirable. A thick, tough, woody or open condition of the necks, or a visible portion of the stem indicates seedstem development which causes excess waste in utilization.

Misshapen onions are objectionable only because of probable waste in preparation for use. The most common forms of off-shape are "splits," "doubles," and "bottle necks"—terms which are largely self-explanatory.

Moisture at the neck of an onion is an indication of decay which may not be visible but may cause the onion to be entirely unfit for use. Decay may also appear on the outer scales as wet, discolored, or moldy areas.

UTILIZATION. Many recipes call for chopped onions, which may be prepared without tears by either (1) putting the onions in a freezer for a short time before chopping them, or (2) chopping the vegetable while it is held under water. The eye-irritating substance in onions is released as a result of the enzyme action brought about by rupturing of cells in the onion. Freezing retards the enzyme action, whereas water dissolves and dilutes the irritant. Also, much of the pungency of raw onions is reduced by cooking.

Chopped or sliced raw onions go well with roasted meats and poultry, and with other raw vegetables in relishes and salads.

Stewed onions may be served with butter, cheese sauce, or white sauce.

Broiled onions are a good accompaniment to broiled fish, fried liver, hamburger, and steak.

Large onions may be stuffed with breadcrumbs, cooked kasha (buckwheat groats), fish, meat, poultry, and/or rice and baked like other stuffed vegetables.

Dehydrated onions may be used in place of either raw or cooked fresh onions, provided that they are rehydrated sufficiently.

Onion powder or onion salt makes an excellent seasoning, but some of the flavor components of fresh onion are missing.

Finally, the various forms of onions may be added to a wide variety of casseroles, soups, and stews.

CAUTION: The use of excessive amounts of either dehydrated onions or onion powder may result in (1) a strong laxative effect, and (2) irritation of the digestive tract, because these products are highly concentrated sources of the irritants present in fresh onions.

Green Onions. These onions are usually early white or bulbless varieties that are harvested when the partially developed bulbs reach the desired size. Good quality green onions should have green, fresh tops, medium-sized necks well blanched for 2 or 3 in. (*5 to 8 cm*) from the root; and should be young, crisp, and tender. Yellowing, wilted, or discolored tops may indicate flabby, tough, fibrous necks or other undesirable qualities. Except for appearance, bruised tops are unimportant in utilization.

Green onions may be served raw as an appetizer, or they may be chopped and added to cottage cheese, cream cheese, salads, and salad dressings. They are also good when pickled, stewed and served with a sauce, or when added to casseroles, soups, and stews.

NUTRITIONAL VALUE. The nutrient composition of various forms of onions are given in Food Composition Table F-36.

Some noteworthy observations regarding the nutrient composition of onions follow:

1. Dry, mature onions are high in water content (89%) and low in calories (38 kcal/100 g), protein (1.5%), and most other nutrients. They are a fair source of potassium, but they contain barely enough vitamin C to prevent scurvy (about 10 mg of vitamin C per 100 g).

2. Dehydrated onion flakes and onion powder contain almost ten times the solids content of fresh onions. Hence, the flakes and powder are much better sources of calories, protein, and other nutrients than the fresh bulbs. However, the dehydrated products may have a strong laxative effect and produce irritation of the digestive tract and gas (flatulence) when used in excessive amounts.

3. The leafy tops of green onions are nutritionally superior to the green bulbs and to mature bulbs in that the tops are (a) a better source of potassium, (b) an excellent source of vitamin A, and (c) a good source of vitamin C. Hence, green onions should be eaten with the tops whenever feasible.

4. Europeans have long believed that onions have medicinal effects such as (a) prevention of colds, (b) loosening of phlegm, (c) correction of indigestion, (d) inducement of sleep, and (e) stimulation of the appetite. In China, it is said that people who eat lots of onions seldom get stomach cancer. Furthermore, onions have often been added to food preparations to retard spoilage. So far, there has been only limited scientific documentation for these beliefs, consisting mainly of findings that onions (a) have a mild antibacterial effect, and (b) contain a substance (adenosine) which stimulates the breakdown of fibrinogen to fibrin, a protein in the blood which is involved in blood clotting.

(Also see VEGETABLE[S], Table V-6 Vegetables of the World.)

ON-THE-HOOF

A term applied to a live animal; for example, the on-the-foot weight would be liveweight.

ON-THE-RAIL

A term applied to carcasses on the rail.

OPHTHALMIA

Severe inflammation of the conjunctiva (the membrane that lines the inner surface of the eyelids) or of the eyeball.

OPOSSUM

A marsupial, reaching the size of a rabbit, which abounds in certain regions of North America. The flesh is esteemed as a food in some sections and resembles that of rabbit.

OPSIN

A protein compound which combines retinal (vitamin A) to form rhodopsin (visual purple).

(Also see VITAMIN A, section headed "Functions," Fig. V-22.)

OPSOMANIA

Indicates a craving for special or certain foods—the pickles and ice cream appetite of pregnancy. In some cases, it may signal a deficiency of some essential element, for instance the periodic craving of chocolate may mean an insufficiency of chromium in the diet.

(Also see APPETITE; CISSA; and PICA.)

ORAL

Pertaining to the mouth.

ORANGE, BLOOD *Citrus sinensis*

Varieties of the sweet orange (a fruit of the *Rutaceae* family) in which the flesh of the fruit has a reddish tint due to the presence of anthocyanin pigments. It appears that the blood coloration develops only when the fruit is grown under hot, dry conditions such as those of the Mediterranean region. Hence, the major areas of production are Italy, Spain, Algeria, Morocco, and Tunisia. Blood oranges are usualy consumed fresh, since the variability of the pigmentation presents difficulties in juice production and canning.

(Also see ORANGE, SWEET.)

ORANGE BUTTER

A mixture of butter or margarine, orange juice, grated orange peel, and/or other seasonings that is used as a sauce for dressing, cooked fish, meats, and poultry.

ORANGE JUICE

The fluid obtained from ripened oranges. Usually, it has been strained to remove excess pulp and seeds. Commercially canned orange juices may also contain juices from mandarin oranges (not more than 10%) and sour oranges (not more than 5%).

CAUTION: Some products may contain allergenic substances from the peel, but those made for infants contain little or none of these substances.

The nutrient compositions of various forms of orange juice are given in Food Composition Table F-36.

Some noteworthy observations regarding the nutrient composition of orange juice follow:

1. A 1-cup (*240 ml*) serving of fresh orange juice provides 112 Calories (kcal) and 26 g of carbohydrates. It is

an excellent source of potassium and vitamin C, and a fair to good source of vitamin A.

2. Canned, unsweetened orange juice is similar in composition to the fresh juice, except that it is about 20% lower in vitamin C.

3. Frozen orange juice concentrates contain over 3 times the nutrient level of the unconcentrated juice. Hence, it may make a significant nutritional contribution when added undiluted to sauces and toppings.

(Also see CITRUS FRUITS, section headed "Processing"; and ORANGE, SWEET.)

ORANGE PEKOE

This refers to the grade of tea leaves from which a black tea is made. Orange pekoe leaves are the smallest grade of leaves, and they are generally from the tips of the branches of the tea plant.

(Also see TEA.)

ORANGE, SWEET *Citrus sinensis*

This citrus species is by far the leading fruit crop of the United States, and it is the second leading one of the world. (Grapes are first, and bananas, watermelons, and plantains follow in that order.) The sweet orange, like the other citrus fruits, is a member of the rue family (*Rutaceae*).

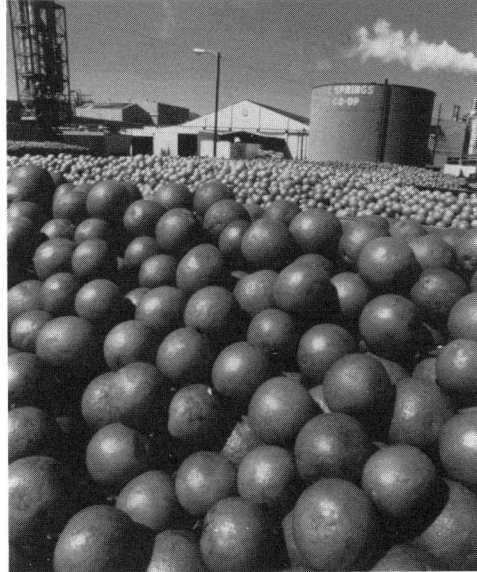

Fig. O-21. Sweet oranges, a leading fruit crop in the United States and the world. (Courtesy, USDA)

ORIGIN AND HISTORY. The sweet orange originated in the area extending from southern China to Indochina. Oranges and other citrus fruits have been grown in China for thousands of years. However, mandarin oranges were more favored by the Chinese, who grew them extensively but produced relatively small amounts of sweet oranges. It is uncertain when traders first brought the sweet orange to India. However, it might have been grown there before the early Christian era.

Sometime around the 10th century A.D., the Arabs brought the sweet orange westward and grew it on the Arabian peninsula, where they had introduced the sour orange (*Citrus aurantium*) a century or two earlier. (The famous Renaissance paintings which show oranges at the Last Supper are in error because the fruit was not likely to have been found in the Holy Land at the time of Christ. Crusaders had seen sweet oranges growing around Jerusalem and had concluded that the fruit was native to the area.)

The sweet orange appears to have been introduced into Europe at various times and places during the 15th century. Many historians believe that one or more varieties were brought into Europe by way of (1) Spain, by the Arabs; (2) Portugal, by Vasco da Gama and other Portuguese explorers and traders returning from India or the Orient; and (3) Italy, by Genoese traders who had brought the fruit from the Holy Land.

Columbus brought orange seeds to Haiti on his second voyage to the New World in 1493. Shortly thereafter, the fruit was planted on the neighboring islands of the Caribbean. Oranges were introduced into Florida by the Spanish explorers sometime between the first landing of Ponce de Leon in 1513 and the establishment of the settlement of St. Augustine in 1565. By 1577, oranges had been planted at the place that is now Parris Island, South Carolina. Two centuries later, Spanish Franciscan monks from Mexico established the mission in San Diego (1769) and planted orange trees there.

Florida was ceded to the United States by Spain in 1821. Shortly thereafter, the new settlers to the territory found many untended groves of oranges (that had been established by the Spaniards in the 16th century) which they used to start a commercial orange industry. The fruit was shipped north to coastal cities, where it brought the best prices. (These cities are still the nation's leading centers for the marketing of citrus fruits.)

California orange production was stimulated by the gold rush of 1849 which brought many people to the state. However, almost all of the fruit was grown in the area around Los Angeles for the 2 decades that followed. The next momentous event of that era was the introduction of the Washington or Bahia navel orange into the Riverside area. In 1870, Mr. and Mrs. F. I. C. Schneider (a Presbyterian minister and his wife who were missionaries to Bahia, Brazil) sent navel orange trees to the U.S. Department of Agriculture in Washington, D.C., where they were propagated, then distributed to nurserymen in California and Florida. The trees planted by Mr. L. C. Tibbets of Riverside, California, bore fruit which were far superior to the Australian navel oranges that had been introduced earlier. In a short time the Washington navel orange became one of the major varieties grown in the citrus producing areas of the world. It is noteworthy that orange production in California increased so rapidly that by the 1880s the resulting surplus of fruit threatened to put most growers out of business. Fortunately, transcontinental railway shipments of oranges were soon initiated and the industry survived.

For a long time, fresh oranges were too expensive to be used regularly by most people. Hence, the fruit was consumed only on special occasions such as Christmas. This situation began to change around the beginning of the 20th century after large scale breeding and cultural experiments were initiated at (1) the U.S. Department of Agriculture's research facilities in Florida in 1893, and (2) the University of California at Riverside in 1914. The U.S. production of oranges increased steadily between World Wars I and II and an ever-increasing proportion of the crop was canned in the forms of fruit and juice. However, the greatest surge in U.S. orange production occurred after the development and promotion of frozen orange juice concentrate in the early 1950s.

In recent years, the prices of orange juice products have remained low in relation to those of other foods because (1) large quantities are produced and consumed, and (2) there is an efficient utilization of such byproducts of juice production as bioflavonoids (vitaminlike substances), citric acid, citrus molasses and dried citrus pulp (livestock feeds), essential flavoring oils, and pectin.

PRODUCTION. The world production of sweet oranges amounts to over 52 million metric tons each year.

About 14% of the world's orange crop comes from the United States. Florida is the leading state by a wide margin.

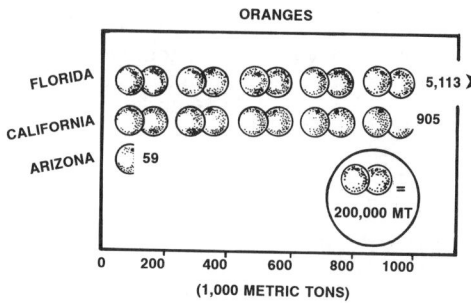

Fig. O-23. The leading orange-producing states of the United States. (Based on data from *Agricultural Statistics*, 1991, USDA, p. 189, Table 278)

Sweet oranges grow best in subtropical climates. Hence, commercial orange production in the United States is limited to Florida, California, Arizona, and Texas.

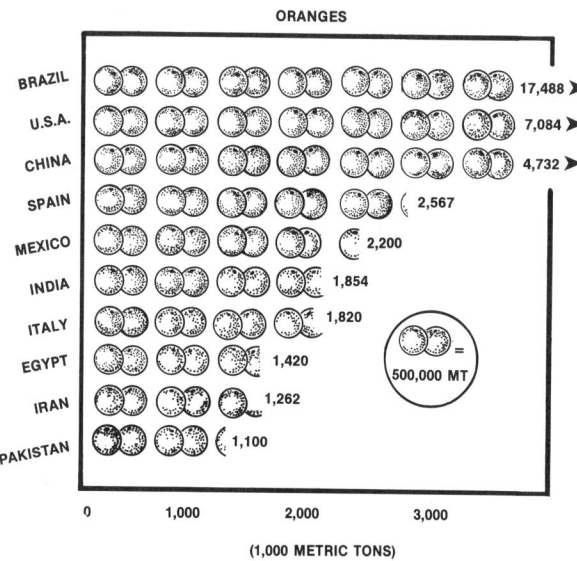

Fig. O-22. The leading orange-producing countries of the world. (Based upon data from *FAO Production Yearbook*, 1990, FAO/UN, Rome, Italy, Vol. 44, p. 163, Table 71)

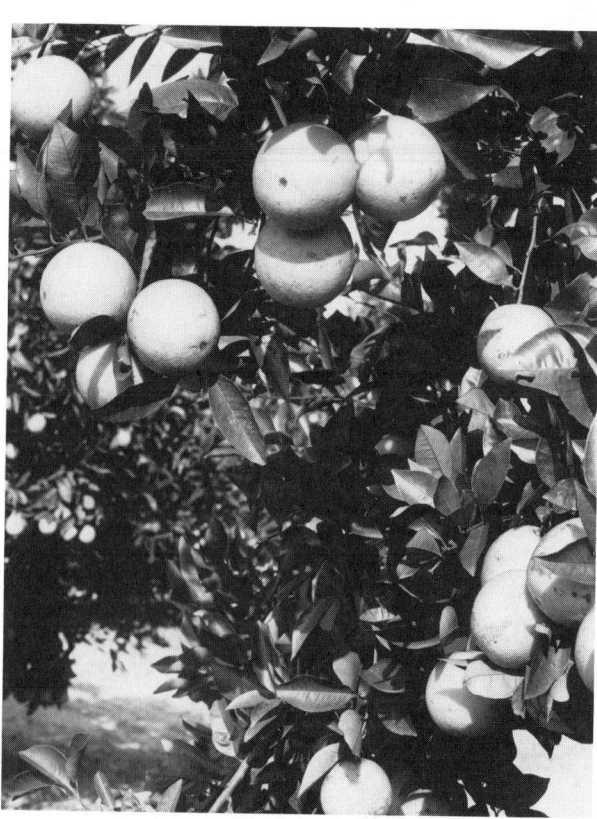

Fig. O-24. An orange tree of the Parson Brown variety growing in Florida. (Courtesy, J. C. Allen & Son, West Lafayette, Ind.)

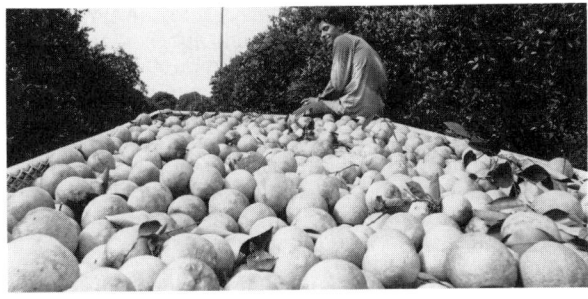

Fig. O-25.   A picker, after filling a trailer which holds the equivalent of 25 field boxes of oranges, takes a break while awaiting a tractor which will pull the trailer from the grove. (Courtesy, USDA)

Each orange-producing state has established standards that specify the contents of sugar, acid, and juice which should be present in the fruit before picking. The fruits are usually sampled and analyzed to determine when they are ready for harvesting. However, the color of the peel is *not* a good indicator of maturity because most oranges will remain green as they mature unless they are exposed to cool night temperatures. Hence,

much of the fruit may be picked green and "degreened" by exposing it to ethylene gas in a warm room. (Ethylene is produced naturally by certain fruits during ripening.)

The general details of citrus fruit growing are given elsewhere.

(Also see CITRUS FRUITS, section headed "Production.")

PROCESSING. About 84% of the U.S. orange crop is processed. The leading item is frozen orange juice concentrate, which utilizes almost 80% of the oranges that are grown for processing.

An additional 15% of the orange crop is used to make chilled fresh orange juice that is packed in glass bottles, plastic bottles, and paperboard cartons; while the remainder is converted into canned orange juice and orange juice blends, canned orange sections, and chilled fresh orange sections packed in glass or plastic containers. Descriptions of these and other products are given elsewhere.

(Also see CITRUS FRUITS, section headed "Processing.")

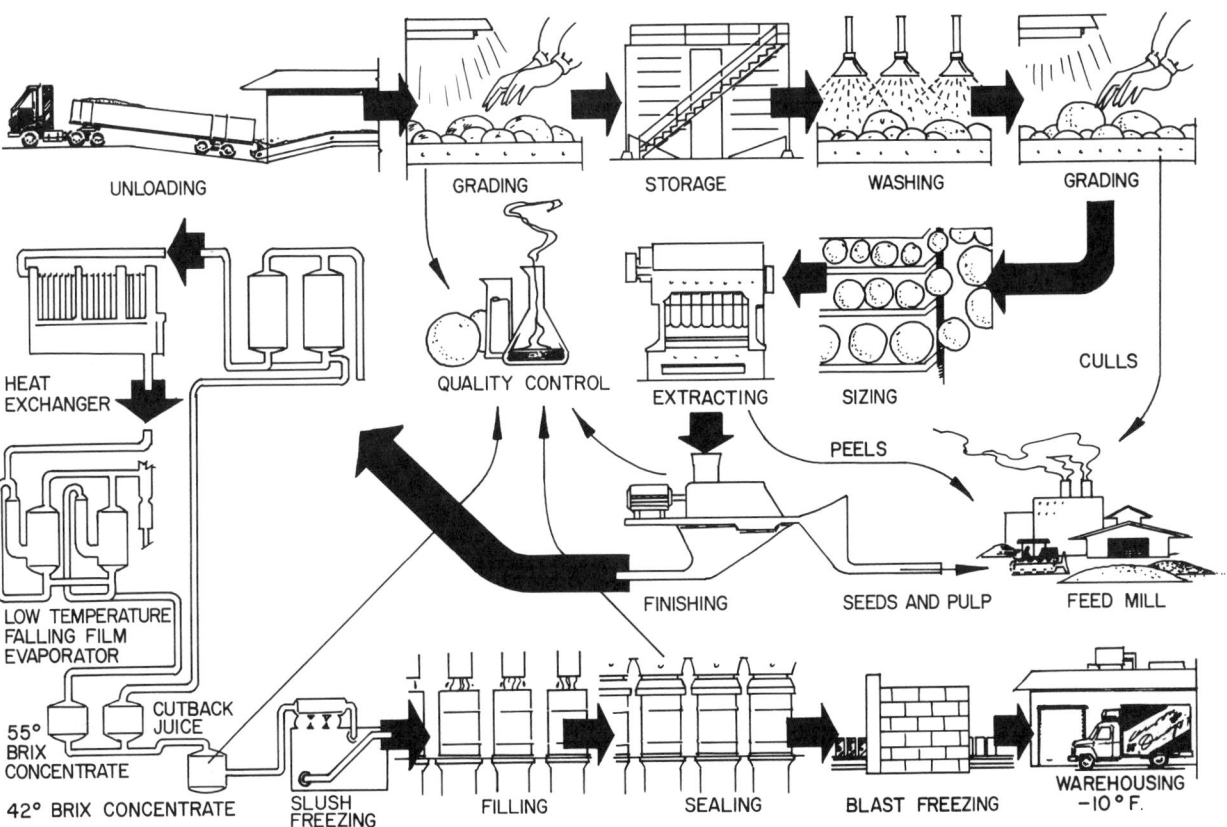

Fig. O-26.   Flowsheet for the production of frozen orange juice concentrate. (Courtesy, USDA)

SELECTION. Fresh oranges of the best quality are firm, heavy, have a fine-textured skin for the variety and are well-colored. Such fruits (even with a few surface blemishes, such as scars, scratches, and slight discolorations) are much to be preferred to oranges that have a badly creased skin, or are puffy or spongy, and light in weight. Puffy oranges are likely to be lacking in juice, and of generally poor quality. When present, decay is usually in the form of soft areas on the surface of the fruit that appears to be water-soaked. These areas may be covered by a mold. In the early stages of development, the skin in the affected area may be so soft and tender that it breaks easily under pressure. Oranges that have been mechanically injured should be carefully examined. Decay may be present at the point of injury, and decay organisms may easily find entrance to the flesh of the fruit.

Wilted, or shriveled, or flabby fruit is sometimes found. Age or injury may cause these conditions. Oranges so affected are not desirable.

Guidelines for the selection of processed orange products are given elsewhere.

(Also see CITRUS FRUITS, section headed "Selection and Preparation.")

PREPARATION. Fresh orange sections and freshly squeezed orange juice have tangy flavors that may not be present in processed orange products because heating during processing drives off some of the aromatic constituents of the fruit. Furthermore, certain types of processing also reduce the content of vitamin C and bioflavonoids (vitaminlike substances). Therefore, some suggestions for using fresh fruit and juice follow:

1. Orange sections go well with other, more bland-flavored fruits such as apples, apricots, avocados, bananas, blueberries, cherries, figs, melons, peaches, and pears. It might also be a good idea to add some orange juice to the fruit mixtures to prevent cut pieces of certain fruits from darkening.

2. The flavor of oranges or orange juice also enhances such vegetables as beets, carrots, squash, and sweet potatoes. A little honey with butter or margarine helps to bring about the blending of the citrus and vegetable flavors.

3. Weight watchers may make a low calorie snack or a light meal by combining orange sections with lowfat cottage cheese or plain (unflavored) yogurt. The fruit also goes well with custard, ice cream, ices, puddings, and sherbets.

4. More nutritious gelatin desserts and salads may be prepared from fresh oranges, orange juice, and unflavored gelatin than from flavored gelatin dessert mixes.

5. The fruit sections may be added to sauces for fish, meats, poultry, and seafood, or to salads which contain these ingredients.

6. Orange juice may be mixed into thick jams and marmalades in order to (a) make them more spreadable and (b) raise their nutrient levels.

CAUTION: Some people are allergic to one or more constituents of citrus peel. When such allergies are suspected, neither the peel nor products containing it should be consumed, and fruit juice should be extracted gently to avoid squeezing the oil and other substances from the peel into the juice. (It is noteworthy that some of the commercially prepared orange juices and orange drinks may contain peel and/or substances extracted from it, but that prepared citrus juice products for infants contain little or none of the peel constituents.)

Additional suggestions for preparing dishes from citrus fruit and other citrus products are given elsewhere.

(Also see CITRUS FRUITS, section headed "Selection and Preparation.")

NUTRITIONAL VALUE. The nutrient compositions of various forms of oranges are given in Food Composition Table F-36.

Some noteworthy observations regarding the nutrient composition of oranges and orange products follow:

1. Fresh oranges are low in calories (47 kcal per 100 g), but they are a good source of fiber, pectin, potassium, vitamin C, inositol, and bioflavonoids (vitaminlike substances). They are also a fair source of folic acid.

2. Fresh orange juice contains about the same levels of most of the nutrients present in fresh oranges, except for fiber, pectin, and the bioflavonoids, which are present mainly in the peel and the membranes which surround the segments of fruit.

3. More vitamin C and folic acid is likely to be retained in chilled fresh orange juice packed in bottles or cartons than in canned orange juice which is heated strongly during canning, then stored at room temperature for an extended period of time.

4. Frozen orange juice concentrate contains from 3 to 4 times the levels of calories and nutrients of an equal amount of fresh orange juice. Hence, the concentrate may make a significant nutritional contribution when it is added undiluted to various beverages, salad dressings, sauces, and toppings.

5. Dehydrated pure orange juice crystals contain over 8 times the levels of calories and nutrients of equal amounts of fresh orange juice. At the present time the crystals are sold mainly by institutional food service suppliers. (The dry mixes sold in retail groceries usually contain considerable amounts of added sugar.)

6. Orange and apricot drink (contains 40% fruit juices) supplies about 3 times the vitamin A of orange juice, but less than half as much potassium and vitamin C.

7. Citrus peel also contains citral, an aldehyde which antagonizes the effects of vitamin A. Hence, people should make certain that their dietary supply of the vitamin is adequate before consuming large amounts of orange peel.

(Also see BIOFLAVONOIDS; FIBER; and VITAMIN C.)

ORGANIC

Substances derived from living organisms. Carbon-containing compounds.

ORGANIC ACID

Any organic compound that contains a carboxyl group (COOH).

ORGANICALLY GROWN FOOD

Organically grown food, organic food, organic gardening, organic farming, natural foods, and health foods are all related, carrying similar implications. Natural and health foods are often the products of organic farming or gardening methods.

At present, there is no national definition of *organic*, and no nationwide program to monitor produce labeled *organically grown*. However, 25 states have established their own definitions. Also, the Farm Bill of 1990 requires that by October 1993, plans for national certification be in effect.

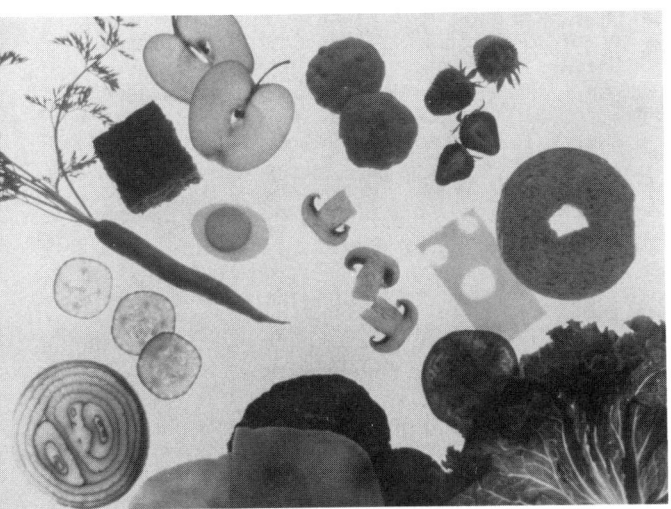

Fig. O-27. Organically grown foods. (Courtesy, USDA)

Although the term organic traditionally refers to compounds of carbon, J. I. Rodale, the "father" of the organic farming and food movement in the United States, defined organic as meaning "production of crops without using pesticides and chemical fertilizers." Recently, the USDA defined organic farming as follows:

"Organic farming is a production system which avoids or largely excludes the use of synthetically compounded fertilizers, pesticides, growth regulators, and livestock feed additives. To the maximum extent feasible, organic farming systems rely upon crop rotations, crop residues, animal manures, legumes, green manures, off-farm organic wastes, mechanical cultivation, mineral-bearing rocks, and aspects of biological pest control to maintain soil productivity and tilth, to supply plant nutrients, and to control insects, weeds, and other pests."[65]

Often, the meanings for *organic*, *natural*, and *health* which people imply or conjure up in their minds, are misleading, harmful, and tend to polarize people. The growing interest of consumers in the safety and nutritional quality of the American diet is a welcome development. Regrettably, however, much of this interest has been colored by those who state or imply that the American food supply is unsafe or somehow inadequate to meet our nutritional needs.

The Food and Drug Administration (FDA) has taken no position on use of the terms *organic*, *natural*, and *health* in food labeling, since the terms are often used loosely and interchangeably. The Federal Trade Commission in its proposed Food Advertising Rule would prohibit use of the words *organic* and *natural* in food advertising because of concern about the ability of consumers to understand the terms in the conflicting and confusing ways they are used. FTC also proposes to prohibit the term *health food* in advertising because it is undefined and may fool consumers into thinking one particular food will provide good health.

ORGANIC VS CONVENTIONAL. Amid the confusion, a comparison of organic and conventional methods, foods, and cost will provide knowledge for choosing foods for health. Perhaps the differences between organic and conventional are not as great as they appear.

Methods. Organic and conventional food producing methods are similar in many respects but differ in their use of the products of modern chemical technology.

• **Fertilizer**—Nitrogen and other nutrients are returned to the soil in animal manure in both conventional and organic farming, but manure returns only a part of the nutrient removed by crops. The total amounts of

---

[65]*Report and Recommendations on Organic Farming*, USDA, 1980.

nitrogen, phosphorus, and potassium added in manure are small in comparison with the amounts of these nutrients supplied in commercial fertilizers. Manure application does, however, have the advantage of supplying organic matter to the soil which improves soil tilth, increases water-holding capacity, lessens water and wind erosion, improves aeration, and has a beneficial effect on soil microorganisms. Also, due to the slower availability of its nitrogen and to its contribution to the soil humus, manure produces rather lasting benefits, which may continue for several years. On a smaller scale, organic gardeners employ mulches of such material as grass clippings, corn cobs, wood shavings, sawdust, and straw.

To meet nitrogen needs, organic farmers prefer to use leguminous crops, which have the capability to remove nitrogen gas from the atmosphere and convert it to nitrogenous compounds useful to the crop. The nitrogen left behind by the leguminous crops supplies part of the needs of the succeedng nonleguminous crops, and the cropping system is built around the legumes as a source of nitrogen. Conventional farmers used to follow the same practice because commercial nitrogen fertilizer was too expensive to compete with legume nitrogen. After World War II, fertilizer nitrogen became available in increasing quantities at relatively low prices. To meet the nitrogen requirements of their nonleguminous crops, many conventionl farmers then substituted fertilizer nitrogen for a part or all of the legume nitrogen and added extra fertilizer nitrogen to the extent that seemed economically advantageous. The result has been a more than tenfold increase in amount of nitrogen fertilizer used per year and a decrease in the use of legumes to supply nitrogen.

Organic farmers prefer to use phosphate rock and potassium salts as mined to provide supplemental phosphorus and potassium, whereas conventional farmers use mostly processed forms in commercial fertilizers. Commercial phosphorus fertilizers have greater solubility and availability to plants than does phosphate rock, and they often contain phosphorus in higher concentration. Commercial potassium fertilizers contain potassium in higher concentration than do potassium salts as mined, but both are relatively soluble and available to plants.

• **Weed control**—Weeds are a problem on all farms. Both conventional and organic farmers use a variety of weed control practices, but conventional farmers make extensive use of herbicides. Organic farmers prefer not to use herbicides. Where used, herbicides are applied both to prevent weeds from emerging and to kill those that have already emerged. Herbicides are most useful for controlling weeds that cannot be killed by mechanical cultivation—weeds that grow in crop rows and crops that are not cultivated. Weed control by herbicides is especially important for small-seeded crops that would otherwise require hand labor to remove the weeds growing in the rows. Weed control on organic farms is achieved primarily by crop rotation, cultivation, mowing, and hand weeding. Conventional farmers also practice crop rotation and cultivation.

• **Insect, nematode and disease control**—Both conventional and organic farmers use a variety of methods to control insects. Insecticides are usually used by conventional, but not organic, farmers to control insect infestations that have already developed. The desirable practice is to make applications only when the infestations are sufficient to cause significant economic losses if not checked. Among conventional farmers, emphasis is now on integrated pest management (IPM) which couples biological control with judicious use of pesticides. Many organic farmers feel that insects can be adequately controlled by selective rotation of crops and natural insect predators.

Nematodes that attack crop roots can be controlled to some degree by crop rotation and suitable tillage, but use of nematicides often results in increased crop yields that could not have been achieved by any alternative method.

The most important biological means of controlling insect, disease, and nematode pests is development of resistant crop varieties. This technique has had greatest success in controlling diseases, and it is used by both conventional and organic farmers. Some vegetable crops are susceptible to diseases for which there is no feasible control except fungicidal sprays, and only conventional farmers can grow these crops successfuly. Also, treating seed with a small amount of an appropriate fungicide improves seedling establishment, especially in years when the soil is cool and wet at planting time. At present there is no effective substitute for such seed treatment.

• **Animal Production**—In conventional farming, extensive use is made of nutritional supplements in animal feeds. Minerals, vitamins, and other nutritional supplements increase animal productivity, and they are of greatest importance in feeds for poultry and swine. In cattle feeding, considerable use is made of urea as an economical, nonprotein source of nitrogen, which is eventually converted to animal protein. Such use of urea upgrades low-quality roughages, and spares protein from other sources. Although urea is a normal metabolic by-product, and the first organic chemical synthesized in a test tube, individuals practicing organic methods shun its use.

The minerals and nonprotein nitrogen used to improve the nutritional quality of animal diets in conventional farming improve also the quality of the manure as fertilizer because much of the quantity of the nutrient elements supplied in the feed is excreted in the manure.

Further increases in production efficiency are achieved in modern conventional animal agriculture by use of hormonally active substances. Some of these substances increase the rate of gain and reduce the amount of feed required per pound of body weight gained by 10 to 15%.

Other drugs are now approved by the Food and Drug Administration for use to protect animal health and to increase production efficiency. Drugs are useful in both conventional and organic systems of farming, but organic farmers prefer not to use them.

Some of the drugs and hormones employed in animal production are naturally-occurring organic compounds, while others are synthesized. The use of drugs and hormones in livestock is controlled by the Food and Drug Administration (FDA) who assures that they are used safely, and that hazardous residues do not occur in edible products.

• **Energy**—Both conventional farming and organic farming are largely powered by fossil fuels, but conventional farmers use more energy per acre than do organic farmers, largely because conventional farmers use fertilizers and pesticides. These products, mainly nitrogen fertilizers, consume about 1% of the energy used nationally but about 40% of the energy used in agricultural production. However, the overall use of energy by agriculure for production represents only about 3% of the total amount of energy used in the United States. About four times this amount of energy is used to get food from the farmers to the consumer; hence, energy savings of organic food production contribute a small part to the overall energy consumption.

(Also see ENERGY REQUIRED FOR FOOD PRODUCTION.)

Food Quality. Much of the promotion of organically grown food, natural and health foods included, comes from the idea that these foods are nutritionally superior to foods grown by conventional agricultural methods. Moreover, organically grown foods are promoted as containing no pesticides or additives, while conventionally grown foods are pictured as being poisoned with pesticides and additives. The truth is, that once organically grown and conventionally grown foods are removed from the field they cannot be identified as to their origin. Plants convert inorganic compounds to organic compounds. Therefore, it is relatively immaterial whether conventional methods or organic methods are followed. Inorganic ions—nitrates, potassium, iron, phosphate—are taken up by the plant roots and manufactured into new organic materials. The nutrient content of a crop—the amount of protein, carbohydrate, fat, vitamins, and most minerals—is largely determined by plant genetics, weather, and time of harvest. Scientific experiments at the Michigan Experiment Station for 10 years; at the United States Plant, Soil and Nutrition Laboratory in Ithaca, New York for 25 years; and as well as a 34-year investigation of organic and chemical agriculture on a British experimental farm failed to show a nutritional superiority of organically grown foods compared to conventionally grown foods.

Organically grown foods contain pesticide residues just as often as do conventional foods, although they may be present in smaller amounts. However, all residues are within Federal tolerance levels, which are set low enough to protect consumers. As for poisons in the food supply, many common foods contain naturally-occurring toxicants, but these are usually present in low levels and pose no health hazards. Poison is a matter of dosage. Further, a poisonous substance made by a plant is no different than the same substance made in a laboratory.

(Also see ADDITIVES; POISONOUS PLANTS; and POISONS.)

Food Quantity. The use of chemical fertilizers has been partly responsible for the abundance of food available. If all farmers were to adopt organic methods, there would be a decline in productivity as shown in Table O-7.

TABLE O-7
ESTIMATED NATIONAL AVERAGE CROP YIELDS UNDER CONVENTIONAL AND ORGANIC FARMING[1]

Crop	Bushels per Acre	
	Conventional	Organic
Corn	98	49
Wheat	43	20
Soybeans	40	20
Other grains	57	17

[1]*Organic and Conventional Farming Compared,* Council for Agricultural Science and Technology (CAST), Report No. 84, October 1980, p. 24, Table 6.

In a 1980 report issued by the Council for Agricultural Science and Technology (CAST), it was estimated that if organic farming were widely adopted the cost of food would increase since the total production from the land under cultivation would decrease. Those now practicing organic methods realize their yields are less, but they receive higher prices for their goods since they sell to a specialty market.

Cost. One major difference between organically grown food and conventionally grown food is that it is often sold at relatively high prices to persons who are willing to tolerate imperfections in return for the suggestion that commercial fertilizers, pesticides, and additives have not been used. Numerous surveys have indicated that people will pay 30 to 100% more for organically produced foods than for their regular counterparts.

Individuals who desire organic foods—foods grown without the use of modern chemical technology—seem to be left with two choices: (1) purchase organic foods from a reputable dealer and pay the price; or (2) engage in organic gardening and grow their own. As for organic gardening, it is probably more feasible than organic farming since organic methods are more easily practiced on a small scale. Moreover, when an organic garden fails due to insects, disease, or weeds, the economic impact is not as great as when a farming operation fails.

Good farmers have always incorporated many of the so-called organic methods, and they have also incorporated new methods such as chemical fertilizer, pesticides, and the other chemical methods which ensure more food for all and at a reasonable price. Undoubtedly, world food production of the future will make use of a combination of both organic and inorganic fertilizers, with the nature and proportions of the combination for different farms and for different countries dependent on their access to fossil fuels, the availability and price of fertilizers, their soils, their food production requirements, their environmental control problems, and many other factors. Regardless of the combination of organic and inorganic fertilizers used, feed and food plants of adequate nutritional quality can be produced.

Furthermore, to meet world food needs, pesticides and other chemical methods cannot be altogether abandoned. Even with the use of pesticides, about one-third of the food produced is lost to pests.

All foods are organic, and all edible foods, when properly selected for a balanced diet, are conducive to physiologic and psychological health regardless of whether they are organically grown (as defined) or conventionally grown.

(Also see ADDITIVES; DELANEY CLAUSE; HEALTH FOODS; MEAT[S], section headed "Meat Myths"; PESTICIDES; and POISONS.)

ORGAN MEAT

Any edible part of a slaughter animal that consists of, or forms a part of, an internal organ, such as the liver, kidney, heart, or brain; distinguished from carcass meat.

ORGANOLEPTIC

It describes the employment of one or more of the special senses. Subjecting food to an organoleptic test employs the sensations of smell, taste, touch and vision. We accept or reject food based on its organoleptic properties. The food industry sells food based on its organoleptic properties. First the consumer assesses the appearance (vision) and aroma (smell), but most important are the in-the-mouth properties—flavor, texture and consistency.

(Also see TASTE.)

ORGEAT

• A nonalcoholic beverage prepared from the sweetened juice of almonds and other flavorings (such as orange blossom essence, or rose water), usually served cold.

• A sweet almond-flavored nonalcoholic syrup used as a cocktail ingredient or food flavoring.

ORINASE

A brand name for a form of sulfonylurea called tolbutamide, a short-acting oral drug used to stimulate the pancreatic cells to release insulin. The drug is only effective for the treatment of diabetes when some insulin-secreting ability remains in the pancreas. Other brand names are Artosin, Diaben, Diabesan, Diabetamid, Diabuton, Dolipol, Ipoglicone, Mobenol, Orabet, Oralin, Oterben, Pramidex, Rastinon, Tarasina, Tolbet, Tolbusal, Tolbutone, Toluina, and Willbutamide.

(Also see DIABETES MELLITUS, section headed "Oral Drugs;" DIABINASE; and DYMELOR.)

ORNITHINE-ARGININE CYCLE (UREA CYCLE)

A cyclic sequence of biochemical reactions in protein metabolism in which citrulline is converted to arginine, thence urea splits off from arginine, producing ornithine.

(Also see METABOLISM; and UREA CYCLE.)

ORTANIQUE *Citrus reticulata X C. sinensis*

A citrus fruit (of the family *Rutaceae*) that was discovered growing in Jamaica, West Indies in 1920. It is believed to be the result of a natural crossbreeding (hybridization) between the mandarin orange (*C. reticulata*) and the sweet orange (*C. sinensis*). It is about the size of an average orange and it is flattened at both ends like certain tangerines. The fruit is quite juicy and its flavor is distinctive. Also, the rind adheres tightly, but is readily peelable.

(Also see CITRUS FRUITS; MANDARIN ORANGE (TANGERINE); and ORANGE, SWEET.)

OSMOPHILIC YEAST

Food preservation by high concentration of sugars or salts, such as in jams and pickles, takes advantage of the inability of most types of microorganisms to grow under this condition—high osmotic pressure. Some yeasts—osmophilic yeasts—are adapted. They thrive under the condition of high osmotic pressure.

(Also see PRESERVATION OF FOOD.)

OSMOSIS

The passage of a solvent such as water through a semipermeable membrane from the side of the membrane where the solution is dilute, to the side where the solution is more concentrated.

OSMOTIC PRESSURE

The force acting upon a semipermeable membrane placed between two solutions of differing concentrations.

OSSEIN

When the mineral salts of bone are dissolved by a dilute acid, the remaining organic material is called ossein.

(Also see PROTEIN[S].)

OSSIFICATION

The process of bone formation.

OSTEITIS

Inflammation of a bone.

OSTEO-

Prefix meaning bone.

OSTEOARTHRITIS (DEGENERATIVE JOINT DISEASE; HYPERTROPHIC ARTHRITIS)

Resulting from the wear and tear on joints, osteoarthritis is the most common type of arthritis. Most persons over the age of 50 have it to some degree, for which reason it is often called "old-age rheumatism." However, it often follows injuries, infections and/or disease afflicting the joints. Affected joints are painful, and they may "creak" or grate on movement. Weight-bearing joints—the knees, hips, ankles and spine—are most often involved. Overweight and stress can aggravate the disease.

(Also see ARTHRITIS, section headed "Osteoarthritis"; OBESITY; and STRESS.)

OSTEOBLAST

Bone-forming cells.

OSTEODYSTROPHY (OSTEODYSTROPHIA)

Defective ossification of bone, usually associated with disturbed calcium and phosphorus metabolism and renal insufficiency.

OSTEOMALACIA

A bone disease of adults caused by lack of vitamin D, inadequate intake of calcium or phosphorus, or an incorrect dietary ratio of calcium and phosphorus.

(Also see DEFICIENCY DISEASES, Table D-1 Major Dietary Deficiency Diseases; and RICKETS.)

OSTEOPOROSIS

A loss of bone mass which generally occurs with aging is called osteoporosis. When such loss is significant (such as one-third of the original adult bone mass), bones will fracture easily and heal poorly. Recent research has shown that osteoporosis often occurs in the skeleton in the following order:[66]

1. **The alveolar bone in the jaw is lost first.** This can be a serious problem because it means a reduction in the amount of support given to the teeth, with the result that they may wobble in the gums, causing gum damage and loss of teeth.

2. **Next in order of bone loss is the spinal column.** Such loss leads to compression fractures which are difficult to heal and cause the person to shrink in height with aging.

3. **Last in order of bone losses are the long bones of the body.** The most common fracture occurring in elderly women is usually called a broken hip. However, the bone which breaks most frequently is the femur bone in the leg, and the actual breaking point is at the head of the neck of the femur, which is likely to thin out during the development of osteoporosis.

CAUSES OF OSTEOPOROSIS. Many investigations conducted in man and animals have led to tentative explanations of why osteoporosis is a problem in the United States where, on the average, dietary calcium intakes are higher than elsewhere in the world. Some of the theories concerning this problem follow.

Dietary Deficiencies of Calcium. Although the Recommended Dietary Allowances (RDA) for calcium for adults in the United States[67] are almost twice as high as the recommended level for adults established by other countries of the world, metabolic balance studies have shown that, for reasons not fully understood, Americans have much greater urinary losses of calcium. Therefore, there may be cause for concern based on the findings

---

[66]Lutwak, L., "Continuing Need for Dietary Calcium Throughout Life," *Geriatrics*, Vol. 29, 1974, p. 171.

[67]*Recommended Dietary Allowances*, 9th rev. ed., 1980, NRC- National Academy of Sciences.

of the most recent dietary survey in the United States by the Department of Agriculture,[68] which showed that adult females had calcium intakes around two-thirds of their RDA (800 mg of calcium per day).

Explanations for the high urinary losses of calcium by Americans may lie in other theories which follow.

Dietary Imbalances of Calcium and Phosphorus. Diets in the United States are believed to contain disproportionately high ratios of phosphorus to calcium (about 5 to 1) which have been shown in animal studies to result in significant loss of bone minerals.[69] Several groups of investigators have theorized that high dietary levels of phosphate reduce calcium absorption and lower blood levels of ionized calcium and parathyroid hormone (PTH). Secretion of the latter is stimulated by blood levels of calcium ions, and it acts on bone to cause demineralization and release of calcium ions in order to bring blood calcium back to normal. PTH also causes increased urinary excretion of phosphate. Thus, chronic ingestion of high levels of phosphate apparently results in a mild form of hyperparathyroidism and a slow, but continuous, demineralization of bone.

(Also see CALCIUM-PHOSPHORUS RATIO; and VITAMIN D.)

High Protein Intakes. Investigators at the University of Wisconsin found that the amounts of calcium needed to balance urinary and fecal losses in young adult males increased as their dietary protein levels were raised.[70] Their data showed that the protein intakes and the corresponding requirements for calcium were as follows: 47 g protein, 500 mg calcium; 95 g protein, more than 800 mg calcium; and 141 g protein, more than 1,400 mg calcium. Thus, it appears that, on the average, these young men required about 10 mg of calcium for every gram of protein.

Similar findings were obtained by researchers at the University of California at Berkeley, who also noted that the elevations in urinary calcium caused by high levels of dietary protein appeared to be independent of the levels of dietary calcium.[71] However, high protein intakes imply high phosphate intakes, because most of the non-dairy sources of proteins contain liberal amounts of phosphate, but only small amounts of calcium. Thus, there is likely to be an imbalance in the ratios of phosphate to calcium in these diets.

Deficiencies of Vitamin D. People who have moderate intakes of calcium, but who live in northern areas, seem to have more osteoporosis than people who eat diets low in calcium, but live in sunny, tropical areas. Furthermore, considerable effort is made in most countries to provide infants and children with adequate levels of the vitamin by either diet or exposure to sunlight, but there is often a lack of attention to the needs of adults, many of whom are kept indoors by either their occupations or the circumstances under which they live.

Recently, a dramatic effect of the vitamin on the utilization of calcium by elderly men was observed in a study conducted at an old soldiers' home in Boston.[72]

The elderly men remained indoors in the winter, during which time the study showed that they absorbed about 40% of their dietary calcium. After 4 more weeks of winter, the calcium absorption of a control group of these men had dropped to 30% of their intake, while that of an experimental group who were exposed daily to radiation from a special lamp rose to 46% of intake. Thus, the group whose skins were stimulated by light to synthesize vitamin D had at the end of the 4-week period about a 50% greater absorption of calcium than the untreated group.

Stresses. Many stresses—such as trauma, chilling, starvation, dehydration, surgery, and fear—are accompanied by great increases in the secretions of adrenal cortical hormones. The net effect of the hypersecretion of these hormones on bone is dissolution of both the mineral and protein components. Catabolism of bone components also occurs in diabetes and Cushings' syndrome, both of which are characterized by hypersecretion of adrenal cortical hormones. However, little is understood concerning the effects of diet on the secretion of these hormones in normal people, other than the fact their levels are elevated during fasting.

Lack of Sufficient Exercise. Immobilization due to fractures, and sitting still for several days in space travel, have been shown to result in significant losses of both calcium and nitrogen in the urine. Patients who are bedridden, or in casts for months at a time, might, therefore, lose large amounts of bone mass as a result of immobilization. There is also some evidence that sedentary persons lose more calcium from their bones than active persons eating essentially the same diet. It has recently been discovered that mechanical forces on bone, such as those which occur during exercise, produce a surface charge (a piezoelectric effect) which may stimulate the building up of bone.[73] Therefore, exercise may be an important factor in the development and maintenance of strong bones.

Postmenopausal Loss of Calcium. Most cases of osteoporosis are diagnosed in women who are more than 50 years of age. Until recently, it has been assumed

[68]*Dietary Levels of Households in the United States, Spring, 1965*, Ag. Res. Serv. Bull. No. 62, 1968.

[69]Krook, L., *et al.*, "Reversibility of Nutritional Osteoporosis: Physiochemical Data on Bones from an Experimental Study in Dogs," *Journal of Nutrition*, Vol. 101, 1971, p. 233.

[70]Linkswiler, H. M., C. L. Joyce, and C. R. Anand, "Calcium Retention of Young Adult Males as Affected by Level of Protein and of Calcium Intake," *Transactions of the New York Academy of Sciences*, Vol. 36, 1974, p. 333.

[71]Margen, S., *et al.*, "Studies in Calcium Metabolism. 1. The Calciuretic Effect of Dietary Protein," *The American Journal of Clinical Nutrition*, Vol. 27, 1974, p. 584.

[72]Wurtman, R. J., "The Effects of Light on the Human Body," *Scientific American*, Vol. 233, 1975, p. 68.

[73]Marino, A. A., and R. O. Becker, "Piezoelectric Effect and Growth Control in Bone," *Nature*, Vol. 228, 1970, p. 473.

that the cessation of estrogen secretion after the menopause resulted in a loss of stimulation of bone remineralization. Now, it is not certain whether estrogen has more than a temporary effect in this regard.

The more rapid development of osteoporosis in women than in men might also be explained by the observation that women generally eat less calcium than men; therefore, they are more likely to have a chronic deficiency of the mineral, since the allowance is the same for both sexes. Both men and women consume, on the average, 30 mg of calcium per 100 Calories (kcal), but women consume far fewer calories.

Bone Loss—A Natural Accompaniment of Aging.

Some researchers have concluded that, irrespective of diet, bone loss is a general phenomenon which accompanies aging in man and may start as early as age 30.[74] There even appears to be an explanation of the physiological basis for such a phenomenon. It is well known that mineralization and demineralization of bone occur in cycles in response to rises and falls in blood levels of calcium ions. There are two hormones which have opposing effects: calcitonin, which is secreted by certain cells within the thyroid, acts to promote deposition of calcium in bone when the blood level of the mineral is high; and PTH, from the parathyroid gland, which causes the release of calcium and phosphate from bone when blood calcium is low.[75] Although calcitonin has a strong effect on blood calcium in young people, this effect is greatly reduced in older persons. Furthermore, the effect of PTH is very strong since it may persist from 12 to 24 hours, although the half-life of the hormone in the blood is only 20 minutes. But there is a ray of hope in this bleak picture since calcium administration has been shown to depress the activity of the parathyroid glands.

SIGNS OF OSTEOPOROSIS.

It has long been thought that the initial signs of this disorder are the occurrence of bone fractures when there has been little or no trauma. Since the long bones of the body do not readily lose bone mass until there has been loss in the jaw and the spinal column, it is difficult to detect early stages of osteoporosis by x rays of the long bones. However, research conducted at Cornell University showed that the early stages of this disorder might readily be observed in x rays of the jaw.[76] Thus, it would seem that dentists might be able to detect early stages of this disorder, particularly when patients seek treatment of periodontal disease caused by loss of bone in the jaw.

TREATMENT AND PREVENTION OF OSTEO-POROSIS.

A variety of therapeutic and prophylactic measures have been suggested, but each of them has its merits and demerits. Therefore, separate discussions of these measures follow:

- **Supplementation of dietary calcium**—It has been suggested that 1,000 mg of calcium per day might be an optimal intake for both the treatment of the early stages of the disease (when bone loss is detectable only in the jaw) and the prevention of the more severe stages.[77] However, the administration of calcium alone has not been shown to be effective in reversing the advanced stages of this disorder, where there have been large reductions of mass in the spinal column and the long bones.

- **Administration of fluoride**—This treatment has been tested as a preventative measure because fluoride-containing bones are more resistant to demineralization. However, a large-scale (460 aged persons), double-blind study in Finland showed that this treatment (25 mg of fluoride ion per day) resulted in an increased incidence of fractures and disorders of joints (arthrosis).[78] The investigators believed that their patients consumed adequate calcium since they drank an average of a liter of milk a day, which provided about 1,200 mg of calcium. However, they suggested that the administration of fluoride should be monitored by the measurement of blood levels of the ion, so that overdoses of fluoride might be avoided. There seems to be some variation in the rates at which different people absorb, utilize, and excrete fluoride.

- **Combined therapy with fluoride, vitamin D, and calcium**—The supplementation of fluoride therapy with vitamin D and calcium apparently produced normal bone in patients with osteoporosis.[79] Dietary calcium has long been known to protect man and animals against the toxic effects of fluoride. However, it is not clear why the results obtained in this trial were superior to those obtained in the Finnish trial. Perhaps the extra vitamin D had a role in the repair of the osteoporotic bones.

- **Estrogen replacement therapy**—At one time it was thought that this therapy offered promise for the treatment of osteoporosis, but recent studies show that the beneficial effects of these hormones on bone may only be temporary.[80] Furthermore, physicians are cautious about the administration of estrogens for fear that long-term treatment with high doses of these hormones may lead to cancer in aging, estrogen-sensitive tissues.

[74]Garn, S. M., C. G. Rothman, and B. Wagner, "Bone Loss as a General Phenomenon in Man," *Federation Proceedings*, Vol. 26, 1967, p. 1729.

[75]Copp, H. D., "Endocrine Control of Calcium Homeostasis," *Journal of Endocrinology*, vol. 43, 1969, p. 137.

[76]Lutwak, L., *et al.*, "Calcium Deficiency and Human Periodontal Disease," *Israel Journal of Medical Sciences*, Vol. 7, 1971, p. 504.

[77]Lutwak, L., "Dietary Calcium and the Reversal of Bone Demineralization," *Nutrition News*, Vol. 37, 1974, p. 1.

[78]Inkovaara, J., *et al.*, "Prophylactic Fluoride Treatment and Aged Bones," *British Medical Journal*, Vol. 3, 1975, p. 73.

[79]Jowsey, J., *et al.*, "Effect of Combined Therapy with Sodium Fluoride, Vitamin D and Calcium in Osteoporosis," *American Journal of Medicine*, Vol. 53, 1972, p. 43.

[80]Riggs, B. L., *et al.*, "Short- and Long-Term Effects of Estrogen and Synthetic Anabolic Hormone in Postmenopausal Osteoporosis," *Journal of Clinical Investigation*, Vol. 51, 1972, p. 1659.

Health Hints for Preventing Bone Fractures.
Every safe measure for the prevention of osteoporosis should be considered, because bone fractures are painful, incapacitating, and costly; and immobilization of the patient during recovery may result in other serious problems, such as further weakening of bones, formation of blood clots, and atrophy of muscles. Some practical recommendations for normal, healthy people follow:

1.   Exercise regularly. This practice results in the improved utilization of calcium for bone remineralization.
2.   Avoid exercises where sharp impacts are transmitted to bones and joints. For example, some joggers run in hard-soled shoes on hard pavement. It has been shown that this practice puts considerable force on the hip joints. Learn to be light on your feet and wear appropriate footwear.
3.   Eat sufficient dairy foods and dark-green vegetables to obtain at least 800 mg of calcium per day (the amount in 3 cups [720 ml] of milk).
4.   Keep your protein intake down to around the RDA (63 g per day for males, and 50 g per day for females).
5.   Calcium supplements, such as dolomite, may be necessary when either the protein intake is considerably higher than the RDA (like 90 g or more per day), or when circumstances prevent the consumption of adequate calcium in foods.
(Also see BONE MEAL; CALCIUM; and DOLOMITE.)
6.   Obtain sufficient vitamin D by either diet or regular exposure to sunlight. Some persons are very sensitive to sunlight, so they need to limit their exposure. It is noteworthy that use of an oral contraceptive may heighten the light sensitivity of some women, which may result in dermatitis after exposure to sunlight.
(Also see DEFICIENCY DISEASES, Table D-1 Major Dietary Deficiency Diseases; CALCIUM, section headed "Calcium Related Diseases"; and VITAMIN D.)

OTAHEITE APPLE (AMBARELLA) *Spondias cytherea.*

The fruit of a tree (of the family *Anacardiaceae*) that is native to Polynesia. Otaheite is an old name for Tahiti. Otaheite apples are yellow, round fruits that range from 2 to 3 in. (5 to 7 cm) in diameter and contain a large stone. The fruit is usually eaten fresh, but is sometimes made into jam and jelly.

Otaheite apples are fairly low in calories (46 kcal per 100 g) and carbohydrates (12%). They are a good source of fiber and vitamin C.

OTAHEITE GOOSEBERRY (GOOSEBERRY TREE) *Phyllanthus acidus*

The fruit of a small tropical tree (of the family *Euphorbiaceae*) that is native to India and Madagascar.

Otaheite gooseberries are small, greenish, sour-tasting fruit about ¾ in. (2 cm) in diameter. They are usually eaten cooked with sugar and made into jam, jelly, pies, and tarts.

The fruit has a high water content (91%) and a low content of calories (37 kcal per 100 g) and carbohydrates (5%). It is an excellent source of iron, but only a fair source of vitamin C.

OVALBUMIN

This is egg albumin, the major protein of egg white representing 75% of the total egg white protein.
(Also see EGG[S].)

OVERWEIGHT

Persons who are 10 to 20% above the ideal weight for their height, age, build and sex are said to be overweight. A person, especially an athlete, may be overweight without being obese since overweight does not imply fatness. Nevertheless, some use obesity and overweight interchangeably.
(Also see OBESITY.)

OVOMUCOID

A minor protein component of egg white containing large amounts of carbohydrate in its structure.
(Also see EGG[S].)

OXALIC ACID (OXALATE; $C_2H_2O_4$)

A naturally occurring toxicant present in such plants as beet leaves, cabbage, peas, potatoes, rhubarb, and spinach. There is some concern that oxalic acid may render calcium as well as some trace minerals less available for absorption from the gut. However, it is doubtful that oxalates pose a problem to man unless the intake of a mineral is marginal, and unusually large amounts of the oxalate-containing food are eaten. Poisoning could occur from the accidental ingestion of some cleaning compounds containing oxalic acid. Interestingly, oxalic acid is a normal constituent of urine derived from the metabolism of ascorbic acid (vitamin C) or glycine (an amino acid).
(Also see POISONOUS PLANTS.)

OXALOACETIC ACID

A 3-carbon ketodicarboxylic acid; an intermediate in the Krebs cycle.
(Also see METABOLISM, Fig. M-78 The Krebs cycle.)

OXALURIA

The presence of an excess of oxalic acid or of oxalates in the urine.

OXIDATION

Chemically, the increase of positive charges on an atom or the loss of negative charges or electrons. It also refers to the combining of oxygen with another element to form one or more new substances. Burning is one kind of oxidation.
(Also see METABOLISM.)

OXIDATIVE PHOSPHORYLATION

The principal function of the oxidation of carbohydrates and fatty acids is to make available to the cells the free energy released in the oxidation process, in a form physiologically usable for cellular energy processes, viz, ATP. This is accomplished by the process known as oxidative phosphorylation, whereby adenosine triphosphate (ATP) with three phosphate groups, two of which are held by high energy bonds, is formed from adenosine diphosphate (ADP) by the addition of phosphate.

(Also see METABOLISM, section headed "Carbohydrates, Catabolism, • ATP—energy currency.")

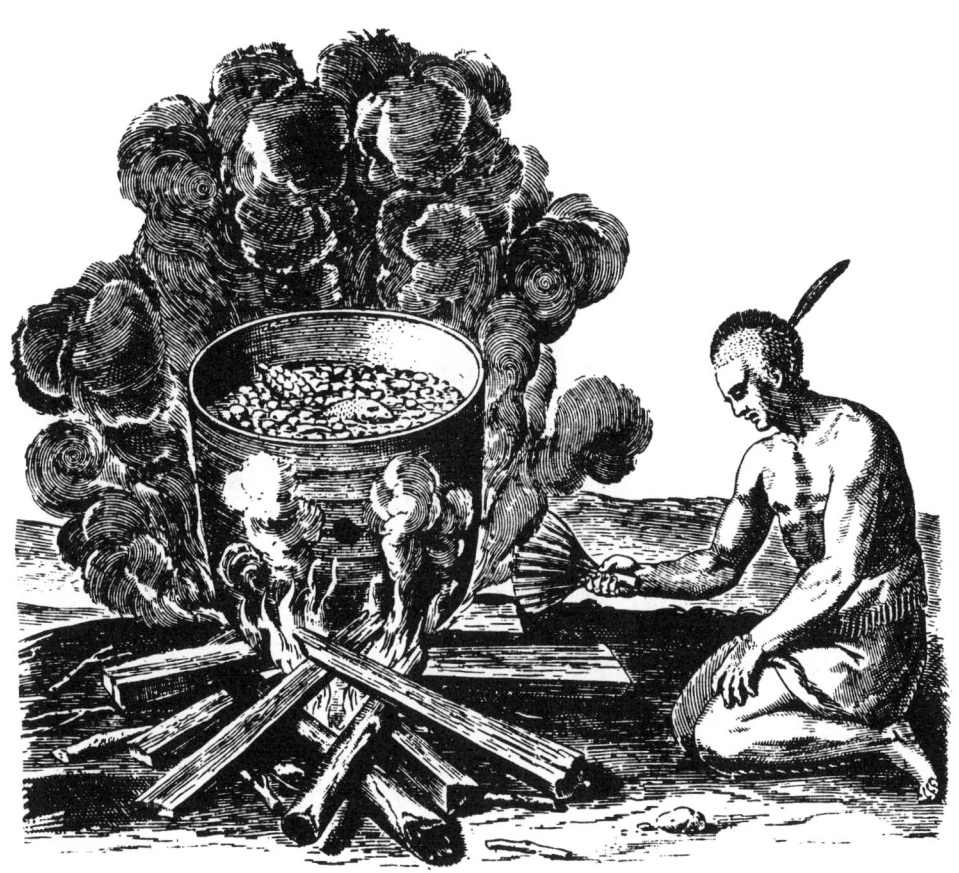

Indian boiling a kettle of seafood. From de Bry's *Travels To America*. Copper engraving. (Courtesy, The Bettmann Archive, Inc., New York, N.Y.)

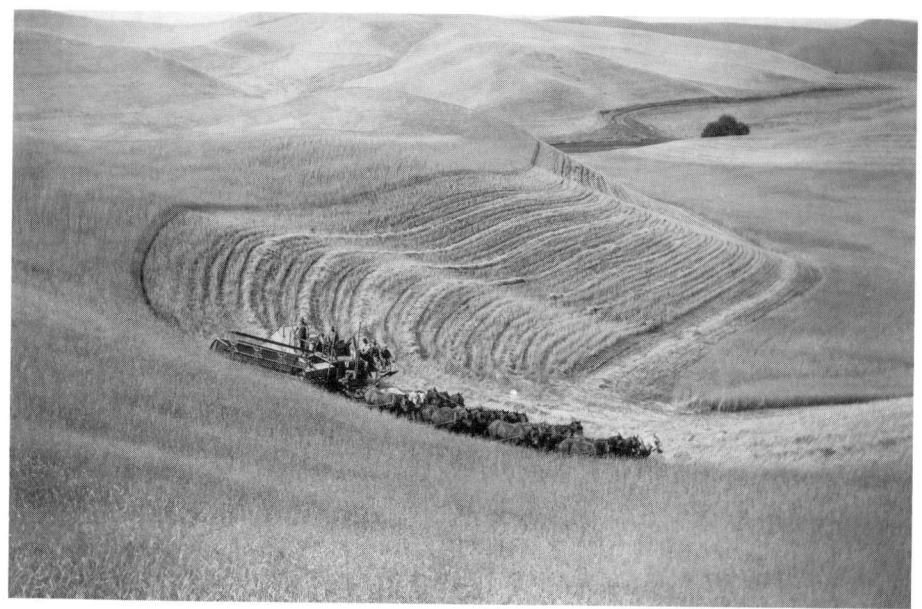

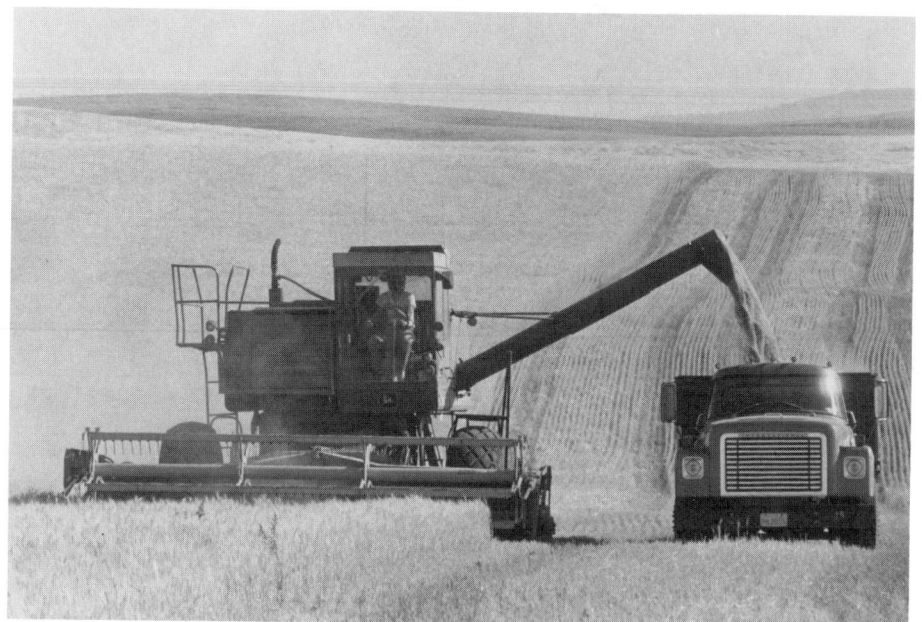

Consumers—all have benefited from the unfinished miracle of American agriculture. Modernization and mechanization have brought bountiful production at reasonable cost.

Two scenes from the famous Palouse wheat area of Washington:

Upper: How it used to be done! Big team hitch shown drawing a combine prior to the advent of tractor power. (Courtesy, Northern Pacific Railway)

Lower: John Deere self-propelled combine that cuts an 18-ft. wide swath and is capable of harvesting over 300 bushels of wheat per hour. (Photo by Henry Fisher, Oaksdale, Wash.)

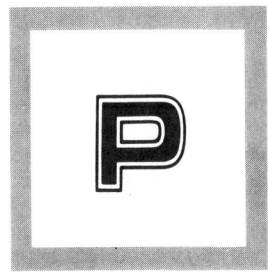

PALATABILITY

If they don't eat it, it won't do them any good. And that applies to all people.

The palatability of a food is the result of the following factors: taste, smell, texture, temperature, sound, and appearance. These factors are affected by the physical and chemical nature of foods.

The sensation of taste is described in terms of sweet, sour, salty, or bitter. This sense is more highly developed in some individuals than in others; for example, foods may be too salty for one person but just right for another. Some persons can detect slight differences in taste, others cannot. It is noteworthy, too, that the taste buds diminish in number later in life, with the result that the elderly often prefer more highly flavored foods. Also, taste sensitivity is decreased by smoking or chewing tobacco.

The smell and taste of foods are closely linked. If one were to hold the nose while eating, much of the enjoyment would be lost. The stimulation of the olfactory organs (the sense of smell organs) is brought about by certain volatile oils. Some foods may be relished because of their pleasing aromas, others may be rejected because of their repulsive odors.

Texture affects the highly developed sense of touch of the tongue. Children may reject foods because they are slippery. Older folks may reject foods because they are stringy, sticky, or greasy.

Some like steaming hot foods. Others prefer foods that are lukewarm. And still others like it cold.

Sound is important in some cases, as in eating popcorn.

Palatability is also conditioned by the attractiveness of the food, and by the surroundings in which it is consumed.

(Also see FLAVORINGS AND SEASONINGS.)

PALM family _Palmae_

Palms are an ancient group of plants. Fossil (buried remains) palm leaves have been found that date from the age of dinosaurs.

The family _Palmae_ embraces more than 2,600 kinds of palms, varying greatly in size and kind of flowers, leaves, and fruits they produce. They are of great economic importance; furnishing food, shelter, clothing, timber, fuel, building materials, sticks, fiber, paper, starch, sugar, oil, wax, wine, tannin, dyeing material, resin, and a host of other products, all of which render them most valuable to the natives and to tropical agriculture. Palms thrive in warm climates, especially in the tropics. They are most common in Southeast Asia, the Pacific Islands, and in tropical America. They grow wild along the coast of North Carolina, in Arizona, and in the deserts of southern California.

Most palms grow straight and tall, but a few do not. The trunks of some palms lie on the ground. Others have most of the trunk buried in the soil. Still others have slender, vinelike stems that are from 10 to 250 ft (_3 to 76 m_) long.

Because of their importance in food production, the following three palms are treated separately in this book:

Coconut (_Cocos nucifera_)
Date(s) (_Phoenix dactylifera_)
Oil Palm (_Elaeis guineensis_)

PALMITIC ACID

A 16-carbon saturated fatty acid.
(Also see FATS AND FATTY ACIDS.)

PALM OIL

A red oil derived from the oil palm tree. It is one of the world's most important edible and soapmaking oils. Moreover, the yield per acre is higher than can be obtained by any other vegetable oil. The oil palm tree is indigenous to West Africa.

(Also see OILS, VEGETABLE, Table O-6 Vegetable Oils, "Palm Oil"; and OIL PALM.)

PANCREAS

A large, elongated gland located near the stomach. It produces pancreatic juice which is secreted into the upper small intestine via the pancreatic duct.

(Also see DIGESTION AND ABSORPTION; and ENDOCRINE GLANDS.)

PANCREATIC JUICE

A thick, transparent liquid secreted by the pancreas into the upper small intestine. It contains three enzymes; pancreatic amylase, pancreatic lipase and trypsin.

(Also see DIGESTION AND ABSORPTION.)

PANCREATIN

A commercially available preparation containing the enzymes of the pancreas of cattle or pigs. It is capable of breaking down starch, lipids, and proteins. Pancreatin may be used as an aid to digestion. However, the stomach environment destroys it; hence, coated pills are used to allow it to reach the small intestine.

(Also see DIGESTION AND ABSORPTION.)

PANCREATITIS

An acute or chronic inflammation of the pancreas whose cause is poorly understood. Cases may be mild to severe, and some may even cause death. Often its occurrence is associated with other diseases such as alcoholism, gallbladder disease, peptic ulcer, an infectious disease or an accident. Symptoms of pancreatitis consist of a severe upper abdominal pain radiating into the back and stimulated by eating, tenderness above the stomach, distention, constipation, nausea and vomiting. The basis of treatment is to limit pancreatic secretion to a minimum. Hence, during the first few days of treatment intravenous feeding is employed, followed by a soft, bland or low residue diet. When medical treatment is ineffective, surgery may be needed.

(Also see MODIFIED DIETS; DIGESTION AND ABSORPTION; DISEASES; and INTRAVENOUS FEEDING.)

PANCREOZYMIN

A hormone secreted by the lining of the duodenum in response to stimulation by partially digested fats and proteins, stomach acid or calcium ions. It is also called cholecystokinin or cholecystokinin-pancreozymin.

(Also see CHOLECYSTOKININ-PANCREOZYMIN; and ENDOCRINE GLAND.)

PANDANUS FRUIT (SCREW-PINE FRUIT)
Pandanus adoratissimus

The fruit of a tree (of the family Pandanaceae) that grows throughout southeast Asia and the Pacific Islands. Pandanus fruits are usually yellow to red in color, round or pear-shaped, and range from 6 to 10 in. (15 to 25 cm) in diameter. The fleshy base of the fruit is usually the only part that is eaten. Some of the Polynesian peoples mix the fruit and coconut milk or grated coconut and bake the pasty mixture into flat cakes. The pandanus-coconut paste may also be made into a refreshing drink by diluting it with water.

Pandanus fruit is rich in calories (150 kcal per 100 g), carbohydrates (18%), fat (8%), protein (5%), and fiber (7%), but it is low in vitamin C.

PANGAMIC ACID (VITAMIN B-15)

Contents

The authors make this presentation for two primary purposes: (1) informational, and (2) stimulation of research.

The nutritional status and biological role(s) of pangamic acid await clarification. Its stimulation of such fundamental processes of transmethylation, cellular respiration, etc. may have physiological application. Certainly, there is sufficient indication of the value of pangamic acid as a therapeutic agent to warrant further study. In the meantime, pangamic acid should not be taken unless prescribed by a physician.

Pangamic acid (also known as vitamin B-15, calcium pangamate, and dimethylglycene) is a chemical substance of an organic nature. It is sometimes classed as a vitamin or vitaminlike substance. Obviously, however, pangamic acid does not meet the classical definition of a vitamin, which is: "A substance, organic in nature, necessary in the diet in small amounts to sustain life, in the absence of which a specific deficiency disease develops." The proponents counter with the argument that: "It's not essential, strictly speaking, but it's helpful biologically under many circumstances."

The FDA classifies pangamic acid as a food additive, and, therefore, subject to the regulations requiring proof that it is nontoxic.

Pangamic acid has been widely studied and accepted in the U.S.S.R. as a necessary food factor with important physiological actions.

HISTORY. In 1951, Krebs *et al.* reported the presence of a water-soluble factor in apricot kernels, which they subsequently isolated in crystalline form from rice bran and polish. Later, it was extracted from brewers' yeast, cattle blood, and horse liver. The name *pangamic acid* (*pan*, meaning universal; *gamic*, meaning seed) was applied to the substance to connote its seeming universal presence in seeds; and it was assigned the fifteenth position in the vitamin B series by its discoverers.

The claim that pangamic acid is a B vitamin is based primarily on its presence in B-vitamin rich foods and on the broad spectrum of physiological functions attributed to it. However, it is not known whether man or other animals have the capacity to synthesize pangamic acid, and no specific disease can be attributed exclusively to a deficiency of the substance. Thus, the designation of pangamic acid as a vitamin is not accepted by most U.S. scientists.

CHEMISTRY, METABOLISM, PROPERTIES.

• **Chemistry**—the chemical structure of pangamic acid is given in Fig. P-1.

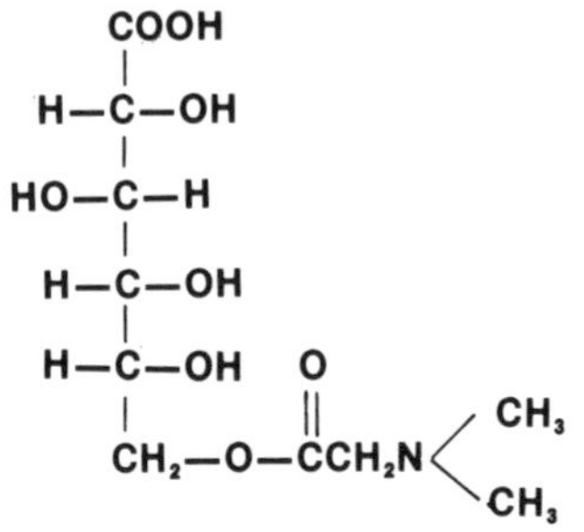

```
        COOH
          |
     H—C—OH
          |
   HO—C—H
          |
     H—C—OH
          |
     H—C—OH      O              CH₃
          |      ‖             /
     CH₂—O—CCH₂N
                               \
                                CH₃
```

Fig. P-1.   Pangamic acid ($C_{10}H_{19}O_8N$).

But the chemical composition of pangamic acid varies from brand product to brand product, and even within the same brand. This, within itself, makes the substance controversial. Some products are a mixture of sodium (or sometimes calcium) gluconate, glycine, and diisopropylamine dichloroacetate. However, the Russians confine their product to pangamic acid, i.e., the form of vitamin B-15 in which it occurs in nature.

• **Metabolism**—Little is known about the metabolism of pangamic acid. Within 10 to 15 minutes after subcutaneous injection of the substance, it is found in the blood, brain, liver, heart, and kidney; the site of its highest concentration and longest duration in the body is the kidney, where it persists for at least 4 days.

Excessive amounts of pangamic acid are excreted in urine, feces, and perspiration.

• **Properties**—Pangamic acid is a white crystalline compound, very soluble in water.

MEASUREMENT/ASSAY. The content of pangamic acid is usually expressed in milligrams (mg).

Chromatographic and spectrophotometric techniques have been developed for the quantitative determination of pangamic acid in biological material.

FUNCTIONS. Numerous functions have been attributed to pangamic acid; among them, the following:

1. **Stimulation of transmethylation reactions.** Pangamic acid possesses methyl groups (-CH₃) which are capable of being transferred from one compound to another within the body, resulting in the stimulation of creatine synthesis in muscle and heart tissue. In turn, when ATP (adenosine triphosphate), a transitory form of energy, is in excess of immediate requirements, creatine forms phosphocreatine, a more permanent form of energy for storage in muscle. Then when the supply of ATP is insufficient to meet the demands for energy, more ATP is produced from phosphocreatine by the reverse reaction.

2. **Stimulation of oxygen uptake.** Pangamic acid stimulates tissue oxygen uptake, thereby helping to prevent the condition called *hypoxia*—an insufficient supply of oxygen in living tissue, especially in heart and other muscles. It does not add to the overall oxygen supply of the body; rather, it increases the efficiency with which the oxygen is delivered from the bloodstream to the cells.

3. **Inhibition of fatty liver formation.** Oral or injection of pangamic acid to rats and rabbits exerts a protective effect against fatty infiltration of the liver induced by starvation, protein-free diets, anesthetics, carbon tetrachloride, or cholesterol.

4. **Adaptation to increased physical activity.** Pangamic acid enables animals to adapt to increased exercise. After periods of enforced swimming, animals previously treated with pangamic acid demonstrate a better maintenance of oxidative metabolism and energy levels than untreated controls; moreover, these effects persist for several days.

Some horse trainers have been known to administer pangamic acid to racehorses because of its reputed, but undocumented, quality of enabling animals to run faster and tire less. Also, athletes have been taking it for years.

5. **Control of blood cholesterol levels.** In most cases, the administration of pangamic acid causes a fall in both cholesterol biosynthesis and blood levels.

DISORDERS TREATED WITH PANGAMIC ACID.
Most treatments with pangamic acid have been conducted in the U.S.S.R., where the principal field of application of the drug has been in the treatment of cardiovascular disorders associated with insufficiency of oxidative metabolism. The Russians also report good results in treatment of liver disorders, a number of skin diseases, and some toxicoses. In the U.S.S.R. and/or elsewhere pangamic acid has been reported to be successful in treating the following disorders:

1. **Cardiovascular disease.** Pangamic acid is considered to be safe and effective in the treatment of—

a. **Atherosclerosis (hardening of the arteries),** characterized by headaches, chest pains, shortness of breath, tension, and insomnia. In patients with arteriosclerosis, pangamic acid strengthens the action of the heart muscles.

b. **Cardiopulmonary (heart-lung) insufficiency,** characterized by shortness of breath.

c. **Angina pectoris,** characterized by chest pain, due to the arteries being incapable of supplying sufficient oxygen-rich blood to the heart muscle.

d. **Congestive heart failure,** characterized by shortness of breath on slight exertion and dropsy (swelling around the ankles with pitting edema). This is a disease complex and group of symptoms caused by a failing heart, with congestion either in the lungs or the systemic circulation, or both. The chief causes are weakness of the heart muscles, high blood pressure, hardening of the arteries, and rheumatic or syphilitic disease of the heart valves. Treatment of patients suffering from congestive heart failure with pangamic acid increases diuresis (urination) and reduces high blood pressure and edema.

e. **Patients recovering from serious heart attacks,** as an aid in speeding their recovery.

It is noteworthy, too, that pangamic acid increases the effectiveness of strophanthin (a heart tonic) on heart function of patients with congestive failure and reduces the incidence of side effects associated with digitalis therapy.

2. **Fatigue.** Pangamic acid is used to reduce fatigue and increase energy—to alleviate that tired feeling. According to the proponents, it accomplishes this by extracting more oxygen from the bloodstream for better metabolism in the cells. Some athletes, both professionals and amateurs, claim that it increases their physical endurance.

3. **Hypoxia.** Pangamic acid is effective in treating hypoxia, characterized by an insufficient supply of oxygen in tissues. It increases the efficiency with which oxygen is delivered from the bloodstream to the cells.

4. **High cholesterol.** Several workers have observed significant reductions in serum cholesterol levels as a result of daily treatment with pangamic acid for 10 to 30 days.

5. **Liver function.** As supportive treatment for infectious hepatitis in children, pangamic acid given orally for 10 to 20 days leads to a more marked and rapid decline in fever, liver size, jaundice and serum transaminase levels and a 5 to 10 day shorter hospitalization period. Similar findings have been reported in adults with acute or chronic hepatitis treated with pangamic acid.

6. **Skin disorders.** It is claimed that pangamic acid is effective in the treatment of various skin diseases. It is reported that patients with scleroderma ("hidebound skin"), a chronic disease in which the skin and subcutaneous tissues become fibrous, rigid, and thickened, respond to daily treatment with pangamic acid for 45 days—relief is associated with softening of the affected skin and often with new hair growth. Also, a reduction of inflammation, edema, and itching has been reported in cases of eczema, psoriasis (a chronic skin disease that disfigures the face and body with recurrent red scaly patches), hives, and other skin disorders treated daily for 15 to 30 days with 100 to 150 mg of pangamic acid.

7. **Tumors.** Pangamic acid offers promise in the treatment of certain kinds of tumors. When given to rats with experimentally induced solid tumors, it did not interfere with the effectiveness of standard chemotherapeutic agents, but it significantly reduced the incidence and severity of the toxicity produced by certain drugs. Also, in preliminary work with rats, it has been reported that pangamic acid reduced both the incidence and latency of drug-induced mammary cancer. These limited studies await confirmation.

DEFICIENCY SYMPTOMS. There is indication that a deficiency of pangamic acid may cause fatigue (a tired feeling), hypoxia (an insufficient supply of oxygen in blood cells), heart disease, and glandular and nervous disorders.

DOSAGE. The usual dosage of pangamic acid is from 150 to 300 mg daily. But pangamic acid should not be taken unless prescribed by a physician.

TOXICITY. Despite initial caution regarding the use of pangamic acid in conditions of hypertension and glaucoma, "it is now regarded that the substance is without demonstrable toxicity in these or other disease states."[1] It is noteworthy, too, that, beginning in 1965, the U.S.S.R. Ministry of Health approved widespread manufacture and distribution of pangamic acid. One of the largest U.S. purveyors of pangamic acid—Da Vinci Laboratories, a subsidiary of Food Science Laboratories—cites several studies in which laboratory rats were fed quantities of B-15 equivalent to more than 100,000 times the recommended dosage for human consumption, without any ill effects.[2]

Perhaps the toxicity of pangamic acid depends on the particular formula. On the basis of available evidence, the so-called "Russian formula" appears to be relatively free of toxicity. Nevertheless, the U.S. Food and Drug Administration does not consider pangamic acid safe for human consumption.

Until the product is standardized (potency, quality, and chemical composition) and the question of toxicity is resolved, the authors recommend that pangamic acid be taken only under the direction of a physician.

TOP FOOD SOURCES OF PANGAMIC ACID. The best natural sources of pangamic acid are sunflower seed, pumpkin seed, yeast, liver, rice, whole grain cereals, apricot kernels and other seeds. Evidence suggests its occurrence wherever B-complex vitamins are found in natural foods.

CONCLUSION. Until more conclusive evidence on the role of pangamic acid is available, the authors subscribe to the view so well expressed by biochemist Richard A. Passwater, Ph.D., as follows:

"While the processes through which vitamin B-15 works are being elucidated, natural wisdom suggests that we take care to see that our diets are rich in vitamin B-15."[3]

(Also see VITAMIN[S], Table V-9)

PANTOTHENIC ACID (VITAMIN B-3)

[1]Stacpoole, Peter W., "Pangamic Acid (Vitamin B-15)," *World Review of Nutrition and Dietetics—Some Aspects of Human Nutrition*, S. Karger, Basel, Munchen, 1977, p. 153.)

[2]Grosswirth, Marvin, "B-15: Is it Superpill?," *Science Digest*, September 1978, p. 12.

[3]Passwater, Richard A., Ph.D., "B-15—New Ally In The Fight Against Major Diseases," *The Health Quarterly*, Vol. 3, No. 5, 1979, p. 16.

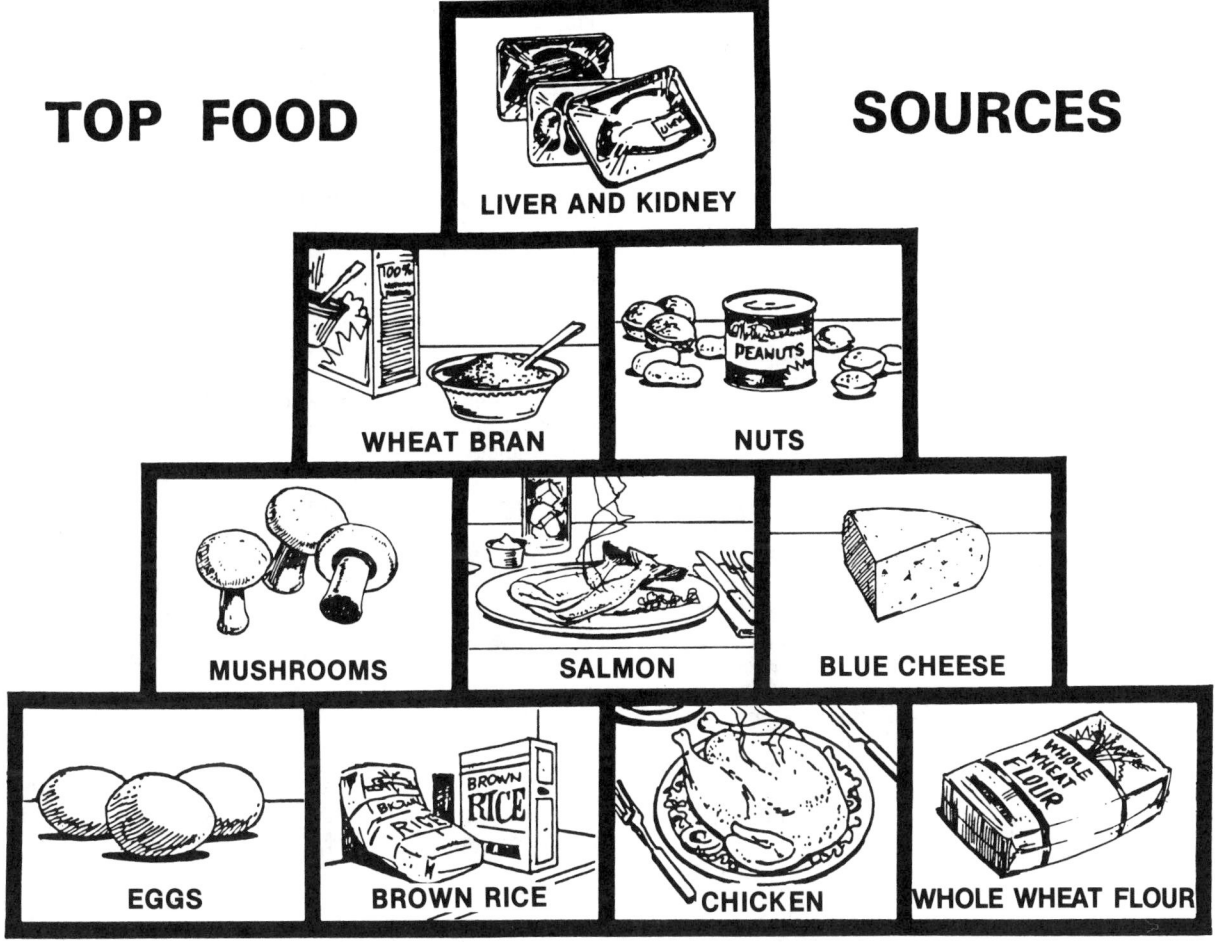

TOP FOOD **SOURCES**

LIVER AND KIDNEY

WHEAT BRAN

NUTS

MUSHROOMS

SALMON

BLUE CHEESE

EGGS

BROWN RICE

CHICKEN

WHOLE WHEAT FLOUR

Fig. P-2. Top food sources of pantothenic acid.

Pantothenic acid, a member of the vitamin B complex, is a dietary essential for man and animals; and, as an important constituent of coenzyme A (CoA), it plays a key role in body metabolism.

In recognition of its wide distribution in foods, the name "pantothenic acid," derived from the Greek word *pantothen*—meaning everywhere, was first given to it in 1933, by R. J. Williams, then of Oregon State, later at the University of Texas.

Before its structure was known, pantothenic acid was called by several other names, now obsolete, including: filtrate factor, chick antidermatitis factor, bios factor, the antigray hair factor, pantothen, factor H, factor 2, vitamin B-x, vitamin B-2, vitamin B-3.

HISTORY. The existence of pantothenic acid and its nutritive significance for the proliferation and fermen-

tative activity of yeast cells first emerged from the studies of R. J. Williams, beginning in 1919. In 1933, Williams fractionated this compound from yeast and called it pantothenic acid; and in 1939, he isolated pantothenic acid from liver. In 1939, Jukes concluded that the antidermatitis factor isolated from liver was one and the same thing as the factor found in yeast. In 1940, pantothenic acid was synthesized by Williams and two other laboratories, all working independently. Also, in 1940, pantothenic acid received widespread attention as a possible preventive for gray hair, since it had been observed that the black hair of a rat would turn gray when the animal was deprived of the vitamin; but subsequent studies did not reveal any such benefits to accrue to humans. In 1946, Lipmann and co-workers showed that coenzyme A is essential for acetylation reactions in the body; and in 1950 reports from the same laboratory showed pantothenic acid to be a constituent of coenzyme A.

CHEMISTRY, METABOLISM, PROPERTIES.

• **Chemistry**—Pantothenic acid is composed of pantoic acid and the amino acid beta-alanine, as shown in Fig. P-3.

PANTOTHENIC ACID

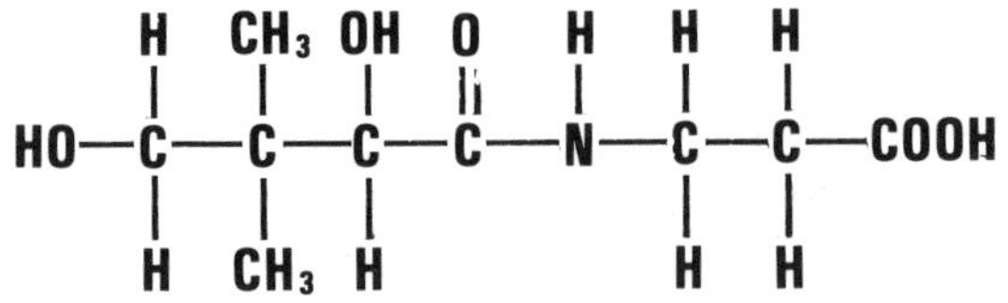

$$HO-\overset{\overset{\displaystyle H}{|}}{\underset{\underset{\displaystyle H}{|}}{C}}-\overset{\overset{\displaystyle CH_3}{|}}{\underset{\underset{\displaystyle CH_3}{|}}{C}}-\overset{\overset{\displaystyle OH}{|}}{\underset{\underset{\displaystyle H}{|}}{C}}-\overset{\overset{\displaystyle O}{||}}{C}-\overset{\overset{\displaystyle H}{|}}{\underset{\underset{\displaystyle H}{|}}{N}}-\overset{\overset{\displaystyle H}{|}}{\underset{\underset{\displaystyle H}{|}}{C}}-\overset{\overset{\displaystyle H}{|}}{\underset{\underset{\displaystyle H}{|}}{C}}-COOH$$

Fig. P-3.   Structure of pantothenic acid.

• **Metabolism**—Pantothenic acid, like the other B vitamins, is readily absorbed through the mucosa of the small intestine and enters the portal circulation. Within the tissues, most of the panothenic acid is used in the synthesis of coenzyme A (CoA); but a significant amount found in the cells is bound to a protein in a compound known as acyl carrier protein (ACP).

Pantothenic acid is present in all living tissue, with high concentrations in the liver and kidney. (Large amounts of CoA are found in the liver, with lesser amounts in the adrenal glands.)

The vitamin is excreted from the body by way of the kidneys.

• **Properties**—In pure form, pantothenic acid is a viscous yellow oil, soluble in water, quite stable in neutral solutions, but destroyed by acid, alkali, and prolonged exposure to dry heat (2 to 6 days—far longer than the usual cooking or baking procedures). Calcium pantothenate, the form in which it is commercially available, is a white, odorless, bitter, crystalline substance, which is water-soluble and quite stable. (Pantothenic acid is also available as the sodium salt.)

MEASUREMENT/ASSAY.   The activity of pantothenic acid is expressed in grams and milligrams of the chemically pure substance.

Pantothenic acid content may be determined by chemical methods (including gas chromotography), microbiologic procedures, and the chick and rat bioassay.

FUNCTIONS.   Pantothenic acid functions in the body as part of two enzymes—coenzyme A (CoA) and acyl carrier protein (ACP).

ACP is composed of a panthetheine linked through a phosphate group to protein. It, along with CoA, is required by the cells in the biosynthesis (the manufacture, or building up) of fatty acids (CoA, without ACP, is involved in their breakdown.)

Coenzyme A, meaning a coenzyme for acetylation, is one of the most important substances in body metabolism. It is a complex molecule containing the vitamin combined with adenosine 3-phosphate, pyrophosphate, and beta-mercaptoethylamine (a compound containing an -SH group), as shown in Fig. P-4.

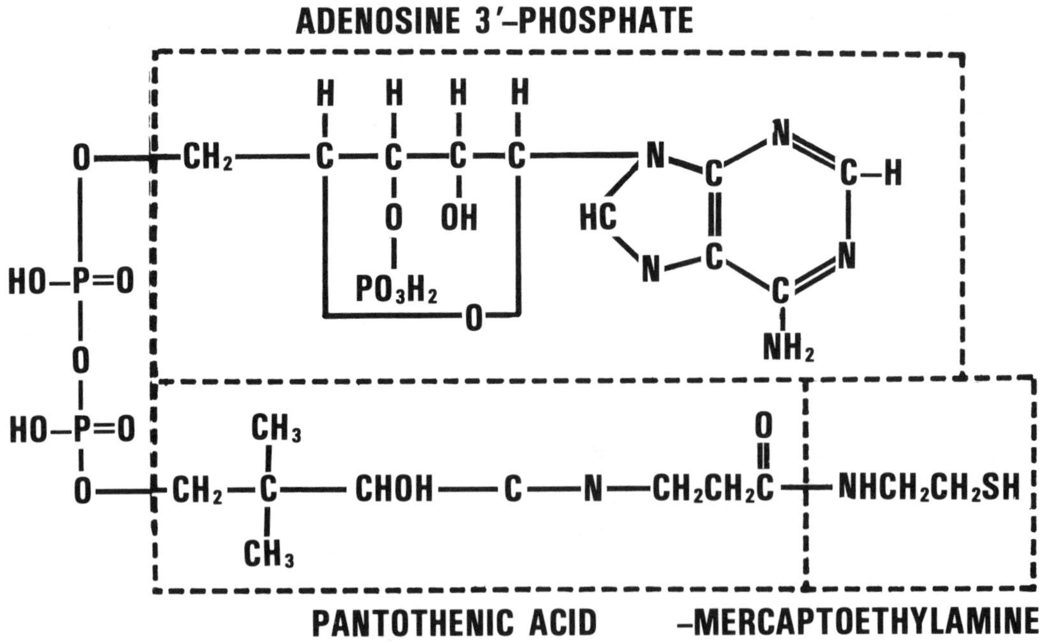

Fig. P-4.   Structure of CoA.

The way in which pantothenic acid is incorporated in the molecule of coenzyme A is shown in fig. P-4. The sulphydryl (-SH) group of the molecule is extremely active, but the other groups are also involved in some of the functions of coenzyme A.

CoA functions in any reaction in which an acetyl group (-CH$_3$CO) is formed or is transferred from one substance to another. In addition to acetyl, other acyl radicals require coenzyme A; it is required whenever succinyl, benzyl, or fatty acid radicals are formed or transferred.

Coenzyme A participates in several fundamental metabolic functions; these include the following:

1. **The synthesis (the building up) of fatty acids.** The most important function of coenzyme A (and, hence, of pantothenic acid) in metabolism is the transfer of radicals of acetic acid (or C$_2$) in the synthesis of fatty acids. During the process of digestion, the triglycerides which are present in the food are split by lipases of the pancreas and of the intestinal wall into glycerol, monoglycerides, and fatty acids which are simultaneously emulsified by the bile acids. The degree of absorption of the fatty acids through the wall of the small intestine depends on the length of the chain; the shorter the chain, the more complete the absorption. After passing through the intestinal wall, the short chain fatty acids are converted into longer chain fatty acids, the major step in the process being the combination of coenzyme A with acetic acid to form "activated acetic acid" or acetyl-coenzyme A.

Acetyl-coenzyme A is next converted to malonyl-coenzyme A (which contains one more carbon atom), a reaction which is catalyzed by an enzyme which contains biotin. Malonyl-coenzyme A then reacts with another activated fatty acid (the chain of which has also become longer by one carbon atom) yielding a product which is a fatty acid with a chain which has been lengthened by two carbon atoms. In this manner, for example, stearic acid (C$_{18}$) is formed from palmitic acid (C$_{16}$) in the body.

2. **The degradation (the breaking down) of fatty acids.** In metabolism, both the synthesis and the degradation of fatty acids are required. Pantothenic acid, as a constituent of coenzyme A, participates in this breaking down process. The energy which is released in this process of degradation is gathered and transferred elsewhere by another system which is based on the (reversible) formation of adenosine triphosphate (ATP), which is high in energy, from two compounds having lower levels of energy, adenosine diphosphate (ADP) and monophosphate (AMP).

3. **The citric acid cycle.** A very large part of the energy required in metabolism is supplied by the citric acid cycle (or the "Krebs' cycle"), in which compounds high in energy (carbohydrates, fats, and proteins) are continually being converted into compounds which are lower in energy; the energy released is again contained in the form of ATP.

Pantothenic acid, as a constituent of coenzyme A, is involved in several of the steps of the citric acid cycle; these include the synthesis of citric acid from oxalacetic acid and its salts, and the oxidation by decarboxylation of *a*-keto-acids.

4. **The acetylation of choline.** Pantothenic acid is necessary for the formation of acetylcholine, the transmitter of nerve impulses.

5. **The synthesis of antibodies.** Pantothenic acid stimulates the synthesis of those antibodies which increase resistance to pathogens.

6. **The utilization of nutrients.** Coenzyme A is essential for the metabolism of fats, carbohydrates, and proteins; hence, a deficiency of pantothenic acid will necessarily impair the utilization of digestible nutrients. The function of coenzyme A is in the endogenous metabolism, not in the digestive tract. Hence, it cannot affect the digestible or metabolizable energy; only its utilization—the net productive energy which is most simply measured in terms of the retention of nutrients. This is true not only for those nutrients which supply energy, but also for those which supply protein.

7. **Other functions.** Pantothenic acid also affects the endocrine glands, and the hormones they produce. Thus, a deficiency of pantothenic acid in rats reduces not only the rate of gain in weight but also the rate of basal metabolism. Also, it has been postulated that the influence which pantothenic acid exerts on the fertility of various animals may be due to some relationship between pantothenic acid and the synthesis of steroid hormones.

Other functions attributed to pantothenic acid (or coenzyme A) are:

    a. It is necessary in the synthesis of porphyrin, a precursor of heme, of importance in hemoglobin synthesis.

    b. It is necessary for the maintenance of normal blood sugar levels.

    c. It may facilitate the excretion of sulfonamide drugs.

    d. It influences the metabolism of some of the minerals and trace elements.

    e. It can be used for detoxification of drugs, including the sulphonamides.

DEFICIENCY SYMPTOMS. A deficiency of pantothenic acid has been associated with the "burning foot syndrome" that occurred in Japan and the Philippines among prisoners during World War II.

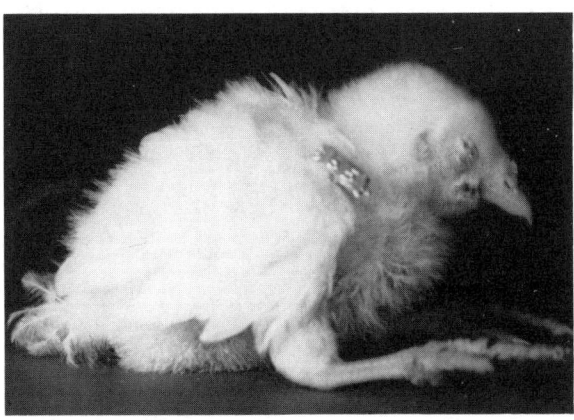

Fig. P-5. Pantothenic acid deficiency in chick. Note the lesions at the corners of the mouth and on the eyelids and feet. (Courtesy, Department of Poultry Science, Cornell University)

Pantothenic deficiency has been produced in human volunteers (1) by feeding them semisynthetic diets low in pantothenic acid for a period of 10 to 12 weeks; and (2) by feeding them diets to which the pantothenic acid antagonist omega-methylpantothenic acid was added. (A vitamin antagonist is a substance so similar in structure to the vitamin that the body accepts it in place of the vitamin, but the antagonist is unable to perform the functions of the true vitamin.) The subjects developed a wide variety of symptoms including: irritableness and restlessness; loss of appetite, indigestion, abdominal pain, nausea; headache; sullenness, mental depression; fatigue, weakness; numbness and tingling of hands and feet, muscle cramps in the arms and legs; burning sensations in the feet; insomnia; respiratory infections; rapid pulse; and a staggering gait. Also, in these subjects there was increased reaction to stress; increased sensitivity to insulin, resulting in low blood sugar levels; an increased sedimentation rate for erythrocytes; decreased gastric secretions; and marked decrease in antibody production. All symptoms were cured by the administration of pantothenic acid.

A lack of pantothenic acid results in premature graying of the hair in piebald rats, foxes, and dogs. But, neither pantothenic acid nor any other nutritional factor has been shown to be involved in the graying of hair in humans.

RECOMMENDED DAILY ALLOWANCE. The amount of pantothenic acid required by human beings has not been determined; so, a recommended daily allowance for pantothenic acid has not been made by the Food and Nutrition Board of the National Research Council. Nevertheless, they do give "estimated safe and adequate intakes" based on proportional energy needs (see Table P-1). Further, they suggest that a higher intake may be needed during pregnancy and lactation.

TABLE P-1
ESTIMATED SAFE AND ADEQUATE DAILY DIETARY INTAKE OF PANTOTHENIC ACID[1]

Group	Age	Pantothenic Acid
	(yr)	(mg)
Infants	0 - .5	2
	.5- 1.0	3
Children and adolescents . .	1.0- 3.0	3
	4.0- 6.0	3-4
	7.0-10.0	4-5
	11.0 +	4-7
Adults		4-7

[1]*Recommended Dietary Allowances*, 10th ed., NRC–National Academy of Sciences, 1989, p. 284.

NOTE WELL:

1. Processing of food can, in some instances, result in appreciable losses of pantothenic acid. Thus, it is possible that unrecognized marginal deficiencies may exist, along with deficiencies of other B-complex vitamins.

2. Deficiencies of pantothenic acid occur in farm animals (especially chickens and swine), fed *natural rations.* As a result, pantothenic acid is commonly added to commercial poultry and swine rations.

These two facts point up the need for more studies on the pantothenic requirement of humans, and perhaps the need for dietary supplementation for buoyant good health.

• **Pantothenic acid intake in average U.S. diet**—The average American diet provides 5 to 10 mg of pantothenic acid per day, with an average of 6 mg.

TOXICITY. Pantothenic acid is a relatively nontoxic substance. As much as 10 g of calcium pantothenate per day was given to young men for 6 weeks with no toxic symptoms; other studies indicate that daily doses of 10 to 20 g may result in occasional diarrhea and water retention.[4]

PANTOTHENIC ACID LOSSES DURING PROCESSING, COOKING, AND STORAGE. Losses up to 50%, and even more, of the pantothenic acid content of foods may occur from production to consumption. Here are some of them:

1. About 50% of the pantothenic content of grains is lost in milling.

2. Up to 50% of the pantothenic content of fruits and vegetables is lost in canning or freezing, and storage, of fruits and vegetables.

3. From 15 to 30% of the pantothenic acid content of meat is lost in cooking or canning.

4. Losses in pantothenic acid from dry processing of foods may exceed 50%.

Pantothenic acid is reasonably stable in natural foods during storage, provided that oxidation and high temperature are avoided. Cereal grains may be stored for periods up to a year without appreciable loss.

Henry A. Schroeder, M.D., of the Dartmouth Medical School, conducted an extensive survey of the pantothenic acid content in hundreds of common foods, and found that modern processing was causing massive losses of the vitamin. His studies showed pantothenic acid losses as follows: From milling wheat and making all-purpose flour, 57.7%; from canning vegetables, 56 to 79%; from freezing vegetables, 48 to 57%; from canning meat and poultry, 26.2%; and from canning seafood, 19.9%.[5]

SOURCES OF PANTOTHENIC ACID. Pantothenic acid is widely distributed in foods, with considerable variation in content according to food, and processing. A grouping and ranking of foods according to pantothenic content follows:

• **Rich sources**—Organ meat (liver, kidney, and heart), cottonseed flour, wheat flour, wheat bran, rice bran, rice polish

[4]Committee on Dietary Allowances, Food and Nutrition Board, *Recommended Dietary Allowances*, 9th ed., 1980, National Research Council, National Academy of Sciences, Washington, D.C., p. 123.

[5]Schroeder, Henry A., M.D., "Losses of Vitamins and Trace Minerals Resulting From Processing and Preservation of Foods," *The American Journal of Chemical Nutrition*, Vol. 24, May 1971, pp. 562-573.

• **Good sources**—Nuts, mushrooms, soybean flour, salmon, blue cheese, eggs, buckwheat flour, brown rice, lobster, sunflower seeds

• **Fair sources**—Chicken, broccoli, sweet peppers, whole wheat flour, avocados

• **Negligible sources**—Butter, corn flakes, white flour, fats and oils, margarine, precooked rice, sugar

• **Supplemental sources**—Synthetic calcium pantothenate is widely used as a vitamin supplement. Yeast is a rich natural supplement.

Intestinal bacteria also synthesize pantothenic acid, but the amount produced and the availability of the

vitamin from this source are unknown.

For additional sources and more precise values of pantothenic acid, see Food Composition Table F-36 of this book.

TOP FOOD SOURCES OF PANTOTHENIC ACID. The top food sources of pantothenic acid are listed in Table P-2.

NOTE WELL: This table lists (1) the top sources without regard to the amount normally eaten (left column), and (2) the top food sources (right column); and the caloric (energy) content of each food. When using this table, however, cognizance should be taken of the fact that the pantothenic content of many foods has not been determined.

(Also see VITAMIN[S], Table V-9.)

TABLE P-2
TOP SOURCES OF PANTOTHENIC ACID AND THEIR CALORIC CONTENT[1]

Top Sources[2]	Pantothenic Acid	Energy	Top Food Sources	Pantothenic Acid	Energy
	(mg / 100 g)	(kcal / 100 g)		(mg / 100 g)	(kcal / 100 g)
Yeast, brewers', debittered	12.0	283	Beef liver, fried	7.7	222
Yeast, torula	11.0	277	Beef heart, lean braised	2.5	179
Egg, chicken, dried, yolk	8.2	687	Peanut butter	2.5	585
Calf liver, fried................	8.0	261	Peanuts.....................	2.4	581
Beef liver, fried	7.7	222	Mushrooms (*Agaricus*		
Egg, chicken, dry, whole	6.7	609	*campestris*), raw	2.2	28
Whey, acid, dry	5.6	339	Soybean flour, low, high,		
Whey, sweet, dry	5.6	354	full or defatted	2.0	386
Chicken liver, simmered........	5.5	157	Salmon, steamed	1.8	197
Kidneys, lamb, raw	4.5	105	Cheese, natural, blue	1.8	359
Egg, chicken, raw, yolks, fresh ..	4.4	369	Egg, chicken, hard cooked......	1.7	157
Cottonseed flour	4.3	356	Pecans, unsalted	1.7	739
Kidneys, calf, raw	4.0	113	Buckwheat flour, dark	1.5	357
Pancreas beef (lean only), raw ...	3.7	141	Rice, brown, cooked	1.5	119
Milk, cow's, dry, skim, solids,			Lobster, boiled	1.5	119
instant	3.6	353	Sunflower seed kernels, dry,		
Rice, polish	3.3	265	hulled	1.4	560
Buttermilk, dried (made from			Cashew nuts, salted or unsalted .	1.3	596
skim milk)	3.2	387	Broccoli spears, cooked	1.1	26
Kidneys, hog, raw	3.2	106	Chicken, stewed	1.2	183
Chicken, broilers or fryers,			Peppers, sweet, immature,		
giblets simmered	3.0	157	green, boiled, drained........	1.1	18
Wheat bran	3.0	353	Wheat flour, whole (from		
Rice bran...................	2.8	276	hard wheats)	1.1	361
Beef heart, lean, braised	2.5	179	Avocados, raw, all varieties	1.1	167

[1]These listings are based on the data in Food Composition Table F–36 of this book. Some top or rich sources may have been overlooked since some of the foods in Table F–36 lack values for pantothenic acid.

Whenever possible, foods are on an "as used" basis, without regard to moisture content; hence, certain high-moisture foods may be disadvantaged when ranked on the basis of pantothenic acid content per 100 g (approximately 3½ oz) without regard to moisture content.

[2]Listed without regard to the amount normally eaten.

PAPAIN (VEGETABLE PEPSIN)

This is an enzyme obtained from the green fruit and leaves of the papaya. It is proteolytic; it breaks down proteins such as the digestive enzymes pepsin and trypsin.

Papain can be employed to tenderize meats, clear beverages, prevent adhesions during wound healing, and aid digestion.

(Also see ADDITIVES, Table A-3.)

PAPAYA (MAMAO) *Carica papaya*

The papaya tree is a fast-growing, short-lived, tree native to tropical America. It is a soft wooded palmlike evergreen with palmate leaves clustered at the top. In

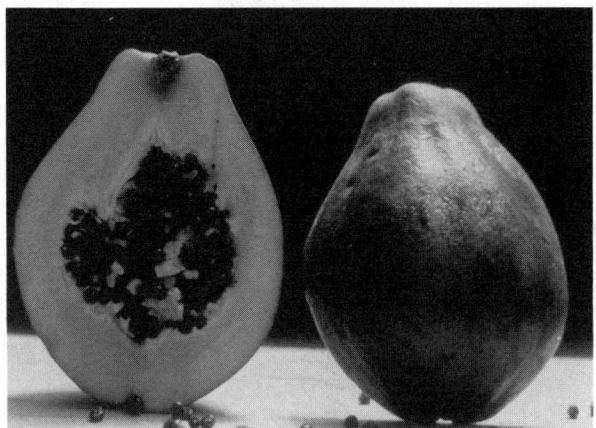

Fig. P-6. The papaya—fruit of a tropical tree that looks like a palm tree with a tuft of large leaves at the top. (Courtesy, USDA)

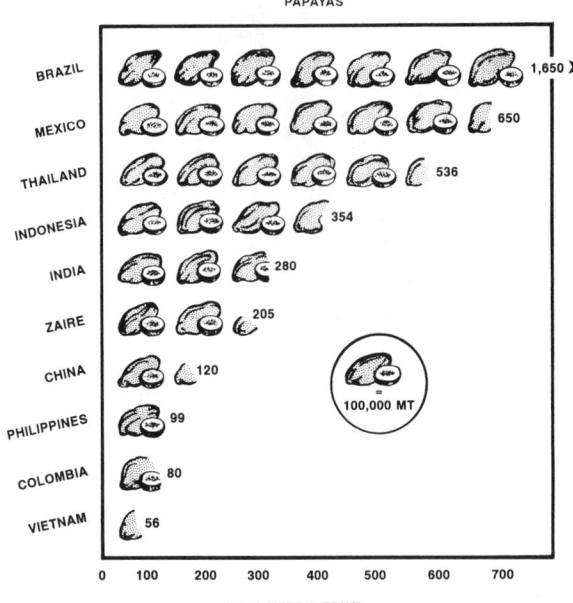

Fig. P-7. Leading papaya-producing countries of the world. (Based on data from *FAO Production Yearbook*, 1990, FAO/UN, Rome, Italy, Vol. 44, p. 169, Table 74)

tropical countries around the world, the papaya is cultivated for its edible melonlike fruit, the papaya, which is round to oblong and may weigh as much as 20 lb (*9.1 kg*). Ripening papayas turn from green to yellowish or orange on the outside and yellow to reddish-orange on the inside. Numerous black, pea-sized seeds are attached to the walls of the inside cavity. The edible inside flesh of the papaya fruit is the consistency of butter and mildly sweet with a slight musky tang. Dried latex obtained from the immature fruit is the source of the protein digestion enzyme papain which is used commercially as a meat tenderizer.

Some people call the papaya *papaw* or *pawpaw*, which tends to confuse the papaya with the edible wild papaw of the United States.

ORIGIN AND HISTORY.
The papaya is native to Central America. Since it grows readily from seed, the papaya was distributed quite early by man all over the tropical and subtropical areas of the world. In the 1500s, the seeds were carried to the West Indies, then to Manila and Africa, and then to India sometime before the 17th century.

PRODUCTION.
Since papayas require a tropical climate for growth and since they are difficult to transport, much of the papaya crop is consumed in the area where it is produced. There are, however, sufficient papayas produced that they rank about nineteenth among the top 20 fruits of the world. Their yearly production averages about 4.4 million metric tons and the leading papaya-producing countries are shown in Fig. P-7.

In the United States, the production of papayas has gradually increased in Hawaii to over 30,000 metric tons each year with a value of almost $15 million.

Propagation and Growing. Papayas are normally propagated by seeds, which are started in a nursery, and then the young plants are transplanted to the field. Papaya trees are placed 8 to 12 ft (*2.4 to 3.7 m*) apart, and a few male trees are necessary in each field. There are, however, some hermaphroditic cultivars. After 9 to 14 months the trees start bearing fruit and trees may be 7 to 33 ft (*2 to 10 m*) high. Yearly yields per tree vary from 30 to 150 fruits, and up to 15 tons of fruit can be produced from an acre of trees.

The peak productive life of papayas is only a few years; hence, rotation planting ensures a continuous supply of bearing trees. They require full sun, windbreaks, well-drained, fertile soil and a warm humid climate. Low temperatures produce fruits with poor flavor. In some dry areas papayas are grown under irrigation. Weeds are controlled and fertilizing increases yields.

Harvesting. When the first traces of yellow appear on the papaya fruits they are picked. Papayas then ripen within 4 to 5 days.

Papain is extracted commercially by making vertical scratches in the green immature fruit from which a latex oozes and drips into a collecting tray. This latex coagulates, then it is dried. Papaya trees are producers of papain for only 3 years.

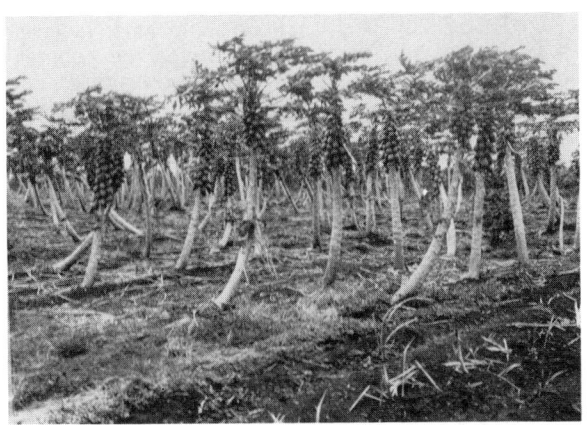

Fig. P-8.   A field of papayas on the island of Kauai, Hawaii. (Photo by A. H. Ensminger)

PROCESSING AND PREPARATION.   Papayas are usually consumed fresh like a cantaloupe or in salads, pies, and sherbets. There is little processing involved. However, they can be squeezed for juice, pickled, candied or made into jellies. In some areas, the unripe fruits are cooked and used like a squash.

Most fresh fruit is consumed in the tropics since it is not very tasty unless eaten at just the proper stage. Some fresh fruits are transported from Hawaii to the mainland, and some are being canned for marketing.

NUTRITIONAL VALUE.   Papayas are listed in Food Composition Table F-36. They contain about 89% water and only 39 Calories (kcal) per 100 g (about 3½ oz) or about 120 Calories (kcal) per medium-sized fruit. Papayas are rich in vitamin A and contain some vitamin C.

(Also see FRUIT[S], Table F-47 Fruits of the World.)

PAPIN'S DIGESTER

The ancestor of today's modern pressure cooker invented in 1679 by Denis Papin, a French physicist. Papin even designed his digester with a safety valve to relieve the pressure before it became hazardous. In 1681, he published an instruction manual describing its uses—cookery, voyages at sea, confectionery and drink making. The application of the pressure cooker to canning was one of the determinants in the evolution of the modern food industry.

PARA-AMINOBENZOIC ACID (PABA)

Para-aminobenzoic acid (PABA) is a constituent of foods, which is sometimes listed with the B vitamins.

In addition to having activity as a growth factor for certain bacteria, PABA has considerable folacin activity when fed to deficient animals in which intestinal syn-

thesis of folacin takes place. For example, for rats and mice, it can completely replace the need for a dietary source of folacin. This explains why para-aminobenzoic acid was once considered to be a vitamin in its own right.

For man and other higher animals, PABA is an essential part of the folacin molecule. But it has no vitamin activity in animals receiving ample folacin, and it is not required in the diet; hence, it can no longer be considered a vitamin, contrary to its listing in many vitamin preparations on the market.

HISTORY.   PABA was first identified as an essential nutrient for certain microorganisms. Later, it was shown to act as an antigray hair factor in rats and mice (but not people) and as a growth-promoting factor in chicks.

CHEMISTRY, METABOLISM, PROPERTIES.

• **Chemistry**—The chemical structure of PABA is given in Fig. P-9.

| *Para*-AMINOBENZOIC ACID |

$$NH_2$$

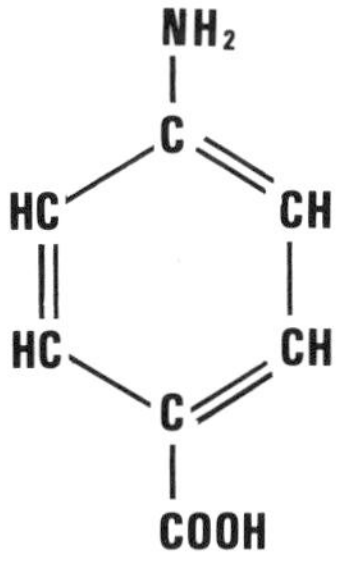

Fig. P-9.   Structure of *para*-aminobenzoic acid.

• **Metabolism**—The body will manufacture its own PABA if conditions in the intestines are favorable.

• **Properties**—PABA is a yellow, crystalline, slightly water-soluble substance.

MEASUREMENT.   The activity of PABA, and of its sodium and potassium salts, is ordinarily expressed in grams of chemically pure substances.

FUNCTIONS.   For man and other higher animals, PABA functions as an essential part of the folacin molecule.

As a coenzyme, PABA functions in the breakdown and utilization of proteins and in the formation of blood cells, especially red blood cells.

• **Human pharmaceutical uses**—PABA is sometimes used as a human pharmaceutical, not as a vitamin, in the following: as an antirickettsial; to counteract the bacteriostatic action of sulfonamides; and as a protective agent against sunburn.

1. **Antirickettesial.** PABA is sometimes used in the treatment of certain rickettsial diseases—diseases in man and animals caused by microscopically small parasites of the genus *Rickettsia*, notably typhus and Rocky Mountain spotted fever.

The therapeutic use of PABA in the treatment of rickettsial diseases is based on the concept of metabolic antagonism. PABA acts as an antagonist to a material essential to these organisms, para-oxybenzoic acid; hence, the rickettsial organisms are killed because PABA blocks their essential metabolite.

2. **Sulfonamide antagonist.** PABA has the ability to reverse the bacteriostatic effects of sulfonamides, thereby counteracting their action. This is an antimetabolite action, explainable on the basis of similarity of structures (see Fig. P-10). According to this theory, sulfonamides suppress bacterial growth by replacing their chemical analog PABA in bacterial enzyme systems; PABA in excess reverses the effect.

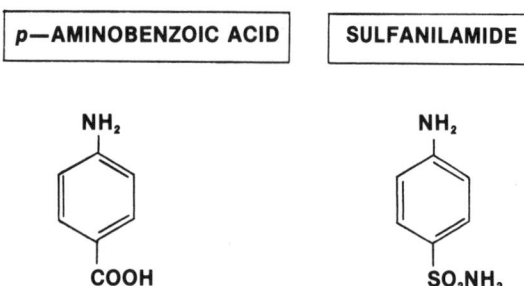

Fig. P-10. The similarity of the structures of PABA and sulfanilamide is obvious.

3. **Sunscreen agent.** PABA is used for protection against sunburn; usually about 5% PABA is incorporated in an ointment, to be applied over exposed parts of the body. Currently, some dermatologists are recommending other sunscreen lotions; so, for protection against sunburn, see your dermatologist.

DEFICIENCY SYMPTOMS. Sulfa drugs may induce a deficiency of not only PABA, but of folic acid as well. The symptoms: fatigue, irritability, depression, nervousness, headache, constipation, and other digestive disorders.

(Also see DISEASES, section headed "Infectious Diseases and Parasitic Infestations," Table D-13 Infectious and Parasitic Diseases Which May Be Transmitted By Contaminated Foods and Water—"Parastic Diseases"; and MALARIA.)

RECOMMENDED DAILY ALLOWANCE OF PABA. The need for PABA has not been established; hence, it follows that there is no recommended daily allowance. The ordinary dose of PABA is 2 to 6 g, but even larger doses have been administered, in a variety of disorders.

TOXICITY. It has generally been considered that PABA is essentially nontoxic in man. But continued high doses may be toxic, causing nausea and vomiting.

SOURCES OF PABA. Food composition tables do not list PABA, but the following foods are generally recognized as the richest sources: brewers' yeast, fish, soybeans, peanuts, beef liver, eggs, wheat germ, lecithin, and molasses.

(Also see FOLACIN; and VITAMIN[S], Table V-9.)

PARABENS

This is a general term referring to the methyl, ethyl, propyl or butyl esters (acid alcohol combination) of *p* hydroxybenzoic acid (parabens)—a group of antimicrobial agents used in foods, cosmetics, and drugs. Specifically, these compounds may be called methyl, ethyl, propyl, or butyl hydroxybenzoic acid, or methyl, ethyl, propyl, or butyl paraben.

(Also see ADDITIVES.)

PARAPLEGIA

Commonly found in spinal cord diseases, or accidents in which the spinal cord is severed in the lumbar region, it is the paralysis or weakness of both legs. Nutritionally, paraplegia is known to occur in humans who ingest Lathyrus seeds over a long period of time. Some dietary modification may be necessary due to reduced activity.

(Also see LATHYRISM; and MODIFIED DIETS.)

PARASITE INFECTIONS

People may harbor a wide variety of internal and external parasites (organisms that live in or on people). They include fungi, protozoa (unicellular animals), arthropods (insects, lice, ticks, and related forms), and helminths (worms). Some parasites require only one host—an animal or person serving as residence—while others need more in order to complete their life cycle.

While in residence, parasites usually seriously affect the host, but there are notable exceptions. Among the ways in which parasites may do harm are (1) absorbing food, (2) sucking blood or lymph, (3) feeding on the tissue of the host, (4) obstructing passages, (5) causing nodules or growths, (6) causing irritation, and (7) transmitting diseases. Two common infestations of man by parasites from undercooked meats are trichinosis and beef tapeworm.

(Also see DISEASES, section headed "Infectious Diseases and Parasitic Infestations," Table D-13 Infectious and Parasitic Diseases Which May Be Transmitted By Contaminated Foods and Water—"Parasitic Diseases"; and MALARIA.)

PARASITES

Broadly speaking, parasites are organisms living in, on, or at the expense of another living organism.

(Also see PARASITE INFECTIONS.)

PARATHYROID GLAND

As its name implies, the parathyroid is in the neck in close association with the thyroid gland. Both are endocrine glands. Normally, there are four very small (each weighs only 0.02 g) parathyroid glands lying behind the thyroid gland. They secrete the hormone parathormone, which controls blood calcium levels.

(Also see ENDOCRINE GLANDS; and PARATHYROID HORMONE.)

PARATHYROID HORMONE

The hormone of the parathyroid gland, which controls calcium and phosphorus metabolism by (1) stimulating the intestinal mucosa to increase calcium absorption, (2) mobilizing calcium rapidly from the bone, and (3) causing renal (kidney) excretion of phosphate.

(Also see CALCIUM, section headed "Absorption of Calcium"; and PARATHYROID GLAND.)

PARBOIL

Partial cooking which is sometimes done before finishing the cooking in the oven. Bagels are parboiled before baking in the oven. Some of the cereals that are partially cooked are parboiled.

PARENTERAL

Introduction of nutrients other than by mouth; it may be accomplished (1) subcutaneously (beneath the skin), (2) intramuscularly (into the muscle), or (3) intravenously (into the vein).

PARESTHESIA

A sensation of burning, numbness, pricking, or tingling, usually associated with an injury or irritation of a sensory nerve or nerve root.

PARIETAL CELLS

The cells of the gastric glands of the stomach which secrete hydrochloric acid (HCl).

PARKIN

This is a popular cake in Scotland. It is made with oatmeal, butter, molasses, baking powder, and spiced with ginger.

PARSLEY *Petroselinum crispum*

The leaves of this vegetable are much used as a garnish and a flavoring. The seeds were once used as a condiment, and an edible root which resembles a parsnip is produced by a European variety called Hamburg parsley (*P. crispum* var. *tuberosum*). Parsley is a member of the parsley family (*Umbelliferae*) of vegetables. Other well-known members of this family are caraway, carrots, celery, dill, fennel, and parsnips. The type of parsley that is most familiar to Americans and the British is the one with the small, curly leaves which is shown in Fig. P-11.

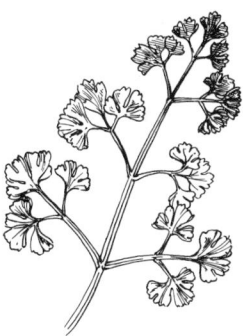

Fig. P-11. A sprig of parsley, a highly nutritious green vegetable that is used mainly as a garnish and a flavoring.

However, there is also a type of parsley that has larger, flat leaves. This type is now sold in the produce sections of many American supermarkets.

ORIGIN AND HISTORY. Parsley is native to the Mediterranean areas. It is believed to have been cultivated for more than 2,000 years, and to have been used medicinally before it was consumed as a food. Ancient Greek tradition associated this herb with death. Hence, it was used in funeral wreaths. Later, athletic contests were held to commemorate deceased heroes and garlands of parsley were awarded to the winning athletes. Around this time, the Greeks and Romans initiated the practice of using parsley as a garnish and a flavoring.

It is not certain when the use of parsley as a food spread throughout Europe. During the Middle Ages, there was a superstition that the plant was once owned by the devil and that anyone who uprooted it could expect the sudden death of a family member, whose soul would go to hell. It was permissible to pick leaves from the plant as long as the crown and roots were left undisturbed. English gardeners believed that the curly-leaved types might be produced by bruising the seed before planting, or by flattening the young plants under a heavy roller. An important reason for the preference for curly-leaved parsley was that the flat-type resembled the poisonous weed called fool's parsley (*Aethusa cynapium*). Parsley was also thought to prevent drunkenness if it was consumed before drinking wine. (Perhaps the latter belief stems from the observation that the eating of parsley helps reduce the odors of garlic and wine which are on the breath after eating and drinking.)

Hamburg (turnip-rooted) parsley appears to have been developed recently in Germany, although some botanists expect that it was used there on a small scale for 200 years or more. More recently, a hybrid of parsley and celery was developed which shows promise of providing one or more new types of vegetables.

PRODUCTION.   Although complete production data are not readily available, it appears that this crop accounts for only a very small part of U.S. vegetable production, since only 7.3 thousand metric tons of parsley were shipped within the country during 1990, compared to 4.8 million metric tons of all vegetables and melons.[6]

Parsley seed may be sown directly in the field in early spring, or it may be started during the winter in a greenhouse or in hotbeds because it germinates very slowly. A rich, moist soil is required. Hence, compost or manure may be added with or without an inorganic fertilizer that supplies nitrogen, phosphorus, and potassium.

Normally, two or more successive crops of parsley may be produced during the growing season which may extend from early spring to fall. However, the plant does not tolerate prolonged periods when the temperature exceeds 90°F (32°C). Hence, the crops are grown during the winter and spring in the southern United States. There is no need to replant parsley during the growing season if (1) the temperature remains favorable, and (2) care is taken to harvest the outer leaves without disturbing the crowns, which will then continue to produce new leaves. Growers in California harvest large fields mechanically by cutting the plants at about an inch above the ground in order to permit the continuous growth of the leaves.

PROCESSING.   Much of the U.S. parsley crop is either marketed fresh or dried for use as a condiment. However, small amounts are frozen.

SELECTION AND PREPARATION.   Parsley of best quality should be bright, fresh, green, and free from yellowed leaves or dirt. Wilting and yellowing denote age or damage. Slightly wilted parsley can be revived to freshness in cold water, but badly wilted leaves are unattractive and otherwise undesirable.

Fresh raw parsley, which is the most commonly-used form of this vegetable, may be used as a garnish or added to casseroles, butter and cheese spreads, Chinese stir-fried dishes, salads, soups, and stews. Sometimes, dried parsley is used in lieu of fresh parsley for these dishes, but the dried leaves are not as flavorful as the fresh leaves.

NUTRITIONAL VALUE.   The nutrient compositions of fresh and dried parsley are given in Food Composition Table F-36.

Some noteworthy observations regarding the nutrient composition of parsley follow:

1.   Fresh parsley has a lower water content (85%) and

---

[6]*Agricultural Statistics 1991*, USDA, pp. 167, 168, Tables 242, 243.

a higher calorie content (44 kcal per 100 g) than most other green leafy vegetables. It is exceptionally rich in protein, calcium, iron, potassium, vitamin A, and vitamin C. For example, 1 cup (*60 g*) of chopped parsley supplies almost as much protein as a cup of cooked cornmeal, but contains only one-fifth as many calories.

2.   Dried parsley has about 6 times the calorie and protein contents of fresh parsley and is correspondingly richer in other nutrients. Hence, small amounts of the dried leaves may make a significant nutrient contribution.

(Also see VEGETABLE[S], Table V-6 Vegetables of the World.)

PARSNIP *Pastinaca sativa*

Contents

This plant is grown for its edible, carrotlike taproot. Parsnips belong to the parsley family (*Umbelliferae*), which also includes carrots, celeriac, celery, caraway, dill, and fennel.

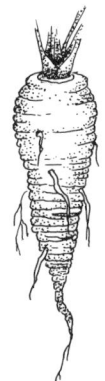

Fig. P-12.   The parsnip, a root vegetable that develops a sweeter flavor after exposure to a frost.

ORIGIN AND HISTORY.   The parsnip is believed to be native to the Mediterranean area. Wild plants were consumed by the ancient Greeks and Romans, but the varieties with fleshy roots were not developed until the Middle Ages, when the vegetable was much used by the English during Lent.

During the early part of the 16th century the colonists from England brought parsnips to Massachusetts and Virginia. Shortly thereafter, both white men and Indians grew this crop. However, the vegetable has not been very profitable for farmers in the United States because (1) it grows too slowly to make optimal use of the land that is required, and (2) few people enjoy the taste sufficiently to pay a price that would make the crop more profitable.

PRODUCTION. Few statistics are kept on the production of parsnips because this crop is not very important from a commercial standpoint.

Parsnips do not grow well in very hot weather. In the southern United States they are planted in the early fall for harvesting the following spring, but in the areas with frigid winters they are planted as soon as the ground can be worked in the spring.

A deeply-cultivated, fine soil that is rich in organic matter is required. Lime may be added to correct soil acidity. An excess of seed is planted because germination is slow and uncertain. Some growers cover the soil with sheets of plastic film to keep it moist and warm until the plants emerge. From 2 to 4 weeks are required for the germination of the seed. Periodic weeding is required until the plants are well established. The plants usually require thinning to make adequate space for the remaining plants. However, a moderate amount of crowding of the plants may be desirable in that it results in more slender and tender roots.

The roots are ready for harvesting within 3 to 4 months after planting. The roots become woody if they are allowed to grow too long. If harvest time is near to the onset of the first frost the roots may be left in the ground all winter since they are not likely to be damaged much by freezing. Low temperatures improve the flavor of parsnips by inducing the conversion of starch to sugar. It is noteworthy that a similar result may be obtained by storing the harvested roots for 2 or more weeks at 34°F (1°C).

PROCESSING. Parsnip roots are generally processed as a cooked food for man. However, they are also used for livestock feed and for making parsnip wine.

SELECTION AND PREPARATION. Smooth, firm, clean, well-shaped parsnips of small to medium size are generally of best quality. Soft, flabby, or shriveled roots are usually pithy or fibrous. Softness may also be an indication of decay, which usually appears as a gray mold or a soft rot. Misshapen roots are objectionable because of waste in preparation for use. Large, coarse parsnips are apt to have tough, woody cores that will have to be discarded.

The skin of young parsnips may be removed by scraping with a knife or scrubbing with a stiff vegetable brush. Older parsnips require about 10 minutes of boiling before the skin may be peeled off. The latter should also be cut lengthwise and the tough core removed.

Some of the most common ways of utilizing cooked parsnips are (1) pureed and whipped with milk, butter or margarine, and seasonings; (2) mashed, and shaped into cakes that are floured and fried; (3) sliced and french fried; (4) served cold with a seasoned dressing; (5) candied or glazed by simmering with butter or margarine, brown sugar or honey, and various spices; (6) roasted with meats; (7) added to casseroles, soups, and stews; and (8) sliced and served hot with butter or margarine, salt, and pepper.

NUTRITIONAL VALUE. The nutrient composition of raw and cooked parsnips are given in Food Composition Table F-36.

Parsnips are very similar to Irish potatoes in nutritional value. Both vegetables contain about 80% water, furnish 76 Calories (kcal) per 3½ oz (100 g) serving, are good sources of potassium, but only fair sources of vitamin C. However, parsnips contain only about 80% as much protein and vitamin C as potatoes.

(Also see VEGETABLE[S], Table V-6 Vegetables of the World.)

PARTS PER BILLION (PPB)

It is an expression of extremely minute quantities. One part per billion equals 0.0000001%, 0.907 mg/ton, 1 mcg/kg, and 1 mcg/liter.

PARTS PER MILLION (PPM)

It is an expression of minute quantities. One part per million is equivalent to the following: 0.454 mg/lb; 0.907 g/ton; 0.0001%; 0.013 oz/gal; 1 mg/liter; and 1 mg/kg.

PARTURITION

Giving birth.

PASTA

Pasta consists of pieces of dough that have been formed in various shapes, then dried.

(Also see MACARONI AND NOODLE PRODUCTS.)

PASTEURIZATION

This is a method of processing food by destroying the microorganisms that cause disease and spoilage. The process was developed by and named for Louis Pasteur, the French scientist who in the early 1860s demonstrated that wine and beer could be preserved by heating above 135°F (57.2°C). In the United States, milk, cheese, egg products, wine, beer, and fruit juice are pasteurized.

(Also see MILK AND MILK PRODUCTS, "Processing Milk"; PRESERVATION OF FOOD, Table P-25 Methods of Food Preservation; and ULTRAHIGH TEMPERATURE STERILIZATION.)

PÂTÉS

• The most common meaning for pâté is a meat or liver dish which has been finely minced and mixed with other ingredients to form a spread for crackers.

• A pastry filled with meat or fish.

PATH-, PATHO-, -PATHY

Each meaning disease; for example, pathological, apathy.

PATHOGENS

Those microorganisms responsible for producing disease. Many microorganisms are harmless.
(Also see DISEASES.)

PATHOLOGY

The science dealing with diseases; their essential nature, causes, and development, and the structural and functional changes produced by them.

PAVLOV POUCH

This is an experimental, surgical technique introduced by the famous Russian physiologist-psychologist, Ivan Petrovich Pavlov. A portion of the stomach is brought to the body wall and formed into a pouch from which samples may be taken. Secretions in the pouch are the same as those in the stomach.

PBI TEST

This test is a measure of thyroid activity by determining the amount of iodine that is bound to thyroxin and in transit in the plasma. The test is based upon the fact that the level of protein-bound iodine circulating in the blood is proportional to the degree of thyroid activity.

Since the hormone thyroxine constitutes the most important single factor influencing the rate of tissue oxidation, or basal metabolism, determination of the level of thyroid hormone in the bloodstream is used to detect the relative rate of basal metabolism. Good correlation with basal metabolism tests have been obtained by this method.

Thyroxine (tetraiodothyronine) is circulated in the blood in temporary union with blood proteins; hence, what the chemical test actually measures is the protein-bound iodine content of the blood, which, in turn, serves as an index of relative activity of the thyroid in releasing its hormone into the blood—hence, the approximate basal metabolic rate.

The PBI test has largely replaced the measurement of oxygen consumption by respiration apparatus (1) because it is much simpler for both patient and technician, and (2) because many doctors feel that it is better suited to clinical purposes. However, the basal metabolism test is still the method of choice for nutritional studies.

PCB

Abbreviation commonly used for polychlorinated biphenyls. They are chlorinated hydrocarbons which may cause cancer when taken into the food supply.
(Also see POISONS; and POLYCHLORINATED BIPHENYLS.)

PEACH AND NECTARINE *Prunus persica*

Contents

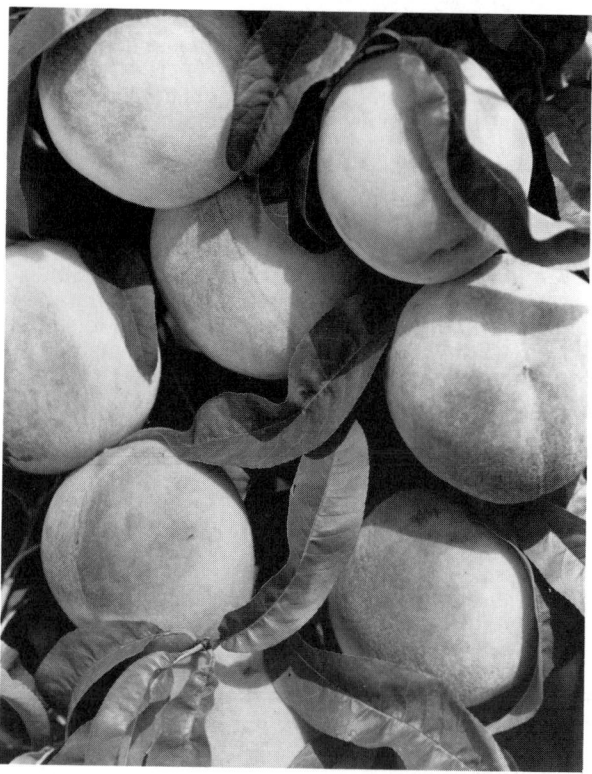

Fig. P-13. A cluster of peaches, the juicy, but fuzzy, fruit. The peach is second only to the apple in distribution around the world; hence, the peach can be called "queen of the fruits." (Photo by J. C. Allen & Son, West Lafayette, Ind.)

The peach is the fruit of a tree bearing the same name. Botanically, a peach is classified as a drupe—a fruit whose seed is contained in a hard pit or stone surrounded by soft, pulpy flesh with a thin skin. As the genus name, *Prunus*, suggests, peaches are close relatives of the apricot, almond, cherry, and plum.

Peaches are round with yellow skin and edible flesh, though the skin may have areas of red. The edible flesh is either soft or quite firm. Peaches are classified as freestone or clingstone, according to how difficult it is to remove the pit from the fruit. Probably the best known freestone variety is the Elberta. Other well-known freestones include J. H. Hale, Redhaven, Hiley, Halehaven, July Elberta, and Golden Jubilee. Some important clingstone varieties include Fortuna, Paloro, Johnson, Gaume, and Sims.

• **Nectarine**—The peach and the nectarine are essentially alike. Only the fuzz-free skin, the usually smaller size, greater aroma, and distinct flavor separate the two. Their trees exhibit similar appearance, growth responses, bearing habits, and other general characteristics. Moreover, some peaches occasionally mutate to a nectarine and some nectarines can mutate to peach. The scientific name for nectarine is *Prunus persica*—the same as the peach. Nectarines have been called smooth-skin peaches. Herein, comments made regarding peaches also apply to nectarines, unless stated otherwise.

ORIGIN AND HISTORY. Scientists believe that the peach is native to China, where it probably grew over 4,000 years ago according to references in Chinese writings. Next, the peach made its way to Persia (Iran) where it was known as the Persian apple. Gradually the peach spread over Europe. Then, as different groups came to America they brought the peach. The peach was grown in Mexico during the era of Cortes. Colonists planted peaches in Virginia sometime before 1629. The Indians helped spread the peach, and peaches soon grew wild over the southern part of the United States. These wild peaches are known as Spanish or Indian peaches. Today, peaches are grown in most states.

PRODUCTION. Worldwide, an average of 8.7 million metric tons of peaches and nectarines are produced each year. The United States and Italy are by far the leading producers. Other leading peach- and nectarine-producing countries are indicated by their yearly production in Fig. P-15.

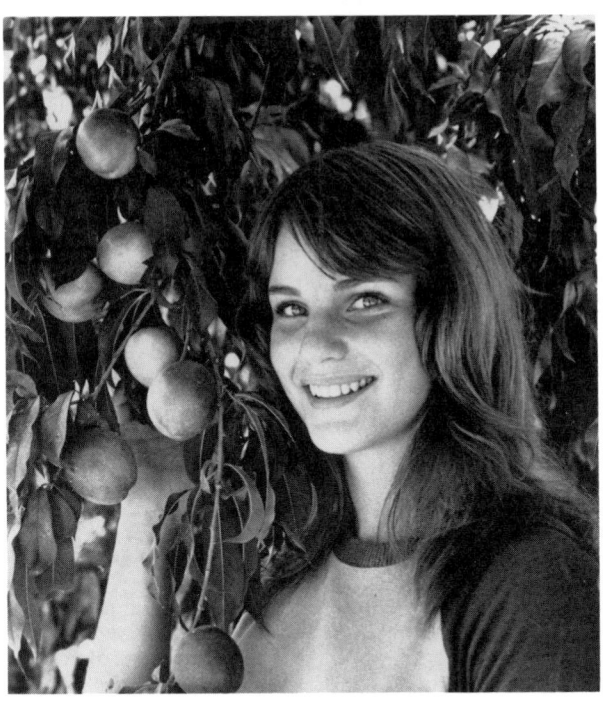

Fig. P-14. Nectarines. (Courtesy, California Tree Fruit Agreement, Sacramento, Calif.)

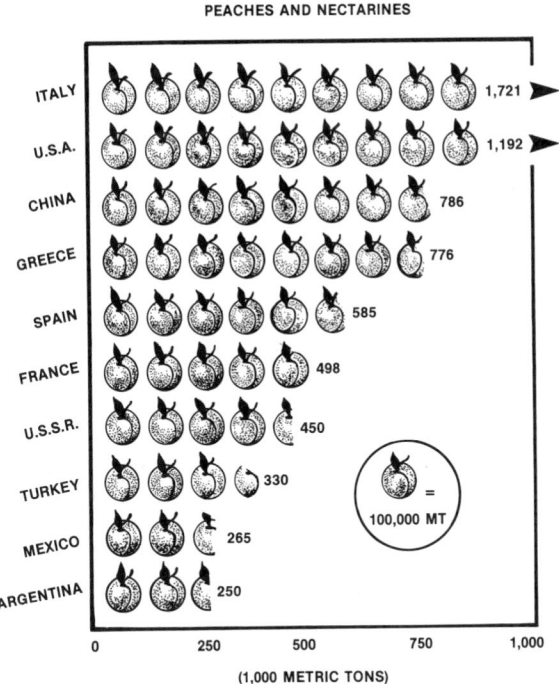

Fig. P-15. Leading peach- and nectarine-producing countries of the world. (Based on data from the *FAO Production Yearbook*, 1990, FAO/UN, Rome, Italy, Vol. 44, p. 162, Table 70)

Peach trees grow to heights of 15 to 25 ft (*4.6 to 7.6 m*). Their leaves are slender with toothed edges. Flowers appear in the spring before the leaves. Frosts can injure the delicate pink blossoms. If the temperature drops below 15°F (*-26°C*) peach trees are often killed. However, peach trees need a certain number of days of sustained temperatures below 50°F (*10°C*) in order to leaf and bloom in the spring. Cultivars (varieties) vary in their climatic requirements.

In North America, peaches are commercially produced in 32 states and Canada. The yearly peach crop in the United States averages 1.3 million tons (*1.2 million metric tons*) with a value of about $365 million. California is by far the leading peach-producing state. It produces 72% of all the peaches grown in the United States. Clingstone varieties comprise about two-thirds of California's crop. Other leading states are indicated by their yearly production in Fig. P-16.

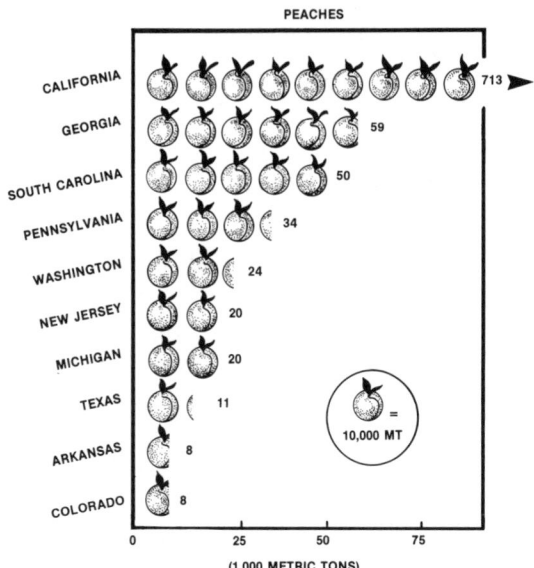

Fig. P-16.   Leading peach-producing states. (Based on data from *Agricultural Statistics 1991*, USDA, p. 201, Table 303)

California is the only state with a commercial crop of nectarines, producing an average of 211 thousand tons (*190 thousand metric tons*) each year. This California crop is valued at around $64 million.

Propagation and Growing.   Peach trees are propagated by budding desired varieties onto 1-year-old peach seedling rootstalks. Standard-sized trees are usually planted 18 to 25 ft (*5.5 to 7.6 m*) apart in the orchard, while dwarfed types are planted 12 to 15 ft (*3.7 to 4.6 m*) apart. Peaches grow best in sandy or sandy-loam soils with a clay subsoil where there is good drainage. Trees begin to bear a large crop 4 to 5 years after planting, and they may be profitable until they are 18 to 20 years old. Peak production is reached when the peach tree is 8 to 12 years old. A single tree produces from 192 to 485 lb (*87 to 220 kg*) of peaches.

Proper orchard management techniques are necessary to ensure a consistent, good crop. Correct fertilization, pruning, and fruit thinning are important. Peach trees must be watered regularly, and peach orchards are kept free of weeds. Diseases of peach trees—brown rot, peach leaf curl, and other fungi—are controlled by regular spraying. Several viral diseases of peaches require that the trees be uprooted and destroyed. Furthermore, several insects damage peach trees. Insects are controlled with sprays, often in combination with the sprays for the diseases.

Harvesting.   Peaches are harvested when they are ripe but firm. Since they mature unevenly, it may be necessary to make two or more pickings, depending upon the variety, crop, weather, and market. It is important that the fruit not be picked too soon. Quality increases only while the fruit is on the tree. Both fruit color and firmness are used as guides for picking ripe fruits. The degree of ripeness depends on the eventual market.

Peaches are picked by hand for sale as fresh fruit. With increased labor cost, mechanical shakers and catching frames have been used with success when fruit is destined for the cannery, or when fruit is picked as "hardripe" for shipment purposes.

Following harvesting many growers hydrocool their peaches to remove field heat. This rapidly cools the fruit to retard ripening, deterioration of quality and the growth of rot organisms. In hydrocooling, peaches are subjected to an ice water drench or spray which usually includes a germicidal agent. Also, many packinghouses defuzz peaches by a brushing machine and water spray.

Peaches may be stored for short periods of time at temperatures of 30° to 32°F (*-1 to 0°C*). Freestone peaches are not stored longer than 2 weeks.

PROCESSING.   Most of the U.S. peach crop is either marketed as fresh or canned produce. Sixty-seven percent is marketed as fresh fruit, while 28% is canned. The remaining 5% of the crop is distributed among the following processes: dried, 1%; frozen, 3%; and jams, preserves, brandy, and some other miscellaneous products, 1%. Nearly all nectarines are marketed as fresh fruit.

Fresh peaches can be found in markets from May through September, and nectarines are in markets from June through September.

Before freezing or canning, peaches are inspected, graded, pitted, and peeled. Automatic pitters can remove pits from either freestone or clingstone varieties. Peaches are canned in water pack, juice pack, or in syrup from light to extra heavy. Frozen peaches are generally frozen in a syrup with a small amount of ascorbic acid to prevent browning.

Dried peaches are halved, pitted, peeled, sulfured, and then dried in the sun or in dehydrators. It takes 6 to 7 lb (*2.7 to 3.2 kg*) of fresh peaches to make 1 lb (*0.45 kg*) of dried fruit.

SELECTION.   Fresh peaches should be fairly firm or becoming slightly soft. The skin color between the red areas should be red or at at least creamy. Reddish skin color alone is not a sign of ripeness, but a mark of certain varieties. At home, peaches should be kept at room temperature 3 or 4 days until fully ripe, then refrigerated.

Immature peaches are very firm or hard with a distinctly green ground color, and in all likelihood will not ripen properly. Very soft fruits are overripe. Bruised peaches will have large areas of discoloration in the flesh. Decay starts as a pale tan spot which expands in a circle and gradually turns darker in color.

PREPARATION.   Peaches and nectarines can be enjoyed when eaten fresh out of the hand or they can be cooked in a variety of baked goods. Sliced fresh or canned peaches can be eaten alone as a dessert dish or in combination with other fruits in salads, or in fruit plates. Also, peaches are a component fruit of canned fruit cocktail. Dried fruit can be eaten as a snack or cooked. Peach jam is a good bread spread.

NUTRITIONAL VALUE. Fresh peaches contain 89% water. Additionally, each 100 g (about 3½ oz or one medium-sized peach) contain 38 Calories (kcal) of energy, 202 mg potassium, 1,330 IU vitamin A, and only 1 mg of sodium. The calories in fresh peaches are derived primarily from the natural sugars (carbohydrate) which give them their sweet taste. Canned peaches are slightly higher in calories due to the addition of syrup, and their vitamin A content is lower. Dried peaches contain only 33% water; hence, most of the nutrients are more concentrated, including calories. Each 100 g of dried peaches contain 237 Calories (kcal) of energy, 983 mg potassium, 3.9 mg of iron and 2,142 IU of vitamin A. Fresh nectarines are 82% water, and they contain 64 Calories (kcal) of energy, 294 mg potassium, 1,650 IU vitamin A, and 13 mg vitamin C in each 100 g (about two medium-size nectarines). More complete information regarding the nutritional value of fresh, canned, dried, and frozen peaches and fresh nectarines is presented in Food Composition Table F-36.

(Also see FRUIT[S] Table F-47 Fruits of the World.)

PEACH PALM (PEJIBAYE) *Guilielma gasipaes*

The fruit of a palm tree (of the family *Palmae*) that is native to Central America and northern South America, but is presently underutilized, considering that its production might be as profitable as that of the cereal grains in the temperate climates.

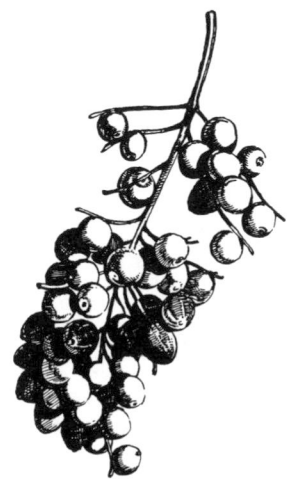

Fig. P-17.   Peach palm (pejibaye).

It is noteworthy that the egglike peach palm fruit develops a nutlike flavor when boiled in saltwater. The oily seeds of the fruit are also edible. They may also be made into flour or fermented into chicha (an alcoholic beverage made by allowing the previously chewed nuts to ferment).

The fruit is rich in calories (196 kcal per 100 g) and carbohydrates (42%). It also contains 2.6% protein (much more than most fruits), and is a good source of iron, vitamin A, and vitamin C.

PEACOCK (PEAFOWL)

This magnificent bird is prized for both its ornamental qualities and its gastronomical value.

In the Middle Ages, the peacock held sway at great state banquets. Its cooking called for all the skill of an experienced master-cook; and only the noblest at the feast had the right to carve it.

Peacocks are still regarded as a delicacy for special occasions. Culinary preparation is similar to pheasant.

PEA, FIELD *Pisum arvense*

Although the field pea (*Pisum arvense*) appears to be very closely related to the garden pea (*Pisum sativum*), it is almost always grown for its mature seeds, whereas the latter is often grown for its immature pods and seeds. Some plant scientists believe that the field pea is one of the ancestral species from which the garden peas was developed by cross breeding, since the former grows wild in the Georgian Republic of the U.S.S.R., whereas the latter is not found in the wild state. Other characteristics which distinguish the field pea from the garden pea are: (1) the flowers are usually purple in color, whereas the flowers of the garden pea are white; (2) the pods and seeds are smaller than those of the garden pea, and (3) the seeds have a greyish brown color, whereas the seeds of the garden pea are green. It is noteworthy that the production of the field pea for food has steadily declined, while the production of the garden pea has risen.

(Also see PEA, GARDEN.)

Fig. P-18 shows the flower, pods, and seeds of the field pea.

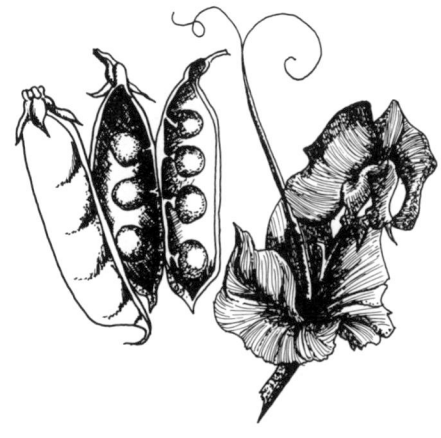

Fig. P-18.   The field pea.

ORIGIN AND HISTORY. It is believed that the field pea originated in Central Asia and Europe, with possibly secondary developments in the Near East and North Africa, as evidenced by 9,000-year-old buried pea seeds found at various archaeological sites in these areas. At that time, and for a long period thereafter, only dried pea seeds were used as food.

Sometime later, the pea was dispersed westward throughout Europe, southward into Africa, and eastward to India and China. One of the major reasons for the spread of this crop to such distant parts of the world might have been that dried pea seeds were nonperishable and served as excellent foods for travelers.

Immature (green) pea pods and seeds appear to have been used as food in China long before the practice was adopted in Europe. French royalty is credited with introducing the use of the green pea in the menus of Europe in the 16th century. Since then, people in the developed countries have increasingly utilized the more tender garden pea at the expense of the field pea. However, the latter is still an important food crop in Africa.

PRODUCTION. Much of the world crop of field peas for food is grown in the African countries of Rwanda and Uganda. Elsewhere, field peas are grown for green manure and/or fodder. Field peas, like garden peas, thrive where the temperature ranges between 50°F (10°C) and 86°F (30°C). Hence, they may be grown as a winter crop in the tropics or subtropics, and as a summer crop in cool temperate climates or at the cooler high elevations in the tropics and subtropics.

The Africans who grow this legume for food invest little in its care and cultivation. Fortunately, it survives the lack of attention because it is hardier than the garden pea in its resistance to drought and high temperatures. At harvest time, the plants are cut, dried, and threshed.

PROCESSING. Field peas are not processed on a commercial scale. However, they can be converted into a flour or a protein concentrate if there should be a future demand for such products.

SELECTION AND PREPARATION. There is little or no use of these legumes as food in the United States. The canned "field" peas sold in the southeastern part of the country are a variety of cowpea. Should one wish to prepare them for human consumption, they should be soaked and cooked like the major types of dried beans. For example, field peas may be soaked overnight, then boiled or baked until tender.

NUTRITIONAL VALUE. The nutrient content of field peas is given in Food Composition Table F-36.

The nutrient composition of dried mature field peas is similar to that of dried navy beans. It follows that the nutritional values of the two species of cooked legumes are similar. Based upon data from the navy bean, the important nutritional characteristics of the field pea are as follows:

1. A 3½ oz (100 g) serving (about ½ cup) of cooked field peas provides about 120 Calories (kcal) and 7 g of protein. This is about double the caloric value and approximately equal to the protein value of 1 oz (28 g) of cooked lean meat.

2. Field peas contain less than half as much calcium as phosphorus. Hence, other foods that contain proportionately more calcium and less phosphorus (dairy products and green leafy vegetables) should also be eaten.

Protein Quantity and Quality. Certain African tribes rely on field peas to supply much of their dietary protein. Therefore, certain aspects of the quantity and quality of pea protein are noteworthy:

1. The grams of protein per 100 Calories (kcal) provided by field peas compared to other selected foods follow:

Food	Grams of Protein per 100 Calories (kcal)
	(g)
Field peas	7.6
Cottage cheese	13.2
Lean meat	12.7
Eggs	8.6
Navy beans	6.6
Sweet corn	3.9
Brown rice	2.1

The above figures indicate that the use of field peas as a protein source in lieu of animal foods is likely to result in an increased consumption of calories unless other dietary items are curtailed. However, the replacement of cereal grains by field peas results in an increase in the amount of protein supplied per calorie.

2. The protein in field peas is moderately deficient in the amino acids methionine and cystine, which are supplied in more liberal amounts by the protein in cereal grains. However, the field pea protein supplies ample quantities of the amino acid lysine, which is deficient in the cereal protein. Therefore, the protein present in mixtures of field peas and grain products provides a more balanced pattern of amino acids than either food alone.

(Also see LEGUMES, Table L-2 Legumes of the World.)

PEA, GARDEN *Pisum sativum*

This legume is among the top ten vegetable crops of the world. It is closely related to the field pea (*Pisum arvense*); yet, it may be distinguished from it as follows: (1) the flowers are white, whereas the flowers of the field pea are purple; (2) the pods and seeds are larger than those of the field pea; and (3) the seeds have a green color, whereas the field pea has tan-colored or mottled seeds. The highly desirable features of the garden pea have resulted in a steady increase in its cultivation at the expense of the field pea.

(Also see PEA, FIELD.)

Fig. P-19 shows freshly harvested pods and seeds of the garden pea.

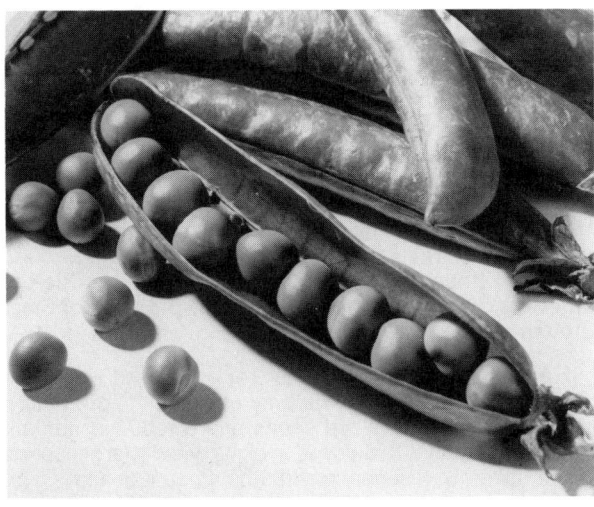

Fig. P-19. Close up of peas in a pod. (Photo by J. C. Allen & Son, Inc., West Lafayette, Ind.)

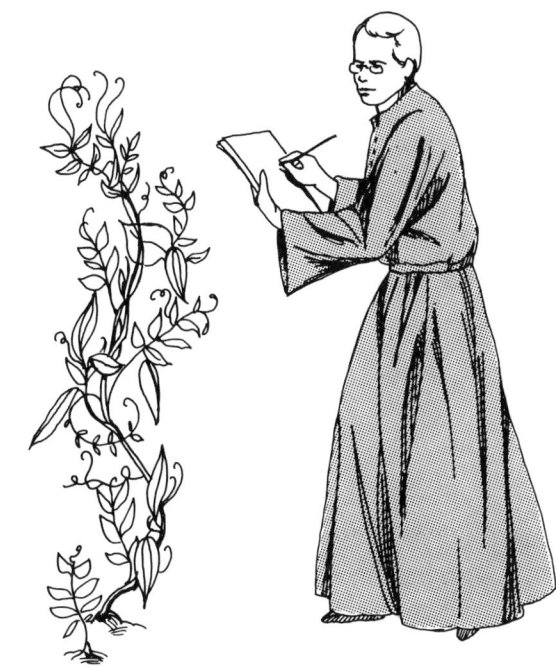

Fig. P-20. The Austrian monk Mendel (1822-1884) noting the characteristics of a pea plant during his research on the transmission of hereditary characteristics.

ORIGIN AND HISTORY.

The garden pea appears to have been derived from the field pea by centuries of cultivation and selection for certain desired characteristics. Credence to this theory is lent by the fact that the garden pea is not found in the wild state, whereas the field pea grows wild in the Georgian Republic of the U.S.S.R.

The garden pea, like the field pea, is thought to have originated in Central Asia and Europe, with possibly secondary developments in the Near East and North Africa. Through the centuries, it spread westward and northward throughout Europe, southward into Africa, and eastward to India and China.

Peas were known to and used by the Chinese in 2000 B.C.; and the Bible mentions peas. For many years, they were used only in the dry form. In England, during the late 1600s, green peas were not considered fit food. One writer of the time remarked, "It is a frightful thing to see persons so sensual as to purchase and eat green peas." Apparently, the Chinese were the first to use the green pods and seeds as food. (They also used other legumes similarly.) However, green peas did not appear on European menus until the 16th century, when they were popularized by French royalty. About this time, the agricultural writings began to distinguish between field peas and garden peas.

The Europeans found the garden pea to be much more appealing for use as a green vegetable than the field pea. Furthermore, peas appear to be the first crop that was scientifically bred to produce new varieties with more desirable characteristics. By the end of the 19th century, many cross breeding trials had been made, the most notable of which were those conducted by the Austrian monk Mendel. Fig. P-20 shows Mendel busy at his work.

The observations made by Mendel in his monastery garden at Brunn (now Brno, in Czechoslovakia) provided the foundation for the science of genetics. Unfortunately, the astute monk did not receive deserved credit during his lifetime, since his results were published in 1866, but were not recognized until 1900, 16 years after this death.

Peas were brought to America about 1800.

Today, some varieties of garden peas are best suited for marketing fresh or frozen, while other varieties are preferred for canning and soups.

PRODUCTION.

Almost 4/5 of the world's pea crop is utilized in the form of dry peas, and only about 1/5 as green pea. Fig. P-21 shows the leading dry pea producing countries, while Fig. P-22 shows those which supply most of the green peas.

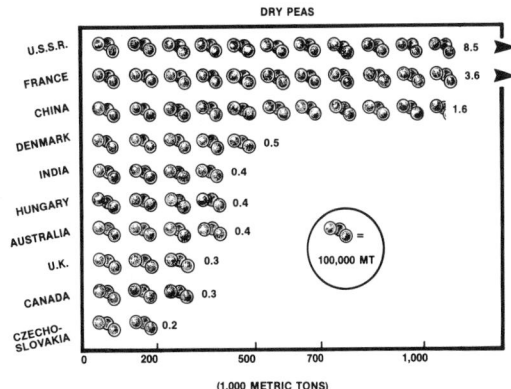

Fig. P-21. Dry pea production around the world. (*FAO Production Yearbook*, 1990, FAO/UN, Rome, Italy, Vol. 44, p. 103, Table 34)

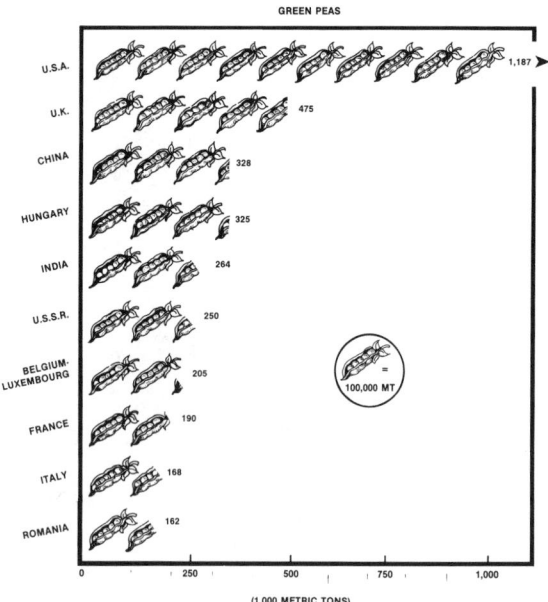

Fig. P-22. Green pea production around the world. (*FAO Production Yearbook*, 1990, FAO/UN, Rome, Italy, Vol. 44, p. 146, Table 61)

The U.S. utilization of dry and green peas differs from that of the world as a whole because dry peas are produced from less than 10% of the U.S. pea crop. Idaho and Washington produce virtually all of the dry peas, which amounts to about 100 thousand metric tons. It is noteworthy that the United States is the world's leading producer of green peas. Production data for green peas is illustrated in Fig. P-23.

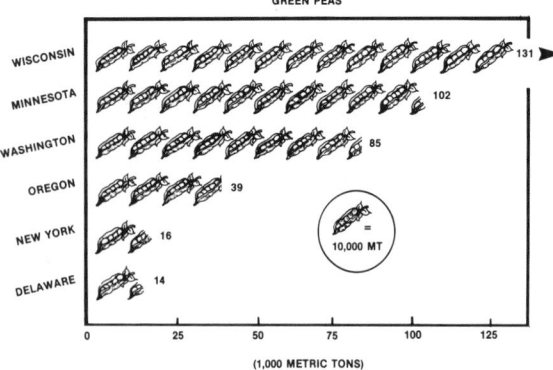

Fig. P-23. The leading states in U.S. green pea production. (*Agricultural Statistics 1991*, USDA, p. 158, Table 225)

Propagation and Growing.

Garden peas are not as hardy as field peas; they are more susceptible to high temperatures and drought. Therefore, they are usually planted as early in the growing season as the climate permits, in order that they will have sufficient time to mature before the warm weather arrives. The crop grows best when the temperature is between 50°F (*10°C*) and 86°F (*30°C*). When the seeds are first planted in areas where they have not been grown previously, they should be inoculated with the appropriate species of nitrogen-fixing bacteria since the soil may not contain sufficient amounts of these microorganisms to promote optimal growth.

Harvesting.

Green (immature) peas must be picked at just the right stage of maturity because (1) premature picking yields small sized seeds and a reduced amount of product, and (2) delayed picking yields large seeds which have a low sugar content (the amount of sugar converted to starch increases with maturity). When most of the crop has reached the desired degree of maturity the vines are cut and hauled to a vining station where a machine is used to separate the seeds from the pods. The average yield of shelled green peas in the developed countries is about 4,824 lb per acre (*5,416 kg/ha*), but higher yields have been obtained in the state of Washington.

Dry (mature) peas are usually left in the field until full maturity is reached, then they are cut, dried, threshed. Yields of dry peas run about 2,000 lb per acre (*2,240 kg/ha*).

In China and in certain other countries, the pods are picked at a very immature stage so that they may be used as a green vegetable.

PROCESSING.

Almost all of the U.S. crop of green peas is processed, since fresh peas spoil rapidly and there is little demand for them. Over half the crop is canned; most of the rest is frozen.

Dried peas may be utilized in the production of canned or dehydrated pea soups, or to a limited extent to make products such as those which follow:

• **Instant pea soup mixes**—These products are made by (1) cooking dried split peas with various other ingredients, (2) drying and flaking the cooked mixture, (3) mixing the flakes with flavorings and thickening agents, (4) steaming the flaked mixture to cause the ingredients to clump together, and (5) drying and grinding the clumped particles. Instant soup mixes are ready to eat within about a minute after mixing with boiling water.

• **Quick-cooking dried peas**—This convenience food is prepared by soaking the peas in an enzyme solution, followed by steam and drying. Normally, dried split peas require at least 25 minutes cooking time, but quick-cooking dried peas require only about half as much time.

• **Pea flour**—The idea of using a pea flour in baking is not new, since ground dried peas were often used to extend wheat and barley flours in Medieval Europe when bad weather reduced the yields of the grain crops. At the present time, the legume flour is utilized experimentally in the production of protein-fortified breads, cakes, noodles, and snacks. There is no esthetic problem in using green pea flour, because the color is bleached out during baking. Also, the tastes and textures of the products are acceptable.

Pea flour contains double the protein content of wheat flour. Hence, the replacement of 15% of the cereal flour with the legume flour results in a 15% increase in the protein content of the product. Furthermore, the amino acid patterns of the two types of flours complement each other so that the protein quality is also increased.

(Also see FLOURS, Table F-26 Special Flours.)

• **Pea protein concentrate**—This product, which contains from 55 to 60% protein, is made from pea flour by using streams of air to blow the lighter particles of starch away from the heavier protein-containing particles. The developers of the protein concentrate have suggested that it be used to increase the protein content of such items as biscuits, breads, cakes, cookies, imitation dairy beverages, macaroni and noodle products, muffins, pancakes, and similar items. It has also been used experimentally in the production of meat analogs similar to those made from soy protein.

SELECTION AND PREPARATION.

Fresh peas of the best quality are young tender, and sweet. The pods should be fresh, uniformly light-green in color, slightly velvety to the touch, and filled with well developed peas. Those containing excessively immature peas are usually flat, dark green in color, and may have a wilted appearance. Pods that are swollen, noticeably light in color, or flecked with grayish marks may be in an advanced stage of maturity and contain tough and poorly flavored peas.

Yellowing or whitish-green colored pods indicate age or damage and should be avoided. Water-soaked pods or those affected with mildew indicate poor quality peas, and the probability of excessive waste in preparation for use.

Most homemakers use canned and/or frozen green peas (the leading frozen vegetable in the United States) in preparing meals for their families, since (1) the cooking of dried peas (the most economical form of this vegetable) at home has declined steadily over the past 3 decades, and (2) fresh green peas are sold in pods and require shelling. Nevertheless, it might be rewarding to try each of the forms of this appetizing vegetable in a variety of dishes, since each one varies with respect to color, taste, texture, and succulence. For example, some people prefer canned peas to the fresh or frozen forms.

Some suggestions for preparing the different products follow:

1. Canned peas need no further cooking since they are already too tender. Therefore, they might be added to cold salads, or to piping hot dishes that are ready to be served.

2. Frozen peas are usually sufficiently tender after thawing to be used without cooking, but most people enjoy them more after a very brief cooking, followed by the addition of butter or margarine. Only the minimal amount of water to prevent burning or sticking to the pan should be used in cooking.

3. Fresh green peas should be cooked from 10 to 15 minutes after the water comes to a boil. (About 1 lb [*0.45 kg*] of peas in pods yields a cup [*240 ml*] of shelled peas.)

4. Dried peas may be cooked much more quickly than dried beans, so it is necessary to use care not to convert the peas to a mushy consistency by overcooking

them. For example, peas require only about 5 minutes of cooking in a pressure cooker (provided that the pressure is allowed to drop without opening the cooker after the cessation of heating), whereas most types of dried beans require at least 25 minutes of pressure cooking.

5. Each pound (about 2 cups, or *0.45 kg*) of dried peas yields about 3 lb (6 cups, or *1.4 kg*) of cooked peas. Usually, this form of peas is the most economical for use in preparing soups.

Peas go well with most other food items such as cereal products, cheeses and other dairy products, fish and seafood, meats, poultry, and vegetables. They may be used in casseroles, salads, soups, stews, and vegetable side dishes. The number and types of pea dishes need be limited only by the imagination of the cook and the ingredients on hand. A typical dish is shown in Fig. P-24.

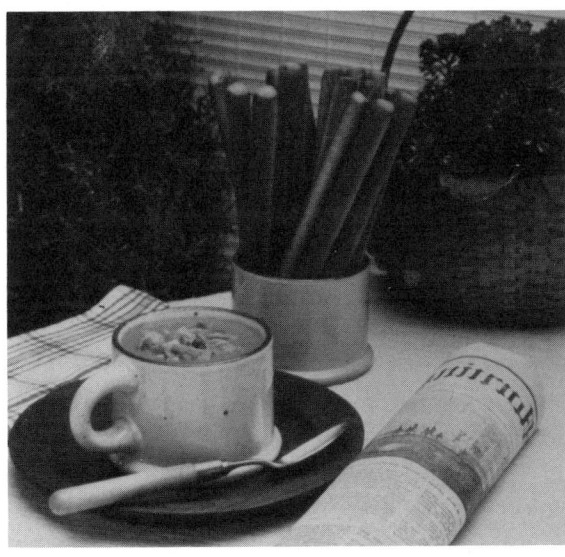

Fig. P-24. Split pea soup made from dried peas. (Courtesy, USDA)

NUTRITIONAL VALUE.

The nutrient composition of peas is given in Food Composition Table F-36.

Some noteworthy observations regarding the nutrient composition of garden peas follow:

1. Cooked dry (mature) peas provide about twice as much solids, calories, carbohydrates, and proteins as cooked green (immature) peas. However, the green peas are a good to excellent source of vitamin A, and a good source of vitamin C, whereas dried peas are a poor source of both vitamins.

2. A 3½ oz (*100 g*) portion (about ½ cup) of cooked dry peas or about 1 cup of cooked green peas provide an amount of protein (*8 g*) equivalent to 1 oz (*28 g*) of cooked lean meat. However, the peas provide about twice as many calories per gram of protein.

3. Peas are much lower in calcium and phosphorus

than beans. Additional calcium may be obtained from dairy products and a wide variety of green leafy vegetables. The items richest in phosphorus are animal protein foods, legumes, and nuts. People whose diets contain ample amounts of these foods should be certain to obtain sufficient calcium, because a high intake of phosphorus may limit the utilization of calcium, which is likely to be furnished in limited amounts.

4. Both dry and green peas are good sources of iron and potassium.

Protein Quantity and Quality. Many people may not realize that peas are a good vegetable source of protein. Therefore, certain facts regarding the quantity and quality of pea protein are noteworthy:

1. The grams of protein per 100 Calories (kcal) provided by green and dry peas compared to other selected foods follows:

Food	Grams of Protein per 100 Calories (kcal)
	(g)
Green peas	7.5
Dry peas	7.0
Cottage cheese	13.2
Lean meat	12.7
Eggs	8.6
Navy beans	6.6
Sweet corn	3.9
Brown rice	2.1

As noted, peas have almost as much protein as eggs. The above figures also show that the amount of protein per calorie in pea dishes may be increased by the addition of a high protein animal food. Similarly, peas may be used to raise the protein content of cereal dishes.

2. Pea protein is moderately deficient in the amino acids methionine and cystine, which are supplied in ample amounts by cereal proteins. However, the legume protein contains sufficient lysine to cover the deficiency of this amino acid in grain proteins. Hence, combinations of peas and cereal products supply higher quality protein than either food alone.

(Also see LEGUMES, Table L-2 Legumes of the World; and VEGETABLE[S], Table V-6 Vegetables of the World.)

PEANUTS (GROUNDNUTS; EARTH NUTS; GOOBERS; GOOBER PEAS; GROUNDPEAS; PINDAS; MONKEY NUTS; CHINESE NUTS)
Arachis hypogaea

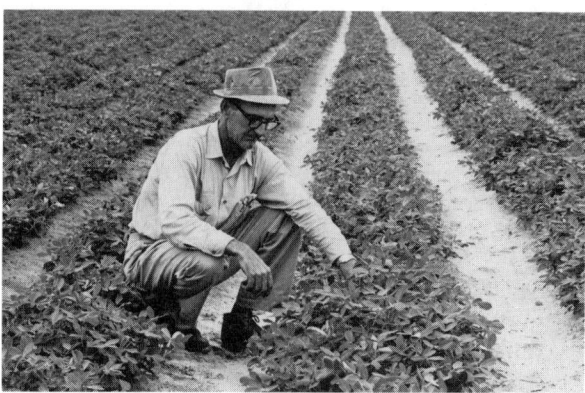

Fig. P-25. Peanut crop being inspected by Georgia farmer, K. C. Wilkinson. (Courtesy, USDA)

The peanut is the strange fruit of the peanut plant. It begins as a fertilized flower aboveground, but the pod and the seed mature in the ground; it's the plant with an aerial flower and subterranean fruit.

Unlike the soybean, peanuts are highly esteemed for human food in the United States; and they are standard fare at American sporting events, circuses, and cocktail parties; and, in the form of peanut butter, they have nourished millions of American youths.

ORIGIN AND HISTORY. Peanuts evolved thousands of years ago in South America. They are known to have existed as early as 950 B.C. But the exact area of origin is unknown. Some scientists claim that the plant originated in Brazil; others say that it is native to Bolivia. Despite obscure and mystery-shrouded beginnings, peanuts had already become an important food item from Mexico through South America when the Spanish and Portuguese explorers set sail for South America in search of gold in the 16th century. These Mediterranean adventurers sampled and savored peanuts growing in Peru as early as 1550.

From South America, Spanish and Portuguese traders took peanuts to Africa, where they exchanged them for spices and elephant tusks. In Africa, peanuts thrived and became a favorite food. The natives even worshiped them along with certain other species of plant life which they believed had souls. Peanuts became so well identified with Africa that, until quite recently, many believed, that they were native to the continent.

When peanuts were first introduced and grown in the United States has not been fully documented. It is known that when black men were transported from Africa to America to be sold as slaves, precious peanuts were put on board to provide food, and possibly assurance, for the long voyage. But there is reason to believe that the Indians were growing peanuts at the time the colonists arrived early in the 17th century. Nevertheless, Americans did not take to peanuts for a number of years; they considered them to be food for the slaves and the poor. It took the Civil War, the circus, and baseball to spark the national appetite for peanuts. The cotton boll weevil, Dr. George Washington Carver, and a St. Louis physician were also instrumental in the expansion of peanuts. When the boll weevil wiped out the cotton crop following the Civil War, Dr. Carver (1864 to 1943), Director of the Department of Agriculture at Tuskegee Institute, a noted black scientist, urged that farmers plant peanuts. Not only that, he led the way by finding over 300 uses for peanuts. Then, in 1890, a St. Louis physician gave peanuts another big boost; he ground the nuts and produced a product called "peanut butter," which he prescribed for his patients as a nutritious, easily-digested food, high in protein and low in carbohydrates.

WORLD AND U.S. PRODUCTION. Peanuts are an important crop, especially in the warm regions of the world. World production in the shell averages 23.1 million metric tons each year. More than 89% of the global production is in Asia and Africa. Ten leading peanut-producing countries of the world, by rank, are: India, China, United States, Nigeria, Indonesia, Senegal, Myanmar, Zaire, Argentina, and Vietnam (see Fig. P-26).

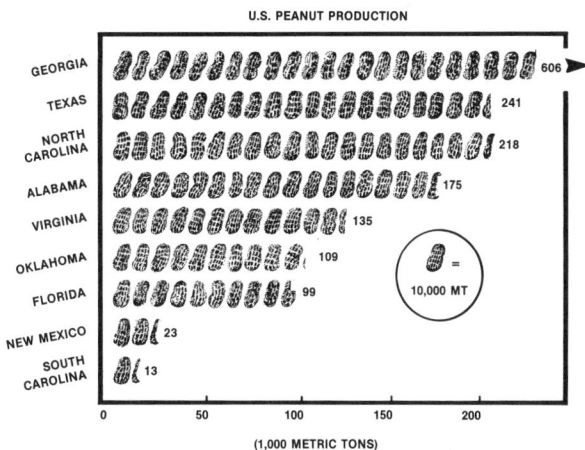

Fig. P-27. Leading peanut-producing states of the United States, in pounds. (Source: *Agricultural Statistics 1991*, USDA, p. 118, Table 160)

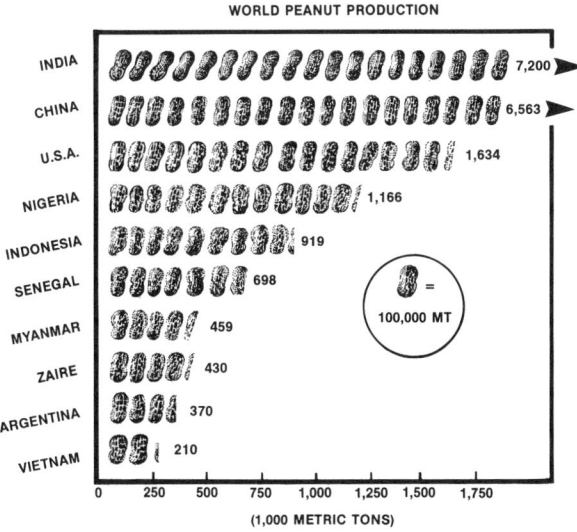

Fig. P-26. Leading peanut-producing countries of the world, in metric tons in the shell. (Source: *FAO Production Yearbook*, 1990, FAO/UN, Rome, Italy, Vol. 44, p. 109, Table 38)

THE PEANUT PLANT. Cultivated peanuts are genus *Arachis,* species *A. hypogaea.* The peanut plant is an annual legume, adapted to warm climates. It may grow to a height of 2½ ft (*76 cm*) and a width of 3 to 4 ft (*91 to 122 cm*). It bears small, yellow, pealike flowers where the leaves are attached to the stems. The plants blossom continuously for 2 or 3 months. Flower buds open at sunrise; fertilization takes place during the morning and the flowers usually wither and die by noon; within a few days, the flower pegs (the stalklike stems) elongate, bend down, and push into the soil to a depth of 1 to 3 in. (*3 to 8 cm*) then the tips of the pegs, which contain the developing seeds, swell and mature into peanut pods (see Fig. P-28).

Although United States peanuts represent only 3.7% of the world's peanut acreage, the United States produces about 7% of the world's supply due to its high yield per acre. The leading peanut-growing states of the United States, by rank, are: Georgia, Texas, North Carolina, Alabama, Virginia, Oklahoma, Florida, New Mexico, and South Carolina.

Globally, the average yield per acre is 1,030 lb (*1,157 kg/ha*). The U.S. average yield per acre is 1,997 lb (*2,242 kg/ha*).

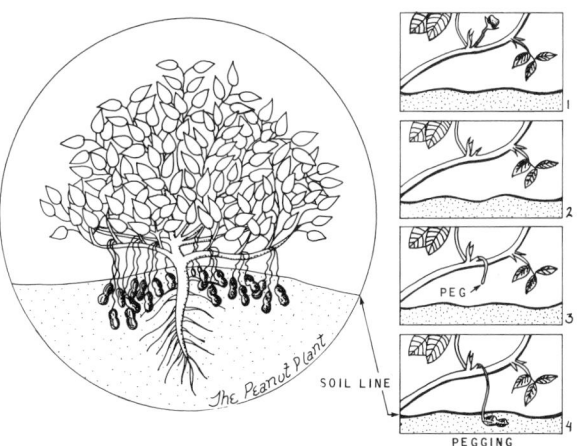

Fig. P-28. How a peanut grows: (1) The flower bud opens at sunrise; (2) fertilization takes place during the morning, and the flower withers and dies by noon; (3) the base of the fertilized flower begins to grow, forming a peg (a stalklike stem) and bending down; and (4) the peg pushes into the ground, then its tip swells and grows into a peanut pod.

The fruit is a pod, which commonly bears 2 to 3 kernels. Each kernel is made up of two large seed-leaves (cotyledons), and between them lies the germ; and the whole is covered by a thin coat (skin). The empty pod is called the shell.

PEANUT CULTURE. Peanuts are grown in tropical and subtropical climates. They need much sunshine, warm temperature, moderate rainfall, and a frost-free growing period of 4 to 5 months. They thrive best in light, well-drained, sandy soil.

The seedbed should be prepared by plowing deeply. Loose soil is important so that the pegs can penetrate the ground easily. The seeds are generally planted about 2 to 3 in. (5 to 8 cm) deep, at intervals of 4 to 6 in. (10 to 15 cm), and in rows 24 to 36 in. (61 to 91 cm) apart.

Peanuts are subject to a number of diseases, which are controlled by fungicides or by selecting resistant varieties.

When the seeds are mature, the inner lining of the pod changes from white to brownish. At harvest, peanuts are generally dug with a combination two-row digger-shaker-windrower; an operation which (1) loosens the plants and cuts the taproots, (2) lifts the plants from the soil and gently shakes them, and (3) puts the plants in fluffy windrows for drying. When dry, the pods are removed from the plants (by combine machines in the United States) and stored. Sometimes the pods are picked when they are half dry, then dried artificially. The pods are cleaned and graded before they are shelled.

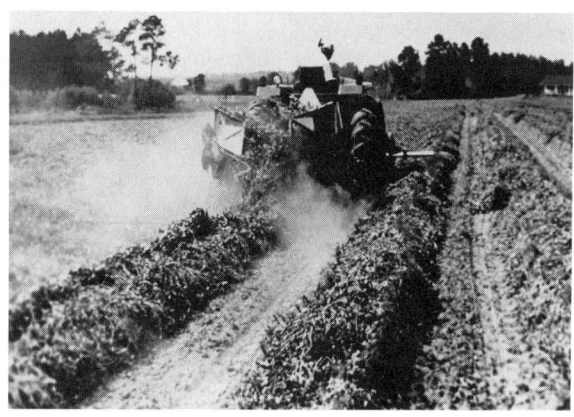

Fig. P-29. Digging peanuts with a combination digger-shaker-windrower. (Courtesy, National Peanut Council, Washington, D.C.)

In most of the Old World, planting, cultivation, and harvesting are still done by hand.

• **Aflatoxin**—Moldy peanuts may contain aflatoxin, a poison, produced by the fungus *Aspergillus flavus*. Because aflatoxin has been shown to be a carcinogen, the Food and Drug Administration enforces an administrative guideline of 20 parts per billion as the maximum of aflatoxin permitted in all foods and feeds, including peanuts and peanut products.

The fungus grows when the temperature is between 86° and 95°F (30° and 35°C) and when the moisture content in the peanut kernel is above 9%. *Aspergillus flavus* in peanuts can be prevented by careful harvesting and by quick drying and storage.

(Also see POISONS, Table P-11 Some Potentially Poisonous [Toxic] Substances—Mycotoxins.)

KINDS OF PEANUTS. There are two main types of peanuts based on characteristics of plant growth—*bunch* and *runner*. The bunch type grows upright, whereas the runner type spreads out on or near the ground. Most modern varieties in the United States are intermediate between these two extremes.

Growers group peanut plants into four market types: (1) large-seeded Virginias; (2) small-seeded Virginias (called *Runners*); (3) Spanish; and (4) Valencia. Both the large-seeded and the small-seeded Virginias include bunch and runner plants. Spanish and Valencia types are bunch. Practically all peanuts retailed in the shell are Virginias; Runners lead in peanut butter; and Spanish peanuts predominate in candy.

The large kernel peanuts come chiefly from the Virginia-Carolina area; the Spanish nuts come from the deep South; and Valencias are grown in limited quantities in the Southwest.

PROCESSING PEANUTS. Following picking, peanuts are delivered to warehouses, where they remain until processed. Processing varies somewhat according to market use, with the following operations involved:

• **Cleaning**—The cleaning operation consists of removing sticks, stems, small rocks, and faulty nuts by a series of screens and blowers.

• **Storing**—Cleaned peanuts are either (1) stored unshelled in silos or warehouses for subsequent shelling and delivery to users; or (2) shelled, then stored in refrigerated warehouses at 32° to 36°F (0° to 2°C) and 65% relative humidity, so as to protect against insects and rancidity.

• **In the shell**—Large, unshelled peanuts may be cleaned, polished, whitened, then marketed in the shell.

Some peanuts are salted and roasted in the shell. This involves soaking in salt water under pressure, then drying and roasting.

• **Shelling**—This consists of breaking the shells by passing the nuts between a series of rollers. Then, the shells (along with small, immature pegs) are separated by screens and blowers; and the discolored kernels are removed by hand and by electric eye. Although varying according to variety, shelling reduces the weight of peanuts by 30 to 60%, the space occupied by 60 to 70%, and the shelf life by 60 to 75%.

• **Blanching**—This consists of removing the skins or seed coats, (and usually the hearts) prior to use in peanut butter, bakery products, confections, and salted nuts.

Blanching may be done with heat or with water:

1. Blanching with heat consists of embrittling the skins by exposure to 259 to 293°F (126 to 145°C) heat for

5 to 20 minutes, followed by rubbing the kernels between soft surfaces and removing the skins by blowers and the hearts by screens.

2. Blanching with water is accomplished in different ways. The newest and most rapid method consists of wetting the nuts with 140°F (60°C) water and removing the skins by rapidly revolving spindles. The kernels are dried to 7% moisture prior to storage or conversion into peanut products.

• **Dry roasting**—Peanuts for use in peanut butter, confections, or bakery products are dry-roasted to develop desirable color, texture, or flavor. Dry roasting is accomplished by heating unblanched peanuts to 399°F (204°C) for 20 to 30 minutes, followed by cooling and blanching.

• **Oil roasting**—Peanuts for salting are first roasted in coconut oil or partly hydrogenated vegetable oil at 300°F (148.9°C) for 15 to 18 minutes.

• **Salting**—Either blanched or unblanched peanuts are roasted in oil and salted. Finely ground salt and an oil-base binder are mixed with freshly cooked nuts, which are then placed in flexible bags and canned under vacuum.

• **Extraction of oil**—The oil from peanuts is extracted by one of three methods:

1. **Hydraulic extraction.** The peanuts are broken between rollers; the shells are removed by blowers; and the meats are crushed and heated under 25-lb steam pressure for 10 minutes, stabilized at 7% moisture, and pressed at 280°F (137.8°C). Hydraulic pressing results in (a) a yield of oil of 41 to 47%, and (b) a press cake containing 42 to 45% protein, 7 to 8% oil, and 5 to 6% moisture.

2. **Expeller extraction.** Hydraulic presses for oil extraction predominated until about 1945; since then, the use of expellers has increased. Expeller extracting consists of (a) tempering (heating); and (b) feeding the peanuts into the expeller apparatus, in which pressure is created and the oil is extracted. Generally, expeller-extracted peanut meal contains 4 to 5% oil.

3. **Solvent extraction.** Solvent extraction results in (a) a yield of oil of 48 to 50%, and (b) a meal containing 50 to 52% protein, 1 to 2% oil, and 1 to 2% moisture.

One hundred pounds of peanuts in the shell will yield about 32 lb of crude oil, 45 lb of meal, and 25 lb of hulls.

NUTRITIONAL VALUE OF PEANUTS. The nutritive value of the different forms of peanuts and peanut products is given in Food Composition Table F-36.

Peanuts are a healthful food. The energy value in 1 lb (0.45 kg) of peanuts (containing about 2,558 Calories (kcal) is about equal to any of the following: 14 oz (397 g) of cooked round steak, 15 oz (425 g) of natural Cheddar cheese, 3 qt (2.8 liter) of milk, or eight eggs.

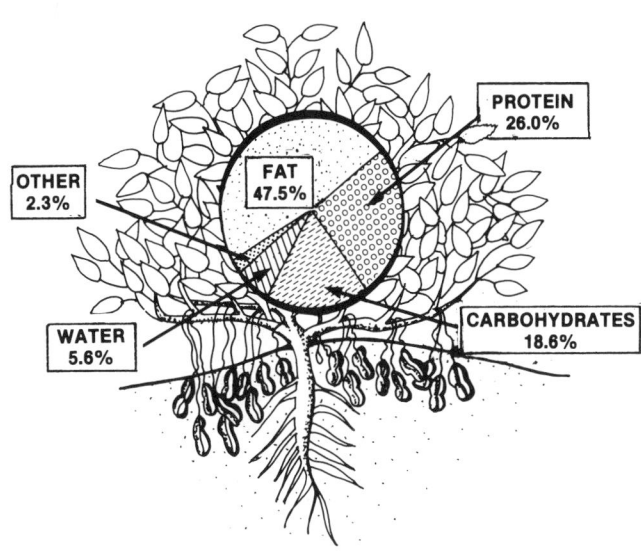

Fig. P-30. Food value of the peanut—the nut with skin.

Peanuts are also a good source of protein, containing about 26% and a fair balance of essential amino acids. They make a good complementary protein. Table P-3 presents the essential amino acid profile of peanuts in comparison to cow's milk—a high-quality protein.

TABLE P-3
PROFILE OF ESSENTIAL AMINO ACIDS IN PEANUTS COMPARED TO MILK—A HIGH-QUALITY PROTEIN

Amino Acid	Peanuts[1]	Cow's Milk[2]
	(mg/g protein)	
Histidine	27	27
Isoleucine	48	47
Leucine	70	95
Lysine	41	78
Methionine and cystine	27	33
Phenylalanine and tyrosine	99	102
Threonine	31	44
Tryptophan	13	14
Valine	58	64

[1]Values from Table P-37, Proteins and Amino Acids in Selected Foods.
[2]Recommended Dietary Allowances, 10th ed., 1989, NRC-National Academy of Sciences, p. 67, Table 6–5.

Raw or processed peanuts are excellent sources of riboflavin and niacin, and peanut skins are high in the B vitamins.

PEANUT PRODUCTS AND USES. Peanuts have much to contribute to the world's food supply, whether the need be for calories, fats, proteins, or certain vitamins.

In the United States, peanuts are almost entirely a human food and not an oilseed crop as such, since so small a proportion of the crop is processed for oil and protein concentrate. The per capita consumption of peanuts and peanut products in the United States in 1976 totaled 8.4 lb (*3.8 kg*), with a breakdown as follows: peanut butter, 3.8 lb (*1.7 kg*); salted peanuts, 1.6 lb (*0.7 kg*); peanut candy, 1.5 lb (*0.7 kg*); roasted in the shell, 0.8 lb (*0.4 kg*); peanut butter sandwiches, 0.1 lb (*45 g*); and all other uses, 0.6 lb (*272 g*).

In the rest of the world, peanuts are primarily processed for their separate constituents—oil and protein. Fortunately, some of the highest peanut-producing countries are in greatest need of their food value. The biggest problem in these countries is to protect the peanuts from molds, rodents, insects, and rancidity. In such countries where there coexists protein deficiency and availability of peanuts, there is much interest in incorporating peanut protein concentrate in the diet of children (see Table P-4, section on "Fortified Foods, Based on Peanut Products, For Developing Countries"). The main deterrent to this program to date has been the cost of peanut protein.

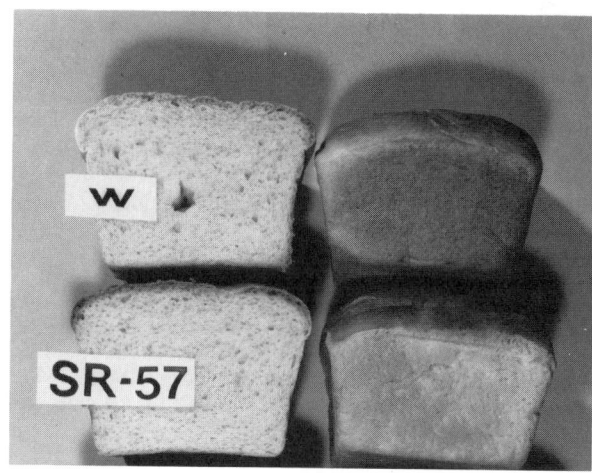

Fig. P-32.   Breads. W = bread made from wheat flour. SR-57 = bread made from wheat flour fortified with white-skinned peanut protein. (Courtesy, USDA)

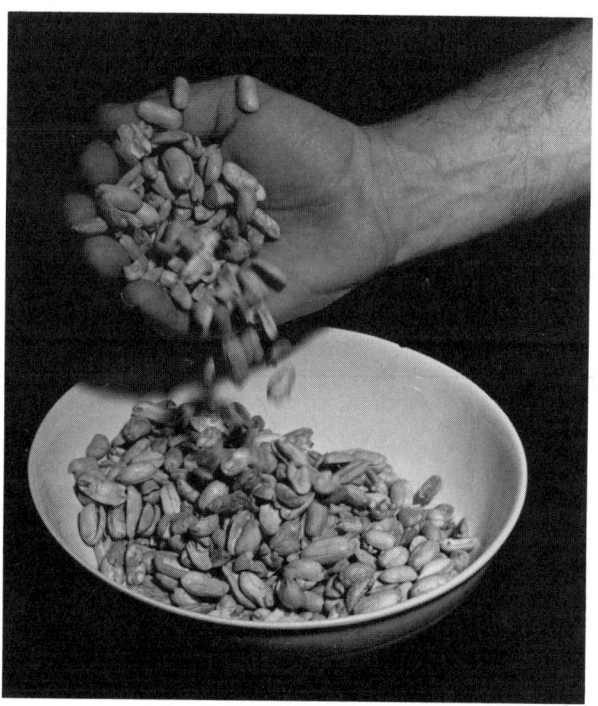

Fig. P-31.   Pressed and reconstituted defatted peanuts. (Courtesy, USDA)

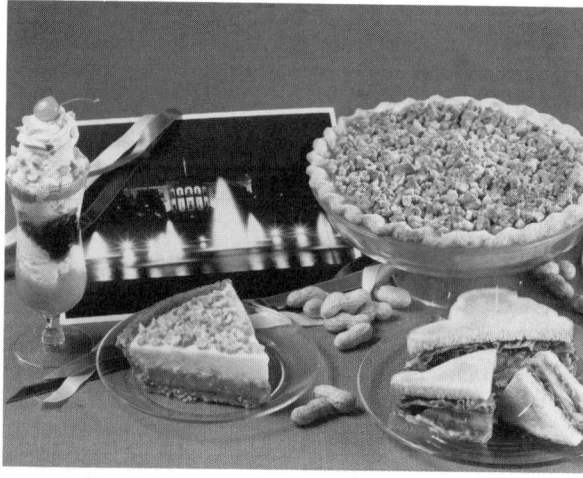

Fig. P-33.   Here are three examples of peanut foods: (1) Presidential Peanut Pie; (2) peanut butter, lettuce, and tomato sandwich; and (3) peanut butter parfait. (Courtesy, National Peanut Council, Washington, D.C.)

Table P-4 presents in summary form the story of peanut products and uses. In addition to the products listed therein, the following human food products are among those that have not yet reached wide distribution: peanut protein, peanut milk, peanut cheese, boiled fresh peanuts, canned boiled peanuts—shelled and unshelled, frozen boiled peanuts, peanut bread, peanut cereals, and numerous products that may be developed from these.

(Also see FLOURS, Table F-26 Special Flours; LEGUMES, Table L-2 Legumes of the World; NUTS, Table N-8 Nuts of the World; and OILS, VEGETABLE, Table O-6.)

TABLE P-4
PEANUT PRODUCTS AND USES

Product	Description	Uses	Comments
HUMAN FOODS			
Whole, roasted-in-shell peanuts	Peanuts roasted inside the shells.	Snacks	About ¼ of the peanuts marketed in the U.S. are in the form of roasted peanuts, primarily following shelling.
Defatted peanuts	This process removes 60 to 80% of the oil and ¾ of the calories, leaving intact a high protein peanut with a flavor that is generally acceptable. Defatted peanuts are prepared as follows: shelled peanuts are reduced to a specific moisture content, then placed in a hydraulic press where most of the oil and calories are removed. Although the kernels are distorted due to the hydraulic pressure, they return to their original shape and size when soaked in water. Salt, sugar, spices and other flavors may be added during the reconstruction period. These low calorie nuts are then dried.	Defatted peanuts are consumed raw, roasted, or used in candy and confectionery products.	
Flour mix (In Congo)	A mixture of fish flour, millet, and peanut flour (50% protein). Made into biscuits.	For children ages 2 to 6 years.	These biscuits, which have a good nutritive value and can be recommended for the prevention of malnutrition, are readily accepted by children.
Flour mix (In India)	A mixture of either (1) 25% roasted Bengal gram, 74% peanut flour (low fat), and 1% (alfalfa) lucerne powder; or (2) 25% roasted Bengal gram, 49% peanut flour, 25% low-fat sesame, and 1% alfalfa (lucerne) powder.	These mixtures are eaten with bread and jaggery (an unrefined brown sugar made especially from palm sap).	These vegetable protein diets are nearly as effective in controlling clinical manifestations of malnutrition as diets based on skim milk, but they are somewhat inferior to milk in restoring the level of blood protein (albumen) to normal.
Flour mix (In Senegal)	A mixture of 60% millet, 30% peanut flour, and 10% fish flour. Baked products.	Food for infants.	This is a satisfactory food for infants.
Fresh peanuts	Fresh peanuts, not dried or roasted.	As a vegetable.	In tropical countries, peanuts are usually consumed in this form.
Granulated (chopped), artifically flavored peanuts	These are granulated, artificially flavored peanuts that have the identical flavor and taste of other nuts, especially black walnuts, almonds, and pecans.	Widely used for ice cream toppings, pies, cakes, and other confectionery products.	These artifically flavored nuts are now commercially available in many food stores.

(Continued)

TABLE P-4 *(Continued)*

Product	Description	Uses	Comments
HUMAN FOODS *(Continued)*			
High protein food (In India)	A mixture of equal parts of peanut protein isolate and skim milk powder.	A high protein food suitable for treatment of protein malnutrition.	
Peanut butter	A cohesive, finely ground product prepared from dry roasted, clean, sound, mature peanuts from which the seed coats and "hearts" are removed, and to which salt, hydrogenated fat, sugars (optional), antioxidants, and flavors have been added. About 90% of the peanut butter is stabilized with hydrogenated oil and antioxidants; 10% is unstabilized (and more flavorsome). Peanut butter contains about 50 to 52% fat, 28 to 29% protein, 2 to 5% carbohydrate, and 1 to 2% moisture.	Sandwiches, salads, desserts, ice cream, custards, confections, and in many baked goods.	Peanut butter, consisting of shelled, ground, and parched peanuts, was first prepared as a kitchen product about 1890, as food for infants and invalids. Today, about half the peanuts consumed in the U.S. are made into peanut butter. By federal regulation, 90% of peanut butter must be peanuts in order to be labeled peanut butter. One pound (*0.45 kg*) of peanut butter has as much total food energy as any of the following: 1⅜ lb (*0.6 kg*) cheese, 2¼ lb (*1 kg*) of steak, 4 qt (*3.8 liter*) of milk, or 32 eggs. Peanut butter is an excellent source of protein (7.8 g per ounce), contains no cholesterol and the fat (14.4 g per ounce) is mostly unsaturated. An ounce of peanut butter contains 6.4 g of carbohydrate, making it acceptable for most diabetic diets. In a diabetic diet, 2 Tbsp (*30 ml*) of peanut butter will be equivalent to one meat exchange, two fat exchanges, or one B vegetable exchange. However, as with any food, it should not be used indiscriminately.
Peanut flakes	After peanuts are blanched (skin removed) and cooked, they are ground to a slurry, then dehydrated. In the process of dehydration, most peanut flavor constituents volatize, leaving a "tasteless–faceless" peanut product.	Peanut flakes, which contain essentially the same nutritive value (protein and calories) as the peanut, offer virtually unlimited potential as a bland high protein extender for meat and bakery products without adversely affecting the flavor of the finished product.	The processing equipment for making peanut flakes is quite expensive. The worldwide demand for this new product is expected to increase substantially.
Peanut flour	In processing peanut flour, a high proportion of the oil is removed, leaving a product that contains about 60% protein, 22% carbohydrates, 5% minerals, and less than 1% fat.	When commercially available, it is expected that peanut flour will be widely used as a highly digestible protein extender in bakery and confectionery products.	Research has also demonstrated the possibility of using peanut protein fibers for manufacturing meat product substitutes.

(Continued)

TABLE P-4 *(Continued)*

Product	Description	Uses	Comments

HUMAN FOODS *(Continued)*

Product	Description	Uses	Comments
Peanut oil	The oil obtained by crushing the nuts in hydraulic presses, or by using chemicals to dissolve the oil out of the nuts. The cold press method gives the lowest yield but the highest quality of edible oil.	Nearly 90% of the peanut oil used in the U.S. is for food uses. For frying foods. It smokes only at high temperatures and does not absorb odors easily. In salad oils and dressings, margarine, and other vegetable shortenings.	About ⅔ of the world's peanut crop is crushed for oil. Peanuts supply about 6% of the world's edible oil production. India produces 31% of the world's peanuts. The large-podded, large-seeded varieties grown in the U.S. contain about 45% oil, and the small-podded, small-seeded kinds up to 50%. From the two types, a ton of nuts in the shell will yield about 480 lb and 580 lb *(218 and 263 kg)* of oil, respectively. Peanut oil contains at least eight nutritionally essential fatty acids and 76 to 82% unsaturated fatty acids, of which 40 to 45% is unsaturated oleic acid and 30 to 35% polyunsaturated linoleic acid. The major portion of the characteristic peanut aroma and flavor is imparted by the oil.
Roasted peanuts	Whole nuts, following shelling and roasting. They are usually salted to improve their flavor, except where they go into peanut butter.	As snacks, eaten alone. In candies, salads, desserts, cookies, pies, and in other ways. In mixed, salted nuts. Peanut bread is made from ground peanuts.	There is a preference for the larger nuts for salted peanuts. About ¼ of all edible peanuts in the U.S. find their way into candies. Some of the most flavorsome, nutritious, and popular candies contain peanuts. Peanut candies are mostly bars and brittle.

FORTIFIED FOODS, BASED ON PEANUT PRODUCTS, FOR DEVELOPING COUNTRIES

Product	Description	Uses	Comments
Biscuit (In Uganda)	A mixture of 41% peanuts, 26% corn meal, 12% sucrose, 6% cottonseed oil, and 15% dried skim milk. Baked into a biscuit containing 20% protein.	It can be mixed with water (1) into a gruel, or (2) into a drink (by adding more water).	When fed to infants and preschool children, it gave the same weight gain as a milk biscuit.

LIVESTOCK FEEDS

Product	Description	Uses	Comments
Peanuts in shell	Peanuts inside the shell, and usually in the ground; they contain about 25% protein and 45 to 50% fat, but they are deficient in carotene, vitamin D, and calcium, and only fair in phosphorus.	Hogging off (turning pigs into the field to root out and eat the nuts).	Even where the peanuts are harvested for human food, hogs may be used to glean the fields. Pigs should have free access to salt and a calcium supplement when hogging off peanuts. Feeding large quantities of peanuts will produce soft pork unless restricted to pigs weighing under 85 lb *(39 kg)*.

(Continued)

TABLE P-4   *(Continued)*

Product	Description	Uses	Comments
LIVESTOCK FEEDS (*Continued*)			
Peanut skins (bran)	The outer covering of the peanut kernel, exclusive of the hulls.	Used chiefly in mixed feeds.	The skin comprises about 3% by weight of the seed. Peanut skins are bitter in taste; hence, only small quantities can be used in a mixed feed.
Peanut hulls	The outer hull—the peanut shell.	As a roughage for beef cattle.	The hulls amount to 20 to 30% of the weight of the whole pod. Peanut hulls average about 6 to 7% protein and 60% fiber.
Peanut meal	The ground product remaining after the oil has been extracted from the kernels mechanically or by solvent. It contains about 50% protein, and it must not contain more than 7% crude fiber.	For all classes of livestock.	The quality of the protein of peanut meal is good, ranking close to soybean meal. But it is usually lower in lysine than soybean meal. It is very palatable. Pigs will eat more of it than necessary to balance their ration when self-fed cafeteria style (allowed to choose between peanuts and other ingredients, with each fed separately). It tends to become rancid if stored too long.
Peanut meal and hulls	Ground peanuts, which contain a small amount of peanut hull residue or to which peanut hulls have been added.	Generally for cattle and sheep, especially if the hull content is high.	The feeding value of peanut meal and hulls depends on the proportion of hulls present.
Forage: Peanut hay	The tops of the plants after picking the nuts from the vines, although the entire plant may be so used. Sometimes it is ground or chopped.	Fed to beef cattle, dairy cattle, and sheep.	The feeding value of peanut hay varies greatly, depending on quality.
OTHER USES			
Peanut oil	The lower grades of oil extracted from the nuts.	Machinery oil, and as an ingredient in soaps, face powders, shaving creams, shampoos, and paints. In making nitroglycerin, an explosive. As a carrier for penicillin and adrenalin, and as the base for cosmetics.	
Peanut-shell powder	Shells ground into powder.	As an ingredient in plastics, cork substitutes, wallboard, and abrasives.	
Peanut shells	The outer hull.	As bedding for all classes of livestock. As a soil conditioner for fertilizers, for which purpose it is ground. Processed into "fireplace logs." Grinding and polishing abrasives, floor sweeping compounds, sound insulators, and wallboarding.	

PEAR(S) *Pyrus* spp

Contents   Page

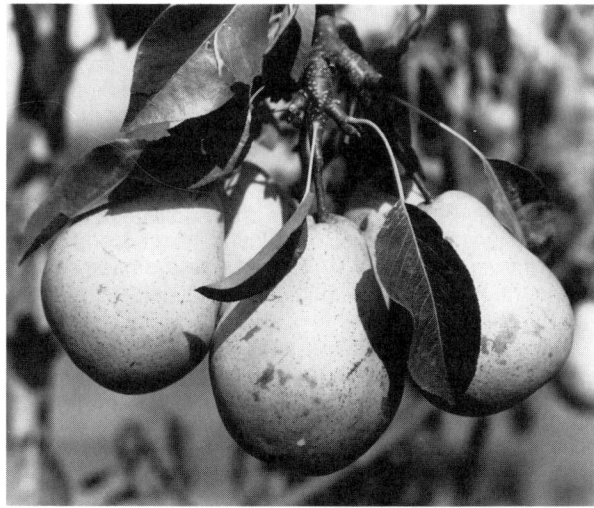

Fig. P-34.   Pears—fruit of the ages and relative of the apple. Color may be yellow, russet, or red. (Photo by J. C. Allen & Son, West Lafayette, Ind.)

The pear is a fruit classified as a pome, and it is closely related to the apple and the quince. Generally pears are large and round at the bottom, tapering inward toward the stem. However, some are almost completely round and others are as small as a cherry. Pears are covered with a smooth thin skin that may be yellow, russet, or red when ripe. Its edible flesh is juicy, sweet, and mellow. The flesh of some pears has a sandy texture due to the presence of grit cells. Enclosed within the center of the fleshy portion is a core which contains as many as 10 seeds. There are hundreds of pear varieties. Depending upon variety, pears vary in shape, size, color, texture, flavor, aroma, time of ripening and keeping qualities.

Mature pear trees may reach a height of 45 ft (*14 m*) and spread to 25 ft (*8 m*) wide. Often trees live to be 75 years old. Leaves of the pear tree are almost oval but they are sharply pointed at the tip. Also, leaves usually have toothed edges and prominent veins.

TYPES OF PEARS. Pears grown in North America belong to one of three botanical groups: (1) the common European pear, *Pyrus communis;* (2) the Oriental (Japanese or Chinese) sand pear, *Pyrus pyrifolia;* and (3) various cultivars (varieties) that are crosses between the two species. European pears are known collectively as butter pears, but this species is very susceptible to the pear disease, fire blight. Oriental pears were found to be resistant to fire blight and at one time plantings of Oriental pears spread through North America. However, the fruit of the Oriental pear is less desirable because it is gritty. Therefore, crosses between the European and Oriental pear were encouraged so a pear could be produced which was resistant to fire blight and desirable for eating. The best known of these hybrid varieties are Kieffer, LeConte, and Garber. Despite the threat of fire blight most pears grown in the United States are varieties originating from the European pear as listed in Table P-5. The Bartlett is probably the most familiar variety.

TABLE P-5
COMMON PEAR VARIETIES

Variety	Origin	Picking Date	Size	Shape	Quality	Use
Anjou	France; intro. to U.S. 1842.	August 10	Medium	Roundish, pyriform, short, thick stem.	Good	Shipping
Bartlett	Chance seedling; intro. to U.S. 1797.	Late June to middle of September.	Medium to large	Oblong pyriform	Good	Shipping, canning
Bosc	Belgium; intro. to U.S. 1832.	August 15	Large	Pyriform, long tapering neck.	Very good	Shipping
Comice	France, 1849	August 10	Large	Roundish to obovate.	Considered best of pears.	Shipping, holiday trade.
Hardy	France, 1820	Late June to middle of September.	Large	Obtuse pyriform	Very good	Shipping, fruit cocktail.
Seckel	Chance seedling, 1800.	Month after Bartlett.	Small	Obovate	Very good	Home orchard
Wilder	N.Y., 1884	June 10	Large	Oblong pyriform	Good	Shipping
Winter Nelis	Belgium; intro. to U.S. 1823.	September 1	Small	Roundish obovate	Good	Shipping

ORIGIN AND HISTORY. The pear is indigenous to western Asia; and it has long been cultivated there and in Europe. Some have speculated that Stone Age men discovered and ate the pear. There is evidence that pears were being cultivated as early as 1000 B.C. About 300 B.C., the Greek botanist, Theophrastus mentioned the pear in his work. A Belgian priest, Nicolas Hardenpoint (1705-1774), developed the first of the pears having soft juicy flesh. Then between 1780 and 1850 A.D. a number of European plant breeders were trying to grow better varieties of pears. Pears made their way to America with some of the first colonists, and most pears in colonial America came from France. Supposedly John Endicott of Massachusetts planted the *Endicott pear* in 1630. Pears gradually moved westward to California in the 1700s when Franciscan Fathers planted rows of pear trees in mission gardens. Now pears are grown in home gardens and on farms in almost every state.

PRODUCTION. Worldwide, the average yearly production of pears is around 9.8 million metric tons, with Italy, the United States, China, and the U.S.S.R. leading in pear production. Other leading pear-producing countries are indicated in Fig. P-35.

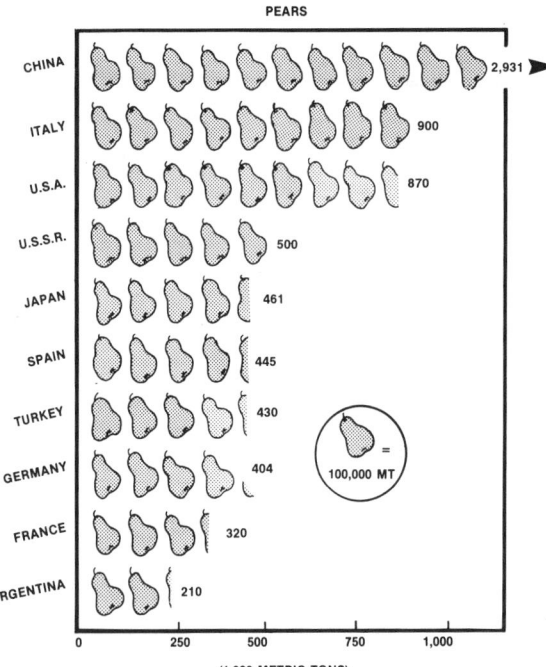

PEARS

CHINA	2,931 ▶
ITALY	900
U.S.A.	870
U.S.S.R.	500
JAPAN	461
SPAIN	445
TURKEY	430
GERMANY	404
FRANCE	320
ARGENTINA	210

= 100,000 MT

0   250   500   750   1,000

(1,000 METRIC TONS)

Fig. P-35. Leading pear-producing countries of the world. (Based on data from the *FAO Production Yearbook*, 1990, FAO/UN, Rome, Italy, Vol. 44, p. 162, Table 70)

In the United States, the commercial crop of pears averages 963,800 tons (*867,420 metric tons*) each year, and it is valued at $264 million. Washington, California,

and Oregon produce 97% of this crop. The nine leading pear-producing states, by rank, are Washington, California, Oregon, New York, Pennsylvania, Michigan, Colorado, Utah, and Connecticut. Bartlett pears dominate among pear varieties grown in the United States, and California dominates in the production of Bartletts.

Propagation and Growing. Pears are propagated by budding the desired variety into seedling stock of European (French) pears or Oriental pears. Quince (*Cydonia oblonga*) rootstock is used to produce dwarf pear trees.

Standard sized pear trees are planted about 18 to 25 ft (*5 to 8 m*) apart while dwarf trees are planted 10 to 15 ft (*3 to 4.6 m*) apart. Trees begin to produce after 5 to 7 years, and reach full production by 12 to 15 years. Pear trees grow in heavy soils, tolerating wetter soil than some other fruits. At the time the trees bloom, cross-pollination of varieties may or may not be necessary depending upon variety and region. Some varieties always need cross-pollination. Bee colonies can be brought into the orchard so bees can help in the cross-pollination. Proper orchard management also includes fertilization, irrigation, spraying, and pruning to encourage a pear crop of the best quality and quantity.

Harvesting. Many Bartlett pears reach the market in July, but the time of marketing pears ranges from May to October depending upon the variety and the producing region.

Pears for both fresh market and processing are picked green and hard. Tree-ripened pears are frequently of inferior quality, often with coarse or gritty flesh. Pears are hand picked with the utmost care since they bruise easily. For storage purposes fresh picked pears should be cooled down to 34°F (*1°C*) soon after picking. Some varieties can be stored all winter. Pears will ripen when exposed to temperatures between 65 and 75°F (*18 and 24°C*).

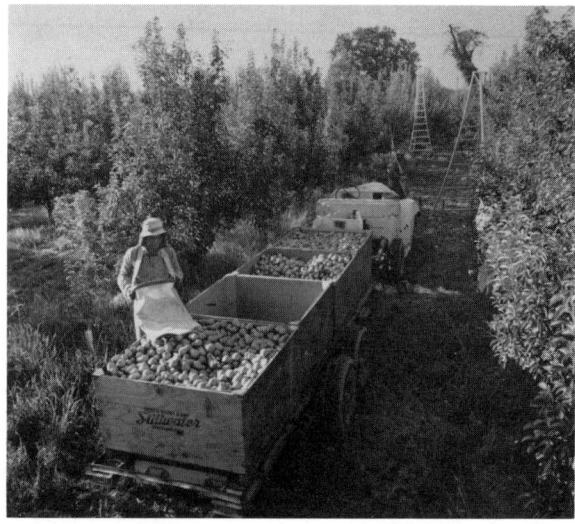

Fig. P-36. Harvesting pears. Pears bruise easily, so skilled, careful workers are required. (Courtesy, California Tree Fruit Agreement, Sacramento, Calif.)

PROCESSING. About 48% of the pear crop is sold as fresh pears for consumption as fresh fruit and for home use. The remaining 52% is processed as canned or dried fruit. There are no recent estimates available as to the amounts canned or dried, though in past years the amount dried has been less than 1% of the crop. Therefore, around 51% of the pear crop is probably canned.

Preservaton of pears by canning includes pears canned in water pack, juice pack, light syrup, heavy syrup, or extra heavy syrup.

• **Perry**—The Europeans use pears to make a drink called *perry*—a beverage somewhat resembling hard (fermented) apple cider.

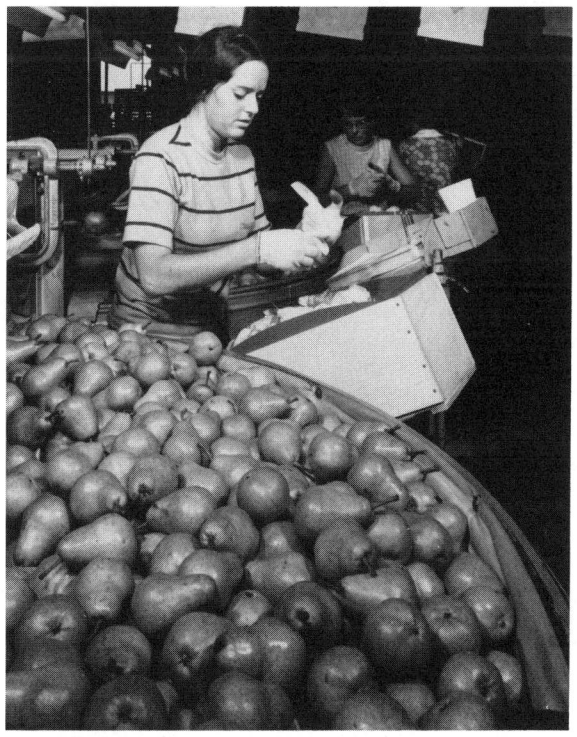

Fig. P-37. Packaging fresh pears for shipment. (Courtesy, California Tree Fruit Agreement, Sacramento, Calif.)

SELECTION. As pears ripen their skin color changes from green to the color characteristic for the variety. Bartlett pears turn yellow. Fresh pears are best when they yield to gentle palm pressure. If still green skinned when purchased, pears can be ripened at home by storing them at room temperature, preferably three or more together in a closed paper bag. When pears begin to turn colors and pass the palm pressure test they should be refrigerated. Bartlett pears can be held in the refrigerator for several days either before or after ripening.

PREPARATION. Pears can be enjoyed by eating fresh out of the hand like an apple, or they may be used in salads, main dishes or desserts, limited only by the imagination. Canned pears are used alone as a dessert dish or in combination with other fruits and/or in gelatin dishes. Some pears are canned with other fruits in fruit cocktails. Dried pears are eaten as a snack or they may be cooked.

NUTRITIONAL VALUE. Fresh pears contain 83% water. Additionally, each 100 g (about 3½ oz) provides 61 Calories (kcal) of energy, 130 mg of potassium, and only 2 mg of sodium. The calories in pears are derived primarily from the sugars (carbohydrate) which give pears a sweet taste. Pears canned in a syrup contain more calories due to the addition of sugar. Also, canning decreases the concentration of some minerals and vitamins. Dried pears contain only 26% water; hence, many of the nutrients, including calories, are more concentrated. More complete information regarding the nutritional value of fresh, canned, and dried pears is presented in Food Composition Table F-36.

(Also see FRUIT[S], Table F-47 Fruits of the World.)

PEARLED

Dehulled grains reduced to smaller smooth particles by machine brushing.

PECAN *Carya illinoensis*

The nut-bearing pecan is a type of hickory, native to North America. Pecan trees may grow to 180 ft (*55 m*) high, but most are 75 to 90 ft (*25 to 30 m*) high. The trend in planting is toward smaller, more highly productive orchard-type trees. Leaves of the pecan are 12 to 20 in. (*30 to 51 cm*) long and they are comprised of 9 to 17 lance-shaped leaflets. Flowers of the pecan tree are separate male and female flowers. Many varieties cannot pollinate

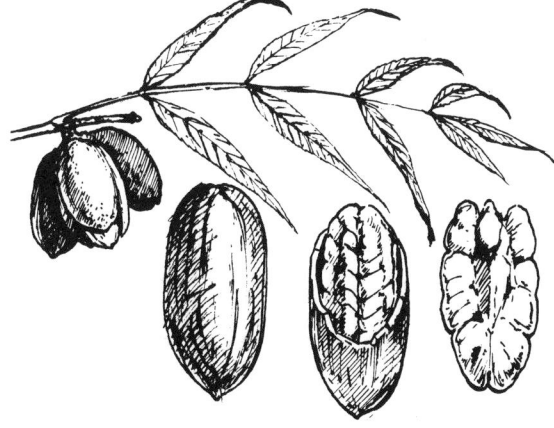

Fig. P-38. Pecans, an American crop requiring patience. Newly planted trees do not bear enough nuts to be profitable until they are about 11 years old.

their own kind, so orchards contain several varieties. Pollination is via windblown pollen. To produce nuts, the trees require a growing season of over 200 days with mid-summer average temperatures of 79°F (*26°C*) or higher. Pecans bear best in warm moist regions. Also nuts are best where the coldest winter month averages less than 61°F (*16°C*). The nuts that form are encased in a leathery husk that splits into four sections when the fruit is mature. Pecans are usually shaped like large olives, though some are nearly round, and others are sharply pointed or oblong. Two kernels (halves) are contained within each shell.

ORIGIN AND HISTORY.   Pecans are native to North America in the valleys of the Mississippi River and tributaries as far north as Iowa and southward, and in the river valleys of Oklahoma and Texas, and northern Mexico. To the Indians and early settlers of these areas, pecans were an important food source. Pecans have been introduced to a few other regions; namely, South Africa, Israel, Brazil, Peru, Australia, and China. Beginning in 1890, grafted trees were planted in orchards within the United States, but outside of the native area. Since 1950, research by the USDA has developed new varieties of pecans which come into production early and produce 7 to 8 g nuts with over 60% kernel content. This helped make orchards profitable sooner and doubled or tripled yields.

PRODUCTION.   Very few pecans are produced out-side the United States. Although some varieties of pecan are adapted to northern climates, most of the pecans are grown in the South. Georgia produces 32% of the U.S. crop which amounts to about 92 thousand metric tons each year with a value of around $248 million. Wild or native trees produce 30% of the pecan crop, while im-proved varieties (cultivars) bred for the thinness of shell produce 70% of the U.S. pecan crop. These thin-shelled pecans are called *papershell*, and they are popular because they can be cracked between the fingers. Fig. F-39 shows the pecan-producing states and the propor-tion of their crop derived from native trees. New Mexico is the only state almost all of whose crop comes from improved varieties.

Propagation and Growing.   Pecan orchard trees are usually grown by grafting improved stock—thin shell varieties—onto the seedlings of native pecans at about 1 year of age. Then these trees are set in the orchard at 2 to 4 years of age. The trend in pecan production is away from native stands and toward planted grafted trees of proven performance.

The first commercial varieties were selections from native stands, whereas most new selections are from breeding programs. The U.S. Department of Agriculture's Pecan Research Center at Brownwood, Texas, has been a leader in releasing new varieties, all distinguished by their Indian names.

Optimum conditions for growing pecans include deep, well-drained soils and a warm growing season. Different varieties are adapted for frost-free growing seasons of 150 to 210 days. Pecan trees flower in April or May and nuts mature from September to November. Some trees may produce 500 lb (*230 kg*) in a year, but yields fluctuate widely from year to year. The tendency is for alternating good and bad years.

Harvesting.   Pecans are harvested after they drop to the ground, usually leaving the husks behind. Light poles may be used to brush some nuts from the branches to the ground. In some large orchards with small trees, mechanical shakers are used, but large native trees are not suited for this method. Nuts are then picked up from the ground by hand or sweeping-vacuuming.

PROCESSING.   Following harvest, pecans are often dried or "cured" for a few weeks. At processing centers the nuts are cleaned, graded, and packaged. More than 90% of the pecans are marketed as shelled nuts. Pecans stored in the shell may be stored at 25°F (*-4°C*) or lower for 2 years or more.
Pecan processing equipment for shelled pecans can size, crack, and separate meats and shells. After separa-tion from the shells, meats are dried to 3 to 4% moisture for better storage. Meats are graded by electric eye and by hand whereupon they are packaged for distribution to bakeries, retail outlets, confectioners, and ice cream manufactures. Some pecans are salted.

SELECTION.   Pecans in shells should be free from splits, cracks, stains, or holes. Moldy nuts may not be safe to eat. Nutmeat should be plump and fairly uniform in color and size. Limp, rubbery, dark, or shriveled kernels are likely stale. If antioxidants are added to delay the onset of rancidity, thus extending the shelf life of pack-aged nutmeat, they are listed on the package. Pecans keep better if stored in tightly closed containers in the refrigerator or freezer.

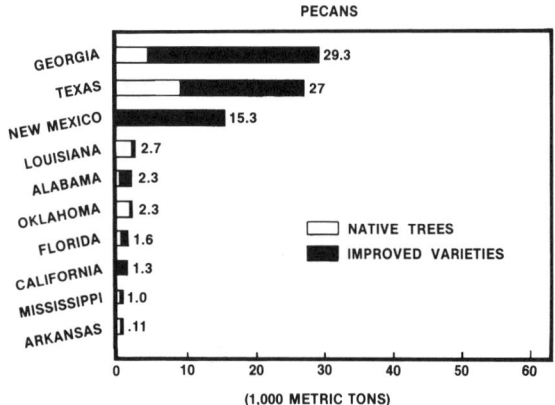

Fig. P-39.   The pecan-producing states, showing the proportion of their yearly crop derived from native trees and improved varieties. (Based on data from *Agricultural Statistics 1991*, USDA, p. 222, Table 346)

PREPARATION. Delicately flavored, sweet tasting pecans are eaten alone or in an array of dishes and products. One estimate places 1,200 uses for pecans in prepared dishes.

Pecans are used to impart their qualities to such foods as baked goods, dairy products, confections, salads, desserts, fowl stuffings, puddings, souffles, meat combinations, cereals, and vegetable dishes. Pralines and pecan pie originated in the South where most pecans grow. The flavor of pecans is compatible with that of most foods, so that they may be used natural, sweetened, salted, or spiced. The texture is such that they may be used as halves or pieces of any desired size. They may be eaten raw or toasted.

NUTRITIONAL VALUE. Pecans are extremely nutritious. They contain only 3 to 4% water and they are loaded with energy. Each 100 g (about 3½ oz) of pecans contains 739 Calories (kcal), primarily due to their fat (oil) content of 71%. Additionally, each 100 g provides 9 g protein, 15 g carbohydrate, 2.4 mg of iron, and 4.1 mg of zinc. More complete information regarding the nutritional value of pecans is provided in Food Composition Table F-36.

(Also see NUTS, Table N-8 Nuts of the World.)

PECTIN

Most plant tissue, fruits in particular, contain pectin—a polysaccharide which functions as a cementing material. Lemon or orange rind is one of the richest sources of pectin, containing about 30% of this substance. Pectin, hemicellulose, and cellulose comprise a part of the diet which is often referred to as fiber or roughage. It is not digestible.

Chemically, pectin is a mixture of methyl esterified galacturonan—long chains of the uronic acid of galactose joined by methyl alcohol—plus some galactan and araban, depending upon the plant source. Hence, the complete breakdown of pectin into component parts yields galacturonic acid, methyl alcohol, and small amounts of the sugars arabinose and galactose.

In a pure form extracted from plant material, pectin is a powder, yellowish-white in color, almost odorless, and with a mucilaginous taste. Due to its ability to form gels in a water solution, pectin is an important commercial product used as a food additive by commercial and household food processors.

Many plant materials could be employed for the production of pectin, but apple pomace and citrus peel (lemon, lime, orange, and grapefruit) are the sources for the commercial extraction of pectin.

The type of pectin, hence, its uses in food, is governed by the amount of methyl alcohol joined to the galacturonic acid within the pectin molecule. Therefore, pectin is generally classified as high methoxyl pectin or low methoxyl pectin. Each type possesses different properties.

• **High methoxyl pectin**—When the degree of methylation is more than 50% for the high methoxyl pectin, half or more of the galacturonic molecules are associated with methyl alcohol. High methoxyl pectin requires 55 to 85% sugar and a pH of 2.5 to 3.8 (acid) to gel. This limits the use of high methoxyl pectin as a gelling agent in sweetened fruit products such as jams and jellies at a concentration of 0.1 to 1.5%.

• **Low methoxyl pectin**—Processing techniques can de-esterify pectin (remove methyl alcohol) and create low-methoxyl pectin. This type of pectin requires no sugar or acid to gel. Therefore, low methoxyl pectin is used as a gelling agent in fruit products with a low sugar content or products containing no added sugar. The low methoxyl pectin has more and varied uses than high methoxyl pectin.

Pectin is a food additive, and since it is found naturally in plant material, and has always been part of man's diet, the Food and Drug Administration (FDA) accepts it as a generally recognized as safe (GRAS) additive. Moreover, pectin may be a beneficial constituent of the diet, even though it is not digested, since it has been shown to lower blood cholestrol levels.

(Also see ADDITIVES, Table A-3; CARBOHYDRATE[S]; and FIBER.)

PECTINASES

Like all living things, plants contain enzymes—protein molecules which catalyze chemical reactions. Pectinases are enzymes in plants or plant products which cause the chemical breakdown of the polysaccharide pectin, resulting in softening and viscosity changes in fruit products. Depending upon the food product, this may be desirable or undesirable. For example, pectins are desirable in tomato, orange, and apricot juices as they make the juice viscous and hold dispersed solids in solutions; hence, pectinase must be destroyed by heat during production. On the other hand, the fruit juices, such as apple and grape juice, a clear juice is desired so commercial pectinase is added. This ensures the production of a clear juice. Vinegar and jelly produced from depectinized juices are a brighter color. Pectinases are also used in making wines. Most commercial pectinases are derived from *Aspergillus niger* fungi.

(Also see PECTIN.)

PEDIATRICS

Relating to the study and treatment of disease in children. A specialist in pediatrics is called a pediatrician. He is trained in both the medical and surgical diagnosis of the illnesses and disorders of infants and children.

(Also see CHILDHOOD AND ADOLESCENT NUTRITION.)

PEKOE

This is a grade of tea leaves, from which a black tea is derived. Pekoe leaves are the middle-sized tea leaves, while orange pekoe leaves are the smallest.

(Also see TEA.)

PELLAGRA

Contents | Page

This dietary deficiency disease is due to lack of the vitamin niacin or of the amino acid tryptophan (which is converted in the body to nicotinic acid). It usually afflicts people whose dietary protein comes mainly from maize (which is deficient in both nicotinic acid and tryptophan). Also, it occurs in areas of India where the diet consists mainly of a millet called *jowar* (*Sorghum vulgare*) without any animal foods. Some alcoholics and persons with disorders of absorption have also been found to have the disease.

HISTORY OF PELLAGRA.   There is no mention of pellagra in early medical writing in Europe. It appears that the first cases in Europe were observed after the cultivation of maize, taken there from the Americas. Casal first described the disorder in Spain in 1730; and by the end of the 18th century, the disease had spread through Europe, North Africa, and Egypt. Casal found that a milk diet cured the disease. Cerri demonstrated the dietary cure of Italian pellagra victims in 1795; and in the early 1800s Buniva showed, by inoculation of humans with material from diseased persons, that pellagra was not infectious. Most of the European investigators recognized the importance of diet in the prevention and treatment of the disease. In general, the dietary prescription was to eliminate corn from the diet and to replace it with foods of animal origin such as meat, milk, and eggs.

The first reported cases of pellagra in the United States were in New York and Massachusetts in 1864. By the early 1900s, it was found to be prevalent in the southeastern United States, with around 100,000 cases per year resulting in up to 10,000 deaths per year. Funk, a Polish scientist working in England, suggested in 1912 that pellagra might be a vitamin deficiency disease like beriberi. It is ironic that he isolated, without realizing it, the antipellagra vitamin while trying to isolate the antiberiberi factor. Funk had tested the material he isolated on the victims of beriberi where it proved not to be effective, but he did not test his material on patients suffering from pellagra. It was difficult to establish in the United States that pellagra was a dietary deficiency disease. Theories as to its cause ranged from an infectious agent to the suggestion that persons of Anglo-Saxon ancestry in the South had genetic weaknesses, particularly with respect to mental disorders. (These persons in the South were descendents of essentially the same Anglo-Saxon stock as the Northerners.)

From 1914 to 1922 Goldberger and his associates, of the U.S. Public Health Service, conducted a series of studies which showed without doubt that the disease was due to diet rather than to an infectious agent. First, they showed that the disease might be cured or prevented by providing diets containing ample quantities of meat, milk, and eggs. Then he and some volunteers ingested feces, had their throats swabbed with nose and throat secretions, and were inoculated with blood from victims of pellagra. None of these human subjects came down with the disease.

Chittendon and Underhill, in 1917, produced a deficiency disease in dogs which very closely resembled pellagra in humans; and Goldberger and Wheeler showed, in 1928, that the disease could be produced in dogs by feeding a diet similar to the type known to cause pellagra in humans. The disease in dogs was called "blacktongue" by veterinarians, and so efforts were made to isolate the blacktongue preventive factor. Experimentation with dogs by Elvehjem and his colleagues at the University of Wisconsin, in 1937, led to the identification of the antiblacktongue factor as nicotinic acid (niacin) and nicotinamide (niacinamide). They also showed that the substance which was isolated earlier by Funk from rice polishings was identical to the factor they had isolated from liver. It was later shown that the administration of niacin resulted in the cure of pellagra.

Niacin, however, is not the complete answer to the prevention of pellagra since it is known that in some areas of the world where there is no pellagra the diets are lower in nicotinic acid than the corn diets which are shown to cause pellagra. Krehl and his co-workers, at the University of Wisconsin, showed, in 1945, that supplements of either niacin or tryptophan were effective in restoring growth to rats made deficient by feeding a high level of corn. The administration of tryptophan was shown to cure pellagra in humans by Vilter and co-workers, in 1949, and by Sarett and Goldsmith, in 1950.

In the decade that followed, Gopalan and his associates in India presented evidence that the utilization of the amino acid tryptophan in corn and sorghum is lowered by excess amounts of the amino acid leucine, present in these foods. (This phenomenon is known as an amino acid imbalance.)

CAUSES OF PELLAGRA.   Although pellagra had long been associated with reliance on corn as a dietary staple, it took investigators over 200 years to identify the specific nutritional conditions which caused this disease. Discussion of these conditions follows:

• **Deficiencies of niacin (nicotinic acid)**—Diets based on corn processed by the methods used in the United States do not contain enough available niacin to prevent pellagra. (The niacin in corn and other grains is in part bound to the indigestible portion of the grains. Therefore, it is not completely available to man. The native Indians of Latin America rely heavily on corn, but do not develop pellagra because they soak the grain in limewater, which frees the bound niacin.)

• **Deficiencies of tryptophan**—It has been shown that about one-sixtieth of the dietary tryptophan is converted in the body to niacin. Thus, this amino acid may help to meet some of the need for niacin. However, the conversion of tryptophan to niacin may not be the complete explanation for the antipellagra role of this amino acid. Recent research has shown that diets based mainly on corn may produce subnormal levels of an important neurotransmitter (serotonin) in the brain.[7] The investigators explain that serotonin is synthesized in the brain from tryptophan, which is supplied by the diet. Therefore, they suggest that dietary deficiencies of tryptophan alone might account for some of the neurological disorders seen in pellagra victims. However, there are still unanswered questions concerning the effects of niacin on brain serotonin levels and other aspects of brain biochemistry.

• **Amino acid imbalances which reduce the utilization of tryptophan**—Corn and a millet called *jowar* (*Sorghum vulgare,* which is used as a staple food in some parts of India) have both been shown to have disproportionately low levels of tryptophan, and unusually high levels of another amino acid, leucine. It has been suggested that these imbalanced ratios of amino acids might result in reductions in the utilization by man of tryptophan from these grains.[8]

• **Chronic alcoholism**—Overindulgence in alcohol results in the diversion of the limited supply of niacin coenzymes from the metabolism of essential nutrients to that of alcohol.[9]

Thus, the chronic abuse of alcohol increases the risk of developing pellagra when diets low in niacin and tryptophan are consumed. However, not as much of this disease is seen today in alcoholics as was once seen in these people. Perhaps the reduction in the disease is due to improved opportunities for obtaining food and medical treatment.

SIGNS OF PELLAGRA.   Clinical signs of pellagra are the characteristic three D's—dermatitis, diarrhea, and dementia. The skin disorder is usually one of the first clear-cut signs of the development of the disease. There is reddening of the areas exposed to the sun or of those areas subjected to friction (such as the elbows). A characteristic dermatitis around the collarbone is called Casal's necklace after the man who first described the condition in Spain. Another very early sign in development of the disease is soreness of the tongue which is swollen, raw, and extra sensitive to hot or seasoned foods (apparently part of an irritation of the entire gastrointestinal tract). The diarrhea, which is not always present, may contain blood and mucus. The mental symptoms range from irritability, anxiety, and depression to psychosis. (In the days of endemic pellagra in the southeastern United States, there were many admissions of pellagra victims to mental hospitals.) A victim of pellagra is shown in Fig. P-40.

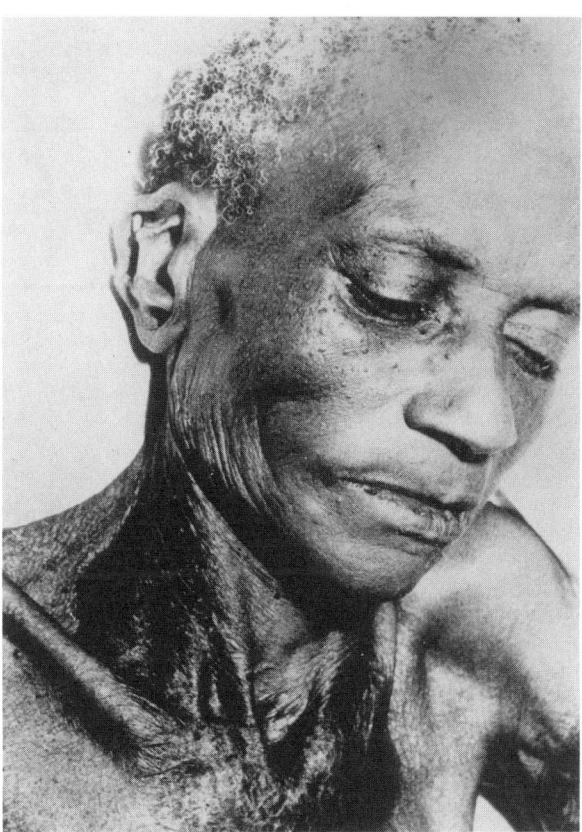

Fig. P-40.   An East African victim of pellagra. Note the inflammation and darkening of the skin around his neck. (Courtesy, FAO, Rome, Italy)

[7]Fernstrom, J. D., L. D. Lytle, "Corn Malnutrition, Brain Serotonin and Behavior," *Nutrition Reviews,* Vol. 34, No. 9, September 1976, p. 257.

[8]Gopolan, C., "A report on the First Fifty Years of the Nutrition Research Laboratories, Hyderabad," *Nutrition Reviews,* Vol. 28, No. 1, January 1970, p. 3.

[9]Iber, F. C., "In Alcoholism, The Liver Sets the Pace," *Nutrition Today,* Vol. 6, No. 1, January/February 1971, p. 2.

TREATMENT AND PREVENTION OF PELLAGRA.   Persons suffering from severe forms of the disease may be given either nicotinamide (a derivative of niacin) or nicotinic acid in oral doses as high as 100 mg every 4 hours. Such high doses of nicotinic acid often cause flushing, which does not result when similar doses of nicotinamide are given. Niacin is well absorbed, even when gastrointestinal disorders are present. Often, a pellagra victim suffers from multiple vitamin and nutrient deficiencies, and, therefore, may require supplemental sources of the vitamin B complex and protein. Brewers' yeast has often been used as such a supplement.

Diets used for the treatment and prevention of pellagra should include abundant sources of animal protein such as meat, fish, eggs, and milk since these foods are good sources of both niacin and tryptophan. Vegetable protein sources high in tryptophan are peanuts, sesame seeds, sunflower seeds, and whole wheat. The refining of grains results in the loss of much of the niacin content, so it is wise to use either whole grain products or those which have been enriched. It should be noted that gelatin, and meats which are high in connective tissue (such as chitterlings, ham hocks, hog jowls, and maws), are very low in tryptophan. It is noteworthy, too, that these were the types of meats commonly used in the South in the years when pellagra was endemic.

(Also see DEFICIENCY DISEASES, Table D-1 Major Dietary Deficiency Diseases; and NIACIN.)

PELLAGRINS

Individuals suffering from pellagra.
(Also see NIACIN.)

PENTOSAN

A pentose-based polysaccharide (like xylan or araban) with the general formula $(C_5H_{10}O_5)_n$ that is widely distributed in plants, such as wheat bran, oat hulls, and mesquite gum.

(Also see CARBOHYDRATE[S].)

PENTOSE

A 5-carbon monosaccharide (as xylose and ribulose) having the formula $C_5H_{10}O_5$. Not abundant in the free form in nature.

(Also see CARBOHYDRATE[S].)

PEPPERONI (PEPERONI)

A highly seasoned dry sausage made with beef, or with pork and beef. Also, poultry and turkey may be added to pepperoni provided it is properly labeled.

PEPPERS *Capsicum* spp

The species of peppers which are native to the Americas have been enthusiastically adopted as commercial crops around the world. These shrubby plants, which are called capsicums to distinguish from the viny pepper plants (*Piper* spp.) of the Old World, are members of the nightshade family (*Solanaceae*). Hence, the capsicum peppers are close relatives of the eggplant, Irish potato, and tomato. Although many botanists believe that the different types of capsicums are simply different varieties of a single species, it is customary to classify most types as either (1) chilies (*C. frutescens*), which are usually very pungent; or (2) sweet peppers (*C. annuum*), which have milder flavored, larger fruits.

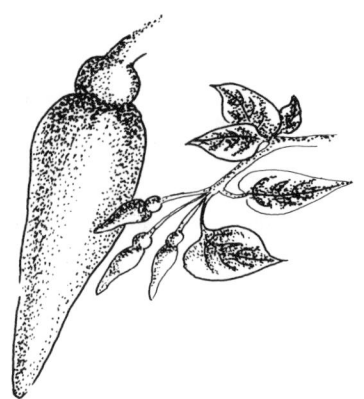

Fig. P-41. Chili peppers, the pungent type of capsicum pepper which is grown in the warm regions of the world.

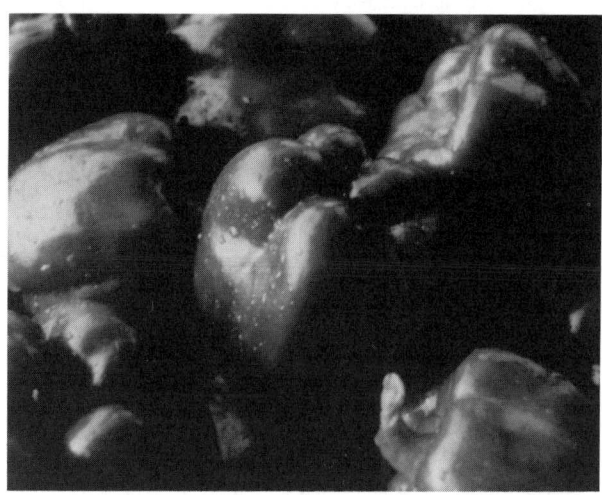

Fig. P-42. A sweet pepper, the type of capsicum pepper which has a mild flavor and grows in temperate climates. (Courtesy, USDA)

ORIGIN AND HISTORY. It seems likely that the prehistoric peoples of Latin America gathered wild capsicum peppers in much the same way as certain varieties are gathered today, since pepper seeds dated before 5000 B.C. were found by archaeologists at Techuacan, Mexico. The seeds are believed to have come from wild varieties of sweet peppers. More recent ruins in the same area contained evidence that these varieties were first cultivated at some time prior to the dawn of the Christian era.

Chili peppers may also have been domesticated independently between 2000 and 1000 B.C. by the Indians living on the Peruvian coast. It is noteworthy that the seeds of these varieties have often been spread over large areas by migratory birds. Chilies had reached the

Caribbean before Columbus discovered the Americas. Hence, he and other explorers brought them back to Europe as a substitute for the expensive black pepper which was then imported from Asia. Within a century of their introduction to the Old World, chilies had become an important export crop of India.

The rapid spread of sweet and chili peppers around the world was due in large part to the Spanish and Portuguese explorers who introduced them wherever they went on their ocean voyages. Today, the capsicums rank among the top 2 dozen vegetable crops of the world.

PRODUCTON. Most of the world production of chili and sweet peppers, which totals about 9.1 million metric tons, comes from the countries listed in Fig. P-43.

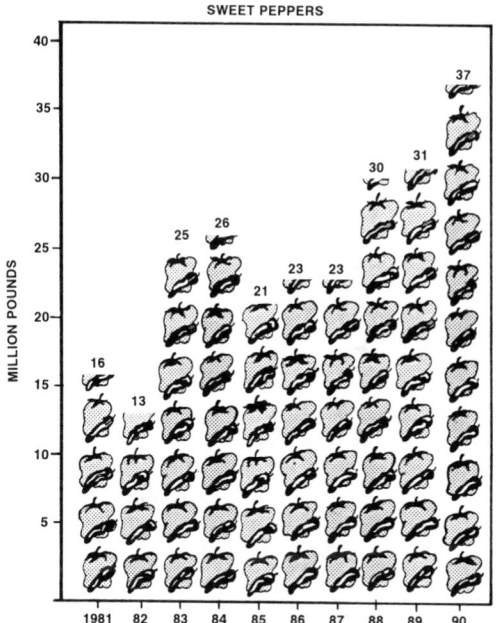

SWEET PEPPERS

Fig. P-44. Commercial frozen pack 1981–90.(From *Agricultural Statistics 1991*, USDA, p. 172, Table 248)

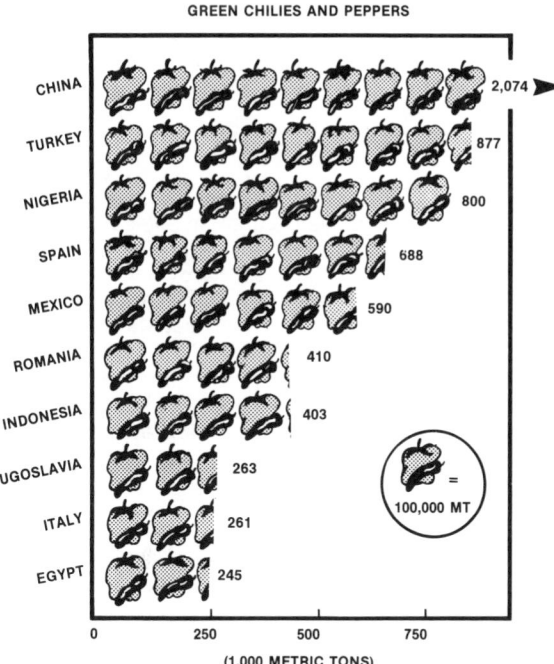

GREEN CHILIES AND PEPPERS

Fig. P-43. The leading pepper-producing countries of the world. (Based upon data from *FAO Production Yearbook*, 1990, FAO/UN, Rome, Italy, Vol. 44, p. 139, Table 57)

About 230 thousand metric tons of sweet peppers are produced in the United States. Most of this crop is eaten fresh, however, an increasing volume is being put into frozen vegetable mixtures, as shown in Fig. 44

The only variety of chili pepper produced commercially in the United States is the Tabasco, a variety that is grown in Louisiana for making Tabasco sauce.

Peppers, like eggplant and tomatoes, are warm weather crops. Therefore, the planting of seeds in open fields is limited to mild climates. Elsewhere, the seeds are planted in greenhouses or hotbeds, then transplanted in the field when the night temperature is not likely to drop below 55°F (*13°C*). The soil should be well-drained and not overly acid. Excess acidity is usually neutralized by the addition of lime. Many commercial growers also apply mixed fertilizer containing nitrogen, phosphorus, and potassium. However, an excessive application of nitrogen should be avoided because it encourages an overgrowth of foliage at the expense of fruit. It is noteworthy that the setting of fruit occurs only when the night temperatures range between 60 and 75°F (*16 and 24°C*). Furthermore, the blossoms may drop before the fruit is set if the plants are stressed by lack of water and/or temperatures over 90°F (*32°C*). Hence, irrigation is always required in dry climates and it may even be needed in moist areas where the pattern of rainfall is erratic.

Most of the sweet peppers which are destined for the fresh market are picked when they have reached their full size, but while they are still green. (This stage is reached at 60 to 80 days after transplanting.) Sweet peppers intended for processing are usually allowed to reach red-ripeness before picking as are chili peppers and some of the sweet peppers for the fresh market. (The ripened ones are ready from 70 to 90 days after transplanting.) The worldwide average yield of chilies and sweet peppers per acre is about 7,300 lb (*8,176 kg/ha*), but yields as high as 49,500 lb (*55,440 kg/ha*) have been obtained in Bahrein. Similarly, the average U.S. yield of green peppers per acre is about 9,800 lb (*10,976 kg/ha*), but yields as high as 21,000 lb (*23,520 kg/ha*) have been obtained in California.

PROCESSING. Much of the U.S. pepper crop is utilized as a fresh vegetable because refrigerated storage and transportation facilities make it possible for the vegetable to be marketed around the country with a minimum of spoilage. Most of the remainder is utilized in such items as (1) canned products—corn and peppers, pimientos, sauces, stuffed peppers, and tomatoes and peppers; (2) dehydrated or dried preparations for reconstitution with water, or for making condiments; (3) frozen items—chopped peppers, pizza, and stuffed peppers; and (4) pickles which utilize chilies or sweet peppers. Some are also used in the preparation of prepackaged salads and in making the stuffed peppers sold in the meat sections of certain supermarkets.

Good cooks often enliven their dishes with various condiments made from chilies and/or sweet peppers. Some of the more popular peppers are:

• **Cayenne pepper**—A "hot" seasoning made by grinding a dried chili pepper that originated in the area around the Cayenne River in French Guiana.

• **Chili powder**—Although this moderately pungent product may be made solely by grinding dried, red-ripe chilies, it is usually prepared from 83% red pepper, 9% cumin, 4% oregano, 2.5% salt, and 0.5% garlic powder.

• **Chili sauce**—Many sauces bearing this name are essentially tomato sauces that contain tomato seeds and various seasonings. However, sauces rich in pulp from chili peppers are usually designated as "hot chili sauces."

• **Dried chilies** ("hot" peppers)—Dried red-ripe chili peppers may be used as a seasoning when whole or in the form of small flakes such as those sprinkled on pizza and similar dishes.

• **Paprika**—A powdered seasoning made by grinding a dried, red-ripe sweet pepper of a variety grown specifically for this purpose. It is mild-flavored and adds a bright orange-red color to dishes such as Hungarian goulash.

• **Pimiento**—A type of red-ripe sweet pepper which is often canned. Diced pimiento is often mixed into soft cheese spreads.

• **Red pepper**—This powdered seasoning is made by grinding dried, red-ripe chilies. It adds a hot, biting taste to dishes.

• **Tabasco sauce**—A pungent sauce prepared from the fresh red-ripe Tabasco variety of chili by macerating the flesh of the pods in vinegar.

SELECTION. Good quality sweet peppers are fresh, firm, bright in appearance, thick fleshed, and have a fresh, green calyx. Immature peppers are usually soft, pliable, thin-fleshed and pale green in color. A firm pepper may yield to slight pressure, but it is not shriveled, limp, or pliable. Peppers that are not fresh may be shriveled or soft, and dull in appearance. Constricted, crooked, or deformed peppers of otherwise good quality are objectionable only because of possible waste, or because the shape is unsuited to a particular use. Injuries which penetrate the flesh wall should be avoided due to susceptibility to decay. Decay may appear as water-soaked, bleached, or blackened areas that may or may not be noticeably sunken.

The pungent or hot varieties are sold in either the green or red stage of maturity, and vary in size from the small chili peppers to sizes nearly as large as the bell type. Red-colored pods are generally the most desired. Chili and Cayenne peppers are sometimes threaded on strings and dried prior to sale, or dried on the plant and displayed for sale with peppers and plant as a unit. The same quality characteristics noted for sweet peppers also apply to fresh hot peppers.

PREPARATION. Many people remove the seeds from peppers, but some leave them in and eat them right along with the fleshy part of the vegetable. However, it may be wise for all but the most hardy souls to remove the seeds from the pungent chilies, because the seeds often contain more of the irritating substance than the fleshy part.

Fresh, frozen, or pickled peppers may be (1) served without cooking in relishes, salads, and sandwiches; or (2) cooked in casseroles; Chinese stir-fried dishes; fried onion garnishes for fish, meats, and poultry; omelets; pizzas; soups; and stews. Sweet peppers are also good when stuffed with bread crumbs, fish, meat, poultry, or rice, and baked. Chilies are suitable for making *rellenos* by stuffing them with cheese and either baking them in a sauce, or dipping them into an egg batter and deep-frying.

CAUTION: Certain types of hot chilies may contain potentially harmful amounts of a highly irritating substance called capsaicin, which can raise blisters on sensitive tissues or even cause ulceration. Hence, the reckless ingestion of these items may result in "chili burns" anywhere along the entire length of the digestive tract. It is said that such injuries to the mouth, esophagus, or stomach may be soothed somewhat by eating ice cream, cold milk, or yogurt. Furthermore, the hands should be washed with soap and water after handling hot chilies in order to avoid the accidental introduction of capsaicin into the eyes.

A recent research report suggests that the consumption of vegetables of the nightshade family (capsicum peppers, eggplant, the Irish potato, and the tomato) may aggravate arthritis in susceptible people. Therefore, it may be a good idea for arthritis-prone people and others who are unaccustomed to eating these vegetables to try eating only small amounts of each vegetable alone until it is certain that there is no sensitivity to one or more of them.

NUTRITIONAL VALUE. The nutrient compositions of various forms of peppers and pepper products are given in Food Composition Table F-36.

Some noteworthy observations regarding the nutrient composition of peppers and pepper products follow:

1. All types of raw peppers have a high water content (74 to 94%) which decreases with maturity, and a low caloric content which increases with maturity. These fresh vegetables are excellent sources of vitamin C and fair to excellent sources of vitamin A. The levels of both vitamins increase with the degree of ripeness. Red peppers have a significantly higher vitamin content than green peppers. Furthermore, chili peppers are richer in these vitamins than sweet peppers at comparable stages of ripeness. Canned, cooked, and dried peppers contain significantly less vitamin C, but approximately the same amount of vitamin A as raw peppers (on a moisture-free basis.)

2. An average stuffed green pepper that weighs about 6½ oz (*185 g*) and is filled with a mixture of meat and bread crumbs is literally a nutritious meal in itself—supplying 314 kcal, 24 g protein, 78 mg calcium, 224 mg phosphorus, 477 mg potassium, 3.9 mg iron, 518 IU vitamin A and 74 mg of vitamin C.

3. A 3½ oz (*100 g*) portion of canned pimientos contains 27 kcal, 2,300 IU of vitamin A, and 95 mg of vitamin C. Hence, this item makes an excellent addition to preparations based upon cereal products, cheeses, eggs, fish, meats, legumes, and poultry because it supplies the vitamins not furnished by the other foods.

4. The chili sauces made from chili peppers (the ones designated as "Hot chili sauces") usually contain only about one-fifth as many calories as the mild sauces made from tomato puree. Furthermore, the vitamin A content of the former preparations is usually several times that of the latter ones (about 1,630 IU vitamin A per Tbsp. vs 238 IU vitamin A per Tbsp.).

5. A teaspoon of paprika furnishes 1,212 IU of vitamin A, compared to the 800 to 900 IU provided by the same amount of chili powder or red pepper.

6. Although it is not shown in Food Composition Table F-36, it is noteworthy that peppers are excellent sources of bioflavonoids.

(Also see VEGETABLE[S], Table V-6 Vegetables of the World.)

PEPSIN

The proteolytic enzyme present in the gastric juice. It acts on protein to form proteoses, peptones, and peptides.
(Also see DIGESTION AND ABSORPTION.)

PEPSINOGEN

The inactive precursor of pepsin, produced in the mucosa of the stomach wall and converted to pepsin by hydrochloric acid.
(Also see DIGESTION AND ABSORPTION.)

PEPTIDE BOND

The bond between carbon and nitrogen in the amide group, resulting in the elimination of water and formation of a CO.NH-linkage. Amino acids of proteins are joined in this manner.
(Also see PROTEIN[S].)

PEPTONE

An intermediate product of protein digestion.
(Also see DIGESTION AND ABSORPTION; and PROTEIN[S].)

PERILLARTINE

This is the purified oil component of the plant *Perilla namkinensis*. It was reported in 1920 to be 2,000 times sweeter than sugar. The oxime of perillartine is employed as a sweetening agent in Japan.
(Also see SWEETENING AGENTS.)

PERINATAL

The period from just before to about 100 hours after birth.

PERISTALSIS

An advancing wave of circular constriction preceded by an area of relaxation in the wall of the gastrointestinal tract. This advancing wave propels the food from the esophagus to the anus. It is similar to the action obtained by wrapping one's fingers tightly around a plastic tube of shampoo and then sliding the fingers forward to expel the shampoo that is forced forward in front of the fingers.
(Also see DIGESTION AND ABSORPTION.)

PERNICIOUS

Denoting a severe disease that is usually fatal.

PERNICIOUS ANEMIA

A severe form of anemia caused by a vitamin B-12 deficiency due to (1) inadequate amounts of B-12 in the diet or (2) lack of the intrinsic factor which is essential for the absorption of B-12. It is more common among strict vegetarians who do not eat any animal food, and among the aged who lack the intrinsic factor. Symptoms of the disease include inflammation of the tongue and mouth, degeneration of the nervous system and abnormal brain wave patterns.

Pernicious anemia was truly pernicious (fatal) until the 1920s, when it was discovered that symptoms were relieved by feeding large amounts of liver and liver extract. Today, the disorder is successfully treated by injecting vitamin B-12 intramuscularly.

(Also see ANEMIA, PERNICIOUS; and DEFICIENCY DISEASES, Table D-1 Major Dietary Deficiency Diseases—"Pernicious Anemia.")

PER ORAL

Administration through the mouth.

PER OS

Oral administration (by the mouth).

PEROXIDATION

Oxidation to the point of forming a peroxide—a compound (oxide) which contains an -0-0- group.

PEROXIDE VALUE

As fats decompose peroxides are formed. Chemically, peroxides are capable of causing the release of iodine from potassium iodide (KI). Therefore, the amount of iodine released from potassium iodide added to a fat is a rancidity test. The more peroxide present, the more iodine released; hence, the higher the peroxide value.

PERSIAN BERRY

The name given to the yellow to green dyes obtained from the native American fruits of the buckthorn family *Rhamnaceae*. Some of these berries are poisonous and have an extremely strong cathartic effect.

PERSIMMON, AMERICAN *Diospyros virginiana*

The fruit of a tree (of the family *Ebenaceae*) that grows wild in the eastern United States. It is grown on a small

scale in the South, where it is usually made into jam and jelly because it is more puckery (astringent) than the Japanese persimmon (*D. kaki*). The fruit is unpalatable

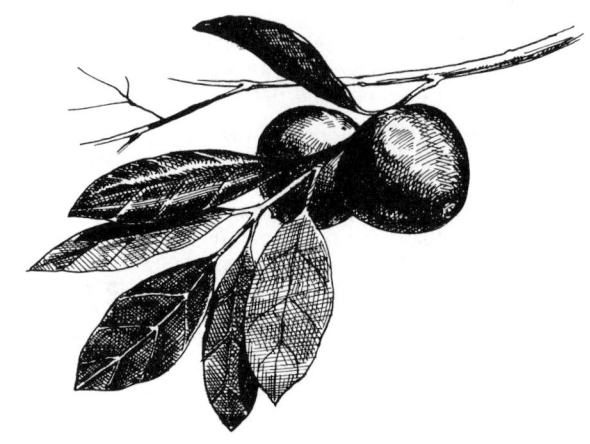

Fig. P-45.   The American persimmon.

unless it is allowed to ripen fully. The American persimmon is orange-yellow and ranges from 1 to 2 in. (*2.5 to 5 cm*) in diameter, which is smaller than the Japanese species.

The nutrient composition of the American persimmon is given in Food Composition Table F-36.

Some noteworthy observations regarding the nutrient composition of the American persimmon follow:

1.   The raw fruit is moderately high in calories (127 kcal per 100 g) and carbohydrates (33.5%).

2.   American persimmons are an excellent source of vitamin C and a good source of potassium.

(Also see FRUIT[S], Table F-47 Fruits of the World—"Persimmon"; and PERSIMMON, JAPANESE.)

PERSIMMON, JAPANESE (KAKI) *Diospyros kaki*

The fruit of a tree (of the family *Ebenaceae*) that is believed to have originated in China and Japan. It is now also grown in Japan, where it is the third most important fruit crop (after mandarin oranges and grapes), and in China, Korea, Hawaii, and California.

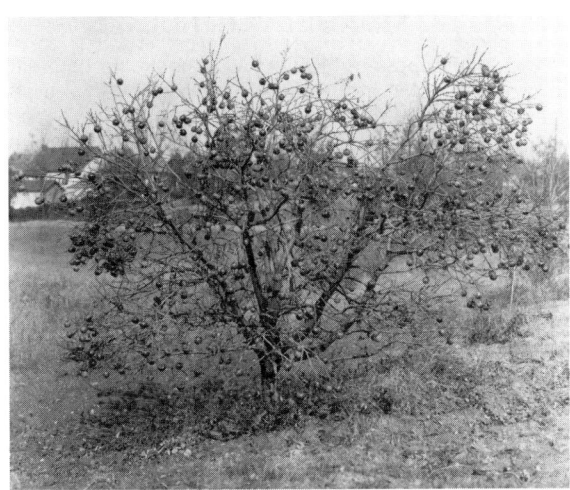

Fig. P-46. A Japanese persimmon (kaki) tree. (Courtesy, USDA.)

The Japanese persimmon is usually orange or red, apple-shaped, and from 2 to 3 in. *(5 to 7.5 cm)* in diameter. Japanese persimmons are not as puckery (astringent) as the native American persimmon. Hence, they may be eaten fresh.

The nutrient composition of the Japanese persimmon is given in Food Composition Table F-36.

Some noteworthy observations regarding the nutrient composition of the Japanese persimmon follow:

1. The raw fruit is moderately high in calories (77 kcal per 100 g) and carbohydrates (20%).

2. Japanese persimmons are an excellent source of vitamin A, a good source of fiber, and a poor to fair source of vitamin C.

(Also see FRUIT[S], Table F-47 Fruits of the World—"Persimmon"; and PERSIMMON, AMERICAN.)

PESTICIDES

Pesticides are chemicals used to destroy, prevent, or control pests of which there are six main groups: (1) insects including mites, ticks, and spiders; (2) snails and slugs; (3) vertebrates, including rats, mice, and certain birds; (4) weeds; (5) plant disease agents; and (6) nematodes. Also, pesticides include chemicals used to attract and repel pests, and chemicals used to regulate plant growth or remove or coat leaves.

When properly used, pesticides are beneficial; when improperly used, they may be hazardous.

As a result of pesticides—along with better technology, breeding better plants and animals, farm mechanization, and the greater use of fertilizers and growth regulators—U.S. consumers enjoy the world's most abundant food supply, with quality and variety second to none. Yet, pesticides can be toxic (poisonous) to man, other animals, and plants.

(Also see POISONS.)

PESTICIDES AS INCIDENTAL FOOD ADDITIVES

The use of synthetic chemical pesticides increased dramatically after World War II because these new materials were highly effective against many of the hundreds of pests attacking fruit and vegetables. It follows that increased American food output is in part due to increased pesticide use.

Some pesticides produce unplanned and undesirable side effects, particularly when they are not used properly. Among such effects are: reduction of beneficial species; drift; wildlife losses; honeybee and other pollinating insect losses; and pollution of air, soil, water, and vegetation. Farmers know that unless they follow federal and state regulations they risk having their products seized and condemned, or refused by food processors. It is, of course, essential that pesticide residues remaining on food following harvesting and processing be at levels that do not constitute a health hazard. Each pesticide is issued a tolerance for residues that may result from its use on food or feed crops. To this end, the Environmental Protection Agency (EPA) sets pesticide residue tolerances and the Food and Drug Administration (FDA) routinely monitors foods in an effort to enforce safe levels of pesticides on domestic food.

In recent years, several programs have evolved in both the public and private sectors to reduce the dependency on synthetic chemicals. These include:

1. Breeding by both traditional and bio-engineered methods for crop resistance to pests.

2. Integrated pest management, which stresses minimal use of pesticides.

3. Organic production, which eliminates all synthetic chemical pesticides.

4. Biological controls, which use either living organisms or toxic extracts from them.

5. Low input sustainable agriculture, which applies integrated pest management principles to all areas of crop production.

No pest control system is perfect; and new pests keep evolving. So, research and development on a wide variety of fronts should be continued. We need to develop safer and more effective pesticides, both chemical and nonchemical. In the meantime, there is need for prudence and patience.

(Also see POISONS, Table P-11 Some Potentially Poisonous [Toxic] Substances.)

PETITGRAIN OIL

An essential oil extracted from the leaves and twigs of the bitter orange tree, the lemon tree, or the tangerine tree. Petitgrain oils are employed for flavoring purposes and are on the GRAS (generally recognized as safe) list of approved substances.

(Also see ADDITIVES.)

pH

A measure of the acidity or alkalinity of a solution. Values range from 0 (most acid) to 14 (most alkaline), with neutrality at pH 7.

(Also see ACID-BASE BALANCE.)

PHAGOCYTE

A cell capable of ingesting bacteria or other foreign material.

PHAGOMANIA

An unusual or unreasonable fondness for eating.

(Also see APPETITE.)

PHEASANT

The pheasant, which originated in the Orient, is classed as both a game bird and an ornamental bird. Connoisseurs of this savory bird prefer hen pheasants about 1 year of age. Pheasants are similar to chickens; so, they may be processed and cooked in a similar manner.

PHENFORMIN

This drug slows the rate of glucose absorption from the intestine; hence, it results in (1) slowing the rise of blood sugar after meals, and (2) increasing the utilization of carbohydrates. Therefore, it is sometimes used in the treatment of diabetes mellitus. The disadvantages of phenformin are that its effects are short lived (4 to 6 hours), it may irritate the gastrointestinal tract, and, occasionally, it may be the cause of lacticacidosis. Hence, the dosage level of this drug has to be limited. However, it works well in combination with the sulfonylureas since the antidiabetic effects of the two agents are additive. Several brand names of phenformin are available. Brand names include Azucaps, D Bretard, Debeone, Debinyl, Diabis, Dibein, Dibiraf, Dibotin, Feguanide, Glucopostin, Glyphen, Inosal, Lentobetic, Normoglucina, Retardo.

(Also see DIABETES MELLITUS, section headed "Oral Drugs.")

PHENOL OXIDASES (PHENOLASES)

A group of copper-containing enzymes responsible for the browning of the cut surfaces of certain fruits and vegetables. Browning reduces the acceptability of a food due to the off-color and off-flavor. Depending upon the intended use of a food, five different methods may be employed to prevent enzymatic browning by the action of phenol oxidases: (1) heat inactivation, blanching; (2) chemical inhibition with sulfur dioxide; (3) reducing agents such as ascorbic acid; (4) exclusion of oxygen during packaging; and (5) alteration of the phenol oxidase substrates by adding another enzyme.

(Also see PRESERVATION OF FOOD.)

PHENYLALANINE

One of the essential amino acids.

(Also see AMINO ACID[S].)

PHENYLKETONURIA (PKU)

A rare inborn error in the metabolism of the essential amino acid phenylalanine. Affected individuals lack the liver enzyme phenylalanine hydroxylase which normally converts excess phenylalanine to the amino acid tyrosine. Hence, phenylalanine builds up in the blood, some of which is metabolized to phenylpyruvic acid, a keto acid which spills over into the urine. The disease derives its name from the appearance of this keto acid in the urine, which gives the urine a musty odor.

Infants appear normal at birth, but if the disease is untreated or undetected, symptoms such as irritability, hyperactivity, and convulsive seizures develop around 6 to 18 months of age. In addition, the infant will become moderately to severely mentally retarded. It is obvious that early detection is necessary for successful treatment. Fortunately most states require screening for PKU by a blood test or the "diaper test."

Treatment consists of a phenylalanine restricted diet. However, phenylalanine is an essential amino acid, and the diet must be planned to meet the requirement for phenylalanine without providing an excess. The diet must be continuously revised as the infant grows and the requirements change, and it must always provide an adequate intake of protein and energy. This is difficult since phenylalanine is present in all proteins. Therefore, a nutritionally complete synthetic preparation is given—a product that contains proteins low in phenylalanine, plus vitamins and minerals. The diet is supplemented by fruits, vegetables, and low protein cereals.

There is no real agreement as to what age dietary measures should be relaxed. Frequently, the restricted diet is discontinued about the time the child begins school. However, phenylketonuric women may require some restriction of phenylalanine during the childbearing years.

(Also see DISEASES, section headed "Congenital and Genetic Disorders"; and INBORN ERRORS OF METABOLISM.)

PHENYLPYRUVIC ACID

An intermediate product in phenylalanine metabolism.

PHEOPHYTIN

A waxy, olive-brown pigment which results from the treatment of chlorophyll with an acid such as oxalic acid. The magnesium atom in the chlorophyll molecule is replaced by two hydrogen atoms. This accounts for the color change when green vegetables are cooked.

PHOSPHATE BOND, ENERGY RICH

Energy is required for practically all life processes— for the action of the heart, maintenance of blood pressure, muscle tone, transmission of nerve impulses, kidney function, protein synthesis, fat synthesis, secretion of milk and muscular contraction. In the body, fats, proteins and carbohydrates represent potential energy sources. However, releasing all of the energy contained in these sources in one step would result in lost and wasted heat energy. Instead, energy is released in steps by a series of metabolic reactions. As the energy is released, it is captured and stored for use in the form of adenosine triphosphate (ATP). When this ATP is formed from ADP (adenosine diphosphate), 8 kcal/mole (molecular weight) must be put into the system. The ATP then acts as an energy rich storage compound. When energy is required for body functions, ATP is broken down to ADP and 8 kcal/mole of ATP are liberated.

(Also see METABOLISM.)

PHOSPHOLIPIDS

These are similar to triglycerides except one of the fatty acids attached to the glycerol molecule is replaced by phosphate and a nitrogen-containing compound. Lecithin, cephalin, phosphatidyl inositol and phosphatidyl serine are all classified as phospholipids. Functionally, phospholipids are (1) structural components of membranes; (2) potential energy sources; (3) involved in the blood clotting mechanism; and (4) components of certain enzymes.

(Also see FATS AND OTHER LIPIDS.)

PHOSPHOPROTEIN

A conjugated protein that contains phosphorus; for example, casein found in milk.

PHOSPHORUS (P)

Contents .... Page

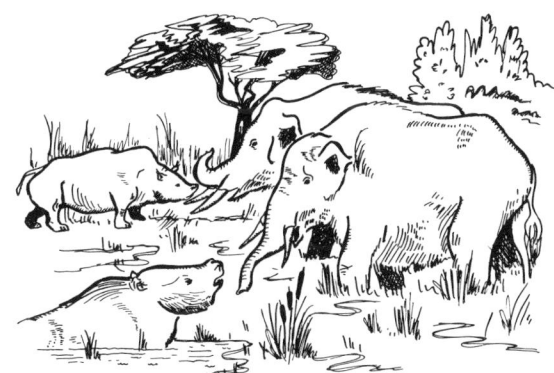

The era of phosphate formation

Fig. P-47. Primeval giants, such as rhinoceros (left) and mastodons (right) roamed Florida during the phosphate forming era.

Phosphorus is the Dr. Jekyll and Mr. Hyde of mineral elements—it can deal life or death. As white phosphorus, it's the flame of incendiary bombs; as red phosphorus, it's the heart of the common match; as organic phosphate, it's nerve gas and insecticides; and as organic combinations, it's a constituent of every cell and fluid of the body. Without phosphorus, no cell divides, no heart beats, and no baby grows.

Phosphorus is closely associated with calcium in human nutrition—to the extent that a deficiency or an overabundance of one may very likely interfere with the proper utilization of the other. Also, both calcium and phosphorus occur in the same major food source—milk; both function in the major task of building bones and teeth; both are related to vitamin D in the absorption process; both are regulated metabolically by the parathyroid hormone and calcitonin; both exist in the blood serum in a definite ratio to each other; and both, as the chief components of bone ash, were used in many ancient medieval remedies.

Phosphorus comprises about 1% or 1.4 lb (650 g) of the adult body weight. That's about ¼ the total mineral matter in the body. Eighty percent of the phosphorus is in the skeleton (including the teeth) in inorganic combination with calcium, where the proportion of calcium to phosphorus is about 2:1. The remaining 20% is distributed in the soft tissues, in organic combination, where the amount of phosphorus is much higher than calcium. In the soft tissues, it is found in every living cell, where it is involved as an essential component in inter-relationships with proteins, lipids, and carbohydrates to produce energy, to build and repair tissues, and to act as a buffer. Whole blood contains 35 to 45 mg of phosphorus per 100 ml; of this, about ½ is in the red cells, and, in adults, 2.5 to 4.5 mg per 100 ml is in the serum. In children, the serum phosphorus level is somewhat higher, ranging from 4 to 7 mg per 100 ml; the higher level during the growth years reflecting its role in cell metab-olism. Four to nine mg of the whole blood phosphorus is inorganic phosphorus, which is readily affected by dietary intake and is in constant exchange with the organic phosphate of the blood.

HISTORY. Phosphorus, a nonmetallic element, was first identified in urine by Hennig Brand, a German alchemist, in 1669. It created much interest because, in the unnatural free form, it glowed in the dark and took fire spontaneously upon exposure to the air. Eventually, the name phosphorus (from the Greek for "light-bringing") was appropriated to this element. Fortunately, phosphorus exists in nature only in combined forms, usually with calcium, in such sources as bone and rock phosphates.

ABSORPTION OF PHOSPHORUS. Phosphorus is more efficiently absorbed than calcium; 70% of the ingested phosphorus is absorbed and 30% is excreted in the feces, whereas only 20 to 30% of the ingested calcium is absorbed and 70 to 80% is excreted in the feces.

Since much of the phosphorus in foods occurs as a phosphate compound, the first step (prior to absorption) is the splitting off of phosphorus for absorption as the free mineral. The phosphorus is then absorbed as inorganic salts.

Phosphorus is absorbed chiefly in the upper small in-testine, the duodenum. The amount absorbed is depen-dent on several factors, such as source, calcium: phosphorus ratio, intestinal pH, lactose intake, and dietary levels of calcium, phosphorus, vitamin D, iron, aluminum, manganese, potassium, and fat. As is the case for most nutrients, the greater the need, the more effi-cient the absorption. Absorption increases, although not proportionally, with increased intake.

METABOLISM OF PHOSPHORUS. Phosphorus absorbed from the intestine is circulated through the body and is readily withdrawn from the blood for use by the bones and teeth during periods of growth. Some in-corporation into the bones occurs at all ages. It may be

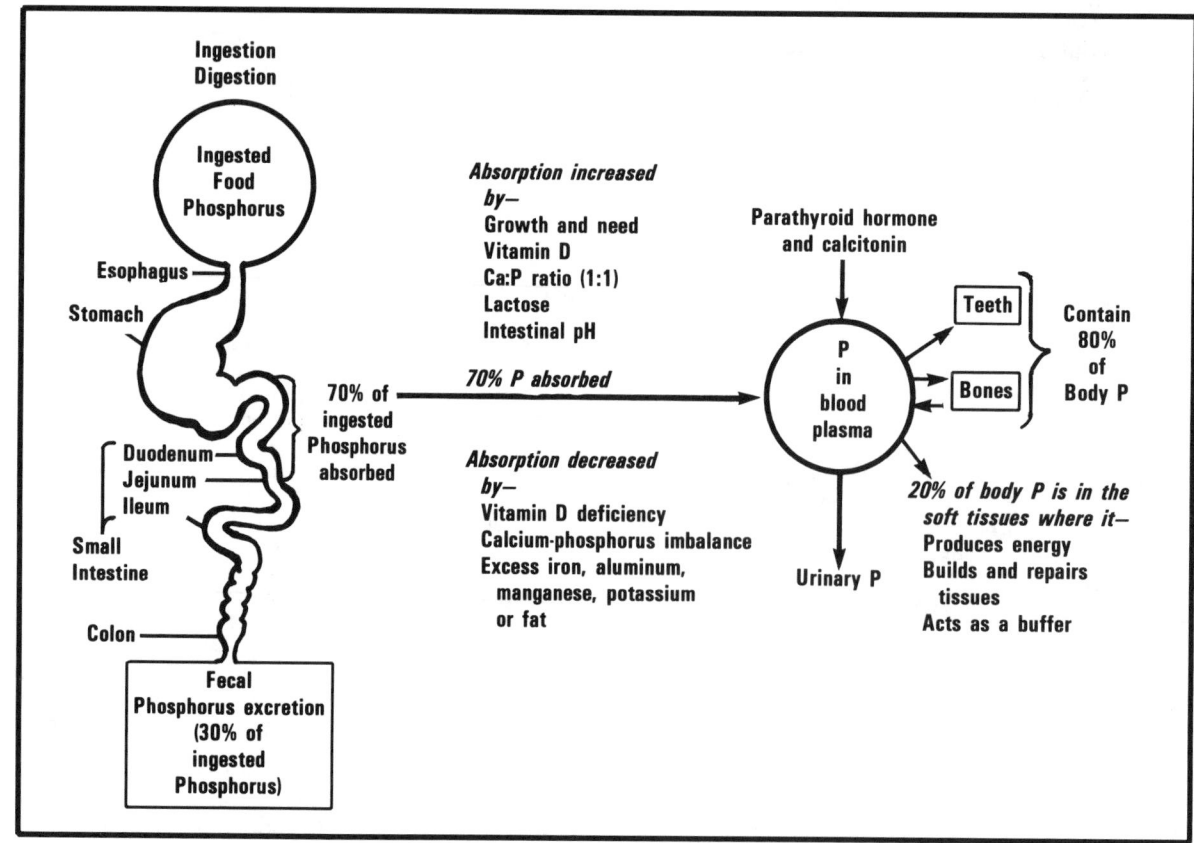

Fig. P-48. Phosphorus utilization. Note that healthy adults absorb 70% of the phosphorus in their food, and that 30% is excreted in the feces. Note, too, the factors that increase and decrease absorption.

withdrawn from bones to maintain normal blood plasma levels during periods of dietary deprivation.

The plasma phosphorus level (which generally falls within the range of 2.5 to 4.5 mg per 100 ml in adults—higher in children), along with calcium, is regulated by the parathyroid hormone and thyrocalcitonin (calcitonin) and is inversely related to the blood calcium level.

Phosphorus metabolism can be disturbed in many types of disease, notably those involving the kidneys and bone.

EXCRETION OF PHOSPHORUS. The kidneys provide the main excretory mechanization for regulation of the serum phosphorus level. All of the plasma inorganic phosphate is filtered through the renal glomeruli. If the serum phosphorus level falls, the renal tubules return more phosphorus to the blood; if the serum phosphorus level rises, the renal tubules excrete more. Also, when the diet lacks sufficient phosphorus, the renal tubules conserve phosphorus by returning it to the blood. On an average diet, an adult excretes from 0.6 to 1.0 g of phosphorus every 24 hours.

FUNCTIONS OF PHOSPHORUS. Among the mineral elements essential to life none plays a more central role than phosphorus. It is found throughout the body in every cell; and it is involved in almost all, if not all, metabolic reactions. Among the diverse and most important functions of phosphorus are the following:

1. It is essential for bone formation and maintenance.
2. It is important in the development of teeth.
3. It is essential for normal milk secretion.
4. It is important for building muscle tissue.
5. It is a component of the nucleic acids, RNA (ribonucleic acid) and DNA (deoxyribonucleic acid), which are important in genetic transmission and control of cellular metabolism.
6. It combines with other elements to maintain osmotic and acid-base balance.
7. It is important in many metabolic functions:

   a. **Energy utilization.** Carbohydrates, such as glucose, are absorbed from the intestinal mucosa as phosphorylated compounds. Glucose-6-phosphate and triose-phosphate are vital intermediates to the glucose scheme of energy metabolism. Energy transfer in most metabolic systems involves phosphate compounds such as ATP (adenosine triphosphate) and creatine phosphate.

   b. **Phospholipid formation.** This is one of the major means by which fatty acids are transported throughout the body.

   c. **Amino acid metabolism; protein formation.** Phosphorus is essential for amino acid metabolism and protein formation.

   d. **Enzyme systems.** Phosphorus is a component and activator of many key enzyme systems, including cocarboxylase, where it is combined with the vitamin, thiamin.

DEFICIENCY SYMPTOMS. Dietary deficiencies of phosphorus in man are unlikely, since this mineral is present in nearly all foods. However, deficiencies are seen in people in certain clinical conditions; in persons receiving excessive antacids over long periods, and in certain stress conditions such as bone fractures. Persons with deficiencies show general weakness, loss of appetite, muscle weakness, bone pain, demineralization of bone, and loss of calcium.

Vegetarian diets, especially those low in milk products, may be deficient in phosphorus as well as in other elements. In support of this concern, it is noteworthy that phosphorus deficiency is common among grazing animals in areas where the soil, and thus the forage, is very low in phosphorus. Afflicted animals become very emaciated and show loss of appetite and even a depraved appetite, frequently referred to as *pica*, which is exhibited by the eating of bones, wood, hair, dirt, and other materials to which they may have access.

Severe and prolonged deficiencies of phosphorus may be manifested in rickets and phosphorus related diseases (see subsequent section headed "Phosphorus Related Diseases").

INTERRELATIONSHIPS. Phosphorus is involved in certain relationships, the most important of which follow:

• **Calcium-phosphorus ratio and vitamin D**—Adequate phosphorus and calcium nutrition is dependent upon three factors: a sufficient supply of each element, a suitable ratio between them, and the presence of vitamin D. Generally, human nutritionists recommend a calcium-phosphorus ratio of 1.5:1 in infancy, decreasing to 1:1 at 1 year of age, and remaining at 1:1 throughout the rest of life; although they consider ratios between 2:1 and 1:2 as satisfactory. With plenty of vitamin D, the ratio becomes of less importance, and more efficient utilization is made of the amounts of the element present.

• **Excess of calcium over phosphorus; excess of phosphorus over calcium**—If the diet contains an excess of calcium over phosphorus (that is, more calcium than can be absorbed in the first part of the small intestine) free calcium will be present at the points where phosphorus is absorbed. This excess calcium will combine with the phosphorus to form insoluble tricalcium phosphate, and thus interfere with the absorption of phosphorus.

An excess of dietary phosphorus over calcium will in the same way decrease the absorption of both calcium and phosphorus.

• **Excess intakes of iron, aluminum, and magnesium**—Large intakes of iron, aluminum, and magnesium may bind phosphorus in insoluble salts and inhibit its absorption.

• **Phosphorus present as phytin or phytic acid**—There is evidence that man utilizes phytin phosphorus poorly—that phytin is incompletely broken down in the digestive tract. As a result, the undigested phytate may depress the absorption of calcium and iron.

RECOMMENDED DAILY ALLOWANCE OF PHOSPHORUS. The National Research Council recommended daily dietary allowances, with provision for individual variation, of phosphorus are given in Table P-6.

Note that the recommended daily allowances for phosphorus range from 300 mg to 1,200 mg. Note, too, that the allowances vary according to age.

**TABLE P–6
RECOMMENDED DAILY
PHOSPHORUS ALLOWANCES[1]**

Group	Age	Weight		Height		Phos-phorus
	(years)	(lb)	*(kg)*	(in.)	*(cm)*	(mg)
Infants ..	0.0–0.5	13	*6*	24	*60*	300
	0.5–1.0	20	*9*	28	*71*	500
Children .	1–3	29	*13*	35	*90*	800
	4–6	44	*20*	44	*112*	800
	7–10	62	*28*	42	*132*	800
Males ..	11–14	99	*45*	62	*157*	1,200
	15–18	145	*66*	69	*176*	1,200
	19–24	160	*72*	70	*177*	1,200
	25–50	174	*79*	70	*176*	800
	51+	170	*77*	68	*173*	800
Females .	11–14	101	*46*	62	*157*	1,200
	15–18	120	*55*	64	*163*	1,200
	19–24	128	*58*	65	*164*	1,200
	25–50	138	*63*	64	*163*	800
	51+	143	*65*	63	*160*	800
Pregnant						1,200
Lactating						1,200

[1]*Recommended Dietary Allowances*, 10th ed., 1989, NRC-National Academy of Sciences, p. 285.

The recommended allowance of phosphorus in milligrams per day is the same as that for calcium, except for the young infant.

The British report that a primary deficiency of phosphorus is not known to occur in man; hence, there is no recommended phosphorus intake in Britain.

• **Phosphorus intake in average U.S. diet**—The intake of phosphorus in ordinary diets is usually higher than that of calcium and is thought to be adequate.

In recent years, the widespread use of phosphate food additives (mainly sodium salts of orthophosphates, pyrophosphates, and polyphosphates) as acidifiers, emulsifiers, chelators, leavening agents, and water-binders has significantly increased the phosphorus content of the food supply. Such additives currently appear to contribute an additional 0.5 to 1.0 g phosphorus per day to the diet of U.S. adults.

The average available phosphorus for consumption per capita per day in the United States is approximately 1,540 mg, the primary sources of which are: dairy products, 34.3%; meat, poultry, and fish, 29.2%; and flour and cereal products, 14.1%. Thus, except for unusual circumstances, a deficiency in man is unlikely.

TOXICITY. There is no known phosphorus toxicity *per se.* However, excess phosphate consumption may cause hypocalcemia (a deficiency of calcium in the blood) and result in enhanced neuroexcitability, tetany, and convulsions.

PHOSPHORUS RELATED DISEASES. Phosphorus is present in nearly all foods, with the result that a dietary deficiency is extremely unlikely to occur in man. Intake of this mineral is almost always, if not invariably, higher than that of calcium and is entirely adequate under most conditions. However, phosphorus deficiencies may occur (1) when there is excess intake of nonabsorbable antacids, (2) when infants are on cow's milk, and (3) when vegetarians are on high fiber diets produced on phosphorus-deficient soils. Phosphorus related diseases include:

• **Rickets**—This is a children's disease, which may be caused by a lack of either phosphorus, calcium, or vitamin D; or an incorrect ratio of the two minerals.

• **Osteomalacia**—This is the adult counterpart of rickets. Osteomalacia is caused by a prolonged deficiency of phosphorus, calcium, and/or vitamin D; or an incorrect ratio of the two minerals.

• **Phosphorus depletion due to prolonged and excessive intake of nonabsorbable antacids**—The frequency of this syndrome is unknown. It is characterized by weakness, anorexia (reduced appetite), and pain in the bones. Treatment consists in discontinuing antacids and providing adequate dietary phosphorus.

• **Hypocalcemic tetany of infants**—Where infants are raised on cow's milk, the Ca:P ratio in cow's milk may contribute to the occurrence of hypocalcemic tetany during the first week of life. This postulation is based on the fact that the Ca:P ratio in cow's milk is approximately 1.2:1, compared with 2:1 in human milk. Because of this situation, the current recommendation is that in infancy the Ca:P ratio in the diet be 1.3:1, decreasing to 1:1 at 1 year of age.

• **Phosphorus deficiency of vegetarians on a high fiber diet produced on phosphorus-deficient soils**—Presently, this is without proof in humans, but there is abundant evidence that this condition occurs in animals.

Phosphorus deficiency is the most widespread and economically important of all mineral disabilities affecting grazing animals on high forage diets. There are two primary reasons for this: (1) The existence of soils low in available phosphorus throughout the world (including the United States), which, in turn, produce plants low in phosphorus content; and (2) the phosphorus deficiency in grass being accentuated by droughts and weathering.

Animals on phosphorus-deficient diets (characteristic of high forage rations produced on phosphorus-deficient soils) may show the following deficiency symptoms: decreased milk production, more milk fever, more breeding problems, lowered feed intake and efficiency, loss of appetite and unthriftiness, stiffness, fragile bones, retarded growth of young stock, and depraved appetite—chewing of wood, bones, hair, soil, and other objects.

At Washington State University, in a study with rabbits, the effect of soil phosphorus on plants, and, in turn, the effects of these plants on animals, was established.[10] Generation after generation, rabbits were fed on alfalfa, with one group receiving hay produced on low-phosphorus soils and the other group eating alfalfa grown on high-phosphorus soils. The rabbits in the low-

[10]Heinemann, W. W., M. E. Ensminger, W. E. Ham, and J. E. Oldfield, "Phosphate Fertilization of Alfalfa and Some Effects on the Animal Body," *Wash. Ag. Exp. Sta., Tech. Bull. 24*, June 1957.

phosphorus soil-alfalfa group (1) were retarded in growth—with 9.8% lower weaning weights, (2) required 12% more matings per conception, and (3) had a 47% lower breaking strength of bones than the rabbits on the high-phosphorus soil-alfalfa group. There is reason to believe that a phosphorus deficiency can affect people similarly, and that some people are consuming suboptimum levels of phosphorus—especially vegetarians on a high fiber diet produced on phosphorus-deficient soils.

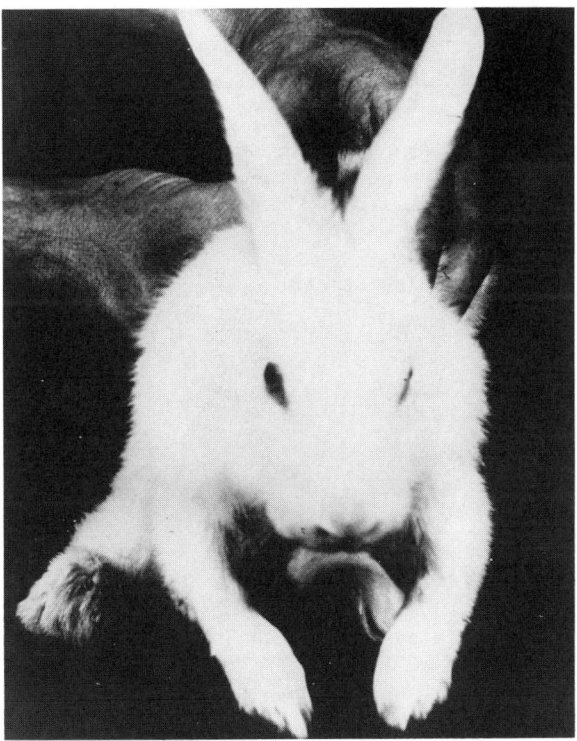

Fig. P-49. Rabbit with bowed legs and enlarged joints resulting from eating alfalfa produced on low-phosphorus soils. There is reason to believe that vegetarians on high fiber diets may suffer similar consequences. (Courtesy, Washington State University)

In addition to the conditions noted above, a phosphorus deficiency may also interfere with the utilization of vitamin A and, in growing children, teeth as well as bones will be less dense and less completely mineralized.

• **Excess phosphorus syndrome**—Excess phosphorus may also create problems. For example, an inhibitory effect of excess dietary phosphorus on bone development in domestic animals has long been recognized. Chronic ingestion of high phosphate diets causes secondary hyperparathyroidism, bone resorption, and, in some cases, calcification of kidney and heart tissue. The level of dietary phosphate required to produce these effects is dependent upon the concentrations of calcium, magnesium, and other ingredients. Excess phosphate also causes the effects of magnesium deficiency to be more severe and increases the intake of calcium required to maintain normocalcemia.

The demonstration that adult animals fed high phosphorus diets, even in the presence of normally adequate concentrations of calcium, undergo an enhanced rate of bone resorption and a net loss of bone mass has raised the possibility that diets high in phosphorus, particularly those that are concomitantly low in calcium, may contribute to "aging bone loss" or osteoporosis in man.

CALCIUM-PHOSPHORUS RATIO AND VITAMIN D. The proportional relation that exists between calcium and phosphorus is known as the calcium-phosphorus ratio. When considering the calcium and phosphorus requirements, it is important to realize that the proper utilization of these minerals by the body is dependent upon (1) a suitable calcium-phosphorus ratio (Ca:P), (2) an adequate supply of calcium and phosphorus in an available form, and (3) sufficient vitamin D to make possible the assimilation and utilization of the calcium and phosphorus. Generally speaking, a rather wide variation in Ca:P ratio in the diet is tolerated. However, nutritionists generally recommend a calcium-phosphorus ratio of 1.3:1 in infancy, decreasing to 1:1 at 1 year of age, and remaining at 1:1 throughout the rest of life; although they consider ratios between 2:1 and 1:2 as satisfactory. If plenty of vitamin D is present (provided either in the diet or by sunlight), the ratio of calcium to phosphorus becomes less critical. Likewise, less vitamin D is needed when there is a desirable calcium-phosphorus ratio.

It is noteworthy that there is much evidence indicating that calcium-phosphorus ratios of 1:1 to 2:1 for nonruminants (hogs and horses) and 1:1 to 7:1 for ruminants are satisfactory; but that ratios below 1:1 are often disastrous.

The dietary Ca:P ratio is particularly important during the critical periods of life—for children, and for women during the latter half of pregnancy and during lactation.

SOURCES OF PHOSPHORUS. Good sources are meat, poultry, fish, eggs, cheese, nuts, legumes, and whole-grain foods. It is noteworthy, however, that much of the phosphorus in cereal grains occurs in phytic acid, which combines with calcium to form an insoluble salt that is not absorbed. Vegetables and fruits are generally low in phosphorus.

Groupings by rank of common sources of phosphorus follow:

• **Rich sources**—Cocoa powder, cottonseed flour, fish flour, peanut flour, pumpkin and squash seeds, rice bran, rice polish, soybean flour, sunflower seeds, wheat bran.

• **Good sources**—Beef, cheeses, fish and seafood, lamb, liver, nuts, peanut butter, pork, poultry, whole grain flours.

• **Fair sources**—Breads and cereals, cottage cheese, dehydrated fruits, eggs, ice cream, kidneys, milk, molasses, most vegetables, mushrooms, sausages and luncheon meats, white flour, yogurt.

• **Negligible sources**—Fats and oils, juices and beverages, raw and canned fruits, some vegetables (lettuce, celery, carrots, tomatoes), sugar.

• **Supplemental sources**—Ammonium phosphate, bone meal, calcium phosphate, dicalcium phosphate, lecithin, monosodium phosphate, wheat germ (toasted), yeast (Brewers', torula).

For additional sources and more precise values of phosphorus, see Food Composition Table F-36.

TOP PHOSPHORUS SOURCES. The top phosphorus sources are given in Table P-7.

NOTE WELL: This table lists (1) the top sources without regard to the amount normally eaten (upper section), and (2) the top food sources (lower section). Note, too, that the calcium content, the calcium-phosphorus ratio, and the caloric (energy) content of each food is given.

TABLE P-7
TOP PHOSPHORUS SOURCES[1]

Top Sources[2]	Phosphorus	Calcium	Calcium-Phosphorus Ratio	Energy
	(mg/100 g)	(mg/100 g)	(Ca:P)	(kcal/100 g)
Baking powder, commerical[3]	10,505	1,677	.2:1.0	122
Fish flour from filet waste	4,060	6,040	1.5:1.0	305
Fish flour from whole fish	3,100	4,610	1.5:1.0	307
Baking powder, home use[4]	1,972	5,077	.4:1.0	102
Yeast, brewers', debittered	1,753	210	.1:1.0	283
Yeast, torula	1,713	424	.2:1.0	277
Rice, bran	1,386	76	.05:1.0	276
Whey, acid dry	1,348	2,054	1.5:1.0	339
Yeast, baker's, dry (active)	1,291	44	.03:1.0	282
Wheat bran, crude, commercially milled	1,276	119	.09:1.0	353
Cereal, bran/sugar and malt extract	1,176	70	.06:1.0	240
Pumpkin and squash seed kernels, dry	1,144	51	.04:1.0	553
Cottonseed flour	1,112	283	.3:1.0	356
Rice polish	1,106	69	.06:1.0	265
Wheat germ, toasted	1,084	47	.04:1.0	391
Milk, cow's, dry, nonfat, calcium reduced	1,011	280	.3:1.0	354
Milk, cow's, dry, skim, solids, instant	985	1,231	1.2:1.0	353
Cereal, bran/sugar and defatted wheat germ	977	73	.07:1.0	238
Eggs, chicken, dried, yolk	946	275	.3:1.0	687
Buttermilk, dried, made from skim milk	933	1,184	.8:1.0	387

Top Food Sources	Phosphorus	Calcium	Calcium-Phosphorus Ratio	Energy
	(mg/100 g)	(mg/100 g)	(Ca:P)	(kcal/100 g)
Wheat bran, crude, commercially milled	1,276	119	.09:1.0	353
Cereal, bran/sugar and malt extract	1,176	70	.06:1.0	240
Cheese, pasteurized process, American	745	616	.8:1.0	375
Soybean flour, defatted	655	265	.4:1.0	326
Cheese, natural, Swiss (domestic)	605	961	1.6:1.0	372
Liver, calf, fried	537	13	.02:1.0	261
Cheese, natural, Cheddar (domestic American)	510	718	1.4:1.0	402
Eggs, chicken, raw, yolks, fresh	508	152	.3:1.0	369
Almonds, dried, shelled, whole	504	234	.5:1.0	598
Sardines, Atlantic, canned in oil, drained solids, skin and bones	499	437	.9:1.0	203
Cheese, natural, Colby	456	685	1.5:1.0	394
Nuts, mixed, shelled	446	94	.2:1.0	626
Salmon, broiled or baked	414	—	—	182
Turkey, all classes, dark meat, cooked, roasted	400	30	.08:1.0	203
Wheat flour, whole (from hard wheats)	372	41	.1:1.0	361
Pork, fresh, loin, broiled	324	12	.04:1.0	391
Trout, cooked	272	218	.8:1.0	196
Herring, smoked, kippered	254	66	.3:1.0	211
Beef[5]	250	11	.04:1.0	250
Chicken, broiler/fryer, light meat, w/o skin, fried	231	12	.05:1.0	197

[1]These listings are based on the data in Food Composition Table F-36. Some top or rich food sources may have been overlooked since some of the foods in Table F-36 lack values for phosphorus.

Whenever possible, foods are on an "as used" basis, without regard to moisture content; hence, certain high-moisture foods may be disadvantaged when ranked on the basis of phosphorus content per 100 g (approximately 3½ oz) without regard to moisture content.

[2]Listed without regard to the amount normally eaten.

[3]Average for all commercial baking powders.

[4]Average for all home use baking powders.

[5]Includes lean choice stew meat, round cubes, round steak, cube steak, and sirloin steak.

The following pertinent deductions relative to the calcium-phosphorus ratios of, and contents in, some foods can be made from Table P-7:

1. Cheeses are rich in calcium but low in phosphorus.

2. Some fish have an acceptable calcium-phosphorus ratio, and are rich sources of both minerals.

3. Cottonseed, soy flour, and wheat flour have an imbalanced calcium-phosphorus ratio. They are fair sources of calcium, but extremely high in phosphorus. A desirable calcium-phosphorus ratio, along with adequate calcium and phosphorus, may be achieved by combining blackstrap molasses with each of these flours.

4. Meats and poultry are excellent sources of phosphorus, but poor sources of calcium. A desirable calcium-phosphorus ratio, along with adequate calcium and phosphorus, may be achieved by combining meats with vegetables which contain calcium.

5. Egg yolks are a fair source of calcium, but a rich source of phosphorus, resulting in a calcium-phosphorus imbalance.

If the diet is low in phosphorus, the element is usually added in the form of an inorganic salt such as monosodium phosphate, calcium phosphate, dicalcium phosphate, or ammonium phosphate.

(Also see MINERAL[S], Table M-67; and CALCIUM.)

PHOSPHORYLATE

To introduce a phosphate grouping into an organic compound; for example, glucose monophosphate produced by the action of phosphorylase.

PHOSPHORYLATION

The chemical reaction in which a phosphate group is introduced into an organic compound.

PHOTOSYNTHESIS

Life on earth is dependent upon photosynthesis. Without it, there would be no oxygen, no plants, no food, and no people.

As fossil fuels (coal, oil, shale, and petroleum)—the stored photosynthates of previous millennia—become exhausted, the biblical statement, "all flesh is grass" (Isaiah 40:6), comes alive again. The focus is on photosynthesis. Plants, using solar energy, are by far the most important, and the only renewable, energy-producing method; the only basic food-manufacturing process in the world; and the only major source of oxygen in the earth's atmosphere. Even the chemical and electrical energy used in the brain cells of man are the products of sunlight and the chlorophyll of green plants. Thus, in an era of world food shortages, it is inevitable that the entrapment of solar energy through photosynthesis will, in the long run, prove more valuable than all the underground fossil fuels—for when the latter are gone, they are gone forever. So, all food comes directly or indirectly from plants which have their tops in the sun and their roots in the soil. Hence, we have the nutrition cycle as a whole—from the sun and soil, through the plant, thence to animals and people, and back to the soil again. In summary form, the story is—

Green factories + 4-stomached animals $\xrightarrow[\text{(store)}]{\text{(convert)}}$ energy
(Plants)

Technically, green factories are known as photosynthetic plants, and 4-stomached animals are called ruminants; together, they convert and store energy in a form available to man. Not only that! They are relatively free from political control; they are universally available on a renewable basis; and, properly managed, they enhance the quality of the environment. Besides, they're free of cancer-laden carcinogens.

The energy required by every living creature, man included, is derived from the photosynthetic process occurring in green plants in which light energy from the sun is converted to chemical energy, then trapped in newly made sugar molecules.[11] Ultimately, all the energy in our food comes from this source.

Nearly 2,400 years ago, Aristotle postulated that plants withdrew food from the soil. For centuries this thinking, known as the "humus theory," prevailed; scholars believed that green plants derived all their nourishment from the organic materials of the soil. Finally, in about 1630, Jean van Helmont, a Belgian physician and experimental scientist, performed a revealing experiment which proved this belief false. He placed exactly 200 lb of completely dried soil into a vessel; planted a 5-lb willow shoot in the container; and added rainwater, but no fertilizer, to the soil at regular intervals. At the end of 5 years, he removed the willow tree, now grown large; carefully scraped the soil from the roots and returned it to the container; dried the willow tree and weighed it; and dried and weighed the soil. He found that the willow tree weighed 169 lb and 3 oz—a gain of approximately 164 lb during

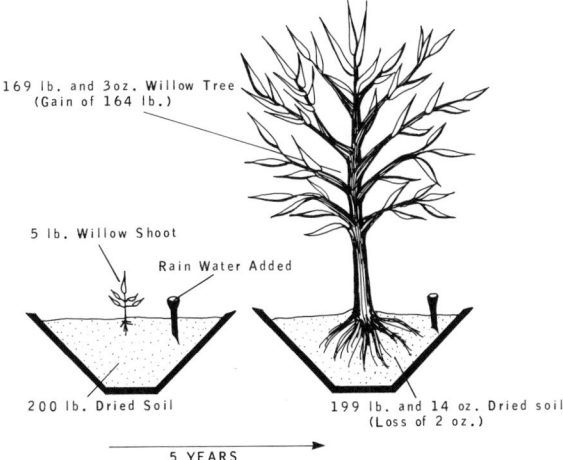

169 lb. and 3oz. Willow Tree
(Gain of 164 lb.)

5 lb. Willow Shoot

Rain Water Added

200 lb. Dried Soil

199 lb. and 14 oz. Dried soil
(Loss of 2 oz.)

5 YEARS

Fig. P-50. Diagram of van Helmont's willow shoot experiment.

[11]Certain types of microorganisms, termed chemoautotrophs, get their energy from inorganic compounds, but aside from this minor exception, the energy that runs the life support system of the biosphere comes from photosynthesis.

the 5-year period, and that the soil weighed 199 lb and 14 oz—indicating a loss of only 2 oz during the same period. Van Helmont concluded that the willow tree built its substance from water alone. This classic experiment proved the falsity of the humus theory, even though van Helmont's explanation was only partially correct, since he did not know of the role of carbon dioxide in the synthesis of organic matter by plants.

More than 100 years later, the English clergyman and chemist, Joseph Priestley, did his classical experiment work with air. He reasoned that the food produced in plants must have something to do with air. To prove his point, in a celebrated experiment, he placed a green plant under an airtight glass container, a live mouse under another, and both a green plant and a live mouse under a third. Within a few days, the isolated plant and the isolated mouse were dead. But the mouse and the plant, placed together, remained alive and thrived. From this and other work, Priestley surmised that breathing exhausted the air, whereas plants revitalized it.

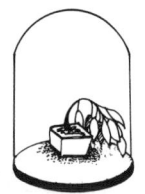 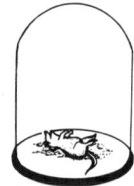 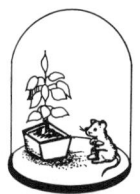

1) DEAD PLANT   2) DEAD MOUSE   3) LIVE GREEN PLANT
                                     & LIVE MOUSE

Fig. P-51.   Diagram of Joseph Priestley's classic experiment showing the relationship of air, plants, and mice.

A contemporary of Priestley's, the Dutch physician, Jan Igenhousz, demonstrated that when plants were exposed to light, they made their own food. He also showed that this occurred in the green portion of the plant.

A summary of these early contributors to our present-day knowledge of photosynthesis is presented in the following formulas:

Aristotle
(384-322 B.C.)   Soil ——→ Food in
                                            Plants

Van Helmont   Water ——→ Food in
(A.D. 1577-1644)   Plants

Priestley H_2O + Exhausted ——→ Food in + Revitalized
(A.D. 1733-1804)   Air   Plants   Air

Igenhousz H_2O + Exhausted ─Light→ Food in + Revitalized
(A.D. 1730-1799)   Air   Green   Plants   Air
                                 Portion
                                 of the
                                 Plant

And so it went! Scientists probed deeper and, in one discovery after another, brought to light and added many new details to the basic information left to us at the beginning of the 19th century. For example, it was learned that Priestley's exhausted air was carbon dioxide, and that his revitalized air was oxygen.

But more than two centuries elapsed after van Helmont's experiment before the concept of chemical energy developed sufficiently to permit the discovery (in 1845) that light energy from the sun is stored as chemical energy in products formed during photosynthesis. Subsequent studies added to the store of knowledge. Today, scientists know that green plants fashion most of their solid materials from the water of the soil and the carbon dioxide of the air through the process of photosynthesis, and that green plants absorb relatively small amounts of solid substances (mineral nutrients) from the soil.

The word photosynthesis means putting together with light. More precisely, photosynthesis may be defined as *the process by which the chlorophyll-containing cells in green plants capture the energy of the sun and convert it into chemical energy; it's the action through which plant synthesize and store organic compounds, especially carbohydrates, from inorganic compounds—carbon dioxide, water, and minerals, with the simultaneous release of oxygen.*

Photosynthesis is dependent upon the presence of chlorophyll, a green pigment which develops in plants soon after they emerge from the soil. Chlorophyll is a chemical catalyst—it stimulates and makes possible certain chemical reactions without becoming involved in the reaction itself. By drawing upon the energy of the sun, it can convert inorganic molecules, carbon dioxide (CO_2) and water (H_2O), into an energy-rich organic molecule such as glucose ($C_6H_{12}O_6$), and at the same time release free oxygen (O_2). It transforms solar energy into a form that can be used by plants, animals, and man. Because of this capability, chlorophyll has been referred to as the link between nonliving and living matter, or the pathway through which nonliving elements may become part of living matter.

Through the photosynthetic process, it is estimated that more than a billion tons of carbon per day are converted from inorganic carbon dioxide (CO_2) to organic sugars ($C_6H_{12}O_6$—glucose), which can then be converted into carbohydrates, fats, and proteins—the three main groups of organic materials of living matter.

Photosynthesis is a series of many complex chemical reactions, involving the following two stages (see Fig. P-52):

Stage 1 —The water molecule (H_2O) is split into hydrogen (H) and oxygen (O); and oxygen is released into the atmosphere. Hydrogen is combined with certain organic compounds to keep it available for use in the second step of photosynthesis. Chlorophyll and light are involved in this stage.

Stage 2—Carbon dioxide (CO_2) combines with the released hydrogen to form the simple sugars and water. This reaction is energized (powered) by ATP (adenosine triphosphate), a stored source of energy. Neither chlorophyll nor light is involved in this stage.

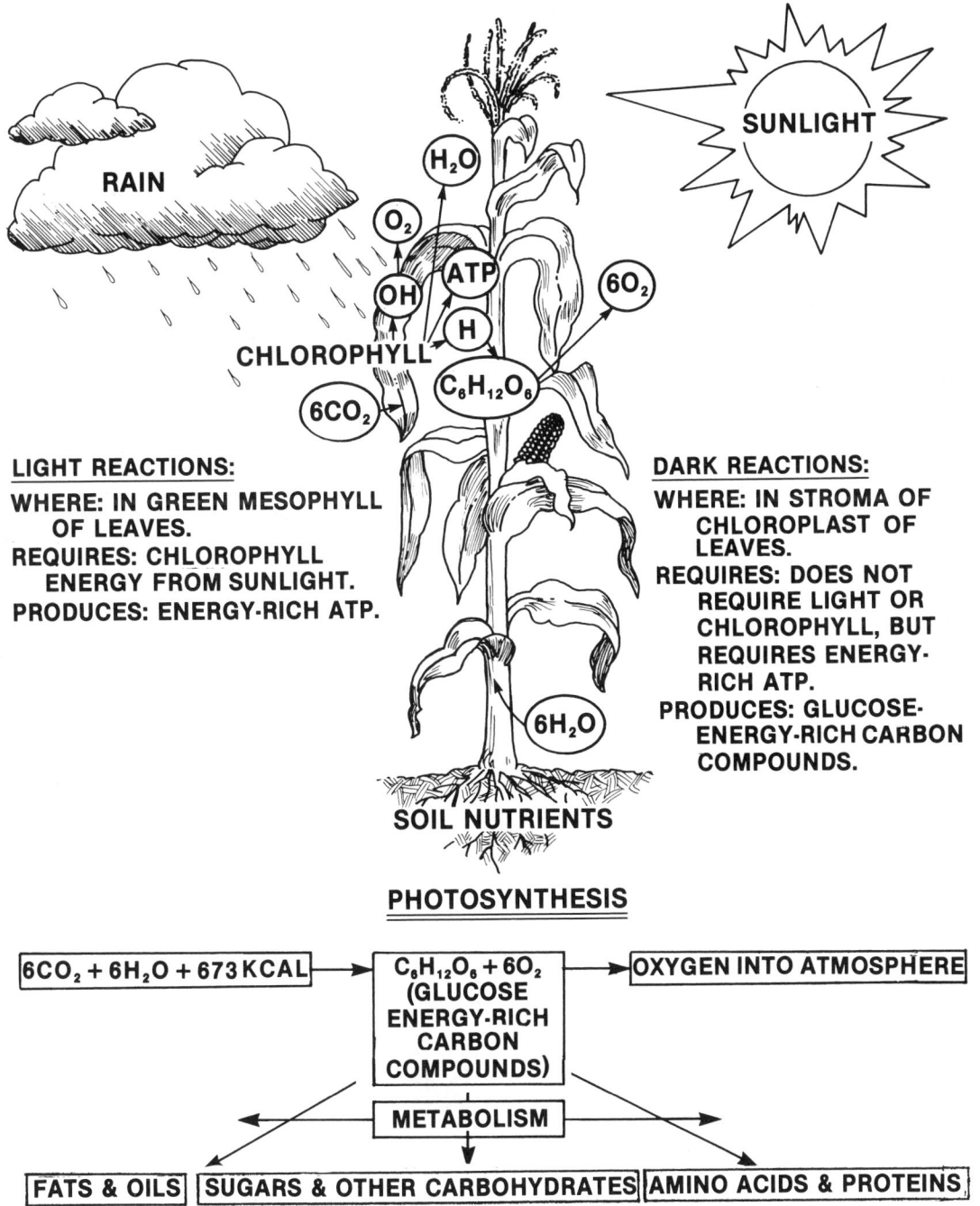

PHOTOSYNTHESIS

LIGHT REACTIONS:

WHERE: IN GREEN MESOPHYLL OF LEAVES.
REQUIRES: CHLOROPHYLL ENERGY FROM SUNLIGHT.
PRODUCES: ENERGY-RICH ATP.

DARK REACTIONS:

WHERE: IN STROMA OF CHLOROPLAST OF LEAVES.
REQUIRES: DOES NOT REQUIRE LIGHT OR CHLOROPHYLL, BUT REQUIRES ENERGY-RICH ATP.
PRODUCES: GLUCOSE-ENERGY-RICH CARBON COMPOUNDS.

$$6CO_2 + 6H_2O + 673\,KCAL \longrightarrow C_6H_{12}O_6 + 6O_2 \text{ (GLUCOSE ENERGY-RICH CARBON COMPOUNDS)} \longrightarrow OXYGEN\ INTO\ ATMOSPHERE$$

METABOLISM

FATS & OILS | SUGARS & OTHER CARBOHYDRATES | AMINO ACIDS & PROTEINS

Fig. P-52.   Photosynthesis fixes energy. Diagrammatic summary of (1) photosynthesis, and (2) the metabolic formation of organic compounds from the simple sugars. This diagram shows the following:
1.   Carbon dioxide gas from the air enters the green mesophyll cells of plant leaves.
2.   Plants take up oxygen from the air for some of their metabolic processes and release oxygen back to the air from other metabolic processes.
3.   Plants take up water and essential elements from the soil.
4.   The energy essential to photosynthesis is absorbed by chlorophyll and supplied by sunlight.
5.   For a net input of 6 molecules of carbon dioxide and 6 molecules of water, there is a net output of 1 molecule of sugar and 6 molecules of oxygen.
6.   The process is divided into light and dark reactions, with the light reactions building up the energy-rich ATP required for the dark reactions.
7.   In the process, 673 Calories (kcal) of energy are used.
8.   The sugar (glucose) manufactured in photosynthesis may be converted into fats and oils, sugars and other carbohydrates, and amino acids and proteins.

The chemical reactions through which chlorophyll converts the energy of solar light to energy into organic compounds is one of nature's best-kept secrets. Man has not been able to unlock it, as he has so many of life's other processes. Moreover, photosynthesis is limited to plants; animals store energy in their products—meat, milk, and eggs—but they must depend upon plants to manufacture it. Additional facts pertinent to an understanding of photosynthesis follow:

1.   During the earth's very long geological past, green plants, growing in warm climates in the presence of more carbon dioxide than the atmosphere now contains, grew faster than they were consumed. As a result, vast quantities of carbon, in the form of organic matter now represented by the fossil fuels (coal, oil, shale, and petroleum), accumulated beneath the earth's surface. The combustion of these fuels provides much of the energy now used in homes, factories, and transportation.

2.   Photosynthesis is an energy-requiring process, which uses light as the source of energy. Hence, it can occur only when light shines upon green plant tissues.

3.   Plant species and genetics (the inherited set of directions) determine whether or not a plant will form high or low levels of specific proteins, carbohydrates, minerals, vitamins, etc. For example, alfalfa always contains more calcium than corn even though they grow side by side.

4.   Environmental factors—including the amount of sunlight, the temperature of the air and of the soil, the humidity of the air, and the moisture content of the soil—may also have an important bearing on the concentration of nutrients in a plant. The impact of environmental factors on plant nutrients is of concern to nutritionists, as evidenced by the following example: The amount of vitamin C in a ripening tomato is primarily controlled by the amount of sunlight that strikes the tomato.

5.   Physiological factors of plants—health, maturity, and whether or not the plant is a flower—also exert an effect on the rate of photosynthesis.

From the above, it is apparent that the concentration in plants of the different nutrients required by man is controlled by several processes that depend on the genetics of the plant, the fertility of the soil, and the environment in which the plant grows. Any one of these factors may affect the level of different essential nutrients or of toxic substances in foods.

A classic example of a "green factory" is sugarcane. The cut cane is moved to the mill, where it is crushed and separated into juice and bagase; thence, the juice is made into sugar and alcohol. The growing and milling of sugarcane constitute a self-contained "energy factory." Here's how: The plants capture and store the energy of the sun as sugar and cellulose (bagasse); the energy in bagasse is used to power the mill and generate surplus electricity; and two concentrated energy products, sugar and alcohol, are made from the juice.

Although photosynthesis is vital to life itself, it is very inefficient in capturing the potentially available energy. Of the energy that leaves the sun in a path toward the earth, only about half ever reaches the ground. The other half is absorbed or reflected in the atmosphere. Most of that which reaches the ground is dissipated immediately as heat or is used to evaporate water in another important process for making life possible. Only about 2% of the earthbound energy from the sun actually reaches green plants, and only half of this amount (1%) is transformed by photosynthesis to energy storage in organic compounds. Moreover, only 5% of this plant-captured energy is fixed in a form suitable as food for man.

With such a small portion of the potentially useful solar energy actually being used to form plant tissue, it would appear that some better understanding of the action of chlorophyll should make it possible to increase the effectiveness of the process. Three approaches are suggested: (1) increasing the amount of photosynthesis on earth, (2) manipulating plants for increased efficiency of solar energy conversion, and (3) converting a greater percentage of total energy fixed as chemical energy in plants (the other 95%) into a form available to man. Ruminant (4-stomached) animals are the solution to the latter approach: they can convert energy from such humanly inedible plant materials as grains and other high-energy feeds and protein supplements, crop residues, pasture and range forages, and harvested forages into food for humans (see Fig. P-53). Also, it is noteworthy that animals do not require fuel to graze the land and recover the energy that is stored in the grass. Moreover, they are completely recyclable; they produce a new crop each year and perpetuate themselves through their offspring. It would appear, therefore, that there is more potential for solving the future food problems of the world by manipulating plants for increased solar energy conversion ("genetic engineering") and by using ruminants to make more plant energy available to man than from all the genetic and cultural methods combined.

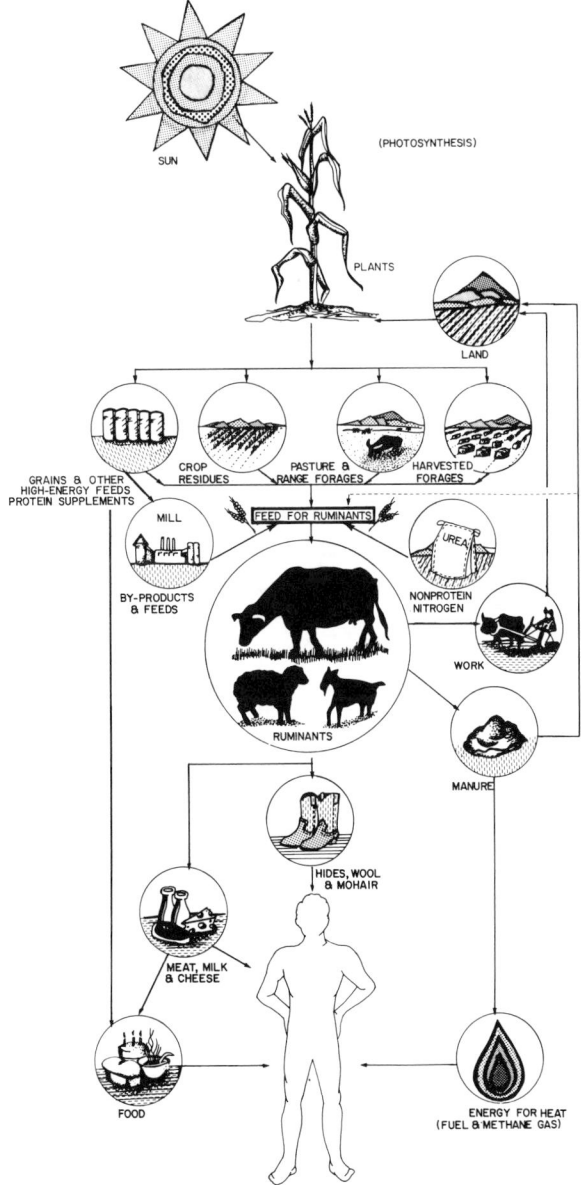

Fig. P-53. Ruminants step up energy. Their feed comes from plants which have their tops in the sun and their roots in the soil. Hence, we have the nutrition cycle as a whole—from the sun and soil, through the plant, thence to the ruminant (and man) and back to the soil again.

PHRYNODERMA *Follicular hyperkeratosis*

A skin condition that is often associated with a vitamin A deficiency. However, it is not a specific manifestation of vitamin A deficiency. In general, it is encountered in malnourished individuals. It is sometimes referred to as "toad-skin" since there is atropy of the subaceous glands resulting in the formation of dry papules with protruding cornified plugs. These lesions appear on the buttocks, arms and legs.

(Also see DEFICIENCY DISEASES, Table D-2 Minor Dietary Deficiency Disorders—"Follicular hyperkeratosis, toad skin or phrynoderma.")

PHYLLOQUINONE

A form of vitamin K—K_1, which occurs in nature and is fat soluble.
(Also see VITAMIN K.)

PHYSICAL ACTIVITIES

The need for continuous, quick and strenuous movement of the body—physical activity—has declined over the years in our society. From youth to old age, we now spend most of our time engaged in moderate to very light activities. However, there has been a heightened interest in the need for physical activity coupled with sound nutrition as the two chief components of health.

The following major points indicate the need for physical activities:

1. Physical activity more than any other body process raises the body's energy requirements, and thus provides a means of weight maintenance and weight reduction.

2. Muscular tone and strength are increased by physical activity. This includes the heart and blood vessels.

3. A psychological benefit is derived from physical activities; it provides an outlet for tension and restlessness, and gives the individual a sense of well-being.
(Also see CALORIC [ENERGY] EXPENDITURE; and PHYSICAL FITNESS AND NUTRITION.)

PHYSICAL FITNESS AND NUTRITION

Many people equate fitness with the ability to perform either athletically or in feats of endurance and strength. However, health professionals consider it to be much broader in scope and to include functions such as (1) performance of work and other physical activities, (2) resistance to degenerative and infectious diseases, and (3) adaptation in beneficial ways to emotional and physical stresses.

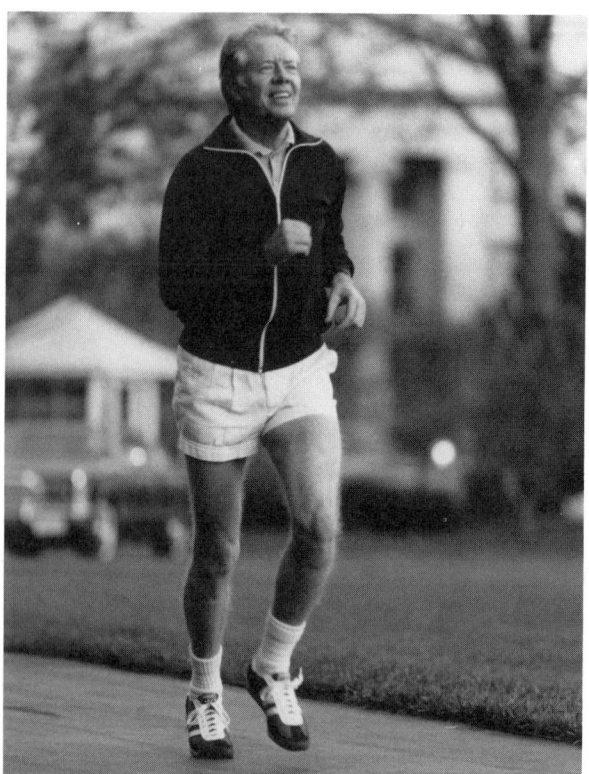

Fig. P-54. When he was President, Jimmy Carter kept fit by jogging. (Courtesy, Karl Schumacher of the Carter White House)

Therefore, the treatment of nutrition as it relates to athletics is presented elsewhere in this book.

(Also see ATHLETICS AND NUTRITION.)

Today, our survival depends not only upon our personal fitness, but upon that of our leaders and various other people upon whom we depend (such as airline pilots, doctors, nurses, etc.).

THE AGE-OLD STRUGGLE TO SURVIVE.

Although there have been many speculations, it is difficult to determine whether the almost legendary peoples of prehistoric times would have rated high on our present day measures of fitness since our relics of the past consist mainly of a few pieces of weathered bones and artifacts, such as stone tools and drawings on the walls of certain caves. Many anthropologists believe that, prior to the establishment of the first settled agricultural communities, small bands of nomadic peoples roamed the earth in search of the wild animals and plants that were edible.

Although it is now quite certain that the first humans shared the meats, fish, and birds obtained by hunting, only the strongest members of the group survived to mate and reproduce themselves because considerable vigor was required to cope with the rugged conditions of life. For example, it seems likely that babies who grew poorly on their mother's milk were allowed to die, and the older people whose strength had waned were left behind to starve or become the prey of animals.

The first agricultural communities were apparently established between 10,000 and 12,000 years ago. Since then, the world population has increased by leaps and bounds. However, evidence unearthed by archaeologists suggest that the average level of fitness of farming cultures in some parts of the world were inferior to that of nomads because the farmers were hampered by (1) survival of sickly infants and older people that would have died under the rigors of nomadism, (2) more mouths to be fed from a limited supply of food, and (3) a reduced variety of foods due to dependence upon those produced within the vicinities of the settlements. These circumstances apparently induced the agricultural peoples to invent implements and develop practices that helped them to obtain much more food from the available lands and waters.

In time, the need for physical strength and endurance lessened as the more developed societies came to rely increasingly on craftsmanship and mental ability to meet their needs. It seems likely, that the early civilizations in Babylon, China, Egypt, and India were the first cultures to have considerable numbers of obese people since less effort was required to obtain the necessities of life. The political and religious leaders of these ancient societies often recognized the dangers that resulted from their people growing soft since barbaric neighboring groups were likely to invade and conquer them. This concern has been passed down to us through the ages in the accounts of the rise and fall of various civilizations presented in our history books. Hence, our present leaders and well-informed people everywhere continue to search for means of improving the fitness of themselves and their fellow humans so that we may benefit from the lessons of the past.

PHYSICAL FITNESS AROUND THE WORLD.

Each time and place requires certain types of fitness for survival. Other types may not be as essential under some circumstances. For example, people living in the tropics have to be able to tolerate high temperatures, but they rarely have need for resistance to chilling. Therefore, people who are seeking models of fitness with which to pattern their lives should pick ones that correspond closely to their own circumstances.

Some examples of exceptionally fit peoples in recent times and in various parts of the world are given in Table P-8.

TABLE P-8
HEALTHY PEOPLE OF THE WORLD

Group of People	Time, Place, and Observer	Cultural Characteristics	Comments
Bulgarians	During the early 1900s, in the rural areas of Bulgaria, by the Russian microbiologist, Elie Metchnikoff.	Peasant farmers who consumed liberal amounts of yogurt, cereals and grain products, vegetables, and limited amounts of meats, poultry, fish, and eggs appeared to be vigorous and long lived.	Metchnikoff theorized that the *Lactobacilli* in yogurt prevented the growth of harmful toxin-producing bacteria in the intestine.
Canadian Indians	In the 1930s, in northern Canada near the Arctic Circle by the American dentist and anthropologist, Weston Price.	Hunting and fishing tribes remained in good health despite scarcity of plant foods because they consumed certain mineral- and vitamin-rich tissues of animals and fish.	Iodine was obtained from the thyroid glands of male mooses, vitamin A from fish heads, and vitamin C from adrenal glands and a brew made from the growing tips of pine or spruce trees.
Equadorians of Vilcabamba	Visits in the early and late 1970s, to Vilcabamba in the Andes of southern Ecuador, by the American gerontologist, Alexander Leaf.	Subsistence farmers living at 4600 ft *(1400 m)* who had a low caloric intake from mainly vegetable foods. The older people, most of whom smoked, appeared to have been healthy.	Reports of very long-lived Vilcabambans appear to have been exaggerated due to confusion over the names listed in baptisimal records.
Eskimos of the Arctic	Throughout the 1900s by many American and foreign researchers.	The groups that still live the hunting and fishing life have an exceptionally high aerobic capacity[1]. Females retain their strength longer than males because their activity is sustained, whereas the males have bursts of activity interspersed with periods of inactivity.	Eskimos who live in settlements and eat the white man's food develop rampant tooth decay, a diabeticlike blood sugar, tuberculosis, and arteriosclerosis.
Georgians and neighboring peoples of the U.S.S.R.	After World War II to the present, in the southern Caucasus mountains of the Soviet Union, by investigators from around the world.	These workers on the Soviet collective farms eat dairy products, meats, plenty of vegetables, and some sweets such as halvah. Their culture emphasizes strong family ties, strict discipline, and fortitude in performing difficult tasks. Premier Josef Stalin (1879-1953) was born in the Georgian republic.	Although the Georgians were once thought to be the longest-lived people on earth, it now appears that ages were exaggerated in order to avoid military service under the Czars and Soviets. Furthermore, aged people are regarded highly in the U.S.S.R.
Hunzas of Pakistan	Throughout the 1900s, in the Himalayas of northeastern Pakistan, by explorers, medical teams, and others from various countries of the world.	These people use primitive agricultural techniques to grow fruits and vegetables on a mountainous terrain. They rarely have meat and dairy products and are rather lean and agile due to the combination of a scarcity of food and strenuous physical activity.	The vigorous old Hunzas represent the survivors of very rigorous living conditions, since 30% of the children die before age 10, and an additional 10% die before age 40.
Masai tribesmen of Africa	From the time of European colonization in Africa to the present, in the Great Rift Valley of Kenya and Tanzania, by people from many countries.	Nomadic cattle herdsmen that live mainly on the blood, milk, and occasionally meat from their animals. They are tall and slender and walk from 10 to 12 mi per day. Their aerobic capacities match those of champion athletes.	Few Masai men develop heart disease because any atherosclerosis which develops in their coronary arteries is offset by the exercise-induced enlargement of the blood vessels.

Footnote at end of table.

(Continued)

TABLE P-8 (Continued)

Group of People	Time, Place, and Observer	Cultural Characteristics	Comments
Mormons	During the 1970s, public health surveys were made in Alameda County, California and in the state of Utah.	Beneficial practices include abstinence from alcohol, coffee and tea, and smoking; consumption of whole grain products, fruits, vegetables, and limited amounts of meat; adequate work, recreation, and rest; family harmony; and an extensive involvement in church affairs.	Mormons have ⅓ fewer cancer deaths and from ⅓ to ½ fewer fatal heart attacks than other Americans. Also, many stay active in business, farming, and church affairs well into their 80s and 90s.
Polish farmers	In the 1970s, in selected agricultural and industrial regions in Poland.	People living in the low mountains of South Poland were well-fed, performed heavy physical work, and lived in a favorable climate.	The people of the mountains retained their fitness much longer than other Poles who lived in various rural and industrial regions.
Seventh-Day Adventists	From the 1950s to the 1970s various investigators studied disease rates in American Adventists.	Most of the people in this group are lacto-ova-vegetarians, who abstain from alcohol, coffee, tea, and smoking. They also have above average concern for health and fitness, and many engage in exercise on a regular basis.	Adventist men live an average of 6 years longer than other American men, and the women live 3 years longer than their counterparts. The death rates from cancer, heart disease, and stroke among Adventists are only 50 to 60% of those for other Americans.
Swiss dairy farmers	During the 1930s, in the Loetschental Valley in Switzerland, by the American dentist and anthropologist, Weston Price.	This group of dairy farmers and their families consumed considerable amounts of the milk and cheeses produced from cows grazed on lush alpine meadows.	These people appeared to be strong and healthy. Furthermore, many of the Pope's Swiss Guards have come from this region.
Tarahumara Indians	At various times from the 1960s to the present, in the Sierra Madre mountains of northwestern Mexico, by various health- and sports-minded investigators.	These people are exceptionally good runners and have unusually high aerobic capacities. Their diet is mainly vegetarian.	Only a small percentage of Tarahumaras survive to adulthood (80% of the children die before age 5). Hence, the survivors represent those with very strong constitutions.

'The aerobic capacity is the volume of oxygen which can be inspired per units of body weight and time.

It may be seen from Table P-8 that the health practices of some of the fittest groups of people around the world are characterized by (1) diets comprised of fresh, minimally processed foods, such as meats and fish, dairy products, fruits and vegetables, and whole grain breads and cereals; (2) limited consumptions of potentially harmful items such as strong alcoholic drinks, coffee and tea, and refined fats, starches, and sugars; and (3) engagement in moderate to vigorous physical activities.

IMPORTANT ASPECTS OF PHYSICAL FITNESS. Although good overall fitness is to be desired by everyone, the particular circumstances that are unique to each person's life make it necessary to emphasize certain aspects, such as those which follow:

Ability to Perform Physical Work. Certain types of jobs, such as construction work, firefighting, the harvesting of crops, military combat, and police work, require considerable physical exertion. Therefore, it is noteworthy that both the maximum rates of performing work and the times during which maximum performance may be sustained tend to decline with increasing age. Some quantitative data on this decline which was obtained in a study of U.S. military personnel is shown in Figs. P-55 and P-56.

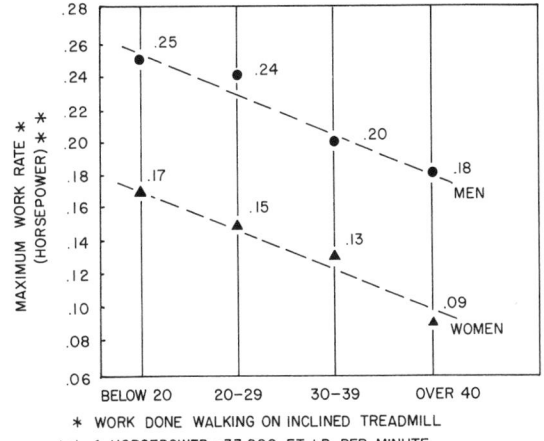

Fig. P-55. Decline in the maximum work rate with age. (Based on data from Consolazio, C. F., et al, "Nutritional Status in Relation To Work Performance, Body Composition and Age," *Proceedings of the Seventh International Congress of Nutrition*, Hamburg 1966, Friedrich Vieweg & Son, Braunschweig, West Germany, Vol. 4, p. 5, Table V)

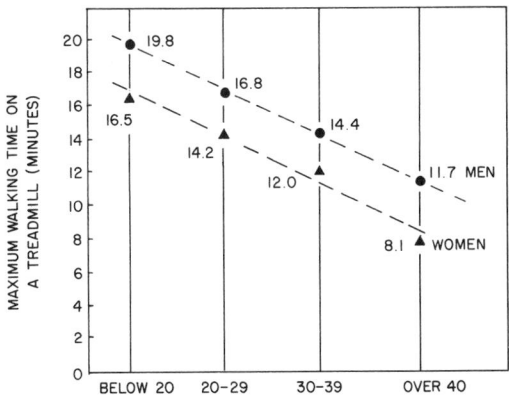

Fig. P-56. Decline in maximal work time with age. (Based on data from Consolazio, D. F., et al, "Nutritional Status in Relation to Work Performance, Body Composition and Age," *Proceedings of the Seventh International Congress of Nutrition*, Hamburg 1966, Friedrich Vieweg & Son, Braunschweig, West Germany, Vol. 4, p. 5, Table VI)

Figs. P-55 and P-56 show that the declines in maximal work performances occurred at about the same rates for men and women. Perhaps, the levels of physical activity over the years were too low to maintain high levels of fitness, since the body fat content of men aged 45 to 49 was double that of men under 20. Furthermore it appeared that muscle mass was lost steadily over the years, since most of the gain in body fat occurred while there was little or no gain in body weight. Other groups of people, such as Masai tribesmen and certain Polish farmers

(see Table P-8, Characteristics of Exceptionally Fit Groups of People Around the World), retain their endurance and strength much longer. Hence, rather strenuous activity may be required on a steady basis to retard the deterioration in work capacity that often occurs during adulthood.

Athletic Prowess. Many sports require agility, speed, and sufficient strength to make the required movements without excessive strain on the various organs and tissues. Therefore, the athletes who perform best owe their success to factors such as (1) development of the requisite neuromuscular coordination, (2) optimal cardiovascular functioning, (3) a high aerobic capacity, (4) well developed muscles, (5) a minimal accumulation of excess body fat, and (6) willpower to persevere.

It is generally believed that optimal nutrition somehow enhances these performance factors although hard data is often difficult to obtain since the effects of mediocre nutrition may not be evident in early adulthood. (Most athletes attempt to eat a moderately good diet, but some are food faddists.) Furthermore, some athletes are sufficiently motivated to achieve high level performances while in poor health. Finally, the most stressful events have usually attracted young adult competitors because most older working adults have little opportunity to engage in the requisite training. Fortunately, increased opportunities for the participation of older adults have developed recently, as certain "master's class" events have been established. Research studies of these older participants have provided a few insights into the prolongation of vigor through diet and exercise.

(Also see ATHLETICS AND NUTRITION.)

Bearing of Healthy Children. Even primitive tribes have long recognized the importance of the maternal diet to the successful outcome of pregnancy, as evidenced by the practices which follow:

1. Eskimos, Peruvian Indians, Polynesians, and other peoples living near the sea or inland lakes gave expectant mothers fish eggs and other aquatic foods.
2. Dairying tribes in Africa did not allow young women to marry until the season when the cattle were fed on lush, green pastures.
3. Papuans of New Guinea reserved special foods such as dried large snakes for their expectant mothers.

Fortunately, mothers-to-be may now skip the fish eggs and snakes since much is known about meeting the nutritional requirements with other types of foods.

(Also see PREGNANCY AND LACTATION NUTRITION.)

Emotional Well-Being. For many people, peace of mind depends upon their feeling well, since symptoms of an illness may provoke anxiety, depression, and other distressful emotions. Recent research on the effects of diet on the nervous system has shown that mental depression may also arise from a subnormal brain content of the nerve transmitter, serotonin, which in turn may result from (1) lack of sufficient amounts of the amino acid tryptophan in the diet, or (2) excessively high levels of dietary fat and/or protein that interfere with the entry of tryptophan into the brain where it is converted to serotonin. Another factor which affects the emotional state and sense of well being is the level of blood sugar, since the brain requires a continuous supply of glucose for optimal functioning, and subnormal blood sugar makes many people feel poorly. Hence, erratic and imbalanced dietary patterns may be responsible for poor mental health.

In general, people who are physically fit appear to be more optimistic and more able to accomplish both mental and physical tasks. Hence, they may have a greater sense of self-sufficiency than those who have let themselves become weak, flabby, and overly dependent on others. For example, the attitudes of male executives who were very anxious about their jobs improved markedly after they started on a program of jogging and other exercises.

Sometimes, the emotional well-being and ability to work are also impaired by chronic disorders such as adrenal cortical insufficiency, allergies, anemia, depression, high or low blood pressure, hypochondriasis (an exaggerated sensitivity to minor discomfort that may be accompanied by unfounded fear of developing a deadly disease), insufficient flow of blood to the brain, nutritional deficiencies, and thyroid diseases. Therefore, a person who feels poorly much of the time should see a doctor to rule out the possibility of a chronic disease before resorting to the excessive use of stimulants such as caffeine and various mood elevating drugs.

Mental Acuity.   This type of fitness is closely related to overall physical fitness because the brain and nerves are very sensitive to changes in the blood chemistry. For example, the performance of tasks which require mental and sensory acuity is enhanced by meal patterns which maintain the blood sugar level at normal throughout the day. Skipping breakfast or having only coffee in the morning usually lowers the quality of work. Other dietary factors, particularly those relating to depression and emotional well being are also important.

Notable changes in a person's mental acuity may result from conditions or factors such as alcoholism, antihypertensive drugs, atherosclerosis, chronic stress, dehydration, depression, diabetes, fatigue, head injuries, insuffient blood flow to the brain, low blood pressure, low blood sugar (hypoglycemia), nutritional deficiencies, sedative or tranquilizer drugs, small strokes, and starvation. Sometimes these possibilities have been overlooked and the patient has been diagnosed as neurotic, psychotic, or senile and confined to an institution. However, some amazing improvements have resulted from the proper types of corrective measures.

Resistance to Infectious Diseases.   Both under nutrition and overnutrition impair the functioning of the body defenses against infection which are collectively called the immune system. Similarly, immunity may be reduced in disorders such as cancer and diabetes; and during severe emotional stress. Finally, some people fail to obtain the immunizations which are now available.

Scientists are now exploring the interactions between these and other factors that affect immunity. For example, there is evidence that the production of optimal immunity requires ample amounts of dietary selenium, zinc, vitamin A, and vitamin C; but only moderate amounts of dietary calories and proteins. Too little or too much of the latter nutrients may impair the functioning of the body's defense system. Hence, it should be possible in the near future to promote optimal functioning of the immune system by a balanced program of dietary measures, immunizations, medical treatment, and psychological counseling.

Slowing of the Physical Decline in Adulthood. Mental and physical faculties must be used fully, but wisely, if they are to be kept operative at high levels of performance throughout adulthood. Furthermore, a vigorous life style helps to prevent obesity, which may hasten physical decline if not corrected soon enough. Finally, the progress of the various degenerative diseases that impair the faculties can be retarded by the proper diet and the use of corrective therapies when needed. This means that regular physical examinations and laboratory tests should be obtained to detect any early warning symptoms of degenerative diseases. It might also be a good idea to have tests of physical performance such as aerobic capacity and endurance.

Some of the symptoms that warrant dietary modification and/or other types of therapies are: diabetic glucose tolerance; high blood levels of cholesterol, triglycerides, and/or uric acid; low blood levels of hemoglobin, iron, red cells, and/or certain vitamins; and subnormal capacity for physical exertion, as evidenced by an electrocardiogram or stress testing on an exercise bicycle or a treadmill. Means of correcting these problems are described in the sections that follow.

DIETARY GUIDELINES.   In order to be certain of obtaining sufficient amounts of each of the required nutrients, one should consult a table showing the best food sources of these essential substances, such as the one given in Table N-6 of this encyclopedia.

Furthermore, meals can be planned with the aid of a food guide that groups commonly used items according to the nutrients which are furnished (see Food Groups).

Finally, it appears that it would be beneficial to the fitness of many Americans to eat more food for breakfast and less at the evening meal. For example, breakfast should contain one or more sources of animal protein such as cheese, eggs, milk products, and meats, plus ample amounts of fresh fruit and whole grain breads or cereals. Lunch should also contain a good source of proteins, plus a milk product, one or more vegetables and whole grain bread. When two good meals have already been consumed, supper may consist of only small servings of protein foods with a bread or a cereal product, plus a large serving of vegetables in a salad or a freshly prepared soup. (Most canned soups have rather high salt contents, which may be harmful to people with tendencies to retain fluids and develop congestive heart failure or high blood pressure.)

(Also see FOOD GROUPS; NUTRIENTS: REQUIREMENTS, ALLOWANCES, FUNCTIONS, SOURCES; and RDA.)

Modified Diets and Nutritional Supplements.
The decision to make a radical change in one's dietary pattern should not be made without first consulting a doctor and/or a dietitian because many factors have to be considered before the appropriate changes can be made. For example, it may be dangerous for people with a family history of gout to lose weight rapidly.

PHYSICAL ACTIVITY AS AN ADJUNCT TO DIETARY PRACTICES. The need for following a carefully controlled diet is lessened somewhat by exercising enough to burn off at least 300 to 500 extra Calories (kcal) daily. Fig. P-57 shows that women who engaged in recreational physical activities were able to keep trim while consuming more calories than those whose activity levels were lower.

Physical activity is also valuable as a means of rehabilitation from various degenerative conditions. For example, the cardiovascular fitness of seven patients with heart disease was improved greatly by a 6-week program of intensive physical training that was supervised by doctors.[12]

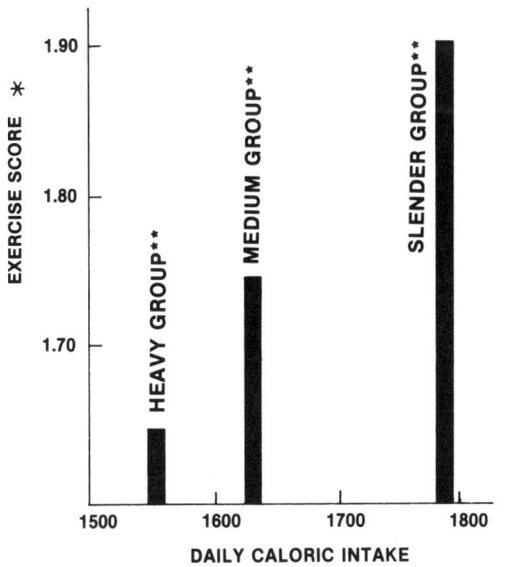

* AVERAGES OF REPORTED RECREATIONAL ACTIVITY (LITTLE OR NONE = 1, MODERATE = 2, MUCH = 3)

** ASSESSMENT OF BODY FATNESS FROM AVERAGE MEASUREMENTS OF TRICEPS SKINFOLD (13.5 MM = SLENDER, 20.8 MM = MEDIUM, 30.8 MM = HEAVY)

Fig. P-57. The effects of caloric intake and recreational exercise on a measure of body fatness in women. (Based on data from Habicht, J-P, testimony before the U.S. House of Representatives Committee on Science and Technology, July 28, 1977, p. 376, Fig. 2)

[12]Redwood, D.R., *et al.*, "Circulatory and Symptomatic Effects of Physical Training in Patients with Coronary Artery Disease and Angina Pectoris." *The New England Journal of Medicine*, Vol. 286, 1972, pp. 959-965.

SUMMARY. Studies around the world have shown that most people can remain fit well into middle age and beyond, providing that they consume a wholesome diet and engage in sufficient exercise. In fact, it is even possible to have a dramatic recovery from disabling heart disease when suitable measures are taken.

PHYSIOLOGICAL SALINE

A salt solution (0.9% NaCl) having the same osmotic pressure as the blood plasma.

PHYTATE

A salt or ester of phytic acid containing inositol and phosphates as the base; they are especially abundant in the outer layers of cereal grains. Phytates decrease the absorption of calcium from the intestine.
(Also see PHYTIC ACID.)

PHYTIC ACID

It is a hexaphosphoric acid ester of inositol present mainly in cereal grains, nuts, and legumes.
(Also see MINERAL[S], section headed "Naturally Occurring Mineral Antagonists in Foods.")

PHYTOCHEMICALS

Phytochemical ("phyto" is derived from the Greek word for plant) is a new term embracing a host of plant chemicals which offer hope and help for the prevention of cancer. They are abundant in fruits and vegetables. In the mid-1990s, the race was on to find, isolate, and study them; hopefully, to find a magic pill that would go beyond vitamins.

Among the multitude of phytochemicals, their sources, and their claims, are the following:

• **Allylic sulfide**—Plentiful in onions and garlic, which detoxifies carcinogens.

• **Capsaicin**—Abundant in hot peppers, which keeps toxic molecules from attaching to DNA.

• **Ellagic acid**—Present in strawberries, grapes, and raspberries, which neutralizes carcinogens before they can invade DNA.

• **Flavonoids**—Present in berries, citrus, yams, and cucumbers, which keeps cancer-causing hormones from attaching to the surface of cells.

• **Genistein**—Abundant in soybeans, which prevents breast, prostate, and other lumps from growing and spreading.

• **Indole-3-carbinol**—Present in cauliflower and cabbage, seems to lessen breast cancer by acting on a precursor to the female hormone estrogen and producing a harmless form of estrogen rather than the form linked to breast cancer.

- **P-coumaric acid and chlorogenic acid**—Found in many fruits and vegetables, including tomatoes, green peppers, pineapples, strawberries, and carrots, which prevents the formation of cancer-causing nitrosamines from nitric acids and amines.

- **Phenethyl isothiocyanate (PEITC)**—Found in cabbage and turnips, which inhibits lung cancer.

- **Sulforaphane**—Found in broccoli, cauliflower, Brussels sprouts, turnips, and kale, which lessens breast cancer in animals.

But phytochemicals are not omnipotent! Remember, too, that lifelong vegetarians get cancer. Much more research is needed before the role of phytochemicals can be established. In the meantime, a balanced diet, including fruits and vegetables, is recommended for buoyant good health.

PICA

An abnormal craving of appetite for substances not usually considered food—starch, clay, hair, dirt, chalk, and wood.

(Also see APPETITE; CISSA; and GEOPHAGIA.)

PIGMENTATION

This refers to melanin, the pigment which imparts color (1) to the skin, hair, and eyes, and (2) to bile and blood.

In sunburn, the skin darkens due to the ultraviolet rays of the sun. In albinos, melanin is absent. Certain skin diseases manifest excessive or unevenly distributed pigment, including freckles, liver spots, melanosis, vitiligo, and leukoderma.

Bile and blood color are due to melanin formed in the body. The two main bile pigments are bilirubin (red) and biliverdin (green). The red blood pigment is hemoglobin, from which the pigments hemosiderin, methemoglobin, bilirubin, and biliverdin are derived.

PIG SOUSE (PIG'S-FOOT JELL)

Made from pig's feet (free from hair and with toes removed), along with hearts, tongues, and shoulder hocks, by boiling in water until the meat separates from the bones; removing the bones; cutting the meat into small chunks; placing the meat back in the broth in which it was cooked; seasoning to taste with salt, pepper, and vinegar; pouring into shallow pans and setting away to chill and jell.

PINEAPPLE *Ananas comosus*

Pineapple is a tropical plant, which grows from 2 to 3 ft *(61 to 91 cm)* tall, and produces a fruit weighing 4 to 8 lb *(2 to 4 kg)*. Leaves of the plant are blue-green and sword shaped. They grow around a thick stem. In some varieties the leaves have sharp spines along the edges. When plants are 14 to 16 months old, a flower stalk with tiny flowers attached—an inflorescence—appears in the

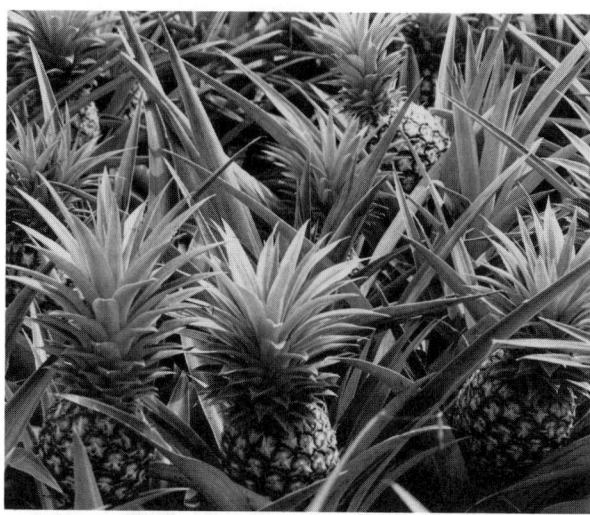

Fig. P-58. Pineapples almost ready for harvesting. Pineapples are a combination of numerous fruitlets that present the appearance of a large pinecone. (Courtesy, Maui Pineapple Company, Ltd., Kahului, Maui, Hawaii)

center. It resembles a pink-red cone. Shortly thereafter, numerous blue-violet flowers bloom for 1 day each, all blooming within 20 to 30 days. Each of these flowers forms a fruitlet, whose fleshy parts unite with the stalk. This combination of 100 or more fruitlets and stalk forms the yellow center of the pineapple. A thick, hard, yellowish-brown shell forms on the outside. The shell is developed from leaflike structures called floral bracts. The fruit is topped with a group of small leaves called the crown.

The edible flesh of the pineapple is firm, pale yellow or white, and the flavor is a mixture of sweetness and tartness. Its flavor has been described as apple, strawberry, and peach mingled all at once.

ORIGIN AND HISTORY. Pineapples are native to South America, possibly originating in Brazil. Columbus observed pineapples on the island of Guadelupe in 1493. Eventually, exploring Europeans took the curious fruit home and grew it in hothouses during the 1700s. In Europe, it became a favorite fruit of the wealthy and royalty; and attempts were made to improve the plant. Then, from the mid-1800s to the early 1900s pineapple plantations were established in tropical colonies; in Australia, the Azores, South Africa, and Hawaii. Pineapples were produced in Florida from the 1860s until about 1914.

PRODUCTION. Worldwide, an average of 9.7 million metric tons of pineapple are produced each year. Thailand is the leading producer. The United States also ranks among the top producers, though pineapples are only produced in Hawaii.

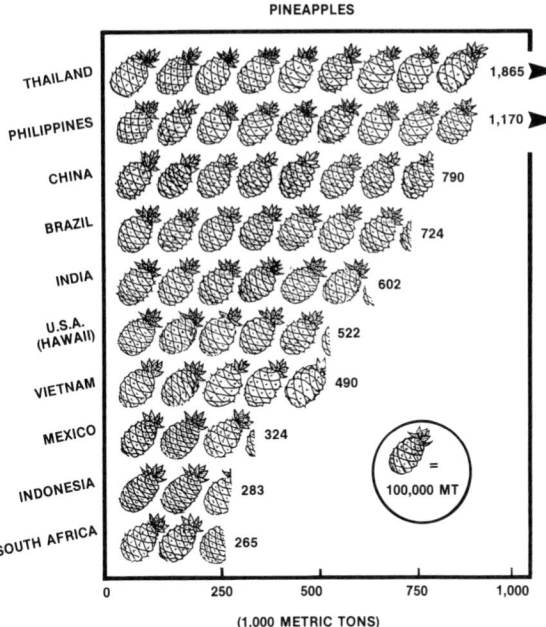

THAILAND 1,865
PHILIPPINES 1,170
CHINA 790
BRAZIL 724
INDIA 602
U.S.A. (HAWAII) 522
VIETNAM 490
MEXICO 324
INDONESIA 283
SOUTH AFRICA 265

= 100,000 MT

0   250   500   750   1,000

(1,000 METRIC TONS)

Fig. P-59. Leading pineapple-growing countries of the world. (Based on data from *FAO Production Yearbook*, 1990, FAO/UN, Rome, Italy, Vol. 44, pp. 167–168, Table 73)

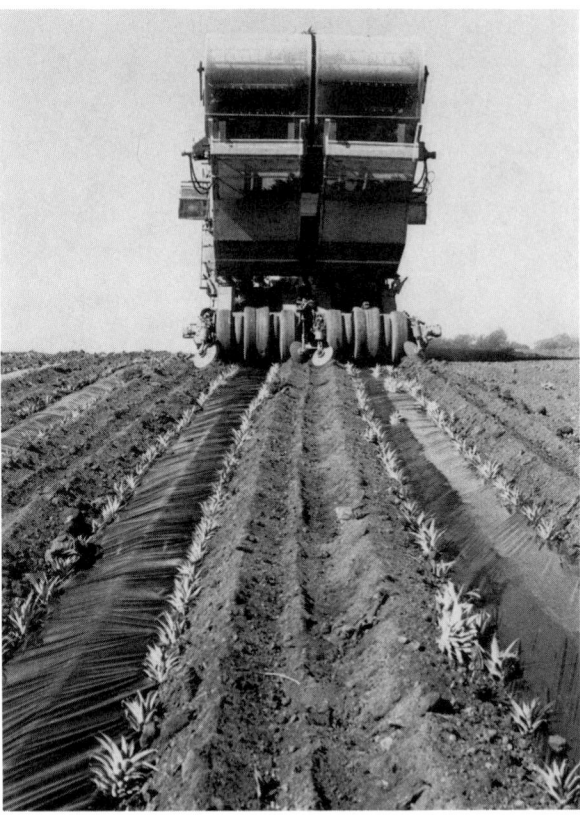

Fig. P-60. Mechanical planter planting crowns from the fruit for the next pineapple crop. Note the strips of black plastic which conserve moisture, warm the soil, and discourage weed growth. (Courtesy, Maui Pineapple Company, Ltd., Kahului, Maui, Hawaii)

Propagation and Growing. Pineapples are propagated from any of three parts of the plant: (1) shoots, (2) slips, and (3) crowns. Shoots or suckers grow from the main stem just beneath the soil or between the lower leaves. Slips grow from the stem just below the fruit. Crowns are the group of small leaves on the top of the fruit. Most pineapple produce seedless fruit, though wild forms were quite seedy.

Prior to planting, the land is plowed deeply, fertilized, and chemicals may be used to kill harmful worms called nematodes. In Hawaii strips of black plastic are laid along the rows at the time of planting. This prevents chemicals from escaping, conserves moisture, warms the soil, and discourages weed growth.

Pineapples grow well in semiarid conditions. Too much water is detrimental to pineapples.

The basis of most commercial crops is the "Cayenne" variety, which have sharp spines only on the tips rather than all along the edges of the leaves.

After about 20 months of growing, pineapples are ready for harvesting. During the first year of production, each plant produces only one pineapple, but each plant may bear 2 or 3 fruits on the second and third harvest.

However, with each harvest the fruits are smaller, and most growers replant fields after 2 or 3 harvests, though plants may be productive for 8 to 10 years.

Harvesting. Ripe pineapples are hand picked by breaking or cutting the stem just below the fruit. Hand harvesting is necessary since all pineapples do not ripen at the same time. However, harvesting has been mechanized as far as possible. A conveyor belt built into a long boom, which extends over many rows, is pulled through the field by a tractor. Pickers, wearing heavy clothing and gloves, walk behind the boom selecting ripe pineapples and placing them on the conveyor belt. The conveyor transports them to a truck, which drives through the field alongside the harvester-conveyer.

In many countries, pineapple harvesting is not as mechanized. Pickers walk through fields and place fruits in large baskets strapped to their backs or in canvas bags carried over their shoulder.

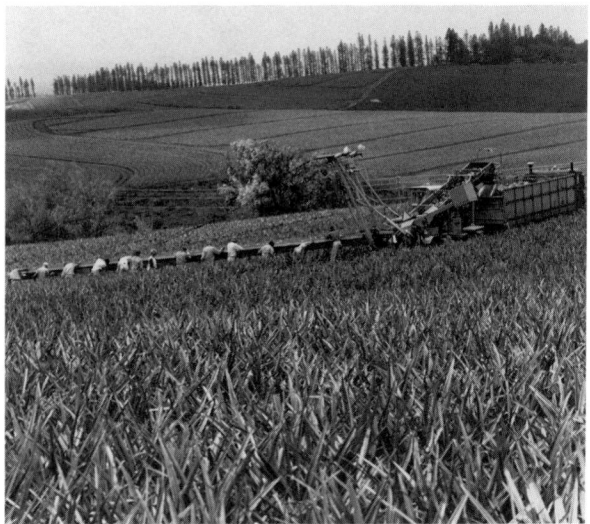

Fig. P-61.   Mechanized pineapple harvesting. A conveyor in the long boom transports the hand selected pineapples to the truck. (Courtesy, Maui Pineapple Company, Ltd., Kahului, Maui, Hawaii)

PROCESSING. A considerable amount of pineapple is consumed fresh. However, most exports are canned. Every part of a pineapple is used in the canning process. The flesh is canned as sliced, chunked or crushed pineapple. The juice is also canned.

At the cannery, pineapples are first washed and graded. Once graded, a machine called a *Ginaca* cuts the core from the fruit, removes the shell, and cuts off both ends. The flesh left on the shell is then scraped by machine so that it may be used for crushed pineapple and juice.

The trimmed fruit is carefully inspected, sliced by machine, and placed in cans. Broken pieces are sent to the shredder to be crushed. The shells and other trimmings are shredded, pressed, and dried to make pineapple bran to feed livestock. Other by-products of the canning process are sugar, alcohol, and vinegar. Sugar is recovered by ion exchange purification of the juice pressed from the cannery waste. However, alcohol and vinegar, instead of sugar, may be produced from the by-product juice through fermentation.

• **Bromelin**—Another by-product in some operations is the enzyme, bromelin, which is used to tenderize meat, to chillproof beer, and to produce protein hydrolyzates. Bromelin is found in the stem and fruit of the pineapple.

(Also see MEAT, section headed "Meat Tenderizing.")

In some areas of the world, namely the Philippines, the fibers of the pineapple are woven into a cloth called *pina*.

SELECTION.   Pineapple varieties vary in color, but most are yellowish. Ripe pineapples have a fruity, fragrant aroma. Usually the heavier the fruit is for its size, the better the quality. Pineapples with decayed or moldy spots should be avoided.

PREPARATION.   Pineapple may be served, fresh or canned, by itself, or it may be used in pies, ice cream, puddings, baked goods, and salads, or with meats. The flavor blends well with other flavors. Cookbooks contain long lists of ideas for the uses of pineapple. The fresh fruit cannot be used in molded gelatin, because it contains the enzyme bromelin that digests and softens the gelatin. This enzyme is destroyed by heating; hence, canned pineapple can be used in gelatin dishes.

NUTRITIONAL VALUE.   Fresh pineapple is 85% water and each 100 g (about 3½ oz) contains 58 Calories (kcal) as well as 70 IU of vitamin A and 17 mg of vitamin C. The calories in pineapples are derived primarily from the sugar (carbohydrate) present. They contain approximately 15% sugar. Canned and frozen pineapples are similar to fresh pineapples, but those canned in a heavy syrup contain more calories, and some vitamin A and C is lost during the processing. The nutrient composition of pineapple juice is very similar to the fresh fruit.

Further information regarding the nutritional value of fresh, canned, frozen, and candied pineapple, and pineapple juice is presented in Food Composition Table F-36.

(Also see FRUIT[S], Table F-47 Fruits of the World.)

PINEAPPLE GUAVA (FEIJOA)
Feijoa sellowiana

The fruit of a small South American tree (of the family *Myrtaceae*) that is related to the common guava (*Psidium guajava*).

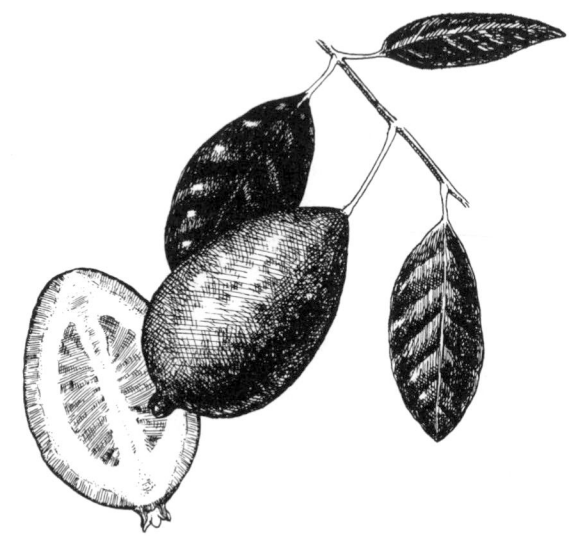

Fig. P-62.   The pineapple guava or feijoa, a fruit of the American tropics.

Feijoa is green outside and white inside, and has a tart sweet flavor somewhat like unsweetened pineapple. As a fresh fruit, it is good in fruit salads; or when made into jam.

PINEAPPLE JUICE

The fluid extracted from fresh pineapple by pressing the pulverized fruit pulp, filtering the juice, adding back some of the pulp, heat processing at 140-145°F (*60-63°C*), pressure homogenizing to keep the pulp suspended, filling into cans, and pasteurizing at 190°F (*88°C*).

The nutrient compositions of various forms of pineapple juice are given in Food Composition Table F-36.

Some noteworthy observations regarding the nutrient composition of pineapple juice follow:

1. A 1-cup (*180 g*) serving of canned pineapple juice supplies 138 Calories (kcal) and is a good source of potassium and a fair to good source of vitamin C. However, some pineapple drinks and juice products contain sufficient added vitamin C to make them much better sources of this vitamin.

2. Frozen pineapple juice concentrate contains over 3 times the caloric and nutrient contents of the single strength canned juice. Hence, it may make a significant nutritional contribution when added undiluted to dishes such as ice cream and sauces for ham and other meats.

(Also see PINEAPPLE.)

PINOCYTOSIS

The process by which liquid droplets are taken into the cell through invagination and subsequent dissolving of part of the cell membrane. This process enables cells to absorb certain lipids and dissolve proteins intact. As can be seen in Fig. P-63, the material to be engulfed comes into contact with the cell membrane. The membrane then invaginates to surround the material. Once the material has been completely surrounded, the membrane fuses, and the invaginated section of the membrane is dissolved by lysosomal enzymes. Absorptive cells in the small intestine are capable of using this mechanism during digestion.

(Also see DIGESTION AND ABSORPTION.)

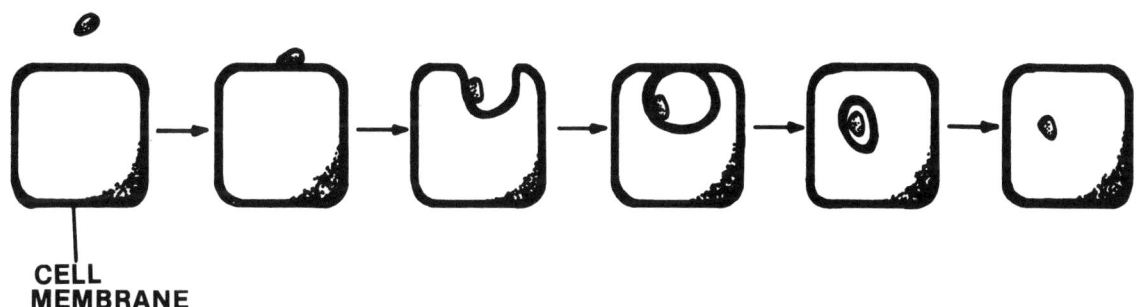

CELL MEMBRANE

Fig. P-63. Pinocytosis involves the invagination of the cell membrane around the liquid to be engulfed. Once the liquid droplet has been completely engulfed, the membrane surrounding the material disintegrates and the material is incorporated into the cell.

PINTAIL (PINTAILED DUCK)

A river duck—a game bird.

PITH

In botany, this word has the following meanings:

• Soft white spongy material found in the center of certain plant stems. It is not usually consumed as a food. However, the natives of New Guinea have long used the starchy pith of sago palms to make a flour and "pearls" which resemble tapioca by (1) pulverizing the pith with water to make a slurry, (2) sieving the slurry to remove the fibrous matter, (3) drying the starchy suspension to obtain a flour, and (4) making tasty granules from the flour and drying them on a hotplate.

• Another name for the albedo of citrus fruits, which is the white fibrous matter that lies between the fruit segments and the outer pigmented portion of the peel (flavedo). Citrus pith is rich in (1) bioflavonoids, and (2) pectin, a gelling agent and an ingredient in diarrhea remedies.

PITS

Stones or seeds of fruits such as cherries, plums, peaches, apricots, dates, or similar fruits.

PITUITARY GLAND

An endocrine gland, located at the base of the brain, which produces a number of hormones and regulates a large portion of the endocrine activity.

(Also see ENDOCRINE GLANDS.)

PIZZA

This is an Italian word meaning pie, which a pizza resembles. Pizza, the creation of which is credited to Naples, is flat leavened bread topped with a variety of such good things as tomatoes, mozzarella and parmesan cheeses, sausages, mushrooms, anchovies, olives, capers, and a profusion of herbs and spices. A pizza is actually an open sandwich.

Although pizza varies nutritionally according to the ingredients, typical pizza contains about 15% protein, 27% fat, and 58% carbohydrate; hence, it's a reasonably well balanced food.

(Also see CONVENIENCE AND FAST FOODS.)

PLACEBO

An inert preparation given for its psychological effect; especially (1) to satisfy the patient, or (2) to serve as a control in an experiment.

PLACENTA

The organ of communication between the fetus and the mother. It is the means by which the fetal blood receives oxygen and nourishment and gives up waste material; hence, the placenta performs the functions of respiration, nutrition, and excretion.

PLANTAINS *Musa paradisiaca*

A type of banana that is more likely to be used as a vegetable than as a fruit. Plantains are similar in most respects to the types of bananas used as fruit, except that they have a lower sugar content and a higher starch content. Hence, they are not as likely to be eaten raw, but rather after cooking by baking, boiling, frying, roasting, or steaming.

The nutrient composition of plantains is given in Food Composition Table F-36.

(Also see BANANA; and FRUIT[S], Table F-47 Fruits of the World.)

PLANT PROTEINS

Those proteins derived from plant sources. This consists of proteins from the seeds, nuts, fruits, vegetables, leaves, stalks and roots. Common sources of plant proteins are the cereal grains and their products, and legumes, oil seeds, and green leafy vegetables. Plant proteins are less concentrated than animal proteins, and often lack some essential amino acids giving them a lower biological value.

(Also see PROTEIN[S].)

PLAQUE

Any patch; for example, atherosclerotic plaque refers to a deposit of lipid material in the blood vessel.

PLASMA

The colorless fluid portion of the blood in which corpuscles are suspended. It is often used as a basis for measurement of bloodborne nutrients and their metabolites.

PLATELETS

Small, colorless, round or rod-shaped bodies in the circulating blood of mammals.

PLUCK

• The organs that lie in the thoracic cavity, consisting of the heart, lungs, gullet, and windpipe.

• To remove the feathers of poultry before cleaning.

PLUM AND PRUNE *Prunus* spp

The plum is the fruit of a tree bearing the same name. Botanically, a plum is classified as a drupe—a fruit whose seed is contained in a hard pit or stone surrounded by soft, pulpy flesh with a thin skin. As the genus name, *Prunus,* suggests, plums are close relatives of the apricot, almond, cherry, and peach.

Plums vary in size from those as small as a cherry to those as large as a small peach. Their shape may be round or oval, and their smooth skin may be colored green, yellow, red, blue, or purple. The edible flesh is thick, juicy, and sweet.

Plum trees range from low, shrubby type to trees 30 ft (*9 m*) high. Its white flowers blossom in the spring before the leaves appear. Since there are many species and hundreds of varieties, plums enjoy widespread distribution in different climates and soil conditions.

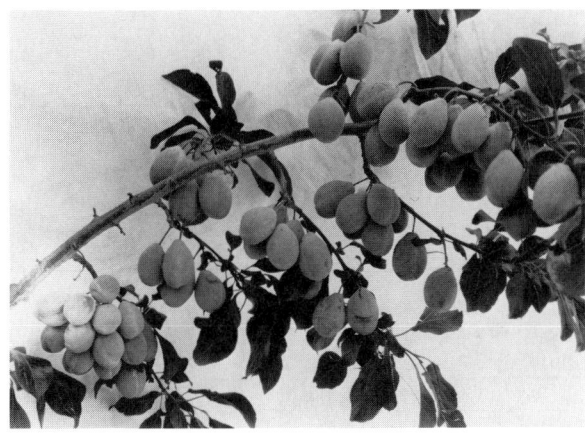

Fig. P-64. A fruiting branch of a plum tree growing in fertile irrigated soil. The thick juicy flesh of plums can be covered with skin which is green, yellow, red, blue, or purple. (Courtesy, USDA)

• **Prune**—A prune is a dried plum, but more than this a prune is a variety of plum that is satisfactory for drying without removing the pit. Growers use the term prune to refer to both the fruit in its fresh state and to the dried product. Also the following saying helps make the distinction between plum and prune: "The prune is always a plum—but a plum is not always a prune." Prune plums generally have firmer flesh and a higher sugar content. Popular varieties of the European plum, *Prunus domestica*, used for prunes include: French or Agen (most

popular), Imperial, Sugar, Robe de Sergeant, Burton, and Contes.

TYPES OF PLUMS. There are five main types of plums from which the important varieties are derived. These five types include the following: European, Japanese, American, damson, and ornamental.

• **European plum**—This plum is also called the garden or common plum. Its scientific name is *Prunus domestica*. Its fruits are blue or red and medium to large in size and may be eaten fresh or canned, though most are dried. European plums grown in the United States include: French or Agen, President, Tragedy, and Grand Duke.

• **Japanese plum**—This plum is also called the salicina plum. The fruits are yellow, crimson and purple, ranging in size from small to large. They are all very juicy and sweet, and they are eaten fresh, cooked, or canned—but never as prunes. The scientific name for the Japanese plum is *Prunus salicina*, and some common varieties include: Beauty, Burmosa, Santa Rosa, Wickson, Redheart, Duarte, Red Rosa, Kelsey, and Burbank.

• **American plum**—This group includes several species such as (1) the cold-resistant *Prunus americana* with amber skin and flesh; (2) the bushy and thorny Hortulan plum, *Prunus hortulana;* and (3) the sand cherry plum, *Prunus besseyi*, which grows in the Middle West and Canada. Some common names include De Soto, Pottawattomi, and Golden Beauty.

• **Damson plum**—These trees resemble the European type, but they are smaller and more cold resistant. Their fruits are tart and blue—favorites for jellies and jams. The scientific name for the damson plum is *Prunus insititia*. Several common varieties include Bullaces, St. Juliens, and Mirabelles.

• **Ornamental plum**—These trees produce red foliage and red fruit which is suitable for jams and jellies. The scientific name for the ornamental plum is *Prunus cerasifera* which is also the myrobalan plum. The major value of the myrobalan plum is its use as a rootstock for other stone fruits.

Table P-9 which follows compares the characteristics of some of the commercial plum varieties from the European and Japanese types.

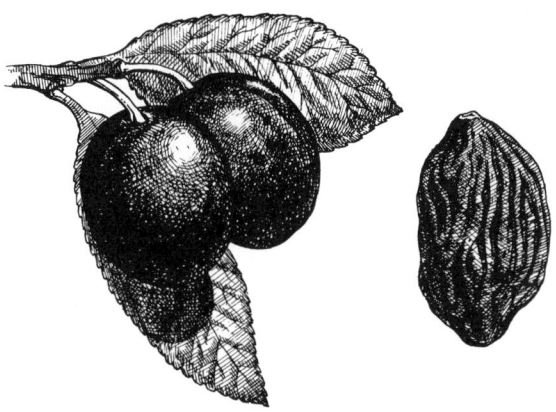

Fig. P-65. A prune (right) is a dried plum (left), but a plum is not always a prune.

TABLE P-9
CHARACTERISTICS OF SOME COMMERCIAL PLUM VARIETIES

Variety	Origin	Approximate Shipping Dates	Size	Shape	Skin Color	Flesh Color
Beauty	Burbank, 1911.	Last week May	Small to medium	Heart	Crimson	Amber
Burbank	Burbank, 1888.	1st week July	Medium	Round	Yellow, red blush	Yellow
Burmosa	Cal. Exp. Sta., 1951.	1st week June	Medium	Round	Greenish, red blush	Light amber
Duarte	Burbank, 1900.	1st week July	Medium	Heart	Dull red, brown spots.	Dark red
French (Agen)	France	Late August	Small to medium	Oval	Purple	Golden yellow
Grand Duke	England	2nd week August	Large	Oval	Purple	Greenish yellow
Kelsey	Intro. from Japan, 1870.	Last week July	Large	Heart	Green to purplish red.	Greenish yellow
President	England, intro. by Millard Sharpe, 1909.	Last week July	Medium to large	Oval	Purple	Yellow
Redheart	Cal. Exp. Sta., 1951.	3rd week June	Medium	Heart	Dull red, brown spots.	Dark red
Santa Rosa	Burbank, 1906.	2nd week June	Medium	Heart	Purplish red dots.	Amber to red at skin
Tragedy	Chance seedling, 1820.	1st week July	Medium	Oval	Dark purple	Greenish yellow
Wickson	Burbank, 1892.	1st week July	Large	Heart	Greenish yellow to light red.	Amber

ORIGIN AND HISTORY. The European or garden plum has been grown in Europe for more than 2,000 years. Some writings of the 6th century B.C. are said to mention the plum in Greece. Whatever its exact origins in Europe, the garden plum came to America with some of the first pilgrims (around 1620). Then, by the late 1700s these trees were planted in larger numbers, and they moved westward with the pioneers. Damson plums were also domesticated in Europe before coming to America. The Japanese plum originated in China, but the Japanese cultivated it for many years before it came to the United States in 1870. Then there are a group of plums, such as *Prunus americana,* which are native to America. The latter are not of any real commercial importance.

PRODUCTION. Worldwide, an average of 5.7 million metric tons of plums are produced each year. Leading plum-producing countries by rank are the U.S.S.R., China, Romania, the United States, and Yugoslavia. Other leading plum-producing countries and their yearly production are indicated in Fig. P-66.

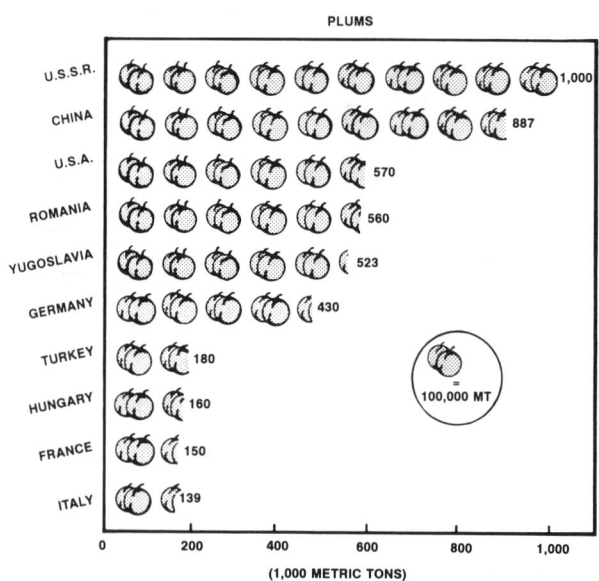

Fig. P-66. Leading plum-producing countries of the world. (Based on data from the *FAO Production Yearbook,* 1990, FAO/UN, Rome, Italy, Vol. 44, p. 162, Table 70)

California produces 89% of the U.S. crop, but plums are also an important commercial crop in Oregon, Washington, Idaho, and Michigan. The value of the plum crop amounts to approximately $143 million, and about two-thirds of the crop is dried to prunes.

PLUMS AND PRUNES

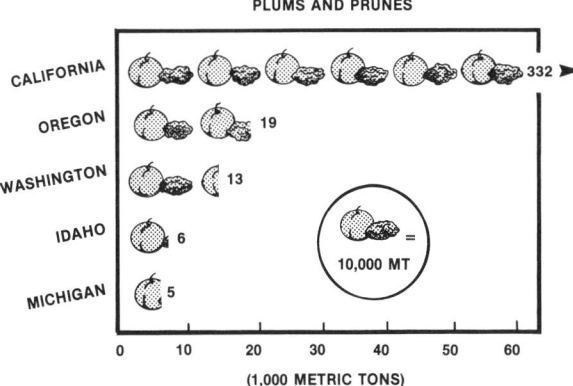

Fig. P-67. Leading plum- and prune-producing states, on a fresh basis. (Based on data from *Agricultural Statistics 1991*, USDA, pp. 207–208, Table 316, 318, and 319)

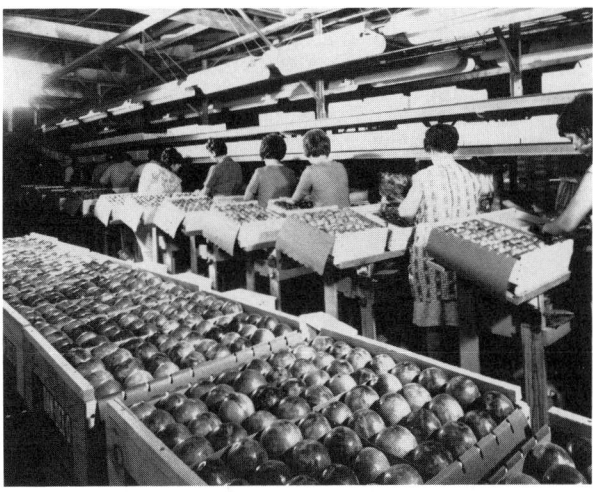

Fig. P-68. Fresh plums being packed for shipment. (Courtesy, California Tree Fruit Agreement, Sacramento, Calif.)

Propagation and Growing. Plums are propagated by budding the desired variety on seedling rootstocks of primarily the myrobalan plum (*Prunus cerasifera*), and less commonly the peach and certain strains of the European plum (*Prunus domestica*).

Depending upon the type of plum, trees are planted 15 to 25 ft (*4.6 to 7.6 m*) apart. Pruning plum trees also varies for each type of plum. When trees are in blossom cross-pollination is probably beneficial for all varieties, though some are self-fruitful. With proper orchard management techniques consisting of fertilization, irrigation, pruning, and possibly thinning of the green fruit, yields of 6 to 10 tons per acre can be expected.

Harvesting. Harvesting of plums may extend from May to October depending on the region. Generally, plums ripen unevenly over the tree, and 2 or 3 pickings may be necessary, though some varieties may require only 1 or 2 pickings. The best indicator of the readiness of plums for prunes is their sugar content.

Wholesalers and retailers prefer firmer, or "greener" plums which hold up better during shipping and handling. These plums must be packed properly, handled carefully, and precooled promptly. Most of this handling of fresh fruit is accomplished in central packing houses which are replacing field packing.

Nearly all of the plum crop is harvested mechanically with tree shakers, mechanical catchers or pickups, and lifting equipment. There are, however, some smaller growers who rely on hand labor for picking plums.

The storage period for fresh plums at 31° to 32°F (*-0.6 to 0°C*) is 3 to 4 weeks, depending upon the variety.

PROCESSING. Plums are marketed as fresh, dried (prunes), and canned or frozen fruit. Approximately 56.3% is marketed fresh, 20.6% dried, 22.2% canned, and 0.9% frozen. In California, about 66% of the plum crop is dried for prunes, and the majority of the remaining crop is utilized fresh.

• **Prunes**—A few prunes are still sun dried, but most are dehydrated. Sun drying requires more than 1 week for completion, and may be hampered by bad weather. Prior to dehydration, plums are immersed in hot water for a few seconds to remove the natural wax, and then dipped in lye to prevent fermentation. Next, the plums (prunes) are placed in single layers on trays, and placed in the dehydrator where temperature, air movement, and humidity are controlled. In efficient operations drying in a dehydrator is completed in 3 to 4 days, when the fruit reaches 18 to 19% moisture. Some larger dehydrators may only require 12 to 24 hours. The drying ratio is approximately 2½ lb (*1.13 kg*) of fresh fruit to 1 lb (*0.45 kg*) of dried fruit.

Canned plums and prunes are canned in water pack, light syrup, heavy syrup, or extra heavy syrup. Prune juice is a by-product of prune dehydration. It is made by leaching prunes with hot water or by using pectic enzymes on a slurry of whole ground prunes. Prune juice is canned, and yearly production is about 7,000,000 cases of No. 2 cans. Plums are frozen primarily in large containers for remanufacture into jams and preserves at a later date.

In the United States, there are no fermented plum products which are popular, but *Slivovitz* or plum brandy has been popular in eastern Europe for sometime.

SELECTION. With so many varieties which differ widely in appearance and flavor, it is best to buy a few of the fresh fruits and be certain that the taste and appearance is appealing. Fresh plums should be selected on the basis of their color characteristic for the type. Additionally, ripe plums are firm to slightly soft, and taste juicy and sweet. Slight softening at the tip is also a good sign of maturity. Fresh fruits with skin breaks, punctures, or brownish discoloration should be avoided. Immature fruits are hard, poorly colored and very tart, while overmature fruits are excessively soft, and possibly leaking or decaying.

If not quite ripe when purchased, keep plums at room temperature a day or so, but watch closely. Plums can turn overripe very quickly. Ripe plums should be refrigerated.

PREPARATION. Plums can be eaten fresh out of the hand or prepared in a variety of fruit dishes. Plums make good jelly, preserves, plum butter, and jam. Canned prunes can be served alone as a side dish or a dessert or in combination with other fruits, or in baked goods.

Prunes are used in baked goods, confections, desserts, salad, and meat dishes. Many prunes are served as a breakfast or dessert fruit, stewed and served with or without cream. Prunes are an excellent ready-to-eat snack.

NUTRITIONAL VALUE. Fresh plums contain 78 to 87% water, depending upon the variety. Additionally, each 100 g (about 3½ oz) provides 48 to 75 Calories (kcal) of energy, 170 to 299 mg potassium, 250 to 300 IU of vitamin A, and only 1 to 2 mg of sodium, depending upon the type of plum. The calories in plums are derived primarily from natural sugars (carbohydrates) which give them their sweet taste. Some canned plums contain more calories due to the addition of sugar, but some canned varieties are also excellent sources of vitamin A, containing, 1,180 to 1,250 IU per 100 g. Dried plums (prunes) contain only 32% water; hence, many of the nutrients, including calories, are more concentrated. Prunes contain 239 Calories (kcal), 754 mg potassium, 2.5 mg iron, and 1,994 IU vitamin A in each 100 g. More complete information regarding the nutritional value of fresh plums, canned plums, prunes and cooked prunes is presented in Food Composition Table F-36.

(Also see FRUIT[S], Table F-47 Fruits Of The World.)

POACH

A method of cooking eggs in a shallow amount of near-boiling water. A favorite method for cooking breakfast eggs.

POI

This is a Hawaiian food made from the root of the taro which is baked, pounded, moistened, and fermented. Poi tastes slightly sour; hence, some individuals trying poi for the first time find it unpleasant.

(Also see TARO.)

POISONING

The act of administering a substance which, in sufficient quantities and/or over a period of time, kills or harms living things. Many substances are poisonous in massive doses while other substances require only minute amounts to be lethal.

(Also see POISONS.)

POISONOUS PLANTS

Contents	Page

Herbal medicine enthusiasts and stalkers of the wild edible plants beware! Plants can be dangerous. But one does not have to be a herbal medicine enthusiast or stalker of the wild to encounter poisonous plants. Many poisonous plants grow in homes, gardens, and recreational areas. Some of the most prized cultivated ornamentals are extremely poisonous. However, this does not mean that poisonous plants should be destroyed, or that laws should be passed to ban their use. Many valuable plants, some of them edible plants, would require destruction or legislation. Rather, people should familiarize themselves with the hazards in their immediate environment, and develop a respectful attitude toward the potential hazards of unfamiliar plants.

Poisonous plants are those plants that contain substance(s) which in sufficient quantities and/or over a perior of time kill or harm man or animals. Primarily, the effects of poisonous plants are noted when the poisonous plant parts are eaten. However, there are some plants whose poisons may be inhaled or contacted by the skin.

HISTORY. Man's experience with plants over the ages has helped him to identify, use, and avoid poisonous plants. Primitive people obtained toxins from plants to use for hunting. African hunters tipped their arrows with ouabain from *Strophanthus gratus*—a poison powerful enough to stop an elephant. American Indians tipped blow gun darts with the powerful muscle relaxant curare from *Strychinos toxifera.*

Men used their knowledge of poisonous plants on other men. Plotters poisoned their enemies with deadly nightshade, *Atropa belladonna.* Some primitive tribes provided drinks from toxic plants to accused individuals as a trial—a survivor was held as innocent. Other cultures used poisonous plants to carry out death sentences. Socrates, about 400 B.C., was condemned to die by drinking a cup of poison hemlock.

The effects of some poisonous plants includes hallucinations. Through the ages men have used these plants for religious rites and to escape from everyday ills. The Aztecs revered a mushroom, *Psilocybe mexicana,* for its hallucinogenic properties, while the priests of India deified a toadstool, *Amanita muscaria,* for its intoxicating juices. Here in the United States, the Navajo Indians and other tribes employed the peyote cactus, *Lophophora williamsii,* to send users into a euphoric state.

No doubt, men watched their livestock get sick or die after eating certain plants. Stories of the Old West have made locoweeds famous because of their effects on livestock. White snakeroot eaten by dairy cows, transfers its poisonous alcohol, tremetol, to their milk. This created the outbreaks of "milk sickness" in the Appalachians and the Midwest, and resulted in the loss of numerous lives during the 19th century.

Gradually, men learned to be cautious, to avoid and treat plant poisonings, and to identify poisonous plants.

PRECAUTIONS AND CAUTIONS. Even in a modern society, that has to a large extent removed itself from the natural vegetation, poisonous plants may still be a hazard. Therefore, the following precautions and cautions will help avert the hazards of poisonous plants:

1. Become familiar with the poisonous plants in your home, garden, yard, and recreational areas. Know them by sight and name.

2. Bright seeds, berries, and flowers attract the curiosity of small children. Be certain to keep these out of their reach.

3. Teach older children to keep unknown plants and plant parts out of their mouths. Instruct them as to the potential dangers of poisonous plants.

4. Know the plants that children use or are apt to use as play things.

5. Do not eat wild plants without *positive* identification.

6. Avoid all mushrooms and toadstools growing in the wild. Their identification is too risky.

7. Never suppose a plant to be edible because it resembles a well-known edible plant.

8. Just because animals eat a plant, it is no guarantee that the plant is harmless to humans.

9. Some plants concentrate or confine the toxic substance to one part of the plant.

10. Cooking, in some cases, destroys or removes the poisonous substance, but this is not a general rule.

11. Some herbal and health food stores carry toxic herbs which are safe to use in proper amounts. Also, the preparation of homemade herbal remedies from native or cultivated plants should be approached with caution.

12. There are *no* absolute "tests" or "rules of thumb" which can be applied to distinguish edible from poisonous plants.

Fortunately, many poisonous plants must be eaten in relatively large amounts, and many are quite unpalatable and therefore will not be eaten in sufficient amounts to cause poisoning. Still, there are some plants that are very toxic and require only a bite or two, or a seed or two, to cause death. Also, some poisonous plants are not at all distasteful and may be eaten easily in large enough quantities to cause serious disturbances and even death.

AID FOR POISONED PERSONS. Despite everything, people will be poisoned by plants. When this occurs, time is the most important factor. The toxic substance must be removed from the body before it is absorbed. When possible the first step should be immediately to call a physician or the Poison Control Center. The person calling should be able to (1) identify or describe the plant that was eaten, (2) tell when and how much was eaten, and (3) describe any observable symptoms. When the victim is transported, a sample of the plant should be taken for identification or verification. Also, it is important to keep parts of a plant that may be present in the stool or vomit, if there is a question about which plant part was eaten. Samples—fruits, flowers, and leaves—of the plants in the area should be quickly collected and taken with the victim.

When a physician is not available, first aid should be administered and the victim transported to a hospital. The first-aid treatment will be determined by the poison. If no other advice has been given by a doctor or a Poison Control Center, take the following emergency steps:

1. If the victim is unconscious, administer artificial respiration if necessary, and head for the hospital immediately.

2. If the swallowed poison is a noncaustic substance (not a strong alkali or strong acid), proceed as follows:

a. Dilute the poison by getting the victim to drink lukewarm soapsuds, soda water made with common baking soda, or salt water (2 Tbsp of salt in a glass of warm water); but *beware of the danger of choking.* It may be necessary to give six or more glasses of the liquid. A poison diluted with a large amount of liquid is absorbed less quickly than a concentrate, and vomiting can be induced more easily when the stomach is filled.

b. Induce vomiting by (1) using the fingers to stimulate gagging, (2) giving 1 tsp of syrup of ipecac (which should be in every medicine cabinet) every 5 minutes for 3 or 4 doses, or (3) giving either soda water made with baking soda, or salt water. When the victim vomits, lay him on his stomach with his head hanging over the edge of the bed or over your knees. If possible, catch any material thrown up in basin or bowl and save for laboratory analysis.

c. After the stomach has been thoroughly emptied by vomiting, give an antidote (a substance to counteract the poison), such as an all-purpose product containing activated charcoal, magnesium hydroxide, or tannic acid.

3. If the poison is a strong alkali, a strong acid, or a petroleum distillate rather than a poisonous plant, *do not induce vomiting* because of the danger of perforating the stomach or esophagus and/or aspirating the corrosive fluid into the lungs. Instead, neutralize and dilute with a weak acid such as dilute lemon juice or vinegar, or with an alkali, such as baking soda, lime water, milk of magnesia, or chalk, then give milk, olive oil, egg white, or an all-purpose antidote.

4. As soon as possible, transport the victim via private car, ambulance, police or paramedics to the nearest hospital and/or physician. Be sure to take samples of the suspected poisonous plant.

(Also see POISONS.)

POISON CONTROL CENTERS. Centers have been established in various parts of the country where doctors can obtain prompt and up-to-date information on treatment of poison cases, if desired. Poison Control Centers have information relative to thousands of poisonous substances, cross-indexed by brand name as well as generic or chemical name, and can give prompt, responsible advice about antidotes.

Local medical doctors have information relative to the Poison Contol Centers of their area, along with their telephone numbers. When the phone number is not known, simply ask the operator for the Poison Control Center. If this information cannot be obtained locally, call the U.S. Public Health Service at either Atlanta, Georgia, or Wenatchee, Washington.

SOME IMPORTANT POISONOUS PLANTS OF NORTH AMERICA. A list and description of all plants that are potentially poisonous is not within the scope of this book. Almost all plants are poisonous if the wrong part is consumed or if too much is consumed. For example, the stalks of rhubarb are a wholesome and delicious food while the leaves contain poisonous levels of oxalic acid; or large quantities of apple seeds, peach pits, or apricot pits may cause cyanide poisoning. Therefore, the table which follows includes some of the most important, and often the most common, poisonous plants in North America.

NOTE WELL: Table P-10 is not meant to serve for the identification of poisonous plants. Rather, it is presented for informational purposes and in the hopes of stimulating the reader's interest to learn more about the poisonous plants in his environment. More can be learned through the advice of experts and publications dealing with poisonous plants common to a specific area.

(Also see MEDICINAL PLANTS; and WILD EDIBLE PLANTS.)

TABLE P-10
SOME IMPORTANT POISONOUS PLANTS OF NORTH AMERICA

Common and Scientific Name	Description; Toxic Parts	Geographical Distribution	Poisoning; Symptoms	Remarks
Baneberry *Actaea* sp.	**Description:** Perennial herb growing to 3 ft (*1 m*) tall from a thick root; compound leaves; small, white flowers; white or red berries with several seeds borne in short, terminal clusters. **Toxic parts:** All parts, but primarily roots and berries.	Native in rich woods occurring from Canada south to Georgia, Alabama, Louisiana, Oklahoma, and the northern Rockies; red-fruited western baneberry from Alaska to central California, Arizona, Montana, and South Dakota.	**Poisoning:** Attributed to a glycoside or essential oil which causes severe inflammation of the digestive tract. **Symptoms:** Acute stomach cramps, headache, increased pulse, vomiting, delirium, dizziness, and circulatory failure.	Only 6 berries can cause symptoms persisting for hours. Treatment may be a gastric lavage or vomiting. Bright red berries attract children.
Buckeye; Horsechestnut *Aesculus* sp.	**Description:** Shrub or tree; deciduous, opposite, palmately, divided leaves with 5 to 9 leaflets on a long stalk; red, yellow, or white flowers; 2- to 3-valved, capsule fruit; with thick, leathery husk enclosing 1 to 6 brown, shiny seeds. **Toxic parts:** Leaves, twigs, flowers, seeds.	Various species throughout the United States and Canada; some cultivated as ornamentals, others growing wild.	**Poisoning:** Toxic parts contain the glycoside, *esculin.* **Symptoms:** Nervous twitching of muscles, weakness, lack of coordination, dilated pupils, nausea, vomiting, diarrhea, depression, paralysis, stupor.	By making a "tea" from the leaves and twigs or by eating the seeds, children have been poisoned. Honey collected from the buckeye flower may also cause poisoning. Roots, branches, and fruits have been used to stupefy fish in ponds. Treatment usually is a gastric lavage or vomiting.

(Continued)

TABLE P-10 — *(Continued)*

Common and Scientific Name	Description; Toxic Parts	Geographical Distribution	Poisoning; Symptoms	Remarks
Buttercup *Ranunculus* sp.	**Description:** Annual or perennial herb growing to 16 to 32 in. *(41 to 81 cm)* high; leaves alternate, entire to compound, and largely basal; yellow flowers borne singly or in clusters on ends of seed stalks; small fruits, 1-seeded pods. **Toxic parts:** Entire plant.	Widely distributed in woods, meadows, pastures, and along streams throughout temperate and cold locations.	**Poisoning:** The alkaloid, *protoanemonin* which can injure the digestive system and ulcerate the skin. **Symptoms:** Burning sensation of the mouth, nervousness, nausea, vomiting, low blood pressure, weak pulse, depression, convulsions.	Sap and leaves may cause dermatitis. Cows poisoned by buttercups produce bitter milk or milk with a reddish color.
Castor bean *Ricinus communis*	**Description:** Shrublike herb 4 to 12 ft (1.2 to 3.7 m) tall; simple, alternate, long-stalked leaves with 5 to 11 long lobes which are toothed on margins; fruits oval, green, or red, and covered with spines; 3 elliptical, glossy, black, or white or mottled seeds per capsule. **Toxic parts:** Entire plant, especially the seeds.	Cultivated as an ornamental or oilseed crop primarily in the southern part of the United States and Hawaii.	**Poisoning:** Seeds, pressed cake, and leaves poisonous when chewed; contain the phytotoxin, *ricin.* **Symptoms:** Burning of the mouth and throat, nausea, vomiting, severe stomach pains, bloody diarrhea, excessive thirst, prostration, dullness of vision, convulsions; kidney failure, and death 1 to 12 days later.	Fatal dose for a child is 1 to 3 seeds, and for an adult 2 to 8 seeds. The oil extracted from the seeds is an important commercial product. It is not poisonous and it is used as a medicine (castor oil), for soap, and as a lubricant.
Chinaberry *Melia azedarach*	**Description:** Deciduous tree 20 to 40 ft (6 to 12 m) tall; twice, pinnately divided leaves and toothed or lobed leaflets, purple flowers borne in clusters; yellow, wrinkled, rounded berries which persist throughout the winter. **Toxic parts:** Berries, bark, flowers, leaves.	A native of Asia introduced as an ornamental in the United States; common in the southern United States and lower altitudes in Hawaii; has become naturalized in old fields, pastures, around buildings, and along fence rows.	**Poisoning:** Most result from eating pulp of berries; toxic principle is a resinoid with narcotic effects. **Symptoms:** Nausea, vomiting, diarrhea, irregular breathing, and respiratory distress.	Six to eight berries can cause the death of a child. The berries have been used to make insecticide and flea powder.
Death camas *Zigadenus paniculatus*	**Description:** Perennial herb resembling wild onions but the onion odor lacking; long, slender leaves with parallel veins; pale yellow to pink flowers in clusters on slender seedstalks; fruit a 3-celled capsule. **Toxic parts:** Entire plant, especially the bulb.	Various species occur throughout the United States and Canada; all are more or less poisonous.	**Poisoning:** Due to the alkaloids, *zygadenine, veratrine,* and others. **Symptoms:** Excessive salivation, muscular weakness, slow heart rate, low blood pressure, subnormal temperature, nausea, vomiting, diarrhea, prostration, coma, and sometimes death.	The members of Lewis and Clark Expedition made flour from the bulbs and suffered the symptoms of poisoning. Later some pioneers were killed with they mistook death camas for wild onions or garlic.

(Continued)

TABLE P-10 — *(Continued)*

Common and Scientific Name	Description; Toxic Parts	Geographical Distribution	Poisoning; Symptoms	Remarks
Dogbane (Indian hemp) *Apocynum cannabinum*	**Description:** Perennial herbs with milky juice and somewhat woody stems; simple, smooth and oppositely paired leaves; bell-shaped, small, white to pink flowers borne in clusters at ends of axillary stems; paired, long, slender seed pods. **Toxic parts:** Entire plant.	Various species growing throughout North America in fields and forest, and along streams and roadsides.	**Poisoning:** Only suspect since it contains the toxic glycoside, *cymarin* and is poisonous to animals. **Symptoms:** In animals, increased temperature and pulse, cold extremities, dilation of the pupils, discoloration of the mouth and nose, sore mouth, sweating, loss of appetite, death.	Compounds extracted from roots of dogbane have been used to make heart stimulant.
Foxglove *Digitalis purpurea*	**Description:** Biennial herb with alternate, simple, toothed leaves; terminal, showy raceme of flowers, purple, pink, rose, yellow, or white; dry capsule fruit. **Toxic parts:** Entire plant, especially leaves, flowers, and seeds.	Native of Europe commonly planted in gardens of the United States; naturalized and abundant in some parts of the western United States.	**Poisoning:** Due to digitalis component. **Symptoms:** Nausea, vomiting, dizziness, irregular heartbeat, tremors, convulsions, and possibly death.	Foxglove has long been known as a source of digitalis and steroid glycosides. It is an important medicinal plant when used correctly.
Henbane *Hyoscyamus niger*	**Description:** Erect annual or biennial herb with coarse, hairy stems 1 to 5 ft (*30 to 152 cm*) high; simple, oblong, alternate leaves with a few, coarse teeth, not stalked; greenish-yellow or yellowish with purple vein flowers; fruit a rounded capsule. **Toxic parts:** Entire plant.	Along roads, in waste places across southern Canada and northern United States, particularly common in the Rocky Mountains.	**Poisoning:** Caused by the alkaloids, *hyoscyamine, hyoscine,* and *atropine.* **Symptoms:** Increased salivation, headache, nausea, rapid pulse, convulsions, coma, death.	A gastric lavage of 4% tannic acid solution may be used to treat the poisoning.
Iris (Rocky Mountain Iris) *Iris missouriensis*	**Description:** Lilylike perennial plants often in dense patches; long, narrow leaves; flowers blue-purple; fruit a 3-celled capsule. **Toxic parts:** Leaves, but especially the root stalk.	Wet land of meadows, marshes, and along streams from North Dakota to British Columbia, Canada; south to New Mexico, Arizona, and California; scattered over entire Rocky Mountain area; cultivated species also common.	**Poisoning:** An irritating resinous substance, *irisin.* **Symptoms:** Burning, congestion, and severe pain in the digestive tract; nausea and diarrhea.	Rootstalks have such an acrid taste that they are unlikely to be eaten.

(Continued)

TABLE P-10 — (Continued)

Common and Scientific Name	Description; Toxic Parts	Geographical Distribution	Poisoning; Symptoms	Remarks
Jasmine *Gelsemium sempervirens*	**Description:** A woody, trailing, or climbing evergreen vine; opposite, simple, lance-shaped, glossy leaves; fragrant, yellow flowers; flattened 2-celled, beaked capsule fruits. **Toxic parts:** Entire plant, but especially the root and flowers.	Native to the southeastern United States; commonly grown in the Southwest as an ornamental.	**Poisoning:** Alkaloids, *gelsemine, gelseminine,* and *gelsemoidine* found throughout the plant. **Symptoms:** Profuse sweating, muscular weakness, convulsions, respiratory depression, paralysis, death possible.	Jasmine has been used as a medicinal herb, but overdoses are dangerous. Children have been poisoned by chewing on the leaves.
Jimmyweed (Rayless goldenrod) *Haplopappus heterophyllus*	**Description:** Small, bushy, half-shrub with erect stems arising from the woody crown to a height of 2 to 4 ft *(61 to 122 cm)*; narrow, alternate, sticky leaves; clusters of small, yellow flower heads at tips of stems. **Toxic parts:** Entire plant.	Common in fields or ranges around watering sites and along streams from Kansas, Oklahoma, and Texas to Colorado, New Mexico, and Arizona.	**Poisoning:** Contains the higher alcohol, *tremetol,* which accumulates in the milk of cows and causes human poisoning known as "milk sickness." **Symptoms:** Nausea, severe vomiting, loss of appetite, constipation, weakness, tremors, jaundice due to liver damage, convulsion, and death.	Other species of *Haplopappus* probably are equally dangerous. White snakeroot also contains tremetol and causes "milk sickness."
Jimsonwood (Thornapple) *Datura stramonium*	**Description:** Coarse, weedy plant with stout stems and foul-smelling foliage; large, oval leaves with wavy margins; fragrant, large, tubular, white to purple flowers; round, nodding or erect prickly capsule. **Toxic parts:** Entire plant, particularly the seeds and leaves.	Naturalized throughout North America; common weed of fields, gardens, roadsides, and pastures.	**Poisoning:** Due to the alkaloids, *hyoscyamine, atropine,* and *hyoscine* (scopolamine). **Symptoms:** Dry mouth, thirst, red skin, disturbed vision, pupil dilation, nausea, vomiting, headache, hallucination, rapid pulse, delirium, incoherent speech, convulsion, high blood pressure, coma, and possibly death.	Sleeping near the fragrant flowers can cause headache, nausea, dizziness, and weakness. Children pretending the flowers were trumpets have been poisoned.
Lantana (Red Sage) *Lantana camara*	**Description:** Perennial shrub with square twigs and a few spines; simple, opposite or whorled oval-shaped leaves with tooth margins; white, yellow, orange, red, or blue flowers occurring in flat-topped clusters; berry-like fruit with a hard, blue-black seed. **Toxic parts:** All parts, especially the green berries.	Native of the dry woods in the southeastern United States; cultivated as an ornamental shrub in pots in the northern United States and Canada; or a lawn shrub in the southeastern coastal plains, Texas, California, and Hawaii.	**Poisoning:** Fruit contains high levels of an alkaloid, *lantanin* or *lantadene A.* **Symptoms:** Stomach and intestinal irritation, vomiting, bloody diarrhea, muscular weakness, jaundice, and circulatory collapse; death possible but not common.	In Florida, these plants are considered a major cause of human poisoning. The foliage of lantana may also cause dermatitis.

(Continued)

TABLE P-10 — *(Continued)*

Common and Scientific Name	Description; Toxic Parts	Geographical Distribution	Poisoning; Symptoms	Remarks
Larkspur *Delphinium* sp	**Description:** Annual or perennial herb 2 to 4 ft (*61 to 122 cm*) high; finely, palmately, divided leaves on long stalks; white, pink, rose, blue, or purple flowers each with a spur; fruit a many-seeded, 3-celled capsule. **Toxic parts:** Entire plant.	Native of rich or dry forest and meadows throughout the United States but common in the West; frequently cultivated in flower gardens.	**Poisoning:** Contains the alkaloids, *delphinine, delphineidine, ajacine,* and others. **Symptoms:** Burning sensation in the mouth and skin, low blood pressure, nervousness, weakness, prickling of the skin, nausea, vomiting, depression, convulsions, and death within 6 hours if eaten in large quantities.	Poisoning potential of larkspur decreases as it ages, but alkaloids still concentrated in the seeds. Seeds are used in some commercial lice remedies.
Laurel (Mountain laurel) *Kalmia latifolia*	**Description:** Large evergreen shrubs growing to 35 ft (*11 m*) tall; alternate leaves dark green on top and bright green underneath; white to rose flowers in terminal clusters; fruit in a dry capsule. **Toxic parts:** leaves, twigs, flowers, and pollen grains.	Found in moist woods and along streams in eastern Canada southward in the Appalachian Mountains and Piedmont, and sometimes in the eastern coastal plain.	**Poisoning:** Contains the toxic resinoid, *andromedotoxin.* **Symptoms:** Increased salivation, watering of eyes and nose, loss of energy, slow pulse, vomiting, low blood pressure, lack of coordination, convulsions, progressive paralysis until eventual death.	The Mountain laurel is the state flower of Connecticut and Pennsylvania. By making "tea" from the leaves or by sucking on the flowers, children have been poisoned.
Locoweed (Crazyweed) *Oxytropis* sp	**Description:** Perennial herb with erect or spreading stems; pealike flowers and stems—only smaller.	Common throughout the southwestern United States.	**Poisoning:** Contains alkaloidlike substances—a serious threat to livestock. **Symptoms:** In animals, loss of weight, irregular gait, loss of sense of direction, nervousness, weakness, loss of muscular control.	Locoweeds are seldom eaten by humans, hence, they are not a serious problem. There are over 100 species of locoweeds.
Lupine (Bluebonnet) *Lupinus* sp.	**Description:** Annual or perennial herbs; digitately divided, alternate leaves; pea-shaped blue, white, red, or yellow flowers borne in clusters at ends of stems; seeds in flattened pods. **Toxic parts:** Entire plant, particularly the seeds.	Wide distribution but most common in western North America; many cultivated as ornamentals.	**Poisoning:** Contains *lupinine* and related toxic alkaloids. **Symptoms:** Weak pulse, slowed respiration, convulsions, and paralysis.	Rarely have cultivated varieties poisoned children. Not all lupines are poisonous.

(Continued)

TABLE P-10 — *(Continued)*

Common and Scientific Name	Description; Toxic Parts	Geographical Distribution	Poisoning; Symptoms	Remarks
Marijuana (hashish, Mary Jane, pot, grass) *Cannabis sativa*	**Description:** A tall, coarse, annual herb; palmately divided and long stalked leaves; small, green flowers clustered in the leaf axils. **Toxic parts:** Entire plant, especially the leaves, flowers, sap, and resinous secretions.	Widely naturalized weed in temperate North America; cultivated in warmer areas.	**Poisoning:** Various narcotic resins but mainly *tetrahydrocannabinol* (THC) and related compounds. **Symptoms:** Exhilaration, hallucinations, delusions, mental confusion, dilated pupils, blurred vision, poor coordination, weakness, stupor; coma and death in large doses.	Poisoning results from drinking the extract, chewing the plant parts, or smoking a so-called "reefer" (joint). The hallucinogenic and narcotic effects of marijuana have been known for more than 2,000 years. Laws in the United States and Canada restrict the possession of living or dried parts of marijuana.
Mescal bean (Frijolito) *Sophora secundiflora*	**Description:** Evergreen shrub or small tree growing to 40 ft (*12 m*) tall; stalked, alternate leaves 4 to 6 in. (*10 to 15 cm*) long, which are pinnately divided and shiny, yellow-green above and silky below when young; violet-blue, pealike flowers; bright red seeds. **Toxic parts:** Entire plant, particularly the seed.	Native to southwestern Texas and southern New Mexico; cultivated as ornamentals in the southwestern United States.	**Poisoning:** Contains *cytisine* and other poisonous alkaloids. **Symptoms:** Nausea, vomiting, diarrhea, excitement, delirium, hallucinations, coma, death; deep sleep lasting 2 to 3 days in nonlethal doses.	One seed, if sufficiently chewed, is enough to cause the death of a young child. The Indians of Mexico and the Southwest have used the seeds in medicine as a narcotic and as a hallucinatory drug. Many necklaces have been made from the seeds.
Mistletoes *Phoradendron serotinum*	**Description:** Parasitic evergreen plants that grow on trees and shrubs; oblong, simple, opposite leaves, which are leathery; small, white berries. **Toxic parts:** All parts, especially the berries.	Common on the branches of various trees from New Jersey and southern Indiana southward to Florida and Texas; other species throughout North America.	**Poisoning:** Contains the toxic amines, *beta-phenylethylamine* and *tyramine*. **Symptoms:** Gastrointestinal pain, diarrhea, slow pulse, and collapse; possibly nausea, vomiting, nervousness, difficult breathing, delirium, pupil dilation, abortion; in sufficient amounts, death within a few hours.	Mistletoe is a favorite Christmas decoration. It is the state flower of Oklahoma. Poisonings have occurred when people eat the berries or make "tea" from the berries. Indians chewed the leaves to relieve toothache.
Monkshood (Wolfsbane) *Aconitum columbianum*	**Description:** Perennial herb about 2 to 5 ft (*61 to 152 cm*) high; alternate, petioled leaves which are palmately divided into segments with pointed tips; generally dark blue flowers with a prominent hood; seed in a short-beaked capsule. **Toxic parts:** Entire plant, especially roots and seeds.	Rich, moist soil in meadows and along streams from western Canada south to California and New Mexico.	**Poisoning:** Due to several alkaloids, including *aconine* and *aconitine*. **Symptoms:** Burning sensation of the mouth and skin; nausea, vomiting, diarrhea, muscular weakness, and spasms, weak, irregular pulse, paralysis of respiration, dimmed vision, convulsions, and death within a few hours.	Small amounts can be lethal. Death in humans reported from eating the plant or extracts made from it. It has been mistaken for horseradish.

(Continued)

TABLE P-10 — *(Continued)*

Common and Scientific Name	Description; Toxic Parts	Geographical Distribution	Poisoning; Symptoms	Remarks
Mushrooms (toadstools) *Amanita muscaria, Amantia verna, Chlorophyllum molybdites*	**Description:** Common types with central stalk, and cap; flat plates (gills) underneath cap; some with deeply ridged, cylindrical top rather than cap. **Toxic parts:** Entire fungus.	Various types throughout North America.	**Poisoning:** Depending on type of mushroom; complex polypeptides such as *amanitin* and possibly *phalloidin;* a toxic protein in some; the poisons ibotenic acid, muscimol, and related compounds in others. **Symptoms:** Vary with type of mushroom but include deathlike sleep, manic behavior, delirium, seeing colored visions, feeling of elation, explosive diarrhea, vomiting, severe headache, loss of muscular coordination, abdominal cramps, and coma and death from some types; permanent liver, kidney, and heart damage from other types.	Wild mushrooms are extremely difficult to identify and are best avoided. There is no simple rule of thumb for distinguishing between poisonous and nonpoisonous mushrooms—only myths and nonsense. Only one or two bites are necessary for death from some species. During the month of December 1981, three people were killed, and two were hospitalized in California after eating poisonous mushrooms.
Nightshade *Solanum nigrum, Solanum elaeagnifolium*	**Description:** Annual herbs or shrublike plants with simple alternate leaves; small, white, blue, or violet flowers; black berries or yellow to yellow-orange berries depending on species. **Toxic parts:** Primarily the unripe berries.	Throughout the United States and southern Canada in waste places, old fields, ditches, roadsides, fence rows, or edges of woods.	**Poisoning:** Contains the alkaloid, *solanine;* possibly *saponin, atropine,* and perhaps high levels of nitrate. **Symptoms:** Headache, stomach pain, vomiting, diarrhea, dilated pupils, subnormal temperature, shock, circulatory and respiratory depression, possible death.	Some individuals use the completely ripe berries in pies and jellies. Young shoots and leaves of the plant have been cooked and eaten like spinach.
Oleander *Nerium oleander*	**Description:** An evergreen shrub or small tree growing to 25 ft (8 m) tall; short-stalked, narrow, leathery leaves, opposite or in whorls of 3; white to pink to red flowers at tips of twigs. **Toxic parts:** Entire plant, especially the leaves.	A native of southern Europe but commonly cultivated in the southern United States and California.	**Poisoning:** Contains the poisonous glycosides, *oleandrin* and *nerioside,* which act similar to digitalis. **Symptoms:** Nausea, severe vomiting, stomach pain, bloody diarrhea, cold feet and hands, irregular heartbeat, dilation of pupils, drowsiness, unconsciousness, paralysis of respiration, convulsions, coma, death within a day.	One leaf of an oleander is said to contain enough poison to kill an adult. In Florida, severe poisoning resulted when oleander branches were used as skewers. Honey made from oleander flower nectar is poisonous.

(Continued)

TABLE P-10 — *(Continued)*

Common and Scientific Name	Description; Toxic Parts	Geographical Distribution	Poisoning; Symptoms	Remarks
Peyote (Mescal buttons) *Lophophora williamsii*	**Description:** Hemispherical, spineless member of the cactus family growing from carrot-shaped roots; low, rounded sections with a tuft of yellow-white hairs on top; flower from the center of the plant, white to rose-pink; pink berry when ripe; black seeds. **Toxic parts:** Entire plant, especially the buttons.	Native to southern Texas and northern Mexico; cultivated in other areas.	**Poisoning:** Contains *mescaline, lophophorine* and other alkaloids. **Symptoms:** Illusions and hallucinations with vivid color, anxiety, muscular tremors and twitching, vomiting, diarrhea, blurred vision, wakefulness, forgetfulness, muscular relaxation, dizziness.	The effects of chewing fresh or dried "buttons" of peyote are similar to those produced by LSD, only milder. In some states, peyote is recognized as a drug. Peyote has long been used by the Indians and Mexicans in religious ceremonies.
Poison hemlock (poison parsley) *Conium maculatum*	**Description:** Biennial herb with a hairless, purple-spotted or lined, hollow stem growing up to 8 ft *(2.4 m)* tall; turniplike, long, solid taproot; large, alternate, pinnately divided leaves; small, white flowers in umbrella-shaped clusters, dry, ribbed, 2-part capsule fruit. **Toxic parts:** Entire plant, primarily seeds and root.	A native of Eurasia, now a weed in meadows, and along roads and ditches throughout the United States and southern Canada where moisture is sufficient.	**Poisoning:** The poisonous alkaloid, *coniine* and other related alkaloids. **Symptoms:** Burning sensation in the mouth and throat, nervousness, uncoordination, dilated pupils, muscular weakness, weakened and slowed heartbeat, convulsions, coma, death.	Poisoning occurs when the leaves are mistaken for parsley, the roots for turnips, or the seeds for anise. Toxic quantities seldom consumed because the plant has such an unpleasant odor and taste. Assumed by some to be the poison drunk by Socrates.
Poison ivy (poison oak) *Toxicondendron radicans*	**Description:** A trailing or climbing vine, shrub, or small tree; alternate leaves with 3 leaflets; flowers and fruits hanging in clusters; white to yellowish fruit (drupes). **Toxic parts:** Roots, stems, leaves, pollen, flowers, and fruits.	An extremely variable native weed throughout southern Canada and the United States with the exception of the west coast; found on flood plains, along lake shores, edges of woods, stream banks, fences, and around buildings.	**Poisoning:** Skin irritation due to an oil-resin containing *urushiol*. **Symptoms:** Contact with skin causes itching, burning, redness, and small blisters; severe gastric disturbance and even death by eating leaves or fruit.	Almost half of all persons are allergic to poison ivy. Skin irritation may also result from indirect contact such as animals (including dogs and cats), clothing, tools, or sports equipment.
Pokeweed (Pokeberry) *Phytolacca americana*	**Description:** Shrublike herb with a large, fleshy taproot; large, entire, oblong leaves which are pointed; white to purplish flowers in clusters at ends of branches; mature fruit a dark purple berry with red juice. **Toxic parts:** Rootstalk, leaves, and stems.	Native to the eastern United States and southeastern Canada.	**Poisoning:** Highest concentration of poison mainly in roots; contains the bitter glycoside, *saponin* and a glycoprotein. **Symptoms:** Burning and bitter taste in mouth, stomach cramps, nausea, vomiting, diarrhea, drowsiness, slowed breathing, weakness, tremors, convulsions, spasms, coma, and death if eaten in large amounts.	Young tender leaves and stems of pokeweed are often cooked as greens. Cooked berries are used for pies without harm. It is one of the most dangerous poisonous plants because people prepare it improperly.

(Continued)

TABLE P-10 — *(Continued)*

Common and Scientific Name	Description; Toxic Parts	Geographical Distribution	Poisoning; Symptoms	Remarks
Poppy (common poppy) *Papaver somniferum*	**Description:** An erect, annual herb with milky juice; simple, coarsely toothed, or lobed leaves; showy red, white, pink, or purple flowers; fruit an oval, crowned capsule; tiny seeds in capsule. **Toxic parts:** Unripe fruits or their juice.	Introduced from Eurasia and widely grown in the United States until cultivation without a license became unlawful.	**Poisoning:** Crude resin from unripe seed capsule source of narcotic opium alkaloids. **Symptoms:** From unripe fruit, stupor, coma, shallow and slow breathing, depression of the central nervous system; possibly nausea and severe retching (straining to vomit).	The use of poppy extracts is a double edged sword—addictive narcotics and valuable medicines. Poppy seeds which are used as toppings on breads are harmless.
Rhododendron; azaleas *Rhododendron* sp.	**Description:** Usually evergreen shrubs; mostly entire, simple, leathery leaves in whorls or alternate; showy white to pink flowers in terminal clusters; fruit a wood capsule. **Toxic parts:** Entire plant.	Throughout the temperate parts of the United States as a native and as an introduced ornamental.	**Poisoning:** Contains the toxic resinoid, *andromedotoxin.* **Symptoms:** Watering eyes and mouth, nasal discharge, nausea, severe abdominal pain, vomiting, convulsions, lowered blood pressure, lack of coordination and loss of energy; progressive paralysis of arms and legs until death, in severe cases.	Cases of poisoning are rare in this country but rhododendrons should be suspected of possible danger.
Rosary pea (precatory pea) *Abrus precatorius*	**Description:** A twining, more or less, woody perennial vine; alternate and divided leaves with small leaflets; red to purple or white flowers; fruit a short pod containing ovoid seeds which are glossy, bright scarlet over ¾ of their surface, and jet black over the remaining ¼. **Toxic parts:** Seeds.	Native to the tropics, but naturalized in Florida and the Keys.	**Poisoning:** Contains the phytotoxin, *abrin* and the tetanic glycoside, *abric acid.* **Symptoms:** Severe stomach pain, in 1 to 3 days, nausea, vomiting, severe diarrhea, weakness, cold sweat, drowsiness, weak, fast pulse, coma, circulatory collapse, death.	The beans are made into rosaries, necklaces, bracelets, leis, and various toys which receive wide distribution. Seeds must be chewed and swallowed to cause poisoning. Whole seeds pass through the digestive tract without causing symptoms. One thoroughly chewed seed is said to be potent enough to kill an adult or child.
Snow-on-the-mountain *Euphorbia marginata*	**Description:** A tall annual herb, growing up to 4 ft (*122 cm*) high; smooth, lance-shaped leaves with conspicuously white margins; whorls of white petal-like leaves border flowers; fruit a 3-celled, 3-lobed capsule. **Toxic parts:** Leaves, stems, milky sap.	Native to the western, dry plains and valleys from Montana to Mexico; sometimes escapes in the eastern United States.	**Poisoning:** Toxins causing dermatitis and severe irritation of the digestive tract. **Symptoms:** Blistering of the skin, nausea, abdominal pain, fainting, diarrhea, possibly death in severe cases.	Milky juice of this plant is very caustic. Outwardly, snow-on-the-mountain resembles a poinsettia.

(Continued)

TABLE P-10 — *(Continued)*

Common and Scientific Name	Description; Toxic Parts	Geographical Distribution	Poisoning; Symptoms	Remarks
Skunkcabbage *Veratrum californicum*	**Description:** Tall, broad-leaved herbs of the lily family, growing to 6 ft (*183 cm*) high; large, alternate, pleated, clasping, and parallel-veined leaves; numerous whitish to greenish flowers in large terminal clusters; 3-lobed, capsule fruit. **Toxic parts:** Entire plant.	Various species throughout North America in wet meadows, forests, and along streams.	**Poisoning:** Contains such alkaloids as *veradridene* and *veratrine.* **Symptoms:** Nausea, vomiting, diarrhea, stomach pains, lowered blood pressure, slow pulse, reduced body temperature, shallow breathing, salivation, weakness, nervousness, convulsions, paralysis, possibly death.	These plants have been used for centuries as a source of drugs and as a source of insecticide. Since the leaves resemble cabbage, they are often collected as an edible wild plant, but with unpleasant results.
Tansy *Tanacetum vulgare*	**Description:** Tall, aromatic herb with simple stems to 3 ft (*91 cm*) high; alternate, pinnately divided, narrow leaves; flower heads in flat-topped clusters with numerous small, yellow flowers. **Toxic parts:** Leaves, stems, and flowers.	Introduced from Eurasia; widely naturalized in North America; sometimes found escaped along roadsides, in pastures, or other wet places; grown for medicinal purposes.	**Poisoning:** Contains an oil, *tanacetin,* or oil of tansy. **Symptoms:** Nausea, vomiting, diarrhea, convulsions, violent spasms, dilated pupils, rapid and feeble pulse, possibly death.	Tansy and oil of tansy are employed as a herbal remedy for nervousness, intestinal worms, to promote menstruation and to induce abortion. Some poisonings have resulted from the use of tansy as a home remedy.
Waterhemlock *Cicuta* sp.	**Description:** A perennial with parsleylike leaves; hollow, jointed stems and hollow, pithy roots; flowers in umbrella clusters; stems streaked with purple ridges; 2 to 6 ft (*61 to 183 cm*) high. **Toxic parts:** Entire plant, primarily the roots and young growth.	Wet meadows, pastures, and flood plains of western and eastern United States, generally absent in the plains states.	**Poisoning:** Contains the toxic resinlike higher alcohol, *cicutoxin.* **Symptoms:** Frothing at the mouth, spasms, dilated pupils, diarrhea, convulsions, vomiting, delirium, respiratory failure, paralysis, and death.	One mouthful of the waterhemlock root is reported to contain sufficient poison to kill a man. Children making whistles and peashooters from the hollow stems have been poisoned. The waterhemlock is often mistaken for the edible wild artichoke or parsnip. However, it is considered to be one of the most poisonous plants of the North Temperate Zone.
White snakeroot *Eupatorium rogosum*	**Description:** Erect perennial with stems 1 to 5 ft (*30 to 152 cm*) tall; opposite oval leaves with pointed tips and sharply toothed edges, and dull on the upper surface but shiny on the lower surface; showy, snow white flowers in terminal clusters. **Toxic parts:** Entire plant.	From eastern Canada to Saskatchewan and south to Texas, Louisiana, Georgia, and Virginia.	**Poisoning:** Contains the higher alcohol, *tremetol* and some glycosides. **Symptoms:** Weakness, nausea, loss of appetite, vomiting, tremors, labored breathing, constipation, dizziness, delirium, convulsions, coma, and death.	Recovery from a nonlethal dose is a slow process, due to liver and kidney damage. Poison may be in the milk of cows that have eaten white snakeroot— "milk sickness."

POISONS

Contents

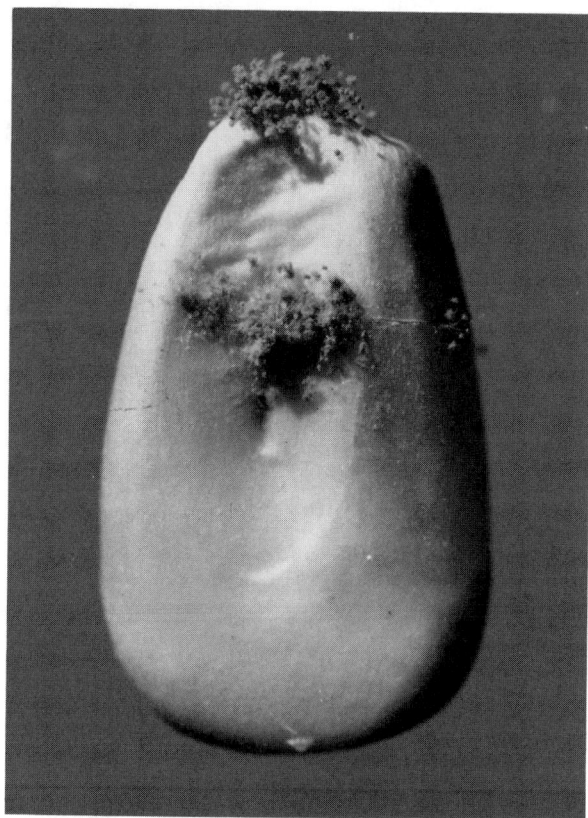

Fig. P-69. Sporulation of *Aspergillus flavus* on a kernel of corn. This fungus produces aflatoxin. Aflatoxin (1) is associated with a high incidence of liver cancer, and (2) may be involved in some types of acute poisoning of children. (Courtesy, C. W. Hesseltine, USDA, Agricultural Research, Peoria, Ill.)

Sola dosis facit venenum, means "only the dose makes the poison." Paracelsus, the noted German-born physician, said it in the 16th century. But it's just as true today as it was four centuries ago. For most food-related poisons, there is both a safe level and a poisonous level; and the severity of the effect depends upon (1) the amount taken, (2) the period of time over which the substance is taken (certain poisons are cumulative), and (3) the age and physical condition of the person.

Take potatoes, for example. They contain solanine, which can be toxic. In consuming an average of 119 lb (*54 kg*) of potatoes per year, the average American ingests 9,700 mg of solanine—enough to kill a horse. Yet it doesn't kill us because we don't eat it all at one time.

Or take lima beans! The average person eats about 1.85 (*0.84 kg*) of these tasty little morsels each year, not realizing that they contain hydrogen cyanide, a deadly poison. But they don't kill us simply because we can't eat enough at any one sitting to be deadly. Besides, most U.S. limas contain little hydrogen cyanide.

And so it goes, on and on through a long list of foods and drinks.

By definition, *a poison is a substance which in sufficient quantities and/or over a period of time kills or harms living things.* Many poisons are called toxins. The study of poisons is called *toxicology.* The discussion that follows and Table P-11 pertain primarily to food-related poisons that are eaten.

There are more than four million chemical compounds, of which more than 60,000 are commercially produced; and about 1,000 new ones are introduced each year. Some of these make their way into food and water. With the growth and use of chemicals, food supplies are subject to contamination from or treatment with chemicals in the course of growing, fertilizing, harvesting, processing, and storing.

Today, there are substantially fewer dangers than formerly from contamination of food and water by

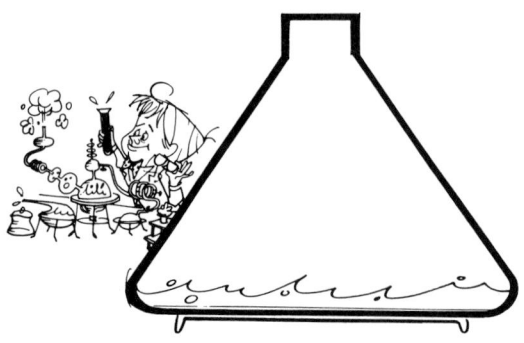

bacteria or from ingesting lead (now that paints are lead-free). Nevertheless, some two million ingestions of potentially dangerous substances occur in the United States each year; and there were 6,226 fatal poisonings in 1985.[13] Despite popular misconceptions, children are no longer the main victims of poisons. Today, only 1% of the deaths from poison involve children under 5 years of age; and poisoning now accounts for only 23% of the accidental deaths among children under age 5.[14] This decline is attributed primarily to the use of childproof safety caps in packaging poisonous agents; the storage of toxic substances separate and apart from other products and out of reach of children; and the banning of lead-containing paints, along with public health screening of children living in old housing areas in which lead-based paints may have been used years ago.

The general symptoms of poisoning are: nausea, vomiting, cramps, and stomach pains. If a corrosive poison (a strong alkali or a strong acid) has been taken, burns and stains may show on and around the mouth and tongue.

POISON PREVENTION AND TREATMENT.

In recent years, physicians, pharmacists, and Poison Control Center personnel have joined forces in advocating the following simple measures to avert poisoning and provide lifesaving aid when poisoning occurs:

1. **Packaging and storing potential poisons with care.** The use of child-resistant containers (opened only with difficulty and know-how), strip packages (with pills and capsules sealed individually in a plastic strip), and safe

---

[13]*Statistical Abstract of the United States 1991*, U.S. Dept. of Commerce, Bureau of the Census, Table 124.

[14]*Healthy People*, the Surgeon General's report on health promotion and disease prevention, U.S. Department of Health, Education, and Welfare, 1979, p. 9-70.

storage have reduced the incidence of accidental poisoning, especially among children.

2. **Keeping a supply of syrup of ipecac on hand at all times.** As a reliable (and usually rapid) means of inducing vomiting, it is the best.

3. **Having an all-purpose antidote on hand.** Antidotes are usually listed on the labels of potentially poisonous products, but finding the ingredients and mixing them takes up valuable time. So, it is best to have an all-purpose antidote readily available. The main ingredients in all-purpose antidotes are powdered activated charcoal, which has a strong capacity to absorb many chemicals; a weak buffering alkali such as magnesium hydroxide to help neutralize an acid poison; and a weak buffering acid such as tannic acid to help neutralize any alkali present. This type of antidote is particularly useful in cases of poisoning in which it is best not to induce vomiting.

EMERGENCY MEASURES IN ACUTE POISONING.

In case of *acute* poisoning, it is important to act swiftly, calmly, and knowledgeably. The following emergency measures, taken in the order listed, may save a life:

NOTE WELL: Although these measures were prepared especially for counteracting the poions listed in Table P-11, they are applicable to all poisons, including those from drugs and household products.

1. **Call a doctor, the nearest Poison Control Center, or a hospital.** Describe over the phone exactly what the poison was (read off the label), provided it is known. If the victim is unable to give information, perhaps a nearby container or the symptoms will identify the poison. Based on this information, the doctor or Poison Control Center may be able to recommend emergency treatment, thereby saving precious time.

2. **Apply first-aid treatment.** The first-aid treatment will be determined by the poison. If no other advice has

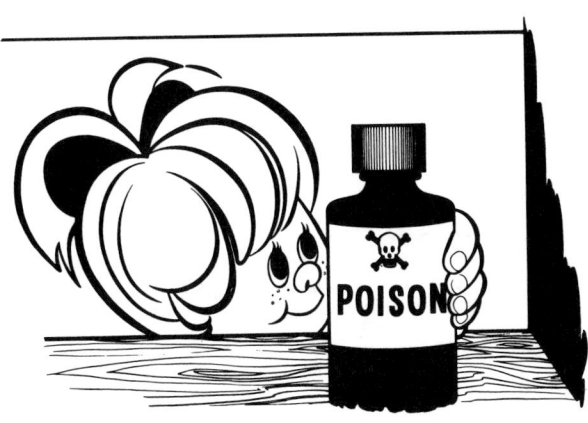

been given by a doctor or a Poison Control Center, take the following emergency steps:

a. If the victim is unconscious, administer artificial respiration if necessary, and head for the hospital immediately.

b. If the swallowed poison is a noncaustic substance (not a stong alkali or strong acid), proceed as follows:

(1) Dilute the poison by getting the victim to drink lukewarm soapsuds, soda water made with common baking soda, or salt water (2 Tbsp of salt in a glass of warm water); but *beware of the danger of choking*. It may be necessary to give six or more glasses of the liquid. A poison diluted with a large amount of liquid is absorbed less quickly than a concentrate, and vomiting can be induced more easily when the stomach is filled.

(2) Induce vomiting by (a) using the fingers to stimulate gagging, (b) giving 1 teaspoonful of syrup of ipecac (which should be in every medicine cabinet) every 5 minutes for 3 or 4 doses, or (c) giving either soda water made with baking soda, or salt water. When the victim vomits, lay him on his stomach with his head hanging over the edge of the bed or over your knees. If possible, catch any material thrown up in a basin or bowl and save for laboratory analysis.

(3) After the stomach has been thoroughly emptied by vomiting, give an antidote (a substance to counteract the poison), such as an all-purpose product containing activated charcoal, magnesium hydroxide, or tannic acid.

c. If the poison is a strong alkali or a strong acid, *do not induce vomiting* because of the danger of perforating the stomach or esophagus and/or aspirating the corrosive fluid into the lungs. Instead, proceed as follows:

(1) For alkali poisoning: (a) neutralize and dilute the alkali with a weak acid such as dilute lemon juice or vinegar, then give milk; or (b) give an all-purpose antidote.

(2) For acid poisoning: (a) neutralize and dilute the poison with an alkali, such as baking soda, lime water, milk of magnesia, or chalk, then (b) give milk, olive oil, egg white, or an all-purpose antidote.

3. **Control shock.** Keep the victim warm.

4. **See the doctor.** A physician should always see a victim of poisoning as soon as possible; with transportation provided by private car, an ambulance, the police, or paramedics (fire department). Also, take the poison container and label along.

POISON CONTROL CENTERS. Centers have been established in various parts of the country where doctors can obtain prompt and up-to-date information on treatment of poison cases, if desired. Poison Control Centers have information relative to thousands of poisonous substances, cross-indexed by brand name as well as generic or chemical name, and can give prompt, responsible advice about antidotes.

Local medical doctors have information relative to the Poison Control Centers of their area, along with their telephone numbers. When the phone number is not known, simply ask the operator for the Poison Control Center. If this information cannot be obtained locally, call the U.S. Public Health Service at either Atlanta, Georgia, or Wenatchee, Washington.

ENVIRONMENTAL CONTAMINANTS IN FOOD. Environmental contaminants include organic chemicals, metals and their derivatives, and radioactive substances that inadvertently enter the human food

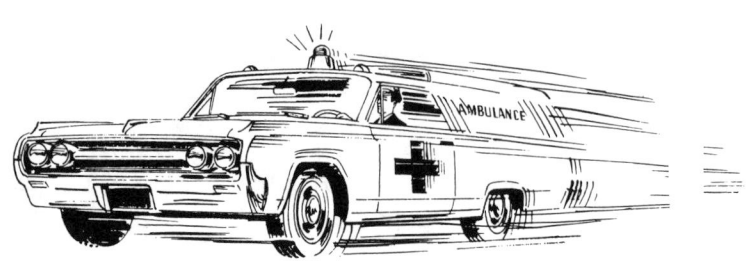

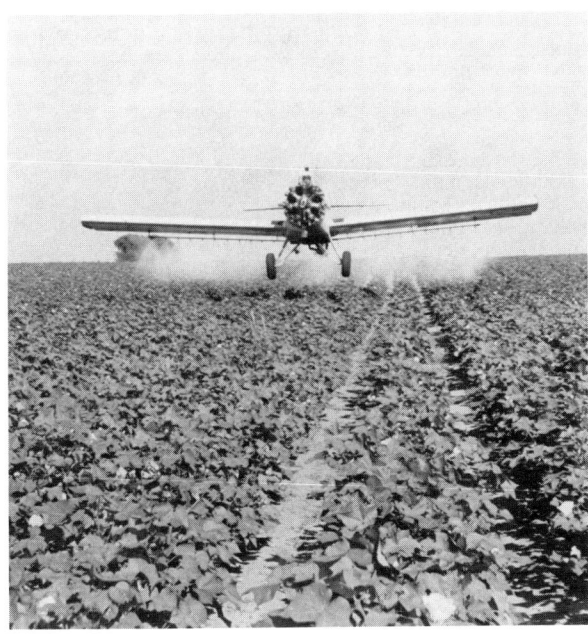

Fig. P-70. Pesticide being applied by airplane. When properly used, consumers benefit greatly from pesticides. It is important, however, to gauge the effect of each pesticide on the ecological food chain and human health.

supply through agriculture, mining, industrial operations, or energy production. To regulate them under the law, the Food and Drug Administration (FDA) defines environmental contaminants as "added, poisonous, or deleterious substances that cannot be avoided by good manufacturing practices, and that may make food injurious to health."

Unlike food additives, environmental contaminants inadvertently find their way into the human food supply (including sports fish and game).

Four factors determine whether and how seriously the environmental contamination of food will affect human health: (1) toxicity of the contaminant, (2) the amount of the substance in the food, (3) the amount of the contaminated food eaten, and (4) the physiological vulnerability of the individual consuming the food.

Although the United States has escaped mass poisonings such as have occurred in most other industrialized nations, between 1968 and 1978, according to an Office of Technology Assessment (OTA) survey, 243 food-contamination incidents were reported in this country. During this same period (1968-1978), at least $282 million in food was lost to contamination—a conservative estimate that included only 30% of the known incidents and ignored such hidden costs as medical expenses and lost workdays.

The FDA sets permissible levels for all known contaminants. Then federal and state regulatory agencies monitor food to ensure that environmental contaminants do not exceed prescribed levels. Consequently, contamination involving an unregulated substance is rarely identified before it becomes a major problem. None of the major environmental contamination incidents in the United States—animal feeds in Michigan contaminated by polybrominated biphenyls (PBBs); the Hudson River contaminated by polychlorinated biphenyls (PCBs); Virginia's James River contaminated by kepone; and fat used to produce meat and bone meal feeds in a meat-packing plant in Billings, Montana, contaminated by PCBs from a damaged transformer—were initially discovered by ongoing monitoring programs. In each case, actual human or animal poisonings alerted authorities to the danger.

SOME POTENTIALLY POISONOUS (TOXIC) SUBSTANCES. Table P-11 is a summary of some potentially poisonous (toxic) substances.
(Also see POISONOUS PLANTS; and BACTERIAL SPOILAGE OF FOOD.)

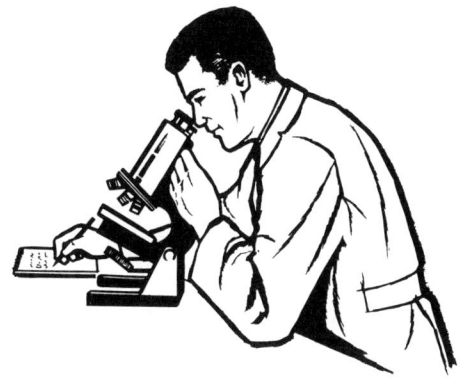

Poison (Toxin)	History	Source	Species Affected
Aflatoxins (See MYCOTOXINS in this table.)			
Aluminum (Al) (Also see MINERAL[S].)	Aluminim, which is the most modern of the common metals, was first produced by Hans Christian Oersted in 1825 and introduced to the public in 1855 at the Paris exposition.	Food additives, mainly present in such items as baking powder, pickles, and processed cheeses. Aluminum-containing antacids. Aluminum cooking utensils.	Man
Arsenic (As)	The alchemists' symbol for arsenic, a menacing coiled serpent, symbolizes very well the element's evil reputation through the ages. Arsenic compounds were the preferred homicidal and suicidal agents during the Middle Ages. A famed case of arsenic poisoning was the alleged attempt to do away with Napoleon Bonaparte on several occasions during his exile on St. Helena. Paris green (copper acetoarsenite) was the first pesticide widely used in modern agriculture.	Consuming foods and beverages contaminated with excessive amounts of arsenic-containing sprays used as insecticides and weed killers. Arsenical insecticides used in vineyards exposing the workers (1) when spraying or (2) by inhaling contaminated dusts and plant debris. Arsenic in the air from three major sources: smelting of metals, burning of coal, and use of arsenical pesticides.	Man All farm animals.
Chromium (Cr) (Also see CHROMIUM; and MINERAL[S].)	Chromium was discovered by the French chemist Vauquelin in 1797. Chromium compounds have long been used in dyeing, in tanning leather, and in corrosion-resistant metals.	Food, water, and air contaminated by chromium compounds in industrialized areas.	Man

(Continued)

(TOXIC) SUBSTANCES

Symptoms and Signs	Distribution; Magnitude	Prevention; Treatment	Remarks
Abnormally large intakes of aluminum irritate the digestive tract. Also, unusual conditions have sometimes resulted in the absorption of sufficient aluminum from antacids to cause brain damage. Aluminum may form non-absorbable complexes with essential trace elements, thereby creating deficiencies of the trace elements.	**Distribution:** Aluminum is widely used throughout the world. **Magnitude:** The U.S. uses more aluminum than any other product except iron and steel. However, known cases of aluminum toxicity are rare.	**Prevention:** Based on the evidence presented herein, no preventative measures are recommended. **Treatment:** This should be left to the doctor.	Currently, not much is known about the amount of aluminum consumed by people or its effects, if any. More experimental work is needed. Because aluminum is dissolved in acid solutions, there is some doubt as to whether it is safe to cook such highly acid foods as rhubarb and tomatoes in aluminum pots and pans. Aluminum toxicity has been reported in patients receiving renal dialysis.
Burning pains in the throat or stomach, cardiac abnormalities, and the odor of garlic on the breath. Other symptoms may be diarrhea and extreme thirst along with a choking sensation. Small doses of arsenic taken into the body over a long period of time may produce hyperkeratosis (irregularities in pigmentation, especially on the trunk); arterial insufficiency; and cancer. There is strong evidence that inorganic arsenic is a skin and lung carcinogen in man.	**Distribution:** Arsenic is widely distributed, but the amount of the element consumed by man in food and water, or breathed, is generally small and not harmful. **Magnitude:** Cases of arsenic toxicity in man are rather infrequent. Two noteworthy episodes occurred in Japan in 1955. One involved tainted powdered milk; the other, contaminated soy sauce. The toxic milk caused 12,131 cases of infant poisoning, with 130 deaths. The soy sauce poisoned 220 people. There are many scattered case reports of subacute to chronic arsenic poisoning.	**Prevention:** Avoid consuming (1) arsenic products, or (2) foods and beverages contaminated with excessive amounts of arsenic. **Treatment:** Induce vomiting and more vomiting, followed by an antidote of egg whites in water or milk. Afterward, give strong coffee or tea, followed by epsom salts in water or castor oil.	Arsenic is known to protect partially against selenium poisoning. The highest residues of arsenic are generally in the hair and nails. Accumulation of arsenic in soils may sharply decrease crop growth and yields, but it is not a hazard to people or livestock that eat plants grown in these fields, provided they do not eat the foliage of sprayed plants.
Inorganic chromium salt reduces the absorption of zinc; hence, zinc deficiency symptoms may become evident in chronic chromium toxicity.	**Distribution:** Chromium toxicity does not appear to be wide spread. **Magnitude:** Chromium toxicity is not very common.	**Prevention:** No special preventative measures are necessary. It is unlikely that people will get too much chromium because: (1) only minute amounts of the element are present in most foods, (2) the body utilizes chromium poorly, and (3) the toxic dose is about 10,000 times the lowest effective medical dose. **Treatment:** Delete chromium sources and follow the treatment prescribed by the doctor.	*Caution:* A person should never take an inorganic chromium compound except on the advice of a doctor because certain types of these compounds are deadly poisons.

(Continued)

TABLE P-11

Poison (Toxin)	History	Source	Species Affected
Copper (Cu) (Also see COPPER; and MINERAL[S].)	Copper has been one of man's most useful metals for more than 5,000 years. Concern about the possibility of copper toxicity is rather recent.	Diets with excess copper, but low in other minerals that counteract its effects Acid foods or beverages (vinegar, carbonated beverages, or citrus juices) that have been in prolonged contact with copper metal may cause acute gastrointestinal disturbance.	Man All farm animals.
Ergot Although ergot is a mycotoxin it is treated separately herein because it differs from the other mycotoxicoses in that it results from the consumption of a considerable amount of fungus tissue in which the toxin is found, whereas in the other mycotoxicoses the toxins are secreted into the substrate on or in which the fungus is growing, and very little fungus tissue as such is consumed. **Cause:** *Claviceps purpurea.* Ergotism is caused by overuse of ergot-containing foods or drugs.	Ergot and its effects have been documented through the ages. Hippocrates, the Greek physician, referred to it; and it is mentioned in the New Testament of the Bible. Ergotism, known as St. Anthony's fire a thousand years ago, formerly killed thousands of people in Europe. It was not until 1673, however, that the discolored grain was recognized as the cause of the disease. The disease continued on a large scale in the USSR in the 1920s and the 1930s. As recently as 1951, an outbreak of ergotism occurred in France.	Rye, wheat, barley, oats and triticale. Ergot replaces the seed in the heads of cereal grains, in which it appears as a purplish-black, hard, banana-shaped, dense mass from ¼ to ¾ in. *(6 to 19mm)* long.	Man Cattle Horses Sheep Swine

(Continued)

(Continued)

Symptoms and Signs	Distribution; Magnitude	Prevention; Treatment	Remarks
Acute copper toxicity: Characterized by headache, dizziness, metallic taste, excessive salivation, nausea, vomiting, stomachache, diarrhea, and weakness. If the disease is allowed to get worse, there may also be racing of the heart, high blood pressure, jaundice, hemolytic anemia, dark-pigmented urine, kidney disorders, and even death. **Chronic copper toxicity:** May be contributory to iron-deficiency anemia, mental illness following childbirth (postpartum psychosis), certain types of schizophrenia, and perhaps heart attacks.	**Distribution:** Copper toxicity may occur wherever there is excess copper intake, especially when accompanied by low iron, molybdenum, sulfur, zinc, and vitamin C. **Magnitude:** The incidence of copper toxicity is extremely rare in man. Its occurrence in significant form is almost always limited to (1) suicide attempted by ingesting large quantities of copper salt, or (2) a genetic defect in copper metabolism inherited as an autosomal recessive, known as Wilson's disease.	**Prevention:** Beware of acid or soft drinking water which has leached the mineral from copper piping. Avoid foods and beverages that have been in prolonged contact with copper metal. Where there is indication of excess copper in the food or water, the doctor may increase the dietary levels of iron, molybdenum, sulfur and zinc. **Treatment:** Vomiting and diarrhea induced by ingesting milligram quantities of ionic copper, prescribed by the doctor, generally protect the patient from serious acute toxicity effects. Where there is severe copper poisoning, the doctor will likely administer special metal-binding (chelating) agents which draw copper out of the body.	Copper is essential to human life and health, but like all heavy metals, it is potentially toxic, also. The blue stains on the surface of sinks where the water drips from the faucet are an indication that drinking water may contain too much copper. Infants are particularly susceptible to copper in tap water because (1) their water needs are high, and (2) their diets may not contain sufficient other minerals to counteract copper, because of being limited in variety. Because copper is absorbed by the lungs, skin, and uterus, as well as by the gastrointestinal tract, studies should be conducted to determine whether any long-term hazard of human toxicosis is possible from copper introduced through inhalation, absorption from the skin, or copper-containing intrauterine contraceptive devices. The total body content of copper in adult mammals is about 2 ppm wet weight.
When a large amount of ergot is consumed in a short period, convulsive ergotism is observed. The symptoms include itching, numbness, severe muscle cramps, sustained spasms and convulsions, and extreme pain. When smaller amounts of ergot are consumed over an extended period, ergotism is characterized by gangrene of the fingertips and toes, caused by blood vessel and muscle contraction stopping blood circulation in the extremities. These symptoms include cramps, swelling, inflammation, alternating burning and freezing sensations ("St. Anthony's fire") and numbness; eventually, the hands and feet may turn black, shrink, and fall off. The amount of ergot in the food consumed determines how rapidly toxic effects will show. Ergotism is a cumulative poison, depending on the amount of ergot eaten and the length of time over which it is eaten.	**Distribution:** Ergot is found throughout the world, wherever rye, wheat, barley, oats, or triticale are grown. **Magnitude:** There is considerable ergot, especially in rye. But, normally, screening grains before processing alleviates ergotism in people.	**Prevention:** Consists of an ergot-free diet Ergot in plants cannot be controlled by treatment; and resistant varieties of cereal grains are not available. Control of ergot in cereal grains consists of using ergot-free seed, following a crop rotation, and using cultural practices which will reduce the incidence of ergot in plants and its spread to other crops. Ergot in food and feed grains may be removed by screening the grains before processing. In the U.S., wheat and rye containing more than 0.3% ergot are classed as "ergoty." In Canada, government regulations prohibit more than 0.1% ergot in feeds. **Treatment:** An ergot-free diet; good nursing; treatment by a doctor.	Six different alkaloids are involved in ergot poisoning. Ergot is used to aid the uterus to contract after childbirth, to prevent loss of blood. It should be used only under the supervision of a doctor. Also, another ergot drug (ergotamine) is widely used in the treatment of migraine headaches.

(Continued)

TABLE P-11

Poison (Toxin)	History	Source	Species Affected
Fluorine (F) (fluorosis) (Also see FLUORINE OR FLUORIDE; and MINERAL[S].)	Airborne fluoride from dusts and gases has been an obvious health risk in many localities since the time of the earliest known volcanic eruptions. However, increased incidence of fluorosis came with industrialization—with factories producing fluorides; steel; aluminum; brick, tile, pottery, and cement (from the clay used in their manufacture); glass, enamel, and fiber glass; phosphate feed supplements; phosphate fertilizers; and similar products.	Ingesting excessive quantities of fluorine through either the food or water, or a combination of these. Except in certain industrial exposures, the intake of fluoride inhaled from the air is only a small fraction of the total fluoride intake in man. Pesticides containing fluorides, including those used to control insects, weeds, and rodents. Although water is the principal source of fluoride in an average human diet in the U.S., fluoride is frequently contained in toothpastes, toothpowders, chewing gums, mouthwashes, vitamin supplements, and mineral supplements.	Man All farm animals, poultry, and fish.
Lead (Pb)	Lead, which has been mined and used for many centuries, was considered by the alchemists to be the oldest metal. Extensive mining and processing of lead dates back to pre-Christian times. The Roman Empire declined and finally fell, according to authoritative speculation, not because of the barbarian hordes, overextended colonization, or because of moral decadence, but mainly as a result of lead poisoning. Eating and drinking from vessels containing lead and dabbing themselves with lead-laden cosmetics, the upper-class Romans unwittingly poisoned themselves, sapping their vitality and the vitality of the society they headed. (The poor people used cheap earthenware utensils and didn't fool with cosmetics.) A study of ancient tombstone inscriptions indicates a life expectancy of 22 to 25 years among upper-class Romans. Their birthrate was ¼ that needed to replace themselves.	Consuming food or medicinal products (including health food products) contaminated with lead. Inhaling the poison as a dust by workers in such industries as painting, lead mining, and refining. Inhaling airborne lead discharged into the air from auto exhaust fumes. Consuming food crops contaminated by lead being deposited on the leaves and other edible portions of the plant by direct fallout. Consuming food or water contaminated by contact with lead pipes or utensils. Old houses in which the interiors were painted with leaded paints prior to 1945, with the chipped wall paint eaten by children. Such miscellaneous sources as illicitly distilled whiskey, improperly lead-glazed earthenware, old battery casings used as fuel, and toys containing lead.	Man All farm animals.

(Continued)

(Continued)

Symptoms and Signs	Distribution; Magnitude	Prevention; Treatment	Remarks
Acute fluoride poisoning: Abdominal pain, diarrhea, vomiting, excessive salivation, thirst, perspiration, and painful spasms of the limbs. **Chronic fluoride poisoning:** Abnormal teeth (especially mottled enamel) during the first 8 years of life; and brittle bones. Other effects, predicted from animal studies, may include loss of body weight, and altered structure and function of the thyroid gland and kidneys. Water containing 3 to 10 ppm of fluoride may cause mottling of the teeth. An average daily intake of 20 to 80 mg of fluoride over a period of 10 to 20 years will result in crippling fluorosis.	**Distribution:** The water in parts of Arkansas, California, South Carolina, and Texas contains excess fluorine. Occasionally, throughout the U.S., high-fluorine phosphates are used in mineral mixtures. **Magnitude:** Generally speaking, fluorosis is limited to high-fluorine areas, for rarely do people or animals in low-fluorine areas have all their food or water transported from high-fluorine areas. Only a few instances of health effects in man have been attributed to airborne fluoride, and they occurred in persons living in the vicinity of fluoride-emitting industries. In the U.S., deaths from fluoride poisoning (suicidal plus accidental) constitute approximately 1% of all deaths by poisoning.	**Prevention:** Avoid the use of food and water containing excessive fluorine. Require that industrial plants producing phosphate fertilizers, steel, brick, ceramics, and similar types of products install equipment to remove both the particulate matter and gases. **Treatment:** Any damage may be permanent, but people who have not developed severe symptoms may be helped to some extent if the source of excess fluorine is eliminated. High dietary levels of calcium and magnesium may reduce the absorption and utilization of fluoride.	Fluorine is a cumulative poison. The total fluoride in the human body averages 2.57 g. Susceptibility to fluoride toxicity is increased by deficiencies of calcium, vitamin C, and protein. Virtually all foods contain trace amounts of fluoride, but the total intake in the average human diet is low. In the U.S., the daily intake of fluoride by an adult in an average diet is estimated to be 0.2 to 0.3 mg, with an added 1.0 mg from drinking water. Most plants absorb very little fluoride from the soil.
Symptoms develop rapidly in young children, but slowly in mature people. **Symptoms of acute lead poisoning:** Colic, cramps, diarrhea or constipation, leg cramps, and drowsiness. The most severe form of lead poisoning, encountered in infants and in heavy drinkers of illicitly distilled whiskey, is characterized by profound disturbances of the central nervous system, and permanent damage to the brain; damage to the kidneys; and shortened life span of the erythrocytes. **Symptoms of chronic lead poisoning:** Colic, constipation, lead palsy especially in the forearm and fingers, the symptoms of chronic nephritis, and sometimes mental depression, convulsions, and a blue line at the edge of the gums.	**Distribution:** Predominantly among children in poverty-stricken neighborhoods, living in dilapidated housing built before 1945, where they may eat chips of lead-containing paints, peeled off from painted wood. Leaded paints are no longer used on the interior surface of houses. **Magnitude:** The Center for Disease Control, Atlanta, Georgia, estimates that (1) lead poisoning claims the lives of 200 children each year, and (2) 400,000 to 600,000 children have elevated lead levels in the blood. Lead poisoning has been reduced significantly with the use of lead-free paint.	**Prevention:** Avoid inhaling or consuming lead. Workers in industries where lead poisoning is an occupational hazard should follow the safety regulations that have been established. **Treatment:** **Acute lead poisoning:** An emetic (induce vomiting), followed by drinking plenty of milk and ½ oz *(14 g)* of epsom salts in half a glass of water. **Chronic lead poisoning:** Remove the source of lead. Sometimes treated by administration of magnesium or lead sulphate solution as a laxative and antidote on the lead in the digestive system, followed by potassium iodide which cleanses the tracts. Currently, treatment of lead poisoning makes use of chemicals that bind the metal in the body and help in its removal.	Lead is a cumulative poison. When incorporated in the soil, nearly all the lead is converted into forms that are not available to plants. Any lead taken up by plant roots tends to stay in the roots, rather than move up to the top of the plant. Formerly, when lead-based paints were used, "painter's colic" was an occupational hazard among painters, but leaded paints are now banned by law. Lead poisoning can be diagnosed positively by analyzing the blood tissue for lead content; clinical signs of lead poisoning usually are manifested at blood lead concentrations above 80 micrograms/ 100 grams. A new, portable device developed by Bell Laboratories can be used as a rapid screening test. The concern today is mainly over the possible hazard that might result from the

widespread dissemination of lead by man into the general environment, and particularly over the insidious effects of long-term exposure.

It is noteworthy that the air over the largest American cities has a concentration of lead 20 times greater than the air over sparsely populated areas of the country and 2,000 times greater than the air over the mid-Pacific Ocean.

(Continued)

TABLE P-11

Poison (Toxin)	History	Source	Species Affected
Mercury (Hg)	In ancient times, mercury was known as "quicksilver," because of its slimy appearance and slippery form. Widespread concern over environmental pollution of mercury did not develop until the 1950s when an epidemic of mercury poisoning occurred in Japan.	Mercury is discharged into air and water from industrial operations and is used in herbicide and fungicide treatments. Mercury poisoning has occurred where mercury from industrial plants has been discharged into water and then accumulated as methylmercury in fish and shellfish. Accidental consumption of seed grains treated with fungicides that contain mercury, used for the control of fungus diseases of oats, wheat, barley, and flax.	Man All farm animals, but especially cattle and hogs.
Mycotoxins ("myco," prefix from the Greek word mykes, meaning fungus), which may produce the toxicity syndromes referred to as mycotoxicoses. There are an estimated 800 species of fungi (yeasts and molds), but fortunately not all fungi produce metabolites that are toxic. Some mycotoxins are carcinogens—capable of causing malignant tumors (cancer). *Cause:* Toxin-producing molds; e.g., *Aspergillus flavus, Aspergillus parasiticus, Penicillium cyclopium, P. islandicum, P. palitans, Fusarium roseum, F. tricinctum* The aflatoxins constitute a family of 14 naturally-occurring toxins. (Also see ERGOT which is presented alphabetically in this table.)	Fungal diseases are very old. Alimentary Toxic Aleukia (ATA), a mycotoxicosis caused by eating grain that had become moldy by overwintering in the field, afflicted thousands of people in the USSR during World War II. Explosive interest in fungus diseases was generated in 1960 when 100,000 turkeys in England died from a mysterious disease. Later, it was discovered that the Brazilian peanut meal incorporated in the turkey feed contained aflatoxin, a toxin produced by the fungus *Aspergillus flavus.* Similar outbreaks of the disease occurred in East Africa and India from local peanuts in those countries.	Contaminated food. Mycotoxins can produce toxic compounds on virtually any food (even synthetic) that will support growth. It is important to know that mycotoxins remain in food long after the organism that produced them has died; thus, they can be present in food that is not visibly moldy. Moreover, many kinds of mycotoxins are relatively stable substances that survive the usual methods of processing and cooking. The possibility of mycotoxicoses resulting from the ingestion of previously contaminated meat and eggs remains uncertain, unless the intake level is extremely high. But there is abundant evidence that lactating cows and lactating mothers consuming diets containing more than 20 ppb of aflatoxin on a dry matter basis will produce milk which contains aflatoxin residues. High levels of phytic acid in soybeans prevents aflatoxin synthesis.	Man Bear Cattle Dog Duckling Guinea pig Hamster Horse Mouse Partridge Pheasant Quail Rabbit Rat Sheep Swine Trout Turkey Young animals are much more susceptible to aflatoxin toxicity than mature animals. Generally, ruminants appear to tolerate higher levels of mycotoxins and longer periods of intake than simple stomached animals. Rainbow trout are extremely sensitive to aflatoxin, developing cancer when fed diets containing less than 1 ppb aflatoxin B_1.

(Continued)

(Continued)

Symptoms and Signs	Distribution; Magnitude	Prevention; Treatment	Remarks
The toxic effects of organic and inorganic compounds of mercury are dissimilar. The organic compounds of mercury, such as the various fungicides (1) affect the central nervous system, and (2) are not corrosive. The inorganic compounds of mercury include mainly mercuric chloride, a disinfectant; mercurous chloride (calomel), a cathartic; and elemental mercury. Commonly the toxic symptoms are: corrosive gastrointestinal effects, such as vomiting, bloody diarrhea, and necrosis of the alimentary mucosa.	**Distribution:** Wherever mercury is produced in industrial operations or used in herbicide or fungicide treatments. **Magnitude:** Limited. But about 1,200 cases of mercury poisoning identified in Japan in the 1950s were traced to the consumption of fish and shellfish from Japan's Minamata Bay contaminated with methylmercury. Some of the offspring of exposed mothers were born with birth defects, and many victims suffered central nervous system damage. Still another outbreak of mercury toxicity occurred in Iraq, where more than 6,000 people were hospitalized after eating bread made from wheat that had been treated with methylmercury.	**Prevention:** Do not consume seed grains treated with a mercury-containing fungicide. Surplus of treated grain should be burned and the ash buried deep in the ground. Control mercury pollution from industrial operations. **Treatment:** This should be left to a medical doctor.	Mercury is a cumulative poison. Ultimate diagnosis depends upon demonstrating the presence of mercury in the hair, kidneys, and liver. Food and Drug Administration prohibits use of mercury-treated grain for food or feed. Grain crops produced from mercury-treated seed and crops produced on soils treated with mercury herbicides have not been found to contain harmful concentrations of this element.
In animals, liver damage is the most characteristic symptom. It is reasonable to assume that man would respond similarly and that liver disease, particularly liver cancer, would be associated with aflatoxin exposure. Studies conducted in Uganda, Thailand, and Kenya have shown that high incidence of liver cancer is associated with high aflatoxin intake. Practically nothing is known about the acute effects of aflatoxins in humans. However, evidence is accumulating that suggests that aflatoxins and mycotoxins may be involved in some types of acute poisoning in children. In the Thailand study mentioned above, it was found that the liver, brain, and other tissues of children dying of a form of acute encephalitis, characterized by degeneration of the liver and other visceral organs (known as Reye's syndrome), contained far higher amounts and frequencies of aflatoxin B₁ than the tissues of children from the same region dying of other causes.	**Distribution:** Mycotoxins are widely distributed throughout the world. It has been known for a long time that liver cancer, which is relatively uncommon in the U.S., and Europe, occurs at much higher frequency in central and southern Africa and in Asia. This prompted several field studies which confirmed that elevated liver cancer incidence is associated with aflatoxin exposure. **Magnitude:** Mass poisoning of human population by mycotoxins occurred in the USSR during World War II. (See column headed "History.") Also, there has long been a high incidence of aflatoxin toxicity in Uganda, Thailand, and Kenya. In contrast to the limited number of documented mycotoxicoses in humans, there has been hundreds of reports of toxicity symptoms in livestock.	**Prevention:** The best way to control aflatoxins is to prevent their production. This calls for the maintenance of food and feed quality during growth, harvest, transportation, processing, and storage. The most important means of controlling mold growth and subsequent aflatoxin production is preventing damage to crops during harvest and reducing post harvest moisture levels below those required for fungal growth. Moisture levels below 18.5% in cereal grains, below 9% in such oilseeds as peanuts, sunflower, and safflower, and below 6% in copra. Organic acids (acetic acid-propionic acid mixture or propionic acid alone) may be applied to high-moisture grains to inhibit the growth of molds. The high aflatoxin risk crops are: peanuts, cottonseed, and copra. Aflatoxin in cottonseed may be inactivated by treating with anhydrous ammonia. Ultraviolet irradiation will also reduce the toxicity of aflatoxin. Certain spices, i.e., pepper	Not all products of fungi are harmful; for example, fungi gave us the antibiotics penicillin, streptomycin, and tetracycline. It is noteworthy, too, that in the Orient, *Aspergillus flavus* has long been used to ripen various vegetable cheeses, to make sake (a fermented product made from rice), and to ferment soy sauce. In the U.S. and some other countries, *A. flavus* is grown on most wheat bran to produce the enzyme diastase, used in various food products. Teranol is being produced commercially for cattle. *Penicillium roquefortii,* a fungus, is used to make Roquefort cheese.

(Continued)

Poison (Toxin)	History	Source	Species Affected
Mycotoxins (Continued)			

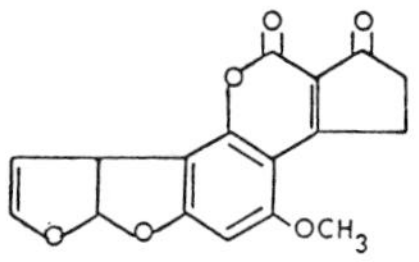

Fig. P-71. The chemical structure of aflatoxin B₁, the most common and the most toxic of the aflatoxins.

Poison (Toxin)	History	Source	Species Affected
Pesticides are chemicals used to destroy, prevent, or control pests. Pesticides also include (1) chemicals used to attract or repeal pests, and (2) chemicals used to regulate plant growth or remove or coat leaves. Pests can be classified into six main groups: 1. Insects (plus mites, ticks, and spiders) 2. Snails and slugs 3. Vertebrates, including rats, mice, and certain birds (starling, linnets, English sparrows, crows, and blackbirds) 4. Weeds 5. Plant disease 6. Nematodes (Also see PESTICIDES AS INCIDENTAL FOOD ADDITIVES.)	Commencing with the passage of the comprehensive Food and Drug Act in 1906, the federal government has played an increasingly important role in protecting consumers against harmful food and drugs. Today, the Environmental Protection Agency (EPA) administers the following acts: 1. The Federal Insecticide, Fungicide, and Rodenticide Act (FIFRA) as amended in 1972. Every pesticide must be registered, and commercial applicators must be certified—showing that they know the safe and correct way to use them. 2. The Toxic Substances Control Act (TOSCA) of 1976, which regulates chemicals that are not presently covered under other federal acts. It might more properly be described as the "chemical health and environmental regulation act."	Pesticides are chemicals. When properly used, they are beneficial; when improperly used, they may be hazards. Pesticide poisoning may be caused by either (1) sudden exposure to lethal quantities, or (2) as a result of repeated exposure to non-lethal quantities (chronic poisoning) during a protracted period of time. Farmers know that unless they follow federal and state regulations they risk having their products seized and condemned, or refused by food processors. Nevertheless, economics dictate that new products be used as soon as they prove useful. On the other hand, food faddists may feel that they are being poisoned; wildlife conservationists may be concerned over possible damage to songbirds and other animals; bee-keepers may become unhappy if insectants kill honeybees; and public health officials may be concerned about contamination of soil and food supplies.	Although pesticides are used to control pests, they can be toxic (poisonous) to man, other animals and plants. Many pesticides are so highly toxic that very small quantities can kill a person and and exposure to a sufficient amount of almost any pesticide can make a person ill. Even fairly safe pesticides can irritate the skin, eyes, nose, or mouth. Pesticides must be used with discretion because they are designed to kill some living organism. But sometimes choices must be made; for example, between malaria-carrying mosquitoes and some fish, or between hordes of locusts and grass-hoppers and the crops that they devour. This merely underscores the need for (1) careful testing of all products prior to use, (2) conforming with federal and state laws, and (3) accurate labeling and use of products.
		Some pesticides produce unplanned and undesirable "side effects," particularly when they are not used properly. Among such effects are: reduction of beneficial species; drift; wildlife losses; honeybee and other pollenating insect losses; and pollution of air, soil, water, and vegetation.	

(Continued)

Symptoms and Signs	Distribution; Magnitude	Prevention; Treatment	Remarks
Aflatoxins interact with DNA and markedly affect transcription of genetic information; they interfere with RNA synthesis.		and cinnamon, have been found to contain potent antifungal agents. Food and feed processors should determine toxin presence by analytical methods. Food and Drug Administration regulations do not permit food or feed containing more than 20 ppb of aflatoxin to be shipped in interstate commerce; but where grain is produced and fed on the farm, this is a difficult regulation to enforce. Food and Drug Administration permits an upper limit of 0.5 ppb of M_1 in milk. (When aflatoxin-contaminated feed is consumed by lactating cows, some aflatoxin is transformed into aflatoxin M_1. Aflatoxin M_1 is as hazardous as aflatoxin B_1.) **Treatment:** People or animals suffering from mold toxicity do not respond to treatmeant with drugs or antibiotics.	
Knowing something of the toxicity and symptoms or signs of poisoning of each type of pesticide may result in getting medical advice quickly and in saving a life. The leading chemical groups along with the toxicity symptoms of each follow:	**Distribution:** In every pursuit of modern agriculture, more and more pesticides are being used. They are the first line of defense against pests that affect human health and well-being and attack crops, livestock, and structures. **Magnitude:** Pesticides are used to control many of the estimated 10,000 species of harmful insects; more than 160 bacteria, 250 viruses, and 8,000 fungi known to cause plant diseases; 2,000 species of weeds and brush; and 150 million rats.	**Prevention:** The first and most important precaution to observe when using any pesticide is to read and heed the directions on the label. In the event of an accident, the label becomes extremely important in remedial measures. For public protection, all chemicals are rigidly controlled by federal laws. Each one is required to be registered by the Environmental Protection Agency before it can be sold in the United States, and each one is issued a tolerance for residues that may result from its use on food or feed crops. **Treatment:** Each label contains a "Statement of Practical Treatment." Read it before handling a pesticide. First aid procedures follow:	Since 1910, total American farm output has increased tenfold, production per man-hour has increased more than tenfold, and yield per acre has increased sixfold. Each person employed on the farm now produces food and fiber for more than 100 people. This revolution in production has been due to a number of factors, including better technology, breeding better plants and animals, farm mechanization, and the greater use of fertilizers, growth regulators, and pesticides. U.S. consumers benefit greatly from the proper use of pesticides. They enjoy the world's most abundant food supply with quality and variety second to none; and they spend only about 10.3% of their income for food, compared with the 50% or more that people in many other countries spend for food. If the world is to "waste not, want not," it must prudently use agricultural chemicals in the future. Pests still cause an estimated 30% annual loss in the worldwide potential production of crops, livestock, and forests. Every part of our food, feed, and fiber supply is vulnerable to pest attack, including domestic and wild animals, marine life, field crops, horticultural crops, and wild plants. Obviously, if these losses could be prevented, or reduced, world food supplies could be increased by a potential of one-third.
Chemical Group: Organophosphates—most toxic; they injure the nervous system Carbamates—safer than the organophosphates Fumigants—make a person seem drunk Plant-derived pesticides—some are very toxic	**Symptoms or signs of toxicity:** *Mild poisoning:* Fatigue, dizziness, sweating, vomiting. *Moderate poisoning:* Inability to walk, constriction of pupil of eye. *Severe poisoning:* Unconsciousness, tremors, convulsions. They produce the same symptoms and signs as the organophosphates, but they respond more easily to treatment. Poor coordination, slurring words, confusion, sleepiness. Technical pyrethrum may cause allergic reaction. Some rotenone dusts irritate the respiratory tract. Nicotine is fast-acting nerve poison.	**Happenstance:** **What To Do:** Pesticide skin contact .... Wash with soap or detergent and plenty of water. Pesticide inhalation .... Get to fresh air right away. Pesticide in eyes .... Flush eyes and face thoroughly with water. Pesticide in mouth or stomach .. Rinse mouth with water. Do not induce vomiting. Go to physician immediately. *Caution:* Take the pesticide label to the physician; it will help him treat the problem.	

TABLE P-11

Poison (Toxin)	History	Source	Species Affected
Polybrominated biphenyls (PBBs), a fire retardant which may cause cancer when taken into the food supply.	Until 1973, PBBs were used without known incident of toxicity, primarily to coat building roofs and to treat clothing for resistance to flammability. Then, a Michigan chemical company, short on bags for their commerical fire retardant, packaged some of it in bags normally used, and labeled, for magnesium oxide, a cattle supplement claimed to increase milk production and butterfat in dairy cattle. Some of the toxic fire retardant found its way into dairy rations. Then something went wrong!	All of the 1973 Michigan toxicity problem was traced to livestock feed which became contaminated with PBB when the fire retardant was shipped by mistake to a feed manufacturer.	Man Aminals, including poultry. Fish Wildlife
Polychlorinated biphenyls (PCBs), industrial chemicals; they're chlorinated hydrocarbons which may cause cancer when taken into the food supply.	The polychlorinated biphenyls (PCBs), a group of chlorinated hydrocarbons, were first used in 1930. PCBs were produced in huge quantities for use as insulation for electrical equipment, and as plasticizers in paints, adhesives, and caulking compounds. Their chief virtue: they are fire resistant; hence, they cut down on fires. Not until tens of millions of pounds of these products were produced and released into the environment was there any realization of their toxicity and persistency. In 1966, scientist Soren Jensen in Sweden detected PCB as an environmental contaminant. Since 1967, monitoring efforts in this country have revealed PCBs in milk, eggs, meat, fish, fats and oils, and cereal products. Despite limited restrictions imposed by industry in the early 1970s to reduce the production and use of PCBs, and the halting of production in 1977, high levels continue to persist in the Great Lakes and other major waters across the nation.	Sources of contamination to man include: 1. Contaminated foods 2. Mammals or birds that have fed on contaminated foods or fish. 3. Residues on foods that have been wrapped in papers and plastics containing PCBs. 4. Milk from cows that have been fed silage from silos coated with PCB-containing paint; and eggs from layers fed feeds contaminated with PCBs. 5. Absorption by human beings of PCBs through the lungs, the gastrointestinal tract, and the skin.	Man Cattle Chickens Ducks Fish Mink Wildlife PCBs have been found in the tissues of humans and in the milk of nursing mothers.

(Continued)

(Continued)

Symptoms and Signs	Distribution; Magnitude	Prevention; Treatment	Remarks
People exposed to PBB in Michigan reported suffering from neurological symptoms such as loss of memory, muscular weakness, coordination problems, headaches, painful swollen joints, acne, abdominal pain, and diarrhea.	In 1973, the accidental contamination of animal feeds exposed many people in Michigan to PBB in dairy products and other foods. The Michigan incident eventually led to the slaughter and burial of nearly 25,000 cattle, 3,500 hogs, and 1.5 million chickens; and the disposal of about 5 million eggs and tons of milk, butter, cheese, and feed.	**Prevention:** Avoid human error such as substituting PBB for a livestock feed supplement. Avoid harmfully contaminated food. **Treatment:** Follow the prescribed treatment of a medical doctor.	PBBs are long-term, low-level contaminants, very stable and resistant to decay.
The clinical effects on people are: an eruption of the skin resembling acne, visual disturbances, jaundice, numbness, and spasms. Newborn infants from mothers who have been poisoned show discoloration of the skin which regresses after 2 to 5 months.	**Distribution:** PCBs are widespread. They have, directly and indirectly, found their way into animal feeds and animal food products through water, paints, sealants used on the interior walls of silos, heat transfer fluids, and plastic and cardboard food-packaging materials.	**Prevention:** Comply with the law; do not use PCBs. Avoid harmfully contaminated food. **Treatment:** People afflicted with PCB should follow the prescribed treatment of their doctor.	Although the production of PCBs was halted in 1977, and the importing of PCBs was banned January 1, 1979, the chemicals had been widely used for 40 years; and they are exceptionally long-lived. So, it is expected that these persistent chemicals will be around for many years to come.

Magnitude: PCB constitutes the first example of a widespread environmental hazard from an industrial chemical not classed as a pesticide. The wide usage and the persistence indicate that PCB will be of considerable concern for many years.

In 1968, the accidental contamination of edible rice-bran oil by PCBs led to a poisoning epidemic among the Japanese families who consumed the oil. The disease, which afflicted 1,291 people, became known as Yusho or rice-oil disease—a condition marked by chloracne (a severe form of acne), eye discharges, skin discoloration, headaches, fatigue, abdominal pains, and liver and menstrual distrubances. In 1972, Japan banned the manufacture of PCB.

The following U.S. incidents dramatically illustrate the potential health hazard and economic harm that can be caused by PCBs: (1) the discharging of PCBs into the Hudson River with waste water from capacitor plants from 1946 to 1976, and the contamination of Hudson River fish; (2) in 1977, a fire in an animal-feed warehouse in Puerto Rico contaminated fish meal, which was subsequently fed to poultry and resulted in the destruction of about 400,000 chickens and millions of eggs in the U.S.; and (3) in 1979, the fat used to produce meat and bone meal feeds in a meat-packing plant in Billings, Montana, contaminated by PCBs from a damaged transformer, resulted (to October 1979) in the destruction of 600,000 to 700,000 chickens, several hundred thousand eggs, and 16,000 lb of fresh pork.

In 1980, the EPA estimated that 91% of Americans carry a measurable quantity of PCB in their fatty tissues.

Most other countries that manufacture PCBs including the USSR, still haven't passed laws restricting their use.

PCBs have been widely used in dielectric fluids in capacitors and transformers, hydraulic fluids, and heat transfer fluids. Also, they have more than 50 minor uses, including plasticizers and solvents in adhesives, printing ink, sealants, moisture retardants, paints, and pesticide carriers.

PCB will cause cancer in laboratory animals (rats, mice, and rhesus monkeys). It is not known if it will cause cancer in humans. More study is needed to gauge its effects on the ecological food chain and on human health.

When fed coho salmon from Lake Michigan with 10-15 ppm PCB, mink in Wisconsin stopped reproducing or their kits died.

In 1977, polar bears at the very top of the Arctic food chain showed PCB levels of up to 8 ppm in their fatty tissue. This indicates that PCBs are spread throughout the biosphere.

(Continued)

Poison (Toxin)	History	Source	Species Affected
Salt (NaCl—sodium chloride) poisoning (Also see MINERAL[S]; and SALT.)	The Bible mentions salt more than 30 times. The Book of Job, written about 300 years before the birth of Christ, says: "Can an unsavory thing be eaten that is not seasoned with salt?" Caesar's soldiers received part of their pay in common salt, which was known as their *salarium;* and it is from this that the word salary comes. The expression "not worth his salt" dates back to the days when workers were paid all or part of their wages in salt.	Table salt (sodium chloride) and foods containing salt.	Man All farm animals.
Selenium poisoning (Also see MINERAL[S]; and SELENIUM.)	The toxic effects of this element were observed long before selenium was identified. In the 13th century, Marco Polo observed that certain forages that grew in the mountains of western China caused the hoofs of grazing animals to drop off. With the opening up of western U.S., the Army surgeon, Madison, observed, in 1856, that cavalry horses in Nebraska lost their hoofs and some of their hair when feeding on the native forage plants. Similar observations were reported by the Wyoming Agricultural Experiment Station in 1893. These disorders were referred to as "Alkali disease" and "blind staggers." However, it was not until the early 1930s that agricultural researchers showed that (1) certain plants contained abnormally high amounts of selenium which had been absorbed from soils that were rich in this mineral, and (2) animals which were fed these plants developed selenium poisoning.	Consumption of high levels of the element in food or drinking water. Presence of malnutrition, parasitic infestation, or other factors which make people highly susceptible to selenium toxicity.	Man All farm animals.
Tin (Sn)	The people of Egypt used tin bronzes to make ornaments and different kinds of utensils as early as 3,000 years before Christ. Most tin cans are made of steel covered with a thin coat of tin.	From acid fruits and vegetables canned in tin cans. The acids in such foods as citrus fruits and tomato products can leach tin from the inside of the can. Then the tin is ingested with the canned food. In the digestive tract tin goes through a methylation process in which nontoxic tin is converted to methylated tin, which is toxic.	Man The danger of methylated metal poisoning is acute in the human fetus. Pregnant women may not suffer the effects themselves; instead, their fetuses may be affected.

(Continued)

(Continued)

Symptoms and Signs	Distribution; Magnitude	Prevention; Treatment	Remarks
Excess dietary salt over a prolonged period of time is believed to lead to high blood pressure in susceptible people. Salt may be toxic (1) when it is fed to infants or others whose kidneys cannot excrete the excess in the urine, or (2) when the body is adapted to a chronic low-salt diet.	**Distribution:** Salt is used all over the world. Hence, the potential for salt poisoning exists everywhere. **Magnitude:** Salt poisoning is relatively rare.	**Prevention:** Do not deplete the body of salt such as can occur (1) when on a strict vegetarian diet without salt, or (2) when there has been heavy and prolonged sweating; followed by gorging on salt. The best preventative against salt poisoning is to provide plenty of water. **Treatment:** Drink large quantities of fresh water.	Even normal salt concentration may be toxic if water intake is low. The Indians and the pioneers handed down many legendary stories about huge numbers of wild animals that killed themselves simply by gorging at a newly found salt lick after having been salt-starved for long periods of time.
Abnormalities in the hair, nails, and skin. Children in a high-selenium area of Venezuela showed loss of hair, discolored skin, and chronic digestive disturbances. However, most of the children were infested by internal parasites, which might have weakened them so that they had increased susceptibility to the toxic effects of selenium. Normally, people who have consumed large excesses of selenium excrete it as trimethyl selenide in the urine, and/or as dimethyl selenide on the breath. The latter substance has an odor resembling garlic. Rates of tooth decay are slightly higher in high-selenium areas.	**Distribution:** In certain regions of western U.S., especially certain areas in South Dakota, Montana, Wyoming, Nebraska, Kansas, and perhaps areas in other states in the Great Plains and Rocky Mountains. Also, in Canada. **Magnitude:** Selenium toxicity in people is relatively rare.	**Prevention:** Abandon areas where soils contain excess selenium, because crops produced on such soils constitute a menace to both man and livestock. **Treatment:** Selenium toxicity may be counteracted by arsenic or copper, but such treatment should be under the direction of a doctor.	Confirmed cases of selenium poisoning in people are rare because (1) only traces are present in most foods, (2) foods generally come from a wide area, and (3) the metabolic processes normally convert excess selenium into harmless substances which are excreted in the urine or breath.
Methylated tin is a neurotoxin —a toxin that attacks the central nervous system, the symptoms of which are numbness of the fingers and lips followed by a loss of speech and hearing. Eventually, the afflicted person becomes spastic, then coma and death follow.	**Distribution:** Tin cans are widely used throughout the world. **Magnitude:** The use of tin in advanced industrial societies has increased 14-fold over the last 10 years.	**Prevention:** Many tin cans are coated on the inside with enamel or other materials. Perhaps such coating should be a requisite when canning acidic fruits and vegetables. **Treatment:** This should be left to the medical doctor.	Currently, not much is known about the amount of tin in the human diet. The presentation herein should merely be accepted as indicative of the need for more experimental work.

POISON, CHEMICAL

Furor created by those living in the housing development over the toxic waste dump at Love Canal suggests the concern for some of the problems created by industrialization. Each year, industry introduces 1,000 new chemicals. Many chemicals or their by-products have found their way into the environment posing the threat of contaminating our food and water. Lead, mercury, cadmium, copper, beryllium, zinc, and silver pollutants can be potential hazards. The numerous insecticides and herbicides, and the toxic organic chemicals such as polychlorinated biphenyls (PCBs) and polybrominated biphenyls (PBBs), have all found their way into the environment. In addition, there is the question of the safety of those chemicals intentionally added to our foods (additives). Hence, the issue of chemical poisons is complicated, and sometimes emotional. We should remember that no chemical is totally safe, all the time, everywhere. Many chemicals, however, help make life more livable; hence, rather than banishing all chemicals, or discouraging the production of new ones, the obvious hazards must be eliminated. Then, our challenge for those chemicals with unknown hazards is their prudent and proper use and disposal coupled with monitoring their levels in food, water, and the environment. If we are able to do this, then we can reap the benefits derived from chemicals without suffering from their misuse.

(Also see PESTICIDES AS INCIDENTAL FOOD ADDITIVES; and POISONS.)

POLISHINGS

A by-product of rice consisting of the fine residue resulting from the brushing of the grain to polish the kernel after the hulls and bran have been removed.

(Also see RICE.)

POLLUTION CONTROL

Today, there is worldwide awakening to the problem of pollution of the environment (air, water, and soil) and its effects on human health and on other forms of life. Much of this concern stems from the sudden increase of animals in confinement.

We must be mindful that life, beauty, wealth, and progress depend upon how wisely man uses nature's gifts—the soil, the water, the air, the minerals, and the plant and animal life.

Certainly, there have been abuses of the environment (and it hasn't been limited to agriculture). There is no argument that such neglect should be rectified in a sound, orderly manner. But it should be done with a minimum disruption of the economy and lowering of the standard of living. Throughout the book, the authors allude to ways in which pollution can be controlled to the maximum.

(Also see PESTICIDES AS INCIDENTAL FOOD ADDITIVES; and POISONS.)

POLY-

Prefix meaning much or many.

POLYARTERITIS NODOSA (KASSMAUL-MAIER DISEASE)

A usually fatal disease affecting the connective tissue in the arteries of the kidneys, heart, lungs, liver, gastrointestinal tract, eyes and joints. Diseased arteries allow blood to clot, become inflamed, and deteriorate. This causes functional impairment of the organs and tissues supplied by the affected arteries. Outward symptoms of the sufferer include fever, weight loss, abdominal and muscular pains, skin disturbances, and high blood pressure. The disease usually occurs in middle age, and affects three times as many men as women. The cause of polyarteritis is unknown, but it belongs to a class of diseases called collagen diseases. If detected early enough, steroids may provide temporary relief and slow the progess of the disease. During steroid therapy, dietary sodium may have to be restricted since many steroid preparations promote sodium retention.

POLYCHLORINATED BIPHENYLS (PCBs)

This is a group of chlorinated hydrocarbons that have been widely used as plasticizers and insulation for electrical equipment, along with a host of other uses. Despite the usefulness of PCB products, there is concern because they will produce cancer in laboratory animals, and because of their persistency. It is not known if they will cause cancer in humans. More study is needed on the PCBs to gauge their effects on the ecological food chain and on human health.

(Also see POISONS, Table P-11, Some Potentially Poisonous [Toxic] Substances.)

POLYCYTHEMIA

Excess blood cells that contain a high concentration of hemoglobin. One type of polycythemia may be caused by an excess of cobalt in the diet of humans, resulting in stimulation of bone marrow accompanied by excessive production of red corpuscles and higher than normal hemoglobin.

POLYDIPSIA

An abnormal or excessive thirst due to the loss of body fluids, as observed in diabetes mellitus.

POLYNEURITIS

Neuritis of several peripheral nerves at the same time, caused by metallic and other poisons, infectious disease, or vitamin deficiency. In man, alcoholism is also a major cause of polyneuritis.

POLYNEUROPATHY

A disease which causes the noninflammatory degeneration of many of the peripheral nerves. It may result from: (1) certain deficiency diseases, (2) metabolic diseases, (3) chemical poisoning, (4) some infective diseases, (5) a carcinoma, or (6) some rare genetic diseases. Symptoms consist of cramps, numbness, weakness, loss of reflexes, loss of positional senses, and partial paralysis. Usually the legs are affected first, and then the arms. Those deficiency diseases exhibiting polyneuropathy are beriberi, pellagra, chronic alcoholism, burning feet syndrome, and pyridoxine or pantothenic acid deficiency.

POLYPEPTIDES

Ten to one hundred amino acids chemically joined by a peptide bond are termed polypeptides. In the body, polypeptides occur as a result of protein digestion or protein synthesis.

(Also see PROTEIN[S].)

POLYPHAGIA

Continuous eating or excessive appetite.
(Also see APPETITE.)

POLYPHOSPHATES

The ability of the phosphates (PO_4) to chemically link up with each other and form long chains gives rise to a variety of phosphate compounds called polyphosphates. They have numerous uses in the food industry as nutrient and/or dietary supplements, sequestrants (chelating agents), flavor improvers in processed meats, and chemical aids to curing meats. The FDA considers most polyphosphates and their sodium, calcium, potassium and ammonium salts as GRAS (generally recognized as safe) additives.

(Also see ADDITIVES, Table A-3.)

POLYSACCHARIDE

Any one of a group of carbohydrates, consisting of a combination of a large but undetermined number of monosaccharide molecules, such as starch, dextrin, glycogen, cellulose, inulin, etc.

(Also see CARBOHYDRATE[S].)

POLYUNSATURATED FATTY ACIDS

Fatty acids having more than one double bond. Linoleic and linolenic acids, which contain two or three double bonds, respectively, are essential in the diet of man.

(Also see FATS AND OTHER LIPIDS; and FATTY ACIDS.)

POLYURIA

A medical term indicating excessive formation and discharge of urine. It is a sign of disease. For example, polyuria is noted in diabetics.

POMACE

The residue of a fruit pulp that remains after the fruit has been pressed to extract the juice. Large amounts of apple, citrus, and grape pomace are produced in the United States during the manufacturing of the respective juices. The apple and citrus pomaces are the raw materials used in the production of pectin, a gelling agent and an ingredient in diarrhea remedies. All three types of pomace are used as animal feed ingredients.

POME

A type of fruit that contains many seeds enclosed within a central cartilagenous core which, in turn, is surrounded by the fleshy portion and skin of the fruit. The best known pome fruits are apples, pears, and quinces.
(Also see FRUIT[S].)

PONDERAL INDEX

A quantity derived from a formula which attempts to express relative leanness as a function of height and weight. The higher the value of the ponderal index, the greater the leanness and the lower the risk of cardiovascular disease.
(Also see OBESITY, section headed "An Index of Slenderness.")

POPULATION, WORLD

Population growth is the major determinant of demand for food.

It took from the dawn of man until 1,600 years after the birth of Christ for the number of people in the world to reach one-half billion. The population of the world first topped 1 billion in 1830. And it took another 100 years—until 1930, for the population to reach 2 billion. In 1960, it was 3 billion; in 1975, it was 4 billion; and in 1982, it was 4.5 billion. Even more frightening in the people-numbers game is the estimation of population experts for the years ahead. By the year 2000, it is predicted that the world will have 6.2 billion mouths to feed; and that by the year 2,045, world population will be doubled (see Fig. P-72).

Assuming 6.2 billion (the estimated population in the year 2000) people standing shoulder to shoulder and oc-

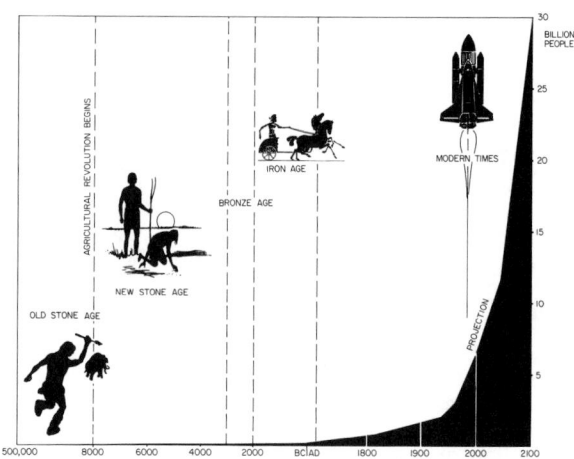

Fig. P-72. Human population growth over the past 1.5 million years, with projections to 2100 A.D.
   NOTE: If the Old Stone Age were in scale, its base line would extend 8 feet to the left.

cupying an average width of 2 ft, 6.2 billion people would circle the world 97 times, or reach to the moon and back (477,750 mi) 5 times. Today's one-year-old baby will likely see the world's population reach 12 billion—three times the present numbers—within his or her lifetime.

Do these population figures foretell the fulfillment of the doomsday prophecy of Thomas Malthus, made in 1798, that world population grows faster than man's ability to increase food production? For almost 200 years, we proved Malthus wrong. Disease had a major role in holding population down; and as population increased, new land was brought under cultivation; and machinery, chemicals, new crops and varieties, and irrigation were added to step up the yields. Now science has given us the miracle of better health and longer life. Malthus was right!

The ominous challenge of our children is that the demand for food will triple in their lifetime. And that's not all! Seventy-five percent of the people of the world live in the developing countries where only 40% of the world's food is produced. Also, this is where most of the world's increase in population is occurring; population in the developing countries is now growing more than 2.1% annually compared to just under 0.6% in the developed countries. The developing countries now account for 89% of the world's annual population increase. More disturbing yet, rate of increased food production per capita in the developing countries is only two-thirds of that in the developed countries. So, people in some of the developing countries will starve to death because of population growth outrunning food production. Increased agricultural production in the developing countries requires more scientific knowledge than the older methods.

(Also see HUNGER, WORLD; MALNUTRITION, PROTEIN-ENERGY; MALTHUS; PROTEIN, WORLD PER CAPITA; and WORLD FOOD.)

PORK

Contents | Page

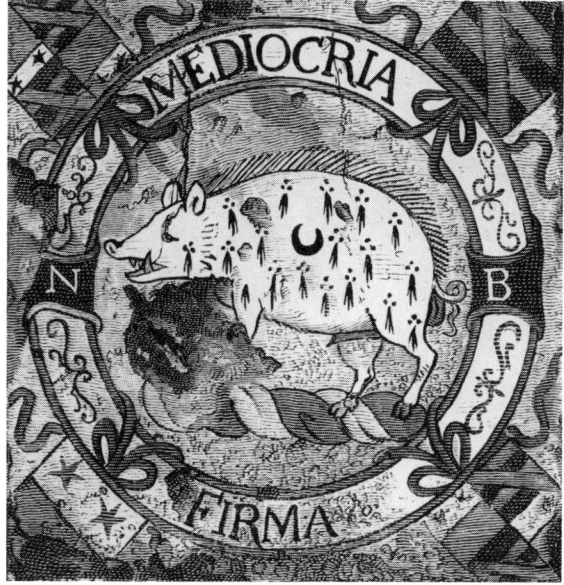

Fig. P-73. The crest of Lord Bacon (1561-1626)—noted English Viscount, lawyer, statesman, politician. According to some authorities, the word "bacon" was derived from Lord Bacon. (Courtesy, Picture Post Library, London, England)

Pork is the flesh of hogs, which are usually slaughtered at about 240 lb liveweight. About 70% of the pork carcass becomes salable retail cuts; the remaining 30% consists of fat trim, sausage trimmings, and feet, tail, and neckbones.

Only about ⅓ of the pork processed in the United States is sold as fresh product, the other ⅔ is cured and smoked. Originally, pork was cured to preserve it, but, today, pork is cured primarily to enhance flavor and provide variety and convenience.

QUALITIES IN PORK DESIRED BY CONSUMERS.
Consumers desire the following qualities in pork:

1. **Quality.** The quality of the lean is based on firmness, texture, marbling, and color.

2. **Firmness.** Pork muscle should be firm so as to display attractively. Firmness is affected by the kind and amount of fat. For example, pigs that are fed liberally on peanuts produce soft pork. Also, pork with small quantities of fat will contain more moisture and tend to be soft.

3. **Texture.** Pork lean that has a fine-grained texture and porous pinkish bones is preferred. Coarse-textured lean is generally indicative of greater animal maturity and less tender meat.

4. **Marbling.** This characteristic contributes to buyer appeal. Feathering (flecks of fat) between the ribs and within the muscles is indicative of marbling.

5. **Color.** Most consumers prefer pork with a white fat on the exterior and a greyish pink lean marbled with flecks of fat.

6. **Maximum muscling; moderate fat.** Maximum thickness of muscling influences materially the acceptability by the consumer. Also, consumers prefer a uniform cover of not to exceed ¼ in. (6 mm) of firm, white fat on the exterior.

7. **Repeatability.** The housewife wants to be able to secure a standardized product; pork of the same eating qualities as her previous purchase.

If these seven qualities are not met by pork, other products will meet them. Recognition of this fact is important, for competition is keen for space on the shelves of a modern retail food outlet.

FEDERAL GRADES OF PORK.
Grades of barrow and gilt carcasses are based on quality-indicating characteristics of the lean and expected yields of the four lean cuts (ham, loin, picnic shoulder, and Boston butt). Quality and yield are combined in one set of grades and are not kept separate, in contrast to the system used with beef and lamb.

From the standpoint of quality, two general levels are recognized—"acceptable" and "unacceptable." Acceptability is determined by direct observation of the cut surface and is based on considerations of firmness, marbling, and color, along with the use of such indirect indicators as firmness of fat and lean, feathering between the ribs, and color. The degree of external fatness is not considered in evaluating the quality of the lean. Suitability of the belly for bacon (in terms of thickness) is also considered in quality evaluation, as is the softness and oiliness of the carcass. Carcasses which have unacceptable quality lean, and/or bellies that are too thin, and/or carcasses which are soft and oily are graded U.S. Utility.

If a carcass qualifies as acceptable in quality of lean and in belly thickness, and is not soft and oily, it is graded U.S. No. 1, 2, 3, or 4, based entirely on projectd carcass yields of the four lean cuts; carcasses not qualifying for these four grades are graded U.S. Utility. The expected yields of each of the grades in the four lean cuts, based on using the U.S. Department of Agriculture standard cutting and trimming methods, are as given in Table P-12.

TABLE P–12
EXPECTED YIELDS OF THE FOUR LEAN CUTS BASED ON CHILLED CARCASS WEIGHT, BY GRADE

Grade	Yield
U.S. No. 1	60.4% and over
U.S. No. 2	57.4% –60.3%
U.S. No. 3	54.4%–57.3%
U.S. No. 4	Less than 54.4%

PIGS ARE NOT ALL PORK CHOPS!

HOG CARCASS BREAKDOWN

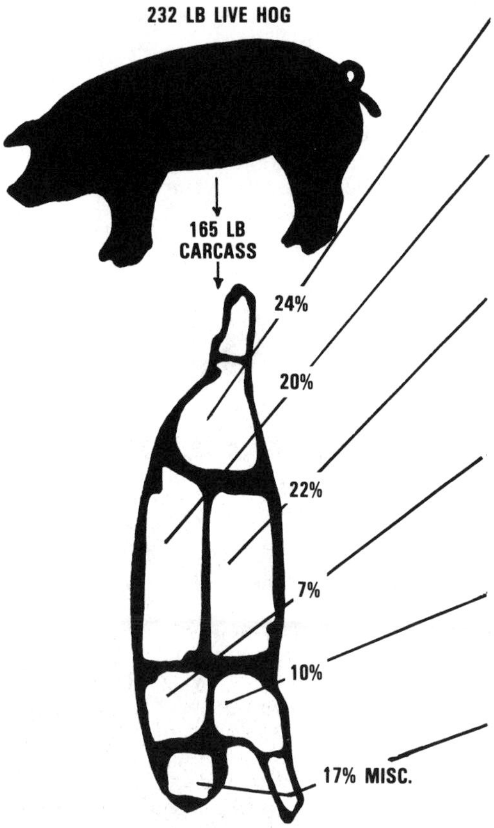

232 LB LIVE HOG

165 LB CARCASS

24%

20%

22%

7%

10%

17% MISC.

	Retail Pork[1] (lb)	Other Products (lb)	Carcass Total (lb)
HAM (39.4 lb)			
Cured Ham	20.1		
Fresh Ham	4.1		
Trimmings	3.0		
Skin, fat, bone		12.2	
Total	27.2	12.2	39.4
LOIN (32.9 lb)			
Blade roast	8.0		
Center chops	17.3		
Sirloin roast	5.6		
Fat		2.0	
Total	30.9	2.0	32.9
SIDE (36.4 lb)			
Cured bacon	18.6		
Spareribs	6.4		
Trimmings	9.4		
Fat		2.0	
Total	34.4	2.0	36.4
SHOULDER (28.0 lb)			
Boston Butt			
Blade steaks	7.0		
Blade roast	4.2		
Trimmings	0.8		
Total	12.0		12.0
Picnic			
Arm roast	7.7		
Trimmings	3.7		
Skin, fat, bone		4.6	
Total	11.4	4.6	16.0
MISCELLANEOUS (28.3 lb)			
Jowls, feet, tails, neckbones, etc.	6.5		
Trimmings	3.9		
Fat, skin, bone		14.4	
Shrink and loss		3.5	
Total	10.4	17.9	28.3
TOTAL	126.3	38.7	165.0

[1]Retail cuts on semiboneless basis. Fully boneless would show lower retail weight.

Fig. P-74. Pigs are not all pork chops! This shows the approximate (a) percentage of yield of carcass in relation to the weight of the animal on foot, and (b) yield of different retail cuts. Note that a 232-lb live hog produces approximately a 165-lb carcass, and ends up with only 126.3 lb of retail pork. Note, too, the small amount of center chops, only 17.3 lb. (Source: Adapted by the author from *Meat Facts*, published by the American Meat Institute, Washington, DC. Data derived from USDA and industry sources.)

The final grade is determined by calculating a preliminary grade based on the backfat thickness over the last rib, then adjusting it up or down one grade for thick or thin muscling.

Pigs are not all pork chops! It is important, therefore, that those who slaughter hogs and the consumer know the approximate (1) percentage of yield of chilled carcass in relation to the weight of the animal on foot, and (2) yield of different retail cuts. Fig. P-74 illustrates these points. As noted, on a liveweight basis only about 7.5% of a pig is center cut pork chops.

PORK CUTS AND HOW TO COOK THEM. The method of cutting pork is practically the same in all sections of the United States. Fig. P-75 illustrates the common retail cuts of pork, and gives the recommended method or methods for cooking each. This informative figure may be used as a guide to wise buying, in dividing the pork carcass into the greatest number of desirable cuts, in becoming familiar with the types of cuts, and in preparing each type of cut by the proper method of cookery.

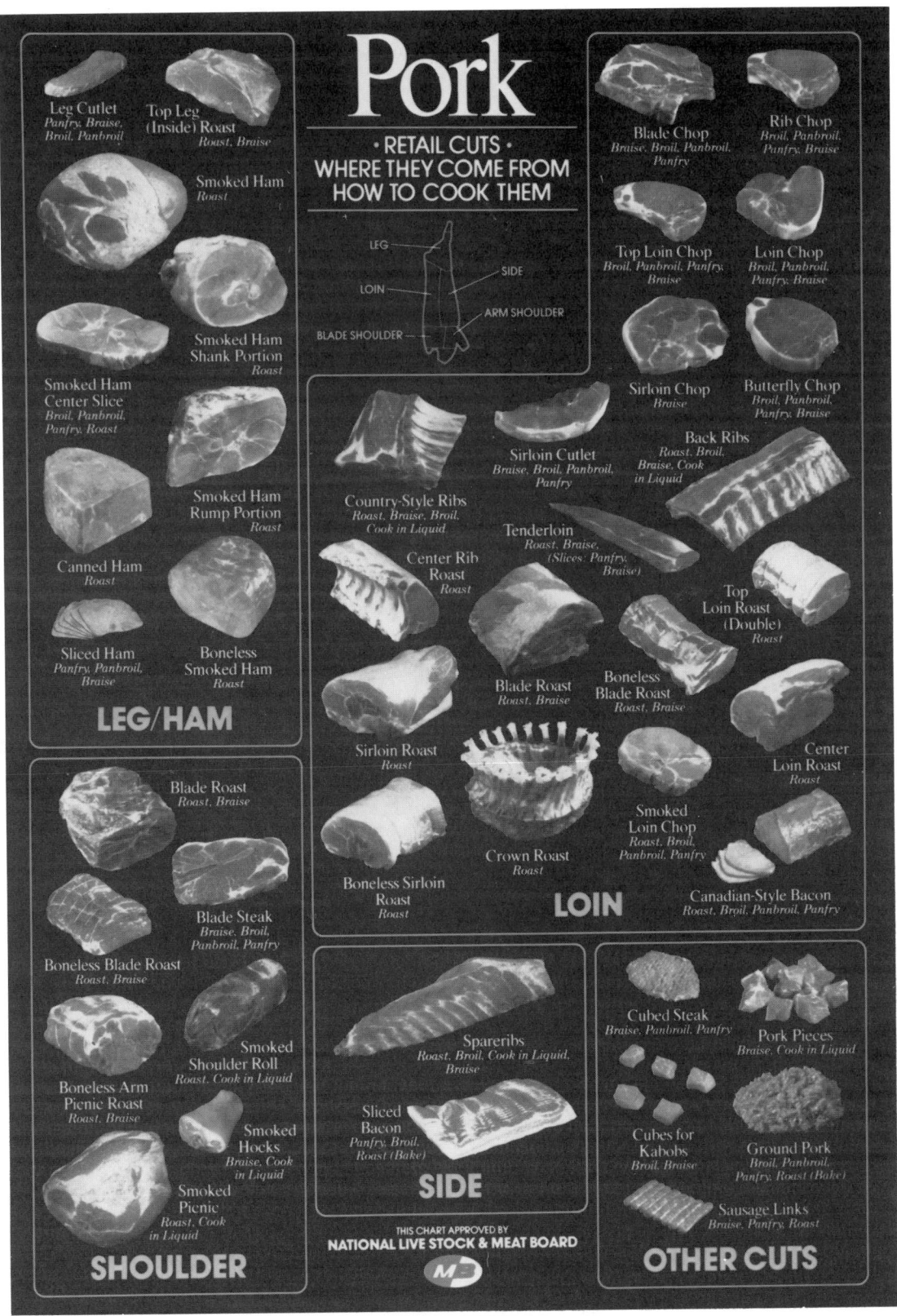

Fig. P-75. PORK, retail cuts, where they come from, and how to cook them. Note, too, that the wholesale cuts are shown in the drawing immediately below the heading. (Courtesy, National Live Stock and Meat Board, Chicago, Ill.)

U.S. PORK PRODUCTION.   On December 1, 1990, there were 54,562,000 hogs in the United States; and 15.3 billion pounds (*7 bil kg*) of pork were produced in the calendar year 1990. In 1990, pork production accounted for 40% of all red meat produced in the United States, while beef accounted for 59%.

PER CAPITA PORK CONSUMPTION.   In 1990, U.S. per capita consumption of pork was 46.3 lb (*21 kg*). That same year, U.S. per capita beef consumption was 112.3 lb (*51 kg*).

Although comprising less than 5% of the world's human population and having only 6.3% of its hogs, the people of the United States eat 10% of the total world production of pork.[15]

In general, pork consumption (and production) is highest in the temperate zones of the world, and in those areas where the human population is relatively dense. In many countries, such as China, pigs are primarily scavengers; in others, hog numbers are closely related to corn, barley, potato, and dairy production. As would be expected, the per capita consumption of pork in different countries of the world varies directly with its production and availability. Food habits and religious restrictions also affect the amount of pork consumed.

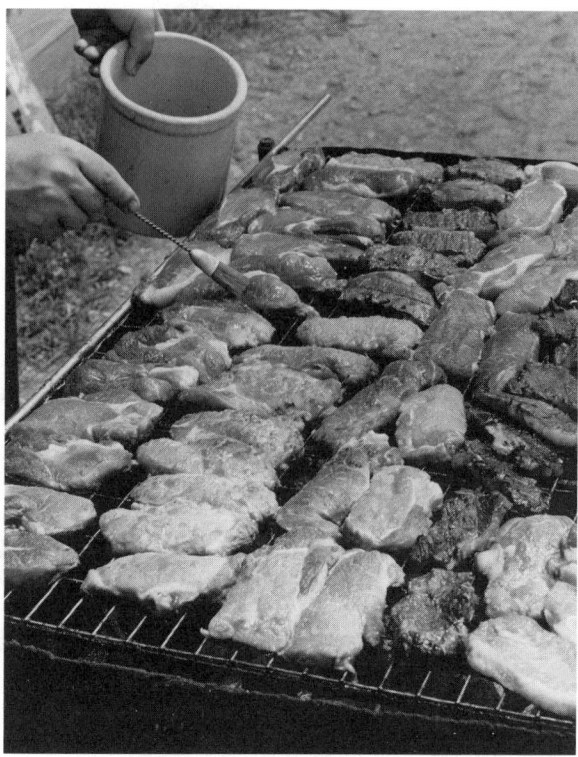

Fig. P-76.   Barbecuing pork tenderloin on grill. (Courtesy, J. C. Allen & Son, West Lafayette, Ind.)

PORK AS A FOOD.   Pork is an important food and a rich source of many essential nutrients. An average 3.5 oz (*99.4 g*) serving of cooked pork ham provides 37 g of protein (that's ⅔ of the recommended daily allowance of protein) and 8.8 g of fat, along with being an excellent source of minerals and vitamins. Its high-quality protein contains all the essential amino acids needed to build, maintain, and repair body tissues. Pork is rich in iron, and the iron is readily used in the formation and maintenance of red blood cells. Also, pork is a major dietary source of the B vitamins, especially thiamin, riboflavin, and niacin. Also pork is about 98% digestible.

Because of its high concentration of several key nutrients, many physicians and nutritionists regard pork as a desirable part of many special diets, such as those for peptic ulcer, diabetes, diseases of the liver, and in geriatric and pediatric conditions where it is important to maintain a good supply of high-quality protein and other body-building and restorative nutrients which patients need. The lean cuts of fresh and cured pork are excellent foods, which afford appetizing variety for the patient.

(Also see MEAT[S].)

---

[15]From *FAO Production Yearbook*, 1990, FAO/UN, Rome, Italy, Vol. 44, pp. 195 and 209.

PORPHYRIN

A derivative of porphin. Porphyrin is present in hemoglobin; heme is ferroprotoporphyrin, a porphyrin combined with iron (ferro- for Fe^{++}).

PORTAL

An entrance. When applied to blood, it may refer to—

• **Portal blood**—The blood in the portal vein passing from the gastrointestinal tract to the liver.

• **Portal circulation**—The circulation within the liver; blood is taken into the liver by the portal vein and carried out by the hepatic vein.

• **Portal system**—The portal vein and its branches through which the portal circulation takes place; the portal system begins and ends in capillaries.

• **Portal vein**—A vein carrying blood from the digestive organs and spleen to the liver where the nutrients are altered by liver cells before passing into the systemic circulation.

POSTOPERATIVE NUTRITION

Major surgery results in a generalized loss of tissue—a catabolic phase—placing the patient in a negative nitrogen balance state. This is in part due to the changes brought about by the neuroendocrine system stimulating the secretion of adrenal cortical hormones. However, the nutritional concerns for most patients immediately following surgery are fluids, electrolytes, and energy. Depending upon the type of surgery these can be given (1) orally, (2) by a nasogastric tube, (3) by a tube placed directly in the small intestine or stomach, or (4) intravenously. As soon as possible the patient should be returned to an adequate oral intake of energy and protein to support a positive nitrogen balance during the time new tissues are being synthesized—the anabolic phase. As normal convalescence proceeds, and if there are no complications, the patient's appetite provides a reliable guide to requirements.

Specific information regarding postoperative situations requiring specialized methods is explained in detail elsewhere.

(Also see MODIFIED DIETS; INTRAVENOUS [Parenteral] NUTRITION, SUPPLEMENTARY; LIQUID DIETS; and TOTAL PARENTERAL [Intravenous] NUTRITION.)

POTASSIUM (K)

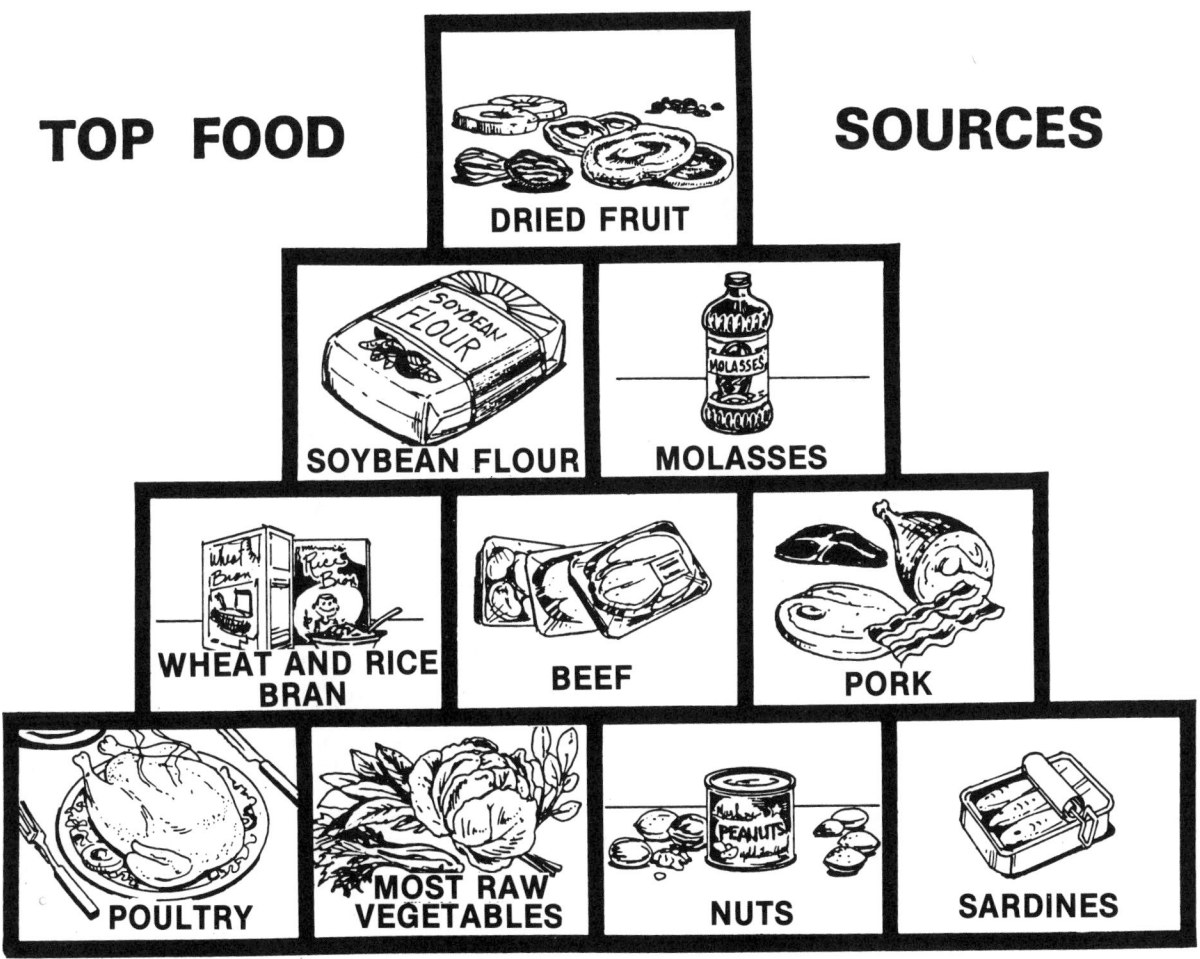

Fig. P-77. Top food sources of potassium.

Potassium is a silver-white metallic element. It is never found as a pure metal—it is always combined with other substances.

Potassium is the third most abundant element in the body, after calcium and phosphorus; and it is present in twice the concentration of sodium.

Potassium constitutes about 5% of the mineral content of the body. It is the primary cation of intracellular (within the cells) fluids. Approximately 98% of the total body potassium is located intracellularly, where its concentration is 30 or more times that of the extracellular (between cells) fluid. The concentration of sodium in blood plasma is much higher than potassium. On the other hand, the potassium concentration in muscle tissue and milk is many times higher than sodium.

HISTORY.

The history of potassium is closely linked to that of sodium. Materials containing their compounds, particularly carbonates and nitrates, were known to some of the earliest civilizations. Records show that they were used in Mesopotamia in the 17th century B.C. and in Egypt in the 16th century B.C. However, the ancient technicians and artisans who used these materials, having no knowledge of the chemical and physical methods of analysis and identification, did not distinguish between them. This problem was finally solved in 1807 by the brilliant young English chemist Sir Humphry Davy, who isolated the metal which he named potassium, and gave it the chemical symbol K, from *Kalium,* the Latinized version of the Arabic word for "alkali." However, more than 100 years elapsed following discovery before McCollum, in 1938—using the rat, obtained positive proof that potassium is an essential nutrient, although this had been suggested earlier.

ABSORPTION, METABOLISM, EXCRETION.

Absorption of dietary potassium is very efficient; more than 90% of ingested potassium is absorbed. Most of the absorption occurs in the small intestine.

Although the digestive juices contain relatively large amounts of potassium, most of it is reabsorbed and the loss in the feces is small.

The kidneys provide the major regulatory mechanism for maintaining potassium balance; and relatively wide variations in intake are not reflected in fluctuations in plasma concentration. Aldosterone, an adrenal hormone, stimulates potassium excretion. Also, alcohol, coffee, and excess sugar increase the urinary excretion of potassium.

Excessive potassium buildup may result from kidney failure or from severe lack of fluid.

FUNCTIONS.

Potassium and sodium are closely interrelated in the maintenance of proper osmotic pressure within cells. Both minerals are involved in the maintenance of proper acid-base balance and the transfer of nutrients in and out of individual cells. The potassium ion relaxes muscle; hence, a high concentration in the heart relaxes the heart—action opposite to that of calcium, which is stimulatory.

Potassium is also required for the secretion of insulin by the pancreas, in enzyme reactions involving the phosphorylation of creatine, in carbohydrate metabolism, and in protein synthesis.

DEFICIENCY SYMPTOMS.

A potassium deficiency may cause rapid and irregular heartbeats, and abnormal electrocardiograms; muscle weakness, irritability, and occasionally paralysis; and nausea, vomiting, diarrhea, and swollen abdomen.

Hypokalemia (decreased serum potassium) of dangerous degree may be caused by a prolonged wasting disease with tissue destruction and malnutrition; by prolonged gastrointestinal loss of potassium as in diarrhea, vomiting, or gastric suction; or by continuous use of diuretic drugs. Finally, the heart muscle may stop.

It should be noted that deficiencies of potassium rarely result from dietary lack of the mineral; rather, they result from crash diets, diarrhea, diabetic acidosis, vomiting, intense and prolonged sweating, body burns, and heavy urine losses induced by diuretic drugs (also known as "water pills").

INTERRELATIONSHIPS.

A magnesium deficiency results in failure to retain potassium; hence, it may lead to a potassium deficiency.

Excessive levels of potassium interfere with magnesium absorption. Also, large excesses of potassium may slow the heart to a standstill when the kidneys are unable to excrete the surplus in the urine.

Because sodium and potassium must be in balance, excessive use of salt depletes the body's potassium supply. Although sodium intake may be the most important dietary determinant of blood pressure, variations in the sodium:potassium ratio in the diet affect blood pressure under certain circumstances.

Potassium is almost a constant component of lean body tissue, so much so that one method of estimating the amount of lean tissue in a person is by measuring the amount of potassium present. (This is accomplished by determining the amount of radioactive potassium that is naturally present in a constant ratio to ordinary potassium.) The need for potassium is increased when there is growth or deposition of lean tissue; and potassium is lost whenever muscle is broken down owing to starvation, protein deficiency, or injury.

Potassium is often prescribed for people with high blood pressure who are required to take diuretics to reduce excess water in the body because of the belief that diuretics deplete the body of potassium. However, newer knowledge indicates that diuretics do not seriously deplete natural potassium levels of the great majority of patients taking these drugs for high blood pressure. Since high blood potassium concentration can cause cardiac arrest (a heart attack) and death, potassium supplements should be taken with caution and only on the advice of a physician.

RECOMMENDED DAILY ALLOWANCE OF PO-TASSIUM.
The exact potassium requirements are unknown. But it is known that the daily intake on typical diets far exceeds the requirements.

Growth (increase in lean body mass) and fecal losses are the major determinants of potassium needs during the early years of life. The Food and Nutrition Board of the National Research Council (FNB-NRC) estimated minimal potassium requirements for the infant and young child are 65 mg per day (*Recommended Dietary Allowances,* 10th ed., 1989, p. 257). Human milk contains 500 mg of potassium per liter, whereas commonly used commercial formulas contains slightly more and cow's milk contains about 1,364 mg per liter. Average intakes of potassium during the first year of life range from about 780 mg per day at age 2 months to about 1,600 mg per day at the end of the first year; hence, normal diets of infants and young children provide a surplus of potassium.

Under ordinary circumstances, the healthy adult can maintain potassium balance with an intake of 1,600 to 2,000 mg.

Estimated safe and adequate intakes of potassium are given in Table P-13.

TABLE P-13
ESTIMATED MINIMUM REQUIREMENTS
OF POTASSIUM[1]

Group	Age	Potassium
	(years)	(mg)
Infants	0.0–0.5	500
	0.5–1.0	700
Children and adolescents	1	1,000
	2–5	1,400
	6–9	1,600
	10–18	2,000
Adults	18+	2,000

[1]*Recommended Dietary Allowances,* 10th ed., 1989, NRC-National Academy of Sciences, p. 253, Table 11–1.

• **Potassium intake in average U.S. diet**—The normal adult dietary intake of potassium is between 1,950 and 5,900 mg per day (3,480 mg per capita), which is more than adequate.

The levels of potassium suggested in Table P-13 were calculated from the sodium intakes in order to achieve equivalent amounts of potassium on a molar basis. Older individuals need relatively less potassium than the rapidly growing infant, but an equivalent intake of potassium appears to be somewhat protective against the blood pressure-elevating effects of a given level of sodium.

TOXICITY. Acute toxicity from potassium (known as *hyperpotassemia* or *hyperkalemia*) will result from sudden increases of potassium to levels of about 18 g per day for an adult, provided the kidneys are not functioning properly and there is not an immediate and sharply increased loss of potassium from the body. Although no significant increase in intracellular potassium content or in total body potassium occurs in this condition, hyperkalemia may prove fatal due to cardiac arrest.

SOURCES OF POTASSIUM. Potassium is widely distributed in foods. Meat, poultry, fish, many fruits, whole grains, and vegetables are good sources. (Although meat, poultry, and fish are good sources of potassium, these items may be restricted when dietary sodium is restricted.)

Groupings by rank of common food sources of potassium follow:

• **Rich sources**—Dehydrated fruits, molasses, potato flour, rice bran, seaweed, soybean flour, spices, sunflower seeds, wheat bran.

• **Good sources**—Avocado, beef, dates, guava, most raw vegetables, nectarine, nuts, pork, poultry, sardines, veal.

• **Fair sources**—Breads, cereals, cheeses, cooked or canned vegetables, eggs, fruit juices, fruits (raw, cooked, or canned), milk, shellfish, whole wheat flour, wine, yogurt.

• **Negligible sources**—Cooked rice, cornmeal, fats and oils, honey, olives, sugar.

• **Supplemental sources**—Potassium gluconate, potassium chloride, seaweed, yeast (Brewers', torula), wheat germ.

NOTE WELL: Sources of potassium other than foods, such as potassium chloride, should be taken only on the advice of a physician or nutritionist.

For additional sources and more precise values of potassium, see Food Composition Table F-36 of this book.

TOP POTASSIUM SOURCES. The top potassium sources are listed in Table P-14.

NOTE WELL: This table lists (1) the top sources without regard to the amount normally eaten (left column), and (2) the top food sources (right column); and the caloric (energy) content of each food.

(Also see MINERAL[S], Table M-67.)

TABLE P-14
TOP POTASSIUM SOURCES[1]

Top Sources[2]	Potassium	Energy	Top Food Sources	Potassium	Energy
	(mg/100 g)	(kcal/100 g)		(mg/100 g)	(kcal/100 g)
Baking powder, commercial, low sodium .	10,948	172	Molasses, cane, blackstrap	2,927	230
Seaweed, raw, Dulse	8,060	—	Soybean flour, defatted	1,820	326
Seaweed, raw, kelp	5,273	—	Apricots, dried, sulfured,		
Coriander leaf, dried	4,466	298	uncooked	1,422	236
Parsley, dried	3,805	276	Peaches, dehydrated, sulfured,		
Baking powder, home use/tartarate	3,800	78	uncooked	1,229	340
Tomato juice, dehydrated (crystals), dry ..	3,518	21	Wheat bran	1,121	353
Basil................................	3,433	251	Wheat germ	827	391
Dill weed, dried	3,308	253	Potatoes, fried from raw	775	268
Tarragon............................	3,020	295	Apples, dehydrated, sulfured,		
Molasses, cane, blackstrap	2,927	230	uncooked	730	353
Seaweed, raw, Irishmoss	2,844	—	Avocados, raw, California,		
Turmeric............................	2,500	354	served w/skin	710	168
Paprika, domestic	2,344	289	Peanuts, roasted/skins, whole .	701	582
Whey, acid dry	2,288	339	Dates, domestic, natural, dry ..	666	271
Cabbage, common, dehydrated,			Beans, lima, mature seeds, dry,		
unsulfited	2,207	308	cooked	612	138
Whey, sweet, dry	2,080	354	Sardines, Atlantic, canned in oil,		
Yeast, torula........................	2,046	277	drained, solids	590	200
Pepper, red.........................	2,014	318	Chard, Swiss, raw............	550	25
Yeast, baker's dry (active)	1,998	282	Veal, all cuts	500	250
			Turkey, all classes, flesh and		
			skin cooked, roasted	490	223
			Spinach, raw...............	470	26
			Squash, winter, all varieties,		
			baked	461	63
			Pork, variety of lean cuts	390	230
			Beef, variety of lean cuts	370	230

[1]These listings are based on the data in Food Composition Table F-36. Some top or rich sources may have been overlooked since some of the foods in Table F-36 lack values for potassium.

Whenever possible, foods are on an "as used" basis, without regard to moisture content; hence, certain high-moisture foods may be disadvantaged when ranked on the basis of potassium content per 100 g (approximately 3½ oz) without regard to moisture content.

[2]Listed without regard to the amount normally eaten.

POTATO (IRISH POTATO) *Solanum tuberosum*

Contents

This vegetable, commonly known as Irish or white potato, is grown around the world and ranks after the major grains (wheat, rice, and corn) in importance as a food. It is a member of the nightshade family of plants (*Solanaceae*), which includes the tomato, red pepper, tobacco plant, and eggplant. However, it is not related to the sweet potato or the yam. The scientific name *Solanum* is derived from the Latin word *solamen*, which means soothing. Fig. P-78 shows a typical potato plant.

The edible part of the potato plant is the tuber, which grows in the ground. Tubers are not part of the roots of the plant, but are formed from underground stems. The

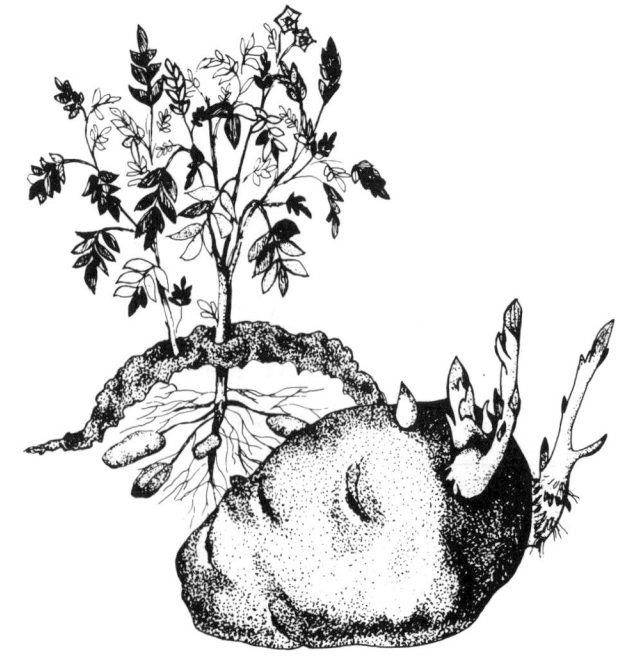

Fig. P-78.   The potato, a vegetable which feeds millions of people around the world.

tubers of the modern types of potatoes range in size from as small as a pea to so large that they can hardly be lifted by a strong man. Fig. P-79 shows an uncommonly large tuber.

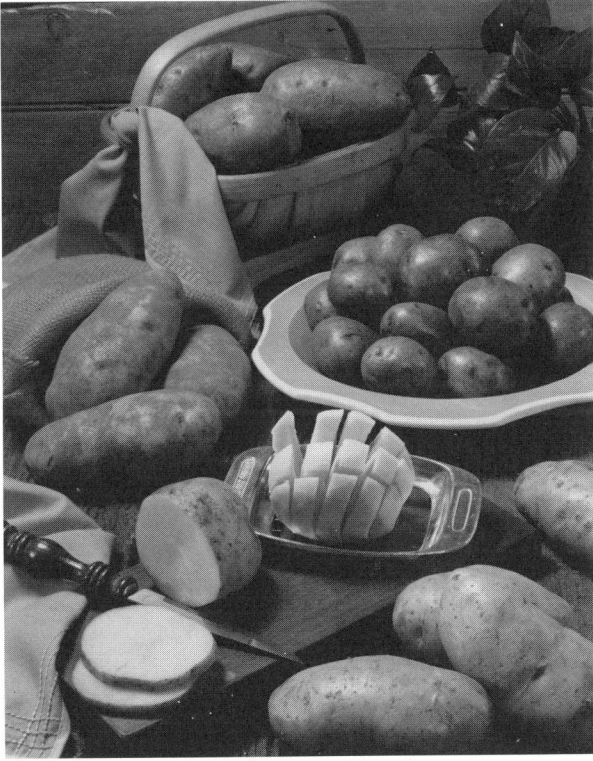

Fig. P-79. Potatoes can be prepared in a great variety of ways. (Courtesy, United Fresh Fruit and Vegetable Assn.)

ORIGIN AND HISTORY. The potato appears to have been first cultivated between 4,000 and 7,000 years ago in the Andes mountains of Bolivia and Peru. Before then, the tubers might have been gathered as a wild food, although the wild varieties were bitter, due to the presence of poisonous substances. Hence, it seems likely that the "seed potatoes" selected for cultivation might have been those that were less bitter. The potato was a major food of the Indians living at high altitudes in the Andes, because few other crops could be grown under such conditions. Fresh potatoes are subject to spoilage or sprouting, but the Indians overcame this difficulty by allowing the tubers to freeze in the cold night air, then tramping on them to squeeze out the moisture when they thawed out during the day. The crude dried product, known as *Chuno*, was the first form of preserved potatoes.

Sometime during the early part of the 16th century, Spanish explorers observed the use of potatoes by the Andean Indians. Within a few years the tubers were car-

ried on Spanish ships because it was found that eating them helped to prevent scurvy during long sea voyages. Hence, potatoes were brought to Europe by way of Spain. Shortly thereafter, this vegetable was being consumed by some of the people in Italy and Germany. (A German cookbook that was published in 1581 gave some recipes for potato dishes.) It is not certain how potatoes were introduced to the British Isles, but it is doubtful that they were introduced by Sir Frances Drake, as was long thought to be the case. The tubers were first grown on a large scale in Ireland, where there was a great need for a food that was easy to grow. However, many Europeans viewed the potato with suspicion for a long time after it was first introduced because (1) they recognized it as a member of the nightshade family, which was then known only for its potent and poisonous drugs; and (2) there was no mention of potatoes in the Bible.

During the 17th century, the Royal Society (a scientific organization) in England and the rulers of Germany attempted to promote greater use of the potato by various means such as the distribution of "seed potatoes" with instructions for planting and cultivation. Still, most of the farmers in these countries were reluctant to produce this crop because the market for it had not developed. Furthermore, many of the French and the Swiss believed that potatoes were the cause of diseases, such as scrofula and leprosy. Therefore, it was not until late in the 18th century that potatoes were grown widely throughout northern Europe. The breaking down of the public's resistance to potato eating came about largely as a result of the events which follow:

1. The French botanist Parmentier, who had first regarded the potato as an emergency crop for famine use only, learned to relish the vegetable while a prisoner of the Germans during the Seven Year's War (1756-1763). When he returned to France, he promoted the potato by means such as (1) allowing the tubers to be stolen from a guarded plot of the king's land, and (2) serving the unidentifiable mashed vegetable with butter and various seasonings.

2. During the early 1800s, Ireland's population grew rapidly, but its economy declined and there was widespread poverty. Because 1½ acres (*0.6 ha*) of potatoes would feed a family of five for a year, most Irish families came to depend on potatoes for food.

3. Count Rumford, who was an American member of the Royal Society, induced the poor of Munich, Germany to accept the potato by having it cooked to a mushy consistency in a soup which also contained barley, peas, and a little vinegar. Hunger finally led the impoverished Germans to concede that the thickened soup was more satisfying than one without the potatoes.

By the 1840s, the potato was grown extensively throughout northern Europe. Ireland was as dependent on the potato crop as China was on rice. All went well until 1845. Then, in 1845 and 1846 most of the crop was ruined by a moldlike blight (*Phytophthora infestans*) and the great potato famine was over all of Ireland. Starvation and disease ran rampant because the poor had no other staple food to substitute for the potato. An estimated 750,000 people died, and hundreds of thousands more left the country. Many of the Irish migrated to the United States. But all was not lost! Out of the tragedy the science of plant pathology was born from the attempts to determine the cause of potato blight.

Little is known about the introduction of the potato into North America. However, the most authenic report shows that potatoes were first brought to the United States in 1719, by Irish immigrants who settled in Londonderry, New Hampshire. It was for this reason, no doubt, that the potato became known as the "Irish potato" in the United States. But Americans, like the Europeans, were slow to adopt the potato, and it was not grown on a large scale until the 19th century.

Ever since the potato was first grown in Europe, agriculturists have been selecting the largest tubers for use as seed potatoes. Hence, the size of potatoes has been increasing steadily. Also, blight-resistant strains from Latin America have been used in many of the potato breeding programs. Efforts are now underway to adapt the crop to some of the warm subtropics and tropics.

PRODUCTION. Potatoes account for 45% of the annual worldwide production of roots and tubers. Fig. P-80 compares the annual tonnage from the leading producing countries.

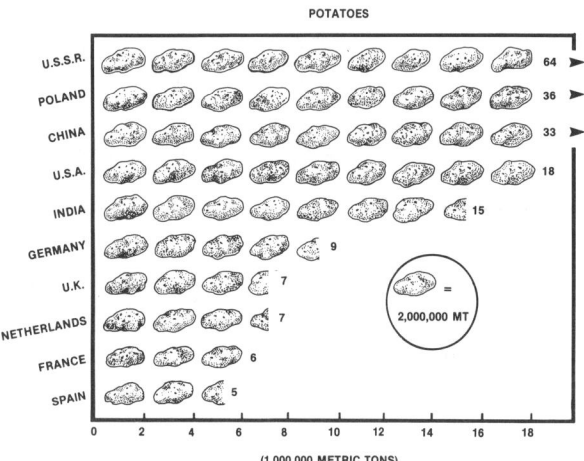

Fig. P-80. Leading potato-producing countries of the world. (Based on data from *FAO Production Yearbook 1990,* FAO/UN, Rome, Italy, Vol. 44, p. 90, Table 26)

Since the 1950s, potato production in the United States has shifted westward. The four top producing states in 1953 were Maine, California, Idaho, and New York, whereas the leaders in 1990 were Idaho, Washington, Colorado, and Wisconsin. (See Fig. P-81.)

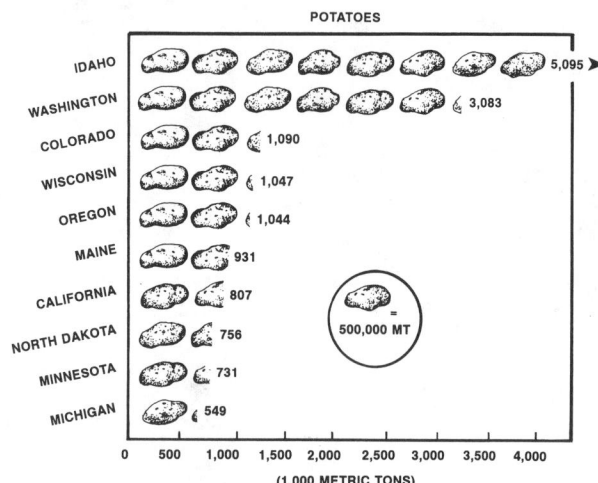

Fig. P-81. The leading potato-producing states. (Based upon data from *Agricultural Statistics 1991*, USDA, pp. 159 and 160, Table 228)

Potatoes are propagated vegetatively from eye-bearing pieces of tubers called "seed potatoes." The seed potatoes are usually grown in disease-free areas. Then, they are harvested and stored until they develop sprouts. Small whole tubers or cut pieces from larger tubers may be planted. The cut pieces should be stored for a few days in a cool, moist environment in order to heal the cut surfaces. Otherwise, the pieces may rot before they sprout.

Seed potatoes are planted as soon as the danger of a hard frost has passed. However, planting should be timed so that tuber formation will occur in cool weather because optimal yields are obtained when the temperature ranges between 60°F and 65°F (*16°C* and *18°C*). Also, the soil should be well drained and rich in organic matter. Fig. P-82 shows a well cultivated field of young potato plants.

FOOD PRODUCTION

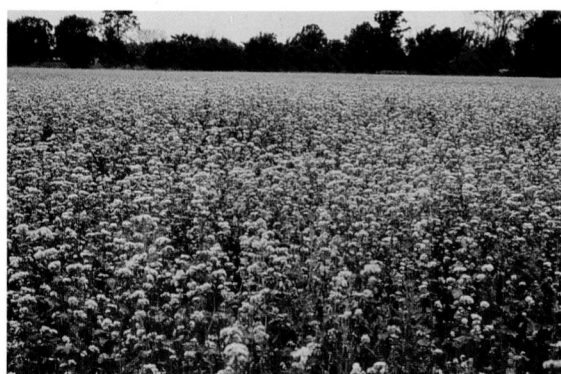

Plate 49. Buckwheat, in full bloom. Buckwheat is used for about the same purposes as the cereal grains, but it is not a cereal; it is related to rhubarb. (Courtesy, University of Minnesota, St. Paul)

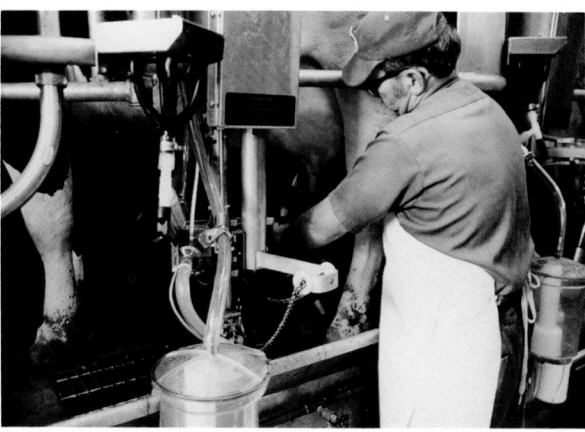

Plate 52. Milking. This shows dairy cows being milked by machine in a milking parlor. (Courtesy, University of Maryland, College Park)

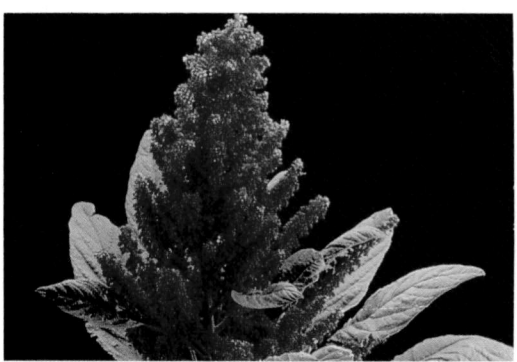

Plate 50. Amaranth. It is grown for the leaves as a green vegetable and for the seed as a grain. (Courtesy, University of Minnesota, St. Paul)

Plate 53. *Below:* Cowpeas. This shows a field of cowpeas in southeastern U.S.A. The plants have a trailing and bushy vine, but do not climb. (Courtesy, University of Minnesota, St. Paul)

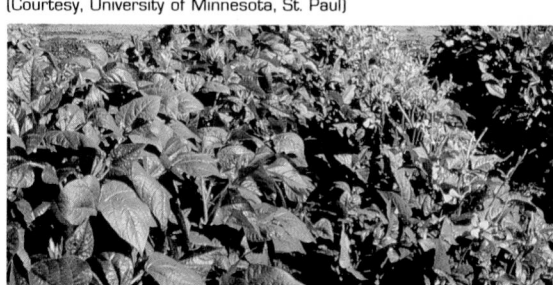

Plate 51. *Below:* Cherries. This shows a cluster of the fruit ready for harvest. (Courtesy, USDA)

Plate 54. Layers in cages. More than 90% of U.S. layers are in cages or on wire. (Courtesy, USDA)

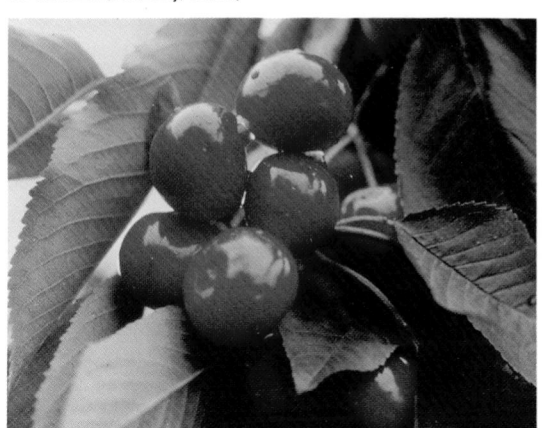

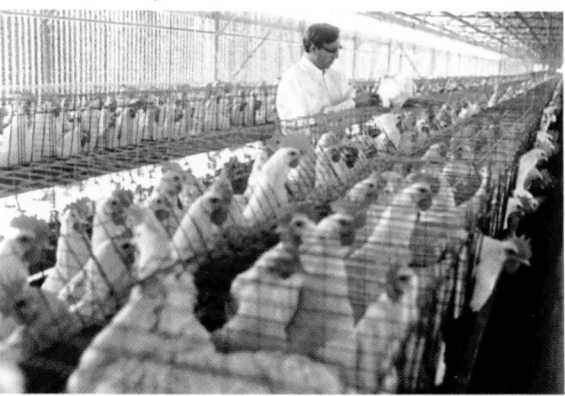

FOOD MARKETING

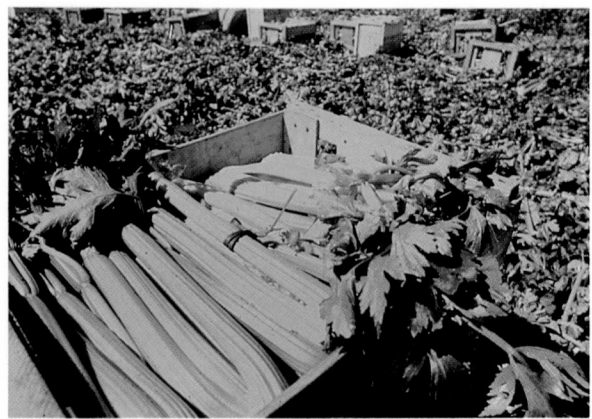

Plate 55. Celery. This shows harvested celery being packed in the field for shipment to market. (Courtesy, USDA)

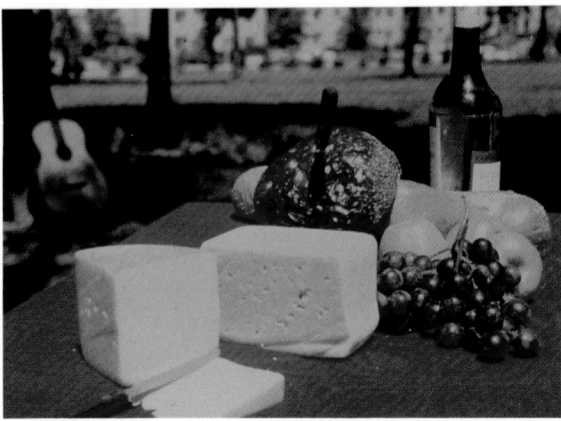

Plate 58. Cheese, bread, and wine—an attractive display. (Courtesy, USDA)

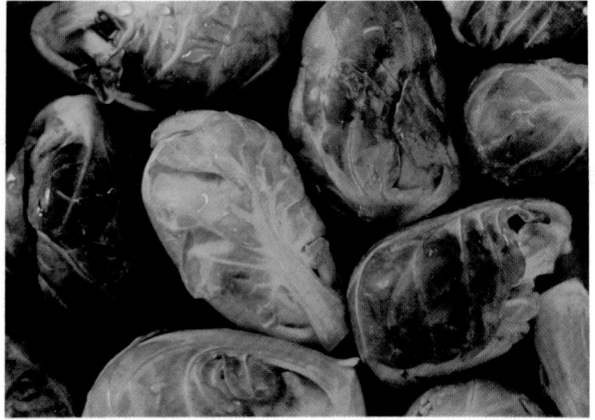

Plate 56. Brussel sprouts in a supermarket. (Courtesy, USDA)

Plate 59. *Below:* Meat, showing customer selecting from a meat display in a supermarket. (Courtesy, USDA)

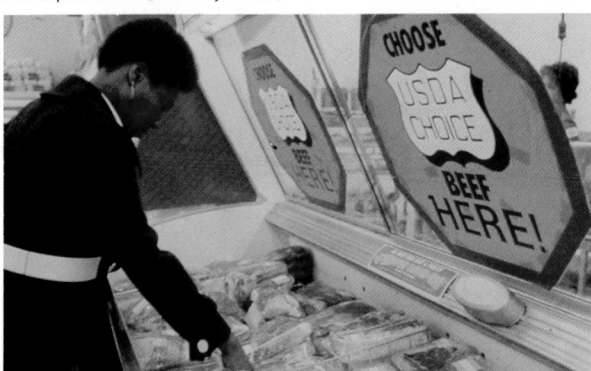

Plate 57. *Below:* Strawberries, fully ripe and glistening in a market. Strawberries are the world's leading berry-type fruit. (Courtesy, USDA)

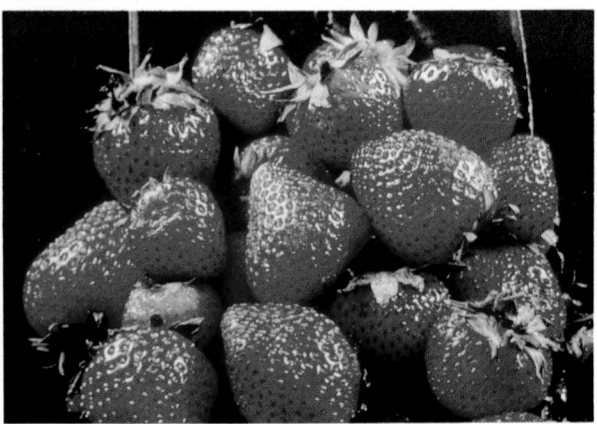

Plate 60. *Below:* Vegetables and fruits—an attractive display. (Courtesy, University of Florida, Gainesville)

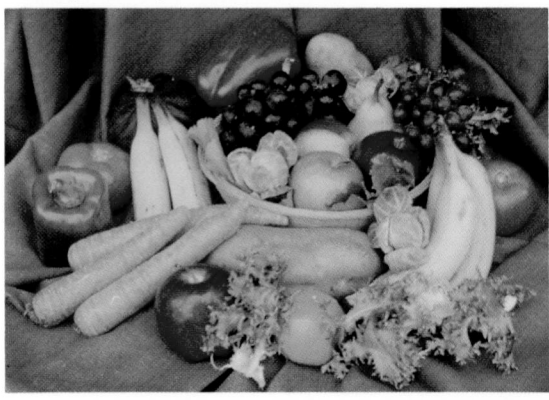

BREAD, CEREAL, RICE, & PASTA GROUP

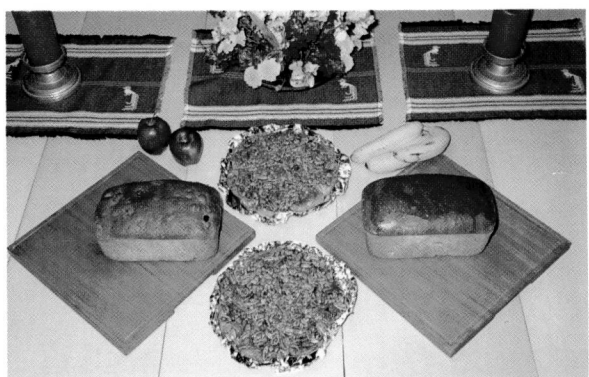

Plate 61. Whole wheat bread—a member of the Bread, Cereal, Rice, & Pasta Group, of which 6-11 daily servings are recommended in the *Food Guide Pyramid.* (Photo by A. H. Ensminger)

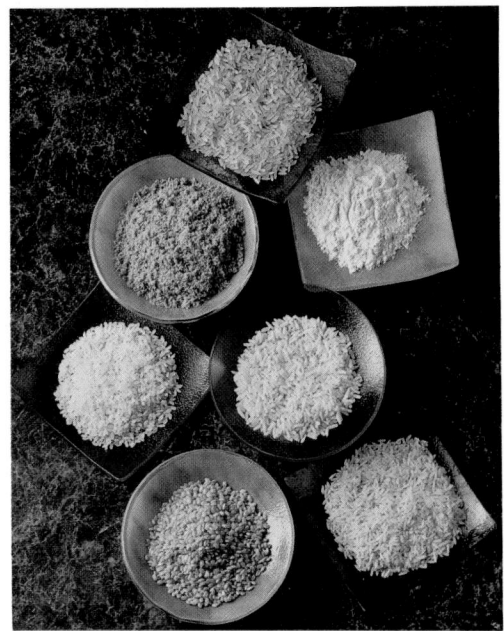

Plate 64. Rice, of which 7 kinds are displayed. Of the thousands of varieties, only about 25 are grown commercially in the U.S.A. (Courtesy, USA Rice Council, Houston, Tex.)

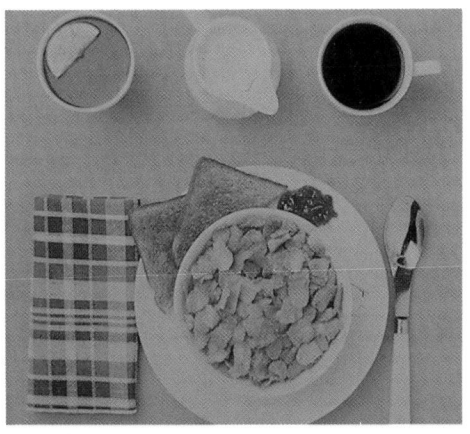

Plate 62. Corn flakes. This ready-to-eat breakfast cereal is manufactured from deskinned, degerminated kernels of soaked dried corn by flavoring, rolling, and toasting. (Courtesy, USDA)

Plate 65. A pita bread sandwich. (Courtesy, USDA)

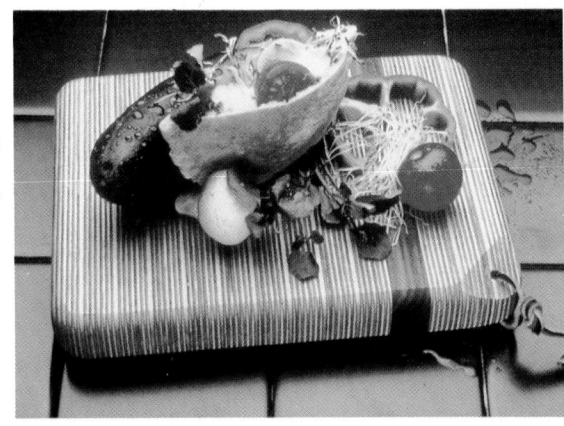

Plate 66. *Below:* Pasta (macaroni). This shows pasta used to extend meat—a high-quality protein. (Courtesy, National Live Stock and Meat Board, Chicago, Ill)

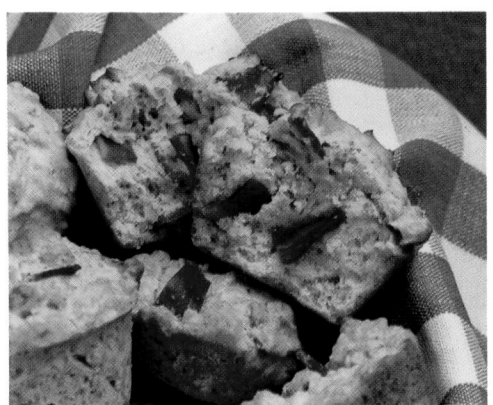

Plate 63. Muffins with turkey bacon. (Courtesy, Oscar Mayer Food Corp., Madison, Wisc.)

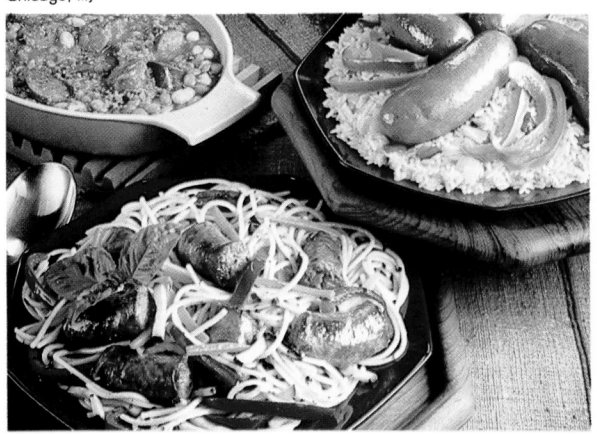

VEGETABLE GROUP

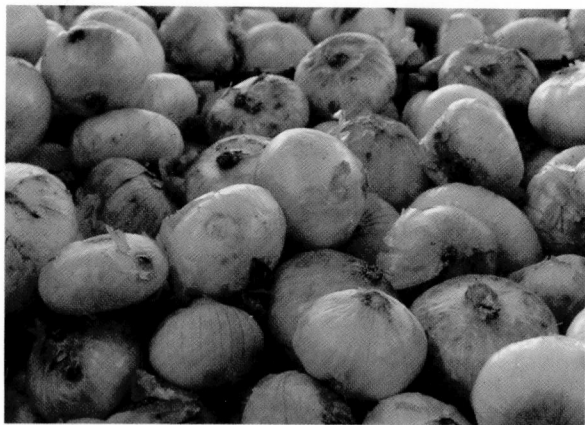

Plate 67. Onions. This vegetable is used primarily for its flavor and appetite appeal. The *Food Guide Pyramid* calls for 3-5 daily servings of the Vegetable Group. (Courtesy, USDA)

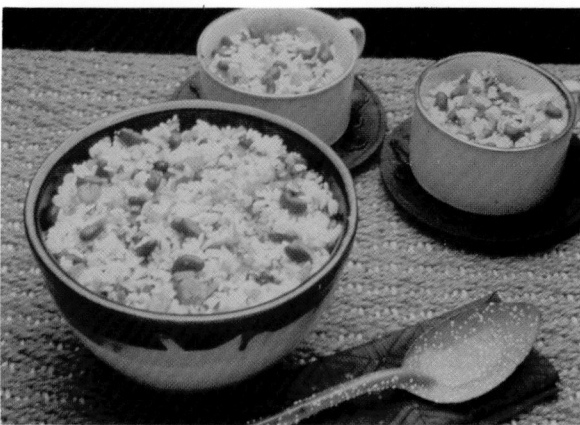

Plate 70. Red beans and rice. A mixture of 50% of each beans and rice has a protein quality that approaches meat, milk, and other animal proteins. (Courtesy, USDA)

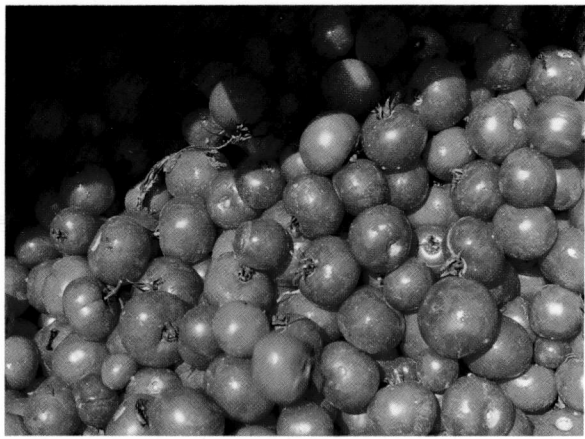

Plate 68. Tomatoes, a member of the nightshade family. Ripe (red) tomatoes are low in calories and a good source of vitamins A and C. (Courtesy, Rutgers University, New Brunswick, N.J.)

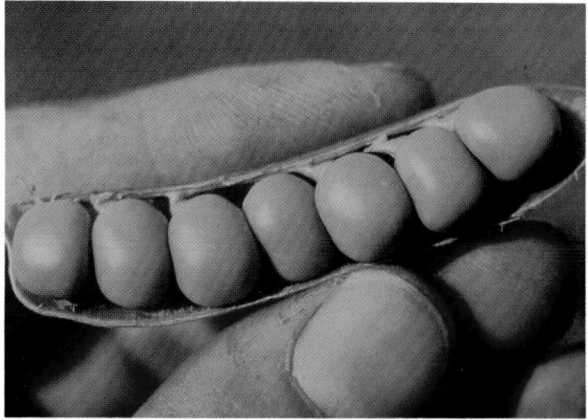

Plate 71. Peas in a pod. Peas are usually picked when immature. They are rich in protein, an excellent source of vitamin A, and a good source of vitamin C. (Courtesy, USDA)

Plate 72. *Below:* Corn-on-the-cob. Three ears of sweet corn-on-the-cob contain about 240 Calories (kcal). Yellow corn is also a fair source of vitamin A. (Courtesy, USDA)

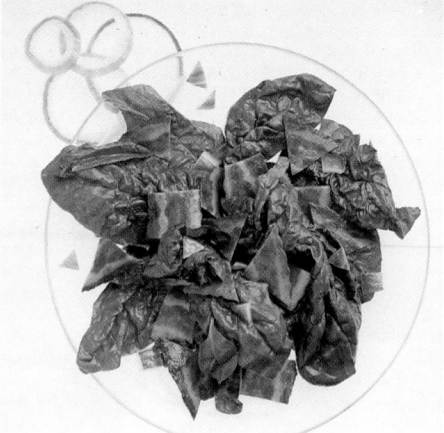

Plate 69. Spinach salad, with turkey and bacon. Spinach has a high water content (90 to 93%), is low in calories, and is an excellent source of magnesium, iron, potassium, and Vitamin A. (Courtesy, Oscar Mayer Food Corp., Madison, Wisc.)

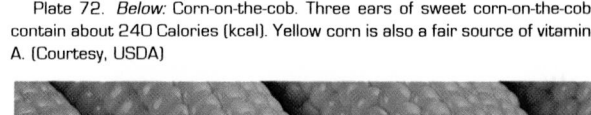

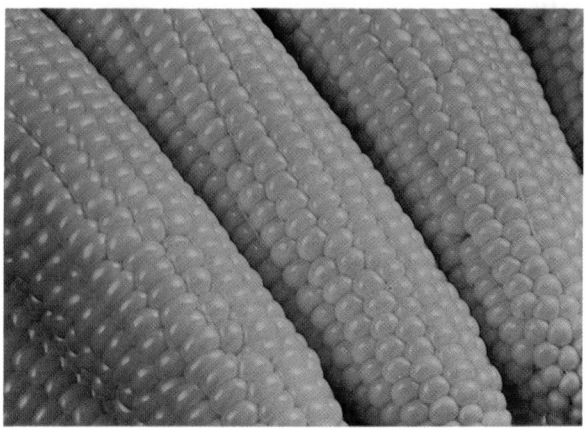

FRUIT GROUP

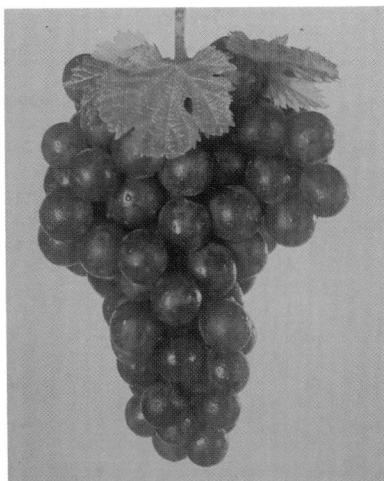

Plate 73. Grapes, the leading fruit crop of the world. Fresh table grapes are one of the richest sources of chromium and a good source of potassium. The *Food Guide Pyramid* calls for 2-4 servings of the Fruit Group daily. (Courtesy, California Table Grape Commission)

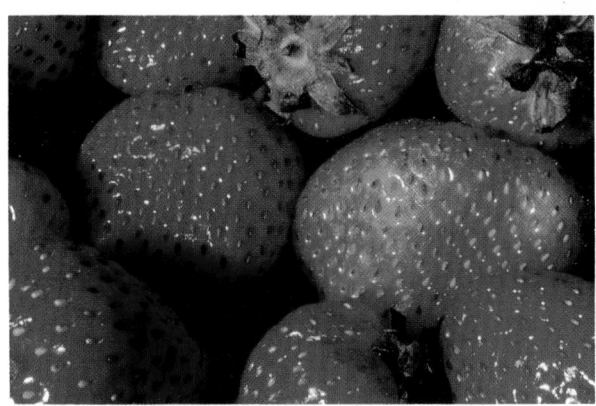

Plate 76. Strawberries, a good source of iron and potassium, and an excellent source of vitamin C. (Courtesy, National Film Board of Canada)

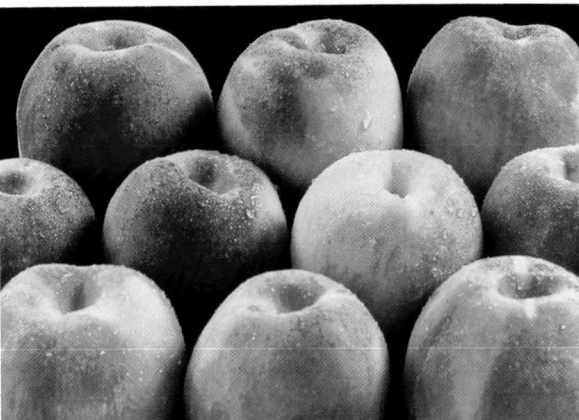

Plate 74. Peaches. Fresh peaches contain 89% water. Additionally, each 100 g (about 3 1/2 oz or I medium-sized peach) contain 38 Calories (kcal) of energy, 202 mg of potassium, 1,330 IU of vitamin A, and only I mg of sodium. (Courtesy, USDA)

Plate 77. *Below:* Fruits for snacks. Fruits provide fiber, few calories, no cholesterol, and little sodium or fat. (Courtesy, North Dakota State University, Fargo)

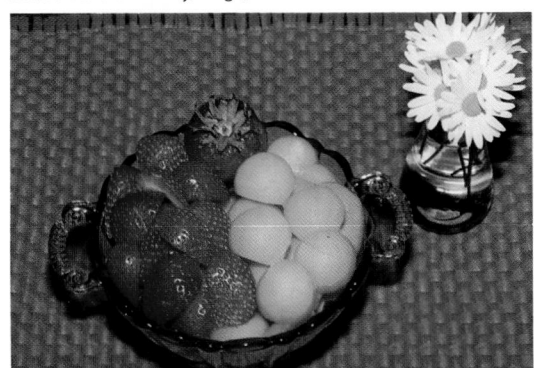

Plate 78. Lemonade, a refreshing beverage and a good source of vitamin C. (Courtesy, Sunkist, Van Nuys, Calif.)

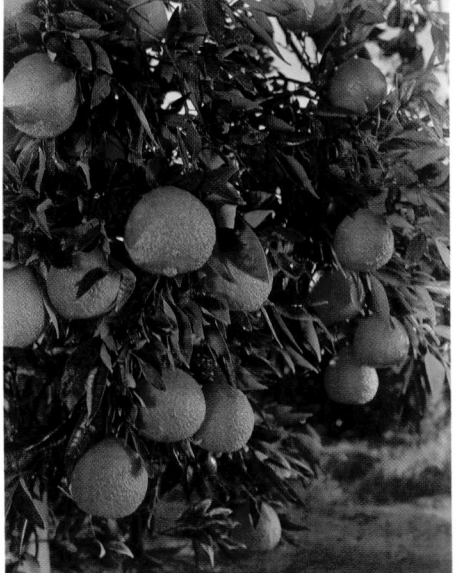

Plate 75. Oranges ready for harvest. Fresh oranges are low in calories (47 kcal per 100 g), but they are good sources of fiber, pectin, potassium, vitamin C, inositol, and bioflavonoids. (Courtesy, Sunkist, Van Nuys, Calif.)

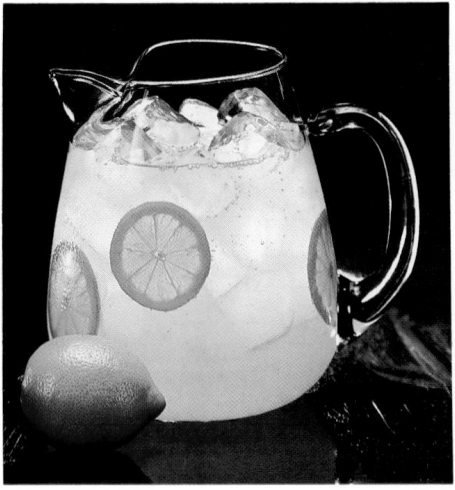

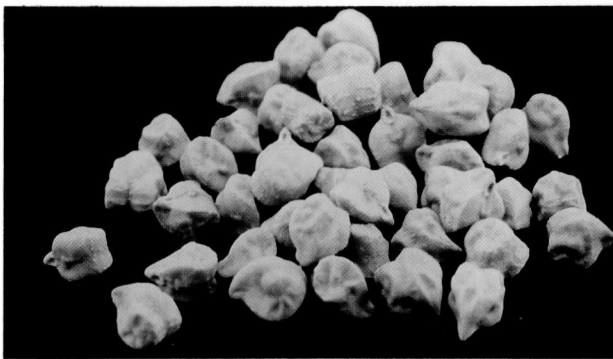

MEAT, POULTRY, FISH, DRY BEANS, EGGS, & NUTS GROUP

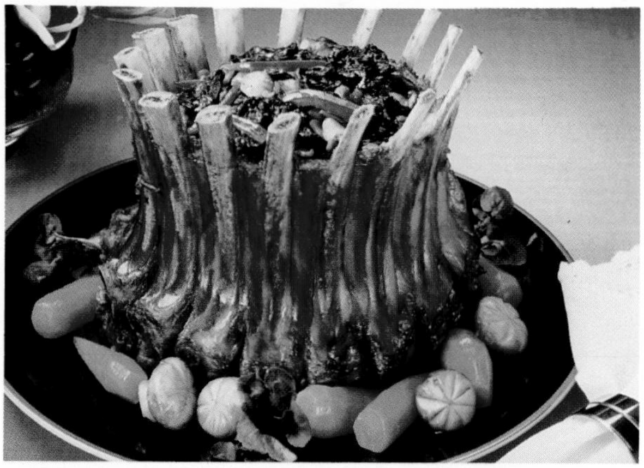

Plate 79. Crown roast of lamb—an elegant dish. Lamb is an excellent source of high-quality protein, a rich source of phosphorus and iron, and an excellent source of vitamins B-12, B-6, biotin, niacin, pantothenic acid, and thiamin. The *Food Guide Pyramid* calls for 2-3 daily servings of the Meat, Poultry, Fish, Dry Beans, Eggs, & Nuts Group. (Courtesy, National Live Stock and Meat Board, Chicago, Ill.)

Plate 82. Garbanzo beans (Chickpeas). Beans may be used (a) to upgrade the protein quantity and quality of diets based mainly on cereals and starchy foods, and (b) to extend and lower the cost of animal proteins. (Courtesy, University of Minnesota, St. Paul)

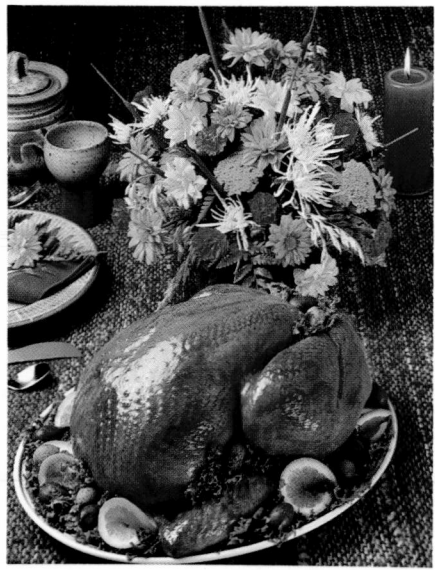

Plate 80. Roasted turkey. Poultry meat is a good source of phosphorus, iron, copper, and zinc; a rich source of vitamins B-12 and B-6; and a fair source of vitamins A, biotin, niacin, pantothenic acid, riboflavin, and thiamin. (Courtesy, Canadian Marketing Agency, Ontario, Canada)

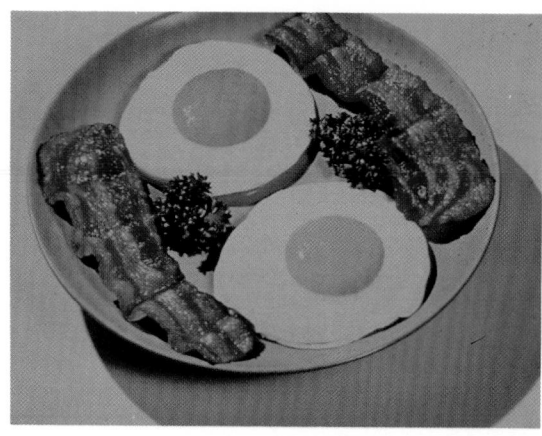

Plate 83. Bacon and eggs, the traditional American breakfast. Bacon contains all the essential amino acids, is rich in iron, and is high in the B-vitamins. Eggs contain an abundance of proteins, minerals, and vitamins. (Courtesy, USDA)

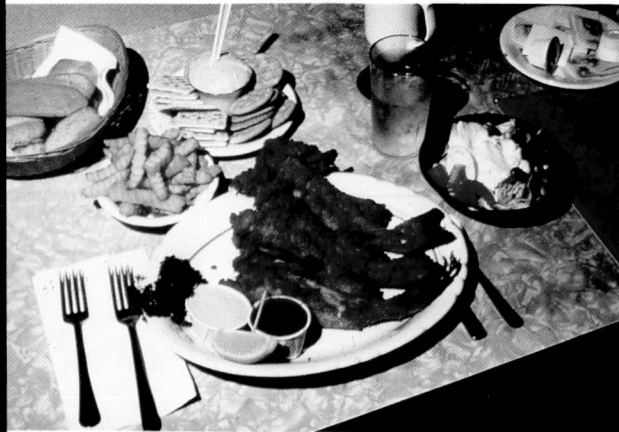

Plate 81. Seafood dinner. Fish and seafood are high in the essential amino acids, and rich in minerals and vitamins. Also, the fatty acids present are polyunsaturated; hence, they can play a major role in low-cholesterol diets. (Courtesy, U.S. Department of Interior)

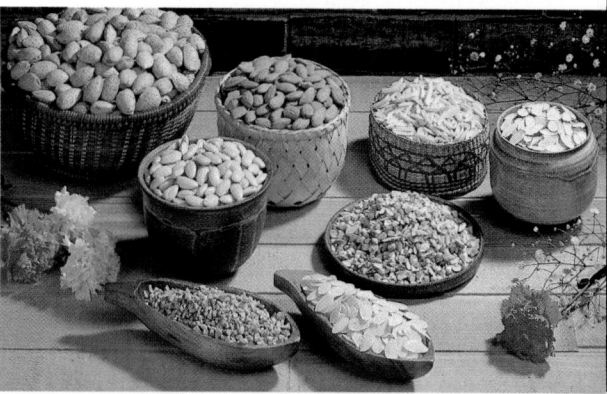

Plate 84. Almonds, which come in more forms than any other nut. Nuts are high in energy and protein; a good source of magnesium, zinc, and copper; and a good source of the B-vitamins. (Courtesy, Almond Board of California, Sacramento)

MILK, YOGURT, & CHEESE GROUP

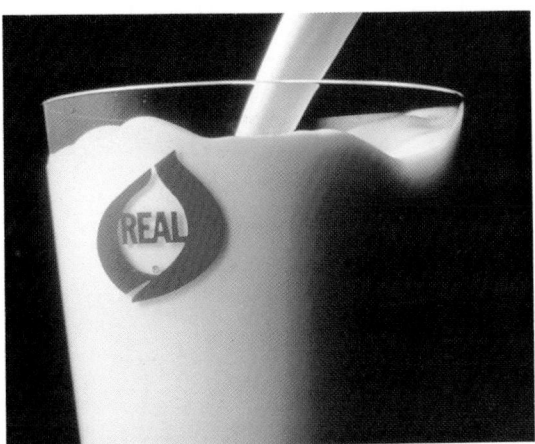

Plate 85. Milk, the major components of which are carbohydrates, fat, and protein. Milk is also a valuable source of certain minerals and vitamins. The *Food Guide Pyramid* calls for 2-3 servings daily of the Milk, Yogurt, & Cheese Group. (Courtesy, American Dairy Assn., Rosemont, Ill.)

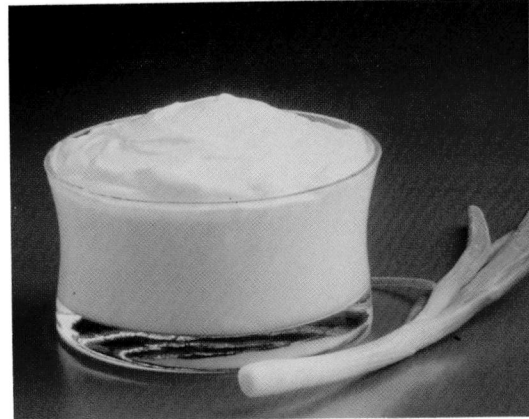

Plate 88. Sour cream. Today, most sour cream is cultured, much the same way as buttermilk. It is a uniformly textured, smooth product which is widely used for flavoring. (Courtesy, American Dairy Assn., Rosemont, Ill.)

Plate 89. Pizzas. This Italian creation is a flat leavened bread topped with such good things as mozzarella and parmesan cheeses, sausages, anchovies, tomatoes, mushrooms, olives, herbs and spices. (Courtesy, USDA)

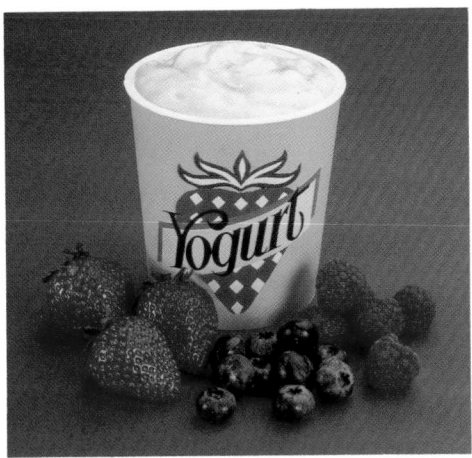

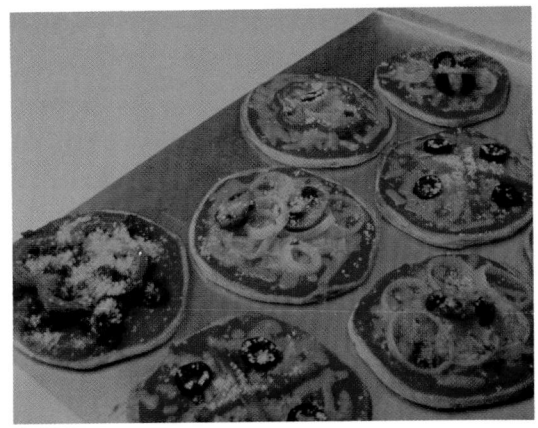

Plate 86. Yogurt, a fermented milk product prepared from lowfat milk, skim milk, or whole milk. (Courtesy, National Dairy Board, Arlington, Va.)

Plate 90. *Below:* Assorted cheeses. Milk can be, and is, processed into many different varieties of cheese. Some are made from whole milk, others from milk that has had part of the fat removed, and still others from skimmed milk. American types of cheese (Cheddar, Colby, Washed curd, Stirred curd, Monterey, and Jack) make up to 60% of the nation's cheese output. (Courtesy, American Dairy Assn., Rosemont, Ill.)

Plate 87. *Below:* Ice cream. Of all the frozen dairy desserts, ice cream contains the most milk solids (about 16 to 24%). (Courtesy, Carnation, Los Angeles, Calif.)

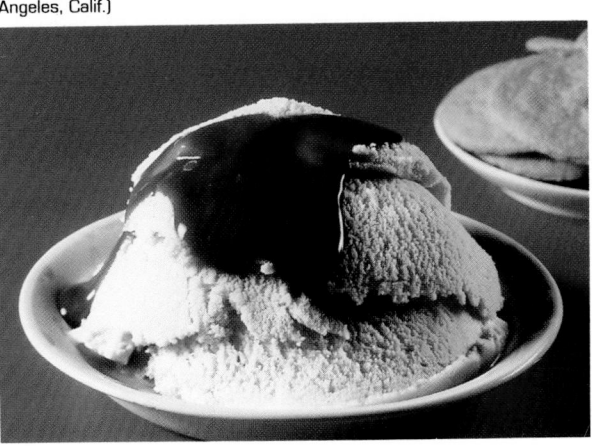

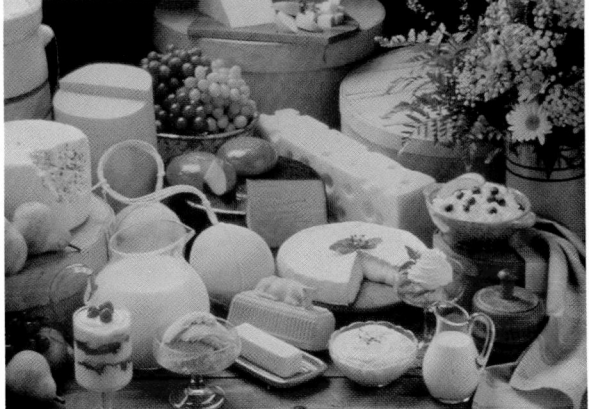

FATS, OILS, & SWEETS GROUP

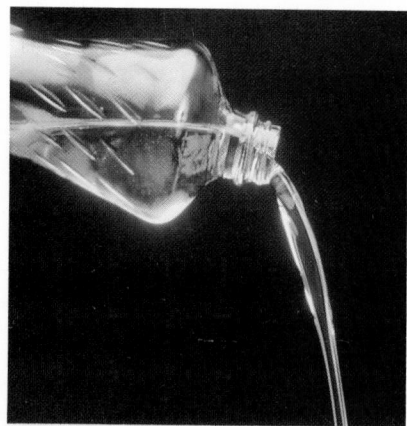

Plate 91. Cooking oil pouring out of a glass bottle. **Caution:** The new *Food Guide Pyramid*, released by the USDA in 1992, lists fats, oils, and sweets at the apex of the pyramid, where they are accorded the least space, along with the admonition to *use sparingly.* (Courtesy, USDA)

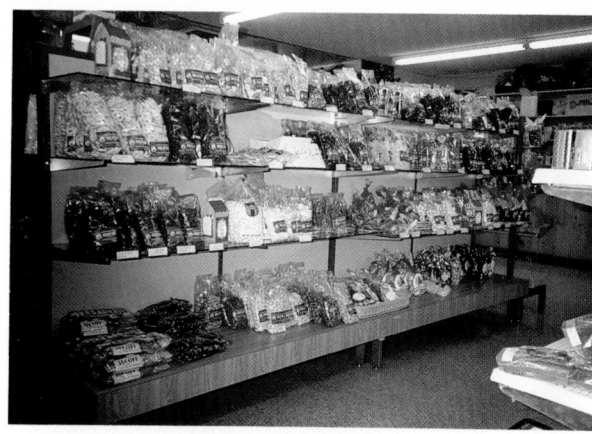

Plate 94. The Candy Store. An assortment of candy and chocolate covered nuts and raisins. **Note well:** The new *Food Guide Pyramid* admonishes that sweets should be *used sparingly.* (Photo by A. H. Ensminger)

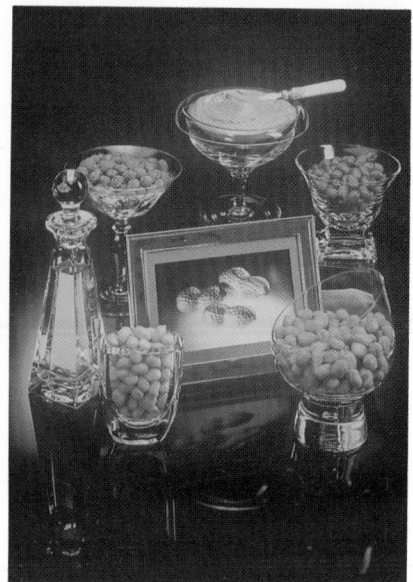

Plate 92. Peanut products. The nuts and skin yield about 47.5% oil. Peanuts supply about $\frac{1}{5}$ of the world's edible oil production. Peanut oil contains 76 to 82% unsaturated fatty acids. (Courtesy, Peanut Advisory Board, Atlanta, Ga.)

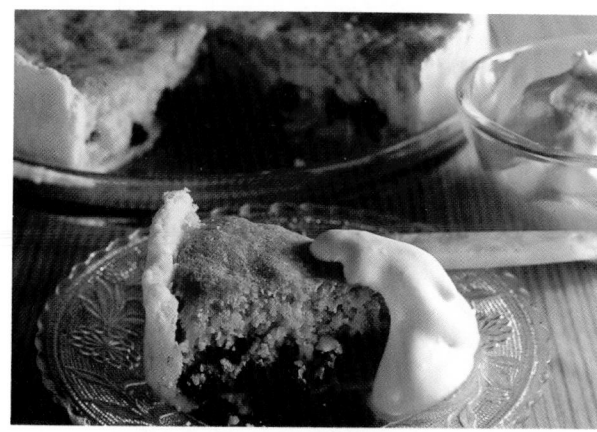

Plate 95. Raisin pie, which is moderately low in sugar, but moderately high in fat because of the crust. The calories in raisins are derived primarily from carbohydrates.

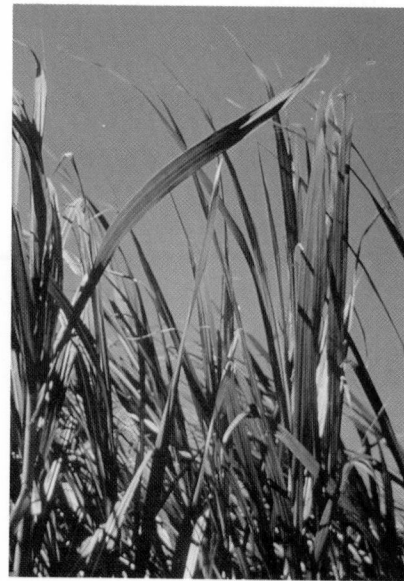

Plate 93. Sugarcane— a coarse grass of tropical and semitropical climates from which refined sugar is derived. (Courtesy, USDA)

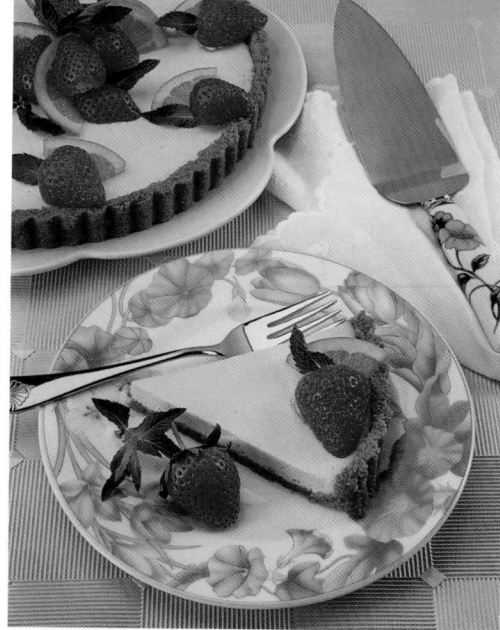

Plate 96. Yogurt cheese tart. Luscious desserts need not be high in fat. This creamy dessert made with lowfat yogurt has only 6 g of fat per serving. (Courtesy, National Dairy Board, Arlington, Va.)

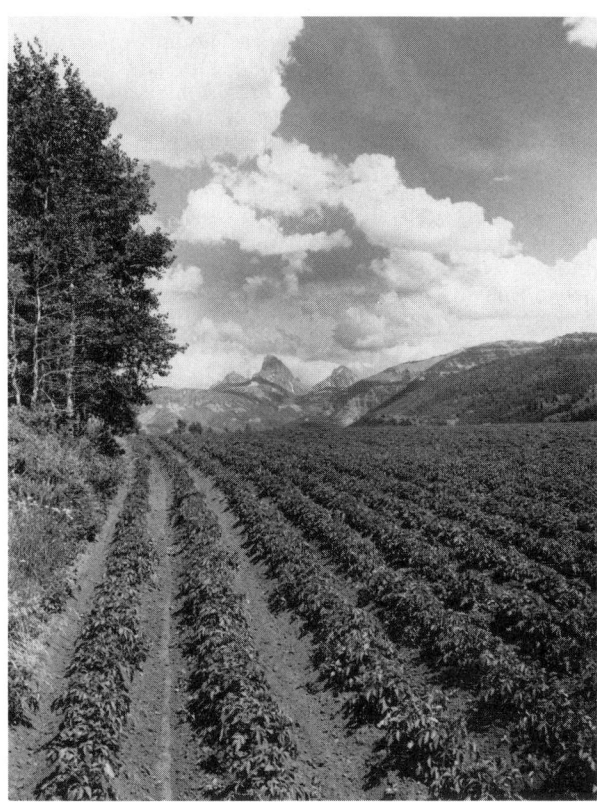

Fig. P-82. A field of potato plants. (Courtesy, Union Pacific Railroad Company, Omaha, Nebr.)

The unfavorable effects of warm atmospheric temperatures may be offset somewhat by keeping the soil cool with irrigation and/or mulching.

Potatoes are subject to several pests and diseases. The most important insect pests that attack potato plants are the potato bug (or Colorado beetle), leafhopper, flea beetle, aphid, and the potato psyllid. The most important fungous and bacterial diseases are late blight, rhizoctonia, scab, and ring rot. Important virus diseases include mosaic, leafroll, and spindle tuber.

Much of the U.S. potato crop is grown in cool areas. Hence, the tubers are harvested mainly in the early fall, although some harvesting is done almost every month of the year somewhere in the country. Most growers plan to harvest potatoes before the onset of high summer temperatures, or before hard frosts which may damage the tubers. Usually, the vines are killed by cutting or

spraying. Then, the tubers are dug up by special machines and collected manually or with harvesters. Fig P-83 shows the mechanical harvesting of potatoes.

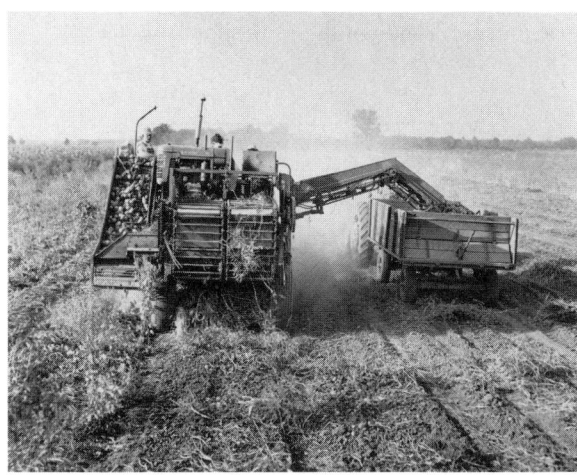

Fig. P-83. Potato digger in operation in Indiana. (Photo by J. C. Allen & Son, Inc., West Lafayette, Ind.)

Potatoes may be stored for 6 months or longer, providing the storage temperature does not exceed 40°F (4.4°C).

Fig. P-84 shows a facility that is filled to the rafters with potatoes.

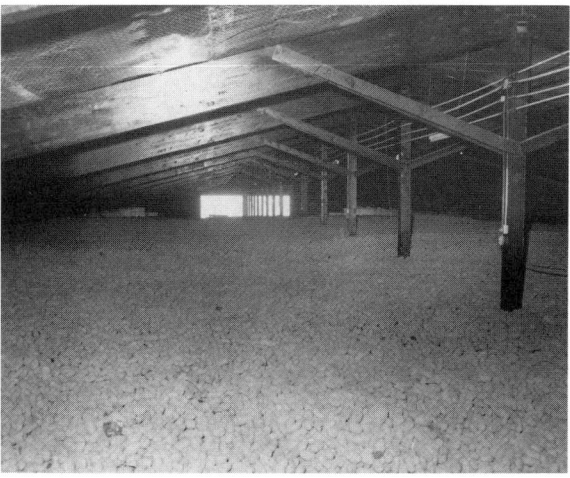

Fig. P-84. A large potato storage house. (Courtesy, Union Pacific Railroad Company, Omaha, Nebr.)

PROCESSING. The consumption of fresh potatoes has declined steadily since World War II, while the use of various forms of processed potatoes has risen to the point where over half the crop is processed. Fig. P-85 shows recent trends in the utilization of potatoes.

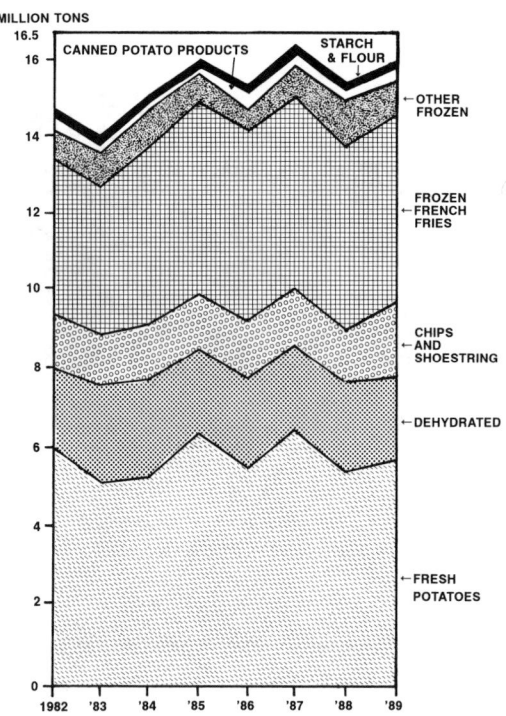

Fig. P-85. Trends in potato utilization during the 1980s. (Based upon data from *Agricultural Statistics 1991*, USDA, p. 161, Table 231)

It may be seen from Fig. P-85 that (1) the utilization of processed forms of potatoes increased steadily throughout the 1980s, and (2) over 97% of these products is represented by chips and shoestring potatoes, dehydrated items (mainly instant mashed potatoes), and frozen french fries and other frozen products. Hence, the following recent developments in the major forms of potato processing are noteworthy.

• **Potato chips and shoestring potatoes**—These items are customarily produced by deep frying blanched potato slices or strips in hot oil. However, a high frying temperature may accelerate the breakdown of the cooking oil (as indicated by a steady darkening of its color) so that it has to be replaced at frequent intervals. Furthermore, the thorough cooking that is required to remove most of the internal moisture from the potato pieces may result in an excessively dark-colored product. To alleviate this problem, the following three new methods of frying potato chips were developed: (1) microwave finish drying of partially fried chips, (2) air drying of partially fried chips, and (3) vacuum finish frying of chips.

• **Dehydrated potato powders**—The mixes used to prepare instant mashed potatoes are usually made by (1) cooking mashed, unpeeled, sulfured (bleached) potato pieces; (2) mashing the cooked potato and mixing it with water to form a slurry; (3) removing the pieces of potato skin from the slurry by passage through a screen; (4) treating the screened slurry with small amounts of additives such as BHA and BHT (antioxidants to prevent the development of off flavors during storage), bisulfites (bleaching agents to stabilize the white color), cellulose derivatives (to impart fluffiness), and monoglycerides and diglycerides (emulsifying agents to promote better mixability of the product with water); and (5) drum drying or spray drying the slurry to produce flakes or granules. Sometimes, milk solids are added to the slurry before drying so that rehydration of the powder will result in a product similar to potatoes mashed with milk. Finally, vitamins such as thiamin, riboflavin, niacin, and ascorbic acid may be added to the slurry prior to drying.

• **French fries (frozen)**—This product is only partially cooked prior to freezing because it is usually baked or fried just prior to serving. The processing steps are likely to consist of (1) washing, cutting, and blanching the potatoes; (2) frying the potato pieces in hot oil for a brief period, then cooling them; and (3) freezing the partially cooked potato pieces. The processor may modify the procedures by (1) coating the blanched pieces with a cellulose gum or gelatinized starch to prevent discoloration during frying, or (2) frying partly dehydrated potato pieces instead of fresh, raw pieces.

• **Rehydration and dispensing equipment for food service operations**—Homemakers rehydrate dried mashed potato products by beating or whipping them with hot water. However, fast food establishments may find that these mixes do not always yield a satisfactory product when large batches of mashed potatoes have to be prepared with ordinary mixing equipment. Therefore, a machine has been developed which mechanically agitates the dehydrated potato with a measured amount of liquid while also fluffing it with compressed air. The machine also has an automatic dispenser for delivering predetermined portions.

SELECTION. Good quality potatoes are sound, firm, relatively smooth, and well shaped. However, shape, size, external color, and cooking qualities may vary according to the degree of maturity, time of the year when harvested, period of storage, variety, and place where grown.

"New" or early potatoes are dug before they reach full maturity and are marketed immediately. Because of immaturity and warm weather at the time they are dug and shipped, they are much more subject to injury from rough handling than potatoes from the "late crop." The immature skins are easily injured and often present a discolored, ragged, feathery appearance. Much of the more mature late crop of potatoes is stored and shipped throughout the period from harvest until spring. Immature late crop potatoes are occasionally seen in the markets. They usually show feathery skins and discoloration not common in the great majority of the late crop shipments. Such potatoes are not necessarily undesirable, but they are not adapted to long keeping.

Several hundred varieties of potatoes are grown in the world. They differ in time of maturity, appearance, skin colors, resistance to insects and diseases, yield, and cooking and marketing qualities. A variety that thrives in one area may do poorly in another area.

Principal round white varieties are: Katahdin, mostly stored and sold as "late crop"; Cobbler, utilized for both "new" and "late crop" purposes; Kennebec, sold both as "new" stock and stored for sale as "late crop," and Sebago, also sold both as "new" stock and as "late crop."

The outstanding long white variety is White Rose, which when shipped from the area of heaviest production, California, is commonly known as "California Long White." This variety is most frequently sold as "new crop," but it may also be stored for later use.

By far the most prominent russet variety, Russet Burbank, widely known for baking quality, is generally elongated in shape, and is marketed from late summer to late spring, primarily from storage stocks. Other principal russet varieties are: Russet Rural, generally round in shape and usually sold as storage stock; and Early Gem, which resembles the Burbank in appearance, and is sold both as "new" and "late crop."

Among the many red varieties, those produced in greatest volume are Red Pontiac, sold both as "new" and storage stock; Red La Soda, also sold as "new" and "late crop"; Red McClure, sold primarily as "late crop" from storage; and Bliss Triumph, sold primarily as "new crop." All of these red varieties are round types.

• **Defects and toxic substances In potatoes**—Wilted, leathery, or discolored potatoes are unsatisfactory for most purposes.

Sometimes, potatoes may be undesirable because of a hollow center known as "hollow heart." Depending on the size of the cavity, the waste may be negligible or excessive. Other internal defects which occasionally affect potatoes are "blackheart" and "internal black spot." Unfortunately, external examination will seldom disclose any of these internal defects, but if shippers, wholesalers, and retailers have been careful to have proper samplings made, seriously affected potatoes should seldom be a problem to the consumer.

In late spring or early summer, old-crop potatoes may be shriveled, spongy, or sprouted. Such conditions may cause considerable waste and unsatisfactory cooking quality. Misshapen potatoes should be judged on the basis of the probable waste in preparation for use. Decay may appear as either a wet or dry rot, affecting either the surface or the interior flesh, or both. It may be so slight that it can be cut away with little waste or it may cause a potato to be completely inedible. Generally, any decay should be avoided.

Damage by "sunburn," caused by field exposure to sun, shows as a definite green to deep-green area on a part of the potato surface. The development of green color, called "Greening" or "Lightburn," may occur in storage, in the market display, or wherever potatoes are exposed for any considerable time to either natural or artificial light. If surface greening has progressed to a noticeable degree, the potatoes may have an undesirable bitter taste and contain significant amounts of the toxic substance *solanine.*

CAUTION: Potatoes that are green, spoiled, or sprouted may contain harmful amounts of the toxic alkaloid solanine. Likewise, potato tops contain this toxic alkaloid. Solanine may cause circulatory and respiratory depression, diarrhea, dilated pupils, headache, loss of sensation, paralysis, shock, stomach pain, subnormal body temperature, and vomiting. Therefore, potato tops and green or spoiled potatoes should not be eaten, and sprouts should be removed completely from otherwise sound tubers that are to be consumed.

PREPARATION. Most supermarkets carry many types of canned, dehydrated, or frozen products that enable homemakers to prepare potato dishes with a minimum expenditure of time. There are even imitations of baked potatoes that consist of frozen pureed potato packed in individual boats made of metal foil or paperboard. (The latter container is designed for heating in a microwave oven.) Nevertheless, people who relish the flavor and texture of baked, fried, or mashed potatoes prepared from the fresh, raw tubers may find that the characteristics of the convenience products leave much to be desired. Fig. P-86 shows a dish made from fresh potatoes that is unmatched by any of the convenience

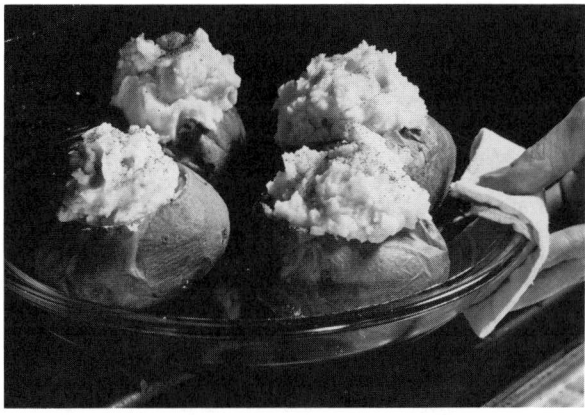

Fig. P-86. Baked and stuffed potatoes being browned in an oven. (Photo by J. C. Allen & Son, Inc., West Lafayette, Ind.)

products. From a health standpoint, it is also wise to cultivate a taste for the natural flavor of potatoes because then only minimal amounts of high-calorie dressings and spreads will be required. Some suggestions for preparing various potato dishes follow:

1.   There is no need to peel potatoes unless dirt is ground into the skins. The outer layer of the tuber is richer in nutrients than the inner layers. However, the skins should be cleaned thoroughly with a vegetable brush.

2.   Microwave heating of baked potatoes is much faster than baking them in an ordinary oven. Also, the use of a microwave oven is a more efficient use of energy because it does not give off heat to the room in which it is located.

3.   Cooking potatoes in a pressure cooker requires only a fraction of the time needed for boiling them in an open saucepan.

4.   The oil or fat used to fry potatoes should *not* be heated to the smoking point because it may break down into bitter tasting and harmful products that are likely to be absorbed by the potatoes. Therefore, people should be wary of eating in establishments where potatoes and other foods are fried in dark-colored or smoking fats.

5.   It is better to cook frozen french fries without any additional fat by placing them in an oven or under a broiler than it is to refry them because the second frying often gives the pieces a tough, poorly digested "skin" that contains more fat than most people need.

6.   The fat content of homemade french fries may be kept low by tossing the raw pieces of potato in a little heated fat or oil (about 1 Tbsp per cup of potatoes), then baking them in an oven.

7.   Yogurt or cottage cheese that has been blended or whipped until smooth may be substituted for butter, cheese, mayonnaise, or sour cream as a dressing for potatoes. The substitution works best when liberal amounts of seasonings such as chives, dried horseradish, mustard powder, oregano, pepper, and/or thyme are used.

NUTRITIONAL VALUE.   The nutrient composition of various forms of potatoes is given in Food Composition Table F-36.

Some noteworthy observations regarding the nutrient composition of potatoes follow:

1.   An average size raw potato (7 oz or *200 g*) contains only about 115 Calories (kcal), 3.2 g of protein, 80 mg of phosphorus, 1 mg of iron, and 30 mg of vitamin C (about the amount in one-half of an average size orange), but only small amounts of calcium and vitamin A. Boiled potatoes have a similar nutrient composition, except that some of the vitamin C is destroyed by cooking.

2.   Baked potatoes contain about 25% more solids and proportionately higher levels of all nutrients than raw or boiled potatoes. Also, an average size baked potato is equivalent in nutritional value to a cup of mashed potatoes, and contains about 4 g of protein, or the amount present in about a cup of cooked cereal such as cornmeal or rice.

3.   French frying reduces the water content of potatoes to the extent that the cooked product contains over twice the solids, 3 to 4 times the calories, and double the protein content of baked or boiled potatoes. Furthermore, each ounce (*28 g*) of french fries contains almost 1 tsp (*5 ml*) of fat.

4.   Potato chips and shoestring potatoes are high in calories because of their very low water content (2%) and high fat content (40%). Therefore, they are concentrated sources of calories (2,400 to 2,600 kcal per lb, or *0.45) kg*, protein (24 to 29 g per lb), and salt (up to 5,000 mg of sodium per lb). However, salt-free potato chips are sold in many health food stores.

5.   Dried potato products, such as instant mashed potato granules and potato flour, are similar in composition to cereal flours. Therefore, they may be used in breads, pancakes, waffles, and similar baked products. Moist forms of potatoes may be used to make these items if the liquid called for in the recipes is reduced somewhat. The Irish have long made potato breads with mashed potatoes.

6.   A 1-cup (*240 ml*) serving of au gratin potatoes made with cheese contains slightly more calcium and protein than a cup of milk, and about twice as many calories.

7.   Potato salads are usually high in calories due to the liberal use of fat-rich mayonnaise or salad dressing in their preparation. Nevertheless, 1 cup of potato salad made with chopped egg usually provides about twice as much protein as a cup of cooked cereal.

The Use of Potatoes as a Staple Food. People living in certain regions where grains do not grow well have long depended upon potatoes as a staple food. Nevertheless, there is a widely held belief that the potato-dominated diets of the Peruvian Indians and the Irish were likely to have led to multiple nutritional deficiencies. Therefore, Fig. P-87 is presented to help dispel such a belief.

NO. OF PEOPLE WHOSE REQUIREMENTS ARE MET BY THE YIELD FROM 1 ACRE OF THE SPECIFIED CROP.

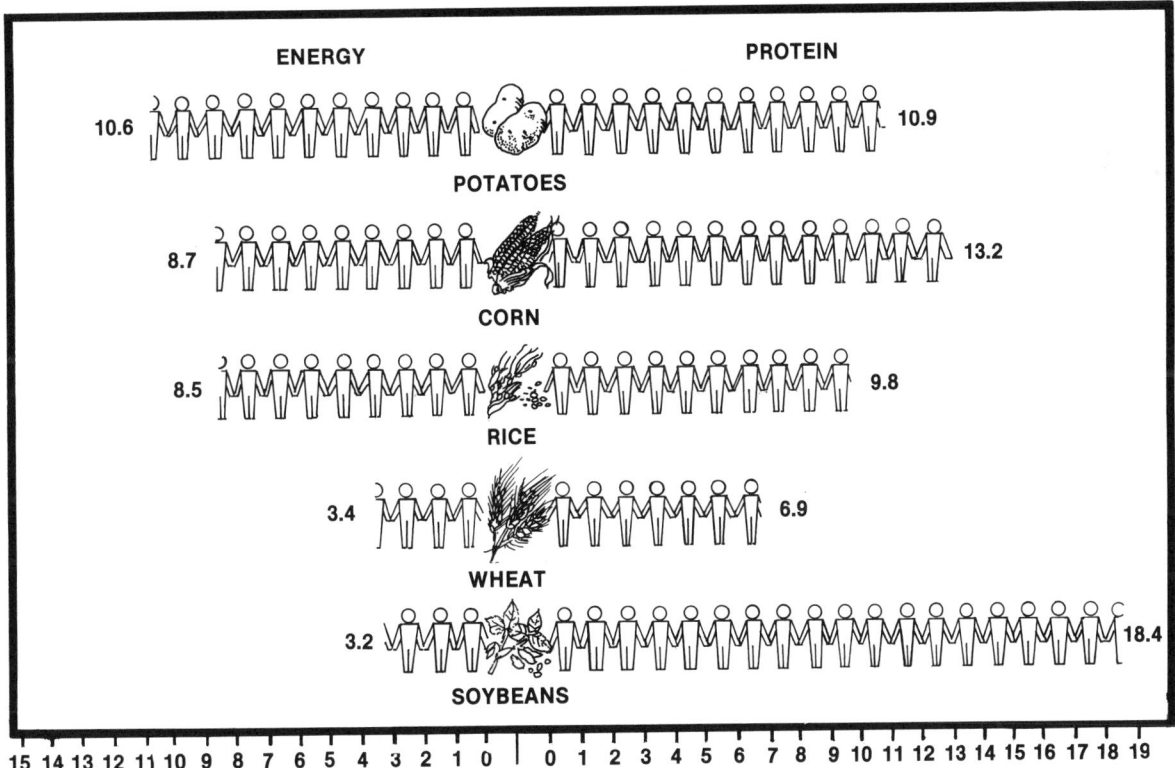

Fig. P-87. The numbers of people whose annual energy and protein needs are met by the yield from 1 acre of potatoes and of various other crops. (Based upon data from *A Hungry World: The Challenge to Agriculture*, University of California Food Task Force, Berkeley, Calif., 1974; and the FAO/UN daily per capita requirements of 2,385 Calories [kcal] and 38.7 g of protein.)

It may be seen from Fig. P-87 that the yield from 1 acre (*0.4 ha*) of potatoes meets both the energy and protein requirements for over ten people, whereas, the other major life-sustaining crops are not as balanced in these nutrients. The requirements for most of the other nutrients may be met if sufficient quantities of potatoes are consumed together with other foods that supply calcium and a vitamin A. Peruvian Indians obtained these supplemental nutrients from the leaves of amaranth (pigweed) and chenopodium (lambs quarters), whereas, it is likely that the Irish received them from Irish moss (a seaweed) and other plants.

Protein Quantity And Quality. Strange as it may seem, potatoes, which contain only 2% protein on a fresh basis, are being tested in Peru and in other countries for use as a protein supplement. Some of the reasons for this interest in the tubers are: (1) dried potato contains 8% protein; (2) the protein-to-calorie ratio of potatoes is 2.3 g per 100 Calories (kcal), which is about the same as that for corn and rice; and (3) potato protein supplies ample lysine, the amino acid that is lacking in cereal grains. Hence, mixtures of potato and cereal proteins contain higher quality protein than either type of food alone.

(Also see FLOURS, Table F-26 Special Flours; and VEGETABLE[S], Table V-6 Vegetables of the World.)

POTATO SYRUP

A clear, viscous, syrup produced by the hydrolysis—splitting—of potato starch with heat and acids, or enzymes. It contains dextrins, maltotetrose, maltotriose, maltose and dextrose (glucose). The amount of each depends upon the conditions and duration of the hydrolysis. Corn syrup, derived in the same manner from corn starch, is more common in the United States.

POULTRY

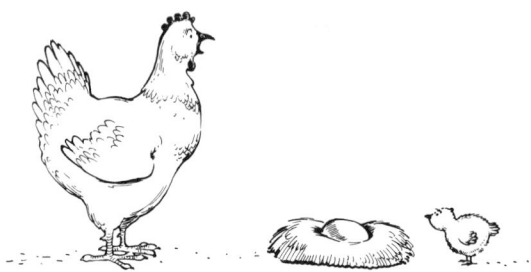

Fig. P-88. That's a good question! But in your case it was the egg.

The term "poultry" applies to a rather wide variety of birds of several species, and it refers to them whether they are alive or dressed.

Poultry appears more frequently in the diet of people throughout the world than any other type of meat. With the exception of strict vegetarians, there are few, if any, social or religious stigmas attached to the use of poultry meat in the diet. Because of its high edible yield, low shrinkage during cooking, ease of cooking and serving, and low cost, it fits well into menus.

KINDS OF POULTRY. The most common kinds of poultry used for meat follow (the respective names of each kind of poultry also refers to the flesh of each of them used for food):

• **Chicken**—The common domestic fowl (*Gallus gallus*).

• **Turkey**—A large American bird (*Meleagris gallopavo*) derived primarily from a Mexican variety of the wild turkey and raised chiefly for their flesh.

• **Ducks**—Swimming birds of the family *Anatidae*, characterized by short neck and legs, usually a broad, flat bill, the sexes differing from each other in plumage, and smaller in size than swans and geese.

• **Geese**—Swimming birds of a distinct subfamily of *Anatidae*, characterized by a high somewhat compressed bill, legs of moderate length, and usually longer-necked and larger than ducks.

• **Guinea fowl**—A West African bird of the subfamily *Phasianidae* (now usually made a separate family, *Numididae*), characterized by a bare neck and head.

• **Pigeon**—A bird of the widely distributed family *Columbidae*, characterized by a stout body with rather short legs, a bill that is horny at the tip but soft at the base, and smooth, compact plumage.

WORLD POULTRY NUMBERS, PRODUCTION, AND CONSUMPTION. Through the ages, poultry meat and eggs have been basic foods throughout the world. In the future, they will become increasingly important for feeding the hungry for the following reasons:

1. Poultry convert feed to food efficiently.
2. The poultry industry can adjust rapidly to a variety of economic factors, e.g., feed availability, demand for animal products, cost, etc.
3. Poultry feeds are not commonly used for human consumption.
4. Layers provide a continuous source of food.
5. Most vegetarians eat eggs.
6. Poultry products are inexpensive.
7. Poultry manure can be used as a fertilizer or as a feed.

• **World poultry numbers**—The production of poultry is worldwide. Figs. P-89, P-90, and P-91 show the leading poultry-producing countries of the world.

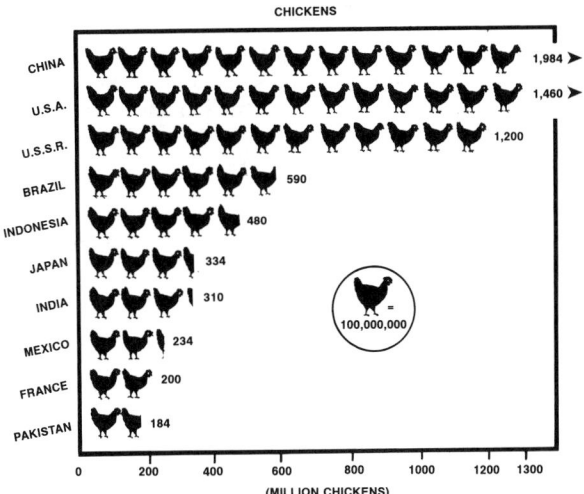

Fig. P-89. Leading chicken producers of the world. (Data from *FAO Production Yearbook*, 1990, FAO/UN, Rome, Italy, Vol. 44, p. 197)

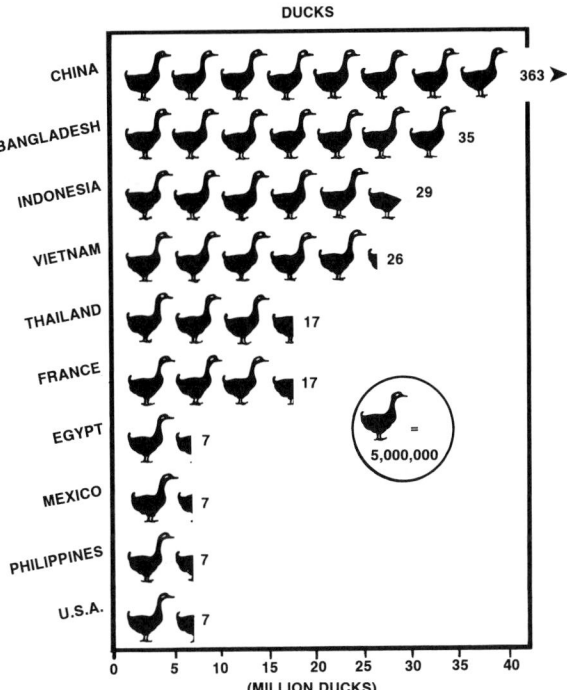

Fig. P-91. Leading duck producers of the world. (Data from *FAO Production Yearbook*, 1990, FAO/UN, Rome, Italy, Vol. 44, p. 198, Table 91)

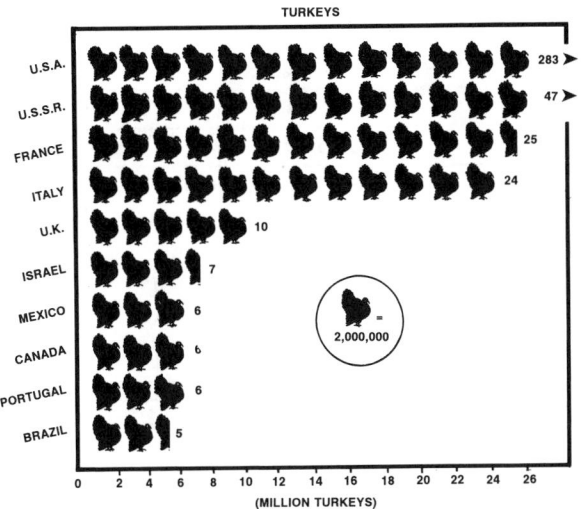

Fig. P-90. Leading turkey producers of the world. (Except for U.S. turkeys raised, data from *FAO Production Yearbook*, 1990, FAO/UN, Rome, Italy, Vol. 44, p. 197. U.S. turkey data, showing turkeys raised, from *Agricultural Statistics 1991*, USDA, p. 347, Table 516)

China holds a commanding lead in chicken numbers, followed by the United States and the U.S.S.R., respectively.

The United States ranks first in turkey production, with the U.S.S.R. second, and France third.

China ranks first in duck numbers, followed by Bangladesh, Indonesia, Vietnam, Thailand, and France, respectively. The duck numbers given in Fig. P-91 are, as shown, from the *FAO Production Yearbook*, 1990, United Nations. Although not shown in the FAO report, it is noteworthy that the annual production of ducks in the United States is approximately 20 million.

• **World poultry meat production**—Table P-15 shows the poultry meat production of the ten leading countries of the world in 1990. With a production of 10,851 metric tons, the United States ranks first in total poultry meat production; that's 27% of the world total.

TABLE P–15
POULTRY MEAT PRODUCTION IN TEN LEADING COUNTRIES OF THE WORLD[1]

Country (leading countries, by rank, of all poultry meats)	Total Poultry Meat Production 1990
	(1,000 MT)
U.S.A.	10,851
China	3,295
U.S.S.R.	3,280
Brazil	2,417
Japan	1,487
France	1,384
Italy	1,104
United Kingdom	981
Spain	825
Canada	699
World Total	39,862

[1]*FAO Production Yearbook*, Vol. 44, 1990, p. 212.

• **World poultry meat consumption**—United States, with a per capita consumption of 91.9 lb (*41.8 kg*), is the leading poultry meat consumer, followed by Singapore with 81.8 lb (*37.2 kg*).

Table P-16 shows the leading poultry eaters of the world.

TABLE P–16
LEADING POULTRY MEAT-EATING COUNTRIES OF THE WORLD 1990[1]

Country (leading countries by rank)	Per Capita Consumption, Dressed Weight Basis	
	(lb)	(kg)
U.S.A.	91.9	41.8
Singapore	81.8	37.2
Israel	77.6	35.3
Hong Kong	70.8	32.2
Canada	61.5	28.0
Saudi Arabia	56.0	25.5
Australia	54.0	24.5
Taiwan	53.8	24.5
Hungary	51.2	23.3
Spain	50.3	22.9

[1]*Statistical Abstract of the United States 1991*, U.S. Dept. of Commerce, p. 843, Table 1452 (with bone in).

U.S. EXPORTS AND IMPORTS OF POULTRY PRODUCTS.

Table P-17 shows the U.S. exports of broilers and turkeys. Broilers constitute the largest segment of poultry exports. The relative values, in percentages, of each group of exports of poultry products in 1990 were: poultry meat, 74.1%; eggs in shell, 7.5%; egg products, 3.4%; live poultry, 11%; and feathers, down and all other products, 4%. In 1990, exports of poultry products totaled $907 million.

The five top markets for U.S. poultry in 1990 were the U.S.S.R., Japan, Hong Kong, Canada, and Mexico. Hong Kong purchased 52% of all U.S. table eggs exported.

U.S. imports of poultry products amounted to $116 million in 1990, 12.8% of the value of U.S. exports of poultry products. The principal import items as a percent of the total value were: shell eggs, 18%; dried eggs, 2.4%; poultry meat, 16.3%; baby chicks, 7.3%; and feathers, 56%. Canada was the principal supplier of shell eggs and baby chicks, while France was the only supplier of goose liver products.

The importation of poultry products into the United States is deterred to some extent by import duties, which change from time to time. More importantly, however, the importation of poultry products is minimal because the United States is an efficient producer of enormous quantities of poultry products.

TABLE P–17
U.S. EXPORTS OF BROILERS AND TURKEYS[1]

Year	Broilers Exports		Turkeys Exports	
	(mil)			
	(lb)	(kg)	(lb)	(kg)
1986	583	265	27	12
1987	767	349	33	15
1988	791	360	51	23
1989	838	381	41	19
1990	1,168	531	54	25

[1]*Agriculture Statistics 1991*, USDA, p. 342, Table 506; and p. 346, Table 514.

TRANSFORMATION OF THE U.S. POULTRY INDUSTRY.

In colonial America, and for many years thereafter, small farm flocks of chickens were tenderly cared for by the farmer's wife, who fed them on table scraps and the unaccounted-for grain from the crib; and turkeys were raised to grace Thanksgiving and Christmas dinners.

Since World War II, changes in poultry production and processing have paced the whole field of agriculture. Practices in all phases of poultry—breeding, feeding, management, housing, marketing, processing, and retailing have become very highly specialized. The net result is that more products have been made available to consumers at favorable prices and per capita consumption has increased.

A brief summary of the changes that have taken place in chicken and turkey production follows:

• **Changes in chicken meat production**—Prior to 1930, chicken meat was mainly the by-product of egg production. Birds which were no longer producing eggs at a satisfactory rate were sold for meat purposes, mainly in the fall of the year. Cockerels raised with the pullets were disposed of as fryers, or roasters, at weights of 3 to 8 lb (*1.4 to 3.6 kg*).

In 1934, 34 million broilers were produced in the United States; in 1990, 5.9 billion broilers were produced, 172 times as many as 56 years earlier. Today, broiler production is so concentrated, and so highly commercialized, that the industry might properly be classed as a poultry or meat factory, rather than a farming operation. In 1990, 3 to 5 lb (*1.4 to 2.3 kg*) broilers were produced in 6 to 8 weeks. The feed required to produce a pound of live bird was reduced from 4 lb (*1.8 kg*) in 1940 to 1.9 lb (*0.87 kg*) on the most efficient broilers in 1990.

• **Changes in turkey production**—The production of turkeys was mostly a small sideline until recent years. In 1929, 18,476,000 turkeys were raised in the United States; in 1990, 283 million turkeys were raised, 15 times as many as 61 years earlier. Today, flocks of 50,000 or more are common. The time needed to pro-

duce a 25-lb (*11.3 kg*) tom has been reduced from 30 weeks 30 years ago to 17 weeks today. The feed required to produce a pound of live market bird has been reduced from 4.5 lb (*2.0 kg*) in 1940 to 2.5 lb (*1.1 kg*) today.

MARKETING POULTRY. It is estimated that 100% of the broilers and 90% of the turkeys are produced under some kind of integrated or contract arrange-

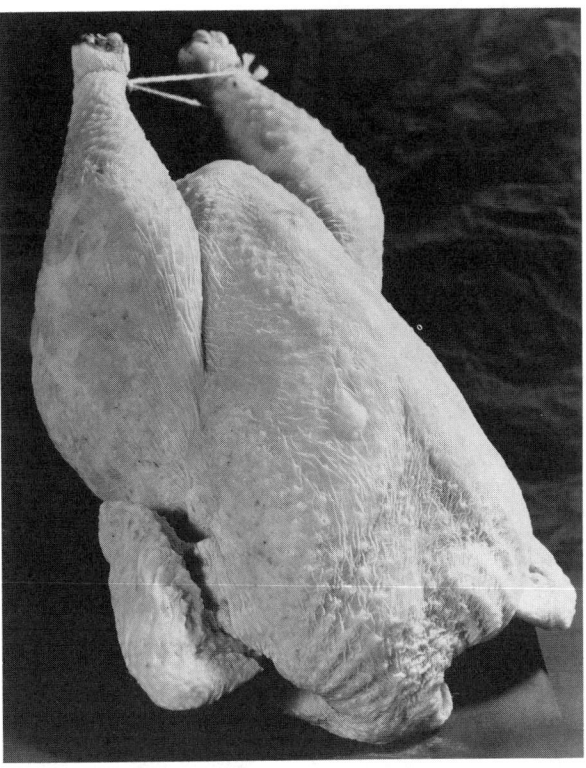

Fig. P-93. Whole broiler, ready to cook. (Photo by J. C. Allen and Son, Inc., West Lafayette, Ind.)

ment. This means that a limited number of big firms are organized in such manner as to control every level of production—all the way from producing broilers and turkeys, through the processing, and finally, the ultimate promotion and marketing of the finished product. However, the chain of events in producing poultry meat (primarily chickens and turkeys) and getting it to the consumer can be broken down into three primary stages: (1) producing, (2) processing, and (3) retailing.

The first stage—producing—has been summarized briefly under the heading "Transformation of the U.S. Poultry Industry." A discussion of each of the other two sections follows.

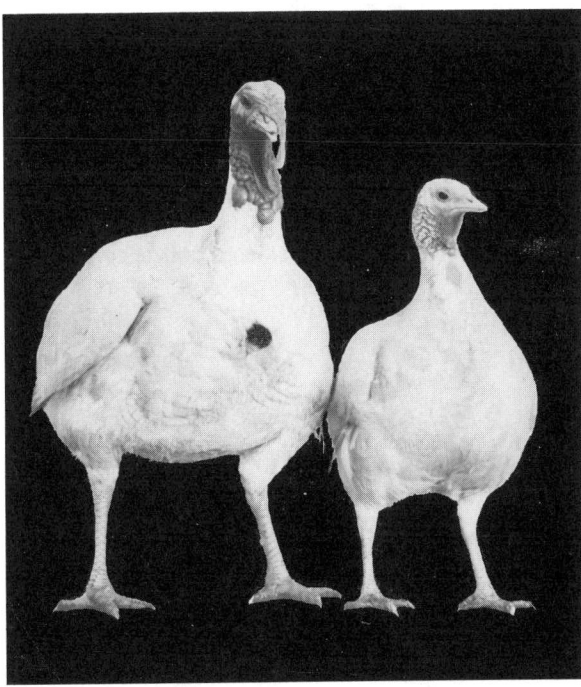

Fig. P-92. Fast-growing, broad-breasted Large White turkeys were developed by Cornell University in the 1950s. This shows a male (left) and a female (right) of the Large White breed. (Courtesy, *Turkey World*)

The first stage—producing—has been summarized briefly under the heading "Transformation of the U.S. Poultry Industry." A discussion of each of the other two sections follows:

Processing, Inspecting, Classifying and Grading.

The slaughter and processing of broilers and turkeys is an assembly line operation conducted under sanitary conditions. Inspecting, classifying, and grading are a part of the processing operation.

Broilers and turkeys are generally processed in separate plants. Although the processing procedure may vary from plant to plant, and between broilers and turkeys, the steps are usually as follows:

1. **Antemortem inspecting.** The birds are inspected before entering the processing plant. Essentially, this is a spot check of each lot of birds, not of each individual bird.

2. **Suspended and shackled.** Each bird is suspended by the leg to a conveying chain, with the feet held in a shackle.

3. **Stunning.** Birds are rendered unconscious by an electric stunner to prevent struggling and relax the muscles that hold the feathers.

4. **Bleeding.** Birds are bled by severing the jugular vein.

5. **Scalding.** The feathers are loosened by scalding in agitated water at 140° to 142°F (60° to 61°C) for 30 seconds to 1 minute.

6. **Picking.** The feathers are picked by machine.

7. **Removing pinfeathers.** The pinfeathers are removed; usually, broiler pinfeathers are removed by machine, whereas turkey pinfeathers are removed by hand.

8. **Eviscerating.** The viscera is removed, following which broilers are singed.

9. **Chilling.** The eviscerated carcass is chilled in ice water or ice slush.

10. **Postmortem inspecting.** This is the after slaughter inspection; it's an inspection of each bird at the time the abdominal cavity is opened and the visceral organs are removed.

11. **Grading.** Next, the carcasses are graded and sorted by weight.

12. **Packaging.** Lastly, carcasses are packaged, frozen, or further processed.

FEDERAL INSPECTION. The Poultry Products Inspection Act was enacted on August 28, 1957, and became fully effective January 1, 1959. It requires inspection of poultry and poultry products by the U.S. Department of Agriculture. Birds are inspected twice: (1) live (antemortem); and (2) after slaughter (postmortem), when the carcasses and entrails are examined. Inspection assures U.S. consumers that the retail meat supply has been inspected to assure wholesomeness; sanitary preparation and handling; and freedom from disease, adulteration, and misbranding.

MARKET CLASSES OF POULTRY. The U.S. Department of Agriculture has established specifications for different kinds, classes, and grades of poultry. *Kind refers to the different species of poultry, such as chickens, turkeys, ducks, geese, guineas, and pigeons. "Class" refers to kinds of poultry by groups which are essentially of the same physical characteristics, such as fryers or hens.* These physical characteristics are associated with age and sex. The kinds and classes of live, dressed, and ready-to-cook poultry listed in the U.S. classes, standards, and grades are in general use in all segments of the poultry industry.

A listing of the various classes of meat birds is given in Table P-18.

TABLE P-18
CLASSES OF POULTRY[1]

Bird-Class	Description
Chickens:	
• Rock Cornish game hen or Cornish game hen	A young, immature chicken (usually 4–6 weeks of age) weighing not more than 2 lb ready-to-cook weight, the progeny of a Cornish chicken or a Cornish chicken crossed with another breed of chicken.
• Broiler or fryer	A young chicken (usually 6–8 weeks of age), of either sex, that weighs 3–5 lb, that is tender-meated with soft, pliable, smooth-textured skin and flexible breastbone cartilage.
• Roaster	A young chicken (usually 9–11 weeks of age), of either sex, that weighs 6–8 lb, that is tender-meated with soft, pliable, smooth-textured skin and breastbone cartilage that may be somewhat less flexible than that of a broiler or fryer.
• Capon	A surgically unsexed male chicken (usually ranges up to 20–24 weeks of age), that weighs 12–14 lb, that is tender-meated with soft, pliable, smooth-textured skin.
• Stag	A male chicken (usually under 10 months of age) with coarse skin, somewhat toughened and darkened flesh, and considerable hardening of the breastbone cartilage. Stags show a condition of fleshing and a degree of maturity intermediate between that of a roaster and a cock or rooster.
• Hen or stewing chicken or fowl	A mature female chicken (usually more than 10 months of age) with meat less tender than that of a roaster, and nonflexible breastbone tip.
• Cock or rooster	A mature male chicken with coarse skin, toughened and darkened meat, and hardened breastbone tip.
Turkeys:	
• Fryer-roaster turkey	A young, immature turkey of either sex, 8–12 lb liveweight, that is tender-meated with soft, pliable, smooth-textured skin and flexible breastbone cartilage.
• Young hen turkey	A young female turkey (usually 14–15 weeks of age) that is tender-meated with soft, pliable, smooth-textured skin, and breastbone cartilage that is somewhat less flexible than in a fryer-roaster turkey.
• Young tom turkey	A young male turkey (usually 17–18 months of age) that is tender-meated with soft, pliable, smooth-textured skin, and breastbone cartilage that is somewhat less flexible than in a fryer-roaster turkey.
• Yearling hen turkey	A fully matured female turkey (usually under 15 months of age) that is reasonably tender-meated and with reasonably smooth-textured skin.
• Yearling tom turkey	A fully matured male turkey (usually under 15 months of age) that is reasonably tender-meated and with reasonably smooth-textured skin.
• Mature turkey or old turkey (hen or tom)	An old turkey of either sex (usually in excess of 15 months of age) with coarse skin and toughened flesh.
Ducks:	
• Broiler duckling or fryer duckling	A young duck (usually under 8 weeks of age), of either sex, that is tender-meated and has a soft bill and soft windpipe.
• Roaster duckling	A young duck (usually under 16 weeks of age), of either sex, that is tender-meated and has a bill that is not completely hardened and a windpipe that is easily dented.
• Mature duck or old duck	A duck (usually over 6 months of age), of either sex, with toughened flesh, hardened bill, and hardened windpipe.
Geese:	
• Young goose	Can be of either sex, is tender-meated, and has a windpipe that is easily dented.
• Mature goose or old goose	Can be of either sex, has toughened flesh, and hardened windpipe.
Guineas:	
• Young guinea	Can be of either sex, is tender-meated, and has a flexible breastbone cartilage.
• Mature guinea or old guinea	Can be of either sex, has toughened flesh, and a hardened breastbone.
Pigeons:	
• Squab	Young, immature pigeon of either sex, and is extra tender-meated.
• Pigeon	Mature pigeon of either sex, with coarse skin and toughened flesh.

[1]*Poultry Grading Manual*, Ag. Hdbk. No. 31, USDA.

MARKET GRADES OF POULTRY. Dressed and ready-to-cook poultry are graded for class, condition, and quality. These are most important since they are the grades used at the retail level. These grades are:

U.S. Grade A
U.S. Grade B
U.S. Grade C

These grades apply to dressed and ready-to-cook chickens, turkeys, ducks, geese, guineas, and pigeons.

Additionally, there are U.S. Procurement Grades, which are designed primarily for institutional use. These grades are: U.S. Procurement Grade 1, and U.S. Procurement Grade 2. In procurement grades, more emphasis is placed on meat yield than on appearance.

The factors determining the grade of carcasses, or ready-to-cook poultry parts therefrom are: conformation, fleshing, fat covering, pinfeathers, exposed flesh, discoloration, disjointed bones, broken bones, missing parts, and freezing defects.

Retailing Poultry. Most of the poultry meat marketed consists of broilers and turkeys, although ducks, geese, guineas, and pigeons are also marketed.

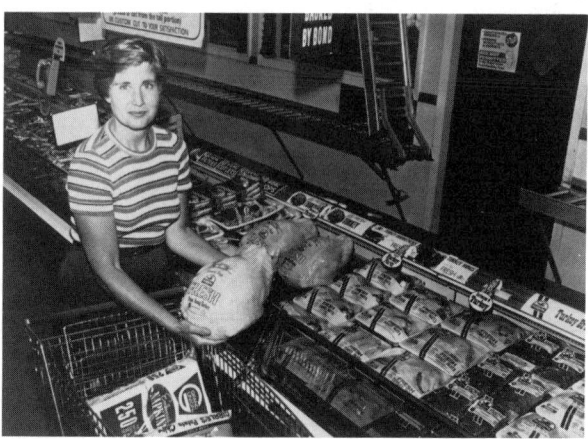

Fig. P-94. Fresh dressed turkey in the supermarket fresh meat case. (Courtesy, Cryovac Division, W. R. Grace & Co., Duncan, S.C.)

• **Broilers**—Today, virtually 100% of the broilers marketed are sold in ready-to-cook form (either whole or cut up) or as processed meat.

In 1989, processors sold 18.3% of their broilers as whole carcasses, 50.4% as cut-up parts, 6.3% as further processed, and 25% in other forms. In 1992, approximately 40% of broilers were further processed.

• **Turkeys**—About 80% of the turkey meat produced today is cut-up or used as further processed product. Whole bird processed turkeys, such as self-basting turkeys, comprise about 20% of the total.

Most turkeys marketed whole are Grade A. To the extent possible, Grades B and C and lower-priced parts are utilized in further processing.

More and more further processed and whole bird turkeys are being marketed directly to retail outlets and institutional outlets.

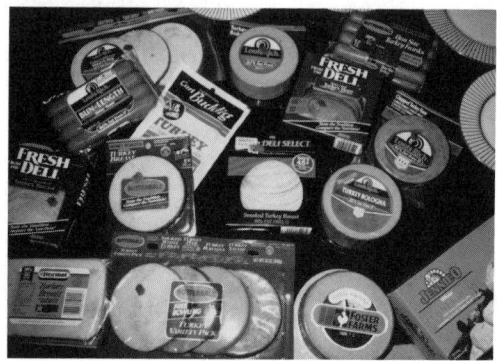

Fig. P-94a. Further processed turkey products. (Photo by A. H. Enmsminger)

HOW TO BUY POULTRY. When buying any kind of poultry—chicken, turkey, duck, goose, guinea, or squab—in addition to price, the buyer should look for and select on the bases of the following:

1. **Look for the inspection mark.** Poultry must be officially inspected for wholesomeness before it can be graded for quality. Often the inspection mark and the grade shield are displayed together, as shown in Fig. P-95.

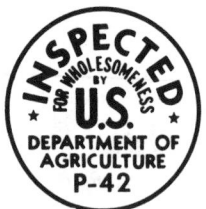
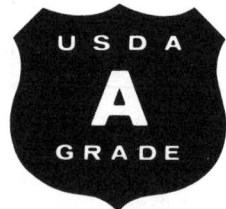

Fig. P-95. *Left:* the mark of wholesomeness. *Right:* the mark of quality.

2. **Select by grade (quality).** Look for the USDA shield, which certifies that the poultry has been graded for quality by a technically trained government grader and is the buyer's assurance of quality (see Fig. P-95, right).

The highest quality is grade A. Grade A birds are—

• fully fleshed and meaty.

• well finished.

• attractive in appearance.

Grade B birds may be less attractive in finish and appearance and slightly lacking in meatiness.

3. **Select by class.** The grade of poultry does not indicate tenderness—the age (class) of the bird determines tenderness. Young birds are more tender than older ones.

a. Young tender-meated classes are most suitable for barbecuing, frying, broiling, or roasting:

• **Young chickens may be labeled**—young chicken, Rock Cornish game hen, broiler, fryer, roaster, or capon.

• **Young turkeys may be labeled**—young turkey, fryer-roaster, young hen, or young tom.

• **Young ducks may be labeled**—duckling, young duckling, broiler duckling, fryer duckling, or roaster duckling.

b. Mature, less-tender-meated classes may be preferred for stewing, baking, soups, or salads.

• **Mature chickens may be labeled**—mature chicken, old chicken, hen, stewing chicken, or fowl.

• **Mature turkeys may be labeled**—mature turkey, yearling turkey, or old turkey.

• **Mature ducks, geese, and guineas may be labeled**—mature or old.

4. **Select to suit the occasion. Poultry can be selected to fill every need.**

• Chilled or frozen ready-to-cook poultry may be purchased in various sizes and forms to suit every occasion.

• Most kinds of ready-to-cook poultry are available as parts and in whole, halved, and quartered form. Some kinds are also available as boneless roasts and rolls.

HOW TO STORE POULTRY. All poultry is perishable. So, it is important that it be properly stored. To this end, the following pointers will be helpful:

For Refrigeration:

• Store poultry in the refrigerator only if you are going to use it within a few days. Temperatures between 35° and 40°F (*2° and 4°C*) should be maintained for refrigerator storage. Keep it in the coldest part of the refrigerator, which is usually near the ice cube compartment or in a special meat keeper.

• Wrap poultry properly for refrigeration. The special wrap on prepackaged poultry is designed to control moisture loss in the refrigerator. Raw poultry wrapped

in paper should be unwrapped, placed on a platter, and then covered for refrigeration. Wrap and store giblets separately.

• Use fresh-chilled poultry within 1 to 2 days.
Follow Table P-19 Poultry Storage Time Chart relative to refrigerating poultry.

**TABLE P-19
POULTRY STORAGE TIME CHART**

Product	Refrigerator 35°-40°F (2°-4°)	Freezer 0°F (−18°C)
	(days)	(months)
Fresh poultry:		
Chicken and turkey (whole) ..	1 to 2	12
Chicken (pieces)	1 to 2	6
Turkey (pieces)	1 to 2	6
Duck and goose (whole)	1 to 2	6
Giblets	1 to 2	3
Cooked Poultry:		
Pieces (covered with broth) ..	1 to 2	6
Pieces (not covered)	1 to 2	1
Cooked poultry dishes	1 to 2	6
Fried chicken	1 to 2	4

For Freezing:

• Keep frozen poultry at 0°F (*-18°C*).

• Keep frozen poultry hard-frozen until time to thaw, then cook promptly after thawing.

• Refreeze poultry only if it still contains ice crystals or if it is still cold and has not been held at refrigerator temperature for more than 1 to 2 days. Remember that refreezing may reduce the quality of a product.

• Follow Table P-19 Poultry Storage Time Chart relative to freezing poultry.

HOW TO HANDLE AND COOK POULTRY.
Care and cleanliness should be used in the preparation, cooking, and serving of poultry products. The following pointers will be helpful:

• Wash poultry before preparing it for cooking.

• Wash your hands often when preparing poultry.

• Completely cook poultry at one time. Never partially cook, then store, and finish cooking at a later date.

• It is safest to cook dressing outside the bird, but if you want to stuff it, do so right before roasting; don't stuff raw poultry and then refrigerate or freeze it. Commercially stuffed frozen poultry should always be cooked without thawing.

• Left-over cooked poultry, broth, stuffing, and gravy should be separated, covered, and refrigerated. Use within 1 to 2 days. Freeze for longer storage.

U.S. PER CAPITA CONSUMPTION OF POULTRY MEAT.

Poultry meat is supplied chiefly by chickens and turkeys, although ducks, geese, guinea fowl, squabs (pigeon), and other fowl contribute thereto. Poultry meat is economical, and quick and easy to prepare and serve.

Fig. P-96 shows the U.S. per capita consumption of ready-to-cook poultry since 1965. Note that most of the increase occurred with broilers. In 1990, poultry meat consumption totaled 63.8 lb (29 kg).

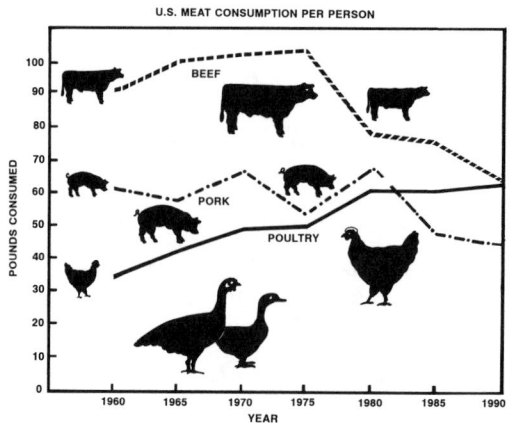

Fig. P-97. U.S. consumption of poultry, pork, and beef.

NUTRITIVE QUALITIES OF POULTRY MEAT.

Poultry meat has a number of desirable nutritional properties. Chicken and turkey meat is higher in quality

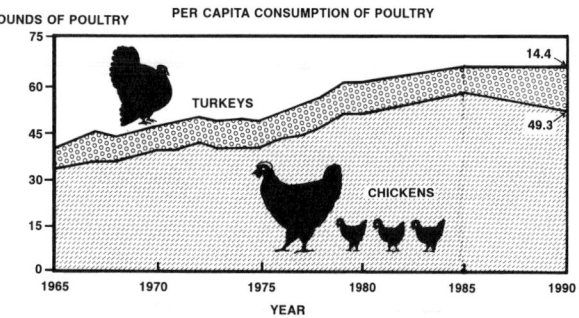

Fig. P-96. Per capita consumption of poultry—boneless, trimmed, or edible weight. (From: USDA)

Fig. P-97 shows how the consumption of poultry meat is fast catching up to beef and pork. From 1960 to 1990, the per capita consumption of poultry almost doubled. During this same period of time, beef and pork consumption both dropped 39%. If the recent trends shown in Fig. P-97 continue, soon Americans will be eating more pounds of poultry meat than of beef or pork.

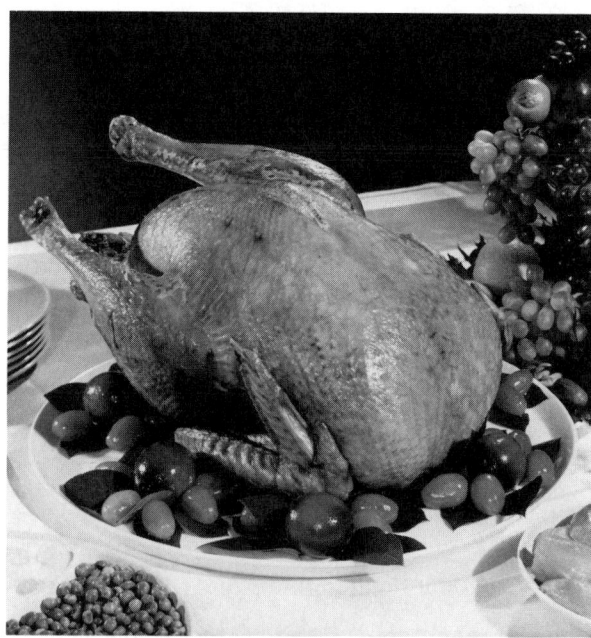

Fig. P-98. Roast turkey. Turkeys produce a higher proportion of edible meat to liveweight than any other species, and compare favorably with other meats as a source of amino acids. (Courtesy, National Turkey Federation, Mount Morris, Ill.)

protein and lower in fat than beef and pork. Additionally, the protein is a rich source of all the essential amino acids. The close resemblance of the amino acid content of poultry meat to the amino acid profiles of milk and eggs serves to emphasize the latter point.

Poultry meat is also a good source of phosphorus, iron, copper, and zinc. Additionally, it is a rich dietary source of vitamin B-12 and vitamin B-6, and it supplies appreciable amounts of vitamin A, biotin, niacin, pantothenic acid, riboflavin, and thiamin.

Poultry is a good, low-fat source of protein. However, poultry skin contains 32.35% saturated fat. Removing the skin reduces the amount of fat by approximately 5 grams per 2.5 oz breast. Because consumers are turning to foods that are lower in cholesterol and saturated fats, beginning in the early 1990s almost all U.S. restaurants included low fat, skinless chicken on their menus.

Table P-20 shows the contribution of meat-poultry-fish combined to meeting the recommended daily nutrient allowance (RDA) of the various nutrients.

Although the RDAs are believed to be more than adequate to meet the requirements of most consumers, it is recognized that individuals vary greatly in their requirements—by as much as twofold. So, Table P-21 presents data showing the contribution of meat-poultry-fish combined toward the total dietary intake of each of the nutrients.

TABLE P–20
CONTRIBUTIONS OF MEAT-POULTRY-FISH, COMBINED
TO THE RECOMMENDED NUTRIENT ALLOWANCES IN THE UNITED STATES[1]

Nutrient	United States Recommended Daily Allowances (RDA)[2]	Contribution from Meat-Poultry-Fish, Combined	
		Total Amount/Day[3]	RDA[4]
			(%)
Energy	2,900 kcal	676.8 kcal	23.3
Carbohydrate	Not established	0.4 g	—
Fat	Not established	53.3 g	—
Protein	63 g	45.5 g	72.2
Calcium	800 mg	34.7 mg	4.3
Phosphorus	800 mg	450 mg	56.2
Magnesium	350 mg	50.8 mg	14.5
Copper	1.5–3 mg	0.30 mg	13.2
Iron[5]	10 mg	3.78 mg	37.8
Zinc	15 mg	5.99 mg	40
Vitamin A[6]	1,000 R.E.	336 R.E.	33.6
Folate	200 mcg	27.8 mcg	13.9
Niacin	19 mg	11.6 mg	61.3
Riboflavin	1.7 mg	0.53 mg	31.3
Thiamin	1.5 mg	0.55 mg	36.7
Vitamin B-6	2.0 mg	0.89 mg	44.6
Vitamin B-12	2.0 mcg	6.93 mcg	346.3
Vitamin C	60 mg	2.6 mg	4.3

[1]From: *Agricultural Statistics 1991*, USDA, pp. 474–478.

[2]National Research Council (1989 for adult male 25-50 years of age).

[3]USDA (1988).

[4]Calculated as follows: % RDA = Avg $\dfrac{\text{daily per capita intake}}{\text{RDA}}$

[5]RDA value used for iron based on adult male, whereas, adult premenopausal female has an RDA of 15 mg/day.

[6]Vitamin A is given in terms of retinol equivalents (R.E.), one R.E. = 3.3 IU of vitamin A activity, which was assumed to be the predominant form in meat, poultry, and fish.

TABLE P–21
CONTRIBUTIONS OF MEAT-POULTRY-FISH COMBINED, TO THE DIETARY INTAKE IN THE UNITED STATES[1,2]

Nutrition	Average Per Capita Consumption Per Day	Total Consumption Contributed by Meat-Poultry-Fish Combined
		(%)
Energy	3,600 kcal	18.8
Carbohydrate . . .	425 g	0.1
Fat	168 g	31.7
Protein	105 g	43.3
Calcium	890 mg	3.9
Phosphorus	1,540 mg	29.2
Magnesium	339 mg	15.4
Copper	1.7 mg	17.5
Iron	17.1 mg	22.1
Zinc	12.7 mg	47.2
Vitamin A (R.E.) .	1,630 mcg	20.6
Folate	284 mcg	9.8
Niacin	26 mg	44.8
Riboflavin	2.4 mg	22.2
Thiamin	2.2 mg	25.0
Vitamin B-6	2.2 mg	40.5
Vitamin B-12	9.1 mcg	76.1
Vitamin C	118 mg	2.2

[1]*Agricultural Statistics 1991*, USDA, pp. 474–479.

[2]The average yearly per capita consumption (carcass basis) amounted to 112.3 lb of red meat, 63.8 lb of poultry, and 15.4 lb of fish that was consumed in 1990.

It should be noted that the values given in both Table P-20 and Table P-21 are calculations based on food disappearance data and may not accurately reflect actual consumption.

In order to illustrate the use of Tables P-20 and P-21, protein will be used as an example.

Table P-20 shows that the RDA for protein for the 25- to 50-year-old man is 63 g, with meat-poultry-fish supplying 72.2% of this amount. Table P-21 shows that meat-poultry-fish supply 43.3%, of the total protein intake.

Similar tables to Table P-20 and Table P-21, along with instructions on how to use the tables, and more complete information relative to the nutritional qualities of meat, are included in the section on MEAT under "Nutritive Composition of Meats"; hence, the reader is referred thereto.

(Also see MEAT[S].)

PRECURSOR

A compound that can be used by the body to form another compound; for example, carotene is a precursor of vitamin A.

(Also see PROVITAMIN A.)

PREGNANCY AND LACTATION NUTRITION

Women who consume a good diet before conception and during pregnancy and lactation greatly improve their chances of successful reproduction, including (1) absence of complications during pregnancy, (2) birth of a healthy full term baby, and (3) having little or no trouble in meeting the nutritional needs of their infants, whether they are breast fed or formula fed. Although even poorly fed mothers may have healthy babies, this result is sometimes achieved at the expense of the mother's tissues and health. Therefore, proper prenatal care is a means of promoting optimal health in both the baby and the mother.

HISTORY. Many ancient cultures appear to have been concerned about the successful result of pregnancy, judging by the many depictions of this condition on the artifacts found at various archaeological sites. Furthermore, students of contemporary primitives, whose practices have changed little over the centuries, have often discovered that the diets which are culturally prescribed for pregnant women have higher nutritional values than some of the food consumption patterns of people in the developed countries. Some of the discoveries of primitive dietary wisdom which were made by the renowned American dentist and anthropologist Weston Price[16] follow:

1. The Coastal Peruvian Indians, the Eskimos in the Arctic, the Gaelic people of the Outer Herbrides Islands, the natives of the South Pacific Islands, and other primitive fishing peoples have long fed expectant mothers fish eggs and other nutrient rich seafoods.

2. Inland dwelling, cattle-raising groups of people in Africa, Central Asia, Central Europe, and India gave their pregnant women ample amounts of milk and other dairy products from cows raised on green pastures. It is noteworthy, too, that certain Masai tribes in Africa did not allow their girls to marry until the season when the cattle had plenty of rapidly growing young grass.

3. Tribes living at the higher elevations of mountainous areas in Africa where goiter is common (due to lack of iodine in the soil) often descended to lower areas to gather iodine-rich plants which they converted to ashes for seasoning their foods. Sometimes, dwellers in mountainous regions elsewhere have traded with coastal dwellers to obtain dried fish eggs.

4. The Indians of Northern Canada near the Arctic Circle relied mainly on hunting and fishing to provide food since there was only a very brief annual period during which edible plants were available. Hence, they obtained their vitamin A by eating the vitamin-rich portion of fish heads just behind the eyes, and they obtained their vitamin C by consuming the adrenal glands from animals they killed. They also ate the thyroid glands from the male moose during the animal's mating season when the glands become exceptionally large.

5. Pregnant and lactating women of certain African tribes have long consumed red millet grains that contain from 5 to 10 times the calcium in other cereals, and seeds from *Chenopodium* species that are reputed to stimulate lactation. The latter seeds were also consumed by Peruvian Indians.

Dr. Price confirmed that substantial benefits were derived from the consumption of nutrient-rich foods in his description of a woman who ate poorly in her first pregnancy and gave birth to an infant with notable dental and facial malformations, but later gave birth to a second child free from defects after eating liberal amounts of milk and dairy products, green vegetables, fish and sea foods, organ meats, and small doses of cod-liver oil in her second pregnancy.

It appears that primitive diets have often deteriorated in both quantity and quality as a result of factors such as (1) rapid growth of the population so that the per capita supply of food decreased greatly; (2) people changing their diets from a wide variety of native foods to a few highly refined imported foods such as flour, lard, and sugar; and (3) migration of the people to new areas where the foods are unfamiliar and likely to have been rejected because of cultural biases. Nevertheless, some groups apparently made a gradual and healthful transition from nomads to settled agriculturalists, as demonstrated by

the outstanding physiques of the Swiss dairy farmers in isolated high Alpine valleys. (Dr. Price observed the people of the Loetschental Valley in Switzerland, which is the region that has supplied many of the Swiss guards who protect the Pope.)

Not much is known about maternal and infant health in the long interval between primitive and modern times because records of birth illnesses, and deaths were seldom kept, except in the cases of certain ruling families. Hence, our knowledge of the past circumstances of pregnancy has been gleaned mainly from the records of European royalty from 1500 to 1899 A.D., which give some indication of the maternal experiences of the ruling classes. (Some of the writers of that period suggest that peasant mothers were healthier and fared better in childbirth than the royal mothers. However, the commoners of the cities probably fared the worst of all.) The most significant improvements in the maternal and infant health of the ruling families which occurred between the beginning of the 16th century and the end of the 19th century were: (1) a great reduction in the mortality rates of older mothers, and (2) a decrease from 10 to 5% in the death rate of infants during the first year. It seems likely that these improvements were due mostly to improved sanitation and better obstetrical care, since little was known about the essential nutrients which were required during pregnancy and lactation.

One of the great advances of the late 19th century was the application of the anti-infectious measures of the Hungarian obstetrician Ignaz Semmelweis (1818-1865) who demonstrated that the high rate of fatal "childbed fever" in hospital maternity wards resulted from the transmission of infectious diseases from patient to patient by attending physicians who failed to scrub their hands between examinations.

A new era in nutrition was ushered in during the early 1900s when the first discoveries of the vitamins were made. Before that time it was assumed that diets were adequate if sufficient amounts of carbohydrates, fats, and proteins were provided. Nevertheless, the application of sound nutritional principles to pregnancy and lactation diets lagged behind the many advances in nutritional science which were made during the first half of the 20th century.

In the 1920s, many doctors believed that a calorie-restricted diet protected pregnant women against toxemia because there was a reduction in the incidence of this condition in Austria, Hungary, and Germany during World War I when scarcities of fats and meats led to smaller weight gains during pregnancy. However, few systematically planned observations were made of (1) the weights of the women before pregnancy, and (2) the effects of dietary restrictions on the health and survival of infants. Evidence concerning the dangers of inadequate diets during pregnancy was provided by studies conducted in the 1930s which showed that toxemia might result from low protein intakes, because subnormal levels of blood proteins sometimes allowed fluid from the blood to accumulate in the tissues.

Additional observations regarding the effects of various diets on the outcome of pregnancy resulted from the experiences of women in certain countries during World War II. Details follow:

---

[16]Price, W. A., *Nutrition and Physical Degeneration*, Paul B. Hoeber, Inc., 1939.

• **England**—There was a rapid decline in the death rates of newborn infants between 1940 and 1945, which resulted in part from giving pregnant and lactating women priority in the distribution of food. Also, sugar was in very short supply and whole grains were more plentiful than refined grains. Hence, the diets of women in the lower socioeconomic classes were improved greatly. Additionally, the very low rate of unemployment during the war was another factor that raised the nutritional plane of working-class diets.

Unfortunately, many of the British mothers who were in Hong Kong during the war had temporary cessations of their menstrual cycles (amenorrhea) due to lack of sufficient dietary calories and protein.

• **Holland**—Food was very scarce in certain parts of the country during 1944 and 1945 because the Nazis used food deprivation as a means of reprisal against the Dutch for collaborating in the unsuccessful invasion attempt by the British at Arnhem. About half of the women of childbearing age developed amenorrhea. However, the other women who became pregnant generally had healthy infants, although the average birth weight was about ½ lb (250 g) below normal. Also, the rates of toxemia and stillbirths dropped during this period. It is believed that the successful outcomes of pregnancy in spite of the food deprivation resulted because the women who conceived had consumed good diets before the period of scarcity. Furthermore, Dutch women may have had a higher rate of complications before the war as a result of habitual overeating and other poor dietary habits.

• **Norway**—Just before food rationing was instituted, about 19% of the pregnant women passed protein in the urine (a sign that toxemia may be present). After rationing was instituted, the incidence of toxemia dropped to about ⅓ of what it had been. The rationing program allowed each woman about 0.5 g of protein per pound (1 g per kg) of body weight and many women received about 1½ oz (40 to 50 g) of dried brewers' yeast daily as a protein and vitamin supplement. It is noteworthy that there were no cases of eclampsia or maternal mortality during the period of rationing.

• **Russia**—The 1942 siege of Leningrad was accompanied by an 18-month period of starvation that resulted in a doubling of the fetal mortality rate and the deaths of about 9% of the full-term infants. Furthermore, the average birthweight was more than 1 lb (500 to 600 g) below normal, and 31% of the low-birth-weight infants died in the first month of life. It is suspected that the Russian women had nutritionally inadequate diets prior to the siege and were therefore affected greatly by the severe deprivation.

After World War II, there was considerable interest in (1) the wartime experiences of pregnant women, and (2) studies which had been conducted in the United States and England during the 1940s. Most of the studies provided evidence that fetal and neonatal deaths, low-birth-weight infants, and congenital malformations were linked to dietary deficiencies during pregnancy. However, interest in the subject waned during the 1950s after other studies failed to find significant relationships between diet and the outcome of pregnancy. One of the main reasons for the contradictory findings in the various studies may have been the failure to obtain information on the eating patterns of the subjects prior to conception. Previously, well-fed women would have had more tissue reserves to carry them through their pregnancies.

Throughout the 1950s and 1960s many American doctors told pregnant women not to gain more than 15 to 20 lb (7 to 9 kg) because they believed that excessive weight gain rendered the women more susceptible to complications such as toxemia. Furthermore, salt was often restricted and diuretics were administered to prevent the buildup of fluids in the tissues. However, this period was also characterized by a growing trend towards prescribing mineral and vitamin supplements for pregnant women. Hence, the latter practice may have offset some of the consequences of dietary restriction.

Starting at about 1960, the birth rates among women in most age groups declined, but in 1965 the rates for girls under age 15 began to rise. These trends are shown in Fig. P-99.

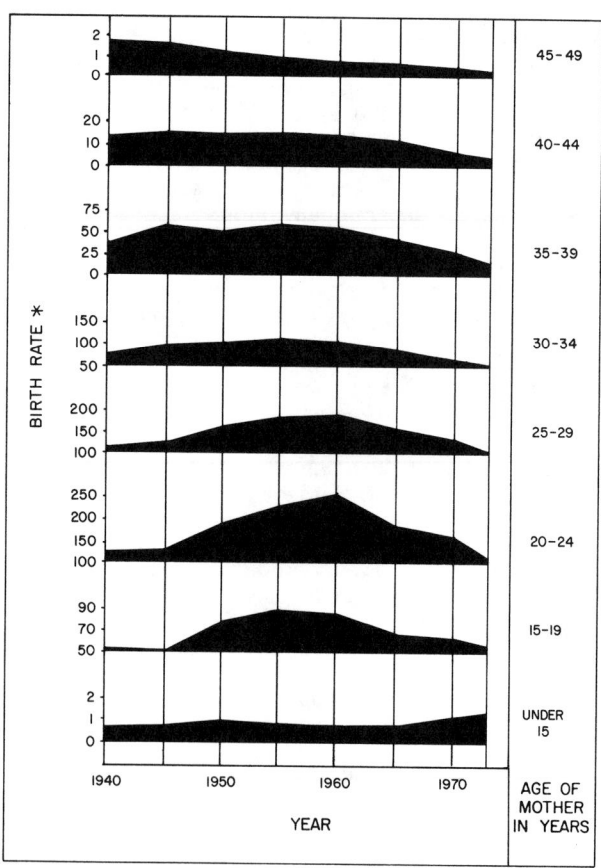

✴ PER 1000 WOMEN IN SPECIFIED GROUP

Fig. P-99. Birth rates for American mothers of various ages during the period from 1940 to 1973. (Based upon data from *Health, United States 1975*, U.S. Dept. HEW, p. 203, Table CD.I.14)

Many of the young adolescent girls had low-birth-weight babies which had high rates of abnormalities and deaths within the first month of life. These unfortunate occurrences, plus reports of similar tragedies among undernourished people in the developing countries rekindled the waning interest in diets during pregnancy. As a result, a committee of experts assembled by the National Academy of Sciences (NAS) published the landmark report *Maternal Nutrition and the Course of Pregnancy* in 1970. The most significant recommendations made in this publication were: (1) the diets of obese women should *not* be restricted during pregnancy; (2) salt (sodium) restriction and the use of diuretics should be avoided; (3) a minimum weight gain of 24 lb (*11 kg*) is usually desirable, since the most successful pregnancies are achieved with gains ranging from 22 to 27 lb (*10 to 12 kg*); (4) daily supplements of iron and folic acid should be used by most women; and (5) a variety of foods from the basic four food groups should be consumed.

In the decade following the NAS report infant mortality in the United States decreased by an average of about 5% annually, thanks to the efforts of an ever-growing number of dedicated doctors, educators, medical researchers, nurses, nutritionists, and public health workers who have applied nutritional principles for the benefit of pregnant and lactating women.

CHANGES IN THE FEMALE BODY DURING PREGNANCY AND LACTATION.

Few people are aware of the amount of tissue growth that occurs in women during their reproductive years. For example, a woman who bears no children has to produce blood and repair uterine lining tissue to cover the loss of menstruation. This task alone is equivalent to the production of

about 110 lb (*50 kg*) of body tissue between ages 15 and 45. However, a woman who bears 6 children and nurses each one for 9 months builds the equivalent of about 220 lb (*100 kg*) of body tissue during her reproductive years.[17]

A depiction of the tissue growth during pregnancy is given in Fig. P-100.

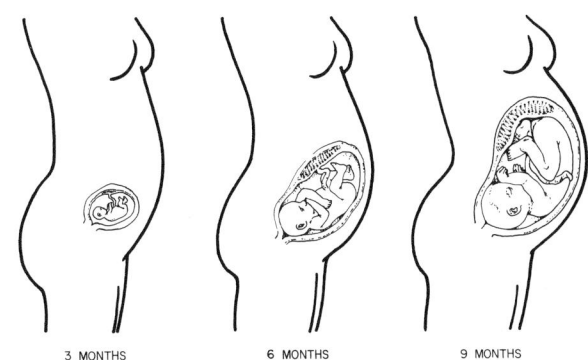

3 MONTHS   6 MONTHS   9 MONTHS

Fig. P-100. The growing fetus depends on its mother for nutrients and removal of wastes. The mother's heart pumps blood through the uterine arteries into the placenta; nutrients and oxygen diffuse through the placental membranes into the fetal bloodstream by way of the umbilical cord; and wastes pass in the reverse direction to the maternal bloodstream through the uterine veins.

Details of the changes during pregnancy and lactation are given in Table P-22.

[17]Toverud, K. U., *et al., Maternal Nutrition and Child Health, An Interpretive Review,* National Academy of Sciences, 1950, p. 116.

TABLE P-22
MAJOR CHANGES IN THE FEMALE BODY DURING PREGNANCY AND LACTATION

Part of the Body	Changes[1]	Biological Significance	Comments
Body Composition Protein	Gain of over 2 lb (*0.9 kg*), which is equal to about 8 lb (*3.6 kg*) of lean body tissue.	Used for enlargement of maternal tissues, production of additional blood plasma and blood cells, and growth of the placenta and fetus.	About ⅓ of the additional protein is converted to fetal tissue. The rest is used for the various "support systems."
Fat	Gain of almost 10 lb (*4.5 kg*), which is equivalent to 47,500 kcal.	Provides reserve energy for both the mother and the fetus, and for subsequent lactation.	A woman may build up considerable fat in several pregnancies, unless it is lost between pregnancies.
Water	Gain of about 15 lb (*7 kg*), or about 60% of the weight gained in pregnancy.	All newly synthesized body tissues in pregnancy contain considerable fluid. A reserve of fluid against blood loss in childbirth.	Over 40% of all pregnant women have some degree of excess fluid retention in their tissues, but it is usually harmless.
Circulatory System Heart	Volume of blood pumped per minute increases by ⅓. Heart rate increases by 40% (from 70 to 85 beats per minute).	The heart has to work harder to pump the extra blood formed during pregnancy to the enlarged body mass of the mother.	Sometimes, there is a temporary enlargement of the heart during pregnancy.
Total blood volume	Increases by about 30% (from 4,000 to 5,250 ml).	Extra blood is needed to serve the tissues added during pregnancy.	The increased flow of blood to the skin causes it to feel warm and moist.
Plasma	Plasma volume increases by about 40%.	Plasma is the vehicle for transporting nutrients and other substances within the body.	This increase occurs early in pregnancy. Hence, the blood is temporarily diluted.

Footnotes at end of table

(Continued)

TABLE P-22 (Continued)

Part of the Body	Changes[1]	Biological Significance	Comments
Red blood cells	Increased by about 18%.	These cells carry oxygen to the tissues.	The ratio of red cells to total blood volume is usually about 10% subnormal in pregnancy.
Digestive System Stomach	Sphincter betwen the esophagus and stomach is relaxed and emptying of the stomach is slowed.	Food is more thoroughly mixed with gastric juice.	Sometimes, the stomach contents pass up into the esophagus, causing "heartburn."[2]
Intestines	Motion is slowed. Towards the end of pregnancy, the fetus presses against the lower bowel.	The slower passage of food results in better digestion and absorption.	Pregnant women tend to be constipated unless the diet is rich in fiber and water.
Endocrine Glands[3] Adrenals	Increased secretion of the adrenal cortical hormone aldosterone.	Promotes sodium and water retention by the body, thereby meeting the special needs of pregnancy.	Progesterone from the placenta prevents the development of excessive fluid retention and high blood pressure.
Kidneys	Increased production of renin, which acts to increase the secretion of aldosterone.	Initiates the chain of events which leads to sodium and water retention by the body.	The renin-initiated reactions may induce high blood pressure in some pregnant women.
Ovary	At the beginning of pregnancy, hormones from the placenta induce the corpus luteum in the ovary to (1) survive much longer than it does in non-pregnant women, and (2) secrete hormones such as the estrogens and progesterone.	The estrogens and progesterone from the ovary help to maintain pregnancy and prevent spontaneous abortion during the first 8 weeks.	After the first 8 weeks of pregnancy, the placenta has usually developed sufficiently to provide the hormones that were secreted by the corpus luteum.
Pancreas	Insulin secretion is usually higher than normal in the second half of pregnancy because the placental hormone HCS[4] antagonizes the effects of insulin and causes an elevation in the blood sugar.	Resistance to the effects of insulin in normal pregnant women results in (1) higher than normal maternal blood levels of nutrients, and (2) a continuously available supply of nutrients for the fetus.	The insulin-secreting capacity of some diabetic women may be overtaxed to the extent that both the mother and the fetus are harmed.
Pituitary	Secretion of prolactin increases throughout pregnancy. Increased secretion of MSH[4]. Increased secretion of TSH[4].	Brings about milk production by the mammary glands. Causes pigmentation in various areas of the body. Stimulates the growth of the thyroid so that it becomes more efficient in the use of iodine.	There is competition between the maternal and fetal thyroids for the supply of iodine. The placenta efficiently takes up iodine and transfers it to the fetus.
Placenta	Secretion of HCG[4] at the onset of pregnancy. Secretion of HCS[4], estrogens, and progesterone throughout pregnancy. (The amounts of the latter hormones increase as the placenta grows larger along with the fetus.)	HCG maintains the functions of of the corpus luteum so that pregnancy is maintained during the first 8 weeks. HCS acts as a growth hormone and stimulates development of functioning mammary glands. Estrogens and progesterone promote many of the maternal adaptations to pregnancy. (After the first 8 weeks, the major source of estrogens and progesterone is the placenta. Hence, poor development and growth of the placenta may lead to a poor outcome of pregnancy.)	
Thyroid	May become a little enlarged.	Enlargement allows the thyroid to use iodine more efficiently.	The formation of a goiter is a sign that the dietary supply of iodine is inadequate.
Fetus	Growth proceeds slowly until about 3 months after conception. The weight of the fetus is tripled during the third trimester (final 13 to 14 weeks).	Optimal growth of the fetus and accompanying placenta are best ensured by a good diet and a maternal weight gain of about 1 lb (0.5 kg) per week in the latter half of pregnancy.	Restriction of the maternal diet may jeopardize the growth of the fetus and placenta.

Footnotes at end of table

(Continued)

TABLE P-22 (*Continued*)

Part of the Body	Changes	Biological Significance	Comments
Fetus (*Continued*) Kidneys	Secrete greater amounts of renin, usually without causing an increase in maternal blood pressure. The flow of blood to the kidneys is increased by about 40%, and the glomerular filtration rate by about 60%.	Renin initiates actions that bring about greater retention of sodium and water in the mother. Waste products are removed with high efficiency so that the fetus is protected against toxic accumulations of substances.	Extra sodium and water is required in the maternal body during pregnancy. The high rate of urination in early pregnancy decreases somewhat in the latter half of this period.
Lungs	Although the rate of breathing remains at the nonpregnant level, the amount of air inspired and expired with each breath increases by more than 40%.	Abundant oxygen is provided for the increased metabolism of pregnancy. However, the blood levels of carbon dioxide become subnormal.	Resting pregnant women may feel lightheaded and have other symptoms that disappear when they increase their activity. (The symptoms are due to the subnormal blood levels of carbon dioxide).
Mammary Glands	Preparation for lactation is stimulated during pregnancy by hormones from ovaries, adrenal glands, pituitary, and the placenta. After childbirth, the hormone prolactin from the pituitary stimulates milk production. Then, suckling by the infant brings about the letdown and release of milk through the action of the hormone oxytocin from the pituitary.	Little is wasted in human lactation because (1) milk production is delayed until after childbirth, (2) suckling stimulates continuation of production, and (3) lactation ceases when mothers either fail to nurse or stop nursing after having done it for a while.	

¹Adapted by the authors from *Maternal Nutrition and the Course of Pregnancy*, National Academy of Sciences, 1970; and *Laboratory Indices of Nutritional Status in Pregnancy*, National Academy of Sciences, 1978.
²Also see HEARTBURN: and HIATUS HERNIA.
³Only the well established endocrine changes are presented. It seems likely that other glandular changes occur in pregnancy, but firm evidence of them is lacking.
⁴HCS is human chorionic somatomammotropin; MSH is melanocyte stimulating hormone; TSH is thyroid stimulating hormone, and HCG is human chorionic gonadotropin.

NUTRIENT ALLOWANCES. Although the nutrition of the fetus is aided by the metabolic alterations that take place in the mother's body during pregnancy, adequate levels of nutrients must be provided in the mother's diet to ensure that (1) the fetus is nourished adequately without depletion of maternal tissues, and (2) maternal reserves for childbirth and lactation are accumulated. Some examples of how certain metabolic changes affect dietary needs follow:

• **Calories**—The requirement for food energy is high during the latter half of pregnancy because the fetus is accumulating a reserve supply of fat for the period after childbirth and the mother is putting on fat in order to be able to supply the necessary food energy in her breast milk. Although some women have given birth to apparently healthy babies after having gained little or no weight during pregnancy, it is likely that there was some withdrawal of fat, protein, and other nutrients from the mother's tissues. Hormones secreted during pregnancy maintain high levels of sugar (glucose), amino acids, and fatty acids in the maternal blood by (1) slowing the rate of nutrient utilization by the maternal tissues, and (2) bringing about the withdrawal of these substances from the maternal tissues when the blood levels decline. However, overweight women should *not* try to lose weight by restricting their diets during pregnancy because harmful conditions such as ketoacidosis may result.

• **Protein**—Most of the growth of the fetus takes place in the latter half of pregnancy, when the rate of protein synthesis is high, as indicated by Fig. P-101.

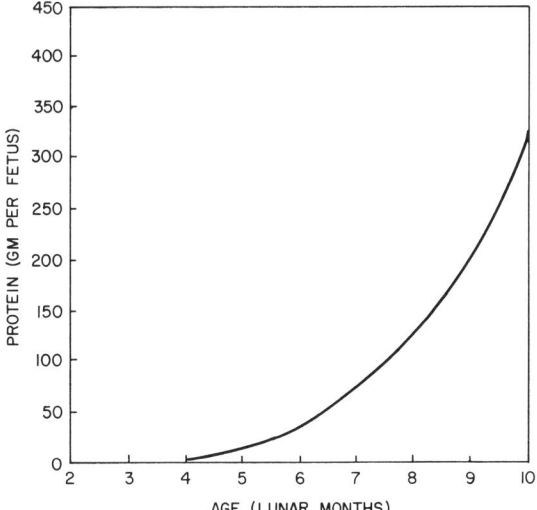

Fig. P-101. Protein accumulation in the fetus during pregnancy. (Adapted by the authors from Toverud, K. U., *et al., Maternal Nutrition and Child Health, An Interpretive Review*, National Academy of Sciences, 1950, p. 36, Fig. 3)

It is noteworthy that the placenta can extract amino acids from the maternal blood so efficiently that the fetal blood levels of these nutrients are usually considerably greater than those of the mother. However, the mother herself has higher than normal needs for protein that is used to enlarge her uterus, mammary glands, and the other tissues that grow to support pregnancy and lactation. Hence, the maternal blood levels of proteins such as plasma albumin may drop to subnormal levels. This condition may be dangerous to both the mother and the fetus because lack of sufficient blood protein may allow fluid from the blood to accumulate in the maternal tissues, causing waterlogging and/or an elevated blood pressure. There appears to be an association between subnormal levels of blood protein and the tendency to develop toxemia of pregnancy.

• **Calcium and phosphorus**—Fetal bone growth proceeds on the same schedule as the growth of the lean body soft tissues, except that the rate of calcium accumulation in the bones literally "skyrockets" during the last 2 months of pregnancy, as is shown in Fig. P-102.

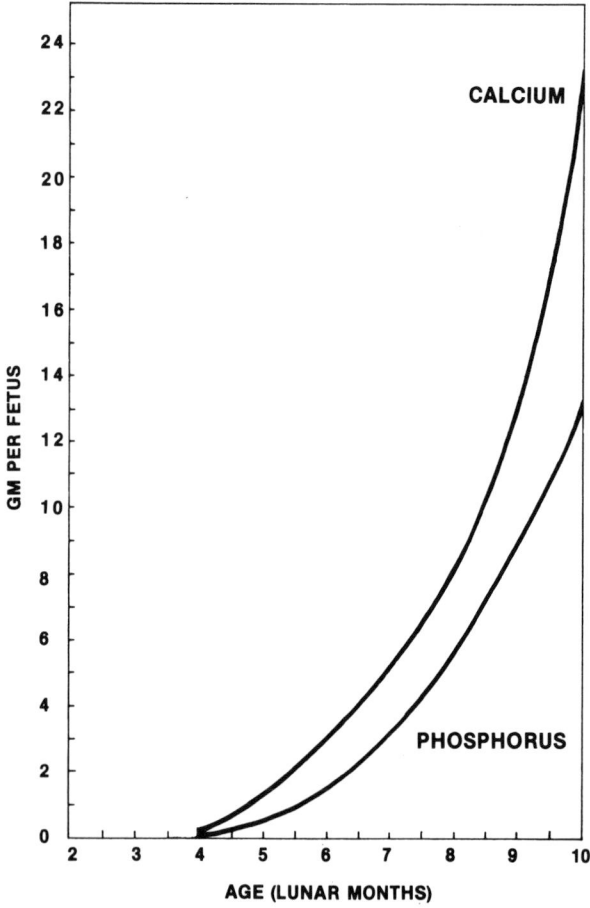

Fig. P-102. Calcium and phosphorus accumulation in the fetus during pregnancy. (Adapted by the authors from Toverud, K. U., *et al.*, *Maternal Nutrition and Child Health, An Interpretive Review*, National Academy of Sciences, 1950, p. 55, Fig. 4)

It is noteworthy that the mother's diet should contain extra calcium from the beginning of pregnancy until the end of lactation, because the early accumulation of the mineral in the maternal tissues provides a reserve for later use, when it becomes almost impossible to consume enough to meet the needs. There is evidence to indicate that (1) dietary calcium is about twice as well absorbed by pregnant women compared to nonpregnant women, and (2) adequate vitamin D during pregnancy enhances calcium utilization. The extra phosphorus that is required is usually provided in diets that contain sufficient protein. Infants that have received adequate calcium while in their mother's womb are less likely to develop rickets.
(Also see MINERAL[S]; CALCIUM; and PHOSPHORUS.)

• **Iodine**—The placenta extracts this essential mineral from the mother's blood so efficiently that fetal blood levels of iodine are usually several times those of the mother. However, the mother may develop a goiter when the supply of the mineral is inadequate to meet her needs. Enlargement of the maternal thyroid gland makes it more efficient in using iodine for the synthesis of thyroid hormones. Goitrous mothers have an increased risk of giving birth to infants that are cretins. Cretinism is a severe form of thyroid hormone deficiency in infants that is characterized by (1) failure of the fetal thyroid to develop, (2) mental retardation, (3) poor mineralization of the bones, and (4) dwarfism. Infants that are born with little or no functioning of the thyroid gland cannot be cured of this condition. Rather, they require the administration of thyroid hormone preparation for the rest of their lives.
(Also see MINERAL[S]; and IODINE.).

• **Vitamin E**—This vitamin does *not* readily pass across the placenta into the fetus. Hence, infants are born with low levels of vitamin E in their tissues. However, the consumption of adequate amounts of this vitamin by the pregnant mother is likely to be reflected in the amounts provided in her breast milk.
(Also see VITAMIN[S]; and VITAMIN E.)

• **Vitamin B-6**—Some pregnant women have developed a diabeticlike condition while consuming diets moderately high in protein, but low in vitamin B-6. Most of them were brought back to normal by giving them a supplement containing the vitamin.[18] It is noteworthy that the placenta concentrates the vitamin in the fetus, which may be a factor in the production of subnormal maternal blood levels of vitamin B-6 during pregnancy. Furthermore, women who have long used oral contraceptives prior to becoming pregnant may need extra amounts of this vitamin.
(Also see VITAMIN[S]; and VITAMIN B-6.)

[18]Coelingh Bennenk, H. T. J., and W. H. P. Schreurs, "Improvement of Oral Glucose Tolerance in Gestational Diabetes by Pyridoxine," *British Medical Journal*, July 5, 1975, pp. 13-15.

Many other nutrients are required in greater amounts by pregnant and lactating women than by nonpregnant women. Hence, the Food and Nutrition Board of the National Academy of Sciences has established the allowances that are given in Table P-23.

TABLE P-23
AVERAGE HEIGHTS, WEIGHTS, AND RECOMMENDED DAILY NUTRIENT INTAKES
FOR PREGNANT OR LACTATING WOMEN OF VARIOUS AGES[1]

Category	Pregnant				Lactating			
	Age				Age			
	11–14 years	15–18 years	19–24 years	25–50 years	11–14 years	15–18 years	19–24 years	25–50 years
Weight[2] ...... lb (kg)	101 (46)	120 (55)	128 (58)	138 (63)	101 (46)	120 (55)	128 (58)	138 (63)
Height ...... in. (cm)	62 (157)	64 (163)	65 (164)	64 (163)	62 (157)	64 (163)	65 (164)	64 (163)
Energy .... kcal	2,500	2,500	2,500	2,500	2,700	2,700	2,700	2,700
Protein .... g	76	76	74	74	66	66	64	64
Minerals								
Calcium .... mg	1,200	1,200	1,200	1,200	1,200	1,200	1,200	1,200
Phosphorus ..... mg	1,200	1,200	1,200	1,200	1,200	1,200	1,200	1,200
Sodium[3,4] .... mg	500	500	500	500	500	500	500	500
Chloride[4] .... mg	750	750	750	750	750	750	750	750
Magnesium ...... mg	320	320	320	320	355	355	355	355
Potassium[4] ...... mg	2,000	2,000	2,000	2,000	2,000	2,000	2,000	2,000
Chromium[4,5] .... mcg	50–200	50–200	50–200	50–200	50–200	50–200	50–200	50–200
Copper[4,5] .... mg	1.5–3.0	1.5–3.0	1.5–3.0	1.5–3.0	1.5–3.0	1.5–3.0	1.5–3.0	1.5–3.0
Fluoride[4] .... mg	1.5–2.5	1.5–2.5	1.5–4.0	1.5–4.0	1.2–2.5	1.5–2.5	1.5–4.0	1.5–4.0
Iodine .... mcg	175	175	175	175	200	200	200	200
Iron[6] .... mg	30	30	30	30	15	15	15	15
Manganese[4,5] ..... mg	2.0–5.0	2.0–5.0	2.0–5.0	2.0–5.0	2.0–5.0	2.0–5.0	2.0–5.0	2.0–5.0
Molybdenum[4,5] .. mcg	75–250	75–250	75–250	75–250	75–250	75–250	75–250	75–250
Selenium[4,5] ..... mcg	65	65	65	65	75	75	75	75
Zinc[8] .... mg	15	15	15	15	19–16	19–16	19–16	19–16
Vitamins, fat-soluble								
Vitamin A ...mcg RE	800	800	800	800	1,300	1,300	1,300	1,300
Vitamin D ...... mcg	10	10	10	10	10	10	10	10
Vitamin E .... mgαTE	10	10	10	10	12	12	12	12
Vitamin K[4] ...... mcg	65	65	65	65	65	65	65	65
Vitamins, water soluble								
Biotin[4] .... mcg	30–100	30–100	30–100	30–100	30–100	30–100	30–100	30–100
Folate[7] .... mcg	400	400	400	400	280	280	280	280
Niacin .... mg	17	17	17	17	20	20	20	20
Pantothenic acid[4] mg	4–7	4–7	4–7	4–7	4–7	4–7	4–7	4–7
Riboflavin .... mg	1.6	1.6	1.6	1.6	1.8	1.8	1.8	1.8
Thiamin .... mg	1.5	1.5	1.5	1.5	1.6	1.6	1.6	1.6
Vitamin B-6 ...... mg	2.2	2.2	2.2	2.2	2.1	2.1	2.1	2.1
Vitamin B-12 .... mcg	2.2	2.2	2.2	2.2	2.6	2.6	2.6	2.6
Vitamin C .... mg	70	70	70	70	95	95	95	95

[1]Adapted by the authors from *Recommended Dietary Allowances,* 10th ed., National Academy of Sciences, 1989.
[2]Average weight of nonpregnant, nonlactating women in each age group.
[3]There is no justification for the restriction of sodium in the diets of healthy women during pregnancy. Hence, the recommended intakes are those for nonpregnant women.
[4]These figures are given in the form of ranges of recommended intakes, because there is insufficient information to determine allowances.
[5]Since the toxic levels for many trace elements may be only several times average intakes, the upper values of the intakes should not be habitually exceeded.
[6]The increased requirement during pregnancy cannot be met by the iron content of habitual American diets nor by the existing iron stores of many women. Therefore, the use of 30 to 60 mg of supplemental iron is recommended. Iron needs during lactation are not substantially different from those of nonpregnant women, but continued supplementation of the mother for 2 to 3 months after childbirth is advisable in order to replenish stores depleted by pregnancy.
[7]The use of a folacin supplement appears to be desirable during pregnancy in order to maintain maternal stores and keep pace with the increased folacin turnover.
[8]For the first 6 mo. of lactation, the recommended allowance is 19 mg; and for the second 6 mo., it is 16 mg.

DIETARY GUIDELINES. If the mother does not have good nutrition during pregnancy, there is a greater chance of having a premature infant or one of low birth weight. There is also a greater chance of problems during pregnancy and delivery, infant death, infant defects, and failure of the infant to grow and develop normally. The benefits of eating well during pregnancy are illustrated in Fig. P-103.

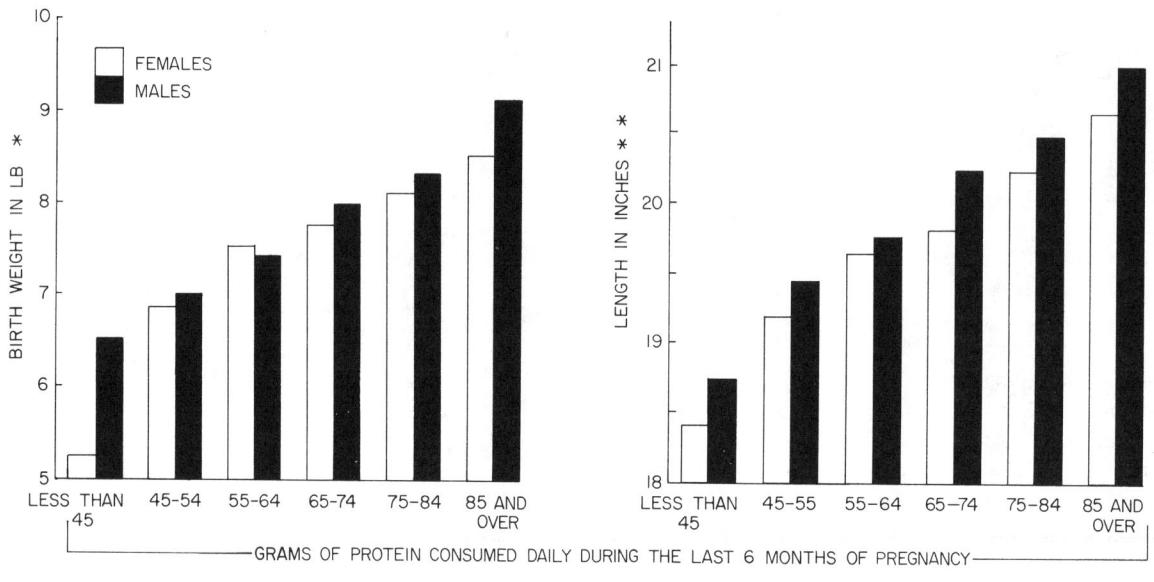

* DIVIDE BY 2.2 TO CONVERT TO KG   ** MULTIPLY BY 2.54 TO CONVERT TO CM

Fig. P-103.   The effect of dietary protein during pregnancy on the weights and heights of newborn infants. (Based upon data from Toverud, K. U., *et al.*, *Maternal Nutrition and Child Health, An Interpretive Review*, National Academy of Sciences, 1950, p. 39, Table 14)

The rate at which the pregnant woman gains weight is also important. Weight should be gained slowly over the entire pregnancy. A good rate of weight gain is 1½ to 3 lb (*0.7 to 1.4 kg*) the first trimester (first 3 months) and then about ¾ lb (*0.3 kg*) a week until the end of pregnancy. Gaining too much weight too quickly may be harmful to mother and baby. Excess weight gain is often due to extra fluid which causes swelling (edema) of the mother's feet, hands, and face.

Excessive weight gain during pregnancy may cause complications or problems for the mother and baby. It also places a strain on the back and leg muscles that may cause pain and fatigue. Too much weight gain will make it difficult to get back to normal size and figure after the baby is born.

Weight reduction is not generally recommended during pregnancy. And crash diets or fad diets should never be used during pregnancy. They may be harmful to mother and baby because essential nutrients may be provided in limited amounts. Low calorie diets should usually be restricted to before pregnancy or following pregnancy.

The mother is eating for two—but that's not two adults! A slight increase of 300 Calories (kcal) per day the last half of pregnancy is recommended for the woman whose activity is light. This is for the growth of the fetus, the placenta, and other maternal tissue. The pregnant woman who is working at a job requiring physical activity or at home with small children may need more than 300 additional calories per day.

Dietary guidelines for pregnancy and lactation are outlined in Table P-24.

(Also see FOOD GROUPS.)

TABLE P-24
BASIC FOUR FOOD GROUPS FOR PREGNANT OR LACTATING WOMEN[1]

Meats, Poultry, Fish, and Beans	Milk and Cheeses	Vegetables and Fruits	Breads and Cereals
Amounts Recommended: 4 servings per day of items from subgroup(s) I and/or II[2].	**Amounts Recommended:** 4 servings per day for pregnant women, and 5 servings per day for lactating women.	**Amounts Recommended:** At least 1 serving daily of an item from subgroup I, 2 servings from subgroup II, and 1 or more from subgroup III.	**Amounts Recommended:** 3 or more servings per day of items from subgroup(s) I (the best choices) and/or II.

I. Meats

A serving is 2-3 oz (60-90 g) cooked (boneless) of the following unless otherwise noted:

Bacon, 6 slices
Beef: ground, cube, roast, chopped
Canned tuna, salmon, crab, etc., ½ c
Cheese (See Milk.)
Chitterlings (tripe)[3]
Clams, 4 large or 9 small
Crab
Duck
Eggs, 2
Fish: filet, steak
Fish sticks, breaded, 4
Frankfurters, 2
Hogmaws[3]
Lamb: ground, cube, roast, chop
Lobster
Luncheon meat, 3 slices
Organ meats: liver, kidney, sweetbreads, heart, tongue[4]
Oysters, 10-15 medium
Pig ears[3]
Pig's feet[3]
Pig snouts[3]
Pork: ham, ground, roast, chop
Poultry: ground, roast
Rabbit
Sausage links, 4
Shrimp, scallops, 5-6 large
Spareribs, 6 medium ribs
Veal: ground, cube, roast, chop

II. Meat Substitutes

A serving is 1 c cooked unless otherwise stated.

Canned garbanzo, lima, kidney beans
Canned pork and beans
Dried beans and peas
Lentils
Nut butters, ¼ c
Nuts, ½ c
Sunflower seeds, ½ c
Tofu (soybean curd)

A serving is 8 oz (1 c or 240 cc) unless otherwise noted.

Cheese: hard and semisoft (except blue, camembert, and cream), 1½ oz
Cheese spread, 2 oz
Cottage cheese, creamed, 1⅓ c
Cow's milk: whole, nonfat, low fat, nonfat dry reconstituted, buttermilk, chocolate milk, cocoa made with milk.
Cream soups made with milk, 12 oz
Evaporated milk, 3 oz
Goat's milk (low B-12 content)
Ice cream, 1½ c
Ice milk
Instant breakfast made with milk, 4 oz
Liquid diet beverage, 5 oz
Milkshake, commercial, 8 oz
Puddings, custard (flan)
Soybean milk (low B-12 content)
Yogurt

Note: Tofu is also a source of calcium; 1 cup tofu may be exchanged for one serving of the above foods.

I. Vitamin C rich items

Fruit juices

Orange, grapefruit, 4 oz
Tomato, pineapple, 12 oz
Fruit juices and drinks enriched with vitamin C, 6 oz

Fruits

Cantaloupe, ½
Grapefruit, ½
Guava, ¼ medium
Mango, 1 medium
Orange, 1 medium
Papaya, ⅓ medium
Strawberries, ¾ c
Tangerine, 2 small

Vegetables

Bok choy, ¾ c
Broccoli, 1 stalk
Brussels sprouts, 3-4
Cabbage, cooked, 1⅓ c
Cabbage, raw ¾ c
Cauliflower, raw or cooked, 1 c
Greens: collard, kale, mustard, swiss chard, turnip greens, ¾ c
Peppers, chili, ¾ c
Peppers: green, red ½ medium
Tomatoes, 2 medium
Watercress, ¾ c

II. Leafy green vegetables

A serving is 1 cup raw, or ¾ cup cooked.

Asparagus
Bok choy
Broccoli
Brussels sprouts
Cabbage
Dark leafy lettuce: chicory, endive, escarole, red leaf, romaine
Greens: beet, collard, kale, mustard, spinach, swiss chard, turnip
Scallions
Watercress

I. Whole grain items

Brown rice, ½ c
Cereals, hot: oatmeal (rolled oats), rolled wheat, cracked wheat, wheat and malted barley, ½ c cooked
Cereals, ready-to-eat: puffed oats, shredded wheat, wheat flakes, granola, ¾ c
Cracked and whole wheat bread, 1 slice
Wheat germ, 1 Tbsp

II. Enriched products

Bread, 1 slice
Cereals, hot: cream of wheat, cream of rice, farina, cornmeal, grits, ½ c
Cereals, ready-to-eat, ¾ c
Cornbread, 1 piece (2 in. square)
Crackers, 4 (all kinds)
Macaroni, noodles, spaghetti, cooked, ½ c
Muffin, biscuit, dumpling, 1
Pancake, 1 medium
Rice, cooked, ½ c
Roll, bagel, 1
Tortilla, corn, 2
Tortilla, flour, 1 large
Waffle, 1 large

(Continued)

TABLE P-24 (*Continued*)

Meats, Poultry, Fish, and Beans	Milk and Cheeses	Vegetables and Fruits	Breads and Cereals

		III. Other Items
		
		Fruits & Vegetables
		
		Apricot, fresh Artichoke
		Nectarine Bamboo shoots
		Peach, fresh Bean sprouts
		Persimmon Beet
		Prunes Burdock root
		Pumpkin Carrot
		Apple Cauliflower
		Banana Celery
		Berries Corn
		Cherries Cucumber
		Dates Eggplant
		Figs Beans: green,
		Fruit cocktail wax
		Grapes Hominy
		Kumquats Lettuce
		Pear Mushrooms
		Pineapple Nori seaweed
		Plums Onion
		Raisins Parsnip
		Watermelon Peas
		            Pea pods
		            Potato
		            Radishes
		            Summer squash
		            Sweet potato
		            Winter squash
		            Yam
		            Zucchini	

Nutritional values: Meats supply calories, fats, proteins, phosphorus, potassium, chloride, sodium, iron, zinc, iodine, and various other essential trace minerals; and the vitamins thiamin, riboflavin, niacin, vitamin B-6 and vitamin B-12. Meat substitutes are similar in nutritive value to meats except that some items are better sources of magnesium and folacin. However, the substitutes furnish little or no vitamin B-12[5].	**Nutritional values:** These items furnish calories, protein, carbohydrates and/or fats, calcium, phosphorus, potassium, chloride, sodium, magnesium, zinc, and various other essential trace minerals; and the vitamins thiamin, riboflavin, niacin, vitamin B-6, vitamin B-12, vitamin A, vitamin D, and vitamin E. *Note:* Calcium supplements in pill form are *not* adequate substitutes for milk and milk products because they do not supply calories, protein, and the other essential nutrients provided by milk. Hence, women who take these pills in lieu of consuming milk products must make certain to obtain the missing nutrients from other foods or supplements that supply them.	**Nutritional values:** The items in group I are rich sources of vitamin C, and in many cases are good sources of substances called bioflavonoids.[6] Leafy green vegetables are good to excellent sources of magnesium, iron and other essential minerals; and the vitamins A, E, riboflavin, B-6, and folacin. The items in group III are generally fair to good sources of the nutrients supplied by the items in groups I and II.	**Nutritional values:** The items from groups I and II supply calories, proteins, carbohydrates, phosphorus, potassium, chloride, sodium, iron, thiamin, riboflavin, and niacin. However, the whole grain products are usually much better sources of fiber, magnesium, zinc, and other essential minerals; and of the vitamin B complex and vitamin E.

[1]Adapted by the authors from *Nutrition During Pregnancy and Lactation,* Revised 1975, California State Dept. of Health, pp. 34-40. To convert to metric, see WEIGHTS AND MEASURES.

[2]Items in subgroup I may be extended with vegetable protein (usually in the ratio of 70% meat to 30% extender) to save money.

[3]These meats have a high content of connective tissue and a low quality of protein. Hence, they should *not* to be used to provide more than one of the daily servings of meats or meat substitutes.

[4]Most organ meats are superior to muscle meats as sources of protein, minerals, and vitamins. The authors recommend serving them at least once or twice each week.

[5]Vegetarians who eat no animal foods should take a vitamin B-12 supplement.

[6]Bioflavonoids act in concert with vitamin C to strengthen the capillaries and provide other beneficial effects. (Also see BIOFLAVONOIDS.)

COMMON NUTRITION-RELATED PROBLEMS OF PREGNANCY.

The physiological changes that occur in the maternal body as a result of conception may bring on or aggravate certain conditions that tend to make pregnancy burdensome to the mother. However, there are nutritional ways of coping with these problems so that the well being of the mother and fetus is promoted.

Anemia.

This condition is characterized by a subnormal blood level of hemoglobin and/or red blood cells. It is usually the result of a chronic dietary deficiency of iron, although it may also result from (1) deficiencies of other nutrients such as protein, copper, folacin, vitamin B-6, vitamin B-12, and vitamin C; or (2) losses of blood that have not been replaced fully.

The need for iron during pregnancy is quite high because it is used to (1) maintain the hemoglobin level of the mother, (2) maintain the mother's store of iron, (3) promote fetal development, and (4) provide a reserve in the infant for blood formation during early infancy before iron-rich foods are added to the diet. Furthermore, the iron stores in women of childbearing age are apt to be inadequate for pregnancy because of (1) loss of blood during menstruation, and (2) failure to consume sufficient amounts of iron-rich foods. Therefore, the Committee on Maternal Nutrition of the National Academy of Sciences has recommended that pregnant women take a daily supplement that contains from 30 to 60 mg of iron.[19]

(Also see IRON.)

One of the benefits of iron supplementation during pregnancy is shown in Fig. P-104.

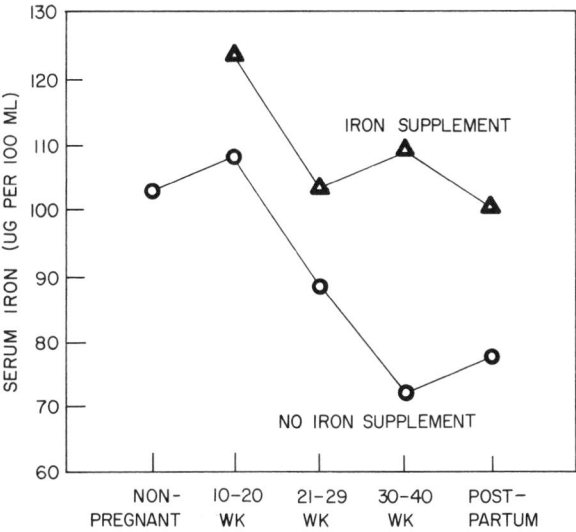

Fig. P-104. The effects of iron supplementation on the serum iron of the mother during and after pregnancy. (The points on the graphs represent averages of the different values given in *Laboratory Indices of Nutritional Status in Pregnancy*, National Academy of Sciences, 1978, p. 161, Table 7-1)

It may be noted from Fig. P-104 that the women who received the iron supplement maintained significantly higher levels of serum iron than the women who did not receive the supplement.

Constipation.

This condition may occur in late pregnancy. It may be due to pressure of the growing fetus on the digestive tract and to a decrease in the firmness (tone) of the muscles in the abdomen which slows down digestion. Thus nutrients remain longer in contact with the walls of the intestines and nutrient absorption is increased.

Constipation may be prevented by drinking plenty of water and eating foods that add bulk to the diet such as fruits and vegetables (preferably raw) and whole grain cereals such as oatmeal, cracked wheat, all bran, etc.

Cravings for Unusual Foods and Nonfood Items (Pica).

Pregnant women sometimes have cravings for unusual items such as starch, clay, plaster, or chalk. The appetite for nonfoods is called pica. Eating of these substances should be discouraged because the practice may result in (1) filling of the digestive tract and reduction of the appetite for nutritious foods, (2) and poisoning by contaminants in the nonfoods. (Some types of plaster contain lead.)

Recently, evidence has been found that pica may be associated with iron deficiency anemia.[20] The abnormal cravings have often been reduced by treatment of the iron deficiency of pregnancy.

It is noteworthy that the craving for pastrami, pickles, or pizza in the wee hours of the morning is not pica and may be satisfied without harm, providing that pregnant women do not overindulge in these foods.

Diabetes.

Diabetes poses a great risk to the developing fetus. The hormones of pregnancy (estrogen, human chorionic gonadotrophin, and human placental lactogen) act to antagonize (counteract) the action of insulin in the body. Because of this antiinsulin activity, women are more prone to display diabetes when they are pregnant. To counteract this situation, the physician may prescribe increased insulin doses and put the mother on a special diet.

Problems with a fetus in a diabetic pregnancy include unexplained stillbirth, placental malfunction, and a large infant (macrosomia).

Excessive Gain in Weight.

Weight, per se, is no indication of nutritional status. Food selections of some pregnant women who have gained weight too rapidly are likely to emphasize foods high in fat or carbohydrate and calories, yet be low in protein, minerals or vitamins. Diets of other heavy women may be low in many nutrients, including calories. For the expectant mother with poor food practices, the prenatal period provides an opportunity to learn better food practices under medical supervision. There is little room in prenatal menus for foods that contribute mainly calories.

[19]*Maternal Nutrition and the Course of Pregnancy,* National Academy of Sciences, 1970, p. 189.

[20]Gibbs, C. E., and J. Seitchik, "Nutrition in Pregnancy," *Modern Nutrition in Health and Disease,* 6th ed., edited by R. S. Goodhart and M. E. Shils, Lea & Febiger, Philadelphia, Pa., p. 748.

The minimal caloric level recommended for the obese expectant mother is 1,500 Calories (kcal). It is very difficult to provide the needed nutrients below this caloric level. If insufficient calories are taken, protein may be used for the mother's energy needs instead of for building new tissue. Even though vitamin and mineral supplements may be given, these supplements do not furnish protein. Major efforts toward weight loss should not be attempted. Weight reduction in pregnancy has been associated with neuropsychological abnormalities in the infant.

Guidelines released by the Institute of Medicine in 1990 indicate that weight gain of 25 to 35 lb during pregnancy is satisfactory.

Fluid Retention (Preeclampsia, Eclampsia).

Many pregnant women accumulate a little fluid in their legs, which in itself is not usually harmful unless it is accompanied by (1) notable fluid retention in other parts of the body, (2) high blood pressure, and (3) passage of protein in the urine. These conditions are signs of toxemia (preeclampsia) which may pose a threat to mother and fetus. However, it is noteworthy that salt restriction and the administration of diuretics may be hazardous in pregnancy and not advisable unless there is a clear-cut threat of toxemia. Some doctors advise pregnant women who have some fluid retention and a moderate elevation in blood pressure to lie down for 30 to 45 minutes several times a day so that an increased amount of fluid is passed in the urine. Furthermore, they may allow the continued use of small amounts of salty foods, but it would be wise to avoid highly salted items such as pizza, potato chips and other similar snacks.

The incidence of toxemia in American women has declined steadily in recent years, thanks to better diets and earlier prenatal care. Also, the condition is more severe when it develops in women who are markedly underweight at conception and who fail to gain weight normally during the early part of pregnancy.

Heartburn.

This condition sometimes occurs when stomach contents are forced back into the esophagus. It usually happens during the latter part of pregnancy when the growing fetus puts pressure on the stomach. As with morning sickness, small, frequent meals may help. It is best to avoid greasy, fried foods and other foods that have previously caused digestive problems.

High Blood Pressure (Hypertension).

Two forms of high blood pressure may be recognized during pregnancy: (1) chronic hypertension, which may cause fetal death and placental malfunction; or (2) acute hypertension, particularly in the last 12 weeks of pregnancy, which is indicative of toxemia. Toxemia can cause stroke, as well as blood-clotting difficulties in the mother, and lead to placental malfunction, separation of the placenta from the uterine wall, and stillbirth.

High blood pressure always warrants the attention of a physician. The blood pressure of the mother before pregnancy is an important factor to be considered in the diagnosis because many teenage girls have low blood pressure when not pregnant so that the rise which occurs may be much greater than suspected. Hence, high blood pressure is declared to be present when (1) the systolic blood pressure is 140 or greater, or the diastolic blood pressure is 90 or greater; or (2) the systolic reading has risen by 30 points or the diastolic reading has risen by 15 points.

Some moderately hypertensive pregnant women benefit by (1) staying off their feet as much as possible and/or (2) lying down for 30 to 45 minutes several times during the day. Many doctors refrain from restricting salt or giving diuretics to pregnant women for fear of creating an even greater problem. However, it would be wise for even a moderately hypertensive woman to avoid eating very salty foods.

(Also see HIGH BLOOD PRESSURE.)

Insufficient Gain in Weight.

Recent studies of pregnant women show that markedly underweight expectant mothers have a greater than average incidence of toxemia and a strikingly increased incidence of prematurity of the infant. In subsequent pregnancies, these same expectant mothers on an adequate diet had a great reduction in the incidence of prematurity over an untreated control group.

This does not mean that the women benefited from an overabundance of calories, but rather that mothers who had various nutritional deficiencies profited from a correction of these shortcomings during pregnancy.

Morning Sickness.

Nausea and vomiting, symptoms often called morning sickness, may occur in early pregnancy. This is usually due to changes taking place in the body. It may also be due to tension or anxiety. Morning sickness usually ends about the third or fourth month.

Morning sickness may be relieved by eating small, frequent meals rather than three large meals. Foods that are fairly dry and easily digested such as toast or crackers may be eaten by the mother before getting out of bed in the morning. Liquids should be taken between meals instead of with food.

THE DECLINE OF TOXEMIA AS A PROBLEM DURING PREGNANCY.

Fortunately, the rate of maternal deaths from toxemia dropped by 88% between 1940 and 1965 (from a rate of 52.2 to 6.2 per 100,000 live births)[21] Nevertheless, many pregnant women may have a fear of becoming toxemic as a result of horror stories told by older female relatives. Therefore, some background on this increasingly uncommon condition follows.

First of all, the term "toxemia" is a misnomer in that there does not appear to be any toxic agent involved in the conditions it designates. Therefore, the Working Group on Nutrition and the Toxemias of Pregnancy (of the National Academy of Sciences Committee on Maternal Nutrition) has suggested that this term be replaced by preeclampsia and eclampsia. They also suggest (1) that the term preeclampsia be used only when the three abnormalities of fluid retention are present—(a) fluid retention throughout the body, not just in the legs, (b) high blood pressure, and (c) passage of protein in the urine; and (2) that the term eclampsia be used to designate the convulsive disorder that sometimes accompanies or

---

[21]*Maternal Nutrition and the Course of Pregnancy*, National Academy of Sciences, 1970, p. 177.

follows the development of preeclampsia. These highly specific criteria for diagnosis are designed to prevent the overreporting of toxemia as a complication of pregnancy. (In the past, women were sometimes diagnosed as toxemic on the basis of a single abnormality such as fluid retention or high blood pressure.)

At one time, toxemia was thought to have resulted from the gain of excessive weight during pregnancy, but recent epidemiological studies have shown that it is much more likely to be associated with the conditions that follow:

1. Underweight at the time of conception, followed by failure to gain sufficient weight by the latter part of pregnancy.

2. Dietary deficiencies of calories and/or protein that produce a marked decrease in the blood level of protein.

3. High blood pressure that was present prior to conception.

4. Little or no prenatal care or counseling prior to the latter part of pregnancy.

5. First pregnancy, or a pregnancy following a multiple birth.

6. Inadequate consumption of calcium during pregnancy.

BREAST-FEEDING (Lactation). Lactation is the period after childbirth when a woman breast-feeds her baby. This is an important time for both the mother and her infant. Maternal nutrition plays a significant role during this time. A good diet is necessary for maternal tissue maintenance and replenishment of nutrient stores. In addition, a high-quality diet helps produce breast milk that is an excellent and natural source of nutrients for growth and development of the infant.

Inadequacies in the maternal diet during lactation may have severe consequences. The woman's health status may deteriorate as a result of large withdrawals of nutrients from her tissues. A poor maternal diet will also result in a decreased volume of breast milk. Also, there will be a reduction in vitamin levels. As a result, the infant may be shortchanged with regard to calories and essential nutrients.

Since human milk has unique properties not found in other milks, it is the best initial food for infants. The use of breast milk will reduce the possibility of allergic reactions to protein or other components of cow's milk formulas. In addition, breast milk contains a smaller amount of casein, and therefore forms smaller and softer curds in the stomach. This makes it easier to digest by the infant whose digestive processes are not fully developed.

Another advantage of breast milk is that it contains antibodies against infectious microorganisms. This helps the infant resist infections during the first few months of life. In addition, breast milk has the advantage of being sterile. Hence, there is no problem with the type of contamination that can occur during formula preparation.

Breast-feeding is an excellent way to prevent overeating during infancy because the breast-fed baby usually consumes fewer calories than the infant who is bottle fed. The lactating woman simply allows her baby to feed at her breast until satisfied. On the other hand, a mother who bottle feeds her infant tends to see that the baby consumes the entire content of the bottle. Excessive caloric intake during infancy can lead to a permanently increased number of fat cells in the body. This can increase the chance of obesity in later life.

Besides its physiological advantages, breast-feeding has a psychological benefit for both mother and infant. Both experience close attachment. This is a natural situation for the mother to provide a soothing and loving atmosphere; it helps the infant develop desirable emotional characteristics.

(Also see BREAST FEEDING.)

Maternal Diet During Lactation. In order to ensure adequate infant nutrition, the maternal diet must meet the nutrient requirements for lactation. (See Tables P-23 and P-24.) Ethnic, social, and economic factors may influence what the mother eats. The health professional should consider these in counseling.

Contrary to a prevalent belief, the diet of a lactating woman must contain an even higher number of calories than during pregnancy. These additional calories are necessary for milk production. Furthermore, the mother should consume the equivalent of 2 to 3 qt (*1.9 to 2.8 liter*) of liquids daily. This fluid is essential to provide the liquid volume for the breast milk and to meet the other needs of the mother.

(Also see BREAST FEEDING.)

Nutritional Supplementation. During lactation, there is a need to supplement the maternal diet with certain nutrients. As in pregnancy, 30 to 60 mg of elemental iron should be taken daily by all women. This supplement should be continued for at least 2 or 3 months after childbirth. Iron supplementation during this period is necessary to replenish maternal iron stores depleted by pregnancy. Doctors may recommend other mineral and vitamin supplements for some patients.

Since breast milk does not contain an adequate amount of vitamin D, it is advisable to give the infant an oral supplement of 7.5 mcg daily.

The fluoride content of breast milk varies with the fluoride concentration of the community's water supply. If the fluoride content of the water exceeds 1.1 ppm, the infant will receive sufficient fluoride through breast milk. However, an oral supplement of 0.5 mg fluoride daily should be given to the infant if the water supply has less than 1.1 ppm fluoride.

(Also see BREAST FEEDING.)

Use of Drugs by the Lactating Mother. If oral contraceptives are taken sooner than 6 weeks after childbirth, the amount of breast milk a woman produces may be diminished. (Hormones such as estrogen and progesterone found in these pills reduce milk production.) Clinical experience shows that the majority of women will not have difficulty producing an adequate amount of milk if they do not use oral contraceptives for 6 weeks after delivery. Hence, they should substitute another form of birth control.

In addition to oral contraceptives, other drugs such as barbiturates (sleeping pills), laxatives, and salicylates (aspirin and similar substances) can be transmitted through breast milk. The taking of any drug during lactation should be done only under a doctor's supervision.

(Also see BREAST FEEDING: and INFANT DIET AND NUTRITION.)

FACTORS THAT MAY WARRANT SPECIAL COUNSELING OF PREGNANT WOMEN.

Experience has shown that even an affluent and educated woman can have nutritional problems throughout her pregnancy. Sufficient money to buy food is not a guarantee that the mother's diet will be nutritionally adequate. In some cases, her diet may consist of a limited variety of foods due to misinformation or adherence to unsound weight reduction diets. For example, the pregnant woman may not drink milk for fear that it will cause leg cramps, or she may eat only low-calorie foods to lose weight. Meals may be infrequent or eliminated with the result that the mother may be vulnerable to nutritional deficiencies. This type of deprivation may have harmful effects on the outcome of her pregnancy. Furthermore, certain factors related to the mother's status may classify her as a higher-than-average risk. These factors may be physiological, socioeconomic, and/or psychological. A high risk pregnant woman needs continuous nutritional assessment and in depth nutritional counseling. Some of the more common risk factors follow.

Adolescence.

Girls younger than 17 years, who are pregnant before completion of their own growth, have greater nutritional requirements than adult women. For these patients, pregnancy creates a dual growth demand—that of the fetus, and of the patient herself. Compounding this, many adolescent girls may restrict their caloric intake in order to lose weight or may have poor dietary habits. Adolescent pregnancies have been associated with low birth weight, premature births, and a high death rate of newborn infants. Fig. P-105 shows how the mother's age is associated with infant death rates.

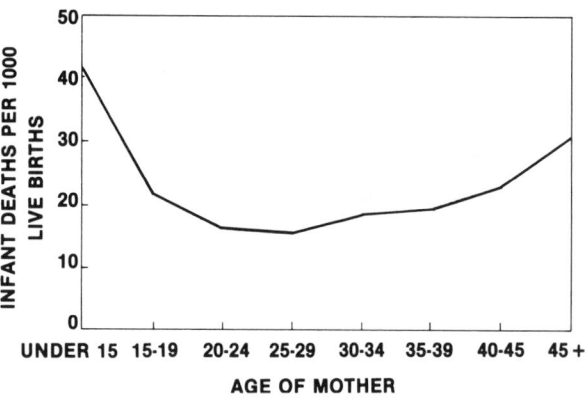

Fig. P-105. Infant mortality rates by age of mother. (Based upon data from *Maternal Nutrition and the Course of Pregnancy*, National Academy of Sciences, 1970, p. 144, Table 3)

Ethnic and/or Language Differences.

The U.S. population is composed of many national, cultural, and regional groups. These groups have a variety of dietary practices, many of which are excellent, that are part of their cultural traditions. However, some families may be unfamiliar with compositions and nutritional values of many foods available in local markets. Unfortunately they frequently adopt poor food practices and replace nutritious foods with ones that contain large amounts of fats, starch, and sugars, but few other nutrients. For example, substituting soft drinks for fruit juice or potato chips for potatoes increases the calories consumed and reduces the intake of essential minerals and vitamins.

For certain individuals, English is not a familiar language. This may present a problem, if the woman is not able to read or understand information about the foods commonly eaten in this country. In many cases, ethnic and/or language differences have been associated with anemia and inadequate or sporadic weight gain during pregnancy.

Therefore, some dietary characteristics and major health problems of three leading ethnic minority groups are presented to illustrate potential nutritional problems of pregnant women. These follow:

• **American Indians (Native Americans)**—Indian diets have become "Americanized" in much the same way that other ethnic food patterns have become assimilated. Everyday meals, usually consisting of breakfast, lunch, and dinner, are a blend of traditional foods and American favorites. For most, traditional meals are only served on special occasions and may incorporate foods having religious and ceremonial significance. Some of the favorite foods include acorn bread, smoked salmon, smoked salmon eggs, deer meat, fried bread, and fruits, leaves, and roots of wild plants.

It is noteworthy that the diet of Native Americans often varies according to the wild foods in the area of residence and the availability of commercial foods at prices they can afford. For example, Indians living in the Northwest eat a wide variety of seafood; on the other hand, those in mountainous areas eat more dried meats and freshwater fish. Finally, the diets of the tribes in the Southwest are similar to those of Mexican-Americans in that tortillas, refried beans (*frijoles refritos*) and fried bread (*sopapillas*) are favorite foods.

The major nutrition related problems of American Indians are obesity, diabetes, dental disease, alcoholism, and iron deficiency anemia. Many of these problems can be eliminated or controlled by better diets. In order to ensure adequate nutrients accompanying dietary calories, more fruits, vegetables, and milk products should be eaten. In addition, high-quality proteins should be incorporated in the meals of the low income groups living on reservations. Sugar should be restricted.

• **African Americans**—Food habits of black families throughout the United States bear some similarities to those of low income people in the South. Certain ethnic foods appear in the diet, such as chitterlings and hot bread with pot liquor. However, these items are not regularly included in the diet. Generally, the foods eaten are more like those in a "typical American" diet. In addition, the diets of many blacks include the frequent use of convenience foods, snacks, and foods sold at carry-out restaurants.

Protein is incorporated in the diet primarily by using meat, fish, and poultry. Beef, pork, and chicken are most popular. Use of traditional "soul foods" such as pig's feet and neck bones appears to be limited. Meat is prepared mainly by frying or simmering. In most cases, the amount of milk product consumed is less than the daily recommended servings for pregnancy and lactation. (See Table P-24.) Too often, carbonated beverages replace milk as a beverage.

Rice is preferred to potatoes and pastas, although, potatoes are still popular and may be substituted for grain products in the diet. Biscuits, cornbread, and white bread are preferred to whole grain products.

Vegetables such as greens, sweet potatoes, okra, cabbage, corn, and green beans are usually boiled for long periods. Salads are not common. Seasonal availability affects the variety of fruits eaten. Although fresh fruits are preferred, canned fruits are also used. Citrus fruits are not consumed very often.

Many water-soluble vitamins are lost when vegetables are boiled. Hence, the intake of vitamin C may be inadequate due to losses in cooking as well as to a limited consumption of citrus fruits. Therefore, the vegetables should be cooked in less water for a shorter period of time or eaten raw. In addition, fruits and vegetables containing more vitamin C should be eaten.

A major nutritional problem of blacks is obesity. This is related to the predominant use of fried foods, fatty meats, breads, rice, and potatoes, and to a limited consumption of other foods such as fruits and vegetables.

Although calories may be adequate, intake of certain nutrients may be low. To improve the diet, a wider variety of foods, different methods of cooking, and smaller amounts of high-calorie foods should be used.

• **Mexican Americans**—The diets of Mexicans in the United States are influenced by the availability of food items, family income, and the region in Mexico from which the family originated.

A variety of meats, poultry, and legumes, as well as eggs are the primary protein foods in their diets. Meat and poultry are usually fried or boiled, and are commonly prepared in combination dishes with vegetables and other foods. Eggs are popular; they may be soft boiled, fried, or scrambled.

Milk is not regularly consumed at meals, but is usually replaced by soft (carbonated) drinks, fruit drinks, or coffee. However, some milk is used in cooking hot cereals or with dry cereals, and in making a very sweet custard (*flan*), rice pudding (*arroz con leche*), or other puddings. Cheese is very common in Mexican cooking. Although Mexican-Americans will eat American-type cheeses, they prefer cheeses produced in Mexico that they can sometimes purchase in local stores.

Tortillas and rice are the staple grain products. Both corn and flour tortillas are used, and may be home-made. The most popular vegetables are tomatoes and chili peppers. Vegetables are sometimes eaten raw, but they are usually boiled for a long time. Potatoes are often fried. Fruit is considered as a dessert in the Mexican diet; it is usually eaten fresh, but sometimes canned. The most popular fruits are oranges, apples, and bananas.

Several inadequacies in the Mexican-American diet may occur. The limited use of milk results in a less than optimal intake of calcium. Although cheese is used, the quantity may not be sufficient to provide enough calcium to meet the Recommended Dietary Allowance (see Table P-23.) In addition, intakes of vitamin D and perhaps riboflavin may be less than adequate. Methods to incorporate more cheese and milk in the diet should be encouraged. Simple dishes such as melted cheese on tortillas (*quesadillas*) can be eaten. Also, nonfat dry milk can be used in preparing tortillas.

Since dark green and yellow vegetables are not regularly eaten, dietary vitamin A and folacin are minimal. To increase the vitamin A content, greater amounts of chiles, carrots, and avocados should be included in the diet. Folacin intake can be improved by eating spinach or dark leafy lettuce. Because vegetables are overcooked, the availability of other B vitamins and ascorbic acid is greatly diminished. Therefore, the vegetables should be prepared in small amounts of water and cooked for shorter periods.

The incidence of obesity among Mexican-Americans is high because the calorie level of the diet may be disproportionately high compared to total nutrient content. The excessive consumption of carbonated beverages, fruit drinks, pastries, and doughnuts (empty calorie foods) contribute excessive calories with little or no protein, vitamins, or minerals. Furthermore, the frequent use of lard or oil to fry foods adds extra calories to a nutritious food. In order to improve the nutrient to calorie ratio, empty calorie foods and fried foods should be limited.

Habituation to Alcohol, Drugs, and/or Smoking.
Some of the current ideas on each of these harmful habits follow:

• **Alcohol**—Dr. David Smith of the University of Washington in Seattle, medical researcher who discovered that alcoholic mothers gave birth to infants with various defects, states that there is no "safe dose" of alcohol for a pregnant woman.[22] It is suspected that the consumption of alcohol during pregnancy may be the greatest single cause of birth defects and the most common cause of mental retardation in infants. Dr. Smith has named the complex of abnormalities the *fetal alcohol syndrome.*

Therefore, anyone who has a role in the counseling of pregnant women should strongly advise against the consumption of alcoholic beverages and help alcoholic mothers find the appropriate therapy means for breaking the habit.

• **Drugs**—The use of addictive drugs such as heroin and morphine by pregnant women has been reported to have neurological effects on their newborn infants. Sometimes, the infants are addicted at birth and have characteristic symptoms of withdrawal such as irritability, sleeplessness, and lack of interest in eating. The symptoms may occur as late as 7 days after delivery.

It is noteworthy that the identification and treatment of drug-addicted mothers early in pregnancy has resulted in great reduction in the harmful effects of the addiction on infants.

• **Smoking**—Women who smoke during pregnancy may give birth to a low birth weight infant. The reduction of

---

[22]Iber, F. L., "Fetal Alcohol Syndrome," *Nutrition Today*, September/October 1980, pp. 4-11.

weight in the fetus is due to the interference of carbon monoxide (from the smoke) with its oxygen supply. Therefore, women of childbearing age or younger should be discouraged from starting to smoke or given assistance in breaking the habit once it is established.

History of Obstetrical Complications.
Previous obstetrical complications reflect potential problems which may recur in subsequent pregnancies. Nutrition related factors in the obstetrical history include inadequate weight gain, preeclampsia and/or toxemia, anemia, diabetes, bleeding prior to delivery, multiple pregnancy, premature or small-birth-weight infant, and fetal or neonatal death.

Low Income.
Women from low income families may find it difficult to obtain sufficient food and to consume adequate diets during pregnancy. Furthermore, the likelihood of prematurity rises sharply with a decrease in nutritional status. The lowest birth weights and larger number of deaths in the neonatal period occur among the infants born to the most poorly nourished mothers.

In order to help improve the nutritional quality of the diet, the low income person should be encouraged to participate in food programs such as Food Stamps and WIC (Special Supplemental Feeding Program for Women, Infants, and Children). These programs increase the buying power or provide specific high-quality foods.

Nutrition education and counseling are important to maximize the benefits from the limited resources available to low income individuals. Information on food buying, storage, and preparation can be extremely useful. In many cases, existing community resources may help provide this support. It is important and valuable to coordinate these efforts.

Psychological Conditions.
Depression, anorexia nervosa, and other mental problems may affect the course and outcome of a patient's pregnancy. These conditions may result in reduced caloric and nutrient intake, which is associated with poor weight gain of the fetus, low-birth-weight infants, and a high death rate of newborn babies.

Rh factor Incompatibility.
This problem, which is also known as erythroblastosis fetalis, has little to do with nutrition, but it is presented here so that it will not be overlooked by prospective parents. (All obstetricians are well aware of this problem and the appropriate preventive measures, but some American women may have their babies with little or no prenatal advice from a doctor.)

The medical name of this condition is actually a description of the effects of the Rh incompatibility on the fetus. During pregnancy, a mother whose blood is Rh negative (from 12 to 15% of Americans have this type of blood) may develop antibodies against a fetus that is Rh positive. Some of the maternal antibodies may cross the placenta into the fetus, where they may destroy some of the red blood cells (this effect is called erythroblastosis). Pigment released from the blood cells may poison the infant's brain before or after birth. It is noteworthy that this condition was the cause of death in 1 of every 400 births at the Chicago Lying-In Hospital in the early 1940s

(most of the deaths occurred within the first few days of life). Since then, the cause of the problem was studied intensively and appropriate preventative measures were developed. Fig. P-106 shows the most common combinations of parental Rh blood types that occur.

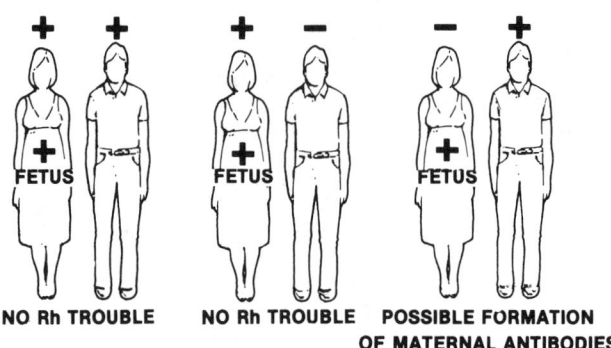

NO Rh TROUBLE   NO Rh TROUBLE   POSSIBLE FORMATION OF MATERNAL ANTIBODIES

Fig. P-106. Combinations of parental Rh blood types and the possibility of Rh factor incompatibility.

It may be seen from Fig. P-106 that only the combination of an Rh-negative mother and an Rh-positive father may lead to incompatibility. Even in these cases, the problem does not occur very often. Nevertheless, all couples should have their blood types checked to rule out the possibility of trouble. (A vaccine may be administered to prevent the formation of maternal antibodies if the potential for incompatibility is discovered early enough.)

Several Previous Pregnancies.
Expectant mothers who have had many pregnancies in rapid succession are often in a depleted nutritional state. For example, if there is not enough time between pregnancies, the losses of iron and other nutrients will not be restored. Careful attention should be given to these dietary needs.

Use of an Oral Contraceptive.
An estimated 10 to 11 million American women use oral contraceptives. Some have used them for many years prior to discontinuing their use in order to have a child. Researchers have found that these agents change the nutritional needs of some women. The levels of several vitamins and minerals in the blood are known to be, or suspected to be, influenced by "the pill." As a result, some oral contraceptive users need increased amounts of certain nutrients in their diets to maintain normal blood levels (a sign of adequate nutrition). Folacin, a B vitamin, is of particular concern since many oral contraceptive users may need a supplement of folacin. In addition, adequate amounts of vitamin C (ascorbic acid), vitamin B-2 (riboflavin), vitamin B-6 (pyridoxine), vitamin B-12, and zinc are needed.

Therefore, pregnant women who previously used an oral contraceptive should ask their doctor whether they should take a vitamin and mineral supplement during pregnancy.

Vegetarianism. The types of diets used by people who abstain from eating meat vary widely in terms of the other foods that are used or not used.

Lacto-vegetarians do not consume meat, poultry, fish, or eggs. However, they do use milk, cheese, and other dairy products. The pure vegetarian (vegan) abstains from all animal protein foods and milk and milk products.

The fruitarian, unlike the majority of vegetarians, eats a more restricted diet of raw or dried fruits, nuts, honey, and oil. Even more restrictive is the macrobiotic diet. This regimen consists of ten diets, ranging from the lowest level which includes cereals, fruits, vegetables, and some animal products, to the highest level made up entirely of brown rice. At all levels, fluids are avoided as much as possible. Individuals who continue to follow the higher levels of this diet are in serious danger of developing nutritional deficiencies.

A vegetarian who eats a wide variety of grains, legumes, nuts, fruits, vegetables, and milk and milk products can have a nutritionally sound diet. However, the vegan and fruitarian diets do not contain any significant amount of vitamin B-12. Lacto-ovo vegetarians will obtain the Recommended Dietary Allowance for this vitamin by consuming the equivalent of four glasses of cow's milk daily. Soybean and goat's milk contain less vitamin B-12 than cow's milk. Therefore, both vegans and vegetarians who do not drink cow's milk will need to take a vitamin B-12 supplement. A deficiency of vitamin B-12 causes an anemia and eventually results in spinal cord degeneration. A high intake of folacin will mask this anemia and thus vitamin B-12 deficiency may go undiagnosed. The irreversible neurological changes will then be the first indication of a deficiency.

The omission of cow's milk or goat's milk from a strict vegetarian diet is also likely to lead to deficiencies of calcium and vitamin D since few other foods contain adequate quantities of these nutrients in forms that are utilized readily. Hence, supplements containing them should be taken.

SUMMARY. Pregnancy and lactation can be great opportunities for the mother to give her child a good start in life, providing a wide variety of nutritious foods are consumed before and during these periods.

(Also see NUTRIENTS: REQUIREMENTS, ALLOWANCES, FUNCTIONS, SOURCES.)

PREGNANCY ANEMIAS

The total iron requirements of pregnancy are considerable; hence, it is not uncommon to detect an iron deficiency anemia during pregnancy because the iron content of habitual U.S. diets is not sufficient. Such an iron deficiency anemia has three contributing factors: (1) low iron storage which may result from iron loss during a previous pregnancy; (2) low dietary iron intake; and (3) greatly increased demand for iron for maternal and fetal hemoglobin synthesis. Iron deficiency anemia during pregnancy can be corrected, and even more important it can be prevented, by appropriate iron supplementation. A daily supplement of 15 mg of iron, averaged over the entire pregnacy, should satisfy the needs of most

women. Also, pregnant women should eat foods rich in iron. Liver contains far more iron than any other food. Other meats, dried beans, dried fruit, green vegetables, eggs, and enriched cereals are good sources of iron.

Although not very common in the United States, megaloblastic anemia due to a folate deficiency does occur during pregnancy. In most cases it appears to be the result of long term use of an oral contraceptive, a marginal diet, vomiting, and increased demands of the developing fetus. Pregnant women have double the requirements of other persons for folic acid. The administration of folic acid causes prompt reversal of the symptoms. If not treated during pregnacy, the baby may show symptoms of megaloblastic anemia and require folic acid supplementation.

(Also see ANEMIA, section headed "Groups of Persons Susceptible to Nutritional Anemias"; ANEMIA, MEGALOBLASTIC; FOLIC ACID; INFANT ANEMIA; IRON; and PREGNANCY AND LACTATION NUTRITION.)

PRENATAL

Before birth.

PRESERVATION OF FOOD

Since the beginning of time, man has searched for ways to protect himself from hunger—for ways to save food in times of plenty for times of scarcity. No doubt, man learned that he could often collect more food than he could eat, but that it soon spoiled and became unfit for consumption—or even poisonous.

There are no records to indicate when some of the first methods of preservation were discovered. Like other discoveries, some of the preservation methods were based on a series of enlightening observations which led to the development of a process. The methods of preservation became refined and more effective as men like Anton van Leeuwenhoek, Lazaro Spallanzani and Louis Pasteur contributed to the understanding of spoilage of food. Until men learned some of the modern methods of preservation, large cities could not develop. Nearby farms were required to feed the city people, since food spoilage was a major problem.

Spoilage of food is caused by growth of microorganisms, enzyme action, oxidation (chemical reactions), extremes in physical surroundings, and/or pests. Insofar as possible, the aim of preservation is to reduce, eliminate, and/or control the causes of spoilage. With the modern methods of preservation, seasonal harvests can be enjoyed year round, and food specifically grown in one area can be shipped across the country or even worldwide. Still, scientists continue to search for better methods of preservation that yield a nutritious, flavorful, and desirable product, with minimal long-term requirements.

Table P-25, which follows, summarizes in a general way the methods of preservation which are applied to food. Often more details concerning the preservation of a food item may be found in the articles dealing specifically with that food. Foods are often preserved by a combination of the methods listed in Table P-25.

(Also see BACTERIA IN FOOD; FRUIT[S]; MEAT[S]; MILK AND MILK PRODUCTS; SPOILAGE OF FOOD; and VEGETABLE[S].)

TABLE P-25
METHODS OF FOOD PRESERVATION

Method(s); History	Description and Principle	Food Application	Length of Storage; Changes in Quality	Remarks
CANNING **History:** A Frenchman, Nicholas Appert, invented canning in response to a prize offered in 1795 by the French government for a food preservation method that would not seriously impair the natural flavor of fresh food. After 14 years of experimenting, Appert won the prize in 1809. His method involved heating foods in glass flasks sealed with corks. Pasteur later explained why the method worked. An Englishman, Peter Durand, conceived the idea of using cans, and by 1839 tin-coated steel containers were widely used.	Properly prepared foods are placed in the glass or can containers and sealed. Then depending upon the type of food (primarily the acidity [pH]), the cans or bottles are heated to a known temperature and then held at that temperature for a specified time. Low acid foods such as meats and vegetables are heated to 240° to 265°F *(116° to 129°C)* while acidic foods such as fruits are heated to about 212°F *(100°C).* The principle of canning is twofold: (1) to destroy spoilage and disease-causing microorganisms, and (2) to keep air away from the food.	Meat, fish, poultry, vegetables, fruits, soups, orange juice, tomato paste, jams, jellies and and other manufactured foods.	**Length of Storage:** Most canned foods keep well for more than 1 year when properly canned. Commercially canned items are dated. **Changes in Quality:** This varies with the food and the process, but some general statements can be made: (1) color and texture often different from fresh product; (2) no practical effect on protein; carbohydrates and fats; (3) no effect on vitamins A, D and riboflavin if protected from oxygen; (4) vitamin C destroyed by heat and exposure to oxygen; and (5) thiamin destruction dependent upon heat treatment and acidity of food.	The chief canning processes are: (1) the conventional retort method for most vegetables, fruits, fish and meat products; (2) preheating and hot filling for very acid foods like orange juice, tomato paste, jams and jellies; and (3) fast canning for foods such as baby foods, sauces, potted meats and cream-style corn. Fast canning uses high temperatures of 250° to 280°F *(121° to 138°C)* for short periods of time. The major concern is proper processing to ensure the destruction of the spores of *Clostridium botulinum*—a toxin-producing bacterium. Commercially canned foods have been free of the botulism hazard for over 30 years.
CHEMICAL ADDITIVES **History:** Man's first uses of salt to preserve foods are lost in antiquity. Sugar has also enjoyed a long-time usage as a preservative. More recently, other chemicals have been tested and used in minute amounts to prevent spoilage and the growth of microorganisms. The uses of chemicals (food additives) in foods for preservative purposes are controlled by the government under the Food Additive Amendment of 1958. (Also see ADDITIVES; and NITRATES AND NITRITES.)	A variety of chemicals will destroy microorganisms. Other than salt and sugar, chemicals used for this purpose must act at low levels. Some common chemical preservatives include ethyl formate, sodium benzoate, sodium and calcium propionate, sodium nitrate or nitrite, sorbic acid, and sulfur dioxide. Some chemicals act by preventing the growth of microorganisms, while others prevent oxidative or enzymatic deterioration of quality during manufacture and distribution.	Depends on the chemical and processing method; ranges from fruits and vegetables to meats to soft drinks; common examples include: BHA (butylated hydroxyanisole) and BHT (butylated hydroxytoluene) in beverages, cereals, chewing gum and oil; calcium propionate in baked goods, and sodium nitrite in meats.	**Length of Storage:** This varies widely depending upon the chemical(s) used and the food product. Some chemical additives merely increase the shelf life a few days or weeks while others may increase storage time to an indefinite period. **Changes in Quality:** The prime reason for the addition of many chemicals is to maintain the quality of the food. Some chemicals may actually increase the value of a food; for example, vitamin C (ascorbic acid) may be added to fruits to prevent browning.	Chemicals may be added to foods for reasons other than preservation. They are also added to enrich, or to improve a food. New chemicals added to food, regardless of the purpose, must undergo rigorous testing for safety.

(Continued)

TABLE P-25 (Continued)

Method(s); History	Description and Principle	Food Application	Length of Storage; Changes in Quality	Remarks
DRYING AND DEHYDRATION **History:** Drying is one of the oldest methods of preserving food and is still a common practice in the world today. Prehistoric man probably dried foods in the sun or near fires. There is evidence that drying foods by the fire was an ancient practice in both the New and Old Worlds. Artificial drying (dehydration) via hot air was developed in France in 1795, where it was used to dry thin slices of vegetables. Technology gained during World War II resulted in the dehydration of more foods.	Drying is accomplished via the sun in hot, dry areas of the world or via dehydrators which produce heat at certain temperatures, maintain humidity and produce a flow of air. Whatever the method, the heated air carries away the moisture. Depending on the food, drying or dehydration may reduce foods to 2% moisture. Drying or dehydrating is effective because microorganisms require water to grow and many enzymatic and nonenzymatic reactions require water to proceed.	Eggs, milk and milk products, fruits, vegetables, juices, meats, spices, soups, coffee, tea, gelatin, dessert mixes, and macaroni.	**Length of Storage:** This varies with the product, storage conditions and the final moisture content. Some very dry items can be stored indefinitely if protected from moisture. Molds can grow on foods with as little as 5 to 16% moisture. Bacteria and yeast usually require a moisture content greater than 30%. **Changes in Quality:** Drying concentrates the nutrients. Protein, fat, and carbohydrate are present in larger amounts per unit weight. Often the reconstituted or rehydrated food is comparable to the fresh food. However, the vitamin content of dried meat is less than that of fresh meat.	Many foods dry as part of the natural process in their production on the plant; for example, legumes, nuts, and grains. Vacuum driers may be used for foods that are especially sensitive to heat. Besides the preservative action of drying, it also reduces the size and weight of foods making them easier to transport and store. There are many methods of drying (dehydrating) foods that are especially adapted to certain food products. Occasionally some toxin producing bacteria may survive the process and cause poisoning when water is added.
FREEZE DRYING (Lyophilization) **History:** First application of freeze drying to a biological sample was reported in 1890 by the German histologist, Altmann. During the 1930s, the technology was applied to blood plasma. World War II stimulated the development of the technology to a commercial basis.	The process removes water from food while the food is still frozen. After cooling food to about −20°F (−29°C), it is placed on trays in a vacuum chamber and heat is carefully applied. Water is evaporated without melting since it goes from the frozen-ice state to the gaseous state without passing through the liquid state— sublimation. The food is not exposed to high temperature until most of the water is removed. Without water, microorganisms cannot grow, and most enzymatic and non-enzymatic reactions cannot proceed.	Any food, raw or cooked, which can withstand freezng.	**Length of Storage:** Freeze-dried foods are often packaged in an inert gas such as nitrogen and they must be packaged in moisture-proof containers. When properly prepared and packaged, most products are acceptable after 1 year of storage at 100°F (38°C)—a temperature much higher than normal storage. Longer storage times can be expected at lower temperatures. **Changes in Quality:** Upon rehydration (adding water), freeze-dried foods are equal in acceptability to their frozen counterparts. There is a substantial retention of nutrients, color, flavor, and texture.	Freeze drying usually produces higher quality foods than the other drying methods, but it costs more. The first significant commercial application of freeze drying was in the production of an improved instant coffee.

(Continued)

TABLE P-25 (Continued)

Method(s); History	Description and Principle	Food Application	Length of Storage; Changes in Quality	Remarks
FREEZING **History:** Since early times, farmers, fishermen, and trappers, living in regions with cold winters, have preserved their meat and fish by freezing and storage in unheated buildings. About 1880, ammonia refrigeration machines were introduced for use in freezing fish. Clarence Birdseye stimulated the development of the business of packaging frozen foods by forming a company that began quick freezing foods in 1924. The frozen food business boomed when home freezers became available after World War II.	Foods are subjected to temperatures below 32° to 25°F (0° to −3°C) where the water in the food turns to ice. Foods are best if rapidly frozen and freezing methods may employ direct immersion in a cooling medium, contact with refrigerated plates in a freezing chamber, freezing with liquid air or nitrogen, or dry ice. Freezing does not kill microorganisms or destroy enzymes, it merely arrests or slows spoilage changes.	Most kinds of fruits and vegetables, meat, fish, poultry, and some dairy products; a variety of precooked foods (convenience foods) from french fries to complete dinners; some foods such as tomatoes, cabbages, bananas, avocados, pears, and some shellfish not well suited for freezing.	**Length of Storage:** Each food has its own recommended storage period, after which time undesirable off-flavors slowly develop. **Changes in Quality:** Many food are pretreated further to ensure quality during frozen storage. In general, freezing promotes the retension of nutrients and does not destroy nutrients. However, some destruction of vitamins may occur during the processing that precedes freezing.	Frozen foods must be kept frozen since partial thawing and refreezing lowers the quality. Freezing and canning are the two most widely used methods of food preservation. Frozen foods must be protected from dehydration and freezer burn during storage.
FERMENTATION **History:** Some of the earliest writings describe the fermentation of grapes and other fruits. Most cultures devised some type of fermented beverage. Fermentation of milk has been known for ages; it is mentioned in the Old Testament. Nomadic tribes fermented milk. Sauerkraut is fermented cabbage—a product of ancient China. (Also see BEERS AND BREWING; MEAT[S], section headed "Meat Processing"; MILK AND MILK PRODUCTS; and WINE.)	In fermentation, the growth of certain bacteria and yeasts which synthesize chemicals that aid in preservation of the food is encouraged. These products of fermentation are primarily lactic acid and ethyl alcohol. Lactic acid is important in the fermentation of cucumbers, olives, cabbage, meats, and milk. Ethyl alcohol is produced by the fermentation of fruits and cereals.	Fruits, vegetables, cereals, meats, and milk.	**Length of Storage:** Fermented products are often subjected to other preservation methods to increase storage time. Milk products are refrigerated while wines are pasteurized. **Changes in Quality:** Fermention changes the quality of both plant and animal products in a marked degree. Some foods are made more edible, others are made more nutritious, and still others are made more flavorful.	Some fermented products require that individuals acquire a taste for their distinctive flavor. Fermentations create wine, beer, rum, hard liquor, breads, cheeses, pickles, salami sausage, olives, Sajur asin (vegetables and rice) poi (taro), yogurt, buttermilk, and acidophilus. Fermentations producing lactic acid are encouraged by the level of salt in the product.

(Continued)

TABLE P-25 *(Continued)*

Method(s); History	Description and Principle	Food Application	Length of Storage; Changes in Quality	Remarks
PASTEURIZATION **History:** The process is named for Louis Pasteur who, in the 1860s, found that heating liquids, especially wines, to a temperature of 140°F *(60°C)* improved their keeping qualities.	This process is the application of mild heat for a specified time to a liquid, food, or beverage. Pasteurization destroys molds, yeasts, and the nonspore-forming bacteria. The lower the temperature the longer the application time, and vice versa. For example, milk can be pasteurized at 143°F *(62°C)* for 30 min. or 162°F *(72°C)* for 15 seconds. Time and temperature vary with the type of food. Foods are rapidly cooled following the heat treatment.	Milk, cheese, wine, beer, and other beverages such as the fruit juices.	**Length of Storage:** This depends upon the type of storage following the pasteurization and upon the type of food. **Changes in Quality:** Since heat is less than boiling temperature and for a short time, the quality of the food is maintained. Foods which are pasteurized include those whose flavor and appearance may be adversely affected by high temperatures.	For milk, the times and temperatures employed are based upon the heat tolerance of *Mycobacterium tuberculosis,* one of the most heat resistant of the nonspore-forming pathogens (disease causing).
PICKLING **History:** Pickling of plant and animal foods is an ancient practice. Sauerkraut was manufactured in ancient China. In the 18th century, scientists recognized that vinegar (acetic acid) was good for preserving biological specimens. The pickling industry has grown rapidly since the 1930s.	Preserving foods in vinegar and salt is called pickling. Vinegar is an acid, and microorganisms are sensitive to acids. Moreover, acids increase in the lethality of heat on microorganisms. There are two methods of pickling: (1) fresh pack pickling, and (2) fermentation pickling. Both rely on brine and vinegar as the primary preservatives. The vinegar needs an acetic acid content of 4 to 6%, and either cider vinegar or white vinegar is acceptable. The addition of spices is a common practice.	Vegetables, fruits, meats, eggs, and nuts; most common include cucumbers, pears, peaches, plums, cured meats, cabbage, mushrooms, cauliflower, onions, tomatoes, beets, peppers, and watermelon.	**Length of Storage:** Pickling alone is not sufficient for long-term storage. Pickled products should be heat treated (canned) unless they are consumed soon after pickling. Even vinegar is often pasteurized for a longer shelf life. **Changes in Quality:** Pickling not only increases the keeping quality of a food, it adds an appealing flavor to the food. The nutritional quality depends on other perservative processes employed on the food.	Pickled foods are not likely to be suspect in a food poisoning incident—at least where sufficient vinegar is used. Vinegar is a chemical preservative used in other foods such as mayonnaise and salad dressing. Cucumbers are the most commonly pickled vegetable. Near perfect produce should be used for pickling.
RADIATION **History:** The first patent related to the radiation treatment of food was taken out in France in 1930. Serious investigations in the U.S. were conducted during the 1950s. Radiation preservation of foods was considered to be in the experimental stages until 1981, when the ban on treating foods with gamma rays was eased by the FDA. (Also see RADIATION PRESERVATION OF FOOD.)	Ionizing radiation—fast moving subatomic particles or energetic electromagnetic waves—is used to treat foods. The radiation prevents the proliferation of microorganisms, insects, and parasites, and inactivates enzymes. The source of radiation may be cobalt-60, cerium-137 or X rays. This process *does not* make the food radioactive.	Very adaptable; considered for use on fruits, vegetables, meats, fish, poultry, eggs, cereals, flours, and dried fruits; many potential foods tested.	**Length of Storage:** Radiation significantly increases the storage of any food in comparison to its preservation by conventional methods. **Changes in Quality:** Only minimal changes in texture, flavor, color, and odor are experienced; and nutrient destruction is no greater than that which occurs when food is preserved by more conventional methods.	At low levels of radiation, the process is comparable to pasteurization; at high levels, it is equivalent to sterilization. Some doses inhibit sprouting and delay ripening in foods. The process has great potential since irradiated foods can be stored for long periods without refrigeration. Also, it is very flexible, adapting to various sizes and shapes of food.

(Continued)

TABLE P-25 *(Continued)*

Method(s); History	Description and Principle	Food Application	Length of Storage; Changes in Quality	Remarks
REFRIGERATION (Cold storage) **History:** In ancient Rome, snow from the mountains was used to pack prawns and other perishables. Root cellars were constructed by many settlers to keep foods cool. The use of ice for refrigeration was introduced toward the beginning of the 19th century. It was not until 1890 that mechanical refrigeration came into use on a large scale.	Refrigeration temperatures may range from 29° to 60°F (−1.6° to 15.5°C). Commercial and household refrigerators run at about 40° to 45°F (4.5° to 7.2°C). Refrigeration retards deterioration by slowing the growth of microorganisms and decreasing the rate of chemical reactions that deteriorate foods.	Meats, poultry, fish, eggs, fruits, vegetables, and all in different stages of processing—cooked, fresh, etc.; baked goods.	**Length of Storage:** The amount of time foods can be stored depends on the type of food and its age. At 40°F (4.5°C), meats, fish and poultry keep for 2 to 10 days depending upon their stage of processing, while some fruits and vegetables keep for weeks or months. **Changes in Quality:** Gradual changes in quality and nutrient composition continue during storage.	Large cold storage warehouses keep huge quantities of apples, apricots, pears, butter, cheese, and eggs for periods of 6 to 10 months. Some fruits and vegetables are harvested at full size, but unripe. These are shipped in refrigerated transports and allowed to ripen or held in cold storage to ripen.
SALT CURING (Brining) **History:** Salting is an ancient method of food preservation. Dry salting and the pickling of meats and fish in brine were practiced before 2000 B.C. (Also see CABBAGE; CUCUMBER AND GHERKIN; MEAT[S], section headed "Meat Processing"; and OLIVE.)	There are four basic methods of salt curing: dry salting, brining, low salt fermentation, and pickling. Dry salting and brining require concentrated amounts of salt. When a food is impregnated with salt, water is drawn out of the cells of microorganisms and their growth is inhibited. Microorganisms vary in their sensitivity to salt, but usually 15 to 20% dissolved in the water phase of a food is highly preservative.	Meat, fish, poultry, and almost any fruit or vegetable by one or more of the salt curing methods.	**Length of Storage:** Most produce will remain fit for consumption 3 weeks to several months when stored at 38°F (3.3°C), though the actual salt-curing process may take several weeks. For longer periods of storage the food needs to be subjected to some other type of preservative process such as canning, drying, or smoking. **Changes in Quality:** Dry salting and brining require the greatest concentrations of salt, and generally the more salt used the better the food is preserved, but the greater the loss in food value. Heavily salted food must be soaked and rinsed to make it palatable—a process which further depletes vitamins and minerals.	Nowadays most people use a salt curing method for the distinctive flavor it imparts to foods such as cucumber pickles, sauerkraut, green olives, and sausage. Low-salt fermentation and pickling ensure that the proper microorganisms develop and suppress the development of undesirable microbial activity.

(Continued)

TABLE P-25 *(Continued)*

Method(s); History	Description and Principle	Food Application	Length of Storage; Changes in Quality	Remarks
SUGAR **History:** Early man used some sugar for preserving. However, sugar (sucrose) availability in the world began increasing after the mid-1750s; hence, more sugar continued to be used in the preservation of foods.	Concentrated sugar solutions draw water out of the microorganisms and bind water, thereby preventing their growth. Microorganisms differ in their sensitivity to sugar, but around 70% sucrose (sugar) is highly preservative.	Preservation of fruits in jellies, jams, conserves, marmalades, preserves, fruit butters, and candied and glaced fruits.	**Length of Storage:** After the addition of sugar, many fruits require further heat processing. When properly bottled or stored, these fruits may be stored a year or more. Some may be stored without hermetic sealing, though such protection is useful to control mold growth, moisture loss, and oxidation. **Changes in Quality:** Due to the addition of sugar, these foods contain more calories than fresh fruit. Also, some of the processing may leach minerals and destroy vitamins. However, some unpalatable fruits may be given a pleasing taste with this method.	Flavoring, coloring agents, and additional pectin may be added to overcome any deficiencies in the fruit. Most fruits contain significant amounts of sugars, and dried fruits are preserved in part by the increased concentration of natural sugars. Sugar is added to meat in some curing processes.
SMOKING **History:** Early settlers relied on curing and smoking of meats for their preservation. The old smokehouse was a common sight on many early farms. This old method led to the development of sausages, hams, and bacon, which are still popular. (Also see MEAT[S], section headed "Meat Processing.")	Chemicals contained in smoke help prevent the growth of microorganisms but, smoking is combined with other preservation methods which cure the product. Curing may be accomplished with salt alone but generally herbs, spices, and sugar are also added. Cured meats are stored in rooms which can be filled with smoke, derived from burning hard woods. The amount of smoke, the temperature, and time of smoking depend upon the desired product.	Meat and fish, and some meat and fish products.	**Length of Storage:** Smoking by itself, as a cool smoke, contributes little to the preservation of meats and fish. In times past, the addition of smoke was associated with heat and drying of the product. Thoroughly cured and smoked meats such as Smithfield hams are reported to keep for years. **Changes in Quality:** The primary use of smoking today is to give the food a desirable smoked taste— an improvement in quality.	Modern refrigeration has opened the way for mild, sweet cures in which the smoked flavor is more important than the long-term preservation by smoke. Many people cure and smoke their game catches.

(Continued)

PRESSED

Compacted or molded by pressure; having fat, oil, or juice extracted under pressure.
(Also see OILS, VEGETABLE.)

PRESSURE COOKING

A pressure cooker is a heavy pan with a tight lid which can be clamped down, a safety valve, and an instrument for measuring the pressure. As the pressure increases, so does the boiling point of water, which means that the food cooks at a higher temperature, thus shortening the length of time required. The pressure cooker is also used for processing canned meats and vegetables.

PRETZELS

The name came from the German word, *brezel*, which originally came from the Latin word, *brachiatus*, meaning *having branches like arms*. Pretzels are brittle, glazed and salted crackers made of ropes of dough typically twisted into forms resembling the letter "B." The dough consists of a mixture of flour, salt, yeast, vegetable shortening, water, and malt. In the final step of their production, they are dipped into a tank of coconut oil maintained at a temperature of about 225°F (107°C), which seals the pretzel and extends its shelf life by 300%. Pretzels are a commercial product, difficult to duplicate in the home kitchen. They are used mainly as a snack food.

PRICKLY PEAR (INDIAN FIG; TUNA) *Opuntia ficus-indica*

The fruit of a cactus (of the family *Cactaceae*) which is native to Mexico and now grows throughout the dry, subtropical areas in the northern and southern hemispheres.

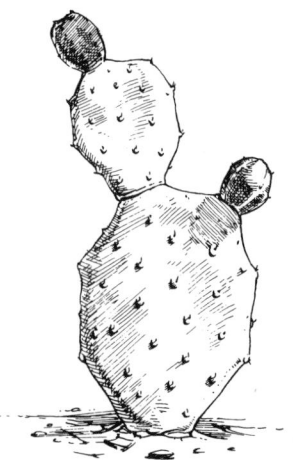

Fig. P-107.   The prickly pear, an appetizing fruit after the thorny skin has been removed.

Prickly pears are a little larger than large plums, but they have a prickly outer skin and a sweet inner pulp. They may be eaten fresh, stewed, or made into jams.

The nutrient composition of the prickly pear (Indian fig) is given in Food Composition Table F-36.

Some noteworthy observations regarding the nutrient composition of the prickly pear follow:

1.   The fresh fruit is moderately high in calories (67 kcal per 100 g) and carbohydrates (17%).

2.   Prickly pears are a good source of fiber and iron, and a fair source of calcium and vitamin C.

PROCESSED FOODS, HIGHLY

Contents   Page

Many species of animals collect and store food, but only *Homo sapiens* processes it. *Processing refers to all the physical and/or chemical operations that are applied to foodstuffs.* Food processing influences the nutritional value of foodstuffs—enhancing some, lowering others.

The term "highly processed foods" designates foods that have been altered significantly in appearance, culinary characteristics, nutritional value, structure, and/or texture as a result of a considerable amount of processing. Some of the reasons why foods are highly processed are: (1) to prevent spoilage; (2) to render them more storable and transportable, by reducing their bulk and water content; (3) to meet special dietary requirements; and (4) to produce concentrated sources of certain nutrients. Often, processing increases the levels of certain nutrients while reducing the levels of others. Hence, selected nutritional and economic aspects of highly processed foods are discussed in the sections which follow.

HISTORICAL BACKGROUND. People have processed foods for thousands of years. One of the first major types of food to be processed was cereal grains, because the hard, hulled seeds of the grassy plants were neither appetizing nor very digestible. The development of grinding and roasting was followed by innovations in cooking such as the baking of pasty grain mixtures into crude breads and the boiling of the dehulled or milled grains to make porridges. Prehistoric peoples also allowed both grains and fruits to ferment, then processed them to make beers and wines.

The domestication of animals led certain nomadic peoples to devise means by which their highly regarded animal foods could be taken on long journeys. For example, the fierce nomadic horsemen who ranged the steppes of Asia from China to the Caucasus mountains, either fermented mare's milk to make a yogurtlike substance or boiled it down to a crude powder. In the New World, the American Indians dried strips of buffalo meat in the sun and wind of the Great Plains. Then, they mixed the dried meat with rendered fat to make pemmican which kept well in storage or on long trips of exploration and trading.

Many of the commercial food processing techniques that are used today have been derived from the primitive practices of ancient peoples. It seems likely that the amount of food processing will increase rather than decrease in the future as efforts are made to provide more food for the many people now lacking even the minimal requirements for sustenance.

CURRENT TRENDS. Some of the most commonly employed types of processing tend to concentrate solids, carbohydrates, fats, and/or proteins at the expense of fiber, certain essential minerals, and certain vitamins. Examples of some highly processed items follow.

Cereal Products. The processing of grains has traditionally yielded products that are higher in starch than the original grains, but lower in most other nutrients. Enrichment of the products results in the restoration of only four of the more than 2 dozen essential nutrients that are depleted significantly by processing. Furthermore, many cereal products are made with substantial amounts of added fats and sugars. However, there has been a recent trend to restore some of the bran and wheat germ that was removed during processing.

Dairy Products And Eggs. These foods were once considered to be ideal for nourishing growing children and hard-working adolescents and adults. Now, many of the traditional items are being modified by (1) replacement of the animal fats with vegetable oil derivatives, (2) removal of much of the fat content without replacement, and (3) extension of certain expensive dairy and egg products with air, emulsifying agents, fillers, gummy binders, water, and less expensive animal or plant products that may possess analogous characteristics. Some noteworthy examples of these trends are cream substitutes (often called "nondairy blends"), filled milks, imitation cheeses, imitation eggs, imitation ice cream, imitation milk (this type of product may contain a soybean derivative plus vegetable oil), margarines, process cheeses, and sour cream substitutes. Producers often capitalize on the current concern over the alleged dangers of animal fats and cholesterol in promoting the modified items as being more beneficial to health than the traditional products.

Fish, Meats, Poultry, And Seafood. These items are steadily becoming more expensive, which makes it increasingly profitable to extend or even replace them with various plant products such as soybean derivatives or wheat gluten. This type of modification usually requires the utilization of additives such as binders, emulsifying agents, flavorings (natural and/or synthetic) and vegetable fats or oils. Stretching these products with less expensive food products is not new, since canned items and sausages have long been produced with ample amounts of fats, starchy fillers, and water.

Fruits And Vegetables. Here again, binders and fillers come to the rescue of food processors beset with rising production costs. "Simulated" pieces of fruits or vegetables may be made from mixtures of fruit or vegetable pulp, vegetable gums, mineral salts, starch, sugar, artificial or natural coloring and flavorings, and water. On the positive side, the use of pulp prevents the wastage which might ordinarily occur, since there is only a limited market for fruit and vegetable purees.

Meal Replacements. These products, which are often in the form of beverage powders or sweetened bars, are designed to be consumed with milk, water, or other beverage in lieu of the various mixtures of foods which usually constitute a meal. Federal regulations require that a typical serving of an item designated as a "meal replacement" provide at least 25% of the Recommended Daily Allowance (RDA) for certain specific nutrients. The macronutrients in these products are provided by various combinations of sugar, nonfat dry milk, soybean derivatives, and peanut butter and/or flour, whereas the required levels of micronutrients are usually met by fortification with selected minerals and vitamins. However, these products usually contain little or no fiber.

NUTRITIONAL ASSETS AND LIABILITIES. Highly processed foods are a mixed blessing in that they have the potential to meet specific nutritional needs, provided that certain pitfalls are avoided.

Assets. The combination of processing with judicious enrichment and fortification makes it possible to provide basically good food to an evergrowing population. Also, "engineered foods" may be designed to meet the special requirements of people with allergies, food intolerances, and/or other health problems that require restriction or even elimination of certain food constituents. Furthermore, compositions of processed foods may be altered in order to provide higher levels of nutrients when required during infancy, childhood, adolescence, convalescence, pregnancy, and lacation.

Liabilities. Highly processed foods that are significantly different in nutrient composition from their minimally processed counterparts may produce certain nutritional imbalances in people who have long been accustomed to eating other combinations of foods. For example, the substitution of a low fiber fortified bar for an ordinary breakfast of fruit, milk, eggs, and toast may contribute to constipation due to lack of bulk.

Also, the replacement of conventional foods by manufactured substitutes raises the question of whether unrecognized, but valuable, nutrients might have been provided by the foods that were replaced. For example, it is noteworthy that the early types of imitation orange drinks contained no potassium and were a source of trouble for people who were advised to drink orange juice for its potassium content.

Another important concern is the widespread addition of phosphate compounds to foods without proportionately increasing the calcium content, since a certain balance between the dietary levels of these essential minerals is necessary for their optimal utilization.

Finally, it is questionable whether fortified vegetable protein replacements for fish, meats, poultry, and seafood are nutritionally equivalent to the animal foods. Meat extractives are well known to be potent stimulators of digestive secretions, while this property does not appear to have been adequately tested in vegetable protein foods.

Limitations Of Enrichment and Fortification.

In theory, it should be possible to add pure forms of the nutrients present in minimally processed foods to highly processed foods in order to obtain nutritional equivalency. However, the U.S. Food and Drug Administration specifies enrichment and fortification levels for only some of the nutrients known to be essential. There are no specified levels for other essential nutrients such as chromium, selenium, and vitamin K. It might even be illegal to add the purified forms of these nutrients to foods.

Secondly, foodborne nutrients may in certain cases be present in combinations which work together. For example, the metabolic activities of the members of the vitamin B complex are interrelated. Hence, the failure to provide sufficient dietary quantities of one or more of these vitamins may impair the functions of other B vitamins in the diet.

SUGGESTIONS.

A large number of people will be affected for better or for worse by the growing trend towards the replacement of minimally processed foods with highly processed, fortified foods. Hence, certain measures should be taken to insure that the effects of this trend are beneficial rather than detrimental; among them, the following:

1. Advise the public regarding mineral and vitamin supplements, when the need for these items is indicated by a careful evaluation of the amounts and types of processed foods that are normally consumed.

2. Require the manufacturers of highly processed foods to supply complete nutritional data on their products to professionals engaged in the dispensing of nutrition information.

3. Revise the basic information given in meal planning guides regularly to incorporate the latest developments in new food products.

4. Consider whether the wholesale extension or replacement of various animal products with vegetable analogs is advisable, since (a) the forms of certain nutrients that are present in animal foods may be utilized better than the forms of the same nutrients which occur in plant foods, and (b) animals raised on grazing lands

are an efficient means of converting the energy and other constituents of pasture plants into the nutrients needed by people.

(Also see NUTRITIONAL SUPPLEMENTS; PROCESSING OF FOOD.)

PROCESSING OF FOOD

Many foods are altered before they reach the table. Grains are ground into flour and other cereal foods. Milk is pasteurized, homogenized or used in making cottage cheese, butter, or yogurt. Meat animals such as cattle and pigs are slaughtered, graded and cut into steaks, ground to hamburger, salted, dried, corned, or cured and smoked. Fruits and vegetables are sold fresh, canned, or frozen. All of these represent some stage or some portion of processing—treatment, preparation, or handling by some special method.

Over the years, man's expanding knowledge of food processing and his inventiveness have successfully extended the period of availability of foods and food combinations in forms that retain their nutritive and esthetic values. This has improved man's health, added variety to his diet, reduced the drudgery of food preparation, and increased his mobility. Furthermore, the technology of processing has greatly expended the markets both at home and abroad for agricultural products of relatively high value.

The increased need for processed food has resulted from the rising standard of living, the desire for a more diversified diet the year round, an expanding urbanization, and an increase in the total population.

Food processing has many goals. Perishable foods are converted into stabilized products that can be stored for extended periods of time. Examples of the basic preserving processes are canning, freezing, dehydrating, and ionizing radiation. Processing can change foods into new or more usable forms. Examples include winemaking, flour milling, olive brining, oil extracting, and butter churning. Processing adds convenience or built-in maid services to products. This phase of processing is typified by bakery products, frozen french fries, frozen TV dinners, frozen meat and fruit pies, canned soups, and instant dehydrated mashed potatoes.

After harvest or slaughter, unprotected food progressively loses quality and then completely deteriorates. Food is suitable for eating if used a relatively short time after harvest, but it becomes inedible and useless if allowed to exist without some kind of processing.

Processing starts on the whole raw material of whatever the food may be. Then, for some foods the whole raw material may be broken into parts which are futher processed, or the parts may be mixed with other components and used to form new products. The final stages of processing includes preservation so that the foods may be stored without spoiling. Finally processing includes some form of packing for shipment, storage, and consumer appeal. Fig. P-108 indicates some of the processes applied to foods by the food-processing industry.

Indeed, food processing is a complex industry, and no one description of food processing can apply. Therefore,

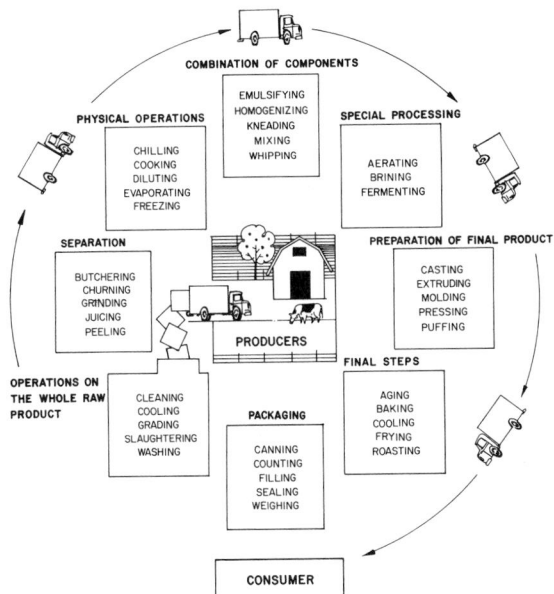

Fig. P-108. Food processing from the producer to the consumer. Not all processes shown are applied to all foods, nor are all food processing methods indicated. These are some major processes grouped according to their similarities.

many of the individual articles provide details of processes specific for individual foods.

(Also see NUTRITIONAL SUPPLEMENTS; and PROCESSED FOODS, HIGHLY.)

PROENZYME (ZYMOGEN)

Inactive form of an enzyme; e.g., pepsinogen.

PROGESTERONE

The hormone secreted by the corpus luteum (yellow substance) of the ovary whose function is to prepare the uterus (by growth of its lining membrane) for reception and development of the fertilized ovum (fertilized female sex egg.)

PROGNOSIS

Prediction of the outcome of an illness based on the person's condition and on scientific knowledge concerning the usual course and results of such illnesses, together with the presence of certain symptoms and signs that indicate the expected outcome.

PROLINE

One of the nonessential amino acids.
(Also see AMINO ACID[S].)

PRONUTRO

A finely ground mixture of corn, skim milk powder, peanuts, soybeans, wheat germ, sugar, salt, minerals, vitamins, and flavoring(s) developed without any governmental or international assistance by Hind Brothers, a private food firm in Natal, South Africa. Pronutro is as effective as skim milk powder in the rehabilitation of infants suffering from severe protein-energy malnutrition (kwashiorkor). Its protein content is about 22%. Pronutro can also be incorporated into cereals, soups, gravies, beverages, and chocolate bars.

(Also see CORN, Table C-45 Corn Products and Uses; MALNUTRITION, PROTEIN-ENERGY; and PROTEIN[S].)

PROPHYLAXIS

Preventive treatment against disease.

PROPYL GALLATE (PG)

An FDA approved food additive which acts as an antioxidant in foods, fats, oils, and waxes. It is often used in combination with butylated hydroxyanisole (BHA) and butylated hydroxytolulene (BHT).
(Also see ADDITIVES.)

PROSTAGLANDINS

These are a class of hormonelike compounds, made in various tissues of the body from arachidonic acid (and other derivatives of linoleic acid), which are important in the regulation of such diverse reactions as gastric secretion, pancreatic functions, release of pituitary hormones, smooth muscle metabolism, and control of blood pressure. Some 16 prostaglandins have been identified.

These highly potent substances have been called local hormones or tissue hormones because they do their work near the area in which they are produced, as distinguished from most circulating hormones which aim at more distant targets. A synthetic prostaglandin is being used to regress the corpus luteum (the growth on the ovary that prevents heat and ovulation). This allows the natural estrous cycle to begin again.

The name "prostaglandin," which is a misnomer, was given to these substances because they were first believed to have originated in the male's prostate gland.

PROSTHETIC GROUP

A protein conjugated with a nonamino acid substance; for example, hemoglobin is a conjugated (joined together) protein—each chain in the protein moiety, globin, is combined with a heme group to form the biologically functional molecule. Proteins are often described in terms of their prosthetic group; thus, hemoglobin is a *heme-protein*, and proteins containing lipid, carbohydrate, or metals are called *lipoproteins*, *glycoproteins*, and *metalloproteins*, respectively.

PROTEASE

An enzyme that digests protein.

PROTEIN(S)

Contents   Page

Chemically, proteins are complex organic compounds made up chiefly of amino acids. For each different protein there are specific amino acids and a specific number of amino acids which are joined in a specific order. Since amino acids always contain carbon, hydrogen, oxygen, and nitrogen, so do proteins. Moreover, the presence of nitrogen provides a tool for chemically estimating the amount of protein in a tissue, food, or some other substance. Crude protein is routinely determined by finding the nitrogen content and multiplying the result by 6.25 since the nitrogen content of all protein averages about 16% (100 ÷ 16 = 6.25). In addition, proteins usually contain sulfur and frequently phosphorus. Proteins are essential in all plant and animal life as components of the active protoplasm of each living cell.

In plants, the protein is largely concentrated in the actively growing portions, especially the leaves and seeds. Plants also have the ability to synthesize their own proteins from such relatively simple soil and air compounds as carbon dioxide, water, nitrates, and sulfates, using energy from the sun. Thus, plants, together with some bacteria which are able to synthesize these products, are the original sources of all proteins.

In animals, proteins are much more widely distributed than in plants. Thus, the proteins of the body are primary constituents of many structural and protective tissues—such as bones, ligaments, hair, fingernails, skin, and the soft tissues which include the organs and muscles. The total protein content of animal bodies ranges from about 10% in very fat, mature animals to 20% in thin, young animals. By way of further contrast, it is also interesting to note that, except for the bacterial action in the rumen of ruminants—cows, sheep, and goats—animals, humans included, lack the ability of the plant to synthesize proteins from simple materials. They must depend upon plants or other animals as a source of dietary protein. Hence, humans must have certain amino acids or more complete protein compounds in the diet.

Animals of all ages and kinds require adequate amounts of protein of suitable quality. The protein requirements for growth, reproduction, and lactation are the greatest and most critical.

The need for protein in the diet is actually a need for amino acids. Proteins in the food are broken down into amino acids by digestion. They are then absorbed and distributed by the bloodstream to the body cells, which rebuild these amino acids into body proteins.

The various amino acids are then systematically joined together to form peptides and proteins. The amino portion of one amino acid will combine with the carboxyl (acid) portion of another amino acid to form a peptide linkage. When several of these junctions occur, the resulting molecule is called a polypeptide. Generally polypeptide chains contain 50 to 1,000 amino acids.

HISTORY. Long ago, man probably divided his foods into two categories: animal derived and vegetable derived. Also, man probably noted that food from these two categories decomposed differently. The animal derived foods putrified, while vegetable derived foods fermented. It was not until 1742 that I. B. Beccari recognized that vegetable (plant) derived foods contained some of the same substances of animal derived foods. Still, this animal portion of foods was not recognized as unique molecules until 1838 when the Dutch chemist Gerardus Johannes Mulder, applied the name "proteins" to a group of complex organic compounds found in both plant and animal materials. It was because of their recognized importance to the structure and function of living matter that proteins were so named from the Greek word *proteios*, meaning "of the first quality."

In 1772, the chemical element, nitrogen, was discovered by Daniel Rutherford in Scotland and by Joseph Priestley in England, but at that time the importance of nitrogen to plant and animal foods was not appreciated. Later, scientists found that proteins contained nitrogen. Justus von Liebig, a German scientist, published a paper in 1841 on the analysis of proteins. Liebig thought that the protein values of different foods could be assessed on the basis of nitrogen content. Then, in 1881, while studying the changes in protein content in grain during germination and fermentation, Johan Kjeldahl, found his progress blocked by lack of an accurate method for determining nitrogen. Kjeldahl concentrated all his efforts on developing an analytical method for determining the nitrogen; hence, protein content of substances. The Kjeldahl method is stil routinely used today.

Gradually, the constituents of proteins—the amino acids—were discovered. In 1902, Emil Fischer, determined the chemical structure of amino acids, the building blocks of protein; and he determined the nature of the chemical bond—the peptide bond—holding the amino acids together.

One of the first recommendations as to protein intake was made by Carl von Voit, a student of Liebig. He suggested in 1881 that 118 g of protein daily was desirable. In 1902, a student of Voit and an American, W. O. Atwater, recommended 125 g per day. However, in 1904, R. H. Chittenden of Yale University recommended only 44 to 53 g of protein per day. Then, between 1909 and 1921, T. B. Osborne and L. B. Mendel conducted numerous experiments on rats which involved protein quantity and quality. Between 1935 and 1955, W. C. Rose conducted experiments in humans to determine how much of each amino acid was needed.

PROTEIN is needed for growth

THREE RATS FROM THE SAME LITTER, 11 WEEKS OLD

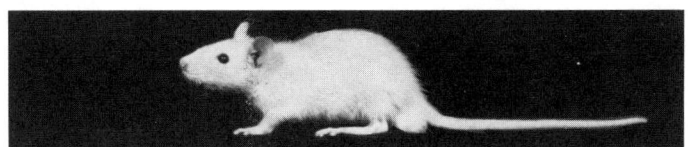

THIS RAT ATE FOODS THAT FURNISHED GOOD QUALITY
PROTEIN, BUT NOT ENOUGH. IT WEIGHED ONLY 70 GRAMS.

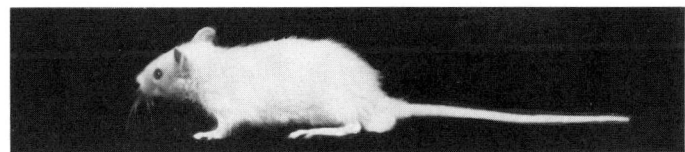

THIS RAT ATE FOODS THAT FURNISHED PLENTY OF PROTEIN,
BUT NOT THE RIGHT COMBINATION TO GIVE GOOD QUALITY.
IT WEIGHED ONLY 65 GRAMS.

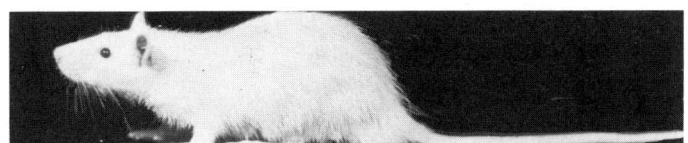

THIS RAT HAD PLENTY OF GOOD QUALITY PROTEIN FROM A
VARIETY OF FOODS. IT HAD GOOD FUR, A WELL-SHAPED
BODY, AND WEIGHED 193 GRAMS.

TOP FOOD SOURCES

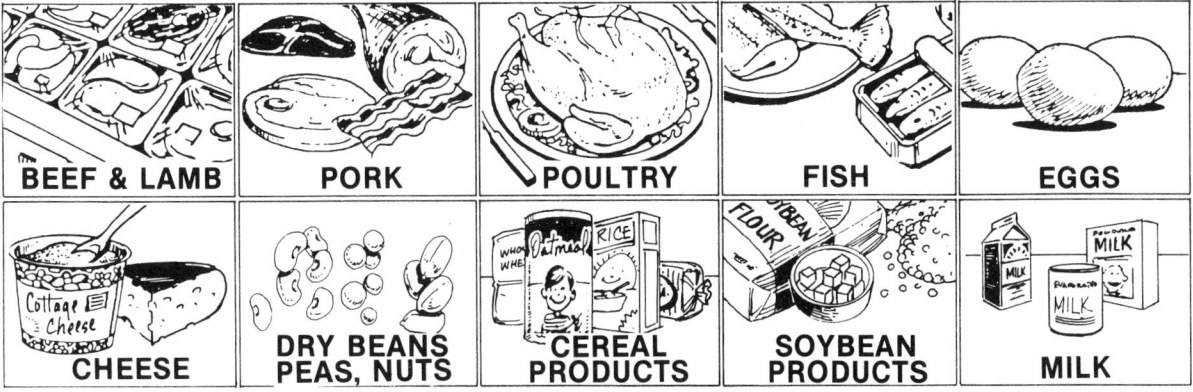

Fig. P-109.   Protein quantity and quality made the difference! The top rat ate too little of a good quality protein. The middle rat ate plenty of poor quality protein, while the bottom rat ate plenty of a good quality protein. (Adapted from USDA sources)

Further studies of actual proteins increased scientists' knowledge of exactly how proteins function in the body. In about 1927, James B. Sumner demonstrated that an enzyme was a protein. Then, during the 1950s, Frederick Sanger made a major discovery when he described the actual amino acid sequence of the protein hormone insulin. Other studies, pointed to the relationships between DNA (deoxyribonucleic acid) and RNA (ribonucleic acid) and protein. In 1953, Francis Crick and James Watson described the structure of the DNA molecule, and gradually scientists have unraveled how cells manufacture specific proteins with specific amino acid sequences. (Also see NUCLEIC ACIDS.)

SYNTHESIS. The basic structural components of protein are amino acids. Many of the amino acids can be synthesized within the body. These are called nonessential amino acids or dispensable amino acids. If the body cannot synthesize sufficient amounts of certain amino acids to carry out physiological functions, they must be provided in the diet; hence, they are referred to as essential or indispensable amino acids. Actually, it is not entirely correct to say that all indispensable amino acids need to be provided in the diet; rather, the requirement is for the preformed carbon skeleton of the indispensable amino acids, except in the case of lysine and threonine.

According to our present knowledge, the following division of amino acids as essential and nonessential seems proper for humans:

Essential (indispensable)	Nonessential (dispensable)
Histidine	Alanine
Isoleucine	Arginine
Leucine	Asparagine
Lysine	Aspartic acid
Methionine (some used for the synthesis of cysteine)	Cysteine
	Cystine
	Glutamic acid
Phenylalanine (some used for the synthesis of tyrosine)	Glutamine
	Glucine
	Hydroxyproline
Threonine	Proline
Tryptophan	Serine
Valine	Tyrosine

NOTE WELL: Arginine is not regarded as essential for humans, whereas it is for animals; in contrast to human infants, most young mammals cannot synthesize it in sufficient amounts to meet their needs for growth. (Also see AMINO ACID[S].)

In order for a protein to be synthesized, all of its constituent amino acids must be available. If one amino acid is missing, the synthesis procedure is halted. When a particular amino acid is deficient, it is referred to as a limiting amino acid because it limits the synthesis of protein. This is why protein quality is so important in human nutrition. Upon digestion, high-quality proteins provide balanced supplies of the various amino acids which can subsequently be absorbed as precursors for protein synthesis. Plant foods often contain insufficient quantities of lysine, methionine and cystine, tryptophan, and/or threonine.

Lysine is the limiting amino acid of many cereals, while methionine is the limiting amino acid of beans (legumes). In general, the proteins of animal origin—eggs, dairy products, and meats—provide mixtures of amino acids that are well suited for human requirements of maintenance and growth.

Protein synthesis is not a random process whereby a number of amino acids are joined together; rather, it is a detailed predetermined procedure. When proteins are formed three requirements must be met: (1) the proper amino acids, (2) the proper number of amino acids, and (3) the proper order of the amino acid in the chain forming the protein. Meeting these requirements allows the formation of proteins which are very specific and which give tissues their unique form, function and character.

Protein synthesis involves a series of reactions which are specific for *each* protein. The directions for manufacturing protein are received in coded form from the genetic material of the cell—the DNA (deoxyribonucleic acid).

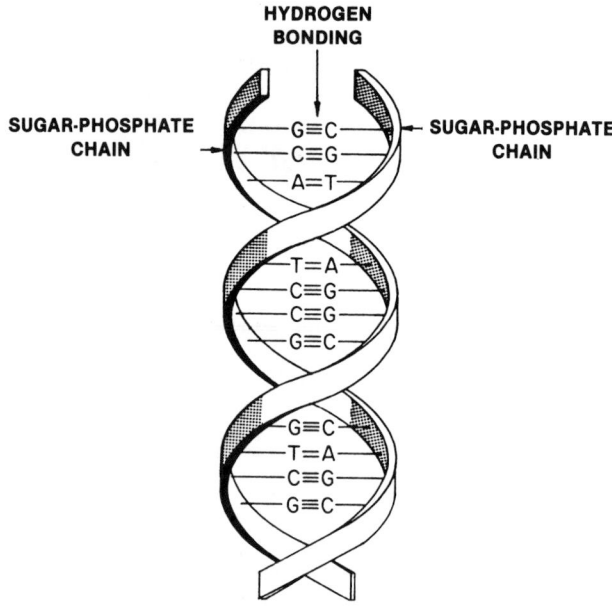

Fig. P-110. Deoxyribonucleic acid or DNA—the code of life. It's a double helix (a double spiral structure), with the sugar (deoxyribose)-phosphate "backbone" represented by the two spiral ribbons. Connecting the "backbone" are four nitrogenous bases (a base is the nonacid part of a salt): adenine (A) paired with thymine (T), and guanine (G) paired with cytosine (C); with the parallel spiral ribbons held together by bonding between these base pairs. The sequence of the bases codes for the synthesis of every protein in the body.

Within the DNA molecules the sequences of the nitrogenous bases adenine, thymine, guanine, and cytosine codes for the synthesis of proteins. The code of the DNA is put into action by ribonucleic acid (RNA). There are three forms of RNA, each one with a special function. Messenger RNA (mRNA) transcribes the information from the DNA and transports it to the cytoplasm of the cell as a single strand. Transfer RNA (tRNA) are small molecules which act as carriers for the specific amino acids. The third type of RNA, ribosomal RNA (rRNA), is a major component of the ribosomes within the cytoplasm of the cell. The site of protein synthesis is ribosomes bound to mRNA. Ribosomes bound to the mRNA translate (decode) the genetic code. As the message from DNA is translated, tRNA, supplies the proper amino acid. These amino acids are then linked by peptide bonds. The amino portion (NH_2) of one amino acid will combine with the carboxyl (COOH) portion of another amino acid releasing water (H_2O) and forming a peptide linkage—like railroad cars joining to form a train. When numerous of these junctions occur, the resulting molecule is called a protein.

Each sequence of amino acids is a different protein. Hence, different proteins are able to accomplish different functions in the body. With 22 amino acids, the different arrangements possible are endless, yielding a variety of proteins. For example, egg albumin, a small protein, con-tains approximately 288 amino acids. Thus, if one assumes that there are about 20 different amino acids in the albumin molecule, then mathematical calculations show that the possible arrangements of this number of amino acids are in excess of 10^{300}. (For comparison, one million is equal to 10^6.)

Since the DNA of each cell carries the master plan for forming proteins, genetic mutations often are manifested by disorders in protein metabolism. Many metabolic defects—inborn errors of metabolism—are the result of a missing or modified enzyme or other protein. The misplacement or omission of just one amino acid in a protein molecule can result in a nonfunctional protein. The disease called sickle-cell anemia results because the blood cells of afflicted individuals contains a faulty pro-tein, with the result that the blood cells often collapse causing anemia.

(Also see INBORN ERRORS OF METABOLISM; METABOLISM, section headed "Proteins"; and NUCLEIC ACIDS.)

CLASSIFICATION. Proteins occur in nature in a number of forms, each one possessing unique chemical properties. Based on chemical compostion, proteins may be divided into two main categories: (1) simple and (2) conjugated. Simple proteins consist of only amino acids or their derivatives, while conjugated proteins are joined to various nonprotein substances. Then, these two main categories are further subdivided. Table P-26 lists the various categories of proteins along with their distin-guishing characteristics.

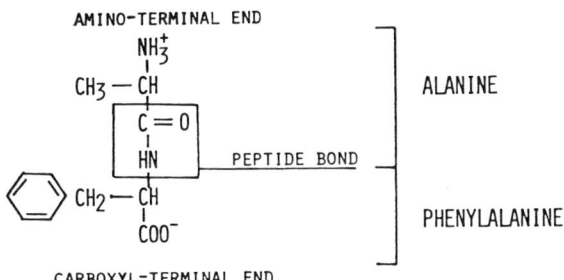

AMINO-TERMINAL END

ALANINE

PEPTIDE BOND

PHENYLALANINE

CARBOXYL-TERMINAL END

Fig. P-111. A peptide bond between two amino acids.

TABLE P-26
CLASSIFICATION OF SOME COMMON PROTEINS

Type	Chemical Properties	General Comments
Simple proteins:		
Albuminoids (scleroproteins)	Insoluble in water; highly resistant to enzymatic digestion; some become gelatinous upon boiling in water or dilute acids or bases	Includes collagen, elastin, and keratin; common in supporting tissues; sometimes referred to as fibrous protein
Albumins	Readily soluble in water; coagulate upon heating.	Present in egg, milk, and serum.
Globulins	Low solubility in water; solubility increases with the addition of neutral salts; coagulates upon heating.	Abundant in nature; examples are serum globu-lins, muscle globulins, and numerous plant globulins.
Glutelins	Insoluble in water; soluble in dilute acids or bases.	Abundant in cereal grains; an example is wheat gluten.
Prolamins	Insoluble in water, absolute alcohol or neutral solvents; soluble in 80% ethanol.	Zein in corn and gliadin in wheat are prolamins.
Conjugated proteins:		
Chromoproteins	Combination of a protein and a pigmented (colored) substance.	Common example is hemoglobin—hematin and protein.
Lecithoproteins	Combination of protein and lecithin.	Found in fiber of clotted blood and vitellin of egg.
Lipoproteins	Water soluble combination of fat and protein.	A vehicle for the transport of fat in the blood; all contain triglycerides, cholesterol, and phospholipids in varying proportions.
Metalloproteins	Proteins that are complexed with metals.	One example is transferrin, a metalloprotein that can bind with copper, iron, and zinc. Various enzymes contain minerals.
Mucoproteins or glycoproteins	Contain carbohydrate such as mannose and galactose.	Examples are mucin from the mucus secretion, and some hormones such as that in human pregnancy urine.
Nucleoproteins	Combination of proteins and nucleic acids.	Present in germs of seeds and glandular tissue.
Phosphoproteins	Compounds containing protein and phophorus in a from other than phospholipid or nucleic acid.	Casein in milk and ovovitellin in eggs, are examples.

Possibly a third category—*derived proteins* may be added to the two above. Essentially derived proteins are the product of digestion. They are fragments of various sizes. From largest to smallest, in terms of the number of amino acids, derived proteins are proteoses, peptones, polypeptides, and peptides.

Proteins may also be classified according to their structure which is very important to their function in the body. Some proteins are round to ellipsoidal and are called *globular proteins*. These include *enzymes*, *protein hormones*, *hemoglobin*, and *globulins*. Other proteins form long chains bound together in a parallel fashion, and are called *fibrous proteins*. These include *collagen*, *elastin*, and *keratin*—the proteins of connective tissue, elastic tissue and hair. Many of the fibrous proteins are not very digestible, and if they are, they are poor-quality proteins.

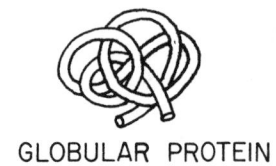

GLOBULAR PROTEIN

FIBROUS PROTEIN

Fig. P-112.   The structure of globular and fibrous protein.

DIGESTION, ABSORPTION, AND METABOLISM.
Protein digestion—the breakdown into smaller units—begins in the stomach and continues to completion in the small intestine. Enzymes from the pancreas and the small intestine eventually split dietary protein into individual amino acids. These amino acids are absorbed from the intestine by the process of active transport whereupon they are distributed to the cells of the body via the blood. In the body, amino acids may be used for primarily protein synthesis or energy production, depending upon the (1) protein quality, (2) caloric level of the diet, (3) stage of development, including growth, pregnancy, and lactation, (4) prior nutritional status, and (5) stress factors such as fever, injury and immobilization.

Occasionally, individuals are born with very specific disorders related to the metabolism of protein or amino acids. These are often referred to as inborn errors of metabolism. Albinism, maple syrup urine disease, and phenylketonuria are examples of some of the more familiar types.

(Also see DIGESTION AND ABSORPTION; INBORN ERRORS OF METABOLISM, Table I-Inborn Errors of Amino Acid Metabolism; and METABOLISM.)

FUNCTIONS.
Each specific protein performs a specific function in the body. One protein cannot and will not substitute for another. Rather broadly, proteins may be classified as performing the following five functions:

1. **New Tissue.** The formation of new tissues—anabolism—requires the synthesis of protein. Such conditions occur during periods of growth—from infancy to adulthood. Wound healing requires the synthesis of new proteins, as do burns, fractures, and hemorrhage. During training, athletes synthesize new proteins which increase muscle mass. Obviously, during pregnancy there is synthesis of new tissue. Not only the fetus but the placenta, uterus, breast, and blood require additional protein synthesis.

2. **Maintenance.** Protein is in a dynamic state even in the adult where overall growth has ceased. It is continually being degraded and resynthesized—a process called protein turnover. Blood cells must be replaced every 120 days, while cells which line the intestine are renewed every 1½ days. Moreover, protein is lost from the body in the perspiration, hair, fingernails, skin, urine, and feces. This constant turnover and loss of protein requires that the body have a "pool" of amino acids upon which it can draw to replace losses. This "pool" is replenished by dietary protein.

3. **Regulatory.** Proteins in the cells and body fluids provide regulatory functions. Hemoglobin, an iron-bearing protein carries oxygen to the tissues. Water balance and osmotic pressure are regulated by the proteins of the blood plasma. Furthermore, the proteins act as buffers controlling the acid-base balance of the body, especially in the intracellular fluids. Many of the hormones which regulate body processes are proteins; for example, insulin, glucagon, growth hormone, and the digestive tract hormones. Enzymes, the catalysts for most all chemical reactions of the body, are proteins. Antibodies, which protect the body from infectious diseases are proteins. The blood clotting mechanism of the body is dependent upon proteins.

Certain amino acids derived from dietary protein or synthesized in the body also perform important regulatory functions. Arginine participates in the formation of the final metabolic product of nitrogen metabolism—urea—in the liver. The process is known as the urea cycle. Cysteine and methionine are the principal sources of sulfur in the diet. Glutamic acid easily loses an amino (NH_2) group and thus participates in the transamination process, which produces other amino acids. Also, glutamic acid is the precursor of gamma-aminobutyric acid, a chemical associated with nervous system function. Glycine participates in the synthesis of purines, porphyrins, creatine, and glyoxylic acid. Glyoxylic acid is of interest because its oxidation yields oxalic acid of which there is increased formation in the genetic disorder oxaluria. Furthermore, glycine conjugates with a variety of substances thus allowing their excretion in the bile or urine. Histamine is formed by decarboxylation—removal of the COOH group—of histidine by the enzyme histidine decarboxylase. Histamine is a powerful blood vessel dilator, and it is involved in allergic reactions and inflammation. Also, histamine stimulates the secretion of both pepsin and acid by the stomach. Lysine provides structural components for the synthesis of carnitine which stimulates fatty acid synthesis within the cell. Tyrosine becomes the parent compound for the manufacture of the hormones norepinephrine and epinephrine by the adrenal gland, and of the hormones thyroxine and triiodothyronine by the thyroid gland. Also, the pigment melanin, which occurs in the skin and retina of the eye, forms from the enzymatic conversion of tyrosine. Finally, an important neurotransmitter of the brain, serotonin, forms from tryptophan. Some niacin can be manufactured from tryptophan, but not sufficient to meet the total niacin requirements of the body.

(Also see AMINO ACID[S]; and NIACIN.)

4. **Milk production.** Each liter of human milk contains about 12 g of protein. Thus, during lactation it is assumed that a woman needs at least as much extra dietary protein as is secreted in the milk. This extra protein should furnish liberal amounts of essential amino acids.

5. **Energy.** Catabolism—breakdown—of amino acids yields energy, about 4 Calories (kcal) per gram of protein.

In order for amino acids to be used for energy, the amino group (NH_2) must first be removed by a process known as deamination. The carbon skeleton remaining following deamination—alpha keto acid residues—may be either (1) converted to glucose—glycogenic, or (2) metabolized in fat pathways—ketogenic. When energy consumption in the form of carbohydrates and fats is low, the energy needs of the body take priority and dietary and tissue proteins will be utilized at the expense of the building or repair processes of the body.

Fig. P-113 summarizes the various functions of protein— its metabolism.

(Also see METABOLISM.)

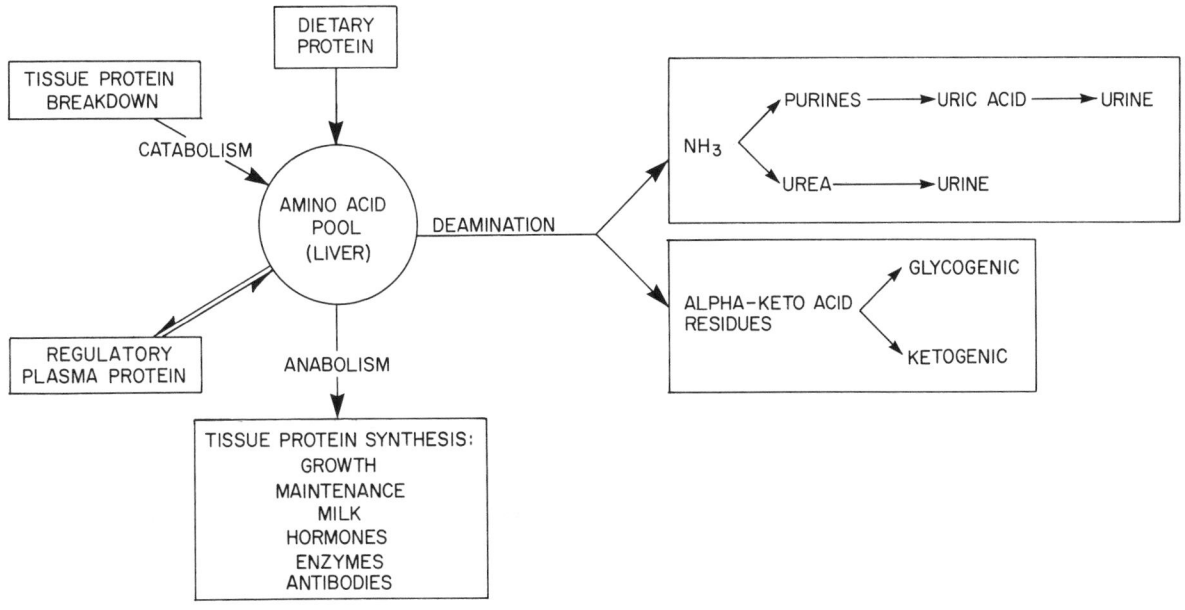

Fig. P-113. Summary of protein functions.

REQUIRED INTAKE. The minimum protein requirement of humans (other animals, too) may be determined by nitrogen balance studies. Nitrogen is obtained from the consumption of protein. As indicated previously, each 100 g of protein contains approximately 16 g of nitrogen. Nitrogen is lost from the body each day in the feces, urine, skin, hair, nails, perspiration and other secretions. Dietary protein (nitrogen) must be sufficient to cover the daily losses. Normal, healthy adults should be in a state of nitrogen equilibrium—intake approximately equals output. When nitrogen intake exceeds nitrogen output, a positive nitrogen balance exists. Such a condition is present in the following physiological states: pregnancy, lactation, recovery from a severe illness, muscular buildup, growth, and following the administration of an anabolic steroid such as testosterone. A positive nitrogen balance indicates that new tissue is being formed. A negative nitrogen balance occurs when nitrogen intake is less than output. Starvation, diabetes mellitus, fever, surgery, burns or shock can all result in a negative nitrogen balance. This is an undesirable state

since body protein is being broken down faster than it is being built up. Table P-27 provides examples of nitrogen balance.

TABLE P-27
THREE EXAMPLES OF NITROGEN BALANCE FOR A 154 LB *(70 KG)* MALE

Nitrogen Intake and Output[1]	Equilibrium	Positive	Negative
	(g/day)	(g/day)	(g/day)
Intake			
Food	9.0	9.0	9.0
Output			
Urine	7.2	4.8	11.3
Feces	1.1	1.0	0.8
Skin[2]	0.4	0.4	0.4
Total output	8.7	6.2	12.5
Balance	+ 0.3	+ 2.8	− 3.5

[1]To convert to protein multiply by 6.25.
[2]This includes losses of nitrogen in perspiration, hair, nails, sloughed skin, saliva, and seminal ejaculation.

For Protein.   Proper nitrogen balance studies are performed over a period of days, and are very time consuming. Often an estimate of nitrogen balance is made by collecting and measuring nitrogen in the urine, since the end products of protein metabolism leave the body mainly via this route. About 90% of the nitrogen in urine is urea and ammonia salts—the end products of protein metabolism. The remaining 10% of the nitrogen in the urine is present as uric acid and creatinine which are products of the metabolism of purines and pyrimidines, and creatine, respectively. The nitrogen lost in the feces consists of unabsorbed dietary proteins, bacteria, and intestinal residues. Small losses of protein from skin, hair, fingernails, perspiration, and other secretions are difficult to measure and are also estimated.

Using nitrogen balance as a tool, the recommended daily dietary allowance for protein may be derived on the following basis:

1.   Obligatory urinary nitrogen losses of young adults amount to about 37 mg/kg of body weight.

2.   Fecal nitrogen losses average 12 mg/kg of body weight.

3.   Amounts of nitrogen lost in the perspiration, hair, fingernails, and sloughed skin are estimated at 3 mg/kg of body weight.

4.   Minor routes of nitrogen loss such as saliva, menstruation, and seminal ejaculation are estimated at 2 mg/kg of body weight.

5.   The total obligatory nitrogen lost—that which must be replaced daily—amounts to 54 mg/kg, or in terms of protein lost this is 0.34 g/kg.

6.   To account for individual variation the daily loss is increased by 30%, or 70 mg/kg. In terms of protein, this is 0.45 g/kg of body weight.

7.   This protein loss is further increased by 30%, to 0.6 g/kg of body weight, to account for the loss of efficiency when consuming even a high quality protein such as egg.

8.   The final adjustment is to correct for the 75% efficiency of utilization of protein in the mixed diet of Americans. Thus, the daily recommended allowance for protein becomes 0.8 g/kg of body weight for normal healthy adult males and females, or 63 g of protein per day for a 174-lb (*79 kg*) man and 50 g per day for a 138-lb (*63 kg*) woman.

The above calculations are summarized in Table P-28.

Growth, pregnancy, and lactation, and possibly work and stress, require an additional intake of protein. Aging may present some special considerations. A discussion of each of these special needs follows:

• **Growth**—During the first year of life, the protein content of the body increases from about 11% to about 15%, and body weight increases by about 15 lb (*7 kg*). By four years of age, body protein content reaches the adult value of 18 to 19%. In estimating protein needs between infancy and maturity, allowances are adjusted upward to ensure a satisfactory rate of growth.

For infants, the allowances are based on the amount of protein provided by a milk intake which ensures a satisfactory rate of growth. This is estimated to be between 2 to 2.4 g/kg/day during the first month of life, gradually declining to 1.5 g/kg/day by the sixth month of

TABLE P-28
CALCULATION OF THE RECOMMENDED DAILY ALLOWANCE FOR PROTEIN

Factor	In Terms Of Nitrogen	In Terms Of Protein
	(g/kg)	(g/kg)
Obligatory urinary loss	.037	.231
Fecal loss	.012	.075
Loss due to perspiration, hair, fingernails, and sloughed skin	.003	.019
Loss due to saliva, menstruation, and seminal ejaculation	.002	.013
Estimated total daily loss . . .	.054	.340
Allowance for individual variation (+30%)	.016	.110
Total	.070	.450
Loss of efficiency (+30%) . .	.020	.150
Total	.090	.600
Correction for the 75% efficiency of utilization of protein in the mixed American diet (divide by .75)	.120[1]	.800

[1]Throughout the calculations, some rounding errors have occurred.

life. For those infants over 6 months of age this 1.5 g/kg/day is adjusted upward to allow for a 75% efficiency of utilization of proteins from a mixed diet, since infants by this time consume foods other than milk. Hence, the allowance for infants between 6 months and 1 year of age becomes 2.0 g/kg/day.

Daily protein allowances for growing children and young adults are calculated from information which has been collected on growth rates and body composition. These allowances assume that the efficiency of protein conversion to tissue for growth is comparable to that observed in adults—about 75%. These allowances decrease gradually between 1 year of age and 18 years of age (see Table P-29).

• **Pregnancy**—The protein allowance for the pregnant woman must cover the needs for both maternal physiological adjustments—expansion of blood volume, uterus and breast—and growth and development of the fetus and placenta. By the end of pregnancy, about 2 lb (*925 g*) of extra protein has been deposited. Still, many uncertainties are involved in the protein requirement of pregnancy. Therefore, a generous allowance of an additional 30 g/day is recommended to prevent the possibility of any adverse effects on the mother or fetus from an inadequate protein intake. This amount is generous in view of the amount of 10 g per day toward the end of pregnancy which can be derived from actual daily accumulation of protein adjusted for individual variability, efficiency of conversion to tissue protein, and mixed dietary protein sources.

According to the RDAs, then, the pregnant adult allowance for protein is 60 g/day. Pregnant adolescents should receive the protein allowance for their nonpregnant body weight plus an additional allowance for pregnancy. Hence, a pregnant female age 11 to 14 should receive 46 g plus 14 g of protein per day.

• **Lactation**—Additional protein needed by the nursing mother is related to the quantity of milk protein produced. The protein content of human milk normally decreases during the first few months of lactation, falling from an average of 1.54 g/100 ml at 14 days to 0.87 g/100 ml at 112 days after birth. Assuming an average content of 1.2 g/100 ml and average daily production of 850 ml, the daily protein yield is approximately 10 g/day.

The efficiency of conversion of dietary protein to milk protein is not known, but it is probably similar to that for protein utilization for other body functions—about 70%. Taking this into account, as well as individual variations such as the possibility of production rates in excess of 850 ml/day, the dietary protein allowance for the lactating woman calls for an addition of 15 g/day to that for the nonpregnant and nonlactating woman.

The Food and Nutrition Board (FNB) of the National Research Council (NRC) recommended daily allowances of protein are given in Table P-29.

TABLE P-29
RECOMMENDED DAILY PROTEIN ALLOWANCES[1]

Group	Age	Weight		Height		RDA
	(years)	(lb)	(kg)	(in.)	(cm)	(g)
Infants	0.0–0.5	13	6	24	60	13
	0.5–1.0	20	9	28	71	14
Children	1–3	29	13	35	90	16
	4–6	44	20	44	112	24
	7–10	62	28	52	132	28
Males	11–14	99	45	62	157	45
	15–18	145	66	69	176	59
	19–24	160	72	70	177	58
	25–50	174	79	70	178	63
	51+	170	77	68	173	63
Females	11–14	101	46	62	157	46
	15–18	120	55	64	163	44
	19–24	128	58	65	164	46
	25–50	138	63	64	163	50
	51+	143	65	63	160	50
Pregnant						60
Lactating						65

[1]*Recommended Dietary Allowances*, 10th ed., 1989, NRC-National Academy of Sciences, p. 284.

• **Work and stress**—Protein needs which may be imposed by work or stress are not included in Table P-29. There is little evidence that muscular activity increases the need for protein, except by the small amount required for the development of muscles during conditioning, especially at energy intakes not adjusted for the increased work done. However, vigorous activity that leads to profuse sweating, such as in heavy work and sports, increases nitrogen loss from the skin. This does not seem to be accompanied by a decrease in urinary nitrogen loss. Calculations indicate that skin losses can be substantial. However, it seems that with acclimatization to a warm environment, the excessive skin loss is reduced. The recommended daily allowances contain a margin of safety; hence, no increment is added for work or training.

Extreme environmental or physiological stress increases nitrogen loss. Moreover, some evidence also suggests that less severe stress may also increase nitrogen loss. Infections, fevers, and surgical trauma can result in substantial urinary nitrogen loss and greatly increased energy expenditure. Severe infections and surgery should be treated as clinical conditions that require special dietary treatment. During convalescence from an illness that has led to protein depletion, requirements for both protein and energy are elevated just as they are during periods of rapid growth.

Day-to-day living may also impose stress on individuals which can cause brief periods of increased urinary nitrogen output. However, it is assumed that the individuals used in the experiments forming the basis for the protein requirement estimates are usually exposed to the same stresses; hence, no added allowance is made for the stress of daily living.
(Also see STRESS.)

• **Aging**—The elderly may require special consideration since their energy intake and needs tend to be low. On the basis of the intakes of protein and energy recommended for persons over 50 years old, some 10% of the calories are provided by the protein allowance. Energy intake per unit of body weight falls progressively with age, but the amount of protein per unit of body weight needed for nitrogen equilibrium may even increase. Furthermore, the elderly often experience recurring episodes of chronic diseases requiring restoration of protein. Therefore, it seems wise to ensure that the elderly receive 12% or more of their energy intake in the form of protein. Assuming 4 Calories (kcal) of energy per gram of protein, Table P-30 presents the recommended protein allowance for the elderly on the basis of their energy intake.

TABLE P–30
RECOMMENDED DAILY PROTEIN ALLOWANCES FOR THE ELDERLY[1]

Group	Age	Weight		Height		Energy Needs	Protein
	(years)	(lb)	(kg)	(in.)	(cm)	(kcal)	(g)
Males	51+	170	77	68	173	2,300	63
Females	51+	143	65	63	160	1,900	50

[1]Based on 12% of the energy intake in the form of protein. Age, weight, height, and energy needs are from *Recommended Dietary Allowances*, 10th ed., 1989, NRC-National Academy of Sciences, p. 284.

For Amino Acids. The requirement for protein carries a restriction. Protein must supply individuals with amounts of the essential amino acids at levels sufficient to meet the protein synthesizing needs of the body. Based on a number of studies on infants, children, and adults, some estimated daily requirements for the essential amino acids have been made; and these are listed in Table P-31.

TABLE P–31
ESTIMATED AMINO ACID REQUIREMENTS OF MAN[1]

Amino Acid	Requirement, mg/kg Body Weight/Day			
	Infants	Children		Adults
	(3–4 mo.)	(2 yr)	(10–12 yr)	
Histidine	16	19	19	11
Isoleucine	40	28	28	13
Leucine	93	66	44	19
Lysine	60	58	44	16
Total S-containing amino acids (methionine and cystine) . . .	33	25	22	17
Total aromatic amino acids (phenylalanine and tyrosine) . .	72	63	22	19
Threonine	50	34	28	9
Tryptophan	10	11	(9)	5
Valine	54	35	25	13

[1]*Recommended Dietary Allowances*, 10th ed., 1989, NRC-National Academy of Sciences, p. 67.

These requirements are adequate only when the diet provides enough nitrogen for the synthesis of the nonessential amino acids so that the essential amino acids will not be used to supply amino groups for the nonessential amino acids via the process of transamination. Even in infants the essential amino acids make up only about 35% of the total need for protein. In adults, essential amino acids account for less than 20% of the total protein requirement. Most proteins contain plenty of dispensable amino acids; usually the concern is to meet the essential amino acid needs, particularly of infants and children.

It should be noted from Table P-31 that on a weight basis infants and children require larger amounts of essential amino acids by virtue of their higher rate of protein synthesis. Currently, there are no specific essential amino acid requirements for pregnancy and lactation, but these are states which involve new protein synthesis.

SOURCES. The protein content of numerous foods is given in Food Composition Table F-36. Furthermore, Table P-32 lists the top food sources of protein.

NOTE WELL: The table lists (1) the top sources without regard to the amount normally eaten or the amino acid content (left column), and (2) the top food sources (right column); and the protein and energy content of each food.

Unfortunately, meeting the protein requirement is more involved than just choosing foods which provide the daily amount of protein. As indicated, the requirement for protein is primarily a requirement for essential amino acids. In terms of amino acid composition, all proteins are not created equal. Some proteins of certain foods are low or completely devoid of some essential amino acids. Hence, meeting the protein requirement demands quality as well as quantity.

Quantity and Quality. Protein values such as those in Table P-32 and Food Composition Table F-36 are crude protein values derived by the Kjeldahl method, which determines the nitrogen content of a substance and then assumes that each gram of nitrogen represents 6.25 g of protein. This procedure estimates protein quantity; and quantity is important. For example, boiled potatoes contain 1.9 g of protein per 3½ oz (*100 g*). To obtain just the extra 30 g of protein daily during pregnancy, a woman would have to consume about 3½ lb (*1.6 kg*) of potatoes, while only 3½ to 4 oz (*100 to 113 g*) of beef, fish, or poultry would supply the extra 30 g of protein. Still, crude protein values may be misleading. For example, Table P-32 shows gelatin ranking second among top protein sources; yet, gelatin contains virtually no tryptophan and very low levels of other essential amino acids. Used as a protein source, gelatin will not support growth or life. Hence, some evaluation of protein quality is necessary.

TABLE P-32
TOP SOURCES OF PROTEIN AND THEIR CALORIC CONTENT[1]

Top Sources[2]	Protein (g/100 g)	Energy (kcal/100 g)	Top Food Sources	Protein (g/100 g)	Energy (kcal/100 g)
Fish, flour from filets	93	398	Soybean flour[3]	45	356
Gelatin, dry	86	335	Veal cutlet, breaded	34	319
Eggs, chicken, dried, white powder .	82	372	Turkey, all classes, light meat,		
Cod, dehydrated, lightly salted	82	375	cooked, roasted	33	176
Fish, flour from whole fish	76	307	Chicken, light meat w/o skin, fried . .	33	197
Eggs, chicken, dried, white flakes . . .	75	351	Beef, separable, lean cooked[4]	31	190
Soybean protein	75	322	Pork, fresh, loin, separable		
Fish, flour from filet waste	71	305	lean cooked	31	260
Eggs, chicken, dried, whole,			Cheese, natural Swiss (domestic) . . .	29	372
stabilized	48	609	Lamb, leg, separable, lean, roasted . .	29	186
Cottonseed, flour	48	356	Cod, broiled	29	170
Peanut, flour, defatted	48	371	Tuna, canned in water, solids/liquid		
Sunflower seed, flour,			with or without added salt	28	123
partially defatted	45	339	Peanuts, redskin	28	608
Soybean, flour[3]	45	356	Beef, hamburger, lean, cooked		
Safflower seed, meal,			w/10% fat	27	219
partially defatted	42	388	Cheese, natural Cheddar		
Soybean, milk powder	41	429	(domestic American)	25	402
Cheese, natural Parmesan, grated . .	41	456	Herring, cooked, Atlantic	24	255
Wheat, flour, gluten (45% gluten/			Trout, cooked	24	196
55% patent flour)	41	378	Nuts, mixed, dry roasted	22	590
Almond, meal, partially defatted	40	408	Cheese, natural cottage (large or		
Yeast, brewers', debittered	39	283	small curd, uncreamed	17	85
Yeast, torula	39	277	Wheat, flour, whole		
			(from hard wheats)	13	361
			Eggs, chicken, hard cooked or		
			poached	13	156

[1]These listings are based on the data in Food Composition Table F-36 of this book, and are listed without regard to amino acid content.
Whenever possible, foods are on an "as used" basis, without regard to moisture content; hence, certain high-moisture foods may be disadvantaged when ranked on the basis of protein content per 100 g (approximately 3½ oz) without regard to moisture content.
[2]Listed without regard to the amount normally eaten, or amino acid content.
[3]Average for defatted, low fat and high fat.
[4]Includes the following cuts: T-bone, Porterhouse, sirloin, hindshank, and chuck.

In 1911, T. B. Osborne, of the Connecticut Agricultural Experiment Station, and L. B. Mendel, of Yale University, formed a brilliant partnership and pioneered in studies of protein quality. They fed rats diets containing 18% protein in the form of either (1) the milk protein, casein; (2) the wheat protein, gliadin; or (3) the corn protein, zein. The rats whose sole protein source was casein remained healthy and grew normally; the rats fed gliadin only maintained their body weight but did not grow; the rats fed zein not only failed to grow but actually lost weight and failed to survive if left on the zein diet. The protein gliadin is very low in the amino acid lysine, and zein is low in both lysine and tryptophan. Subsequently, when the rat's diets were supplemented with adequate lysine and/or tryptophan all rats grew and thrived. Another experiment by Osborne and Mendel demonstrated that adequate amounts of even a good protein like casein were necessary for growth. Rats fed diets containing 9% protein as casein grew only one-half as fast as those receiving 18% protein as casein. Hence, quality and quantity of protein are both important. This early work on the quality of protein resulted in proteins being classified as complete, partially incomplete, and incomplete. Complete proteins contain all of the essential amino acids in sufficient amounts to maintain life and support growth. Partially incomplete proteins can maintain life, but cannot support growth. Incomplete proteins cannot maintain life or support growth. These terms are still used by some when describing protein quality. Following the work of Osborne and

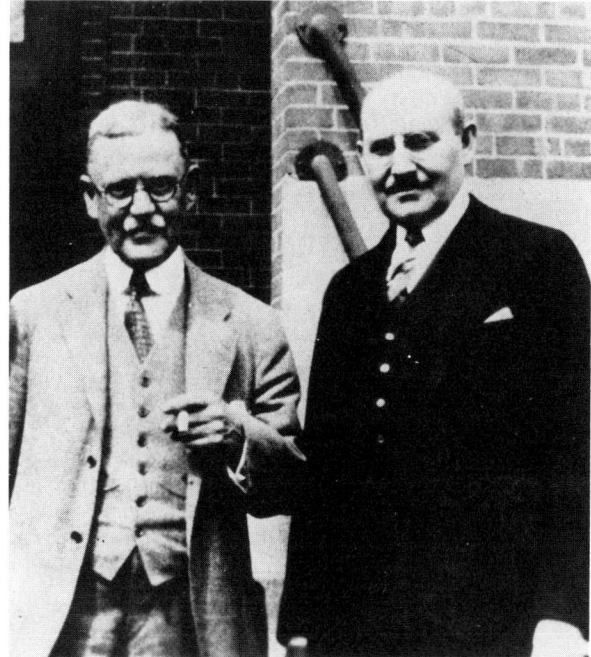

Fig. P-114. Thomas B. Osborne (left) and Lafayette B. Mendel (right), who pioneered in studies of protein quality. (Courtesy, The Connecticut Agricultural Experiment Station, New Haven, Conn.)

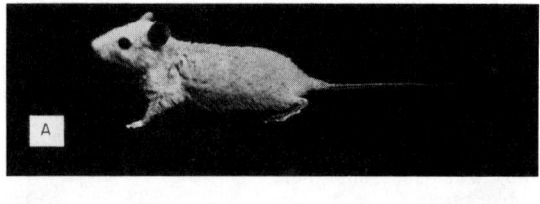

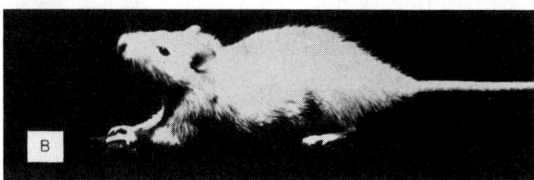

Fig. P-115.   Stunting of growth due to feeding an incomplete protein. The two rats were the same age (140 days old) and were fed the same diets except for the protein. Rat A received gliadin from wheat—an incomplete protein, deficient in the amino acid lysine, whereas rat B received casein from milk—a complete protein. (From experiments by Osborne and Mendel. Courtesy, The Connecticut Agricultural Experiment Station, New Haven, Conn.)

Mendel, there was a quest for some method of evaluating proteins in terms of their ability to meet the needs of the body. The following are descriptions of some of these methods:

• **Biological value**—In a 1924 publication, Karl Thomas and Harold H. Mitchell proposed a method for determining the biological value of a protein—the percentage of the true digestible protein utilized by the body. This method assumes that the retained nitrogen—ingested nitrogen not recovered in the urine or feces—represents a perfect assortment of amino acids utilized by the body. The following equation indicates how the biological value (BV) is determined:

$$\frac{100 \times \text{N intake} - \left(\frac{\text{feces N} - \text{metabolic N}}{\text{urine N} - \text{endogenous N}}\right)}{\text{N intake} - (\text{feces N} - \text{metabolic N})} = \% \text{ BV}$$

In the above equation, N stands for nitrogen, while the metabolic and endogenous nitrogen are determined during a pretest period when a protein-free diet is fed so that the nitrogen retained from the food may be distinguished. Hence, the biological value is estimated from measurements of nitrogen intake and losses made under carefully standardized conditions with protein intakes that are below the requirement level. Biological value is a measure of the efficiency of utilization of absorbed nitrogen, and it depends primarily on the amino acid composition of the dietary protein. Needless to say, determining the quality of protein in the diet by this means is time-consuming, and hence, not often used. Moreover, few animals other than rats will consume protein-free diets long enough to complete the trial. However, biological value is often used to describe protein quality.

• **Net protein utilization (NPU)**—Digestibility is estimated from the quantity ingested that is subsequently not recovered in the feces, expressed as a percentage of the intake. The multiplication of the biological value and the digestibility gives the net protein utilization, a measure of the efficiency of overall utilization of the ingested nitrogen. For proteins that are completely digested, net protein utilization and biological value are the same. For less digestible proteins or for foods containing large amounts of fiber, the biological value does not provide a measure of efficiency of utilization of the protein consumed—only the efficiency of utilization of that absorbed.

• **Protein efficiency ratio (PER)**—This is the simplest test of protein quality, and the one used widely in comparing the nutritive value of proteins in individual foods. The PER is defined as the weight gain of a growing animal divided by its protein intake over the period studied, often 10 days. Although simple in application, it does not provide protein evaluations that are directly proportional to quality, because no account is taken of loss of weight when animals are given no protein in the diet. It assumes that all protein is used for growth and no allowance for maintenance is made.

• **Net protein ratio (NPR)**—This method attempts to correct the fault of the PER by making some allowance for maintenance. The NPR accomplishes this by the inclusion of a control group of animals receiving no dietary protein. Thus, the NPR is the weight gain of a group of animals (rats) fed the test diet plus the weight loss of a similar group fed a protein-free diet, and the total divided by the weight of the protein consumed by the animals on the test diet.

• **Nitrogen balance index**—This method is similar to the biological value but there is no period of feeding a protein-free diet. It is simply the nitrogen in the food minus that in the urine and feces. Nitrogen balance has been used as a means of evaluating protein foods in the human diet and determining the amino acid requirements of humans. When proteins (amino acids) are adequate in the diet, the nitrogen balance is positive. W. C. Rose, using a diet consisting of sugar, starch, fat, and a mixed solution of purified amino acids in known amounts, was the first to determine the amount of each essential amino acid needed for young men. One at a time, the amino acids were left out of the solution and nitrogen balance was noted. When the omitted amino acid was essential, a negative nitrogen balance resulted. The method used for determining the nutritive value of proteins for humans is an extension of nitrogen balance and is termed a nitrogen balance index. The food to be evaluated is fed at several intakes below and slightly above nitrogen equilibrium. Then, values for nitrogen balance versus nitrogen absorbed or nitrogen intake are plotted on a graph, and a straight line connects these points and the slope of the line is determined. When nitrogen intake is used in place of nitrogen absorbed, the values obtained are equivalent to net protein utilization (NPU).

• **Slope ratio method**—This is a modification of the nitrogen balance index wherein various levels of protein are fed *ad libitum* to growing animals. Then growth rate and protein intake are plotted on a graph, and the slope of this line is taken as the measure of protein quality.

• **Chemical score (CS)**—By chemically examining the essential amino acid content of a food, some idea of its nutritive value may be gained. To determine the chemical score one must first have a reference pattern of amino acid concentrations with which to compare the dietary protein. Table P-33 indicates what type of amino acid pattern a high-quality protein should possess in order to meet the body's needs. This amino acid pattern is based on the essential amino acid requirements of children 10 to 12 years of age. Also, Table P-33 shows how the essential amino acid patterns of human milk and eggs compare to that of the requirement of children

TABLE P–33
AMINO ACID REQUIREMENT OF CHILDREN 10–12 YEARS COMPARED TO THE AMINO ACID PROFILES OF HUMAN MILK AND EGGS

Amino Acid	Amino Acid Requirement for Children 10–12 Years[1]	Human Milk[2]	Whole Egg[2]
	(mg/g protein)		
Histidine	19	26	22
Isoleucine	28	46	54
Leucine	44	93	86
Lysine	44	66	70
Methionine and cystine	22	42	57
Phenylalanine and tyrosine	22	72	93
Threonine	28	43	47
Tryptophan	9	17	17
Valine	25	55	66

[1]*Recommended Dietary Allowances*, 10th ed., 1989, National Academy of Sciences, p. 67, Table 6–5.
[2]Values for the protein and amino acid content are from Proteins and Amino Acids in Selected Foods Table p. 37.

10 to 12 years of age. Human milk and eggs are frequently used as standards due to their amino acid patterns. The reference or standard pattern is assigned a value of 100, and the percentage by which each essential amino acid in the food or dietary protein differs from the value of the standard is calculated. The essential amino acid showing the greatest deficit is considered to be the amino acid limiting utilization of the protein. The amount of this amino acid present, expressed as a percentage of that in the standard, provides the chemical score. This score usually shows good agreement with biological evaluation of protein quality but tends to overestimate quality for proteins that are not well digested.

The following equation may be used to calculate the chemical score of each essential amino acid:

$$CS = \frac{\text{mg of amino acid per g test protein x 100}}{\text{mg of amino acid per g reference protein}}$$

Often, only the chemical scores for lysine, methionine and cystine, and tryptophan are calculated as one of these is commonly the limiting amino acid. The following is an example for potatoes:

1. Consider the reference pattern of whole eggs:
   Methionine and cystine   56 mg/g
   Lysine   68 mg/g
   Tryptophan   16 mg/g

2. List the amount of the same amino acids in the protein of potatoes:
   Methionine and cystine   27 mg/g
   Lysine   127 mg/g
   Tryptophan   35 mg/g

3. Calculate the chemical score for these amino acids as indicated by the above formula:
   Methionine and cystine   48
   Lysine   187
   Tryptophan   219

Obviously, the amino acids methionine and cystine—the sulfur-containing amino acids—are limiting in potatoes.

• **Net dietary protein calories percent (NDₚCal%)**—This method of evaluating protein considers the percentage of the calories from protein in the food which is adjusted according to the net protein utilization (NPU) or quality. The following formula describes NDₚCal%:

$$ND_pCal\% = \frac{\text{g of protein x 4 kcal x 100}}{\text{total kcal in food or diet}} \times NPU$$

Table P-34 demonstrates how some of these methods compare when used to estimate the quality of some common foods.

TABLE P-34

COMPARISONS OF VARIOUS METHODS FOR ESTIMATING THE PROTEIN QUALITY OF SOME COMMON FOODS

Food	Protein	Energy	Digesti-bility	Bio-logical Value (BV)	Net Protein Utilization (NPU)	Net Dietary Net Dietary Calories (ND$_p$Cal)	Protein Efficiency Ratio (PER)	Chemical Score (CS)[1]	Limiting Amino Acid
	(g/100 g)	(kcal/100 g)	(%)	(%)	(%)	(%)			
Eggs............	13	163	99	94	94	30	3.92	100	None
Cow's milk, whole .	4	66	97	85	82	20	3.09	61	Methionine and cystine
Fish	19	125	98	83	81	49	3.55	75	Tryptophan
Beef	18	250	99	74	74	21	2.30	69	Valine
Chicken	21	120	95	74	70	49	—	67	Valine
Pork	12	350	—	74	—	—	—	68	Methionine and cystine
Gelatin	86	335	—	—	3	3	−1.25	0	Tryptophan
Soybeans.......	34	403	90	73	66	22	2.32	46	Methionine and cystine
Common dry beans	22	340	73	58	42	11	1.48	34	Methionine and cystine
Peanuts	26	564	87	55	48	9	1.65	43	Methionine and cystine
Brewers' yeast....	39	283	84	67	56	31	2.24	45	Methionine and cystine
Wheat, whole grain	12	330	91	66	60	9	1.50	48	Lysine
Corn, whole grain .	9	355	90	60	54	5	1.12	40	Lysine
Brown rice	8	360	96	73	70	6	—	56	Lysine
White rice	7	363	98	64	63	5	2.18	53	Lysine
Potato	2	76	89	73	5	7	—	48	Methionine and cystine

[1]Using egg as a reference protein.

One must bear in mind that each method for evaluating protein quality is only a tool to aid in identifying foods capable of meeting the protein—amino acid—needs of the body. These protein quality measurements are useful for comparing the nutritive value of different lots of a single protein, such as an infant formula, a processed food, or a uniform diet for man or animals. However, measurements made on individual foodstuffs do not give useful information about the protein quality of complex human diets. The only meaningful measure of the protein quality of a diet is one made on the total diet as consumed. To this end, there are some steps which can be taken to ensure that the total diet provides the needed amino acids.

Complementary Proteins. Fortunately, the amino acid deficiencies in a protein can usually be improved by combining it with another, and the mixture of the two proteins will often have a higher food value than either one alone. In other words proteins having opposite strengths and weaknesses complement each other. For example, many cereals are low in lysine, but high in methionine and cystine. On the other hand, soybeans, lima beans, and kidney beans are high in lysine but low in methionine and cystine. When eaten together, the deficiencies are corrected. Complementary protein combinations are found in almost all cultures. In the Middle East, bread and cheese are eaten together. Mexicans eat beans and corn (tortillas). Indians eat wheat and pulses (legumes). Americans eat breakfast cereals with milk. This kind of supplementation works only when the deficient and complementary proteins are ingested together or within a few hours of each other. For those who are interested, the protein and amino acid content for a variety of foods are given in the Proteins and Amino Acids in Selected Foods Table P-37, at the last of this article. By using the information contained in Table P-34, chemical scores for the various foods may be derived and a better idea of complementary proteins can be gained. Table P-35 shows the weaknesses of some common foods which may serve as protein sources. Some examples of complementary food proteins may include: (1) rice and black-eyed peas; (2) whole wheat or bulgur, soybeans, and sesame seeds; (3) cornmeal and kidney beans; and (4) soybeans, peanuts, brown rice, and bulgur wheat.

TABLE P-35
THE CHEMICAL SCORES, LIMITING AMINO ACIDS, AND NET PROTEIN UTILIZATION (NPU) OF SOME FOODS

Food	Chemical Score Based on the Egg Essential Amino Acid Pattern	Limiting Amino Acid	NPU
Egg	100	—	100
Egg albumin	90	tryptophan	83
Rye	90	threonine	—
Spinach	90	methionine and cystine	—
Beef	80	methionine and cystine	80
Cottonseed meal	80	methionine and cystine	66
Pork tenderloin	80	methionine and cystine	84
Sweet potato	75	methionine and cystine	72
Fish	75	tryptophan	83
Rice	75	lysine	57
Beef heart	70	methionine and cystine	67
Beef liver	70	methionine and cystine	65
Beet kidney	70	methionine and cystine	77
Oats	70	lysine	—
Peanut flour	70	methionine and cystine	48
Soybean flour	70	methionine and cystine	56
Sunflower seed	70	lysine	65
Wheat germ	65	methionine and cystine	67
Casein	60	methionine and cystine	72
Milk (cow's)	60	methionine and cystine	75
Millet	60	lysine	56
Peas	60	methionine and cystine	44
Sesame seed	50	lysine	56
White flour	50	lysine	52
Potato	48	methionine and cystine	71
Cornmeal	45	tryptophan	55
Navy bean	42	methionine and cystine	47
Cassava	40	methionine and cystine	—
Wheat gluten	40	lysine	37

Factors Affecting Amino Acid Utilization. The presence of amino acids in a protein does not assure their utilization. So, in addition to the amino acid content of a food(s), the following related factors must be considered:

• **Digestibility**—The amino acids of most animal proteins are efficiently absorbed, but this is not necessarily so for many proteins of plant origin. Animal proteins are about 90 to 95% digestible, but the digestibility of some plant proteins may be as low as 73% (see Table P-34).

• **Energy**—Protein is used inefficiently when the energy intake is grossly inadequate. When the energy intake is below a certain level, the nutritive value of the protein to the consumer diminishes. For example, an increase in the protein supply to undernourished subjects will not be fully effective if the energy content of the diet is restricted. This principle also applies to replenishment of body protein following malnutrition and during convalescence after injury or disease; full utilization of dietary protein for replenishment is best assured by an adequate calorie intake.

The influence of calorie intake on protein metabolism is shown by the rapid development of a negative nitrogen balance when the energy content of the diet is reduced below requirements—an unfavorable effect which persists if the sub-maintenance diet continues to be fed. From this, it can be concluded that an inadequate intake of energy will, by itself, cause a loss of protein from the body and will consequently aggravate protein deficiency in the diet. Hence, carbohydrates are said to have a protein-sparing effect. A daily intake of 50 to 100 g of digestible carbohydrates is required for protein-sparing.

• **Vitamins and minerals**—Any essential mineral or vitamin whose presence is needed for normal growth and metabolism can be presumed to affect utilization of dietary protein, in so far as deficiency of the vitamin or mineral leads to loss of body substance. For this reason, tests of protein quality are normally performed with diets containing adequate amounts of vitamins and minerals.

In treating persons with protein deficiency, the supply of some vitamins and minerals appears to be more critical than that of others. In particular enough niacin, potassium, and phosphorus should be given to ensure that they are not limiting factors in protein replenishment. Thus, in a niacin deficiency, not only is tryptophan converted to niacin when present in excess but there is evidence that some conversion may occur even when there is insufficient tryptophan for protein synthesis.

(Also see MINERAL[S]; and VITAMIN[S].)

• **Amino acid imbalances**—One type of amino acid imbalance arises when the addition of a single amino acid or mixture of amino acids to a diet reduces the utilization of the dietary protein. Even a small increase in the concentrations of certain amino acids can increase the needs for others when the total protein intake is low.

Utilization of one dietary amino acid may also be depressed by addition to the diet of another structurally related to it. The two best-known examples are the interference of an excess of leucine with the utilization of isoleucine and valine, and the interference of lysine with the utilization of arginine. Large amounts of single amino acids added to experimental diets may induce various toxic reactions, including depression of growth. The most toxic amino acids are methionine, tyrosine, and histidine, and their effect is most serious when the diet is low in protein.

Not enough is presently known about the practical bearing these observations may have in relation to human diets but they must be taken into account in studies of the biological effectiveness of essential amino acid patterns. Circumstances in which amino acid imbalances would occur are unlikely in individuals at normal levels of dietary protein.

• **Nonessential amino acid nitrogen**—The proportion of nonessential amino acid nitrogen has an influence on the essential amino acid requirements. If the ratio of essential amino acids to the total nitrogen in a food is too high, essential amino acids will be used as a source of nitrogen for the nonessential amino acids which, in spite of their being so designated, are necessary parts of the protein molecule and hence, needed for protein synthesis. When the nonessential amino acids are in short supply, some of the essential amino acids furnish nitrogen (NH_2) more readily than others for the synthesis of the nonessential amino acids.

• **Food processing**—Heat and chemicals used during processing can affect amino acid availability. Loss of available lysine can occur from mild heat treatment in the presence of reducing sugars such as glucose or lactose. For example, during mild processing, the sugar reacts with free amino groups of lysine to render lysine unavailable. This may also occur when the protein and sugar are stored together at low temperatures. Under severe heating conditions, in the presence of either sugars or oxidized lipids or even without either of these, food proteins form additional chemical bonds and can become resistant to digestion so that availability of all amino acids is reduced. Small amounts of sugar promote more chemical bonds. When protein is exposed to severe treatment with alkali, lysine and cysteine can be eliminated, with formation of lysinoalanine which may be toxic. The use of oxidizing agents such as sulfur dioxide (SO_2) give rise to a loss of methionine in the protein, through the formation of methionine sulfoxide.

Heating can also have favorable effects. Heating soybean flour improves the utilization of protein by making the amino acid methionine more available, and heating raw soybeans destroys the inhibitor of the protein digestive enzyme trypsin. Cooking eggs destroys the trypsin inhibitor ovomucoid in the white.

PROTEIN MALNUTRITION.   Protein deficiency is common worldwide. This is primarily because in many underdeveloped areas of the world, protein intake is marginal, but energy intake is so low that the protein eaten is not spared for its essential functions. The name, protein-energy (calorie) malnutrition is applied to a whole spectrum of protein and energy deficiencies. At one end of the spectrum is kwashiorkor—a severe clinical syndrome caused by a deficiency of protein. Pertinent protein malnutrition information follows:

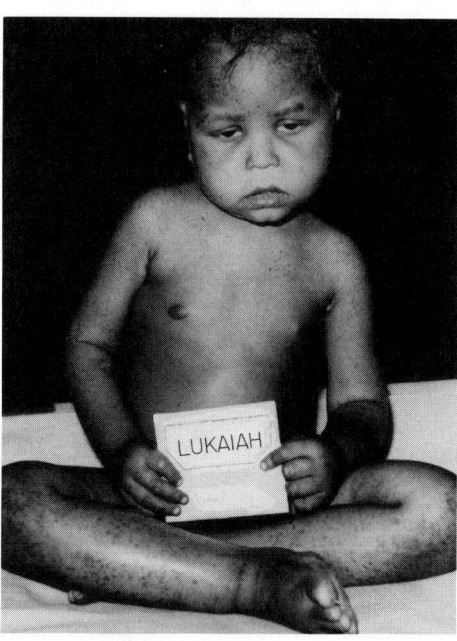

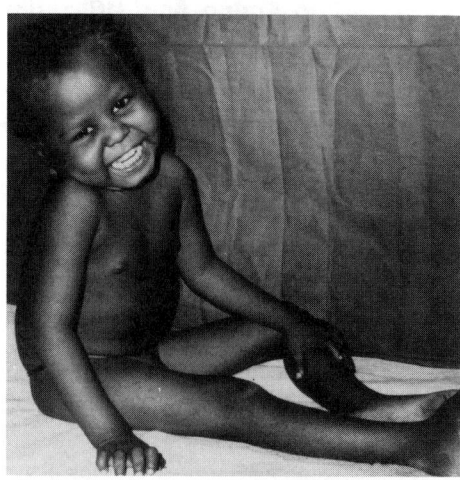

Fig. P-116.   A 4½-year-old child from South India suffering from kwashiorkor. *Top:* Lukaiah before rehabilitation weighed 21½ lb (*9.8 kg*) and was in a state of severe kwashiorkor showing edema, hair and skin changes, and misery. *Bottom:* After 1 month of rehabilitation, Lukaiah weighed almost 24 lb (*10.9 kg*). The edema disappeared; the skin was normal, and the hair was recovering. Furthermore, Lukaiah was happy and full of mischief—like any child. (Courtesy, WHO, Geneva, Switzerland)

• **Kwashiorkor**—Infants fed low-protein, starchy foods such as bananas, yams, and cassava after weaning may develop kwashiorkor. Often, the weaning is not by choice but birth of a new baby. This imbalanced diet, which has a subnormal protein-to-calorie ratio for infants, prevents some of the adaptive mechanisms of the body from operating the way that they do in the case of starvation or marasmus—a wasting condition due to lack of food.

In kwashiorkor there is less breakdown of protein and release of amino acids from muscle than in marasmus since provision of adequate energy in the diet reduces the adrenal gland response and, consequently, the flow of amino acids from muscle is not sufficient to meet the synthesizing needs of the internal organs. Particularly critical is the loss of tissue cells from the gastrointestinal lining which leads to various types of malabsorption. Also, the severe shortage of protein results in a reduction in synthesis of digestive enzymes, normally secreted from the pancreas or present in the intestinal wall. Thus, there is likely to be diarrhea which may cause excessive loss of water or dehydration, loss of mineral salts, and an electrolyte imbalance.

Liver function is greatly reduced due to lack of protein for the synthesis of enzymes. Also, there is likely to be fat accumulation in the liver due to its inability to package fat with protein for transport in the blood. Low blood levels of albumin, along with anemia, result from the scarcity of amino acids for protein synthesis. Edema—swelling—is a consequence of the depletion of plasma proteins and electrolytes.

The production of antibodies is likely to be greatly reduced and the victim, therefore, will be prone to infectious diseases. In chronic cases, there is likely to be delayed eruption of teeth, poor enamel with many caries, and pale gums and mucous membranes due to anemia.

Besides the physical changes there are also some mental changes such as general indifference, irritability, and apathy.
(Also see MALNUTRITION.)

Both dietary protein and energy supplies are adequate in the United States. For the past 70 years, individuals in the United States have derived about 12% of their calories from protein. For a man consuming 2,700 Calories (kcal) daily, or a woman consuming 2,000 Calories (kcal) daily, this converts to 81 g and 60 g of protein, respectively. Furthermore, dietary surveys indicate that in the United States, protein intake is considerably above the recommended allowance. In 1965, the average consumption of protein per person per day was 106 g. Also, the Ten-State Nutrition Survey of 1968-1970 conducted by the U.S. Department of Health, Education and Welfare, indicated that protein intake was adequate in even low-income-ratio states. The USDA Nationwide Food Consumption Survey of 1977 also suggested that 95% of the households met the recommended allowance for protein. In 1979, government surveys indicated that the amount of protein available per person per day in the United States was 105 g—well above the required intake. Moreover, the protein in the United States is consumed from a variety of sources as Table P-36 shows.

TABLE P-36
CONTRIBUTION OF FOOD GROUPS TO ENERGY INTAKE[1]

Food Group	Men 23-34 Years	Women 23-34 Years	Children 6-8 Years
	←– – – (%) – – – – →		
Milk, milk products	11	12	20
Meat, poultry, fish	31	29	22
Eggs	2	3	2
Grain products	25	23	29
Fruit, vegetables	13	14	13
Legumes, nuts	2	2	3
Other[2]	16	17	11

[1]*1980 Handbook of Agriculture Charts,* USDA, Chart 95, p. 41.
[2]Includes fats, oils, sugar, sweets, and alcoholic and nonalcoholic beverages.

Protein malnutrition is generally not considered a problem in healthy individuals in the United States. Still, there are some who run the risk of receiving a low-protein intake due to poor food choices or poverty, but do not develop the characteristic symptoms of protein-calorie malnutrition.

• **Ill and elderly**—Once protein is ingested, an individual's condition may preclude proper digestion of absorption of the intact protein source. Example problems include various types of inflammatory bowel disease, such as pancreatitis or enteritis, or a gastrointestinal fistula or bowel resection, or just the stress of an infection or surgery. Elderly individuals with low incomes, poor health, and poor appetites may not secure food with high-quality protein. In both the ill and the aged, the protein deficiency may be manifested by delayed convalescence or poor wound healing.
(Also see GERONTOLOGY AND GERIATRIC NUTRITION.)

• **Infants**—The diets of infants after weaning should be carefully planned to include a high-quality protein source since infants and children require suitable patterns of amino acids in their diets. This means that if grains are a major dietary staple, there should be supplementation with animal proteins—such as milk, eggs, fish, or if these are unavailable, with such legumes as soybean or peanuts (which may be in the form of a powder). None of the commonly used grains—corn, rice, wheat, and barley—are adequate as the major source of protein for growing children. Mental function disturbances may follow a severe protein deficiency occurring in infancy.
(Also see INFANT DIET AND NUTRITON.)

• **Pregnancy**—Many uncertainties exist concerning the storage and efficiency of protein utilization during pregnancy, but inadequate protein may have adverse effects on the mother and fetus. Pregnant adolescents and women from low-income groups ignorant of the essentials of a good diet may be particularly susceptible.
(Also see PREGNANCY AND LACTATION DIETS.)

• **Vegetarians**—Strict vegetarian diets which offer little variety such as the Zen macrobiotic diet can be dangerous. Some individuals practicing the Zen diet plans eat only brown rice, which fails to provide many essential nutrients. Fruitarians, who eat only raw or dried fruits, nuts, honey, and olive oil may also suffer from an inadequacy of essential nutrients. Although adults may get along through well planned vegetarian diets, the protein needs of infants and growing children may not be met. Indeed, children of some vegetarian cults have demonstrated retarded growth and poor nutrition.

(Also see VEGETARIAN DIETS; and ZEN MACROBIOTIC DIET.)

PROTEIN FOR THE WORLD.   While there is adequate protein and energy available in the United States and other developed countries, many countries are low in calories and low in protein supplies. Moreover, countries low in total protein are also low in animal protein,

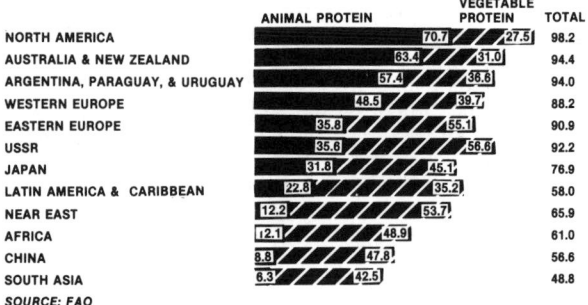

THERE IS PROTEIN AND PROTEIN!
AVERAGE GRAMS CONSUMPTION PER PERSON PER DAY

	ANIMAL PROTEIN	VEGETABLE PROTEIN	TOTAL
NORTH AMERICA	70.7	27.5	98.2
AUSTRALIA & NEW ZEALAND	63.4	31.0	94.4
ARGENTINA, PARAGUAY, & URUGUAY	57.4	36.8	94.0
WESTERN EUROPE	48.5	39.7	88.2
EASTERN EUROPE	35.8	55.1	90.9
USSR	35.6	56.6	92.2
JAPAN	31.8	45.1	76.9
LATIN AMERICA & CARIBBEAN	22.8	35.2	58.0
NEAR EAST	12.2	53.7	65.9
AFRICA	12.1	48.9	61.0
CHINA	8.8	47.8	56.6
SOUTH ASIA	6.3	42.5	48.8

SOURCE: FAO

Fig. P-117. Average grams protein consumption per person per day, with a breakdown into animal and vegetable protein, by geographic areas and countries. (From: *Ceres*, FAO/UN, Vol. 8, No. 3)

which generally has a higher biological value than plant protein. Several approaches have been and are being taken to develop and supply good-quality proteins to undeveloped countries. The aim is to provide acceptable, nutritious, and inexpensive products from the foods available. Some of the approaches to feeding the world include the following:

1. **Food combinations.**   Using foods common to an area, various nutritious food combinations have been developed and tried by agencies and governments throughout the world. Some examples of these include: (a) Incaparina, a mixture of whole grain corn, whole grain sorghum, cottonseed flour, torula yeast, calcium carbonate and vitamin A developed for use in central America; (b) L' aubina, developed in Lebanon and containing chick peas, parboiled wheat, some dried skim milk and bone ash; (c) corn-soy-milk (CSM) fortified with minerals and vitamins; and (d) whey soy drink mix (WSDM)—a mixture of sweet whey, full-fat soy flour, soybean oil, corn syrup solids, and a vitamin and mineral premix.

2. **Genetic improvement of grains.**   Scientists at Purdue University developed a special corn called Opaque-2 in which the incomplete protein, zein, is reduced to one-half the normal amount, while the complete protein glutelin is doubled. Moreover, lysine and tryptophan concentrations are increased about 50%, and leucine and isoleucine are in a better balance. Feeding trials on both animals and humans have demonstrated the increased value of Opaque-2. Breeding programs have also developed (a) high lysine sorghum and barley, (b) high protein rice and wheat, and (c) a cross between wheat and rye, called triticale. These genetic improvements bring plant protein quality closer to that of the animal proteins, and are very promising.

(Also see CEREAL GRAINS; and CORN, section headed "High-Lysine Corn.")

3. **Protein concentrates.**   Isolation of protein from oilseeds, nuts and leaves provides another method of increasing the supply of quality protein. The proteins remaining following the extraction of oil from soybeans, cottonseeds, sunflower seed, peanuts, and coconut have been used as protein supplements in animal feeds for a number of years. For humans, the oil-free residue of soybeans holds great promise since it can be used to make soy grits, soy flour, and soy protein concentrates (SPC). These SPCs are high in protein (see Table P-32) and can be used in a variety of products which include baked goods, dietary foods, meat products, and infant formulas. Moreover, soybean protein may be spun into fine filaments, flavored, and colored to resemble chicken, ham, or beef—a product referred to as texturized vegetable protein (TVP). Also, these proteins may be extruded to form ground meat extenders and meat analogs. Research is being conducted on the similar development of protein isolates from cottonseed and peanuts.

Isolating protein from plant leaves may provide a protein source which could be used as a complementary protein in countries where it is too rainy to dry seed crops. Green leaves are among the best sources of protein. By pressing the leaves, a protein-containing juice can be obtained which may be coagulated and dried forming a product that is 50% protein. This product is called leaf protein concentrate (LPC).

(Also see COTTONSEED; PEANUTS; and SOYBEANS, Table S-22 Soybean Products and Uses, Soybean Protein Isolates, and Textured Soybean Proteins.)

4. **Single-cell protein.** This refers to protein obtained from single-cell organisms or simple multicellular organisms such as yeast, bacteria, algae, and fungi. The most popular and most familiar of these are brewers' yeast and torula yeast, both of which are marketed. The potential for producing single-cell protein (SCP) is tremendous. Furthermore, many of the industrial by-products with little or no economic value may be used as a growing media. Some of these by-products include petroleum products, methane, alcohols, sulfite waste liquor, starch, molasses, cellulose, and animal waste. Still with all its potential, problems such as (a) safety, (b) acceptability,

(c) palatability, (d) digestibility, (e) nutrient content, and (f) economics of production need to be solved.

(Also see ALGAE; and SINGLE-CELL PROTEIN.)

5. **Amino acid supplementation.** Since lysine is the limiting amino acid in wheat and other grains, the addition of limited amounts of lysine to cereal diets improves their protein quality. Indeed, studies in Peru and Guatemala demonstrated that growing children benefited by this addition. However, in most countries there is more to be gained by focusing on increasing the food supply in general.

(Also see LYSINE.)

PROTEINS AND AMINO ACIDS IN SELECTED FOODS. Table P-37, Proteins and Amino Acids in Selected Foods, provides information on a number of foods. This information can be used to select foods and plan diets which yield a high-quality protein.

(Also see MALNUTRITION; MALNUTRITION PROTEIN-ENERGY; ORGANICALLY GROWN FOOD; and VEGETARIAN DIETS.)

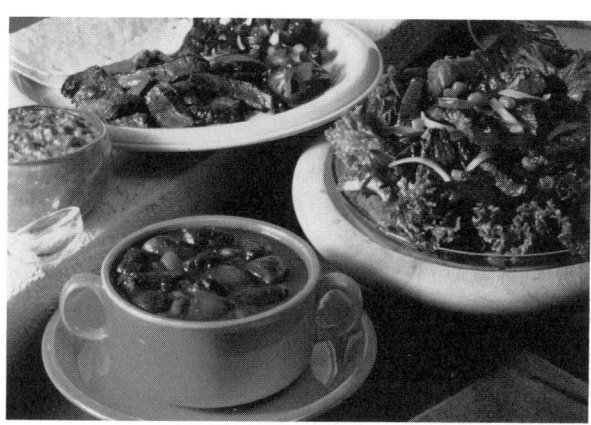

Some attractive dishes made with beef. (Courtesy, National Live Stock and Meat Board, Chicago, Ill.)

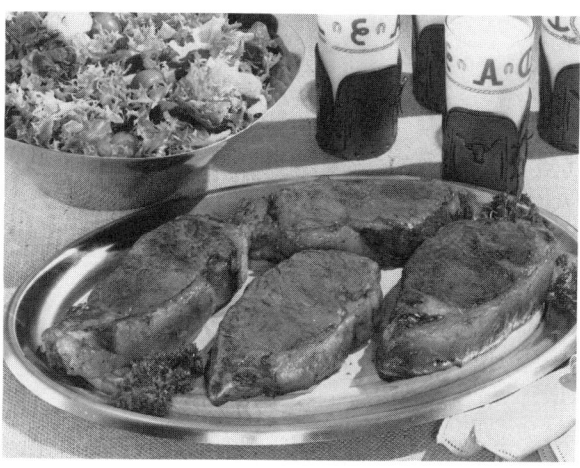

In this country, we are fortunate to have plenty of meat and milk—two of the most complete proteins. (Courtesy, National Live Stock & Meat Board, Chicago, Ill.)

TABLE P-37   PROTEINS & AMINO ACIDS IN SELECTED FOODS[1] (SEE END OF TABLE)

Food Name—100 Gram (3.5 oz) Portion	Water	Food Energy Calories	Total Protein	Animal Protein	Plant Protein	Amino Acids										
						Cystine	Histi-dine	Iso-leucine	Leucine	Lysine	Methi-onine	Phenyl-alanine	Threo-nine	Trypto-phan	Tyro-sine	Valine
	(g)	(kcal)	(g)	(g)	(g)	(mg)	(mg)	(mg)	(mg)	(mg)	(mg)	(mg)	(mg)	(mg)	(mg)	(mg)
BAKERY PRODUCTS																
BREADS																
BREADCRUMBS, dry grated	6.5	392	12.6	0.3	12.4	—	—	593	989	334	170	687	378	151	—	561
CRACKED WHEAT BREAD	34.9	263	8.7	0	8.7	—	—	373	582	234	130	426	252	104	—	400
CRACKED WHEAT TOAST	22.5	313	10.4	0	10.4	—	—	373	582	234	130	426	252	104	—	400
FRENCH BREAD	30.6	290	9.1	0	9.1	—	—	255	695	205	115	495	260	110	—	385
FRENCH BREAD TOAST	19.3	338	10.6	0	10.6	—	—	255	695	205	115	495	260	110	—	385
ITALIAN BREAD	31.8	276	9.1	0	9.1	—	—	255	695	205	115	495	260	110	—	385
RAISIN BREAD	35.3	262	6.6	Trace	6.6	—	—	278	434	173	95	321	130	78	—	300
RAISIN TOAST	22.0	316	8.0	Trace	8.0	—	—	336	526	210	115	389	157	94	—	363
RYE BREAD, DARK (pumpernickel)	34.0	246	9.1	0	9.1	—	—	390	606	371	143	425	334	100	—	471
RYE BREAD, LIGHT	35.5	243	9.1	0	9.1	—	—	391	613	291	139	439	291	100	—	473
RYE TOAST, LIGHT	25.0	282	10.6	0	10.6	—	—	450	705	335	160	505	335	125	—	545
VIENNA BREAD	30.6	290	9.1	0	9.1	—	—	255	695	205	115	495	260	110	—	385
VIENNA TOAST	19.3	338	10.6	0	10.6	—	—	255	695	205	115	495	260	110	—	385
WHITE BREAD, enriched	35.6	270	8.7	0.2	8.5	—	—	417	691	260	126	469	269	104	—	400
WHITE TOAST, enriched	25.1	314	10.1	0.2	9.9	—	—	480	795	300	145	540	310	120	—	460
WHOLE WHEAT BREAD	36.4	243	10.5	—	—	—	—	460	721	308	160	508	313	126	—	491
WHOLE WHEAT TOAST	24.3	289	12.5	—	—	—	—	547	873	373	194	615	378	152	—	594
CAKES																
ANGEL FOOD CAKE	34.0	259	5.7	4.4	1.3	—	—	262	439	131	74	314	165	68	—	245
DOUGHNUTS																
DOUGHNUT, cake type, plain	23.7	391	4.6	1.5	3.1	—	—	240	381	165	81	256	159	59	—	237
DOUGHNUT, raised type, plain	28.3	414	6.3	2.1	4.2	—	—	323	513	223	106	346	216	80	—	320
LEAVENINGS																
YEAST, DRY (active), baker's	5.0	282	36.9	0	36.9	—	—	2280	3970	3160	844	2090	2270	440	—	2900
MUFFINS																
BLUEBERRY	39.0	281	7.3	3.1	4.2	—	—	388	608	305	133	393	265	95	—	393
CORN MEAL	32.7	314	7.1	3.0	4.1	—	—	393	771	340	162	336	307	78	—	433
PLAIN, enriched	38.0	294	7.8	3.3	4.5	—	—	415	650	328	143	420	283	103	—	420
QUICK BREADS																
BAKING POWDER BISCUIT	27.4	369	7.4	0.2	7.3	—	—	342	571	171	97	408	214	88	—	320
BOSTON BROWN BREAD, canned	45.0	211	5.5	1.6	3.9	—	—	257	480	225	97	265	200	57	—	302
CORNBREAD OR JOHNNYCAKE	37.9	267	8.7	—	—	—	—	400	1130	260	160	400	350	52	—	440
POPOVER, home recipe	54.9	224	8.8	4.8	4.0	—	—	514	766	468	200	478	366	124	—	542
ROLLS																
CINNAMON BUN, w/raisins	32.0	275	6.9	1.6	5.3	—	—	315	527	157	88	377	198	82	—	293
DANISH PASTRY, plain w/o fruit or nuts	22.0	422	7.4	—	—	—	—	366	586	220	120	411	240	94	—	357
DINNER TYPE (pan), enriched	31.4	298	8.2	0.2	8.0	—	—	403	655	268	124	437	268	100	—	392
HARD ROLL, enriched	25.4	312	9.8	0.3	9.5	—	—	480	780	320	149	520	320	120	—	469
HOAGIE OR SUBMARINE	30.6	290	9.1	0	9.1	—	—	255	695	205	115	495	260	110	—	385
SWEET ROLL	31.5	316	8.5	2.0	6.5	—	—	436	698	309	142	464	291	109	—	431
CEREALS & FLOURS																
CEREALS																
BARLEY, pearled light, uncooked	11.1	349	8.2	0	8.2	—	—	343	568	279	114	429	279	100	—	411
BULGUR (parboiled wheat) canned, unseasoned	56.0	168	6.2	0	6.2	—	—	—	—	217	148	—	—	347	—	—
CORN GRITS, degermed, enriched, cooked	87.1	51	1.2	0	1.2	—	—	55	155	34	22	54	47	7	—	60
CORN MEAL, white or yellow, degermed enriched, cooked	87.7	50	1.1	0	1.1	—	—	46	131	29	19	45	40	5	—	51
FARINA, quick cooking, enriched, cooked	89.0	43	1.3	0	1.3	—	—	489	689	200	121	521	279	—	—	439
MACARONI, any shape, enriched, cooked	72.0	111	3.4	0	3.4	—	—	171	226	110	51	179	134	41	—	196
NOODLES, EGG, cooked	70.4	125	4.1	2.6	1.5	—	—	202	273	137	70	198	173	46	—	243
OATMEAL, dry	8.3	390	14.2	0	14.2	309	261	733	1065	521	209	758	470	183	524	845

Footnote at end of table

(Continued)

TABLE P-37 *(Continued)*

Food Name—100 Gram (3.5 oz) Portion	Water	Food Energy Calories	Total Protein	Animal Protein	Plant Protein	Amino Acids Cystine	Histi-dine	Iso-leucine	Leucine	Lysine	Methi-onine	Phenyl-alanine	Threo-nine	Trypto-phan	Tyro-sine	Valine
	(g)	(kcal)	(g)	(g)	(g)	(mg)	(mg)	(mg)	(mg)	(mg)	(mg)	(mg)	(mg)	(mg)	(mg)	(mg)
CEREALS *(Continued)*																
OATMEAL OR ROLLED OATS, cooked	86.5	55	2.0	0	2.0	—	—	117	213	94	36	117	87	32	—	135
RICE, BROWN, long grain, cooked	70.3	119	2.5	0	2.5	—	—	119	218	99	45	127	99	28	—	177
RICE, WHITE, enriched, long grain, cooked	72.6	109	2.0	0	2.0	—	—	96	172	78	36	100	78	22	—	140
SPAGHETTI, enriched, cooked	72.0	111	3.4	0	3.4	—	—	170	225	109	51	177	133	41	—	194
WHEAT GERM, dry	11.5	363	26.6	0	26.6	—	—	1270	1840	1650	430	970	1430	270	—	1460
BREAKFAST CEREALS																
SHREDDED WHEAT	6.6	354	9.9	0	9.9	204	236	449	684	331	139	481	405	85	236	577
FLOURS																
CORN FLOUR	12.0	368	7.8	0	7.8	101	161	361	1011	225	145	354	311	47	477	398
FLOUR, WHITE, all purpose, enriched	12.0	364	10.5	0	10.5	210	210	483	809	239	138	577	302	129	359	453
DESSERTS & SWEETS																
GELATIN, unsweetened, dry powder	13.0	335	85.6	85.6	0	77	771	1357	2930	4226	787	2036	1912	6	401	2421
GELATIN, sweetened, dry powder	1.6	371	9.4	9.4	0	—	—	94	207	301	56	150	141	—	—	169
TOPPINGS, DESSERT																
non-dairy powdered	1.5	577	4.9	4.9	0	21	145	301	484	394	149	263	207	68	280	351
non-dairy powdered, made w/whole milk	66.7	189	3.6	3.6	0	28	101	219	354	287	97	180	159	50	185	247
non-dairy pressurized	60.4	264	1.0	1.0	0	4	29	60	97	79	30	53	41	14	56	70
non-dairy frozen, semisolid	50.2	318	1.3	1.3	0	5	37	77	123	101	38	67	53	17	72	89
EGGS & SUBSTITUTES																
EGG WHOLE, fresh & frozen, raw	74.6	158	12.1	12.1	0	289	293	759	1066	820	392	686	596	194	505	874
EGG WHITE, fresh & frozen, raw	88.1	49	10.1	10.1	0	251	230	618	883	625	394	638	451	156	407	759
EGG YOLK, fresh raw	48.8	369	16.4	16.4	0	291	394	939	1396	1110	417	714	890	241	706	1000
EGG WHOLE, FRIED in butter	71.9	180	11.7	11.7	0	278	282	731	1026	789	377	660	574	187	486	841
EGG WHOLE, HARD-COOKED	74.6	158	12.1	12.1	0	289	293	759	1066	820	392	686	596	194	505	874
EGG OMELET, made w/butter & milk	76.3	148	9.3	9.3	0	208	227	581	883	641	294	519	453	147	394	666
EGG WHOLE, POACHED	74.3	157	12.1	12.1	0	288	292	756	1062	816	391	683	594	193	503	870
EGG WHOLE, SCRAMBLED w/butter & milk	76.3	148	9.3	9.3	0	208	227	581	883	641	294	519	453	147	394	666
EGG WHOLE DRIED	4.1	594	45.8	45.8	0	1093	1107	2867	4026	3094	1481	2588	2251	733	1907	3300
EGG WHOLE DRIED, stabilized	1.9	615	48.2	48.2	0	1148	1164	3014	4231	3252	1557	2721	2366	771	2004	3468
EGGNOG	74.4	135	3.8	3.8	0	38	95	230	369	298	87	182	175	54	182	253
DUCK EGG, whole fresh, raw	70.8	185	12.8	12.8	0	285	320	598	1097	951	576	840	736	260	613	885
FATS & OILS																
MARGARINE, regular, soft, whipped, or low sodium	15.5	720	0.6	0	0.6	—	—	50	70	60	20	40	40	10	—	50
FISH & SEAFOODS																
ANCHOVY, pickled, canned	58.6	176	19.2	19.2	0	—	—	1067	1590	1840	607	772	900	209	—	1109
BLUEFISH, baked or broiled	68.0	146	26.2	26.2	0	—	—	1338	1994	2308	760	971	1128	262	—	1390
CAVIAR, sturgeon, granular	46.0	262	26.9	26.9	0	—	—	1510	2210	1920	700	1190	1620	240	—	1650
COD, cooked	64.6	129	28.5	28.5	0	—	—	1400	2084	2421	800	1010	1210	273	—	1463
FLOUNDER, baked	58.1	140	30.0	30.0	0	—	—	1530	2250	2640	870	1110	1290	300	—	1590
HADDOCK, cooked	66.3	90	19.6	19.6	0	—	—	1000	1491	1725	568	725	843	196	—	1039
HALIBUT, cooked	66.6	130	25.2	25.2	0	—	—	1285	1915	2218	731	933	1083	252	—	1336
HERRING, pickled	59.4	223	20.4	20.4	0	—	—	1040	1530	1775	592	755	877	204	—	1081
HERRING, w/tomato sauce, canned	66.7	176	15.8	14.8	1.0	—	—	806	1185	1375	458	585	679	158	—	837
LOBSTER, whole, cooked	76.8	95	18.7	18.7	0	—	—	742	1558	1721	580	852	798	164	—	815
SALMON, broiled or baked	63.4	182	27.0	27.0	0	—	—	1350	2025	2349	783	999	1161	270	—	1431
SALMON, canned, Sockeye (red)	67.2	171	20.2	20.3	0	271	—	1025	1526	1771	588	750	876	200	546	1076
SARDINE, Pacific, canned, w/mustard	64.1	196	18.8	18.8	0	238	—	898	1337	1552	515	657	767	176	479	943
SHRIMP, canned	70.4	116	24.2	24.2	0	—	—	1234	1839	2130	702	895	1041	242	—	1283
SWORDFISH, broiled	64.6	174	28.0	28.0	0	—	—	1428	2100	2464	812	1036	1204	280	—	1484
TUNA, canned w/oil or water	60.6	197	28.8	28.8	0	—	—	1469	2160	2534	835	1066	1238	288	—	1526
WHITEFISH, lake, cooked	63.2	125	13.7	13.7	0	—	—	775	1140	1338	441	562	654	152	—	806
WHITEFISH, smoked	68.2	155	20.9	20.9	0	—	—	1066	1568	1839	606	773	899	209	—	1108

Footnote at end of table

(Continued)

TABLE P-37 *(Continued)*

Food Name—100 Gram (3.5 oz) Portion	Water	Food Energy Calories	Total Protein	Animal Protein	Plant Protein	Amino Acids										
						Cystine	Histi-dine	Iso-leucine	Leucine	Lysine	Methi-onine	Phenyl-alanine	Threo-nine	Trypto-phan	Tyro-sine	Valine
	(g)	(kcal)	(g)	(g)	(g)	(mg)	(mg)	(mg)	(mg)	(mg)	(mg)	(mg)	(mg)	(mg)	(mg)	(mg)
FLAVORINGS & SEASONINGS																
BASIL, ground	6.4	251	14.4	0	14.4	159	287	588	1078	618	202	733	588	221	432	717
DILL SEED	7.7	305	16.0	0	16.0	—	320	767	925	1038	143	670	575	—	—	1120
FENNEL SEED	8.8	345	15.8	0	15.8	222	331	695	996	758	301	647	602	253	410	915
FENUGREEK SEED	8.8	323	23.0	0	23.0	369	668	1241	1757	1684	338	1089	898	391	764	1102
GARLIC POWDER	6.4	332	16.8	0	16.8	172	309	648	1027	578	336	484	468	215	215	712
GINGER, ground	9.4	347	9.1	0	9.1	42	158	266	387	299	67	236	187	63	102	382
MUSTARD SEED, YELLOW	6.9	469	24.9	0	24.9	582	762	1081	1783	1519	480	1067	1095	526	744	1325
ONION POWDER	5.0	347	10.1	0	10.1	181	136	293	327	467	86	249	199	120	232	238
POPPY SEED	6.8	533	18.0	0	18.0	453	528	905	1484	1099	470	882	905	255	681	1287
SESAME SEEDS, decorticated	4.8	588	26.4	0	26.4	523	677	1289	2150	831	896	1528	1180	473	1125	1478
THYME, ground	7.8	276	9.1	0	9.1	274	—	468	430	207	274	482	252	186	482	502
FRUITS																
APPLE, w/skin, raw	84.4	58	0.2	0	0.2	—	—	—	—	—	—	6	—	—	3	—
APPLESAUCE, canned	75.7	91	0.2	0	0.2	—	—	—	—	—	—	6	—	—	3	—
APRICOTS, raw	85.3	51	1.0	0	1.0	—	—	—	—	—	—	24	—	—	—	—
AVOCADO, raw	74.0	167	2.1	0	2.1	—	—	—	—	74	12	—	—	14	—	—
BANANA, yellow, raw	75.7	85	1.1	0	1.1	—	—	—	—	55	11	34	—	18	33	—
CANTALOUPE, cubed, raw	91.2	30	0.7	0	0.7	—	—	—	—	15	2	21	—	1	—	—
CANTALOUPE & HONEYDEW MELON BALLS, frozen in syrup	83.2	62	0.6	0	0.6	—	—	—	—	15	2	—	—	1	—	—
DATES, moisturized or hydrated	22.5	274	2.2	0	2.2	—	49	74	77	65	27	61	61	61	17	94
FIGS, dried, uncooked	23.0	274	4.3	0	4.3	—	—	—	—	—	—	107	—	—	179	—
GRAPEFRUIT, sections, all varieties, raw	88.4	41	0.5	0	0.5	—	—	—	—	6	0	—	—	1	—	—
GRAPEFRUIT, sections, canned	81.1	70	0.6	0	0.6	—	—	—	—	7	0	—	—	1	—	—
GRAPES, GREEN, seedless raw, Thompson	81.4	67	0.6	0	0.6	11	25	6	14	15	23	18	19	3	11	19
GRAPES, canned, water pack, Thompson	85.5	51	0.5	0	0.5	11	25	6	14	15	23	14	19	3	12	19
HONEYDEW MELON	90.6	33	0.8	0	0.8	—	—	—	—	15	2	—	—	1	—	—
LIME, acid type	89.3	28	0.7	0	0.7	—	—	—	—	15	2	—	—	3	—	—
MANGO, raw	81.7	66	0.7	0	0.7	—	—	—	—	93	8	—	—	14	—	—
NECTARINES, raw	81.8	64	0.6	0	0.6	—	—	—	—	—	—	19	—	—	—	—
ORANGE, raw	86.0	49	1.0	0	1.0	—	—	—	—	24	3	12	—	3	21	—
PEACH, raw	89.1	38	0.6	0	0.6	9	17	13	29	30	31	12	27	4	15	40
PEACH, canned, water pack	91.1	31	0.4	0	0.4	—	—	—	—	—	—	8	—	—	10	—
PEAR, canned, water pack	91.1	32	0.2	0	0.2	—	—	—	—	—	—	6	—	—	10	—
PEAR, canned, heavy syrup	79.8	76	0.2	0	0.2	—	—	—	—	—	—	6	—	—	10	—
PINEAPPLE, raw	85.3	52	0.4	0	0.4	—	—	—	—	9	1	8	—	5	8	—
PINEAPPLE chunks, frozen, sweetened	77.1	85	0.4	0	0.4	—	—	—	—	9	1	—	—	5	—	—
PINEAPPLE, canned, water pack	89.1	39	0.3	0	0.3	—	—	—	—	7	1	8	—	4	8	—
PRUNES, dried, uncooked	28.0	255	2.1	0	2.1	—	—	—	—	—	—	88	—	—	—	—
RAISINS, uncooked	18.0	289	2.5	0	2.5	—	—	—	—	—	—	36	—	—	—	—
STRAWBERRIES, fresh	89.9	37	0.7	0	0.7	7	16	18	42	32	1	17	25	9	26	23
TANGERINE, raw	87.0	46	0.8	0	0.8	—	—	—	—	28	4	—	—	5	—	—
WATERMELON, raw	92.6	26	0.5	0	0.5	—	—	—	—	—	—	12	—	—	12	—
JUICES																
GRAPEFRUIT, fresh, all varieties	89.2	41	0.5	0	0.5	—	—	—	—	6	0	—	—	1	—	—
GRAPEFRUIT, canned, unsweetened	90.0	39	0.5	0	0.5	—	—	—	—	6	0	11	—	1	6	—
ORANGE, canned, unsweetened	87.4	48	0.8	0	0.8	—	—	—	—	21	2	—	—	3	—	—
ORANGE, canned, sweetened	86.5	52	0.7	0	0.7	—	—	—	—	—	—	9	—	—	15	—
PINEAPPLE, canned, unsweetened	85.6	55	0.4	0	0.4	—	—	—	—	9	1	—	—	5	—	—
TOMATO, canned or bottled	93.6	19	0.9	0	0.9	—	—	26	37	38	6	25	30	8	—	25
TOMATO, canned or bottled, low sodium	94.2	19	0.8	0	0.8	—	—	23	33	34	6	22	26	7	—	22

Footnote at end of table

(Continued)

TABLE P-37 *(Continued)*

Food Name—100 Gram (3.5 oz) Portion	Water	Food Energy Calories	Total Protein	Animal Protein	Plant Protein	Amino Acids Cystine	Histi-dine	Iso-leucine	Leucine	Lysine	Methi-onine	Phenyl-alanine	Threo-nine	Trypto-phan	Tyro-sine	Valine
	(g)	(kcal)	(g)	(g)	(g)	(mg)	(mg)	(mg)	(mg)	(mg)	(mg)	(mg)	(mg)	(mg)	(mg)	(mg)
MEAT																
BEEF																
dried, chipped, uncooked	47.7	203	34.3	34.3	0	—	—	1795	2809	2996	850	1410	1515	401	—	1903
dried, chipped, creamed	72.0	154	8.2	8.1	0.1	—	—	690	1093	1010	304	590	555	159	—	717
flank steak, braised	61.4	196	30.5	30.5	0	—	—	1793	2808	2999	851	1409	1513	401	—	1904
hamburger (ground beef), cooked	54.2	286	24.2	24.2	0	—	—	1342	2101	2242	636	1055	1132	300	—	1424
kidney, braised	53.0	252	33.0	33.0	0	—	—	942	1678	1402	396	911	858	285	—	1130
liver, fried	—	229	26.4	26.3	0.1	—	—	1246	2197	1781	560	1200	1130	357	—	1495
roast, canned	60.0	224	25.0	25.0	0	316	868	1308	2048	2184	620	1028	1104	292	848	1388
stew w/vegetables, canned	82.5	79	5.8	—	—	—	—	282	427	459	126	235	241	67	—	308
tongue, braised	60.8	244	21.5	21.5	0	—	—	792	1286	1364	356	661	708	196	—	840
CHICKEN																
chicken, canned	65.2	198	21.7	21.7	0	—	—	1100	1507	1830	543	820	887	253	—	1023
liver, simmered	65.0	165	26.5	26.5	0	—	—	1533	2707	2197	690	1480	1393	440	—	1847
LAMB																
ground, cooked	54.0	279	25.3	25.3	0	—	—	1332	1990	2081	617	1045	1176	332	—	1267
leg roast, roasted	54.0	279	25.3	25.3	0	—	—	1332	1990	2081	617	1045	1176	332	—	1267
rib chop, broiled	42.9	407	20.1	20.1	0	—	—	1052	1572	1643	487	825	929	263	—	1000
LUNCHEON MEATS																
BRAUNSCHWEIGER (smoked liver sausage)	52.6	319	15.4	15.4	0	187	458	754	1291	1200	320	700	668	172	471	956
CORNED BEEF, canned	59.3	216	25.3	25.3	0	—	—	1185	1857	1982	560	932	1000	264	—	1260
HEAD CHEESE	58.8	268	15.5	15.5	0	209	278	509	946	907	250	569	418	79	569	617
LIVERWURST	53.9	307	16.2	16.2	0	203	497	818	1400	1301	347	759	724	187	510	1037
POLISH SAUSAGE (kolbassi), cooked	53.7	304	15.7	15.7	0	—	—	1420	1580	1717	507	800	890	147	—	1080
PORK/HAM LOAF type luncheon meat	54.9	294	15.0	15.0	0	241	479	741	1151	1252	362	570	610	143	575	775
POTTED MEAT, beef/chicken/turkey	60.7	248	17.5	17.5	0	—	322	641	1203	1061	361	641	662	149	—	943
SALAMI, beef	29.8	450	23.8	23.8	0	298	642	1159	1713	1923	505	872	979	203	776	1201
SPICED LUNCHEON MEATS, pork/ham type	54.9	294	15.0	15.0	0	241	479	741	1151	1252	362	570	610	143	575	775
VIENNA SAUSAGE	63.0	240	14.0	14.0	0	197	425	766	1133	1272	334	576	647	134	513	794
PORK																
Canadian bacon, cooked	49.9	277	27.6	27.6	0	—	—	1471	2281	2481	719	1129	1210	286	—	1538
loin roast or chops, cooked	45.8	362	24.5	24.5	0	—	—	1279	1833	2044	621	980	1155	323	—	1295
shoulder blade steak, cooked	48.1	353	22.5	22.5	0	—	—	1156	1656	1847	561	886	1044	292	—	1170
VEAL																
cutlet, braised or broiled	60.4	216	27.1	27.1	0	—	—	1751	2429	2769	758	1346	1438	435	—	1714
loin roast or chop, cooked	58.9	234	26.4	26.4	0	—	—	1189	1657	1889	517	919	981	297	—	1169
shoulder arm roast, cooked	58.5	235	27.9	27.9	0	—	—	1562	2169	2471	677	1202	1283	389	—	1530
rib chop, cooked	54.6	269	27.2	27.2	0	—	—	1776	2464	2809	769	1366	1459	441	—	1738
round, cooked	60.4	216	27.1	27.1	0	—	—	1494	2072	2362	647	1148	1227	371	—	1462
TURKEY, canned	64.9	202	20.9	20.9	0	—	—	1109	1611	1904	586	837	900	—	—	1046
MILK & PRODUCTS																
BUTTER, regular or unsalted	15.9	717	0.9	0.9	0	8	23	51	83	67	21	41	38	12	41	57
CHEESE																
AMERICAN, pasteurized process	39.2	375	22.1	22.1	0	142	903	1024	1958	2198	573	1125	719	323	1212	1326
AMERICAN, spread, pasteurized process	47.7	290	16.4	16.4	0	—	509	833	1780	1507	538	931	628	—	890	1366
BLUE	42.4	353	21.4	21.4	0	108	759	1126	1922	1855	585	1089	786	313	1297	1559
BRICK	41.1	371	23.2	23.2	0	131	823	1137	2244	2124	565	1231	882	324	1115	1472
BRIE	48.4	334	20.8	20.8	0	114	716	1015	1929	1851	592	1158	751	322	1200	1340
CAMEMBERT	51.8	300	19.8	19.8	0	109	683	968	1840	1766	565	1105	717	307	1145	1279
CHEDDAR, shredded	36.8	403	24.9	24.9	0	125	874	1546	2385	2072	652	1311	886	320	1202	1663
CHESHIRE	37.7	387	23.4	23.4	0	117	821	1451	2238	1945	612	1231	832	300	1128	1560
COLBY	38.2	394	23.8	23.8	0	119	834	1475	2275	1978	622	1251	845	305	1147	1586
COTTAGE, creamed	79.0	103	12.5	12.5	0	116	415	734	1284	1010	376	673	554	139	666	773

Footnote at end of table

(Continued)

TABLE P-37 *(Continued)*

Food Name—100 Gram (3.5 oz) Portion	Water	Food Energy Calories	Total Protein	Animal Protein	Plant Protein	Amino Acids										
						Cystine	Histidine	Iso-leucine	Leucine	Lysine	Methionine	Phenylalanine	Threonine	Tryptophan	Tyrosine	Valine
	(g)	(kcal)	(g)	(g)	(g)	(mg)	(mg)	(mg)	(mg)	(mg)	(mg)	(mg)	(mg)	(mg)	(mg)	(mg)
CHEESE *(Continued)*																
COTTAGE, creamed w/fruit added	72.1	124	9.9	—	—	92	329	582	1018	801	298	534	439	110	528	613
COTTAGE, dry curd	79.8	85	17.3	17.3	0	160	574	1015	1776	1397	520	931	766	192	920	1069
COTTAGE, lowfat, 2% fat	79.3	90	13.7	13.7	0	127	457	808	1413	1111	413	741	609	153	732	851
COTTAGE, lowfat, 1% fat	82.5	72	12.4	12.4	0	115	412	728	1274	1002	373	668	550	138	660	767
CREAM	53.8	349	7.6	7.6	0	66	271	399	731	676	181	419	321	67	360	443
EDAM	41.6	357	25.0	25.0	0	—	1034	1308	2570	2660	721	1434	932	—	1457	1810
GJETOST, made from goat's & cow's milk	13.4	466	9.6	9.6	0	57	293	519	992	814	318	540	393	135	541	765
GOUDA	41.5	356	24.9	24.9	0	—	1032	1306	2564	2654	719	1431	930	—	1454	1806
GRUYERE	33.2	413	29.8	29.8	0	304	1117	1612	3102	2710	822	1743	1089	421	1776	2243
LIMBURGER	48.4	327	20.0	20.0	0	—	578	1219	2093	1675	619	1116	739	289	1197	1439
MONTEREY	41.0	373	24.5	24.5	0	123	859	1519	2344	2037	641	1289	871	315	1182	1635
MOZZARELLA	54.1	281	19.4	19.4	0	116	731	931	1893	1972	542	1014	740	—	1123	1215
MOZZARELLA, low moisture	48.4	318	21.6	21.6	0	129	813	1036	2106	2194	603	1127	823	—	1249	1351
MOZZARELLA, part skim	53.8	254	24.3	24.3	0	144	913	1164	2365	2464	677	1266	924	—	1403	1517
MOZZARELLA, low moisture, part skim	48.6	280	27.5	27.5	0	164	1033	1318	2678	2790	766	1434	1046	—	1589	1718
MUENSTER	41.8	368	23.4	23.4	0	132	829	1145	2260	2139	569	1240	888	327	1123	1482
NEUFCHATEL	62.2	260	10.0	10.0	0	87	357	526	965	891	239	553	423	89	475	584
PARMESAN, grated	17.7	456	41.6	41.6	0	274	1609	2202	4013	3843	1114	2234	1531	560	2319	2853
PARMESAN, hard	29.2	392	35.8	35.8	0	235	1384	1894	3452	3306	958	1922	1317	482	1995	2454
PIMIENTO, pasteurized process	39.1	375	22.1	—	—	142	902	1023	1956	2196	572	1124	718	323	1211	1325
PORT DU SALUT	45.5	352	23.8	23.8	0	—	686	1446	2482	1987	734	1323	876	343	1420	1707
PROVOLONE	41.0	351	25.6	25.6	0	116	1115	1091	2297	2646	686	1287	982	—	1520	1640
RICOTTA, made w/whole milk	71.7	174	11.3	11.3	0	99	459	589	1221	1338	281	556	517	—	589	692
RICOTTA, made w/part skim milk	74.4	138	11.4	11.4	0	100	464	596	1235	1353	284	562	523	—	596	700
SWISS	37.2	376	28.4	28.4	0	290	1065	1537	2959	2585	784	1662	1038	401	1693	2139
SWISS, pasteurized process	42.3	334	24.7	24.7	0	159	1008	1143	2186	2454	640	1256	802	360	1353	1481
TILSIT, made w/whole milk	42.9	340	24.4	24.4	0	—	704	1484	2548	2039	754	1358	899	352	1458	1752
CREAM																
half & half (milk & cream), fluid	80.6	130	3.0	3.0	0	27	80	179	290	235	74	143	134	42	143	198
heavy whipping	57.7	345	2.0	2.0	0	19	56	124	201	163	51	99	93	29	99	137
light whipping, fluid	63.5	292	2.2	2.2	0	20	59	131	213	172	54	105	98	31	105	145
medium (25% fat), fluid	68.5	244	2.5	2.5	0	23	67	149	242	196	62	119	111	35	119	165
light (coffee or table), fluid	73.8	195	2.7	2.7	0	25	73	163	264	214	68	130	122	38	130	181
whipped cream topping, pressurized	61.3	257	3.2	3.2	0	30	87	194	313	254	80	154	144	45	154	214
CREAM SUBSTITUTES																
non-dairy liquid, w/hydrogenated vegetable oil & soy protein	77.3	136	1.0	0	1.0	18	28	56	85	68	15	55	43	15	37	56
non-dairy liquid, w/lauric acid oil & casein	77.3	136	1.0	1.0	0	4	30	61	99	80	30	54	42	14	57	72
non-dairy, powdered	2.2	546	4.8	4.8	0	21	142	294	473	385	145	257	203	66	274	343
ICE CREAM																
French vanilla ice cream, soft serve	59.8	218	4.1	4.1	0.0	42	109	244	393	317	102	195	188	58	194	269
vanilla ice cream, regular (10% fat) hardened	60.8	202	3.6	3.6	0	33	98	218	354	286	91	174	163	51	174	242
vanilla ice cream, rich (16% fat) hardened	58.9	236	2.8	2.8	0	26	76	169	273	221	70	135	126	39	135	187
vanilla ice milk, soft serve	69.6	128	4.6	—	—	42	124	278	450	364	115	222	207	65	222	307
vanilla ice milk, hardened	68.6	140	3.9	3.9	0	36	107	238	386	312	99	190	178	56	190	264
orange sherbet	66.1	140	1.1	1.1	0	10	30	68	110	89	28	54	51	16	54	75
MILK, (COW'S)																
whole milk, 3.7% fat	87.7	64	3.3	3.3	0	30	89	198	321	260	82	158	148	46	158	220
whole milk, 3.3% fat	88.0	61	3.3	3.3	0	30	89	199	322	261	83	159	149	46	159	220
whole milk, low sodium	88.2	61	3.1	3.1	0	29	84	188	304	246	78	150	140	44	150	207
lowfat milk, 2% fat	89.2	50	3.3	3.3	0	31	90	201	326	264	84	161	150	47	161	223
lowfat milk, 2% fat w/nonfat milk solids added	88.9	51	3.5	3.5	0	32	94	211	341	276	87	168	157	49	168	233
lowfat milk, 2% fat, protein fortified	87.7	56	4.0	4.0	0	37	107	239	387	313	99	191	178	56	191	264
lowfat milk, 1% fat	90.1	42	3.3	3.3	0	30	89	199	322	261	83	159	149	46	159	220
lowfat milk, 1% fat w/nonfat milk solids added	89.8	43	3.5	3.5	0	32	94	211	341	276	87	168	157	49	168	233

Footnote at end of table

(Continued)

TABLE P-37 *(Continued)*

Food Name—100 Gram (3.5 oz) Portion	Water	Food Energy Calories	Total Protein	Animal Protein	Plant Protein	Amino Acids										
						Cystine	Histidine	Isoleucine	Leucine	Lysine	Methionine	Phenylalanine	Threonine	Tryptophan	Tyrosine	Valine
	(g)	(kcal)	(g)	(g)	(g)	(mg)	(mg)	(mg)	(mg)	(mg)	(mg)	(mg)	(mg)	(mg)	(mg)	(mg)
MILK, (cow's) *(Continued)*																
lowfat milk, 1% fat, protein fortified	88.7	48	3.9	3.9	0	36	107	238	385	312	99	190	177	55	190	263
skim milk	90.8	35	3.4	3.4	0	32	92	206	334	270	86	165	154	48	165	228
skim milk, protein fortified	89.4	41	4.0	4.0	0	37	107	240	388	314	99	191	179	56	191	265
skim milk w/nonfat milk solids added	90.4	37	3.6	3.6	0	33	97	216	350	283	90	172	161	50	172	239
chocolate milk, whole, 3.3% fat	82.3	83	3.2	3.2	0	29	86	192	311	251	79	153	143	45	153	212
chocolate milk, 2% fat	83.6	72	3.2	3.2	0	30	87	194	314	255	81	155	145	45	155	215
chocolate milk, 1% fat	84.5	63	3.2	3.2	0	30	88	196	317	257	81	156	146	46	156	217
buttermilk, cultured	90.1	40	3.3	3.3	0	31	95	204	329	277	81	174	158	36	139	243
whole milk, evaporated, canned	74.0	134	6.8	6.8	0	63	185	412	667	540	171	329.	307	96	329	456
skim milk, evaporated, canned	79.4	78	7.6	7.6	0	70	205	457	740	599	189	364	341	107	364	505
sweetened condensed milk, canned	27.2	321	7.9	7.9	0	73	214	479	775	627	198	382	357	112	382	529
whole milk, dry	2.5	496	26.3	26.3	0	243	714	1592	2578	2087	660	1271	1188	371	1271	1762
nonfat dry milk powder, non-instantized	3.2	362	36.2	36.2	0	334	981	2188	3542	2868	907	1746	1632	510	1746	2420
nonfat dry milk powder, instantized	4.0	358	35.1	35.1	0	325	952	2124	3438	2784	880	1694	1584	495	1694	2349
hot cocoa, homemade w/whole milk	81.6	87	3.6	3.6	0	34	99	220	357	289	91	176	164	51	176	244
malted milk powder, natural flavor	2.6	411	13.1	—	—	261	261	391	749	356	180	439	335	140	362	445
malted milk beverage, natural flavor	81.2	89	4.1	—	—	49	103	214	356	269	90	181	163	54	175	238
malted milk powder, chocolate flavor	2.0	396	6.5	—	—	77	121	187	345	186	82	246	176	41	166	222
malted milk beverage, chocolate flavor	81.2	88	3.5	—	—	11	28	61	100	79	26	51	47	14	50	71
milkshake, vanilla flavor, thick type	74.4	112	3.9	—	—	36	105	234	378	306	97	186	174	54	186	258
milkshake, chocolate flavor, thick type	72.2	119	3.0	—	—	28	83	185	299	242	76	147	138	43	147	204
MILK, GOAT'S, whole	87.0	69	3.6	3.6	0	46	89	207	314	290	80	155	163	44	179	240
MILK, HUMAN, whole	87.5	70	1.0	1.0	0	19	23	56	95	68	21	46	46	17	53	63
YOGURT																
plain	87.9	61	3.5	3.5	0	—	86	189	350	311	102	189	142	20	175	287
plain, lowfat	85.1	63	5.3	5.3	0	—	130	286	529	471	155	286	216	30	265	434
plain, skim milk	85.2	56	5.7	5.7	0	—	142	313	577	514	169	313	235	32	289	474
coffee & vanilla varieties, lowfat	79.0	85	4.9	4.9	0	—	122	269	497	442	145	269	202	28	249	408
fruit varieties, lowfat (9g protein/8oz)	75.3	99	4.0	—	—	—	99	217	401	357	117	217	163	22	201	329
fruit varieties, lowfat (10g protein/8oz)	74.5	102	4.4	—	—	—	108	238	440	392	129	238	179	25	221	362
fruit varieties, lowfat (11g protein/8oz)	74.1	105	4.9	—	—	—	120	265	490	436	143	265	200	27	245	402
NUTS & SEEDS																
ALMONDS	4.7	598	18.6	0	18.6	377	517	873	1454	582	259	1146	610	176	618	1124
BRAZIL NUTS	4.6	654	14.3	0	14.3	—	—	593	1129	443	941	617	422	187	—	823
CASHEW NUTS	5.2	561	17.2	0	17.2	—	—	1135	1410	740	327	877	688	430	—	1479
COCONUT, fresh	50.9	346	3.4	0	3.4	62	69	180	269	152	71	174	129	33	101	212
COCONUT, dried, shredded, sweetened	3.3	548	3.6	0	3.6	—	—	190	284	162	75	183	136	35	—	223
FILBERTS OR HAZELNUTS	5.8	634	12.7	0	12.7	165	288	853	939	417	139	537	415	211	434	934
PEANUTS, roasted, Spanish or Virginia	1.6	585	26.0	0	26.0	—	—	1355	2003	1176	290	1666	886	364	—	1639
PEANUTS, roasted in shell	1.8	582	26.2	0	26.2	—	—	1248	1845	1083	267	1534	816	335	—	1510
PEANUT BUTTER	1.8	581	26.1	0	26.1	449	727	1228	1816	1066	263	1510	803	330	1071	1487
PECANS	3.4	687	9.4	0	9.4	216	273	553	773	435	153	564	389	138	316	525
PISTACHIO NUTS	5.3	594	18.9	0	18.9	385	471	881	1523	1080	367	1088	613	—	667	1344
PUMPKIN OR SQUASH SEEDS	4.4	553	29.0	0	29.0	—	—	1624	2291	1334	551	1624	870	522	—	1566
SUNFLOWER SEED KERNELS, hulled	4.8	560	23.0	0	23.0	464	586	1276	1736	868	443	1220	911	343	647	1354
WALNUTS, ENGLISH	3.5	651	15.0	0	15.0	320	405	767	1228	441	306	767	589	175	583	974
PICKLES & RELISHES																
BREAD & BUTTER PICKLES	78.7	73	0.9	0	0.9	—	—	28	39	40	9	21	24	6	—	31
DILL PICKLE, whole	93.3	11	0.7	0	0.7	—	—	22	30	31	7	16	19	5	—	24
OLIVE, ripe	73.0	184	1.2	0	1.2	—	24	53	79	15	17	45	40	—	38	60
PEPPER, HOT CHILI, green. canned	92.5	25	0.9	0	0.9	—	—	34	34	38	12	42	38	6	—	25
PICKLE, SWEET	60.7	146	0.7	0	0.7	—	—	22	30	31	7	16	19	5	—	24
PIMIENTOS, canned	92.4	27	0.9	0	0.9	—	22	37	60	48	6	45	43	—	22	49
SALADS																
COLESLAW, w salad dressing	82.9	99	1.2	0	1.2	—	—	47	48	56	11	25	34	10	—	36

Footnote at end of table

(Continued)

TABLE P-37 (Continued)

Food Name—100 Gram (3.5 oz) Portion	Water	Food Energy Calories	Total Protein	Animal Protein	Plant Protein	Amino Acids										
						Cystine	Histi-dine	Iso-leucine	Leucine	Lysine	Methi-onine	Phenyl-alanine	Threo-nine	Trypto-phan	Tyro-sine	Valine
	(g)	(kcal)	(g)	(g)	(g)	(mg)	(mg)	(mg)	(mg)	(mg)	(mg)	(mg)	(mg)	(mg)	(mg)	(mg)
SNACK FOODS																
POPCORN, plain	4.0	386	12.7	0	12.7	—	—	593	1671	371	243	579	514	79	—	657
POPCORN, popped in coconut oil w/salt	3.1	456	9.8	0	9.8	—	—	461	1300	289	189	450	400	61	—	511
POTATO CHIPS	1.8	568	5.3	0	5.3	—	—	233	265	281	64	233	217	53	—	281
SOUPS & CHOWDERS																
BEEF BROTH, bouillon, consomme, canned, diluted w/water	5.8	13	2.1	2.1	0	—	—	27	70	76	14	47	79	1	—	58
BEEF NOODLE, canned, diluted w/water	92.8	29	1.6	—	—	—	—	80	65	156	56	65	75	14	—	77
CHICKEN NOODLE, canned, diluted w/water	93.1	27	1.5	—	—	—	—	80	75	180	43	75	65	13	—	55
CHICKEN W/RICE, canned, diluted w/water	94.7	22	1.3	—	—	—	—	60	65	176	47	52	50	11	·	40
CHICKEN VEGETABLE, canned, diluted w/water	92.3	30	1.7	—	—	—	—	62	92	87	21	47	53	18	—	56
CREAM OF ASPARAGUS, canned, diluted w/milk	85.2	69	2.7	—	—	—	—	159	254	181	57	119	155	28	—	173
CREAM OF ASPARAGUS, canned, diluted w/water	91.7	35	0.9	—	—	—	—	—	—	—	—	33	—	—	—	—
CREAM OF CHICKEN, canned, diluted w/water	92.2	38	1.4	—	—	—	—	60	60	115	42	53	50	11	—	47
CREAM OF MUSHROOM, canned, diluted w/milk	83.4	92	2.6	—	—	—	—	151	213	227	85	124	109	31	—	152
CREAM OF SHRIMP, frozen, made w/milk	81.8	100	3.8	—	—	—	—	194	316	265	84	165	242	38	—	209
MINESTRONE, canned, diluted w/water	91.2	36	1.6	0	1.6	—	—	68	98	78	16	56	54	17	—	71
ONION, canned, diluted w/water	94.5	24	1.5	—	—	—	—	39	85	86	15	47	99	6	—	58
PEA, green, canned, diluted w/water	85.1	58	3.5	1.1	2.3	—	—	135	167	359	43	141	104	22	—	42
TURKEY NOODLE, canned, diluted w/water	92.7	32	1.6	—	—	—	—	92	108	81	23	53	58	16	—	70
TOMATO, canned, diluted w/water	90.5	36	0.8	0	0.8	—	—	33	28	75	32	37	27	6	—	25
VEGETABLE BEEF, canned, diluted w/water	91.9	33	2.1	—	—	—	—	71	170	234	36	92	94	21	—	124
VEGETARIAN VEGETABLE, canned, diluted w/water	91.8	32	0.9	0	0.9	—	—	38	46	101	37	39	30	6	—	32
VEGETABLES																
ASPARAGUS, green, cooked	93.6	20	2.2	0	2.2	—	—	79	97	103	33	68	66	26	—	106
green, frozen, cooked	92.2	23	3.2	0	3.2	—	—	79	97	103	33	68	66	26	—	106
green, canned	92.5	21	2.4	0	2.4	—	—	68	84	89	28	59	57	22	—	92
green, low sodium, canned	93.6	20	2.6	0	2.6	—	—	94	114	122	39	81	78	31	—	125
white, canned	92.3	22	2.1	0	2.1	—	—	56	68	73	14	48	46	19	—	75
white, low sodium, canned	94.0	19	1.9	0	1.9	—	—	68	84	89	28	59	57	23	—	92
BEANS, common, red (kidney), unsalted, cooked	69.0	118	7.8	0	7.8	—	—	437	671	577	78	429	335	70	—	468
common, red (kidney), canned	76.0	90	5.7	0	5.7	57	162	324	490	423	57	315	247	53	220	346
common, dry, white pea (navy), unsalted, cooked	69.0	118	7.8	0	7.8	—	—	445	671	577	78	429	335	70	—	476
common, white, canned w/pork & sweet sauce	66.4	150	6.2	Trace	6.2	—	—	355	536	462	62	343	269	56	—	381
common, white, canned w/pork & tomato sauce	70.7	122	6.1	Trace	6.1	—	—	346	523	450	61	334	262	54	—	371
common, white, canned w/o pork	68.5	120	6.3	0	6.3	—	—	360	543	468	63	347	272	57	—	386
green, raw	90.1	32	1.9	0	1.9	—	—	86	110	99	28	69	72	27	63	91
green, cut or french style, boiled	92.4	25	1.6	0	1.6	—	—	72	92	83	24	38	60	21	—	76
green, frozen, boiled	92.1	25	1.6	0	1.6	—	—	72	93	83	24	38	61	22	—	77
green, canned	91.9	24	1.4	0	1.4	—	—	64	83	75	21	34	54	20	—	68
green, low sodium, canned	93.2	22	1.5	0	1.5	—	—	67	87	78	22	36	57	21	—	72
baby lima, frozen, cooked	68.8	118	7.4	0	7.4	—	—	348	498	402	96	354	282	54	—	378
lima, frozen, cooked	73.5	99	6.0	0	6.0	—	—	429	614	496	118	437	348	67	—	466
lima, canned	74.7	96	5.4	0	5.4	—	—	313	447	360	86	318	253	48	—	340
lima, low sodium, canned	75.6	95	5.8	0	5.8	—	—	336	481	389	93	342	273	52	—	365
lima, cooked, mature seeds, dry	64.1	138	8.2	0	8.2	—	—	473	678	547	130	482	384	73	—	514
sprouts (mung beans), cooked	91.0	28	3.2	0	3.2	—	—	179	291	218	35	154	99	22	—	189
wax, boiled	93.4	22	1.4	0	1.4	—	—	63	81	73	21	34	53	20	—	67
wax, frozen, boiled	91.5	27	1.7	0	1.7	—	—	76	99	88	26	41	65	24	—	82
wax, canned	92.2	24	1.4	0	1.4	—	—	63	81	73	21	34	53	20	—	67
wax, low sodium, canned	93.6	21	1.2	0	1.2	—	—	54	70	62	18	29	46	17	—	58

Footnote at end of table

(Continued)

TABLE P-37 (Continued)

Food Name—100 Gram (3.5 oz) Portion	Water	Food Energy Calories	Total Protein	Animal Protein	Plant Protein	Amino Acids										
						Cystine	Histidine	Isoleucine	Leucine	Lysine	Methionine	Phenylalanine	Threonine	Tryptophan	Tyrosine	Valine
	(g)	(kcal)	(g)	(g)	(g)	(mg)	(mg)	(mg)	(mg)	(mg)	(mg)	(mg)	(mg)	(mg)	(mg)	(mg)
BEET GREENS, cooked	93.6	18	1.7	0	1.7	—	—	71	109	92	29	99	65	20	—	85
BEETS, red, whole, cooked	90.9	32	1.1	0	1.1	—	—	34	37	59	4	18	22	9	—	33
red, canned	89.3	37	1.0	0	1.0	—	13	22	28	27	9	14	18	8	16	28
BROCCOLI, raw	89.1	32	3.6	0	3.6	—	—	137	176	158	54	131	133	40	124	184
cooked	91.3	26	3.1	0	3.1	—	—	118	152	136	46	112	115	34	—	158
frozen, cooked	91.4	26	3.1	0	3.1	—	—	110	142	128	44	104	107	32	—	148
BRUSSELS SPROUTS, cooked	88.2	36	4.2	0	4.2	—	—	176	185	189	42	151	147	42	86	185
frozen, cooked	89.3	33	3.2	0	3.2	—	—	134	141	144	32	106	112	32	—	141
CABBAGE, raw	92.4	24	1.3	0	1.3	28	25	40	57	66	13	32	39	11	27	43
cooked, small amount water	93.9	20	1.1	0	1.1	—	—	43	44	52	10	23	31	9	—	33
cooked, large amount water	94.3	18	1.0	0	1.0	—	—	31	40	47	9	21	28	8	—	30
CABBAGE, RED, raw	90.2	31	2.0	0	2.0	—	—	78	80	94	18	50	56	16	41	60
CARROT, raw	88.2	42	1.1	0	1.1	29	17	46	65	52	10	36	43	10	17	56
cooked	91.2	31	0.9	0	0.9	—	—	34	48	39	7	31	32	7	14	41
slices, canned	91.2	30	0.8	0	0.8	—	—	30	43	34	6	28	29	6	—	37
CAULIFLOWER, raw, whole flowers	91.0	27	2.7	0	2.7	—	—	116	181	151	54	84	113	35	—	162
cooked	92.8	22	2.3	0	2.3	—	—	99	154	129	46	71	97	30	—	138
frozen, cooked	94.0	18	1.9	0	1.9	—	—	82	127	106	38	59	80	25	—	114
CELERY, raw	94.1	17	0.9	0	0.9	—	1	19	22	25	2	15	16	—	7	26
diced, cooked	95.3	14	0.8	0	0.8	—	—	—	—	12	10	—	—	8	—	—
CHICORY GREENS, raw	92.8	20	1.8	0	1.8	6	24	—	—	52	16	—	—	24	40	—
COLLARDS, leaves & stems, cooked	90.8	29	2.7	0	2.7	—	—	84	151	140	32	86	78	38	—	135
frozen, cooked	90.2	30	2.9	0	2.9	—	—	90	162	151	35	93	84	41	—	145
CORN, sweet, cooked, cut off cob before cooking	76.5	83	3.2	0	3.2	—	—	—	—	—	—	—	—	—	—	—
sweet, cooked on cob, white/yellow	74.1	91	3.3	0	3.3	—	—	122	363	122	63	185	135	20	88	208
sweet, frozen, cut off cob, cooked	77.2	79	3.0	0	3.0	—	—	—	—	—	—	—	—	—	—	—
sweet, whole kernel, canned	75.9	84	2.6	0	2.6	—	—	97	291	97	50	140	108	15	67	16
sweet, whole kernel, low sodium, canned	78.4	76	2.5	0	2.5	—	—	92	275	92	48	140	102	15	—	158
sweet, cream style, canned, white/yellow	76.3	82	2.1	0.4	1.7	—	—	96	286	96	49	146	107	16	—	164
CUCUMBER, raw, pared	95.7	14	0.6	0	0.6	—	—	18	26	26	6	14	16	4	—	20
raw, not pared	95.1	15	0.9	0	0.9	—	—	32	46	44	10	24	28	8	—	34
DANDELION GREENS, raw	85.6	45	2.7	0	2.7	—	—	—	—	—	—	—	—	—	—	—
cooked	89.8	33	2.0	0	2.0	—	—	—	—	—	—	—	—	—	—	—
ENDIVE, curly & escarole, raw	93.1	20	1.7	0	1.7	13	31	72	123	78	22	78	71	—	54	81
KOHLRABI, raw	90.3	29	2.0	0	2.0	—	19	56	68	30	6	43	38	10	38	65
cooked	92.2	24	1.7	0	1.7	—	—	—	—	—	—	43	—	—	—	—
LENTILS, whole seeds, cooked	72.0	106	7.8	0	7.8	—	—	413	554	476	55	359	273	70	—	421
LETTUCE, Bibb or Boston, raw	95.1	14	1.2	0	1.2	—	—	—	—	70	4	—	—	12	—	—
Iceberg, raw	95.5	13	0.9	0	0.9	—	—	—	—	—	—	36	—	—	—	—
Romaine or Cos, raw	94.0	18	1.3	0	1.3	—	—	—	—	70	4	—	—	12	—	—
MUSHROOMS, raw, Agaricus campestris	90.4	28	2.7	0	2.7	—	—	597	316	—	189	—	—	8	—	424
MUSTARD GREENS, leaves w/o stems & midribs, boiled	92.6	23	2.2	0	2.2	—	—	73	59	108	22	70	57	35	—	103
OKRA PODS, cooked	91.1	29	2.0	0	2.0	—	—	76	112	84	24	72	74	20	—	100
ONION, raw	89.1	38	1.5	0	1.5	—	14	21	37	64	13	38	22	21	42	31
boiled	91.8	29	1.2	0	1.2	—	—	18	31	55	11	34	19	18	—	26
PARSLEY, raw	85.1	44	3.6	0	3.6	—	—	—	—	230	18	—	—	72	—	—
PEAS, green, immature, raw	78.0	84	6.3	0	6.3	—	—	290	397	296	44	223	101	50	161	258
green, immature, cooked	81.5	71	5.4	0	5.4	—	—	248	340	254	38	191	86	43	138	221
green, immature, frozen, cooked	82.1	68	5.1	0	5.1	—	—	235	321	240	36	199	82	41	—	209
green, sweet, low sodium, canned	81.8	72	4.4	0	4.4	—	—	202	277	207	31	172	70	35	—	180
PEPPERS, green, sweet, raw	93.4	22	1.2	0	1.2	—	14	46	46	51	16	55	50	9	—	33
green, sweet, immature, cooked	94.7	18	1.0	0	1.0	—	—	38	38	42	13	46	42	7	—	27

Footnote at end of table

(Continued)

TABLE P-37 *(Continued)*

Food Name—100 Gram (3.5 oz) Portion	Water	Food Energy Calories	Total Protein	Animal Protein	Plant Protein	Amino Acids										
						Cystine	Histidine	Isoleucine	Leucine	Lysine	Methionine	Phenylalanine	Threonine	Tryptophan	Tyrosine	Valine
	(g)	(kcal)	(g)	(g)	(g)	(mg)	(mg)	(mg)	(mg)	(mg)	(mg)	(mg)	(mg)	(mg)	(mg)	(mg)
POTATO, baked in skin	75.1	93	2.6	0	2.6	—	101	463	486	330	70	295	225	90	84	420
pared, boiled	82.8	65	1.9	0	1.9	—	—	84	95	101	23	84	78	19	—	101
french fried	44.7	274	4.3	0	4.3	—	—	184	210	222	50	184	172	42	—	222
fried from raw w/vegetable shortening	46.9	268	4.0	0	4.0	—	—	176	200	212	48	176	164	40	—	212
hashed brown in vegetable shortening	54.2	229	3.1	0	3.1	—	—	136	155	164	37	136	127	31	—	164
mashed, plain, w/o milk, fat, or seasonings	82.8	65	1.9	0	1.9	—	—	84	95	101	23	84	78	19	—	101
mashed, w/milk & margarine	79.8	94	2.1	0.6	1.5	—	—	92	105	111	25	92	86	21	—	111
RADISHES, raw	94.5	17	1.0	0	1.0	—	—	—	—	34	2	—	59	5	—	30
SOYBEANS, mature seeds, cooked	71.0	130	11.0	0	11.0	—	—	649	935	759	165	594	423	165	—	638
SPINACH, raw	90.7	26	3.2	0	3.2	—	—	150	246	198	54	145	141	51	116	176
cooked	92.0	23	3.0	0	3.0	—	—	141	231	186	51	136	132	48	109	164
frozen, cooked	91.9	23	3.0	0	3.0	—	—	141	231	186	51	129	132	48	—	165
canned	91.4	24	2.7	0	2.7	—	—	126	206	166	46	122	117	43	98	146
low sodium, canned	91.3	26	3.2	0	3.2	—	—	126	206	166	46	114	117	43	—	146
SQUASH, summer, cooked	95.5	14	0.9	0	0.9	—	—	29	41	34	12	24	21	7	—	33
winter, baked	81.4	63	1.8	0	1.8	—	—	58	81	68	23	49	41	14	—	66
winter, boiled	88.8	38	1.1	0	1.1	—	—	35	50	42	14	30	25	9	—	41
SWEET POTATO, baked in skin	63.7	141	2.1	0	2.1	—	—	101	120	99	38	104	99	36	61	157
boiled in skin	70.6	114	1.7	0	1.7	—	—	—	—	—	—	85	—	—	50	—
canned	71.9	108	2.0	0	2.0	—	—	96	114	94	36	100	94	34	58	150
low sodium, canned	71.9	108	2.0	0	2.0	—	—	96	114	94	36	110	94	34	—	150
candied	60.0	168	1.3	0	1.3	—	—	62	74	61	23	72	61	22	—	98
TOMATO, raw	93.5	22	1.1	0	1.1	—	15	29	41	42	7	28	33	9	24	28
cooked	92.4	26	1.3	0	1.3	—	15	29	41	42	7	33	33	9	28	28
canned	93.7	21	1.0	0	1.0	—	15	29	41	42	7	25	33	9	21	28
low sodium, canned	94.1	20	1.0	0	1.0	—	—	29	41	42	7	25	33	9	21	28
TOMATO, GREEN, raw	93.0	24	1.2	0	1.2	—	15	29	41	42	7	28	33	9	14	28
TOMATO PASTE, canned, w/o salt	75.0	82	3.4	0	3.4	—	58	70	95	98	18	72	78	—	45	78
TOMATO PUREE, canned	87.0	39	1.7	0	1.7	—	—	49	70	71	12	48	56	15	—	48
canned, low sodium	88.0	39	1.7	0	1.7	—	—	49	70	71	12	48	56	15	—	48
TURNIP GREENS, frozen, chopped, cooked	92.7	23	2.5	0	2.5	—	—	81	156	99	40	100	95	35	71	112
TURNIP, raw	91.5	30	1.0	0	1.0	—	8	12	19	21	3	12	12	—	7	17
cooked	93.6	23	0.8	0	0.8	—	—	14	—	42	9	17	—	—	21	—
WATERCRESS OR GARDEN CRESS, raw	89.4	32	2.6	0	2.6	—	—	140	230	160	20	110	150	50	—	150

1 The authors gratefully acknowledge that these food compositions were obtained from the HVH-CWRU Data Base developed by the Division of Nutrition, Highland View Hospital, and the Departments of Biometry and Nutrition, School of Medicine, Case Western Reserve University, Cleveland, Ohio.

PROTEIN, ANIMAL

Generally high quality protein derived from meat, milk, poultry, fish, and eggs, and their products.
(Also see PROTEIN[S].)

PROTEIN AS ENERGY SOURCE

In the body, protein functions in the (1) building of new tissues, (2) upkeep of tissues, (3) regulation of water and acid base balance, (4) production of enzymes, antibodies, hormones, and vitamins, (5) formation of milk, and (6) provision of energy. When more protein is eaten than is needed for the first five functions listed above, the excess protein is metabolized for energy. In addition, protein of the diet, along with tissue proteins, is burned for energy when the diet contains insufficient carbohydrates and fats. When this occurs, the building or repair processes of the body suffer. However, energy needs of the body have a higher priority. As a source of energy, protein yields about 4 kcal/g.

(Also see METABOLISM; PROTEIN[S]; and BIOLOGICAL VALUE [BV] OF PROTEINS.)

PROTEIN-BOUND IODINE (PBI)

The iodine that is bound to thyroxin and in transit in the plasma is known as protein-bound iodine. In the normal individual, PBI values range from 4 to 8 micrograms/100 milliliters of plasma.

PROTEIN, COMPLETE

Casein and egg albumin are examples of complete proteins. They contain all of the essential amino acids in sufficient amounts to maintain life and support growth.

(Also see PROTEIN[S].)

PROTEIN, CRUDE

This refers to all the nitrogenous compounds in a food. It is determined by finding the nitrogen content, as determined by the Kjeldahl process, and multiplying the result by 6.25. The nitrogen content of protein averages about 16% (100 ÷ 16 = 6.25).

(Also see PROTEIN[S].)

PROTEIN EFFICIENCY RATIO (PER)

By definition it is the weight gain of a young growing animal expressed in grams divided by the grams of protein eaten over a 4 week period, or some other predetermined time. It provides a biological means for evaluating protein quantity. Casein and egg albumin yield the maximum values, while proteins like gliadin will not even support growth.

(Also see PROTEIN[S]; and BIOLOGICAL VALUE [BV] OF PROTEINS.)

PROTEIN FACTOR

A number used to convert the Kjeldahl nitrogen content of food to protein, since most of the nitrogen measured by the Kjeldahl method is derived from the protein contained in the food. On the average, protein contains about 16% nitrogen (16 g of nitrogen for every 100 g of protein); however, this can range from 15 to 18%. For most foods, to determine the crude protein content, the Kjeldahl nitrogen value is multiplied by 6.25 (100 ÷ 16). Where greater accuracy is desired, the specific factor for converting nitrogen to protein may be used. For example, the factor for most nuts is 5.30 while for milk and cheese it is 6.38.

(Also see KJELDAHL; and PROTEIN[S].)

PROTEIN HYDROLYSATE

A solution containing the amino acids derived from an artificially digested protein, usually milk or beef protein. Used extensively in medicine and surgery. Usually administered by a stomach tube or intravenous injection.

PROTEIN, INCOMPLETE

A protein that cannot maintain life or support growth is classified as incomplete; for example, zein (corn protein) and gelatin.

(Also see PROTEIN[S].)

PROTEIN MALNUTRITION

When the diet fails to meet the body's needs for protein quality and quantity, impaired function, growth and/or development result. The extreme case of protein malnutrition is kwashiorkor, which develops in infants consuming a deficiency of protein and marginal to adequate amounts of energy. Often there is an inadequate or imbalance of both protein and energy; hence, it is convenient to class the resulting disorders as various types of protein-energy malnutrition (PEM).

(Also see DEFICIENCY DISEASES, Table D-1 Major Dietary Deficiency Diseases—"Protein-energy malnutrition"; MALNUTRITION and MALNUTRITION, PROTEIN-ENERGY.)

PROTEIN, MILK

When the term milk refers to cow or human milk, the proteins involved are casein and lactalbumin, both high quality proteins. In cow milk casein is the predominate protein, while in human milk casein and lactalbumin are present in about equal amounts. However, human milk contains only about one third as much protein as cow milk.

(Also see MILK AND MILK PRODUCTS; and PROTEIN[S].)

PROTEIN, PARTIALLY COMPLETE

Gliadin, a protein found in wheat, is an example of a partially complete protein. It can maintain life, but it cannot support growth.

(Also see PROTEIN[S].)

PROTEIN SCORE (CHEMICAL SCORE)

A chemical means of evaluating a protein on the basis of its amino acid content. More often this is called the chemical score or amino acid score.

(Also see PROTEIN[S], section headed "Quantity and Quality.")

PROTEIN, SINGLE-CELL

Protein obtained from single-cell organisms, such as yeast, bacteria, and algae, and grown on specially prepared growth media. Dried brewers' yeast is one of the most familiar examples.

(Also see PROTEIN[S], section headed "Protein of the World.")

PROTEIN, VEGETABLE

Protein derived from plants. Most vegetable protein supplements, although not all, are the by-products that remain after extracting oil from soybeans, cottonseed,

linseed, peanuts, safflower, sunflower, rapeseed, and coconut. Soybean is by far the most widely used vegetable protein.
(Also see PROTEIN[S].)

PROTEINURIA

Presence of protein in the urine.

PROTEIN UTILIZATION (NET PROTEIN UTIL-IZATION; NPU)

A procedure employed to determine protein quality. It is the proportion of the nitrogen in the food that is retained by the tissues of the body. In other words, it is the amount of nitrogen contained in the food consumed minus the amount lost in the urine and feces divided by the amount of nitrogen in the food.
(Also see PROTEIN[S], section headed "Quantity and Quality.")

PROTEIN, WORLD PER CAPITA

Worldwide, there are about 69 g of protein available each day for every individual—an amount which should be more than adequate. However, each individual does not receive this amount and the following must be considered: (1) distribution of protein, (2) the source of protein, and (3) the calories available.

1. **Distribution.** In developing countries, there are about 57 g of protein available each day for every individual, while in the developed countries there are about 98 g per person per day available. However, within a country, the per capita consumption of total amounts of food and therefore, protein, declines as income declines—as a general rule.

2. **Source.** Worldwide, people in developing countries receive a smaller portion of their daily intake of protein from animal sources than do people of developed countries. In developing countries, the protein from animal sources accounts for about 15% (9 g) of the daily protein intake, whereas in developed countries, animal protein represents an average of about 59% (57 g) of the daily protein in the diet. Therefore, people of the developing countries consume largely protein of plant origin which is often deficient in essential amino acids, especially lysine, methionine, and/or tryptophan. Also, it is important to remember that within any country the poor receive a smaller portion of their daily protein as animal proteins.

3. **Calories.** In many underdeveloped areas of the world, protein intake is marginal and of poor quality (plant origin), but the energy (calorie) intake is so low that the protein eaten is not used for its essential functions. The name "marasmus," resulting from a protein-energy (calorie) malnutrition, is applied to a whole spectrum of protein and energy deficiencies, while the condition resulting from a severe protein deficiency, but adequate energy, is called kwashiorkor.

(Also see HUNGER, WORLD; INCOME, PROPORTION SPENT FOR FOOD; MALNUTRITION; POPULATION, WORLD; PROTEIN[S]; and WORLD FOOD.)

PROTEOLYSIS

The breakdown of proteins or peptides into smaller units—polypeptides tripeptides, dipeptides and amino acids. Digestion of proteins entails proteolysis.
(Also see DIGESTION AND ABSORPTION; and PROTEIN[S].)

PROTEOSE

A derivative of protein formed during digestion.

PROTHROMBIN

One of four blood clotting proteins synthesized by the liver, the manufacture of which is regulated by vitamin K, present in the blood plasma, essential to clotting of blood.
(Also see VITAMIN K.)

PROTHROMBIN ACTIVATOR

A complex substance that splits prothrombin to form thrombin, an essential step in the blood clotting process.

PROTON

A particle of the nucleus of an atom that has a charge of plus one. A proton is a positive hydrogen ion (H^+).

PROTOPLASM

The living matter in all cells.

PROTOPORPHYRIN

The precursor of heme.

PROVITAMIN A

Carotene.
(Also see VITAMIN A.)

PROXIMAL

Next to or nearest the point of attachment or origin.

PROXIMATE ANALYSIS

Developed by workers at the Weende Experiment Station in Germany in 1895, it is the most generally used chemical scheme for evaluating foodstuffs, despite the fact that the information it gives may often be of uncertain nutritional significance or even misleading. According to it, a foodstuff is partitioned into the six fractions: (1) moisture (water) or dry matter (DM); (2) total (crude) protein (CP or TP—N x 6.25); (3) ether extract (EE) or fat; (4) ash (mineral salts); (5) crude fiber (CF)—the incompletely digested carbohydrates; and (6) nitrogen-free extract (NFE)—the more readily digested carbohydrates (calculated rather than measured chemically).

(Also see ANALYSIS OF FOODS.)

PRUNE *Prunus* **spp**

A type of plum that may be dried satisfactorily without removal of the pith. Only a few of the many cultivated varieties of plums can be so dried. Usually, the prune types of plums have a higher than average sugar content.

The nutrient compositions of various forms of prunes are given in Food Composition Table F-36.

Some noteworthy observations regarding the nutrient composition of prunes follow:

1.   Unsweetened, stewed prunes are moderately high in calories (119 kcal per 100 g) and carbohydrates (31%). They are a good source of potassium, iron, and vitamin A, but their vitamin C content is very low.

2.   Sweetened prunes are almost 50% higher in calories and carbohydrates than unsweetened prunes.

3.   Uncooked dried prunes are very rich in calories (344 kcal per 100 g), carbohydrates (91%), potassium, and iron. They are also an excellent source of vitamin A, and a good source of calcium and phosphorus.

(Also see PLUMS AND PRUNES; and PRUNE JUICE.)

PRUNE JUICE

A water extract of dried prunes that is produced by (1) pulverizing the prunes (this may be done with the aid of enzymes that break down the pectin which binds the fruit tissue), and (2) leaching the prune pulp with hot water. The resulting prune juice may be either (1) sweetened, or (2) left unsweetened, because the natural sugar content of prunes is generally high.

The nutrient composition of prune juice is given in Food Composition Table F-36.

Some noteworthy observations regarding the nutrient composition of prune juice follow:

1.   A ½-cup serving (*125 g*) of unsweetened prune juice is moderately high in calories (96 kcal) and carbohydrates (24 g).

2.   Prune juice is an excellent source of iron and potassium, but it is a poor source of vitamins A and C.

3.   Many people find that the consumption of prune juice helps to promote regularity of bowel movement. However, the amounts required to produce this effect vary considerably among different people, from as little as a small glass to as much as a pint or more.

(Also see PLUMS AND PRUNES; and PRUNE[S].)

PSORIASIS

A condition of the skin wherein red, itchy patches frequently appear on the scalp, knees, elbows, chest, abdomen, palms, and soles of the feet. These red patches tend to grow and join together creating extensive, unsightly and umcomfortable areas. However, psoriasis seldom causes long-term physical harm. Its cause is obscure but there is evidence to suggest it runs in families. No single treatment exists which will completely clear up the disease. Some treatments providing relief include ointments containing coal tar derivatives or mercury compounds, cortisone pills or ointment, x-ray and sunbathing. In the past, low taurine—a product of cysteine metabolism and normal constituent of animal protein—diets were designed, and recommended for sufferers of psoriasis.

PSYCHROPHILIC BACTERIA

These bacteria are "cold lovers," but despite their name they actually tolerate cold rather than prefer it. Most bacteria, mesophiles, have optimal growth at 97-111°F (*37-44°C*). Psychrophiles grow and reproduce at the usual refrigeration temperatures. In fact, some types can substantially multiply at 32°F (*0°C*). These bacteria are important as they are responsible for most of the fresh food spoilage that occurs. Low temperatures should not be relied on to destroy bacteria. Even in frozen foods some bacteria survive; hence, after thawing, frozen foods should not be allowed to stand at room temperature.

(Also see BACTERIA IN FOOD; and PRESERVATION OF FOOD.)

PSYLLIUM *Plantago psyllium*

An annual herb grown in southern Europe and India. It bears a seed that has laxative qualities and is used in medicines. When the seed is moistened, it looks like gelatin.

PTOMAINES

The word ptomaine comes from the Greek word *ptoma*, meaning "dead body." It refers to a group of extremely poisonous organic compounds formed during the microbial or enzymatic decomposition of animal proteins. Ptomaines are easily detected by the deteriorated appearance of the material (almost to a liquid state) and the putrid odor. Such food is hardly human fare!

Food poisoning by bacterial toxins, such as salmonellosis or staphylococcal intoxication, is sometimes called "ptomaine poisoning," which is incorrect.

(Also see BACTERIA IN FOOD.)

PUBERTY

The age at which the sex organs begin to function and at which sexual features begin to appear. The average age of puberty in boys is from 13 to 16, in girls from 11 to 14.

PUERPERIUM

The period from delivery of the infant to the time when the uterus regains its normal size, usually about 6 weeks.

PULP

The solid residue remaining after extraction of juices from fruits, roots, or stems.

PULSES

Pulses are the seeds of leguminous plants. The following pulses are commonly used for human food: beans, chickpeas, cowpeas, field peas, peanuts, pigeonpeas, and soybeans.

PUMMELO (POMELO; SHADDOCK) *Citrus grandis*

This fruit is the largest of the citrus fruits (which belong to the family *Rutaceae*) ranging in size between 4 and 12 in. (*10 and 30 cm*) in diameter.

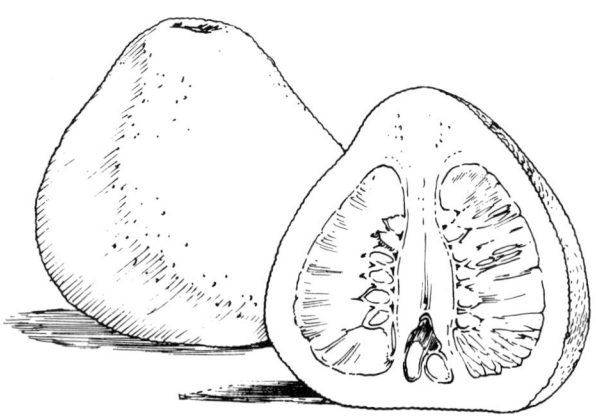

Fig. P-118.   Pummelo, an ancestor of the grapefruit.

The pummelo was brought from its native home of Malaysia to Barbados in the 17th century by Captain Shaddock of the British East India Company. The grapefruit (*C. paradisi*), which was discovered in Barbados in 1750, is believed to have arisen as either a mutation or a natural hybrid of this fruit.

Pummelos are low in calories (34 kcal per 100 g) and carbohydrates (8.5%). However, they are also a good source of vitamin C.

(Also see GRAPEFRUIT.)

PUMPERNICKEL BREAD

This is a sourdough bread made from unbolted (unsifted) rye flour.

PUMPKINS *Cucurbita* spp

The fruits of these plants provide both edible flesh and edible seeds. Also, the flowers are edible. Pumpkins belong to the gourd or melon family (*Cucurbitaceae*), which also includes squashes and cucumbers. The different species of pumpkins are *C. maxima, C. mixta, C. moschata,* and *C. pepo.* Certain varieties of fruits within each of these species are squashes rather than pumpkins. Although there is some confusion between the terms *pumpkin* and *squash,* pumpkins are generally considered to be the large, orange fruits that have a coarse, strongly flavored flesh. They are not usually served as table vegetables, but are used mainly for (1) pies, and (2) decorations during the holidays in the fall. Pumpkins often have been referred to in writings; for example, James Whitecomb Riley mentions them in his poem "When the Frost is on the Punkin."

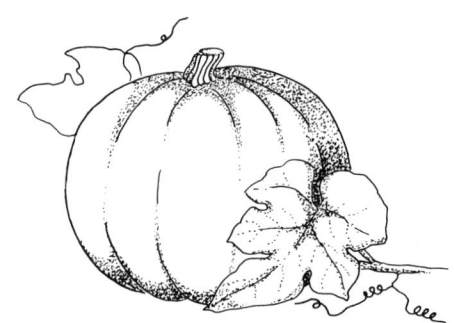

Fig. P-119.   The pumpkin, a sign of autumn in North America.

ORIGIN AND HISTORY. It is believed that the wild ancestors of the pumpkins originated in the region that is now Mexico and Guatemala. The ancient Aztec, Inca, and Maya Indians used pumpkin seeds as food, but they probably discarded the pulp because the wild fruits contained only small amounts of bitter tasting flesh. Most likely the modern varieties with abundant sweet flesh arose when the Indians selected mutant varieties for cultivation.

The European explorers of the New World thought that pumpkins were giant species of melons. By that time, these fruits were seen growing throughout Mexico, North America, and the West Indies, from as far north as southeastern Canada to as far south as Mexico City. They were soon brought back to the Old World to be grown from western Europe to eastern Asia.

Sometimes the Indians' ways of utilizing the crops were adopted and modified by Asians and Europeans. For example, the farmers of Manchuria dried strips of pumpkin in the sun and the Italians ate deep-fried, batter-covered pumpkin flowers. Both practices have been passed down through the ages and are still utilized.

The early American colonists learned much from the Indians after having experienced a severe winter that killed crops, livestock, and people. Later, turkey and pumpkin pie became traditional foods that remind us of the first Thanksgiving when the Indians and Pilgrims shared in a feast comprised mainly of native American foods. However, we seem to have forgotten the early American practice of making beer from pumpkins, maple sugar, and persimmons.

At the present time certain agricultural scientists are engaged in breeding some of the wild, ancestral species of pumpkins in order to develop new varieties that (1) will grow well in arid regions, and (2) will produce large amounts of high-protein seed.

PRODUCTION. Statistics on the production of pumpkins are not readily available, because data for this crop is usually combined with that for squashes. Furthermore, squashes are much more widely grown and utilized than pumpkins. Hence, the combined data reflects mainly the production of the former crop.

(Also see SQUASHES.)

Most commercial growers plant pumpkin seeds directly in the fields because the roots of the young plants are easily injured by transplanting. The seeds are planted in groups called hills. The soil should be fertile, well-drained, rich in organic matter, and only mildly acid to mildly alkaline. Strongly acid soils may require the addition of lime. Often, the soil may be fertilized with various combinations of animal or green manure, and nitrogen, phosphorus, and potassium mixtures. Pumpkins should *not* be watered with sprinklers if it can be avoided because wetting the leaves of the plant may encourage the spread of disease. Hence, drip irrigation and furrow irrigation are more desirable methods of watering.

Pumpkins require 4 months to reach maturity. They may be picked after the rind has hardened, but they may be left on the plant until after the first light frost or when the vines have begun to wither. A light frost makes the fruits sweeter. However, the fruits should be picked before they are likely to be damaged by a hard frost. Pumpkins may be stored at 50° to 55°F (*10° to 13°C*) for several months if they are harvested at full maturity and immediately cured for 2 weeks at 75° to 85°F (*24° to 29°C*).

PROCESSING. Pumpkins are processed by removal of the rind and seeds, followed by cooking of the pulp prior to canning, freezing, or baking into cakes, custards, or pies. However, canned pumpkin pie fillings or even the ready-made pies may often contain winter squash in lieu of pumpkin. Some gourmets believe that the flavor of the squash is superior.

Other noteworthy, but less common, pumpkin products are (1) dehydrated pumpkin flakes that are made by drum-drying cooked pumpkin puree which has been mixed with starch and sugar; (2) dehydrated pumpkin pie mix which contains dehydrated pumpkin flakes, dried milk powder, dried egg, sugar, corn syrup solids, starch, flavorings, and a vegetable gum; (3) pumpkin pickles made from pumpkin cubes that have been cooked briefly, then mixed with sugar, vinegar, water, and spices, and canned in glass jars; and (4) pumpkin seeds that are sold raw or roasted and salted.

SELECTION. The rind of a pumpkin should be hard. Softness of rind may indicate immature, thin flesh, which may be watery and lacking in flavor when cooked. Fruits with cuts, punctures, water-soaked areas, or moldy spots on the rind may have begun to decay. However, slight variations in the color of the skin do not affect the quality.

PREPARATION. Some suggestions for utilizing the various parts of the pumpkin plant follow:

• **Pumpkin flesh**—The fruits should be cut into halves or small sections, the rind, fibrous matter, and seeds removed, and the remaining flesh cut into smaller pieces. Usually, a half hour to an hour of boiling is required to tenderize the flesh, but only 15 minutes of cooking in a pressure cooker is sufficient. Then, the cooked pumpkin may be mashed or pureed in a blender. (The puree may require straining to remove residual fibers.) Cooked pumpkin is usually made into custards, pies, and puddings. (Canned, cooked pumpkin serves these purposes very well.) However, Latin Americans utilize pumpkin mainly in soups and stews.

• **Pumpkin flowers**—These should be picked when open so that no bees will be treapped within the blossoms. The flowers are good when dipped in a batter and fried in deep fat.

• **Pumpkin seeds**—The seeds of pumpkins may be dried for a few days, after which any adhering tissue should be removed. Then, they may be roasted or fried in oil. Some people boil the seeds briefly in salted water before roasting or frying.

NUTRITIONAL VALUE. The nutrient compositions of various forms of pumpkin are given in Food Composition Table F-36.

Some noteworthy observations regarding the nutrient composition of pumpkin follow:

1. Fresh and canned pumpkin contain over 90% water and are low in calories (about 30 kcal per 100 g). However, they are excellent sources of vitamin A. It is noteworthy that pureed squash baby food has a nutrient composition similar to that of canned pumpkin and may be used in lieu of the latter when only small quantities are required.

2. A 4 oz (*114 g*) serving of pumpkin pie plus an 8 oz (*244 g*) glass of milk constitute a nutritious meal for a growing child, except that insufficient iron is provided unless dark molasses is used as the sweetener in the pie.

The pie supplies ample calories and vitamin A, a moderate amount of protein, and fair amounts of calcium and phosphorus; whereas the milk is rich in protein, calcium, phosphorus, and the vitamin B complex.

3. Pumpkin flowers contain 95% water and are low in calories (16 kcal per 100 g) and most other nutrients, except that they provide fair amounts of phosphorus, iron, vitamin A and vitamin C. It is suggested that calorie-conscious people eat pumpkin flowers in a salad, soup, or stew.

4. The seeds from pumpkins are very rich in calories (553 kcal per 100 g), protein (29%), iron (11.2 mg per 100 g), and phosphorus (1,144 mg per 100 g). Hence, the consumption of as little as 1 oz (*28 g*) of the seeds per day will make a significant nutritional contribution to the diet.

(Also see VEGETABLE[S], Table V-6 Vegetables of the World.)

PURGATIVE

A strong laxative.
(Also see LAXATIVE.)

PURINES

These are nitrogen-containing substances with a ring structure like that of Fig. P-120. They are widely distributed in nature, and are components of the nucleic acids.

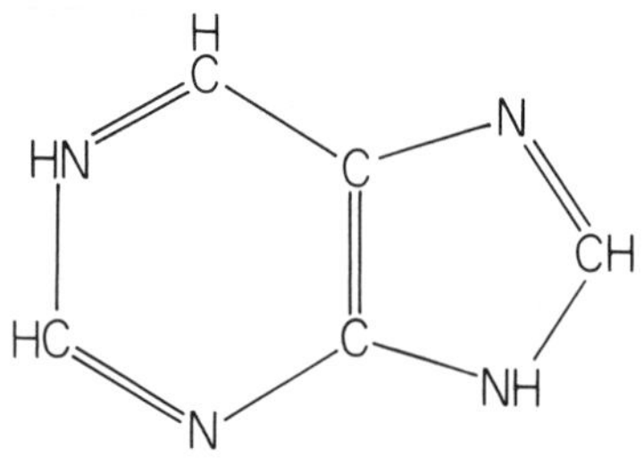

Fig. P-120.   The general structure of a purine.

Important purines are adenine, guanine, xanthine, and uric acid, which is the excretory form of the purines in humans. Another common purine is the stimulant caffeine. Persons suffering from gout or uric acid kidney stones should limit their dietary sources of purines. Some of the richest food sources of purines are anchovies, asparagus, brains, kidney, liver, mincemeats, mushrooms, sardines, and sweetbreads. Foods with a low purine content include breads, cereals, fats, cheese, eggs, fruits, milk, nuts, sweets, and most vegetables.

(Also see ARTHRITIS, section headed "Gout [gouty arthritis]"; CAFFEINE; and NUCLEIC ACIDS.)

PURIS

A puri is a very light, fried wheat cake which originated in India. Butter is the preferred fat in which to fry it. Because it is an expensive dish, it is usually reserved for festive occasions.

PUROTHIONIN

A small easily digested protein of wheat. It has anti-bacterial properties, and in excess it may interfere with the rising of dough.
(Also see WHEAT.)

PUTREFACTION

The decomposition of proteins by microorganisms under anaerobic conditions.

PUTRESCINE

A foul-smelling chemical which arises in the bacterial fermentation of animal protein. It can be formed from ornithine or the amino acid arginine.

PYRIMIDINE

The parent substance of several nitrogenous compounds found in nucleic acids. The principal pyrimidines found in RNA are uracil and cytosine; in DNA they are thymine and cytosine.

PYRUVIC ACID (PYRUVATE; $CH_3COCOOH$)

An organic 3-carbon acid that is a key intermediate in carbohydrate, fat, and protein metabolism. It can participate in several metabolic pathways in the body. These pathways include (1) complete oxidation to water and carbon dioxide in the tricarboxylic acid (Krebs) cycle, (2) formation of fatty acid, (3) reversible conversion to lactic acid, (4) conversion to the amino acid alanine, and (5) formation of glucose by reversal of the enzymatic sequence which normally breaks down glucose.

(Also see METABOLISM.)

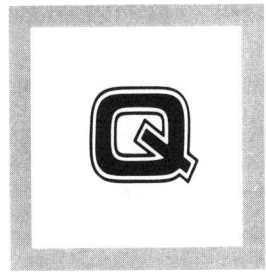

QUADRIPLEGIA

Paralysis of both arms and both legs. It can be caused by disease—poliomyelitis, Landry's acute ascending paralysis (due to an acute infection of the spinal cord), diptheria, leprosy—or injury which severs the spinal cord at the fifth or sixth cervical vertebra. Quadriplegics require some special dietary considerations due to reduced activity and difficulties encountered in preparing and eating food.

(Also see MODIFIED DIETS; and DISEASES.)

QUAIL (CALIFORNIA QUAIL, GAMBEL'S QUAIL, MEARN'S QUAIL, MOUNTAIN QUAIL, SCALED QUAIL)

Quail is the name given to several different kinds of birds. In Europe, it refers to several kinds of game birds of the pheasant family. Americans use the name for the bobwhite.

The bobwhite quail and the Japanese quail are listed in separate sections of this book. Other kinds of American quail are the California quail, Gambel's quail, Mearn's quail, mountain quail, and scaled quail. These birds live in western and southwestern United States.

All of the different quails are highly prized game birds and furnish good eating.

QUALITY OF PROTEIN

A term used to describe the amino acid balance of protein. A protein is said to be of good quality when it contains all the essential amino acids in proper proportions and amounts; and it is said to be of poor quality when it is deficient in either content or balance of essential amino acids. From this it is evident that the usefulness of a protein source for man depends upon its amino acid composition.

QUICK BREADS

This term is usually applied to batters or doughs that are baked (in some cases, boiled, fried, grilled, or steamed) right after mixing, rather than being allowed to rise before baking. Hence, quick breads are not made with yeast. Instead, they are unleavened, or leavened with air, baking powder, a sourdough starter, or steam.

The elimination of the need for yeast leavening allows the use of a wide variety of flours that may contain little or no gluten—the elastic protein in wheat flour that helps to trap the leavening gas. (Weaker flours may be used for quick breads because rising takes place in the oven, as the proteins in the dough are gradually made firm by baking. Furthermore, egg white has a greater strengthening effect on doughs that are baked right after mixing.)

HISTORY. There is archaeological evidence that the first breads baked by primitive peoples were crude, unleavened forms of quick breads similar to those used today. These breads were made by mixing flours or meals with water and baking the dough on hot stones. Fig. Q-1 depicts the making of an early type of quick bread.

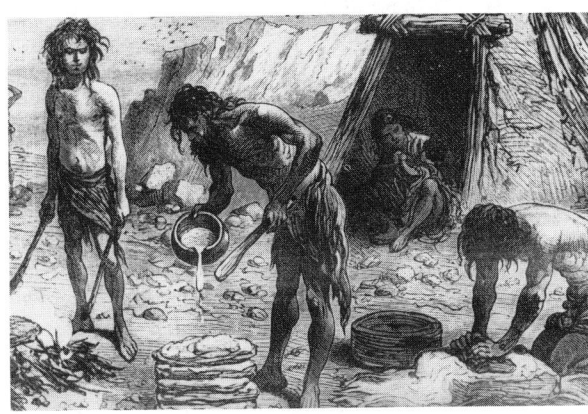

Fig. Q-1. History's first pancake-maker: prehistoric man pouring dough on heated stones. At the right side, a boy is preparing the dough. On the left side, another boy is heating the baking stones. Stones were piled, one upon the other, until sufficient pancakes were made for the whole family. (Courtesy, The Bettmann Archive, Inc.)

The ancient quick breads were likely to be heavy and soggy unless there was some leavening by air and/or steam, which could have occurred when (1) the bread grain(s) was ground to a fine flour, and (2) heating of the dough was rapid due to a high cooking temperature and/or rolling the dough into a thin layer.

Lighter breads were made after the discovery of sourdough and yeast leavening, although the wheat and rye flours which were best suited for this type of leavening were often in short supply. Hence, many people had to eat heavy breads made from acorns, barley, beans, nuts, peas, and seeds of wild plants. It appears that the American Indian always prepared the latter type of bread, because wheat and rye were not native to North America.

Thin, unleavened pancake-type breads became popular in many places around the world, because they could be prepared more rapidly, and they were more palatable after baking. The thicker types of unleavened breads were likely to remain soggy inside even though the outside had been baked until brown, or burned. Some of the thin breads which have remained popular to the present day are: (1) Chinese unleavened pancakes (egg roll wrappers); (2) chapaties made from whole wheat flour in India; (3) tortillas made from corn in Mexico; (4) crepes, usually

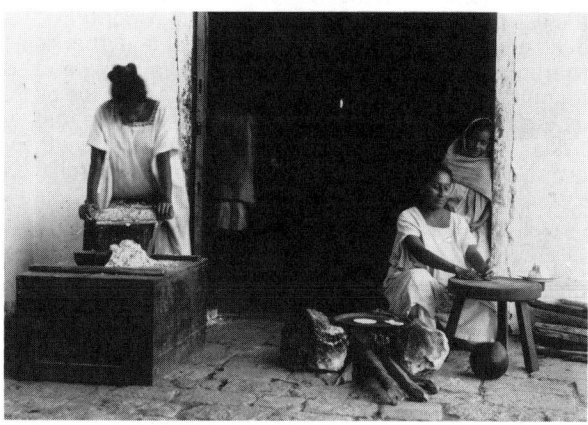

Fig. Q-2.   Crushing maize for tortillas in Mexico. (Courtesy, Field Museum of Natural History, Chicago, Ill.)

made from wheat, in France; (5) the crackerlike matzo—the only form of bread eaten by orthodox Jews during Passover; (6) Swedish crispbreads made by mixing rye meal with snow or powdered ice; and (7) bannocks made from oats and/or barley in Scotland. Even the American pioneers made an unleavened corn bread called a "hoe cake," which was baked on the blade of a hoe placed over hot coals. Wheat was scarce in North America until the Great Plains were settled and hardy Northern European wheats were planted.

The first type of baking powder appears to have been pearl ash, a crude form of potassium carbonate derived from wood ashes, which was invented in America in the 1790s. (Carbonates react with acids and give off carbon dioxide gas, the most commonly used leavener. Sometimes, heating is required to bring about the leavening reaction.) However, pearl ash left an unpleasant taste that had to be masked with sugars and other ingredients.

Later, in 1835, a mixture of cream of tartar (obtained from the residue in wine vats) and baking soda was developed. Shortly thereafter, the mixture was utilized in commercial baking powders. Also, a self-rising flour (one that contains baking powder) was developed in England in 1849. The marketing of these quick acting leavening agents soon led to the development of many new types of baked goods, such as baking powder biscuits, layer cakes, quick muffins, and soda bread. By the early 1900s, many homemakers were using self-rising flour and preleavened pancake mixes. Other preleavened baking mixes, which contained all required ingredients except a liquid, did not become popular until the 1940s, when new products were developed for the use of the military services.

At the present time, most people use preleavened baking mixes for preparing quick breads, cakes, and similar items. Some churches have even dispensed with cake sales to raise money because many of the products cost almost as much to make as the prices they receive.

(Also see BAKING POWDER AND BAKING SODA.)

MAJOR TYPES OF QUICK BREADS.
Fig. Q-3 shows some of the more popular items.

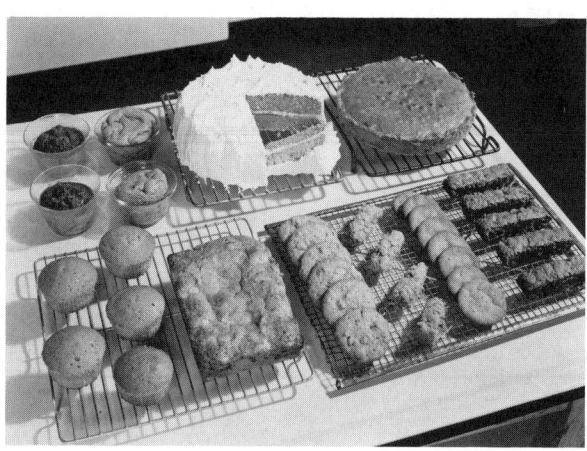

Fig. Q-3.   Cakes, cookies, muffins, and other highly desirable quick breads. (Courtesy, J. C. Allen & Son, West Lafayette, Ind.)

The basic ingredients used in all quick breads are flour, liquid, and a leavening agent. Many also contain shortening, eggs, sugar, salt, flavorings, and other ingredients. However, the characteristics of each baked product are determined mainly by the proportions of the ingredients, and the ways in which they are mixed. Table Q-1 gives brief descriptions of the preparation and characteristics of the more common types of quick breads. The basic proportions of ingredients and baking conditions for most of these products are given in the article BREADS AND BAKING—Table B-17.

TABLE Q-1
PREPARATION AND CHARACTERISTICS OF SELECTED QUICK BREADS

Product	Preparation[1]	Characteristics
Biscuits	(1) Flour, baking powder, and salt are sifted together; (2) fat is mixed in; (3) liquid is added; and (4) the dough is kneaded briefly, rolled out, and cut into rounds that are placed on an ungreased baking sheet. (Batter biscuits contain more liquid and are dropped from a spoon onto the sheet.)	Golden brown outside, moist inside, with a tender and flaky texture. Biscuits used for shortcake may be richer in fat and contain sugar.
Cakes: Angel food	(1) Egg whites are beaten until a foam[2] starts to form; (2) cream of tartar and flavoring are added; (3) beating is continued while sugar and flour are gradually folded in; and (4) the batter is poured into ungreased cake pans.	White, moist, very light, tender, and sweetly flavored.
Chiffon	(1) Flour, sugar, baking powder, and salt are sifted together; (2) oil, egg yolks, liquid, and flavoring are added; (3) the batter is mixed well; (4) egg whites[2] beaten with cream of tartar are folded in; and (5) the batter is poured into an ungreased tube pan, square pan, or rectangular pan.	Light brown outside, yellow inside, light and tender.
Plain	(1) Fat is creamed[3] with sugar; (2) eggs and flavoring are added and the mixture is stirred well; (3) portions of the sifted dry ingredients (flour, sugar, baking powder, and salt) are added alternately with the liquid and mixed gently; and (4) the batter is poured into greased pans.	Light, velvety texture; moist.
Pound	Similar to *Biscuits*, except that (1) considerable sugar is added, (2) eggs are beaten and added with the liquid; and (3) the batter is poured into an ungreased loaf pan.	Golden yellow inside, rich flavored, moist and compact.
Sponge	(1) Egg yolks, sugar, and liquid are beaten together until fluffy; (2) flavoring is added; (3) flour and salt are folded in gently; (4) stiffly beaten egg whites[2] are folded in; and (5) the batter is treated as for *Chiffon* cakes.	Golden yellow inside, very light, velvety texture, mildly sweet.
Coating batter	Similar to *Biscuits*, except that (1) much more liquid is used, and (2) this batter is allowed to stand for about ½ hour before being used to coat items (a stronger coating results when the leavening gas escapes).	Crispy, rich coating. Used mainly for coating fish, poultry, and vegetables that are fried in deep fat.
Cookies	Similar to *Plain Cakes*, except that this batter or dough generally contains more fat and egg, but less liquid and leavening. The dough may be refrigerated overnight before being sliced thin for baking.	Crisp, tender texture, and sweet flavor.
Cornbread	Similar to *Biscuits*, except that (1) more liquid is used, (2) cornmeal is substituted for some of the wheat flour, (3) a little sugar is added to the dry ingredients, (4) eggs are added with the milk and oil, and (5) batter is poured into a greased pan, or into muffin tins.	Moist and crumbly with rich flavor.
Crackers (Soda) Hard tack, Pilot Bread	Similar to *Biscuits*, except that (1) less leavening agent is used, and (2) the dough is rolled into a thin sheet. Hard tack contains the same ingredients but is larger and harder.	Crisp, light, and tender. Hard tack was developed for use on ships, hence, another name for it is ship biscuit.

Footnotes at end of table   *(Continued)*

TABLE Q-1 (*Continued*)

Product	Preparation[1]	Characteristics
Doughnuts	Similar to *Plain Cakes*, except that (1) less liquid is used, (2) this dough is rolled out and cut into doughnut shapes, and (3) the doughnuts are fried in deep fat.	Light brown, tender, with a sweet, rich flavor.
Dumplings	Similar to *Biscuits*, except that (1) more liquid is used, (2) fat is omitted, and (3) the batter is dropped by spoonfuls on the top of soups and stews.	Light and spongy.
Gingerbread	(1) The liquid, molasses, sugar, and fat are heated together with stirring in a saucepan, then allowed to cool, (2) flour, salt, spices, and baking soda are stirred in, and (3) the mixture is poured into a square cake pan.	Dark brown, moist and tender, with a mildly sweet, spicy flavor.
Muffins	Similar to *Biscuits*, except that (1) more liquid is used, (2) eggs and sugar are added, (3) blueberries, nuts, and/or raisins may be added, (4) cornmeal may be substituted for some of the wheat flour, and (5) the batter is poured into muffin pans.	Golden brown outside, tender texture, and slightly sweet flavor.
Pancakes	Similar to *Muffins*, except that the batter is baked on a hot griddle.	Golden brown color, light, tender, slightly sweet flavor.
Pastry: Pie crust	(1) The fat is cut into the mixture of flour and salt, (2) water is added, (3) the dough is rolled thin and placed in a pie pan.	Tender, flaky, and rich flavored.
Puff	(1) The fat is boiled with the water;[4] (2) the flour is added with stirring, and the heating continued until the mixture thickens; (3) the mixture is then allowed to cool before the eggs are added with constant beating; and (4) the batter is dropped on a greased baking sheet.	Rounded, hollow balls of flaky, tender pastry that are usually filled with whipped cream or a custard.
Popovers	Similar to *Biscuits*, except that (1) much more liquid is used, (2) eggs are added, and (3) the leavening agent is the steam generated by rapid baking in a hot oven.	Crisp, crusty, muffin-shaped bread with a hollow center that may be filled with pieces of cooked eggs, fish, meats, etc.
Scones	The original Scotch scones were made of oatmeal or barley flour, w/ or w/o added wheat flour, rolled flat, cut into wedges and baked on a griddle. Now, any flour or mixture of flours can be used, w/ added eggs, sugar, and currants, They may be rolled out or put in a round pan and flattened with the palm of the hand, marked in wedges and baked in the oven.	Scones are best served warm, with butter and jelly.
Soda bread	Similar to *Biscuits*, except that (1) more liquid (usually buttermilk) is used, and (2) baking soda is substituted for baking powder. (Sometimes, raisins may be added.)	Best taste and texture when eaten warm.
Waffles	Similar to *Pancakes*, except that (1) more eggs (best results are obtained when the yolks and the beaten whites are added separately) and fat are used, and (2) the batter is baked in a preheated waffle iron.	Golden-brown, crisp, tender, with a slightly sweet flavor.

[1]The preparation is usually made more simple by the use of preleavened mixes or complete mixes which require only the addition of the liquid. Also, many all-purpose biscuit and pancake mixes have directions on the package for the preparation of a wide variety of quick breads.
[2]Much of the leavening is provided by the air trapped in the egg white foam.
[3]The creaming of the semisolid fat results in the entrapment of considerable air, which provides a leavening effect.
[4]During baking, the water is converted to steam, which provides the leavening.

NUTRITIVE VALUES. Most quick breads are higher in calories than most yeast-leavened breads because they are usually made with more sugar and fat. Since many people have to control their caloric intake in order to avoid becoming obese, careful selection of dietary breads is necessary if one is to obtain the optimal nutritional benefits from these products without putting on excess weight. It is noteworthy that both the American Diabetes Association and the American Dietetic Association have recently advised dieters not to include cakes, cookies, and pies in their meal plans without the permission of a diet counselor.[1] However, certain dessert items such as custard pie may equal or exceed the nutritive values of many plain breads (in terms of nutrients per calorie). What is most important is that portion sizes of high caloric items be chosen within appropriate limits.

The Food Composition Table F-36 presents the nutritive values for many of the most popular baked goods—biscuits, cakes, cupcakes, cookies, crackers, doughnuts, muffins, pancakes, pies, waffles, and wafers.

In general, the information in Food Composition Table F-36 shows that there are wide variations in the values for calories and other nutrients supplied by the various quick breads. However, a dieter should not judge the merits of an item solely by its caloric content because sometimes a rich but nutritious item might be substituted for one or more of the nonbread foods in the diet. For example, two popovers have the protein content of 1 oz (28.4 g) of meat. This type of substitution should not be carried too far, because popovers supply from 2 to 3 times as many calories as the lean types of meat.

A convenient way of assessing the protein contribution of quick breads is to consider items containing less than 2.0 g of protein per 100 Calories (kcal) as poor sources of protein, those supplying from 2.0 g to 2.9 g as fair sources, and those containing 3.0 g or more of protein per 100 Calories (kcal) as good sources. Therefore, some poor choices for dieters are most cakes with icing and/or filling, cookies, doughnuts, gingerbread, and pies. Fair choices are biscuits, uniced angelfood cake, peanut cookies, cheese crackers, muffins, coconut custard and custard pies, and waffles. Some good choices are the items made with plenty of eggs and milk, but with only small amounts of fat and sugar. The best examples of the latter types of products are pancakes and popovers. Dieters might also select whole rye wafers, which contain more than 3 g of protein per 100 Calories (kcal). However, the protein quality of items containing only cereal protein (rye wafers) is lower than those containing a mixture of cereal with eggs and milk (pancakes).

Most quick breads are low in minerals and vitamins because they are made from white flour. Even the use of enriched flour does little to correct these deficiencies because only iron, thiamin, riboflavin, and niacin are restored; whereas more than 2 dozen essential minerals and vitamins are removed during the production of white flour.

Improving The Nutritive Values Of Homemade Quick Breads. The tables of nutritive values in the preceding section clearly showed that most baked goods supply too many calories and too few other nutrients. Hence, it is necessary for modern homemakers to revise recipes for quick breads by (1) reducing fat and sugar content, and (2) adding other ingredients that are low in calories and rich in more essential nutrients. Some suggestions for modifying recipes follow:

1. Muffins and pancakes lend themselves readily to experimentation because (a) wide ranges of consistencies and textures are acceptable in these products, and (b) small amounts may be prepared so that wastage of food is minimized if an experiment is unsuccessful.

2. Low-calorie, high-protein items may be prepared from mixtures of whole wheat flour, nonfat dry milk, beaten egg white, and water.

3. The use of a nonstick frying pan or griddle for making pancakes eliminates the need for oiling the cooking surface.

4. About 1/3 cup of grated cheese may be added for each cup (240 ml) of flour. This addition raises the content of protein, calcium, and phosphorus.

5. Sprouted seeds (usually those of beans or grains) add protein, fiber, minerals, and vitamins (about 1/3 cup per cup of flour).

6. Extra eggs may be added to most baked products, providing that a soft flour is used. Too many eggs toughen doughs.

7. About 1/8 cup of soy flour or nonfat dry milk may be substituted for a cup of wheat flour.

8. The caloric content of dessert items may be reduced by mixing one part of cake or cookie mix with one part of biscuit mix.

RECENT TRENDS IN QUICK BREAD TECHNOLOGY. The continuing rise in the employment of mothers has been accompanied by a reduction in the amount of time available for baking at home. Furthermore, the growing trends of eating out and of buying baked goods from bakeries have brought about a shortage of experienced bakers in certain areas. Hence, food technologists have recently developed some almost foolproof, time-saving products, such as those which follow:

• **Emulsified shortenings for packaged cake mixes**—The need to cream fats has been eliminated by the specially emulsified shortenings used in prepared cake mixes. Air bubbles are trapped by the special shortenings during mixing.

• **Frozen batters**—After thawing, these products may be poured right from the package (which is usually a short,

---

[1]*Exchange Lists for Meal Planning*, American Diabetes Association, Inc., and The American Dietetic Association, 1976, p. 4.

squat cardboard container like those used for cream or milk) onto a pancake griddle or a waffle iron.

• **Frozen quick breads**—These items are available in the forms of unbaked doughs and frozen baked products. The state of the art is such that few people can tell the difference between frozen and unfrozen products once they have been heated.

• **Fruit pie fillings**—Thickened fillings containing pieces of fruit have long been available in grocery stores. Now, a new line of pie fillings is made from gums, starches, sugar, and fruit purees. The new types of fillings make more efficient use of available fruit, so, hopefully, the cost of these products may be lower than those of the former types of fillings.

• **Gums**—These ingredients are often added to commercial baked goods and to packaged mixes because they strengthen weak flours without causing excessive toughening. Some other functions of these additives are: (1) thickening pie fillings and jellied ingredients, and (2) reducing the fat absorption of fried doughnuts.

• **Prebaked items**—Most prebaked products require only a little warming and/or browning in an oven prior to serving. Hence, they are being utilized increasingly by both homemakers and commercial and institutional food service establishments.

• **Prepackaged items for microwave baking**—Certain items packaged in cardboard trays may be heated in microwave ovens, but *not* those that are sold in metal foil pans. Metal foil may cause damage to microwave ovens.

• **Refrigerated doughs**—Most of these products require only (1) their placement in a suitable pan, and (2) baking. Cookie doughs also require slicing. The most popular items in this line are ready-to-bake biscuits, pastry, and rolls.

• **Separation of flours into high-protein and low-protein fractions**—In the past, high-protein hard wheats were used to make flours suitable for yeast-leavened doughs, and low-protein soft wheats yielded flours for quick breads. Now, either type of wheat may be milled and separated into high-protein and low-protein fractions by swirling streams of air in a process called air classification. This procedure enables millers to produce flours to meet customers' requirements.

QUILLAJA (SOAP BARK)

This is the inner dried bark of *Quillaja saponaria*, which grows in Peru and Chile. It contains quillaic acid, quillajasaponin, sucrose, and tannin. Soap bark is used to manufacture saponin, and to produce foams in various products. It is also approved as a natural flavor which can be used in foods.

QUINCE, PINEAPPLE *Cydonia oblonga*

A variety of pear-shaped quince that originated in California.

(Also see FRUIT[S], Table F-47 Fruits of the World—"Quince.")

QUINOA *Chenopodium quinoa*

This is a small annual herb of the goosefoot family, which is very similar to the common lamb's quarter. It is native to Bolivia, Chile, and Peru where it has been cultivated since 3000 B.C. The plant produces a great abundance of very small seeds, which are ground into meal and made into cakes or gruel or boiled like rice. The green parts are used as a pot herb like spinach. The ancient Incas called it "the mother grain" and revered it as sacred. Compared to other grains, it is high in protein (16% vs 7.5% for rice), calcium, and iron. Also, the grain has less than 1% gluten (compared to 15 to 16% in wheat flour); so, most people who are allergic to gluten can tolerate quinoa.

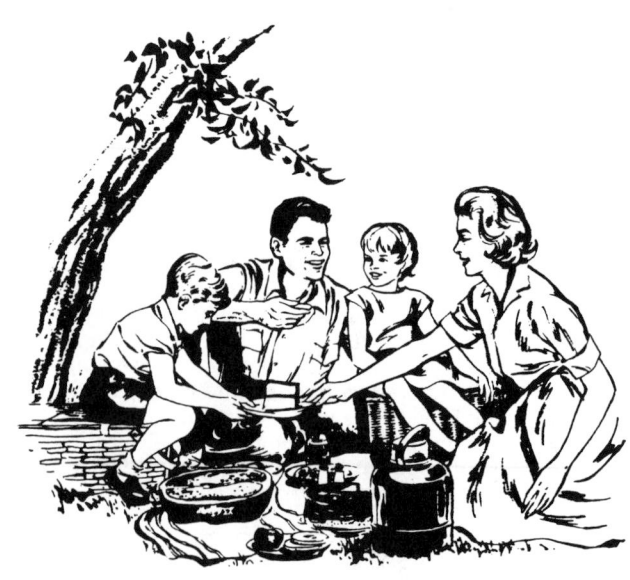

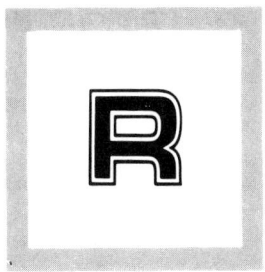

RABBIT

A small grayish brown mammal, native to southern Europe and northern Africa, which has been introduced into various other regions where it is often a pest because of its rapid reproduction. Under domestication, many breeds have been developed, with special adaptation for meat, fur, or show.

Ready-to-cook domestic rabbit is classed as either (1) fryer or young rabbit, or (2) roaster or mature rabbit. Fryers weigh from 1 ½ to 3 ½ lb (0.7 to 1.6 kg) and are usually less than 12 weeks of age; and the flesh is fine grained, tender, and a bright pearly pink color. Roasters usually weigh more than 4 lb (1.8 kg) and are 8 months of age or older; and the flesh is more coarse grained, slightly darker, less tender, and the fat more creamy in color than fryers.

RABBIT FEVER

The common name applied to the disease tularemia, since it is often contracted by man from infected rabbits.
(Also see TULAREMIA.)

RACCOON (RACOON)

A small wild animal, with longish grey fur, living in the forests of America. It is edible and cooked like wild rabbit.

RAD

In relation to radiation, it is a unit for measuring the radiation energy absorbed by a substance. One rad equals the absorption of 100 ergs of energy per gram.
(Also see RADIATION PRESERVATION OF FOOD.)

RADIATION (IRRADIATION)

The emission and propagation of energy in the form of waves or particles through space or matter.

• **In food**—It refers to ionizing radiation which kills off various microorganisms—so-called cold sterilization. Irradiation for the preservation of food has been used experimentally, but, to date, it has not developed as an acceptable method of commercial food preservation for three reasons: (1) the high cost, (2) the radiation changes the characteristics of the food, and (3) the problem of safety. However, these problems may be overcome, with the result that foods will be commercially preserved by irradiation in the future.

• **In health and disease**—It refers to the process in which any one or a combination of rays—sunshine, radioactive particles, x rays, for example—are used for diagnostic or therapeutic purposes.

RADIATION PRESERVATION OF FOOD (COLD STERILIZATION; IRRADIATION; RADAPPERTIZATION; RADICIDATION; RADURIZATION)

Ionizing radiation—fast moving subatomic particles or energetic electromagnetic waves which are strong enough to strip electrons from atoms or molecules—provides the basis for a new method of food preservation. By subjecting foods to ionizing radiation a number of desirable storage characteristics—sprouting inhibition, slowed ripening, pasteurization, and complete sterilization—may be induced, depending upon the dose of radiation. Since the radiaton must not make the food radioactive, the sources of radiation are limited to the isotopes cobalt-60 and cesium-137, and to x rays. The doses of ionizing radiation to which these sources subject foods are expressed by a unit called the rad—the energy absorption of 100 ergs per gram. Since one million rads only increases the temperature of food by about 2°C, radiation processing of foods is sometimes called cold sterilization. Table R-1 indicates some of the potential uses of this process.

TABLE R-1
POTENTIAL APPLICATIONS OF RADIATION TO FOOD PROCESSING

Use	Foods	Action of Radiation	Rads of Exposure
Extension of storage life	Potatoes, onions, and other tubers and bulbs	Inhibits sprouting	Less than 20,000
	Fruits and some vegetables	Delays ripening and reduces the yeast and mold population	100,000 to 500,000
	Meat, fish, poultry, and other highly perishable foods	Reduces the population of microorganisms capable of growth below 37°F (3° C)	50,000 to 1 million
	Cereals, flours, dried fruits, and any other food prone to insect infestations	Kills or sexually sterilizes the insects preventing loss during storage or spread of the pests	10,000 to 50,000
	Meat, fish, poultry, and other highly perishable foods	Complete sterilization, destruction of any organism capable of causing spoilage thus preparing food for long-term storage when properly packaged.	4 to 6 million
Prevention of *Salmonella* food poisoning	Frozen meat, eggs, poultry, and other foods liable to contamination	Destroys *Salmonella* bacteria	300,000 to 1 million
Prevention of parasitic diseases	Meat or any other parasite-carrying food	Destroys parasites such as *Trichinella spiralis* and *Taenia sagnata*	10,000 to 30,000

As Table R-1 demonstrates, irradiation can be applied to a wide variety of foods and will yield numerous processing benefits. In addition, there are other attractive advantages. Irradiation of foods is extremely flexible, adapted to processing a variety of sizes and shapes of foods—from crates of potatoes and fruit to packaged flours, to large roasts, to slices of meat and sandwiches. Increased shelf life can be measured in terms of days or weeks for fruits, vegetables and milk, and in years for meat and poultry.

Along with the advantages there are also some problems. Not all foods can be preserved by exposure to ionizing radiation. In some foods, the possibility exists that all organisms except *Clostridium botulinum* would be destroyed, thus providing an environment for its growth without the conventional signs of spoilage. Also, radiation high enough to sterilize food sometimes causes undesirable changes in color, flavor, and texture; cooked meats (normally brown or gray) turn pink, lettuce wilts, egg whites thin, and baked products are reduced in volume. Moreover, modifications of nutritive value may occur; Vitamins A and E, ascorbic acid, and thiamin are especially sensitive. Packaging of some food for irradiation requires a substance able to withstand radiation and low temperatures like -40°F (-40°C). Above all, the greatest problems is that of providing convincing evidence of the absence of toxicity and carcinogenicity in radiation processed foods to health regulating bodies at the consumer level.

The first patent related to irradiated foods was taken out in France in 1930. Irradiation of food was first approved in the United States by the FDA in 1963, for use on bulk wheat and canned bacon, largely on the basis of extensive test data submitted by the U.S. Army Quartermaster Research Organization; gamma radiation was used to kill insect life in bulk wheat, and the electron beam was used to sterilize bacon. However, in the United States it was considered to be in the experimental stage until 1981, when control of the Mediterranean fruit fly caused the Food and Drug Administration to ease the ban on treating food with gamma rays. Under the Food, Drug, and Cosmetic Act as amended in 1958, ionizing radiation is legally defined as a food additive. Hence, each food processed by radiation requires the FDA's approval. Outside of the United States, the Joint Expert Committee of the Food and Agriculture Organization (FAO), the International Atomic Energy Agency (IAEA), and the World Health Organization (WHO) influence legislation in various countries on the control of production and the use of irradiated foods. The committee has given unconditional acceptance to the irradiation (1) of stored wheat and ground wheat products to control insect infestation, (2) of potatoes to control sprouting during storage, and (3) of chicken to prolong storage life and reduce the number of pathogenic microorganisms in eviscerated chicken stored below 50°F (10°C). Other foods are being evaluated by the joint FAO/IAEA/WHO Expert Committee.

Despite the fact that some people are somewhat squeamish about accepting irradiated products, irradiation under approved processes does not make food radioactive; hence, it poses no danger to consumers.

The possible use of radiation preservation is especially important in tropical and subtropical countries, where the temperature is high and the humidity is often excessive. In India, for example, 10 to 50% of the food production is often lost because of spoilage.

RADIATION THERAPY

The therapeutic use of x rays or radioactive substances such as radium and radioactive cobalt-60 isotope in the treatment of disease, primarily of a malignant nature.

RADIOACTIVE FALLOUT (CONTAMINATION)

Often, the mention of radioactivity creates alarm among people; conjuring up fear of cancer, genetic defects, and death. It is true that the advent of the nuclear

bomb and the use of nuclear power has increased the amount and chance of exposure to radioactivity. However, our exposure to man-made radioactivity is still small when compared to naturally occurring radiation. Nevertheless, our awareness of radioactivity and the increased chances of exposure make for concern lest the foods we eat contain harmful levels of radioactivity.

From radioactive fallout, man may become contaminated directly from the atmosphere, or indirectly through plant and animal products and water (see Fig. R-1). As noted, man may be contaminated (1) from the atmosphere, (2) from consuming contaminated plants (especially leafy vegetables and grains) and water, and (3) from consuming contaminated milk, meat, and eggs from exposed animals feeding on contaminated plants and water.

Of the several radioactive isotopes that enter the food chain, three—*strontium-90*, *cesium-137*, and *iodine-131*—are important from a health standpoint. In

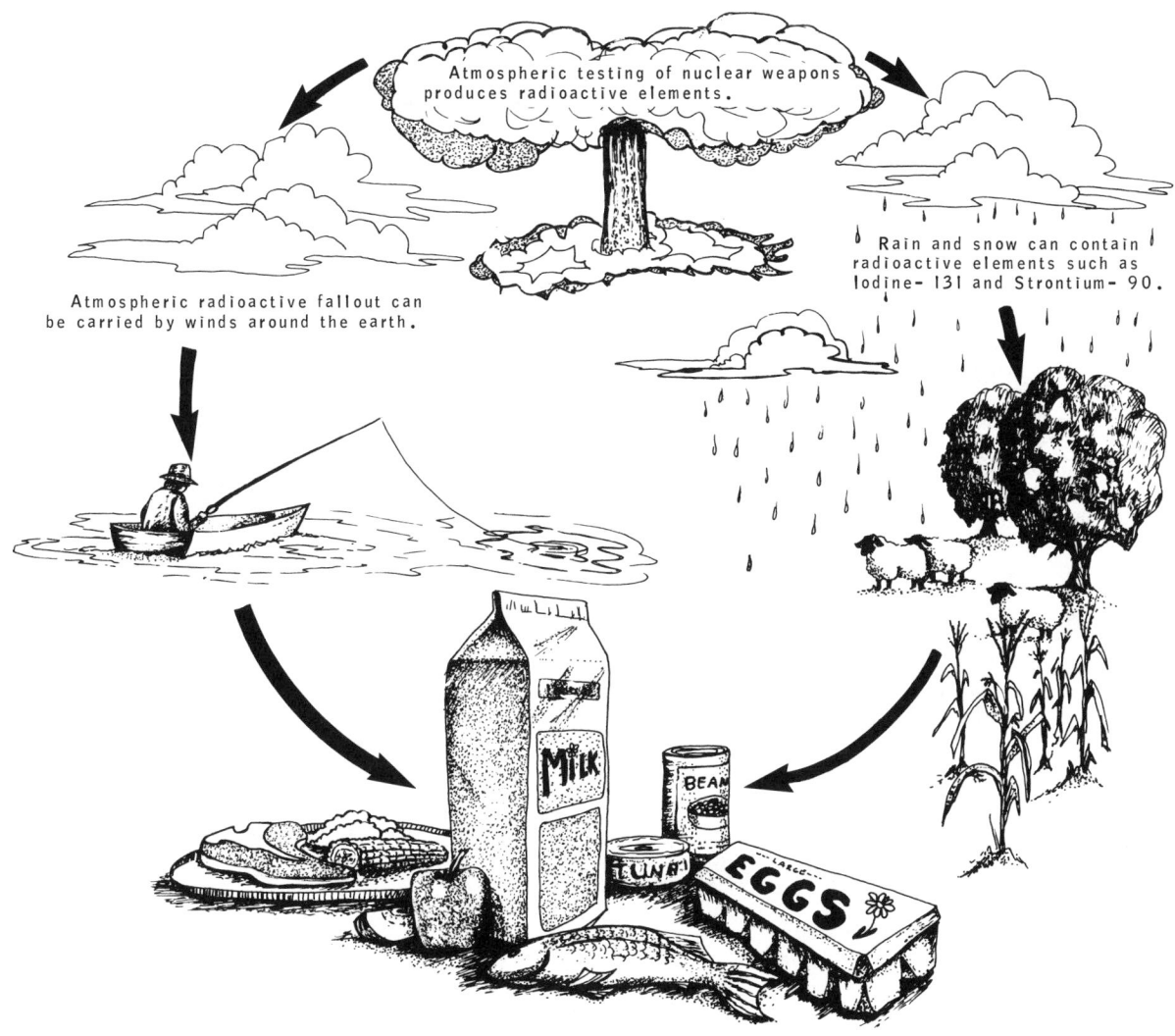

Fig. R-1. Pathways of radioactive fallout.

the body, strontium-90 (half-life 28 years, which means that it takes 28 years for half of the radioactivity of the element to decay) behaves like calcium. It is absorbed from the intestine in the same manner, and is deposited and concentrated in the bones and teeth where it may remain for years. When both strontium and calcium are present, calcium is absorbed in preference to strontium. Hence, high dietary calcium levels provide some protection against the absorption of strontium. At high levels in the bone, strontium-90 damages the bone marrow. Cesium-137 (half-life 30 years) presents less of a hazard since it becomes widely distributed throughout the soft tissues of the body. In addition, cesium is eliminated from the body faster than strontium-90. Virtually all iodine-131 concentrates in the thyroid gland; hence, high levels can have a carcinogenic effect on the thyroid. Fortunately, iodine-131 has a very short physical half-life of eight days. Both strontium-90 and iodine-131 are especially harmful to infants and children. These isotopes are not likely to present a health hazard unless nuclear testing increases, nuclear warfare begins, or a nuclear power plant accident occurs.

Of the naturally occurring radioactive substances, the two major food contaminants are (1) *potassium-40*, formed at the time of the earth's creation, and (2) *carbon-14*, continually formed by the interaction of the cosmic rays with the upper atmosphere. Due to their long half-life—1,260 million years for potassium-40, and 5,570 years for carbon-14—they are potentially dangerous. However, carbon-14 is absorbed into the body in small amounts lessening its danger. The danger of potassium-40 is reduced by the rapid rate at which it leaves the body. However, a 160 lb man contains about 31 mg of potassium-40 in his body.

As a safeguard to our health, the Food and Drug Administration (FDA), the U.S. Department of Agriculture (USDA), the U.S. Public Health Service (USPHS) and the Federal Radiation Council (FRC), are among the groups that periodically monitor the level of radioactivity in the food supply. The FRC has stipulated the lower levels of radioactive contamination of foods. Should the level exceed these limits, the Agency will recommend actions which should be taken.

Also, it is noteworthy that a "Food For Survival" publication is available from the U.S. Department of Agriculture, suggesting a two weeks' food and water stockpile to alleviate fallout radiation in case of an atomic or hydrogen bomb attack.

(Also see HALF-LIFE; MINERAL[S], section headed "Contamination of Drinking Water, Foods, or Air With Toxic Minerals.")

RADIOACTIVE ISOTOPES

An isotope is an element which has the same atomic number as another element but a different atomic weight. A radioactive isotope is one that decomposes spontaneously, emitting alpha or beta particles or gamma rays through the disintegration of its atomic nuclei. Usually, when fed or injected, its course and concentration can be traced and tagged by use of a special instrument, a Geiger counter. More than 150 radioactive isotopes are used (some experimentally) in the treatment of various diseases; among them, radioactive iodine (sodium iodide I-131)—used in the treatment of hyperthyroidism and other ailments, radioactive gold, radioactive phosphorus, and radioactive iron.

RADIOACTIVE ¹³¹I TEST

This is a test of thyroid function by using a radioactive isotope of iodine, ¹³¹I. After administering the test dose, the uptake and utilization of iodine by the thyroid gland is measured by tracing the ¹³¹I.

RADIOGRAPHY

The diagnostic, production, development, viewing and interpretation of x-ray films.

RADIOLOGY

The medical speciality which deals with x-ray diagnosis, and the therapeutic application of x rays, radium, cobalt, and other radioactive substances.

RADIOTHERAPY

The use of x rays, radium, cobalt and other radioactive substances in the treatment of various conditions in which they are believed to be helpful, particularly inoperable cancer.

RADISH *Raphanus sativus*

This tangy-flavored vegetable is a member of the mustard family *Cruciferae*, grown for its edible root. Fig. R-2 shows a typical radish plant.

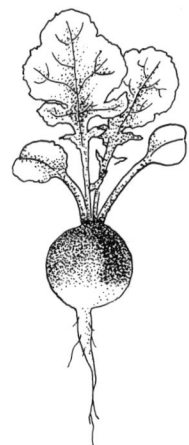

Fig. R-2.   Radish. Both the roots and green leaves of this plant may be eaten.

The roots vary in shape, size, and color, according to the variety. In the United States, round red radishes, ranging in size between a ping-pong ball and a golf ball, are most popular. However, Oriental people utilize varieties, such as daikon, which may weigh up to 5 lb (*2.3 kg*), and which they use as a vegetable or for making pickles. Also, certain other radishes may produce enormous roots that weigh as much as 50 lb. (*23 kg*), like the one shown in Fig. R-3.

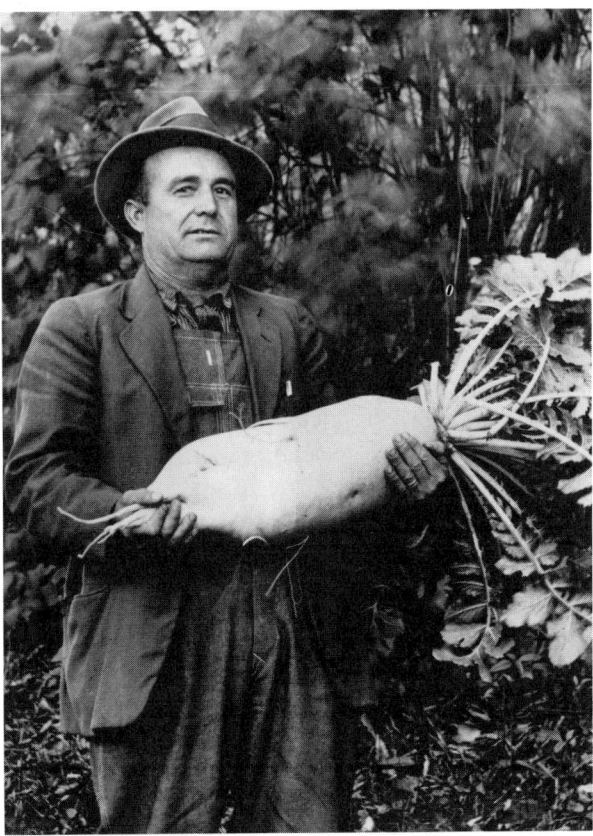

Fig. R-3. A farmer holding a giant radish. (Courtesy, The Bettmann Archive, Inc.)

ORIGIN AND HISTORY.
The radish is believed to have originated east of the Mediterranean, in Western Asia. Ancient writings show that it was used about 4,000 years ago by the Babylonians and the Egyptians. Apparently, the vegetable was brought to China about 500 B.C. It is noteworthy, too, that the Chinese developed new varieties, particularly those with the elongated large roots that have a much milder flavor than the small spherical ones most westerners know so well.

The Greeks and Romans regarded radishes highly because they are ready for harvesting sooner than any other vegetable. (The scientific name *Raphanus*, is derived from the Greek word *raphanos*, which means easy to rear. However, the English name is derived from the Latin word *radix*, which means root.) Greek artists showed their appreciation for the vegetable by making gold replicas of it, whereas Roman farmers cultivated a wide range of varieties.

PRODUCTION.
Statistics on radish production are not readily available. However, the USDA reports that each year more than 87.8 million pounds (*39.9 thousand metric tons*) of radishes are shipped within the United States.

Radishes grow best in cool weather. Hence, the spring varieties are planted during the winter in the southern states, and in the spring in the north. The large Oriental varieties, such as daikon, are usually planted in the late summer or early spring, although they may be grown throughout the year near the California coast, where the weather is always mild.

The small spring radishes are usually ready for harvesting in 3 to 5 weeks after planting, but the larger varieties require about 3 weeks longer to grow to optimal size. However, radishes which are left in the ground too long are likely to become woody.

After harvesting, the leafy tops are trimmed off and the roots washed and packed for shipping. The large mild-flavored varieties store much better (under cool and humid conditions) than the small sharp-flavored ones.

PROCESSING.
There is little or no processing of radishes except in the Orient, where they may be made into fermented or pickled preparations.

SELECTION AND PREPARATION.
People who grow their own radishes may wish to use the leafy tops as a green vegetable. They may be cooked briefly, then served with a white sauce or a cream sauce. Also, radish tops may be added near the end of the cooking period to casseroles, soups and stews.

Good quality radish roots are well formed, smooth, firm, tender, crisp and mild in flavor. Those which show signs of age, wilting, or decay are undesirable. Americans usually serve the small, red radishes raw in relish trays and salads after they have been scrubbed with a vegetable brush and rinsed in water. Sliced raw radishes are also good with sweet butter on whole grain rye or wheat bread, or after marination in a sweet-sour sauce.

Radishes may be steamed, as the Chinese and Japanese frequently do with the larger varieties. (Cooking eliminates some of the peppery flavor.) After cooking, they may be served with a cheese sauce or a cream sauce.

NUTRITIONAL VALUE.
The nutrient composition of radishes is given in Food Composition Table F-36.

Some noteworthy observations regarding the nutrient composition of radishes follow:

1. Radishes are very low in calories (17 to 19 kcal per 100 g) because they have a high water content (94%).

2. Oriental radishes, which have a milder flavor and can be eaten in larger quantities than common radishes,

are lower in potassium and higher in vitamin C than common radishes.

(Also see VEGETABLE[S], Table V-6 Vegetables Of The World.)

RADIUM

A highly radioactive element found in pitchblend and other minerals in the earth's crust, identified by Pierre and Marie Curie in 1898. Its radioactive rays have an effect on the growth of human tissue. Radium is generally used in the form of one of its salts, because they are more stable than the element itself. The radium salts are used in the treatment of malignant tumors (especially inoperable cancer), leukemia, polycythemia (increased red blood cells), and certain nonmalignant conditions.

RAFFINOSE

A trisaccharide containing the three hexoses, glucose, fructose, and galactose. Raffinose is found in molasses, cottonseed meal, and Australian manna.

(Also see CARBOHYDRATE[S].)

RAGOUT

This dish is essentially the same as a stove-top stew. The meat is browned, then the onion, garlic, parsley, stock and vinegar are added along with seasonings, and the mixture is simmered until the meat is tender. Duck, chicken, rabbit, hare, lamb, or young partridge maybe prepared in this way. The gravy is usually thickened at the end. The name comes from the French word *ragouter*, which means "to awaken the senses."

RAISIN(S)

These are the dried fruit produced from certain varieties of grapes. The word raisin comes from the Latin *racemus*, which means "a cluster of grapes or berries." All of the U.S. production, and nearly half of the world's supply of raisins comes from the San Joaquin Valley in California. Other raisin-producing countries include Turkey, Australia, Greece, Iran, South Africa, and Spain.

Mankind has enjoyed raisins since ancient times. Prehistoric drawings, such as the famous murals in Lascaux, France, show that raisins were in existence in France and the Mediterranean area at that time. Raisins were used for necklaces and decorations; cave dwellers attributed religious or magic power to the fruit. By 1000 B.C., the Israelites paid their taxes to King David with raisins. Armenia had a flourishing raisin business by 400 B.C., but 500 years later Asia Minor was the center of production. The Persians and Egyptians grew raisin-type grapes 200 years before Christ was born. Nero included raisins on many of the elaborate menus he served at Bacchanalian feasts during his reign between A.D. 54 and 68. In early Rome, the value of slaves was quoted in raisins, and for hundreds of years raisins were scarce and a sign of wealth. Not until the 14th century did raisins become more plentiful. In fact, shortly after 1450, they were shipped to England in such large quantities that many had to be returned.

The grape industry of California was started by Spanish missionaries, who planted grapevines around the missions. However, legend has it that nature, not man, produced California's first raisin crop. Just before the harvest in September 1873, a devastating heat wave struck the San Joaquin Valley. Before growers could complete the harvest, most of the grapes shriveled on the vine. Hoping to salvage what he could from this disaster, one enterprising grower took his accidental raisin crop to San Francisco. He found a grocer who was willing to sell the raisins to customers unfamiliar with this ancient and tasty delicacy. Raisins quickly became popular and soon there was a sizeable market for them.

Many varieties of grapes are produced in California, but only four principal varieties have been found suitable for drying into raisins. These four varieties are the Thompson Seedless, Muscat, Sultana, and Zante Currant, and they are either sun-dried or mechanically dehydrated.

• **Sun-dried**—When clusters of raisin variety grapes are fully ripened, they are picked by hand and spread on paper trays between the vine rows to dry in the sun. It takes 2 to 4 weeks, depending on weather conditions, to dry the grapes into raisins and change their color to the brownish-purple of sun-dried raisins. Harvesting operations generally commence during late August and are concluded by late September for Thompson Seedless, Sultanas, and Currants. Muscats, which are later in maturing, generally follow about 3 weeks later.

• **Golden seedless**—These raisins are Thompson seedless grapes which are picked, washed, and then placed on trays and exposed to the fumes of burning sulfur in a closed chamber. Following this treatment, the grapes are dehydrated in forced draft heating chambers. Their finished color is green to golden yellow to amber, since the sulfur dioxide treatment prevents the oxidative darkening that occurs with the sun drying of fruit.

Each type of raisin is compared in Table R-2.

Raisins contain only 17% water whereas grapes contain about 80% water. Therefore, many of the nutrients in grapes are more concentrated in raisins. Each 100 g (about 3 ½ oz) of raisins provides 289 Calories (kcal) of energy, 2.8 mg of iron, and 678 mg of potassium. The calories in raisins are derived primarily from the naturally occurring sugars (carbohydrates). More complete information regarding the nutritional value of raisins is presented in Food Composition Table F-36.

(Also see FRUIT[S], Table F-47 Fruits Of The World—"Grape"; and GRAPE[S].)

TABLE R-2
TYPES OF RAISINS

Generic Name	Variety of Grape	Preparation	Description	Availability	Uses
Sun dried natural seedless	Thompson Seedless	Dried under the sun. No chemical treatment used.	Seedless; dark brown color; average size.	93% of the total U.S raisin crop. Found in all food stores all year round.	The most popular raisin for cooking, baking, salads, desserts, and eating out of hand.
Golden seedless or Goldens	Thompson Seedless	Mechanically dehydrated. Specially treated with sulfur dioxide to preserve the golden color.	Seedless; golden-amber color; average size.	5% of the total U.S. raisin crop. Available in most food stores, especially in the fall and winter.	Used wherever a light colored raisin is desirable. Popular for fruit cakes and confections.
Sun ripened natural seedless	Thompson Seedless	Sun ripened. Bathed in hot water and mechanically dehydrated. No chemical treatment used.	Seedless; light brown color; more plump than standard seedless.	Limited availabilty. Found in large food stores.	Used in cooking, baking, salads, desserts, and for eating out of hand.
Seeded or "puffed" Muscat	Muscat	Dried under the sun. No chemical treatment used. Seeds removed mechanically during processing.	Large, dark, and extra sweet. Distinctive fruity flavor; seeds removed.	Limited availability. Found in food stores, especially in the fall and winter.	Prized for baking, especially in fruit cakes.
Zante currants or currants	Black Corinth	Dried under the sun. No chemical treatment used.	Seedless, mini-raisin, 1/4 average size. Very dark color; tart, tangy flavor.	Limited availability. Found in large food markets.	Popular for baking; traditional in hot cross buns.
Sultanas	Sultana	Dried under the sun. No chemical treatment used.	Similar to natural seedless raisins; tart in flavor.	Primarily available in bulk to bakers and other industrial user.	Commercial and institutional uses.

RAISINE

A preserve made with either pears or grapes plus quinces and cooked slowly in sweet wine or cider.

RAISIN OIL

The oil that is extracted from the seeds of muscat grapes before they are dried to make raisins. It gets its name from its use as a coating on raisins to prevent them from (1) sticking together, (2) becoming excessively dried out, and (3) being attacked by insects.

(Also see GRAPE[S]; and RAISIN[S].)

RAMP (WILD LEEK) *Allium tricoccum*

This native American species of wild onion has a folklore of its own. The mountain people of West Virginia hold annual ramp festivals in the spring, when the bulbs are ripe for eating. Fig. R-4 shows a typical ramp.

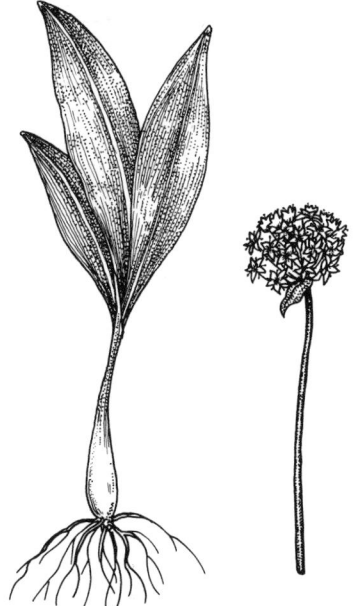

Fig. R-4.   The ramp, a wild leek that is native to North America. An onionlike odor is emitted by the leaves, which are often eaten with the bulbs.

ORIGIN AND HISTORY. The ramp is native to a broad area of eastern North America which extends southward from eastern Canada to the Carolinas, and as far west as Illinois and Wisconsin. It is found most abundantly in the forested areas of foothills and mountains. The consumption of the wild plant appears to have started among the British settlers of West Virginia and the surrounding areas since other species of wild leeks had long been used as a spring tonic in Europe.

Today, "ramp romps" are held early in the spring, when the emergence of the tender young leaves is induced by the first mild weather. The festivities include the preparation and consumption of ingeniously concocted ramp dishes, which are accompanied by storytelling and plenty of good old mountain music.

PRODUCTION. Ramps are not usually planted, but the self-propagating wild plants are systematically harvested on a small scale in some areas. The plants appear to thrive on woodland soils that are rich in organic matter and that receive plenty of rain.

It is best to pull up the plants soon after the leaves have emerged, because the leaves usually wither away before the flowers appear in the early summer.

PROCESSING. All of the ramps that are harvested are consumed fresh, so there is no processing. However, it appears that it might be feasible to can, dry, or freeze them so that one may enjoy their flavor all year. Freezing may be the best means of preserving the pungency of the vegetable.

SELECTION AND PREPARATION. The best ramps are those with dark green leaves tightly rolled together at their bases, and with crisp, tender bulbs. Yellowing, wilted, or discolored leaves indicate plants that are past their prime and which are likely to be tough.

Ramps are prepared by removing the outer skin and root tendrils from the bulbs and the top 3 in. *(8 cm)* of the leaves. Then, the trimmed plants should be washed thoroughly to remove any adhering soil.

The washed raw vegetable may be chopped and added to cheese spreads, relishes, salad dressings, salads, and sandwiches. It is also good when sliced and eaten on buttered bread.

Ramps may be cooked in appealing dishes such as baked beans and ramps, casseroles, gravies, meaty pot pies, soups, and stews. The boiled vegetable is enhanced by butter or margarine, cheese sauce, cream sauce, or white sauce.

NUTRITIONAL VALUE. Data on the nutrient composition of ramps is not readily available. However, it is believed that they are a fair to good source of vitamin C, and that the green leaves may supply valuable amounts of vitamin A.

RAMPION *L. rapa*

This now-neglected vegetable is of the same family as the turnip. It has an edible root which can be eaten raw in salads and tastes like a walnut. The leaves are used raw in salads, or cooked like spinach.

RANCID

A term used to describe fats that have undergone partial decomposition.
(Also see FATS AND OTHER LIPIDS.)

RANCIDITY

The oxidation (decomposition) primarily of unsaturated fatty acids resulting in disagreeable flavors and odors in fats and oils. This process occurs slowly and spontaneously, and it is accelerated by light, heat, and certain minerals. Rancidity may be prevented through proper storage and/or the addition of antioxidants such as sodium benzoate.
(Also see ADDITIVES; FATS AND OTHER LIPIDS; OILS, VEGETABLE; and PRESERVATION OF FOOD.)

RANGPUR RANGPUR LIME; MANDARIN-LIME) *Citrus limonia*

A highly acid citrus fruit (of the family *Rutaceae*) that is native to India and which (1) resembles the mandarin orange (*C. reticulata*) and (2) is highly acid. It is *not* related to the lime (*C. aurantifolia*). Rather, it is thought to be a sour mutant of the mandarin orange. The rangpur is used mainly as an ornamental plant and a rootstock for bearing the grafts of other citrus fruit trees.
(Also see CITRUS FRUIT, section headed "Production.")

RAPE (CANOLA) *Brassica napus; B. campestris*

Rape is a general term applied to members of the *Cruciferae* family. It ranks number three among the oilseeds globally; and it is the only oilseed grown successfully in all parts of the world.

Development of new varieties of rape which contain little or no erucic acid and glucosinolate, two antinutritional factors, will make for expanded production and utilization of rapeseed, a cool climate oilseed. This will have a significant impact on producer countries, thereby lessening their dependence on soybeans, sunflowers, peanuts, or cottonseed.

• **Canola**—The name "canola" is registered by the Western Canadian Oilseed Crushers Association; it stands for CANadian Oil Low Acid. To qualify as canola, rapeseed must yield oil with less than 2% erucic acid and meal with less than 30 micromoles of glucosinolate per gram.

• **Origin and history**—It is probable that the primary types of rape came from Asia, the Mediterranean, and western Europe. It has a long history, with earliest references found in Indian Sanskrit writings of 2000 to 1500 B.C.

• **World and U.S. production**—In 1990, world production of rapeseed totaled 24.5 million metric tons. That

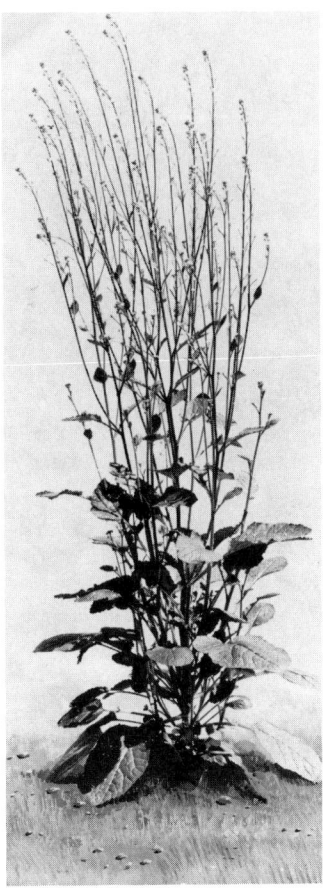

Fig. R-5.   Rape, the only oilseed grown successfully worldwide. (Courtesy, USDA)

year, the leading producers, by rank, and the million metric tons produced by each were: China, 6.9; India, 4.1; Canada, 3.3; Germany, 2.2; and France, 2.0.

U.S. production of rapeseed in 1990 totaled 67,000 metric tons.

• **The rape plant**—The two main species of rape are: *Brassica napus* and *B. campestris*. Both may be grown as annuals or biennials, depending on the variety and time of sowing. Both plants are 2 to 3 ft (*0.6 to 0.9 m*) high and have thick succulent stems and leaves.

• **Rape culture**—Rape is better adapted to cooler, shorter growing seasons than any other major edible oil seed crop. But it does well in such subtropical areas as northern India, Japan, and Mexico, where it is grown as a cool season or winter crop. Rape grows well on a wide variety of soils.

• **Kinds of rape**—The two leading species of rape, *B. napus* and *B. campestris*, have both winter and summer forms. There are numerous varieties.

• **Processing rapeseed**—The processing of rapeseed to obtain oil and meal is similar to that of other oilseeds. There are three methods: (1) mechanical pressing, (2) straight solvent, or (3) prepress solvent extraction. The latter is the method of choice. In the prepress solvent extraction method, a large portion of the oil is removed from the seeds by mechanical presses (expellers), then the remaining oil is extracted by using the organic solvent n-hexane. After discharging from the extracter, the meal, which contains about 1% oil, is dried to about 10% moisture, cooled, and placed in storage. The crude oil must still be refined.

• **Nutritional Value of rape**—The seeds contain 40 to 45% oil and 25% protein, along with about 4% glucosinolates. When processed, rapeseed yields about 40% oil and 50% oil meal which ranges from 32 to 40% protein.

In the past, rapeseed characteristically possessed two nutritional substances that were undesirable: (1) the oil was high (it contained 40 to 45%) in the long chain fatty acid, erucic acid, and (2) the meal was high (about 4%) in glucosinolates. Nutritional studies have indicated that these substances can be detrimental to human and animal health if consumed in substantial quantities. This stimulated plant breeders to try to make genetic changes in the composition of rapeseed—to lower or eliminate erucic acid and glucosinolate.

Rapeseed oil from most species formerly contained 40 to 45% of the long chain fatty acid, erucic. As a result, they were well suited for such industrial uses as engine lubricant, grease, and lubricant for cold rolling steel, but not desirable for human consumption. Fortunately, strains that produce seed oil with less than 1% erucic acid were isolated. So, plant breeders changed most commercial rape from high to low erucic acid. This change has proceeded at different rates in different countries, but is now nearly completed in Canada—the leading rapeseed producer of the world. The new oil contains only those fatty acids found in oils traditionally used for edible purposes. Rapeseed oil is listed in Food Composition Table F-36.

High glucosinolate rapeseed meal can cause goiter—an enlargement of the thyroid gland. Here again the best solution to the problem is to lower or eliminate the causative substance from the seed. This has been accomplished.

Plant breeders in Canada and northern Europe have been highly successful in changing rapeseed species to meet consumer needs. It is noteworthy that the reduction or elimination of glucosinolates from rapeseed meal also results in more effective use of the favorable amino acid balance of rapeseed protein.

Tower, the first Canadian rape variety both low in the erucic acid content of the oil and low in the glucosinolate content of the meal, was released in 1974.

Oil made from the new varieties of rape is almost free of the long chain fatty acid, erucic acid, while the oleic acid content is significantly higher. Except for the presence of linolenic acid, the composition of the new oil greatly resembles olive oil.

Rapeseed meal, the residue remaining after removal of oil from the seed, contains 35 to 40% protein, 20 to 25% carbohydrate, 12 to 16% crude fiber, and 5 to 7%

ash. Due to its high content of lysine,methionine, and cysteine, rapeseed protein has a higher nutritive value than any other known vegetable protein. Based on growth studies with rats and on a nitrogen balance study on student volunteers, the nutritive value of rape protein is as high as that of good animal protein.[1] With the exception of a negative effect on the zinc balance in rats, which can be compensated, no negative findings have been recorded.

• **Rapeseed products and uses**—The primary use of rapeseed oil is for human food. Its relatively low linolenic acid content permits it to compete with other vegetable oils in shortenings, margarines, salad oils, and frying oils. Oils which are almost free of erucic acid will open up new uses of rapeseed oil.

Until now, rapeseed meal has been used almost solely as a protein supplement for animals. With the development of glucosinolate-free rapeseed meal, it is expected that rapeseed protein will join soybean protein as an ingredient in meat analogs, meat extenders, dairy products, bakery goods, and other processed foods.

(Also see CANOLA [RAPE]; and OIL, VEGETABLE, Table O-6.)

RASHER

A portion, usually 2 or 3 slices, of bacon.

RASPBERRY *Rubus* **spp**

These species of fruits (of the family *Rosaceae*) usually grow on thorny bushes or trailing vines. Raspberries are similar to blackberries, except that in the case of the former the core of the fruit remains on the plant when the berry is picked, whereas blackberry cores come off with the fruit when it is picked. Both fruits are classified as "aggregate fruits" because each berry is made up of many tiny drupes or druplets, each of which is considered to be a fruit.

Raspberries may be red, yellow, black, or purple. Reds are by far the major type grown in the United States, whereas yellows are an uncommon mutant variety of the reds. Blacks (blackcaps) and purples (hybrids of reds and blacks) have similar characteristics, which differ somewhat from those of reds and yellows.

ORIGIN AND HISTORY. It appears that the ancestor(s) of modern types of raspberries came from eastern Asia, where the largest number of varieties are now found. However, native species of this fruit are also found in both the Eastern and Western Hemispheres. Perhaps the berry was brought to the New World by the people and/or animals which crossed the Bering Strait in ancient times. New World raspberries grow wild from the Arctic Circle to northern South America.

The distribution and evolution of raspberries over the ages was influenced to some extent by prehistoric

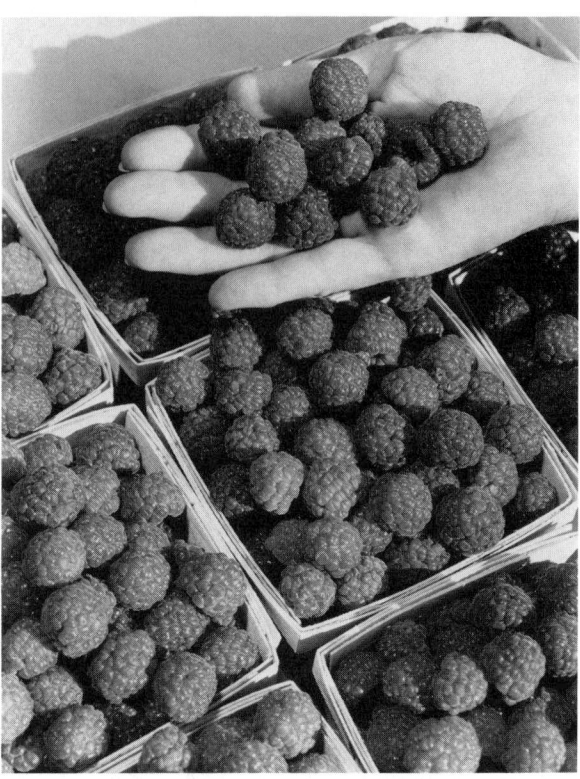

Fig. R-6. Boxes of red raspberries.

peoples who gathered the wild fruits and brought them back to their settlements. It seems likely that the largest and most succulent berries were collected and the remains of the fruit distributed over the areas traversed by the collectors. For example, evidence of the use of raspberries as food has been found at the site of the ancient lake dwellings in Switzerland, which were occupied thousands of years before the Christian Era.

There is no evidence that raspberries were cultivated before recent times. The first written reference to the growing of the fruit in gardens was in an English herbal published in 1548. It is noteworthy that the first raspberry species to be domesticated in Europe was the red-colored *Rubus idaeus*, which the Crusaders found growing in the vicinity of Mount Ida, Turkey. Black raspberries were not cultivated until the 19th century.

The widespread growing of raspberries in Europe and North America began in the 1800s. Many new varieties of the fruit arose from the accidental and intentional crossbreeding of the domesticated species with the wild ones which grew near the cultivated plots. For example, the *loganberry (Rubus loganbaccus)* was discovered growing in the garden of Judge Logan of Santa Cruz, California in 1881. This fruit apparently resulted from the spontaneous crossing of a domesticated red raspberry with a western wild blackberry. Similarly, the *boysenberry (Rubus loganbaccus)* was discovered in California by Rudolph Boysen in 1923. The latter fruit appears to be closely related to the loganberry.

[1]Ohlson, R. and K. Anjou, "Rapeseed Protein Products," *Journal of the American Oil Chemists' Society*, Vol. 56, No. 3, March 1979, p. 431.

Recently, plant geneticists have been hard at work developing new varieties which will bear large, early-ripening fruit that is firm enough for machine harvesting, while possessing a considerable resistance to disease and pests.

PRODUCTION. The world production of raspberries, which varies considerably from year to year, averages over 352,000 metric tons annually. Fig. R-7 shows the amounts contributed by the major producing countries.

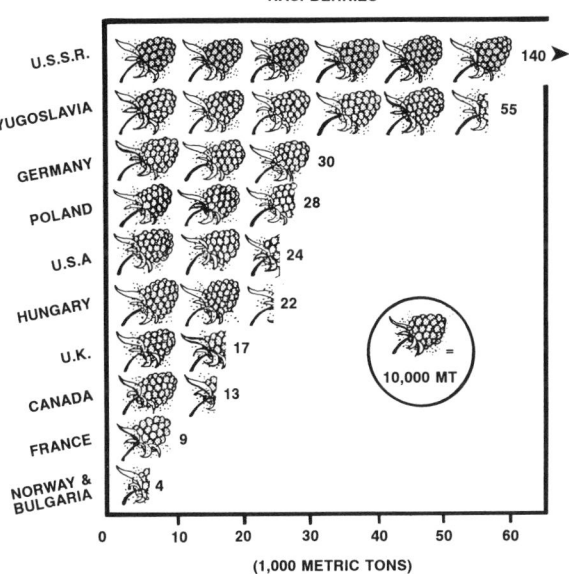

RASPBERRIES

Country	(1,000 METRIC TONS)
U.S.S.R.	140 ▶
YUGOSLAVIA	55
GERMANY	30
POLAND	28
U.S.A	24
HUNGARY	22
U.K.	17
CANADA	13
FRANCE	9
NORWAY & BULGARIA	4

= 10,000 MT

0   10   20   30   40   50   60
(1,000 METRIC TONS)

Fig. R-7. The leading raspberry-producing countries. (Based upon data from *FAO Production Yearbook*, 1990, FAO/UN, Rome, Italy, Vol. 44, p. 171, Table 75)

In recent years the U.S. raspberry production averaged about 23,000 metric tons annually. About 92% of the crop is red raspberries and the rest is black raspberries. Washington and Oregon are the major red raspberry growing states.

Most of the U.S. crop of black raspberries is produced in Oregon. Other important black raspberry-producing states are Michigan, New York, Washington, Ohio, Pennsylvania, New Jersey, and Minnesota.

Raspberries are hardier and can be grown farther north than blackberries. Furthermore, they require a certain amount of winter chilling to bring about the fruit-bearing (reproductive) phase of growth. Hence, most of the U.S. raspberry crop comes from the northern two-thirds of the country. The stems and side branches of raspberries and blackberries grow vegetatively the first year, go into rest during the winter, and develop fruit-bearing shoots on the first year's growth during the second year.

Red raspberries have erect stems (canes) and are usually propagated by root suckers (shoots), whereas black raspberries have stems that bend over and propagate themselves by rooting in the ground. The latter means of propagation is called "tip layering." Cuttings from the parent plants are often grown in nurseries until they are suitable for transplanting in the field.

In the East, raspberry cuttings are planted in the spring, whereas the milder climate of the Pacific Coast allows them to be planted there in the winter. A fertile, well-drained, and slightly acid soil is required. Most commercial growers fertilize their fields with nitrogen, phosphorus, and potassium because raspberries take large amounts of these nutrients from the soil. In the days when horses were kept on farms, stable manure was used to fertilize raspberry fields.

Young raspberry plants are usually tied to stakes or trellises to keep them from spreading over the field to form a dense, thorny thicket. The lanes between the rows of plants are kept free of weeds, grasses, and raspberry suckers in order to ensure that (1) only the tended plants receive the limited supply of water and soil nutrients, and (2) the harboring of diseases and pests is minimized.

Irrigation water must be used judiciously to prevent the (1) waterlogging of poorly-drained soils, and (2) growth of mold on the leaves and fruits. Therefore, drip irrigation systems are the most satisfactory.

Various machines are used to pick raspberries in the Pacific Northwest, but mechanical picking results in considerable wastage of the more tender berries. Hence, much of the eastern raspberry crop is still picked by hand.

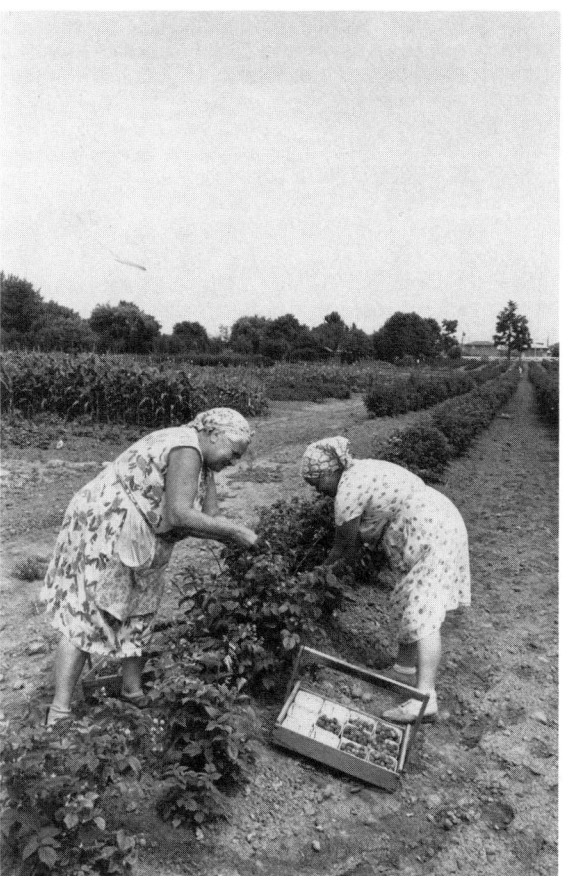

Fig. R-8. Picking raspberries in the Ottawa Valley of Ontario, Canada. (Courtesy, National Film Board of Canada, Ottawa, Ontario, Canada)

PROCESSING. In the United States, over 90% of the red raspberry crop, and almost all of the blackberries are processed. Most of the processed berries are quick frozen, but some are canned, and the remainder are used in baked goods, desserts, jam, jelly, pie, and syrup.

SELECTION AND PREPARATION. High quality raspberries are firm, plump, and fresh. Soft, mushy berries that leak juice are likely to be overripe and/or spoiled.

Fresh raspberries are likely to be available only at harvest time in the areas where the fruit is grown because the tender fresh berries are highly susceptible to damage and spoilage. When available, they should be rinsed briefly, but never soaked, just prior to their use. They make an excellent topping for ready-to-eat breakfast cereals, ice cream, plain cake, and vanilla pudding; or, they may be served in a bowl with a little cream and sugar. Of course, they are excellent when made into jam, jelly, or a pie.

Canned berries are extremely soft and should be used only in dishes that require no additional heating. The packing medium may be used as a flavoring for refreshing drinks.

The frozen berries are a good substitute for the fresh berries when they are thawed, then served raw or in various cooked dishes. However, it should be noted that frozen berries have already been cooked partially by the blanching step in the freezing process. Therefore, it might be a good idea to use unthawed frozen berries in dishes such as pies that require a moderately long cooking period.

NUTRITIONAL VALUE. The nutrient compositions of various raspberry products are given in Food Composition Table F-36.

Some noteworthy observations regarding the nutrient compositions of the more commonly available raspberry products follow:

1. The raw fruit is moderately high in calories (57 kcal per 100 g for red raspberries and 73 kcal per 100 g for black raspberries) and carbohydrates (14% for reds, and 16% for blacks). Raspberries are rich in fiber and are a fair to good source of potassium, iron, vitamin C, and bioflavonoids.

2. Canned raspberries packed in water contain only about two-thirds the caloric and nutrient levels of the raw fresh fruit.

3. Frozen sweetened raspberries contain about 50% more calories and carbohydrates than the raw fresh berries. Hence, no sugar need be added to this product.

4. Raspberry turnovers are rich in calories (405 kcal per 100 g), carbohydrates (42%) and fats (25%), but low in most other nutrients.

5. The color of raspberries is due mainly to anthocyanin pigments (which are also classified as bioflavonoids).

(Also see FRUIT[S], Table F-47 Fruits of the World.)

RATAFIA

A liqueur made by infusing and usually not distilled, flavored with plum, peach, and apricot kernels and bitter almonds, and supplied with a base of brandy and fruit juices. There are many different ratafias in different countries; obviously, they are of great potential value to cooks.

RAVIOLI

This is a favorite pasta dish of Italy, and Italians around the world. It is made by rolling out the pasta dough and dropping a spoonful of special cheese filling on each 2-inch square (13cm²) of pasta. This is covered with another sheet of pasta, sealed, and cut with a ravioli cutter. These little squares are cooked in rapidly boiling water and served with or without a tomato sauce, grated Parmesan cheese, or butter.

RAW SUGAR

This is the stage in cane sugar manufacturing at which sugar is transferred from the sugar mills to the refineries. Raw sugar is about 96 to 98% sucrose covered with molasses, but containing extraneous materials which prevent its use without further refining. FDA regulations prohibit the sale of raw sugar unless impurities such as dirt and insect fragments are removed.

Usually, tranportation from sugar mills to refineries is by oceangoing vessels, and the refineries are located at seaports.

Unlike sugarcane, sugar beets are put through a single, continuous process; all at the same location, and they produce no raw sugar.

(Also see SUGAR.)

RDA (RECOMMENDED DIETARY ALLOWANCES)

The first edition of *Recommended Dietary Allowances* was published in 1943. It was a product of the then newly established (1940) Food and Nutrition Board of the National Research Council–National Academy of Sciences whose first assignment was to determine dietary standards for people of different ages. At that time, it was recognized that the recommendations were judgments—not final—based on the available scientific knowledge. Hence, these recommendations were revised in 1945, 1948, 1953, 1963, 1968, 1974, 1980, and 1989.

Ideally, these allowances should be determined through experimentation on humans. However, for a number of reasons—some quite obvious—this is not always possible. Therefore, estimates of nutrient requirements are determined by the following six methods, some rather indirect: (1) determination of nutrient intake in apparently normal, healthy people; (2) biochemical studies; (3) studies of clinical cases of nutrient deficiencies; (4) balance studies that determine nutrition status in relation to nutrient intake; (5) experiments that maintain individuals on diets low or deficient in a nutrient followed by correction of the deficiency; and (6) animal studies.

The RDAs are estimates, not standards, and should be employed as a goal—not ideal nor optimal, but acceptable—for meeting the nutritional needs of a group of people. If nutrients are consumed at the level of the RDA, the needs of nearly all healthy members of the group will be satisfied, since the RDAs are not averages (except energy), but calculated for individuals with the highest requirements. However, the RDAs do not allow for the special needs of inherited metabolic disorders, infections, and chronic diseases. Furthermore, the RDAs are not intended for use to evaluate individual nutritional status.

In the 1989 edition of *Recommended Dietary Allowances,* compiled by the Committee on Dietary Allowances and the Food and Nutrition Board, nutrient allowances are given by age, weight, height, sex, pregnancy, and lactation.

• **Dietary recommendations for Americans**—The National Academy of Sciences has also called on the American public to make the following changes in its eating habits:

1. Reduce total fat consumption to 30% or less of total daily calorie intake.
2. Reduce cholesterol intake to less than 300 mg a day.
3. Increase the amount of starches and other complex carbohydrates in the daily diet.
4. Increase the amount of fiber in the diet.
5. Increase the amount of fruits and vegetables eaten daily.
6. Avoid drinking alcohol, especially during pregnancy. If abstaining is impossible, drink in moderation.
7. Reduce daily intake of sodium to 6 g or less.
8. Maintain desirable body weight through prudent

diet and regular exercise.

NOTE WELL: Table N-6 in section headed "Nutrients: Requirements, Allowances, Functions, Sources" of this encyclopedia gives the United States Recommended Daily Allowances (RDA) of each nutrient, *plus* its major function(s) in the body and best food sources; hence, the reader is referred thereto. A comparison of United States RDAs with the recommended daily dietary guidelines of selected countries and FAO follows.

RECOMMENDED DAILY DIETARY GUIDELINES OF SELECTED COUNTRIES AND FAO.

Table R-3 gives a comparison of the daily dietary guidelines for adults in selected countries and in all countries as made by the Food and Agriculture Organization (FAO) of the United Nations. The FAO dietary guidelines are intended to apply to people in all countries when translated in terms of local foods. These recommendations differ primarily for the following reasons:

1. They are set for population groups that live under different environmental conditions (climate, occupation, and activity) and that have different dietary practices. For example, more calories need to be allowed for people in a country where considerable physical activity is involved in daily work than in a country that is highly mechanized and activity is sedentary. In turn, the increased calorie allowances call for increased allowances of some of the B-complex vitamins such as thiamin.

2. Those who prepare the standards give varied interpretations to scientific data; differences which have narrowed with increased research and knowledge of the nutrient needs of human beings.

All the standards include recommended intakes of only those nutrients for which the requirements for human beings have been established. In order to assure that the

TABLE R–3
COMPARATIVE DAILY DIETARY GUIDELINES FOR ADULTS IN SELECTED COUNTRIES AND FAO[1]

Country	Sex	Age	Weight		Activity[2]	Calories	Protein	Calcium	Iron	Vitamin A (retinol eq.)	Thiamin	Ribo-flavin	Niacin eq.	Vitamin C
		(yr)	(lb)	(kg)			(g)	(g)	(mg)	(mcg)	(mg)	(mg)	(mg)	(mg)
United States (1989)	M	25–50	174	79	MA	2,900	63	0.8	10	1,000	1.5	1.7	19	60
	F	25–50	138	63	MA	2,200	50	0.8	15	800	1.1	1.3	15	60
Canada	M	19–35	154	70	MA	3,000	56	0.8	10	1,000	1.5	1.8	20	30
	F	19–35	123	56	MA	2,100	41	0.7	14	800	1.1	1.3	14	30
United Kingdom	M	18–34	143	65	MA	2,900	63	0.5	10	750	1.0	1.6	18	30
	F	18–34	120	55	MA	2,150	54	0.5	12	750	0.9	1.3	15	30
FAO	M	25	143	65	MA	3,000	37[3]	0.4–0.5	5–9	750	1.2	1.8	19.8	30
	F	25	120	55	MA	2,200	29[3]	0.4–0.5	14–28	750	0.9	1.3	14.5	30

[1]Daily dietary guidelines for Canada, United Kingdom, and FAO provided by Z. I. Sabry, Director, Food Policy and Nutrition Division, Food and Agriculture Organization of the United Nations, Rome, Italy.

[2]Moderate activity.

[3]Expressed in reference protein.

nutrients that are known to be essential, but for which the requirements are as yet unknown, will be included in the diet, the selected diet should include as much variety of foods as practical, acceptable, and palatable.

The dietary allowances or standards of each country may be used in the following ways:
1. To establish a ration for an individual or group.
2. To evaluate the diet of an individual or group.
3. To serve as a guide in teaching.
4. To formulate regulations for the composition of foods, dietary supplements, or drugs.

(Also see NUTRIENTS: REQUIREMENTS, ALLOWANCES, FUNCTIONS, SOURCES.)

RECTAL FEEDING

A discontinued practice of administering nutrient solutions into the rectum, a type of enema. Only limited amounts of nutrients are absorbed, and frequently the rectum is irritated. When patients are unable to take sufficient foods and fluids by mouth, nasogastric feeding, intravenous feeding, or surgical placement of a tube into the stomach or small intestine provide better methods for administering nutrients.

(Also see INTRAVENOUS FEEDING; and TUBE FEEDING.)

RECTUM

The last 6 in. (*15 cm*) of the large intestine (colon) before ending at the anal opening. It functions to store the products of digestion prior to defecation. Crescent-shaped valves inside the rectum support the weight of fecal material until distention initiates the desire to defecate. The rectum is surrounded and supported by a group of veins which may dilate and produce hemorrhoids (piles).

(Also see DIGESTION AND ABSORPTION.)

RED MEAT

Meat that is red when raw. Red meats include beef, veal, pork, mutton, and lamb.

(Also see MEAT[S].)

REDUCING DIETS

The principle is to decrease the calorie intake. However, a good reducing diet must still provide the required nutrients. At the same time it should be acceptable and palatable, offer a variety, be economically feasible, and promote a sense of well-being.

Basically, the modifications which are usually made in low-calorie diets involve reduction in the number of items high in carbohydrates and fats, but retention of those which are good sources of minerals and vitamins. However, it is often necesary to calculate caloric requirements so that the dietary calorie content may be low enough to produce the appropriate caloric deficit.

Generally a weight loss of 1 to 2 lb (*0.45 to 0.91 kg*) per week is ideal. This requires a caloric deficit of 500 to 1,000 Calories (kcal) per day.

(Also see FOOD GROUPS; and OBESITY, section headed "Treatment of Obesity.")

REFERENCE MAN

A healthy man of specified age, weight, environmental temperature, and physical activity permitting the formulation of standard calorie allowances. In the 1968 edition of *Recommended Dietary Allowances*, a reference man was 22 years old, weighed 154 lb (*70 kg*), and presumed to live in an environment with a mean temperature of 68°F (*20°C*). His physical activity was considered light, 120 to 240 kcal/hr. In the 1989 *Recommended Dietary Allowances*, the average mature male used for the basis of energy recommendation is engaged in light activity, and presumed to live in an area where the mean environmental temperature is 68°F (*20°C*), and has the desirable weight of 174 lb (*79 kg*). However, the energy requirements for the average mature male are given for two age groups: (1) 25 to 50 years of age; and (2) 51 years and over.

REFERENCE PROTEIN

Proteins differ in nutritive value mainly due to their amino acid composition. A reference protein provides all of the essential amino acids in sufficient quantities and balances so as to meet the body's requirements without an excess. Table R-4 shows the amino acid requirements

TABLE R–4
AMINO ACID REQUIREMENT OF CHILDREN
10–12 YEARS COMPARED TO THE AMINO ACID
PROFILES OF HUMAN MILK AND EGGS

Amino Acid	Amino Acid Requirement for Children 10–12 Years[1]	Human Milk[2]	Whole Egg[2]
Histidine	19	26	22
Isoleucine	28	46	54
Leucine	44	93	86
Lysine	44	66	70
Methionine and cystine	22	42	57
Phenylalanine and tyrosine	22	72	93
Threonine	28	43	47
Tryptophan	9	17	17
Valine	25	55	66

[1]*Recommended Dietary Allowances*, 10th ed., 1989, NRC-National Academy of Sciences, p. 67, Table 6-5.

[2]Values for the protein and amino acid content are from the Protein and Amino Acids in Selected Foods, Table P-37.

of children 10 to 12 years of age. Also Table R-4 shows how the essential amino acid patterns of eggs and human milk compare to that of the requirements of children 10 to 12 years of age. Eggs and human milk are frequently used as reference proteins due to their amino acid patterns. As reference proteins they are used to assign a chemical score to other proteins in an effort to gain some idea of their nutritive value. The amount of limiting amino acid present in a protein, expressed as a percentage of that in the reference pattern, provides the chemical score.

(Also see AMINO ACID[S]; CHEMICAL SCORE; and PROTEIN[S].)

REFERENCE WOMAN

A healthy woman of specified age, weight, environmental temperature, and physical activity permitting the formulation of standard calorie allowances. In the 1968 edition of *Recommended Dietary Allowances*, a reference woman was 22 years old, weighed 128 lb (*58 kg*), and presumed to live in a climate with a mean temperature of 68°F (*20°C*). Her physical activity was considered light, 120 to 240 kcal/hr. Still, in the 1989 *Recommended Dietary Allowances,* the average mature female used for the basis of energy recommendation is engaged in light activity, and presumed to live in a climate where the mean environmental temperature is 68°F (*20°C*). However, the average mature female has a desirable weight of 138 lb (*63 kg*), and her energy requirements are given for two age groups; (1) 25 to 50 years of age; and (2) 51 years and over.

REGURGITATION

The return of food from the stomach, gullet, or duodenum (first portion of the small intestine) after eating, without vomiting. Patients with this afflication can usually lessen regurgitation (1) by sleeping with the head and chest higher than the rest of the body, and (2) by drinking lots of water.

REINDEER

The flesh of the reindeer provides venison, which, however, is inferior to that of the roebuck or deer. The venison from reindeer is prepared in the same way as venison from roebuck or deer. The meat of young reindeer is delicate; the meat from old reindeer is less tender and needs marinating.

RELAPSE

The return of the symptoms of a disease after convalescence has begun.

RELIGIONS AND DIETS

Religion is difficult to define, but, stated simply, *religion is the belief in and/or worship of God or gods.* As far back as primitive tribes can be studied, records reveal that most of them had a set of beliefs that made up a form of religion. In one way or another all religions imply that man does not and cannot stand alone, that he is vitally related to and even dependent upon powers and forces in nature and society beyond himself. Probably, man's acquaintance with death and disaster was largely responsible for his realization of this. As men shared their fears, feelings, and beliefs, religion developed around common sets of fears, feelings, and beliefs. Religion became "the tie that bound." Along with the development of religion, food has always played an important role in the lives of men. Often, food was the most precious and scarce of man's possessions. Not surprisingly, religious rituals or customs became associated with food. Religions have (1) decreed what foods man could or could not eat, (2) prescribed the preparation of foods, (3) indicated what food may or may not be eaten on certain days or certain occasions, and (4) symbolized foods and drink, and their ingestion. Furthermore, the religious idea of defiling or polluting objects influenced food choices. Since food is taken into the body, many religions held beliefs that certain foods and drinks were polluting or defiling.

Due to the diversity of mankind, religious beliefs and practices are varied and perhaps the least understood aspects of other people. Through the ages, man has had many religious ideas. Man has worshipped departed ancestors, animals, humanlike animals, wind, fire, inanimate objects, unseen objects, nature, and other men. Religious beliefs surrounding the religions have included casting spells, singing chants, foretelling the future,

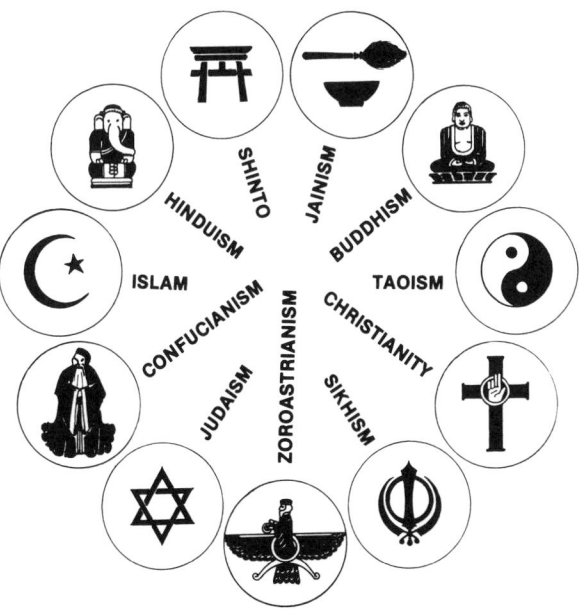

Fig. R-9. Symbolic representation of man's religions.

using protective charms, endowing objects with power, praying, and offering sacrifices.

Religious thought of each passing civilization has in some way influenced that of the civilization that followed. Although religions of such groups as the Incas, Aztecs, Egyptians, Greeks, and American Indian have passed, no doubt they left their imprint on the thoughts of men. However, from the history of mankind 11 religions have survived. While there are countless religious groups in the world, the broad grouping represented by these surviving 11 religions seems to represent the wellsprings of religious thought. Casual study of the various religions of the world would suggest that they are all very different; and, in many respects, they are different. However, a close inspection of the world's religions also reveals a large number of similarities.

These religions developed from various areas of the world and then spread. Hinduism, Buddhism, and Jainism originated in India. Confucianism and Taoism originated in China. Shintoism started in Japan. Christianity, Islam, Judaism, and Zoroastrianism arose from the Middle East. Sikhism is a hybrid of Islam and Hinduism from India. Some of these religions prescribe very specific dietary practices while others do not appear to do so. Nevertheless, the philosophy of a religion may have subtle influences over food selection. For this reason, Table R-5 presents the basic tenets of the 11 religions as well as foods or drinks which are specifically taboo or encouraged by the religion.

(Also see DIETS OF THE WORLD.)

TABLE R-5
LIVING RELIGIONS OF THE WORLD, AND THE DIET PRESCRIBED BY EACH

Religion; Adherents	Origins; Chief Scripture(s); Basic Tenets	Food Taboos	Foods Encouraged by Beliefs	Remarks
Religion: **Buddhism** Adherents: About 245 million in primarily Southeast Asia, Sri Lanka, Korea, China, Japan, and Tibet; and about 60,000 in the United States.	Origins: More than 2,500 years ago in India with the teachings of Prince Siddhartha Gautama, the Buddha, which means "the wise one" or "the enlightened one" Chief Scriptures: The *Pali Canon* Basic Tenets: The way beyond sorrow and suffering is a middle path between striving and spiritual contemplation. Buddhists believe in the rebirth of persons through the transmigration of soul. What a person is today is the result of past karma—action or deed. The object of Buddhist life is to achieve nirvana—a state of complete redemption which frees an individual from the cycle of rebirth. The Buddhist teachings are embodied in the Four Noble Truths: 　1. Existence is suffering. 　2. This suffering is due to selfish desires. 　3. The cure of suffering is to destroy these selfish desires. 　4. This cure can be accomplished by practicing the Eight-Fold Path: right belief, right thought, right speech, right action, right means of livelihood, right exertion, right remembrance, and right meditation.	Strict Buddhists are vegetarians. They will not eat the flesh of any animal and many will not eat milk and eggs. Part of right action includes a vow to abstain from intoxicating beverages.	Buddhist monks do not eat after midday but they are allowed to drink tea and coconut milk. Every morning Buddhist monks make the rounds in the village with their beggar's bowls and receive the very best of the rice, curry, or fruit available. Abstaining from taking life limits the use of any livestock, but encourages the growing of rice and the introduction of new food crops. Eating fish is not viewed as killing but simply removing the fish from water. Ritual vegetarian feasts may be held for a variety of reasons. For some, the sin is not in eating the animal flesh but in killing.	Buddhism has ceased to be an important influence in India. Buddhist associations have been established in Europe and the United States. In 1942, the Buddhist Churches of America were incorporated. Part of right action includes a vow to abstain from killing or injuring any living being. Buddhism is difficult to discuss in terms of diet because it lacks unity.

(Continued)

TABLE R-5 (*Continued*)

Religion; Adherents	Origins; Chief Scripture(s); Basic Tenets	Food Taboos	Foods Encouraged by Beliefs	Remarks
Religion: **Christianity** *Adherents:* About 1 billion throughout the world and about 135 million in the United States.	*Origins:* Began with the birth of Jesus Christ about 2,000 years ago, though Judaic teachings taught of the birth of a promised savior for hundreds of years. *Chief Scriptures:* The *Bible* (Old and New Testament) *Basic Tenets:* Jesus Christ—the Savior—was the Son of God. He suffered for man's sins. He was crucified and then resurrected. Jesus Christ will return. Teachings and life of Christ are contained in the New Testament of the Bible. Primarily, Christ taught love of God and love for fellow men.	Overall, Christianity does not teach that any specific foods are taboo, but several of the major Christian religions prohibit some foods: • **Greek Orthodox**— On Fridays and Wednesdays, the use of meat, fish, poultry, eggs, and dairy products is restricted. These foods are also restricted during the first and last weeks of the Greek Orthodox Lent. Devout members may abstain from olive oil. • **Mormons (Latter-day Saints)**—The Mormons prohibit the use of alcoholic beverages, tea, coffee, and tobacco, and encourage the sparing use of meat. • **Roman Catholic**— Historically, the most notable dietary law in Christianity was the Roman Catholic ban on eating meat on Friday. During the reign of Pope John XXIII, this ban was lifted. • **Seventh-day Adventists**— Adventists are taught to avoid meat, fish, poultry, alcohol, tea, coffee, ripened cheese, excess sugar, and excess refined grains, as well as irritating spices and too much salt.	Several of the major Christian religions encourage certain types of foods or diets: • **Greek Orthodox**— Dietary laws have been interpreted more liberally in recent years. On fast days— days meat and dairy products are restricted—shell fish may be eaten. Koliva, a boiled whole wheat dish, is important in memorial services for the dead. • **Mormons (Latter-day Saints)**—The Mormon "Word of Wisdom" encourages the use of grains, fruits, and vegetables. • **Roman Catholic**— Local customs vary with regard to foods allowed on fast days and days of abstinence. • **Seventh-day Adventists**—In general, Adventists are ovo-lactovegetarians, and allow the use of eggs and milk. Furthermore, they encourage the use of nuts, legumes, and whole grains. The Adventists have encouraged the development of meat analogs such as the soy protein products.	The Roman Catholic Church centralized under the authority of the Pope in Rome, is the largest Christian body. The numerous Protestant churches are the product of the Reformation of the 1500s. Through missionary activity, Christianity has spread to most parts of the world. Major holidays are Christmas, the Epiphany, All Saints' Day, Ash Wednesday, Palm Sunday, Good Friday, Easter Sunday, Ascension Day, and Pentecost. Christian religions use bread to symbolize the body of Christ and wine (water) to symbolize the blood of Christ.

(*Continued*)

TABLE R-5 (Continued)

Religion; Adherents	Origins; Chief Scripture(s); Basic Tenets	Food Taboos	Foods Encouraged by Beliefs	Remarks
Religion: **Confucianism** Adherents: About 276 million, primarily in China and Taiwan.	Origins: Developed around the philosophy of Confucious (K'ung Fu-tzu) who lived in China from 551 to 479 B.C. Chief Scriptures: The *Analects* (Conversations or sayings) Basic Tenets: Confucianism is primarily a group of ethics or proper conduct: kindness, righteousness, decorous behavior, wisdom, and uprightness. The chief ethic is benevolence. Confucianism does not restrict itself to any formalized theology—no teachings of a god, heaven, or life after death. Confucianism does encourage ancestor worship, and at one time Confucious was worshipped.	Confucianism does not seem to have any specific food taboos.	Confucianism does not seem to encourage the use of any certain foods, other than those that may be part of ancestor worship.	Mencius (Meng Tse), who lived around 400 B.C., propagated and elaborated on Confucianism. Confucianism waned in China with the overthrow of China's monarchy in 1911 to 1912. Then, during the 1970s the communist government tried to wipe out Confucianism in China. However, Confucianism has returned to an accepted position in China.
Religion: **Hinduism** Adherents: Over 500 million in India or in Indian communities throughout the world.	Origins: No founder, but developed gradually over 5,000 years. Chief Scriptures: The *Vedas* which includes the *Rig Veda*, the *Upanishads*, the *Bhagavad-Gita*, and many other writings Basic Tenets: Hinduism does not have a common creed or one doctrine to bind Hindus together. Membership in an Indian caste is encouraged by Hinduism. Brahman is the unifying spirit and Hindus may worship many gods that represent different sides of Braham. Hindus believe in reincarnation or rebirth. All living things are caught in a cycle of becoming and perishing, which gives hope to those whose position seems hopeless. Where the soul of a dead person goes for rebirth depends upon his actions or karma. Release from the cycle of rebirth and redeath and a state of happiness is called nirvana.	Some Hindus reject pork because of the value they place on life and because of the filth of pigs. Hindus view the cow as sacred; hence, beef is not a food, though there are numerous cows in India. Both eggs and poultry are rejected by Hindus. Strict Hindus will eat the flesh of no animal. Strict Hindus also avoid onions, garlic, turnips, and mushrooms, and for some, the association of blood with the color of some lentils and tomatoes has made these vegetables unacceptable.	Strict Hindus are vegetarians. Ghee (clarified butter) and milk from the cow are sacred foods. The coconut is also considered sacred. To insure success, new enterprises may be started by breaking a coconut. Following a fast, which may be either a complete fast or at least abstaining from cooked foods, a Brahmin—high priest of Hinduism—can be fed ghee, coconuts, fruits, or some uncooked food.	Hindus have complete freedom of belief in a deity. A Hindu may be a monotheist, polytheist, or atheist. Since Hindus believe that the most important part of every living thing is its soul or spirit uniting us all, Hindus will not injure or kill an animal. Hindus come from all over India to bathe in the Ganges River, which is sacred and supposed to wash away the impurity of sin. The practice of Hinduism consists of rites and ceremonies performed within the framework of the caste system. Hindu temples are dwelling places of Hindu gods, to which people bring offerings.

(Continued)

TABLE R-5 (*Continued*)

Religion; Adherents	Origins; Chief Scripture(s); Basic Tenets	Food Taboos	Foods Encouraged by Beliefs	Remarks
Religion: **Islam** Adherents: About 700 million worldwide, with about 1 million in the United States.	Origins: Founded by Mohammed, who was born in Mecca (now Saudi Arabia) and who lived from about 570 to 632 A.D. Chief Scriptures: The *Koran* Basic Tenets: The simple article of faith of Islam is that they worship one God (Allah) and Mohammed was his messenger. The *Koran* is a compilation of revelations Mohammed received from Allah. Good deeds will be rewarded in paradise and evil deeds will be punished in hell. Islam means commitment or dedication to Allah. Duties of Islam include: 5 daily prayers, observance of Ramadan, giving of alms, and a pilgrimage to Mecca at least once in a lifetime.	Eating pork and drinking intoxicating beverages is forbidden. The observance of the month of Ramadan involves fasting during the daylight hours. With the exception of fish and locusts, no animal food is considered lawful unless it has been slaughtered according to the proper ritual. At the instant of slaughter, the person killing the animal must repeat, "In the name of God, God is great."	During the month of Ramadan, nights are often spent in feasting, possibly beginning with an appetizer like dates and a sherbetlike drink. Then following Ramadan there may be a feast lasting up to 3 days. This is called Eid-al-Fitr, where chicken or veal sauteed with eggplant and onions and simmered in pomegranate juice and spices may be served. But the highlight is a whole lamb stuffed with a rich dressing of dried fruits, cracked wheat, pine nuts, almonds, onions, and spices. The feast is concluded with rich pastries and candies, some of which are taken home and used over a period of time as reminders of the festival.	Mohammed is believed to have been a descendent of Abraham. Followers of Islam are called Moslems. Jesus Christ is not considered the Son of God, but merely a prophet sent to warn the people and tell what God desired. Major holidays are Eid-al-Fitr which occurs after the day fasting, the night feasting month of Ramadan, and Eid-al-Azha which is the feast of sacrifice on the last day of Hajj.
Religion: **Jainism** Adherents: About 2 1/4 million, mostly in the western part of India.	Origins: Founded in the 6th century B.C. in India by Prince Vardhamana who later became known as Mahavira or "the Great Hero." Chief Scriptures: None Basic Tenets: Jainism stresses nonviolence to all living creatures, a doctrine called *ahismsa*. This requires extreme caution during all activities. Jainism emphasizes stern asceticism to conquer the appetites of the body. Vows taken by Jain monks are very strict. Jains also believe in reincarnation or transmigration of the soul. Jainism does not recognize a supreme deity.	Since Jainism stresses nonviolence to all living creatures, any food that requires the taking of life is forbidden. Also, Jains refrain from eating certain fruits, honey, wine, and root vegetables which carry organisms on their skins.	Jains are vegetarians.	The Jains figure Mahavira as the last of 24 founders or Terlhamkaras. A Jain monk carries a broom representing the sacredness of a life and a bowl for begging. The broom is used to sweep insects from his path so he will not step on them, and the bowl for begging represents the asceticism or self denial. Jains cannot take part in war nor any other activity or profession in which they must kill or injure any living thing.

(Continued)

TABLE R-5 (*Continued*)

Religion; Adherents	Origins; Chief Scripture(s); Basic Tenets	Food Taboos	Foods Encouraged by Beliefs	Remarks
Religion: **Judaism** *Adherents:* Worldwide about 15 million, in the United States about 6 million.	*Origins:* From the time of Abraham in about 1800 B.C. *Chief Scriptures:* The *Torah*, containing the first 5 books of the *Old Testament*, and the *Talmud*. *Basic Tenets:* The Jews believe in one God. Their life is guided by the commandments contained in the *Torah*. Judaism teaches that man is responsible for his actions and that he has a choice between right and wrong. The Jewish Sabbath is from sunset Friday to sunset Saturday. Judaism is a way of life, which assumes that life is significant, has value, and that the individual is important. Life has a divine purpose. In traditional synagogues·worship services are held 3 times daily. Jews look forward to the coming of the Messiah—Savior.	Eating unclean animals is forbidden. The *Torah* provides the distinction between animals considered as clean and those which are unclean (see Leviticus Chapter 11 and Deuteronomy Chapter 14). Unclean foods include pork, camel, horse, most winged insects, reptiles, creeping animals such as the mouse, and birds of prey. All shellfish and eels are eliminated from the diet. Blood is taboo for human consumption, as is the internal fat from an animal. Meat and dairy foods cannot be eaten in the same meal. Meat of animals dying of natural causes or disease is unfit. Trefah is the term used to indicate an unclean food or a food not correctly prepared.	Clean foods which are permitted to be eaten include cow, sheep, and goat, and fish (see Leviticus Chapter 11 and Deuteronomy Chapter 14). Dietary laws are further expanded in the *Talmud* which contains the Laws of Kashrut. Kosher foods are those which are permitted according to the *Torah* (*Bible*) and foods which have been processed in a prescribed manner. A rabbi must supervise the killing of all animals which is performed by a trained person called a shohet. A swift deep slash at the throat renders the animal unconscious and allows blood to drain from the animal. Then truly kosher meat is soaked in cold water, drained, sprinkled with salt, washed in cold water, and cooked. The *Talmud* forbids Jews to eat certain sinews of the hindquarters which presents some prob-	Throughout the ages, the Jews have been persecuted from Roman days through the days of Nazi Germany. Judaism is a cultural heritage. Jewish congregations are classified as Orthodox, Conservative, or Reform, depending on their degree of adherence to ancient religious customs and dietary laws. Major holidays in Judaism are Pesach (Passover), Shavuot (Pentecost), Sukkot (Tabernacles), Rosh Hashanah (New Year), Yom Kippur (Day of Atonement), and Hanukkah (Festival of Lights).

lems since the sinews are difficult and costly to remove.
Many of the processed foods contain the symbols U or K on the label which refers to the Union of Orthodox Jewish Congregations and O.K. Laboratories, respectively. These symbols indicate that the food is kosher.
Food plays a major role in the symbolism of the Jewish holidays and festivals. Familiar foods during these times include honey, honey cake, carrot tzimmes, holishkes, strudel, potato latkes, potato krugel, St. John's Bread, fruits, nuts, raisins, pastry, wine, cheese blintzes, cheese kreplach, eggs, and unleavened wheat bread (matzo).
(Also see MEAT, section headed, "Kosher Meats.")

(Continued)

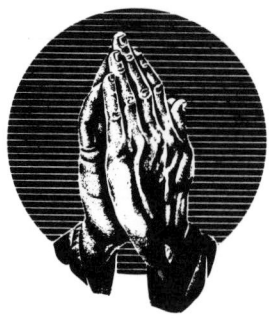

TABLE R-5 *(Continued)*

Religion; Adherents	Origins; Chief Scripture(s); Basic Tenets	Food Taboos	Foods Encouraged by Beliefs	Remarks
Religion: **Shinto** *Adherents:* About 63 million Japanese.	*Origins:* Originated in ancient times with the beginnings of the Japanese culture. *Chief Scriptures:* None *Basic Tenets:* The word shin-to or in Japa- nese Kami-no-michi means "the way·of the gods." The gods and goddesses that are worshipped are the forces of nature which may reside in rivers, trees, rocks, moun- tains, certain animals, and particularly in the sun and moon. The worship of ances- tors, heroes, and dead emper- ors was started later. The highest deity is the sun god- dess who is known as the Ruler of Heaven. Until Emperor Hirohito disavowed his divinity after World War II, the Emperor was believed to have the immortal status of a deity. Today, Shinto sects stress world peace and broth- erhood but no universal pro- phetic message.	No foods seem to be forbidden by the Shinto religion.	The only foods that may be considered as encouraged are those associated with ceremonies dealing with abundant harvest or good health. Gifts of cakes are offered at some public shrines. In traditional villages, the diet tends to be largely vegetarian with an occasional fish or chicken, and milk con- tinues to be consid- ered as dirty. These food habits may be the influence of Shinto and/or other religions which entered Japan over the years.	Shinto gradually borrowed ethi- cal principles from Buddhism and Confucian- ism, but did not evolve an ethi- cal system of its own. Worship takes place in shrines or temples approached through gate- ways called *torii.* Acts of worship consist of pray- ers, hand clasp- ing, purification acts, and offerings. Japanese homes have a god shelf which is a small wooden shrine containing the tablets with the names of ancestors.
Religion: **Sikhism** *Adherents:* About a million worldwide, primarily in India, but some small communi- ties in the United Kingdom, Canada, the United States, Malaysia, and East Africa.	*Origins:* Founded by Guru Nanak about 1500 A.D. *Chief Scriptures:* *Granth Sahib* *Basic Tenets:* Sikhism combines the beliefs of Islam and Hinduism. Nanak taught that there was one God, thus rejecting the deities of Hinduism and the worship of idols. Nanak opposed the caste system, uniting his fol- lowers into one class.	Sikhs vow not to smoke or to drink alcoholic bever- ages.	No foods seem to be encouraged by the Sikh beliefs. There are certainly some tradi- tional foods which may in part reflect the Hindu and Moslem in- fluence.	Most people who follow Sikhism live in the state of Punjab in northwestern India. Govind Singh, the tenth and last guru formed Sikhs into a mil- itary commun- ity. Then under Ranjit Singh in the 19th cen- tury, the Sikh empire reached its height only to be conquered by the British. Sikhs are chiefly farmers and soldiers. Sikhs are easily identified by their turbans.

(Continued)

TABLE R-5   *(Continued)*

Religion; Adherents	Origins; Chief Scripture(s); Basic Tenets	Food Taboos	Foods Encouraged by Beliefs	Remarks
Religion: **Taoism** *Adherents:* About 30 million worldwide.	*Origins:* Founded about 2,600 years ago by Lao-tzu. *Chief Scriptures:* Tao te ching *Basic Tenets:* In Chinese, the word "tao" means way or path. Taoism stresses quiet contemplation, and the elimination of all striving and strong passions which allows a man to live in harmony with the principles that underlie and govern the universe. Taoism divided all reality into male and female principles of *yang* and *yin*, respectively. *Tao* cannot be comprehended by reason and knowledge. Taoism did develop beliefs of an afterlife with a heaven and hell.	No specific food taboos seem to be taught.	Yang and yin philosophy may have some influence in the food choices, as may the philosophy of living close to nature. Some Taoist groups have included special diets as part of their search for immortality. Early Taoists practiced alchemy—mixing elixirs designed to ensure immortality.	After 500 A.D., Taoism adopted aspects of Confucianism and Buddhism. In China a person may be a Confucian, a Taoist, and a Buddhist all at the same time. At one time Taoism became concerned with magic and also provided the basis for some secret societies. Taoism developed partly as a reaction against Confucianism.
Religion: **Zoroastrianism** *Adherents:* Only about 200,000 primarily in limited areas of Asia.	*Origins:* Founded in the 6th century B.C. by Zoroaster, a religious teacher and prophet of Persia (now Iran). *Chief Scriptures:* The *Avesta* or *Zend-Avesta*. *Basic Tenets:* Zoroaster taught monotheism—the belief in one god. The supreme being or god of Zoroastrianism is Ahura Mazda. Also this religion teaches that the world is ruled by two forces—good and evil. Therefore, the rituals of Zoroastrianism center on devotion to good and the battle against evil. A lie is a great evil in Zorastrianism.	No specific foods are limited by the teachings of Zoroastrianism.	Zoroastrians have a ritual drink called haoma. There may be traditional foods which are associated with religious festivals. Zoroaster encouraged people to till the soil, raise grain, grow fruits, irrigate and weed crops, reclaim wasteland, and to treat animals kindly.	The Moslem conquest of the 7th century A.D. marked the beginning of a steady decline. Zoroastrians consider fire the most perfect symbol of their god. There is a Zoroastrian sect in Iran called Ghebers, who worship fire. Part of the *Avesta*, the *Vendidad*, contained some of the best hygienic laws existing before the start of modern medicine.

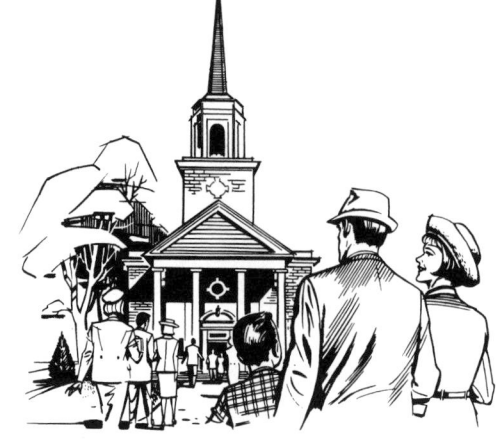

RELISH, CHUTNEY, PICCALILLI

All three of these words mean essentially the same thing: a mixture of chopped vegetables, with a blend of spices and vinegar.

REMISSION

An interval in the course of a disease in which the symptoms subside or abate.

RENAL GLUCOSURIA

A term which implies the excretion of glucose (sugar) in the urine while blood glucose remains within the limits of normal concentrations. It is caused by a disorder in kidney (renal) function and is sometimes called renal diabetes. Glucosuria or the excretion of sugar in the urine is often, but not always, associated with diabetes mellitus. However, in diabetes mellitus the blood sugar is elevated far beyond normal concentrations.
(Also see DIABETES MELLITUS.)

RENAL THRESHOLD

The level of concentration of a substance in the blood beyond which it is excreted in the urine. For example, the renal threshold of glucose is about 180 mg per 100 ml; diabetics excrete glucose because this level is exceeded.

RENDERING

• The process of liberating the fat from the fat cells, as in the production of lard and tallow.

• The processing of inedible animals and meats into livestock feeds, industrial fats and oils, and fertilizers.

RENNET

An extract of the stomach of certain mammals, which contains the enzyme rennin. It is used in making most cheeses and junkets.

RENNET, VEGETABLE

The name given to proteolytic enzymes derived from plants, such as bromelin (from the pineapple) and ficin (from the fig).

RENNIN (CHYMOSIN)

The milk-coagulating enzyme found in the gastric juice of the fourth stomach compartment of certain mammals.

REPLETION

To fill up; the act of overeating or the state of being overfed.

RESECTION

Removal of part of an organ.

RESERPINE

An active alkaloid that is extracted from the root of shrubs of the genus *Rauwolfia*, and used as a tranquilizer or sedative. It is also used as an antihypertensive drug, in the treatment of high blood pressure, various mental diseases, and tension.

RESIDUE

Left over, remaining; dietary residue refers to the content remaining in the intestinal tract after digestion of food—including fiber and other unabsorbed products.

RESORPTION

A loss of substance; for example, the withdrawal of calcium from bone.

RESPIRATION (BREATHING)

Commonly used to mean the taking in of oxygen and the throwing off of carbon dioxide and water vapor through the lungs, but it also includes the metabolism of the cells.

RESPIRATORY CHAIN (ELECTRON TRANSPORT SYSTEM)

The series of chemical reactions in the oxidation system of the cell that transfer hydrogen ions or electrons to produce ATP (high-energy phosphate compounds.)
(Also see METABOLISM, section on "Catabolism,
• **ATP**—energy currency.")

RESPIRATORY QUOTIENT (RQ)

A ratio indicating the relation of the volume of carbon dioxide given off in respiration to that of the oxygen consumed. The RQ is used to indicate the *type* of nutrient being metabolized. This is possible because carbohydrates, fats, and proteins differ in the relative amounts of oxygen and carbon contained in their molecules. Thus, the RQ is near 1 when the body is burning chiefly carbohydrates; near 0.7 when chiefly fats; near 0.8 when chiefly proteins; and sometimes exceeding 1 when carbohydrates are being changed to fats for storage.

(Also see CALORIC [Energy] Expenditure, section headed "Respiratory Quotient.")

RESPIRATORY SYSTEM

The body's apparatus for inhaling oxygen and exhaling carbon dioxide and water vapor; it consists mainly of the lungs and bronchial tubes, and its movements are activated by the midriff and the muscles between the ribs.

RETICULOCYTE

A young red blood cell.

RETICULOENDOTHELIAL SYSTEM

Groups of cells, except leukocytes, with phagocytic properties, functioning to rid the body of debris.

RETINAL

Retinal (or retinene) is the aldehyde form of retinol (formerly called vitamin A); it is one of the three biologically active forms of retinol (retinol is also active as an alcohol and as an acid).

(Also see VITAMIN A.)

RETINOIC ACID

Retinol (formerly called vitamin A) is biologically active as an alcohol, as an aldehyde, and as an acid. The acid form is usually referred to as retinoic acid. Retinoic acid can partially replace retinol in the rat diet; it promotes growth of bone and soft tissues and sperm production, but it cannot be used in the visual process and will not permit maturation of embryos. Retinoic acid is converted by the rat to an unknown form that is several times as active as the parent compound in the usual vitamin A nutritional assays.

RETINOL

One of the two forms of vitamin A as such; the other form is dehydroretinol. Retinol (formerly called vitamin

A), which is found as an ester (retinyl palmitate) in ocean fish oils and fats, and in liver, butterfat, and egg yolk, is biologically active as an alcohol, as an aldehyde, and as an acid. The alcohol, the most common form, is usually referred to as retinol, the aldehyde as retinal or retinene, and the acid as retinoic acid.

(Also see VITAMIN A.)

RETINOPATHY

Degenerative disease of the retina.

RETROGRADATION

Starch is insoluble in cold water, but in a heated suspension the granules swell and form a paste or gel. However, upon aging or freezing, the amylose portion of starch aggregates, forming an insoluble substance and reducing the water-holding ability of the starch. This process, which is termed retrogradation, is undesirable in foods. In the food industry, monoglycerides are added to starch to reduce the tendency of retrogradation.

(Also see STARCH.)

RHAMNOSE

A hexose monosaccharide found combined in the form of plant glycosides. It occurs in free form in poison sumac.

RHEUMATIC FEVER

A childhood disease that is always preceded by an infection of *Streptococcus* bacteria or scarlet fever. It occurs in acute and chronic forms, and it is one of the leading causes of chronic illness in children. Rheumatic fever belongs to a class of diseases termed collagen diseases.

Rheumatic fever occurs following about one out of every hundred cases of throat infection by *Streptococcus* bacteria, as a result of the body's defense system against infection going awry, so that the antibodies generated to fight the bacteria also attack the healthy tissue at the joints, tendons, and heart valves. This happens because the bacteria contain substances (antigens) very similar in composition to components in the tissues that are attacked. This is accompanied by a sudden onset of a high fever, and the development of intensely painful, swollen, hot joints. Characteristically, this condition migrates from joint to joint. The chief danger of rheumatic fever, however, is the destruction to heart valve tissue. When the valves become inflamed, scar tissue forms as they heal, leaving the victim with the condition known as rheumatic heart disease.

The best treatment for rheumatic fever is the early detection and treatment of a streptococcal infection. Unfortunately, mild strep infections can go unnoticed and result in rheumatic fever. Once acquired, the disease requires bed rest during the acute stage, and antibiotic therapy. Aspirin may be prescribed to help relieve the symptoms, and sometimes hormone therapy—ACTH, or cortisone—is employed to prevent or lessen heart damage. Nutritional support is important.

(Also see MODIFIED DIETS.)

RHODOPSIN (VISUAL PURPLE)

The pigment in the rods of the retina that contains vitamin A. When light strikes the normal retina, this pigment is bleached to another pigment known as retinaldehyde (visual yellow). As a result of this change, images are transmitted to the brain through the optic nerve. Vitamin A is required for regeneration of rhodopsin.

(Also see VITAMIN A, section headed "Functions • Vision.")

RHUBARB (PIEPLANT) *Rheum rhaponticum*

Rhubarb is believed to be a native of Asia minor. It is a perennial plant which forms large fleshy rhizomes and large leaves with long, thick petioles. It is one of the few vegetables in which the petiole is the part consumed. The leaf portion contains a toxic substance. Rhubarb's popularity in preserves, pies, and desserts causes many people to think of it as a fruit; however, it is a vegetable.

RIBOFLAVIN (B-2)

Riboflavin is present in virtually all living cells; and, like niacin, it has an essential role in the oxidative mechanisms in the cells.

As early as 1879, the existence of a yellow-green fluorescent pigment in milk whey was recognized. Subsequently, other workers found this pigment in such widely varying sources as liver, heart, and egg white. This pigment, which possessed fluorescent properties, was called *flavin*. But, at the time, the biological significance of the pigment was not understood.

By 1928, it became evident that what had been called vitamin B was not a single vitamin. Numerous investigators found that a growth-promoting substance re-

RIBOFLAVIN
PROMOTES HEALTH BY HELPING BODY CELLS USE OXYGEN TO RELEASE ENERGY FROM AMINO ACIDS, FATTY ACIDS, AND CARBOHYDRATES.

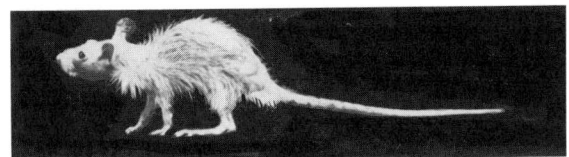 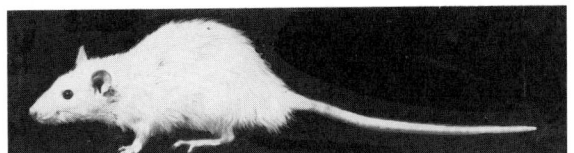

RIBOFLAVIN MADE THE DIFFERENCE! SAME RAT BEFORE (LEFT) AND AFTER (RIGHT). LEFT: THIS RAT 28 WEEKS OLD, HAD NO RIBOFLAVIN. IT SOON BECAME SICK, AND LOST HAIR, ESPECIALLY ABOUT THE HEAD. IT WEIGHED ONLY 63 g. RIGHT: THE SAME RAT 6 WEEKS LATER, AFTER RECEIVING FOOD RICH IN RIBOFLAVIN. IT RECOVERED ITS FINE FUR AND WEIGHED 169 g. (COURTESY, USDA.)

TOP FOOD SOURCES

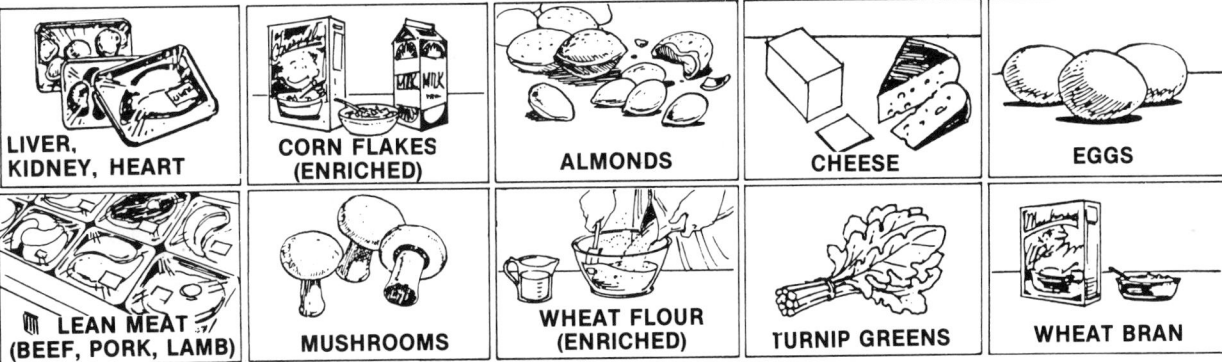

Fig. R-10.   The riboflavin story.

mained after heat had destroyed the beriberi-preventive factor (thiamin, or vitamin B-1) in yeast. This unknown substance was called *vitamin G* by U.S. research workers and *vitamin B-2* by British scientists. At the time, it was thought to be only one vitamin; later, it was found that the heat-stable fraction was composed of several vitamins.

HISTORY. The first serious attempts to isolate the long-known and widely-distributed fluorescent pigment was undertaken by workers in Germany and Switzerland in the early 1930s. In 1932, two German scientists, Warburg and Christian, isolated the "yellow enzyme," part of which was later identified as flavin mononucleotide (FMN)—riboflavin phosphate. In the following year (1933), Kuhn, working at the University of Heidelberg, isolated pure riboflavin from milk; and, in 1935, he elucidated the structure and synthesized the vitamin. Independently, Swiss researchers, Karrer and co-workers, accomplished the same feat that year (in 1935). Karrer[2] named it riboflavin, because it was found to have a pentose side chain —ribitol (similar to the sugar, ribose)—attached to a flavinlike compound; and, in 1952, the name was adopted by the Commission on Biochemical Nomenclature.

Riboflavin is widely distributed in both plant and animal tissues. It is formed by all higher plants, chiefly in the green leaves. Also, the bacteria in the intestinal tract may be a considerable, but variable, source of it for man and other animals, just as with thiamin. So, higher animals must rely on food for their vitamin.

CHEMISTRY, METABOLISM, PROPERTIES.

• **Chemistry**—Chemically, riboflavin is composed of an alloxazine ring linked to an alcohol derived from the pentose sugar ribose (see Fig. R-11).

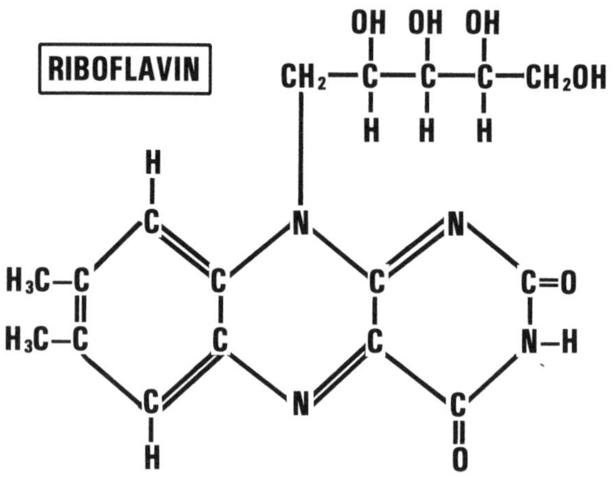

Fig. R-11.   Structure of riboflavin.

---

[2]Karrer, who died in 1971, was also the first to synthesize carotene. In 1937, he was awarded the Nobel Prize for his important discoveries in nutrition.

• **Metabolism**—Riboflavin is absorbed in the upper part of the small intestine by passive diffusion, which controls the amount of the vitamin taken up by the cells of the intestinal mucosa. It is phosphorylated in the intestinal wall and carried by the blood to the tissue where it may occur as the phosphate or as a flavoprotein.

The body has limited capacity for storing riboflavin, although higher concentrations are found in the liver and kidneys than in other tissues. So, day-to-day tissue needs must be supplied by the diet. Excretion is primarily via the urine, with the amount excreted related to uptake. When the intake is high, urinary excretion is high; when the intake is low, excretion is low. Some riboflavin is excreted in the feces. All mammals secrete riboflavin in their milk,

• **Properties**—In pure form, riboflavin exists as fine orange-yellow crystals, which are bitter tasting and practically odorless. In water solutions, it imparts a greenish-yellow fluorescence. It is sparingly soluble in water. (It is much less soluble in water than thiamin.) It is heat-stable in neutral or acid solutions, but it may be destroyed by heating in alkaline solutions. It is easily destroyed by light, especially ultraviolet light; for example, it may be destroyed by sunlight striking milk kept in glass bottles. (Milk in cartons is protected against such losses.) Synthetic riboflavin should always be kept in dark bottles. Because of its heat stability and limited water solubility, very little riboflavin is lost in processing and cooking foods.

MEASUREMENT/ASSAY. Riboflavin is measured in terms of the metric weight of pure riboflavin; human requirements are expressed in milligrams, and food content in milligrams or micrograms.

Although the growth of rats and chicks may occasionally be used to assay riboflavin in mixed diets, the biologic method of assay has been generally superseded by microbiological and chemical methods.

The assessment of riboflavin nutriture in man is determined by urinary excretion or by blood analysis.

FUNCTIONS. Riboflavin functions as part of a group of enzymes called flavoproteins. *Flavin mononucleotide (FMN)* and *flavin adenine dinucleotide (FAD)* operate at vital reaction points in the respiratory chains of cellular metabolism. The structure of these two compounds is shown in Fig. R-12.

FMN and FAD function as coenzymes in a number of different flavoprotein systems. They play a major role with thiamin- and niacin-containing enzymes in a long chain of oxidation-reduction reactions by which energy is released. In the process, hydrogen is transferred from one compound to another until it finally combines with oxygen to form water. Thus, riboflavin functions in the metabolism of amino acids, fatty acids, and carbohydrates. During this process, energy is released gradually and made available to the cell. In addition, riboflavin, through its role in activating pyridoxine (vitamin B-6), is necessary for the formation of niacin from the amino acid tryptophan. Also, riboflavin is thought to

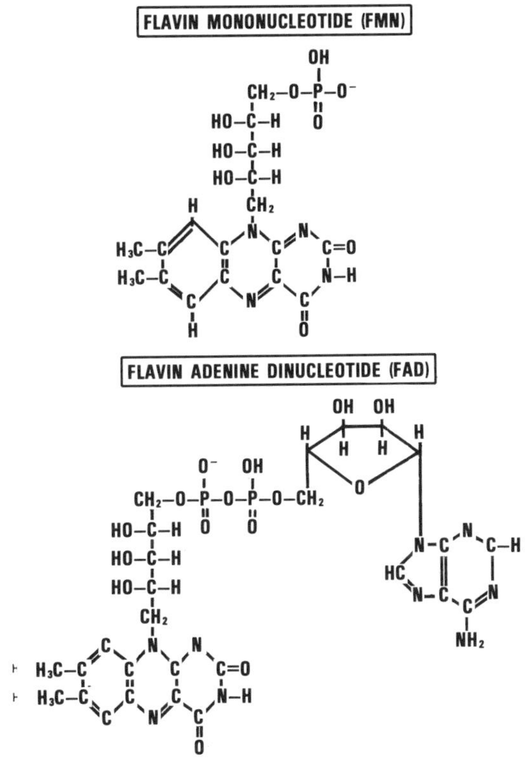

FLAVIN MONONUCLEOTIDE (FMN)

FLAVIN ADENINE DINUCLEOTIDE (FAD)

Fig. R-12.   The structure of FMN and FAD.

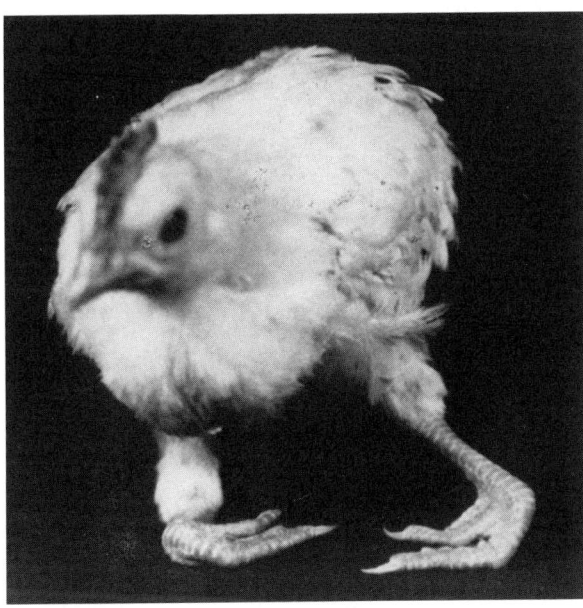

Fig. R-13.   Riboflavin deficiency in a young chick. Note the curled toes and the tendency to squat on the hocks; this condition known as "curled toe paralysis," is caused by degenerated nerves. (Courtesy, Department of Poultry Science, Cornell University)

be (1) a component of the retinal pigment of the eye; (2) involved in the functioning of the adrenal gland; and (3) required for the production of corticosteroids in the adrenal cortex.

DEFICIENCY SYMPTOMS.   Unlike some of the other vitamins, riboflavin deficiency does not cause any serious disease in human beings; nevertheless, clinical signs associated with riboflavin deficiencies are found among persons of all ages in developing countries.

Manifestations of riboflavin deficiency center around the following symptoms:

1.   **Fatigue.**   The most important of the nonspecific symptoms is fatigue and inability to work.

2.   **Wound healing.**   Even minor wounds become aggravated and do not heal easily.

3.   **Mouth.**   Cheilosis (sores around the mouth) develops. The lips become swollen, reddened, and chapped, and characteristic cracks develop at the corners of the mouth (angular stoma).

4.   **Nose.**   Cracks and irritation develop at nasal angles.

5.   **Tongue.**   Glossitis (inflammation of the tongue) develops. The tongue becomes swollen, reddened, fissured, and painful.

6.   **Eyes.**   Extra blood vessels develop in the cornea (the eyes become bloodshot), and the eyes become sensitive to light and easily fatigued. There is also blurring of the vision, and the eyes burn, itch, and tear. Cataracts have been observed in rats, mice, chickens, pigs, and monkeys after prolonged deficiency of riboflavin.

7.   **Skin.**   Seborrheic dermatitis (oily crusts and scales) may develop. The skin may become scaly, and greasy eruptions may develop—especially in the skin folds, around the nose, and on the scrotum in males.

8.   **Anemia.**   Anemia has been produced experimentally in human subjects given galactoflavin, a riboflavin antagonist. The anemia, along with other symptoms, responded rapidly to riboflavin therapy.

9.   **Pregnancy.**   Deficiency of riboflavin during pregnancy leads to skeletal abnormalities of the fetus, including shortened bones; deformed growth between ribs, toes, and fingers; and short fingers with fewer joints.

All of the above conditions are common, especially in children in the developing countries where the supply of meat, milk, and eggs is poor. The same conditions are sometimes seen among the elderly in well-fed countries.

Also, it is noteworthy that riboflavin deficiencies seldom occur alone. Instead, they are apt to be found along with deficiency diseases of the other members of the B complex.

RECOMMENDED DAILY ALLOWANCE OF RIBOFLAVIN.

Prior to 1980, the Recommended Dietary Allowances of the Food and Nutrition Board (FNB), National Research Council, National Academy of Sciences, related the allowances for riboflavin to (1) protein allowances (1958), (2) energy intake (1964), and (3) metabolic body size (1968). In the ninth edition, 1980, the FNB concluded that the information available does not support strongly any one of these over another. In the tenth edition, 1989, the FNB listed the following factors as being known to affect the riboflavin requirements: nitrogen balance, energy (work) expenditure, and pregnancy and lactation.

Table R-6 gives the current FNB Recommended Daily Riboflavin Allowances.

TABLE R-6
RECOMMENDED DAILY
RIBOFLAVIN ALLOWANCES[1]

Group	Age	Weight		Height		Riboflavin
	(years)	(lb)	(kg)	(in.)	(cm)	(mg)
Infants	0.0–0.5	13	6	24	60	0.4
	0.5–1.0	20	9	28	71	0.5
Children	1–3	29	13	35	90	0.8
	4–6	44	20	44	112	1.1
	7–10	62	28	52	132	1.2
Males	11–14	99	45	62	157	1.5
	15–18	145	66	69	176	1.8
	19–24	160	72	70	177	1.7
	25–50	174	79	70	176	1.7
	51+	170	77	68	173	1.4
Females	11–14	101	46	62	157	1.3
	15–18	120	55	64	163	1.3
	19–24	128	58	65	164	1.3
	25–50	138	63	64	163	1.3
	51+	143	65	63	160	1.2
Pregnant						1.6
Lactating						1.8

[1]*Recommended Dietary Allowances*, 10th ed., 1989, NRC-National Academy of Sciences, p. 285.

• **Adults and children**—The riboflavin allowances in Table R-6 have been computed on the basis of 0.6 mg/1,000 Calorie (kcal) for people of all ages. However, for elderly people and others whose calorie intake may be less than 2,000 Calories (kcal), a minimum intake of 1.2 mg/day is recommended.

• **Pregnancy**—The recommended allowances call for an additional 0.3 mg/day of riboflavin during pregnancy.

• **Lactation**—An additional daily intake of approximately 0.5 mg is recommended during lactation.

• **Riboflavin intake in average U.S. diet**—According to the U.S. Department of Agriculture, in 1988 the riboflavin available for civilian consumption in the United States was 2.4 mg per person per day. Further, 79.5% of the riboflavin in the U.S. diet was supplied by three food groups: (1) meat, fish, and poultry; (2) milk and dairy products; and (3) flour and cereal products.

A U.S. enrichment program for white flour (with standards for riboflavin, thiamin, niacin, and iron) was initiated in 1941. Subsequently, several other products have been designated for enrichment, and the levels of added nutrients have been changed.

Currently, the riboflavin supplementation of flour and cereal products from synthetic and/or fermentation sources contributes an average of 0.33 mg of riboflavin per person per day, which is about one-fifth of the requirement of an adult male—a very significant amount. However, not all states require an enrichment program; hence, where products are not involved in interstate commerce, they need not be enriched. Besides, average consumption figures do nothing for those persons whose consumptions are below the recommended allowances, or who have higher than normal requirements. Chronic or borderline riboflavin deficiencies are most likely to occur to a variable extent in persons with inadequate intake of animal proteins (especially among those not consuming adequate milk) and enriched foods, in alcoholics, in the aged, in women taking oral contraceptives or who are pregnant or lactating. Also, it is recognized that riboflavin deficiencies, usually along with deficiencies of vitamin A, folacin, calcium, iron, and sometimes vitamin D, are commonplace in many other countries.

TOXICITY.

There is no known toxicity of riboflavin.

RIBOFLAVIN LOSSES DURING PROCESSING, COOKING, AND STORAGE.

The two properties of riboflavin that may account for major losses are (1) that it is destroyed by light, and (2) that it is destroyed by heat in alkaline solution. The following facts relative to riboflavin losses during processing, cooking, and storage are noteworthy:

• **Milk**—As much as 20% of the riboflavin content of fluid milk is destroyed in pasteurization, evaporation, or drying. Also, one-half or more of the riboflavin in milk may be lost in 2 hours if it is exposed to light; as happened prior to 1960 when clear glass bottles of milk were delivered on the doorsteps of U.S. homes—a practice still common in many countries. The use of opaque cartons or dark bottles for the distribution of milk markedly reduces the loss of riboflavin.

• **Blanching**—In the blanching processes used prior to canning or freezing certain foods, losses of 5 to 20% of riboflavin occur.

• **Drying**—Dehydration and freeze-drying processes have little effect on the vitamin content of foods. However, the practice of sun-drying of foods, such as fish and vegetables in tropical countries, results in considerable destruction of riboflavin.

• **Cooking**—Because riboflavin is heat stable and only slightly soluble in water, little of it is lost in home cooking or commercial canning. Average losses of riboflavin in cooking are 15 to 20% in meats, 10 to 20% in vegetables, and 10% in baking bread.

• **Alkali**—Riboflavin may be destroyed by heating in alkaline solutions; hence, sodium bicarbonate should not be used in the cooking of vegetables.

SOURCES OF RIBOFLAVIN.
Riboflavin is widely distributed in most foods. However, there is wide variation in levels, due primarily to source, harvesting, processing, enrichment, and storage. For example, whole cereal grains contain useful amounts, but much of this is removed in milling; hence, highly milled cereals and breads contain very little riboflavin unless they are enriched. Riboflavin is the only vitamin present in significant amounts in beer; beer drinkers may find consolation in knowing that 1 liter (*1.06 qt*) of beer daily almost meets the recommended intake. Green leafy vegetables vary greatly, but some are fair sources of riboflavin. Fruits, roots and tubers, with few exceptions, contain relatively small amounts of riboflavin. Pure sugars and fats are entirely lacking in riboflavin.

A grouping and ranking of foods according to normal riboflavin content follows:

• **Rich sources**—Organ meats (liver, kidney, heart).

• **Good sources**—Corn flakes (enriched), almonds, cheese, eggs, lean meat, (beef, pork, lamb), mushrooms (raw), wheat flour (enriched), turnip greens, wheat bran, soybean flour, bacon, cornmeal (enriched).

• **Fair sources**—Chicken (dark meat), white bread (enriched), rye flour, milk, mackerel and sardines, green leafy vegetables, beer.

• **Negligible sources**—Fruits (raw), roots and tubers, white sugar, fats and oils (butter, margarine, salad oil, shortening).

• **Supplemental sources**—Yeast (brewers', torula).

Riboflavin is the only vitamin present in significant amounts in beer.

The average person is not apt to get an optimum amount of riboflavin unless he consumes a generous amount of milk. Each quart (*950 ml*) of milk contains 1.66 mg of riboflavin, which just meets the recommended daily allowance of adult males. Of course, the addition of riboflavin in the enrichment of flour, bread, and certain other products has helped to raise the average intake.

For additional sources and more precise values of riboflavin (B-2), see Food Composition Table F-36 of this book.

TOP FOOD SOURCES OF RIBOFLAVIN.
The top food sources of riboflavin are listed in Table R-7.

NOTE WELL: This table lists (1) the top sources without regard to the amount normally eaten (left column), and (2) the top food sources (right column); and the caloric (energy) content of each food.

(Also see VITAMIN[S], Table V-9.)

TABLE R-7
TOP SOURCES OF RIBOFLAVIN AND THEIR CALORIC CONTENT[1]

Top Sources[2]	Riboflavin	Energy	Top Food Sources	Riboflavin	Energy
	(mg/ 100 g)	(kcal/ 100 g)		(mg/ 100 g)	(kcal/ 100 g)
Yeast, baker's dry (active)	5.41	282	Liver, beef or calf, fried	4.18	242
Liver, lamb, broiled	5.11	261	Cheese, pasteurized, process American	3.53	375
Yeast, torula	5.06	277	Liver, chicken, simmered	1.75	165
Kidneys, beef, braised	4.58	252	Corn flakes, w/added nutrients	1.40	380
Liver, hog, fried in margarine	4.36	241	Almonds, shelled	0.93	598
Yeast, brewers', debittered	4.28	283	Cheese, natural, Roquefort	0.59	369
Liver, beef or calf, fried	4.18	242	Eggs, chicken, fried	0.54	210
Brewers' yeast, tablet form	4.04	—	Beef, tenderloin steak, broiled	0.46	224
Cheese, pasteurized, process American	3.53	375	Mushrooms, raw	0.46	28
Turkey, giblets, cooked (some gizzard fat), simmered	2.72	233	Cheese, natural Swiss (American)	0.40	372
Kidneys, lamb, raw	2.42	105	Wheat flour, all-purpose, enriched	0.40	365
Kidneys, calf, raw	2.40	113	Turnip greens, raw	0.39	28
Eggs, chicken, dried, white powder	2.32	372	Cheese, natural Cheddar	0.38	402
Whey, sweet, dry	2.21	354	Wheat bran	0.35	353
Eggs, chicken, dried, white flakes	2.16	351	Soybean flour	0.35	333
Liver, turkey, simmered	2.09	174	Bacon, cured, cooked, drained, sliced, medium	0.34	575
Whey, acid dry	2.06	339	Pork, loin, lean, broiled	0.33	391
Heart, hog, braised	1.89	195	Lamb, leg, good or choice, separable lean roasted	0.30	186
Milk, cow's, dry, skim, solids, instant	1.78	353	Cornmeal, degermed, enriched	0.26	362
Liver, chicken, simmered	1.75	165	Chicken, dark meat w/o skin, fried	0.25	220
			Bread, white, enriched	0.24	270
			Milk, cow's, whole, 3.7% fat	0.17	66

[1]These listings are based on the data in Food Composition Table F-36. Some top or rich food sources may have been overlooked since some foods in Table F-36 lack values for riboflavin.

Whenever possible, foods are on an "as used" basis, without regard to moisture content; hence, certain high-moisture foods may be disadvantaged when ranked on the basis of riboflavin content per 100 g (approximately 3 1/2 oz) without regard to moisture content.

[2]Listed without regard to the amount normally eaten.

RIBONUCLEIC ACID (RNA)

Molecules in cell cytoplasm which serve for the transfer of the amino acid code from nuclei and the synthesis of protein.

(Also see METABOLISM, section headed "Anabolism"; and NUCLEIC ACIDS.)

RIBOSE

A 5-carbon sugar—a pentose—synthesized by the body in all animals, including man. Hence, it is not essential in the diet, but in the body ribose plays an important role. When it is joined with pyrimidines—cytosine, thymine, and uracil; and purines—adenine and guanine—nucleosides are formed. When phosphoric acid is esterified with the nucleosides, nucleotides are formed. These compounds are then used in the formation of ribonucleic acid (RNA) and deoxyribonucleic acid (DNA). The nucleotides of adenosine monophosphate (AMP), adenosine diphosphate (ADP), and adenosine triphosphate (ATP) are compounds that are essential to cellular metabolism. Ribose is also a constituent of the vitamin riboflavin.

(Also see CARBOHYDRATE[S]; and METABOLISM.)

RIBOSOMES

The site of protein synthesis in the cell.
(Also see METABOLISM.)

RICE *Oryza sativa*

Rice is one of the most important cereal grains of the world. It provides most of the food for over half the human population of the earth, most of them living in the Orient where some 94% of the world's rice is produced and consumed. In some countries of the Orient, the per capita consumption of rice is 200 to 400 lb (*90 to 180 kg*) per year; by contrast, the yearly per capita consumption of rice in the United States is less than 8 lb (*3.6 kg*). In several national languages and local dialects, the word "eat" means "to eat rice". American children associate rice with chopsticks.

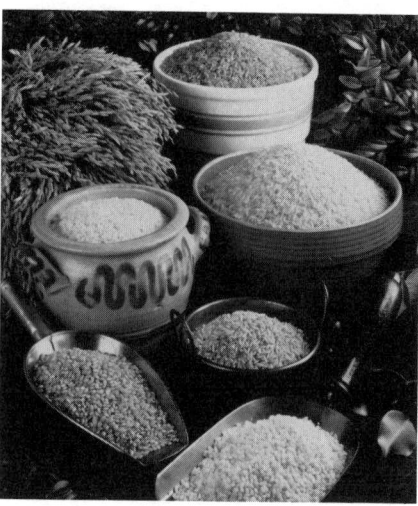

Fig. R-14. Kinds of rice. (Courtesy, USA Rice Council, Houston, Tex.)

Oriental peoples often eat rice cakes at certain festivals as symbols of happiness and long life. In Japan, the Emperor, who is the patron of all agriculture, joins in the ritual harvest of rice. In the Orient, rice is the symbol of life and fertility; hence, the origin of the widespread custom of throwing rice on bridal couples.

Rice is the only major cereal that is largely consumed by man directly as harvested (after hulling, and usually polishing). Wheat is usually milled to flour, then baked; and corn (maize) is largely fed to animals for the production of meat, milk, and eggs.

(Also see CEREAL GRAINS.)

ORIGIN AND HISTORY. Rice originated from wild species indigenous to southeastern Asia, where wild types still persist, although there is some evidence of an African center of domestication. Primitive man collected wild rice. Eventually, he cultivated it and selected mutant types with larger nonshattering grains. Hybridization with various wild species followed, contributing to great variability in the plant.

The antiquity of rice culture in China is indicated by a ceremony dating back 3,000 years before Christ, in which the Emperor and Princess honored rice planting by sowing a handful of seed with their own royal hands. Professor Ting Yeng, China's foremost rice scientist, is authority for the statement that China began to grow rice as early as the 27th century B.C., and that by the 12th century B.C. paddy rice was widely grown in the Yellow River Valley. The word *paddy,* along with recorded predictions of bad and good harvests, has been found in the inscriptions on the oracle-bones unearthed from the tombs of the Yin Dynasty (16th to 11th century B.C.).[3]

Archaeological evidence of rice in Thailand dates to 5000 to 3500 B.C. Rice is mentioned in early Hindu scriptures. It was taken to Greece by the Arab traders; and it was taken to India by Alexander the Great, when he invaded India around 326 B.C. The scientific name *Oryza* comes from the Greek word for rice. The Moors intro-

---

[3]Ensminger, M. E., and Audrey Ensminger, *China—the impossible dream*, Agriservices Foundation, 1973, p. 47.

duced the crop to Spain during their conquest of that country about 700 A.D. The Spanish colonists took it to the West Indies and South America in the early 1600s. Rice was first introduced into the United States, in the Carolinas, in 1647, where it became an important crop before the end of the century, and from which it spread throughout southeastern United States.

WORLD AND U.S. PRODUCTION.   Rice is a cheap and abundant crop, easy to grow on little land, and well adapted to the climatic conditions of the East Indies and the Asian Coast from India to Japan. Asia produces 92.3% of the world's rice crop. China and India lead the world in rice production. Fig. R-15 shows the ten leading rice-producing countries of the world.

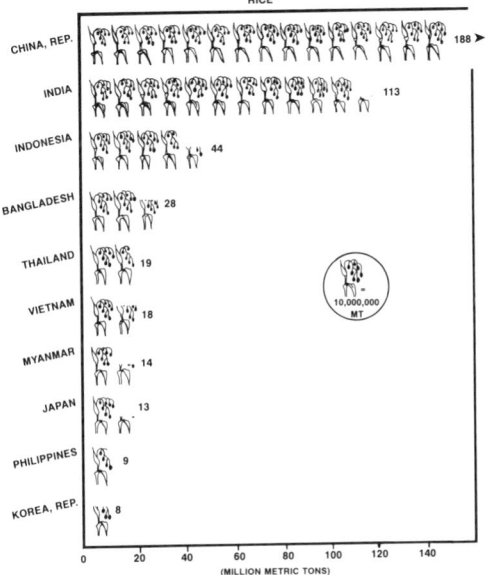

Fig. R-15. Leading rice-producing countries. (Source: *FAO Production Yearbook*, 1990, FAO/UN, Rome, Italy, Vol. 44, p. 72. Table 17)

The United States, which produces little more than 1% of the world crop, usually accounts for a third of the world rice trade. Over half of the U.S. crop is exported, largely to the Asian countries. Rice is largely concentrated in selected areas of Arkansas, California, Louisiana, Texas, Mississippi, and Missouri (see Fig. R-16). The U.S. average yield of 3.3 metric tons per acre is slightly more than the world figure.

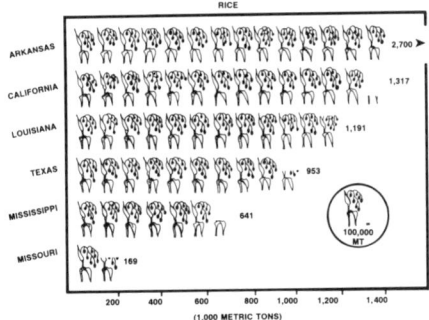

Fig. R-16.   Leading U.S. rice-producing states. (Source: *Agricultural Statistics 1991*, USDA, p. 22, Table 29)

THE RICE PLANT   Rice is an annual grass of the family, *Gramineae*, genus *Oryza*, species *O. sativa*. It varies in height from 2 to 6 ft (*0.6 to 1.8 m*). Plants develop

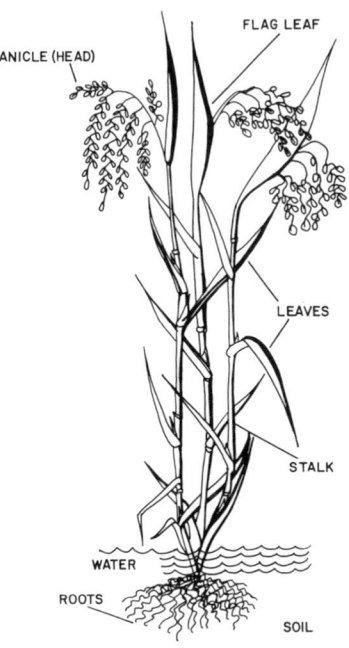

Fig. R-17.   The rice plant.

new shoots (tiller), with the number of shoots depending upon spacing and soil fertility. At first a single shoot appears; then, one, two, and often many more offshoots develop. Each stalk has five or six, or more, hollow joints; and there is a leaf for each joint. The leaf blades are long, pointed, flat, and rather stiff. The highest joint grows a branched head (panicle), much like an oat plant—but it is more compact and it droops more. Each head bears from 50 to 300 flowers (spikelets) from which the grains develop.

The Green Revolution—the development of short, stiff-stemmed varieties of rice, coupled with increased fertilization and improved irrigation and management—is resulting in greatly increased production in Asia.

RICE CULTURE.   Rice does not have to grow in water. But, because it is a water-tolerant plant, flooding rice fields is the most efficient and desirable method of weed and insect control. Also, yields of flooded rice are higher than those of upland rice. Consequently, more than 90% of the rice is grown in water in the important rice-producing areas. The farmer prepares the seed bed by plowing and cultivating, in much the same manner as for wheat or barley. Additionally, the land must be leveled, since rice must be kept evenly flooded. Also, there must be provision for an inflow and outflow of water, because the water should not become stagnant.

• **Oriental rice culture**—Oriental methods of growing rice (called *paddy*) are in sharp contrast to the mechanized production in the United States. With an abundance of labor, most Asian rice farmers still use the same primitive methods and crude tools of their ancestors, although sim-

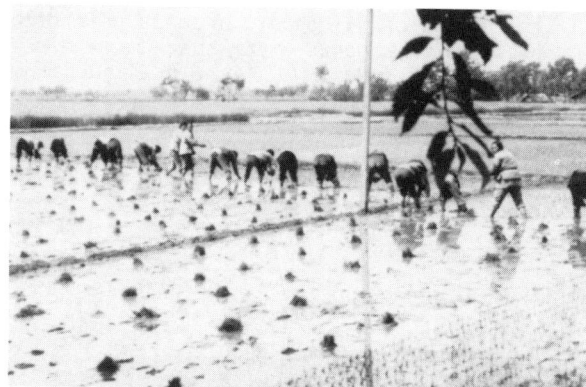

Fig. R-18. Rice is a great agricultural industry, as well as the chief food, of the Asian nations. Because it needs a great deal of water, most rice is grown in flooded lowlands or higher ground that is easily irrigated. The carabao, or water buffalo, often provide motive power for cultivation; planting is done by hand. (Photo by A. H. Ensminger)

ple machines are gradually replacing hand labor. Typically, the land is plowed with a wooden plow (called a stick plow) drawn by a water buffalo; manure or sewage is applied to the soil; the seedbed is smoothed by dragging a log over it; the dikes are repaired; and river water, hand-dipped with buckets or lifted by a human-powered water wheel, is used to flood the fields in areas where there is not sufficient rainfall. The rice is then planted; either by broadcasting dry or previously germinated seed, or

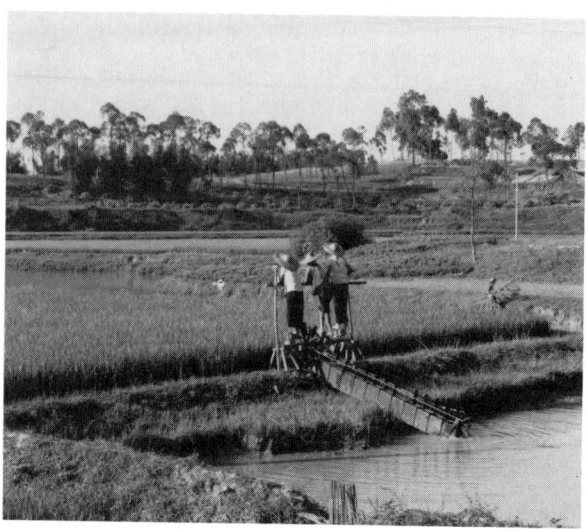

Fig. R-19. Water lifted by a human-powered water wheel to flood rice fields in the People's Republic of China. Today, most of this work is mechanized. (Photo by A. H. Ensminger)

by transplanting seedlings or young plants that have been grown in a nursery bed. Transplanting, which is backbreaking work that requires much stooping, is usually done by the women and children. weeding is done by hand. From 4 to 6 in. (*10 to 15 cm*) of water are kept on the field until the grain begins to ripen. Then the water

is drained from the fields so that the soil will dry by harvest time. Harvesting is done by hand, with the stalks cut by sickles or knives and tied into sheaves. After dry-

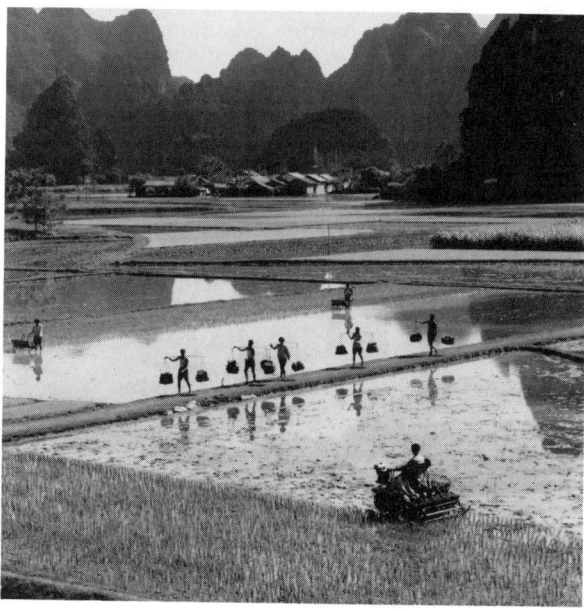

Fig. R-20. Something old, something new. Rice seedlings being tranported with carrying poles, but transplanted by machine. (Courtesy, *China Pictorial*)

ing in the sun, the grain is threshed. Some use simple foot- or gasoline-powered threshing machines. Others use animals or barefooted humans to tread upon the seed heads; or they flail the grain by hitting the sheaves against wide-spaced screens with the separated grain falling through the openings. Winnowing to remove the chaff from the grain is often accomplished by tossing the rice from bamboo or rattan trays and allowing the wind to blow away the lighter chaff while the grain settles nearby.

One of the most important by-products of much oriental rice farming does not come from the plant itself, for paddy fields are frequently used for fish farming. The fish (primarily carp) thrive, control the mosquitoes, and augment high rice diets with an excellent protein.

• **U.S. rice culture**—In the United States transplanting is impractical because of high labor costs. Two methods of seeding are practiced: (1) seed is drill-planted on dry land, then when the seedlings are a few inches tall, the fields are irrigated; or (2) low-flying airplanes broadcast sprouted seeds onto flooded fields. The water is kept at the 4- to 6-in. (*10 to 15 cm*) depth until the land is drained about 2 weeks before harvest. Airplanes spray chemicals to kill certain weeds and grasses. When the moisture content of the rice grains is from 23 to 28%, it is harvested with large self-propelled combines similar to those used for wheat and other grain crops; the straw is either left in the field to decay and serve as fertilizer, or baled for livestock feed and bedding. The grain is dried artificially to 14% moisture.

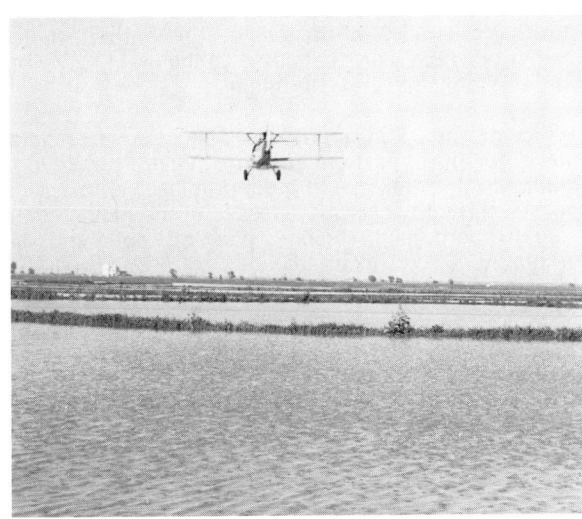

Fig. R-21. Low-flying airplane broadcasting sprouted rice seeds onto flooded fields in California. This assures a quick, efficient, uniform distribution of seed. In this "going-away" view of the airplane, thousands of tiny splashes can be seen as the rice seeds hit the water in the flooded fields. (Courtesy, Rice Growers Association of California, Sacramento, Calif.)

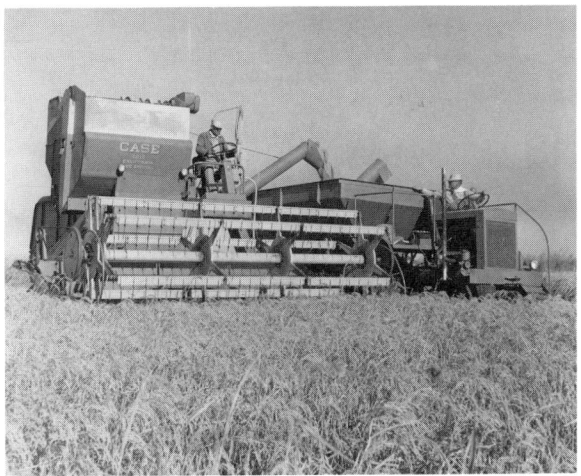

Fig. R-22. Harvesting rice with a large self-propelled combine. This shows the combine unloading the paddy rice into a self-propelled "bankout wagon." (Courtesy, Rice Growers Association of California, Sacramento, Calif.)

KINDS OF RICE.

There are about 25 species of *Oryza*, but one species, *Oryza sativa*, furnishes virtually all the rice of the world. The species *O. glaberima* is cultivated in Africa. Thousands of strains or varieties of rice are known. Today, there are about 40,000 strains of rice in China alone, with variations in characteristics and adaptations; and the crop is being grown from the low-lying coastal regions to the highlands of Tibet, and from the warm areas of south China where three crops a year are harvested to the northern areas where early-maturing strains with growing periods as short as 90 to 100 days must be used. The International Rice Research Institute in the Philippines has collected more than 30,000 varieties, but they report that relatively few of these are widely grown. In the United States, only about 25 varieties are grown commercially.

The types of cultivated rices are:

1. **Upland or lowland.** Upland types, which produce relatively low yields, grow in areas of Africa, Asia, and South America, which have plentiful rainfall and are too hilly to be flooded. The lowland types, which are high yielding, are grown submerged in water the greater part of the season. All rice in the United States is of the latter type.

2. **Long-grain, medium-grain, and short-grain.** This refers to the length/width ratio of kernels of rice that are unbroken. Most long-grain rices have high amylose content, which causes them to cook dry, with the kernels separated from each other. But long-grain rice costs more because many of the long kernels break during milling and must be removed. Most short-grain rices have lower amylose content and are sticky when cooked. Medium-grain rices have cooking qualities similar to short-grain varieties.

3. **Glutinous or waxy.** Some Asian people have a preference for glutinous or waxy rice, the milled kernels of which appear white and waxy. It cooks to a sticky paste and is used for cakes and confections. This rice is called "glutinous" because of having the sticky quality of glue, but neither it nor any other rice contains gluten.

4. **The "shorty" varieties.** The International Rice Research Institute (IRRI) began its work in the Philippines in 1962, under the joint sponsorship of the Ford Foundation and the Rockefeller Foundation. Through hybridization, IRRI plant breeders were successful in developing varieties of rice that combined high yields, vigor, and disease resistance, along with short straws and the ability to stand erect (without lodging) until harvest. Additionally, the IRRI improved other aspects of rice growing—including fertilization, irrigation, and an inexpensive threshing machine. Thus, in a few short years, rice yields increased dramatically and were a major force in the *green revolution*.

Wild Rice *Zizania aquatica.* Wild rice (Indian rice, water oats) is native to eastern North America, and was an important food crop of the Great Lakes region, especially in what is now Minnesota, Wisconsin, and Manitoba. It is an annual grass, not closely related to true rice, *Oryza*; it belongs to a different genera and even a different tribe of the grass family. Formerly, wild rice was not cultivated. It grew wild in lakes and was harvested in canoes. Even today, about 10% of Minnesota's crop is collected by the Indians for their own use and as a cash crop. Seed is harvested by "ricing," which to the Indians means harvesting from canoes by bending the stems over the boat and beating the heads with a stick. Following harvesting, the moist seed is dried by parching in a heated rotating drum or in an open kettle with constant stirring to prevent burning.

(Also see WILD RICE.)

PROCESSING RICE. The main parts of the rice grain are the hull (husk, lemma), the seed coat (pericarp), the embryo (germ), and the endosperm (starchy en-

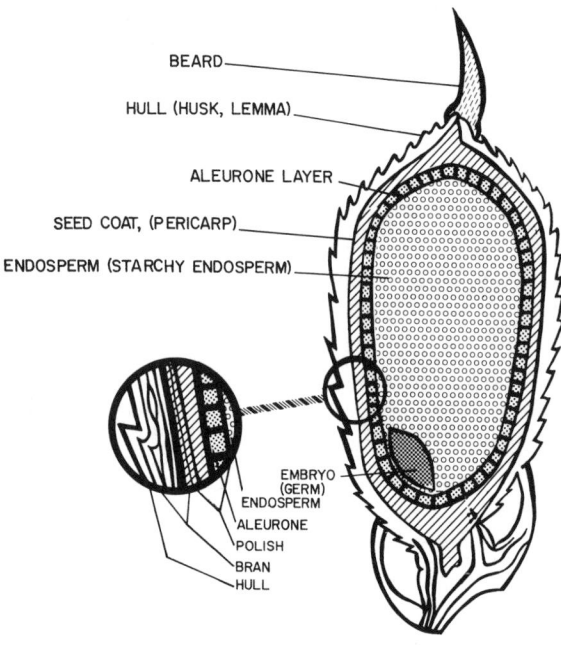

Fig. R-23.   Structure of the rice grain.

dosperm). The seed coat consists of six layers of differentiated types of cells, the innermost one of which is the aleurone layer.

Table R-8 shows that, together, the pericarp, aleurone, and scutellum (which is part of the germ) contain 79%

TABLE R-8
THIAMIN CONTENT OF FRACTIONS OF THE RICE GRAIN[1]

Part of Grain	Proportion of Grain	Thiamin Content	Proportion of the Total Thiamin of the Grain
	(%)	(mcg)	(%)
Pericarp and aleurone	5.95	31	} 35.2
Covering to germ ..	.20	12	
Epiblast	.27	78	3.9
Coleorhiza.........	.20	94	3.5
Plumule	.31	46	2.7
Radicle	.17	62	2.0
Scutellum	1.25	189	43.9
Outer endosperm	18.80	1.3	} 8.8
Inner endosperm ..	73.10	.3	

[1]Davidson, Sir Stanley, *et al., Human Nutrition and Dietetics,* 7th ed.,The Williams and Wilkins Company, Baltimore, Md., 1979, p. 173, Table 17.5.

of the total thiamin present in the grain, although constituting only 6.2% of the weight. By contrast, the endosperm, which represents 92% of the grain by weight, contains only 8.8% of the thiamin.

• **Rice milling**—The purpose of milling rice is to separate the outer portions from the inner endosperm with a minimum of breakage. In modern mills, the rough rice passes through several processes in the mill: cleaning (usually parboiling), hulling, pearling, polishing, and grading (see Fig. R-24).

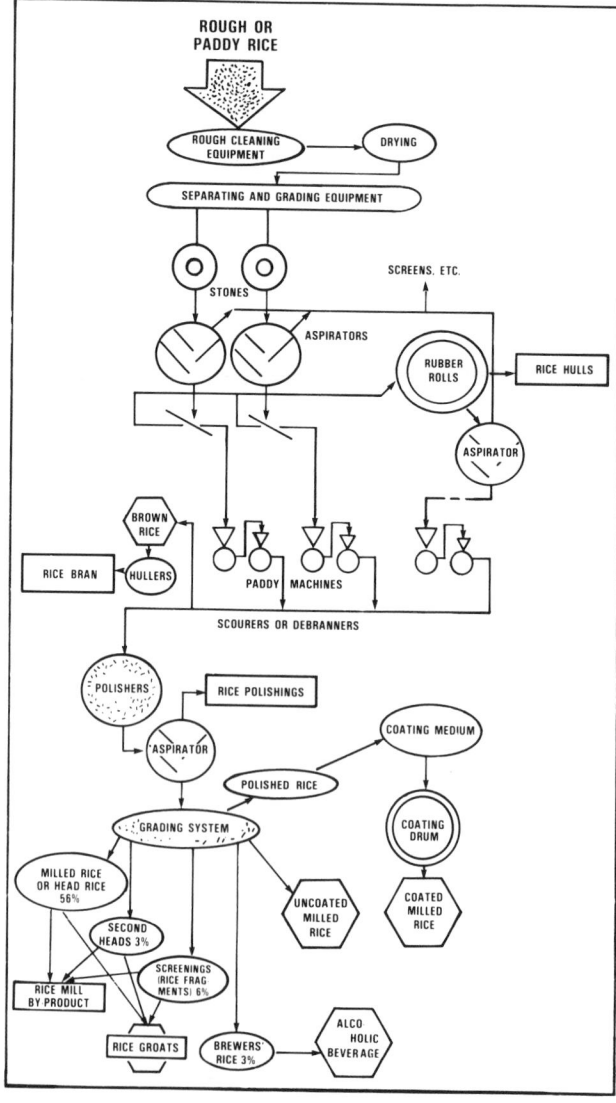

Fig. R-24.   Rice milling flow chart. Six-sided shapes are used for human food and the oval shapes are used for animal feeds.

Dramatic changes of immense health importance occur when rice is milled, the most important of which is the loss of much of the thiamin. Fig. R-25 shows the thiamin content of rice at different stages of milling. As noted, highly milled rice is almost devoid of thiamin. This loss has been responsible for much beriberi among people whose diet consists almost entirely of white rice.

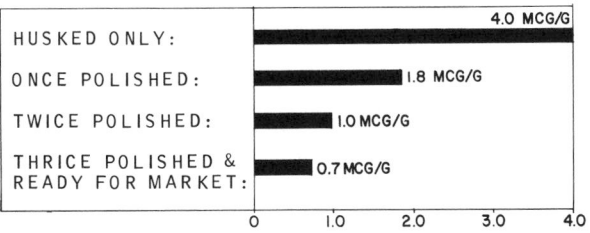

Fig. R-25.   Thiamin content of rice at different stages of milling.

In the United States, most rice undergoes a polishing process, during which the outer, colored, protein-rich parts (12%) become livestock feed, and the starchy white endosperm alone is left for human consumption. Polished rice is approximately 92% carbohydrates and has only 2% additional materials of nutritional value.

Dried rice that still has its hull is referred to as "rough" or "paddy" rice. Following the removal of foreign material by means of vibrating sieves and air currents, the rough rice passes into an awning machine where the awns are removed from the grain. The grain then passes through a series of shellers, and the hulled grain is separated from the unhulled in the paddy machine—a complex sifter. At this stage, the hulled rice, which represents approximately 79% of the weight of rough rice, is referred to as *brown rice.*

In the next milling step, the brown rice is conveyed to the hullers, which scour off the outer bran coats and germ from the rice kernels. The term "hullers" is a misnomer because these machines remove the bran, not hulls, from the rice kernel. Loosened bran and smaller pieces of kernel pass through the huller screen and are later separated by aspiration and screening. The rice bran is sold as a by-product for livestock feed.

Thence, the undermilled rice is passed through the brushing machine (polisher) which removes most of the inner bran coat or polish, producing a by-product known as rice polishings; which is sold for animal feeds, and sometimes as an ingredient of baby foods. The rice resulting from this operation is termed *polished rice,* which consists of the white, starchy endosperm, together with fragments of the aleurone layer.

Rice may be sold either as (1) polished or uncoated rice, or (2) coated with talc and glucose, an inert, harmless coating used to give it a high gloss or sheen, which is desired by the Puerto Rican market.

Throughout the entire milling process, a number of kernels are unavoidably broken. So, a series of machines classify the different size kernels as head rice (whole and ¾ kernels), second heads (¾ to ⅓ size grains), screenings ⅓ to ¼ length grains), or brewers' rice (under ¼ length fragments).

In the United States, there are the following grades of rice: U.S. No. 1, U.S. No. 2, U.S. No. 3, U.S. No. 4, U.S. No. 5, U.S. No. 6, and U.S. Sample grade. The grades are determined by size of kernels, number of heat-damaged kernels and objectionable seeds, percent of red rice and damaged kernels, percent of chalky kernels, percent of broken kernels, and color.

The yields of products and by-products obtained from rough rice in the milling process are approximately as shown in Fig. R-26.

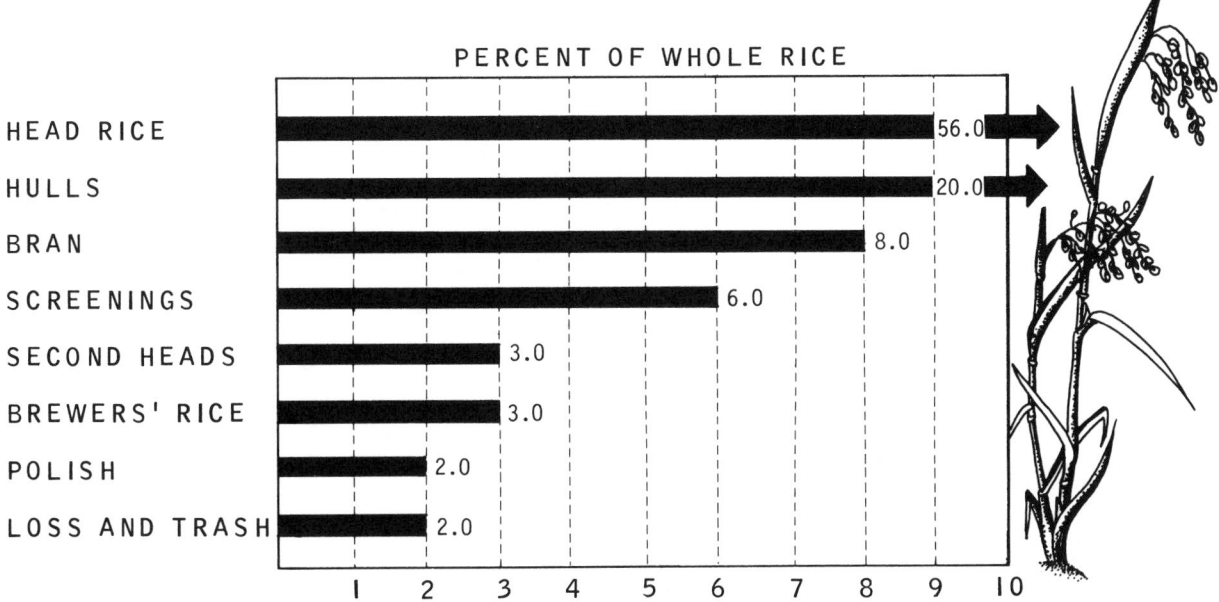

Fig. R-26.   Products obtained from milling rice.

• **Parboiled rice**—In southern Asia, rice is parboiled before milling. Approximately 20% of the world's rice is treated in this manner. Essentially, the process consists of soaking dry rough or paddy rice (in the hull) in warm water, steaming under pressure, and drying before milling.

In the United States, there are several patented methods of parboiling. When parboiled, the rice retains more minerals and vitamins (some of the minerals and vitamins present in the bran and embryo move into the grain proper), breaks less in subsequent processing, and stores better.

After parboiling, rice is milled in the conventional manner. It requires a longer cooking period (25 min) than regular rice (20 min). Because parboiling eliminates the surface starch common to regular rice, it ensures a separateness of grain that's especially desirable for kitchens preparing rice in large quantities.

NUTRITIONAL VALUE.   Rice without hulls contains about 80% starch, 8% protein, and 12% water.

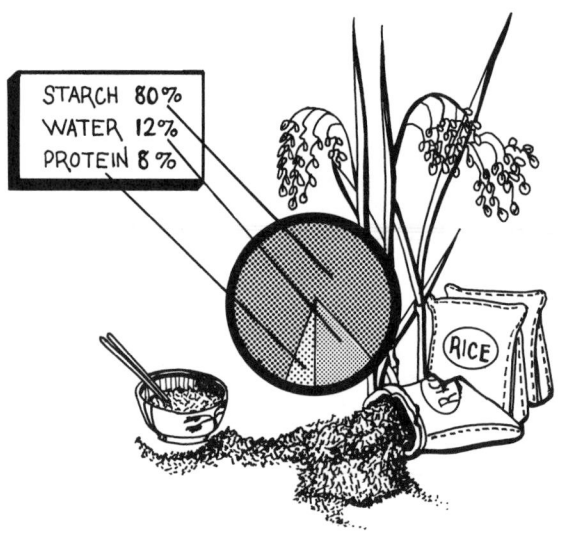

Fig. R-27.   Food value of rice.

Because rice is such a predominant food in the diets of Oriental people, its nutrient composition is relatively more important than the nutritional composition of wheat in Western countries. In most wheat-eating countries, the cereals contribute only 30 to 40% of the average food-caloric consumption, whereas in the rice-eating nations some 60 to 80% of the calories come from rice. Thus, at best, the Oriental diet includes only 20 to 40% vegetables, meats, fish, fruits, and all other foods that could furnish the missing vitamins and minerals. Under such dietary conditions, it is easy to understand how the nutrient composition of rice determines the health of those who subsist largely on it.

In its natural state, rice has good nutritional values, comparing favorably with those of the other major cereals used as food staples around the world. It is better than corn and approximately as good as wheat. Brown rice—

rice freed only of its chafflike hulls—has about the same caloric content, vitamins, and minerals as whole wheat; somewhat less proteins, but better quality proteins; and more fats and carbohydrates. Compared with corn, it has the advantage of carrying liberal amounts of the antipellagra vitamin, niacin. White rice—brown rice that has been milled and polished to remove the bran and germ—loses a portion of its best protein and most of its fat, vitamins, and minerals, especially if it is cooked in an excess of water which is discarded. Thus, where white rice is the main food, growth retardation, kwashiorkor, marasmus, vitamin A deficiency, and beriberi (thiamin deficiency) are commonplace.

Nutritional Losses.   In most of the rice-eating areas of the world, there is chronic undernourishment, malnutrition, low vitality, impairment of general health and physical development, and a high incidence of diseases resulting from insufficient and improper diet. Ranking high among these diseases as a killer of mankind is beriberi.

(Also see BERIBERI.)

High beriberi death rates and high consumption of rice, occurring in the same areas, are not the result of coincidence. The kind of rice most of the people prefer is white—the kind that deprives them of the natural food substances that would prevent or cure beriberi.

The rice grown by these people has many of the vitamins and minerals they need, but by the time it is milled and polished, then washed and cooked, it has lost most of them. The taste of cooked white rice appeals to their palates; the bulk appeases their hunger; the protein, carbohydrate and calorie content give them the strength to live and work; but the grain, robbed of many of its health-giving elements and reinforced with little other food, brings disease and death.

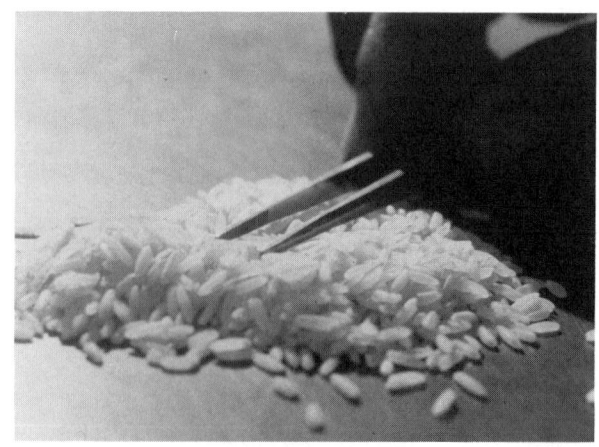

Fig. R-28.   Rice—the chief food of the Asian nations.

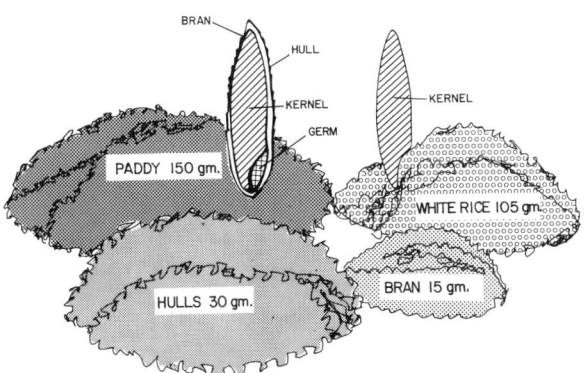

Fig. R-29. Rice nutrients lost in milling. Paddy rice has high nutritional value, mainly in the layer of bran and the germ which lie under the hull. With only the hull removed, it becomes brown rice; when milled and polished, it is white rice. Paddy rice yields 70% of its weight as white rice, 20% as bulky hulls that are inedible for man or beast, and 10% as bran, germ, and polish. Although the latter contain the better protein and most of the fat, vitamins, and useful minerals, they are lost to the white-rice eater.

As early as 1897, Eijkman, working in Java, showed that beriberi was due to the continued consumption of polished rice. Thus, it might seem that the rice-eating nations of the world have been either negligent or indifferent. This is not the case, however, for many of the nations have made intensive studies of the problem. Some have attempted to reform milling practices or to bring about wider consumption of other foods, only to find that these solutions could not be effected because of very real economic or human factors. Important among these is the cost of other and more varied foods. Even more important is the extraordinary resistance of the people to changes in their established dietary habits and food practices.

Occasionally, resistance to change in food habits works to the advantage of the consumer's health, as in some remote areas where rice, grown largely for home use, is milled by hand, often by pounding in wooden mortars. Fortunately, the labor required is a deterrent to complete removal of the bran; some of the bran stays on the rice, and beriberi does not appear.

However, with the industrialization of the Far East, rice is increasingly grown and milled as a specialized, commercial undertaking. So, on the average, Asian rice is now probably whiter than ever before in history. Nevertheless, efforts to increase the use of undermilled rice should continue. It is the natural solution—just to keep the bran on the rice.

Washing and cooking practices in many Asian countries are also obstacles to better rice. In general, the more water used in cooking, and the more water thrown away, the more vitamins and minerals lost—whether from brown, parboiled, white, or enriched rice. However, somewhat more thiamin, riboflavin, niacin, and iron are retained in all improved forms of rice, even with the worst cooking practices. Fortunately, the Filipinos, Cantonese, and Malays customarily cook rice with relatively small amounts of water which is fully absorbed by the swelling of the grains. Elsewhere, it is to be hoped that education may in time improve cooking methods so that the vitamin-laden water will not be thrown away.

• **Parboiled rice**—There are some areas where the rice most in demand and most acceptable is not white. These regions, mainly in India, traditionally prefer parboiled rice—rough rice steeped in water, steamed under pressure, and dried in the sun to loosen the hulls, followed by milling. While this practice probably originated in man's attempts to lessen the labor of hulling, it has had far-reaching health benefits for it drives some of the vitamins and minerals from the bran into the kernel. Thus, when parboiled rice is milled, greater portions of the health-giving elements remain in the grain, and beriberi rates are low among the people in such areas.

But rice parboiled by primitive methods has a slightly different color, taste, and odor; factors which have discouraged its use by those unaccustomed to it. Certainly where it is already established in public favor, as in much of India, it should be assiduously fostered as another natural approach to better rice and better health.

In the United States, and in certain other countries, better parboiling processes have been perfected so that the rice retains even more of its health-giving elements after milling. Although these Western methods require more elaborate machinery and produce processed rice that is somewhat yellow in color, the rice whitens during cooking and has been successfully introduced on a commercial scale.

Enrichment.   Enrichment is another possible solution for the rice-eating peoples who insist on the pure white product. Enrichment of white rice is a process in which selected vitamins and minerals are sprayed on rice grains. The treated rice is then coated with a film of edible substances, which protects the added elements against deterioration and reduces losses of vitamins during washing prior to cooking. The "premix" thus produced is as white as the untreated milled grain. When it is mixed with white rice in the proportion of one part of the premix to 200 parts of ordinarily milled rice, the resulting enriched rice contains approximately the same amounts of thiamin, niacin, and iron as brown rice.

While the addition of riboflavin, another vitamin lost in milling, is perfectly feasible, it is presently being omitted because it colors the premix grains. Confirmed white-rice eaters would undoubtedly be suspicious of these yellow grains, and sort them out and throw them away. However, in those rice-eating countries where it is desirable, riboflavin or other nutrients can be included. With proper public education, the occasional yellow grain might become the hallmark of enrichment.

Table R-9 shows the enrichment levels for rice in the United States.

TABLE R-9
ENRICHMENT LEVELS FOR MILLED RICE

Nutrient	Level			
	(mg/lb)		(mg/100 g)	
Thiamin	2.0-	4.0	.44-	.88
Riboflavin[1]	1.2-	2.4	.26-	.53
Niacin	16 -	32	3.53-	7.05
Iron	13 -	26	2.87-	5.73
Calcium[2]	500	-1,000	110	-220

[1]The addition of riboflavin is feasible but the practice was stopped many years ago since its addition colors the rice yellow; hence, rice may or may not be enriched with riboflavin.
[2]The addition of calcium is optional.

Protein Quality. Table R-10 presents a comparison between the essential amino acid content of brown rice, white rice, and milk—a high-quality protein. Like the other cereal grains, rice—brown and white—is deficient in the amino acid lysine; hence, lysine is the limiting amino acid. Infants and small children in particular need their essential amino acid requirements fulfilled. Therefore, due to the amino acid deficiency, and other vitamin and mineral deficiencies, brown or white rice alone is not a diet on which children will thrive, or even survive.

(Also see PROTEIN[S], section headed "Sources.")

TABLE R–10
PROFILE OF THE ESSENTIAL AMINO ACIDS OF BROWN RICE AND WHITE RICE COMPARED TO MILK—A HIGH-QUALITY PROTEIN[1]

Amino Acid	Brown Rice	White Rice	Cow's Milk
	(mg/g protein)		
Histidine	26	25	27
Isoleucine	40	46	47
Leucine	86	89	95
Lysine	40	39	78
Methionine and cystine	36	40	33
Phenylalanine and tyrosine	91	87	102
Threonine	41	36	44
Tryptophan	13	13	14
Valine	57	63	64

[1]*Recommended Dietary Allowances*, 10th ed., 1989, NRC-National Academy of Sciences, p. 67, Table 6–5. The essential amino acid requirement of infants can be met by supplying 0.79 g of high-quality protein per pound of body weight (1.7 g/kg of body weight per day).

The nutritive value of 1 cup (*240 ml*) of each of the different forms of rice is given in Food Composition Table F-36. Of the whole rice forms, brown rice ranks highest and unenriched white rice lowest. Of course, enriched rice can be fortified to any desired level. As shown, rice polish is a rich source of thiamin, which explains why it will prevent and cure beriberi.

BETTER RICE FOR MILLIONS.
While the dramatic results of the Bataan experiment—a full-scale enrichment program which reduced beriberi among a rice-eating population—gave world health authorities another means for bringing better rice and better health to millions of people, the difficulties of actually adopting this measure should not be underestimated. Most of these are the obstacles which have stood in the way of adopting undermilling and parboiling, the earlier known measures. Principal among them have been the lack of popular understanding of the need for better rice (as portrayed in Fig. R-30), inadequately financed governments, authorities too busy with other problems to enforce the necessary inspection systems, and an inadequate supply of technically trained and administratively effective personnel to perform required services for the protection of the masses.

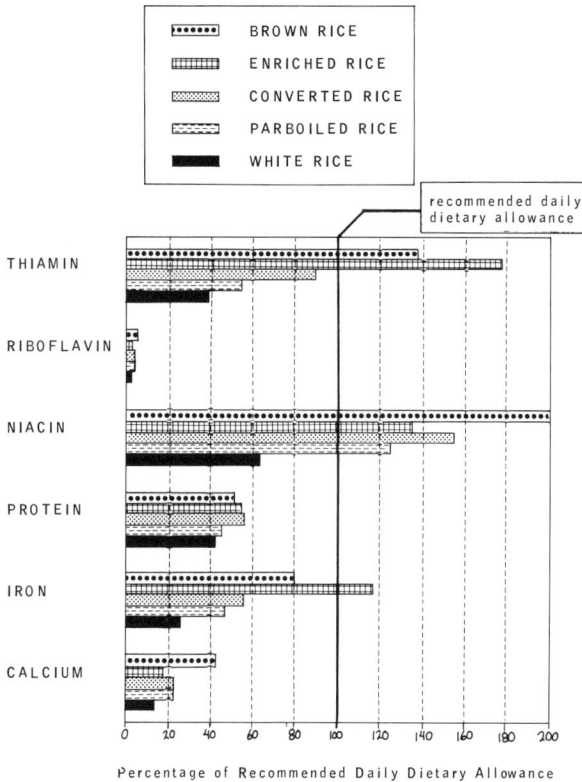

Fig. R-30. Nutritional value of rices. One pound per day of any of the rices shown here will yield these proportions of recommended daily dietary allowances. Of the "natural" forms, brown rice ranks highest, milled white rice lowest, with undermilled rice (not shown) ranging between in direct proportion to the degree of undermilling. The enriched rice is of the strength used in the Philippines, but the formula is adjustable to any level. "Converted" rice is a patented method of parboiling in the United States; it is highly milled, polished rice of greatly improved nutritive value.

Enrichment avoids one additional barrier that has hindered adoption of undermilling and parboiling—the distaste of many people for any but white forms of rice This is an enormous gain, but the money shortage may be a serious deterrent to importing vitamins for fortification.

Perhaps the greatest significance of the Bataan project was to point up the possibility of doing something about beriberi immediately. The ready and rapid introduction of enrichment in the Philippines produced far more striking evidence than could be cited for any measure which by its nature requires slow introduction, bit by bit, over a period of years. This success furnishes a basis for reconsidering the merits of all the possible measures.

Where the difficulties of undermilling or parboiling appear insurmountable, rice enrichment may be the answer, as was demonstrated in the Philippines.

(Also see ENRICHMENT [Fortification, Nutrification, Restoration], section headed "The Bataan Experiment.")

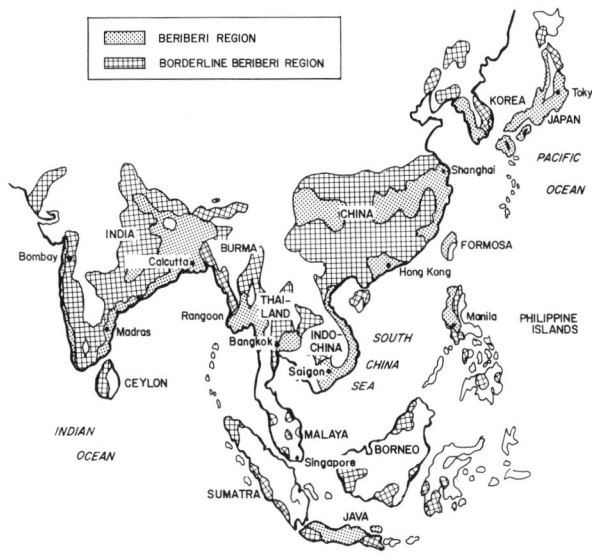

Fig. R-31. Probable beriberi regions of the world. The field for action in the fight against beriberi is most of the rice-growing and rice-eating area of the Orient. Although health statistics are largely lacking, there are probably high death rates from beriberi in all the regions where ordinary white rice is the chief food.

• **For a healthier world**—Since it is fully established that there are several remedies which mean better health for white-rice eaters, and more especially now that positive, measurable reductions in beriberi mortality and incidence have been shown through better rice, there is a basis for action to bring better rice to other parts of the world.

Although recognizing that rectifying the deficiencies of white-rice eaters will be a difficult task, in 1950 the Williams-Waterman Fund concluded that it would be worthwhile in terms of human lives saved and human suffering alleviated. To the latter end, it recommended the following action program:

1 **That adequate beriberi surveys be made in each rice-eating nation**, in order to establish the presence of beriberi.

2. **That public information programs for rice betterment be strengthened where beriberi is known to exist**, for no solution will be fully effective unless cooperation is obtained from all interested governmental and private agencies and from the people themselves. Legislated programs will be effective only if preceded by such cooperation.

3. **That the results of the Bataan experiment be studied.** Public health officials of the rice-eating nations, government officials, and members of international nutritional bodies are strongly urged to study the full report carefully.

4. **That representatives of other rice-eating nations visit the Philippines**, to inspect the methods, clinical, mechanical, chemical and commercial, which are being used.

5. **That the solution for each country be fitted to that country's needs.** Attempts should not be made to force on one nation a program not adjusted to it. Where parboiling is practiced, it should be extended as fully as possible. Where undermilling is presently acceptable, it

should be expanded. Where converting promises to be the solution, it should be inaugurated. Where artificial enrichment is economically feasible, it should be introduced.

6. **That improvement of rice-cooking practices is of utmost importance.** Where the prevailing custom is to cook rice in an excess of water which subsequently is drained off, it is essential to correct it by popular reeducation. Water so discarded carries off much of the vitamins and minerals from any form of rice. If the water is used for soups or for feeding babies, these nutrients will be saved; if used to starch clothes, it will hardly benefit the individual's health.

Rice can be cooked in small amounts of water to perfect tenderness and still remain loose and whole grained, not a sticky mess. The best practice is to use about 1 cup (*240 ml*) of water to 1 cup of wet, washed rice, then to cook the mixture in a thick-walled metal or clay pot over a slow fire until all the water is absorbed. The Filipinos, who are rice connoisseurs, have always cooked it in this manner.

7. **That a minimum content of thiamin, in all rice offered for sale be required by law.** Adopting such a standard for all forms of improved rice would protect everyone from beriberi, yet permit each element of the population to follow its own preferences within the limits set by the individual pocketbook. Provision of such a latitude of choice will greatly soften the opposition to the enforcement of restrictive measures for the common good. In the long run, the method or methods most acceptable will win out.

• **FAO report**—An international team of experts from FAO and WHO made a study of the Philippine experiment. The following General Comments and Conclusions are taken from their report:[4]

Great credit is due to those responsible for introducing enriched rice into the Philippines and for conducting extensive trials of enriched rice under difficult conditions. These efforts represent a pioneer attempt to solve a serious nutritional problem by novel methods. In principle, the enrichment of rice with nutrients needed by a population must lead to improvement in nutrition. Rice enrichment has the important advantages that it can be introduced fairly rapidly, that it benefits the whole community, that it does not affect the flavor of rice and that the amount and kind of nutrients added can be controlled to some extent.

The team fully recognized these advantages but, at the same time, noted serious obstacles to the successful introduction of rice enrichment by the present method into many countries where rice is a staple food. Unless these obstacles can be overcome, enrichment by present methods may be found, in practice, to be of less general value for the nutritional improvement of the diet in these countries than might theoretically be expected. The reasons for this conclusion which take into account various factors existing in the coun-

[4]Aalsmeer, W. C., *et al.*, *Rice Enrichment in the Philippines*, FAO Nutritional Studies No. 12, Food and Agriculture Organization of the United Nations, Rome, Italy, March 1954.

tries concerned are as follows: (1) the present dependence of rice-eating countries on external sources for synthetic vitamins and other necessary chemicals and the considerable expense involved in paying for these; (2) the difficulty of ensuring that premix is added to rice in correct proportion in the mills; (3) the need for an elaborate system of control, the cost of which must be added to the cost of manufacture; (4) the need for appropriate standards and suitably equipped laboratories to secure legal conviction in the case of non-compliance with the regulations; (5) the slightly greater cost of enriched rice compared with that of ordinary rice, which affects its sale to the lower income groups; (6) the complications arising from the inclusion or otherwise of home-pounded rice in rice enrichment programs; (7) the losses of added vitamins which may occur when enriched rice is cooked in excess water, subsequently discarded, according to current practice in some rice-eating countries; (8) the need for inter-governmental agreements and standards when enrichment programs are undertaken in countries not self-sufficient in rice and depending to a varying extent on imports; (9) the present lack of knowledge of loss of added nutrients during storage under tropical conditions of temperature and humidity.

Obstacles to the successful introduction of rice enrichment must, however, be considered in relation to those encountered in popularizing other measures, such as the use of under-milled or parboiled rice.

It is pointed out that further research and investigation may result in modifications and improvements of present methods of rice enrichment, through which many of these disadvantages may be overcome.

• **Conclusions**—The authors' conclusions are: The rewards are high, for human life is at stake. Despite the very considerable obstacles, pointed out in both the body of this report and in the FAO report, rice can be enriched for the multitudes and beriberi can be alleviated. As evidence of the latter assertion, the following two examples are cited:

1. **Iodine fortification.** The iodization of salt is a classical example of food fortification which has produced obvious benefits in those areas of the world where soil, water, and vegetation are so lacking in iodine that endemic goiter is a major health problem.

2. **Enrichment of bread.** Today, almost all bread in the United States and Canada is enriched and labeled as such. Enrichment of white bread with three B vitamins was inaugurated in the United States in 1941 as a medical measure to improve the health of the population by using a common food as a carrier for the essential nutrients. Standards for enrichment were carefully determined to meet known deficiencies in the average American diet. It has been estimated by the U.S. Department of Agriculture that the enrichment program has added $1/3$ more thiamin, $1/5$ more iron and niacin, and $1/10$ more riboflavin to the general diet than would be available if bread and other cereal foods were not enriched. To satisfy labeling regulations in the United States, enriched bread must be made from flour to which the following minimum mg/lb have been added: thiamin, 2.9; riboflavin, 1.8; nicotinamide, 24.0; and iron, from 13.0 to 16.5. Vitamin D and calcium are sometimes added, also. These are usually added by the baker. There is general agreement that enrichment of bread in the United States has been a major factor in the control of deficiency diseases and the improvement of health.

Most thinking people in the Western nations agree that something should be done to prevent beriberi's waste of human life. But the remoteness of the Orient in terms of distance and customs tends to make the problem seem less important or immediate than it is to the people of the rice-eating nations. However, the world has grown far smaller than it used to be, and no nation can afford to be unconcerned about saving needless suffering and deaths from the preventable disease beriberi, for each of us is our brother's keeper.

RICE PRODUCTS AND USES.

The whole grain of rice, with the hulls on, is known as rough rice or paddy rice. Milled rice (raw or parboiled), consisting of the kernels, is the major rice product. But rice milling produces a number of other products (see Table R-11).

Milled rice is used mainly for human food; it may be sold as raw, quick-cooking, or canned rice. Rice is also used extensively as breakfast food—as puffed rice, rice flakes, or rice crispies. Broken rice is used as food or in the manufacture of alcoholic beverages. Rice flour is used in various mixes. Hulls are used as fuel, insulation, and certain manufactured products. The bran is used mainly as livestock feed. The products and uses of rice are summarized in Table R-11.

TABLE R-11
RICE PRODUCTS AND USES

Product	Description	Uses	Comments
		HUMAN FOODS	
Brown rice	Rice with the hulls removed, but with the bran left on.	To provide more protein and more of the anti-pellagra vitamin, thiamin, than can be obtained from white rice. The use of brown rice is the natural way to prevent beriberi.	Because of its color and relatively long cooking period (45-60 min), this highly nutritious rice is a specialty food in the U.S. It is available in many health food stores and in some supermarkets.
Milled rice	The kernels, after the milling is completed and the hulls, bran layers, and germ are removed.	Cooking, mostly by boiling.	The U.S. per capita consumption of milled rice averages about 7.5 lb (3.4 kg). Milled rice with the hulls removed, either polished or parboiled, is the major rice product.
Polished rice	Kernels from which the outer bran coats and germ have been removed, followed by polishing. Polished rice consists of the white, starchy endosperm, with fragments of the aleurone layer.	Cooking, mostly by boiling.	For the Puerto Rican market, polished rice is coated with talc and glucose, an inert, harmless coating to give it a high gloss or sheen.
		Quick-cooking rice (instant rice), a convenience food, some types of which can be cooked in 5 min.	There are many approaches to making raw milled rice into a quick-cooking product. Essentially, the process consists of selecting premium grade rice, and, under carefully controlled conditions, soaking, cooking, cooling, and drying it. More recently, some processors have imparted quick-cooking properties to rice by soaking and cooking, followed by freezing, thawing, and dehydrating or drying. In still other processes, the puffing-gun and pressure vacuum methods are employed to produce quick-cooking products.
		Canned rice.	The canning process consists of (1) soaking the rice to a moisture of 30 to 35%; (2) cooking in excess water for 4 to 5 min; (3) draining and packing the rice in cans; and (4) vacuum sealing and retorting. "Clumping" of the kernels and difficulty in emptying the contents of the can have been overcome by using surface-active agents to produce a free-flowing product, or freeze-processing, with the processed rice frozen in the can, then thawed prior to labeling.
Parboiled rice	Rough or paddy rice (in the hull) soaked in warm water, steamed under pressure, and dried before milling. Since parboiled rice is milled in the usual manner, it is similar to polished rice, except (1) it is precooked, and (2) the kernels are a rich cream color, but they cook to the snowy whiteness of polished rice.	Parboiled rice is used in cooking much the same as polished rice. Parboiling retains higher portions of the vitamins and lessens beriberi among people eating it.	Parboiled rice differs from raw milled rice in that the treatment (1) gelatinizes the starch; (2) makes for better consistency, greater hardness, and better vitreousness of the kernel; (3) diffuses the soluble vitamins from the exterior to the interior of the grain; (4) makes for greater resistance to mechanical breakage during milling; and (5) lengthens the period of storage. In the U.S., there are several patented methods of parboiling.
Enriched rice	Polished or parboiled rice enriched by spraying with a watery solution of vitamins (usually thiamin and niacin, and sometimes riboflavin) and sometimes iron and other minerals.	In rice-eating areas to prevent beriberi and other nutritional diseases.	The federal standard for enriched rice is; <table><tr><td>*Ingredient*</td><td>*Required/lb of Rice*</td></tr><tr><td>Thiamin</td><td>2.0- 4.0 mg</td></tr><tr><td>Riboflavin</td><td>1.2- 2.4 mg</td></tr><tr><td>Niacin</td><td>16.0-32.0 mg</td></tr><tr><td>Iron</td><td>13.0-26.0 mg</td></tr><tr><td>Calcium</td><td>500-1000 mg (optional)</td></tr></table>

(Continued)

TABLE R–11 (Continued)

Product	Description	Uses	Comments
		HUMAN FOODS (Continued)	
Ang-khak	A product prepared in China by culturing a red pigment-producing fungus (*Monascus purpureus*) on whole rice kernels until they are thoroughly permeated with mycelia which produce the color. They are then dried and powdered. The powder imparts a red color to whatever food to which it is added.	Used as a food coloring agent in China, Taiwan, and the Philippines, for coloring cheese, fish, red wine, and other foods.	The Chinese are very secretive about the method of preparation of ang-khak. Apparently the amount of water used in producing ang-khak is quite critical; the secret of success is to have the rice grains just moist enough to permit the fungus to grow.
Bran	Rice bran is the layer beneath the hull, containing outer bran layers and parts of the germ.	As a water-soluble fiber, similar to oat bran. Cholesterol responds to water-soluble fibers, which combine with bile acids and decrease the body's absorption of fat. Rice bran is also used as a livestock feed.	In addition to being high in water-soluble fiber, rice bran is rich in protein and B-vitamins. Rice oil is extracted from rice bran.
Breakfast foods: Puffed rice Rice crispies Rice flakes	Made from quality milled rice, usually of the short-grain type, which is generally precooked, dried, flaked, foamed and/or puffed or expanded, then toasted.	Ready-to-eat breakfast cereals.	Preparations of different products vary in cooking time, steam pressure, temperature, and the addition of malt and nutrients.
Brewers' rice (Chipped rice, broken rice)	Small, broken rice segments, separated out in the grading process.	Much of it is mixed back with whole grain rice and sold as low-grade rice. As the raw material for rice flour.	Brewers' rice has the same chemical composition as polished rice.
Flour, of which there are two types:			
1. Flour made from regular rice, raw or parboiled.	Fine, powdery, white particles.	Primarily as a thickening agent in gravies and sauces.	Because rice protein does not contain gluten, its use for confectionery and baking purposes is limited.
2. Waxy rice flour. (Also see FLOURS, Table F-25 Major Flours.)	Waxy rice flour is made from waxy or glutinous rice. It has little starch or amylose; it is essentially amylopectin.	As a thickening agent for white sauces, gravies and puddings—preventing liquid separation (syneresis) when these products are frozen, stored, and subsequently thawed.	Both types of rice flour are available commercially in the U.S.A.
Rice baby foods	Flaked rice.	Baby foods.	Most rice baby foods are prepared by cooking ground, broken rice kernels and rice polishings; adding nutrients; and drum drying the rice slurry.
Rice oil	A high-grade oil extracted from rice bran, followed by refining and bleaching.	Rice oil is used in margarine, salad oil, and cooking oil.	Rice bran contains 14 to 18% oil. When refined, bleached, and deodorized, rice oil has greater stability than other vegetable oils.

(Continued)

TABLE R-11 *(Continued)*

Product	Description	Uses	Comments
		HUMAN FOODS *(Continued)*	
Rice polishings	Inner white bran, protein-rich aleurone layers, and starchy endosperm; obtained in the milling operation by brushing the grain to polish the kernel.	In many baby foods. To prevent and cure beriberi.	Rice polishings are easily digested, low in fiber, rich in thiamin, and high in niacin.
Wild rice	The kernels are slender, round, purplish black, and starchy. It's high in protein and low in fat.	Highly esteemed for its unique taste.	Normally, wild rice sells at 2 to 3 times the price of regular white rice.
		FORTIFIED FOOD, BASED ON RICE PRODUCTS, FOR DEVELOPING COUNTRIES	
Protex	Defatted mixture of rice bran, germ, and polish. Contains between 17% and 21% protein, plus minerals and vitamins present in the outer layers of the rice grain.	Acceptable at levels of 5%, 10%, and 15% in yeast-leavened breads and quick breads. Base for breakfast cereals, pasta, and milklike beverages.	The process for producing Protex commercially was developed by Riviana Foods, Inc. at their Abbeville, La. plant.
		BEVERAGES (Also see BEERS AND BREWING; DISTILLED LIQUORS)	
Brewers' rice (chipped rice, broken rice)	Small, broken rice segments, separated out in the grading process.	Used by the brewing industry, where it is mixed with barley. Used for the production of arrak in the Orient, a liquor of high alcoholic content distilled from a fermented mash of rice and molasses.	
Polished rice	Cooked, whole grains of white rice.	Japanese rice beer (sake), which has an alcohol content of 14 to 16%. (It is sometimes called "rice wine.")	Sake is prepared by (1) conversion of the starch in cooked rice to sugar by the fungus *Aspergillus oryzae*; (2) a multistage conversion of the rice sugar to alcohol; (3) filtration, settling, heating, and aging; and (4) bottling for distribution. It is usually warmed before serving.
		ANIMAL FEEDS	
Rough rice or paddy rice	The whole grain, including the hulls.	Occasionally, rough rice or paddy rice is ground and fed to animals as a substitute for other grains. Ground rough rice may replace up to 50% of the corn in the ration of cattle and pigs, but the feed conversion is somewhat depressed. For laying hens, rough rice should not exceed 20 to 30% of the diet.	Generally, the highest and best use for rough rice or paddy rice is for milling for human food. Because of the hardness of the kernels, and the abrasiveness of the hulls, it should always be ground, except possibly for poultry. Rice is used almost entirely for human food. It is fed to livestock only when off grade or low in price.
Brown rice	Rice with the hulls removed.	As ground brown rice for livestock feed, for all classes of animals.	Brown rice contains less fiber and silica than rough rice, and more protein and vitamins than polished rice.

(Continued)

TABLE R-11 (Continued)

Product	Description	Uses	Comments
		ANIMAL FEEDS (Continued)	
Brewers' rice (chipped rice, broken rice)	Small, broken rice segments, separated out in the grading process.	As a palatable, high-energy feed for all classes of animals, including pets. It is of special value for growing chickens.	Brewers' rice is used chiefly in the brewing industry.
Rice bran	The layer directly beneath the hull, consisting of the bran layer (or pericarp) and parts of the germ. It must not contain more than 13% crude fiber.	Rice bran may constitute up to 40% of cattle and sheep rations, and up to 25% of poultry rations. Rice bran should not exceed 30 to 40% of the growing ration of pigs, and even less in the final weeks of finishing; otherwise, soft pork will be produced.	Rice bran is the most important by-product of rice; it is a good source of B vitamins (especially thiamin and niacin) and fairly palatable to animals. Rice bran may turn rancid in storage due to the high oil content. When the calcium carbonate exceeds 3% (Ca 1.2%), the percentage must be declared in the bran name; i.e., rice bran with calcium carbonate not exceeding _____%.
Rice bran, solvent extracted	Rice bran after removing part of the oil by the use of solvents. It must contain not less than 14% crude protein and not more than 14% crude fiber.	**For all classes of livestock.** **Rice bran is also used as a human food.**	De-oiled rice bran can be fed at higher levels than ordinary rice bran.
Rice hulls	The outer covering of rice.	For cattle; (1) as a low-quality roughage in high-concentrate rations for finishing cattle, or (2) as a replacement for straw in areas with a shortage of roughage. As ammoniated rice hulls for ruminants; prepared by adding monocalcium phosphate, removing silica, ammoniating under pressure, and toasting. For animal litter (bedding).	Rice hulls have a very low value as a feed; they furnish only about ¼ as much energy as oat straw and practically no digestible protein. When the nonprotein nitrogen of ammoniated rice hulls is incorporated in ruminant rations at low levels, nitrogen is used rather efficiently.
Rice mill by-product	The total mixture obtained in the milling of rice; it consists of the rice hulls, rice bran, rice polishings, and broken rice grains. Its crude fiber must not exceed 32%.	Rice mill by-product is fed chiefly to ruminants, because of its high fiber content.	The description given in the second column conforms to the specifications for rice mill by-product as given by the American Feed Control Officials.
Rice polishings	Finely powdered material obtained in the milling operation of brushing the grain to polish the kernel.	In swine and poultry rations.	Rice polishings are rich in thiamin and high in niacin.
Rice straw	The stalk that remains after threshing the grain.	Ruminant feed, as a replacement for other cereal straw in areas with a shortage of roughage.	Rice straw is a low-quality roughage.

(Continued)

TABLE R-11 (*Continued*)

Product	Description	Uses	Comments
		OTHER USES	
Rice hulls	The outer covering of rice.	Industrial purposes; as an abrasive in polishing castings, as conditioners for commercial fertilizers, in the manufacture of hand soaps and furfural, and as fuel and insulation.	
Rice oil	Oil extracted from rice bran.	Cosmetics and paints.	
Rice straw	The rice stalk without the grain.	Thatching roofs; for making paper, mats, hats, and baskets; for weaving into rope; and as cordage for bags.	

RICE PAPER

A thin delicate material resembling paper made by cutting the pith of the rice-paper tree into one roll or sheet and flattening under pressure. It is edible; so, macaroons and similar biscuits are baked on it and the paper can be eaten with the biscuit.

RICE, WHITE (POLISHED RICE)

Brown rice from which the outer bran layers up to the endosperm and germ have been removed.
(Also see RICE.)

RICKETS

Contents   Page

The most common disorder of bone formation in growing children is rickets. It is characterized by softening and deformation of the bones. The adult counterpart of rickets is called *osteomalacia*. Both of these conditions result from subnormal mineralization of the protein structure of bone, which is also called the bone matrix.

A third bone disorder, *osteoporosis*, differs from rickets and osteomalacia in that it is characterized by a normal amount of mineralization of the bone matrix, but there is a reduction in the total bone mass and a tendency for fractures rather than deformation of bone.
(Also see OSTEOPOROSIS.)

HISTORY OF RICKETS. In the 1st century A.D., Soramus of Ephesus gave a full description of rickets in Roman children as part of his treatise on the diseases of women. He thought the disease was caused by children sitting indoors on damp floors. The first time that the disorder was mentioned in Britain was in 1645 in the D.M. (Doctor of Medicine) thesis of Whistler at Oxford. By the time the industrial revolution was underway (in the 19th century), rickets were widespread as the urban residents lived under clouds of black smoke from the burning of soft coal, with the result that the ultraviolet rays of the sun were largely screened out and were insufficient to produce vitamin D. Whistler's thesis was not as well known as the 1650 account of the disease by Glissin, a London physician. The latter account gave the clinical signs of rickets when it occurred by itself and when it was complicated by the coexistence of scurvy.

An understanding of the pathology of rickets, however, required the development of better chemical methods for the analysis of bone. An accurate analysis of the proportion of calcium and phosphorus in bone was reported by Berzelius in 1801. Knowledge of bone was enhanced by two major German publications in 1858. Muller gave a lengthy description of bone growth and the healing process for rickets, while Pommer described in detail features of rickets, osteomalacia, and osteoporosis. Cod-liver oil was used throughout the 19th century in England for the treatment of tuberculosis and rickets, but many physicians were uncertain of its value. Some of these doubts were dispelled in 1889 by the report of the British physician Bland-Sutton, who cured the deformed bones of animals at the London zoo by feeding dietary supplements of crushed bones and cod-liver oil.

Around the end of the 19th century, in Britain there emerged two distinct schools of thought as to the cause of rickets. One school, with its investigators centered around Glasgow, believed strongly in the prevention of rickets by sunlight and fresh air, while the other school, centered at London, postulated the existence of an anti-rickets factor present in foods such as cod-liver oil. Both schools soon had at their disposal abundant observations to support their theories. Kassowitz of Germany commented in 1884 that the seasonal variation in rickets might be due to keeping infants indoors during the winter months, since rickets usually appeared in late winter and early spring. In 1906, Hansemann observed at autopsy that all German children who were born in the fall and died in the spring had rickets, while those that were born in the spring and died in the fall did not have the disease. Findlay, at the University of Glascow, in 1908, experimentally produced rickets in puppies by confining them in cages; and, in 1918, he showed that animals allowed out of doors in the country did not develop rickets as did his caged animals. Both groups of animals were fed essentially the same diet. In 1919, the Germany pediatrician, Huldinsky, showed that children with advanced rickets could be cured by exposure to ultraviolet light from a mercury-vapor quartz lamp.

Comprehensive controlled studies on the dietary cause of rickets were conducted in London by Mellanby who reported his results in 1919 and the years following. His experimental animals were puppies, which was a fortunate choice, since the bone physiology of the young dog is similar to that of the growing child. (Rats remain free of rickets for as long as they receive adequate amounts and proportions of calcium and phosphorus, even though the diet may have a significant deficiency of vitamin D. However, rats are useful for the bioassay of vitamin D potency, which is measured by the degree of healing of rickets produced in these animals by diets high in calcium and low in phosphorous.) Mellanby found that cod-liver oil was the most effective of the dietary fat sources in the prevention and cure of rickets of puppies. He thought that rickets were prevented by the presence in cod-liver oil of fat-soluble vitamin A. But, in 1922, McCollum and his coworkers, at Johns Hopkins, demonstrated that when vitamin A was destroyed in cod-liver oil by heating there remained a second fat-soluble factor which was shown to be an antirickets factor. This factor was named vitamin D, since it was the fourth vitamin to be discovered.

In 1924, Steenbock and Black, of the Wisconsin Experiment Station, discovered that irradiation of liver and a rickets-producing diet with ultraviolet light transformed these materials into cures for rickets. In 1936, the German chemist, Windaus, demonstrated that provitamin D (7-dehydrocholesterol) is found in the skin, and that it is converted into vitamin D (calciferol) by the action of sunlight. This discovery brought together the two British schools of thought through explaining the relationship between the effects of sunlight and cod-liver oil. However, the demonstration of Windaus led to an argument as to whether vitamin D might better be considered a hormone, rather than a vitamin, since its effect on bone is like that of a hormone. There are present in the body some related hormones, such as parathormone and calcitonin, which act on bones; and these hormones, together with vitamin D, regulate the net flow of calcium in and out of bones. It might also be argued that vitamin D is not actually a vitamin since it can be made in the body when the skin is exposed to ultraviolet light. In the absence of sufficient sunlight, however, it is necessary to provide an adequate source of vitamin D in the diet.

CAUSES OF RICKETS AND OSTEOMALACIA.
These disorders may result from dietary deficiencies and/or poor utilization of calcium, phosphorus, and/or vitamin D; or from an incorrect ratio of the two minerals. However, different circumstances may be responsible for the development of each disorder. Also, rickets is a disease of children, while osteomalacia occurs in adults. Therefore, separate discussions of these disorders follow.

Rickets.   This disease is most commonly caused by lack of vitamin D since it is usually found in children whose skin has had only a limited exposure to sunlight. The ultraviolet rays in sunlight convert provitamin D on the surface of the skin to vitamin D. Even children living in tropical areas may not have sufficient exposure to sunlight if clothing covers most of their skin, or they are kept indoors by their parents. In some areas, it is desirable to have a light-colored skin, so parents try to protect their children from the skin-darkening effects of sunlight.

Only in recent times have different peoples of the world relied on foods, such as cod-liver oil and the livers of edible animals, as sources of vitamin D. However, it is said that the taking of cod-liver oil by Norwegian fishermen and sailors goes back to the Vikings in the 8th and 9th centuries. Unfortunately, these food sources of the vitamin are not well liked, so their usefulness in preventing rickets is limited. Also, there may be poor absorption of dietary vitamin D in disorders such as pancreatitis, celiac disease, sprue, etc.

Recently, it has been found that even when sufficient vitamin D may be obtained from the diet and/or its synthesis in the body, some persons may be unable to convert efficiently the vitamin to its physiologically active forms.[5] Vitamin D is converted to its 25-hydroxy derivative in the liver; then, the derivative is carried through the blood to the kidneys, where it is converted to 1, 25-dihydroxy-vitamin D. Sometimes rickets occurs in conditions such as uremia where the kidney fails to synthesize the 1, 25-dihydroxy form of the vitamin.

Exposure to sunlight or oral administration of the vitamin may fail to be effective in preventing or curing the disease when there are great reductions in the amount of calcium absorption from the gastrointestinal tract (either as a result of severe dietary deficiencies of the mineral, or due to malabsorption). For example, diets consisting mainly of whole grain cereals which contain phytates (phosphorus compounds found in the brand) may result in reduced absorption of dietary calcium, due to the binding of calcium by the phytates.

The physiology of rickets and osteomalacia is outlined in Fig. R-32.

---

[5]"Recent Developments in Vitamin D," *Dairy Council Digest*, Vol. 47, No. 3, May-June 1976, p. 13.

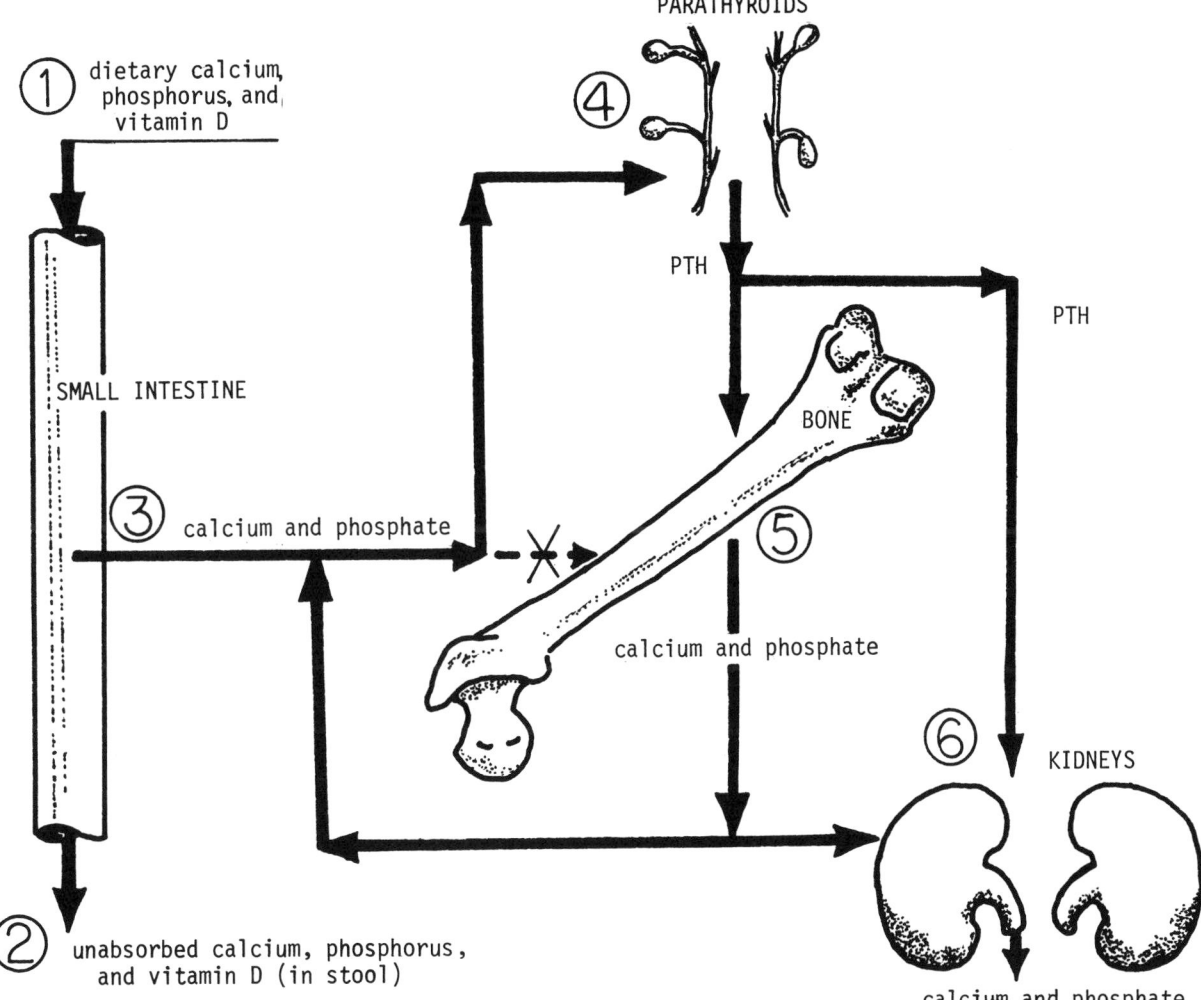

PARATHYROIDS

① dietary calcium, phosphorus, and vitamin D

④

PTH

SMALL INTESTINE

PTH

BONE

③ calcium and phosphate

⑤

calcium and phosphate

② unabsorbed calcium, phosphorus, and vitamin D (in stool)

⑥

KIDNEYS

calcium and phosphate

Physiological Factors In The Development Of Rickets And Osteomalacia

1. <u>Dietary deficiencies or imbalances</u> of calcium, phosphorus, and/or vitamin D (lack of sunlight may limit synthesis in the body)
2. <u>Unabsorbed calcium, phosphorus, and vitamin D</u> are lost in stool.
3. <u>Low blood level of calcium</u> (due to diet or malabsorption) prevents calcification of bone.
4. <u>Stimulation of parathyroid secretion</u> of parathyroid hormone (PTH) by low blood level of calcium
5. <u>Demineralization and softening of bone</u> (PTH causes release from bone of calcium and phosphate)
6. <u>PTH acts on kidneys</u> to produce urinary phosphate loss and conservation of calcium by reabsorption.

Fig. R-32.   Development of rickets and osteomalacia.

In rare cases, there may be rickets of urinary origin, where there are excessive urinary losses of either calcium or phosphorus.

Vitamin D-resistant rickets is, in most cases, a genetic disorder where excessive phosphate is lost in the urine which reduces the supply available for mineralization of bone.

Osteomalacia. This disease is more likely to be found in women than men because (1) women usually wear more clothing than men, with the result that they have less synthesis of vitamin D in their skin; (2) pregnancy and lactation greatly increase the requirements of women for calcium (it is mobilized from their bones when it is not provided in adequate amounts in the diet); and (3) the average bone mass of an adult woman is about one-third less than that of an adult man, so women have a lower margin of safety against deformation of bone due to physical stresses.

Like rickets, osteomalacia may also be caused by interference with calcium absorption by phytates in cereals, disorders of absorption, excessive excretion of calcium and/or phosphate in the urine, and subnormal synthesis of the physiologically active form of vitamin D.

An Iatrogenic Cause of Rickets and Osteomalacia. Epileptics, who have been treated with anticonvulsant drugs, have higher incidences of rickets and osteomalacia. It appears that there may have been in these cases a deficiency of vitamin D since exposure to ultraviolet light or oral administration of vitamin D corrected the problem in some of the patients.

SIGNS AND SYMPTOMS OF RICKETS AND OSTEOMALACIA.

Although these two disorders have essentially the same causes, the features of the two diseases differ somewhat because rickets occurs while the bones are still growing, while osteomalacia develops after growth of the long bones has ceased. Therefore, the signs and symptoms of these conditions will be considered separately.

Rickets. The characteristic signs of rickets are protruding abdomen, beaded ribs or "rachitic rosary," bowed legs, knock knees, cranial bossing (thickening of parts of the skull), pigeon chest (the breastbone or sternum is pushed backwards as it descends, forming a depression between the ribs), and enlargement of the epiphyses.

The epiphyses are the regions at the ends of the long bones which are separated from the shaft of bone or diaphysis by a layer of cartilage called the epiphyseal plate. These regions are mineralized during growth and eventually become part of the shaft of bone. (See Fig. R-33.)

Teeth may erupt in an abnormal manner and the enamel may be defective. Malformed pelvic bones in women cause serious difficulties in childbirth. Permanent crippling results if severe cases are not treated. Other abnormalities associated with rickets are weak and flabby muscles, and muscle spasms (in severe cases). The deformities of rickets (curving and twisting of the bones from their normal shapes) are likely to be found in the bones that bear the most weight or stress, such as the legs.

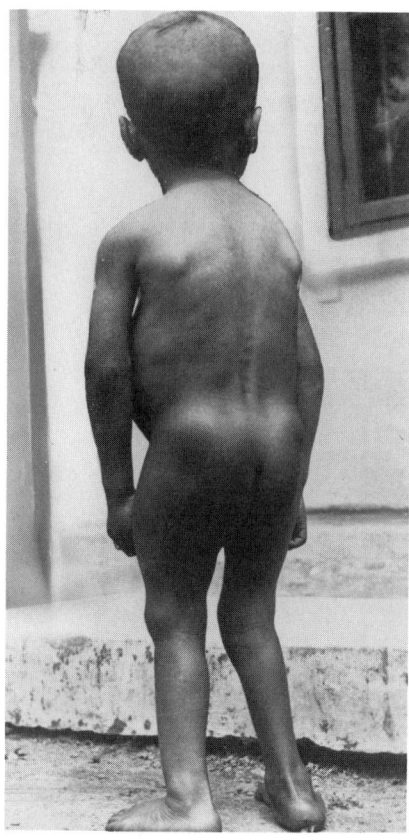

Fig. R-33. An Indian boy suffering from rickets. Note the protruding abdomen, knock knees, enlarged skull, and enlarged wrists. (Courtesy, FAO, Rome, Italy)

Osteomalacia. One of the worst features of this disorder in a woman is the deformation of the pelvic bones so that she has great difficulty in childbirth. Another common feature of this disorder is a curvature of the spine (kyphosis) which gives the person a bent or hump-backed shape. Other features are pains in the bones, muscle weakness, a waddling gait, and muscle spasms (a mild form of tetany due to a subnormal level of serum calcium).

TREATMENT AND PREVENTION OF RICKETS AND OSTEOMALACIA.

Treatment of these disorders is based upon the administration of therapeutic doses of vitamin D (1,000 to 5,000 IU per day) together with the provision of adequate levels of dietary calcium (ranging from 800 mg [milligrams] per day for infants and children, to 2,400 mg per day for adults suffering from severe osteomalacia). Periodic X-rays may be used to determine whether healing is taking place as expected. There may be cases of either rickets or osteomalacia that are resistant to therapeutic doses of vitamin D. It has sometimes been necessary to administer massive doses of the vitamin (50,000 to 100,000 IU per day). However, prolonged administration of such large doses of the vitamin may result in toxic effects.

Prevention of rickets and osteomalacia is usually achieved by the provision of adequate dietary calcium (a daily amount equivalent to that in 1½ pints [*720 ml*] of milk) and making certain that vitamin D is obtained from the diet or from the effect of sunlight on the skin. There is usually sufficient phosphorus present in the diets of people that a deficiency occurs only when there is an abnormally high level of urinary excretion of this element. Therefore, there have been worldwide efforts to promote the fortification of all milk with 400 IU of vitamin D per quart (*950 ml*). Should this prophylactic measure be unfeasible in some instances, calcium and vitamin D might be administered in the form of a mineral and vitamin supplement. It is noteworthy that in some areas of the Middle East, infants are fitted with miniature goggles (to protect their eyes) and placed out in the sun in bassinets.

(Also see DEFICIENCY DISEASES, Table D-1 Major Dietary Deficiency Diseases.)

RICKETTSIAL DISEASES

Serious diseases—including Rocky Mountain spotted fever, Q fever, trench fever, and typhus—caused by the genus *Rickettsiaceae*, most of which are rod-shaped organisms intermediate in size between the larger bacteria and the smaller viruses. The rickettsiae are transmitted from the infected person to others by an intermediate host such as blood-sucking ticks, mites, lice, fleas, and spiders.

RIGOR MORTIS

Within a few hours after death the muscles become stiff and rigid. Since the blood no longer delivers oxygen to the tissues, anaerobic metabolism produces lactic acid which lowers the pH. As the ATP (adenosine triphosphate) is depleted, the muscles harden—contract.

RISSOLES

• These are like little turnovers, filled with a highly seasoned mixture of chopped chicken, ham, or other tender meat moistened with a little sauce, dropped onto pastry, which is sealed, then fried in deep fat.

• A patty of ground meat or fish, rolled in crumbs and dipped in egg, and more crumbs, then fried. The English name for the American croquette.

ROASTED GRAIN DRINKS (CEREAL COFFEE, CEREAL BEVERAGE, COFFEE SUBSTITUTE)

By roasting certain grains and grain products in combination with other flavor sources, a product may be obtained which can be mixed with hot water yielding an aromatic beverage similar to coffee. These cereal beverages are commercially available or they may be homemade. One popular product, developed over 75 years ago by C.W. Post, helped form the foundation for the General Foods Corporation.

Grains and grain products in the commercially prepared products are generally barley, wheat, rye, malt and bran, while additional flavor is contributed by molasses, chicory, carob, cassia bark, allspice, and star anise, depending upon the manufacturer. A homemade roasted grain drink can be prepared by baking a combination of wheat bran, eggs, cornmeal, and molasses. There are even those cereal beverages which can be percolated like coffee. Several such percolated types were recently introduced by Celestial Seasonings.

Roasted grain drinks are caffeine-free. With the recent publicity involving the health effects of coffee and caffeine, these cereal grain beverages have gained in popularity.

ROASTERS (ROASTING PIGS)

Roasters are fat, plump, suckling pigs, weighing 30 to 60 lb (*14 to 27 kg*) on foot. They are dressed shipper style (with the head on), and are not split at the breast or between the hams. When properly roasted and attractively served with the traditional apple in the mouth, roast pig is considered a great delicacy for the holiday season.

ROCAMBOLE *Allium scorodoprasum*

European leek, usually cultivated like the shallot and used in the same way.

ROLLS

These can be defined as yeast-leavened miniature loaves of bread. There are as many kinds of rolls as the cook can devise. Some are the same basic recipe, but formed into different shapes. Others have slight variations in the proportion of fat or sugar to flour; and eggs may or may not be added. And the choices of added ingredients such as raisins, other fruits, spices, nuts, and poppy, sesame, or caraway seeds give added dimensions. A good basic roll recipe is like a good basic suit in the wardrobe—it can be used for all occasions. Any bread recipe can be used for rolls. Some of the more familiar rolls are:

Bagels: Doughnut-shaped rolls which are boiled first, cooled, then baked in an oven.

Bread sticks: The dough is shaped into pencil-thin sticks and baked until dry and crisp. Bread sticks are very popular in Italy.

Brioche: This is a French word meaning *bun* or *cake*. These rolls have added eggs and more sugar and therefore, are richer than plain rolls.

Butterflake: These are made by rolling dough ¹/₈-in. (*3 mm*) thick and spreading with soft butter; cutting six long strips and stacking them; then cutting into 1-in. (*25* *mm*) pieces and placing cut-side-down in greased muffin cups.

Cinnamon: These popular rolls are made by rolling out the dough; spreading with butter, cinnamon, and sugar; and rolling up like a jelly roll, which is then cut crosswise.

Clover-leaf: These rolls are made by putting three tiny balls of dough in muffin tins, allowing the dough to rise, then baking.

Crescents (butterhorns): To make crescents, triangles of dough are rolled up, shaped into crescents, raised, and baked.

Croissants: This is the French word for *crescents*. These are the traditional rolls that are served, along with fruit juice and coffee, as the Continental Breakfast, which one finds around the world. These rolls are richer because they are rolled out, dotted with butter or shortening, and folded over several times, which gives them a flaky texture bordering on a pastry.

English muffins (crumpets): A misnomer, because they are not muffins. The dough is cut in rounds and baked on an ungreased griddle or baked in the oven, but whichever method is used they should be brown on both sides with lots of "nooks and crannies" to hold the butter. In England, these are called *crumpets*, but they are thinner and spongier than the American counterpart.

Hamburger buns: These are made with a basic roll recipe and shaped to produce the round, flat hamburger bun.

Hot Cross buns: It is an English tradition in the spring, at Eastertime, to serve these rolls which contain added raisins and spices and have a cross marked on the top, either with pastry or icing.

Parker House (pocket rolls): The dough is rolled out, cut with a biscuit cutter, brushed with butter and folded over.

Pecan: Cinnamon rolls can be used for these. Cover the bottom of a baking pan with melted butter, brown sugar, and pecans, then place the rolls on top, allow to rise, bake, then turn out upside down on a platter.

Submarine: These rolls are shaped to resemble a boat, and snipped on top. They are used to make the increasingly popular submarine sandwiches which are meal-sized sandwiches, with any kind of filling desired.

Twists: The dough is worked into a rope and twisted into little braids or knotted and tied.

Wiener buns: These are plain rolls shaped in large, long fingers which are used for splitting and serving with frankfurters (wieners).

Rolls are as nutritious as the ingredients in them. See Table F-36, Food Composition Table, under "Bakery Products," for the nutritive qualities of rolls.

(Also see BREADS AND BAKING.)

ROPE

A condition in breads caused by *Bacillus mesentericus* or *Bacillus subtilis*. Spores of these bacteria can survive baking and then germinate under proper moisture and temperature surroundings. The bread develops sticky yellow patches that can be pulled into ropelike threads; hence, the name rope. Obviously, the bread is inedible. Food additives such as calcium acetate, calcium propionate and sodium diacetate retard this bacterial growth.

(Also see ADDITIVES; and BREADS AND BAKING.)

ROSE APPLE (POMARROSA) *Eugenia jambos*

The fruit of a small tree (of the family *Myrtaceae*) that is native to the Indo-Malaysian region, and which was introduced into the New World tropics where it now grows wild. The rose-centered fruits are egg-shaped, about 1½ in. (*4 cm*) in diameter, yellowish-white or pink with a yellow flesh and one or two seeds. The fruit is eaten fresh or made into jam or pies.

The nutrient composition of rose apples is given in Food Composition Table F-36.

Some noteworthy observations regarding the nutrient composition of rose apples follow:

1 .The raw fruit is low to moderately high in calories (56 kcal per 100 g) and carbohydrates (14%).

2. Rose apples are a good source of iron and a fair to good source of vitamin C.

ROSE HIPS *Rosa* spp

The fleshy fruit at the base of the rose bloom of plants of the family *Rosaceae*.

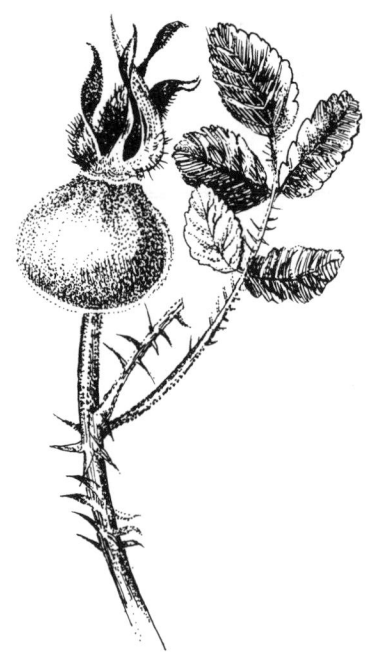

Fig. R-34. Rose hips, a fruit that is an excellent source of vitamin C.

Rose hips are not eaten as such; rather, they are concentrated as a powder, made into jams, jellies, and syrups, or brewed as a tea. Rose hips are used as an ingredient of many vitamin C products, often in combination with ascorbic acid.

(Also see VITAMIN C.)

ROSELLE

An East Indian herb, cultivated for its fleshy calyxes, which are used to make tarts and jellies, and a very acid drink.

ROUX

A mixture of fat and flour which is used as a base for thickened sauces. It is prepared by melting the butter or other fat, adding the flour, and stirring until it is browned. This produces some dextrin which gives the sauce an enjoyable flavor, which gourmet cooks feel is superior to other methods of making white or other sauces.

ROWE ELIMINATION DIETS

Widely used elimination diets formulated by Dr. Albert H. Rowe. These diets are used to determine food allergies by removing certain types of foods from the diet. In general, elimination diets are tedious and time-consuming and should be employed only when dietary history, skin tests, and provocative food tests fail to detect the causative food. Rowe diets are organized on the basis of food items that have proven the least likely to produce an allergic response.

(Also see ALLERGIES, Table A-7 Rowe Elimination Diets.)

ROYAL JELLY

This is the milky white food that is prepared exclusively for the queen bee in a beehive. Royal jelly, which is available as a supplement in capsule form, is a rich source of the B-complex vitamins, along with 20 amino acids. But about 3% of this substance made by bees still defies analysis.

Queen bees look different from worker bees: they are about twice the size; they live up to 8 years—fully 40 times longer than the normal lifespan of worker bees; and they lay about 2,000 eggs per day, whereas female worker bees are infertile. What makes queen bees so different? All the eggs start out the same, fed on a rich protein diet secreted from the glands of the worker bees. After 2 days, the eggs that are to become worker bees are changed to a diet of honey. Meanwhile, the egg that is to become the queen is fed royal bee jelly throughout her growth stage. Royal jelly makes the difference!

The implication of the promotors of royal jelly is that it will do as much for humans as for queen bees; that it will increase size, longevity, and fertility.

No effect has been demonstrated in humans, except a tendency to produce wakefulness. Royal jelly is judged to be of no practical value in human nutrition because of the very large amounts required for any definite effect.

RUMEN (PAUNCH)

The large first compartment of the stomach of a ruminant from which the food is regurgitated for cud-chewing and in which cellulose is broken down by bacterial and protozoan symbionts.

RUSKS (ZWIEBACK)

Zwieback is the German word meaning *twice-baked*. Originally, rusks were developed to take on ships for long voyages. They are made from either plain or sweet bread which is baked, then sliced and baked again to produce a hard crisp product. Rusks are a favorite food on which the infant can chew. They are also good for taking on camping or fishing trips, instead of trying to keep fresh bread on hand.

RUTABAGA (SWEDISH TURNIP; SWEDE)
Brassica napobrassica

This vegetable should be called the "super turnip" because it is bigger and better than the ordinary turnip in several ways. The rutabaga belongs to the mustard family of vegetables (*Cruciferae*). Fig. R-35 shows a typical rutabaga.

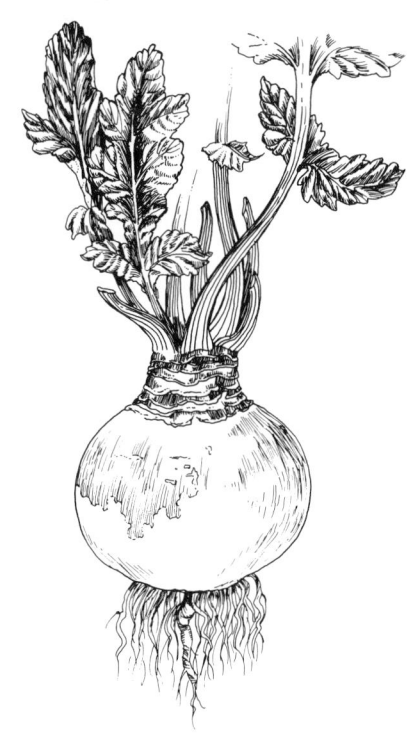

Fig. R-35. The rutabaga (swede), a cross between the common turnip and a variety of kale.

ORIGIN AND HISTORY. It is suspected that the ancestor of the rutabaga originated from an accidental crossing (hybridization) between kale and turnips in one or more areas where the two crops were planted side by side. The first hybridization may have occurred as early as the Middle Ages in Europe, but the rutabaga was not identified as a distinct type of vegetable until the 17th century. Furthermore, it seems likely that the early types of rutabagas were repeatedly crossed with turnips in the course of development of the enlarged root.

After the modern form of the rutabaga (which the Europeans call a swede) had been developed, stockmen found it to be a more nutritious fodder than the turnip. (Rutabaga contains about 50% more dry matter, which is responsible for the higher feeding value.) Also, rutabagas store better through the winter than turnips. Hence, swedes became an important feedstuff throughout northern Europe.

PRODUCTION.   Statistics on rutabaga production are not readily available. However, the U.S. Department of Agriculture reports that each year 18 to 19 million pounds (*8.2 to 8.6 thousand metric tons*) of rutabagas and turnips are shipped within the United States. Most of the U.S. crop of rutabagas is grown in Minnesota, Washington, Wisconsin, and other northern states.

This vegetable must be planted so that it will reach maturity in cool weather, because prolonged periods of temperatures over 80°F (*27°C*) cause irregular root growth. However, exposure of the growing plants to temperatures below 50°F (*10°C*) may cause them to go to seed. Hence, rutabagas are usually planted in June and harvested in October and November. Also, the plants require a soil containing ample amounts of nitrogen, phosphorus, potassium, and organic matter.

The roots are harvested when they are three or more inches in diameter. Home gardeners may leave some of the roots in the ground until they are needed. Rutabagas store better than turnips, particularly if they are first coated with a layer of wax or paraffin.

PROCESSING.   Rutabagas that are to be used as a human food are not processed beyond waxing them for storage. However, those intended for the feeding of livestock may be dried so that the animals will be able to consume greater quantities of them.

SELECTION AND PREPARATION.   High-quality rutabagas are usually large and elongated, with yellow flesh and a slightly sweet flavor. Those which have been stored may be covered with a thin layer of paraffin or wax that should be removed before using them. The leafy tops of home-grown rutabagas should be removed and discarded, because they are not as edible as turnip greens.

The most common way of preparing this vegetable is to (1) cut off the peel, (2) dice or slice the pared root, (3) cook the pieces in lightly salted boiling water for 12 to 15 minutes, and (4) mash and serve them with butter and seasonings. Rutabagas are also good when (1) mashed together with boiled potatoes, (2) used in souffles, (3) served in various sauces, or (4) cooked in casseroles, soups, and stews.

CAUTION: Rutabagas and other vegetables of the mustard family (*Cruciferae*) contain small amounts of substances called *goitrogens* that interfere with the utilization of iodine by the thyroid gland. Hence, people who eat very large amounts of these vegetables while on an iodine-deficient diet may develop an enlargement of the thyroid, commonly called a goiter. The best insurance against this potentially harmful effect is the consumption of ample amounts of dietary iodine. This element is abundantly present in iodized salt, ocean fish, seafood, and edible seaweeds.

NUTRITIONAL VALUE.   The nutrient composition of rutabaga is given in Food Composition Table F-36.

Some noteworthy observations regarding the nutrient composition of rutabaga follow:

1.   A 1-cup (*240 ml*) serving of mashed cooked rutabaga, which provides more than ½ lb (*227 g*) of food, contains only 84 Calories (kcal), whereas a cup of mashed potatoes (about ⅓ lb) supplies 118 Calories (kcal).

2.   The solids content of the rutabaga is about 50% greater than that of the turnip, which is why the former has greater nutritional value for man and animals.

3.   Rutabagas are a good source of vitamins A and C, although the cooked vegetable contains lower levels than the raw form. Hence, cooking should be limited to that needed to produce tenderness.

FUTURE PROSPECTS FOR THE RUTABAGA.
The attempts to improve the rutabaga by crossbreeding continue, since the root is a valuable food that may be stored outdoors for several months during the winter. Therefore, it is noteworthy that a retired plant breeder named Meader has developed a Colbaga, which is a hybrid of the cabbage and the rutabaga.[6] The new vegetable has cabbagelike leaves and a rutabaga-type of root which may be eaten raw or cooked. Perhaps this hybrid will prove to be profitable to growers and appealing and nutritious to consumers.

(Also see VEGETABLE[S], Table V-6 Vegetables of the World.)

RYE *Secale cereale*

Contents   Page

Rye is a bread grain, second only to wheat in importance. It is the main bread grain of the Scandinavian and eastern European countries. Although nutritious, and palatable to some people, rye bread is not comparable to wheat bread in crumb quality and bold appearance of the loaf. As living standards rise, the consumption of rye bread falls, and the consumption of wheat bread rises.

(Also see CEREAL GRAINS.)

ORIGIN AND HISTORY.   Rye was domesticated relatively recently, about the 4th century B.C., in Germany, and later in southern Europe. According to N. I. Vavilov, the Russian plant scientist, cultivated rye originated from wild species that occurred as weeds in wheat and barley crops, and rye was introduced into cultivation simultaneously and independently at many localities in central Asia or Asia Minor.

[6]Chapline, J., "The Fruitful Inventor," *Blair & Ketchum's Country Journal*, Vol. VII, 1980, p. 43.

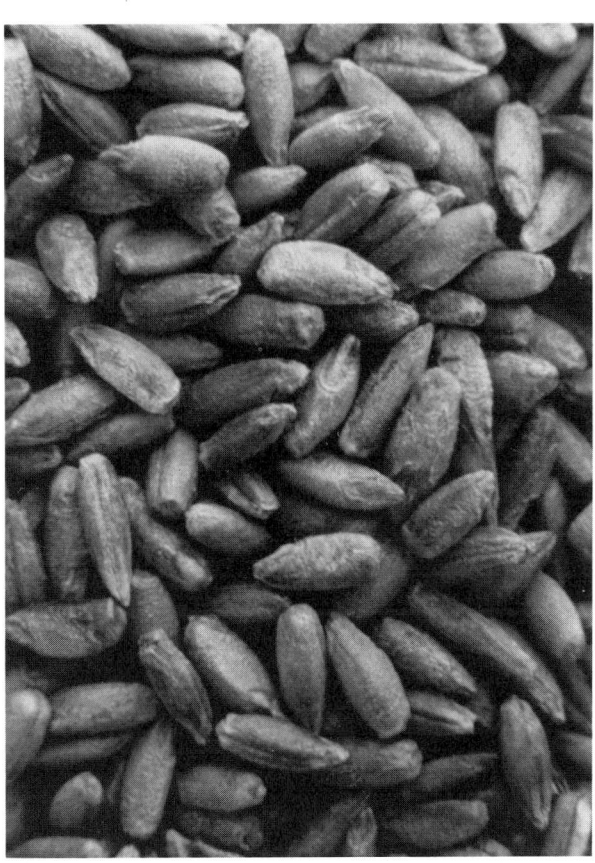

Fig. R-36. Rye grains. (Courtesy, USDA)

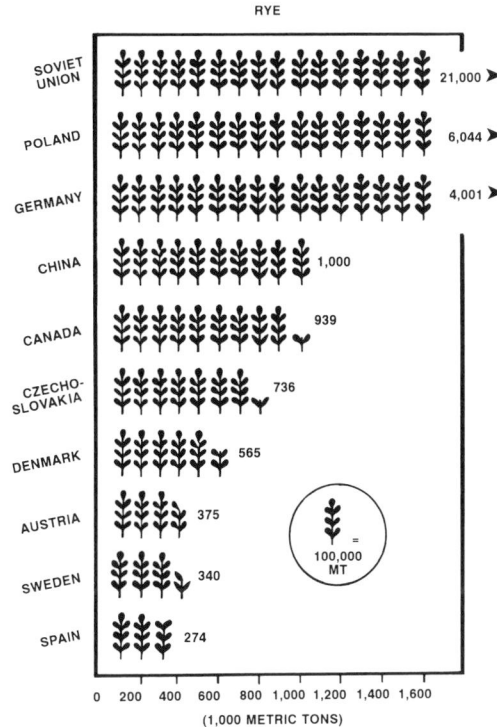

Fig. R-37. Leading rye-producing countries. (Source: *FAO Production Yearbook*, 1990, FAO/UN, Rome, Italy, Vol. 44, p. 81, Table 21)

No trace of rye have been found among the Egyptian ruins or Swiss lake dwellings. It was, however, known to the Romans, to whom it was introduced by the Teutonic invaders.

During the Middle Ages, the poorer people of England ate bread made from rye, or from a mixture of rye and wheat, known as maslin.

WORLD AND U.S. PRODUCTION. World production of rye is about 37 million metric tons, only about 6% of the world production of wheat, and only 2% of the world production of cereals. Rye is more important in Europe and Asia than in the western hemisphere. The Soviet Union is the leading world producer, followed by Poland, Germany, China, Canada, Czechoslovak, Denmark, Austria, Sweden, and Spain (see Fig. R-37).

Rye production in the United States has steadily declined since World War I. Annually, about 245 thousand metric tons are harvested from about 373,000 acres, with an average yield of 27.1 bu per acre. The U.S. wheat crop averages 36.7 bu per acre (*2,069 kg/ha*). The leading rye-producing states, by rank, are: South Dakota, Georgia, Minnesota, North Dakota, Nebraska, South Carolina, Michigan, Wisconsin, and North Carolina (see Fig. R-38).

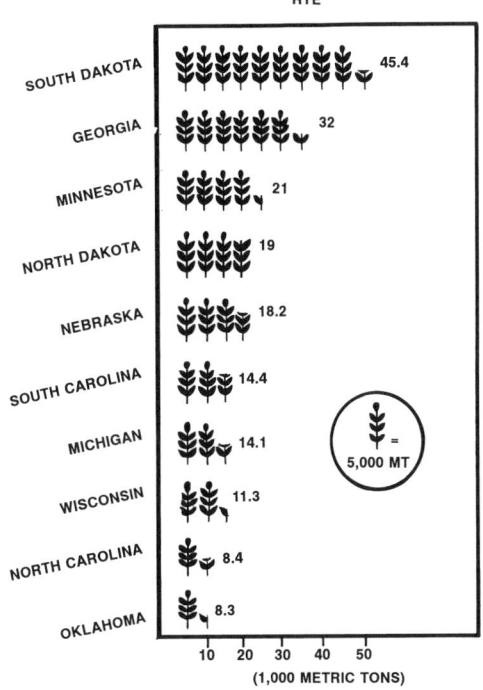

Fig. R-38. Leading U.S. rye-producing states. (Source: *Agricultural Statistics 1991*, USDA, p. 16, Table 19)

THE RYE PLANT.   Rye belongs to the grass family, *Gramineae*. It is a member of the genus *Secale* and of the species, *S. cereale*.

The rye plant is an annual under cultivation, although at times tending to maintain itself by sprouting anew from the stubble. The abundant, fibrous root system penetrates downward more deeply than other cereals.

Rye has the tallest and strongest straw of all the small grain crops. At maturity, the plants may attain a height of 7 to 8 ft (*2.1 to 2.4 m*) on fertile soils, although they are usually under 5 ft (*1.5 m*). The leaves are long, narrow, and thin.

The plant has slender seed heads (spikes) with long, stiff beards. The grains fall free from the chaff when threshed. The mature grain is more slender than wheat, and is usually grayish yellow. Because the flowers are largely self-sterile, cross pollination occurs almost completely.

RYE CULTURE.   The culture of rye is similar to that of wheat, but rye grows better on poorer, dryer soils and in colder climates than other cereal grains. Also, it is less exacting in seedbed and seeding requirements than the other small grains, although, like other crops, it responds to favorable treatment. Rye can be seeded from late summer to October 1 and even later in the southern states. It is usually seeded at the rate of 1¼ to 2 bu per acre (*77 to 124 kg/ha*), and the seed is covered to a depth of 1½ to 2 in (*3.8 to 5.1 cm*).

When the plants are ripe and thoroughly dry, rye is harvested in the same manner as wheat and the other small grains.

FEDERAL GRADES.   The Official United States Standards For Grain, established by the U.S. Department of Agriculture, designate the following five grades of rye: U.S. No. 1, U.S. No. 2, U.S. No. 3, U.S. No. 4, and U.S. Sample Grade. Grades are determined by test weight per bushel, damaged kernels (including heat damage), and foreign matter other than wheat.

KINDS.   Both winter and spring varieties of rye are grown in the United States. However, the spring varieties are less productive than the winter varieties and are grown only to a limited extent.

Unlike the other small grains, rye is self-sterile. Thus, for seed to be produced on one plant, pollen must be provided by another plant. For this reason, it is much more difficult to keep varieties of rye pure than with the other small grains.

Varieties of rye differ considerably in hardiness, productivity, and habit of growth.

PROCESSING.   The processing of rye involves cleaning, conditioning, and milling.

The cleaning principles and machinery are similar to those used in wheat cleaning, complicated by two primary differences: (1) The grain is more variable in size; and (2) the grain is more subject to ergot (a poisonous fungus), which should be separated out before it is broken up and rendered difficult to remove.

Conditioning, or tempering, consists of bringing the grain to a moisture content of about 14.5%.

Rye is milled by grinding the grain on a succession of pairs of rollers, most of which are fluted, and sifting out the flour from the grind. The process resembles wheat flour milling, but it deviates from the latter because of two important differences between the grains; (1) the endosperm of rye breaks up into flour fineness more readily than the endosperm of wheat, and (2) the separation of the endosperm from the bran of rye is more difficult.

A yield of 64 to 65% of reasonably pure flour can be obtained from rye. At higher extraction rates, the flour becomes progressively darker in color and more fibrous, and the characteristic rye flavor becomes more prominent.

Rye whole meal refers to ground, dry whole rye grain, whereas rye meal may be of any extraction rate.

• **Ergot**—A poisonous fungus, called ergot, often replaces the grain of rye. Ergot is a hornlike blackish body several times longer than the normal grain. It will poison human beings and livestock that eat infested grain or products, producing a disease called ergotism. Ergot may cause pregnant sows to abort.

But ergot supplies a valuable drug! Doctors prescribe small doses of the drug made from ergot to ease migraine headaches, control bleeding, and aid in childbirth.

(Also see POISONS, Table P-11 Some Potentially Poisonous [Toxic] Substances.)

NUTRITIONAL VALUE.   Food Composition Table F-36 gives the nutrient compositions of rye grain and rye products.

The food value of rye is similar to wheat. It is a good source of starch (carbohydrates) and a fair source of protein. However, the protein, in terms of essential amino acids, falls short in lysine compared to cow's milk—a high-quality protein, as shown in Table R-12. Therefore, like wheat and the other grains lysine is the limiting amino acid. Of the vitamins, rye is devoid of vitamins A, C, and B-12.

TABLE R–12
PROFILE OF THE ESSENTIAL AMINO ACIDS IN RYE COMPARED TO MILK—A HIGH-QUALITY PROTEIN

Amino Acid	Rye	Cow's Milk[1]
	← (mg/g protein) →	
Histidine	21	27
Isoleucine	39	47
Leucine	59	95
Lysine	35	78
Methionine and cystine	29	33
Phenylalanine and tyrosine	69	102
Threonine	31	44
Tryptophan	11	14
Valine	46	64

[1]*Recommended Dietary Allowances*, 10th ed., 1989, NRC-National Academy of Sciences, p. 67, Table 6–5.

As a livestock feed, numerous feeding trials show that rye has only about 95% the feeding value of wheat, primarily because of lack of palatability and the tendency to be laxative if fed in large amounts.

PRODUCTS AND USES. Rye is used for human food, livestock feed, fermented products, and certain other uses. Although American farmers feed a major portion of the rye crop to livestock, it must be remembered that, indirectly, it enters the human diet primarily as meat and milk.

The uses of rye and rye products are summarized in Table R-13.

(Also see CEREAL GRAINS, Table C-18 Cereal Grains of the World; and BREADS AND BAKING.)

TABLE R-13
RYE PRODUCTS AND USES

Product	Description	Uses	Comments
HUMAN FOODS			
Rye	Whole grain, unground.	Hot breakfast cereal. Starchy vegetable.	The whole grains may be cooked like rice by (1) soaking overnight in water (2–3 C of water per C [*240 ml*] of rye), then boiling until tender; or (2) cooking in a pressure cooker, using a standard recipe.
Rye	Ground, dry whole rye grain. Rye meal, consisting of any extraction rate less than 100%.	Rye crisp. Rye crisp.	Rye crisp is a popular bread served with most meals in Sweden. Traditionally, rye crisp bread in Sweden is made by mixing rye meal with snow or powdered ice, then the expansion of the small air bubbles in the ice-cold foam raises the dough when it is placed in the oven.
Rye flakes	Rolled whole rye.	Hot breakfast cereal.	
Rye flour (Also see FLOURS, Table F-25 Major Flours.)	Produced by milling rye, much like milling wheat. It does not contain as much gluten as wheat flour.	Bread. In the U.S., rye bread is usually made from a combination of rye flour and wheat flour. Biscuits and crackers (usually made from mixtures of about 10% rye flour and 90% wheat flour). Rye pancakes. Filler for sauces, soups, and custard powders.	In most countries, rye is used as a bread grain—for human food. Yeast does not raise rye dough as easily as wheat dough, because of lack of gluten in rye flour. When bread is made from straight rye flour, it is black, soggy, and rather bitter. For centuries, a large portion of the population of Europe lived mainly on schwarzbrot, made from rye flour, which is still rather common in rural Germany, Poland, and the U.S.S.R. Whole rye and mixed rye-wheat breads have a longer shelf life than wheat bread. Rye contains more pentosans than other cereals; hence, it is used in reducing diets because: (1) the pentosans gelatinize and swell in the stomach, imparting a feeling of satisfaction; and (2) digestion of the polysaccharides is slow, with the result that the blood sugar level rises slowly but is maintained for 5 to 6 hours, thereby controlling appetite.
FERMENTED BEVERAGES			
Rye grain	Cleaned whole grain.	Rye whiskey. Industrial alcohol.	Rye whiskey is made from a fermented mash containing a minimum of 51% rye.
Rye bread	Brown rye bread.	Russian rye bread beer (kvass or quass).	A mash made by pressure cooking the bread is treated with rye malt, then fermented by a mixture of yeast and *Bacillus lactis*. The beer, which contains only about 0.7% alcohol, is usually dispensed cold from tank trucks.

(Continued)

TABLE R-13 (*Continued*)

Product	Description	Uses	Comments
LIVESTOCK FEEDS			
Rye grain	Ground whole grain.	Fed to cattle, sheep, and swine.	American farmers feed a major portion of the rye crop to livestock. Limit to 15-20% of the ration because of lack of palatability. Rye has about 95% the feeding value of wheat. Rye is seldom fed to poultry because it tends to depress growth and cause sticky, pasty droppings when used at moderate to high levels.
Rye middlings	Rye feed and red dog flour combined in the proportions obtained in the usual process of milling rye flour. It must not contain more than 8.5% crude fiber.	Fed to beef cattle, dairy cattle, sheep, and swine.	For beef cattle, dairy cattle, sheep, and swine, rye middlings are a satisfactory partial substitute for wheat middlings, but the amount fed had best be limited to 20% of the concentrate mixture.
Rye mill run	The outer covering of the rye kernel and the rye germ, along with small quantities of rye flour and aleurone. It must not contain more than 9.5% fiber.	Fed to beef cattle, dairy cattle, sheep, and swine.	For beef cattle, dairy cattle, sheep, and swine, rye mill run is a satisfactory partial substitute for wheat mill run, but the amount had best be limited to 20% of the concentrate mixture.
Rye forages: Rye plant	The green, growing plant.	Pasture (especially for winter grazing.	Rye is sometimes seeded for pasture to provide supplemental grazing during the fall, winter, and spring when permanent or rotational pastures are unproductive.
Rye straw	The straw following threshing.	Roughage for cattle. Animal bedding.	Because rye straw is usually long, it should be chopped for bedding.
OTHER USES			
Rye plant	The green, growing plant.	Cover crop and green manure.	Cover crops are grown for the purpose of protecting the soil from leaching and erosion. Green manure crops are turned under to add organic matter to the soil.
Rye starch	Derived from the endosperm of the seeds.	Adhesives	Rye starch for adhesives is of 70% extraction.
Rye straw	The straw following threshing.	Mats, mattresses, thatching for roofs, hats, and paper.	Rye has the longest and strongest straw of all the small grains.

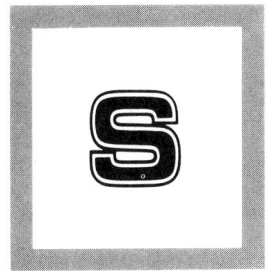

SACCHARIMETER

An apparatus for determining the concentration of sugar in a solution, based on the optical activity of the sugar; especially a polarimeter adapted for distinguishing different kinds of sugar in a solution.

SACCHARIN

A nonnutritive, noncaloric synthetic sweetener which is 300 to 500 times sweeter than table sugar. Mainly, the sodium and calcium salts of saccharin have found widespread use in dietetic foods and diet soft drinks since 1900. It was on the first GRAS (generally recognized as safe) list published in 1959. However, in 1972, following the ban on cyclamates, saccharin was removed from the GRAS list and given a provisional food additive status.

Today, saccharin is still being used on a limited basis.

(Also see ADDITIVES, Table A-3 Common Food Additives; ARTIFICIAL SWEETENERS; CANCER; and DELANEY CLAUSE.)

SACCHAROMETER

A floating apparatus, a special hydrometer, used to determine the specific gravity of sugar solutions. It can be graduated to read directly the percentage of sugar in solution. It is distinct from a saccharimeter.

SAFETY OF FOOD

Food safety involves a number of concerns, the most important of which are: (1) pesticides, and (2) harmful bacteria.

1. Pesticide residues in and on foods are the public's number one food safety fear. Because pesticides cannot be seen or smelled, consumers feel that they have little control over their level of exposure. So, we need to develop safer and more effective pesticides, and to use less pesticides on fruits and vegetables.

(Also see PESTICIDES AND INCIDENTAL FOOD ADDITIVES; and POISONS.)

2. Without bacteria in food there would be no yogurt, no blue cheese, and no sourdough bread. However, other bacteria left to grow unchecked can cause spoilage and even food-related illness. Making sure that this does not happen is the job of producers, workers, supervisors, and quality control specialists from farm to food counter, and finally to the consumer. Despite some concerns and scares from time to time, America's cornucopia of foods remains the envy of the world, both in quantity and quality.

(Also see DISEASES, sections on "Sanitary Measures Which Help to Prevent the Spread of Diseases" and "Health and Nutrition Functions of Government Agencies"; FOOD—BUYING, PREPARING, COOKING, AND SERVING; BACTERIA IN FOOD; and FOOD POISONING.)

SAFFLOWER *Carthamus tinctorius*

The ancients used safflower primarily as a dye plant; its flowers were used to make a red dye for silk and toilet rouge. Also, oil from safflower seeds lighted the lamps of Egypt's pharaohs and the meal fattened the cattle of the peasants.

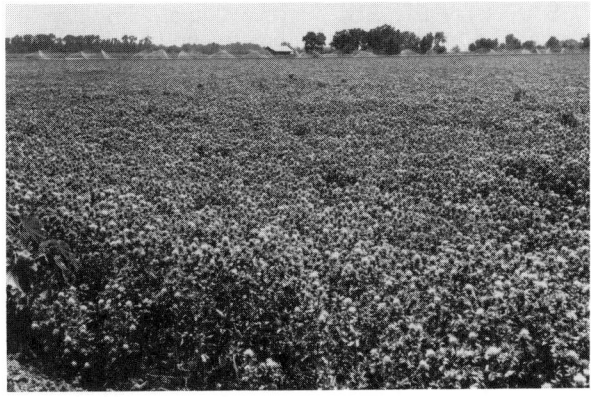

Fig. S-1. Field of safflowers in bloom in the Sacramento Valley of California. The safflower is a relative of the thistle family. (Courtesy, Pacific Oilseeds Incorporated, Woodland, Calif.)

In the 1950s, interest in safflower oil as a food ingredient skyrocketed as a result of studies relating saturated fats in the diet to atherosclerotic heart disease.

Safflower's unique fatty acid composition places it highest in polyunsaturates and lowest in saturates of all commercial fats and oils. As a result, safflower oil was (1) extolled as a preventative of cholesterol build-up in the blood; and (2) recommended in the diets of persons suffering from heart disease and hypertension, although the value of polyunsaturated fatty acids for such treatment remains a matter of controversy.

ORIGIN AND HISTORY. Safflower is native to Southeastern Asia, but it has long been cultivated in India, Egypt, China, and Northern Africa. It was taken to Mexico by the early Spanish explorers. Although the crop was introduced into the United States earlier, it was not considered established until the late 1950s.

WORLD AND U.S. PRODUCTION. The world production of safflower seed totals almost 1 million metric tons. India is far in the lead globally with a production of about 491,000 metric tons—53% of the world production. The United States with a production of about 170,000 metric tons ranks second, and Mexico with 159,000 metric tons ranks third. Lesser quantities are produced in Ethiopia and Australia.

Total U.S. seed production reached a high of 350,000 metric tons in 1967, but has since declined to around 170,000 metric tons.

THE SAFFLOWER PLANT. The safflower belongs to the composite family, *Compositae*. It is classified as genus *Carthamus*, species *C. tinctorius*. It is an annual, thistlelike plant that grows about 3 ft (*91 cm*) high, sends down a taproot that may penetrate to 6 to 8 ft (*183 to 244 cm*) or more, and has coarse branching stems and broad leaves that are usually spiny. The blooms vary in color—they may be red, orange, yellow, or white, or a combination of colors. The seed, which resembles a small sunflower seed, is composed of a thick fibrous white hull encasing a yellow kernel.

SAFFLOWER CULTURE. Climatically, the safflower is adapted to a dry climate and is salt-tolerant. Generally speaking, it thrives under about the same conditions as barley. In the United States, it is grown chiefly in the Southwest and in the northern Great Plains. Harvesting is accomplished with the same type of combine as is used in harvesting small grains. Yields of seed normally range from 350 to 1,200 lb per acre (*392 to 1,344 kg/ha*), although as high as 4,000 lb per acre (*4,480 kg/ha*) can be attained under irrigation.

KINDS OF SAFFLOWER. There are numerous varieties of safflower. Breeding programs are giving emphasis to the development of varieties having a lower percentage of hull and higher oil and protein content. Higher yields are being achieved by use of hybrids.

PROCESSING SAFFLOWER SEED. Normally, the steps in processing consist of: (1) cleaning the seed by screening and aspiration; (2) grinding the seed; (3) cooking under steam pressure; (4) extracting the oil by the continuous screw press-solvent extraction method; (5) grinding and screening the cake to produce meal; and (6) refining the oil.

NUTRITIONAL VALUE OF SAFFLOWER SEED. The commercial varieties of safflower grown in the United States average 35 to 40% hull and yield 39 to 40% oil and 15% protein. However, varieties with up to 50% oil content have been developed.

The oil is extremely variable, perhaps reflecting its mixed heredity. California studies on safflower procured from many parts of the world showed great variation in the content of polyunsaturated fats, with iodine numbers ranging from 87 to 149. It averages about 6.6% saturated acids and 93.4% unsaturated acids, with the latter consisting of 77.0% linoleic acid and 16.4% oleic acid (The high linoleic acid content makes the oil susceptible to rancidity). Linolenic acid is absent. Genetically modified varieties of safflower with greater resistance to rancidity have been introduced that contain 80% oleic, 15% linoleic, and 5% saturated fatty acids. Safflower oil is listed in Food Composition Table F-36 and Table F-9, Fats and Fatty Acids in Selected Foods.

The extracted cake is ground to yield a 20 to 42% protein meal, with the higher protein content obtained from decorticated (dehulled) seed. Meal produced by the solvent method contains about 1% fat vs 5% when the expeller process is used. Safflower meal is of good quality, although somewhat deficient in lysine and methionine.

SAFFLOWER PRODUCTS AND USES. Safflower oil is a bland, almost colorless product. Due to its susceptibility to oxidation, care is taken to exclude air during storage, transport, and packaging. Interest in the oil as a food ingredient stems largely from its high percentage of unsaturated (polyunsaturated) fatty acids.

Safflower oil is used principally in the production of margarine, salad oils, mayonnaise, shortening, and other food products. The oil is also used as a drying agent in varnishes and paints. Because of its high linoleic acid content and the absence of linolenic acid, varnishes and white paint made with safflower oil do not yellow with age.

High protein content safflower meal, made from dehulled seed and containing about 42% protein, is now considered a protein source for human consumption. However, most safflower meal is used as a protein supplement for livestock. The meal is not very palatable when used alone.

(Also see OILS, VEGETABLE, Table O-6.)

SAINT ANTHONY'S FIRE

A thousand years ago, this name was given to the condition known now as ergotism—a poisoning due to the consumption of foods containing the fungus ergot.

Symptoms of ergotism include alternating burning and freezing sensations; hence, the name Saint Anthony's Fire.

(Also see POISONS, Table P-11 Some Potentially Poisonous [Toxic] Substances, "Ergot.")

SAINT JOHN'S BREAD (CAROB)

The carob pod is sometimes called Saint John's bread because of the widely held belief that the "locusts" that John the Baptist ate while in the wilderness were really carob pods (Matthew 3:4).

The carob tree is a dark evergreen tree which grows wild in the countries that border the Mediterranean Sea. It produces brown, leathery pods 4 to 10 in. (*10 to 25 cm*) long. The pods contain a sticky pulp, consisting of about 50% sugar, which is fed to horses and cattle and is sometimes eaten by people.

(Also see CAROB.)

SALAMI

A highly seasoned sausage made of pork and beef in various proportions; either (1) air-dried, hard, and of good keeping qualities, or (2) fresh, soft, and requiring refrigeration until consumed.

SALEP

A starchy foodstuff from the Middle East which consists of the dried tubers of various orchids. It is easily digested and highly esteemed in the East.

SALINE

It refers to anything containing or consisting of salt. Physiological saline is a solution containing 0.9% NaCl (salt). Since it is compatible with the blood, it is sometimes administered intravenously.

SALIVA

A clear, somewhat viscid solution secreted into the mouth by three pairs of salivary glands—the parotid, the sublingual, and the submaxillary.

The functions of saliva are manyfold including the following:

1. **Lubricant.** These secretions act as aids in mastication and swallowing. Without this moisture, swallowing would be extremely difficult. This lubricating ability is attributed to the presence of a glycoprotein.

2. **Enzymatic activity.** The enzyme alpha-amylase (ptyalin) is found in the saliva. It acts to break alpha 1, 4 glucosidic linkages in starch.

3. **Buffering capacity.** A large quantity of bicarbonate is secreted in saliva, thus serving as a buffer in the ingesta, and in the mouth.

4. **Taste.** Saliva solubilizes a number of the chemicals in the food which, once in solution, can be detected by the taste buds.

5. **Protection.** The membranes within the mouth must be kept moist in order to remain viable. Saliva provides one means by which this is accomplished. In addition, the saliva may also possess some antibacterial action, which protects the teeth against dental caries.

Secretion of saliva is stimulated by the sight, the smell, and even the mere thought of food.

(Also see DIGESTION AND ABSORPTION.)

SALLY LUNN

This bread came to America from Bath, England, the home of Sally Lunn. It is baked in a tube-center pan, and it should have a porous, cakelike texture.

SALMONELLA

A genus of bacteria responsible for one of the most common foodborne infections in the United States—salmonellosis. *Salmonella* bacteria grow rapidly in cooked foods such as meats, eggs, custards, and salads which have been left unrefrigerated for several hours. It may also be transmitted by sewage-polluted water. The bacteria produce diarrhea, abdominal cramps, and vomiting which usually last for 2 to 3 days. Mortality is very low. The best treatment is prevention which can be accomplished by refrigeration of foods, hand washing by food handlers, and scrupulous cleaning of food processing equipment. *Salmonella* in foods is destroyed by a temperature of 140°F (*60°C*) for 20 minutes, or 149°F (*65°C*) for 3 minutes. Flies, cockroaches, and rodents should be prevented from coming in contact with food.

(Also see BACTERIA IN FOOD, Table B-5 Food Infections [Bacterial]—"Salmonellosis.")

SALSIFY (OYSTERPLANT)
Tragopogon porrifolius

The major edible part of this plant is the taproot, which has a flavor like that of oysters. However, the young leaves are also edible. It is better known in Europe than in the United States. Salsify is a member of the sunflower family (*Compositae*), which also includes the artichoke, chicory, dandelion, endive, Jerusalem artichoke, and lettuce.

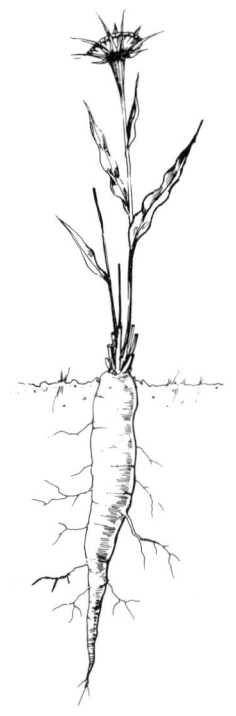

Fig. S-2. Salsify, a vegetable with a white carrotlike root that has an oyster taste when cooked.

ORIGIN AND HISTORY.
Salsify is native to the Mediterranean region. It does not appear to have been grown as a food plant until the beginning of the 17th century. However, it was one of the vegetables that Thomas Jefferson grew in his garden. Recently, the plant has been considered to be useful in the diets of diabetics and of people trying to lose weight because most of the carbohydrate present in the fresh roots is in the form of inulin, which is not utilized by the human body. Hence, the root may be substituted for starchy vegetables when it is necessary to restrict the biologically available carbohydrate in the diet.

PRODUCTION.
Salsify is of little commercial importance at the present time. Hence, data on the amounts produced are not readily available.

This crop requires a long period of growth. Hence, it is often planted as soon as the ground can be worked in the spring. However, the long periods of hot summer weather in the southern United States may cause bolting (the premature production of seedstalks). The bolting problem in this region is overcome by planting the seed in the summer so that most of the growth occurs during the fall and early winter.

The soil should be rich in organic matter, deeply-cultivated, loose, and crumbly so that there is little interference with the growth of the roots. Sometimes, the newly-seeded soil is covered with sheets of transparent plastic film to keep it moist and warm until the plants emerge. Home gardeners seem to get the best results when they grow the crop in specially prepared, raised beds that are enclosed on the sides with wooden boards and are filled with a mixture of fine soil and other materials such as compost, peat moss, perlite, and/or vermiculite. The newly-emerged plants usually require thinning because it is customary to plant an excess of seed to cope with the slowness and uncertainty of germination.

The roots are ready for harvesting in about 5 months after planting the seed. They may be left in the ground until after the first frost, which improves their flavor. The low temperature brings about the conversion of the stored carbohydrate inulin to the sugar fructose, which is the sweetest of the common sugars.

PROCESSING.
There is little or no processing of salsify at the present time. However, its content of inulin makes it potentially valuable for (1) low-calorie dietetic foods because the carbohydrate is not utilized by the body, and (2) chemical and/or enzymatic conversion of inulin to the sugar fructose, which is much in demand at the present time.

SELECTION AND PREPARATION.
Firm, clean, well-shaped salsify roots are generally of best quality. Soft, flabby, or shriveled roots are usually pithy or fibrous. Softness may also be an indication of decay, which appears as a gray mold or a soft rot. Misshaped roots are objectionable because of waste in preparation for use.

The skin of the roots may be scraped off with a knife, or scrubbed off with a stiff vegetable brush. It is noteworthy that cut pieces of root may turn dark unless discoloration is prevented by wetting the pieces with lemon juice or vinegar.

Raw salsify roots may be cut into strips lengthwise and served with dips; or they may be grated, dipped in lemon juice or vinegar, and added to salads. Also, the young leaves are good when served raw in salads.

The cooked vegetable may be prepared in ways such as (1) boiled and served with butter, margarine, seasonings, or a special sauce; (2) sliced and added to a soup; (3) dipped in batter and fried in deep fat; or (4) boiled, mashed, formed into patties, floured, and browned in fat or oil.

NUTRITIONAL VALUE.
The nutrient compositions of raw and cooked salsify roots are given in Food Composition Table F-36.

Some noteworthy observations regarding the nutrient composition of salsify roots follow:

1. Salsify has about the same water content (78%) as parsnips and potatoes but supplies much fewer calories because its carbohydrate content is comprised mainly of inulin, a substance that is not metabolized by the body. (The predominant carbohydrate in parsnips and potatoes is starch, which is readily utilized for its calorie content.) Fresh salsify roots provide only a few calories, whereas those that have been left in the ground during the winter or stored in a cold environment have approx-

imately the caloric values shown in Table F-36, because low temperatures bring about the conversion of inulin to fructose.

2. A 1-cup (*150 g*) serving of cooked salsify roots provides about the same amount of protein as a cup of cooked cornmeal or cooked rice, but the roots contain much fewer calories. Also, salsify supplies about one-third more protein than potatoes. Hungry dieters might consider substituting salsify for starchy vegetables because they would be able to eat much larger quantities of the former without exceeding their caloric allowances.

3. Salsify roots are a good source of iron and potassium; a fair source of calcium, phosphorus, and vitamin C; and a very poor source of vitamin A. However, a salad containing salsify leaves should provide the vitamin A and other nutrients which are lacking in the roots.

(Also see VEGETABLE[S], Table V-6 Vegetables of the World.)

SALT (SODIUM CHLORIDE; NaCl)

Salt is created by the combination of the soft silvery-white metal sodium (Na), and the yellow poisonous gas chlorine (Cl). Sodium and chlorine are vital elements found in the fluids and soft tissues of the body. Salt also improves the appetite, promotes growth, helps regulate the body pH, and is essential for hydrochloric acid formation in the stomach.

HISTORICAL IMPORTANCE OF SALT. Throughout history, salt has occupied a unique position. Wars have been fought over it, empires have been founded on it and have collapsed without it, and civilizations have grown up around it.

Mosaic law prescribed the use of salt with offerings made to Jehovah; and there are frequent Biblical references to the purifying and flavoring effects of salt. The Greeks used salt as the medium of exchange in buying and selling slaves; a good slave was said to be "worth his weight in salt." The word salary is derived from the Latin *salarium*, referring to the salt which was part of a Roman soldier's pay. In medieval England, royal banquet halls had imposing salt cellars; and the seating arrangement in relation thereto served as a status symbol. Important persons were invited to "sit above the salt," where they could use the salt on their food freely; those of lesser importance were seated "below the salt." In some parts of Africa, gold was once evaluated in terms of how much salt it would buy—rather than the reverse. Salt caravans, part of the ancient lore of Africa, still ply certain desert areas to this day. By common use, the expression "salt of the earth" refers to a really good person. These and other salt lore give ample evidence that in olden times salt was a valuable and relatively scarce commodity.

FUNCTIONS OF SALT. Most people think of salt as a seasoning, but it is probably used in greater quantities and for more applications than any other chemical. In fact, it is estimated that over 14,000 uses are made of salt.

Physiological. Sodium (Na) and chlorine (Cl) are essential parts of the human diet. (Salt as such isn't essential, since other sources of Na and Cl are satisfactory; for example, Na_2CO_3 and KCl.)

In body solution, salt dissociates into two ions—sodium and chloride, both of which are normal and necessary constituents.

• **Sodium (Na)**—Sodium is the major positively charged ion in the fluid outside the cells (extracellular), where it helps to maintain the balance of water, acids, and bases. It is a constituent of pancreatic juice, bile, sweat, and tears. Also, sodium is associated with muscle contraction and nerve function, and it plays a specific role in the absorption of carbohydrates. In part, the sodium concentration in the blood acting on centers in the hypothalamus controls the formation of urine and the sensation of thirst. Secretion of aldosterone from the adrenal cortex acts to salvage sodium ions during the formation of urine, while it promotes the release of potassium ions into the urine.

For the estimated daily requirements of sodium, the reader is referred to SODIUM, section headed "Recommended Daily Allowances of Sodium."

• **Chloride (Cl)**—The dietary source of nearly all chloride is table salt. In the body, the highest concentrations of chloride are found in the cerebrospinal fluid and in secretions into the gastrointestinal tract. It is an important negatively charged ion in the maintenance of fluid and electrolyte balance and it is a component of stomach acid—hydrochloric acid. Rapid movement of the chloride ion across the red blood cell membrane helps to minimize fluid shifts, and enhances the ability of blood to carry carbon dioxide to the lungs.

For the estimated daily requirements of chloride the reader is referred to CHLORINE or CHLORIDE, section headed "Recommended Daily Allowance of Chlorine." The estimated safe and adequate dietary intakes of chloride are figured on the basis of sodium intake, because losses of chloride and intakes of chloride are closely tied to sodium. Only in cases of dietary salt restriction—sodium restricted diets—would it be necessary to provide other sources of chloride.

One important, but often overlooked, physiological function of salt is that it provides a vehicle for meeting the body's iodine requirement. Until 1924, when iodized salt was introduced, iodine-deficiency goiter was common in certain inland areas of the United States. Iodized salt contains 0.01% potassium iodide or 76 mcg of iodine per gram. Thus, the average use of 3.4 g of iodized salt per person per day adds approximately 260 mcg to the daily intake, more than meeting the normal requirement of about 150 mcg.

SALT DEFICIENCY. Salt deficiency is rarely a problem since most Americans consume ten times more salt than is recommended. Fortunately, the body adjusts. If there is a high intake of salt (sodium), the rate of excretion is high. On the other hand, if there is a low intake the excretion rate is low. However, deficiencies may occur from strict vegetarian diets without salt, or when there has been heavy, prolonged sweating, diarrhea, vomiting, or adrenal cortical insufficiency—Addison's disease.

A deficiency of salt (sodium) may cause reduced growth, loss of appetite, loss of body weight due to loss of body water, reduced milk production of lactating mothers, muscle cramps, nausea, diarrhea, and headache. In cases of prolonged or severe vomiting, or indiscreet use of diuretics, chloride losses may exceed that of sodium—resulting in a state of metabolic alkalosis. To restore the acid-base balance of the body, adequate chloride must be provided.

SALT TOXICITY. Excess dietary salt, over a long period of time, is believed to contribute to the development of high blood pressure in susceptible individuals. While the connection between the development of high blood pressure and salt intake is not clear, there are no known benefits derived from excessive salt consumption by healthy individuals. Possibly by adapting to a low salt intake early in life, the risk of developing high blood pressure later in life may be lessened.

In addition, salt may be toxic (1) when ingested in large quantities, especially with a low water intake; (2) when the body has been depleted by a salt-free vegetarian diet or excess sweating, followed by gorging on salt; (3) when large amounts are fed to infants or others afflicted with kidney diseases, whose kidneys cannot excrete the excess in the urine; or (4) when the body is adapted to a chronic low-salt diet, followed by ingesting large amounts.

(Also see HIGH BLOOD PRESSURE; MINERAL[S]; POISONS, Table P-11 Some Potentially Poisonous [Toxic] Substances; and SODIUM.)

Commercial. As important as salt is to the body, the majority of the millions of tons produced each year is used by a variety of industries and businesses.

FOOD INDUSTRY. Its first uses in man's foods are lost in antiquity. Thus, not surprisingly, salt is on the FDA list of GRAS (generally recognized as safe) food additives. In foods, salt performs three primary functions: (1) as a flavor enhancer or seasoner; (2) as a preservative; and (3) as a solubilizing agent.

Salt alters both the taste and the smell of food, and, used in high enough concentrations, it can change the "feel" of a food. Salt is used to season most processed meats such as frankfurters, corned beef, luncheon meats, sausage, ham, and bacon. In canned vegetables, salt is added during processing to improve their flavor. Salt enhances the flavor of breads; indeed, the taste of salt-free breads is not generally popular. Popular snack food items—pretzels, potato chips, and popcorn—are characterized by salt on their surface. Overall, small amounts of salt increase the sweetness of food products and beverages, while a very sugary taste can be lessened by a small amount of salt. At the dinner table, many consumers further modify the taste of their food with the salt shaker.

For centuries, the preservative nature of salt has been recognized. In early times salted meat and fish were an important part of the diet. Other types of fresh produce have been stored in salt for future use or further processing. The most familiar example is the cucumber which is pickled in a salt brine. Also, as part of the preservative action of salt, it controls the growth of microorganisms in foods which depend upon microbial action. In the production of sauerkraut, pickles, fermented sausages, and cheese the proper amount of salt provides an environment for the growth of the desirable bacteria. Even in the production of bread, salt controls the rate of growth of desirable yeast and prevents the development of undesirable types of yeast.

As a solubilizing agent, the use of salt goes back to 3000 B.C. Varying concentrations of brine are used to dissolve the different muscle proteins of meat in making sausage. This protein dissolved in a salt solution forms the "glue" which combines the meat, moisture, and fat into a gel texture—sausage. The name "sausage" comes from the Latin world "*salsus*," meaning salt.

CHEMICAL INDUSTRY. Much of the salt is utilized in the manufacture of other chemicals. By passing an electric current through salt—electrolysis—it can be broken up into sodium metal and chlorine gas. The sodium can be used as a catalyst, or it can combine with other elements to form new chemicals such as sodium carbonate, sodium bicarbonate, and lye (sodium hydroxide). The chlorine formed by electrolysis can also be used to make other chemicals, or it can be employed in bleaching paper and textiles, or in disinfecting water supplies. Many of the chemicals derived from salt find their way into numerous other industries.

OTHER INDUSTRIES AND BUSINESSES. Salt is important to a number of other industries and businesses. The leather industry uses salt for the preservation of hides. Salt can be employed to soften water. Railroads use salt to keep their switches from icing up. Highway departments use salt on icy roads, and on secondary roads to stabilize the soil and control the dust. Farmers feed salt to livestock. It is also employed in heat-treating, smelting, and refining metals. The list of uses seems endless for this basic chemical.

EXCESS SALT; LABELING. For years, the subject of salt and its relation to hypertension has been debated by consumers, federal officials, and food industry representatives. Finally, in 1981, for the first time, the food industry was asked by the Food and Drug

Administration to lower the salt content in foods, voluntarily and not by regulation. In support of the request, Richard S. Schweiker, Secretary of Health and Human Service, had the following to say:

"Sixty million Americans suffer from hypertension, which can lead to strokes and heart attacks. Hypertension can be significantly controlled."

At about the same time, a bill was introduced in the U.S. Congress that would *require* food processors and manufacturers to disclose through a label the salt content of their products if the salt is above a certain level. Also, it was revealed that the FDA had drafted a regulation that would *require* sodium labeling, but it would have to be approved by the Office of Management and Budget before it could be instituted.

The FDA, which has jurisdiction over about 80% of all processed foods, indicated that labeling would apply to both natural and added salt in a product.

Simultaneously, the U.S. Department of Agriculture announced that the department plans to encourage sodium disclosure for meat products under its jurisdiction through similar action to that of the FDA.

(Also see SODIUM, section headed "Recommended Daily Allowance of Sodium.")

SOURCES OF SALT. The United States is by far the leading salt-producing country. The states of Louisiana, Texas, New York, and Ohio produce 88% of U.S. salt. In 1985, 39.5 million tons of salt, worth $741.8 million, were taken from the seas, mines, and wells in the United States.

Sea Salt. About 13% of the salt in the United States is taken from the seas which contain about ¼ lb of salt per gallon (*30 g/liter*). However, large inland seas like the Great Salt Lake, the Dead Sea, and the Red Sea contain a higher concentration of salt. Salt from the seas is obtained by collecting the sea water in holding areas and then allowing the water to evaporate off leaving behind the salt and other minerals. This is called the solar process, and it is thousands of years old. Salt is harvested from the Great Salt Lake in this manner. Impurities in solar salt make it unsatisfactory for commercial food use.

Mine Salt. About 34% of the U.S. salt production comes from mines, which are mined in much the same way as deep coal mines. Shafts are sunk to the deposit of salt, and miners break the rock salt loose before it is transported to the surface for refining processes.

Brine Well Salt. Most of the salt, 53%, produced in the United States comes from brine wells. To obtain salt, two pipes are driven into the underground salt deposit. Water is pumped down to the salt bed via one pipe, and after dissolving some salt, the brine is pumped to the surface via the other pipe. The brine is then evaporated during refining processes, or used in industry as a brine.

Due to the abundance of salt today, a person would be offended if he received part of his salary in salt as did the Roman soldiers. Nevertheless, salt still holds a respected position among the chemicals, and it is the major source for two of the major electrolytes of the body. (Also see ADDITIVES; MINERAL[S]; and SODIUM.)

SALT DIET, LOW

Low salt diet is a rather misleading term. Since table salt is by far the most important source of sodium in the diet, most sodium-restricted diets begin with the elimination or at least restricted use of table salt on food. Hence, sodium-restricted diets are sometimes called low salt diets. A mild sodium restriction which is used as a maintenance diet in cardiac and renal diseases limits daily sodium intake to 2,000 to 3,000 mg. This means no salty foods and no salt used at the table. Other sodium-restricted diets include moderate sodium restriction (1,000 to 1,500 mg daily), strict sodium restriction (500 mg), and severe sodium restriction (250 mg). All of these diets require limited or no use of salt at all stages of food preparation. The strict and severe sodium restriction necessitates careful selection of foods for all sources of sodium, not just salt.

(Also see MODIFIED DIETS.)

SALT FOODS, LOW

Table salt—sodium chloride—is the most important source of sodium in the diet. Salt may be added to foods during processing, during cooking, and at the table by the consumer. When an individual requires the restriction of daily sodium intake, the first step involves limiting the intake of salt. Depending upon the level of sodium restriction, foods may need to be carefully selected in regards to the amount of salt used in processing. However, salt is not the only source of sodium in foods, so if a strict or severe restriction of sodium is needed, all sources of sodium in foods must be considered. Other sodium sources include baking soda, baking powder, sodium benzoate, sodium citrate, monosodium glutamate (MSG), sodium propionate, and sodium alginate. When selecting foods for sodium restricted diets, labels should be noted for the words "salt" and "sodium." Furthermore, some foods possess a naturally high level of sodium and must be used in measured amounts in sodium restricted diets.

(Also see MODIFIED DIETS; SALT; and SODIUM.)

SALT-FREE DIETS

A more accurate description of these diets is sodium restricted or low sodium. Since much of the sodium added to foods comes from table salt—sodium chloride—the first step in a sodium-restricted diet is the elimination of table salt. Hence, these diets are commonly called salt-free.

Sodium-restricted diets, varying in the amount of sodium restriction, are prescribed for the elimination, control, and prevention of edema—water accumulation in the tissues—which accompanies such things as congestive heart failure, cirrhosis, kidney disorders, and corticosteroid therapy. Sodium restriction is also helpful in control of some cases of high blood pressure.

For persons on sodium restricted diets, a 1:1 mixture of table salt (NaCl) and potassium chloride (KCL) for salting foods will lessen the sodium intake without a change in taste. However, excessive use of dietary potassium should be avoided due to toxic effects at high levels.

(Also see MODIFIED DIETS; HIGH BLOOD PRESSURE; and SODIUM.)

SALTINE

This is a thin crisp cracker covered with salt. All saltines are soda crackers, but not all soda crackers are saltines.

SALTPETER

A name sometimes applied to potassium nitrate; sodium nitrate is called Chile saltpeter.
(Also see NITRATES.)

SAMBAL

A condiment common to Indonesia and Malaya, eaten with curry and rice. Typically, it contains peppers, pickles, grated coconut, salt fish, or fish roe.

SAMP

Coarse hominy or a boiled cereal made from it.

SAPONIFICATION

The formation of soap and glycerol from the reaction of fat with alkali.

SAPONINS

A group of heart-stimulating glycosides derived from plants such as foxglove, squill, and legumes. They can be broken down into a sugar and a steroid. All saponins foam when shaken with water, and all are surface-active agents. When injected into the bloodstream they are capable of bursting (hemolyzing) red blood cells. Saponins are used as an emulsification agent for fats and oils, as a soap or detergent, and as a subject of research on steroid sex hormones.
(Also see POISONOUS PLANTS.)

SAPOTE, GREEN *Calocarpum viride*

The fruit of a tree (of the family *Sapotaceae*) that is native to Central America and Mexico. Green sapotes are 3 to 6 in. (*7.5 to 15 cm*) long and have a rich sweet flavor. They may be eaten fresh or used to make jam, jelly, or juice.

The nutrient composition of green sapotes is given in Food Composition Table F-36.

Some noteworthy observations regarding the nutrient composition of green sapotes follow:

1.   The peeled and seeded fruit is moderately high in calories (107 kcal per 100 g) and carbohydrates (27%).

2.   Green sapotes are a good source of vitamins A and C.

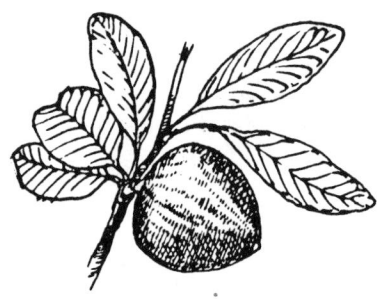

Fig. S-3.   The green sapote.

SARCOMA

A tumor of fleshy consistency—often highly malignant.

SATIETY

Full satisfaction of desire; may refer to satisfaction of appetite.
(Also see APPETITE.)

SATSUMA

This is a type of Japanese pottery, but it has lent its name to a particular type of mandarin orange, and also to one of the plums.

SATURATED

A state in which a substance holds the most of another substance that it can hold.

SATURATED FAT

A completely hydrogenated fat—each carbon atom is associated with the maximum number of hydrogens; there are no double bonds.

(Also see FATS AND OTHER LIPIDS.)

SAUCES

The word *sauce* comes from the Latin word *salsa* meaning *salted. A sauce can be defined as a liquid food, which is poured over a solid food.* It can appear on the menu from appetizer to dessert. It can range from liquid to very thick; from no seasoning to highly seasoned; from cold to piping hot; from sour to extremely sweet; from simple to complicated and rich; and from the same every time to never the same way twice.

Sauces do not take any great amount of time to make. Nevertheless, they should not be a neglected art, for, in the final analysis, the sauce often lifts up the dish: it glamorizes the simplest food; it gives the recipe distinction; it increases the appetite appeal; it is the crowning touch.

There are so many kinds of sauces that it is difficult to organize them into any kind of order; for instance, a white sauce can be used either for fish or for dessert, depending on the added flavorings and seasonings. Some of the basic sauces are presented in Table S-1, along with the most common ingredients and the popular ways to use them.

TABLE S-1
SAUCES FOR EVERYTHING

Name of Sauce	Basic Ingredients	Instructions and/or Popular Uses
For hors d'oeuvres and salads **French dressing**	Oil, vinegar, and seasonings.	French dressing is almost exclusively used for salads, either vegetable or fruit, depending on the seasonings.
Mayonnaise	Egg yolks, vinegar, oil, and seasonings.	Although mayonnaise and dressings are not called sauces, they may be so classified. Besides mixing with salad greens, mayonnaise can be mixed with minced meats, nuts, or cheese and used in sandwiches, canapes, or appetizers. Some casseroles call for the use of mayonnaise, also.
Salad dressings	Egg, milk, flour, vinegar, butter, seasonings.	Salad dressings are cooked. Because they contain considerably less oil than mayonnaise, they are lower in calories. They can be used interchangeably with mayonnaise.
For main dishes **Barbecue sauce**	Ketchup, onion, vinegar, Worcestershire sauce and other seasonings. Green pepper optional.	Barbecue sauce is a favorite for serving with steaks, hamburgers, shish kebab, barbecued ribs, etc. What would a barbecue be without barbecue sauce?

Name of Sauce	Basic Ingredients	Instructions and/or Popular Uses
Butter sauce	Butter, lemon juice, chopped parsley.	This is a simple, but good, sauce for fish dishes. There are many variations of butter sauces.
Cheese sauce	1. White sauce with cheese added. 2. Melted cheese with cream or milk added.	Used for egg dishes, fondus, pasta dishes, and vegetables.
Fruit sauces	Apple . . . . . . Cranberry. . Currant jelly Orange w/ or w/o pineapple Orange-currant . . Raisin . . . . . . Added ingredients: sugar, water, cornstarch, etc.	For game, goose, or pork. For turkey, of course. For game. For ham or tongue. For chicken, duck, ham, and lamb. For ham or tongue.
Gravies	Meat stock or juice; flour; added liquid if needed—water for beef or lamb, milk for chicken,	The juices extracted from meat during the cooking process are tasty and nutritious. They can be served either just as they come from the pan, or with some added water if necessary to dissolve the browned juices, or with some

(Continued)

TABLE S-1 (Continued)

Name of Sauce	Basic Ingredients	Instructions and/or Popular Uses
Gravies (Continued)	pork or ham; seasoning.	of the fat skimmed off. These are called *pan gravy* or *au jus*. Those who desire thickened gravy can have it as thin or as thick as desired. Do not add too much water; otherwise, the flavor will be lost.
Hollandaise sauce	Butter, egg yolks, boiling water, seasoning, lemon juice.	The butter is melted, the well-beaten eggs are added gradually, then the boiling water is stirred in slowly. This is an emulsion similar to mayonnaise, and in this case, if it is overcooked the emulsion will break down. At that point it must be beaten vigorously until smooth and creamy. This aristocrat of sauces is used mostly for fish, asparagus, broccoli, and cauliflower.
Tartar sauce	Mayonnaise, capers, olives, parsley, chopped pickles.	This is a favorite sauce for fish. There are many different recipes.
Tomato sauce and ketchup	Tomatoes, onion, cloves, flour, fat, salt and pepper.	It can be homemade or commercially produced. Tomato sauces have a wide variety of uses with pasta dishes and meats—especially hamburgers and wieners, and Mexican dishes.
White sauce	Butter, flour, milk, salt and pepper.	This is a basic sauce which can be as thin or as thick as desired, and can have any kind of added in-

Name of Sauce	Basic Ingredients	Instructions and/or Popular Uses
White sauce (Continued)		gredients. It can be used for fish, meats, poultry, and vegetables. Many casseroles have a white sauce as part of the recipe.
For desserts Chocolate sauce	Chocolate, water and/or milk, vanilla, sugar.	Chocolate sauce is used for cakes, ice cream, and parfaits.
Custard sauce	Eggs, milk, flavoring.	The custard is stirred while it is cooked in a double boiler. It can be served with a wide variety of desserts.
Fruit sauces	Mostly mashed berries and sugar. Optional: egg white, butter.	Usually, fruit sauces are not cooked. They are served over ice cream, cottage cake, cheese cake, or in parfaits, etc.
Hard sauce	Butter, powdered sugar, vanilla.	Cream butter and sugar, and add vanilla or other flavoring. This sauce can be used with any hot pudding, especially steamed plum pudding at Christmastime.
White sauce	Variations of white sauce are used for caramel, butterscotch, lemon, honey, and other sauces.	These sauces are used for ice creams, steamed puddings, cottage pudding, souffles, and bread puddings.

SAUERKRAUT

This is salted sliced cabbage that has undergone fermentation by lactic acid bacteria. In the fermentation process, the sugars of the cabbage are converted primarily to lactic and acetic acids, ethyl alcohol, and carbon dioxide.

The first description of sauerkraut manufacture, comparable to the methods used commercially today, was given by James Lind in 1772, in his treatise on scurvy. Barrels, kegs, and stone crocks were the common containers. Wooden vats were introduced in the United

States about 1885. Recently, reinforced concrete with plastic coatings and glazed tile vats have been introduced.

In most modern kraut factories, salt is weighed and applied at a 2.25% level to the shredded cabbage. Ordinarily, sauerkraut is left in the vats until completely fermented.

Very little kraut is retailed in bulk today. Most of it is canned, although the use of plastic and glass containers is increasing.

Sauerkraut is often eaten as an adjunct to other foods,

thereby making them more appetizing and digestible. It is generally recognized that when sauerkraut is cooked with other foods, particularly meats, it enhances their palatability.

(Also see CABBAGE, section headed "Preparation".)

SAUSAGE

Highly seasoned finely ground meat (usually pork or beef, but other meats may be used), most of which is stuffed in casings, used either fresh or cured.

(Also see MEAT[S], section headed "Sausage Making".)

SAUSAGE CASINGS

Natural casings are made from the middle wall of the small and large intestines of cattle, hogs, sheep, and goats. Also, the lung, bladder, and (in the case of hogs) the stomach are used as containers for special sausages.

Additionally, there are: cellulose casings, made from cotton linters; collagen casings, made from a collagen source, such as the corium layer of beef hide; and plastic netting made of polyethylene threads.

SCARLET RUNNER BEAN
Phaseolus coccineus

People in the European countries are fond of this legume from the Americas. The scarlet runner bean is similar in many respects to the common bean (*Phaeolus vulgaris*) to which it is closely related. Fig. S-4 shows the attractive bean plant.

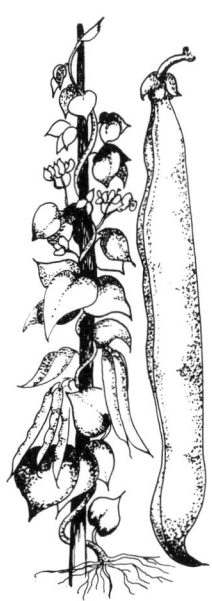

Fig. S-4. Scarlet runner bean.

ORIGIN AND HISTORY. There is archaeological evidence that the ancient American Indians in Mexico may have used this bean as food as early as 9,000 years ago, when the only source was wild plants. It is uncertain when the plant was first cultivated, but it is thought that domestication took place by 2000 B.C.

The bean was brought to England in the 17th century, where it was long grown as an ornamental plant. It was not until the 18th century that the Europeans utilized the scarlet runner for food. Today, it is a popular food plant in the cooler climates, which it tolerates better than the common bean.

PRODUCTION. Statistics for the annual production of this vegetable are not readily available because (1) commercial production is limited to Great Britain, (2) it is grown mainly on a small scale in home gardens in Europe, and (3) it is planted among other crops such as corn (maize) in the highlands of Central America. It is noteworthy that the scarlet runner bean is planted from seed each year in the cooler climates, but that it is a perennial in Central America. Also, the Europeans generally harvest the immature pods and seeds for utilization like snap beans, whereas the crop is allowed to grow to fuller maturity in Central America, where the green seeds, mature seeds, and fleshy tubers are consumed. Yields as high as 30,000 lb per acre (*33,600 kg/ha*) may be obtained when the soil has optimal fertility and the green beans are picked by hand throughout the growing season.

PROCESSING. Little commercial processing is done, because most of the crop is marketed fresh. However, European gardeners sometimes can some of the crop.

SELECTION AND PREPARATION. Any of the scarlet runner beans that are available in the United States are likely to have been grown in home gardens. Usually, they are utilized in the same ways as snap beans, which are very appetizing when cut lengthwise and sauteed with chopped bacon, onions, and/or garlic. However, some gardeners allow the seeds to mature in order to utilize them like kidney beans.

(Also see BEAN, COMMON.)

NUTRITIONAL VALUE. The nutrient composition of scarlet runner beans is given in Food Composition Table F-36.

Some noteworthy observations regarding the nutritive value of scarlet runner beans follow:

1. The dried mature seeds of the scarlet runner bean are very similar in composition to the seeds of the kidney bean. Therefore, it might be assumed that the nutritive values of the cooked dry beans of the two species are similar, and that 1 cup (*240 ml*) of the cooked mature runner beans contains about 14 g of protein (the amount in 2 oz [*57 g*] of lean meat) and 218 kcal (about twice the calories furnished by the equivalent amount of meat).

2. Immature pods and seeds are low in calories and other nutrients because of their high water content. However, they are a fair to good source of vitamins A and C.

3.   The dried mature seeds contain only about one-third as much calcium as phosphorus. (It is suspected that low dietary calcium to phosphorus ratios sometimes result in the poor utilization of calcium by the body.) Hence, foods higher in calcium and lower in phosphorus, such as dairy products and green vegetables, should also be consumed.

4.   Both the mature and the immature beans provide ample amounts of iron per calorie.

Protein Quantity and Quality.   Some of the people in the highlands of Central America utilize the dried mature beans as a staple food. Hence, certain facts concerning the bean protein are noteworthy:

1.   A 3½ oz (*100 g*) portion (about ½ cup) of the cooked beans furnishes about 118 Calories (kcal) and about 7 g of protein, the amount provided by 1 ¾ oz of cottage cheese (*53 kcal*) or 1 large egg (*82 kcal*).

2.   The protein quality of the dried beans is inferior to that of most animal proteins, because the bean protein is deficient in the sulfur-containing amino acids methionine and cystine.

3.   A cup of cooked dried beans (*about 185 g*) supplies from 14 to 15 g of protein, which ranges from 2 to 4 times the protein content of similar amounts of cooked cereal grains.

4.   The amino acid deficiencies of the beans are compensated for by the amino acid contents of most cereals, and vice versa. Hence, mixtures of beans and cereals have higher quality protein than either food alone.

(Also see BEAN[S], Table B-10 Beans of the World; and LEGUMES, Table L-2 Legumes of the World.)

SCHOOL LUNCH PROGRAM

Contents   *Page*

This program, which is administered by the U.S. Department of Agriculture (USDA), was established for the purposes of (1) safeguarding the health and well-being of American children and (2) encouraging the consumption of nutritious agricultural commodities and other foods. It operates by assisting the states, through grants-in-aid and other means, in the establishment, maintenance, conduct, and expansion of nonprofit school lunch pro-

grams. Hence, the costs of providing lunches are shared by the USDA, state and local government, and the recipients of the meals. The cost to the federal government of the school lunch program is shown in Fig. S-5.

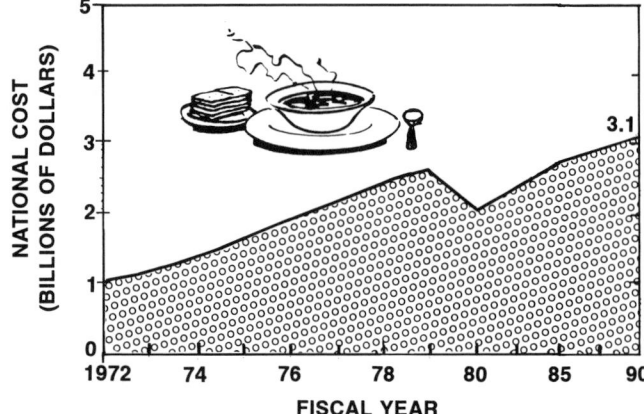

Fig. S-5.   The cost to the federal government for the school lunch program. (Source: *Statistical Abstract of the United States 1991*, Dept. of Commerce, p. 358, Table 584)

The school lunch program has expanded rapidly in response to (1) more children being transported to schools greater distances from their homes, (2) more mothers working away from home, (3) the desire of people and governments to provide improved nutrition to the children of the poor, and (4) low-cost, subsidized meals.

A good understanding of the school lunch program is important to parents and teachers who influence the child's eating habits.

HISTORY.   In the 1800s, Germany, France, and other European countries began to serve lunches in their public schools. From Europe, the program spread across the Atlantic.

The first organized school lunch program on record in the United States was started by the Children's Aid Society of New York in 1853, when the Society opened the first of its vocational schools for the poor. The next well-known program was established in 1894 by the Star Center Association of Philadelphia, in elementary schools. Later, the Philadelphia school board assumed responsibility for its support and operation.

By 1910, many American cities had penny-lunch programs in elementary schools, which were often started by voluntary organizations and later operated by the school administrations. In these programs, they usually served small portions of bread and butter, cocoa, and soup, at a total cost of 1 to 3¢.

It is noteworthy that a USDA bulletin published in 1916 suggested that milk, breads and cereals, butter, vegetables and fruits, and desserts be furnished in the schools so that the pupils would not be tempted to spend their lunch money in poorly kept shops that offered less wholesome items such as pickles, pies, starchy foods and sweets. The bulletin also noted that the school lunch was a "silent lesson" in food and nutrition for the pupils who were served.

The operation of the lunch programs in the rural areas in the first few decades of the 1900s differed from those in the cities in that (1) cold lunches were usually brought from home, (2) supplemental hot dishes were sometimes contributed by people in the community and prepared on a wood-burning stove by the teacher or volunteers, and (3) menu plans and recipes for the dishes served at lunch were often developed by federal and state extension home economists.

During the depression, assistance in feeding school children was provided by contributions from teachers, funds from voluntary organizations such as the American Friends Service Committee and the American Red Cross, and by appropriations from state and local governments. For example, in 1934 the State of New York appropriated $100,000 for free lunches and milk for poor children. One year later, federal funds from the Works Progress Administration (WPA) were provided to pay the cooks and servers of food in the schools.

Surplus agricultural commodities were distributed on a limited basis for free lunches as early as 1932. In 1935, the USDA was authorized by law to purchase and distribute the commodities on a much larger scale. By 1942, surplus foods were used to feed 6.2 million children.

The supplies of surplus agricultural commodities were greatly reduced by 1943 as a result of wartime demands. Hence, the USDA started a cash reimbursement program to pay schools for a part of the food purchased locally. However, the participating schools were required to (1) meet certain nutritional standards in the lunches served, (2) provide free meals for the children unable to pay, and (3) operate their lunch programs on a nonprofit basis. These provisions formed much of the basis for the National School Lunch Act of 1946, which placed the basic responsibility for the administration of school lunch programs in the hands of state educational agencies. Since then, the provisions of the original act have been modified several times by new laws that were enacted to bring about the serving of greater numbers of free and reduced-price lunches to needy children. Participating schools are provided (1) cash assistance, (2) donation of surplus food commodities, and (3) technical assistance in the purchase and use of foods and in the equipping and managing of the school lunchroom.

During the 1970s, authorizations and regulations were established for a Nutrition Education and Training Program (NET) that had the objectives of (1) teaching students about the relationships between food, nutrition, and health, (2) training food service personnel in the principles and skills of food service management, and (3) instructing teachers in sound principles of nutrition education.

At the present time, more than 90% of all elementary and secondary children attend schools that participate in the National School Lunch Program. On a typical day in 1990, lunches were served to 24.6 million children and adolescents. That year, the federal cost of school lunches was $3.2 billion. It is noteworthy, however, that more and more critics—who are concerned about the ever-increasing taxes needed to pay for the free and reduced-price lunches and other aspects of the program—are asking whether the benefits justify the costs. Hence, the future prospects of these services will depend in part on how well administrators answer this question.

PROVISIONS OF THE NATIONAL SCHOOL LUNCH ACT. The enactment of the National School Lunch Act of 1946 placed the school lunch program of the USDA on a firmer foundation, since up to that time the funds for its operation came mainly from customs receipt funds (import duties collected under Section 32 of the Agricultural Act of 1935) that were originally intended for the expansion of domestic and export markets for agricultural commodities. (The lunch program fulfilled this mission to a limited extent by utilizing surplus commodities.) Furthermore, it was felt that the new law would encourage the states to increase their commitments to the program. Therefore, the major provisions that formed the basis for policies which remained in effect for over 4 decades are noteworthy.

Funds for each of the states were allocated according to a formula based upon (1) the number of children in the state between the ages of 5 and 17, and (2) the state's per capita income. (It was felt that the states with large numbers of children from low-income families needed more assistance than those with few children and a high per capita income.) In addition to cash assistance, participating schools received donations of surplus food commodities and technical assistance in menu planning, purchasing food and equipment, sanitation practices, and management. However, eligibility for participation in this program is contingent upon (1) operating the program on a nonprofit basis, (2) providing free or reduced-price lunches to needy children, (3) making lunches available without regard to race, color, or national origin, (4) providing kitchen and dining facilities, (5) avoiding public identification or segregation of needy children, and (6) serving nutritious lunches that conform to USDA guidelines. "Type A" and "Type B" patterns for school lunches were established by the Secretary of Agriculture to provide guidance for lunchroom managers. Type B guidelines, which covered supplements for lunches brought from home, were later discontinued.

Guidelines for the well-known Type A lunches are given in Table S-2.

TABLE S-2
A TYPE-A   SCHOOL LUNCH[1,2]

Item	Quantity and Description
Fluid whole milk	1/2 pint (*240 ml*), served as a beverage.
Protein-rich food	2 oz (*57 g*) of cooked or canned lean meat, fish, or poultry; or items equivalent in protein value, such as 2 oz (*57 g*) cheese, 1 egg, 1/2 cup (*120 ml*) cooked dry beans or peas, 4 Tbsp (*60 ml*) peanut butter, or an equivalent of any combination of these foods in a main dish.
Vegetables and fruits	3/4 cup (*180 ml*), consisting of two or more servings. (One serving of full strength juice may be counted as not more than 1/4 cup (*60 ml*) of the requirement.)
Bread	1 slice of whole grain or enriched bread; or muffin, cornbread, biscuit, or roll made from enriched or whole grain flour.
Butter or fortified margarine	2 tsp (*10 ml*), as a spread, as a seasoning, or in food preparation.

[1]Adapted by the authors from *National School Lunch Program*, Bull. PA-19, USDA, 1959.

[2]It is also recommended that an ascorbic acid-rich food be served daily and that a vitamin A-rich food be served at least twice a week. Several sources of iron should be included each day.

BENEFITS OF THE SCHOOL LUNCH.   Some of the main benefits of the National School Lunch Program follow:

1.   For over 2 decades most of the children attending public and private schools in all 50 states, the District of Columbia, Puerto Rico, the Virgin Islands, and Guam have had the opportunity to obtain a school lunch.

2.   Many needy children have been served nutritious lunches which they would not likely have received through other means. Fig. S-6 shows that the numbers of children receiving free or reduced-price lunches increased steadily throughout the 1980s.

3.   School lunches have provided about one-third of the Recommended Dietary Allowances for school children on a daily basis.

4.   Recent modifications in the food patterns have provided pupils with experiences in (1) eating foods used mainly by minority ethnic groups (items such as bulgur wheat and corn grits), and (2) new types of food preparations (such as meat dishes extended with soy protein).

Children in the National School Lunch Program

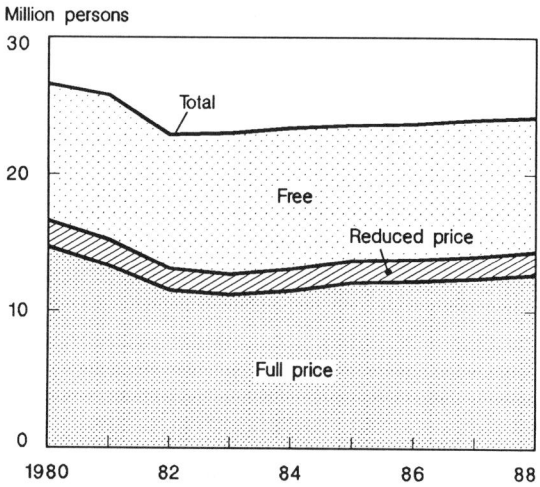

Fig. S-6.   The number of children in the National School Lunch Program during the 1980s. (Source: *1989 Agricultural Chartbook*, USDA Ag. Hdbk. No. 684, p. 70)

5.   Teachers have been motivated by students' comments on their lunches to spend more time discussing foods, health, and nutrition subjects.

6.   Children, parents, teachers, and community groups have had opportunities to contribute viewpoints regarding the types of foods served. Some of these groups have been successful in making significant improvements in their local programs. For example, whole wheat pizza, sprouts, yogurt, and other highly nutritious foods are now served in certain local schools.

7.   Poorly equipped and staffed schools have received both financial and technical assistance in developing better cooking and serving facilities and in upgrading the education and training of their personnel.

8.   Surplus commodities have been utilized profitably and have helped to keep the prices of the lunches within the means of the students.

9.   Local food suppliers have benefited from the purchases made for the program.

10.   States have been induced to contribute some of their revenues to the program. At first, the state contributions came mainly from the payments of school children for the lunches.

PROBLEMS.   Some of the main problems that have long plagued the lunch program follow:

1. Local communities may decide not to participate, or not to serve any food whatever to pupils. For example, it was largely through the efforts of mothers that certain cities in Michigan established lunch programs in the 1970s.

2. Students may spend their money on competitive foods instead of on school lunches. Fig. S-7 shows the factors present in or around various types of schools that tend to reduce the purchasing of school lunches.

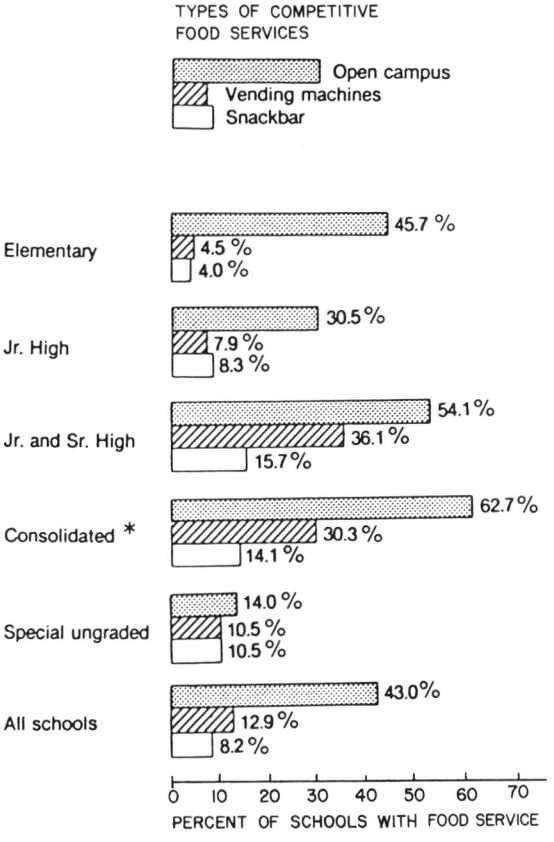

TYPES OF COMPETITIVE
FOOD SERVICES

  Open campus
  Vending machines
  Snackbar

Elementary
45.7 %
4.5 %
4.0 %

Jr. High
30.5%
7.9 %
8.3 %

Jr. and Sr. High
54.1 %
36.1 %
15.7 %

Consolidated *
62.7 %
30.3 %
14.1 %

Special ungraded
14.0 %
10.5 %
10.5 %

All schools
43.0%
12.9 %
8.2 %

0 10 20 30 40 50 60 70
PERCENT OF SCHOOLS WITH FOOD SERVICE

* CONSOLIDATED SCHOOLS ARE THOSE OFFERING ELEMENTARY THROUGH SENIOR HIGH AND SPECIAL SCHOOLS.

Fig. S-7.   The average prevalences of food services that compete with school lunches. (Source: *1980 Handbook of Agricultural Charts*, USDA, p. 59, Chart 148)

For example, an open campus (students are allowed to leave the school grounds during lunchtime) means that foods may be bought from local food establishments. Unfortunately, the prices of balanced meals outside of the school often are beyond the means of many students. Hence, they are likely to purchase various types of snacks and soft drinks. This type of competition is also present within the schools in the form of vending machines and snack bars that may be favored by school administrations because they generate an income for supporting various activities. Sometimes, parents, teachers, and community groups have been able to have nutritious foods served by the competitive food services.

3. The amounts of waste food left on the plates of children are much greater than they should be, since in most cases the portions are small to moderate in size compared to what many pupils are served at home. It seems that the fullest garbage pails result from the serving of the highly nutritious vegetables such as broccoli. Often, the reduction of waste comes down to catering to the tastes of the students, which may strengthen poor eating habits that have already been formed.

4. Kitchens in each of the schools within a district may be wasteful because an average of only 8 to 12 lunches per worker hour is prepared in the smaller schools, whereas districts with central kitchens that utilize trucks to deliver meals to individual schools ("satellite systems") average 18 to 24 lunches per worker hour.

5. The sudden availability of certain surplus commodities has often taxed the ingenuity of school food service managers to utilize the foods in ways that are both acceptable to students and within the guidelines of the USDA.

RECENT CHANGES IN POLICIES.   During the late 1960s and early 1970s, Congress increased the appropriations for the school lunch program by considerable amounts to ensure that every needy child would be able to receive a free or reduced-price lunch. Furthermore, legislation passed in 1975 made more children eligible for reduced-price lunches. However, efforts in the late 1970s to curtail federal spending and to balance the national budget led to investigations of how funding for the program might be reduced. It seems likely that substantial changes in funding will be made in the near future. Therefore, only the recent policy changes which affect the types of food served in the schools will be presented here. An outline of recently published USDA guidelines is given in Table S-3.

TABLE S-3
SCHOOL LUNCH GUIDELINES[1]
(Minimum amounts of foods listed by food components to serve students of various age/grade groups)

Food Component and Description	Preschool Children		Elementary School Students		Secondary School Students
	Group I (1 and 2 years of age)	Group II (3 and 4 years of age)	Group III (5, 6, 7, and 8 years of age; or Grades 1 to 3)	Group IV (9, 10, and 11 years of age; or Grades 4 to 6)	Group V (12 years of age and over; or Grades 7 to 12)
	(amount per day)	(amount per day)	(amount per day)	(amount per day)	(amount per day)
Meat and meat alternates[2] Meat—a serving (edible portion) of cooked lean meat, poultry, or fish. Alternates: The following meat alternates may be used alone or in combination to meet the meat/meat alternate requirement:[3] Cheese (1 oz = 1 oz of meat), eggs (1 large egg = 1 oz of meat), cooked dry beans or peas (1/2 cup [120 ml] = 1 oz meat),[4] peanut butter (2 Tbsp [30 ml] = 1 oz of meat)	1 oz (28 g)	1 1/2 oz (43 g)	1 1/2 oz (43 g)	2 oz (57 g)	3 oz (85 g)
Vegetables and fruits 2 or more servings consisting of vegetables or fruits or both (A serving of full strength vegetable or fruit juice can be counted to meet not more than 1/2 of the total requirement.)	1/2 cup (120 ml)	1/2 cup (120 ml)	1/2 cup (120 ml)	3/4 cup (180 ml)	3/4 cup (180 ml)
Bread and bread alternates[5] 1 serving (1 slice) of enriched or whole-grain bread, or a serving of biscuits, rolls, muffins, etc. made with whole-grain or enriched meal or flour, or a serving (1/2 cup [120 ml], of cooked enriched or whole-grain rice, macaroni, noodles, and other pasta products[6]	5 servings per week	8 servings per week	8 servings per week	8 servings per week	10 servings per week
Milk, fluid[7] Unflavored fluid lowfat milk, skim milk, or buttermilk must be offered as a beverage. If a school serves whole or flavored milk, it must offer unflavored fluid lowfat milk, skim milk, or buttermilk as a beverage choice.	3/4 cup (180 ml)	3/4 cup (180 ml)	1/2 pint (240 ml)	1/2 pint (240 ml)	1/2 pint (240 ml)

[1]Adapted by the authors from *Code of Federal Regulations*, Title 7, Revised January 1, 1980, Part 210, Sec. 210.19b.

[2]It is recommended that in schools not offering a choice of meat/meat alternate each day, no one form of meat (ground, sliced, pieces, etc.) or meat alternate be served more than three times per week. Meat and meat alternates must be served in a main dish, or in a main dish and one other menu item.

[3]When it is determined that the serving size of a meat alternate is excessive, the particular meat alternate shall be reduced and supplemented with an additional meat/meat alternate to meet the full requirement.

[4]Cooked dry beans or peas may be used as the meat alternate or as part of the vegetable/fruit component, but not as both food components in the same meal.

[5]One-half or more slices of bread or an equivalent amount of bread alternate must be served with each lunch with the total requirement being served during a 5-day period. Schools serving lunch 6 or 7 days per week should increase the quantity specified for a 5-day week by approximately 20% for each additional day.

[6]Enriched macaroni products with fortified protein may be used as part of a meat alternate or a bread alternate, but not as both food components in the same meal.

[7]One-half pint of milk may be used for all age/grade groups if the lesser specified amounts are determined by the school authority to be impractical.

GOAL OF THE SCHOOL LUNCH PROGRAM.

The goal of the school lunch program should be twofold:

1. The lunches offered to children should be nutritionally adequate and designed to develop and encourage the child's liking for a wide variety of the protective foods which frequently are not included in home diets.

2. The meals should be closely linked to the school's education program for better health.

These objectives merit further implementation. They need to be carried out by informed food service managers, cooks, and helpers in thousands of participating schools in every section of the country.

In addition to school lunches, it is noteworthy that, today, more and more children eat at least one meal outside the home—in day nurseries, child-care centers, day-care centers, or nursery schools. Usually, the noon meal is provided.

A sound school lunch program can help to improve the diets and food habits of children, and, thus, eventually lead to better diets and food habits for the population as a whole. This goal merits the support of federal, state, and local governments, and of parents and school officials.

SCLERODERMA

One of the first signs of scleroderma is tight, firm skin, and eventually a diffuse thickening and rigidity of the skin and subcutaneous tissue. These changes in the skin are reflected in the name of this disease, which means "hard skin." Sometimes the disease is called "hidebound skin." As the disease progresses, it involves the internal organs, specifically the intestinal tract, the heart, and the kidneys.

The cause of scleroderma is unknown. It belongs to a larger group of diseases sometimes classed as collagen diseases. In scleroderma, the changes in the skin and internal organs seem to be due to the overproduction of collagen—connective tissue.

There is no specific treatment for scleroderma. Corticosteroid therapy may slow the disease, or produce improvement in the early stages. This may require a sodium-restricted diet to prevent sodium retention during corticosteroid therapy. As the disease progresses, swallowing difficulties and a malabsorption syndrome may be encountered, which require some dietary adjustments.

(Also see MODIFIED DIETS.)

SCRAPPLE

Made from head meat, feet, hearts, tongues, shoulder spare ribs, fresh picnic shoulders, or any pork trimmings that contain some fat. Liver may be used if desired. Twenty percent of the meat may consist of beef or veal, but all pork is preferable.

Cook the meat in sufficient water to keep it covered; drain off the liquid when the meat separates readily from the bones. Remove the bones, then grind the meat. Place the ground meat and the liquor in which it was cooked together in a kettle and bring it to a boil.

Mix meal or flour (cornmeal, oatmeal, buckwheat flour, or soybean flour) with some water or some of the meat juice, add slowly and work the cereal to avoid lumps. Pour the diluted meal or flour into the cooked meat, season with condiments and herbs, and cook for another 30 minutes. Pour into a mold to cool, and serve sliced and fried.

SCREENED

A ground material that has been separated into various-sized particles by passing over or through screens.

SCREENINGS

By-products obtained from screening grains and other seeds.

SCURVY

Contents   Page

A severe deficiency of ascorbic acid (vitamin C) results in a specific disease called scurvy. The major lesions of scurvy are believed to be due to an impairment in the formation of connective tissue which requires ascorbic acid for its synthesis and repair. This impairment leads to pathologies of bone, teeth, skin, muscle, joints, adrenal glands, and blood vessels. Also, scurvy may be accompanied by hemorrhages of the adrenal glands and a gross impairment of adrenal function. If scurvy is not promptly treated, internal hemorrhages of increasing severity occur and death may follow.

HISTORY OF SCURVY. Although disorders resembling scurvy were described in ancient medical writings (such as *Papyrus Ebers* in Egypt about 1550 B.C., and in Greek and Roman writings), the causative agent was frequently attributed to a plague or other infectious diseases. Perhaps this happened because scurvy may be accompanied by lesions that resemble those associated with certain contagious diseases. The northern European cities, where the main foods during the winter were meat and bread, had high incidences of scurvy in the late winter and early spring. Countryfolk, however, were more fortunate in having preserved from their land some vegetables for winter food.

Most long sea voyages suffered large losses of men from scurvy. The greatest number of outbreaks occurred, however, after the change from oar-driven vessels which traveled only short distances from land, to sail-powered ships which traversed the high seas. There was not enough time during short voyages for depletion of the vitamin C stored in the tissues. Fresh fruits were not generally carried aboard such ships, since it was feared that they might spoil, and thereby cause diarrhea.

There were many reports of scurvy in overseas explorations during the 16th, 17th, and 18th centuries. For example, many men with the French explorer, Cartier, came down with scurvy during his second voyage to Newfoundland in 1535; but fortunately the Indians showed his crew how to cure the disease with a drink made from spruce needles. About this time, physicians and nava commanders tried various remedies. In 1564, Ronsseas, a Dutch physician, recommended that oranges be provided to protect sailors against scurvy.

The tragic experiences of British Admiral Hawkins (deaths of thousands of his sailors from scurvy) led him to give lemon juice to his men in 1593 (it cured the disease). In the *Surgeon's Mate*, written by Woodall in 1617, it was recommended that lemon juice, sweetened with sugar and mixed with brandy, be used as a medicine against scurvy. Cockburn's book, *Sea Diseases or A Treatise of Their Nature, Cause, and Cure* (1696), suggested a number of remedies for scurvy, such as fresh fruits and vegetables, dilute sulfuric acid, vinegar, salt water, cinnamon, and whey. Thus, the idea of using citrus fruits did not originate with the Scottish naval surgeon, Lind. However, Lind conducted the first controlled experiment in the treatment of scurvy in 1753, by giving different groups of sailors supplements of either cider, dilute sulfuric acid, vinegar, sea water, or oranges and lemons. The citrus fruits were found to be the only effective prevention and cure for scurvy. It was not until over 50 years later, however, that British sailors came to be known as "limeys," due to the suggestion of another Scottish physician, Blane, who managed to put Lind's findings into practice.

In three long sea voyages between 1758 and 1779, the British explorer, Captain Cook, demonstrated that scurvy could be prevented if the use of greens and fruits was strenuously enforced. In spite of all these demonstrations, it was tragic that, in the American Civil War, both sides suffered from scurvy and, in 1912, half of the British polar expedition under Captain Scott died of scurvy at the South Pole.

The first production of scurvy in an experimental animal was accomplished in 1907 by Holst and Frolich. These Norwegian investigators showed that it was necessary to supplement a ration of oats, rye, and rice, with vegetables and fruits, in order to protect guinea pigs against scurvy. This was a landmark experiment because only guinea pigs, monkeys, and man require vitamin C in their diets; other species are able to synthesize this substance in their livers. These investigators also found that substances which did not normally protect against scurvy (dried grains and legumes—such as oats, barley, peas, beans, and lentils) developed the ability to protect against scurvy when they were germinated into sprouts.

The concept of vitamins was born in 1912 when Hopkins, in England, showed that animals apparently required in their diet small amounts of what he called "accessory food factors." At the same time, Funk, a Polish scientist working in London, developed the concept of special organic compounds called "vitamines" (later changed to vitamins). In 1928, Szent-Gyorgyi, a Hungarian biochemist, working in Hopkin's laboratory, isolated "hexuronic acid" from orange and cabbage juices and adrenal glands of animals. That same year, King, at the University of Pittsburgh, showed that hexuronic acid was vitamin C. In 1933, the British chemist, Haworth, determined the structure of ascorbic acid and Reichstein, of Switzerland, synthesized ascorbic acid. These investiga-

tions made possible the development of a commercial synthesis of vitamin C from glucose. As a result, vitamin C can now be made in very large quantities and at a low cost.

CAUSES OF SCURVY. Today, this disease is more likely to be found in infants than in adults because (1) the requirements of infants for ascorbic acid are proportionately higher than those of adults due to the special role of the vitamin in the growth of tissues; (2) cow's milk, which is the main food of infants, has much of its ascorbic acid destroyed during pasteurization, whereas mother's breast milk contains sufficient amounts of the vitamin to prevent scurvy; and (3) other foods usually fed to infants, such as cereals and meats, also are low in vitamin C.

Some adults do not eat any vegetables or fruits, while others eat only overcooked vegetables with most of the vitamin C destroyed during cooking. There is less likelihood of these persons developing scurvy now than formerly, since there are presently many fruit drinks which are fortified with ascorbic acid. Even cocktail mixes may contain the vitamin.

Older persons, living on reduced incomes, may be susceptible to scurvy if they fail to eat fresh produce. These persons are more likely to be depleted of the stores of the vitamin than others due to the greater chances of their being subjected to stresses such as chronic diseases, injuries, and surgery. It appears that the destruction of vitamin C within the body is hastened by stress since the secretion of stress hormones, such as ACTH from the pituitary and corticosteroids from the adrenal cortex, is accompanied by a marked decrease in the amounts of ascorbic acid present in the adrenals.

In recent times, very few persons are known to have died from scurvy, except, perhaps, prisoners of war and malnourished infants. However, mild cases of scurvy might render people more susceptible to other disorders which may lead to death.

SIGNS AND SYMPTOMS OF SCURVY. Prior to the appearance of specific signs of the disease, the victim may feel feeble and listless, be short of breath, and have slow healing of wounds. Next, there develops the characteristic feature of swollen, bleeding gums (gingivitis), which may become at least slightly infected and impart a foul odor to the breath. Sometimes, there is loosening or loss of teeth. Another early sign of scurvy is the minute hemorrhages (petechiae) which appear around the hair follicles on the abdomen, buttocks, arms, and legs. As the disease progresses, these petechiae merge into larger hemorrhagic areas or bruises, which are unusual in that they occur in the absence of trauma. At this stage of the disease, the victim usually experiences severe pain in his or her bones, joints, and muscles.

Fig. S-8 depicts the afflictions which often accompany scurvy.

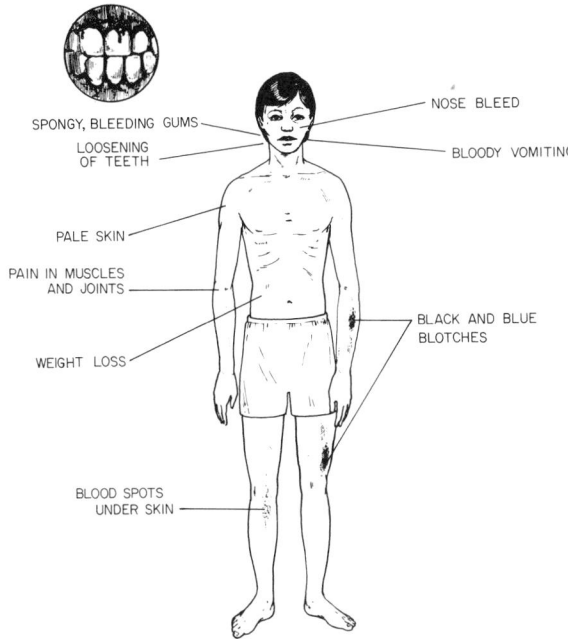

Fig. S-8. Signs and symptoms of scurvy.

Special Features of Scurvy In Infants. The first signs and symptoms of scurvy in infants differ from those in adults because the infant has special requirements for ascorbic acid to sustain growth and development. Thus, early features of infant scurvy may be retarded growth, irritability, lack of appetite, and shrinking from the touch of others in anticipation of pain. Soon, the infant may assume the "frog-legs" position (lying on its back, with the thighs spread widely apart and the legs flexed at the knees). There may also be bone malformations such as "bayonet chest" (a condition in which the breastbone or sternum gradually slopes out from the collarbone, then is indented sharply at its tip due to the sinking of the chest wall just above the belly) and beading of the ribs like that which occurs in rickets. Sometimes, there may be bloody stools or urine and discoloration of the eyelids.

TREATMENT AND PREVENTION OF SCURVY. Sudden death sometimes occurs in severe scurvy, so prompt and aggressive treatment is necessary. The usual treatment consists of ascorbic acid in doses as high as 250 mg each, four times a day, for a week. The purpose of such high levels is to achieve rapid saturation of the body fluids with ascorbic acid so as to hasten the healing of diseased tissues. Excesses of the vitamin are excreted in the urine, so there is little danger of large doses over a *short* period of time. The long-term effects of such dosage may be hazardous. When the crisis has passed, sufficient amounts of the vitamin may be provided by diets which contain one or more servings per day of fresh fruits or vegetables. Vitamin tablets may need to be provided for persons who do not eat such foods.

Although it has been estimated that as little as 10 mg per day of ascorbic acid will prevent scurvy, such a low intake is not likely to provide a reserve against such unexpected stresses as disease, trauma, and chilling. The Recommended Dietary Allowances (RDAs)[1] are 60 mg per day of ascorbic acid for adult males and for adult females who are neither pregnant nor lactating.

Infants should receive 30 mg of vitamin C from birth to 6 months of age, and 35 mg from 6 to 12 months of age. Therefore, at least one rich source of ascorbic acid (such as orange juice) should be given to a baby each day. In the event that citrus juices are not tolerated well, there are vitamin C drops which may be put in the drinking water.

(Also see DEFICIENCY DISEASES, Table D-1 Major Dietary Deficiency Diseases; and VITAMIN C.)

SEAFOOD

This refers to marine fish and shellfish used as food. A great variety of food is prepared from many species of fish and shellfish. Seafood products are preserved by refrigerating, freezing, canning, salting, smoking, pickling, dehydrating, or by combinations of these processes. In many countries, seafoods serve as a principle source of protein and an important source of fat, minerals, and vitamins in the diet.

(Also see FISH AND SEAFOOD[S].)

SEA KALE *Crambe maritiima*

This is a European perennial herb that has a fleshy branching rootstalk and is sometimes cultivated for its large ovate long-stalked leaves which are used as a potherb.

SEAWEED (KELP)

Any plant that grows in the sea is a seaweed. Botanically, seaweeds are algae.

For centuries, seaweed has been used as a food for humans and animals; prized for its minerals and vitamins.

The ancient Chinese thought highly of seaweed and made offerings of it as a food to their ancestors; and, in 800 B.C., mention was made of seaweed in a Chinese book of poetry. In his *Natural History*, in the 1st century A.D., Pliny the Elder referred to the use of seaweed. The Greeks are known to have used seaweed to treat intestinal disorders and to counteract goiter, despite knowing nothing about iodine. On his first voyage to America, Columbus' ships passed through masses of seaweed floating in the Atlantic Ocean.

[1]*Recommended Dietary Allowances,* 10th rev. ed., Food and Nutrition Board, NRC-National Academy of Sciences, 1989.

• **Many names and varieties of seaweed**—One of the most confusing things about seaweed is the various names by which it is known; among them, seaweed, agar-agar, algae, carrageenan, dulse, Iceland moss, Irish moss, kelp, laver, rockweed, and sea lettuce. It has been estimated that there are some 2,500 varieties of marine plants; so, seaweed embraces a great variety of plants of many hues, shapes, and sizes. It is noteworthy, too, that seaweed is one of the few members of plant life that has remained unchanged for centuries, since its cultivation and growth is still controlled by the elements—not man.

Seaweeds are algae, of which there are four principal groups:

> Brown algae
> Red algae
> Green algae
> Blue-green algae

When the botanist speaks of seaweed, he usually means one of the larger brown or red algae. The seaweeds of cold waters are chiefly brown algae; those of the tropics are mainly red algae.

Although seaweeds occur at depths of up to 100 ft (*30 meters*), certain red algae grow as deep as 600 ft (*180 meters*).

The giant seaweed of the Pacific, a type of brown algae, is commonly known as *kelp*. The "stems" of these huge weeds sometimes grow more than 200 ft (*61 meters*) long. There are said to be over 800 species of kelp.

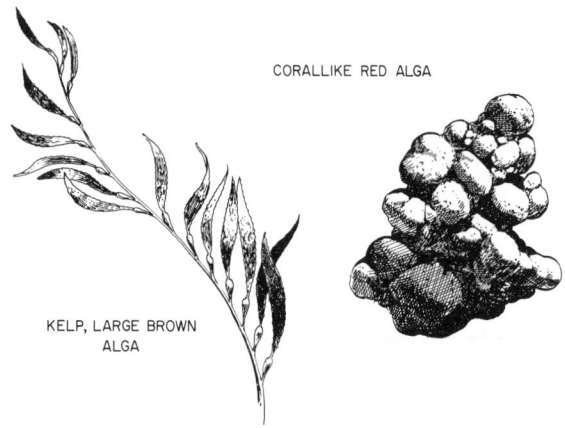

CORALLIKE RED ALGA

KELP, LARGE BROWN ALGA

Fig. S-9.   Kelp, the large brown alga of the Pacific ocean; and corallike red alga, of subtropical waters.

• **Processing**—The giant seaweed (kelp) off the coast of California is mechanically harvested by specially equipped barges, following which it is unloaded by a mechanical fork, artifically dried, then ground. After grinding, the resultant meal is olive green in color. The best of the harvest is reserved for the production of kelp tablets and seaweed powder for human consumption, while the bulk of the crop is marketed for livestock feed.

• **Composition of seaweed**—The Norwegian Seaweed Institute reports the following proximate analysis of seaweed:

Component	Percent
Protein	5.7
Fat	2.6
Fiber	7.0
Nitrogen-free extract	58.6
Ash	15.4
Moisture	10.7
	100.0

Contrary to claims that are sometimes made, seaweeds are low in protein, and the protein is of very low biological value.

The Norwegian Seaweed Institute has found an assortment of 60 different mineral elements in seaweed, all harnessed from the sea (see Table S-4). Additionally, seaweed contains carotene, vitamin D, vitamin K, and most of the water-soluble vitamins, including vitamin B-12.

The nutritive value of seaweed is affected by species, geographic area, season of the year, and temperature of the water. But it is always a rich source of iodine. Moreover, seaweed cumulates iodine; the iodine content of seaweed can be as much as 20,000 times more than that of the sea water in which the plants grew. Dried kelp (seaweed) contains 62,400 mcg of iodine per 100 g, whereas iodized salt contains only 7,600 mcg per 100 g; hence, dried seaweed contains more than 8 times as much iodine as iodized salt.

CAUTION: Dried kelp (seaweed) is so rich in iodine that consumption of a large amount for a prolonged period may be harmful; hence, it should be taken according to directions.

(Also see IODINE, section headed "Toxicity.")

• **Uses**—Seaweed has many important uses. Mention has already been made of seaweed as a staple food for humans and animals. For human food, kelp can be used in a variety of ways. In powdered form, it can be added to soups, salads, cottage cheese, tomato juice, fruit juices, or sprinkled on baked potatoes. Some persons use it as a salt substitute. Also, it is made into tablets and sold as a mineral-vitamin supplement in health food stores. About 25% of all food consumed in Japan consists of one form or another of seaweed (sea-vegetable), prepared and served in many forms.

Seaweed has many important uses, in addition to food. It has long been harvested and made into fertilizers. During World War I, giant kelp was harvested and made into explosives. Chemists extract large amounts of iodine and algin from seaweeds. Algin has many commercial uses because it can hold several different liquids together. In ice cream, it keeps the water in the milk from forming crystals. In the food and bakery industry, it is used for thickening, gelling, or binding products. It is also used in salad dressings, chocolate milk, aspirin, and in other foods and drugs.

TABLE S-4
MINERAL ELEMENTS IN DRIED SEAWEED[1]
(Average Analysis, Norwegian Brown Variety)

Element	Percent	Element	Percent
Ag Silver	.000004	Mg Magnesium	.213000
Al Aluminum	.193000	Mn Manganese	.123500
Au Gold	.000006	Mo Molybdenum	.001592
B Boron	.019400	N Nitrogen	1.467000
Ba Barium	.001276	Na Sodium	4.180000
Be Beryllium	Trace	Ni Nickel	.003500
Bi Bismuth	Trace	O Oxygen	Undeclared
Br Bromin	Trace	Os Osmium	Trace
C Carbon	Undeclared	P Phosphorus	.211000
Ca Calcium	1.904000	Pb Lead	.000014
Cb Niobium	Trace	Pd Palladium	Trace
Cd Cadmium	Trace	Pl Platinum	Trace
Ce Cerium	Trace	Ra Radium	Trace
Cl Chlorin	3.680000	Rb Rubidium	.000005
Co Cobalt	.001227	Rh Rhodium	Trace
Cr Chromium	Trace	S Sulphur	1.564200
Cs Caesium	Trace	Se Selenium	.000043
Cu Cupper	.000635	Sb Antimony	.000142
F Fluorin	.032650	Si Silicon	.164200
Fe Iron	.089560	Sn Tin	.000006
Ga Gallium	Trace	Sr Strontium	.074876
Ge Germanium	.000006	Te Tellurium	Trace
H Hydrogen	Undeclared	Th Thorium	Trace
Hg Mercury	.000190	Ti Titanium	.000012
I Iodine	.062400	Tl Thallium	.000293
Id Indium	Trace	U Uranium	.000004
Ir Irridium	Trace	V Vanadium	.000531
K Potassium	1.280000	W Tungsten	.000033
La Lantanum	.000019	Zn Zinc	.003516
Li Lithium	.000007	Zr Zirconium	Trace

[1]Data from the Norwegian Seaweed Institute, as reported in *Review of Seaweed Research*, Research Series No. 76, Clemson University, 1966.

Seaweed is sometimes promoted for its therapeutic properties in alleviating constipation, gastric catarrh, mucous colitis, and other disorders. But these claims need to be substantiated by more properly conducted and controlled experiments.

Some years ago, scientists became interested in the longevity of the population of Hizato situated in the Nagano province of Japan. Nearly 10% of the villagers were over 70 years of age; and a survey showed that there were 250% more 70-year-olds than in any other Japanese village. After extensive study, the conclusion was reached that the diet of the inhabitants of Hizato was a contributing factor to their longevity. The food consumed by these villagers consisted of all kinds of vegetables, including dried seaweed.

• **Sea farming and world food shortage**—There exist almost unlimited opportunities for increased sea farming. The water area of the world is many times greater than the land space; and phenomenal yields of seaweed are obtained—as much as 60 tons per acre. Not only that, seaweed farming does not suffer from drought or loss of crop through pests and disease; and seaweed requires no planting, weeding, or fertilizing. Some scientists predict that by the turn of the century the world's sea crops will have to be farmed to ensure the survival of our teeming population.

With one of the world's densest populations and a long coastline, the Japanese already have great expertise in the art of sea farming. Teams of girls, all expert swimmers and skin divers, play a part in this form of cropping, which is also known as aqua-culture. These underwater laborers are specially trained and equipped to carry out the cutting of seaweed from cultivated beds off the seashores.

(Also see ALGAE; and CARRAGEENAN.)

SECRETIN

A digestive hormone secreted by the duodenum of the small intestine in response to the presence of acid and protein in the digestive tract. It acts on the pancreas stimulating the secretion of an aqueous fluid high in bicarbonates that can neutralize the acid mixture from the stomach.

(Also see DIGESTION AND ABSORPTION; and ENDO-CRINE GLANDS, Table E-14 Hormones of the Endocrine Glands.)

SEEDS

Lots of seeds are eaten for human nutrition. A seed is the primary reason for which whole plants exist. It is the next generation of plants, since it contains a new plant in the form of an embryo plus stored food to nourish the embryo as it develops. Since the plant embryo requires proper nutrition from the stored food, seeds are good sources of protein, carbohydrate, fat (oil), minerals, and vitamins.

Seed types are as diverse as the plant kingdom. Seeds come in all shapes and all sizes, from the dustlike seeds of the orchid to the large seed contained in the coconut.

Man has learned to use a variety of seeds for the food stored in them. For example, rice and wheat feed millions of people. Beans, peas, corn, oats, soybeans, barley, buckwheat, rye—all seeds—are good foods. Coffee and chocolate are made from seeds. Many seeds are used for flavoring and seasoning; among them, vanilla, caraway, dill, mustard, black pepper, and nutmeg. Some nuts are seeds while others are fruit. Such seeds as cottonseed, linseed, castor, sunflower, soybean, peanut, coconut, and palm are sources of oils which have a multitude of uses—foods, cooking, soaps, inks, paints, perfumery, varnishes, and numerous other items. Other seeds are roasted and salted and consumed as snack food; for example, sunflower seeds, pumpkin seeds, and watermelon seeds.

Specific information about seeds consumed by humans can be located under individual articles or in Food Composition Table F-36.

SELECTIVE PERMEABILITY

When only certain substances are permitted to pass through the membrane, and others are rejected.

SELENIFEROUS

Areas in which the soil is high in the mineral selenium. (Also see SELENIUM.)

SELENIUM (Se)

Contents	Page

This comparatively rare, nonmetallic element, which makes up less than 0.0001% of the earth's crust, has recently been found to be essential. Fortunately, it is needed only in minute amounts, because (1) only traces are present in most foods, and (2) poisoning may result when the dietary level of this element is 0.0003% or greater. However, it seems that adequate dietary selenium is one of the keys to the maintenance of health under stressful conditions such as (1) prematurity at birth, (2) protein-energy malnutrition, and (3) the tissue disorders which accompany aging. An extended coverage is given to this mineral because of the limited information which is available to the American public regarding their needs for extra dietary selenium. Closely related to this concern is the issue of selenium supplementation of feeds for various species of livestock.

HISTORY. The toxic effects of selenium were observed long before the existence of this element was known. Around the end of the 13th century, the famous world traveler Marco Polo noted that certain forages which grew in the mountains of western China caused the hoofs of grazing animals to drop off. However, such observations were few and far between for many centuries after his travels, because there are only a few places in the world where there are toxic levels of selenium in the soils and plants.

This element also occurs as a trace contaminant of substances which contain sulfur, because the chemical properties of the two elements are similar. Therefore, it is noteworthy that in 1817 the Swedish chemist Berzelius discovered the element selenium while testing the residue which remained after sulfur had been burned to make sulfuric acid.

The opening up of the West led to the observation by the Army surgeon, Madison, in 1856 that cavalry horses in Nebraska lost their hoofs and some of their hair when feeding on the native forage plants. Similar observations were reported from the Wyoming Agricultural Experiment Station in 1893. The disorders in livestock, which were called "alkali disease," and "blind staggers," were traced to the consumption of plants such as locoweeds and poison vetches (generally, these common names refer to various species of *Astragalus* and *Oxytropis*). However, it was not until the early 1930s that agricultural researchers showed that (1) certain poisonous plants contained abnormally high amounts of selenium which had been absorbed from soils that were rich in the mineral, and (2) animals which were fed these plants developed selenium poisoning. About the same time, selenium compounds were developed for use in insecticides, but some scientists, including Nelson of the U.S. Food and Drug Administration (FDA), warned that residues of these products on fruits might be hazardous to people. Later, in 1943, Nelson produced nonmalignant liver tumors in rats by feeding them selenium. Since then, the FDA has been very wary of this element, and even now it is very cautious about permitting its use as a nutritional supplement for people or animals.

In the 1950s, indirect evidence of the beneficial effects of dietary selenium accumulated slowly, but steadily. During the 1940s, German scientists had tested the European type of brewers' yeast for use as a protein supplement and found that it sometimes produced a liver disease in rats which was prevented by feeding wheat germ or other sources of vitamin E. Then, in 1951, the German medical researcher Schwarz, who at the time was a visiting scientist at the National Institutes of Health (NIH), discovered that the American types of brewers' yeast contained an unidentified "Factor 3" which apparently acted along with vitamin E and sulfur-containing amino acids in protecting the liver against damage due to certain types of diets. Schwarz stayed in the United States to continue his research, and, in 1957, he and a co-worker, Foltz, reported that Factor 3 contained selenium.

Other studies by the group at NIH, and by Scott and his co-workers in the Department of Poultry Husbandry at Cornell, showed that the addition of selenium salts to the diets of chicks prevented certain disorders which resulted from vitamin E deficiencies. The pace of discovery quickened as other investigators showed that selenium protected calves and lambs against white muscle disease (nutritional muscular dystrophy). Finally, in 1973, Rotruck and his co-workers at the University of Wisconsin reported that selenium acted as a cofactor for a recently discovered enzyme (glutathione peroxidase) which breaks down toxic peroxides, most of which are formed from the oxidation of polyunsaturated fats. Hence, the link between selenium and vitamin E was shown; with selenium participating in the breaking down of these highly toxic compounds, and with vitamin E pre-

venting their formation. Nevertheless, it may be that new chapters will be added to the story on selenium, as recent research suggests that there are other roles for this essential element.

SELENIUM IN SOILS. In large areas of the United States, the soils contain little available selenium. Plants produced in these areas are low in this element, and selenium deficiency in livestock (and perhaps in people) is a serious problem. It would appear, therefore, that if foodstuffs grown in these areas are to exert their maximum benefit, some means of combatting their selenium deficiency must be achieved, and this must be accomplished without hazard.

In the Great Plains and Rocky Mountain States (especially in parts of the Dakotas and Wyoming), however, some of the soils are so rich in available selenium that the plants produced thereon are so high in selenium that they are poisonous to animals that eat them.

Fig. S-10 is a map showing areas of the United States where forages and grains have been found (1) low, (2) variable, and (3) adequate or high in selenium. As noted, deficient and high regions are scattered around the country, and some states contain two or more levels of concentration.

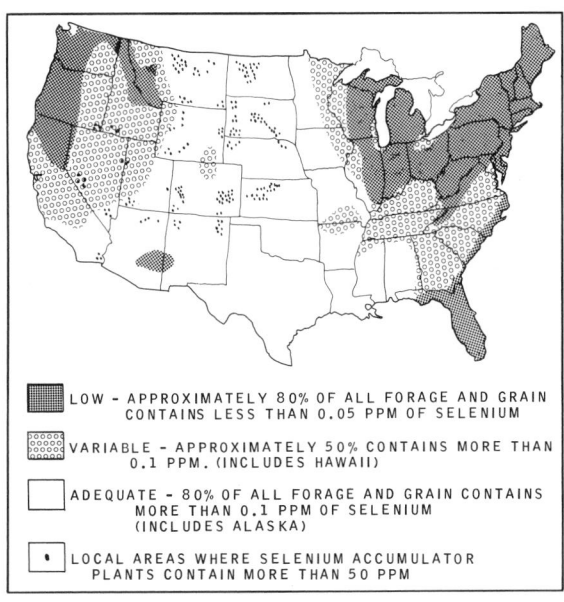

LOW – APPROXIMATELY 80% OF ALL FORAGE AND GRAIN CONTAINS LESS THAN 0.05 PPM OF SELENIUM

VARIABLE – APPROXIMATELY 50% CONTAINS MORE THAN 0.1 PPM. (INCLUDES HAWAII)

ADEQUATE – 80% OF ALL FORAGE AND GRAIN CONTAINS MORE THAN 0.1 PPM OF SELENIUM (INCLUDES ALASKA)

LOCAL AREAS WHERE SELENIUM ACCUMULATOR PLANTS CONTAIN MORE THAN 50 PPM

Fig. S-10. Geographic distribution of low, variable and adequate or high selenium areas in the United States. (Source: Kubota, J. and W. H. Allaway, "Geographic Distribution of Trace Element Problems," *Micronutrients in Agriculture*, Soil Science Society of America, 1972.)

Regional Differences in the Selenium Content of Foods.

The average selenium content of the crops used for human foods and livestock feeds is highest in the region of the United States which lies west of the Mississippi River and east of the Rocky Mountains. On the other hand, the areas which yield the crops that are very low in selenium are (1) the northern states between the Atlantic Ocean and the Mississippi River; (2) the southeastern coastal plain, including most of the state of Florida; and (3) the western sections of Washington, Oregon, and northern California. Hence, it is noteworthy how these regional differences affect the selenium content of grains and meats, which are the main sources of the mineral in the American diet.

• **Corn**—Feed corn from South Dakota contained 11 times as much selenium as similar corn from Michigan (34.5 mcg/100 g vs 3.2 mcg/100 g).[2] The sweet corn which is eaten by people might be expected to have a similar variation in its selenium content, because it is grown in places where the levels of selenium in the soil vary.

• **Wheat Flour**—Standard white flour milled from a sample of hard red spring wheat grown in a high-selenium area of Montana contained 45 mcg of selenium per 100 g, compared to only 1 mcg per 100 g in flour produced from soft red winter wheat grown in Indiana.[3] Hence, it would not be surprising to find substantial differences in the selenium content of breads made from wheats grown in different parts of the country.

• **Beef and lamb raised on high- or low-selenium corn**—The muscle meats and livers from steers and lambs which were fattened on high-selenium corn from South Dakota contained twice as much selenium as those fed low-selenium corn from Michigan.[4] However, the very high content of selenium in the kidneys of each species remained about the same, regardless of the level of the mineral in the ration.

• **Pork produced on corn-based rations**—The fresh muscle meat from pigs fattened on corn in South Dakota contained 15 times as much selenium as pigs raised on corn-based rations in Virginia.[5]

Some nutritionists maintain that the wide variations in the selenium contents of grains and meats from different parts of the United States do not result in similar variations in the selenium content of the diets of Americans because most people eat a variety of foods which have been produced in both high-selenium and low-selenium areas of the country. However, there are some rough correlations between the incidences of certain diseases in various regions and the levels of selenium in the foods produced in these regions.

METABOLISM OF SELENIUM.

Ingested selenium is absorbed in the intestine, mainly in the duodenum. Thence, it is bound to a protein and transported in the blood to the tissues, where it is incorporated into tissue protein as selenocysteine and selenomethionine; in the latter process, selenium replaces the sulfur in the amino acids cysteine and methionine. Excretion of selenium is largely by way of the kidneys, although small amounts are excreted in the feces and in sweat.

Many factors may affect dietary selenium; some enhancing it, others reducing it. These factors are elucidated in the section that follows:

Factors Which May Affect Dietary Selenium.

It is not surprising that deficiencies of selenium are sometimes hard to detect, because vitamin E and the sulfur-containing amino acids (cysteine and methionine) may act as partial substitutes for the mineral in some of its functions. Other nutrients, such as fat and protein, may also affect the body's need for selenium. Therefore, some of the major factors which influence selenium nutrition follow:

• **Biological availability of selenium from various foods**—All of the selenium in wheat appears to be biologically available whereas only about one-third of that in herring and tuna is available.[6] It might be that the selenium in certain species of ocean fish—which contain more of this element than most other foods—has a reduced availability because some of it is chemically bound to mercury. This idea is supported by the following evidence: (1) Many ocean fish contain small amounts of methylmercury; (2) selenium compounds have been shown to bind tightly with methylmercury; and (3) the toxicity of the methylmercury in tuna appears to be reduced greatly by the presence of selenium.[7]

• **Dietary protein**—Increasing the dietary protein intake reduces the chances of selenium poisoning when foods containing potentially hazardous amounts of the mineral are consumed. (High-selenium foods are produced only in the areas of the United States around the Rocky Mountains and in the Upper Missouri River Valley of the Dakotas.) However, most people are more likely to consume too little selenium rather than too much; so, protein foods are also valuable in this regard, because they are generally the best sources of selenium.

• **Form and source of the mineral**—Although seafood has a high selenium content, its value as a dietary source is reduced because of the poor availability of its

[2]Ullrey, D. E., "Selenium for Ruminants and Swine," *Feedstuffs*, June 6, 1977, p. 18.

[3]*Millfeed Manual*, The Millers' National Federation, Chicago, Ill., 1967, p. 47.

[4]Ullrey, D. E., "Selenium for Ruminants and Swine," *Feedstuffs*, June 6, 1977, p. 18.

[5]Ku, P. K., *et al.*, "Natural Dietary Selenium, alpha-Tocopherol and Effect on Tissue Selenium," *Journal of Animal Science*, Vol. 34, 1972, p. 211, Table 3.

[6]*Selenium and Interrelationships in Animal Nutrition*, Hoffman-La Roche, Inc., Nutley, N.J., 1974, p. 4.

[7]*An Assessment of Mercury in the Environment*, National Academy of Sciences, 1978, pp. 84-86.

selenium. For example, the selenium in tuna is only 33 to 50% available, possibly because it tends to bind to heavy metals such as mercury.

The selenium content of plant foods reflects the content of the soil in which they are grown. The soil content also influences the amount of selenium in muscle, eggs, or milk of animals raised on crops grown in the soil. Organ meats, muscle meats, cereals, and dairy products rank in descending order as good sources of selenium. The amount of selenium present in food tends to parallel the protein content of the food. Selenium is reduced in the milling process and is lost as vegetables are boiled.

Inorganic salts of selenium, called selenites, should be taken only under the direction of a medical doctor.

• **Intestinal microorganisms**—*E. coli, Streptococcus faecalis* and certain species of *Clostridia* and *Salmonella* metabolize selenium by (1) incorporating it into their enzymes, (2) utilizing selenium amino acids instead of sulfur amino acids, and/or (3) converting soluble forms of selenium into insoluble forms. The insoluble selenium is not likely to be absorbed, if it is produced in the intestines of people who harbor these microorganisms. Therefore, the dietary allowances for selenium should take into account the possibility that intestinal bacteria might somehow interfere with the utilization of selenium by animals and man.

• **Iron-deficiency anemia**—This disorder may be accompanied by a reduction in the activity of a selenium enzyme (glutathione peroxidase) in human red blood cells. Supplementation of the diet with iron sometimes restores the enzyme activity to normal, providing that the dietary supply of selenium is adequate. Hence, the optimal utilization of selenium may depend upon adequate iron nutrition.

• **Malnutrition**—Certain malnourished children who were given therapeutic formulas based upon skim milk powder did not respond well and had (1) subnormal blood levels of selenium, (2) a persistent anemia, and (3) very poor growth; all of which were corrected by giving them a selenium supplement.[8] However, one of the children required extra vitamin E to bring about the restoration of red blood cells. These findings show the need for (1) administering selenium supplements when rehabilitation diets contain only minimal amounts of this mineral; and (2) providing sufficient vitamin E, which enhances some of the effects of selenium.

• **Polyunsaturated fats from vegetable oils**—A diet rich in polyunsaturated fatty acids (PUFA) but poor in vitamin E might raise the requirement for selenium because (1) PUFA may be readily converted to toxic peroxides by various metabolic processes unless there is sufficient vitamin E to prevent this conversion, and (2) selenium is needed to activate the enzyme (gluthathione peroxidase) which destroys the peroxides.

• **Processing and preparation of foods**—The losses of selenium during the milling of grains into flours are smaller than those for the other essential minerals, because selenium is distributed throughout the kernel, whereas the other minerals are concentrated in the outer layers of the grain which are removed during milling.

Most cooking procedures have been found to cause little loss of selenium from most foods, except that the boiling of asparagus and mushrooms resulted in significant losses of the mineral (29% and 44%, respectively).[9]

• **Stresses**—Pigs which had been subjected to social and environmental stresses such as crowding, chilling, and overheating developed the severe disorders associated with selenium deficiency much sooner than unstressed animals.[10] Hence, it seems likely that highly stressed people might have above average requirements for selenium, since pigs and people are very similar in the ways that their bodies respond to various stresses.

• **Sulfur-containing amino acids**—Certain disorders which result from selenium-deficient diets are prevented in part by the sulfur-containing amino acids methionine and cysteine because they are converted in the body to glutathione, a substance that has a limited ability to carry out some of the functions of the selenium enzyme glutathione peroxidase. Hence, the need of the human body for selenium is greater when the dietary levels of the sulfur-containing amino acids are low. It is noteworthy that vegetarian diets may be low in the amino acids and low in selenium, unless large amounts of high-selenium wheat are consumed.

• **Vitamin E**—The metabolic roles of selenium and vitamin E overlap, so that each nutrient may replace the other to a limited extent in preventing certain types of disorders. However, there are also unique functions for each nutrient, so each must be supplied in the diet to ensure good nutrition. Furthermore, the experimental supplementation of animal feed with vitamin E resulted in an improvement in selenium absorption, and a doubling of the amount of the mineral which accumulated in the liver.[11]

FUNCTIONS OF SELENIUM. The essential functions of selenium have been proven conclusively in many species. Hence, most of our knowledge on this subject has been derived from studies on farm animals which have metabolic processes that are similar, but not strictly identical, to those in man.

The best known biochemical function of the element is its role as part of the enzyme glutathione peroxidase,

[8]Hopkins, L. L., Jr., and A. S. Majaj, "Selenium in Human Nutrition," *Selenium in Biomedicine*, edited by O. H. Muth, The Avi Publishing Company, Inc., Westport, Conn., 1967, pp. 205-206.

[9]Higgs, D. J., V. C. Morris, and O. A. Levander, "Effect of Cooking on Selenium Content of Foods," *Journal of Agricultural and Food Chemistry*, Vol. 20, 1972, p. 678.

[10]Ullrey, D. E., "The Selenium-Deficiency Problem in Animal Agriculture," *Trace Element Metabolism in Animals-2*, edited by W. G. Hoekstra, *et al.*, University Park Press, Baltimore, Md., 1974, pp. 276-277.

[11]Combs, G. F., Jr., "Influences of Vitamin A and Other Reducing Compounds on the Selenium-Vitamin E Nutrition of the Chicken,"*Proceedings of the 31st Distillers' Feed Conference*, 1976, p. 44, Table VIII.

which protects vital components of the cell against oxidative damage. Additionally, selenium functions as a protective agent against toxic substances, and in an interrelationship with vitamin E. Details relative to each of these functions follow.

Component Of The Enzyme Glutathione Peroxidase.
This enzyme—which depends upon the presence of selenium for its activity—is present in vital tissues such as the liver, heart, lung, pancreas, skeletal muscles, lens of the eye, white blood cells, and the blood plasma. Its metabolic role is to promote the breakdown of the toxic peroxides which are formed during the normal course of metabolism—before they have the opportunity to cause damage to the vital membranes of cells. However, tissues which are low in this enzyme—such as the brain—are very dependent upon receiving enough vitamin E to prevent the formation of peroxides, since a means of breaking them down once they are formed is lacking.

Protective Agent Against Toxic Substances.
In addition to its role as a component of the enzyme glutathione peroxidase, selenium functions apart from the enzyme in protecting tissues from damage by certain poisonous substances. It appears that inorganic forms of selenium somehow bind with toxic minerals such as arsenic, cadmium, and mercury—and render them less harmful. However, the detoxification of these poisonous elements might tie up some of the selenium which would ordinarily be utilized by the body. This effect may be desirable when dietary selenium is excessive, but not when it is marginal or deficient.

• **Arsenic**—The administration of trace amounts of arsenic and selenium to experimental animals resulted in the two elements counteracting each other, as evidenced by (1) the lowering of the liver levels of both elements to about half of those found in the animals given either element alone; and (2) an increased excretion of both elements in the bile.[12] This means that not only does selenium reduce the toxicity of arsenic, but also that abnormally large amounts of dietary arsenic might reduce the utilization of selenium. (About the only foods rich in arsenic are fish, oysters, mussels, and shrimp.)

A diet rich in arsenic might also be hazardous to people who have long had a high selenium diet because (1) the body rids itself of excessive selenium by forming derivatives of the element which usually are excreted in the breath and in the urine, and (2) animal studies have shown that arsenic reacts with the selenium derivatives to form highly toxic substances.[13] However, it is not known whether there are any circumstances under which this reaction occurs in people.

• **Cadmium**—This element, which is a common environmental pollutant in highly industrialized areas, is dangerous when it gets into the body by means of drinking water and/or food because it may damage the kidneys and the reproductive glands. Furthermore, cadmium damage to the kidneys has been shown to raise the blood pressure in experimental animals. Hence, it is noteworthy that selenium, if given soon enough and in large enough doses, counteracts various types of cadmium poisoning.

• **Mercury**—The organic form of this mineral which is most toxic to man—methylmercury—is produced by the action of aquatic microorganisms on inorganic mercury that is present in the water. Then, methylmercury travels up the food chain as ever larger aquatic organisms eat smaller ones, until it becomes concentrated in the tissues of large carnivorous fishes such as the swordfish and the tuna. Fortunately, ocean fish often contain sufficient selenium to combine with whatever amounts of methylmercury might be present.[14]

On the other hand, foods which contain more than minute traces of inorganic mercury might be hazardous to people who have been chronically exposed to excesses of selenium, because (1) the body detoxifies selenium by methylating it, and (2) methylated forms of selenium—which are normally harmless—become highly toxic when they react with inorganic mercury.[15]

Interrelationship of Selenium and Vitamin E.
During the 1950s, an interrelationship between selenium and vitamin E was established. It was found that selenium prevented exudative diathesis in vitamin E-deficient chicks and liver necrosis in vitamin E-deficient rats. Subsequent research demonstrated that both selenium and vitamin E protect the cell from the detrimental effects of peroxidation, but each takes a distinctly different approach to the problem. Selenium functions throughout the cytoplasm to destroy peroxides, while vitamin E is present in the membrane components of the cell and prevents peroxide formation. This explains why the biological need for each nutrient can be offset, at least partially although not totally, by the other. Simplified diagrammatically, this relationship is shown in Fig. S-11.

---

[12]Levander, O. A., "Factors That Modify the Toxicity of Selenium," *Newer Trace Elements in Nutrition*, edited by W. Mertz and W. E. Cornatzer, Marcel Dekker, Inc., New York, N.Y., 1971, pp. 67-70, Tables V and VIII.

[13]*Selenium*, National Academy of Sciences, 1976, p. 66.

[14]"Mercury Toxicity Reduced by Selenium," *Nutrition Reviews*, Vol. 31, 1973, p. 26.

[15]*Selenium*, National Academy of Sciences, 1976, p. 65.

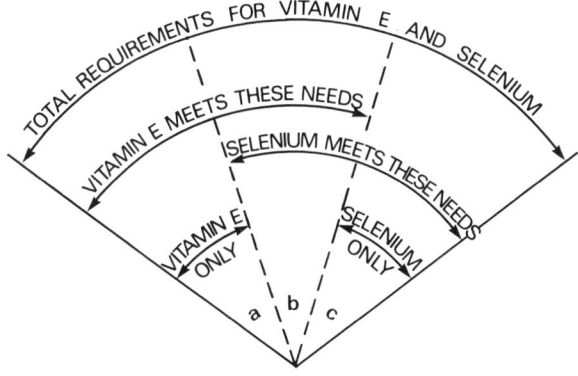

Fig. S-11. Diagram of the nutritional interrelationship of selenium and vitamin E.

TABLE S-5
SELECTED VALUES FOR BLOOD LEVELS OF SELENIUM IN SICK AND HEALTHY PEOPLE

Description of Blood Donor(s)	Whole Blood	Plasma	Red Blood Cells
	◄------(mcg/ml)------►		
Healthy adults in Oregon[1]	0.150-0.300	—[2]	—
Malnourished children[3]	0.100	0.060	0.210
Healthy children[3]	0.230	0.150	0.410
Infants who died suddenly[4]	0.100	0.069	—

[1]Data cited as a personal communication from P. H. Weswig in *Selenium*, National Academy of Sciences, 1976, p. 92.

[2]A blank indicates that value was not given in the source that is cited.

[3]Data which was reported by Burk, R., W. N. Pearson, and F. Viteri in the discussion at the end of the article by Hopkins, L. L., Jr., and A. S. Majaj, "Selenium in Human Nutrition," *Selenium in Biomedicine*, edited by O. H. Muth, The Avi Publishing Company, Inc., Westport, Conn., 1967, p. 212, Table 93.

[4]Data from Rhead, W. J., *et al.*, "The Vitamin E and Selenium Status of Infants and the Sudden Infant Death Syndrome," *Bioinorganic Chemistry*, Vol. 1, 1972, pp. 289-294.

Fig. S-11 depicts the requirements for vitamin E and selenium by means of a large sector which is subdivided into subsectors a, b, and c. The total requirements for the two nutrients are met when the needs represented by all three subsectors are filled by the appropriate combinations of these nutrients. Consequently, the only sure means of preventing deficiencies are (1) providing enough vitamin E to meet all of the needs represented by subsector *a* and a good part of those in subsector *b*; and (2) supplying sufficient selenium to fill the needs in subsector *c*, plus much of those in subsector *b*. Hence, some overlapping of vitamin E and selenium in meeting the needs represented by subsector *b* is desirable in order to guarantee that the total requirements for both nutrients are met.

DEFICIENCY SYMPTOMS. There are no clear-cut signs or symptoms which indicate when people are mildly to moderately deficient in selenium. However, many tests on diverse species of animals and man have shown that blood and tissue levels of selenium are in most cases accurate reflections of the selenium nutritional status. At the present time, the most practical tests for use in man appear to be those which follow.

NOTE: The interpretation of laboratory findings and the diagnosis of selenium deficiency are strictly jobs for health professionals, even though certain laboratories may analyze specimens for lay persons. Hence, the information which follows is presented so that the patient and his or her doctor might consider whether such tests are advisable.

• **Blood tests**—The selenium content of red blood cells is higher than the levels in either whole blood or plasma, because more of the selenium enzyme glutathione peroxidase is present in the red cells than in the other fractions of blood. Table S-5 gives some normal and deficient values for blood selenium.

• **Analysis of hair and fingernails**—The selenium contents of the hair and fingernails appear to be rough indicators of the selenium content of the rest of the body, so clippings of these materials might be a painless way of testing people for their nutritional status. However, the tests may be invalid if the patient has recently used a shampoo or a medication which contains selenium. Selenium is the active ingredient in preparations used to treat dandruff and fungus infections of the skin.

EVIDENCE OF SELENIUM DEFICIENCIES. There is no hard evidence of human selenium deficiency in the United States. Nevertheless, a growing number of nutrition researchers believe that the well-documented and severe disorders which occur in all species of selenium-deficient farm animals show the need for closer examination of the circumstantial evidence for human deficiencies. Also, it is noteworthy that several studies have shown that there are low levels of selenium in the diet and/or in the blood of severely malnourished children in developing countries.

Associations Between Certain Diseases And Selenium. Studies of the geographical distribution of certain diseases have shown that the disease rates are lower in areas where the selenium content of crops is higher than average. Such findings do not necessarily prove that selenium prevents the diseases, or that high rates of the diseases indicate selenium deficiencies; although they give reason to probe further into the association between certain diseases and selenium.

According to the National Research Council, National Academy of Sciences, "One could reasonably suppose that selenium is involved in such human medical problems as cancer, cataract, diseases of the liver, cardiovascular or muscular diseases, and the aging process."[16] Additional health problems which appear to result from a selenium deficiency are discussed in this section, also.

Selenium participates in some of the important metabolic processes which take place in many of the body's tissues. Therefore, the disruption of these processes by deficiencies of selenium might be expected to result in various disorders if the deficiencies are not corrected promptly.

NOTE: This is *not* to say that selenium deficiency is the one and only cause of the disorders which follow, but rather that the possibility of such a deficiency ought to be taken into account in the planning of measures to prevent or to treat these conditions.

• **Cancer**—Certain forms of this disease might result from both the effects of potent carcinogens and the weakening of the body's defenses by deficiencies of nutrients such as selenium. One of the current theories regarding the prevention of cancer by selenium postulates that this element acts by (1) counteracting poisonous substances which may cause cells to mutate; and (2) stimulating the defenses of the body that act against abnormal cells.[17]

Some human population data and laboratory experiments indicate that selenium may have anticancer properties. An increased incidence of cancer in human beings has been correlated with decreased levels of selenium in the blood. Also, selenium has been found to have some inhibitory effect on the development of tumors in rodents given certain carcinogens.

The cancer rates for 1959 were generally higher in the states which had low levels of selenium in their crops.[18] In many cases, however, the states which had high cancer rates had other potentially health-threatening conditions such as (1) heavy industrialization, (2) mining and ore processing, and/or (3) large populations.

In 1969, Shamberger and Frost reported that human cancer mortality might bear an inverse relationship to selenium distribution.[19] Also, controlled animal studies conducted by Shamberger at the same time showed an inhibitory effect of selenium on cancer.[20]

Other studies showed that (1) certain male cancer patients had subnormal blood levels of selenium; and (2) administration of supplemental selenium slowed the growth of tumors which were induced in animals by various carcinogens.[21]

Dr. Daniel Medina, Baylor College of Medicine in Houston, who has been studying the effects of selenium on animals for 3 years, adding it to their drinking water, reported that in rats and mice exposed to special viruses that cause breast cancer selenium reduced the expected number of tumors between 42 and 85%, depending on the dose of the virus and the type of animal. Yet he cautioned, "There's not enough known about the appropriate levels in the diet to warrant running down and buying a bunch of it."[22]

Further studies along these lines are needed. Both epidemiologic and laboratory approaches should be taken.

• **Heart disease and selenium**—A review of the effects of selenium deficiency reveals a repetitious undercurrent of vascular-type lesions suggesting a heart involvement in selenium disorders. Sudden death associated with selenium deficiency in newborn or rapidly growing lambs and calves apparently results from weakening of the heart muscle, commonly called white muscle disease. Selenium-deficient monkeys also have heart lesions. This disorder is characterized by white streaks in muscles, and in some cases, by abnormal electrocardiograms. Often, the animals affected with this disease die suddenly when they are subjected to moderate stresses.

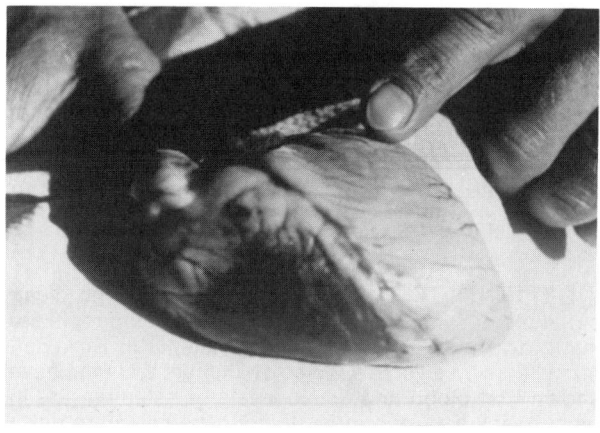

Fig. S-12.   Heart of a 6-week-old calf afflicted with white muscle disease. Note abnormal white areas in the heart muscles. (Courtesy, Oregon Agricultural Experiment Station, Corvallis, Ore.)

Some researchers have suggested that combined deficiencies of selenium and vitamin E might contribute to heart disease in man because these nutrients help maintain adequate levels of coenzyme Q in the heart muscle. *(Coenzyme Q is a vital cofactor in energy metabolism.)* If this cofactor is lacking, the production of energy in the heart and in other muscles may fall off to the extent that

[16]*Selenium,* Subcommittee on Selenium, National Research Council, National Academy of Sciences, Washington, D.C., 1976, p. 152.

[17]Schrauzer, G. N., "Trace Elements, Nutrition and Cancer: Perspectives of Prevention," *Inorganic and Nutritional Aspects of Cancer,* edited by G. N. Schrauzer, Plenum Press, New York, N.Y., 1978, p. 330, Scheme 1.

[18]*Ibid,* p. 326, Fig. 1.

[19]Shamberger, R. J., and D. V. Frost, "Possible Protective Effect of Selenium Against Human Cancer," *Canadian Medical Association Journal,* Vol. 100, 1969, p. 682.

[20]Shamberger, R. J., "Relation of Selenium to Cancer. 1. Inhibitory Effect of Selenium on Carcinogenesis," *Journal of National Cancer Institute,* Vol. 44, 1970, pp. 931–936.

[21]"Selenium and Cancer," *Nutrition Reviews,* Vol. 28, 1970, pp. 75-80.

[22]Medina, Daniel, Common, Maybe Crucial, Cancer-Fighter, *Star-Bulletin,* Honolulu, June 19, 1981.

these tissues can no longer carry their workloads. This hypothesis is supported by the finding that biopsy samples from the hearts of people with heart disease had subnormal levels of coenzyme Q. Hence, it is noteworthy that the administration of selenium to farm animals raised the levels of coenzyme Q in their hearts.

A sure sign of a dietary deficiency of selenium and/or of vitamin E in poultry and pigs is damaged blood vessels that leak into the surrounding tissues.[23] It is believed that this disorder is prevented by (1) selenium which circulates in the blood as part of the enzyme glutathione peroxidase, and (2) vitamin E which protects the membranes in the cells lining the blood vessels. While it does not appear that people develop the acute disorder which occurs in farm animals, it may be that the development of atherosclerosis is hastened by selenium deficiency, because the selenium-containing enzyme has been found to break down the cholesterol complexes that build up in lesions within the walls of arteries.

The following studies indicate that selenium is likely involved in heart disease:

1. The death rates from heart disease have consistently been highest in the low-selenium states.[24] However, these states are also the most densely populated and heavily industrialized states—so this evidence is open to other interpretations.

2. A comparison of the maps of early heart mortality and cardiovascular-related deaths of different areas of the United States revealed an inverse relationship between selenium levels and the mortality pattern.[25]

3. It has been hypothesized that selenium deficiency (rather than manganese deficiency as was first thought), which is prevalent all over Finland, may contribute to the unusually high death rates from heart disease and cancer in Finland.[26]

4. Lesions of selenium deficiency in rats have been associated with vascular abnormalities.[27]

5. Selenium is required by the enzyme that breaks down toxic peroxides which may damage the heart muscle.[28]

6. In May 1980, in a report before the Second International Symposium in Biology and Medicine, held at Texas Tech University, Lubbock, Texas, Dr. G. R. Yang, Chinese Academy of Medical Sciences, Peking, reported that selenium was effective in preventing heart muscle disease in certain parts of China. The malady, known as keshan, is common to certain areas of China where the soil is low in selenium. In a study involving 45,000 Chinese—the most massive study ever done on selenium deficiency in people—supplementation with selenium wiped out a heart disorder affecting 40 out of every 1,000 children in certain areas of China. Although there is no question that selenium was a pivotal factor in the Chinese study, Dr. Yang hastened to add that it is unlikely that it is the only factor.

• **Cloudiness in the lens of the eye (cataracts)**—Normally, the selenium content of the lens of the eye increases steadily from birth to death, but it has been found that lenses with cataracts may contain less than one-sixth of the normal amounts of this element.[29] It is suspected that lack of selenium to activate the enzyme glutathione peroxidase impedes the destruction of peroxides in the lens of the eye, and that the peroxides may then accumulate in amounts sufficient to damage the lens.

It is noteworthy, too, that cataracts are one of the selenium deficiency symptoms noted in rats.[30] Many other injurious agents and nutrient deficiencies might also be associated with the formation of cataracts, so it is uncertain whether selenium deficiency is a frequent cause of this disorder.

• **Growth failure during the rehabilitation of malnourished children**—So far, no evidence has been found to indicate that any normal, apparently healthy children suffer from a deficiency of selenium. However, several groups of children who were suffering from protein-energy malnutrition were found to have very low blood levels of selenium.[31] Selenium and protein are found together in both the diet and the body, so it is not surprising that children who lacked protein were also deficient in selenium. The standard rehabilitation procedures —which are based upon providing a good source of protein such as skim milk, extra fat and/or sugar, and certain vitamins and minerals—produced only limited improvement until selenium supplements were given.

• **Hemolytic anemia of newborn infants**—Newborn infants are more prone than other people to have abnor-

[23]*Selenium*, National Academy of Sciences, 1976, pp. 84-88.

[24]Sauer, H. I., and F. R. Brand, "Geographic Patterns in the Risk of Dying," *Environmental Geography in Health and Disease*, edited by H. L. Cannon and H. C. Hopps, The Geological Society of America, Inc., Boulder, Colo., 1971, p. 137.

[25]Frost, D. V., "Selenium Has Great Nutritional Significance for Man; Should Be Cleared for Feed," *Feedstuffs*, Vol. 44 (8), 1972, pp. 58-59.

[26]Marjanen, H., and S. Soini, "Possible Causal Relationship Between Nutritional Imbalances, Especially Manganese Deficiency and Susceptibility to Cancer, in Finland," *Ann. Agric. Fenn.*, Vol. 11, 1972, pp. 391-406.

[27]Sprinker, L. H., *et al.*, "Selenium Deficiency Lesions in Rats Fed Vitamin E Supplemented Rations," *Nutr. Rep. Int.*, Vol. 4, 1971, pp. 335-340.

[28]Hoekstra, W. G., "Biochemical Role of Selenium," *Trace Element Metabolism in Animals-2*, edited by W. G. Hoekstra, *et al.*, University Park Press, Baltimore, Md., 1974, p. 61.

[29]Ganther, H. E., *et al.*, "Selenium and Glutathione Peroxidase in Health and Disease—A Review," *Trace Elements in Human Health and Disease*, edited by A. S. Prasad and D. Oberleas, Academic Press, Inc., New York, N.Y., 1976, p. 205.

[30]*Selenium*, Subcommittee on Selenium, National Research Council, National Academy of Sciences, 1976, p. 143.

[31]Hopkins, L. L., Jr., and A. S. Majaj, "Selenium in Human Nutrition," *Selenium in Biomedicine*, edited by O. H. Muth, The Avi Publishing Company, Inc., Westport, Conn., 1967, pp. 203-214.

mally short-lived red blood cells because blood levels of vitamin E—which together with selenium protects the membranes of red cells from premature disintegration—are often subnormal at birth.[32] Hence, it is suspected that selenium deficiency might tend to aggravate this condition, since the selenium enzyme glutathione peroxidase protects against this disorder. It is noteworthy, therefore, that cow's milk contains only half as much selenium as human milk, and that both types of milk are relatively poor sources of the mineral.

• **Increased susceptibility to infections**—The germ-eating (phagocytic) white blood cells constitute one of the body's major defenses against infectious disease, because their formidable cells ingest living microorganisms, enclose them in killing chambers (phagocytic vacuoles) and kill them with blasts of highly potent forms of oxygen. The selenium enzyme glutathione peroxidase might extend the lifespan of these white blood cells by breaking down the toxic peroxides which may escape from the "killing chambers" into the more vulnerable parts of the cells. It is noteworthy that phagocytic white cells from selenium-deficient rats had a reduced ability to kill yeast cells, even though they had no difficulty ingesting the yeast.

So far, it has been difficult to confirm that selenium deficiency might be responsible for chronic susceptibility to infections in man, because many other factors affect this condition.

• **Infertility**—Studies on various species of farm animals and laboratory animals have shown that selenium deficiency causes infertility which is characterized in the male by fluid accumulation in the testicles, and feeble and broken sperm cells; and in the female by death of the fetus during early embryonic development. Although no similar investigations have been made in man, it is well known that people are subject to most of the disorders of fertility which have been observed in selenium-deficient animals.

• **Liver disease**—The liver is vulnerable to damage by the toxic peroxides generated during fat metabolism, unless it is supplied with sufficient amounts of selenium, vitamin E, and/or sulfur-containing amino acids (methionine and cysteine) to prevent the buildup of peroxides.

• **Pancreatic disease**—The reason for the degeneration of the pancreas in selenium-deficient animals is not clear. It does *not* appear to be related to the level of activity of the selenium enzyme glutathione peroxidase. Furthermore, an abundant dietary supply of vitamin E does not protect the pancreas when selenium is lacking. Eventually, deficiencies of vitamin E and other fatborne nutrients may develop, when the damage to the pancreas is great enough to interfere with the secretion of enzymes which digest the fatty components of foods.

• **Poisoning by normally harmless amounts of toxic substances**—In addition to the counteraction of the toxic effects of arsenic, cadmium, and methylmercury by inorganic selenium, selenium in the enzyme glutathione peroxidase may protect against the effects of poisonous organic compounds such as carbon tetrachloride (a common dry-cleaning agent) and certain drugs.

• **Sudden infant death syndrome (crib or cot death)**—Several researchers have put forward the hypothesis that combined deficiencies of selenium and vitamin E in cow's milk may be contributory to "crib death," where an infant that had appeared to be healthy is found to have died suddenly in its bed.[33] It seems that certain infants that were fed cow's milk received only ½ as much selenium and $1/10$ as much vitamin E as infants that were breast-fed.

However, the tentative explanation of crib deaths which is entertained by many doctors is that (1) an infant may develop antibodies (become sensitized) to cow's milk after bringing up part of a feeding and inhaling it into its bronchial tubes (the air passages which lead from the windpipe into the lungs), and (2) repetitions of these episodes lead to such a severe allergy to cow's milk that eventually one such event leads to a fatal allergic shock. Other doctors believe that the severe allergic shock may be triggered by a variety of allergens, or perhaps even by a virus.

The explanations are all compatible because severe allergic reactions are accompanied by (1) a marked enlargement (dilation) of the blood vessels, and a great drop in the blood pressure; and (2) a speeding up of the heart rate as the heart attempts to maintain the normal circulation of blood. Deficiencies of selenium and vitamin E may weaken the heart muscle so that it cannot cope with the increased workload brought about by a state of allergic shock.

TREATMENT AND PREVENTION OF SELENIUM DEFICIENCY. As a result of extensive animal experiments, the Food and Drug Administration (FDA) approved the use of selenium for livestock as follows:

1. In 1974, FDA approved the addition of selenium as either sodium selenite or sodium selenate at the rate of 0.1 parts per million (ppm) to complete feed (total ration) for swine, growing chickens to 16 weeks of age, breeder hens producing hatching eggs, and nonfood animals; and at the rate of 0.2 ppm in complete rations for turkeys.

2. In 1979, FDA amended the food additive regulations for selenium to include beef cattle, dairy cattle, and sheep; with the addition of selenium approved at the rate of 0.1 ppm of complete feed, along with stipulations on how to incorporate it into the ration.

3. In 1987, FDA provided an increase in the maximum allowance of selenium in complete feeds for cattle (beef and dairy), sheep, swine, chickens, turkeys, and ducks from 0.1 ppm to 0.3 ppm.

---

[32]Fomon, S. J., *Infant Nutrition*, 2nd ed., W. B. Saunders Co., Philadelphia, Pa., 1974, p. 220.

[33]*Selenium*, National Academy of Sciences, 1976, pp. 93–94.

In 1989, for the first time ever, the Food and Nutrition Board, National Research Council, included selenium in its *Recommended Dietary Allowances*, 10th Edition (see Table S-6).

INTERRELATIONSHIPS.
The major selenium relationships are:

1. The functions of selenium are closely related to those of vitamin E and the sulfur-containing amino acids.
2. Selenium protects against the toxic effects of arsenic, cadmium, copper, mercury, and silver. Likewise, these elements counteract the toxic effects of selenium.
3. A diet high in protein or high in sulfate provides some protection against selenium poisoning.
4. The optimal utilization of selenium may depend upon adequate iron nutrition.
5. Diets rich in polyunsaturated fatty acids but poor in vitamin E may raise the requirements for selenium.

RECOMMENDED DAILY ALLOWANCE OF SELENIUM.
Table S-6 gives recommended selenium intakes that the FNB–NRC deems to be appropriate for various age groups.

TABLE S-6
RECOMMENDED SAFE AND ADEQUATE
DAILY DIETARY INTAKES OF SELENIUM[1]

Group	Age	Selenium Intake
	(years)	(mcg)
Infants	0.0–0.5	10
	0.5–1.0	15
Children	1–3	20
	4–6	20
Adolescents	7–10	30
	11+	40
Adults		55–70

[1]Adapted by the authors from *Recommended Dietary Allowances*, 10th ed., 1989, NRC-National Academy of Sciences, p. 285.

Certain researchers, such as Dr. Schrauzer and his co-workers at the University of California at San Diego, believe that many cases of cancer might be prevented by selenium intakes that are approximately double the level recommended by the Food and Nutrition Board.[34] They have found that (1) the rates of cancer in man decrease as blood levels of selenium increase, and (2) the minimum disease rates are those for the high-selenium areas. Hence, these researchers believe that

people should consume enough selenium to bring their blood levels up to those of people living in the low-cancer, high-selenium areas. This would require allowances which are at least double those given in Table S-6.

• **Selenium intake in average U.S. diet**—Analyses of national food composites in the United States indicate that the overall adult mean dietary selenium intake was 108 mcg/day between 1974 and 1982. The daily mean for each year ranged from 83 to 129 mcg.

TOXICITY.
Confirmed cases of selenium poisoning in man are not often found because (1) the foods and beverages which are consumed by people are not likely to contain toxic excesses of the element, and (2) well-nourished people are protected by metabolic processes that convert selenium into harmless substances which are excreted in the urine, or in the breath. Nevertheless, a few cases of poisoning sometimes occur under unusual circumstances such as (1) very high levels of the element in drinking water, or (2) the presence of malnutrition, parasitic infestation, or other factors which may make people highly susceptible to selenium toxicity. Therefore, descriptions of some poisonous effects of selenium follow:

• **Abnormalities of the hair, nails, and skin**—It appears that some of the toxic effects of selenium might be due to its interference with the normal structures and functions of proteins rich in sulfur-containing amino acids. Hence, poisoning by this element is characterized by abnormalities in the hair, nails, and skin; which are tissues rich in sulfurous proteins. For example, a group of children living in a high-selenium area of Venezuela had loss of hair, discolored skin, and chronic digestive disturbances.[35] However, most of the children were infested with intestinal parasites, which might have weakened them so that they had increased susceptibility to the toxic effects of selenium.

• **Garlic odor on the breath**—Normally, people who have consumed large excesses of selenium excrete it as trimethyl selenide in the urine, and/or as dimethyl selenide on the breath. The latter substance has an odor resembling garlic.

• **Intensification of selenium toxicity by arsenic or mercury**—Usually, the toxicity of selenium is reduced by the presence of either arsenic or mercury. However, the methyl derivatives of selenium—which are formed when animals or people are chronically exposed to excessive amounts of the mineral—may become highly toxic when they react in the body with arsenic or mercury. So far,

[34]Schrauzer, G. N., "Trace Elements, Nutrition and Cancer: Perspectives of Prevention," *Inorganic and Nutritional Aspects of Cancer*, edited by G. N. Schrauzer, Plenum Press, New York, N.Y., 1978, pp. 330-331.

[35]Burk, R. F., "Selenium in Man," *Trace Elements in Health and Disease*, edited by A. S. Prasad and D. Oberleas, Academic Press, Inc., New York, N.Y., 1976, p. 121.

these reactions have been observed only in animals in laboratory experiments. Hence, it is not certain whether there are circumstances under which they might occur in man.

• **Promotion of tooth decay**—Various studies have shown the rates of tooth decay to be slightly higher in high-selenium areas than in low-selenium areas. Research on laboratory animals has produced evidence that excesses of selenium interfere with the formation of the protective tooth enamel. However, this research has usually been conducted with much higher levels of the mineral than are likely to be encountered by man.

SOURCES OF SELENIUM.
The selenium content of plant products varies according to the amounts and availability of the mineral in the soil. Likewise, the selenium content of animal products depends upon the content of the element in livestock feeds; for example, the Ohio Station reported that the addition of 0.1 ppm selenium to the animal's diet increased the selenium content of beef liver by 72%.[36] Also, there are cooking losses in some cases, although these are minor for most foods. Hence, the data regarding the amounts of the mineral supplied by various foods *cannot* be taken to indicate a constant content of selenium for any particular food. Nevertheless, such data are useful in that they show which foods are likely to be good sources of the mineral. Fortunately, food eaten in the United States is generally varied in nature and origin. Nevertheless, it appears likely that most diets barely meet minimal requirements; hence, many diets are bound to be deficient.

Groupings by rank of some common food sources of selenium follow:

• **Rich sources**—Brazil nuts, butter, fish flour, lobster, smelt.

• **Good sources**—Beer, blackstrap molasses, cider vinegar, clams, crab, eggs, lamb, mushrooms, oysters, pork kidneys, spices (garlic, cinnamon, chili powder, nutmeg), Swiss chard, turnips, wheat bran, whole grains (wheat, barley, rye, oats).

• **Fair sources**—Cabbage, carrots, cheese, corn, grape juice, most nuts, orange juice, whole milk.

• **Negligible sources**—Fruits and sugar.

• **Supplemental sources**—Sodium selenate, sodium selenite. *Note well:* Do not take separate selenium supplements without medical advice.

Many drug stores and health food stores now carry special types of yeast which were grown on media rich in selenium; hence, they contain much greater amounts of the mineral than ordinary yeast. Tablets made from high-selenium yeast are also available.

---

[36]Moxon, A. L. and D. L. Palmquist, "Selenium Content of Foods Grown or Sold in Ohio," *Ohio Report*, Ohio State University, Columbus, Ohio, January-February 1980, pp. 13-14, Table 1.

For additional sources and more precise values of selenium, see Table S-7, Selenium Content of Some Foods, which follows.

TABLE S-7
SELENIUM CONTENT OF SOME FOODS

Food	Selenium
	(mcg/100 g)
Fish flour	193
Butter	146
Eulachon (smelt)	123
Torula yeast	123
Wheat germ	111
Lobster	104
Brazil nuts	103
Brewers' yeast	91
Cider vinegar	89
Pork kidneys	64
Wheat, whole grain	63
Wheat bran	63
Clams	55
Whole wheat flour	53
Crab	51
Oysters	49
Pork	42
Rye, whole grain	37
Kidney beans	36
Lamb	30
Soybean flour	30
Turnips	27
Swiss chard	26
Blackstrap molasses	26
Garlic	25
Oats, whole grain	21
Beer	19
Barley, whole grain	18
Eggs	16
Skim milk (dehy)	13
Mushrooms	13
Soybeans	11
Cheese	8
Corn	7
Orange juice	6
Grape juice	4
Cow's milk, whole 3.7% fat	3
Pecans	3
Filberts (hazelnuts)	2
Almonds	2
Carrots	2
Cabbage	2

SUMMARY. It might be desirable for people who live in low-selenium areas of the United States—which are generally located east of the Mississippi River and west of the Rocky Mountains—to make certain that they get enough selenium by eating ample amounts of foods rich or good in selenium. However, undesirable effects or toxicities might result from consuming too much selenium, so one should consult with a doctor or a dietitian before taking special, selenium-rich supplements.

(Also see MINERAL[S], Table M-67; and POISONS, Table P-11 Some Potentially Poisonous [Toxic] Substances.)

SEMIDISPENSABLE AMINO ACID

An amino acid which is essential only under certain circumstances or which may replace part of one of the essential amino acids. Arginine, cystine, and tyrosine fall into this group.
(Also see AMINO ACID[S].)

SEMIPERMEABLE MEMBRANE

A membrane that is permeable to some small molecules (like water and inorganic salts) but bars the passage of larger particles (like protein molecules).

SEPTICEMIA

A diseased condition resulting from the presence of pathogenic bacteria and their associated poisons in the blood.

SERENDIPITY BERRY
Dioscoreophyllum cumminsii

A very sweet tasting berry that is native to West Africa. The substance which is responsible for the sweet taste has been isolated and named monellin.

SERINE

One of the nonessential amino acids.
(Also see AMINO ACID[S].)

SEROTONIN

A derivative of the essential amino acid tryptophan which plays a role in brain and nerve function.

SERUM

The colorless fluid portion of blood remaining after clotting and removal of corpuscles. It differs from plasma in that the fibrinogen has been removed.

SERUM CHOLESTEROL

The level of the sterol cholesterol in the blood.

SERUM TRIGLYCERIDE

The level of fat in the blood.

SESAME *Sesamum indicum*

Sesame has been grown in tropical countries since time immemorial, primarily to obtain seed for use on bakery goods and food delicacies and for edible oil production. It appears to be the earliest condiment used and

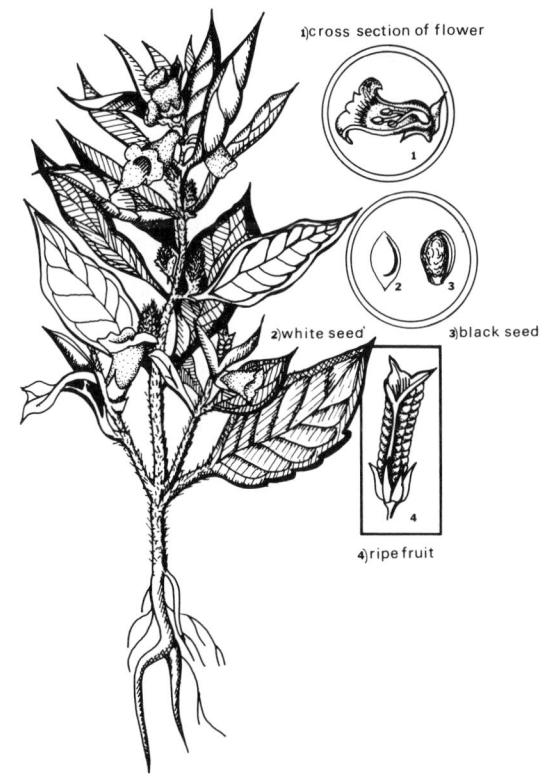

1) cross section of flower

2) white seed   3) black seed

4) ripe fruit

Fig. S-13. Sesame plant.

the oldest crop grown for edible oil. The magic words "open sesame" found in the Arabian Nights are thought to have been inspired by the characteristic bursting open of the sesame pods when the grain is ripe, a nettlesome trait that has necessitated hand harvesting of the crop.

Production of sesame is limited to countries where labor is plentiful and inexpensive, and will so remain until and unless nonshattering varieties with satisfactory yields and/or improved mechanical harvesting techniques are developed. Intense breeding and engineering research programs to alleviate these problems are in progress.

ORIGIN AND HISTORY.   Although sesame has not been identified in the wild state, it is believed to have originated in the Indian archipelago. A series of tablets now in the British Museum giving the Assyrian account of the creation of the world tell of a meeting of the gods in their council chambers where they refreshed themselves with sesame wine prior to creating the world. Later, the seed was often the subject of contracts and accounting as shown by references to sesame on the tablets and deeds now in the Babylonian Room of the British Museum. Sesame was the symbol of immortality in early Hindu legend. Archaeological evidence indicates that sesame was cultivated in Palestine and Syria around 3000 B.C., and by the civilization of Babylonia in 1750 B.C. An Egyptian tomb bears a 4,000-year-old drawing of a baker adding sesame to bread dough. Archaeologists have found sesame seed mash in the ruins of the Old Testament Kingdom of Ararat. In 1298, Marco Polo observed the Persians using sesame oil for cooking, body massage, medicinal purposes, illumination, cosmetics, and lubricating primitive machinery.

According to some historians, sesame seed was taken from the Sundae Islands to India several thousand years ago. From India, it spread to Egypt, China, Japan, Africa, South America, Central America, and Mexico. Sesame was introduced into the United States in the late 17th century by slaves who brought the seed from Africa to the plantations along what is now the South Carolina coast.

WORLD AND U.S. PRODUCTION.   In 1990, the world production of sesame seed totaled 2 million metric tons. That same year, the six leading nations, by rank, with the metric tons produced by each, were: India, 550,000; China, 420,000; Myanmar, 207,000; Mexico, 71,000; Nigeria, 70,000; and Sudan, 66,000. Globally, the average yield in 1990 was only 302 lb per acre (*339 kg/ha*). Sudan is the largest exporter of seed, and the Mediterranean countries, Japan, and the United States are the chief importers.

THE SESAME PLANT.   The sesame plant belongs to the family *Pedaliaceae*; genus *Sesamum*; species *S. indicum*. Sesame is an annual herb that grows 2 to 4 ft (*61 to 122 cm*) high, has oblong leaves and tiny pink or white flowers, and produces flat seeds that range from white to brown in color and are encased in a small pod which bursts open when the grain is ripe.

SESAME CULTURE.   Most sesame is produced in tropical areas that are not agriculturally mechanized, and where harvesting is usually done by hand—by flailing pods with a stick. Plant breeders are trying to develop a strain that will lend itself to commercial harvesting with a minimum of shattering, yet yield well; but they have not been too successful to date.

KINDS OF SESAME.   There are numerous varieties of sesame. Two common varieties are the Sudanese White and Indian Black.

PROCESSING SESAME SEED.   In those areas where sesame is primarily processed for its oil content, the seed is not dehulled; rather, the entire seed is crushed. However, in areas such as India, where the meal is an important food, dehulling is necessary.

There is a U.S. patented process for extraction of oil from crushed sesame seed with hot calcium hydroxide solution. A similar acqueous processing technology was developed at the Food Protein Research and Development Center, Texas A&M University, to isolate a sesame protein fraction containing 78.2% protein with less than 2.1% crude free lipid.

NUTRITIONAL VALUE OF SESAME.   The hull accounts for 15 to 20% of the total weight of the unhulled seed. Dehulling of sesame for human consumption is important because the hull contains 2 to 3% oxalic acid, which chelates calcium and has a bitter flavor. Sesame averages about 50% oil, which is highly resistant to oxidation, and 25% protein, which has a unique balance of amino acids. Dehulled, defatted meal contains 50 to 60% protein and is bland. Food Composition Table F-36 gives the nutrient composition of sesame seeds and sesame oil.

Table S-8 compares the chemical composition of two varieties of sesame, Sudanese White and Indian Black. In general, Indian varieties tend to be lower in protein and higher in oil than Sudanese varieties such as generally appear in the export market and are commonly used in the United States.

TABLE S-8
COMPOSITION OF SESAME SEED PRODUCTS[1]
(Moisture-free Basis)

	Unit	Sudanese White		Indian Black Variety				
		Whole Seed	Dehulled Seed	Whole Seed	Dehulled Seed	Hull	Dehulled Expeller-Pressed	Dehulled Hexane-Extracted
Fat (ether extractable)	%	53.28	57.50	54.25	63.36	10.65	10.62	.43
Protein (N x 6.25)	%	25.02	29.90	20.20	23.44	8.35	57.75	60.22
Ash	%	5.42	3.46	6.18	2.41	23.80	6.58	6.53
Crude fiber	%	4.08	3.04	4.49	2.46	19.31	5.41	5.29
Oxalic acid	%	2.71	.36	2.51	.13	14.93	.25	.28
Calcium	%	.98	.23	1.31	.22	10.18	.33	.37

[1]Johnson, L. A., T. M. Suleiman, and E. W. Lusas, "Sesame Protein: A Review and Prospectus," *Journal of the American Oil Chemists' Society*, Vol. 56, No. 3, March 1979, p. 465, Table 2.

The unique quality of sesame protein is the presence of a high level of the sulfur-containing amino acids, methionine and cystine. The limiting amino acid of sesame protein is lysine (Table S-9). It is also noteworthy that sesame does not contain some of the objectionable characteristics found in soy protein, particularly with regard to the trypsin inhibiting factor.

Table S-10 shows the average analysis of crude sesame oil. Due to the presence of natural antioxidants in the crude oil, sesame oil is the most stable naturally-occurring liquid vegetable oil. It will keep for several years without turning rancid. Sesame oil is classified as polyunsaturated; it contains approximately 44% of the essential fatty acid, linoleic acid, and 40% oleic acid.

(Also see FATS AND OTHER LIPIDS; and OILS, VEGETABLE, Table O-6.)

TABLE S-9
**PROFILE OF ESSENTIAL AMINO ACIDS
IN DEHULLED SESAME PRODUCTS
COMPARED TO MILK—A HIGH-QUALITY PROTEIN[1]**

Amino Acid	Meal	Isolate	Cow's Milk[2]
	←——— (mg/g protein) ———→		
Histidine	24	21	27
Isoleucine	47	36	47
Leucine	74	66	95
Lysine	35	21	78
Methionine and cystine ..	56	37	33
Phenylalanine and tyrosine	106	79	102
Threonine	39	33	44
Tryptophan	19	18	14
Valine	46	46	64

[1]Adapted from Johnson, L.A., T. M. Suleiman, and E. W. Lusas, "Sesame Protein: A Review and Prospectus," *Journal of the American Oil Chemists' Society*, Vol. 56, No. 3, March 1979, p. 465, Table 3.
[2]*Recommended Dietary Allowances*, 10th ed., 1989, National Academy of Sciences, p. 67, Table 6–5. The essential amino acid requirements of infants can be met by supplying 0.79 g of a high-quality protein per pound of body weight (*1.7 g/kg body weight*) per day.

TABLE S-10
ANALYSIS OF CRUDE SESAME OIL (AVERAGE)[1]

Free fatty acid (as oleic)	1.3%
Color	35y/1.2r
Iodine Value	110
Peroxide Value	13
AOM	24 hr
Percent unsaponifiable	2.3%
Smoke point	330°F
Specific gravity @ 25°C	.918
Saponification Value	185.8
Fatty acids (natural oil)	**(%)**
Oleic..	40
Linoleic.....................................	44
Other unsaturates...........................	1
Palmitic.....................................	9
Stearic......................................	5

[1]Source: USDA Southern Regional Laboratories.

SESAME PRODUCTS AND USES. Sesame in many forms is now offered to the food industry for human consumption; among them, the following:

> Dry, cleaned, unhulled sesame seed
> White, hulled sesame seed
> Toasted sesame seed
> Toasted, flaked sesame seed
> Partially defatted sesame flour
> Solvent extracted sesame flour
> Sesame butter made from toasted sesame
>   seed

In the United States, sesame is used primarily in the bakery industry, where whole, hulled sesame seed is used as a decoration and flavoring agent on specialty breads, rolls, buns, candies, and other delicacies. Sesame is also used in high-protein snack foods and granola.

The protein (meal) of sesame has become increasingly important for human food due to the following unique properties: (1) the presence of a high level of the sulfur-containing amino acids, methionine and cystine; (2) its freedom from the trypsin inhibiting factor, an objectionable characteristic of soy protein; and (3) its pleasant flavor. The meal is very palatable to humans. In India, it is used extensively in human foods; and in India and Java, it is sometimes fermented for food. In the United States, most of the meal is used for livestock feed.

Sesame oil (also known as gingili, benne, or til) is straw-colored, with a pleasant, mild taste and remarkable stability. It is a natural salad oil requiring little or no winterization and is one of the few vegetable oils that can be used without refining. These are factors of increasing importance as energy costs escalate. It is popular because of the presence of a natural antioxidant, sesamol, and because of its high content of polyunsaturated fatty acids, 43% oleic and 43% linoleic. The oil is used as a substitute for olive oil—primarily as a salad and cooking oil and for margarine and soap. Also, a significant quantity of oil is used by the cosmetic industry for softening and soothing purposes, and by the pharmaceutical industry as a carrier for medicines.

In addition to the uses listed above, sesame is being used to enhance the flavor of fried or baked snacks, high-protein beverages, cereals, seasoning blends; and as a garnish for vegetables, high-protein breads, and pies.

In the Orient, sesame is used in various ways. Dehulled seed may be fried and mixed with sugar to form a sweetmeat or soup ingredient. A peanut butter counterpart, called *tachini*, is made from seed and honey. *Halvah*, a candy made with tachini, sugar, egg albumen, gelatin, and Panama root juice, is the traditional food of Greek, Turkish, and other Near Eastern people. Also, the natives of the areas where sesame is grown use the seeds and leaves for soothing and medicinal purposes.

Blends of peanut/chickpea, wheat/chickpea, rice/chickpea, peanut/soybean, sunflower/maize, and cowpea/rice have all shown improved nutritional qualities with supplementation of sesame meal. Even more significant, however, is the finding that a simple blend of one part sesame and one part soy protein has about the same protein nutritive value as casein, the main protein of milk. The high-lysine and low-methionine content of soy protein is complementary to sesame protein.

(Also see OILS, VEGETABLE, Table O-6 Vegetable Oils.)

SEVEN FOODS PLAN (BASIC 7 FOODS PLAN)

The different types of foods are sometimes divided into the following seven groups: *Group 1*—Green and yellow vegetables; *Group 2*—Oranges, tomatoes, grapefruit, or raw cabbage or salad greens; *Group 3*—Potatoes and other vegetables, and fruits; *Group 4*—Milk and milk products; *Group 5*—Meat, poultry, fish, or eggs, or dried beans, peas, nuts, peanut butter; *Group 6*— Bread, flour, and cereals; and *Group 7*—Butter and fortified margarine. A well-balanced diet should include food from each group every day. A more common plan is the selection of foods from the basic four food groups—(1) the meat, poultry, fish, and beans group; (2) the milk and cheese group; (3) the vegetable and fruit group; and (4) the bread and cereal group.

(Also see FOOD GROUPS.)

SEVILLE ORANGE (SOUR ORANGE) *Citrus aurantium*

This citrus fruit is rarely seen in the fresh form in the United States because it is grown mainly in Seville, Spain, for making marmalade. The Seville orange, like the other citrus fruits, belongs to the rue family (*Rutaceae*). It is distinguished from the Sweet orange (*C. sinensis*) by its much rougher skin and very sour taste.

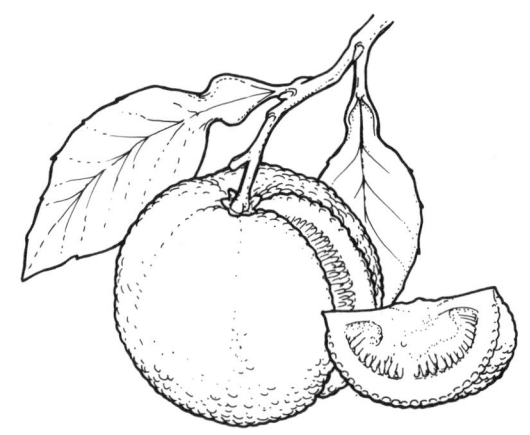

Fig. S-14.   The Seville orange, a sour-flavored fruit which is used mainly for making marmalade and flavorings.

ORIGIN AND HISTORY. The sour orange originated in Indonesia and was brought to India in ancient times. Sometime around the 9th century A.D., the Arabs brought it to the Middle East. The first orchards were planted on the Arabian peninsula in the beginning of the 10th century. Later, the trees were planted in Mesopotamia and Syria. The spread of Islam and Arabic culture across North Africa and into Spain led to the introduction of the sour orange into Seville, Spain, in the 11th century. Shortly thereafter, the Crusaders brought the fruit from Palestine to France and Italy.

Spanish colonists introduced the sour orange to the West Indies in the 16th century. The trees were transplanted in Florida soon after the region was settled in 1565. However, the production of the sour orange in North America declined sharply after the sweet orange was introduced. Nevertheless, it still serves as a hardy rootstock for bearing grafts of the sweet orange and other citrus fruits.

PRODUCTION. Most of the world's crop of sour oranges is produced in the area around Seville, Spain. Production statistics are not readily available. It is noteworthy that Spain has more injurious frosts than the other major citrus fruit producing countries of the world. Hence, the sour orange is the most suitable citrus species for large-scale production, because it is one of the hardiest citrus trees.

In the other citrus-producing countries, sour orange trees are grown mainly for use as rootstocks that will receive the grafts of other citrus species.

Details of citrus fruit growing are given elsewhere.

(Also see CITRUS FRUITS, section headed "Production.")

PROCESSING. Most of the sour orange crop is processed because the fruit is too sour to eat raw. Large quantities of the oranges are exported to Great Britain, where they are used to make a marmalade that has a strong distinctive flavor that is not found in similar products made from sweet oranges.

In Spain, the peel is scraped from the oranges and pressed to yield an oil that is much used as a flavoring agent. The clarified juice is used to impart a strong orangy flavor to highly diluted beverages such as orangeades and other fruit drinks. The U.S. Standards of Identity permit the use of up to 5% sour orange juice in the production of frozen orange juice concentrate. Finally, the by-products of sour orange processing are usually dried and fed to cattle.

SELECTION AND PREPARATION. One is not likely to see fresh sour oranges in the United States except in a few orchards in Florida. If some of the fresh fruit is obtained, it is best to use small amounts of the juice, peel, and/or pulp for flavoring various preparations that would ordinarily utilize fresh oranges.

CAUTION: Some people are allergic to one or more constituents of citrus peel. When such allergies are suspected, neither the peel nor the products containing it should be consumed, and fruit juice should be extracted gently to avoid squeezing the oil and other substances from the peel into the juice. It is noteworthy that some of the commercially prepared orange juices and orange drinks may contain peel and/or substances extracted from it, but that prepared citrus juice products for infants contain little or none of the peel constituents.

Guidelines for the selection and preparation of processed citrus products are given elsewhere.

(Also see CITRUS FRUITS, section headed "Selection and Preparation.")

NUTRITIONAL VALUE. The fruit and juice of the sour orange are rarely consumed alone, but are usually mixed with other citrus products. Hence, data on the nutrient composition of this fruit are not readily available. However, it might be expected to be similar to the sweet orange in its content of potassium, vitamin C, and bioflavonoids.

Citrus peel contains citral, an aldehyde which antagonizes the effects of vitamin A. Hence, people should not consume large amounts of peel-rich products such as candied peel and marmalade without making certain that their dietary supply of this vitamin is adequate.

(Also see CITRUS FRUITS; and FRUIT[S], Table F-47 Fruits of the World.)

SHALLOT *Allium cepa* **variety** *aggregatum*

This variety of onion differs from the common variety in that (1) it forms smaller bulbs which are shaped like large cloves of garlic; (2) the bulbs have a mild garlic flavor; and (3) a cluster of shallot bulbs is formed, whereas, the common onion forms only a single bulb. Therefore, the shallot has been designated as a cluster (*aggregatum*) variety of onion. The shallot and its close relatives in the *Allium* genus belong to the *Alliaceae* family of plants. Fig. S-15 shows the bulbs and a flower of a typical shallot.

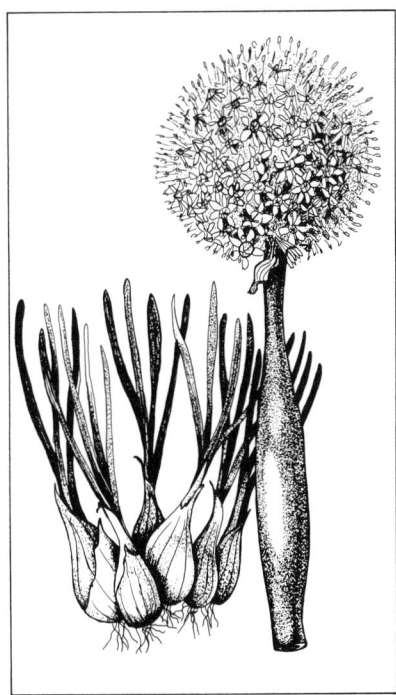

Fig. S-15. The shallot, a mild tasting variety of onion which forms a cluster of bulbs.

ORIGIN AND HISTORY. For a long time it was thought that the shallot and the common onion were different species. However, it has been confirmed by breeding experiments that the two vegetables are merely different varieties of the same species. Therefore, the place of origin of the shallot is suspected of being near to that of the common onion, which originated in central Asia. Some botanists and historians believe that the shallot was taken to Europe in the 12th and 13th century by crusaders returning from the Near East.

It is not known for certain when the shallot became popular in Europe, but it appears to have been adopted most enthusiastically by the French, who developed a variety of sauces based upon the simmering of the minced bulbs in white wine. After America was discovered, French cooking became established in New Orleans, which became part of the United States with the Louisiana Purchase in 1803. Hence, the use of shallots became part of a regional American cooking tradition which survives to this day.

PRODUCTION. Few statistics are available regarding the production of shallots in the United States and elsewhere. Nevertheless, it is believed that the annual U.S. commercial production ranges between 1,000 and 2,000 metric tons, and that the vegetable is also grown in many home gardens. Shallots are also produced in France and other European countries.

The optimal conditions for growing shallots are very similar to those for onions. That is, the bulbs should be planted in a well-cultivated organic (muck) soil and irrigated when the rainfall is inadequate. Shallots grown on clay soils usually have a bitter taste. It is noteworthy that cool weather favors the growth of the tops of the plant, whereas, warm (not hot) weather stimulates enlargement of the bulbs. Hence, shallots grown for "green onions" (immature bulbs and stems) are usually planted in the fall and early winter for harvesting in the spring, provided that there is no likelihood of a heavy frost during the growing period. Most of the U.S. crop is grown in the South. However, shallots grown for bulbs are planted in late winter or early spring for harvesting in the summer.

Immature shallots are harvested by pulling up the plants when the bulbs are about ¼ in. (*6 mm*) in diameter, whereas mature bulbs are harvested after the leaves turn yellow and start to wither.

PROCESSING. There is little or no processing of shallots because most of the crop is marketed as a fresh vegetable.

SELECTION. Immature shallots should have green, fresh tops, medium-sized necks well blanched for 2 or 3 in.(*5 to 8 cm*) from the bulb; and should be young, crisp, and tender.

Young, firm shallot bulbs with the skin unbroken are the most desirable. Soft or spongy shallot bulbs may have begun to sprout, and are undesirable. Split or broken skins of bulbs may also indicate sprouting. Decay may appear as mold, dry rot, or soft rot.

PREPARATION. Immature shallots may be served raw as an appetizer, or they may be minced and added to casseroles, hors d'oeuvres, relishes, salad dressings, salads, sandwiches, soups, and stews. They are also good when pickled.

Mature shallot bulbs may be chopped finely and used as a condiment. Certain French sauces are made by simmering the pieces in ample amounts of white wine until the volume of fluid is reduced greatly.

NUTRITIONAL VALUE. The nutrient composition of shallots is given in Food Composition Table F-36.

Some noteworthy observations regarding the nutrient composition of shallots follow:

1. Shallot bulbs are similar in nutrient composition to the Irish potato, in terms of the levels of calories, protein, and potassium provided. However, only small amounts of shallots are usually consumed.

2. The flavor of shallots is more delicate than that of either garlic or onions. Furthermore, shallots are believed to be more digestible.

(Also see VEGETABLE[S], Table V-6 Vegetables of the World.)

SHEA BUTTER

This is a fat obtained from the kernel of the fruit of the African tree, *Butyrospermum parkii*, also called butter tree or shea tree. Natives use the fat as a substitute for butter.

SHEARER (SHEARLING)

Yearling sheep, 12 to 18 months of age, intended for shearing and further finishing prior to slaughter.

SHIGELLOSIS (BACILLARY DYSENTERY)

A disease which may be transmitted by food and water contaminated with the *Shigella* bacteria from the feces of infected individuals. Houseflies are also active in its spread. Symptoms consist of fever, loss of appetite, vomiting, severe abdominal cramps, and massive diarrhea. Shigellosis is especially dangerous to young children and frail adults since they may become dehydrated. Epidemics are common where large groups are crowded together without adequate sanitation.

(Also see BACILLARY DYSENTERY; BACTERIA IN FOOD, Table B-5 Food Infections; and DISEASES, Table D-13 Infectious and Parasitic Diseases Which May Be Transmitted by Contaminated Food and Water—"Bacillary Dysentery [Shigellosis].")

SHORTENING

Fat substances given this name are used to "shorten foods." Their function is accomplished by forming films or clumps of fat throughout the food thereby preventing the protein and carbohydrate from cooking into one continuous hard mass. Thus, shortenings tenderize foods. Also, cake batters and icings often contain tiny air bubbles trapped in shortening that help to develop a fine delicate structure. It is the plastic consistency of shortenings that helps hold air in the food. The amount of shortening varies according to the product. Breads and rolls contain 1 to 2%, cakes 10 to 20%, and piecrusts contain over 30%. When shortenings are used in frying they serve for heat transfer and as antisticking agents, and provide some tenderness and richness of flavor.

Rendered animal fats and butter are shortening agents, but the term generally refers to fats which have been especially processed. For a number of years, lard or beef tallow were the main shortenings. Then with the development of hydrogenated vegetable oils came the increased use and acceptance of vegetable shortenings. Hydrogenation—adding hydrogen to the unsaturated fatty acids—can convert naturally liquid fats to semisolids. These shortenings may be prepared in all degrees of stiffness, from liquid to solid, depending upon their melting point. Melting point is determined by their degree of saturation. Then, in order to achieve specific physical, chemical, and biological properties, it is common to blend three or more different fats. Vegetable oils used include corn oil, cottonseed oil, soybean oil, olive oil, palm oil, peanut oil, safflower oil, and sesame oil. Thus, there are several general types of shortening meeting different needs.

• **General purpose**—These shortenings meet a variety of uses and are the household shortenings sold in grocery stores in metal containers. General purpose shortenings are semisolids when temperatures range from 60 to 90°F (*16 to 32°C.*) They may be employed by the home cook in biscuits, cookies, pie crusts, breads and rolls, pancakes, and pan frying. Also, these shortenings usually contain monoglycerides (glycerol molecules with only one fatty acid) so they may also be employed in cakes, icings, frostings, and other recipes wherein relatively large amounts of fat and water must be mixed without danger of separation. Monoglycerides act as emulsifiers.

• **Frying**—Shortenings used in frying must resist oxidation at high temperatures. Oxidation causes fat to darken, become thicker, foam during frying, and develop unpleasant flavors and odors. To resist oxidation at high temperatures, frying fats are composed of saturated fatty acids—low iodine value, and cannot contain mono- or diglycerides as these produce smoke at high frying temperatures. Moreover, fats whose fatty acids are short chain such as coconut oil are not suitable for deep fat frying because they breakdown and foam. Frying fats generally contain some antioxidants and antifoaming agents.

• **Special emulsifying**—These shortenings contain at least four emulsifying agents which complement each other and provide some particular characteristic. They provide the special properties necessary in prepared baking mixes, whipped toppings, icings, fillings, and the like.

• **Liquid oils**—Vegetable oils are required in mayonnaise and salad dressings, and may be used as a shortening agent in rolls, breads, and other fairly hard baked goods. They are a notable convenience in many kitchens. Also, the vegetable oils are the basis of margarine which may also be a shortening agent.

(Also see ADDITIVES; FATS AND OTHER LIPIDS; LARD; MARGARINE; and OILS, VEGETABLE.)

SHORTS

A by-product of flour milling consisting of a mixture of small particles of bran and germ, the aleurone layer, and coarse flour.

(Also see FLOURS.)

SHREDDED

Cut into long, narrow pieces.

SICKLE CELL ANEMIA

An inherited blood disease in which a defect in the manufacture of hemoglobin causes the blood cells to be sickle-shaped rather than round, and to be destroyed in the bloodstream with consequences that are frequently fatal. It is estimated that approximately 10% of all American blacks carry the sickle cell trait.

SIFTED

Materials that have been passed through wire sieves to separate particles of different sizes. The common connotation is the separation of finer material than would be done by screening.

(Also see FLOURS.)

SILICON (Si)

Silicon is one of the most abundant elements on earth—present in large amounts in soils and plants. The highest concentrations in animal tissue are found in the skin and its appendages; for example, the ash of feathers is more than 70% silicon.

HISTORY.   Although the early chemists considered silica (SiO_2) an elementary substance, Antoine Lavoisier, founder of quantitative chemistry, suspected in 1787 that it was an oxide of an undiscovered element. In 1823, Jons J. Berzelius, the Swedish chemist, discovered the element. The name *silicon* is derived from the Latin *silex* or *silicis*, meaning flint—appropriately indicating its hardness.

In 1972, Dr. E. Carlisle, Nutritionist at the University of California, Los Angeles, reported that the trace element silicon (Si) is needed in microgram amounts for normal growth and skeletal development of chicks and rats.

The free element silicon is not found in nature, but it occurs either as the oxide silica (SiO_2) in such forms as sand and quartz, or as silicates in such materials as granite. Silicon is important in plant and animal life; it is present in the ashes of plants and in human skeletons.

ABSORPTION, METABOLISM, EXCRETION. Silicon is absorbed readily. Even over a wide range of intake, the concentration in the blood remains relatively constant—not more than 1 mg per 100 ml. It is excreted easily—via both the feces and urine.

FUNCTIONS OF SILICON.   Silicon appears to be essential for chicks and rats; its absence from the diet impedes normal growth and skeletal development. These findings suggest that it may also have essential functions in man.

DEFICIENCY SYMPTOMS.   The production of deficiencies in chicks and rats, characterized by growth retardation and skeletal alterations and deformities, especially of the skull, depends on strict control of dietary and environmental contamination; this suggests a low requirement that is easily met by the amount in the environment.

Deficiencies of silicon have not been produced in man. However, it has been found that the silicon content of the aorta, skin, and thymus decrease significantly with age; this is probably related to the fact that the mucopolysaccharide (the substance that binds with water to form the thick gelatinous material which cements cells together and lubricates joints and bursas) content of body tissues also declines with aging.

INTERRELATIONSHIPS.   Silicon appears to take part in the synthesis of mucopolysaccharides and is a component of the mucopolysaccharide-protein complexes of connective tissue.

Normally, urinary silicon is eliminated efficiently. However, high levels of silicon in the diet of farm animals may be detrimental. In a manner not yet fully understood, part of it is sometimes deposited in the kidney, bladder, and urethra to form calculi (stones).

A common nondietary form of silicon toxicity is a lung condition known as silicosis, due to inhalation of airborne silicon oxide dust. The amount of silicon in the blood and urine increases in silicosis.

RECOMMENDED DAILY ALLOWANCE OF SILICON.   A human requirement of silicon cannot be established on the basis of available knowledge.

• **Silicon intake in average U.S. diet**—Human intake of silicon has been estimated at approximately I g per day.

TOXICITY.   Silicon does not appear to be toxic in the levels usually found in foods.

SOURCES OF SILICON.   Because of the abundance of silicon in all but the most highly purified foods, it is of little concern in human diets.

The best sources of silicon are the fibrous parts of whole grains, followed by various organ meats (liver, lungs, kidneys, and brain) and connective tissues. Much of the silicon in whole grains is lost when they are milled into highly refined products.

(Also see MINERAL[S], Table M-67.)

SIMPLE SUGARS

The *monosaccharides.* The most important simple sugars are *fructose, galactose, glucose,* and *mannose.*

SINGLE-CELL PROTEIN (SCP)

This refers to protein obtained from single-cell organisms, such as yeast, bacteria, and algae, that have been grown on specially prepared media. Production of this type of protein can be attained through the fermentation of petroleum derivatives or organic waste, or through the culturing of photosynthetic organisms in special illuminated ponds.

Historically, algae was a staple food of the Aztecs of Mexico. The high-protein algae was carried as rations by warriors. Today, Mexico exports 700 tons of algae to Japan, annually. For centuries, the natives of Lake Chad in Africa have dried and eaten algae from the lake. Of course, yeast and bacteria have long been used in the baking, brewing, and distilling industries, in making cheese and other fermented foods, and in the storage and preservation of foods. Dried brewers' yeast, a residue from the brewing industry, and torula yeast, resulting from the fermentation of wood residue and other cellulose sources, are currently marketed.

A wide variety of materials can be used as substrates for the growth of these organisms. Current research deals with the use of industrial by-products which otherwise would have little or no economic value. By-products from the chemical, wood and paper, and food industries have shown considerable promise as sources of nutrients for single-cell organisms; among them, (1) crude and refined petroleum products, (2) methane, (3) alcohols, (4) sulfite waste liquor, (5) starch, (6) molasses, (7) cellulose, and (8) animal wastes.

The potential of single-cell protein as a high-protein source for both man and livestock is enormous, but many obstacles must be overcome before it becomes widely used. It has been calculated that a single-cell protein fermenter covering ⅓ square mile *(0.8 km²)* could yield enough protein to supply 10% of the world's needs. To put this potential in a different perspective, a 1,000-lb steer will produce about 1 lb *(0.45 kg)* of protein per day. One thousand pounds of single-cell organisms might well produce up to 50 tons of protein per day. This is not to imply that we have solved the world's protein needs with single-cell protein because serious problems involving palatability, gastrointestinal disturbances, uric acid-accumulation, and simple economics must be solved before widescale production of single-cell protein becomes a reality. There is a limited amount of single-cell protein on the market in the form of brewers' yeast and torula yeast, but these products are generally too expensive to use as a major protein source.

TYPES OF SINGLE-CELL PROTEIN.

Single-cell protein can be produced by nonphotosynthetic and photosynthetic organisms. Of the nonphotosynthetic organisms, yeasts are the most popular sources, but bacteria and fungi are also currently being investigated, as potential sources. The photosynthetic organisms—algae—are grown in ponds that are illuminated and fortified with simple salts such as carbonates, nitrates, and phosphates.

Nonphotosynthetic Organisms.

Traditionally, yeasts have been used as sources of vitamins and uniden tified factors. They are easily harvested and pose few consumer resistance problems. One disadvantage to the utilization of yeasts as protein sources is that they are deficient in the sulfur amino acids. Fortunately, methionine hydroxy analog (MHA) is a cheap commercial product that can make up for this deficiency.

Bacteria grow very rapidly and tend to have a more balanced amino acid profile than yeasts. Additionally, they generally contain more protein. Since humans will probably avoid this type of protein for esthetic reasons, this type of single-cell protein, in all likelihood, will be developed as livestock feed. Currently, two serious problems exist with the culture of bacterial protein: (1) susceptibility to phages (bacteria-destroying agents) and (2) high ribonucleic acid content.

Until recently, the fungi have received little attention as single-cell protein. Since fungi can be harvested with relative ease and possess considerable enzymatic activity, they will likely be intensively studied in the near future.

Photosynthetic Organisms.

Photosynthetic organisms, such as algae, provide nutrients in relatively large quantities in a limited area. They convert sun energy directly into food. Depending on the type of organism, temperature, and latitude, yields of harvested protein can be attained on the order of 4 to 16 tons per acre yearly.

These organisms contain 5 to 15% dry matter. Nutrient composition (moisture-free) tends to be rather variable, with protein ranging from 8 to 75%, carbohydrate from 4 to 40%, lipids from 1 to 86%, and ash from 4 to 45%. The protein obtained from this type of single-cell protein is deficient in the sulfur amino acids, methionine and cystine. The biological value of algae protein has been estimated to range from 50 to 70. Additionally, algae provides a means of recycling animal wastes and renovating waste water

CURRENT PROBLEMS ASSOCIATED WITH SINGLE-CELL PROTEIN.

Although single-cell protein appears to be an excellent alternative or supplemental source of protein, several problems must be overcome before it becomes a widely used food; among them, palatability, digestibility, nucleic acid content, toxins, protein quality, and economics. A discussion of each of these problems follows:

• **Palatability**—Microbial cells must be processed to some extent if they are to be palatable. Otherwise, people will not eat them. Yeasts are bitter tasting, and algae and bacteria have characteristically unpleasant tastes which can depress intake. At the present time, processes making single-cell protein tasteless are being developed so that this souce of protein can be used as a supplement to more conventional foods.

• **Digestibility**—Ways of making single-cell protein more digestible must be developed if it is to be competitive with traditional protein foods. Digestibility among single-cell product sources tends to be extremely variable. When eaten alone, the digestibility of algae is low, while mixing algae with other foods improves digestibility. If the organisms are not killed prior to being used as a food, digestibility is dramatically reduced. Certain forms of processing can improve the digestibility of some single-cell protein products. For example, if algae are cooked prior to use, digestibility can be doubled in many cases. However, processing beyond the killing of yeasts does little to improve digestibility.

• **Nucleic acid content**—Much of the nitrogen found in single-cell organisms is in the form of nucleic acids. When the purines of the nucleic acids are metabolized, uric acid is formed. In man, uric acid is relatively insoluble with the result that uric deposits accumulate and lead to kidney stones or gout. Some of the current research is aimed at reducing the nucleic acid concentration.

Although the feeding of SCP to livestock may not produce physiological problems, it will be necessary to demonstrate to the consuming public that problems will not arise from the consumption of animal products produced from the feeding of SCP.

• **Toxicities**—Toxicities arising from the use of single-cell protein can result from two sources: (1) from toxins produced by the microorganisms themselves, and (2) from contaminated microorganisms. The second type of risk is probably the most likely to occur. Much of the single-cell protein will be derived from processes whereby by-products of industry are used as substrates. Thus, the microorganisms will in some ways reflect the chemical composition of the by-product. For example, if chemical residues, such as pesticides, or large amounts of trace minerals are present in the by-product substrate, the microorganism will, in all likelihood, absorb these chemicals. When livestock consume these contaminated microorganisms, toxicities may result. Hence, before widespread use can be made of single-cell proteins, there is the problem of convincing people and agencies of their wholesomeness.

• **Protein quality**—Research to date has indicated that SCP is deficient in the sulfur-containing amino acids, and possibly in lysine and isoleucine. While the amino acid profile of SCP is more balanced than that of the cereal grains, it is clearly inferior to the traditional protein supplements. However, this inferiority can often be overcome through the addition of commercially available methionine, or combination with other protein sources. Also, the advances in genetic engineering offer hope of developing new microorganisms capable of producing ideal amino acid profiles.

• **Economic problems**—As long as the more traditional sources of protein—such as the oilseed meals, meat, fish, eggs, and milk—are readily available at reasonable prices, single-cell protein will remain a relatively obscure alternative.

As the world's human population increases, there will be an increasing demand for cheap protein. This demand could dry up the sources of traditional protein, thereby opening the way for intensive development of alternative sources of proteins.

We are also entering an era of concern for the maintenance of the quality of our environment. This means that greater emphasis will be placed on the transformation of industrial by-products into usable commodities for both livestock and man. Single-cell protein is one way that this challenge can be met.

It is noteworthy that full-scale production of high protein animal supplement, made up of dried cells from a microorganism that lives on methanol, is now under way at Bellingham, in northern England, with a projected production of 50,000 tons annually. (Sherwood, Martin, Science News, Vol. II)

SIPPY DIET

A type of diet offered to bleeding peptic ulcer patients, originated by an American physician, Bertram Sippy, in 1915. It broke the previous practice of initial starvation treatment and established the beginning principles of continuous control of gastric acidity through diet and alkaline medication. To start with, the Sippy Diet consists of hourly feedings of 3 oz (*150 ml*) of whole milk, skim milk, or equal parts of cream and milk. After 2 or 3 days, up to 3 oz (*85 g*) of soft eggs, or strained cereals are added to the milk. Bland, easily digested foods may be occasionally added to break the monotony. Never does the total bulk of one feeding exceed 6 oz (*300 ml*).

(Also see LENHARTZ DIET; MODIFIED DIETS; and ULCERS, PEPTIC.)

SKIMMED

Material from which floating solid material has been removed. It is also applied to milk from which fat has been removed by centrifuging.

SKIN

• *Outer coverings of fruits or seeds, as the rinds, husks, or peels.*

• *Dermal tissue of man and animals.*

SKIN TEST (PATCH TEST) IN ALLERGY

A test used to diagnose allergies. It is a valuable diagnostic tool when used by an allergist. The test is conducted by injecting into the skin or rubbing into a scratch a minute quantity of an extract of the food or other substance suspected of causing the allergic reaction. If temporary hivelike wheals of varying sizes appear, it is indicative of sensitivity to the substance in question. Before accepting the results of the skin test two factors should be considered. First, if positive, it does not necessarily follow that a patient is sensitive to the same protein when taken by mouth. Second, the skin test may be negative to a protein which is producing allergic reactions elsewhere; for example, in the gut.

(Also see ALLERGIES.)

SLOE (BLACKTHORN) *Prunus spinosa*

A small, wild European plum (of the family *Rosaceae*) that is blackish purple with a very sour, green-colored flesh.

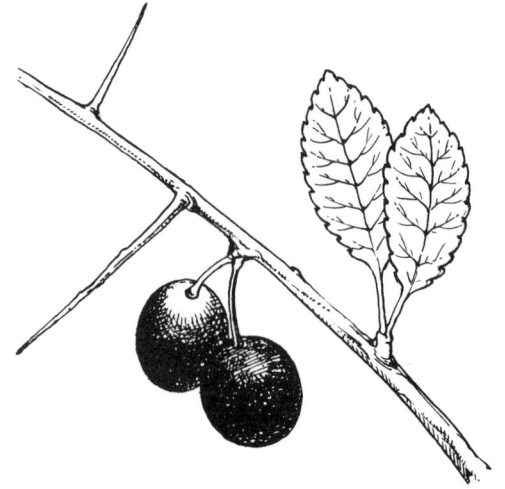

Fig. S-16.   Sloe, a very sour little plum that is used to make highly esteemed alcoholic beverages.

The sloe plum is used mainly in the production of sloe gin, jam, and a highly esteemed liqueur. Few people care to eat it raw.

SNACK FOODS

Snacks are those small portions of food eaten between meals; hence, no certain food is really a snack food. Individuality and need determine snack foods.

Snacking can be good or bad, depending upon the snack food and the frequency of snacking. Unfortunately, many people choose foods loaded with sugar and fat—calories—but low in protein, vitamins, and minerals. In keeping with the objective of good nutrition for good health, it just makes sense to eat nutritious snacks; for example, an orange, an apple, peanut butter and crackers, milk, nuts, raw vegetables, juice, etc. However, the type of snack depends on age and activity. Small children often fail to consume the amount of food in regular meals that will add up to their nutritional needs. A slice of cheese, a wheat cracker, or a banana at various times helps supply the added energy they need. The active growing bodies of teenagers need nutritious snacks which provide extra protein, vitamins, minerals, and energy; for example, nuts, yogurt, milk, fruit salads, and leftovers. Senior citizens often have chewing or digestion problems which interfere with regular eating habits. Here again nutritious snacks are helpful to meet daily needs.

Nutritious snacks are, however, no excuse for overindulgence. A calorie is still a calorie, and lots of little snacks add up. If more energy is consumed than used, the excess is stored as fat. Dieters should choose nutritious, but filling, snacks such as fresh fruits and raw vegetables.

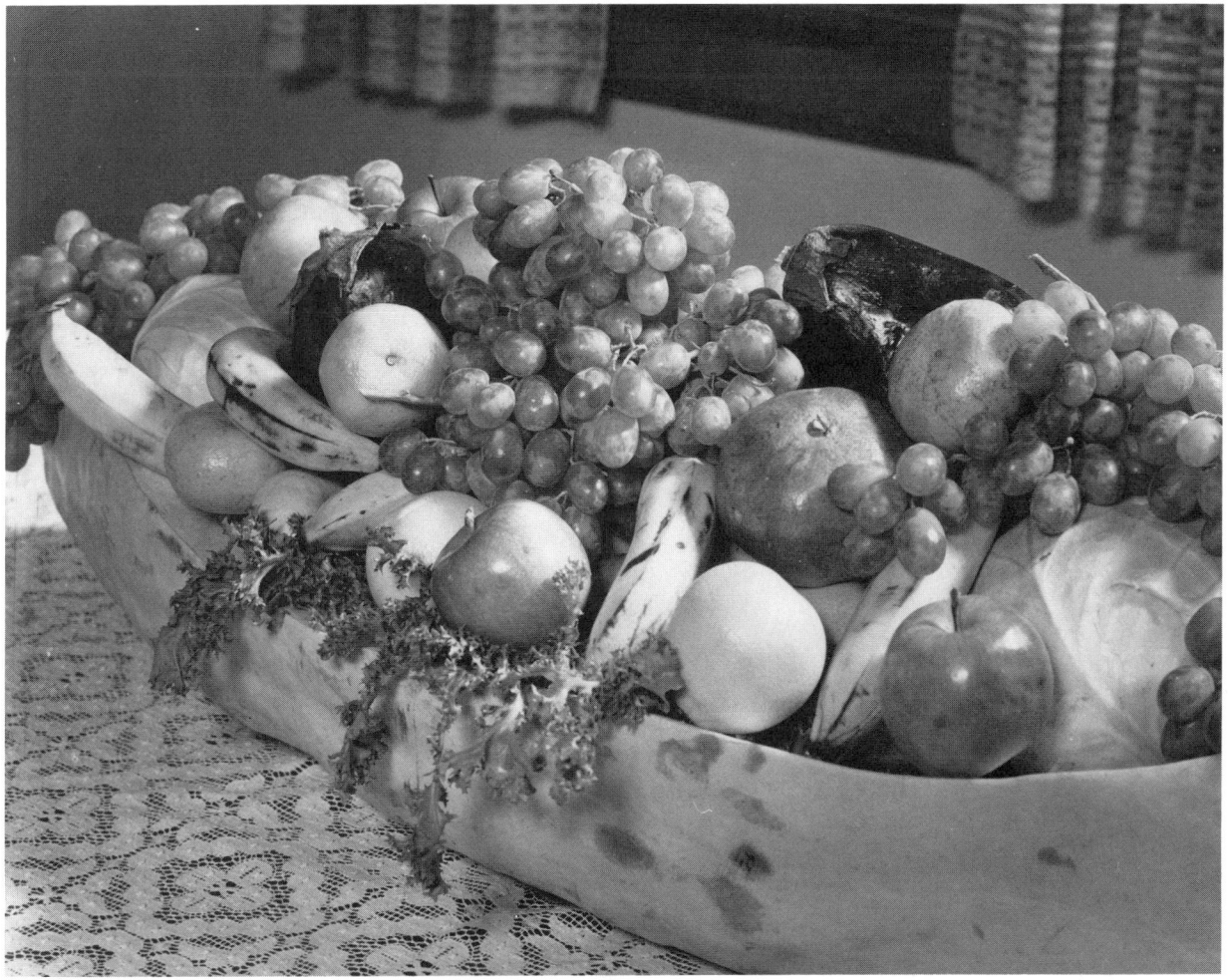

Fig. S-17.   America is blessed with a distribution system that provides a wide variety of fresh fruits and vegetables the year round. (Photo by J. C. Allen and Son, West Lafayette, Ind.)

The best way to ensure nutritious snacking is to keep the nutritious snacks on hand and available. Ideas for nutritious snacks are endless, and may be chosen by evaluating foods in terms of energy, protein, mineral and vitamin content as given in Food Composition Table F-36 of this book.

Table S-11 lists some of the common snacks—some are nutritious, others are not. Nevertheless, they are often used as snacks, and Table S-11 shows how the snacks compare calorie (energy) wise. Many individuals would do well to cut down on high calorie snacks.

(Also see CONVENIENCE AND FAST FOODS; and FAST FOODS.)

TABLE S-11
CALORIES CONTAINED IN
SOME COMMON SNACK FOODS[1]

Food	Approximate Measure	Weight	Calories	Food	Approximate Measure	Weight	Calories
		(g)	(kcal)			(g)	(kcal)
Bakery products				**Juices**			
Angel food cake...	1 piece	45	121	Apple cider	1 cup	249	125
Apple pie	1 average piece	118	302	Grape juice	1 cup	250	165
Assorted cookies..	1 average	20	96	Orange juice	1 cup	250	113
Cinnamon roll	1 average	55	174	Tomato juice......	1 cup	200	38
Cherry pie	1 average piece	118	308				
Chocolate cake ...	1 piece	40	146	**Milk and products**			
Doughnut	1 average	30	124	Cheddar cheese...	1 oz	28	113
Graham cracker...	1 average	7	27	Chocolate milk....	1 cup	250	175
Oatmeal cookie ...	1 average	13	60	Chocolate milk			
Pecan pie.........	1 average piece	103	431	shake	1 cup	345	413
Ritz cracker.......	1 average	3	16	Cottage cheese ...	1 cup	225	233
Rye wafer, whole				Ice cream	1 cup	135	282
grain	1 average	7	24	Swiss cheese	1 oz	28	104
Soda cracker	1 average	7	31	Yogurt, plain	1 cup	227	139
Beverages				**Nuts and seeds**			
Beer, 4, 5% alcohol.	1 cup	240	101	Almonds..........	1 average	1	6
Beer, natural light..	1 cup	240	67	Hazelnut..........	1 oz	28	107
Cola...............	1 cup	240	86	Peanut butter	1 Tbsp	32	190
Cream soda.......	1 cup	240	103	Peanuts	1 average	3	18
Root beer.........	1 cup	240	98	Sunflower seeds ..	1 cup	145	812
Desserts and sweets				**Snack foods[2]**			
Banana split	Individual	411	581	Corn chips........	1 cup	40	220
Caramel candy....	1 medium	10	40	Popcorn, popped			
Chewing gum	1 piece	3	10	with oil	1 cup	9	41
Chocolate bar.....	1 oz	28	148	Potato chips	1 cup	20	114
Chocolate-coated				Pretzels	1 average	13	51
fondant	1 oz	28	115				
Chocolate fudge ..	1 piece	25	100	**Vegetables**			
Gelatin dessert....	1 cup	240	147	Carrot, raw	1 large	100	42
Hard candy	1 piece	5	19	Cauliflower, raw...	1 cup	100	27
Jams or jelly	1 Tbsp	20	55	Celery, raw	1 small	20	3
Jelly beans	1 piece	3	11	Cucumber, raw ...	1 medium	100	14
Licorice	1 oz	28	97	Kohlrabi, raw	1 cup	149	43
Marshmallows	1 average	8	26	Lettuce, raw	1 cup	66	12
Rice pudding	1 cup	260	369	Mushroom, raw ...	1 small	10	3
Tapioca pudding..	1 cup	260	312	Radish, raw	1 small	10	2
				Tomato, raw	1 small	100	22
Fruits							
Apple, dried	1 oz	28	67				
Apple, raw	1 medium	150	84				
Banana, raw	1 average	115	112				
Cantaloupe	1 whole	770	231				
Grapefruit, raw....	1 whole	482	198				
Grapes, raw.......	1 cup	153	106				
Orange, raw	1 small	100	49				
Peach, dried	1 cup	160	379				
Peach, raw........	1 medium	100	38				
Pear, raw	1 average	200	122				
Prunes, dried	1 large	10	24				
Raisins	1 Tbsp	10	29				

[1]Foods are from the Food Composition Table F-36; hence, the food categories in the left column are those appearing in Table F-36.

[2]Snack foods are different for every individual, so it would be impossible to include all snack foods in this category. Nevertheless, this category appears in Food Composition Table F-36 of this book.

SNAP BEANS

The immature pods and seeds of the common bean. Also called string beans or green beans.

(See BEAN[S], Table B-10 Beans of the World; and BEAN, COMMON.)

SNIPE

Any of several game birds (genus *Capella*) that are widely distributed in the New and Old Worlds, especially in marshy areas. The snipe is best prepared by roasting.

SOAP

Chemically, soap is the alkali salt of fatty acids. It is formed by a process called saponification. Specifically, soap is a mixture of the sodium salts of the following fatty acids: stearic acid ($C_{17}H_{35}COOH$); palmitic acid ($C_{15}H_{31}COOH$); and oleic acid ($C_{17}H_{33}COOH$). Soft soaps are the potassium salts of these fatty acids. Hence, saponification is accomplished with either sodium hydroxide or potassium hydroxide. Glycerin or glycerol is a by-product of saponification, since the fatty acids are triglycerides—three fatty acids joined to glycerol. Saponification releases the fatty acids from glycerol. During World War II, housewives saved used cooking fats to be used in making soap, and more importantly glycerin for explosives. In a broad sense, soap is any salt of long-chain fatty acids. In the body, fatty acids which leave via the feces are almost entirely soaps.

(Also see FATS AND OTHER LIPIDS.)

SODA WATER

Water charged with carbon dioxide is termed soda water. It bubbles and fizzes as the gas is released. Soda water is added to syrups in soft drinks and to mixed alcoholic drinks. It does not possess any medicinal properties.

(Also see SOFT DRINKS [Carbonated Beverages] and WATER.)

SODIUM (Na)

Contents	Page

Most of the sodium in the diet is in the form of sodium chloride (NaCl), a white granular substance used to season and preserve food. It is created by combining the elements sodium (Na), a soft silvery-white metal, and chlorine (Cl), a poisonous, yellow gas; neither of which is desirable for use alone.

The need for sodium in the diet has been recognized since the classic experiment of Osborne and Mendel, reported in 1918.[37]

---

[37]Osborne, T., and L. Mendel, "Inorganic Elements in Nutrition," *Journal of Biological Chemistry*, Vol. 34, 1918, p. 131.

The body contains about 0.2% sodium, or about 100 g in a 154-lb (*70 kg*) person. About 50% of the sodium is in the extracellular (between cell) fluids, 40% is in the skeleton, and only about 10% is within the cells. In the blood, most of the sodium is in the plasma, which contains 320 mg per 100 ml.

HISTORY. Compounds of sodium were known and used extensively during ancient times, but the element was not isolated until 1807, when Sir Humphrey Davy, the English chemist used electricity (in a process called electrolysis) to extract the pure metal from sodium hydroxide. Although sodium had long been believed to be a dietary essential, final proof was not obtained until 1918 when Osborne and Mendel conducted laboratory animal experiments.

ABSORPTION, METABOLISM, EXCRETION. Virtually all sodium ingested in the diet is readily absorbed from the gut, following which it is carried by the blood to the kidneys, where it is filtered out and returned to the blood in amounts needed to maintain the levels required by the body.

Excess sodium, which usually amounts to 90 to 95% of ingested sodium, is, for the most part, excreted by the kidneys as chloride and phosphate and controlled by aldosterone, a hormone of the adrenal cortex. A deficiency of aldosterone, known as Addison's disease, leads to excessive losses of sodium in the urine.

The levels of sodium in the urine reflect the dietary intake; if there is high intake of sodium the rate of excretion is high, if there is low intake the excretion rate is low.

In hot weather, sodium excretion through the skin is important because each liter of sweat contains 0.5 to 3.0 g of sodium.

FUNCTIONS OF SODIUM. Sodium is the major positively charged ion in the fluid outside the cells, where it helps to maintain the balance of water, acids, and bases. Also, it is a constituent of pancreatic juice, bile, sweat, and tears.

Sodium is associated with muscle contraction and nerve functions. Sodium also plays a specific role in the absorption of carbohydrates.

DEFICIENCY SYMPTOMS. Deficiencies of sodium are rare because nearly all foods contain some sodium. However, deficiencies may occur from strict vegetarian diets without salt, or when there has been heavy prolonged sweating, diarrhea, vomiting, or adrenal cortical insufficiency. A deficiency of sodium may cause reduced growth, loss of appetite, loss of body weight due to loss of water, reduced milk production of lactating mothers, muscle cramps, nausea, diarrhea, and headache.

Excess perspiration and salt depletion may be accompanied by heat exhaustion. Salt tablets taken with a liberal amount of water may be advised under these conditions.

INTERRELATIONSHIPS. Sodium, potassium, and chlorine are closely related metabolically. They serve a vital function in controlling osmotic pressures and acid-base equilibrium; and they play important roles in water metabolism. Both sodium and potassium ions occur in the body chiefly in close association with the chloride ion; therefore, a sodium or potassium deficiency is rarely found in the absence of a chlorine deficiency.

Excess dietary salt, over a long period of time, is believed to lead to high blood pressure in susceptible people. Also, excess sodium may cause edema, evidenced by swelling of such areas as the legs and face. The simplest way to reduce sodium intake is to eliminate the use of table salt.

RECOMMENDED DAILY ALLOWANCES OF SODIUM. The salt requirements of the infant and young child are estimated to be about 58 mg per day. Human milk contains 161 mg of sodium per liter, whereas commonly used bottle formulas contain between 161 and 391 mg per liter and cow's milk contains about 483 mg per liter. Average intake of sodium during the first year of life ranges from about 300 mg per day at 2 months of age to about 1,400 mg per day at 12 months—far in excess of needs.

The healthy adult can maintain sodium balance with an intake of little more than the minimal requirements of the infant. When doing hard physical labor in high ambient temperatures, an adult may lose 8.0 g of sodium in sweat. Whenever more than 3 liter of water per day are required to replace sweat losses, extra salt (NaCl) should be provided; somewhere between 2 and 7 g of sodium chloride per liter of extra water loss, depending on the severity of losses and the degree of acclimatization. For those with a family history of high blood pressure, the food intake of salt should be limited to 1 to 2 g per day.

Pregnancy increases the sodium requirement, by an estimated 69 mg of sodium per day.

Estimated safe and adequate intakes of sodium are given in Table S-12.

TABLE S–12
ESTIMATED SAFE AND ADEQUATE
DAILY DIETARY INTAKES OF SODIUM[1]

Group	Age	Sodium
	(years)	(mg)
Infants	0.0–0.5	120
	0.5–1.0	200
Children and adolescents	1–3	225
	4–6	300
	7–10	400
	11+	500
Adults		500

[1]*Recommended Dietary Allowances*, 10th ed., 1989, NRC-National Academy of Sciences, p. 253, Table 11–1.

• **Sodium intake in average U.S. diet**—The average daily American intake of salt is 10 to 15 g, or about 5 g of sodium (salt is approximately 40% sodium and 60% chlorine by weight).

• **Salt intake and high blood pressure**—There is strong evidence linking too much salt to high blood pressure, which affects 20 million Americans. Also, there is evidence that high salt intake increases the incidence of hypertension among various societies and cultures of the world (Altschal, A. M. and J. K. Grommet, "Sodium Intake and Sodium Sensitivity," *Nutrition Reviews*, Vol. 38, December 1980, No. 12, pp. 393-402).

Under ordinary circumstances, children and adults require no more than 0.2 g—about 1/10 tsp—of salt per day. With strenuous exercise or labor accompanied by profuse sweating, only 2 g—just under 1 tsp— is necessary. Normally, therefore, an allowance of 1 g of salt per day is sufficient. Yet, studies reveal that the average American consumes about 10 g of salt per day—ten times more than the recommended allowance.

People with high blood pressure should drastically curtail their salt intake. Fortunately, salt appetite can be readily revised downward, for there are no withdrawal pains from giving up salt. This can be accomplished by using the salt shaker sparingly, both in the kitchen and in the dining room; and by avoiding salty foods, such as olives, popcorn, potato chips, french fries, and sauerkraut.

It is noteworthy that cultural factors appear to determine the salt consumption. For example, the Japanese commonly consume 25 to 50 g of salt per day, whereas the Eskimos, Lapps, Australian aborigines, numerous tribes of New Guinea, South America and Africa, and many midwestern American Indian tribes consume from a few hundred milligrams to no more than 5 g of salt per day.

(Also see SALT.)

TOXICITY. Salt may be toxic when (1) a high intake is accompanied by a restriction of water, (2) when the body is adapted to a chronic low salt diet, or (3) when it is fed to infants or others whose kidneys cannot excrete the excess in the urine.

SOURCES OF SODIUM. In addition to salt (sodium chloride) used in cooking, processing and seasoning, sodium is present in all foods in varying amounts. Generally more sodium is present in protein foods than in vegetables and grains. Fruits contain little or no sodium. The salt added to these foods in preparation could be many times that found naturally in foods. Also, the sodium content of the water supply varies considerably; in some areas of the country, the amount of sodium in the water is of sufficient quantity to be of significance in the total daily intake.

Generally speaking, the need is for low sodium diets, rather than high sodium diets; especially by people with high blood pressure. Table S-13 has been prepared to meet this need.

TABLE S-13
GROUPINGS OF SOME LOW SODIUM FOODS[1]

Sodium Level				
0-5 mg/100 g	**5-10 mg/100 g**	**10-20 mg/100 g**	**20-40 mg/100 g**	**40-60 mg/100 g**
Almonds	Apples, dried	Avocados	Artichokes	Arrowroot
Apples	Apricots, dried	Broccoli	Brown sugar	Black pepper
Asparagus	Chestnuts	Brussels sprouts	Chinese cabbage	Beef
Apricots	Cucumbers	Cabbage	Coconut	Carrots
Banana	Dock	Cantaloupe	Cream	Chicken giblets
Blackberries	Green onions	Cauliflower	Hot chili peppers	Dandelion greens,
Cherries	Honey	Collards	Passion fruit	cooked
Currants	Kohlrabi	Dried figs	Potato flour	Egg yolks
Dates	Lettuce	Endive	Red cabbage	Kale
Eggplant	Nectarine	Garden cress	Sunflower seeds	Milk
Figs	Parsnips	Garlic	Turnips	Parsley
Fresh fruit juices	Peaches, dried	Mangos		Pork pancreas
Grapefruit	Peanut flour	Mature onions		Rabbit meat
Grapes	Peanuts	Molasses		Red beets, boiled
Green beans	Pears, dried	Mushrooms		Sablefish
Green peas	Persimmons	Mustard greens		Sole
Guavas	Pigeonpeas	Pecans		Sunflower seed flour
Lard	Waxgourd	Prunes		Tamarinds
Lima beans	Wheat bran	Radish		Tuna
Oils		Raisins		Turkey
Okra		Split peas		Walleye pike
Oranges		Sweet potatoes		Watercress
Peaches		Turnip greens		Yogurt, whole milk
Pears		Yeast		
Pineapple				
Potatoes				
Raspberries				
Rhubarb				
Rye flour				
Shortening				
Soybean flour				
Squash				
Strawberries				
Sugar				
Sweet corn				
Tomatoes				
Walnuts				
Watermelon				
Wax beans				
Wheat flour				
Wheat germ				
Whole wheat flour				

[1]These listings are based on data from the Food Composition Table F-36. The above foods contain no added salt or other sodium source, and are listed without regard to the amount normally eaten.

Often there is also need to know what foods are particularly high in sodium, so that they may be avoided. Groupings of common food sources of sodium in descending order follow:

• **Rich sources**—Anchovy paste, bacon, bologna, bran cereal, butter and margarine, Canadian bacon, corned beef, cornflakes cereal, cucumber pickles, cured ham, dehydrated cod, dried squid, frankfurters, green olives, luncheon meats, oat cereal, parmesan cheese, pasteurized process cheese, potato chips, pretzels, sausages, seaweed, shrimp, smoked herring, soda crackers, soy sauce, tomato catsup, wheat flakes cereal.

• **Good sources**—Breads and cookies, canned vegetables, cheeses, condensed soups, many prepared foods and mixes, peanut butter, pickled foods, salad dressings, seafoods.

• **Fair sources**—Beef, desserts and sweets, eggs, lamb, milk, pork, poultry, salt-loving vegetables (spinach, beets, chard, celery, carrots), some fish (cod, haddock, salmon, tuna) depending upon preparation, veal, yogurt.

• **Negligible sources**—Lard, legumes, most fresh fruits and vegetables, rye flour, shortening, soybean flour, sugar, vegetables oils, wheat bran, wheat flour.

• **Supplemental sources**—Salt (sodium chloride), baking soda, monosodium glutamate (MSG), sodium-containing baking powders.

NOTE WELL: Many processed foods contain high levels of sodium due to the addition of salt and other sodium-containing additives; among them, sodium alginate, sodium aluminum sulfate, sodium benzoate, sodium citrate, sodium diacetate, sodium erythorbate, sodium nitrate, sodium nitrite, sodium propionate, and sodium sorbate.

For additional sources and more precise values of sodium, see Food Composition Table F-36.

HIGH SODIUM SOURCES. In order that consumers may intelligently cut back on sodium intake, it is important that they know which foods are high in sodium. Table S-14 lists some of the high sodium foods and gives the precise sodium content of each.

(Also see MINERAL[S], Table M-67; and SALT.)

TABLE S-14
SOME HIGH SODIUM FOODS[1]

Food	Sodium
	(mg/100 g)
Canadian bacon	2,555
Olives, green	2,400
Shrimp, canned	2,300
Caviar	2,200
Corned beef	1,740
Pretzels	1,680
Parmesan cheese	1,602
Pasteurized process cheese	1,430
Cucumber pickles	1,428
Bologna	1,300
Oat cereal	1,267
Luncheon meat	1,200
Soda crackers	1,100
Cured ham	1,100
Frankfurters	1,084
Wheat flakes cereal	1,032
Bacon	1,021
Bran cereal	1,012
Corn flakes cereal	1,005
Potato chips	1,000
Rice flakes cereal	987
Sausage	958

[1]Data from the Food Composition Table F-36.

SODIUM BICARBONATE (NaHCO₃)

A chemical compound which is known to function as a buffer and pH agent, maintaining sufficient alkaline reserves (buffering capacity) in the body fluids to ensure normal physiological and metabolic functions.

(Also see ACID-BALANCES; ADDITIVES, Table A-3; and ANTACIDS.)

SODIUM CHLORIDE (NaCl)

The chemical term for ordinary table salt which is composed of the two elements, sodium and chlorine.

(Also see ADDITIVES, Table A-3; SALT; and SODIUM.)

SODIUM DIACETATE

An antimicrobial food additive which controls both rope (bacterial action) and mold in breads. The FDA allows flour used in bakery goods to contain 0.4% sodium diacetate.

(Also see ADDITIVES, Table A-3; and ROPE.)

SODIUM PHYTATE

A chelating agent that is formed from phytic acid. In the past, it has been employed as part of a treatment for calcium phosphate kidney stones.

(Also see PHYTIC ACID.)

SODIUM-POTASSIUM RATIO

Sodium and potassium are closely interrelated. Although sodium intake may be the most important dietary determinant of blood pressure, variations in the sodium: potassium ratio in the diet affect blood pressure under certain circumstances. In rats with high blood pressure due to a high intake of sodium, blood pressure may be lowered to a more normal level by increasing the potassium intake and lowering the sodium intake. It seems that a 1:1 ratio may be somewhat protective against the blood pressure-elevating effects of a given level of sodium. This ratio can be achieved by increasing the intake of potassium, or lowering the intake of sodium, or both. Good dietary sources of potassium include meats, milk, dried dates, bananas, cantaloupe, apricots, tomato juice, and the dark green leafy vegetables.

(Also see HIGH BLOOD PRESSURE; POTASSIUM; and SODIUM.)

SOFT DRINKS (CARBONATED BEVERAGES)

This name is given to the familiar American beverages, often called *soda pop* or *pop.* The name "soft" is used to distinguish these beverages from "hard" or alcoholic beverages. Soft drinks are generally, but not always, carbonated, and contain a sweetening agent, edible acids,

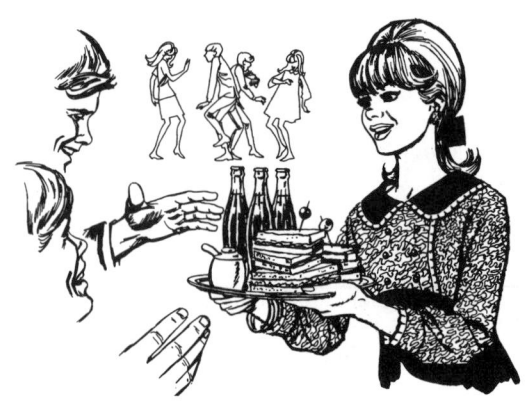

Fig. S-18. In moderation, the occasional soft drink at a party can be part of the fun.

and natural or artifical flavors. Today, everywhere people work or play, soft drinks are available and their yearly consumption reflects their availability—and the advertising budget of the major producers.

HISTORY.

In 1772, the Englishman, Joseph Priestley, described a pleasant-tasting, sparkling water which he produced by introducing carbon dioxide (CO_2) into the water. Thus, carbonated beverages were born; however, Priestley is better known for his discovery of oxygen.

In 1806, the real business of selling soft drinks was started by Benjamin Silliman, a chemistry professor at Yale College in Connecticut. In New Haven, he bottled and sold soda water—water charged with carbon dioxide. Sometime after 1830, flavored soda water became popular, and by 1860, the census reported 123 plants producing carbonated drinks. During the Civil War the following soda water flavors were promoted: pineapple, black cherry, orange, apple, strawberry, raspberry, gooseberry, pear, melon, lemon, cherry, plum, grape, apricot, and peach. In 1886, a druggist and former Confederate soldier named John Styth Pemberton created a drink which is still favored. He added an extract from the African kola nut to an extract from cocoa. Another enterprising pharmacist named Hires, introduced bottled root beer in 1893. Currently, the popular flavors are cola, lemon-lime, orange, ginger ale, root beer, and grape, but every conceivable type of flavor has been produced. Cola drinks are the most popular.

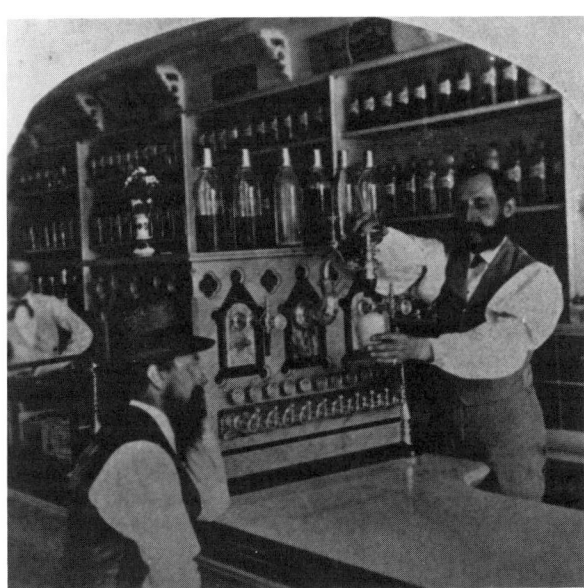

Fig. S-19. An American soda fountain, part of the beginnings of the profitable soft drink industry. (Photo of The Bettmann Archive, Inc., New York, N.Y.)

Now, the soft drink industry is one of the most profitable American businesses, with the wholesale value of soft drinks over $23.3 billion, annually.

CONSUMPTION. In 1850, the United States per capita consumption of soft drinks was only about 1 pt per year. In 1990, the per capita consumption was about 47.5 gal—more than 3.5 times the consumption in 1960 (see Fig. S-20). But that's not all! Ponder these figures:

• In 1990, the average man, woman, and child in the United States drank 760 8-oz soft drinks (in comparison to only 25.4 gal of milk)—that's an average of 1½ 12-oz cans per day.

• Soda pop now provides about 8% of the calories consumed daily by the average person, with virtually all these calories coming from sugar.

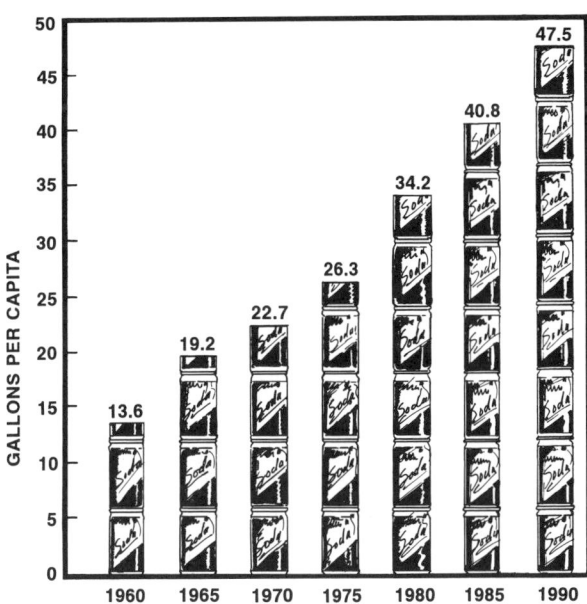

Fig. S-20. The rise in soft drink—carbonated beverage—consumption. (Sources: USDA; J. C. Maxwell, *Beverage Industry*, February 1991)

Yearly, consumption of soft drinks surpasses milk, beer, or coffee. This popularity is probably due to their availability and the tremendous advertising efforts of the major companies. The ad expenditures of the soft drink companies total over $200 million each year—all for convincing people to drink "the real thing," "the uncola," or to join a certain "generation" or to become a "pepper."

INGREDIENTS AND PRODUCTION. The precise formulaton of most soft drinks is not well known. However, certain aspects of soft drinks are governed by standards of identity enforced by the Food and Drug Administration (FDA).

• **Soda water**—According to the standards of identity, soda water is the class of beverages made by absorbing carbon dioxide in potable water. The amount of carbon dioxide used is not less than that which will be absorbed by the beverage at a pressure of one atmosphere and at a temperature of 60°F (15.5°C). It either contains no alcohol or only such alcohol as is contributed by the flavoring ingredient used not in excess of 0.5% by weight of the finished beverage.

• **"Cola" or "pepper"**—Soda water designated by any name which includes the word "cola" or "pepper" shall contain caffeine from kola nut extract and/or other natural caffeine-containing extracts. Also, caffeine may be added to any soda water. The total caffeine content in the finished food shall not exceed 0.02% by weight.

Soda water may contain any safe and suitable optional ingredient, except that vitamins, minerals, and proteins added for nutritional purposes and artificial sweeteners are not suitable for food encompassed by this standard.

The optional ingredients include: sweetening agents, acids, flavors, colors, preservatives, emulsifying, stabilizing or viscosity-producing agents, and foaming agents. Sweetening agents may consist of the following nutritive sweeteners (calorie-containing): dry or liquid sugar (sucrose), invert sugar, dextrose, fructose, corn syrup, glucose syrups, or sorbitol, singly or in combination. Presently, the nonnutritive sweetener aspartame is used in diet soft drinks. Flavoring agents in a carrier of ethyl alcohol, glycerin, or propylene glycol may include fruit juices, including concentrates and natural flavoring derived from fruits, vegetables, bark, roots, leaves, and similar plant materials. Artificial flavoring may also be used, as well as natural or artificial color. The edible acids which may be used singly or in combination are acetic, adipic, citric, fumaric, gluconic, lactic, malic, tartaric, and phosphoric acids. Table S-15 shows how some of these ingredients make up the familiar soft drinks.

Even with all of the ingredients in Table S-15, water is in the greatest quantity, representing 86 to 92%, when nutritive sweeteners are used, and nearly 100% in the diet soft drinks. In drinks containing nutritive sweeteners, these sweeteners comprise most of the remaining 9 to 14%, leaving a very small portion for the flavoring, preservatives, color, acid, etc.

(Also see ADDITIVES; ASPARTAME; SUGAR; and SWEETENING AGENTS.)

Fig. S-21 provides a generalized scheme for the production of soft drinks.

The following salient points apply to the production of soft drinks:

1. Water is usually subjected to some additional processing including chlorination, treatment with lime, coagulation, sedimentation, and sand filtration, followed by treatment with activated carbon, with some adaptation to the properties of the particular water.

2. The syrup is the complete mixture of all ingredients necessary to make the carbonated beverage, with the exception of the carbonated water.

3. Carbonation is accomplished by a presyrup or premix process. In the presyrup process, a measured amount of syrup is placed in the washed **bottle**, carbonated water is added, a constant counter-pressure

TABLE S-15
SOFT DRINK INGREDIENTS

Soft Drink	Flavors	Color	Sugar (%)	Edible Acid	Carbon Dioxide (CO_2) (volume of gas)[1]
Cola	Extract of kola nut, lime oil, spice oils, caffeine.	Caramel	11-13	Phosphoric	3.5
Orange	Oil of orange and orange juice.	Sunset yellow FCF with some Tartrazine.	12-14	Citric	1.5-2.5
Ginger ale	Ginger root, oil or ginger, and lime oil.	Caramel	7-11	Citric	4.0-4.5
Root beer	Oil of wintergreen, vanilla, nutmeg, cloves or anise.	Caramel	11-13	Citric	3
Grape	Methyl anthranilate and oil of cognac, sometimes grape juice.	Amarinth and Brilliant Blue FCF.	11-13	Tartaric	1.0-2.5

[1]A volume of gas is equivalent to 15 lb per square inch at sea level and 60°F (15.5°C). Correct carbonation results in pungent taste.

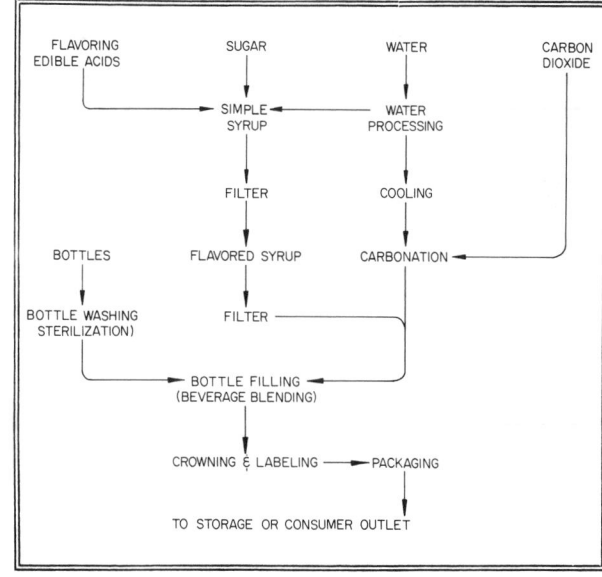

Fig. S-21. How carbonated beverages are made.

prevents the loss of carbon dioxide before crowning, whereupon the bottle is whirled to mix the contents. The premix system eliminates the whirling (mixing) step by combining the proper volumes of syrup and water which are carbonated in a specific type of carbonator and then bottled.

For a number of years, carbonated beverages were packaged predominantly in glass bottles of 6 to 32 oz (*120 to 960 ml*). Recently, there has been an increase in the use of nonreturnable bottles—glass and plastic. These bottles eliminate the washing operation. However, resource-saving and pollution control may dictate the type of bottle in the future. Furthermore, since the early 1950s more and more cans have been used for carbonated beverages. Now most cans are aluminum and recycling is encouraged. Most soft drinks are sold in bottles or cans, but many are also prepared in fast food operations and dispensed in glasses or cups.

Soft drink plants are subject to state and federal laws and regulations which are designed to protect the consumer and to serve as an operational guide for the manufacturer.

NUTRITIONAL VALUE. Probably the best thing that can be said about soft drinks is that their flavor encourages people to drink water. Soft drinks containing nutritive sweeteners contribute empty calories to the diet. Each 12-oz (*360 ml*) can supplies about 147 Calories (kcal); hence, excessive usage may contribute to tooth decay and overweight. Diet soft drinks, which became popular during the 1960s, are essentially flavored water. Also, sparkling water (club soda) is carbonated water without sugar (calories), and sometimes with added sodium bicarbonate or sodium sulfate in an effort to simulate natural mineral water. Despite the nutritional shortcomings of carbonated beverages, many people indulge primarily because they enjoy the taste, the tingling sensation of the carbonation, and the mildly stimulating effects. Food Composition Table F-36 compares some of the common soft drinks.

Considering the alternatives, water costs less and quenches the thirst, and milk provides a few more calories but better nutrition. Moreover, 12 oz of milk costs less than 12 oz of a soft drink. Fruit juices are also viable alternatives providing substantially more nutrition at a cost comparable to soft drinks.

(Also see BEVERAGES; DENTAL HEALTH, NUTRITION, AND DIET; MILK; and WATER.)

SOLANINE

A naturally occurring toxicant found in the nightshade family, which includes such useful plants as the potato, tomato, ground cherry, red pepper, and eggplant. In large enough doses it acts on the nervous system since it is an inhibitor of acetylcholinesterase, an enzyme involved in the transmission of nervous impulses. Potatoes contain the highest levels of solanine. However, a person would have to eat, at one sitting, 4.5 lb (*2.0 kg*) of potatoes containing 200 mg (100 ppm) of solanine to produce the initial effects of poisoning—drowsiness and itchiness behind the neck.

CAUTION: Potatoes that are green, spoiled, or sprouted may contain harmful amounts of solanine.

(Also see POISONOUS PLANTS; and POTATO, section headed "Selection.")

SOLIDS, MILK

The solids, or total solids, of milk includes all the constituents of milk except water. Milk contains an average of 12% total solids.

(Also see MILK AND MILK PRODUCTS, section headed "Nutrients of Milk.")

SOLIDS-NOT-FAT, MILK

This includes the carbohydrate, protein, minerals, and water-soluble vitamins of milk—it excludes the fat. Milk contains an average of 8.6% solids-not-fat.

(Also see MILK AND MILK PRODUCTS, section headed "Nutrients of Milk.")

SOLUTES

Particles in solution in body water. Three types of solutes influence internal shifts and balances of body water: (1) electrolytes, (2) plasma proteins, and (3) organic compounds of small molecular size.

SOLVENT-EXTRACTED

Fat or oil removed from materials (such as oilseeds) by organic solvents. Also called "new process."

(Also see OILS, VEGETABLE; and FATS AND OTHER LIPIDS.)

SORBIC ACID (SORBATE; $C_6H_8O_2$)

A food additive possessing antimicrobial activity especially toward yeast and molds. It is commonly used in the form of *sodium sorbate* and *potassium sorbate*. In the body, all evidence indicates that sorbate is metabolized like other fatty acids. It is on the GRAS (generally recognized as safe) list of approved food additives. Food applications or sorbic acid are numerous, but they include: baked goods, beverages, cheese and cheese products, dried fruits, fish, fruit juices, jams, jellies, meats, pickled products, salads, and wines.

(Also see ADDITIVES, Table A-3.)

SORBITOL (HEXITOL; $C_6H_{14}O_6$)

A naturally occurring 6-carbon sugar alcohol or polyol that tastes about 60% as sweet as table sugar (sucrose). In nature, it occurs in many berries, cherries, plums, pears, apples, and blackstrap molasses. Sorbitol is a

GRAS (generally recognized as safe) food additive. For commercial use, it is prepared by the hydrogenation of glucose.

Due to a variety of unique properties, sorbitol enjoys widespread use by the food industry. It has the following applications: (1) viscosity or bodying agent; (2) crystallization modification; (3) humectant; (4) dietetic foods; (5) sequestrant; (6) rehydration aid; (7) solvent; (8) softening or plasticizing agent; and (9) bulking agent. Hence, the consumer will find sorbitol in confections, chewing gum, dried roasted nuts, meat products, pet foods, icings, toppings, coconut, dairy products, brown sugar, and beverages. Furthermore, because of its sweetness and unique metabolism—burned to CO_2 without ever appearing as blood sugar, glucose—sorbitol is used to replace sugar in numerous special dietary foods. These foods often carry the label "sugarless" or "sugar free." This is somewhat misleading since this leads many consumers to believe that the product or food contains fewer or no calories. This is not true. Sorbitol contains the same number of calories per gram as does table sugar (sucrose). It is just metabolized differently.

(Also see ADDITIVES, Table A-3.)

SORGHUM (GUINEA CORN: KAFFIR: MILO)
Sorghum vulgare

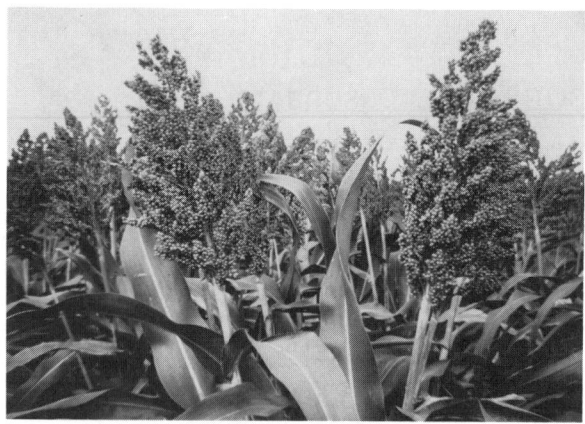

Fig. S-22. Hybrid grain sorghum, headed out and nearing harvest. (Courtesy, National Grain Sorghum Producers Assn., Abernathy, Tex.)

Sorghum is widely scattered throughout the world and known under a variety of names. It's called guinea corn in West Africa; kaffircorn and mealies in South America; mtama in East Africa; durra in the Sudan; Egyptian corn in Egypt; juar, jowar, and cholam in India; koaliang in China; and kaffir and milo in America. By whatever name, it is the staple food in parts of Asia and Africa. In the United States, where it is used primarily as an animal feed, it is the third ranking cereal crop in acreage harvested, being exceeded only by corn and wheat.

(Also see CEREAL GRAINS.)

ORIGIN AND HISTORY. Sorghum has been cultivated in Africa and Asia for 4,000 years.

Under the name "chicken corn," sorghum was introduced along the southern Atlantic Coast of the United States in colonial times. But it was not successfully cultivated at that time. Subsequently, grain sorghums and Sudangrass were reintroduced from Africa.

WORLD AND U.S. PRODUCTION. Sorghum is a tropical or subtropical plant, grown mainly in hot, dry regions where corn, rice, and wheat cannot be produced successfully. Although well adapted to semiarid conditions, sorghum makes efficient use of irrigation.

Sorghum is the fifth ranking cereal food crop of the world, being exceeded by wheat, rice, corn, and barley. The world sorghum crop averages 58 million metric tons. The ten leading producing countries, by rank, are: United States, India, Mexico, China, Nigeria, Argentina, Sudan, Ethiopia, Australia, and Burkino Faso (see Fig. S-23).

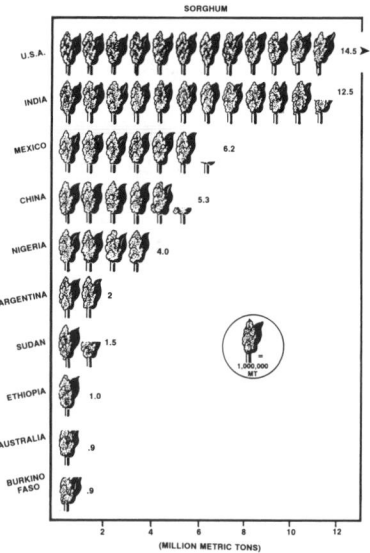

Fig. S-23. Leading sorghum-producing countries of the world. (Source: FAO Production Yearbook, 1990, FAO/UN, Rome, Italy, Vol. 44, p. 85, Table 24)

The United States produces about 25% of the world's sorghum grain. The U.S. sorghum belt is the Southern Great Plains. The ten leading states, by rank, are: Kansas, Texas, Nebraska, Missouri, Arkansas, Oklahoma, Illinois, South Dakota, Colorado, and Louisiana. Kansas and Texas account for 56% of the nation's production (see Fig. S-24).

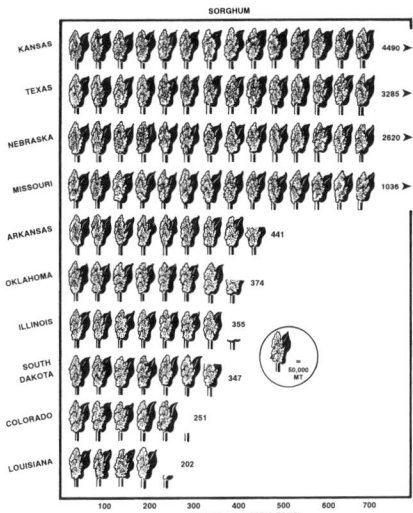

Fig. S-24. Leading sorghum-producing states of the United States. (Source: *Agricultural Statistics 1991*, USDA, p. 52, Table 67)

THE SORGHUM PLANT.

Sorghum is a member of the grass family, *Gramineae*. Grain sorghum, sweet sorghum, broomcorn, and Sudangrass are classified as genus *Sorghum*, species *vulgare*.

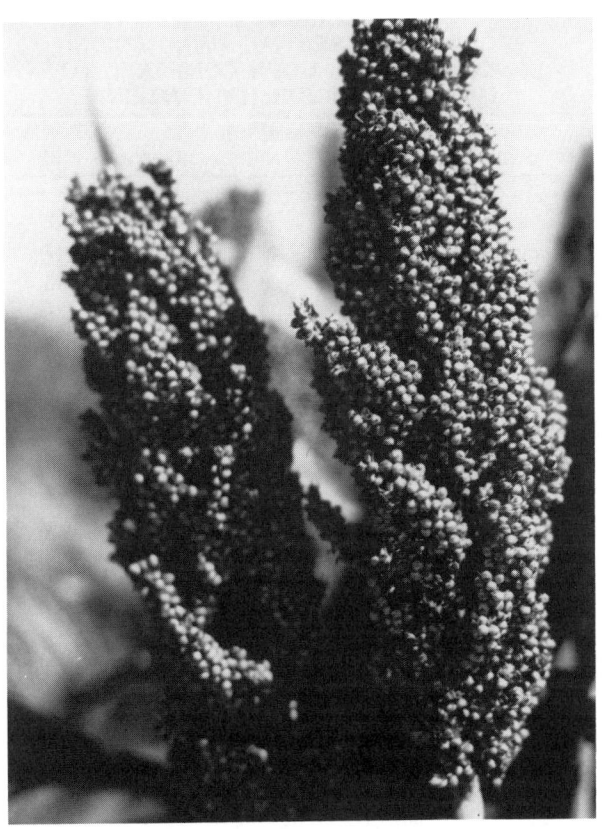

Fig. S-25. Heads of grain sorghum. (Courtesy, Funks Seeds International, Bloomington, III.)

In its early growth stages, grain sorghum is difficult to distinguish from corn. Later, it becomes strikingly different. Sorghum plants may tiller (put out new shoots), producing several head-bearing culms from the basal nodes. The head varies from a dense to a lax panicle. Mature grain varies in size according to varieties, and in color from white to cream, red, and brown. Color pigments are located in the pericarp (outer covering) of the grain or in a layer of cells beneath the pericarp called the testa. The endosperm (starch portion of the seed) is either white or yellow.

SORGHUM CULTURE.

Good seedbed preparation is essential for full stands and weed control.

Being tropical in origin, sorghum should not be planted in the spring until the soil temperature is 70°F (*22°C*) at planting depth. A seeding depth of 1 in. (*2.5 cm*) is acceptable in moist, friable soil, but 2 in. (*5.1 cm*) may be necessary under dry land conditions. The distance between rows depends on whether or not cultivation is intended. Seeding rate ranges from 3 to 5 lb per acre (*3.4 to 5.6 kg/ha*) in dry-land farming up to 10 lb per acre (*11.2 kg/ha*) when planted under more favorable moisture conditions and irrigation. A rotary hoe may be used in controlling weeds when the plants are small, with a cultivator used later; or minimum tillage may be practiced, with weeds controlled by herbicides.

Nearly all grain sorghum in the United States is harvested with a combine. The grain threshes freely from the head when the moisture content is under 22%. The grain should not contain more than 12 to 13% moisture for safe storage. Grain dryers may be used when newly harvested grain is not dry enough for safe storage.

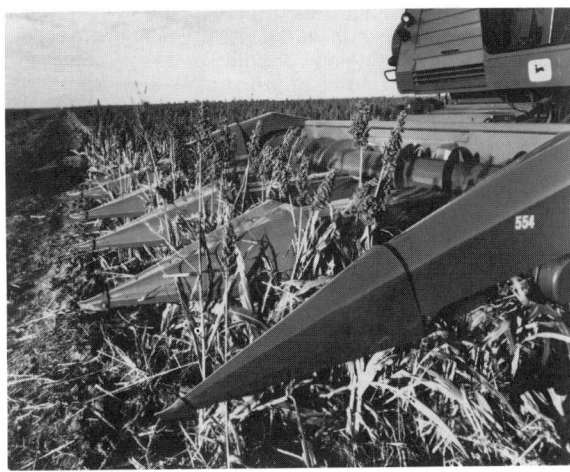

Fig. S-26. Harvesting grain sorghum with a combine. (Courtesy, Deere & Company, Moline, III.)

KINDS.

The cultivated sorghums can be classified into the following four broad classifications according to use:

1. **Grain sorghums.** These sorghums are bred specially for grain production. Most types in the United States are less than 5 ft tall. Common grain varieties include kaffir, milo, leterita, Durra, shallu, koaliang, and hegari.

2. **Grass sorghums.** These have thin stems, narrow leaves, and numerous tillers—characteristics which make them useful for hay or grazing by animals. Sundangrass and Johnsongrass belong to this group.

3. **Sweet sorghums (sorgos).** These have tall, sweet, juicy stalks that are used for forage, syrup, and sugar production.

4. **Broomcorn sorghums.** These have panicle branches which are suitable for making brooms.

Today, most of the sorghums grown in the United States are hybrids, developed by crossing varieties. For grain production, crosses involving kaffir and milo are most common.

FEDERAL GRADES. The U.S. Department of Agriculture recognizes four classes of grain sorghums: yellow, white, brown, and mixed. Within each class, there are five grades: U.S. No. 1, U.S. No. 2, U.S. No. 3, U.S. No. 4, and U.S. Sample grade. Grades are based on moisture, damaged kernels (including heat damage), broken kernels, foreign material, and other grain.

PROCESSING. As with corn, sorghum may be either dry milled or wet milled. However, most sorghum is dry milled, simply because it is easier to accomplish.

• **Dry milling**—The objective in dry milling of sorghum grain is to separate the endosperm, germ, and bran from each other.

To facilitate milling, the sorghum grain is first conditioned by tempering with water. The dry milling processes consist of roller milling and pearling or decortication procedures. The yield, degree of refinement, and separations are determined by the efficiency of the operation.

The endosperm is processed into grits and flour. The other products of dry milling are bran, germ, and hominy feed. Sorghum grits from dry milling are used for brewing and industrial purposes.

(Also see CORN, section headed "Dry Milling.")

• **Wet milling**—The wet milling of sorghum closely resembles the wet milling of corn. However, sorghum is more difficult to wet mill than corn because (1) it is difficult to separate the starch and protein, (2) it is difficult to extract the sorghum germ from the kernel, (3) pigments discolor the starch and must be removed by bleaching, and (4) recovery of starch is lower than with corn. It is noteworthy, however, that new hybrids with improved wet milling qualities have been developed.

(Also see CORN, section headed "Wet Milling.")

NUTRITIONAL VALUE. Generally speaking, sorghum and corn are interchangeable in the diet; with corn preferred and grown where adapted, and sorghum grown in hot, dry regions where corn cannot be grown success-

fully. So, both the nutritionist and the consumer need to compare the two foods. Tables S-16 and S-17 compare selected nutrients and essential amino acids of sorghum grain and corn. Also, Food Composition Table F-36 gives the nutrient compositions of corn and sorghum, and their products.

TABLE S-16
COMPARISON OF SELECTED NUTRIENTS IN SORGHUM GRAIN AND CORN

Nutrient		Sorghum Grain	Corn
		◄----(per 100 g) ----►	
Calories	kcal	366.0	348.0
Carbohydrates	g	73.0	71.1
Fat	g	3.3	3.9
Protein	g	11.0	9.6
Calcium	mg	28.0	30.0
Phosphorus	mg	287.0	270.0
Iron	mg	4.4	2.0
Niacin	mg	3.9	3.0
Riboflavin	mg	.15	.13
Thiamin	mg	.38	.21

TABLE S–17
PROFILE OF ESSENTIAL AMINO ACIDS IN SORGHUM AND CORN COMPARED TO MILK—A HIGH-QUALITY PROTEIN

Amino Acid	Sorghum Grain	Corn	Cow's Milk[1]
	◄——— (mg/g protein) ———►		
Histidine	21	27	27
Isoleucine	40	38	47
Leucine	129	133	95
Lysine	22	27	78
Methionine and cystine	30	41	33
Phenylalanine and tyrosine	86	92	102
Threonine	33	37	44
Tryptophan	13	9	14
Valine	47	46	64

[1]*Recommended Dietary Allowances*, 10th ed., 1989, NRC–National Academy of Sciences, p. 67, Table 6–5.

It is recognized that compositional data provide only an approximate comparison because the influence of environment is very striking, affecting both the physical and chemical properties of both sorghum and corn. Nevertheless, the following comparisons of the two grains appear to be justified: sorghum grain is higher in protein but lower in fat than corn.

The amino acid composition of sorghum grain and corn is strikingly similar. The most limiting amino acid is lysine —a feature common to all grains.

Although not shown in Tables S-16 and S-17, the authors take cognizance of the following additional differences between sorghum and corn: corn contains more carotene (vitamin A) than sorghum; sorghum has slightly more starch than corn; sorghum contains 0.1 to 0.3% waxes, which is 50 times the quantity of waxes in corn; tannins are present in the pericarp and testa of sorghums, especially in bird-resistant varieties, but absent in corn; and high yields of sorghum are generally inversely related to the protein content of the grain.

Other than the differences noted above, the nutrient composition of sorghum grain and corn are similar.

PRODUCTS AND USES. Sorghum is used for food, fermentation products, feed, and industrial purposes.

The sweet stalks of sorghum are chewed by the natives in various countries; and sorghum is the staple food and basis of beverages in much of Asia and Africa. It is usually consumed as a porridge or stiff paste prepared by adding pounded flour to hot water. Sometimes a flat cake is prepared. Also, the grain may be parched, popped, or boiled whole.

In the United States, the vast majority of grain sorghum is used as livestock feed; in 1990, 450 million bu were so used. So, sorghum enters the human diet primarily as meat, milk, and eggs. Some sorghum is also used for industrial products.

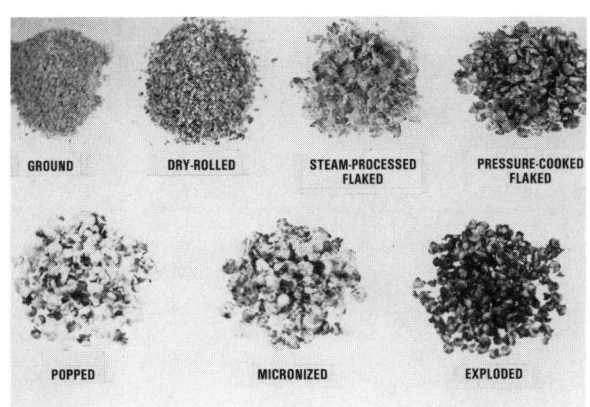

Fig. S-27.   Sorghum grain processed for livestock by several different methods. (Courtesy, W. H. Hale, Department of Animal Science, University of Arizona.)

Table S-18 presents in summary form the story of sorghum products and uses.

(Also see BEERS AND BREWING; BREADS AND BAKING; CEREAL GRAINS, Table C-18 Cereal Grains of the World; and OILS, VEGETABLE, Table O-6.)

TABLE S-18
SORGHUM PRODUCTS AND USES

Country/Product	Description	Uses	Comments
HUMAN FOODS			

In the United States:
Sorghum flour—
  wheat flour,
  blended
	An off-white flour.	Muffins, bread, and griddle cakes.	Only about 1.4% of U.S. sorghum grain is used for food, alcohol, and seed; the rest is used for livestock feed. Nevertheless, sorghum has many potential uses in food products.

Sorghum oil	Oil extracted from the germ of the grain.	Cooking oil; and in such products as margarine and shortenings.	
Sorghum starch	An off-white powdery material (varieties with dark colored outer layers may stain the starch).	Thicken puddings, gravies, and sauces.	
Sorghum syrup	A distinctly flavored, mild, sweet, light amber-colored syrup.	A specialty product, especially in southeastern U.S.	The technology for satisfactorily converting sweet sorghum beyond the syrup stage—into sugar—is known. Thus, when the price is right, sweet sorghum can serve as a supplementary crop for the sugar cane and sugar beet industries.

(Continued)

TABLE S-18   (*Continued*)

Country/Product	Description	Uses	Comments
		HUMAN FOODS (*Continued*)	
Africa and Asia: East Africa	Pounded sorghum flour.	Porridge, made by adding pounded sorghum flour to hot water.	
Ethiopia, Sudan	Sorghum flour. Sorghum grain, whole.	Flat cakes. Parched, popped, or boiled whole.	
India	Sorghum grain, ground or cracked.	Prepared into a dough and baked as flat, unleavened bread (called rotti), or cooked like rice.	White, pearly grains are preferred for bread.
	Sorghum grain.	Whole grain is parched or "fried" in a hot pan, then ground and mixed with salt, buttermilk, or molasses. Special sorghums for popping or roasting are grown in small quantities.	
Nigeria	Sorghum flour.	A food called "tuwo," prepared by stirring flour in hot water, then allowing the thick paste to cool and gel.	Pieces of the cooled gel are eaten with soup.
	Immature sorghum heads.	Roasted, much like sweet-corn in the U.S.	
	Sorghum (special varieties).	Popped, similar to popcorn.	
Uganda	Sorghum grain, whole.	The grain is malted and sprouted, the radicle (root portion) removed, and the grain dried.	Some of the pigment and the bitter principle are removed. The sugars produced make the porridge sweet.
West Africa	Sorghum flour.	Porridge or stiff paste made from stirring flour in hot water. These may be allowed to cool and gel, or the paste may be fried to make pancakes.	

(*Continued*)

TABLE S-18 (*Continued*)

Country/Product	Description	Uses	Comments
		FERMENTATION PRODUCTS	
Country and beverage: United States Alcohol	The whole grain is ground, cooked, hydrolyzed by enzymes or acid, fermented by yeast, and the alcohol distilled off. Beverage alcohol production is similar, except malt enzymes are preferred for hydrolysis.	1. Ethyl alcohol for beverages. 2. Denatured alcohol for industrial purposes. 3. Gasohol (10% anhydrous ethanol/90% gasoline)—a motor fuel.	In the U.S., the use of sorghum for fermentation depends on its price relative to other grains.
Sorghum grits	The starchy portion of the endosperm.	Brewing and distilling, making industrial alcohol.	
Sorghum starch	An off-white powdery material.	Brewing and distilling, making industrial alcohol	
Africa Bantu (tribe or family)	Sorghum beer.	Beer, made by malting and brewing sorghum (preferably red grains).	It differs from beer made from barley malt in that it is an opaque reddish-colored liquor, contains 5 to 6% solids, has a yeasty sour taste, has a low alcohol content, and is high in nutritional value.
Central Africa; tribes in Zambia, Zaire, and the Central African Republic.	Homemade sorghum beer; made from sorghum alone, or from a mixture of sorghum with maize (corn) and/or millet.	As a nutritious beer.	The grain is soaked in water, sprouted, dried, ground, mixed with water, and allowed to ferment in clay pots. The crude beer may or may not be filtered prior to consumption. Sprouting and fermentation of sorghum results in a more nutritious product than the original grain because additional amounts of the vitamin B complex are produced during these processes.
China Mao-tai	About a 53% alcoholic beverage made from grain sorghum.	At Chinese banquets, Mao-tai is used for toasts.	The Chinese claim that "it's easy on the throat, and it doesn't go to the head." But "first timers" are admonished to approach it with caution. It's potent! As a result of experiencing the traditional Chinese toasts on three different visits to China, two of the authors of this book, the Ensmingers, concluded that the only reason Mao-tai is not used for airplane fuel is that it is too readily combustible.

(Continued)

TABLE S-18 (Continued)

Country/Product	Description	Uses	Comments
		LIVESTOCK FEEDS	
Sorghum grain	The hard grain processed by numerous methods, including: grinding, dry rolling, steam rolling, extruding, micronizing, popping, roasting, cooking, exploding, steam flaking, pressure flaking, crumbling, high moisture (early harvested), and reconstituted (water added).	All classes of livestock. However, sorghum lacks the yellow pigments (such as found in yellow corn) needed to produce yellow-skinned boilers and colored yolks.	Grain sorghum by-products are very much like the counterpart by-products of corn, except they do not contain carotene. When properly processed, sorghum has 90 to 100% the value of corn for livestock. The U.S. exports large quantities of sorghum grain to Japan and Israel for feeding poultry, swine and cattle. In 1989, the U.S. shipped 2,634 metric tons to Japan, which accounted for 32% of our total sorghum grain exports that year.
Gelatinized sorghum grain flour	The endosperm of sorghum grain which has been gelatinized and reduced to a finely ground meal. It must not contain more than 1% crude fiber.	Primarily in poultry and swine rations.	
Grain sorghum germ cake or **grain sorghum germ meal**	The germ of the grain from which part of the oil has been pressed.	Primarily in poultry and swine rations.	
Grain sorghum gluten feed	That part of the grain that remains after the extraction of the larger part of the starch and germ by the wet milling manufacture of starch or syrup.	As a medium protein feed for beef cattle, dairy cattle, sheep, and swine. It is not very palatable.	
Grain sorghum gluten meal	That part of the grain that remains after the extraction of the larger part of the starch and germ and the separation of the bran by the wet milling manufacture of starch and syrup.	As a high protein feed for beef cattle, dairy cattle, sheep, and swine. It is not very palatable.	
Grain sorghum grits	The hard flinty portions of sorghums containing little or no bran or germ.	Dog food.	
Grain sorghum mill feed	A mixture of grain sorghum bran, germ, part of the starchy portion of grain sorghum kernels, or a mixture thereof as produced in the manufacture of grain sorghum grits and refined meal and flour. It must not contain more than 5% crude fat and 6% crude fiber.	All classes of livestock.	

(Continued)

TABLE S-18 (*Continued*)

Country/Product	Description	Uses	Comments
LIVESTOCK FEEDS *(Continued)*			
Partially aspirated gelatinized sorghum grain flour	Whole sorghum grain which has been partially aspirated and has been gelatinized and reduced to a finely ground meal. It must not contain more than 2.5% crude fiber.	Primarily in poultry and swine rations.	
Sorghum Forages: Sorghum fodder and stover	The whole stalks with the heads on are called fodder. The stalks without the heads are called stover.	Beef cattle.	
Sorghum hay	A coarse hay.	Primarily beef cattle.	
Sorghum pasture	A rank-growing, warm weather pasture.	Primarily beef cattle.	Care should be exercised in grazing sorghum forage because of the danger of prussic acid (hydrocyanic acid) poisoning, which disappears after the fodder is cured.
Sorghum silage	Fermented sorghum forage.	Primarily beef cattle and dairy cattle.	When of comparable quality and grain content, sorghum silage and corn silage are equal in feeding value. The sorghums are more dependable than corn in dry areas. Also, the sorghums are higher in sugar content than corn forage.
OTHER USES			
Sorghum grain	The processed grain.	Wax, lactic acid, riboflavin, microbial polysaccharides, antibiotics, and citric acid.	
Broomcorn sorghum	Long fiber, suitable for brooms.	Brooms	
Sorghum grits	The hard flinty portions of ground sorghum containing little or none of the bran or germ.	Paper making, aluminum ore refining, building materials, mineral processing, charcoal briquettes, oil-well drilling, foundry binders.	
Sorghum starch	An off-white powdery material (varieties with dark colored outer layers may stain the starch).	Adhesives, and paper and cloth sizings.	

SORGHUM SYRUP AS A CARBOHY-DRATE SOURCE

Sweet sorghum, or sorgo, is grown mainly in south central and southeastern United States. Its juice contains about 12% sugar and may be used to manufacture syrup. Sorghum syrup is distinctly flavored, mild, sweet, and light amber color. It contains about 68 g of carbohydrates per 100 g (257 kcal/100 g) of syrup as well as significant amounts of calcium, potassium, and iron. (See Food Composition Table F-36.)

As a carbohydrate source, sorghum syrup is about equal to table syrups, maple syrup, and molasses.

(Also see SORGHUM.)

SORRELS (DOCKS; SOUR-GRASSES) *Rumex* spp

The edible leaves of these plants are much more esteemed as vegetables in Europe than they are in the United States, where sorrels are often considered to be undesirable weeds. In Europe, the roots and flowers of the plants are used in various herbal preparations. Sorrels belong to the buckwheat family (*Polygonaceae*), which also includes rhubarb. Although there are seven or more sorrels or docks which belong to the *Rumex*

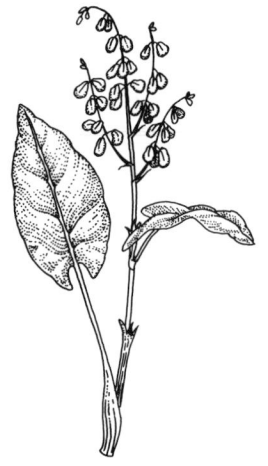

Fig. S-28.   Common sorrel, one of several closely-related species that are both garden crops and hardy weeds.

genus, the most commonly used ones are (1) common or garden sorrel (*R. acetosa*), which has pointed leaves and may grow up to 3 ft (*91 cm*) tall; (2) French or round-leaved sorrel (*R. scutatus*), that is only about 2 ft (*61 cm*) tall; and (3) spinach dock or patience (*R. patientia*), which may grow as high as 5 ft (*152 cm*). It is noteworthy that French sorrel has a milder flavor than common sorrel.

ORIGIN AND HISTORY.   Sorrels of the *Rumex* genus are native to Asia and Europe. The domesticated varieties were selected for large leaves that were milder-flavored than the small sour ones of the wild plants. Certain wild species have a high content of oxalic acid. The ancient Egyptians and Romans believed that the acidic leaves aided the digestion when heavy, rich meals were consumed. The entry of acid into the small intestine brings about the secretion of digestive juices from the pancreas. Hence, the ancient belief may have been correct.

In Medieval Europe, sorrel leaves were crushed in a mortar to make green sauces that were served with goose or pork. Herbalists of those days noted that the eating of the leaves prevented scurvy, a disease that results from a severe deficiency of vitamin C. Scurvy was widespread in northern Europe during the late winter and early spring, when the supplies of fresh fruits and vegetables from the preceding harvest were exhausted or spoiled and it was still too early for the new crops. Therefore, it is noteworthy that sorrel leaves appeared in the early spring before any of the other green leafy vegetables.

Sorrel seeds were brought to North America by the first English colonists, who planted them in their gardens in New England. From there, the sorrels escaped from cultivation and spread as weeds across a wide area from Canada to New Jersey and Pennsylvania. Consequently, American gardeners were warned not to plant these vegetables because they were hard to eradicate once they had become established. However, it is now known that careful management prevents the uncontrolled spreading of the plants.

PRODUCTION.   Sorrels and docks are grown only on a small scale. Hence, production statistics are not available.

Seeds may be planted in the field as early as 1 month before the average date of the last frost. The plants require a rich, moist soil and plenty of sunlight. Most growers thin the plants so that each one will have adequate room for growth. Spinach dock requires more space per plant because it grows much taller than either common sorrel or French sorrel. Leaves may be cut from the plants throughout the growing period. A stainless steel knife should be used because contact with iron gives the leaves a metallic taste. It is noteworthy that the leaves may develop a bitter taste during a spell of hot weather, but that this effect may be minimized by mulching so that the soil is kept moist. Furthermore, the flavor usually improves when the weather becomes cooler. Flowering stalks should be removed as soon as they appear because this action (1) encourages the growth of more leaves, and (2) prevents the plant from going to seed and spreading to places where it is not wanted.

PROCESSING.   Almost all of the sorrels grown at the present time are consumed fresh. Hence, little or none is processed. However, it is easy to dry or can the leaves. Their acid content makes them safer to can than most other vegetables. Furthermore, a variety of good sauces and soups could be produced commercially if there were sufficient demand.

SELECTION AND PREPARATION.   High quality sorrel leaves are fresh, young, tender, and green. Those which show insect injury, coarse stems, dry or yellowing leaves, excessive dirt, or poor development, are usually lacking in quality and may cause excessive waste. Flabby, wilted leaves are generally undesirable.

Sorrel leaves that are to be used raw in salads should be young and tender, because older leaves are more likely to be too bitter or too sour. Some of the ways in which the leaves may be used in cooked dishes are (1) minced and added to casseroles, omelets, soups, and stews; (2) boiled briefly and served with butter, margarine, or a special dressing; (3) pureed, heated briefly with butter or margarine, and served as a sauce with eggs, fish, meat, or poultry; (4) in salad dressings (little vinegar is needed because the sorrel has a sour flavor); and (5) as an ingredient of stuffings for fish, meat, or poultry.

CAUTION: From time to time there have been reports of people having been poisoned from eating the leaves of sorrel or those of its close relative rhubarb, *Rheum rhaponticum*.[38] The cause(s) of toxicity has been suspected as being due to the oxalates and/or the anthraquinone glycosides that are present in both plants. Nevertheless, many people have eaten ample amounts of sorrel leaves without showing any signs of even a mildly toxic effect. Some possible explanations of the apparently unpredictable occasions of toxicity might be as follows:

1. Some people are unduly sensitive or even allergic to one or more constituents of sorrel leaves.
2. Certain varieties of sorrel contain greater quantities of the offending substance(s) than other varieties.
3. The growing conditions affect the composition of the leaves. For example, the addition of extra calcium and nitrates to the soil increases the oxalate content of spinach, which may also be the case for sorrel. Furthermore, the bitterness that develops in sorrel leaves during hot weather may be due to an increased content of anthraquinone glycosides.

Therefore, people who develop dermatitis from handling sorrel should not eat the leaves. Furthermore, leaves that are either very bitter (possibly due to elevated levels of anthraquinone glycosides) or very sour (perhaps resulting from a high content of oxalates) should either be discarded or used only in very small amounts.

NUTRITIONAL VALUE. The nutrient composition of raw and cooked sorrel are listed under "dock" in Food Composition Table F-36.

Some noteworthy observations regarding the nutrient composition of sorrel follow:

1. Raw sorrel leaves contain 91% water and only 28 Calories (kcal) per 100 g portion. They are an excellent source of vitamin A (better than carrots) and vitamin C (the content is about twice that of oranges), a good source of iron and potassium, and a fair source of calcium and phosphorus.

2. A 1-cup (*200 g*) serving of cooked and drained sorrel leaves supplies only 38 Calories (kcal), but it furnishes as much protein as a cup of cooked cornmeal or cooked rice, as much calcium as 3 oz (*90 ml*) of milk, and more than a 4-day's supply of vitamin A for adults.

NOTE: Some nutritionists have expressed concern that the heavy consumption of oxalate-rich foods such as sorrel, rhubarb, and spinach may result in mild to moderate deficiencies of calcium and other essential minerals because certain of these elements form insoluble oxalates that are poorly absorbed. However, various research studies have shown that adequate levels of dietary calcium, phosphorus, and vitamin D prevent the development of oxalate-induced calcium deficiencies, but little is known about the effects of oxalates on other essential minerals.

(Also see VEGETABLE[S], Table V-6 Vegetables of the World.)

SOUCHONG

Souchong tea is a fine black tea derived from the largest grade of tea leaves.
(Also see TEA.)

SOUPS

Probably the first dish ever cooked in a kettle over the open fire was a soup, and because this method of cooking was the only one for countless years, soups were standard fare.

In France, the evening meal is called *la soupe*; and in English, our word *supper* came from the word *soup*. Soup is always available in restaurants; however, we have gotten away from serving soup in the home, largely because, without a domestic servant to serve three courses, the busy housewife of modern America has eliminated the soup course. For a light supper, sometimes a soup containing meat and vegetables, which is a meal in itself, is served. On a cold winter evening by the fire, there is no better dish.

Each nation has its own special soups, rich in meat, chicken or fish; health-giving vegetables; and nourishing barley, rice, or macaroni. At one time, soups were thought to be restorative of one's health, and in 16th-century France, one enterprising person advertised his soup establishment as a "restaurant"—alluding to its reputed health-restoring properties. Soon others copied him. Eventually, the name *restaurant* came to be used for all establishments that serve any kind of food.

The purpose of soup in the meal is twofold: (1) to improve digestion and stimulate appetite; and (2) to increase the variety of foods served at the meal. The clear, stock soups serve the first purpose, and the cream soups serve the latter. A heavy meal such as steak or roast, should be preceded by a clear soup, but a light meal of fish, eggs, or salad, is best with a heartier soup.

A generation ago, before the era of commercially canned soups, all sorts of nutritious things which other-

[38]Fassett, D. W., "Oxalates," in *Toxicants Occurring Naturally in Foods*, 2nd ed., National Academy of Sciences, 1973, pp. 346-362.

wise would have been thrown out went into the soup pot; for instance, the liquid from cooking vegetables and the bones from a roast of turkey or chicken were simmered and strained for soup. Sometimes leftovers made good additions to the soup of the day. Now, there are countless varieties of canned, frozen, or dried soups available. Therefore, the cook has the choice between the commercial or the homemade product.

Basically, there are two kinds of soups: (1) clear soups, and (2) cream soups. Either may have added ingredients. Soups are usually served hot, but on a warm summer day, there are several delicious cold soups such as jellied bouillon, the famous French potato-and-leek soup called Vichyssoise, or even a fruit puree.

The number of good soup recipes would, literally speaking, stretch around the world. Usually the soup is named after the ingredients, but there are some world-famous soups with which everyone should become acquainted, unless they are already old friends. Some of these, the recipes for which can be found in the local cookbook library, follow:

• **Bird's nest soup (Chinese)**—The Asian swiftlets coat their nests with a translucent gelatinous material (their saliva), which is high in protein (11.9 g/100 g). It is packaged and available in Chinese specialty shops. First, the nest is soaked, then simmered in chicken stock. "Chicken velvet" is added and it is served garnished with ham. The chicken velvet is made by finely mincing the chicken and mixing it with cornstarch and beaten egg whites. When added to soup, this becomes light and frothy. Bird's nest soup is considered a delicacy.

• **Bisque**—A cream soup made from fish.

• **Borsch (Russian)**—This soup, of which there are several different recipes, is popular in both the U.S.S.R. and in Poland. Basically, it is a beet soup which is thickened with cornstarch. It may or may not have added vegetables and meats.

• **Bouillabaisse (French)**—This is a fish soup with a hot pepper sauce.

• **Bouillon**—Meat and/or meat scraps are simmered slowly to produce the stock or bouillon. It is usually served clear, but it can also be served with added vegetables and pieces of meat.

• **Chowder**—This word comes from the French word, *chaudiere*, meaning *caldron*. The chowder of today has not changed much from the chowder of yesterday. It consists of pieces of different vegetables, or of fish and potatoes, with seasonings, all cooked in milk, and with crackers added just before serving.

• **Cock-a-leekie**—This soup is made by boiling chicken and leeks together.

• **Consumme**—From the French word meaning *to boil down*. Basically, there is little difference between consumme and bouillon. But bouillon is usually thought of as strictly beef stock, whereas consumme may be beef, veal and/or chicken stock.

• **Cream soups**—A thin white sauce is combined with any desired vegetables or meats. When vegetables or meats are pureed to make a soup, this can be classified as a cream soup, also.

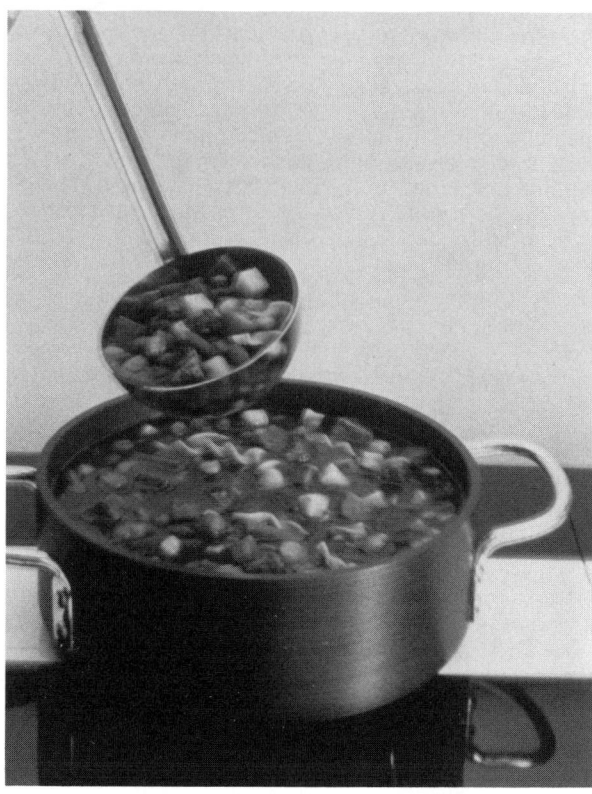

Fig. S-29. Beef and vegetable soup. (Courtesy, USDA)

• **Egg drop soup (Chinese)**—A clear stock soup, into which is dropped a slightly beaten egg. The egg is cooked in the soup the same way that a poached egg is cooked.

• **Gazpacho (Spain)**—This soup, which originated in Spain, and is popular in Mexico and the southwestern United States, is a highly-seasoned tomato soup with added vegetables, which is served chilled. It may also be jellied.

• **Minestrone (Italy)**—A mixed vegetable soup with beans and macaroni.

• **Mulligatawny (East Indies)**—Chicken, carrots, green pepper and apple are cooked together. The vegetables and apple are pureed and returned to the pot, seasonings, including curry, cloves, and mace, are added.

• **Printanier soup**—This name comes from the French word *printemps*, meaning *spring*. The soup is made from fresh spring vegetables.

• **Vichyssoise (French)**—Potatoes and leeks are cooked together in a chicken broth, then blended, or put through a sieve. Thick cream is added and the mixture is served chilled with a garnish of chopped chives.

Soups can be served with innumerable garnishes, plus a raft of soup accessories. All good cookbooks will furnish the recipes for these.

The nutritive value of soups depends on the ingredients. See Table F-36 Food Composition Table, under the section, "Soups and Chowders" for the analysis of some of the more popular soups.

SOYBEAN *Glycine max*

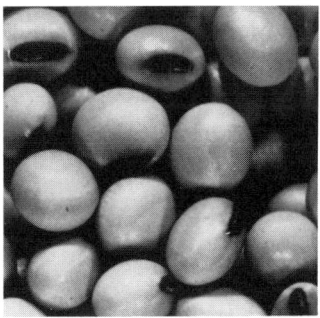

Fig. S-30. Soybeans, precious beans of the Orient.

Soybeans were cultivated in China long before written history. The ancient Chinese used the soybean as food and made medicines from it.

Today, U.S. soybeans supply food for human beings, feed for animals, and many raw materials for industry. The following facts attest to the importance of the U.S. soybean crop.

1. In 1990, soybeans ranked number 2 in U.S. acreage harvested, with corn leading by about 10 million acres.

2. In dollar value to U.S. farmers, corn leads, soybeans are the number 2 crop, and wheat and cotton rank third and fourth, respectively.

3. Soybeans are the nation's largest single source of vegetable oil for human food and of protein meal for animal feed.

4. The United States is the world's largest supplier of soybeans and soybean products; the annual sales abroad account for about 10% of the total economic value of all goods exported by the United States.

ORIGIN AND HISTORY. The soybean plant was native to eastern Asia. It emerged as a cultivated crop in China in the 11th century B.C. Records of methods of culture, varieties for different purposes, and numerous usages indicate that the soybean was among the first crops grown by man. The Chinese Emperor Shung Nang described the soybean plant in a publication in 2838 B.C. The ancient Chinese considered the soybean their most important crop, and one of the five sacred grains necessary for living. Soybeans were taken from China to Japan in the 7th century.

The German botanist Kaempfer first took soybeans to Europe in the 17th century. They were introduced into the United States in 1804. However, scant attention was given to soybeans in North America until the 1930s. At that time, the U.S. Department of Agriculture and the agricultural experiment stations of the states and the Canadian provinces cooperated in developing improved soybean varieties through hybridization and selection. These improved varieties increased yield and oil content and were more suitable to modern farming methods. They contributed greatly to the rapid expansion of the crop.

WORLD AND U.S. PRODUCTION. Soybeans are one of the world's most important oilseed crops and a staple food of the Orient. Although indigenous to the Far East, it is now cultivated elsewhere—particularly in the United States.

World production in 1990 totaled 107,767,000 metric tons. Fig. S-31 compares the ten leading soybean-producing countries. The United States is, by far, the leading soybean producing country, producing more than 49% of the world's soybeans.

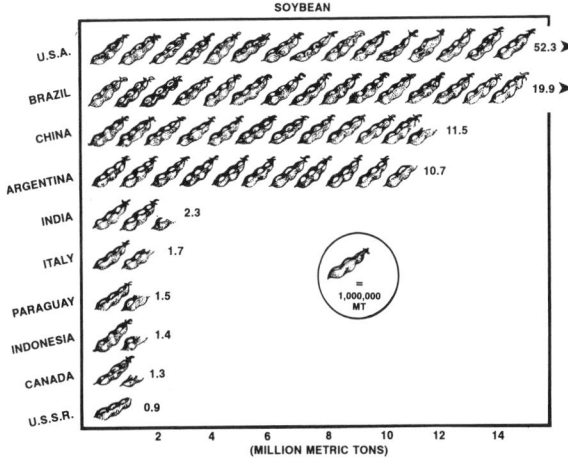

Fig. S-31. Leading soybean-producing countries of the world. (Source: *FAO Production Yearbook*, 1990, FAO/UN, Rome, Italy, Vol. 44, p. 107, Table 37)

The United States produced 1.9 billion bu of soybeans in 1990. The ten leading states, by rank, were: Illinois, Iowa, Minnesota, Indiana, Ohio, Missouri, Arkansas, Nebraska, South Dakota, and Kansas (see Fig. S-32). In yields, the leading states and the number of bushels that each of them produced per acre in 1990 were: Indiana, 41 bu; Iowa, 41 bu; Pennsylvania, 41 bu; Wisconsin, 41 bu; Illinois, 39 bu; Minnesota, 39 bu; Ohio, 39 bu; Michigan, 38 bu; New Jersey, 37 bu; and Maryland, 36 bu.

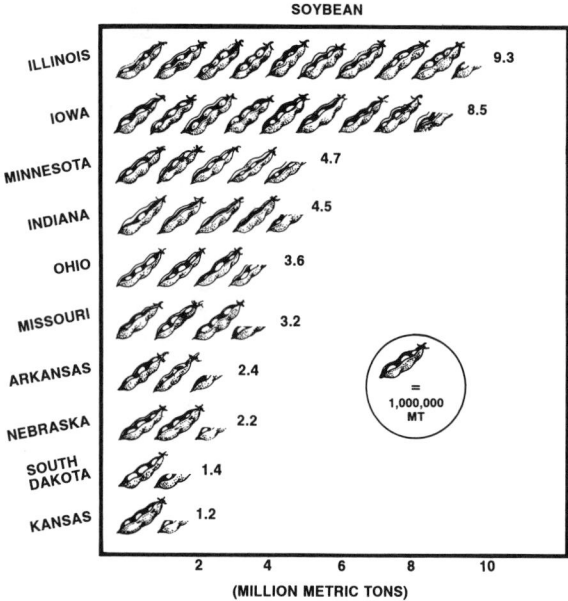

Fig. S-32.   Leading soybean-producing states of the United States. (Source: *Agricultural Statistics 1991*, USDA, p. 123, Table 169)

THE SOYBEAN PLANT.   Soybeans belong to the pea family, *Leguminosae*. It is classified as genus *Glycine*, species *G. max*.

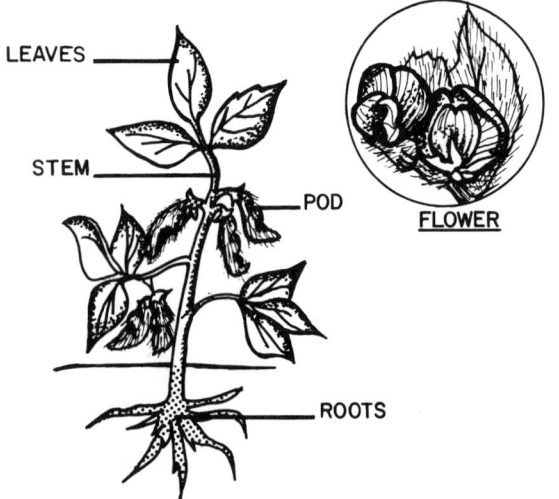

Fig. S-33.   The growing soybean plant.

The plant is an erect annual, 1 to 5 ft (*30 to 152 cm*) tall, with trifoliolate leaves and small white or purple flowers borne in clusters where the leaf joins the stem. The stems, leaves, and pods are covered with short, fine, brown or gray hairs. The bean pods range in color from very light yellow to shades of gray, brown, or black, each containing 1 to 4 round or oval seeds. The seeds themselves may be colored in shades of yellow, green brown, black, or they may be speckled. Most food soybeans are yellow. As a legume, the soybean is able to use free nitrogen from the air, provided the proper bacteria (*Rhizobium japonicum*) are present in the roots to change the nitrogen into a form that can be used by the plant.

The number of days from planting to maturity of soybeans ranges from 90 to 180.

SOYBEAN CULTURE.   Soybeans produce maximum yields in soils where residual soil fertility has been maintained at a high level and the pH is between 6.0 and

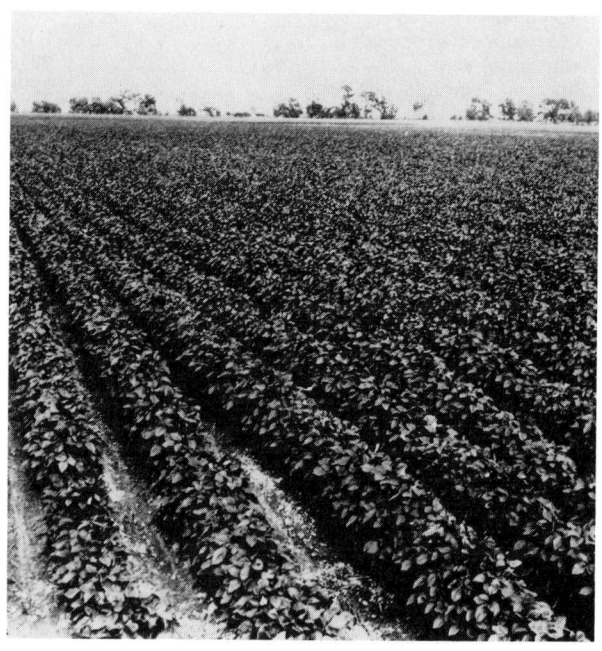

Fig. S-34.   A field of soybeans. (Courtesy, USDA)

6.5. Like other legumes, soybeans obtain part of their nitrogen enrichment from the air through the action of certain nodule-forming bacteria living on the roots of the plant. Thus, where soybeans are being grown in a field for the first time, the seed should be inoculated with a fresh, viable type of bacteria called *Rhizobium japonicum*. With optimum conditions and the *Rhizobium* bacteria present, over 140 lb of nitrogen per acre—more than half the nitrogen requirements of the soybean plants—can be fixed from the air.

which threshes as it reaps, when the plants are mature, the leaves have fallen, the pods are dry, and the seed has dried to a moisture content of around 13 to 14% or less, at which time the crop can be stored safely.

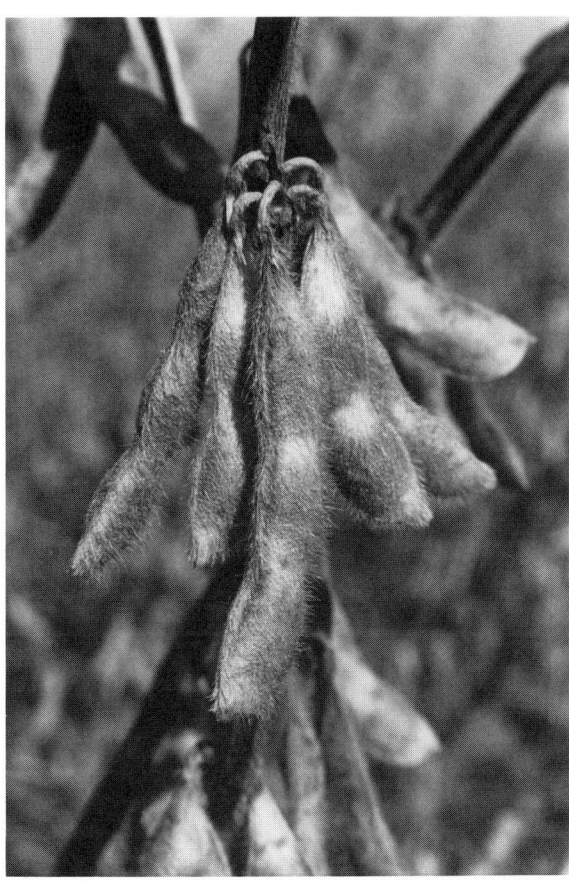

Fig. S-35.   Cluster of ripe soybean pods, covered with hair. Note that each pod contains 2 to 3 seeds. (Courtesy, American Soybean Association, St. Louis, Mo.)

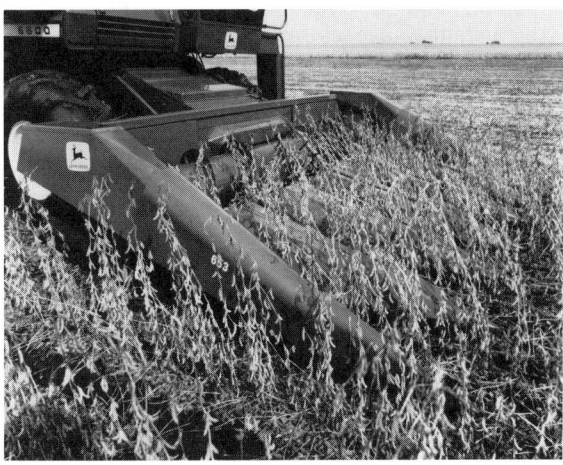

Fig. S-36.   Soybeans being harvested by a combine. (Courtesy, Deere & Company, Moline, Ill.)

In the United States, soybeans are usually planted in a well prepared seedbed in May or early June, to a depth of 1 to 2 in. (*2.5 to 5.1 cm*), in rows 21 to 42 in. (*53 to 107 cm*) apart, at a planting rate of 40 to 80 lb per acre (*45 to 90 kg/ha*). Chemical weed control is a part of almost every weed control program, but supplementary cultivation is recommended. Early cultivation is usually done with a rotary hoe. Later cultivation may be done with row equipment similar to what is used for corn or cotton.

Over 50 diseases affect soybeans, reducing yields an estimated 12% per year. Fortunately, some varieties have delayed resistance against certain soybean diseases; so, resistant varieties are the most practical and economical means of controlling soybean diseases. Additionally, the following practices can be applied for disease control if the situation so warrants: removal or destruction of crop residue, crop rotation, good fertility, proper soil preparation, good drainage, and use of pathogen-free vigorous seed.

Many insects attack soybeans, but few can be considered serious economic threats. The extensive use of insecticides is not usually recommended since they also kill parasite and predator insects which control many soybean-damaging insects naturally.

Most soybeans are harvested by means of a combine,

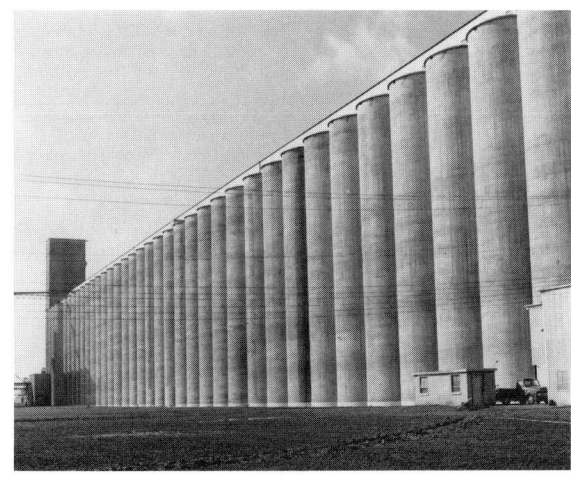

Fig. S-37.   Marketing and storage come next. This shows the huge soybean elevators of the Arkansas Grain Corp., Stuttgart, Ark. (Courtesy, American Soybean Association, St. Louis, Mo.)

KINDS OF SOYBEANS. Soybeans are generally classified into three groups or classes according to their use: (1) commercial or seed, (2) vegetable, and (3) forage. Most varieties grown for commercial or seed purposes and used for oil have yellow seeds. Varieties grown for use as a vegetable cook easily, possess a nutty flavor, and are usually straw-yellow or olive-green. The forage and commercial varieties have a poor flavor and are rather difficult to cook. Commercial varieties can also be used for forage production provided the planting rate is increased.

More than a hundred useful varieties of soybeans have been developed in the United States. Many important new varieties have been produced by hybridization (crossing varieties). In selecting a variety for a particular area or field, consideration should be given to the following: use, adaptation, maturity, yield potential, plant height, lodging resistance, disease resistance, shatter resistance, and genetic vigor.

FEDERAL GRADES OF SOYBEANS. The United States Standards for Soybeans, established by the U.S. Department of Agiculture, provide for five classes: yellow soybeans, green soybeans, brown soybeans, black soybeans, and mixed soybeans.

There are five official grades of soybeans. The grades and grade requirements are given in Table S-19.

TABLE S-19
GRADE AND GRADE REQUIREMENTS OF SOYBEANS[1]

Grade	Minimum test weight per bushel	Maximum limits of—					
		Moisture	Splits	Damaged kernels		Foreign material	Brown, black, and/or bicolored soybeans in yellow or green soybeans
				Total	Heat damaged		
	(lb)	(%)	(%)	(%)	(%)	(%)	(%)
U.S. No. 1	56.0	13.0	10.0	2.0	0.2	1.0	1.0
U.S. No. 2	54.0	14.0	20.0	3.0	.5	2.0	2.0
U.S. No. 3[2]	52.0	16.0	30.0	5.0	1.0	3.0	5.0
U.S. No. 4[3]	49.0	18.0	40.0	8.0	3.0	5.0	10.0
U.S. Sample grade	U.S. Sample grade shall be soybeans which do not meet the requirements for any of the grades from U.S. No. 1 to U.S. No. 4, inclusive; or which are musty, sour, or heating; or which have any commercially objectionable foreign odor; or which contain stones; or which are otherwise of distinctly low quality.						

[1]Adapted from *The Official United States Standards For Grain*, Agricultural Marketing Service, Grain Division, USDA, January 1974, p. 84, Table 26.603.
[2]Soybeans which are purple mottled or stained shall be graded not higher than U.S. No. 3.
[3]Soybeans which are materially weathered shall be graded not higher than U.S. No. 4.

PROCESSING SOYBEANS. About 59% of the soybeans produced in the United States are crushed and processed domestically, 35% are exported as whole beans, 5% are used for seed, and 1% have miscellaneous uses.

The processing of soybeans into oil and meal began in the Orient. The oil was used primarily for human food, while the meal was used for animal feed.

In the United States, soybeans are processed primarily to obtain (1) oil for use in shortenings, margarines, and

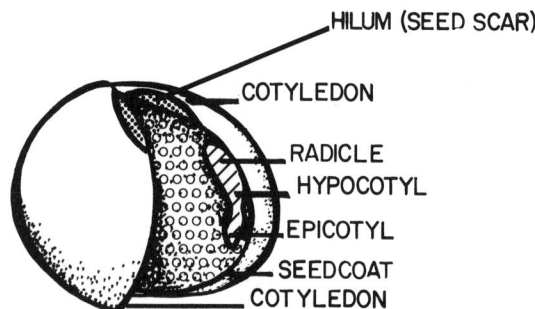

Fig. S-38.   The soybean seed. There are three basic parts: (1) the seedcoat, which protects the embryo from fungi and bacteria before and after planting; (2) the embryo, consisting of (a) the radicle (which becomes the primary root), (b) the hypocotyl (which lifts the cotyledons above the soil surface), and (c) the epicotyl (which is the main stem and growing point); and (3) the cotyledons, which account for most of the bulk and weight of the seed and contain nearly all the oil and protein.

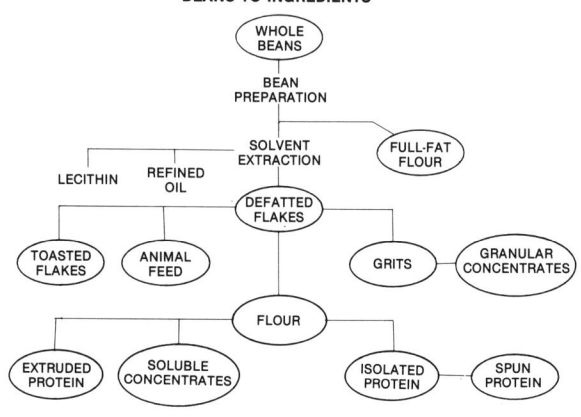

Fig. S-39.   Processing soybeans.

salad dressings; (2) soybean protein products for direct human consumption; and (3) soybean meal for use as a protein supplement for livestock. Processing of soybeans, and the production of soybean oil and meal, began in a small way in the early twenties; but the real impetus came in 1928 when the American Milling Company agreed to purchase on contract all soybeans produced from 50,000 acres in Illinois at a guaranteed minimum of $1.37 per bushel. Following this, soybean acreage continued to expand. Today, the United States produces about one-half of the world's soybeans.

There are three basic processing methods: solvent extraction, hydraulic extraction, and expeller extraction. Today, almost all of the oil is extracted by the solvent process. Soybean meal normally contains 41, 44, 48, or 50% protein, depending on the amount of hull removed. Because of its well-balanced amino acid profile, the protein of soybean meal is of better quality than other protein-rich supplements of plant origin. However, it is low in calcium, phosphorus, carotene, and vitamin D.

SOYBEAN OIL MEAL PROCESSING

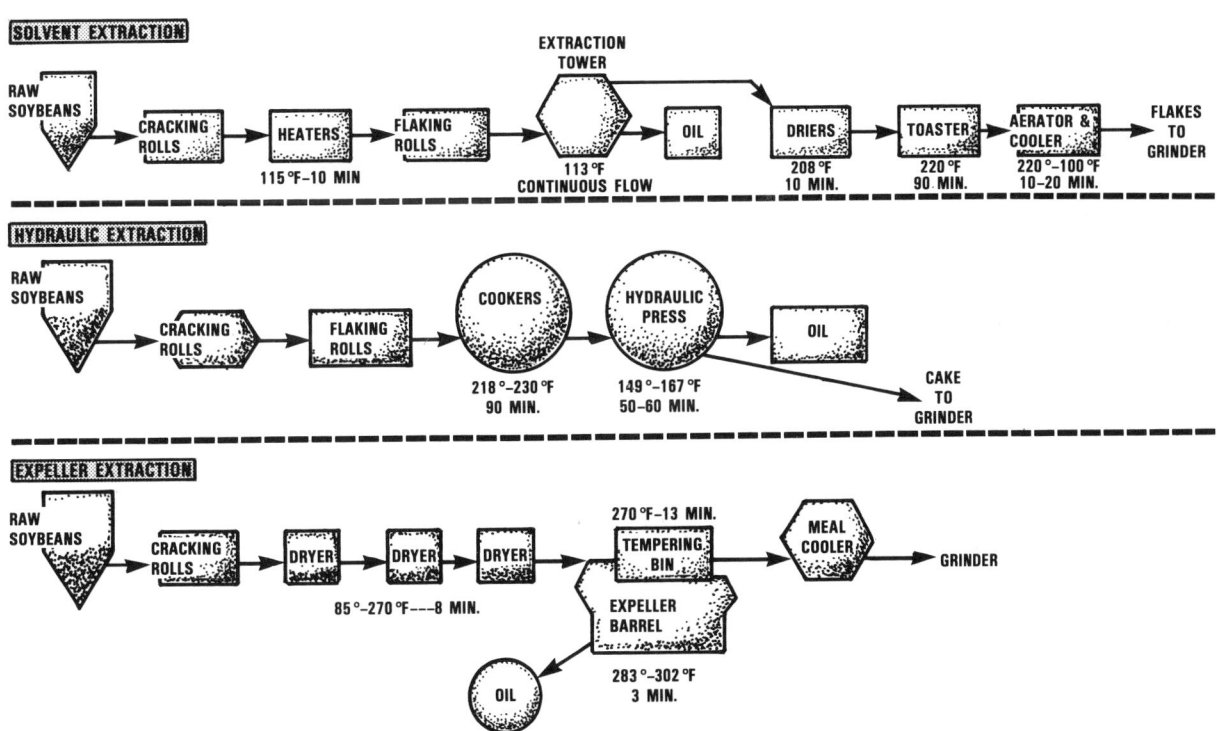

Fig. S-40.   Three methods of processing soybeans.

Solvent Extraction. In this method, the soybeans are first cracked, then heated to 140°F (60°C) for about 10 minutes. After the cracked seeds are heated, they proceed through a series of grinding rollers where they are flaked. The flakes are allowed to cool to about 113°F (45°C) and are then moved to the extraction equipment where the oil is removed by a petroleum solvent—usually hexane.

The extracted flakes then proceed to driers where the solvent is completely volatilized. From the drier, the flakes are conveyed to a toaster, thence they are cooled and ground.

The normal processing yields are: crude oil, 17 to 19.3%; and meal and feed products, 80.7 to 83%. One bushel (60 lb) of soybeans gives approximately 48 lb (22 kg) of meal and 11 lb (5 kg) of oil. The maximum yield of crude oil is always sought. Generally, less than 2% oil remains in the meal after solvent extraction. The hulls, accounting for about 5% of the beans, are ground and may be added back to the meal for the production of meal of a specific protein content.

Hydraulic Extraction.   In the hydraulic extraction procedure, raw soybeans are cracked, ground, and flaked. The flakes (called meats) are then transported to cookers where they are exposed to both dry and steam heat. The cooking stage takes about 90 minutes.

After cooking, the meats are formed into cakes and wrapped in heavy cloth whereupon they are placed in hydraulic presses for the mechanical extraction of the oil. This procedure takes about 1 hour. Following extraction, the cakes are ground. Hydraulic press cake may have 5 to 8% residual oil.

Since this form of extraction is labor intensive and inefficient in the removal of oil, very few soybeans are processed by this method today.

Expeller Extraction.   In this type of extraction, raw soybeans are initially cracked and dried to about 2% moisture. The dried soybeans are then transported hot to a steam-jacketed tempering apparatus which is directly above the expeller apparatus. The tempering apparatus stirs the cracked soybeans for about 10 to 15 minutes so that the seeds are heated uniformly.

From the tempering bin, the soybeans are fed into the expeller barrel (screw presses). A central revolving worm shaft creates pressure within the expeller barrel thereupon extracting the oil from the ground soybeans. The extracted soybeans leave the expeller in the form of flakes, which are subsequently ground.

The expeller process tends to extract less oil than the solvent process; consequently, it is used less frequently. Generally, expeller-extracted soybean meal contains 4 to 5% oil while solvent-extracted soybean meal contains less than 1%.

Soybean Oil Processing.   About 93% of soybean oil is used for food. To be suitable for human consumption, the extracted crude oil must undergo further processing, which is generally referred to as refining (see Fig. S-41).

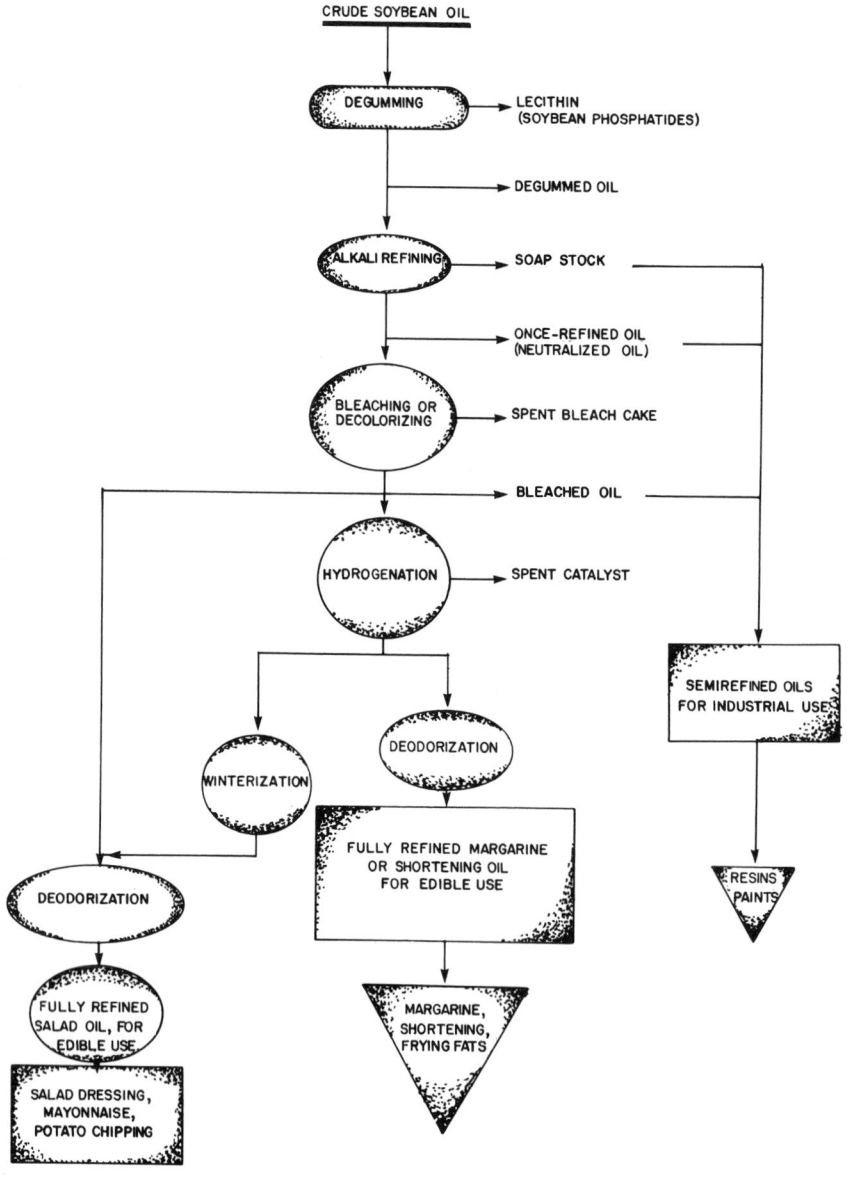

Fig. S-41.   Soybean oil refining process.

The steps in processing are:

1. **Degumming.** This consists in the removal of the soybean phospholipids, which are dried and sold as soybean lecithin. The crude lecithin, which is dark colored, may be bleached with hydrogen peroxide to produce a light, straw-colored product. Fatty acids may be added to make a fluid product, or the lecithin may be treated with ammonia to form a firm, plastic consistency. More refined grades (pharmaceutical lecithins) are produced by acetone extraction of the entrained soybean oil. (For uses of soybean lecithin, see [1] Table S-22 and [2] ADDITIVES, Table A-3 Common Food Additives.)

2. **Alkali refining.** The degummed soybean oil is next alkali-refined (treated with caustic soda, soda ash, or a combination of the two) to neutralize the free fatty acids. The neutralized free fatty acids, known as soap stock, may be removed from the oil and sold to soap manufacturers, fatty acid industries, or feed manufacturers in either (a) the alkaline form, or (b) the acidulated form after treatment with acid.

3. **Bleaching (decolorizing).** Bleaching agents (activated earth or carbon) are used to remove the pigments present in the oil.

4. **Hydrogenating.** Hydrogenation is achieved by treating the oil with hydrogen gas at an elevated temperature and pressure in the presence of a catalyst.

5. **Winterizing.** Hydrogenated soybean oil that is to be used as a salad oil must remain clear at refrigerator temperatures. This is accomplished by winterization—cooling the oil and filtering off the cloudy haze that forms.

6. **Deodorizing.** Undesirable flavors and odors are removed under high temperature and vacuum, with steam injected to assist volatization of the undesirable components.

NUTRITIONAL VALUE. The nutritive value of different forms of soybeans and soybean products is given in Food Composition Table F-36.

The soybean seed is 13 to 25% oil, 30 to 50% protein, and 14 to 24% carbohydrate. The fatty acid composition of the oil is: linoleic acid, 55%; oleic acid, 21%; palmitic acid, 9%; stearic acid, 6%; and other fatty acids, 9%. The ratio of polyunsaturated to saturated fatty acids (P/S ratio) is 82:18, which is conducive to lowering blood cholesterol. The soybean contains more protein than beef, more calcium than milk, and more lecithin than eggs. Also, it is rich in minerals, vitamins, and amino acids.

In terms of essential amino acids—those not produced by the body and must be eaten—soybeans are an excellent source as shown in Table S-20. Indeed soybeans and soybean products are good complementary protein sources when the diet consists of largely cereal grains.

TABLE S–20
PROFILE OF ESSENTIAL AMINO ACIDS
IN SOYBEANS COMPARED TO MILK—
A HIGH-QUALITY PROTEIN

Amino Acid	Soybeans	Cow's Milk[1]
	← (mg/g protein) →	
Histidine	28	27
Isoleucine	50	47
Leucine	85	95
Lysine	70	78
Methionine and cystine	28	33
Phenylalanine and tyrosine	88	102
Threonine	42	44
Tryptophan	14	14
Valine	53	64

[1]*Recommended Dietary Allowances*, 10th ed., 1989, NRC–National Academy of Sciences, p. 67, Table 6–5. The essential amino acid requirements of infants can be met by supplying 0.79 g of a high-quality protein per pound of body weight (1.7 g/kg body weight) per day.

Fig. S-42 compares the levels of essential amino acids of soybeans and other foods.

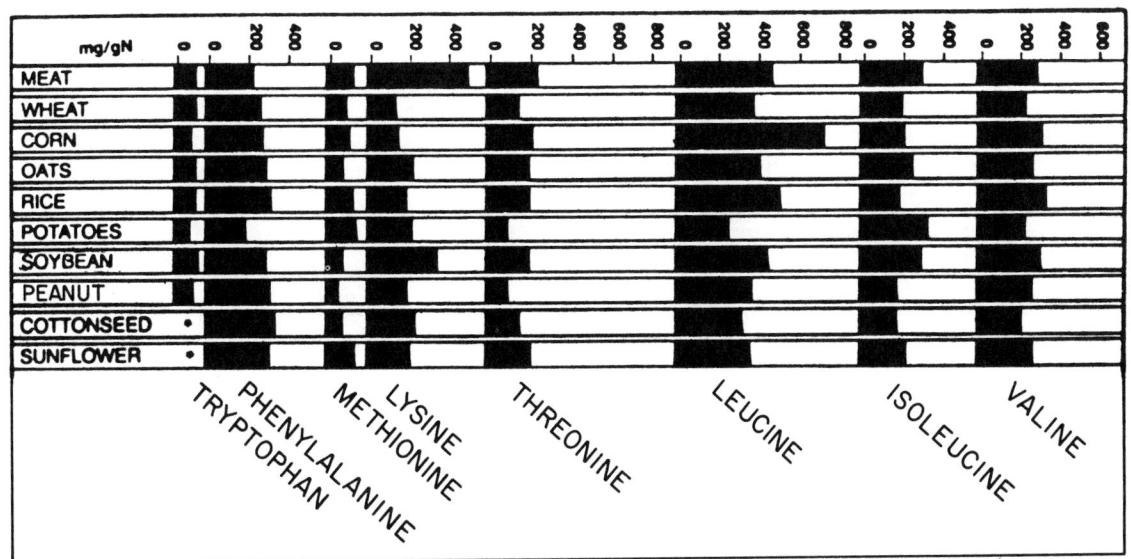

Fig. S-42. Comparative levels of essential amino acids (in mg/g of nitrogen) of soybeans and other foods. (Source: *Vegetable Protein: Products and the Future*, Food Protein Council, Washington, D.C.)

V. R. Young and N. S. Scrimshaw, Clinical Research Center and Department of Nutrition and Food Science, Massachusetts Institute of Technology, make the following authoritative statement relative to the nutritional value of processed soy protein in human nutrition:

> When well processed soy products serve as the major or sole source of protein intake, their protein value approaches or equals that of foods of animal origin, and they are fully capable of meeting the long term essential amino acid and protein needs of children and adults... For feeding of the newborn, the limited data available suggest that supplementation of soy-based formulas with methionine may be beneficial.[39]

Perhaps more important than the individual nutritional strength of soy protein is its ability to complement the biological quality of other protein sources. For example, corn meal, which is the basis of many human diets around the world, is of low protein quality when used alone because of certain amino acid deficiencies. But, when blended with soy flour, the resulting nutritive value is comparable to milk protein (casein). This is accomplished because the low lysine content of corn meal is offset by the naturally high lysine content of soy protein. Conversely, the limited methionine content in soy products is offset by the excess of methionine in corn products. The results, when the two are combined at levels that do not inhibit palatability, is a combined meal nutritionally superior to corn meal alone. This same complementary relationship occurs when soy products are used with wheat and other foods (see Fig. S-42).

The cereals and meals based on corn and wheat are a vital basis of diets in the less developed countries. But these grains do not provide adequate nutrition. If combined with soybeans, however, these grains can boost the general nutritional value of the foods eaten in the less developed countries.

Different nutritional needs prevail in industrialized economies. For the affluent, meat analogs made from textured soy protein are largely free of cholesterol and are high in polyunsaturates. For example, one kind of sausage made from textured soy protein contains 40% more polyunsaturated fats than saturated fats, while traditional pork sausage contains 400% more saturated than polyunsaturated fats.[40]

Evidence relative to the effectiveness of a soy protein diet in reducing serum cholesterol concentrations was dramatically corroborated by an Italian research team, whose work was reported in *The Lancet*, a respected British journal of medicine, in February 1977. A group of patients found to have high blood serum cholesterol levels was put consecutively on two kinds of diets: (1) a low-fat animal protein diet, and (2) a predominantly soy protein diet. The study showed that the soy protein reduced serum cholesterol concentrations in the patients by about 20%.[41]

It is noteworthy, too, that among the leading users of soy protein products are mass feeding institutions, including schools, hospitals, and military units, where nutritional standards must be maintained in the face of cost restrictions. The Federal Government's National School Lunch Program is the largest consumer of soy protein for food served in institutional settings. Hydrated soy protein may constitute up to 30% by weight of meat products served in that program. Over 50 million lb of soy protein are used each year in the school lunch program.

• **Savings in protein costs**—Savings realized by food service operators and feeding institutions explain why the applications of soy protein continue to expand and diversify. Also, the individual consumer is becoming increasingly aware of these savings. (See Table S-21.)

TABLE S-21
RELATIVE COST INDICATORS
FOR LEADING PROTEIN FOODS

	Approximate Percent Protein	Cost Multiplying Factor
Soy isolates	90	1
Sodium caseinate	90	1
Soy concentrates	65	1.5
Soy flour	50	2
Dried skimmed milk	36	3
Cheese (Cheddar)......	25	4
Dried beans	22	5.5
Fish/chicken	20	5.5
Beef (chuck—35% fat)..	16	6
Dried whey.............	13	8
Wheat flour	12	8.5
Corn meal (whole)	9	11
Rice...................	7	15
Whole milk	3.5	28.5

---

[39]Young, V. R., and N.S. Scrimshaw, "Soybean Protein in Human Nutrition: An Overview," *Journal of the American Oil Chemists' Society*, Vol. 56, No. 3, March 1979, p. 110.

[40]*Vegetable Protein: Products For the Future*, Food Protein Council, Washington, D.C.

[41]*Ibid.*

To determine relative protein costs from Table S-21, multiply the cost of a product by its cost multiplying factor. *Example:* Soy flour at 20¢ per pound has a protein cost of 40¢ per pound (20¢ x 2); whereas beef at 80¢ per pound has a protein cost of $4.80 per pound (80¢ × 6).

• **Improved nutritive value of infant products**—Soy protein-based infant formulae are a universal staple for babies who are (1) allergic to milk protein, or (2) unable to utilize lactose. Soy protein infant products provide the same order of growth and weight gain as cow's milk. Also, soy protein is used in baby cereal blends and canned baby foods to improve nutritive value.

• **Improved nutritive value of breakfast cereals and pastas**—New emphasis on nutrition in breakfast cereals has meant more use of soy protein to increase their protein quantity and value. Today, soy proteins are used extensively as additives to hot cereal mixes, and as components of granola bars and compound breakfast bars. Also, U.S. standards of identity for pasta products permit fortification with soy protein.

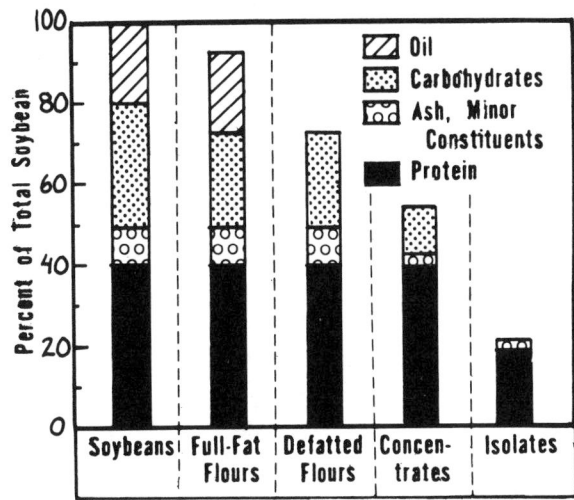

Fig. S-43.   Proximate compositions (dry basis) and yields of the major protein forms obtained from soybeans (Source: Wolf, W. J., "Kinds of Soy Products," *Edible Soy Protein*, FCS Research Report 33, USDA, 1976, p. 3, Fig. 1)

SOYBEAN PRODUCTS AND USES.   In the People's Republic of China, Taiwan, Japan, Korea, and Indonesia, soybeans are a regular part of the diet and a major source of protein and oil. Soybean milk, soybean curd, soy sauce, fermented soybean paste, soybean sprouts, immature green seed, and deep-fried mature seed are common foods in the Orient.

Soybean oil is widely used throughout the world for human consumption as margarine, salad and cooking oils, and shortening.

In the United States, about 30% of the soybean production is used for food and industrial products, and soybean products are the leading protein supplements for livestock. In addition to the use of soybean oil, soy protein is revolutionizing the modern food system; its use as an ingredient, extender, and analog has spread to products in every category of food available to the public—in home and away from home.

Soy protein is available to the food industry in a multitude of forms, most of which may be classified according to protein content as: (1) soy flour and grits, containing 40 to 50% protein; (2) soy protein concentrates, with about 70% protein; (3) soy protein isolates, with 90 to 95% protein; and (4) textured soy protein, which is made from one or more of the other three types. Fig. S-43 shows the proximate compositions of yields of flours, concentrates, and isolates in relation to soybeans.

• **Soy proteins in foreign-feeding programs**—Soy flour is included in many commodities used in foreign-feeding programs, such as soy-fortified bulgur, soy-fortified bread flour, corn-soy milk, corn-soy blend, and wheat-soy blend. In particular, soy protein fortification improves the amino acid composition of the foods to which it is added.

Low cost, good nutrition, and functional versatility account for the ever-increasing quantities of soy proteins in food programs in the less-developed countries. Soy flour is the major ingredient in blended foods with flour and grits added to corn, sorghum, and oat products distributed overseas. Whey-soy drink mix is a new product recently added to the list of commodities available for distribution in feeding programs. It was developed as a replacement for dry milk. The finished product—41.4% sweet whey, 36.5% full fat soybean flour, 12.1% soybean oil, and 9.5% corn sugar—when mixed with water at 15% solids, provides a drink with nearly the same energy and protein content as whole milk.

Table S-22 presents in summary form the story of soybean products and uses.

(Also see BEAN[S], Table B-10 Beans of the World; FLOURS, Table F-26 Special Flours; LEGUMES, Table L-2 Legumes of the World; OILS, VEGETABLE, Table O-6; and VEGETABLE[S], Table V-6 Vegetables of the World.)

TABLE S-22
SOYBEAN PRODUCTS AND USES

Product	Description	Uses	Comments
		HUMAN FOODS	
Soybeans	Whole soybeans.	As mature, dry soybeans used (1) in recipes like other dry beans, or (2) as roasted soybeans—a snack food. As immature green seed served hot as a vegetable, like peas or corn.	In the Orient, soybeans (including whole soybeans) are the principal source of protein in the diet. Soybeans are also rich in minerals, vitamins, and amino acids. Direct food usage of soybeans is expected to increase dramatically around the world due to population pressure on the food supply.
Chee-fan	A type of sufu made by salting small cubes of soybean curd, inoculating with a species of *Mucor*, and allowing them to ferment for about 7 days. After fermentation, are allowed to age in yellow wine for a year.	Consumed much like cheese is eaten in the western world.	
Fermented soybeans	Prepared from black soybeans in China, using a species of *Mucor* as the fermentation organism. After fermentation, they are aged for 6 months or longer in sealed earthenware jars, then seasoned with salt, spices, and wine or whiskey.	As an appetizer.	
Hamanatto (A similar product called Meitanza or tu su is prepared in China. In the Philippines, it is known as taosi)	A liquid, fermented soybean product prepared from whole soybeans by using a starter (koji) made from roasted wheat or barley treated with spores of the mold *Aspergillus oryzae*.	For flavoring many foods.	Hamanatto is expensive and very dark in color. Nagoya University, in Japan, reported the following analyses of hamanatto: water, 38%; protein, 25%; carbohydrate, 25%; salt and calcium, 12%.
Ketjap	A type of soy sauce made from black soybeans in Indonesia.	As a flavoring agent for many foods.	
Metiauza	A product prepared from the insoluble protein and other materials which are separated out from the soybean milk in the preparation of tofu. These residual solids are pressed into cakes; fermented with *Actinomucor elegans* for 10 to 15 days; then sun dried.		

(Continued)

TABLE S-22 (*Continued*)

Product	Description	Uses	Comments
		HUMAN FOODS (*Continued*)	
Miso	A fermented food paste; made by inoculatig trays of rice with *Aspergillus oryzae*, and leaving it to mold abundantly. Then a ground preparation of cooked soybeans and salt is mixed in, and the mass is allowed to ferment and age for several days before being ground into a paste of the consistency of peanut butter.	As a food in Japan. It is used primarily as a flavoring material, added to soups and vegetables. Miso is also spread thinly on cucumbers or substituted for meat sauce on spaghetti.	Miso originated in China. A Japanese missionary who was sent to China in the 7th century learned how it was made and modified it into a product suited to the Japanese taste. The entire process of making miso requires from 10 to 40 days, varying according to the temperature at which the yeast fermentation is conducted. The qualities and proportions of amino acids in miso compare quite favorable with those of casein and soybean meal.
Natto	A fermented whole protein food, fermented by *Bacillus natto*. In this product, the shape of cooked whole soybeans is retained.	Natto is served with soy sauce (shoya) and mustard.	Natto originated in Japan. In 1087, a ruler in the northern part of Japan discovered natto to be part of the local farmers' diets.
Soybean flour	An extremely fine powdered product, containing 40 to 50% protein, the particles of which are 100 or finer mesh size (U.S. standard screen.	Bakery products: breads, rolls, and buns; doughnuts; sweet goods; cakes and cake mixes; pancake and waffle mixes; specialty crackers and cookies. Meat products: sausages, luncheon loaves, patties, canned meats in sauces. Breakfast cereals. Infant and junior foods. Confectionery items. Dietary foods.	Soybean flour is produced like soybean meal, except that the hulls are carefully removed before extraction. Flours are differentiated from grits on the basis of particle size. In Israel, 10% soybean flour is included with wheat flour in baking bread.
Soybean grits	A granular product, containing 40 to 50% protein, the particles of which range from 10 to 80 mesh size (U.S. standard screen).	Bakery products: bread, rolls, and buns; doughnuts; sweet goods; cakes and cake mixes; pancake and waffle mixes; specialty crackers and cookies. Meat products: sausages, luncheon loaves, patties, canned meats in sauces. Breakfast cereals. Infants and junior foods. Confectionery items. Dietary foods.	Soybean grits are produced like soybean meal, except that the hulls are carefully removed before extraction.
Soybean lecithin	The phospholipids which are removed from the crude oil during the degumming process.	Baked goods, cake mixes, instant foods, candies, and drugs. As an antioxidant, emulsifier, and softener in food manufacturing.	Crude soybean oil contains 1 to 3% lecithin.

(*Continued*)

TABLE S-22 (Continued)

Product	Description	Uses	Comments
HUMAN FOODS (Continued)			
Soybean milk	The product obtained by soaking beans in water, grinding the soaked beans, and filtering the insoluble pieces out.	Consumed primarily by the Chinese. As the starting material for the preparation of a soybean curd, probably the most important and popular soybean food in the Orient. In soybean-milk-based infant formulas.	The soft cheeselike curd, known as "toufu," "tofu," "tubu," and other local names, contains about 53% protein, 26% fat, 17% carbohydrate, and 4% fiber, minerals, and vitamins. Curd has a bland taste and can be flavored with seasonings or blended with other foods. It is made into a variety of products by frying, dehydrating, or freezing and is consumed daily in the same manner as high-protein foods in the U.S.
Soybean oil	The crude oil which is extracted from soybeans, then refined.	Margarine, shortening (cooking oil), and salad oil. The hydrogenated oil finds much use in restaurant chains and institutions for deep fat frying of foods. In the Far East, oil is consumed extensively as a food.	About 1/5 the bean is oil. More than 90% of the oil is refined and used for foods—for margarine, shortening, and salad oil. All edible oils are deodorized. Hydrogenation varies, depending upon the final use of the oil.
Soybean protein concentrates	Soybean protein products containing 70% protein. They are prepared from defatted flakes or flours by removing water-soluble sugars, ash, and other minor constituents.	Bakery products: bread, biscuits, and buns; cakes and cake mixes. Meat products: sausages, luncheon loaves, poultry rolls, patties, meat loaves, canned meats in sauces. Breakfast cereals. Infant foods. Dietary foods.	
Soybean protein hydrolysates	Soybean proteins that are partially hydrolyzed by a number of agents such as enzymes, acids, alkalis, or steam, or by yeasts, molds, or bacteria. Hydrolysates are soluble in water over the entire pH scale.	Soy sauce and other flavorings, foaming agents, and whipping agents.	
Soybean protein isolates (Also see "textured soybean proteins")	Soybean protein isolates, which contain 90 to 95% protein, are the purest form of soybean protein marketed. They are produced by (1) washing out the proteins from dehulled, defatted soybean flakes, (2) precipitating the protein out of the liquid solution with a mild alkali, and (3) drying by a spray process.	As the basic ingredient of spun fiber types of meat analogs. Meat products: sausages, luncheon loaves, poultry rolls. Dairy-type foods: whipped toppings, coffee whiteners, frozen desserts, beverage powders. Infant foods. Dietary foods.	Soybean protein isolates are required for spinning.

(Continued)

TABLE S-22 (*Continued*)

Product	Description	Uses	Comments
HUMAN FOODS (*Continued*)			
Soybean sprouts	Sprouts of soybeans about 4 in. (*10 cm*) long. Prepared by germinating whole soybeans under optimum moisture conditions at a temperature of 72-86°F (*22-30°C*) for 4 to 7 days.	As a fresh vegetable, or in soup.	Soybean sprouts are a rich source of vitamin C. On a moisture-free basis, soybean sprouts run about 50% protein content.
Soy sauce (shoyu in Japan, chiang-yu in China)	A salty brown sauce made by fermenting soybeans—a liquid food. The "starter" (koji) for making soy sauce is prepared from rice inoculated with the spores of the molds of either *Aspergillus oryzae* or *Aspergillus soyae*. In Japan, about equal quantities of soybeans and wheat are used in making soy sauce. In China, more soybeans and less wheat are used.	As a flavoring agent for many foods—especially in Chinese and Japanese cooking.	Soy sauce originated in China some 2,500 years ago and was introduced in Japan in the 7th century by Buddhist priests. The average annual per capita consumption in Japan is about 3 gal. (*11.4 liter*). Good soy sauce contains large amounts of amino acids, especially glutamic acid.
Tao-cho	Prepared from light colored soybeans. They are soaked, dehulled, and boiled, then mixed with rice flour and roasted. Next, they are inoculated with *Aspergillus*, then fermented for 3 days and sun-dried. The cakes are dipped in brine, arenga sugar and a paste of glutinous rice, following which they are exposed to the sun for a month or more.	As an appetizer	
Tao-si	A soybean product, made from unhulled beans. Soybeans are soaked and boiled; wheat flour is added; the mix is inoculated with *Aspergillus oryzae* and incubated for 2 to 3 days; thence placed in earthenware jars and salt brine is added; and the product is finished in about 2 months.	An Appetizer	

(*Continued*)

TABLE S-22 (*Continued*)

Product	Description	Uses	Comments
HUMAN FOODS (*Continued*)			
Taotjo	A soybean product of the East Indies. Boiled soybeans are mixed with roasted wheat meal or glutinous rice; inoculated with *Aspergillus oryzae* for 2 to 3 days; then placed in brine for several weeks, with palm sugar added to the brine at intervals.	A condiment.	
Tempeh	An Indonesian food made entirely from soybeans, prepared by using a phycomycete, *Rhizopus oliogosporus*.	Tempeh is used as a main dish, rather than as a flavoring agent for other foods. Raw tempeh is sliced and then fried or baked.	A similar product called *tempeh bongkrek* is sometimes made from coconut meat. Tempeh made from coconut meat may become poisonous, but tempeh made from soybeans never does. The *Rhizopus* mold synthesizes vitamin B-12; hence, tempeh is one of the few vegetable products that contain significant amounts of this vitamin.
Textured soybean proteins (analogs) (Also see "soybean protein concentrates" and "soybean protein isolates.")	Further processing of the basic forms—flours and grits, concentrates, and isolates—is now practiced to give soybean proteins a texture that resembles specific types of meat; these items range from extenders to be used with ground meats to complete meat analogs. Two basic types of textured soybean protein products are now available: 1. *Extruded*, made by cooking soybean flour and other ingredients and forcing the mixture through small holes into a chamber of lower temperature and pressure. Granules of these expanded materials are available in both colored and uncolored and flavored and unflavored forms.	Ground meat extenders. Meat analogs (baconlike bits, etc.)	Textured items, mainly of the extruded type, are the fastest growing segment of the edible soy protein business. Production of meat analogs either by extruding soybean flour or by spinning protein isolate into fibers results in products that look and taste like beef, pork, and other kinds of meat. Soy protein can augment whole fish, improve the texture and eating characteristics of finished consumer fish products, and replace the functional fish protein. It can, for example, build the visual content of processed shellfish without altering the distinctive flavor and mouthfeel of such products. Soy protein seems assured of increased use in dairy product analogs made for people who have special health or religious diet requirements. The extruded soy process is patented and licensing is required.
	2 *Spun*, made by spinning the fibers and then flavoring, coloring, and forming them in shapes which resemble pieces of meat, poultry, and fish.	Meat analogs: baconlike bits, simulated sausages, simulated ham chunks, simulated chicken chunks, simulated bacon slices. Meat extenders.	The basic patent for spun protein isolates has expired, but companies now engaged in this business hold patents on improved methods for converting the fiber into meat analogs.

(Continued)

TABLE S-22 (*Continued*)

Product	Description	Uses	Comments
		HUMAN FOODS (*Continued*)	
Tofu and Sufu (soybean cheese)	In producing sufu, a product called tofu, the Oriental equivalent of curdled milk, is produced. It is	Both tofu and sufu are sliced and eaten much like cheese is consumed in the western world.	Tofu has been one of the most important foods in the Orient for centuries. Sufu, which originated in China in the 5th century, is widely used in China today.

made by soaking, grinding, and straining soybeans to produce soybean milk; then boiling to coagulate the proteins and pressing to remove water. At this stage, which is prior to inoculation with fungi, it is called tofu; hence tofu is not fermented.

Sufu, a fermented soybean product, often referred to as Chinese cheese, because it closely resembles cheese of the western world. At least five species of fungi have been isolated from sufu, but *Actinomucor elegans* appears to be the organism of choice.

Product	Description	Uses	Comments
		BEVERAGES	
Soy protein shake	A beverage containing soy protein.	As shakes at fast food outlets.	Shakes with soy protein have been widely marketed.
Whey-soy drink	A beverage containing whey and soy protein. The base product (41.4% sweet whey, 36.5% full fat soybean flour, 12.1% soybean oil, and 9.5% corn sugar) is mixed with water at 15% solids.	As a drink with nearly the same energy and protein content as whole milk.	This is a new product available for distribution in the developing countries.
		LIVESTOCK FEEDS	
Soybeans: 1. Ground soybeans	Ground or cracked whole soybeans without cooking or removing any of the oil.	Cattle, sheep, and horses.	Raw whole soybeans are seldom fed to livestock. Rather, they are processed and utilized as either oil meal or whole, heat-processed beans. Limit soybeans to the amount needed to balance the ration. Too large an allowance may be unduly laxative and throw the animals off feed. Feeding a large proportion of soybeans tends to produce soft butter. Today, most soybeans are fed in oil meal form; but as the cost of energy increases, the cost of soybean meal will likewise increase. As a result of these increased processing costs, the use of heat-processed whole soybeans will play an increasing role in livestock nutrition. Whole soybeans must be heated to deactivate the anti-nutritional factors of the seeds; but once properly heated, the whole seed provides a valuable source of energy and protein. Many of the problems associated with feeding this high-oil feed, such as soft pork, have been overcome by adjustments in feed formulations.
2. Heat processed soybeans (dry roasted soybeans)	The product resulting from heating whole soybeans without removing any of the component parts. It may be ground, pelleted, flaked, or powdered.	Swine and poultry.	

(*Continued*)

TABLE S-22 (*Continued*)

Product	Description	Uses	Comments
		LIVESTOCK FEEDS (*Continued*)	
Condensed soybean solubles	The product obtained by washing soybean flour and soybean flakes with water and acid at pH of 4.2 to 4.6. The wash water is then concentrated to a solid content of not less than 60%.		
Ground extruded whole soybeans	The meal product resulting from the extrusion by friction heat and/or steam of whole soybeans without removing any of the component parts.		
Kibbled soybean meal	The product obtained by cooking ground, solvent-extracted meal, under pressure and extruding from an expeller or other mechanical pressure device. It must not contain more than 7% crude fiber.		
Soybean feed, solvent-extracted	The product remaining after partial removal of protein and nitrogen-free extract from dehulled solvent-extracted soybean flakes.		
Soybean grits or soybean flour	The screened and graded product remaining after removal of most of the oil from selected, sound, cleaned, and dehulled soybeans by a mechanical or solvent-extraction process.		It must contain not more than 3% crude fiber.
Soybean hulls	The outer covering of the soybean.	In commercial feeds.	
Soybean meal, dehulled, solvent-extracted	The product obtained by grinding the flakes remaining after removal of most of the oil from dehulled soybeans by a solvent-extraction process. Heat must be applied during the process.	In mashes for chicks and broilers and in pig starters.	It must contain not more than 3.3% crude fiber. It may contain up to 0.5% of a conditioning agent to reduce caking and improve flowability, with the name of the conditioning agent shown as an added ingredient. This product is high in protein and low in fiber.

(Continued)

TABLE S-22 (*Continued*)

Product	Description	Uses	Comments
LIVESTOCK FEEDS (*Continued*)			
Soybean meal, mechanically extracted	The product obtained by grinding the cake or chips which remain after removal of most of the oil from soybeans by a mechanical extraction process. Heat must be applied during the process.	For all classes of livestock.	It must contain not more than 7% crude fiber. It may contain up to 0.5% of a conditioning agent to reduce caking and improve flowability, with the name of the conditioning agent shown as an added ingredient.
Soybean meal, solvent-extracted	The product obtained by grinding the flakes which remain after removal of most of the oil from soybeans by a solvent-extraction process. Heat must be applied during the process.	For all classes of livestock.	It must contain not more than 7% crude fiber. It may contain up to 0.5% of a conditioning agent to reduce caking and improve flowability, with the name of the conditioning agent shown as an added ingredient.
Soybean mill feed	The soybean hulls and the offal from the tail of the mill which result from the manufacture of soybean grits or flour.	For ruminants, as a hay replacement.	It must contain not less than 13% crude protein and not more than 32% crude fiber.
Soybean mill run	The soybean hulls and such bean meats as adhere to the hulls which result from the normal milling operations in the production of dehulled soybean meal.		It must contain not less than 11% crude protein and not more than 35% crude fiber.
Soybean phosphatide or soybean lecithin	The mixed phosphatide product obtained from soybean oil by a degumming process.		
Soybean protein concentrate	The product remaining after removing most of the oil and water-soluble nonprotein constituents from high-quality, sound, clean, dehulled soybean seeds.	In calf milk replacers.	It must contain not less than 70% protein on a moisture-free basis.

(*Continued*)

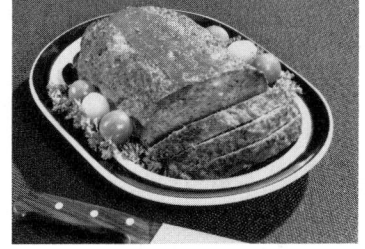

Meatloaf, using soybean extender with ground beef. (Courtesy, Worthington Foods, Worthington, Ohio)

TABLE S-22 (*Continued*)

Product	Description	Uses	Comments
LIVESTOCK FEEDS (*Continued*)			
Soybean protein product, chemically modified	The product resulting from the chemical modification of dehulled solvent-extracted soybean materials (soybean flour, soybean flakes, soybean grits, soybean meal, soybean protein concentrate) utilizing acids, alkalis, or other chemicals with or without heat processing, without removing any of the component parts.	For all classes of live-stock.	It must contain a minimum of 48% crude protein, and it may be ground, flaked, or powdered.
Forages: Soybean hay, ground	The ground soybean plant, including the leaves and beans.	Cattle and sheep.	It must not contain more than 33% crude fiber. Digestive disturbances may result from feeding soybean hay alone.
Soybean pasture	Green growing plants.	For swine.	Not a good cattle pasture, as trampling damages the plants.
Soybean silage	The chopped, fermented whole plant.	For cattle and sheep.	Soybeans are seldom ensiled alone. They make a better silage when ensiled with corn.
Soybean straw	The residue that remains after threshing the beans from the plants.	For dry cows and replacement heifers.	It is a relatively poor roughage; high in fiber and low in protein.
OTHER USES			
Soybean oil	The oil extracted from the seed.	Paints, enamels, soaps, varnishes, linoleum, pharmaceuticals, cosmetics, core oil, synthetic rubber, and printing ink.	

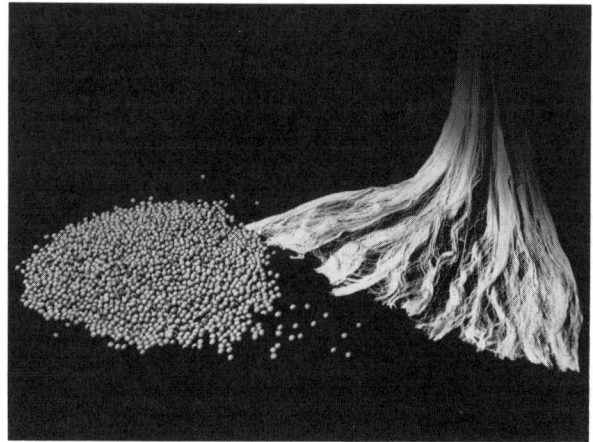

Fig. S-44.   Soybeans and spun soy fiber. After spinning the fibers, they may be flavored, colored, and formed into shapes which resemble pieces of meat, poultry, and fish. (Courtesy, Worthington Foods, Division of Miles Laboratories, Inc., USA, Worthington, Ohio)

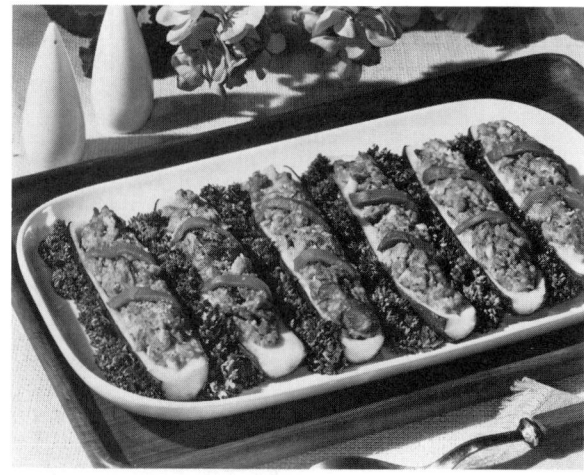

Fig. S-45.   Chickenlike pieces of meat made from spun soy fiber. (Courtesy, Worthington Foods, Division of Miles Laboratories, Inc., USA, Worthington, Ohio)

SOYBEAN PROTEIN

The protein of soybean, after suitable processing. It has the highest nutritive value of any plant protein source. Foods made from soybeans include soy flour, soy milk, spun fiber, soy sauce, tofu and tempeh (fermented cheese and curd), and soy butter. Also, soybeans may be cooked as green or dried beans, canned in sauce, or roasted (like peanuts). Soybean meal is the leading protein supplement for animals.
(Also see SOYBEAN.)

SOY FLOUR

May be used in many baked products. Some 6 to 8% of soy flour added to wheat flour and used for bread and pastries will significantly improve the protein value of the product without making much change in texture and appearance.
(Also see SOYBEAN.)

SOY MILK

Food from soybeans made by soaking soybeans 4 to 5 hours, grinding them in a hot water slurry (1 part of soaked beans to 3 parts of water), then straining out the insoluble residue. It has been consumed for centuries in China and in some other countries of the Far East. A 200-milliliter bottle of soy milk will supply at least 6 g of high-quality protein, 50% of a child's daily requirement.
(Also see SOYBEAN.)

SPANISH GOAT

The primary meat-type goat, represents a cross of many dairy goat breeds. The meat from this type of goat is known as "cabrito," meaning little goat in Spanish.
(Also see LAMB AND MUTTON.)

SPANISH LIME (MANONICILLO) *Melicocca bijuga*

The fruit of a tropical American tree (of the family *Sapindaceae*) that is related to the litchi of Asia. Spanish limes, which are not related to the citrus fruits, are greenish plumlike fruits that have a tart sweet flesh and a large pith. They may be eaten fresh or when made into preserves.
The fruit is moderately high in calories (59 kcal per 100 g) and carbohydrates (20%). It is a poor source of vitamin C.

SPECIAL DIETS

Those diets altered to meet specific body requirements under different conditions of health or disease. Diets may be altered in a variety of ways: consistency, specific nutrient content, flavor, preparation method, or frequency of feeding. The purposes behind special diets include: (1) maintenance of good nutritional status, (2) correction of deficiencies, (3) adjustment of food intake to the body's ability to metabolize the nutrients, and (4) alteration of body weight if necessary. Some special diets have specific names while others may be described by the terms high, low, restricted or free.
Also see MODIFIED DIETS.)

SPECIFIC DYNAMIC ACTION (SDA)

The increased production of heat by the body as a result of a stimulus to metabolic activity caused by ingesting food.

SPECIFIC GRAVITY

The ratio of the weight of a body to the weight of an equal volume of water.

SPECIFIC HEAT

• The heat-absorbing capacity of a substance in relation to that of water.

• The heat expressed in calories required to raise the temperature of 1 g of a substance 1°C.

SPHINCTER

A muscle surrounding and able to contract and close a bodily opening or channel (the anal).

SPHINGOMYELIN

A lipid composed of a fatty acid such as stearic or palmitic, phosphate, choline, and the amino alcohol, sphingosine. It is found primarily in nervous tissue.
(Also see FATS AND OTHER LIPIDS.)

SPICES

The word *spice* is of French origin, meaning "fruits of the earth." *Spice is the name given to food seasonings made from plants.* They have a sharp taste and odor— they're more pungent than herbs. Some spices are valued for their taste, others for their smell. Common spices include pepper, nutmeg, cloves, ginger, allspice, mace, mustard, and cinnamon.
Spices have little in common except for their use. They usually come from tropical plants; and different parts of various spice plants may be used. For example, cloves

come from the bud, cinnamon comes from the bark, pepper comes from the fruit, ginger and horseradish come from the root, and mustard comes from the seed.

Some people grow spice plants such as sage, marjoram, thyme, and others in their gardens; others grow them in pots in sunny windows. They then dry the plants for later use.

Spices have little food value, but they do increase the appetite and stimulate the organs of digestion. Before foods were canned or refrigerated, spices were used to make tainted foods taste better.

• **Spice trade**—Since ancient times, spice trade routes have existed between Arabia, India, and the Far East. The value placed on spices was often greater than that of gold and jewels; and ancient cities like Palmyra (in modern Syria) were founded on the wealth of Muslim spice merchants whose camel caravans and ships brought spices from India and China. The first major monopoly arose in the 9th century among Indian traders operating from Java. Marco Polo's 13th-century account of spices in the Far East generated interest in establishing independent spice trade between European and Asian countries. The cities of Genoa and Venice became powerful because they were the center of the spice trade with the East. When Columbus set sail across unknown seas, he was interested in discovering an all-water route to the spice lands of the East. The Portuguese, after rounding South Africa and reaching India, captured Melaka in 1512 and dominated the trade for the rest of the century. Dutch and British fleets drove Portugal from Asian waters after 1600, but the Dutch seized Melaka in 1641 and denied the British access to Moluccas (the Spice Islands, a famous source of spices). They established the profitable Dutch East India Company and—except for intervals of British domination—controlled the spice trade into the 20th century.

(Also see FLAVORINGS AND SEASONINGS.)

SPINACH *Spinacia oleracea*

This vegetable, which is grown for its highly nutritious leaves, is a member of the Goosefoot family (*Chenopodiaceae*). Hence, it is related to the various types of beets, chards, and hardy weeds which belong to the same family. Typical spinach leaves are shown in Figs. S-46 and S-47.

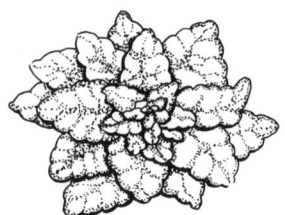

Fig. S-46.   A cluster of spinach leaves in the form of a rosette.

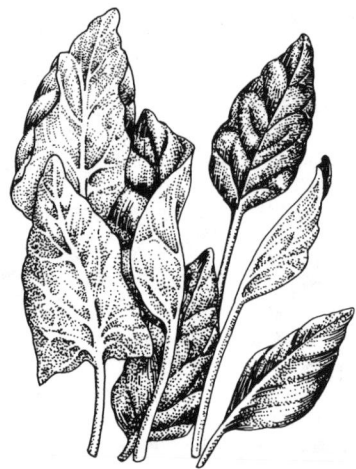

Fig. S-47.   Individual leaves of spinach.

ORIGIN AND HISTORY.   Spinach is believed to have originated in Persia or neighboring areas of southwestern Asia. It was introduced into China in the 7th century, A.D., when some plants were sent as a gift from the king of Nepal. Somewhat later (about 1000 A.D.), the Moors brought the vegetable to Europe. However, it was not grown throughout northern Europe until the 18th century.

PRODUCTION.   The United States, the Netherlands, and the Scandinavian countries are the major producers. Each year, about 174,000 metric tons of spinach are produced in the United States. Much of the crop is grown in California, but significant amounts are also produced in Texas and Oklahoma.

Spinach does best in cool weather because it has a tendency to go to seed when daytime temperatures reach 75°F (24°C) or more. Furthermore, it withstands freezing much better than most other vegetables, although it is likely to be injured by night temperatures below 25°F (-4°C). Therefore, it is planted when it will have at least 6 weeks of cool, but not frigid, growing weather. In warm climates, spinach is sown throughout the late fall, winter, and early spring; but in cooler climates it is planted only in the early spring or late summer.

Generally, spinach plants have either male flowers or female flowers. Female forms are slower to bolt, a characteristic that led to the development of warm-weather varieties in which the plants are primarily female.

The soil should not be too heavy, and it should range in pH from 6 to 8 (mildly acid to mildly alkaline). Acid soils may require the addition of lime to bring them closer to neutrality. Most spinach growers fertilize the soil with nitrogen, phosphorus, and potassium.

Spinach leaves are harvested when they are full size, but before the plant develops a seed stalk. However, it is not wise to cut the leaves right after a rain or a heavy dew because they are likely to be very crisp and susceptible to breaking. The average yield of spinach per acre in the United States is about 13,500 lb (*15,120 kg/ha*), but yields as high as 20,400 lb (*22,848 kg/ha*) have been obtained in California.

PROCESSING. About three-quarters of the spinach crop is processed. The major types of processing are canning and freezing, although small quantities are used to make baby foods, spinach noodles, and other special items.

SELECTION. Good quality spinach plants should be well developed and relatively stocky. Straggly overgrown plants or plants with seedstems are generally undesirable. Leaves should be clean, fresh, and tender, and of good green color. Yellow, discolored, wilted, bruised or crushed leaves should be avoided. Small yellowish-green, undeveloped heart leaves are natural and should not be considered objectionable. Decay appears as a soft, slimy disintegration.

PREPARATION. Spinach leaves should be washed under running water to remove adhering particles of soil. Then, the vegetable may be served raw in salads or cooked in as little water as possible. Steaming in a metal basket above boiling water is another suitable means of cooking. Usually, 5 to 10 minutes of cooking is sufficient to make the leaves tender. The cooked vegetable is often served with butter or a cheese sauce. Canned spinach is overcooked during processing. Hence, it should be used in dishes requiring little or no heating. The can liquor is rich in minerals and vitamins and should be used in soups or other preparations. Some other tasty ways of serving spinach follow:

• **Casseroles**—Spinach goes well wth eggs, fish, meats, poultry, and seafood in casseroles. Usually, these dishes are well seasoned and may also contain thickened gravies or sauces.

• **Custards and souffles**—These baked dishes are usually made from chopped spinach, cheese and/or milk, eggs, and various seasonings.

• **Fillings**—Chopped spinach mixed with crumbled cooked bacon, shredded cheese, bread crumbs, seasonings, and/or other ingredients may be used as a filling or a stuffing for fish filets, green or red peppers, popovers, ravioli, and timbales.

• **Frittata**—This Italian crustless pie is made from finely chopped spinach, eggs, onions, cheese, and seasonings.

• **Greek spinach pie**—The special *fila* pastry which serves as the bottom and top crusts of this pie makes it different from *frittata*.

• **Poached eggs and spinach**—The cooked eggs are usually placed on cooked whole spinach leaves and dressed with a cream sauce and paprika.

• **Soups**—Chopped or pureed spinach may be used in a wide variety of tasty soups, ranging from those made with heavy cream to those which owe their body to a thick spinach puree.

NUTRITIONAL VALUE. The nutient composi- tions of various forms of spinach are given in Food Com- position Table F-36.

Some noteworthy observations regarding the nutrient composition of spinach follow:

1. Spinach has a high water content (90 to 93%) and is low in calories. It is an excellent source of magnesium, iron, potassium, and vitamin A; a good source of calcium and vitamin C (only when raw, because cooking may destroy as much as half the content of this vitamin); and a fair to good source of phosphorus, zinc, pantothenic acid, and pyridoxine (vitamin B-6). Considerable amounts of the minerals and vitamins in raw spinach may be leached into the cooking water. Therefore, only a mini- mum of water should be used. Also, nutrient-rich cook- ing water and can liquor should not be discarded, but should be used whenever it is feasible.

2. The protein-to-calorie ratio (12.3 g per 100 kcal) of spinach is almost equal to that of creamed cottage cheese. Hence, significant amounts of dietary protein may be supplied by this vegetable if sufficiently large quantities are consumed. For example, ¾ cup (*180 ml*) of cooked spinach supplies the calories and protein con- tent of 1 oz (*28 g*) of cottage cheese.

3. Spinach contains more than twice as much cal- cium as phosphorus. Hence, this vegetable complements such foods as eggs, fish, legumes, meats, nuts, and sea- foods which contain much more phosphorus than cal- cium. (A balance between the dietary levels of calcium and phosphorus is necessary to insure optimal utiliza- tion of both essential elements.)

CAUTION: Spinach is rich in *oxalates*, which may be harmful if consumed in excessive amounts because (1) they interfere with the utilization of calcium and iron, and (2) under certain circumstances oxalate stones may form in the urinary tract. However, it is not likely that these effects will result from the consumption of spinach alone. Rather, they may be caused by an excessive intake of a combination of oxalate-rich foods such as almonds, cashew nuts, cocoa, rhubarb, spinach, and tea.

(Also see VEGETABLES[S], Table V-6 Vegetables of the World.)

SPOILAGE OF FOOD

Although food spoilage is often thought of as some- thing caused by bacteria, molds, or yeast, it is actually any change which renders a food unfit for human con- sumption. Here a distinction should be drawn between unfit and undesirable. Food may be undesirable due to the dislikes of an individual, but this does not mean it is unfit for everyone. Furthermore, food spoilage cannot be equated to danger to the consumer. Spoilage results in abnormal colors, flavors, odors, texture, or other unac- ceptable changes. The causes of food spoilage can be grouped into five broad categories: (1) microbial spoilage, (2) enzymatic spoilage, (3) chemical spoilage, (4) physical spoilage, and (5) pest spoilage. A discussion of each groups follows:

1. **Microbial spoilage.** Three different groups of microorganisms may be responsible for food spoilage: bacteria, yeasts, and mold. These microorganisms are

found everywhere. Examples of bacterial spoilage include the spoilage of meat, milk, eggs, and often canned goods. Fresh fruits and vegetables, dried foods, and foods with a high sugar content are frequently spoiled by yeast and molds. Characteristically, molds grow on the surface and appear as fuzzy growths on bread, cheeses, jams, jellies, fruits, and vegetables. Yeast may spoil food by fermentation or by the formation of slime. Most microorganisms like warm moist conditions.

2. **Enzymatic spoilage.** Natural enzymes, organic catalysts within the food itself, cause widespread spoilage, but most often this is manifest as a loss of quality rather than outright spoilage. Frozen vegetables develop a haylike flavor due to enzymatic action during long or improper storage. Enzymatic action is responsible for the softening and overripeness which develops during storage. Some enzymes even survive processing methods and can create odors and flavors even when microorganisms have been eliminated.

3. **Chemical spoilage.** Chemical reactions causing spoilage include oxidation of fats, hydrogen production by the action of food acids on metal containers, or the discoloration of a food by metal ions from the container. These chemical reactions can be prevented by using the proper lining in cans and by use of antioxidants.

4. **Physical spoilage.** Exposure to extremes in heat, cold, or light can lead to spoilage. A rise in temperature increases the rate of enzymatic and nonenzymatic reactions, and excessive heat denatures proteins, breaks emulsions, dries out food, and destroys some vitamins— all increasing the chance of an unfit food. Excessive cold may crack fresh foods, disrupt texture, deteriorate some liquid foods, cause the development of off-color, and produce surface pitting. Proper temperatures for storage vary according to the product. For some food items, excessive light causes the development of off-flavor; for example, the light struck flavor of milk and "skunky" beer.

5. **Spoilage by pests.** Food products containing such items as insects, rat hair, and animal droppings are unfit for consumers for aesthetic reasons as well as health reasons (disease). These items in foods generally indicate unsanitary processing conditions. The Food and Drug Administration checks the sanitation of a product by examining it for rat hairs, droppings, insects, insect fragments, and mold hyphae. Presence of these items can lead to confiscation or prohibition of shipments until unsanitary conditions are corrected.

The aim of modern food production, processing, and preservation is to, so far as is possible, reduce and/or eliminate all sources of food spoilage. By the time a food reaches the consumer proper heat and/or chill treatments, canning, drying, freezing, sanitation, and food additives may all play a role in eliminating spoilage. Then the control of spoilage is passed on to the consumer who must exercise proper storage and preparation methods.

(Also see ADDITIVES; BACTERIA IN FOODS; POISONS; and PRESERVATION OF FOOD.)

SPORE

A resting reproductive form of certain microorganisms.

SPRAY-DEHYDRATED

Material which has been dried by spraying onto the surface of a heated drum. It is recovered by scraping it from the drum.

SPRING LAMBS

Lambs marketed in the spring of the year. Usually they are born in the fall or in the early winter and marketed prior to July 1. After July 1, animals of like birth are designated as lambs on the market.

SPRUCE BEER

This is a fermented drink made from an extract of spruce needles and twigs boiled with molasses or sugar. At one time it was used as a diuretic and antiscorbutic.

SPRUE

A collective term for a group of nutritional deficiency diseases characterized by impaired absorption of nutrients from the small intestine, especially fats, glucose, and vitamins. Although all sprues exhibit the same general clinical manifestations of intestinal malabsorption and steatorrhea (fatty diarrhea), the following three etiologic classifications are presented in this book:

1. **Celiac disease,** a rare metabolic disorder of children, which results from a sensitivity to gluten.

2. **Nontropical sprue,** the term commonly applied to adults exhibiting a sensitivity to gluten.

3. **Tropical sprue,** caused by a deficiency of folic acid and vitamin B-12.

(Also see CELIAC DISEASE; SPRUE, NONTROPICAL; and SPRUE, TROPICAL.)

SPRUE, NONTROPICAL (CELIAC-SPRUE)

The term nontropical sprue is commonly applied to adults exhibiting a sensitivity to gluten. It is due to an intolerance to wheat gluten, a main constituent of wheat flour, which is also present to a small extent in rye, barley, and oats, but not in rice. Symptoms are provoked by the ingestion of any of the numerous foods containing wheat gluten. Characteristic symptoms of sprue include steatorrhea (fatty diarrhea), weight loss, and lesions of the small intestine. As the disease progresses, a multitude of other symptoms may appear due to the loss of fat and other nutrients in the stool.

Treatment consists of a gluten-free diet. This means the exclusion of all cereal grains except corn and rice and the use of potato and soy flours. This is easier said than done, since wheat flour is used in such a variety of products. However, familiarity with these products, and careful label reading should help ensure a gluten-free diet. If the disease progresses to the point that malnutrition is present, then the diet should be high in proteins and calories, and probably minerals and vitamins, also.

(Also see ALLERGIES, section headed "Wheat Allergy"; MODIFIED DIETS; MALABSORPTION SYNDROME; and SPRUE.)

SPRUE, TROPICAL

A malabsorption syndrome affecting mainly individuals living in the West Indies, Central America, and the Far East. Even individuals from temperate climates visiting these countries may develop tropical sprue during or after their visit. Although somewhat similar to nontropical sprue, tropical sprue responds to different therapy. Both types of sprue are characterized by the typical flat mucosa of the small intestine, secondary enzyme deficiencies in the intestinal mucosa, and steatorrhea. However, in tropical sprue, a macrocytic anemia occurs as a manifestation of folic acid and vitamin B-12 deficiencies. Indeed, marked improvement of the sufferer is noted following the administration of folic acid and vitamin B-12. Diet therapy consists of a diet high in calories and protein to counteract the malnutrition, restricted in fiber and fat; and rich in bananas. Substitution of fat with medium-chain triglycerides has resulted in the disappearance of steatorrhea (fatty diarrhea), and weight gain. Contrary to nontropical sprue, response to a gluten-free diet is minimal. Although no infective agent has been demonstrated, broad-spectrum antibiotics have proven beneficial.

(Also see ANEMIA, MEGALOBLASTIC; MODIFIED DIETS; FOLACIN; MALABSORPTION SYNDROMES; and SPRUE.)

SQUAB

A young pigeon that is about 4 weeks old and weighs 1 lb. Squabs should be slaughtered just before leaving the nest. They are processed and cooked much like any other poultry.

SQUASHES *Cucurbita* spp

The fruits of these plants provide both edible flesh and edible seeds. Also, the flowers are edible. Squashes belong to the gourd or melon family (*Cucurbitaceae*), which also includes pumpkins and cucumbers. The different species of squashes are *C. maxima, C. mixta, C. moschata,* and *C. pepo.* Certain varieties of fruits within each of these species are pumpkins rather than squashes. The characteristics which may be used to distinguish between the two closely related types of fruits are (1) summer squashes are immature, soft, and watery; (2) winter squashes are mature, hard-skinned, and have a mildly-flavored, finely-grained flesh; and (3) pumpkins are mature, hard-skinned, and have a strongly-flavored, coarsely-grained flesh.

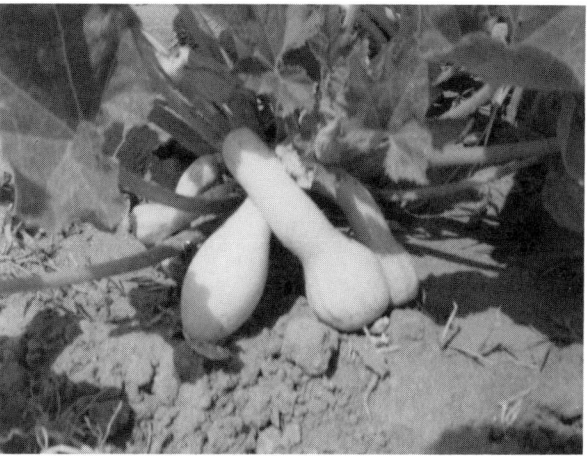

Fig. S-48.   Summer squashes. (Photo by Audrey Ensminger)

ORIGIN AND HISTORY. The wild ancestors of the squashes appear to have originated in the vicinity of the border between Mexico and Guatemala. From there they spread to North America and South America. The first use of these vegetables as food appears to have occurred around 8000 B.C. in Mexico. At that time the Indians gathered the wild plants mainly for the seeds because the fruits contained only small amounts of bitter-tasting flesh. Over the centuries, mutant plants with more fleshy, milder-flavored fruits appeared and were grown along with beans and corn by the Aztec, Inca, and Mayan Indian civilizations of Latin America.

Columbus was the first white man to see these fruits when he observed them growing in the West Indies. Other early explorers of the Americas noted the widespread practice of growing squashes between rows of corn. Often, the squash vines climbed upon the cornstalks or upon the trunks of small trees that the Indians had killed by girdling. Later, the French missionary priest Marquette (1637-1675) noted that the Indians of Illinois dried strips of winter squashes in the sun in order to preserve them. Some Indians even cooked the flowers of the plants in meat stews.

Shortly after the discovery of America, pumpkins and squashes were brought back to the Old World, where the production of these vegetables eventually surpassed that of the New World.

At the present time certain agricultural scientists are engaged in breeding some of the wild, ancestral species of squashes in order to develop new varieties that (1) will grow well in arid regions, and (2) will produce large amounts of high-protein seed.

PRODUCTION. The world production of squashes, pumpkins, and gourds combined is about 5.2 million metric tons. (Much of this production is comprised of squashes which are much more widely grown and utilized than pumpkins and gourds.) Fig. S-49 shows the amounts contributed by each of ten top producing countries.

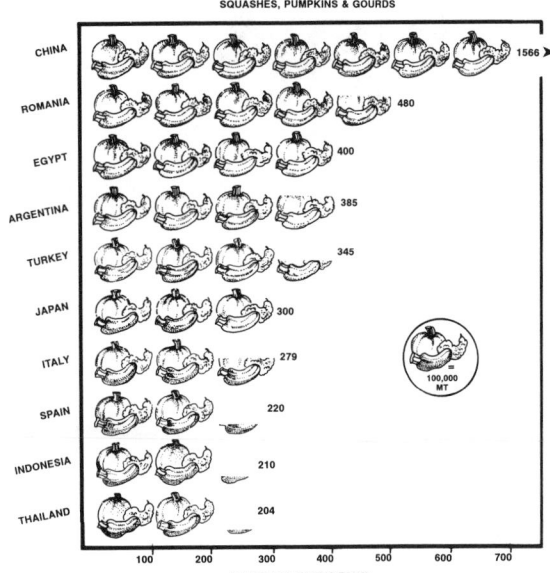

SQUASHES, PUMPKINS & GOURDS

CHINA 1566 ➤

ROMANIA 480

EGYPT 400

ARGENTINA 385

TURKEY 345

JAPAN 300

ITALY 279

SPAIN 220

INDONESIA 210

THAILAND 204

100,000 MT

100   200   300   400   500   600   700
(THOUSAND METRIC TONS)

Fig. S-49.   Ten top contributors to the world production of squashes, pumpkins, and gourds. (Based upon data from *FAO Production Yearbook*, 1990, FAO/UN, Rome, Italy, Vol. 44, p. 134, Table 54)

Statistics on the total U.S. production of squashes and pumpkins are not readily available, but it is estimated that over 31 thousand metric tons of these vegetables are frozen and that about the same amount are canned.[42]

Most commercial growers plant squash seeds directly in the fields because the roots of the young plants are easily injured by transplanting. Home gardeners sometimes start their plants indoors in peat pots or other special containers that can be planted in the field when the danger of frost has passed and the soil temperature is at least 60°F (16°C). It is noteworthy that summer varieties of squash may be planted in the spring and harvested in the summer, whereas winter squashes should be planted later in the season since they do not tolerate hot summer weather. Furthermore, some varieties of winter squash do not set much fruit during the summer because long, hot days promote the production of a preponderance of male flowers. On the other hand, short, cool days stimulate the formation of female flowers in these varieties.

The soil should be fertile, well-drained, rich in organic matter, and only mildly acid to mildly alkaline. Strongly acid soils may require the addition of lime. Often, the soil may be fertilized with various combinations of animal or green manure, and nitrogen, phosphorus, and potassium mixtures. Squashes should *not* be watered with sprinklers if it can be avoided because wetting the leaves of the

[42]*Agricultural Statistics 1991*, USDA.

plant may encourage the spread of disease. Hence, drip irrigation and furrow irrigation are more desirable methods of watering.

It is usually necessary to thin the plants after they have become established in order to prevent stunting due to overcrowding. Home gardeners who have only a limited amount of space for these crops often train the vines to climb trellises or other supporting structures. However, most structures are not designed to carry the larger squashes. Therefore, it is usually best to allow the vines to spread along the ground unless it is feasible to support the fruits by means of slings made of cheesecloth or a similar material.

Summer squash is usually ready for harvesting 2 to 3 months after planting. They should be picked when they are small and tender and before the rind has hardened. Home gardeners often pick summer squash as it is needed, because it does not keep well after it has been picked.

Winter squashes require about 3 months to reach maturity. They are picked after the rind has hardened; they may be left on the plant until after the first light frost or when the vines have begun to wither. A light frost makes the fruits sweeter. However, the fruits should be picked before they are likely to be damaged by a hard frost. One of the many merits of winter squashes is that they may be stored at 50° to 55°F (10° to 13°C) for several months if they are harvested at full maturity and immediately cured for 2 weeks at 75° to 85°F (24° to 29°C).

The worldwide average yield of squashes is about 8,400 lb per acre (*9,408 kg/ha*), compared to the U.S. average of 14,000 lb (*15,680 kg/ha*). However, yields as high as 31,000 lb per acre (*34,720 kg/ha*) have been obtained in Bahrain.

PROCESSING.   Summer squashes are often sliced and cooked briefly in preparation for canning or freezing, whereas winter squashes are usually cooked much longer before being similarly processed. Canned pumpkin pie fillings or even the ready-made pies may often contain winter squash in lieu of pumpkin. Some gourmets believe that the flavor of the squash is superior.

SELECTION.   The culinary characteristics of the different varieties of these vegetables vary considerably. Hence, a good cook should know the differences between each type.

Types of Squashes.   Each country has its native names for these vegetables. Hence, some designations that are applicable in the United States follow:

• **Summer squash**—A bush-type cucurbit that produces many fruit which are usually harvested in the summer, while they are immature (the rind is still quite soft) and very watery.

The most common white or creamy-white variety of this type is the White Bush Scallop which is disk-shaped and smooth with scalloped edges. It is also called Cymling and Patty Pan.

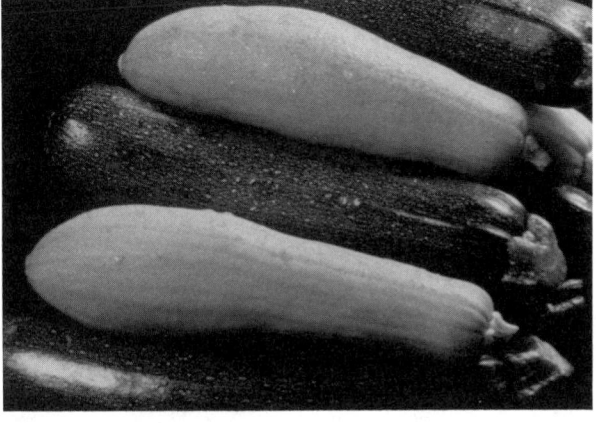

Fig. S-50. Summer squash. (Courtesy, USDA)

Most yellow summer varieties are elongated-bulbous in shape with a rough warty rind and are designated as either Straight or Crookneck.

Green, green-black or green-striped varieties, such as Zucchini and Italian Marrow, are elongated-cylindrical in shape.

• **Winter squash**—A bush-type, semivining, or vining cucurbit that is harvested in the fall when fully mature. The flesh of these squashes is usually less coarse and less fibrous, darker in color, milder flavored, and sweeter than that of pumpkins. They are often used in baked vegetable dishes and are sometimes used instead of pumpkin in making custards and pies.

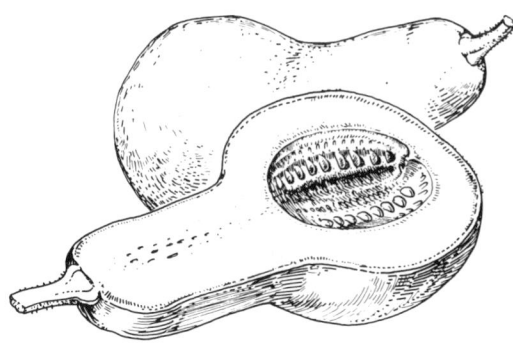

Fig. S-51. Winter squash, a highly nutritious vegetable that is very appetizing when baked and served with butter.

Common fall and early winter varieties are the green-colored corrugated Des Moines, Acorn, or Danish, the buff-colored Butternut, and the green or golden Delicious.

Vegetable spaghetti is an unusual variety of winter squash that has a large cylindrical fruit which contains a spaghettilike pulp.

Most of the late winter squash varieties are relatively large and may have either a light-green, dark-green, bluish-green, or orange-colored rind.

Indicators of Quality. Summer squash should be fresh, fairly heavy in relation to size, free from cuts or noticeable bruises, crisp, and tender. Summer squash which has developed to a hard-rind stage usually has hard or semihard seeds. Since for many uses seeds and rind are not discarded, both the hard rind and well developed seeds are generally undesirable. Also, the flesh of hard-rind summer squash is apt to be stringy.

The rind of winter squash should be hard. Softness of rind may indicate immature, thin flesh, which may be

watery and lacking in flavor when cooked. Winter squash is susceptible to decay and should be carefully examined. Decay usually appears as a water-soaked area which may show brown or black mold growth.

PREPARATION. Some suggestions for utilizing the various forms of squashes follow:

• **Squash flowers**—These should be picked when open so that no bees will be trapped within the blossoms. The flowers are good when dipped in a batter and fried in deep fat.

• **Squash seeds**—The seeds of winter squashes may be dried for a few days, after which any adhering tissue should be removed. Then, they may be roasted or fried in oil. Some people boil the seeds briefly in salted water before roasting or frying.

• **Summer squash**—Usually these fruits are left unpeeled and cooked whole, sliced, cubed, or grated. The cooked item may be served with butter, margarine, or a special sauce. Some other ways in which summer squash may be prepared are (1) stuffed with ingredients such as bread crumbs, cheese, chopped eggs, ground meat, nuts, seasonings, and/or sour cream, and then baked; (2) peeled, grated, mixed with eggs, flour, baking powder, salt, and seasonings, shaped into patties, and fried on a griddle or baked in a bread; (3) sliced, dipped in batter, and fried in deep fat; (4) cooked, pureed, and used as a soup stock; or (5) sliced and baked in casseroles with cheese and other ingredients.

• **Vegetable spaghetti**—This special type of winter squash is usually baked or boiled whole until the rind softens, then it is cut open lengthwise, and the spaghetti-like strands removed for serving alone with butter or margarine as a substitute for spaghetti, or it may be added to sauces or soups.

• **Winter squash**—These fruits, should be cut in half and the fibrous matter and seeds removed. Then, they may be baked, broiled, or steamed and served with butter, margarine, and/or seasonings. Most varieties are equal or superior to pumpkin in recipes calling for the latter. The mashed, cooked vegetable is also good when it is (1) uséd to make breads, cakes, muffins, and pancakes, and (2) added to soups and stews near the end of the cooking periods to give them more body and to enhance their nutritional values. (Pureed squash baby food might be convenient to use in some of these dishes.)

NUTRITIONAL VALUE. The nutrient composi-tions of various forms of squashes are given in Food Composition Table F-36.

Some noteworthy observations regarding the nutrient composition of squashes follow:

1. Squash flowers contain 95% water and are low in calories (16 kcal per 100 g) and most other nutrients, ex-cept that they provide fair amounts of phosphorus, iron, vitamin A and vitamin C. It is suggested that calorie-conscious people eat squash flowers in a salad, soup, or stew.

2. The seeds from winter squashes are very rich in calories (553 kcal per 100 g), protein (29%), iron (11.2 mg

per 100 g), and phosphorus (1,144 mg per 100 g). Hence, the consumption of as little as 1 oz (*28 g*) of the seeds per day will make a significant nutritional contribution to the diet.

3. Summer squashes contain more than 95% water and are very low in calories (14 kcal per 100 g) and most other nutrients. However, they are fair sources of potassium, vitamin A, and vitamin C. (The yellow and dark green varieties are generally richer in vitamin A than the white and pale green varieties.)

4. Baked winter squashes have a lower water content (81%) than most other cooked vegetables. They contain more than 4 times the calories, twice the potassium, and 10 times the vitamin A content of summer squashes. Although all winter squashes are excellent sources of vitamin A, the content is greatest in the varieties with deeply-colored yellow-orange flesh.

(Also see VEGETABLE[S], Table V-6 Vegetables of the World.)

SQUIRREL

A rodent of the family *Sciuridae*, characterized by a bushy tail and long strong hind limbs. In some countries, squirrel is highly esteemed as game. It is cooked in the same way as rabbit.

STABILIZED

Made more resistant to chemical change by the addition of a particular substance.

STABILIZER

Any substance which tends to make a compound, mixture or solution resistant to changes in form or chemical nature. In the food industry stabilizers are used to thicken, to keep pigments and other components in emulsion form, and to prevent the particles in colloidal suspensions from precipitating. Algin, methyl cellulose, carrageenan, and propylene glycol alginate are but a few of the stabilizers utilized.

(Also see ADDITIVES; and EMULSIFYING AGENTS.)

STACHYOSE

A tetrasaccharide composed of two molecules of galactose and one molecule of fructose and glucose. It occurs in many beans, beets, peas, soybeans, and tubers. Since the intestinal tract does not produce enzymes able to split stachyose, bacteria in the intestine act on it— forming gas. Hence, it is believed to be responsible for the gas producing properties of beans.

(Also see CARBOHYDRATE[S]; and BEAN[S], COMMON, section headed "Dried Beans."

STALING

This term generally relates to bakery products where it is characterized in breads by (1) a firming of the crumb due to loss of water, (2) loss of flavor, and (3) loss of crispness in the crust resulting in leatheriness. The staling of breads is a complex combination of changes. Methods have been developed to detect these changes. However, the method most commonly employed to study staling is the detection of changes in the compressibility of a loaf of bread, since consumers associate softness with freshness. Softness of a bread may be increased by the inclusion of monoglycerides (emulsifiers), but this does not necessarily retard staling. Storing bread at refrigerator temperature increases the rate of staling while freezing bread arrests staling. Furthermore, staling can be reversed by heat; hence, stale bread makes good toast. No bakery products stale as fast as bread, but even rich cakes stale if kept long enough. Also, dry bakery goods like crackers stale, but they stale because they pick up moisture from the air.

STAPHYLOCOCCAL POISONING

By far the most common form of food poisoning observed in the United States. It is caused by a toxin formed primarily by the bacteria *Staphylococcus aureus* before the contaminated food is ingested. Symptoms which follow the ingestion of contaminated food by 2 to 4 hours include abdominal cramps, severe nausea, vomiting and diarrhea. Fortunately, the illness passes in only 1 to 3 days and mortality is low. Control of this type of food poisoning is mainly a matter of educating food handlers to proper preventative techniques—cleanliness, storage, and preparation.

(Also see BACTERIA IN FOOD, Table B-6 Food Infections [Bacterial Toxins]—"Staphylococcal Food Poisoning.")

STAR-APPLE (CAINITO) *Chrysophyllum cainito*

The fruit of a tree (of the family *Sapotaceae*) that is native to the West Indies and Central America. The fruit is applelike, purple, round, up to 4 in. (*10 cm*) in diameter, with a white, sweet, edible pulp. The pulp is usually eaten fresh after removal of the skin.

The ripe fruit pulp is moderately high in calories (68 kcal per 100 g) and carbohydrates (14.5%). It is a fair source of vitamin C.

STARCH

Contents	*Page*

Starch is a polysaccharide—long chains of the simple sugar, glucose—formed by the process of photosynthesis. It is the storage carbohydrate, stored as granules in seeds, roots, tubers, or stems of the higher plants. The chemical formula of starch is $(C_6H_{10}O_5)_n$. The "n" outside of the parentheses indicates an indefinite number of repeating glucose molecules. Furthermore, these glucose units may be linked in either of two patterns: (1) a straight-chained pattern called amylose; or (2) a highly branched pattern called amylopectin. The amount of amylose and amylopectin in starch depends on the source, but on the average starch is about 27% amylose and 73% amylopectin. Fig. S-52 illustrates the structures of amylose and amylopectin.

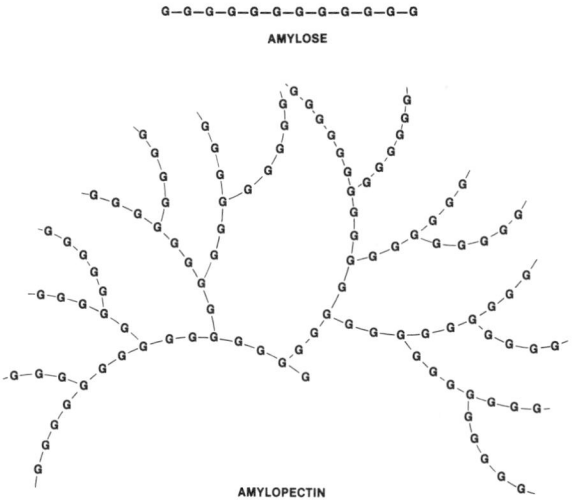

Fig. S-52.   The structures of amylose and amylopectin of starch. Each "G" represents a glucose molecule.

Unlike cellulose, which is also a long chain of glucose molecules, starch can be split by the digestive enzymes of the body. When either amylose or amylopectin are split, dextrins are formed. Dextrins may vary in length from five or more glucose molecules, and the final product of enzymatic splitting of starch is glucose.

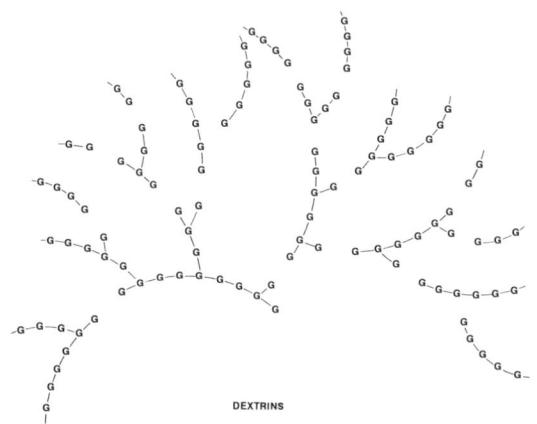

Fig. S-53.   The formation of dextrins from amylopectin. Each "G" represents a glucose molecule.

IN THE DIET.   Since starch is a product of photosynthesis, many foods contain starch. It is the primary digestible carbohydrate in foods. Furthermore, starch and starch products are employed in many foods to facilitate processing or to give foods specific properties. Hence, starch and starch products are food additives.

Natural Starch.   Very little of the available carbohydrate occurring naturally in foods occurs as the dissaccharides sucrose, lactose, or maltose or as the monosaccharides glucose or fructose. Cereal grains, roots, tubers, legumes, nuts, and some fruits and vegetables provide carbohydrate to the diet mainly as starch. The major sources of starch are the seeds of corn, rice, rye, sorghum, and wheat. Potatoes, which are tubers, are also a good source of starch. Dry mature beans and peas also contain starch, while fresh beans and peas contain starch but at much lower levels. Carbohydrate values given in Food Composition Table F-36 for the cereal grains, roots, tubers, nuts, dried beans and peas can be considered as approximating the starch content of these foods.

Worldwide, natural starch is an important energy food. The staple food of a country provides the primary source of starch; for example, corn in Mexico; roots, tubers, and sorghum in parts of Africa; and rice in India, China and Indonesia. Starch is an economical food; hence, it contributes a large portion to the diets where income is low. As income increases, the amount of starch in the diet decreases while consumption of fat, animal protein and sugar increase, as shown in Fig. S-54.

Aside from the starch which is natural in many foods, starch is an important commercial product, and it is extracted from several plant sources which produce it in sufficient quantities.

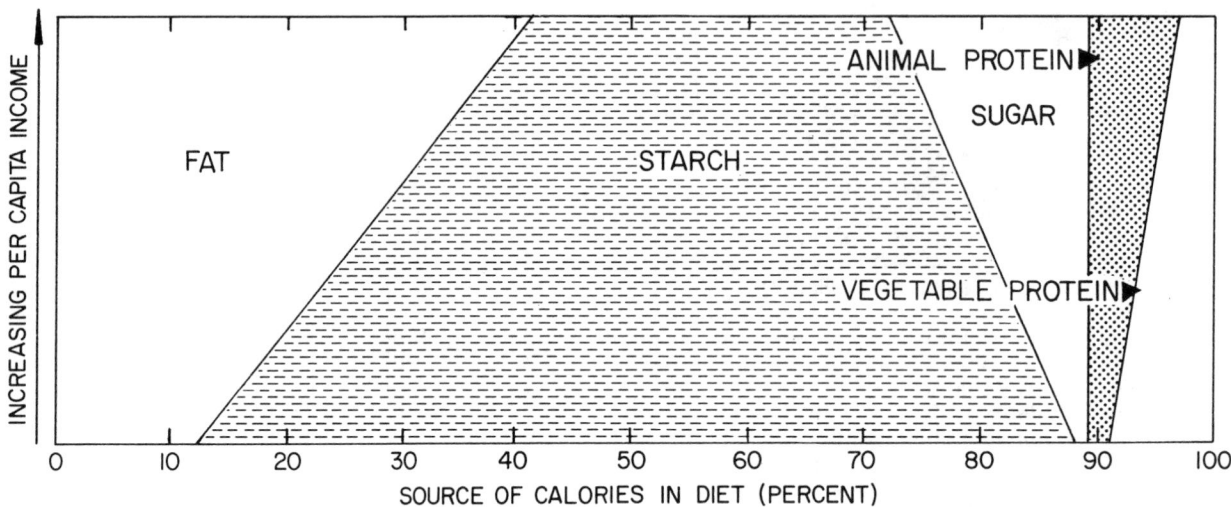

Fig. S-54.   Dietary patterns for fat, starch, sugar, and protein as per capita income increases.

Commercial Starch. Commercially extracted starch, due to some unique chemical and physical properties, low cost, and availability, may be added to foods during processing—a food additive. While many plants produce starch, only a few produce it in quantities to make extraction feasible.

PRODUCTION. Corn is the major source of commercial starch in the United States, followed by sorghum, wheat, and rice. Other sources include oats, barley, rye, potato, sago, arrowroot, and tapioca (cassava).

Starch production from corn is achieved by the wet milling process. Corn kernels are soaked in warm water containing sulfur dioxide until they become soft. Then, the kernels are cracked and the germ is removed. Next, the kernel fragments are ground and screened down to starch granules and gluten. The gluten is removed, and the starch is filtered, washed, dried, and packaged.

A newer process for obtaining wheat starch involves the milling of wheat into flour, followed by preparing a flour and water dough. Starch granules are then washed from the dough.

Starch is obtained from rice by soaking the grain in an alkaline chemical which dissolves the gluten, leaving the starch.

Starch from roots and tubers such as potato, arrowroot and cassava is prepared by grinding the root or tuber to free the starch granule, screening to remove the fiber and skins, soaking, and separating the starch from other water-soluble material by settling or centrifugation. Starch granules are insoluble in cold water.

(Also see CEREAL GRAINS; CORN; POTATO; SORGHUM; and WHEAT.)

CHARACTERISTICS. Although starch is a white powder to the unaided eye, it appears as granules or grains under the microscope, which vary in size and shape depending upon the plant source. Furthermore, the content of amylose and amylopectin vary depending upon the source. Table S-23 presents these characteristics for some of the common starches. These charac-

TABLE S-23
CHARACTERISTICS OF SOME COMMON STARCHES

Source	Starch Content on a Dry Weight Basis	Amylose	Amylopectin	Shape of Granules	Diameter of Granules
	←----------(%)----------→				(microns)
Corn	72	28	72	Polygonal and rounded.	5-25
Waxy hybrid	72	less than 1	99	Polygonal and rounded.	5-25
High amylose	72	52-80	20-48	Polygonal and rounded.	5-25
Potato	75	23	77	Oval and egg-shaped.	15-100
Rice	82	14-32	68-86	Polygonal, tending to cluster.	3-8
Sorghum	69			Polygonal and rounded.	5-25
Tapioca (cassava)	86	17	83	Kettledrum-shaped.	5-35
Wheat	68	26	74	Flat, round, or elliptical with small and large tending to cluster.	2-38

teristics of the starches affect their gelatinization, modification, and uses.

Gelatinization. Starch gelatinizes, when mixed with water and heated beyond 133° to 167°F (*56° to 75°C*)—the critical temperature. This temperature differs depending upon the type of starch. As starch is heated, the chemical bonds (hydrogen bonds) holding the granules together start to weaken. This permits the water to penetrate the granules causing them to swell to many times their original size—a change referred to as gelatinization. As gelatinization occurs the clarity and the viscosity (thickness) of the solution increases, and the starch granules lose their unique microscopic shape by rupturing and releasing amylose and amylopectin.

The characteristics of these cooked viscous solutions vary from starch to starch. After cooling to room temperature, the starch from roots are clearer and more fluid, while starch from the cereal grains yield a cloudy less fluid paste that tends to be jellylike. These characteristics are dependent upon the amylose and amylopectin content of the starch and upon the size of the amylose and amylopectin molecule. Some hybrids—waxy hybrids—of corn and sorghum have been developed which yield starch that is almost entirely amylopectin, while other hybrids have a high amylose content. Table S-24 summarizes the gelatinization properties of some important starches. Overall, the tendency to thicken or gel upon cooling, and to become opaque is caused by the presence of amylose.

TABLE S-24
GELATINIZATION OF STARCH

Starch Source	Critical Temperature (°F)	(°C)	Characteristics of Cooked Starch
Cereal grains (corn, sorghum, rice and wheat)	144-167	62-75	Form viscous, short-bodied pastes; set to opaque gel upon cooling.
Roots and tubers (potato and tapioca)	133-158	56-70	Form viscous, long-bodied, relatively clear pastes; weak gel upon cooling.
Waxy hybrids (corn and sorghum)	145-165	63-74	Form heavy-bodied, stringy, clear pastes; resistant to gelling upon cooling.
High amylose hybrids (corn)	212-320	100-160	Form short-bodied paste; set to very rigid opaque gel upon cooling.

Modifications. Besides the property of gelatinization, starch may be modified to yield some unique and useful properties which are used advantageously by the food industry and others. Some methods of modifying starch follow:

• **Conversion**—Acids and/or heat, or chemical oxidizers, are used on starch to reduce the viscosity, alter the cooking behavior, increase the cold water solubility, or to modify the tendency to form pastes or gels. These modifications of raw starch allow it to be used in foods at higher concentrations. The products formed by conversion include: British gums, white dextrins, yellow dextrins, and oxidized starches.

• **Cross-linking**—In general, the period of maximum viscosity of a starch is very brief. To overcome this, chemical bridges—cross-links—are formed in starch molecules which prevent rupture of the starch granule during heating. Chemicals such as anhydrides of acetic and citric acid, metaphosphates, phosphorus oxychloride, and epichlorohydrin are used to form cross-links in the starch. Then these chemicals are washed out and the starch is dried. Upon cooking the cross-linked starch maintains its maximum viscosity longer and may even demonstrate increased viscosity.

• **Derivatives**—This process consists of adding other chemicals to the starch molecules thereby modifying the physical properties of the starch. Starch derivatives such as acetates, carboxyls, carboxylates, phosphates, succinates, and hydroxypropyl demonstrate, resistance to retrogradation—aggregation of the amylose molecules to an insoluble precipitate—lowered gelatinization temperature, increased cooking rate, increased viscosity, and emulsion-stabilizing properties.

• **Pregelatinized**—Any of the starches may be precooked, and then dried yielding a starch which will swell in cold water.

• **Syrups and sugars**—Starch from any starch source—rice, corn, or other grains, or potatoes—may be broken down into its component sugar either enzymatically or with dilute acids. The most familiar example in the United States is corn syrup (Karo). Complete hydrolysis of starch yields glucose—dextrose.

Corn syrup is the product of the incomplete hydrolysis of starch. It is a viscous liquid containing dextrose, maltose, and dextrins. Unlike sugar, it has a distinct flavor other than sweetness. The degree of conversion is expressed by the "dextrose equivalent" (D.E.) which is, in effect, the measure of sweetness in the syrup, or in other words the amount of starch converted to glucose. Even high conversion syrups are substantially less sweet than sugar. A special corn syrup on the market is a "high fructose corn syrup" (HFCS) which is made by treating high conversion corn syrup with enzymes. The enzymes convert some of the glucose to fructose, which is much sweeter than glucose.

Corn sugar is glucose (dextrose) recovered by crystallization from hydrolyzed starch. Two types of refined dextrose are commercially available: dextrose hydrate, containing 9% by weight of water of crystallization, and anhydrous dextrose, containing less than 0.5% of water. Dextrose hydrate is most often used by food processors.

USES. Starch and modified starches are considered food additives, and they are employed in a wide variety of foods. As additives they contribute calories to foods, but starch and modified starches are primarily used in foods to facilitate processing or impart specific properties to foods. The following are some examples of the uses of starch in its various forms:

• **Dry granular starch**—One pound of cornstarch granules has a surface area of about 3,500 sq ft (315 m²). Dried starch or modified starch serve as moisture absorbing agents in many products. Starch is added to baking powder to absorb moisture and keep the ingredients from losing their activity. Confectioners sugar is protected from lumping during storage by the addition of cornstarch. Aside from food, the absorbing capacity of starch is sometimes employed on the human body as a substitute for powder, including baby diapers.

Candy and gum molds are formed from powdered cornstarch or modified starch.

Dry starch derivatives are used in foods to maintain their flow properties.

Starch powders are used as bulking or diluting agents in enzyme preparations or flavorings so that a larger unit of measurement may be used.

• **Starch pastes**—Most of the uses of starch as a food additive are for thickening and gelling. The proper starch or modified starch is chosen which yields the desirable properties. In the canning industry starches are used in baby foods, soups, sauces, pie fillings, gravies, vegetables in sauces, chow mein, chili, spaghetti, stews and cream style corn. In the baking industry, starch, cross-linked starch and pregelatinized starches are employed in flour, fruit pie fillings, imitation jellies, whipped topping stabilizers, icing stabilizers, cream fillings, custards, salad dressings, candies, and gums.

• **Starch films**—The ability of starch to form films is utilized in covering foods with decorative and protective coatings, binding foods and providing a matrix to carry food substances. Starches are used as binders in meat products, and pet food, while modified starches are used as a matrix to carry flavor oils. Futhermore, starch coatings are oil resistant and can be used on nut and chocolate confections to prevent the migration of oil.

Starch coatings are found on chewing gums or other confections with hard sugar coatings.

• **Starch syrups and sugar**—Since corn syrups can (1) control crystallization, (2) retain moisture, (3) ferment, (4) produce a high osmotic pressure solution for preservation, and (5) aid browning; they are employed in many food products including the following: baby foods, bakery products, canned fruits, carbonated beverages, confections, dry bakery mixes, fountain syrups and toppings, frozen fruits, fruit juice drinks, ice cream and frozen desserts, jams, jellies and preserves, meat products, pickles and condiments, and table syrups (Karo syrup).

Due to its browning, fermentability, flavor enhancement, osmotic pressure, sweetness, humectancy (prevention of drying), hygroscopicity (moisture absorption), viscosity, and reactivity properties, starch sugar—dextrose—is utilized in many food products. The major uses of dextose are the confection, wine, and canning industries.

In medicine, various concentrations of glucose (dextrose) are utilized for intravenous administration.

Nonfood uses of starch are also important. Fabrics are starched and sized. High-quality paper is strong, smooth and glossy due to starch. Pasteboard, cardboard, and plywood manufacturing rely on starch. Some pastes are made of starch. Yearly, about 2 to 3 billion pounds (*1 bil kg*) of starch are produced and sold for nonfood uses, while 5 to 6 billion pounds (*2.5 bil kg*) are used in foods.

NUTRITIONAL VALUE. Starch contributes energy—calories—to the diet. On the average, each gram of starch supplies 4 Calories (kcal) of energy. Upon ingestion, enzymes in the saliva begin breaking starch down to its component sugar, glucose. This process continues in the small intestine where the glucose is absorbed into the bloodstream and used by the cells of the body for energy production, stored as glycogen, or converted to chemicals used in the synthesis of fatty acids. Raw starch, as it occurs naturally in food, is contained in granules, and cooking of starch softens and ruptures these granules making the starch containing food more palatable and more digestible.

Over the past 70 years, the value of starch in American nutrition has been decreasing. As shown in Fig. S-55, starch now supplies about 21% of the calories in the American diet. The decreased intake of starch has been countered by an increase in fat intake, particularly unsaturated fats.

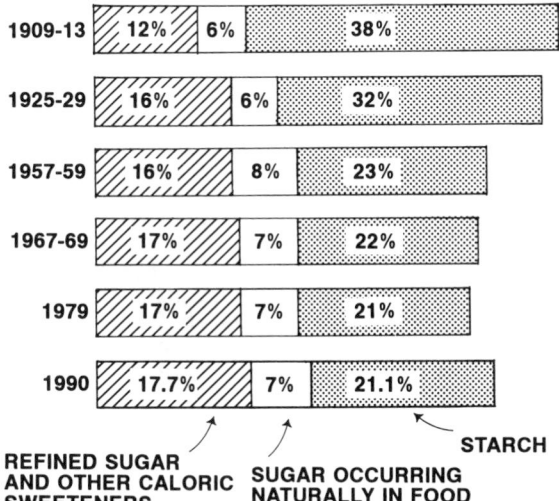

1909-13	12%	6%	38%
1925-29	16%	6%	32%
1957-59	16%	8%	23%
1967-69	17%	7%	22%
1979	17%	7%	21%
1990	17.7%	7%	21.1%

REFINED SUGAR AND OTHER CALORIC SWEETENERS   SUGAR OCCURRING NATURALLY IN FOOD   STARCH

Fig. S-55. Changes in the percentage of calories in the American food supply derived from sugars and starch (Courtesy, USDA)

(Also see ADDITIVES; CARBOHYDRATE[S]; CEREAL GRAINS; DIGESTION AND ABSORPTION; and METABOLISM.)

STARCH EQUIVALENT (SE)

A system that is used in Europe for evaluating animal feedstuffs. This system is based on the amount of starch that produces as much fat as 220 lb (*100 kg*) of the feed being used.

STARCHES, WAXY

Properties of starch are influenced by the ratio of amylose (linear chains of glucose molecules) to amylopectin (branched chains of glucose molecules). Common starches contain 17 to 27% amylose, and 73 to 83% amylopectin. Waxy starches contain nearly 100% amylopectin. These do not form gels except at high concentrations; they remain as relatively clear solutions. Waxy starches can be derived from corn, grain sorghum, and rice.

(Also see STARCH.)

STARCH, PREGELATINIZED

None of the raw starches will form a paste with cold water unless they are precooked and then rolled or spraydried. Therefore, pregelatinized starch is starch which has been cooked and dried. It can then be used in instant puddings, fillings, imitation jellies, whipped toppings, etc.

(Also see ADDITIVES; and STARCH.)

STARCH SUGAR

The complete hydrolysis of starch by enzymes, or by heat and acids, yields the sugar dextrose (glucose) which can be purified by crystallization. Hence, it may be called starch sugar. When corn starch is utilized to produce glucose, it may be called corn sugar.

(Also see CARBOHYDRATE[S]; CORN SYRUP; DEXTROSE; STARCH; and SUGAR.)

STARCH SYRUP

Starch from any source—rice, potatoes, or corn—may be hydrolyzed—split—by dilute acids and heat, or by enzymes, into a syrup containing dextrins, maltotetrose, maltotriose, maltose and dextrose. The composition and characteristics of the syrup depend upon the time and conditions of the hydrolysis. In the United States a familiar example is Karo syrup—a corn starch syrup.

(Also see CORN SYRUP; DEXTROSE; STARCH; and SUGAR.)

STARVATION

This condition usually results from the prolonged and drastic deprivation of food. It is characterized by wasting of tissues and other alterations of normal physiology. If continued sufficiently long, there may be disability, or even death. Situations where large numbers of people starve are called *famines*.

Failure of children to get sufficient food results in growth failure, marasmus, and other serious disorders developing much sooner than in adults because children have proportionately higher requirements for nutrients to support their rapid rate of growth.

(Also see MALNUTRITION, PROTEIN-ENERGY.)

CAUSES OF STARVATION.
The ultimate effect of starvation is the deprivation of the cells of the body of their essential nutrients. Although lack of food is the main cause of this condition, other factors may produce starvation at the cellular level. Therefore, discussions of a variety of causes of cellular starvation follow:

• **Unavailability of food**—This prime cause of starvation has in recent times been associated with catastrophes such as droughts, earthquakes, floods, civil disorders, and wars. However, lack of food may also result from overpopulation, poor agricultural practices, failure to control diseases and pests, lack of storage facilities, inadequate distribution systems, or lack of money to buy food.

• **Restriction of food intake**—Medical procedures such as anesthesia, surgery and other types of treatments may require restriction of food intake. Whether or not such restriction results in starvation depends upon the length of time that food is withheld; the use of support measures, such as intravenous feeding; and the condition of the patient prior to and after the medical treatment.

Another type of food deprivation is that which is imposed for coercion or punishment.

• **Self-denial of food**—This means of self-starvation may be used for purposes of weight reduction, protest, or religious fasting.

• **Failure to eat due to lack of appetite**—Sometimes, for physiological or psychological reasons, people lose their appetites and find it difficult to eat. Such anorexia (lack of appetite) occurs in severe thiamin deficiency, acidosis or ketosis, uremic poisoning which occurs in kidney failure, and when there are emotional aversions to food such as in *anorexia nervosa*.

• **Disorders of the digestive tract**—Even when the food intake seems to be adequate, cells may be starved due to reduced nutrient absorption in conditions such as diarrhea, malabsorption, vomiting, or surgical removal of part of the digestive tract.

• **Metabolic abnormalities**—The cells may fail to fully utilize the nutrients which are available in the body when there are such conditions as fever, diabetes, hyperthyroidism, Cushings' syndrome, extreme stress, or wasting diseases such as cancer.

(Also see MALNUTRITION.)

ADAPTATION TO STARVATION.
Persons, who are otherwise healthy, can adapt to deprivation of nutrients for short periods of time by means of various physiological processes which have helped the human race to survive many famines.

Prolonged dietary deficiency of energy results in an eventual reduction in voluntary activities and in the metabolic rate, so that it is possible to survive on about one-half of the energy which had been the normal intake in the diet. It is thought that the reduction in metabolic rate may be due in part to a shortage of energy-yielding nutrients and in part to subnormal blood levels of thyroid hormones. Likewise, body temperatures of starved persons are often subnormal.

If fluids are limited, the kidneys set into play a mechanism which conserves water. They secrete renin, an enzyme which initiates the conversion of a bloodborne protein (an alpha-globulin) to angiotension II, a hormonelike substance. The latter substance stimulates the adrenal cortex to secrete aldosterone—a hormone which causes the retention of water and sodium by the kidney and a reduction in the amount of urine volume.

Energy is supplied first from stored fat, then from body protein. Stored fat, in the form of triglycerides, is split into fatty acids and glycerol by hormone-sensitive lipase enzymes in adipose tissue. The fatty acids are then released into the blood where they immediately form complexes with plasma albumin, while the glycerol travels free in the blood to the liver where it may be converted to glucose or recombined into triglycerides. Many tissues, such as muscles, are able to utilize fatty acids as their sole sources of energy, although the metabolism of carbohydrates when they are available, requires about 10% less oxygen to produce the same amount of energy.

Blood glucose (critical for the brain and nervous system) is maintained at close to a normal level by the breakdown of protein in muscle to amino acids which travel through the blood to the liver where they are converted to glucose. The breakdown of body protein is limited, however, and so it is fortunate that the brain can adapt to the utilization of ketone bodies which are formed from fat in the liver when glucose becomes scarce.

Catabolism of body tissue for energy results in rapid weight loss, particularly when fat stores have been exhausted, since each pound of protein loss results in a corresponding loss of 3 lb of water which are eliminated from the body.

Starved persons vary in their susceptibility to low blood sugar and ketosis. Some become weak and feel dizzy after only a day of starvation, while others feel few effects after weeks of total fasting; hence, the use of starvation to obtain weight reduction should be done only under the supervision of a physician.

The edema of starvation results from a flow of water from the blood to the tissues because the ability of blood to retain water is reduced when proteins in the blood are depleted.

Diarrhea results from the loss of absorptive cells in the intestine which occurs as part of the wholesale catabolism of body tissues in severe starvation.

Minerals—such as potassium, magnesium, and phosphate ions—are released into the blood from the catabolism of tissues, thereby delaying the appearance of clinical deficiencies of these essential nutrients. However, there are likely to be deficiencies of nutrients which are not stored in the body and need to be provided on a regular basis in the diet, such as water-soluble vitamins, chloride, and other ions. Also, the absorption of vitamins and minerals is increased and their urinary excretion is decreased. Thus, there is more efficient utilization of vitamins and minerals by the body in starvation.

(Also see FASTING.)

EFFECTS OF STARVATION.
The effects of food deprivation are dependent upon the severity and length of the deprivation, and the status of the victim prior to starvation. Thus, one cannot draw up an exact timetable of survival. There have been reports of survival after 8 months of total fasting, but the survivors were obese adult women at the beginning of starvation.

Death results from the loss of function of vital organs such as the digestive tract, which may become almost transparent and nonfunctional due to wasting, and the heart, where muscle wasting often results in circulatory failure.

Some crude generalizations about survival from starvation are as follows: Young adults may survive much longer than chidren (due to the proportionately higher nutrient requirements of the latter) or older persons; women survive longer than men because of their greater proportions of body fat to lean tissue which results from the action of female hormones; and the obese survive longer than lean persons. Thus, the now frowned-upon practice of trying to fatten children had a basis in the more precarious times of our ancestors. Some of the specific effects of starvation follow.

Infants With Low Birth Weights From Deprived Mothers.
In Holland, from the winter of 1944 through spring of 1945, food was very scarce. Although the children of acutely starved mothers did not show any long-term effects of this starvation, serious effects of such deprivation have been reported in areas where malnutrition is more chronic in nature. A follow-up study of children 8 to 10 years of age in North Carolina, who had been low-birth-weight babies, showed that 24% of these children had major physical defects, while only 2 to 3% of children who had a higher birth weight had such defects.[43]

Impairment Of Mental Development.
Most of the recent reports state that nutritional deprivation is most likely to have a lasting effect on children if it occurs during the first year of life. Studies on the brains of infants who died from starvation at less than 1 year of age showed a significant reduction (15 to 20%) in the number of brain cells.[44] Low-birth-weight infants (less than 5 lb, or *2,000 g*) who died under similar circumstances had a reduction of 60% in the total number of brain cells. Smaller head circumferences of children who suffered from marasmus early in life are indicative of proportionate reductions in brain size. Intelligence tests have shown that such children do not seem to catch up in mental development by 6 years of age. When starvation occurs after 2 or 3 years of age, the effect on learning is temporary, since brain tissue is not affected once complete development of the brain has occurred.

Stunted Growth.
Water, calories, and protein are the most essential nutrients for survival and growth in children. Children subjected to acute or chronic deprivation of these nutrients in fetal life, or in the years between birth and school age, may show permanent retardation in growth and development or even disability and death, since the ability of a child to adapt physiologically to such deprivation is much less than that for adults. Autopsies have shown great reductions in the sizes of the vital organs of these children.

Increased Susceptibility to Diseases.
Both children and adults who have been starved are more susceptible to, and suffer more severly from, diseases such as diarrhea, measles, plague, influenza, tuberculosis, and cholera. This is due to the exhaustion of nutrient reserves and concomitant reduced immunity.

Abnormal Behavior.
In the beginning stages of starvation, the victims become preoccupied with food and are increasingly restless, irritable, undisciplined, and nervous. Eventualy there is increasing apathy, depression, and decreasing sociability until the victims become totally withdrawn and inactive. During rehabilitation from severe starvation, the patients go through a rebellious period that may last until recovery. Thus, it seems that, the severely deprived in the world are not as likely to engage in civil disorders and strife as are the moderately deprived, or those partially rehabilitated from severe deprivation.

Reduced Work Capacity.
Studies of worker productivity in the coal mines and steel mills of Germany showed that the average output per worker declined in

---

[43]Lowenberg, M. E., *et al, Food and Man*, 2nd ed., John Wiley & Sons, New York, N.Y., 1974, p. 275.

[44]Winick, M., *Cellular Changes During Early Malnutrition*, Ross Laboratories, Columbus, Ohio, 1971, p. 29.

proportion to the decrease in food energy which occurred as a result of decreasing food supplies during the course of war.[45] The work output returned to the original levels when it became possible for the workers to consume additional food.

SIGNS OF STARVATION.
Signs of this disorder are weight loss, wasting of tissue, loose skin, ketone breath, ketones in urine, dehydration, low blood sugar, weakness, diarrhea, low blood pressure, edema, irritability, and antisocial behavior. It is usually easier to detect starvation in children than in adults, since one can readily observe in the former the great reduction in activity, smaller body weight for height and age, and other signs of malnutrition.

Fig. S-56 shows two children who are suffering from starvation.

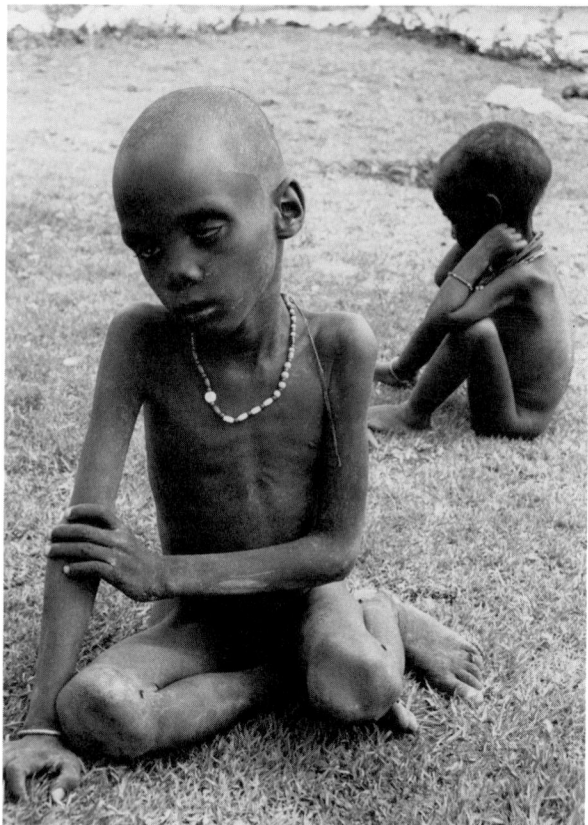

Fig. S-56. African children suffering from starvation. Severe drought for several years led to famine among the Masai in Kenya. These people normally obtain milk from their cattle, and also blood, which is extracted from the necks of the beasts. However, many of the cattle died when their grazing lands were parched by the drought. (Courtesy, FAO, Rome, Italy)

Starvation may be overlooked in cases of adults such as alcoholics, hospital patients, and the elderly, since emaciation and weakness are frequently attributed to conditions other than nutrition. Sometimes the presence of starvation edema masks the wasting which has occurred. A brief study of a group of 130 hospital patients by a group of Boston physicians showed that about half of those surveyed were at least moderately depleted (as indicated by under average measurements of triceps, skin folds, and muscle circumference, and low to marginal levels of serum albumin).[46]

TREATMENT AND PREVENTION OF STARVATION.
Although many victims of starvation are ravenously hungry, their digestive functions may be severely impaired. Therefore, care has to be taken not to feed foods known to cause or aggravate diarrhea (fats, fried foods, beans, and high-fiber foods), which is one of the main causes of death from starvation. It may be necessary to provide small, but frequent feedings of skim milk. Supplements of vitamins and minerals may need to be provided when there is likely to have been depletion of nutrients. Vitamins A and C are needed for optimal healing of tissues, while mineral elements such as potassium, sodium, and magnesium are critical for cardiac function and electrolyte balance. Persons who cannot eat normally by mouth may have to be fed intravenously or by tube feedings.

(Also see INTRAVENOUS FEEDING; and TUBE FEEDING.)

Programs For The Prevention Of Starvation.
Preventing starvation by providing food to those who need it, while simple in principle, may be difficult in practice when large numbers of people must be aided. The supplying of large quantities of food may be closely tied to economic, social, and political factors. While it is beyond the scope of this article to provide in-depth discussions of such factors, it is worthwhile to note briefly some of the programs and problems encountered in the prevention of starvation. Some of these follow:

• **Distribution of food**—Although this is the most direct approach, it may well be the least satisfactory means of long-term assistance for chronically underfed populations, since these people may come to depend upon free or low-cost food from outside sources, rather than developing their own food supply. However, increasing food production takes time; in the meantime, it may be necessary to provide food for such vulnerable groups as infants and children, pregnant mothers, handicapped persons, and the aged.

• **Provision of money or scrip to buy food**—When a local supply of food is available, its sale through commercial channels may help to encourage local enterprises such as farming and marketing. However, the money or scrip may be used to purchase items other than food, as evidenced by abuses of the food stamp program in the United States (for example, their use to purchase liquor

[45]Keller, W. D., and H. A. Kraut, "Work and Nutrition," *World Review of Nutrition and Dietetics*, G. H. Bourne, Editor, S. Karager Ag, Basel, Switzerland, Vol. 3, 1959, p. 69.

[46]Blackburn, G. L., and B. Bistrian, "A Report from Boston," *Nutrition Today*, Vol. 9, 1974, p. 30.

followed by their illicit redistribution at discounts). Furthermore, such doles to the able-bodied unemployed may lead to their rejection of employment when it is available.

• **Price controls**—The government may attempt to control food prices in order to prevent those with more money from buying large quantities of food for resale at higher prices. When controls are stringent, this type of policy sometimes makes food production and distribution unprofitable in the private sector, thereby creating more problems than it solves. Also, just about every attempt at price control or rationing has been accompanied by diversion of foods into "black market" channels. Thus, there must be adequate provision for enforcement of price controls.

• **Planning for the relief of famines**—Famines are often presaged by such events as bad weather during the planting, growing, and harvesting of crops; outbreaks of plant or animal diseases; steady increases in unemployment and reduction of food production; and political unrest. Failure to heed such warnings has frequently resulted in considerable wasted effort and materials as public and private groups have rushed aid to famine-stricken areas.

The preceding discussion shows the need for advance planning against starvation along lines which consider not only nutritional needs of people, but which take into account the various economic, social, and political circumstances in the vulnerable areas of the world.

(Also see DEFICIENCY DISEASES, Table D-1 Major Dietary Deficiency Diseases; and WORLD FOOD.)

STASIS

A slowing or stoppage of the normal flow of fluid or semifluid material in an organ or vessel in the body, as (1) slowing the flow of blood in arteries and veins, or (2) reduced motility of the intestines accompanied by retention of feces.

STEARIC ACID

An 18-carbon saturated fatty acid which occurs in tallow and other animal fats, and in cocoa butter and other hard vegetable fats, and which reacts with glycerol to form stearin.

(Also see FATS AND OTHER LIPIDS.)

STEATORRHEA

Describes a greasy or fatty bowel movement (stool), a characteristic of many malabsorption syndromes such as celiac disease and sprue.

(Also see CELIAC DISEASE; MALABSORPTION SYNDROMES; and SPRUE.)

STENOSIS

A constriction or narrowing of a channel.

STERILIZATION

A process used to destroy all living microorganisms. (Also see PRESERVATION OF FOOD.)

STEROIDS

Any of a group of fat-related organic compounds. They include cholesterol, numerous hormones, precursors of certain vitamins, bile acids, alcohols (sterols), and certain natural drugs and poisons (such as the digitalis derivatives).

STEROL

One of a class of complex, fatlike subtances widely distributed in nature.

(Also see CHOLESTEROL; and FATS AND OTHER LIPIDS.)

STEVIOSIDE

A glycoside obtained from the leaves of the wild shrub *Stevia rebaudiana Bertoni*. It is approximately 300 times sweeter than table sugar. The people of Paraguay have been using it for years to sweeten their drinks. Stevioside has been proposed as a sweetening agent; and, currently, *Stevia rebaudiana Bertoni* is being cultivated in Japan. Stevioside contains calories, it is not noncaloric like saccharin. However, small quantities of stevioside should adequately sweeten, since it is so much sweeter than sugar. Available evidence suggests that stevioside is not toxic to humans.

(Also see SWEETENING AGENTS.)

STILLAGE

The mash from fermentation of grains after removal of alcohol by distillation.

(Also see DISTILLATION.)

STOMACH

That part of the digestive tract lying between the esophagus and the small intestine.

(Also see DIGESTION AND ABSORPTION.)

STOMACH CANCER (GASTRIC CARCINOMA)

For some unexplained reasons, the incidence of stomach cancer, and the reported death rate from stomach cancer, have declined over the past 50 years. However, it is still a major health problem affecting twice as many men as women.

One of the major obstacles of stomach cancer is that of delayed diagnosis, since the onset is so subtle it is often overlooked until too late. Hence, all persistent abdominal discomfort should be investigated, especially when accompanied by lack of appetite, vomiting, weight loss, and bloody stools.

Numerous attempts have been made, and are still being made, to link stomach cancer occurrence and prevention to some specific dietary factors. To date, there are many clues but no definitive scientific evidence. Dietary and nutrient excesses, deficiencies or imbalances may be related to the development of cancer of the stomach, esophagus, colon, pancreas, liver, and breast. Also, the tendency to develop stomach cancer does seem to run in families, and the environment may also play a role.

Diagnosis may involve x-ray examination, gastroscopic examination, and biopsy. Once confirmed, stomach cancer is treated (1) surgically—removal of the tumor-containing tissue—providing the cancer has not involved too many other tissues beyond the stomach, (2) with postoperative x ray, and (3) with chemotherapy. Following recovery from surgery small, frequent feedings of easily digested foods should be given. Types of foods and progression of the diet will depend upon the extent of the surgery. In the event of an inoperable cancer, the diet should support the patient's morale while providing adequate nutrition.

(Also see CANCER; and MODIFIED DIETS.)

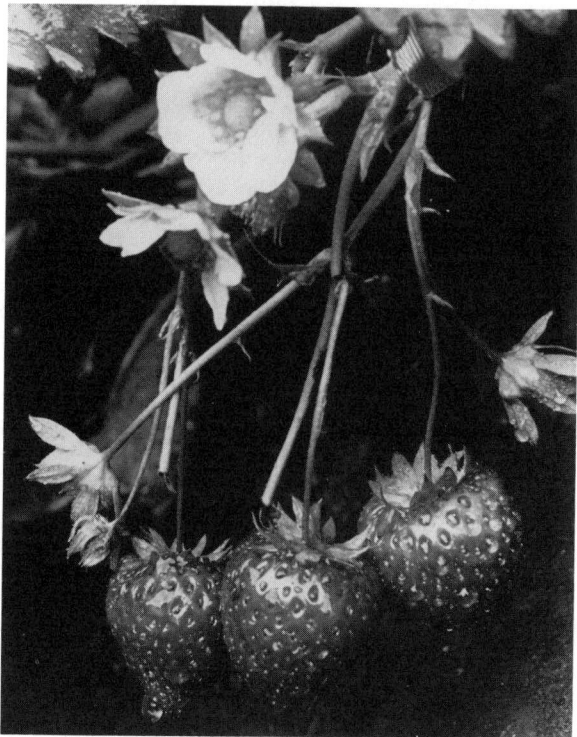

Fig. S-57.   Fully ripe strawberries glistening with morning dew. (Courtesy, Botsford Ketchum, Inc., Advertising and Public Relations for California Strawberry Advisory Board, Watsonville, Calif.)

STOMATITIS

Inflammation of the mucous membrane of the mouth due to a variety of causes, including a riboflavin deficiency.

STOOL

Fecal material; that which is evacuated from the digestive tract following the digestive process.

STRAWBERRY *Fragaria* spp

This fruit is borne by a small herbaceous plant (of the family *Rosaceae*) that grows close to the ground.

Strawberries are the world's leading berry-type fruit, although they are not true berries from a strict botanical point of view because the tiny seeds are carried on the outside of the fleshy part of the fruit, whereas, true berries have seeds enclosed within the flesh.

ORIGIN AND HISTORY.   Some species of strawberry are native to the temperate parts of the Old World, whereas others originated in North America and South America. It seems likely that wild strawberries were gathered for food long before the first plants were cultivated, although there is no archaeological evidence that the fruit was consumed in prehistoric times. The lack of strawberry remains preserved at sites of human habitation may be explained by the fact that this fruit is highly perishable.

Ancient Roman writers have described the growing of the fruit in gardens during the pre-Christian era. Apparently, the wild plants were dug and transplanted to more convenient locations where they might be tended readily. It is said that the Roman statesman Cato (234 to 149 B.C.) was so fond of strawberries that he personally supervised their cultivation on his estate. For many centuries after the fall of Rome, there appears to have been little interest in growing strawberries for food, since there is no mention of the plant by the leading agricultural writers. During the Middle Ages, a few herbalists grew the fruit and its leaves for medicinal purposes.

Strawberry production was apparently revived at some time near the end of the Middle Ages since the fruit was grown in the royal gardens of France in the 14th century. Early attempts to improve the berries by selecting plants with large fruits often resulted in the loss of the flavor and fragrance that characterized the smaller fruits. Native European strawberries tend to be much smaller than those from the Americas. Nevertheless, interest in growing the fruit spread to England, where, within a century, it was produced in market gardens for sale in London and other cities.

Most of the great advances in strawberry culture occurred after certain New World varieties of the fruit were introduced into Europe by the returning explorers. In the latter part of the 16th century, the explorer Cartier brought Canadian strawberries back to France, and Sir Francis Drake brought the Virginia strawberry to England. Both types are believed to have been varieties of *Fragaria virginiana*. About the same time, Spanish explorers discovered the large Chilean strawberry (*F. chiloensis*) and introduced it into Peru and Ecuador, but made no attempt to bring it to Europe. It was only by a major stroke of luck that this South American species fostered the growth of the modern strawberry industry.

In 1712, the French engineer Frezier was sent by his country to spy on the Spanish coastal fortifications in Chile and Peru in the event that a war should break out between France and Spain. While on his mission Frezier, who studied plants as a hobby, observed the large Chilean strawberries and arranged to have some plants brought back to France. Only four plants survived the voyage and were planted in Brittany, where climatic conditions favored their growth. However, the plants bore fruit only rarely, until accidental crossbreeding took place between the Chilean species and some Virginia strawberries that were growing in close proximity. Apparently, the Chilean plants bore only female flowers and required pollination from male flowers in order to set fruit. The large new hybrid, which was an immediate success throughout Europe, became the world's leading type of strawberry by the end of the 18th century.

Strawberries remained a luxury during the first part of the 19th century and only the most affluent could enjoy them. The problem was that they spoiled readily and could not be shipped very far by the means of transport then available. By the middle of the century, this problem had been solved in the United States by the initiation of railway shipment, followed in short order by the development of a high-yielding variety of the hybrid strawberry. Today, fresh strawberries are carried thousands of miles in refrigerated railcars and trucks.

PRODUCTION. The world production of strawberries is about 2.4 million metric tons per year. Fig. S-58 shows the amounts contributed by the leading strawberry-producing countries.

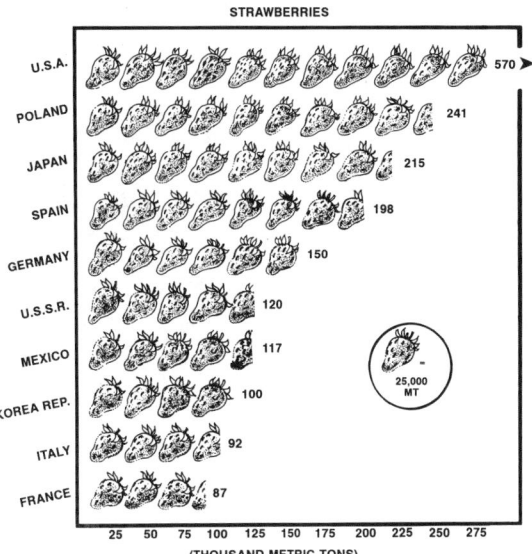

Fig. S-58. The leading strawberry-producing countries. (Based upon data from *FAO Production Yearbook*, 1990, FAO/UN, Rome, Italy, Vol. 44, p. 171, Table 75)

About 79% of the U.S. strawberry crop, approximately 445 thousand metric tons, comes from California. Smaller amounts are produced in Oregon, New York, Michigan, North Carolina, Washington, and Pennsylvania.

Strawberries propagate themselves vegetatively by means of long stems called runners or stolons which grow horizontally along the ground and form new plants by rooting in the soil at their tips. Each new plant in turn forms runners, and if their growth is not checked, the ground will soon be covered with a densely packed mat of strawberry plants.

Most growers start their strawberry beds with disease-free plants produced by a nursery. Some commercial plots are replanted every year, while others are maintained for 2 or 3 years before replanting. Usually, the plants are set in the field in rows during the fall, winter, or spring, depending upon the location and the variety planted.

At the time of planting, the soil is fertilized with a mixture of nitrogen, phosphorus, and potassium and is kept adequately watered. However, excessive watering encourages the formation of a large number of runners which may sap the vitality of the plants and reduce fruit production. Mulches are used for (1) protecting the plants against injury by low temperatures, and (2) keeping the

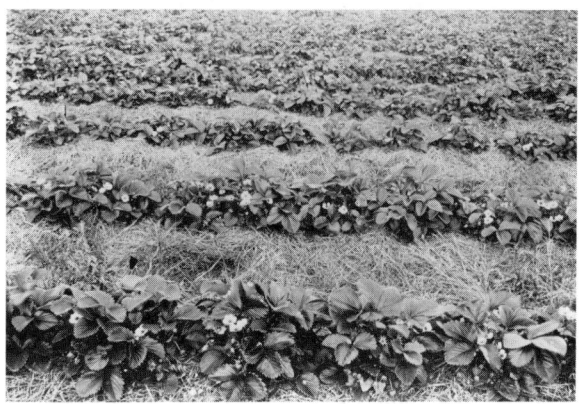

Fig. S-59. Rows of strawberry plants that are mulched with straw. (Courtesy, USDA)

berries clean when rain or watering is likely to cause splashing of the soil on the fruit.

Strawberries that are to be sold fresh in distant markets are often picked before they are fully ripe in order to minimize spoilage during shipment, but the fruit intended for nearby markets or processing plants may be allowed to attain optimal ripeness.

Much of the crop is still picked by hand, although the labor requirement has been reduced somewhat in recent years by the development of mechanical pickers and other harvesting aids. The fruit keeps best during shipment if it is precooled within 2 hours of picking, followed by shipment or storage at a temperature below 40°F (4°C).

PROCESSING. Over one-third of the U.S. strawberry crop is processed. About 95% of processed fruit is frozen and most of the rest is made into preserves. However, it is noteworthy that sometimes freezing merely serves as a means of preserving the highly perishable berries until they can be utilized by the manufacturers of baked goods, ice cream, jams and jellies, and other items.

The most common ways in which frozen strawberries are packed for retail sales are (1) sliced and packed with sugar at a ratio of 80% by weight of fruit to 20% sugar, and (2) frozen whole berries without added sugar.

Frozen strawberries that are destined for manufacturing into various processed food products are usually packed with sugar at the ratio of 80% fruit to 20% sugar.

SELECTION. Fresh strawberries should be bright red, plump, medium size, free from dirt, and well rounded with attached stems and caps. Unripe berries will not ripen after picking. Excessively large berries may have an overly bland flavor, while small, misshapen berries may be bitter. Staining of the fruit container may indicate leakage of juice and possible spoilage. Moldy berries may be found anywhere in the container and are not always evident in the top layers.

Those who wish to freeze or otherwise preserve a large quantity of the fruit are likely to obtain the best buy in the late spring, when a large supply is marketed.

PREPARATION. Some tips from the California Strawberry Advisory Board follow:

1. Fresh strawberries may be kept in a refrigerator for several days if they are removed from their store containers and placed in a single layer in a shallow container.

2. The berries should not be washed until just before using. Then, they should be rinsed with caps and stems intact under a gentle stream of cold water.

3. After washing, the caps and stems may be removed and the berries patted dry with paper towels.

4. Fresh strawberries are good in dishes such as breakfast cereals, cheesecake, compotes, cottage cheese salads, crepes, custards, French toast, gelatin salads, ice cream, milk shakes, pancakes, pies, puddings, sherbets, sundaes, and waffles. Thawed frozen berries may also be used in many of these dishes.

5. The syrup from thawed, sweetened frozen strawberries may be mixed with unflavored carbonated water, or plain water flavored with a little lemon juice, to make a refreshing drink.

6. Some of the flavorings which enhance strawberry dishes are almond extract, brandy, cinnamon, citrus juices (particularly when diluted and sweetened a little), fruit-flavored liqueurs, and vanilla extract.

NUTRITIONAL VALUE. The nutrient compositions of various strawberry products are given in Food Composition Table F-36.

Some noteworthy observations regarding the nutrient composition of the more common strawberry products follow:

1. The raw fruit and the frozen unsweetened berries are fairly low in calories *(37 kcal per 100g)* and carbohydrates (8%). They are good sources of fiber, potassium, iron, vitamin C, and bioflavonoids.

2. Frozen sweetened strawberries contain about 3 times the caloric and carbohydrate levels of the raw fruit and the frozen unsweetened fruit, but the levels of the other nutrients are similar to those of the unsweetened products.

3. Strawberry ice cream is rich in calories *(188 kcal per 100g)* and carbohydrates (24%). It is a good source of calcium, phosphorus, and potassium, and a fair to good source of vitamin A.

4. Pie made from strawberries is rich in calories *(198 kcal per 100g)* and carbohydrates (31%). It is a fair to good source of potassium and vitamin C.

5. The red color of strawberries is due mainly to the anthocyanin pigment pelargonidin 3-monoglucoside (which belongs to the large family of substances called bioflavonoids).

(Also see FRUIT[S], Table F-47 Fruits of the World.)

STRAWBERRY GUAVA *Psidium cattleianum.*

A fruit from a tree (of the family *Myrtaceae*) that is native to Brazil.

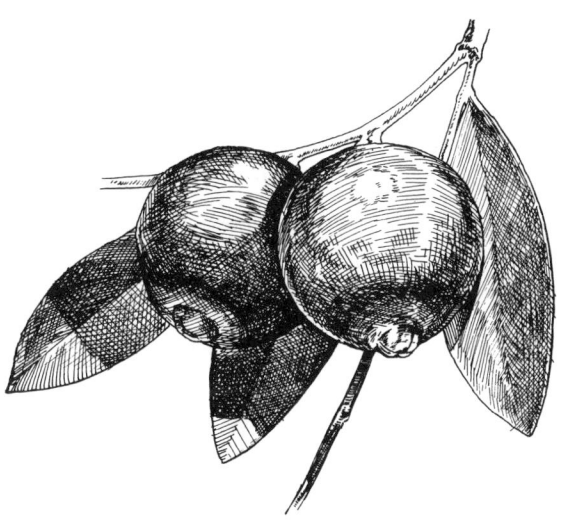

Fig. S-60. Strawberry guava.

It is closely related and similar in appearance to the common guava *(P. guajava)*, except that its fruits are (1) smaller (about 1 1/4 in. *[3 cm]* in diameter), and (2) reddish-purple-colored outside and white inside. They are usually eaten raw, or made into jam or jelly.

The nutrient composition of the strawberry guava is given in Food Composition Table F-36.

Some noteworthy observations regarding the nutrient composition of the strawberry guava follow:

1. The raw fruit is moderately high in calories (65 kcal per 100 g) and carbohydrates (16%).

2. Strawberry guavas are an excellent source of fiber, a good source of potassium and vitamin C, and a fair source of iron.

(Also see FRUIT[S], Table F-47 Fruits Of The World—"Guava"; and GUAVA.)

STRAWBERRY PEAR *Hylocereus undatus*

The red egg-shaped fruit of a cactus that is native to the West Indies. It is fairly low in calories (54 kcal per 100 g) and carbohydrates (13%), and is a good source of iron, but only a fair source of vitamin C.

STRAWBERRY TOMATO (TOMATILLO)
Physalis pubescens

A member of the husk tomato fruits (*Physalis* species of the family *Solanaceae*) which is native to Mexico and is related closely to the Cape Gooseberry and the ground cherry.

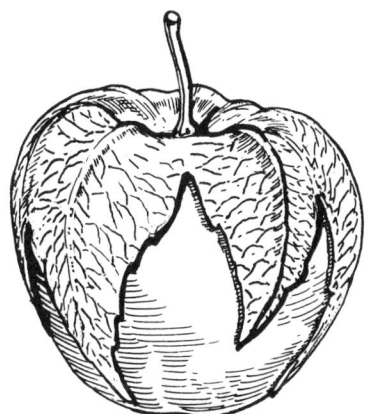

Fig. S-61. The strawberry tomato, a relative of the common tomato.

It is noteworthy that the Indians of Mexico used this plant for food long before they used the related plant that was developed into the common tomato *(Lycopersicum esculentum)*. Some botanists suspect that the latter was eventually domesticated because it resembled the strawberry tomato.

The strawberry tomato is low in calories (40 kcal per 100 g) and carbohydrates (9%). It contains much less vitamin A and vitamin C than the common tomato.

(Also see CAPE GOOSEBERRY; and TOMATO.)

STREPTOCOCCAL INFECTIONS, FOODBORNE

Streptococcus pyogenes may get into foods from infected handlers since they are carried on airborne droplets from the respiratory tract of infected people who may sneeze or cough on food. The disease caused by this bacteria is commonly called strep throat. Other *Streptococcal* bacteria can get into the food and cause scarlet fever. However, this is uncommon in the United States today. These diseases are characterized by fever, vomiting, and sore throat. To prevent their spread, food should be protected from contamination by infected handlers. Once contacted the disease responds to penicillin and other antibiotics. Occasionally streptococcal infections produce complications such as rheumatic fever and glomerulonephritis.

(Also see DISEASES, Table D-13 Infections and Parasitic Diseases Which May Be Transmitted By Contaminated Foods and Water—"Strep Throat" and "Scarlet Fever.")

STRESS

Stress is one of those words often used and assumed to be understood—until one is required to become precise about its meaning. Then stress becomes different things to different people. Stated simply, stress is a strain, a force or a great pressure acting on an individual resulting from physical factors—illness, injury and environment—or psychological factors—prolonged fear, anger, and anxiety.

Stresses of many kinds affect people; among such external forces are previous nutrition, abrupt diet changes,

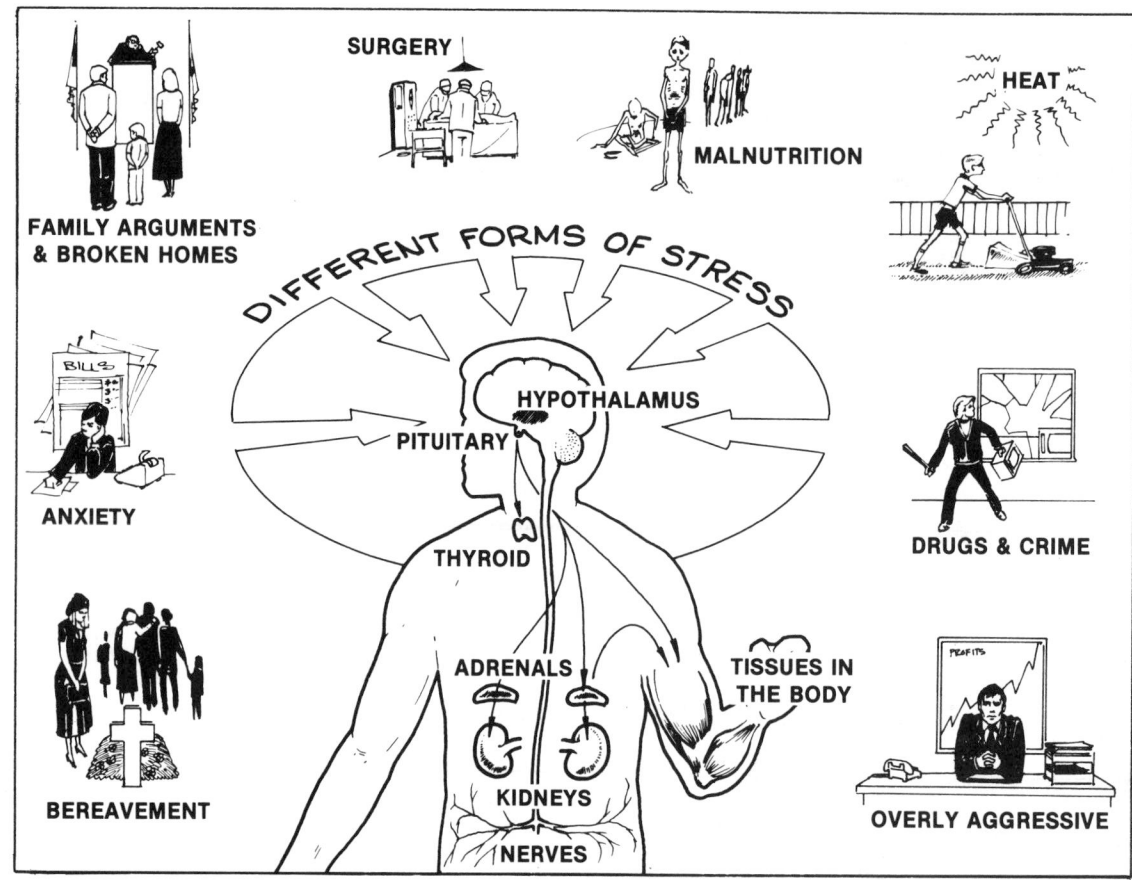

Fig. S-62.   The different forms of stress and the action of stress on the body.

a large number of people crowded together, changing houses or offices, irregularity, travel, excitement, presence of strangers, fatigue, previous illness, temperature, and abrupt weather changes.

Due to our individuality, what stresses one person may have no effect on another. Physiologically, stress is characterized by increased blood pressure, increased muscle tension, rapid heart rate, rapid breathing and altered endocrine gland function. In the whole scheme, the nervous system and the endocrine system are intimately involved in the response to stress and the effects of stress. In turn, changes produced by these two systems—collectively the neuroendocrine system—can alter nutritional processes and increase the needs of

tissues for nutrients. Moreover, stress and nutrition interact since (1) malnutrition itself may produce a stress response, (2) response to stress is determined by the nutritional state of an individual, and (3) stress can produce nutritional deficiencies or aggravate already existing deficiencies. Ultimately, through the neuroendocrine system, the nutrition and stress interactions are mediated via hormones released or inhibited by the body's response to stress.

THE STRESS RESPONSE. Table S-25 summarizes the hormones—the chemical messengers of the body—which may be directly involved in the stress response.

TABLE S-25
HORMONES DIRECTLY INVOLVED IN THE STRESS RESPONSE

Hormone	Origin	Physiological Functions	Comments
Adrenocorticotropic hormone (ACTH)	Anterior pituitary	Synthesis and release of hormones from the adrenal cortex, mainly the glucocorticoids. ACTH acts directly on fat tissue to liberate free fatty acids into the blood.	The effects of stress such as fear, anxiety and injury mediated through the hypothalamus cause increased release.
Aldosterone (mineralocorticoid)	Adrenal gland (cortex)	Stimulates kidneys to excrete potassium into the urine, and to conserve sodium.	Stresses such as anxiety, physical injury, surgery and hemorrhage all stimulate the release of aldosterone.
Epinephrine (adrenaline) **norepinephrine** (noradrenaline), or **catecholamines**	Adrenal gland (medulla)	Both hormones alter heart output; dilate or constrict blood vessels; elevate blood pressure; release free fatty acids into the blood; stimulate the brain to increase alertness; increase metabolic rate; cause rapid release of glucose from the liver.	Responsible for the alarm reaction—the fight or flight preparation. Thyroid hormones are required for action of catecholamines. A variety of nervous stimuli such as surprise, fright, shock, and emotional stresses may cause release. Release results from direct nerve stimulation of the adrenal gland.
Glucagon	Pancreas (alpha cells of islets of Langerhans)	Mobilizes glucose from liver glycogen; increases the formation of glucose from proteins—gluconeogenesis.	The important role of glucogen is to keep glucose high enough to prevent hypoglycemic convulsions or coma. Infections and other stresses stimulate the release. Starvation (fasting) increases secretion. Insulin and glucagon have antagonist actions.
Glucocorticoids (cortisone, **coricosterone**, and cortisol)	Adrenal gland (cortex)	Increase protein catabolism; cause glucose production from protein and fats; elevate blood glucose; make amino acids available for use wherever needed; stimulate protein synthesis in the liver; mobilize fats for energy; antagonistic to action of the hormone insulin.	Necessary for individuals to combat stress; exposure to stress results in increased release of ACTH from the pituitary which stimulates secretion of glucocorticoids. Glucocorticoids necessary for some actions of glucagon and catecholamines.
Growth hormone (GH; somatotropin, STH)	Anterior pituitary	Growth of all tissues; protein synthesis; mobilization of fats for energy while conserving glucose by preventing glucose uptake by some tissues.	Psychologic stresses and infections stimulate increased release.
Prolactin	Anterior pituitary	Formation of milk by the mammary glands by stimulating breast growth and secretory activity.	A variety of stressful stimuli can cause the release of prolactin, but the reason for this is not clear.
Triiodothyronine (T_3)	Thyroid	Both hormones have similar actions; however, triiodothyronine is more potent, and its actions are noted faster. Steps up metabolic rate; increases heart performance; increases nervous system activity; stimulates protein synthesis; increases motility and secretion of gastorintestinal tract; increases absorption of glucose from the intestine.	Increased blood levels during cold adaptation. Decreased blood levels during starvation. Psychologicl stresses may increase or decrease levels depending upon their nature. Release from the thyroid controlled by the hypothalamus of the brain.
Thyroxine (T_4)	Thyroid		
Vasopressin (antidiuretic hormone ADH)	Posterior pituitary	Acts on the kidneys to reduce urine volume and conserve body water thus preventing body fluids from becoming too concentrated; urine becomes concentrated and urine volume decreases.	Pain, injury, and emotional stress may all increase release.

Normally, the secretion of the hormones is not viewed as a single event, but as a concert. As one hormone comes into play, another may fade out; or one hormone may cause the secretion of another, or the action of one may complement the action of another. Furthermore, the brain or nervous system in many cases acts as the conductor by signaling the proper time for increased or decreased secretion of a hormone. In particular, the hypothalamus acts like a "switchboard" by "plugging in" the proper hormone in response to a variety of nervous stimuli received by the brain. Thus, such things as stress, nutritional status, emotions, nursing, time of day, season of the year, etc. may manifest themselves as disruptions in bodily function.

As noted from Table S-25 the hormones involved in the stress response alter the metabolic reactions of the body, and hence, increase the nutritional needs of the body, possibly for protein, energy, fat, carbohydrates, minerals or vitamins.

The response to stress is characterized as occurring in three stages, even when the cause is nonspecific.

1. **Alarm.** The body recognizes a stress and prepares for flight or fight. This preparation occurs via the release of hormones from the endocrine glands, primarily the adrenal medulla. These hormones cause increased heart rate, respiration, blood sugar, perspiration, dilated pupils, and slowed digestion. During the alarm stage, the burst of energy or alertness may be used for flight or fight. However, resistance is down.

2. **Resistance.** During this stage the body adapts to, and the body reaches, a heightened level of resistance or preparedness. The body attempts to repair any damage caused by the stress. The resistance stage cannot be maintained indefinitely; if the stress is not removed, then the body plunges into the third stage.

3. **Exhaustion.** Continued stress depletes the body's energy, and the body may fall victim to other disorders.

NUTRITIONAL DEMANDS OF STRESS.
Nutrient requirements of the stressed individual are affected by the previous nutritional status, and the type and duration of the stress. The 1989 edition of *Recommended Dietary Allowances* (RDAs), compiled by the Committee on Dietary Allowances and the Food and Nutrition Board provide for the nutrient needs of healthy people living under usual environmental stresses. The RDAs do not allow for the special needs of infections and chronic diseases—both forms of stress. Due to the individuality of the response to stress, persons under severe stress must be individually identified. Stress severe enough to increase the body's needs for essential nutrients may come from physical factors, or from psychological or emotional factors.

Physical Stress.   Stress due to physical, tangible, and specific events is well understood, and results in some definite nutritional recommendations.

INJURIES AND INFECTIONS.   Injuries, surgery, burns, and infections result in increased energy expenditure via the neuroendocrine system. The magnitude of the changes elicited depends upon (1) the prestress nutritional status of the individual, (2) age of the individual,

(3) the severity and duration of the stressing event.

Energy and protein requirements of physical stresses have been the prime concern. Little information exists concerning vitamins, minerals, and electrolytes.

• **Energy**—Stress associated with minor surgery increases the energy requirements of the body by less than 10%, while multiple bone fractures may increase energy expenditure by 10 to 30%. Some infections increase the basal metabolic rate (BMR); hence, energy expenditure, by 20 to 50%. The largest energy drain on the body is incurred by third degree burns, where the need for energy increases 40%. When burns are complicated by infection, the requirement for energy is further increased. Some patients may require 4,000 to 8,000 kcal/day.

Often, individuals subjected to injuries, surgery, and/or infections have a depressed food intake which may complicate the nutritive requirements. Once carbohydrate stores of energy (muscle and liver glycogen) are depleted—usually within 24 hours—energy must be provided by fat and protein stores. Amino acids from the catabolism—breakdown—of skeletal muscle are an important energy source. If prolonged this results in massive tissue wasting.

Energy replacement in some cases may be accomplished by oral feeding, tube feeding, or intravenous feeding, thus preventing or lessening tissue catabolism.

• **Protein**—As indicated, protein and energy metabolism are closely related. Injury, burns, surgery, and infection all induce protein breakdown via glucocorticoid secretion. Protein catabolism results in a negative nitrogen balance—the hallmark of stress which stimulates the catabolic mechanism. Adequate protein, with a high biological value, is necessary to prevent tissue wasting during a stressful illness, and to encourage convalescence following diminution of the stress.

• **Vitamins, minerals and electrolytes**—Studies have shown that during moderate to severe stresses, more zinc, copper, magnesium, and calcium are lost in the urine. Furthermore, stress results in altered blood levels of vitamins A and C, and of zinc and iron. Also, part of the response to stress includes water and sodium retention, via vasopressin and aldosterone secretion. As for the water-soluble vitamins—thiamin, riboflavin, niacin, pyridoxine (B-6), pantothenic acid, folic acid, and vitamin C—stress increases their requirement. However, no dietary recommendations are made for these nutrients for individuals under stressful situations. Still, it seems wise to supply some supplementation before deficiency symptoms appear.

Environmental Extremes.   Overall, man has learned to protect himself from extreme heat or cold. However, nutrient requirements are increased during adaptation to environmental temperatures above 97°F (37°C). Protein, energy and water needs are elevated while losses of minerals and electrolytes (calcium, iron, sodium and potassium) may be anticipated, all depending upon the amount of physical work performed. Also, vitamin C requirements may be increased by stress of a hot environment. Exposure to a cold environment increases the metabolic rate and hence the energy requirement of unprotected individuals. Warm clothing and dwellings have minimized the effects of cold on man.

Psychological or Emotional Stress.
Day-to-day psychological or emotional stress is normal, and it is inevitable—a part of life. In our society, stressful situations may include family arguments, death of a loved one, drug addiction, crime, unemployment, broken homes, and executive positions requiring aggressive personalities. The degree each individual is stressed depends on how the individual perceives day-to-day situations. Some individuals react excessively, causing hormonal and metabolic responses which tax the body's protective mechanisms. Indeed, some studies indicate a relationship between emotional stress and diseases such as cardiovascular disease, high blood pressure, peptic ulcers, cancer, and streptococcal throat infections, which in turn may increase or alter nutritional requirements.

Nutritionally, emotional stress may have a variety of effects. Prolonged fear, anxiety, anger, and tension all may stimulate hormonal and metabolic responses thus depleting energy, and increasing the need for energy, protein, vitamins, and/or minerals. Overeating, extreme under eating (anorexia nervosa), and eating binges with self-induced vomiting—bulimarexia—may be the result of psychological stress.

Without question, more research is needed in this area—especially in a society such as ours—so that stressed individuals may be identified and specific recommendations made. It seems reasonable to assume that persons experiencing emotional stresses need nutrient adjustments similar to those of individuals experiencing physical stresses. Most of the hormones altering the metabolism are influenced by either emotional or physical stimuli. Ultimately the brain determines the body's response to any stimuli.

COPING WITH STRESS OR DISTRESS.
Stress is unavoidable. Therefore, the best protection comes from recognizing it, and coping with it. Recognizing stress requires individual evaluation. Stress is different for every individual. Coping with stress involves relaxation, regular exercises, and periodic evaluation of priorities. Moreover, one should recognize that stress may be turned into a positive force since it can stimulate some form of favorable action on the part of an individual. Therefore, people should differentiate between stress and distress in their lives. Thus, distress—not being able to adapt—is responsible for the harmful effects. Health professionals are beginning to recognize stress as a legitimate health concern, which may produce damaging or predisposing responses in the body, though clear cut connections between stress and disease are difficult to establish.

Diet-Stress Connection.
It is noteworthy that most people have certain foods that they instinctively turn to when under stress—foods that create a feeling of security. The most common security food is milk, perhaps as a symbol of the more protected days of childhood and a desire to return to them. But the food or foods that comfort one person may trigger anxiety in another. So, individuals are best advised to study their own responses to stress, and to evaluate the effectiveness of their coping strategies, possibly by keeping a diary. If eating custard makes one feel better able to cope, then custard it should be. But because a certain approach works for one person it should not necessarily be urged upon the entire population. A moderate, well-balanced diet with emphasis on the stress-related nutrients and regular but not excessive meals is one approach that can be recommended for all.

(Also see ANOREXIA NERVOSA; BULIMAREXIA; DISEASES; ENDOCRINE GLANDS; HEART DISEASE; HIGH BLOOD PRESSURE; METABOLISM; and ULCERS, PEPTIC.)

STRING BEANS

Common beans that are picked at a young stage, and both the half-formed seeds and pods are eaten.
(See Bean, Common.)

STROKE (APOPLEXY)

An interruption in the normal circulation of the blood through the brain leading to a sudden loss of consciousness and some degree of paralysis, which may be temporary or permanent depending on the severity of the oxygen deprivation of the brain cells. Most strokes can be traced to previously existing conditions of atherosclerosis, hypertension, or arterial aneurysm.

The three immediate causes of stroke are:

1. *Cerebral thrombosis*, in which normal blood circulation through the brain is cut off from a part of it by a clot in an atherosclerotic artery.

2. *Cerebral embolism*, in which a traveling blood clot, fat, or an embolus of air (a bubble of air) settles in one of the cerebral arteries and chokes off the circulation.

3. *Cerebral hemorrhage*, in which there is a rupture of a blood vessel within the brain, usually an artery with a thin spot (aneurysm) in its wall. The latter type of stroke may be triggered by overexertion, overeating, great stress, or a violent coughing fit.

The most effective prevention of stroke consists in having a complete physical checkup once a year, following the doctor's instructions, and eliminating emotional stress and pressure.

(Also see HEART DISEASE; and HIGH BLOOD PRESSURE.)

STRONTIUM (Sr)

This is a soft, silvery metal with physical and chemical properties similar to those of calcium. There is no evidence as yet that strontium plays an essential role in man and other higher animals; so, it must be considered as a nonessential element at this time. It is noteworthy, however, that it has been reported that (1) the omission of this element from the diet of rats and guinea pigs on a purified diet resulted in growth depression, an impairment of the calcification of bones and teeth (but this report has been neither confirmed nor invalidated); and (2) a higher incidence of carious teeth.

The strontium content of bone has attracted particular interest because of the affinity of this tissue for strontium and, therefore, its relevance to the problem of strontium retention from radioactive fallout.

SUB-

Prefix denoting beneath, or less than normal.

SUBCUTANEOUS

Situated or occurring beneath the skin.

SUBSTRATE

The base on which an organism lives; a substance upon which an enzyme acts; a source of reactive material.

SUCCINIC ACID

An intermediate product in the Krebs cycle.
(Also see METABOLISM, Fig. M-78 the Krebs cycle.)

SUCCOTASH

A mixture of corn and beans with some milk and butter added. The beans may be either string, butter, or lima. It makes a good combination of cereal and beans together, and a more complete protein.

SUCRASE

An enzyme present in intestinal lining cells which acts on sucrose to produce glucose and fructose.
(Also see DIGESTION AND ABSORPTION; and ENZYME.)

SUCROSE

A disaccharide having the formula $C_{12}H_{22}O_{11}$. It is hydrolyzed to glucose and fructose. Commonly known as cane, beet, or table sugar.
(Also see ADDITIVES, Table A-3; CARBOHYDRATE[S]; and SUGARS.)

SUCROSE ESTERS

Sucrose, table sugar, can form esters with fatty acids like lauric acid and stearic acid. These esters are surface active agents—surfactants, used as additives. An example is sucrose monostearate.
(Also see ADDITIVES.)

SUGAR

To most people, sugar is sucrose, the white granular sweetener of commerce sold in 1, 5, 10 and 25 lb bags at the supermarket. It contributes virtually pure energy to the diet—16 Calories (kcal) per teaspoonful. To the chemist, sugar includes many carbohydrates such as ribose, glucose, fructose, galactose, lactose, maltose, and sucrose—the chemical combination of the two sugars glucose and fructose. Since sugar is usually recognized as sucrose, the following discussion deals specifically with sucrose; hence, the terms "sugar" and "sucrose" are used interchangeably. Other sugars, when mentioned, are specified.

SOURCES. Since 1978, the per capita consumption of refined sugar in the United States has been dropping. In 1990, it was 64.5 lb. However, corn sweeteners (corn sugar and corn syrup) have replaced sugar in many sweetened commercial products. The per capita annual consumption of corn sweeteners now amounts to 70.7 lb. Also, aspartame, a low calorie artificial sweetener, is widely used. Although sucrose is widely distributed in nature in green plants, it is obtained commercially in large quantities from the sugar beet and sugarcane plants.

In some countries, sugar is obtained from sugar beets and sugarcane on a grand scale. Ten countries listed in Table S-26 produce over one-half of the world's beet and cane sugar. As a sugar producer, the United States ranks sixth. Sugar production in the United States is rather unique, since both temperate climates for sugar beet

production and tropical and subtropical climates for sugarcane production are available.

TABLE S–26
TOP TEN SUGAR-PRODUCING
COUNTRIES OF THE WORLD[1]

Country	1990 Production
	(thousand metric tons)
India	11,946
U.S.S.R.	9,130
Cuba	8,050
Brazil	7,900
China	6,430
U.S.A.	5,888
France	4,595
Germany	4,279
Thailand	3,641
Australia	3,570
Total	65,429
Percent of World Production	60

[1]*FAO Production Yearbook 1990,* FAO/UN, Rome, Italy, p. 160, Table 69.

Sugarcane. Sixty to sixty-two percent of the world's refined sugar is derived from sugarcane—a coarse grass of tropical and semitropical climates. Sugarcane produces stalks 7 to 20 feet (*2 to 7 m*) high and about 2 in. (*5 cm*) in diameter which contain a sugary juice. Most of the cultivated cane today is probably an ancestor of *Saccharum officinarum,* a native of New Guinea.

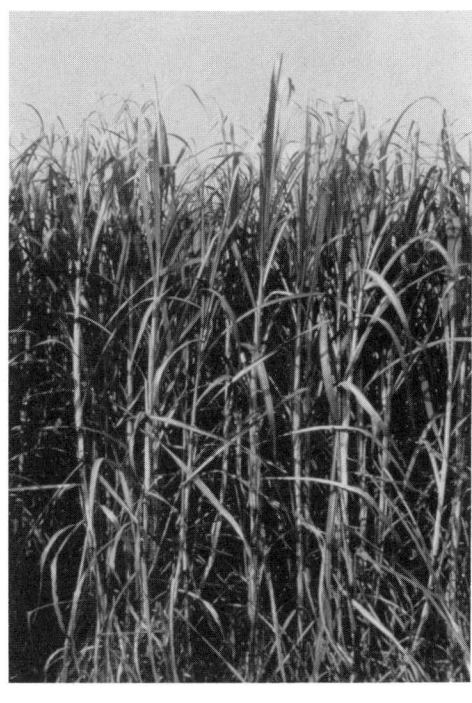

Fig. S-63.   Sugarcane. (Courtesy, USDA)

ORIGIN AND HISTORY.   Mankind has enjoyed a longer relationship with sugarcane than with sugar beets. Although honey was the only sweetening agent of early man, cane sugar was probably in use in India before 400 B. C. On an expedition down the Indus River, an officer in the army of Alexander the Great, noted a grass that produced honey without the help of bees. In his writings, the Roman, Pliny (23-79 A.D.), mentioned a kind of honey that collects in reeds. However, the Romans and Greeks may have only imported cane sugar from the East for use as a medicine. During the Middle Ages cane sugar remained as part of the spice trade from the East—still a scarce commodity. When the Moors overran Spain in A.D. 700s, they brought sugarcane, and for 200 years Spain was the only source of sugar in Europe. From A.D. 900 to 1100, Venice became a center of sugar trade. Sugar was obtained by the Venetians from the Tigris-Euphrates Valley and from Egypt and Syria. The writings of Marco Polo, a Venetian, suggest that he was familiar with sugar. In China, he remarked on its abundance, and indicated that Egyptians taught the Chinese how to refine sugar. Still, for many years, sugar was costly and normally used as a medicine or luxury by kings and the rich.

It is believed that sugarcane culture began in New Guinea. From there, it eventually spread throughout the islands of the South Pacific, and then to Indonesia, Asia, China, and the Philippines. On the second voyage of Christopher Columbus to the New World, he carried sugarcane. However, his transplants failed. But, other explorers who soon followed were able to introduce successfully sugarcane to the West Indies, Brazil, and Mexico. The first sugar mill in the New World was built in 1508 near Santo Domingo. Soon tropical America became the world's greatest sugar producing area. In 175I, Jesuit missionaries brought sugarcane from Haiti to New Orleans, Louisiana. By 179I the commercial production of sugar had begun in a mill set up by Antonio Mendez. Then in 1795, Etienne de Bore produced the first granulated sugar in what was soon to become part of the United States. With the increased planting and processing of sugarcane in the New World and the development of the sugar beet industry, sugar became accessible to everyone.

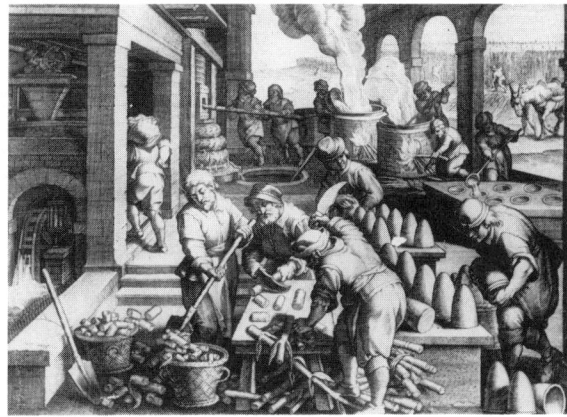

Fig. S-64.   An early "sugar factory" where sugar was made from sugarcane and poured into molds. (Photo of the Bettmann Archive, Inc., New York, N.Y.)

PRODUCTION. In 1990, the worldwide production of sugarcane was about one billion metric tons. Although the United States produces only 2.3% of the total world production, it is still considered a leading sugarcane growing country, as shown in Fig. S-65. In the United States, all of the sugarcane is grown in four states—Florida, Hawaii, Louisiana, and Texas—where the yield per acre is about 35.2 tons (*78 metric tons/ha*) on about 725,000 acres (*293,522 ha*). Worldwide, sugarcane is grown on about 33 million acres (*16.9 mil ha*), and the average yield per acre is about 27 tons/acre (*61.3 metric tons/ha*).

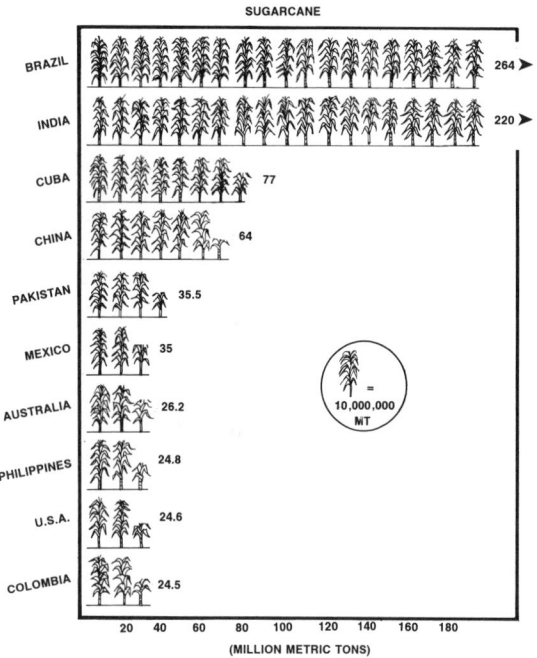

Fig. S-65. Leading sugarcane growing countries. (Source: *FAO Production Yearbook*, 1990, FAO/UN, Rome, Italy, Vol. 44, p. 157, Table 67)

Propagation and Growing. Most sugarcane is propagated asexually with stem cuttings. Sprouts grow from the buds at the nodes, or joints of the stalk, in much the same way as potatoes. Stalk cuttings or whole stalks are laid in furrows 5 to 7 ft (*1.5 to 2.1 m*) apart and covered with soil. Soon leaves appear and then in a few weeks the new plants take on the appearance of sugarcane with nodes and internodes—the jointed grass. Sugarcane stalks grow in bunches called stools.

Sugarcane has a heavy water and fertilizer requirement. Over 60 in.(*152 cm*) of annual rainfall or irrigation is necessary, and large quantities of nitrogen, phosphorus, and potassium are required. The soils of Louisiana, Florida, and Hawaii are well suited for cane production, and yield excellent crops.

Depending upon location, the length of growing time before harvest varies. In general, 11 to 16 months are

necessary in the tropics, while crops in the subtropics are harvested after 8 to 12 months.

Some sugarcane is produced for seed. Every new variety of sugarcane begins as a single stalk that develops from a seed. New varieties are continually developed that are adapted to the major sugarcane producing areas of the world. Currently, most of the commercial varieties of cane are interspecific hybrids of primarily *Saccharum officinarum*, *Saccharum robustum*, and *Saccharum spontaneum*. Development of disease resistant varieties provides the most satisfactory means of controlling disease.

Sugarcane is subjected to over 60 diseases caused by viruses, bacteria, and fungi. Sugarcane diseases are of particular importance for three reasons: (1) the use of stalks for commercial planting easily spreads disease; (2) the small number of varieties grown in a country predisposes large areas to disease; and (3) the production of several crops from one original planting. Losses from disease, if not controlled, can be as high as 50%.

Harvesting. At harvest, canes contain about 12 to 15% sucrose. Sugarcane is harvested by cutting the stalks at the surface of the ground. After a crop of cane is harvested, new shoots appear in the stubble. The first crop of cane is called plant cane, the next is called the first ratoon crop, the next the second ratoon crop, and so on. Fields are allowed to produce 2 to 10 crops, depending upon location. Another crop, such as soybeans, is usually grown between crops of sugarcane.

When the stalks are ready for harvest, they are cut by hand or by machine and piled in windrows for later loading and transport, or in some cases machines cut and load stalks for transport. In many areas of the world, cane is cut by hand with large steel knives—machetes—5 in.(*13 cm*) wide and 18 in.(*48 cm*) long. A hook on the back of the knife is used to strip off the leaves.

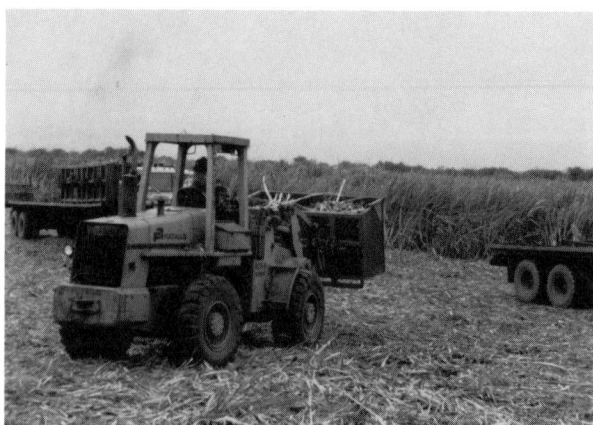

Fig. S-66. Harvesting sugarcane in Hawaii. (Photo by Audrey Ensminger)

PROCESSING. At the sugar mill the cane is washed, shredded, crushed, and passed through a series of heavy rollers(*mills*) under great pressure to extract the cane juice. Fig. S-67 outlines the production of sugar from cane.

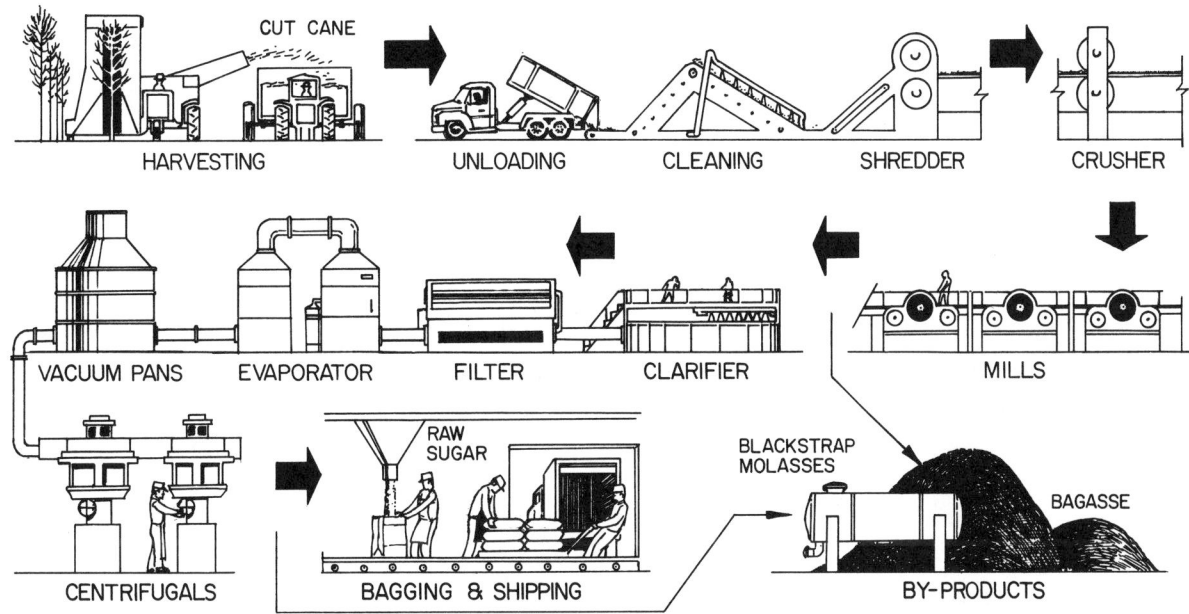

Fig. S-67.   The production of cane sugar from harvest through the separation of blackstrap molasses and raw sugar.

Each set of rollers (*mills*) crushes the mat of cane stalks a little harder, pressing out more juice. At the end of the series of rollers, nothing remains but the fibrous part of the cane, termed bagasse. This is used to fuel the mill furnaces or to produce other by-products. Next, the juice is strained, and then pumped to large tanks for clarification by the addition of lime which precipitates impurities. After clarification, the juice is filtered and then transferred through a series of evaporators which remove water. The resulting syrup is then transferred to heated vacuum pans where it is reduced to a mixture of sugar crystals and molasses—massecuite. After the vacuum pans, the thick syrup is cooled and further crystallization occurs. Next this mass is moved to centrifugals which spin at high speeds and separate the sugar and molasses. The sugar is dried, cooled, weighed and then readied for shipment as raw sugar, about 96% sucrose. The molasses is collected and reworked until no more sugar can be profitably extracted. At this point, usually the third extraction, the molasses—blackstrap molasses—becomes a by-product of the sugarcane industry.

Some raw sugar, in which part of the natural molasses remains in the crystals, is marketed and consumed as raw sugar. But most of it is further refined to produce granulated white sugar.

Raw sugar is an economical form in which to ship sugar in bulk to refineries where it is washed to remove the molasses, and dissolved in water. This syrup is then filtered, decolorized, crystallized in vacuum pans, and centrifuged to remove the sugar crystals which are then dried, screened, and packaged as the familiar granulated white sugar. The crystallization process is repeated as long as extractable sugar remains in the syrup. Brown sugar consists of the sugar crystals in the molasses syrup remaining after the granulated white sugar has been removed, although some commercial brown sugar is prepared by adding molasses back to the refined white sugar. Brown sugar is actually a mass of fine crystals covered with a film of brown, highly refined, molasses-flavored syrup. Brown sugar is not usually made from sugar beets due to the strong flavor of sugar beet molasses.

BY-PRODUCTS.   The principal by-products of sugarcane processing are bagasse and molasses. Bagasse is used as a fuel for the sugar mill furnaces, and for the manufacture of paper products and building boards. In some areas, bagasse has been ammoniated and used as cattle feed. Also, bagasse has been used effectively as a carrier of molasses for cattle feed. Molasses may contain up to 50% sugar. It is used either for livestock feed, for alcohol production, or for yeast production, which is subsequently manufactured into food for humans and livestock. Also, some molasses is sold for human consumption, and some is used to make rum. Cane wax and aconitic acid are also recovered during the processing of sugarcane. Cane wax is used in the manufacture of polishes, cosmetics, and paper coatings, while a derivative of aconitic acid is used in the manufacture of plastics.

(Also see MOLASSES; and SINGLE-CELL PROTEIN.)

Sugar Beet.   Sugar beets rank second to sugarcane as a source of sugar. The sugar beet is a biennial plant. During the first year, it produces the fleshy root which contains 13 to 22% sugar. Hence, sugar beets are harvested and the sugar extracted following the first growing season. The scientific name for the sugar beet is *Beta vulgaris*, a newcomer as a world sugar source.

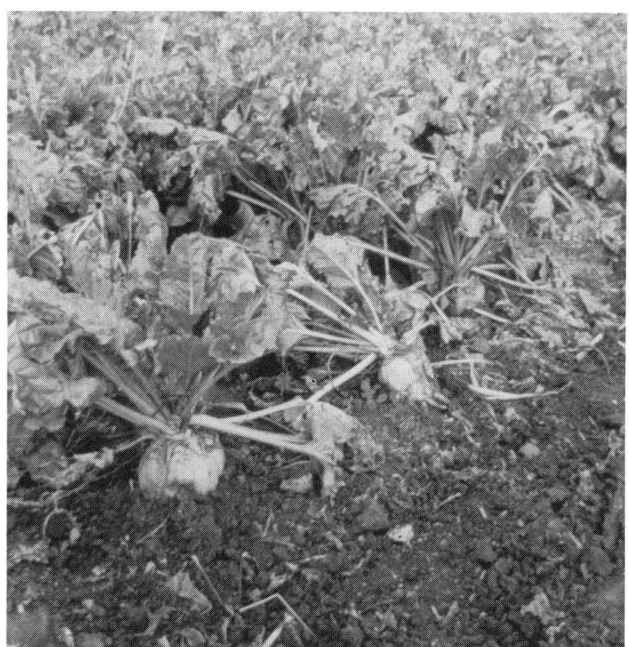

Fig. S-68.   Sugar beets. (Courtesy, USDA)

plowed under. Gradually, curly top was controlled through breeding of resistant varieties. Yields and acreages increased again, and now sugar beets are grown in about 17 states where soil and climate are flavorable. However, sugar production from sugar beets and sugarcane, and sugar importation, have been regulated by acts of Congress since the 1930s.

PRODUCTION.   Worldwide, the United States ranks fourth in sugar beet production as is shown in Fig. S-69.

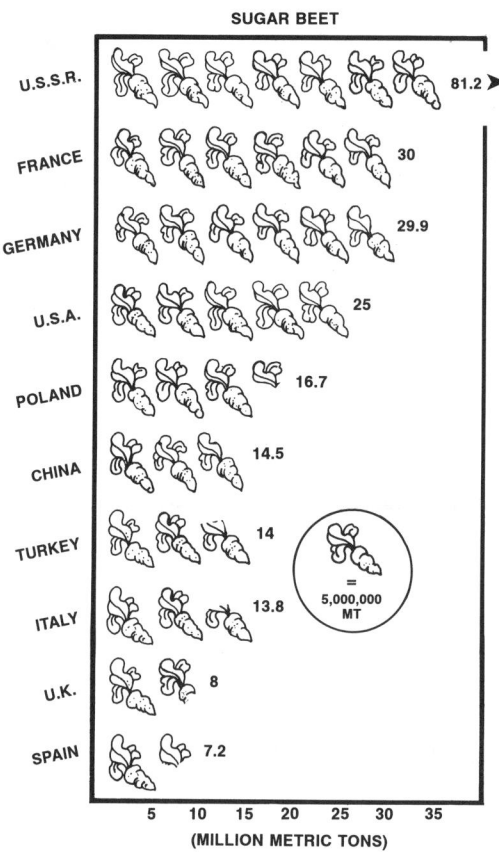

Fig. S-69.   Leading sugar beet growing countries. (Source: *FAO Production Yearbook*, 1990, FAO/UN, Rome, Italy, Vol. 44, p. 159, Table 68)

Interestingly, the Soviet Union produced about 3½ times as many sugar beets as the United States, but the yield per acre was a little over ½ that of the United States.

Sugar beet production, the world over, supplies about 38 to 40% of the refined sugar.

Since 1964 in the United States, 1.2 to 1.6 million acres (*566,801 ha*) of sugar beets have been planted annually and they have yielded 18 to 21 tons per acre, or roughly 5,000 lb of sugar per acre (*5,600 kg/ha*). The leading sugar beet producing states are shown in Fig. S-70. For the three years 1988, '89, and '90, the United States produced an average of 25,845,000 tons (*23,260,000 MT*) of sugar beets yearly. This yielded 3,352,000 tons of refined sugar; hence, 7.7 lb of sugar beets were required to produce 1 lb of refined sugar.

ORIGIN AND HISTORY.   The sugar beet was cultivated in ancient times in southern Europe and North Africa. During the middle of the 18th century, Franz Karl Archard developed a practical method for extracting sugar from beets. He was a student of Andreas Marggraf, a German chemist who discovered that the sugar in sugarcane and sugar beets was the same. Following these discoveries, sugar beet culture spread into France, Austria, Hungary and Russia. The world's first sugar beet factory was built in Germany in 1803. Development of the sugar beet industry in Europe received a stimulus during Napoleon's struggles when ports were closed to ships bearing sugarcane from the tropical regions. The French knew of the work done by Archard, and, in 1811 Napoleon ordered thousands of acres of beets to be planted and factories to be established to produce sugar. Within 2 years over 300 were constructed.

During the middle of the 19th century the sugar beet was brought to the United States, where the first successful beet sugar processing plant was built in 1870 at Alvarado, California, by E. H. Dyer. With the development of some new irrigated districts, sugar beet production increased. Average yields were low at first, but they gradually improved with increasing experience. The acreage was expanded because of the sugar shortage during World War I, until sugar beets supplied about 25% of the sugar needs of the United States. Then came the first outbreak of a sugar beet disease—curly top. From this time, about 1919 until 1935, yields of sugar beets dropped to disastrous levels. Yields were only about 5 to 6 tons per acre (*12 metric tons/ha*) and many acres were

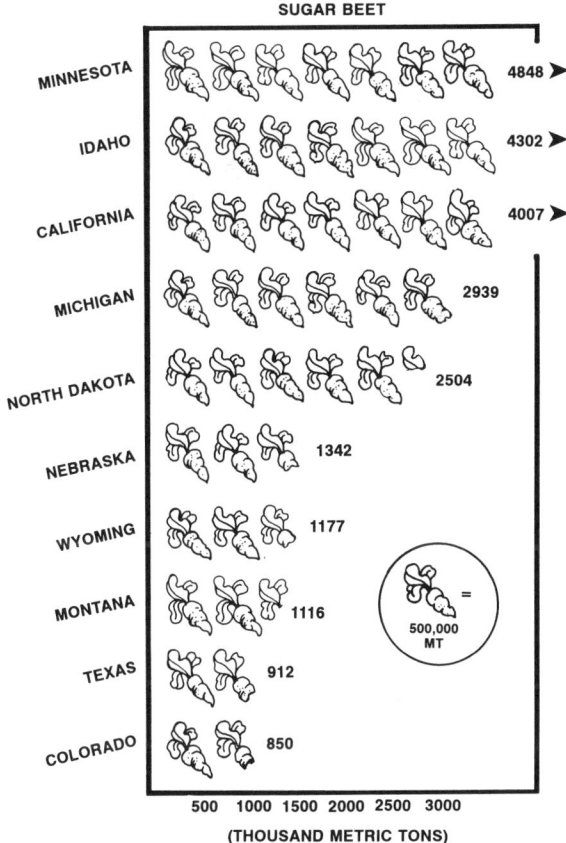

SUGAR BEET

MINNESOTA	4848 ▶
IDAHO	4302 ▶
CALIFORNIA	4007 ▶
MICHIGAN	2939
NORTH DAKOTA	2504
NEBRASKA	1342
WYOMING	1177
MONTANA	1116
TEXAS	912
COLORADO	850

= 500,000 MT

500 1000 1500 2000 2500 3000
(THOUSAND METRIC TONS)

Fig. S-70. Ten leading sugar beet growing states. The numbers in parentheses are short tons. (Source: *Agricultural Statistics 1991*, USDA, p. 74, Table 105)

Propagation and Growing. Originally, sugar beets were propagated from "seedballs", which is a round multiple fruit containing 1 to 7 seeds. Hence, the sugar beets sprouted as clumps and required hand thinning to single plants. In 1948, plant breeders discovered a sugar beet with heritable single seed fruits. Since 1966, all sugar beets planted in the United States have been grown from single seed varieties which reduced the requirement for hand labor 50%, and the seeds per acre by 85%.

Seeds are planted in rows 1 to 2 ft (*27 to 54 cm*) apart with 2 to 6 in. (*4.5 to 13.5 cm*) between seeds, depending on growing conditions and location. The seedlings are thinned to leave plants 10 to 12 in. (*22.5 to 27 cm*) apart. Weed control is provided by cultivation and herbicides.

The sugar beet is biennial; 2 years are required to complete a generation—the formation of flowers and seeds. However, the broad root weighing about 2 lb (*0.9 kg*) and containing the sugar is produced in the first season. Growing sugar beets is most profitable where the average summer temperature is 67°F to 72°F (*19° to 22°C*). Six frost-free months each year and warm days and cool nights are considered favorable growing conditions. About 20 to 30 weeks after planting, the sugar beets are harvested.

Harvesting. Sugar beets were traditionally gathered and topped—leafy top removed—by hand. Now, in the United States nearly all of the sugar beets are harvested mechanically. Machines dig, top, and load beets on trucks for transport to sugar factories where the sugar is extracted. The tops remain in the field.

Time of harvest and length of storage before processing influence the level of sugar in the beets. Lengthy storage reduces the sugar content.

PROCESSING. The major difference between processing sugarcane and sugar beets is that sugar beet processing is a single, continuous process. Upon arrival at a sugar factory the beets are thoroughly washed and then shredded. The shreds are soaked in tanks of circulating hot water. This allows the diffusion of about 97% of the soluble sugar into the water. Next the shreds are pressed to squeeze out all of the sugary water. The squeezed shreds are called pulp, which is a by-product of the sugar beet industry. The sugar solution or "raw juice" contains about 10 to 15% sugar and many non-sugar substances. Clarification of the sugar solution is accomplished by the application of lime, carbon dioxide and eventually sulfur dioxide, the sugar solution is filtered several times to remove sediments. Next the juice is concentrated by boiling, which promotes crystallization of the sucrose. Centrifuges separate the sugar crystals from the liquid portion or molasses. The molasses is subjected to additional crystallizations, but eventually it becomes a by-product. The sugar at this point is raw sugar and it is subjected to further refining which involves repeated washings and recrystallizations and decolorization until it is pure white and nearly 100% sucrose. At this stage, beet sugar and cane sugar are identical. However, for years beet sugar was considered inferior, and sold at a price disadvantage.

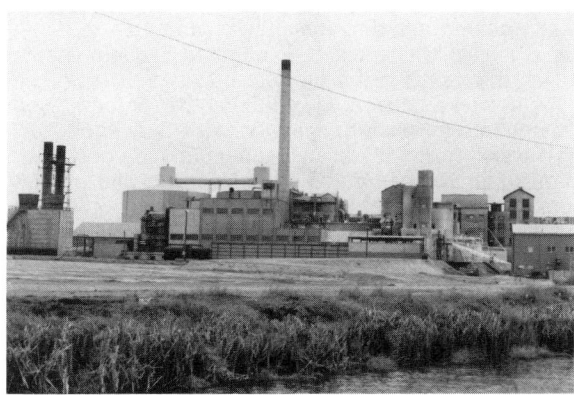

Fig. S-71. A modern sugar beet factory at Paul, Idaho. Following harvest of sugar beets in the fall, the factory operates only during the winter months. (Photo by Jayne Parker)

BY-PRODUCTS. All of the by-products of the sugar beet industry can be used as livestock feeds. The resulting beet pulp can be fed wet, or it can be ensiled or dried. Molasses is often added to beet pulp to increase the energy content. Furthermore, beet tops and crowns—very top portion of the beet—are relished by livestock. These can be fed fresh, dried or ensiled.

NUTRITIONAL VALUE OF SUGAR.

During digestion, sugar—sucrose—is split by the digestive enzyme, sucrase, into its two single sugars, glucose and fructose. Both of these sugars are easily used by the body for the production of energy since fructose is eventually converted to glucose. One ounce (*28 g*) of refined granulated sugar provides the body with 109 Calories (kcal) of energy and little else. Refined sugar is a concentrated form of energy. One ounce of brown sugar also provides nearly as much energy (106 kcal/oz) and small amounts of calcium, phosphorus, sodium, magnesium, potassium, and iron—hardly enough to contribute to our requirements.

Assuming our yearly consumption of sugar to be about 64.5 lb (*29.3 kg*), then each day we supply approximately 306 Calories (kcal) of our daily energy requirement from refined sugar—sucrose. For an average man, that is 10.5% of the recommended daily intake; for an average woman, it is 14%.

OTHER SOURCES OF SUGAR.

Production and consumption of beet and cane sugar are so enormous that other sources are dwarfed, but several other important sugar sources or sweetening agents do exist. Other sugar sources are: maple sugar, palm sugar, sorghum, honey and plant nectar, and starch hydrolysis. A discussion of each of these follows:

• **Maple Sugar**—Making sugar from the sugar maple, *Acer saccharum*, was practiced by the American Indians long before there were any settlers. Early in the spring, the Northeast Indians tapped the hard maple trees by gashing them with their tomahawks, and then collecting the sap in a birch bark dish. By continually adding heated rocks, they evaporated the sap down to a thick, dark syrup. It was a rather crude, but effective, process. Upon arriving in the New World, the early settlers soon learned the skill from the Indians, and improved upon the Indian system by using iron drill bits to tap the tree and copper or iron kettles to evaporate the sap to syrup and sugar.

Even today, in the late winter or early spring when the sap flow begins, sugar maple trees—a common forest tree of the northeastern United States—are tapped. Large stands of maple trees are called a "sugar bush." The sap of the sugar maple is about 95% water, and 15 to 20 gal (*57 to 76 liter*) of sap yields about 2 qt (*1.9 liter*) of maple syrup. Sugar in the sap is mainly sucrose. During the winter, some of the starch that the tree made the previous summer and stored in its roots is converted to sugar. When the sap begins to rise in the spring, the sugar is carried along. Sap flows for an average of 34 days when warm sunny days are followed by cool crisp nights.

Although collecting and processing sap have changed some since colonial days, gathering sugar from the maple is picturesque and truly American. Today, power drills are used to bore holes 2 to 3 in. (*7.6 to 6.8 cm*) deep in the trunk of the maple about 3 ft (*1 m*) above the ground. The number of holes varies with the size of the tree. Large trees, over 2 ft (*0.6 m*) in diameter, can be tapped in four or more locations. These holes usually heal by midsummer. Once the hole is drilled a spike is inserted and a pail hung below it. Sometimes the rate of flow is better than one drop per second. Collection of sap is a daily operation by hand using a sap-yoke with pails hung from its ends, by sleds, by wagons, or by gravity piping using plastic pipes connected to the hole in the tree and transporting to a single collection point.

The final stages of processing occur in the sugarhouse. Immediately after the sap is collected, it is strained. Then it is boiled in shallow aluminum evaporating pans which are 20 to 30 ft (*6.2 to 9.2 m*) long. The sap is boiled down to a specific thickness for maple syrup. Still more boiling produces maple sugar. A good tree yields up to 40 gal (*152 liter*) of sap in a season, but 30 to 50 gal (*114 to 190 liter*) of sap are required to make 1 gal (*3.8 liter*) of syrup, depending upon the quality of the sap. It is the boiling which gives maple syrup its characteristic flavor.

Nowadays, maple sugar and syrup are rather a treat and a luxury, but for the Indians and colonists they were important and abundant. Production of maple sugar increased in the colonies until about 1860, when cane sugar began to take its place. Still, about 1 million gal (*3.8 million liter*) of maple syrup are produced in the United States every year—some for home use and some for commercial use—almost entirely from wild trees. Table S-27 presents the history of maple syrup and sugar production in the United States for the past 75 years.

TABLE S–27
PAST 50 YEARS OF MAPLE SYRUP AND MAPLE SUGAR PRODUCTION AND THE AVERAGE PRICE OF MAPLE SYRUP IN THE UNITED STATES[1]

Year	Production		Season Average Price per Gallon of Syrup
	Syrup[2]	Sugar[3]	
	(1,000 gal)	(1,000 lb)	($)
1940	2,601	21,202	1.65
1945	1,030	8,442	3.21
1950	2,006	16,302	4.12
1955	1,578	12,624	4.68
1960	1,124	8,992	4.96
1965	1,266	10,128	5.04
1970	1,110	8,880	6.83
1975	1,201	9,608	10.60
1980	973	N/A	N/A
1985	1,325	N/A	N/A
1990	1,088	N/A	40–48

[1]*Agricultural Statistics*, 1962 and 1980, USDA, pp. 117 and 91, Tables 143 and 127 respectively; 1991, p. 90.
[2]Includes syrup later made into sugar.
[3]Assumes that 1 gal (*3.8 liter*) of syrup is equivalent to 8 lb (*3.6 kg*) of sugar.

Most of the maple sugar and syrup produced now is sold to large syrup companies and tobacco companies. The remainder is consumed by the producer or marketed independently—for a good price as Table S-27 shows.

The composition of maple sugar and maple syrup are given in Food Composition Table F-36. Maple sugar contains about 98 Calories (kcal) of energy per ounce and several macrominerals, while maple syrup contains about 7l Calories (kcal) of energy per ounce and several macrominerals. Both are slightly less concentrated sources of sugar than refined sugar.

(Also see MAPLE SYRUP.)

• **Palm sugar**—In tropical regions of the world, obtaining sugar from several species of palm is an important village industry. Collecting the sap from the sugar palm is an old practice in India and in the eastern tropics. The sap is collected from the stalk of the male flower rather than from a hole in the trunk as practiced with maple trees. At the time of collection, the sap is 10 to 16% sucrose. To process the sap it is evaporated much the same way as maple sap until it becomes a thick syrup containing sucrose crystals. It may be crudely centrifuged or poured into molds to form small cakes, a product known as jaggery.

• **Sorghum**—Generally, sorghum is considered a grain, forage, or silage crop, but some sorghum is sweet sorghum or sorgo. Sweet sorghum has a tall, sweet, juicy stalk that can be used for syrup and sugar production. In some countries the sweet stalks of sorghum are chewed by the natives. The juice contains about 12% sugar. In the United States, sorghum syrup is a distinctly flavored, mild, sweet, light amber-colored syrup. It is a specialty product of the southeastern United States. Although seldom carried beyond the syrup stage, the technology exists for converting sweet sorghum to sugar. Thus, sweet sorghum could serve as a supplementary crop for the sugarcane and sugar beet industries.

The composition of sorghum syrup is given in Food Composition Table F-36. It contains about 73 Calories (kcal) of energy per ounce, several of the macrominerals and some iron.

(Also see SORGHUM.)

• **Honey and plant nectars**—Honey is essentially an invert sugar, a mixture of equal portions of the monosaccharides, glucose, and fructose. Some honeys, depending on the flower source from which the bees collected nectar, possess more fructose. Bees collect plant nectar which contains sucrose, contribute an enzyme to invert the sucrose, and evaporate the water to produce the honey they store in combs. Man has learned to exploit this instinct of the honeybees.

Nutritionally, honey provides energy—about 86 Calories (kcal) per ounce—plus traces of minerals and vitamins, and 14 to 19% water. The composition of honey is given in Food Composition Table F-36.

In Africa and Asia the nectars of some plants have been consumed directly by man. Plants reportedly used for this include the madhuca tree (family *Sapotaceae*) of India, and the honey flower, Boer honey pots and Proteaceae of Africa.

(Also see HONEY.)

• **Starch hydrolysis**—Starch from any starch source— rice, corn, and other grains, and potatoes—may be broken down into its component sugar, either enzymatically or with dilute acids. The most familiar example in the United States is corn syrup (Karo). Complete hydrolysis

of starch yields glucose or dextrose. Corn syrup and dextrose (corn sugar) are widely used in food products. Crystalized dextrose is pure energy. One ounce supplies 120 Calories (kcal) of energy. Each year, the foods we eat contain about 71.9 lb of corn sugar and 22 lb of corn starch.

(Also see CORN MILLING, WET MILLING AND DRY MILLING; STARCH; and SYRUPS.)

• **Naturally Occurring**—Of course, all sugar occurs naturally in some form or another before being processed. Many raw fruits and some vegetables contain sugar— sucrose, fructose, and glucose—as shown in Table S-28.

TABLE S-28
SUGAR CONTENT OF SOME RAW FOODS[1]

| Food | Sugar | | | Sugar |
	Sucrose	Fructose	Glucose	
	←------ g/100 g ------→			(%)
Apple	3.8	6.0	1.2	11.0
Apricot	3.5	0.8	1.8	6.1
Banana	8.5	5.9	5.2	19.6
Blackberry	0.9	2.9	3.2	7.0
Cauliflower	.03	—	2.8	3.1
Cantaloupe	4.1	1.3	1.1	6.5
Carrot	1.7	—	—	1.7
Dates	—	23.9	24.9	48.8
Dried Fig	9.9	22.1	32.2	64.2
Grapes	0.2	4.3	4.8	9.3
Grapefruit	2.1	1.2	1.9	5.2
Honeydew melon	4.1	—	—	4.1
Mango	7.4	—	—	7.4
Onion	7.9	—	—	7.9
Orange	4.2	1.8	2.5	8.5
Peach	5.5	1.0	1.0	7.5
Pear	1.2	5.0	2.5	8.7
Peas	5.5	—	—	5.5
Pineapple	6.9	1.4	2.3	10.6
Raisin	14.2	—	—	14.2
Raspberry	2.1	1.3	0.9	4.3
Strawberry	1.0	1.8	1.7	4.5
Tangerine	3.8	—	—	3.8
Tomato	—	1.2	1.6	2.8
Watermelon	3.2	—	—	3.2

[1]Data from Carbohydrates and Sugars in Selected Foods, Table C-16.

Also, one other sugar—a nonplant sugar—is derived from an important food source. Milk sugar or lactose is present as 4.5% of whole cow's milk and 7.5% of human breast milk.

(Also see CARBOHYDRATE[S]; and MILK AND MILK PRODUCTS.)

CONSUMPTION AND USE OF SUGAR. Sugar consumption comes from a variety of sources, and the overall consumption of sugar from all sources is about 137.5 lb (*63 kg*) per person per year. However, the consumption of refined sugar makes a major contribution to this amount. While a number of factors influence our consumption of refined sugar, the average yearly consumption per person in the United States has been steadily dropping since 1972. In 1990, it was 64.5 lb per person per year.

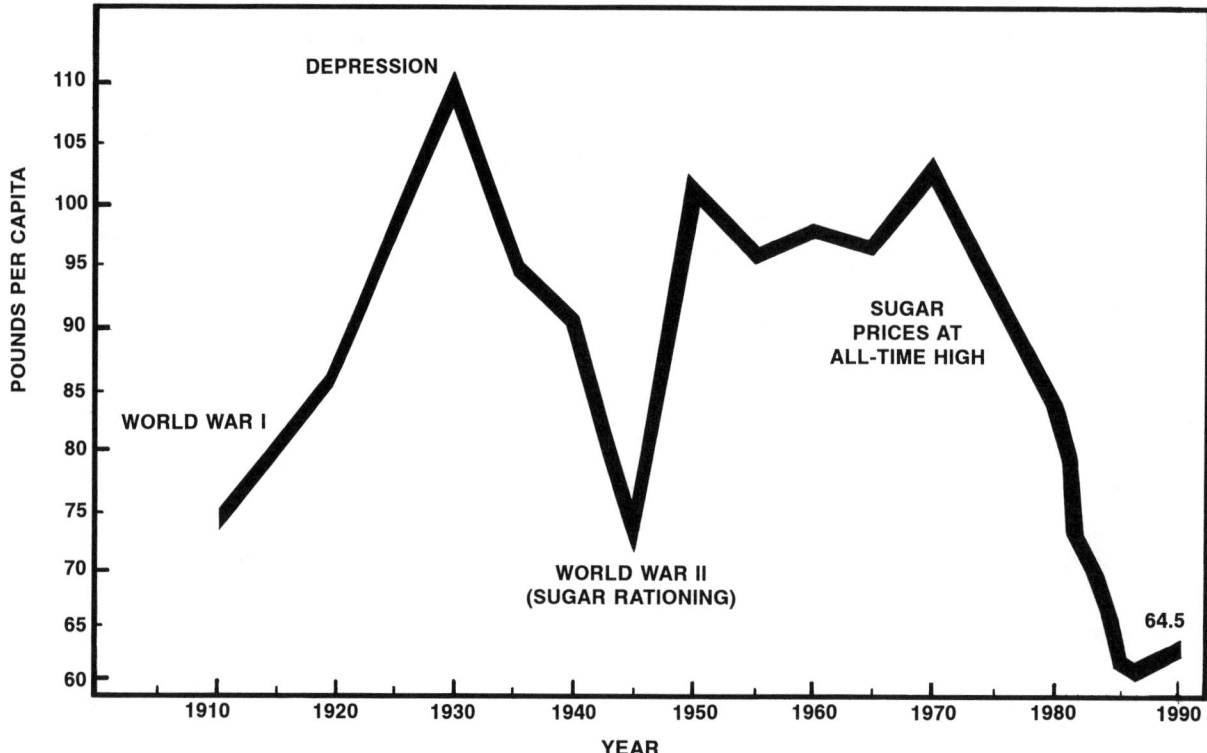

Fig. S-72.   History of refined sugar consumption in the United States. (Source of data: *Statistical Abstract of the United States*, 1940–1990, U.S. Department of Commerce)

Most homes maintain a supply of sugar for use in baking, cooking, and sweetening, but a large share of the sugar consumed is derived from food products. Sugar is classified as a food additive, and on the basis of intake it is the number one food additive. Sugar—glucose, fructose, sucrose, corn syrup, and invert sugar—is employed as a food additive to make the aroma or taste of a food more agreeable or pleasurable. Sugar of one kind or another is commonly used in the following: cereals, baked goods, candies, processed meats, processed foods, and soft drinks. Table S-29 shows the level of sugar contained in some common foods.

Today, the use of sugar in households is less than one-half of what it was at the beginning of this century, but the use of sugar by industry in processing foods and beverages is three times greater. Industry uses about 70% of the refined sugar.

Sugar is available in the variety of forms which follow:

• **Raw sugar**—This is the tan to brown product obtained from the evaporation of sugarcane juice. FDA regulations prohibit the sale of raw sugar unless the impurities—dirt, insect fragments, etc.—are removed.

• **Granulated sugar**—The white, refined sugar used in the home and in commerce comes from sugarcane and sugar beets. It is 99.9% pure, and keeps indefinitely. Granulated sugar is classified according to crystal size

TABLE S-29
SUGAR CONTENT OF
SOME CANNED OR PACKAGED FOODS[1]

Food	Sugar
	(%)
Nondairy creamer	57-65
Ready-to-eat cereals[2]	.1-56
Milk chocolate candy	44-51
Brownies	50
Chocolate cake	36
Salad dressings	7-30
Ketchup	29
Ice cream	21
Peaches, canned	7-18
Yogurt	14
Crackers	12
Fruit juice drink	12
Corn, canned	11
Cola-type beverages	9-10
Peanut butter	9

[1]Values from *CNI Weekly Report*, Vol. 4, May 2, 1974, and *Consumer Reports*, March 1978, pp. 136-141.

[2]For more information also see BREAKFAST CEREALS, section headed "The Breakfast Cereal Sugar Binge."

as: (1) *fine*, the "regular" granulated sugar used in foods and beverages and served at the table; or (2) *ultrafine*, the granulated sugar used in industrial cake-baking, dry mixes and coating confectionery, and packaged for consumer use in cake-making and mixed drinks. Three other forms of granulated sugar are produced mainly for industrial use: (1) *very fine*, for dry mixing with other finely divided materials for food processing; (2) *medium-coarse*, known as a "strong" sugar because it resists color changes and inversion at high temperatures; and (3) *coarse*, sometimes preferred in place of medium-coarse sugar.

• **Powdered sugars**—Powdered sugars are usually classified as (1) *ultra fine* (Confectioners' 10x type), (2) *very fine* (Confectioners' 6x type), (3) *fine* (Confectioners' 4x type), (4) *medium*, and (5) *coarse*. They are used for icings, frostings, uncooked candies, and for dusting on finished products. Confectioners' sugars are usually packed with small amounts of cornstarch to prevent caking.

• **Turbinado sugars**—A partially refined sugar which is similar in appearance to raw sugar. Turbinado sugar is sold for consumption without further refining.

• **Brown sugar**—So called "soft" sugar or brown sugar is a mass of fine crystals covered with a film of highly refined, colored, molasses-flavored syrup. It is valued primarily for flavor and color. Four grades are commonly available for food manufacturing—Numbers 6, 8, 10, and 13. The higher numbers are darker and more flavorful. Lighter types are used in baking and making butterscotch, condiments, and glazes for ham. The dark brown sugar, with its rich flavor, is desirable for gingerbread, mincemeat, baked beans, plum pudding, and other full-flavored foods. A light brown (about No. 8) and a dark brown (about No. 13) are produced for household use.

• **Invert sugar**—When a solution of sugar is heated in the presence of an acid or treated with enzymes, the sugar breaks up into the two sugars of simpler chemical structure that characterize sucrose as a disaccharide. One is glucose, commercially called dextrose. The other is fructose, commercially called levulose. This mixture of dextrose and levulose in equal weights is known as invert sugar. Water combines chemically with sugar to produce the two simpler sugars during inversion. As a result, there is a gain of 5.26 lb (*2.39 kg*) of solids for every 100 lb (*45.4 kg*) of the original sugar. Invert sugar resists crystallization and has moisture-retention properties.

Invert sugar is sold only in liquid form and is sweeter than sucrose. It prolongs the freshness of baked goods and confectionery, and it is useful in preventing food shrinkage. It is used in the form of invert syrups in beverages, preserves, icings, and conserved foods.

$$C_{12}H_{22}O_{11} + H_2O \xrightarrow[\text{OR ENZYMES}]{\text{HEAT + ACID}} C_6H_{12}O_6 + C_6H_{12}O_6$$

SUCROSE   WATER   GLUCOSE   FRUCTOSE

Fig. S-73. The process of inversion.

• **Liquid sugars**—Sugar syrups or liquid sugars are clear solutions that contain a highly purified sugar. There are many grades, but among them are: (1) *water-white (uninverted)*, a sparkling clear syrup for canned foods, confectionery, beverages, baked goods, flavored syrups, frozen fruits, pickles, and ice cream; (2) *light straw (uninverted)*, used for the same purposes as water-white, whenever a small amount of color and a slightly higher percentage of nonsugars will not affect the final product; and (3) *partially and completely inverted grades*.

The following are other commercial sugars or sugar sources employed in food processing or drug manufacturing:

• **Levulose**—Fructose, or levulose as it is known commercially, is one of the two components of invert sugar. It is intensely sweet and highly soluble, and is produced in small quantities mainly for pharmaceutical applications.

• **Dextrose**—Dextrose is the commercial name for glucose, the second component of invert sugar. Dextrose is also called corn sugar. It is made commercially from starch by the action of heat and acids, or enzymes. Two types of refined dextrose are available commercially: dextrose hydrate, containing 9% by weight of water of crystallization; and anhydrous dextrose, containing less than 0.5% of water. Dextrose hydrate is most often used by food processors. It is 74% as sweet as sugar.

• **Lactose**—Milk sugar, or lactose, is generally made from whey and skim milk. Compared to sugar, it is only slightly sweet and markedly less soluble in water. It is used primarily in pharmaceuticals.

• **Maltose**—Malt sugar is formed from starch by the action of yeast. Maltose is much less sweet than sugar. Preparations containing maltose, often in mixture with dextrose, are used in bread-baking and in infant foods.

• **Corn syrup**—This is a viscous liquid containing maltose, dextrin, dextrose and other polysaccharides—glucose chains of various lengths. Unlike sugar, it has a distinct flavor other than sweetness. Corn syrup is the product of the incomplete hydrolysis of starch; it is usually obtained by heating cornstarch with a dilute acid or by enzymatic action. The degree of conversion is expressed by the "dextrose equivalent" (D.E.) which is, in effect, the measure of sweetness in the syrup. Even high conversion syrups are substantially less sweet than sugar. Corn syrup can control crystalization in candymaking, and has moisture-containing properties. A special corn syrup on the market is a "high fructose corn syrup"(HFCS) which is made by treating high conversion corn syrup with enzymes. The enzymes convert some of the glucose to fructose.

• **Molasses**—Molasses consists of concentrates extracted from sugar-bearing plants, such as the thick liquid produced in the refining of sugar. It contains other substances that occur naturally in the plants as well as sugar. The highest grade is edible molasses. It is most often seen as a table syrup or as an ingredient in a blend of table syrups. It is suitable for use in gingerbread, spice and fruit cakes, rye and whole wheat breads, cookies, baked beans, and certain candies. Edible molasses provides nutrition in the form of sugar and certain minerals—primarily iron. Blackstrap molasses is the final molasses in the sugar manufacturing process.

(Also see MOLASSES.)

• **Honey**—Honey is essentially an invert sugar, but it contains a slight excess of fructose. It is used in food products where its distinctive flavor is desired.

• **Maple sugar and syrup**—Both are products of the condensation of the sap of the maple tree. However, their characteristic flavor is not manifested until the sap has been boiled. Maple sugar and syrup are also used in food products for their distinctive taste and smell.

Whether sugar is utilized in the home or in the food industry, its properties have made it (1) the world's most widely used sweetener, and (2) one of the most versatile ingredients in food preparation. Six of sugar's qualities are particularly important; namely—

1. **Sweetening.** In addition to helping satisfy the strong human demand for sweet-tasting food, sugar makes other foods more pleasing. Sprinkled on grapefruit, for example, it takes away the sourness; stirred into chocolate, it offsets the bitterness.

2. **Susceptibility to hydrolysis.** Hydrolysis can be described as a process of splitting of the sucrose molecule that occurs in most sugar cookery. The sugar molecule, when heated in solution, picks up a water molecule. Then splits to form one glucose and one fructose molecule of equal weights, thus forming invert sugar.

3. **Solubility.** Sugar is completely soluble in water and can form unsaturated, saturated, or supersaturated solutions. An unsaturated solution exists when sugar will completely dissolve in it, without increasing the temerature of the solution. A saturated solution exists when undissolved sugar will not dissolve in the solution until the temperature is raised. A super-saturated solution can be obtained only by adding undissolved sugar to a saturated solution, heating it, then permitting the resulting solution to cool to room temperature without stirring or other agitation.

4. **Crystallization.** This is a process that separates excess sugar out of a supersaturated solution. It begins by the formation of minute crystals that act as nuclei for the growth of larger ones. The size of the crystals can be controlled by (a) stirring the solution while still hot, or (b) allowing the solution to grow cold before stirring. The uniform, small crystals in granulated sugar are the result of controlled crystallization.

5. **Caramelization.** Dry sugar melts when heated to about 347°F (175°C). As it melts, the color changes from white to yellow to brown to form the liquid known as caramel. Carmelization contributes to the brown color in the crusts of baked food that contain sugar.

6. **Preservative action.** A preservative is any subtance that prolongs the life of foods by inhibiting the growth of microorganisms. A concentrated sugar solution acts as a preservative. It dehydrates bacteria or yeast cells through the process of osmosis, in which water from their bodies moves toward the sugar syrup. This inactivates the microorganisms.

Primarily due to the popularity of sugar for promoting qualities we desire in foods, Americans may be eating more sugar than they realize, since more than two-thirds of the refined sugar used is added to foods and beverages before they enter the home.

(Also see ADDITIVES; and CARBOHYDRATE[S].)

SUGAR AS A FACTOR IN HUMAN DISEASES.

Recently, charges have been leveled at sugar as a causative factor in some human diseases. Some studies have claimed that sugar intake is related to the development of coronary heart disease, diabetes mellitus, obesity and dental caries. To date, however, any causative role of sugar in coronary heart disease is far from certain, and as for diabetes mellitus no proven direct links exist. As for obesity, any time the amount of energy flowing into our body exceeds the amount flowing out, the remainder is deposited as triglycerides in adipose tissue—fat. Excess energy derived from fats, carbohyrates and proteins may all contribute to the deposition of fat. No reliable evidence exists that implicates any specific nutrient as contributing excess energy—rather, excessive intake creates the problem. Dental caries—tooth decay—is influenced by such factors as structural resistance of the teeth, oral hygiene, oral microflora, salivary flow, and composition of the diet. Nevertheless, indirect proof has been obtained implicating sugar. In China and Ethiopia, where the consumption of sugar is low, the incidence of tooth decay is also very low, while in Australia, Hawaii and French Polynesia where sugar consumption is high, so is the incidence of dental caries. Direct evidence from a number of studies demonstrate a firm link between sugar exposure and tooth decay. However, the manner of exposure and dental hygiene make a large contribution to the development and prevention of dental caries. Frequent exposure to a solid and/or sticky form of sugar between meals has resulted in a high incidence of dental caries, while taking sugar with meals, followed by quick brushing or rinsing, prevents the accumulation of bacteria and plaque, and removes the substrates for acid production by bacteria.

(Also see DENTAL HEALTH, NUTRITION AND DIET; DIABETES MELLITUS; HEART DISEASE; and OBESITY.)

Until more definitive evidence can be gained, the real danger of sugar seems to be its attractiveness to the human taste buds—its palatability. Hence, excesses are often eaten, displacing more nutritious foods from the diet and possibly creating a diet low in other essential nutrients.

(Also see CARBOHYDRATE[S].)

SUGARCANE Saccharum officinarum

Sugarcane, which belongs to the grass family, is commercially grown in the tropics and subtropics for the production of table sugar—sucrose. Following a growing season of 8 to 16 months, sugarcane is harvested and the sugar-bearing juice of the stalk is squeezed out and processed to raw sugar at mills, and then transported to refineries where pure cane sugar is produced. Cane sugar accounts for about 60 to 62% of the world's refined sugar. Four states—Florida, Hawaii, Louisiana and Texas—

produce the sugarcane grown in the United States.
(Also see SUGAR, section headed "Sugarcane.")

SUGAR DOCTOR

Sucrose crystallizes, and many foods, especially confectionery products like creams, fondants, and fudge, are dependent upon a balance between sugar crystals and sugar syrup for their texture characteristics. A sugar doctor helps prevent, or helps control, the degree of sucrose crystallization, thus extending the shelf-life by maintaining the desired consistency of the product. Often invert sugar is employed as a sugar doctor. Invert sugar may be added during the candy making process or developed from sucrose during the candy making process. Invert sugar "doctors" because it crystallizes more slowly and forms smaller crystals than sucrose. Glycerine, sorbitol, and the polyhydric alcohols also are used to control crystal formation.
(Also see ADDITIVES; and INVERT SUGAR.)

SUGAR, ICING

Icing for cakes is made from a grade of sugar termed powdered sugar or confectioners' sugar; hence, the name icing sugar.
(Also see DESSERTS; and SUGAR.)

SUGARING OF DRIED FRUITS

The whitish deposits of sugar that are sometimes seen on the surface of dried fruits are formed during drying when water containing dissolved sugars flows from the inside of the fruit to the surface. Hot air at the surface of the fruit causes the water to evaporate, leaving behind the sugars in the form of tiny crystals.

SUGARING OFF

The process of making maple sugar by boiling off the water from the maple sap. The early spring of the year, when warm days follow cool nights, is the sugaring off season in the northeastern and north central states and eastern Canada. During this time of year, the sap begins to flow and maple trees are tapped for collection. Traditionally, sugaring off gatherings were held at the sugarhouse—the shed where the sap is boiled—there neighbors helped in the making and sampling of the maple sugar. For the production of 1 gal (*3.8 liter*) of maple syrup, 30 to 50 gal (*114 to 190 liter*) of maple sap are required, and 1 gal of maple syrup yields about 8 lb (*3.6 kg*) of maple sugar.
(Also see MAPLE SYRUP.)

SUGAR PALM

In tropical regions of the world, sugar is obtained from several species of palm trees. The sap, which contains 10 to 16% sucrose, is collected from the stalk of the male flower rather than by tapping a hole in the trunk as practiced with the maple tree. Then it is processed by heating until most of the water evaporates and the sucrose crystallizes.
(Also see MAPLE SYRUP; and SUGAR, section headed "Other Sources of Sugar.")

SULFA DRUGS (SULFONAMIDE DRUGS)

Any of a group of compounds characterized by the presence of both sulfur and nitrogen, with high specificity for certain bacteria. Among the best known are sulfanilimide, sulfadiazine, sulfapyridine, sulfamerazine, and sulfasoxazole.

SULFHYDRYL GROUP

The -SH radical that forms high-energy bonds in chemical compounds, which are similar to the high-energy bonds formed by phosphates in compounds such as ATP.

SULFUR

Contents	Page

Sulfur is a nonmetallic element that occurs widely in nature; it is found in every cell of the body and is essential for life itself, mostly as a component of three important amino acids—cystine, cysteine, and methionine. Also, it is a part of two vitamins—thiamin and biotin, and it is present in saliva and bile, and in the hormone, insulin. Approximately 0.25% of the body weight (or 175 g in the adult male) and 10% of the mineral content of the body are sulfur. It is sometimes referred to as nature's "beauty mineral", because it is reputed to keep the hair glossy and the complexion clear and youthful.

HISTORY. The name is derived from the Latin word *sulphurum*. Sulfur has been used since ancient times. It was often called brimstone (burning stone); and ignited sulfur is mentioned in the earlier records of many countries as having been used in religious ceremonies and for purifying (fumigating) buildings. The early medical books of Dioscorides of Greece and Pliny the Elder mention sulfur; and the Romans used it in medicine and in warfare. Alchemists recognized sulfur as a mineral substance that can be melted and burned. It was first classified by Antoine Lavoisier in 1777.

ABSORPTION, METABOLISM, AND EXCRETION.
The small intestine is the major site of sulfur absorption.

During digestion, the sulfur-containing amino acids are split off from protein and taken into the portal circulation. Sulfur is stored in every cell of the body, with the highest concentration found in the hair, skin, and nails.

Excess sulfur is excreted in the urine and in the feces. About 85 to 90% of the sulfur excreted in the urine is in the organic form, derived almost entirely from the metabolism of the sulfur amino acids. Since inorganic sulfates are poorly absorbed, it follows that the fecal excretion of sulfur is about equal to the inorganic sulfur content of the diet.

FUNCTIONS OF SULFUR.
Sulfur has an important relationship with protein. It is a necessary component of the sulfur-containing amino acids methionine, cystine, and cysteine. Sulfur is present in keratin, the tough protein substance in the skin, nails, and hair; and it appears to be necessary for the synthesis of collagen.

As a component of biotin, sulfur is important in fat metabolism; as a component of thiamin and insulin, it is important in carbohydrate metabolism; as a component of coenzyme A, it is important in energy metabolism; as a component of certain complex carbohydrates, it is important in various connective tissues. Insulin and glutathione, regulators of energy metabolism, contain sulfur. Also, sulfur compounds combine with toxic substances such as phenols and cresols and convert them to a nontoxic form, following which they are excreted in the urine.

DEFICIENCY SYMPTOMS.
Sulfur deficiencies are manifested primarily in retarded growth because of sulfur's association with protein synthesis.

INTERRELATIONSHIPS.
Sulfur is related to the amino acids methionine, cystine, and cysteine, and to biotin, thiamin, insulin, coenzyme A, certain complex carbohydrates, insulin, and glutathione.

RECOMMENDED DAILY ALLOWANCE OF SULFUR.
Sulfur requirements are primarily those involving amino acid nutrition.

There are no recommended allowances for sulfur because it is assumed that the sulfur requirements are met when the methionine and cystine intakes are adequate.

TOXICITY.
Except in rare, inborn errors of metabolism where the utilization of the sulfur-containing amino acids is abnormal, excess organic sulfur intake is essentially nonexistent. However, inorganic sulfur can be dangerous if ingested in large amounts.

SOURCES OF SULFUR.
Inorganic sulfur is poorly utilized by man and other monogastrics. So, the sulfur needs of the body are largely met from organic complexes, notably the amino acids of proteins, rather than from inorganic sources. The sulfur content of protein foods varies from 0.4 to 1.6%, depending on the quality of the protein. The average mixed diet contains about 1% sulfur. Good food sources of sulfur are: cheese, eggs, fish, grains and grain products, legumes, meat, nuts, and poultry.

TOP SULFUR SOURCES.
Unfortunately, few foods have been analyzed for sulfur, with the result that sulfur content is not given in Food Composition Table F-36. So, a special table, Table S-30, was prepared for this book; this gives some good sources of sulfur.

(Also see MINERAL[S], Table M-67.)

TABLE S-30
SOME FOOD SOURCES OF SULFUR AND THEIR CALORIC CONTENT

Food	Sulfur	Energy
	(mg/100 g)	(kcal/100 g)
Soybean flour	410	386
Brewers' yeast	380	283
Peanuts, roasted, salted	380	582
Molasses, blackstrap........	350	230
Pork chops, lean, roasted ...	300	254
Brazil nuts	290	715
Turkey, light or dark meat, roasted	290	190
Sardines, canned in oil, drained solids	310	246
Beef, variety of lean cuts...	270	220
Chicken, light or dark meat, fried	255	210
Lamb, shoulder roast, lean...	240	205
Wheat germ	240	391
Navy beans, dry	230	340
Cheese, natural cheddar	230	402
Soybeans, dry	220	405
Wheat bran	220	353
Salmon, canned	220	124
Oats, whole grain	210	283
Beans, lima, dry	200	359
Wheat flour	190	345
Rice bran	180	276
Rice polish	170	265
Wheat, whole grain	160	360
Barley, whole grain	150	305
Almonds....................	150	598
Sorghum, whole grain	150	339
Eggs, chicken	140	157
Corn, whole grain	120	348
Cabbage, raw...............	110	24
Buttermilk, dehydrated	80	387
Alfalfa leaf meal, dehydrated.	60	215
Peas, raw	50	84
Rice, whole grain	50	363
Sweet potato	40	82
Turnip greens, raw..........	40	28
Turnip, raw	40	30
Milk, skim	30	34
Rutabaga, raw	30	46
Beet, common red, raw	20	43
Carrot, raw	20	42
Potato, raw	20	76
Apple, raw	10	58

SULFUR AMINO ACIDS

The two amino acids, cystine and methionine, contain sulfur in their chemical structure. Methionine is an essential amino acid; cystine is not.

(Also see AMINO ACID[S]; and PROTEIN[S].)

SULFUR DIOXIDE (SO₂)

A colorless, nonflammable gas derived from burning sulfur. Its odor is pungent and suffocating. The ancient Egyptians and Romans used the fumes of burning sulfur in their wine making. Thus, they were utilizing the antimicrobial properties of sulfur dioxide. It also prevents enzymatic and nonenzymatic decolorization of some foods. In the food industry, sulfur dioxide is applied to dehydrated fruits and vegetables; to increase storage life, preserve color and flavor, and aid in the retention of ascorbic acid and carotene. In wine making, it is employed first to sanitize the equipment, then at several stages as an antioxidant, and finally during bulk storage to prevent bacterial spoilage.

(Also see ADDITIVES: and PRESERVATION OF FOOD.)

SULTANAS

This term is used differently in the United States and Europe. Hence, the two major meanings follow:

• In the United States, the term designates the raisins produced *without* sulfuring from sultana grapes. They are used mainly by commercial food manufacturers and food service establishments.

• In Europe, this term refers to golden seedless raisins which are produced from Thompson Seedless grapes or a related variety of grape by (1) washing the freshly harvested fruit, (2) dipping it in a solution to crack the skin, (3) sulfuring the grapes by exposure to the fumes of burning sulfur, and (4) drying the sulfured fruit in heating chambers. In the Mediterranean region, a delicate white wine is also made from sultana grapes.

SUN-CURED

Material dried by exposure in open air to the direct rays of the sun.

SUNFLOWER MEAL

The residue which remains after extracting oil from sunflower seed, which is then ground.

SUNFLOWERS *Helianthus annuus*

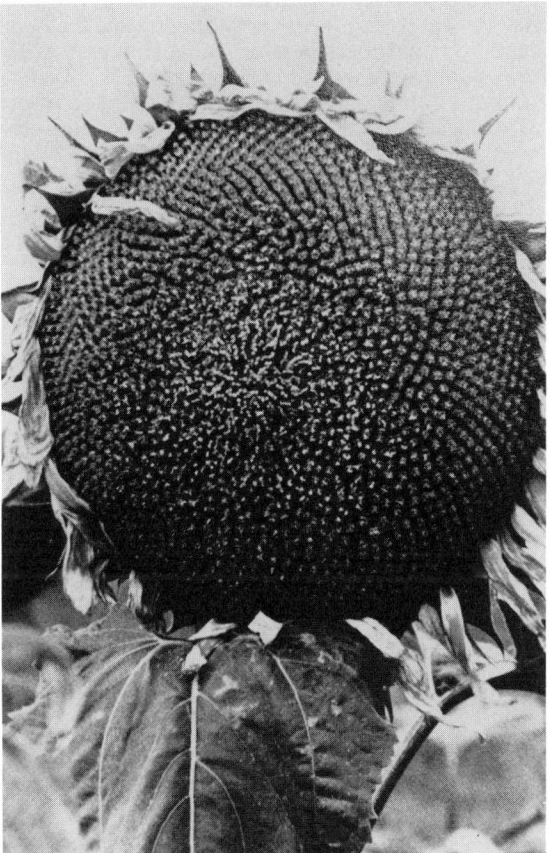

Fig. S-74. Close-up of a sunflower head. (Courtesy, Sunflower Association of America, Fargo, N.D.)

For Peru, the sunflower is the national emblem; for Kansas, it's the state flower; and for farmers throughout the world, it's symbolic of a bright future for sunflower oil.

A Russian agronomist described the sunflower as "a plant that raises its head to follow the sun across the sky." Myth or no myth, the time may come when sunflowers and soybeans will split the market for top U.S. oilseed crop; with sunflowers taking over as the premier oil crop, and soybeans serving as the protein crop. In support of this assertion, it is noteworthy that sunflowers yield over 40% oil, whereas soybeans yield about 18%; and that on a per pound basis oil is more valuable than meal. As a consequence, sunflowers are grown primarily for their oil—which contributes 75% of the crop's proportionate value, compared with 40% for soybean oil. Although sunflower meal is just about as high in protein content as soybean meal when the hulls are completely removed, it is handicapped by its normally high fiber content due to difficulty in removing all of the hulls. Consequently, it is at a disadvantage in the meal market.

United States sunflower production has spiraled in recent years largely because of two breakthroughs which vastly improved oil production: (1) the development in the 1960s of sunflower varieties with an oil content of more than 40%—a one-third increase over earlier varieties; and (2) the development of hybrid sunflowers in the 1970s, which boosted yields another 25%.

The domestic food use of sunflower oil is expected to expand now that there is a dependable supply of U.S. oilseed sunflowers available for crushing.

Sunflower oil is higher in polyunsaturates than corn oil and is much more stable than safflower oil. Thus, it has an edge over these two competitors for use in premium grade margarine and in cooking and salad oils.

ORIGIN AND HISTORY.   The sunflower is one of the few annual cultivated plants which was first domesticated in the United States, although there is evidence that this honor should go to, or be shared with, Peru and Mexico. Its culture for food by the Indians was at an advanced state when the colonists came to America. Nevertheless, sunflower production in the United States was of minor importance until recent years, primarily due to production problems, insects, and the rise of soybean production.

In the Soviet Union, superior varieties were selected, and in the 1830s a method was developed for obtaining oil from the seed. The present-day interest in sunflowers in Europe, and elsewhere, stems primarily from the work of the Russian scientist, Dr. V. S. Pustovoit, at the Sunflower Research Institute, near Krasnodar, U.S.S.R., which two of the authors of this book—the Ensmingers—visited in 1972. Dr. Pustovoit, who began his classic sunflower breeding work in the early 1900s, started with a local variety that contained 28% oil. Today, some of the newer varieties in the Soviet Union produce up to 60% oil, and 95% of the nation's sunflower seed averages 50% oil content. Eighty percent of the vegetable oil produced in the Soviet Union comes from sunflowers.

Although U.S. production of sunflowers for oil started in the 1940s, present-day interest in sunflowers began in 1962 when new high-oil varieties were introduced.

WORLD AND U.S. PRODUCTION.   The global growth in the 1960s of sunflower seed production and of the sunflower seed and oil trade is the most impressive of any in the fat and oil industry. In 1960, sunflowers

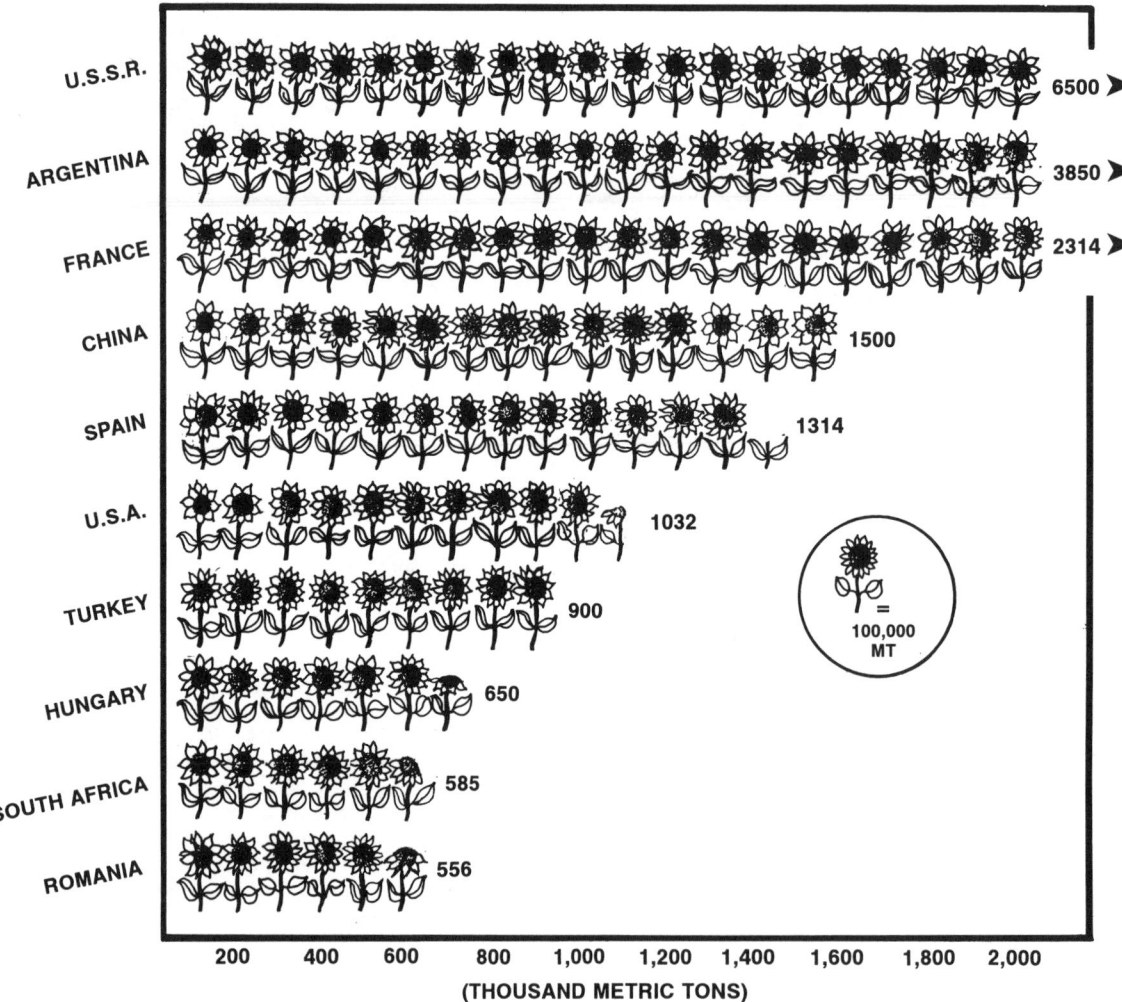

SUNFLOWER

U.S.S.R. 6500 ➤
ARGENTINA 3850 ➤
FRANCE 2314 ➤
CHINA 1500
SPAIN 1314
U.S.A. 1032
TURKEY 900
HUNGARY 650
SOUTH AFRICA 585
ROMANIA 556

= 100,000 MT

200   400   600   800   1,000   1,200   1,400   1,600   1,800   2,000

(THOUSAND METRIC TONS)

Fig. S-75.   Leading sunflower-producing countries of the world. (Source: *FAO Production Yearbook*, 1990, FAO/UN, Rome, Italy, Vol. 44, p. 112, Table 40)

ranked fourth in the world among sources of vegetable oils, exceeded by soybeans, peanuts, and cottonseed. Today, sunflower oil holds undisputed claim to third place, exceeded only by soybean and palm oils.

World production of sunflower seed averages 22 million metric tons, about 29% of which is produced by the U.S.S.R. The ten leading sunflower-producing countries, by rank, are: U.S.S.R., Argentina, France, China, Spain, U.S.A., Turkey, Hungary, South Africa, and Romania (see Fig. S-75).

In addition to being the world's leading producer of sunflower seed, the U.S.S.R. is the world's largest exporter of sunflower oil. Sunflowers are grown throughout a wide geographical area of the country, and generally occupy about 11.4 million acres (*4.6 mil ha*).

THE SUNFLOWER PLANT. Sunflowers belong to the composite family, *Compositae.* The common annual is genus *Healianthus*, species *H. annuus.* The plant has a rough hairy stem 3 to 20 ft (*1 to 6 m*) high; coarse, heart-shaped leaves 3 to 12 in. (*5 to 8 cm*) long; and a flat, disklike head up to 20 in. (*51 cm*) in diameter surrounded by "rays" of yellow petals.

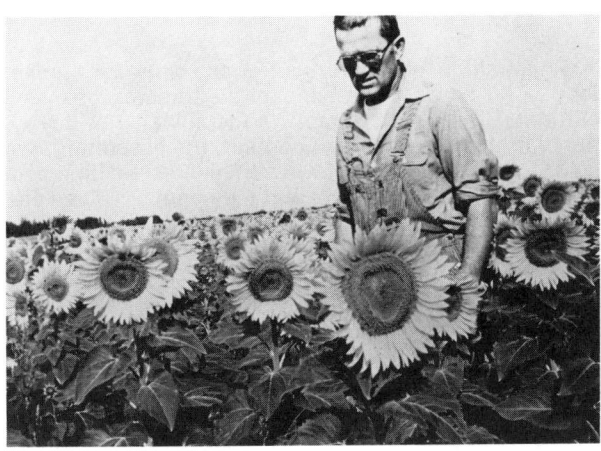

Fig. S-76. Sunflowers at bloom stage. (Courtesy, Sunflower Association of America, Fargo, N.D.)

The Spanish word for sunflower is *girasol*, meaning "turn to the sun," based on the mistaken notion that sunflower blossoms turn all day to keep facing the sun.

Dwarf types that are only a few feet tall have been developed. These can be harvested mechanically with adapted combines. In the Soviet Union, the leading sunflower producer of the world, yields of seed average 1,101 lb per acre (*1,233 kg/ha*).

SUNFLOWER CULTURE. Sunflowers are adapted to most of the climates and cultivated soils of the United States. They are very drought resistant except for the 3-week interval during flower and seed develop-

ment. Sunflowers demand proper management, and they yield poorly when the management practices are not good.

Equipment for sunflower production is similar to that needed for corn. Row spacing of 40 in. (*102 cm*) and plant spacings of 6 to 12 in. (*15 to 30 cm*) permit the use of standard cultivating and planting equipment. The dwarf types can be harvested with a combine, but the standard varieties are too tall and coarse—hence, they must be harvested by hand.

KINDS OF SUNFLOWERS. The genus *Helianthus* contains more than 100 species. But, broadly speaking, sunflowers can be divided into two distinct kinds: (1) the nonoilseed varieties, and (2) the oilseed varieties. The nonoil varieties, which are of North American origin, produce large, striped, low-oil content seeds that are used exclusively for human food and bird feed.

The oilseed varieties, which are primarily of Russian origin, have small seeds with more than 40% oil content.

With the discovery of male-sterile and fertility restorer parental lines, it became possible to produce hybrid sunflower seed in much the same way as hybrid corn and sorghum. In 1977, the year U.S. farmers made a major shift from open-pollinated to hybrids, hybrids took over 90% of the planted area.

GRADES OF SUNFLOWERS. There are no U.S. Department of Agriculture grading standards for sunflower seed. However, the standards shown in Table S-31 were developed by representatives of industry, the grain inspection services of Minnesota and North Dakota, and experiment station and extension service personnel.

TABLE S-31
SUNFLOWER SEED GRADE STANDARDS

| Grade | Minimum test weight per bushel | | | Maximum limits of damaged seed | | | |
| | Class I | | Class II | Mois-ture | Total | Heat dam-aged | De-hulled Seed |
	Large Seed[1]	Small Seed					
(number)	(lb)	(lb)	(lb)	(%)	(%)	(%)	(%)
1	24	27	29	10	5	0.5	2
2	22	25	27	14[2]	8	1.0	3
3	20	24	25	14[2]	10	1.5	5

The classes are:
Class I—Edible and bird seed varieties
Class II—Oilseed varieties
Class III—Mixed class. Seed that contains more than 2% of both Class I and Class II.

Sample grade shall include sunflower seed that does not come within the requirements of the Grades No. 1, No. 2, or No. 3 of Class I, Class II, or Class III; or which contains fire-damaged sunflower seed; or which contains more than 14% moisture; or which is musty, or sour, or heating, or hot; or which has any commercially objectionable foreign odor; or which is otherwise of distinctly low quality; or which shows evidence of chemicals not approved.

[1]30% or more held over 20/64-in. round hole screen.
[2]Tough shall be sunflower seed in Grades No. 2 and No. 3 containing more than 12% but not more than 14% moisture.

PROCESSING SUNFLOWERS. The sunflower seed is a four-sided, flattened fruit or achene. It has a dry, brittle hull which ranges in color from white, white and grey striped, white and black striped, to black. The hull encloses a whitish kernel which has a thin, translucent skin covering or coat.

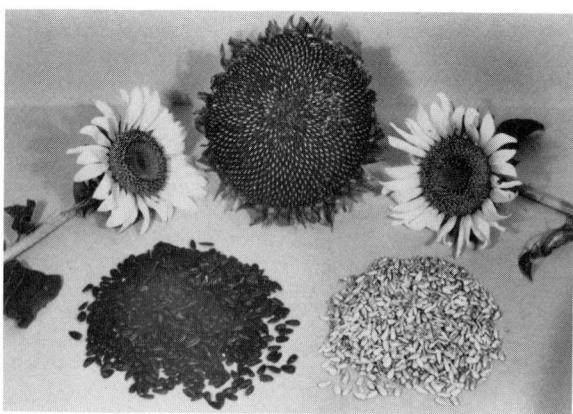

Fig. S-77. Sunflower heads (top) and seeds (below). (Courtesy, Texas A&M University)

High-oil-type sunflower seeds are processed to obtain the oil and meal. The separation of the oil may be achieved (1) by direct solvent extraction, (2) by prepress solvent extraction, or (3) by mechanical means (screw pressing).

The steps in processing are:

1. **Cleaning.** Cleaning seed involves removing foreign materials—such as stems, leaves, heads, chaff, straw, dirt, and stones—by screening and aspiration. Generally, the seed is cleaned at the extraction plant just before processing.

2. **Dehulling.** Since high-oil-type sunflower seed contains 26% hull, dehulling is an important operation in processing the seed. If sufficient hull is not removed before extraction of the oil, a meal high in crude fiber and of questionable feeding value for single-stomached animals is produced.

If sunflower hulls and kernels are carefully separated by hand, the minimum crude fiber is: in the kernels, 2.5%; and in the hulls, 50.5%. But not all the hulls can be removed by the normal commercial process employed; 6 to 8% hulls may be considered as optimum.

In order to produce a sunflower meal of low fiber and high protein content for use in human food formulations and for feeding swine and poultry, sieving and aspiration of hulls from extracted meal is necessary.

3. **Rolling and cooking.** Following cleaning and dehulling, the kernels are crushed by roller mills to facilitate subsequent cooking and extraction.

Cooking is generally carried out in stack cookers, consisting of a series of closed cylindrical steel kettles stacked one on top of the other. The cooking conditions depend on the subsequent extraction procedure. For a typical expeller extraction using a six-high cooker, the temperature in the top kettle should be approximately 160°F (*71°C*), and in the bottom kettle it should be 255° to 265°F (*124° to 129°C*).

4. **Extracting oil.** In the United States, high-oil sunflower seed is processed primarily by the prepress solvent extraction; and only small quantities of seed are dehulled prior to extraction. Small quantities of seed are processed in a straight pressing operation by screw presses (expeller process) and by direct solvent extraction.

After solvent extraction, hexane is removed by indirect heating and by direct steam injection. The desolventized meal from dehulled seed contains approximately 4.0% moisture, 1.0% fat, 44.0% protein, and 12% crude fiber, whereas meal from crushed whole seed contains not less than 1% fat, 28% protein, and not more than 23% crude fiber. The latter type meal is used for ruminant feed.

The crude oil is stored in tanks until further processing.

NUTRITIONAL VALUE OF SUNFLOWERS.

Composition data on sunflower seed kernels, flour, and oil are given in the Food Composition Table F-36.

A few salient features of the nutritional value of sunflower products follow:

• **Composition of nonoil sunflower seeds for human food**—The seeds are a concentrated source of many nutrients. The oil is desirable in the human diet due to the high linoleic fatty acid content, the essential fatty acid. Their protein content is sufficient to recommend them as a meat substitute; and the nonoil varieties are substantially higher in lysine, an essential amino acid, than the high-oil varieties. Sunflower seeds contain 31% more iron than raisins—a popular source of iron; and they are a good source of the vitamins thiamin and niacin.

• **Composition of the hulls**—The fibrous hulls have only a small percentage of oil and crude protein and contain about 50% crude fiber. Chemically, the hulls are largely lignin, pentosans, and cellulosic constituents.

• **Composition of sunflower meal (sun meal)**—The composition of defatted sunflower meal varies considerably, depending primarily on the method of processing. A typical commercial sunflower meal contains approximately 9.0% water, 45% protein, 3.5% fat, 9.5% fiber, 7.0% ash (mineral), and 26% carbohydrate.

Sunflower meal compares favorably with other oilseed meals as a source of calcium and phosphorus; it runs about 0.46% calcium and 1.47% phosphorus.

The meal is superior to other oilseed meals in vitamin content. It is richer in B-complex vitamins than soybean meal; it is equal in nicotinic acid content to peanut meal, which is rated as an outstanding source; the pantothenic content is similar to soybean meal; and it is a rich source of vitamin A. Sunflower flour is similar to sunflower meal.

The toxic compounds present in several vegetable proteins have not been found in sunflower meal. Also, sunflower meal products cause considerably less flatus (gases) in the digestive tract than soybean meal products.

• **Protein quality**—Table S-32 shows the essential amino acid composition of the protein of sunflower seed kernels and of a typical sunflower meal. Kernels and meal are deficient in lysine, but adequate in the other essential amino acids. It is noteworthy, however, that the amino acids of sunflowers vary with varieties and planting locations.

The main disadvantage of sunflower meal as a source of high-protein human food is that it turns off-color (generally to green or brown) during processing. These off-colors are caused by the reaction of chlorogenic acid at high pH values.

The commercial use of sunflower flour for human food is dependent on the development of low chlorogenic acid varieties and hybrids and efficient procedures for dehulling them.

TABLE S–32
PROFILE OF ESSENTIAL AMINO ACIDS IN SUNFLOWER SEEDS COMPARED TO MILK—A HIGH-QUALITY PROTEIN

Amino Acid	Sunflower Seeds		Cow's Milk[1]
	Kernels	Meal	
	◄——— (mg/g protein) ———►		
Histidine	25	17	27
Isoleucine	55	52	47
Leucine	75	62	95
Lysine	38	38	78
Methionine and cystine ..	39	34	33
Phenylalanine and tyrosine	81	80	102
Threonine	40	40	44
Tryptophan	15	13	14
Valine	59	52	64

[1]*Recommended Dietary Allowances*, 10th ed., 1989, NRC–National Academy of Sciences, p. 67, Table 6–5.

• **Composition of sunflower oil (sun oil)**—The fatty acid composition of sunflower oil makes it desirable as an edible oil. Of all oils produced in the United States, sunflower oil strikes the most ideal compromise between the amount of polyunsaturated fatty acids and stability. Its polyunsaturated fatty acid composition is superior to all oils except safflower oil; hence, it offers a popular approach to the prevention and/or cure of cardiovascular diseases. It contains only trace amounts of linolenic acids, which makes it a fairly stable oil. The stability imparts the capacity of the oil to maintain its flavor (not go rancid) and to resist change in viscosity (not congeal or leave deposits on cooking vessels) after prolonged periods of high temperature. The latter characteristic is particularly important to the rapidly growing fast food and snack industries where deep fat frying is used. Oils which can be reused without flavor deterioration and which allow maximum shelf life of products are desired.

TABLE S-33
COMPOSITION OF COMMERCIAL SUNFLOWER OIL

Nutrient		Amount	
		100 g	Tablespoon *(13.6 g)*
Calories	kcal	884	120
Vitamin E	mg	44.9	6.1
Palmitic acid[1]	g	5.9	.8
Stearic acid[1]	g	4.5	.6
Oleic acid[2]	g	19.5	2.7
Linoleic acid[3]	g	65.7	8.9

[1]Saturated fatty acid.
[2]Monounsaturated fatty acid.
[3]Polyunsaturated fatty acid and the essential fatty acid.

As shown in Table S-33 sunflower oil is relatively low in the saturated fatty acids, palmitic and stearic, but it is rich in the unsaturated fatty acids, oleic and linoleic. The lack of linolenic acid is primarily responsible for its good storage qualities. The oleic and linoleic acid contents of sunflower oil are quite variable, ranging from 13.9 to 60.0% for oleic and from 29.9 to 76.4% for linoleic acid. Seeds grown in cold climates (such as those in central U.S.S.R, Canada, and northern U.S.) contain less oleic acid and more linoleic acid than those grown in warmer areas (such as southern U.S.).

The high linoleic acid content and the high ratio of polyunsaturated to saturated fatty acids suggest that sunflower oil may be useful in the prevention of high blood cholesterol and heart disease. It is noteworthy, however, that the degree of unsaturation of sunflower oil is affected by plant location, climatic conditions during the growing season, and genetics.

SUNFLOWER PRODUCTS AND USES. Table S-34 presents in summary form the story of sunflower products and uses.

(Also see FLOURS, Table F-26 Special Flours; and OILS, VEGETABLE, Table O-6.)

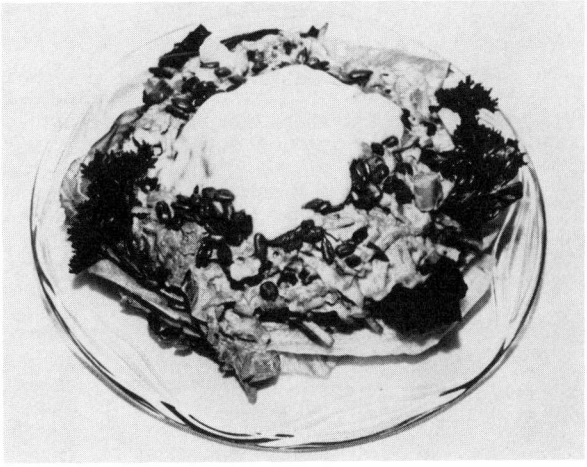

Fig. S-78. Sunflower kernels used in salad. (Courtesy, Sunflower Association of America, Fargo, N.D.)

TABLE S-34
SUNFLOWER PRODUCTS AND USES

Product	Description	Uses	Comments
		HUMAN FOODS	
Whole seed, with hulls	Whole seed may be: 1. Dehulled with fingernails or teeth and eaten raw. 2. Roasted by heating (a) in an oven for 15 min. at 350°F (*177°C*) or (b) in a frying pan while stirring. 3. Salted by— a. soaking the whole seed overnight in salt brine (2 Tbsp salt to 1 cup water), boiled for a few minutes, then dried with heat; b. boiling in brine for at least 20 min.; or c. frying the salted whole seed in edible oil.	Snack food.	Consumers prefer a large seed and kernel with a loose hull to facilitate cracking. Also, they like uniformity, and bright black and white stripes. Roasted seeds have a relatively short shelf life because of high oil content and high proportion of polyunsaturated fatty acids. Many snack foods contribute little to the diet except calories. Raw or roasted sunflower kernels, with or without salt, are nutritious. They are a valuable source of unsaturated fat, quality protein, and some vitamins and minerals. Roasted seeds are very popular in the U.S.S.R.
Whole seed, hulled	Seed dehulled commercially in an impact dehuller, following which the mixed hulls and meats are separated by screening and aspiration. Then the dehulled seed is either— 1. Marketed raw as dehulled sunflower kernels, 2. roasted in sunflower or other vegetable oil, or 3. dry roasted, salted, and vacuum packed.	Considerable attention has been given to the use of hulled seed in candies, salads, cereals, bakery goods, and health foods. As a nut substitute in a number of confectionery and bakery formulas.	Dehulled kernels must be stored under refrigeration.
Sunflower meal and flour	Sunflower meal is the product obtained by grinding the residue that remains after extraction of most of the oil from the seed. Sunflower flour is similar to sunflower meal, except that it is finer and more of the hulls have been removed. Sunflower flour has high protein content, bland flavor, and contains no antinutritive factors.	Sunflower meals and flours have not been used commercially as a protein source for human nutrition in the U.S. Experimentally, sunflower flour has been added to wheat flour at 3 to 20% levels to make breads, griddle cakes, cupcakes, pies, dips, rolls, and candies; without loss in attractiveness, volume, or acceptance, and enhanced by a pleasant distinctive, nutty flavor.	Sunflower proteins are deficient in lysine and isoleucine, but they contain adequate levels of the other essential amino acids for humans. The vitamin B complex content of defatted sunflower seed flour is superior to the products prepared from wheat germ, corn germ, and soya. A major problem in using sunflower meal in human foods is the presence of hulls and chlorogenic acid in the meal, both of which may cause undesirable discoloration. Hulls also cause excessive bulk and fiber in a food product.

(Continued)

TABLE S-34 *(Continued)*

Product	Description	Uses	Comments
		HUMAN FOODS *(Continued)*	
Sunflower oil	Oil of an attractive color and pleasant, faintly nutty flavor.	1. Cooking and salad oil. 2. In Europe, it is used extensively in shortening and margarine. 3. For frying foods, popping corn, and other culinary processes that require a liquid oil with a high smoke point. 4. For blending with other vegetable oils. 5. As a cooking fat for potato chip frying. 6. For producing a modified butter with improved low temperature spreadability.	Sunflower oil is a high-quality edible oil, high in the polyunsaturated acid linoleic acid. The oil is considered equal to olive oil and almond oil for table use. Oil from sunflowers produced in the South has a lower linoleic acid content than oil from sunflowers produced in the North; hence, it is more stable. Because of the high ratio of polyunsaturated to saturated fatty acids, sunflower oil possesses serum cholesterol-lowering abilities.
		LIVESTOCK FEEDS	
Whole seed	Cleaned whole seed.	Bird feed, for both wild and caged birds. Hamsters, squirrels, and other pets.	The Arrowhead variety is used exclusively for bird feed.
Sunflower meal, dehulled, mechanically extracted	The product obtained by grinding the residue remaining after the extraction of most of the oil from dehulled sunflower seed by a mechanical extraction process. Sunflower meal made from dehulled seed runs 41 to 50% protein.	Protein supplement for livestock.	Sunflower meal is low in lysine. Hence, when it is used in nonruminant feed, it should be combined with high-lysine supplements, such as meat scrap or fish meal. Meals with a high fat content tend to produce soft pork and soft butter if fed in large amounts. When limited to about 1/3 of the protein supplement, sunflower meal gives good results with pigs.
Sunflower meal, dehulled, solvent extracted	The product obtained by grinding the residue remaining after extraction of most of the oil from dehulled sunflower seed by a solvent extraction process.	Protein supplement for livestock.	
Sunflower meal, mechanically extracted	The product obtained by grinding the residue remaining after extraction of the oil from the whole sunflower seed by a mechanical extraction process. Sunflower meal made from whole sunflower runs about 28% protein.	Protein supplement for ruminants.	The meal remaining after extracting the oil from whole seed is too high in fiber for monogastric animals, such as the pig and horse.

(Continued)

TABLE S-34 (Continued)

Product	Description	Uses	Comments
LIVESTOCK FEEDS (Continued)			
Sunflower meal, solvent extracted	The product obtained by grinding the residue remaining after extraction of most of the oil from the whole sunflower seed by a solvent extraction process.	Protein supplement for ruminants.	
Sunflower hulls	The outer covering of sunflower seed.	Roughage for ruminants.	
Forage: Sunflower silage	Plants harvested when approximately half of the heads are in bloom, then fermented in a silo.	Ruminant feed.	Sunflower plants were formerly made into silage and used as a ruminant feed in northern U.S. and Canada, but this practice has practically disappeared. Sunflower silage is not too palatable.
OTHER USES			
Sunflower oil	The oil extracted from the seed.	Soap Drying oil in paint.	
Sunflower hulls	The outer covering of sunflower seed.	Alcohol and furfural.	
Sunflower stalks	The hairy stem of the sunflower plant.	Fuel	
Sunflower flowers	The yellow petals that surround the head.	A yellow dye.	

SUPERGLYCINERATED FATS

These are mono- and diglycerides which are the products of interesterification. They are employed as emulsifiers by the food industry.

(Also see ADDITIVES; and INTERESTERIFICATION.)

SUPEROXIDE DISMUTASE (SOD)

An enzyme contained in most cells of the body and in most organisms. It catalyzes the breakdown of superoxide free radicals—oxygen joined by an extra electron—to oxygen and hydrogen peroxide. This protects cells from the toxic effects of oxygen, since these superoxide radicals damage DNA, and age and destroy cells. Deactivation of these superoxide radicals is called dismutation; hence, the name superoxide dismutase. Some chemicals, poor nutrition, shock, and radiation therapy may increase the formation of superoxide radicals. Scientists feel that gaining an understanding of this enzyme may unlock secrets which (1) control the rate of human aging, (2) block tumor formation, and (3) maintain the body's immune system. As an injectable drug, SOD could be used to fight inflammatory diseases. Currently, the FDA has approved SOD for use by veterinarians. Human use is for investigational purposes only. Several European nations permit its use for rheumatoid arthritis, osteoarthritis, urological disorders, and the side effects of radiation treatment. However, in the United States, some health-food stores and mail order businesses sell SOD as a compound to reverse aging and degeneration. Currently, no firm evidence demonstrates that taking SOD will increase the life span.

(Also see ENZYME.)

SUPPLEMENTS

Food supplements are foodstuffs used to improve the value of basal foods.

(Also see NUTRITIONAL SUPPLEMENTS.)

SURFACE AREA

The area covered by the exterior of cubes, spheres and cylinders is fairly easy to calculate. However, the area covered by the exterior of the body is not quite as easy to figure due to the variety of body shapes, heights, and weights. Charts and mathematical formulas are available for determining body surface area in relationship to height and weight. It is the body surface area which determines heat loss from the body and therefore basal metabolism is correlated to surface area.

(Also see BASAL METABOLIC RATE; BODY SURFACE; and METABOLIC RATE.)

SURFACTANT (SURFACE ACTIVE AGENT)

Surface tension is that inward force acting on the surface of a liquid. It is an effect of the forces of attraction existing between the molecules below the surface. Water has a high surface tension compared to alcohol, and mercury has the highest surface tension of any known liquid. The surface tension of a liquid is related to (1) the tendency of a liquid to spread or wet a solid surface, and (2) the ability of a liquid to blend with other liquids. Hence, surface tension plays a role in a variety of processes; for example, emulsification, bubble formation, fabric cleaning, foams, and adhesives. Surface active agents or surfactants reduce the surface tension of a liquid, thereby increasing the wetting or blending ability. There are three categories of surfactants: (1) detergents, (2) wetting

agents, and (3) emulsifiers. A variety of surfactants are employed as food additives by the food industry.

(Also see ADDITIVES.)

SURINAM CHERRY *Eugenia uniflora*

This is another name for the Brazilian cherry.

(Also see BRAZILIAN CHERRY.)

SWEETBREADS (THYMUS GLAND)

The sweetbreads, which are considered to be the most delicate of the variety meats, are located in the neck area of young bovines (veal); as the animal matures, they disappear.

SWEETENING AGENTS

Sweet is a taste sensation—a pleasurable sensation for which man relies upon for his food selection. To satisfy his desire to stimulate the sweet taste sensation, man discovered honey bees, learned to keep bees, and then cultivated sugarcane and sugar beets. Still, man searches for sweet tasting substances. Primarily the search is for a low-calorie or no-calorie substance which satisfies the taste sensation and is safe to eat.

There are over 200 chemicals known to taste sweet, but many sweet-tasting chemicals present problems such as bitter aftertaste, lack of stability, and toxicity. For the individual or the company that discovers a sweet-tasting, low-calorie (no calorie), safe compound, a pot of gold awaits, since there are many people who wish or need to limit their intake of sugar. Not just table sugar (sucrose) but the intake of monosaccharides such as glucose and fructose need to be controlled by diabetic individuals and individuals cutting down on calorie—energy—intake. Any new sweetener should (1) possess a flavor that is clean and without aftertaste, (2) be made for a price competitive with sugar (sucrose) on a cost-per-sweetness basis, (3) be adequately soluble and stable, and (4) be subjected to and pass the lengthy and costly program of rigorous safety testing required by the U.S. Food and Drug Administration. Very few meet all of these requirements. Table S-35 lists chemicals which are, have been, or possibly may be sweetening agents.

TABLE S-35
SWEETENING AGENTS

Name	Chemical Structure	Sweet-ness[1]	Calories	Classi-fication	Uses	Comments
Acesul-fame-K (sold under brand Sunette)		130	(kcal/g) 0	Nonnutri-tive; arti-ficial.	As a tabletop sweetener, chewing gum, dry beverage mixes and puddings.	This is actually the potassium salt of the 6-methyl derivative of a group of chemicals called oxathiazinone dioxides. Approved by the FDA in 1988.
Aspartame (Also see ASPAR-TAME.)		180	4	Nutritive; artificial.	It is in most diet sodas. Also, used in cold cereals, drink mixes, gelatin, puddings, toppings, dairy products, and at the table by the consumer; not used in cooking due to lack of stability when heated.	Composed of the two naturally occurring amino acids, aspartic acid and phenylalanine; results of a serendipitous discovery by a scientist at G. D. Searle and Company, who gained the FDA's approval for marketing; sweeter than sugar, therefore less required, hence fewer calories. Aspartame was introduced in 1981. In 1991, it had 75% of the sweetener market.
Cyclamate		30	0	Nonnutri-tive; arti-ficial.	Used as a tabletop sweetener and in drugs in Canada and 40 other countries.	Discovered in 1937. FDA banned all cyclamate-containing beverages in 1969, and all cyclamate-containing foods in 1970, because of cyclamate being carcinogen in some rat studies. Cyclamate is now being reevaluated by the FDA.
Dulcin (4-ethoxy-phenyl-urea)		250	0	Nonnutri-tive; arti-ficial.	None	Not approved for food use in the United States; used in some European countries. Also called Sucrol and Valzin
Fructose (levulose)		1.7	4	Nutritive; natural.	Beverages, baking, canned goods; anywhere invert sugar or honey may be used.	A carbohydrate; a monosaccharide; naturally occurs in fruits; makes up about 50% of the sugar in honey; commercially found in high-fructose syrups and invert sugars; contributes sweetness and prevents crystallization.

Footnote at end of table

(Continued)

TABLE S-35 (Continued)

Name	Chemical Structure	Sweetness[1]	Calories	Classification	Uses	Comments
Glucose (dextrose) (Also see GLUCOSE; and STARCH.)		.7	(kcal/g) 4	Nutritive; natural.	Primarily in the confection, wine, and canning industries; and in intravenous solutions	Glucose is "blood sugar"— the fuel for the cells of the body. It is commercially produced from the conversion of starch (cornstarch) by the action of heat and acids, or enzymes; glucose in corn syrup may be enzymatically converted to fructose, yielding a high-fructose syrup. Glucose acts synergistically with other sweeteners.
Glycine		.8	4	Nutritive; natural.	Permissible to use to modify taste of some foods.	A sweet-tasting amino acid. Tryptophan is also a sweet-tasting amino acid.
Mannitol (Also see MANNITOL.)		.7	2	Nutritive; natural.	Candies, chewing gums, confections, and baked goods; dietetic foods.	A sugar alcohol or polyhydric alcohol (polyol); occurs naturally in pineapples, olives, asparagus, and carrots; commercially prepared by the hydrogenation of mannose or glucose; slowly and incompletely absorbed from the intestines; only slightly metabolized, most excreted unchanged in the urine; may cause diarrhea
Miraculin	Glycoprotein; molecular weight about 44,000.	—	4	Nutritive; natural.	None	Actually a taste-modifying protein rather than a sweetener; after exposing tongue to miraculin sour lemon tastes like sweetened lemon; responsible for the taste changing properties of miracle fruit, red berries of *Synsepalum dulcificum*, a native plant of West Africa; first described in 1852; one attempt made to commercialize by a U.S. firm but FDA denied approval and marketing was stopped.

Footnote at end of table

(Continued)

TABLE S-35 *(Continued)*

Name	Chemical Structure	Sweet-ness[1]	Calo-ries	Classi-fication	Uses	Comments
			(kcal/g)			
Monellin	Protein; molecular weight about 10,700; about 91 amino acids.	3,000	4	Nutritive; natural.	None; only a potential low-calorie sweetener.	Extract of the pulp of the light red berries of the tropical plant *Dioscoreophyllum cumminsii*; also called Serendipity Berry; first protein found to elicit a sweet taste in man; first extracted in 1969; potential use limited by lack of stability; taste sensation is slow and lingering; everything tastes sweet after monellin
Neohes-peridin dihy-drocha-lone (Neo DHC, NDHC)		1,250	0	Nonnutri-tive; arti-ficial.	None approved; potential for chewing gum, mouthwash, and toothpaste.	Formed from naringen isolated from citrus fruit; slow to elicit the taste sensation; lingering licoricelike aftertaste; animal studies indicate not toxic.
P-4,000 (5-nitro-2-pro-poxyan-iline)		4,100	0	Nonnutri-tive; arti-ficial.	None approved.	Derivative of nitroaniline; used as a sweetener in some European countries but banned in the United States due to toxic effects on rats; no bitter aftertaste; major drawback of P-4,000 is powerful local anesthetic effect on the tongue and mouth. Used in the Netherlands during German occupation and during Berlin blockade
Phyllodul-cin		250	—	Natural	None approved.	Isolated from *Hydrangea macrophylla Seringe* in 1916; displays a lagging onset of sweetness with licorice aftertaste; not well studied; possible market for hard candies, chewing gums, and oral hygiene products

Footnote at end of table

(Continued)

TABLE S-35 *(Continued)*

Name	Chemical Structure	Sweet-ness[1]	Calo-ries	Classi-fication	Uses	Comments
Saccharin (*O* ben-zosul-fimide (Also see CANCER; and SAC-CHARIN.)		500	(kcal/g) 0	Nonnutri-tive; arti-ficial.	Used in beverages, as a tabletop sweetener, and in cosmetics, toothpaste, and cough syrup. Used as a sweetener by diabetics.	Both sodium and calcium salts of saccharin used; passes through body unchanged; ex-creted in urine; origin-ally a generally recog-nized as safe (GRAS) additive. Subsequently, saccharin was classed as a carcinogen based on experiments with rats. However, recent ex-periments indicate that saccharine causes cancer in rats, but not in mice and people.
Sorbitol (Also see SOR-BITOL.)	CH₂OH | HCOH | HOCH | HCOH | HCOH | CH₂OH	.6	4	Nutritive; natural.	Chewing gum, dairy products, meat prod-ucts, icings, toppings, and beverages.	A sugar alcohol or poly-hydric alcohol (polyol); occurs natu-rally in many fruits; commercially pre-pared by the hydrogenation of glu-cose; many unique properties besides sweetness; on the FDA list of generally recognized as safe (GRAS) food addi-tives; the most widely used sugar alcohol; slow intestinal absorption; consump-tion of large amounts may cause diarrhea
SRI Oxime V (Perilla sugar)		450	0	Nonnutri-tive; arti-ficial.	None approved.	Derived from extract of *Perilla namkinensis*; clean taste; needs research; used as sweetening agent in Japan.

Footnote at end of table

(Continued)

TABLE S-35 *(Continued)*

Name	Chemical Structure	Sweet-ness[1]	Calo-ries	Classi-fication	Uses	Comments
Stevioside		300	(kcal/ g) 4	Nutritive; natural.	None approved.	Isolated from the leaves of the wild shrub, *Stevia rebaudiana Bertoni*; used by the people of Paraguay to sweeten drinks; limited evidence suggests non-toxic to humans; Japanese interested in developing. Rebaudioside A is isolated from the same plant, and it is said to taste superior to stevioside. Its chemical structure is very similar to stevioside and it is 190 times sweeter than sugar.
Sucrose (brown sugar, liquid sugar, sugar, table sugar, white sugar) (Also see SUGAR.)		1.0	4	Nutritive; natural.	Many beverages and processed foods; home use in a wide variety of foods.	The chemical combination of the sugars fructose and glucose; one of the oldest sweetening agents; most popular and most available sweetening agent; occurs naturally in many fruits; commercially extracted from sugarcane and sugar beets; per capita yearly consumption about 100 lb (45.5 kg); health concern primarily excessive calories and tooth decay

Footnote at end of table

(Continued)

TABLE S-35 *(Continued)*

Name	Chemical Structure	Sweet-ness[1]	Calo-ries	Classi-fication	Uses	Comments
Thauma-tins	Proteins; molecular weight about 21,000	1,600	(kcal/g) 4	Nutritive; natural.	None	Source of sweetness of the tropical fruit from the plant *Thaumato-coccus daniellii*; enjoyed by inhabit-ants of western Africa; doubtful commercial appli-cations.
Xylitol (Also see XYLITOL.)	CH₂OH | HOCH | HCOH | HOCH | CH₂OH	.8	4	Nutritive; natural.	Chewing gums and dietetic foods.	A sugar alcohol or poly-hydric alcohol (polyol); occurs natu-rally in some fruits and vegetables; pro-duced in the body; commercial produc-tion from plant parts (oat hulls, corncobs, and birch wood chips) containing xylans—long chains of the sugar xylose; can possibly contrib-ute to reduction in tooth decay; possible diarrhea; one British study suggests xylitol causes cancer in animals.

[1]Relative to sucrose, table sugar, which is assigned the value of 1.0.

The search for sweetening agents will continue, since there are so many individuals who wish to "have their cake and eat it too," providing a large market for any new low-calorie sweetener. Within a few years, dieters may be able to choose from many new sweeteners; among them, Alitame, which can be used in baking; Sweetener 2000, with no calories and 10,000 times as sweet as sugar; Sucralose, which is derived from ordinary table sugar.

Whatever the product, the cost, time, and effort getting it to market will be tremendous due to the rigorous re-quirements of the Food and Drug Administration.

(Also see CARBOHYDRATE[S], section headed "Flavor"; and SUGAR.)

SWEET POTATO *Ipomoea batatas*

This tropical plant, which forms nutritious tubers, is the third leading vegetable crop of the world. (Irish potatoes and cassava rank first and second, respectively, as the leading vegetables of the world.) The sweet potato is a member of the morning glory family (*Convolvulaceae*). Fig. S-79 shows a typical sweet potato plant.

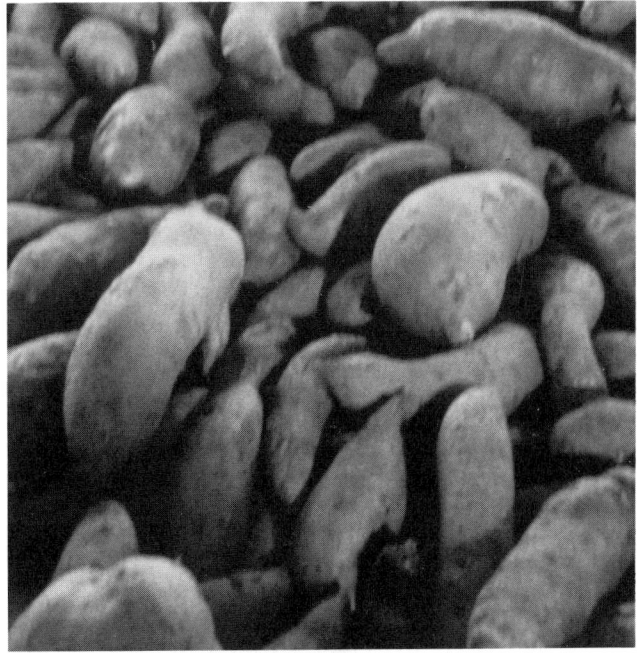

Fig. S-79. Sweet potatoes. (Courtesy, USDA)

ORIGIN AND HISTORY.
Remains of sweet potatoes estimated to be between 10,000 and 12,000 years old were found in a cave in Peru. However, it is not certain whether the ancient tubers had grown wild or been cultivated. The present form of the plant does not grow wild. Hence, it is suspected that these historic sweet potatoes were a hybrid of a wild ancestor which originated somewhere between Mexico and northern South America.

The means by which sweet potatoes spread from Latin America to Polynesia is not known, although it is now fairly certain that they were grown on the South Pacific islands before Columbus discovered America.

Columbus took sweet potatoes from the Caribbean with him when he returned home after discovering America. Shortly thereafter, the English imported the tubers from Spain, because King Henry VIII had acquired a taste for spiced and sweetened sweet potato pie. Also, the English colonists of Virginia grew the crop. Therefore, it is not surprising that cakes and pies made from the tubers are relished by many people of British ancestry now living in southeastern United States.

Other notable spread of the sweet potato during the 16th century involved (1) their transport to Guam and the Philippines by the Spanish, and (2) the carrying of them eastward from the Americas to Africa, India, Southeast Asia, and Indonesia by the Portuguese. By the end of the century, the Chinese had obtained them from the Philippines.

The ease with which high yields of the tuber are produced in warm, humid areas has led to its worldwide cultivation. In many places it has been used for feeding both people and livestock. Commercial sweet potato processing began in the United States near the end of the last century when the mashed cooked tubers were canned. By the late 1930s it was found that varieties which usually became mushy during processing retained their firmness when canned whole in syrup. World War II created a great demand for dehydrated sweet potatoes which led to the establishment of many processers in the South. However, the demand slackened after the end of the war since the canned product had superior characteristics. Nevertheless, research on sweet potato utilization continues, because (1) new varieties which grow in colder climates have been developed in recent years, and (2) high yields of tubers are obtained from this crop.

PRODUCTION.
About 132 million metric tons of sweet potatoes are produced worldwide each year. Fig. S-80 shows the amounts contributed by the ten top producers.

Although the United States produces less than 0.5% of the world's sweet potatoes, the tuber is still an important vegetable crop in certain southern states. Fig. S-81 shows the amounts produced in the states.

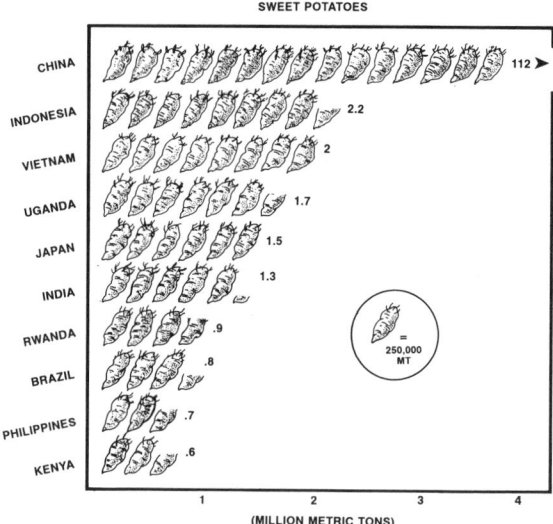

Fig. S-80. The leading sweet-potato-producing countries of the world. (Based upon data from *FAO Production Yearbook*, 1990, FAO/UN, Rome, Italy, Vol. 44, p. 92, Table 27)

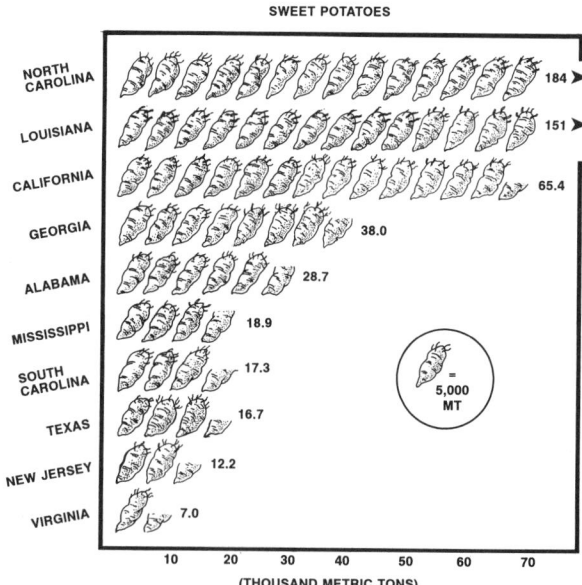

Fig. S-81. The leading sweet-potato-producing states. (Based upon data from *Agricultural Statistics 1991*, USDA, p. 164, Table 237)

Sweet potatoes are propagated vegetatively by planting either (1) plants or sprouts grown from tubers of the previous crop, or (2) cuttings from the vines of the plant. The former method is used mainly in temperate regions with short growing seasons, whereas the latter one is utilized in warm, subtropical areas such as the southern states of the United States and in the tropical countries.

The plant requires a frostfree growing period of at least

4 months and warm nights for most of that time. Also, it grows best in areas which have 4 in. (*10 cm*) or more of rainfall each month of the growing season, or where an equivalent amount of irrigation water is used. The soil should be well drained, slightly to moderately acid, and rich in mineral content. Sandy soils may require fertilization with nitrogen, phosphorus, and potassium. However, the addition of large amounts of nitrogenous fertilizer

should be avoided in order not to overstimulate the growth of the vines at the expense of the tubers.

Sweet potatoes have the highest yields and the best eating quality when they are harvested at full maturity. However, tubers grown in regions with short growing seasons must be dug with the arrival of the first weather that is cold enough to damage or kill the vines, because once the vines are dead the tubers usually decay rapidly. Sweet potatoes should be dug carefully to avoid injuries to the protective skin, since the inner part of the tuber is highly susceptible to darkening and decay. Furthermore, the handling after harvesting should be kept to a minimum for the same reason. The average yield of tubers in the United States is 11,600 lb per acre (*12,992 kg/ha*), but yields in California of about 16,000 lb per acre (*17,920 kg/ha*) are obtained. Even higher yields (22,000 lb per acre, or *24,640 kg/ha*) are obtained on the South Pacific island of Niue, and in parts of Africa.

PROCESSING. Tubers which are to be stored keep better if they are cured after harvesting. Curing consists of holding the sweet potatoes in a facility where the temperature is about 85°F (*30°C*) and the relative humidity is about 85%. These conditions promote the healing of small wounds in the tubers. Even with careful curing, the spoilage of sweet potatoes after 7 months of storage ranges from a low of about 20% to a high of about 80%. Hence, various other means of processing have been developed, the most common of which follow:

• **Canning**—This process is used mainly for small whole tubers or cut pieces of larger tubers, which are first cooked, then packed in syrup. Only small amounts of canned sweet potato puree are produced, most of which is packed in glass jars by baby food manufacturers.

• **Dehydration**—The sun-drying of raw sweet potato chips or slices has long been one of the major means of preservation utilized in the developing countries of the tropics. However, dehydration in the United States usually involves the drum drying of a puree made from the cooked tubers. The retail market for this type of product is limited because most people use either fresh or canned sweet potatoes. Nevertheless, the dried powder is used by the armed forces, in school lunch programs, and by bakers who produce sweet potato cakes and pies.

• **Gelling**—Processors in Argentina mix cooked sweet potato pulp with sugar and a gelling agent such as agar or an Irish moss derivative to make a very firm gel. American food technologists have produced similar products, including a powdered mix which may be rehydrated by adding water and heating, but little has been done to market these products in the United States.

• **Starch, sugar, and syrup production**—This process is most important in Japan, where sweet potatoes rank second only to rice. Starch is extracted by washing the pulp of ground tubers on a series of fine mesh screens. Then, the starch is separated from the wash water by centrifugation or settling. The spent pulp which remains on the screens is dried and used as a livestock feed ingredient. However, superior vegetable starches are usually available for most commercial uses. Hence, much of the sweet potato starch is processed further into sugars and syrups by cooking with one or more enzymes.

SELECTION. There are two general types of sweet potatoes. One type has soft, moist flesh when cooked and a high sugar content (sweet potatoes of this type are commonly, but incorrectly, called yams). The second type, when cooked, has a firm, dry, somewhat mealy flesh, which is usually light yellow or pale-orange in color, as contrasted to the usually deeper-yellow or distinctly orange-red colored flesh of the moist type. The skin of the dry type is usually light yellowish-tan or fawn-colored, while the skin of the moist-fleshed varieties may vary in color from whitish-tan to brownish-red. Varieties of each type vary considerably in shape, but most moist-fleshed varieties are usually more plump in shape than most dry-fleshed varieties. A mixture of types or a mixture of varieties within types is undesirable because of lack of uniformity in cooking, as well as differences in flavor and color of flesh.

Best quality sweet potatoes are clean, smooth, well-shaped, firm and bright in appearance.

Seriously misshapen sweet potatoes and those showing growth cracks or wireworm injury are apt to be undesirable because of the waste entailed in preparation for use. A damp appearance may indicate decay in an adjacent tuber. Decay in sweet potatoes usually progresses and spreads very rapidly and generally imparts a disagreeable flavor to apparently unaffected flesh even if the decayed portion is removed before cooking. Decay may appear as a soft wet rot frequently accompanied by mold growth, or as discolored, shriveled or sunken areas of dry rot. The ends of the tubers are most frequently affected, although decay often develops in other areas. Another type of decay occasionally appears as greenish-black variable-sized circular spots. If occurring in bruised or injured areas, such spots may be irregular rather than circular in outline.

PREPARATION. Many people like sweet potatoes prepared with a sweetener such as honey, molasses, sugar, or a syrup. However, the yam type of tuber provides much of its own sweetening when it is cooked slowly, because it contains an enzyme (beta-amylase) that converts starch to maltose and dextrins. Heating the tuber activates the enzyme, which is eventually inactivated when the internal temperature becomes too high. Prior to cooking, the tubers should be scrubbed well with a vegetable brush so that they may be cooked with the skins intact. Removal of the skin before cooking may result in darkening of the flesh. Also, the skins loosen and are easier to remove after cooking.

Sweet potatoes may be cooked in much the same ways as Irish potatoes, but they require only about half as much cooking time. In addition, they are good in casseroles when accompanied by apple slices or pineapple rings and seasoned with spices such as allspice and cinnamon. Finally, mashed cooked sweet potato may be used to make biscuits, breads, cakes, cookies, custards, muffins, and pies.

NUTRITIONAL VALUE. The nutrient compositions of various forms of sweet potatoes are given in Food Composition Table F-36.

Some noteworthy observations regarding the nutrient composition of sweet potatoes follow:

1. Compared to cooked Irish potatoes, cooked sweet potatoes contain about an equal number of calories, less protein and vitamin C, and much more vitamin A—they are one of the leading plant sources of the latter vitamin.

2. A 1-cup serving (*about 9 oz or 225 g*) of mashed cooked sweet potatoes provides 275 Calories (kcal) and 5 g of protein, which is almost double the calories and about equal to the protein furnished by a cup of a cooked cereal such as corn or rice.

3. Candied sweet potatoes supply almost 50% more calories than the unsweetened cooked tubers.

Protein Quantity And Quality. Some of the people living in certain tropical countries may depend upon sweet potatoes for most of their dietary protein. But when the vegetable makes up most of the diet, the quantity and quality of protein is barely adequate to meet the needs of adults, and is inadequate for the needs of children. Fortunately, many tropical peoples supplement their diets with small amounts of protein-rich foods such as fish, legumes, and wild game.

(Also see VEGETABLE[S], Table V-6 Vegetables of the World.)

SWEETSOP (SUGAR APPLE) *Annona squamosa*

The fruit of a small tree (of the family *Annonaceae*) that is native to the American tropics. The yellowish-green heart-shaped fruit are 3 to 4 in. (*8 to 10 cm*) in diameter, white, and have a sweet granular custardlike pulp. They are used as a dessert fruit, and are closely related to the other *Annona* species of fruit (the most common ones are the cherimoya, custard apple, and soursop). Their flavor is best when fully ripe, a stage at which the fruit is very perishable.

The nutrient composition of sweetsop (sugar apple) is given in Food Composition Table F-36.

Some noteworthy observations regarding the nutrient composition of sweetsop follow:

1. The raw fruit is moderately high in calories (94 kcal per 100 g) and carbohydrates (24%).

2. Sugar apples are a good source of fiber, potassium, and vitamin C, and a fair source of iron.

(Also see FRUIT[S], Table F-47 Fruits of the World.)

SWISS CHARD (CHARD) *Beta vulgaris,* **var** *cicla*

This vegetable is a variety of beet which was developed for its large fleshy leaves rather than for its roots. Chard, like the red beet, sugar beet, and spinach, is a member of the Goosefoot family (*Chenopodiaceae*). Fig. S-82 shows a cluster of swiss chard leaves.

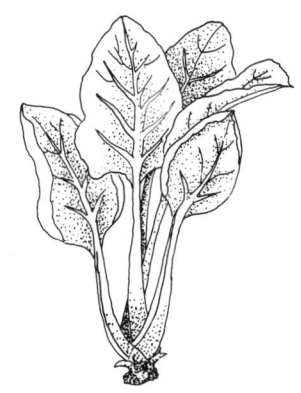

Fig. S-82. Swiss chard, a green leafy vegetable which resembles spinach, but has a milder flavor.

ORIGIN AND HISTORY. It is suspected that Swiss chard was developed from the wild beet which is native to the shores of the Mediterranean. The people who developed this plant apparently sought succulent leaves, rather than the roots which were produced by the red and white varieties of beets. In the 4th century B.C., the Greek writers Aristotle and Theophrastus described varieties of Swiss chard that were dark green, light green, or red. Somewhat later, the Roman naturalist Pliny (23 to 79 A.D.) described a variety which was grown for its long, heavy stems. Eventually, the plant was grown throughout Europe, where it is now highly regarded.

PRODUCTION. Statistics on the production of chard are not readily available. However, it appears that it is more widely grown in Europe than in the United States.

Chard does better in hot weather than most of the other popular green leafy vegetables. The other greens tend to go to seed in the summer. Therefore, it is planted in the spring so that it may be harvested throughout the summer and in the fall until the first hard frost. The vegetable is also grown during the winter in greenhouses. Fertilizer is usually applied to the crop to insure optimal production.

The leaves are harvested while they are still young and tender by cutting them off at 1 to 2 in. (*3 to 5 cm*) from the ground, while taking care not to injure the crowns of the plant. Intact crowns will continue to bear leaves to replace those which have been removed.

PROCESSING. Little or no chard is processed; it is used mainly as a fresh green vegetable. However, it may be canned or frozen like spinach.

SELECTION AND PREPARATION. Chard stalks should be fleshy and turgid, with leaves which are fresh, tender, crisp, and free from insect injury. Wilted stalks may be tough, coarse, and stringy. Yellowed leaves or discolored stalks indicate aging or other injury. Coarse stalks indicate pithiness.

Some varieties of chard have unusually large stems which require longer cooking than the more tender leaf blades. In such cases, the stems and blades of the leaves should be cooked separately. The cooked leaves are good in soups and stir-fried dishes, or they may be served with butter, margarine, or a cheese sauce.

NUTRITIONAL VALUE. The nutrient compositions of raw and cooked chard are given in Food Composition Table F-36.

Some noteworthy observations regarding the nutrient composition of chard follow:

1. Chard has a high water content (91 to 94%) and is low in calories. It is an excellent source of magnesium, iron, potassium, and vitamin A; a good source of vitamin C when raw; and a fair to good source of calcium. Cooking destroys about half of the vitamin C and causes minerals and vitamins to be leached into the cooking water. Therefore, only a minimum of water should be used in cooking, and the cooking water should be utilized whenever it is feasible.

2. The protein-to-calorie ratio (9.6 g per 100 kcal) of chard is about equal to that of skim milk. Hence, significant amounts of dietary protein may be supplied by this vegetable, if sufficiently large quantities are consumed. For example, 2 ¾ cups (*660 ml*) of cooked chard furnish the calories, protein, and calcium content of a cup (*240 ml*) of skim milk.

(Also see VEGETABLE[S], Table V-6 Vegetables of the World.)

SYMPTOM

A complaint by patients which may lead them to seek medical advice.

SYN-

Prefix meaning with, or together.

SYNDROME

A combination of symptoms occurring together.

SYNERGISM

The joint action of agents in which their combined effect is greater than the sum of their separate actions; each agent enhances the action of the other.

SYNTHESIS

The process of building up a chemical compound by a reaction or a series of reactions.

SYNTHETIC

An artificially produced product that may be similar to the natural product.

SYRUPS

Although there is a large variety of syrups, they all contain sugar and water. There are those syrups which come from sources used to manufacture sugar and glucose, such as corn syrup, maple syrup, molasses, and sorghum syrup. Specialty syrups can be created from sugar, water, and a variety of flavors such as almond, cherry, chocolate, currant, orange, strawberry, and other fruit flavors. Plain sugar and water syrups are used for canning fruits. Also, syrup serves as a carrier of medicines as in cough syrup.

(Also see CARBOHYDRATE[S], section headed "Sources"; MAPLE SYRUP; MOLASSES; SORGHUM; and SUGAR.)

SYSTEMIC

Pertaining to the body as a whole, as distinguished from local.

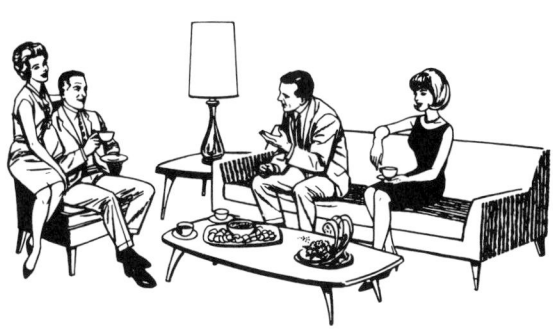

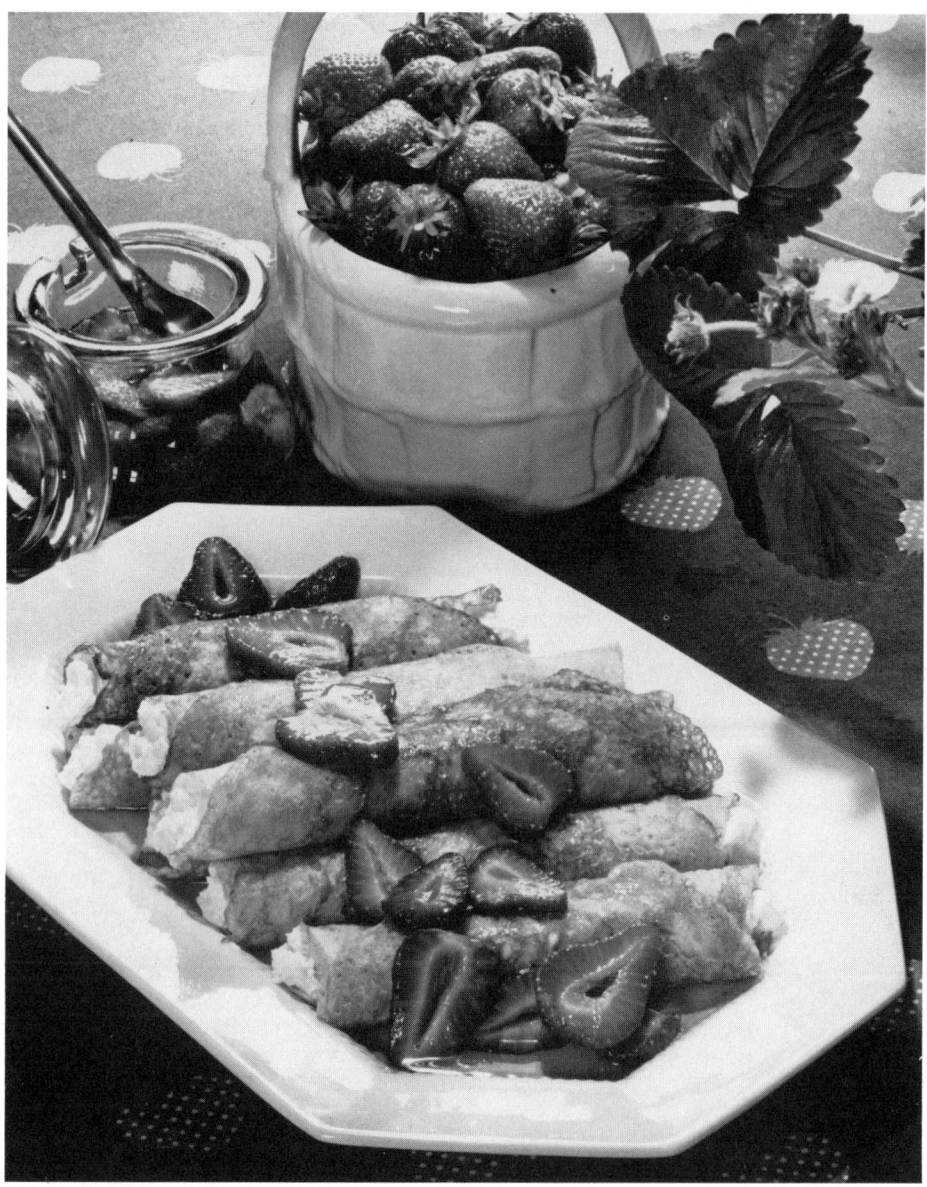

The complete strawberry crepe—an elegant dessert created to dazzle. (Courtesy, California Strawberry Advisory Board)

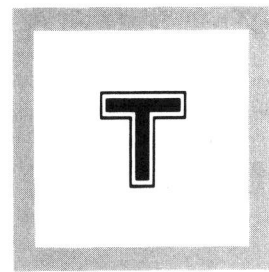

TACHYCARDIA

An abnormally rapid heart beat, faster than 100 beats per minute. It occurs during exercise, in fevers, in certain heart conditions, and in a number of diseases.

TALLOW

The fat extracted from adipose tissue of cattle and sheep.
(Also see FATS and OTHER LIPIDS.)

TANGELO

This name is applied to hybrids of the mandarin orange (*Citrus reticulata*) with either the grapefruit (*Citrus paradisi*) or the pummelo (*Citrus grandis*). Mandarin oranges hybridize easily. Usually, these fruits have the loose skins and sweetness of the mandarin, but the ugli fruit is a tangelo which more closely resembles the grapefruit.

Most of the U.S. crop of tangelos is grown in Florida, where each year about 132,000 tons (*118,800 metric tons*) are produced. The production techniques, processing, and preparation of tangelos are similar to that of the mandarin orange and other citrus fruits.

The nutrient composition of the most common form of tangelo is given in Food Composition Table F-36. It contains only 23 Calories (kcal) per 100 g; and it is a good source of potassium and a fair source of vitamin C.
(Also see CITRUS FRUITS; and MANDARIN ORANGE.)

TANNIA (YAUTIA; MALANGA; COCOYAM)
Xanthosoma sagittifolium

This plant of the aroid family (Araceae) yields edible leaves and tubers. However, it is sometimes confused with taro (another aroid plant) because of certain similar characteristics. Fig. T-1 shows a typical tannia plant.

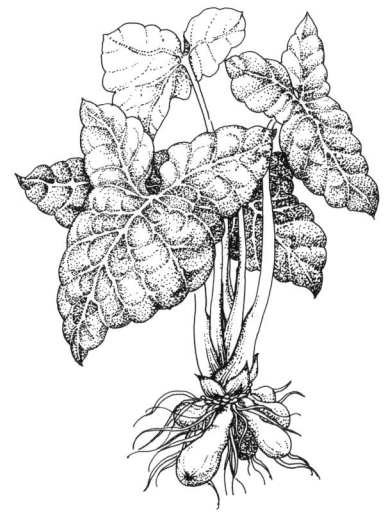

Fig. T-1. Tannia, a tuber-bearing plant from tropical America.

The various names given to the plant are also responsible for cases of mistaken identity. Therefore, some definitions of the more common names follow:

• **Tannia and Yautia**—These common names designate all varieties of the species *X. sagittifolium*.

• **Malanga**—This Latin American name is often applied to tannia, but it may also refer to similar tuberous plants of different species.

• **Cocoyam**—Some people give this general name to various tuberous plants grown alongside cocoa (*Theobroma cacao*) to provide shade for the young plants. Africans distinguish between tannia and taro by calling the former the "new" cocoyam, and the latter the "old" cocoyam.

Only the name tannia will be used in the remainder of this article.

ORIGIN AND HISTORY. Tannia is native to the tropical region which extends from northern South America to the West Indies. It was brought to Africa during the days of slave trading, and to the South Pacific within the past century. Since its introduction into new lands, tannia has become increasingly important at the expense of other similar tubers such as taro, because it is more resistant to certain diseases and pests. Furthermore, the Africans have found that it is one of the most satisfactory substitutes for yams in the preparation of their traditional dish *fufu*.

PRODUCTION. Data regarding the worldwide production of tannia are not readily available since most of the crop is consumed in the areas where it is produced. However, it is known that the major producing areas are the West Indies and other parts of the American tropics, West Africa, and the tropical islands in the southwestern Pacific.

Tannia is propagated by planting either (1) the crowns of large tubers or (2) small whole tubers. The plant requires abundant moisture and warm weather. Hence, its production is limited to the humid tropics. Some of the tubers are ready for harvesting in about 9 months after planting. This is done by carefully digging the soil around the base of the plant and removing the mature tubers, then replacing the soil around the immature tubers so that they will continue to grow. The highest yields of tubers are obtained in Trinidad, where the best varieties produce from 27,000 to 29,000 lb per acre (*30,240 to 32,480 kg/ha*). It is noteworthy that the tubers may be stored for several weeks without refrigeration, and for more than 4 months at 45°F (7°C) and a relative humidity of 80%. Fig. T-2 shows freshly harvested tubers.

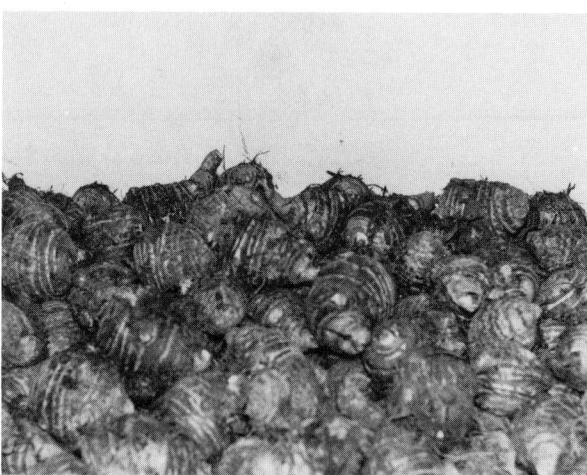

Fig. T-2. Tannia (malanga) tubers in a Cuban market. (Photo by Mrs. Audrey Ensminger)

PROCESSING. There is little commercial processing of tannia, although starch may be extracted from the tubers by grating them and washing the pulp on a fine screen.

PREPARATION. In West Africa tannia is used to prepare *fufu*, a pasty dough made by mashing boiled peeled tubers. People in other tropical areas of the world use the plant in much the same ways as they have long used cassava, taro, and yams. For example, the tubers may be baked, boiled, fried, or roasted; and the cooked young leaves may be used as a green vegetable.

CAUTION: Neither tannia roots nor tannia leaves should be consumed without cooking them thoroughly because some varieties contain high levels of calcium oxalate crystals, which are very irritating to the digestive system. The latter possibility may be alleviated by boiling the roots or leaves for about 15 minutes in water containing a small amount of baking soda (sodium bicarbonate), discarding the used water, rinsing the vegetable thoroughly, and boiling again in clear water.

Based on studies that have been made with both people and pigs, however, it would seem to require a rather improbable combination of circumstances—a very high intake of calcium oxalate-containing food plus a simultaneously low calcium and vitamin D intake over a prolonged period—for chronic toxic effects to be noted.[1]

NUTRITIONAL VALUE. The nutrient compositions of various forms of tannia are given in Food Composition Table F-36. Note that—

1. Compared to Irish potatoes, tannia tubers furnish about twice as many calories, the same amount of protein, and less than half as much vitamin C. The protein to calorie ratio (1.6 g per 100 kcal) of the tubers is barely high enough to meet the protein requirements of adults. So, children fed a tannia-rich diet are likely to develop protein-energy malnutrition unless they are given supplemental protein foods in their diets. Finally, tannia tubers are deficient in many vitamins and minerals.

2. Tannia leaves are nutritionally superior to the tubers with respect to protein, calcium, phosphorus, iron, vitamin A, and vitamin C. They are an excellent source of vitamin A. Hence, they compensate for most of the nutritional deficiencies of the tuber. However, the leaves may contain much higher levels of highly irritating calcium oxalate crystals than the tubers. Therefore, the leaves should not be consumed raw by people or livestock, unless it is certain that they contain little or no oxalates. The leaves may be rendered safe by boiling.

TANNINS

This refers to a complex group of chemicals which occurs naturally in many plants. They are responsible for the astringent taste of coffee and tea. Tannic acid, a commercial tannin, is used widely in industry.

[1]Strong, Frank M., Chairman, Subcommittee on Naturally Occurring Toxicants In Foods, *Toxicants Occurring Naturally in Foods*, National Academy of Sciences, 1973, p. 358.

TAPIOCA

This is a starch derived from the roots of the tropical cassava plant. It is extracted by washing, peeling, and grinding the roots to fine pulp which is passed over a series of screens to remove root fibers. In some processes it may be further refined in settling basins or centrifuges. The moist starchy mass is dried; and, during the drying process, it forms small, uneven milky white balls known as pearl tapioca. High grade tapioca has a brilliant white color.

Tapioca is used like starch from other sources. It swells and thickens the liquid in which it is cooked. It is used in its natural state, as well as in modified and pregelatinized versions like other starches. The most familiar use of tapioca is the popular pudding which contains small lumps or granules. Special cooking, grinding, and screening methods produce this type of tapioca. Pearl tapioca requires prior soaking and yields larger lumps in puddings.

(Also see CASSAVA; FLOURS, Table F-26 Special Flours; and STARCH.)

TAPIOCA-MACARONI

A product developed in India. It may be a mixture (1) of 80 to 90 parts of tapioca flour and 10 to 20 parts peanut flour; or (2) of 60 parts of tapioca, 15 parts peanut, and 25 parts semolina. It is baked into shapes resembling rice grains or macaroni.

TARO (COCOYAM; DASHEEN; EDDOE) *Colocasia esculenta.*

This tropical, tuber-bearing plant of the arum family (*Araceae*) is designated by various common names in different parts of the world. Hence, some designations that are adapted from a leading authority[2] follow:

- **Taro**—This common name designates (1) all varieties of the species *C. esculenta*, and (2) the starchy material obtained from the tubers of this species.

- **Cocoyam**—Some native peoples apply this nonspecific term to the various tuberous plants that are grown to provide shade for young cocoa (*Theobroma cacao*) plants. Generally, cocoyams are considered to be either (1) a variety of taro, or (2) a variety of tannia (*Xanthosoma sagittifolium*). Tannia, which is also an aroid, bears tubers that resemble taro tubers. Africans distinguish between the two by calling the former the "new" cocoyam, and the latter the "old" cocoyam, because taro was grown there long before tannia was brought from the New World.

- **Dasheen**—This term designates the *esculenta* variety of taro, which usually has a large main edible tuber (corm) and few side tubers (cormels).

---

[2]Purseglove, J. W., *Tropical Crops: Monocotyledons 1*, John Wiley & Sons, Inc., New York, N.Y., 1972, p. 61.

- **Eddoe**—This common name refers to the *antiquorum* variety of taro, which usually has a small main tuber and many side tubers.

However, it is often difficult to distinguish between dasheen and eddoe. Therefore, the name taro will be used in the remainder of this article.

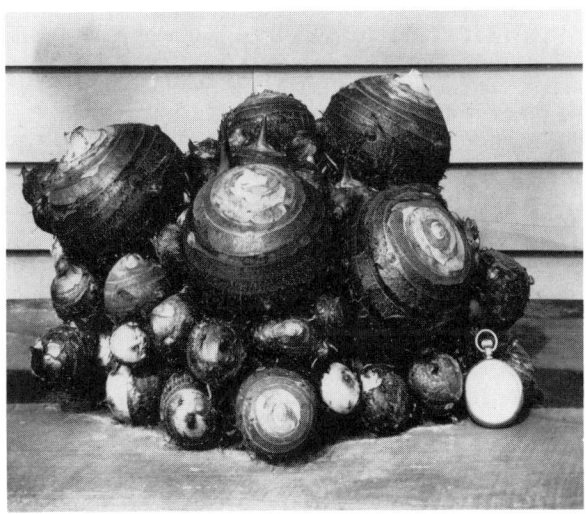

Fig. T-3.   A 22-lb (*10 kg*) hill of Trinidad taro. This cluster of tubers is unusually large, since it is more common to find only 1 or 2 large tubers. (Courtesy, USDA)

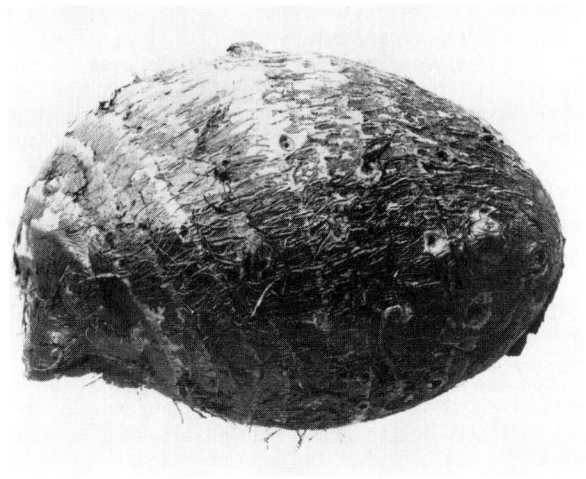

Fig. T-4.   A large tuber of the Ventura taro. (Courtesy, USDA)

ORIGIN AND HISTORY. Taro is native to Southeast Asia, where it grows wild. It is believed to have been first cultivated between 4,000 and 7,000 years ago, and to have been brought by traders eastward to Japan and China, and westward to the eastern Mediterranean and Egypt, 2,500 years ago. Some 500 years later, the tuber had reached West Africa. The spread of taro throughout the southwestern Pacific region was brought about by the peoples who migrated from Southeast Asia to Polynesia about 2,000 years ago. Centuries later, the tuber was taken to both Hawaii and New Zealand. Taro came to the Americas on the slave-bearing ships from Africa.

PRODUCTION.   Much of the taro that is produced in the tropical regions does not enter worldwide commerce, but is consumed locally. Hence, few statistics on the production of the crop are available. However, it is estimated that about 4 million metric tons are produced annually, and that the greater part of the worldwide crop is now grown in Africa.

Most of the U.S. production comes from Hawaii, where about 5.8 million pounds are produced annually.[3]

Taro is propagated vegetatively by planting small tubers that weigh between 2 and 5 oz (*28 and 140 g*). Some varieties will grow where there is at least 5 months of frostfree weather, while others require 8 to 10 months without frost. Also, the plant does best in rich, moist soil that is underlaid by clay so that water does not drain off too readily. In the United States, these conditions are found in California and Hawaii, and in the low-lying coastal lands between South Carolina and Texas. Lighter soils may require fertilization with one or more applications of nitrogen, phosphorus, and potassium.

The crop may be harvested repeatedly, provided that sufficient labor is available at a reasonable cost. In such cases, the larger more mature tubers may be removed while leaving the smaller ones to grow larger. Yields ranging from 13,500 to 17,500 lb per acre (*15,120 to 19,600 kg/ha*) have been obtained from the harvesting of the larger tubers only, and total yields as high as 33,000 lb (*36,960 kg/ha*) were reported when both the first and second crops of tubers were harvested. It is noteworthy that small tubers may be dried more readily and keep better in storage than large ones. When most of the tubers on a plant have matured, it may be uprooted. Sometimes, the leaves are also harvested for use as food.

PROCESSING.   Only small amounts of taro are processed on a commercial scale because most of the crop is consumed near to where it is produced. This situation may change in the near future because food processing industries are being developed in some of the taro-producing countries. Two commodities that are currently manufactured on a limited scale are (1) taro starch, which is extracted by grating the tubers and washing the pulp on a screen; and (2) canned Callaloo soup, an item produced in Trinidad by boiling taro leaves with okra, ham, and crabmeat. Some other potentially profitable products are: (1) poi, a fermented starchy paste made from boiled, peeled tubers; (2) fried taro chips (an item similar to potato chips, except that less fat is picked up by the taro); and (3) taro flour.

PREPARATION.   Taro leaves are usually most palatable when cooked in casseroles, soups, and stews. The tubers may be baked, boiled, fried, or roasted in much the same ways as Irish potatoes.

---

[3]*Agricultural Statistics 1991*, USDA, p. 164, Table 236.

CAUTION: Neither taro leaves nor taro roots should be consumed raw, because some varieties contain potentially hazardous amounts of calcium oxalate crystals. The crystals may cause severe irritation of the digestive tract. Therefore, the leaves and roots should be cooked thoroughly to eliminate the crystals. Some authorities recommend that varieties known to be rich in oxalate be boiled in two or more changes of water. The leaves may require boiling in water that contains a small amount of baking soda (sodium bicarbonate).

NUTRITIONAL VALUE. The nutrient compositions of various forms of taro are given in Food Composition Table F-36.

Some noteworthy observations regarding the nutrient composition of taro follow:

1.   The nutritional value of taro tubers is similar to that of Irish potatoes, except that the taro contains about one-fourth as much vitamin C. Also, the protein to calorie ratio (2.3 g per 100 kcal) of the tubers is high enough to meet the protein requirements of adults. However, children fed a taro-rich diet are likely to develop protein-energy malnutrition unless they are given supplemental sources of protein. Finally, taro tubers are deficient in many minerals and vitamins.

2.   Taro leaves are nutritionally superior to the tubers with respect to protein, calcium, phosphorus, vitamin A, the vitamin B complex, and vitamin C. Hence, they compensate for most of the nutritional deficiencies of the tubers. However, the leaves may contain much higher levels of highly irritating calcium oxalate crystals than the tubers. Therefore, it is unwise to feed the raw leaves to either people or livestock.

(Also see VEGETABLE[S], Table V-6 Vegetables of the World.)

TARTAR

• A mineral deposit on the teeth, mainly calcium phosphate.
• A substance consisting basically of cream of tartar found in the juice of grapes, and often deposited in wine casks during the production of wine.

TARTAR EMETIC

This is another name for the chemical antimony potassium tartrate. Under hospital supervision, its slow intravenous administration is a dangerous but effective treatment used to eliminate certain parasites from the body.

TARTARIC ACID (HOOC(CHOH)₂·COOH)

A strong dicarboxylic acid. It is widely found in plants especially fruits—both free and combined with salts.
(Also see ADDITIVES, Table A-3.)

TARTAZINE

This is an alternate name for the yellow color, FD & C Yellow no. 5, which is approved for use in food, drugs, and cosmetics. It may also be employed to dye wool and silk.

TASTE

This is a chemical sense detected by receptors—the taste buds—in the mouth, primarily on the tongue. Upon entering the mouth, certain dissolved chemicals create nervous impulses in the taste buds. These impulses travel to the brain where they are interpreted as (1) salty, (2) sweet, (3) bitter, or (4) sour. Humans have about 12,000 taste buds, and each taste bud possess a greater degree of sensitivity to 1 or 2 of the taste sensations. In general, the tip of the tongue is the most sensitive to sweet, the sides to sour, the back to bitter, while salt sensitivity is distributed over most of the tongue.

Taste plays a major role in the acceptance or rejection of foods. Most of the time, salty foods are considered pleasant, but very salty foods will be rejected. Sweet is, of course, considered pleasant, and is associated with the sugar content of a food. However, much effort has been directed toward finding substances such as saccharin, which will "fool" the sweet taste buds, without contributing to calories as do the sugars. Foods with a bitter taste are generally rejected. This may have been a protective mechanism for early man, since many poisonous wild plants taste bitter due to alkaloid compounds. The sour taste may be considered as pleasing or objectionable. For example, foods containing dilute vinegar solutions are very palatable, while extremely sour foods are rejected. Sourness is a measure of the degree of acidity—hydrogen ion concentration—of foods. Although, taste is important in food acceptance, most of the pleasurable experience associated with food is known as flavor. The flavor of foods results from the interaction of taste and smell—another chemical sense. Humans can detect as many as 10,000 different smells. Much of what is called taste is actually smell. This is emphasized during a cold when foods seem to lose their "taste."

(Also see SUGAR; and SWEETENING AGENTS.)

TASTE BUDS

The sense organs for taste located in the epiglottis, palate, pharynx, and tongue. Taste buds are excited by chemical substances in the food we eat. We can detect four types of taste: (1) salty, (2) sweet, (3) bitter, and (4) sour. Taste sensations from these taste buds help regulate the diet. Much of what we usually call taste is actually smell.

(Also see TASTE.)

TAURINE ($C_2H_7NO_3S$)

This chemical is present in bile, combined with cholic acid.

TEA

The word *tea* refers to (1) a common drink made by pouring boiling water over the dried and prepared leaves of an oriental evergreen tree, (2) the dried and prepared leaves from which the drink is made, or (3) the tree upon which these leaves grow. Tea may also mean (1) a brew made from kinds of leaves other than tea, (2) an afternoon or early evening meal in Britain, or (3) a large reception at which tea is served. Herein, the word tea will refer to the dried leaves or the plant and the drink made from them. Tea is the most popular beverage in the world.

ORIGIN AND HISTORY. It is believed that the tea plant originated in a region encompassing Tibet, western China, and northern India. The exact origin of tea culture and brewing tea leaves into a drink is obscure. But, according to an ancient Chinese legend, tea was discovered by the Chinese emperor, Shen-Nung, in 2737 B.C. Leaves from a wild tea bush accidentally fell into the water that he was boiling; and he discovered that the drink was good. However, the earliest mention of tea in Chinese literature appeared about 350 A.D. Then, in 780 A.D. Lu Yu's The Classic of Tea, published in China, described the cultivation, processing, and use of tea. By the 9th century A.D., tea was growing in Japan after being introduced by Chinese Buddhist monks. Eventually, tea culture spread to Java, the Dutch East Indies, and other tropical and subtropical areas. Traders from Europe sailing to and from the Far East in the 16th century began to introduce Europeans to the unusual oriental beverage called tea, a word derived from the Chinese local Amoy dialect word "t'e," pronounced "tay." By the 18th century, tea had become the national beverage of England. Tea also was popular in the American colonies, but in 1767 the British government placed a tax on the tea used by the colonists. The rest of the story Americans know as the Boston Tea Party of 1773—a contributing factor to the Revolutionary War.

Several tea innovations originated in the United States. In 1904, Thomas Sullivan, a New York City merchant, sent his customers samples of tea leaves in small silk bags. Customers recognized that these bags could be used for conveniently brewing one cup of tea at a time, and soon began ordering tea leaves in bags. Instant tea is another U. S. contribution to tea drinking. It was first marketed in 1948.

PRODUCTION. No longer is it "all the tea in China," since India ranks as the number one producer of tea. Sri Lanka (previously Ceylon) is, however, the major supplier of tea to the United States. Worldwide about 2.5 million metric tons of tea are produced annually. Fig. T-5 shows the leading tea growing countries.

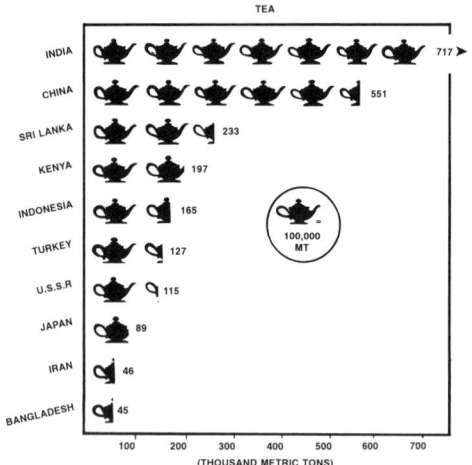

TEA

INDIA 717 ►
CHINA 551
SRI LANKA 233
KENYA 197
INDONESIA 165
TURKEY 127
U.S.S.R 115
JAPAN 89
IRAN 46
BANGLADESH 45

= 100,000 MT

100   200   300   400   500   600   700
(THOUSAND METRIC TONS)

Fig. T-5. The leading tea growing countries indicated by their yearly production. (Based on data from *FAO Production Yearbook*, 1990, FAO/UN, Rome, Italy, Vol. 44, p. 177, Table 80)

Propagation and Growing. The tea plant is an evergreen tree with the botanical name of *Camellia sinensis*. In the wild, the tree may grow to a height of 30 ft (*10 m*), but on tea plantations, or so-called gardens or estates, the tea plants are constantly pruned to keep their height at about 3 ft (*1 m*) to encourage new growth and to keep at a convenient picking height.

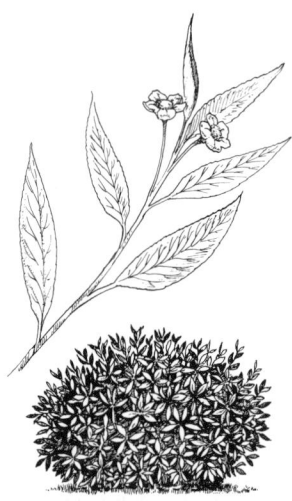

Fig. T-6. A pruned tea plant with abundant foliage, and a twig showing the camellialike flowers. It is the two leaves at the end of the twig which are plucked for tea.

Tea plants grow best in warm climates where the rainfall averages 90 to 200 in. (*220 to 500 cm*) yearly, and the plants grow at altitudes from sea level to 7,000 ft (*2,200 m*). The best teas are produced at the higher altitudes where plants grow more slowly in the cooler air and their leaves yield a better flavor.

Tea plants may be started from cuttings or seeds. The tea seedlings or small plants are placed in the soil about 3 to 5 ft (*1.0 to 1.5 m*) apart, and then, depending upon the altitude, 2 1/2 to 5 years are required before the tea plants produce leaves for commercial production. Young plants are often shaded to protect them from the heat of the sun. Once in production a plant may produce for almost a century.

Harvesting. Tea plants produce abundant foliage, a camellialike flower, and berries containing one to three seeds. However, it is the smallest and youngest leaves that are plucked for tea. Two leaves and a bud at the top of each young shoot are picked. A growth of new shoots is termed a flush. At lower altitudes a new flush may grow every week, while at higher altitudes more time is required. Flushes are picked off the tea plant by hand by workers called "tea pluckers." Good pluckers harvest about 40 lb (*18 kg*) per day, or enough to make 10 lb (*4.5 kg*) of manufactured tea.

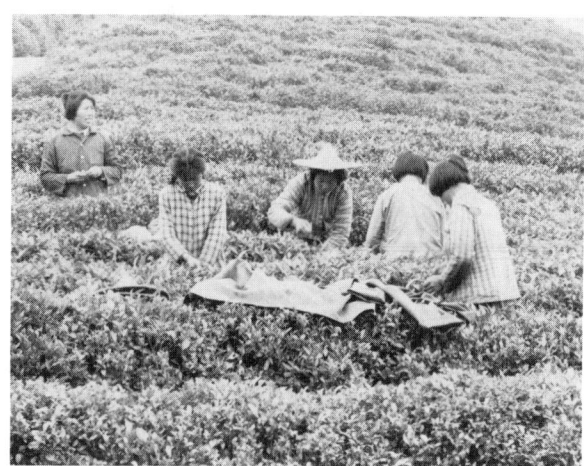

Fig. T-7. Picking tea in Hangchow, China. (Photo by Audrey Ensminger)

PROCESSING. Although the kind and quality of leaves vary somewhat according to the local conditions and particular strains, the real difference in color, aroma, and flavor is caused by the way in which the leaves are processed. There are three different types of tea: black, green, and oolong. Most green and oolong tea comes from China, Japan, and Taiwan, while all tea-producing countries manufacture black tea.

• **Black tea**—First the leaves are transported from the plantation to the factory as rapidly as possible. The leaves are spread on withering racks and air is blown over the leaves to remove excess moisture. This removes about one-third of the moisture, and the leaves become soft and pliable. After this they are rolled to break the cells and release the juices, which are essential for the fermenting process. Then the leaves are spread out and kept under high humidity to promote fermentation, which develops the rich flavor of black tea, and the leaves become a coppery color. Finally, the leaves are hot-air dried (fired) until the moisture is removed, leaving the leaves brownish black.

• **Green tea**—In making green tea, the plucked leaves are steamed as quickly as possible. Steaming prevents the leaves from changing color and prevents fermentation. After steaming, the leaves are rolled and dried in the same way as black tea until they are crisp.

• **Oolong tea**—Oolong tea is somewhat like both green tea and black tea. It is semifermented. Fermentation is stopped before the process is complete. This produces a greenish-brown leaf with a flavor richer than that of green tea but more delicate than that of black tea.

GRADES OF TEA AND BLENDING.
Tea is graded according to the size of the leaf, which has nothing to do with the quality of the tea. Large and small, broken and unbroken leaves are sorted by passing them across screens with different size holes. The largest leaves, classified in order of size, are orange pekoe, pekoe, and pekoe souchong. These large leaves are generally packaged as loose tea. The smaller or broken leaves are classified as broken orange pekoe, broken orange pekoe fannings, and fannings. These smaller grades of tea are generally used in tea bags.

Since tea grown in different countries or even different parts of the same country, varies in taste, flavor, and quality, tea companies employ a tea taster. The tea taster selects the tea to purchase so that a company can sell tea with the flavor for which it is known. To achieve a particular flavor, teas are often blended. Nevertheless, some unblended varieties are popular. Some blended and unblended teas that have achieved fame for their flavor are listed in Table T-1.

TABLE T-1
FAMOUS VARIETIES OF TEA

Name of Tea	Kind of Tea	Where Grown	Flavor
Assam	Black	India	Rich, pungent.
Darjeeling	Black	India	Delicate, sweet.
Earl Grey	Black	India, Sri Lanka	Richly fragrant.
Taiwan Oolong	Oolong	Taiwan	Pleasantly fragrant.
Gunpowder	Green	India, Sri Lanka, China	Delicate
Jasmine	Oolong	China, Taiwan	Delicate, scented.
Keemun (English) breakfast tea	Black	China, Taiwan	Delicately pungent.
Lapsang Souchong	Black	China, Taiwan	Rich, smoky.

Assam and Darjeeling teas are unblended varieties, while teas like Jasmine and Earl Grey contain flavors from other sources.

BREWING TEA.
A cup of tea is brewed by pouring fresh, boiling water over l tsp (5 *ml*) of loose tea or one tea bag. The best flavor is obtained by allowing the tea to steep (soak) for 3 to 5 minutes before being served. If tea is steeped too long, it will have a bitter taste from the excess tannins that are released. Also, the longer steeping times yield tea with a higher caffeine content.

Iced tea is made with 50% more tea leaves, to allow for the melting ice. The tea is poured into tall glasses that are two-thirds full of ice. Sliced lemons are served with it, and each person sweetens the tea to his taste. Flavorings of cloves, grated orange peel, or mint are sometimes added.

• **Instant tea**—Instant tea is an innovation developed in the United States. A strong brew of tea is made in large vats, and then the water is removed by a drying process. Consumers can make hot or cold tea by merely adding water to the powder which remains after the drying process.

TEA DRINKING AROUND THE WORLD.
Tea enjoys worldwide popularity, and the manner in which people prepare and drink their tea differs all over the world. Some people drink plain tea, while others add milk and sugar or lemon juice. A few people add liquor such as rum, scotch, or cognac to their tea.

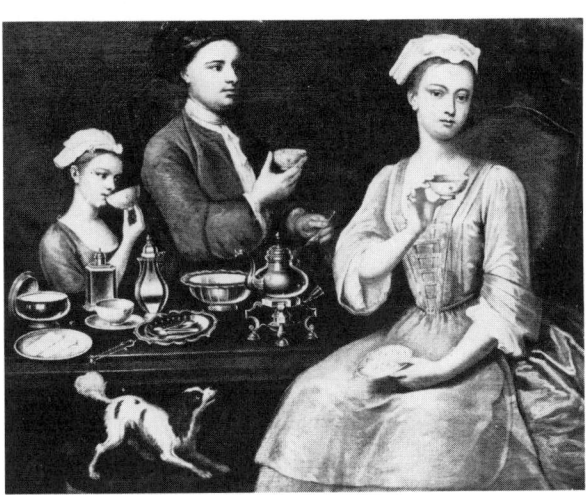

Fig. T-8. Tea for two, or three, or four—the pause that refreshes. (Painting by an unknown master, English. Courtesy, The Bettman Archive, New York, N.Y.)

In China, where tea drinking originated, there are many ways of drinking and preparing tea. The people of Kiangsu and Chekiang Provinces love green tea, but they like it infused and served in cups with lids. In Fukien and Swatow, the tea drinker prefers to sip oolong tea from cups of delicate porcelain. Tea drinkers in Peking champion vigorously scented tea fired with fresh flowers, preferably jasmine. For the Mongolians in the north of China, a meal is not complete without milk-tea, which they make by boiling chipped brick tea in a brass pot or an iron pan and adding milk and salt. For the Tibetans, butter-tea is a daily necessity. They take boiled brick tea, butter, and salt and place them in an oblong receptacle which they churn until the mixture thickens. It is then ready to drink with their tsambie (bread made with barley), beef, or mutton.

In China, tea is a social drink. Chinese custom decrees serving tea to guests as a token of friendship. During the Spring Festival in Kiangsu and Chekiang, hosts place olives in the tea as a token of good luck before serving it to their guests. The butter-tea of the Tibetans is an honor accorded to a visitor.

An old custom once typical in Russia was the use of a samovar—a large, graceful urn made of copper, brass, or silver. The samovar holds about 40 cups of boiling water heated by charcoal, and the top of the samovar is saucer-shaped to hold a teapot. This teapot contains a strong essence of tea which is kept steaming hot. Then when tea is served about one-quarter of a cup of the tea essence is used and the remainder of the cup is filled with boiling water from the samovar.

NUTRITIONAL VALUE. Without sugar, cream, or other additions, tea provides little nutrition other than a few calories, and trace amounts of some minerals as indicated in Food Composition Table F-36. Green tea is, however, an excellent source of vitamin K.

Caffeine in tea accounts for its mildly stimulating properties, while the tannins contribute pungency, slight astringency, and color to tea. An essential oil contributes the flavor. The amount of caffeine in a cup of tea depends upon the steeping time.

(Also see CAFFEINE.)

TEASEED OIL

This is a vegetable oil extracted from *Camellia sinesis*, the tea-oil plant, and cultivated in China. Teaseed oil is used for salad oil and frying. It is claimed to be similar to olive oil.

TEFF *Eragrostis abyssinica*

This is an important cereal food of Ethiopia and the eastern African highlands. It is a leafy, quick-maturing annual plant that grows up to 4 ft in height. Teff is adapted to dry areas with a short rainy season.

The teff of Africa is grown by primitive methods. Fields are cultivated by crude plows drawn by oxen, followed by hand sowing and another tilling to cover the seed. When ripe, the grain is harvested by small hand sickles and threshed by treading with animals.

Women grind the white or black grain (grain color depends on variety) on flat stones to make a flour, which is baked into large, flat pancakes called injara.

Nutritional data on teff grains and meal are listed in the Food Composition Table F-36.

Teff is used as an annual grass hay as well as a food grain. Following threshing, the straw may be mixed with mud for constructing huts.

(Also see CEREAL GRAINS, Table C-18 Cereal Grains of the World.)

Table T-2 tells about *faffa*, a special fortified food based on teff.

TABLE T-2
A FORTIFIED FOOD BASED ON TEFF

Product	Description	Uses	Comments
Faffa	A finely ground mixture of teff, chickpeas, skim milk powder, sugar, salt and vitamins. Contains from 14% to 15% protein.	May be mixed with water to make a porridge for infants. Leavened or unleavened breads. Mixed with the false banana (*Ensete ventricosum*).	The Ethiopian and Swedish governments established the Children's Nutrition Unit in Addis Ababa to conduct the development, production, and test marketing of Faffa. Sufficient vitamins are added to the product to ensure that 3½ oz (*100 g*) supplies the daily allowances for all of the essential vitamins. A large scale feeding trial with children aged 6 months to 10 years produced dramatic decreases in the incidence and severity of goiter, rickets, and skin infections; and a noticeable increase in muscle mass. However, the cereal did not cure anemia as rapidly as it did the other deficiency diseases.

TEG (TEGG)

A 2-year-old sheep.

TEMPLATE

A mold, pattern, or guide.

TENDERLOIN

The most tender muscle of the carcass (beef, lamb, and pork), located inside the loin and running nearly the entire length of the loin.

TEPARY BEAN *Phaseolus acutifolius*

This legume, which is well adapted to hot, dry climates, has long been used as food by the inhabitants of the American tropics.

ORIGIN AND HISTORY. The tepary bean was used over 5,000 years ago in the Tehuacan region of Mexico. It grows wild in northwestern Mexico and Arizona. Recently, the tepary bean was introduced into certain drought-ridden parts of Africa.

PRODUCTION. Most of the world production of tepary beans is limited to small areas in Mexico and Arizona. To date, it has not become popular in Africa.

Tepary beans are a good crop for low rainfall tropical areas, because the seeds germinate rapidly when moistened. Also, they take advantage of the very brief period that the soil is moist by growing very rapidly. However, they do not do well in the rainy tropics. Mature beans are often ready for harvesting within 2 months after planting the seed crop. Without irrigation, the yields range from 450 lb to 700 lb per acre (*504 to 784 kg/ha*); with irrigation, 800 lb to 1,500 lb per acre (*896 to 1,680 kg/ha*) are obtained. Sometimes the plants are grown for fodder, in which case the yields of dry hay range from 5,000 lb to 9,500 lb per acre (*5,600 to 10,640 kg/ha*).

When the beans are mature, the plants are cut and allowed to dry in the field. After drying, the pods are threshed to obtain the beans.

PROCESSING. There is little or no processing of tepary beans other than drying because (1) the crop is small, and (2) the dried beans keep well without further processing.

SELECTION AND PREPARATION. The dried beans may be prepared and served in the same ways as dried kidney beans or dried limas. However, tepary beans are likely to absorb more water during soaking and cooking than the other types of dried beans. Also, they require longer cooking to produce tenderness.

NUTRITIONAL VALUE. The nutrient composition of tepary beans is given in Food Composition Table F-36.

Tepary beans provide about the same amount of calories, protein, minerals and vitamins as the more commonly used types of dried beans.

(Also see BEAN[S], Table B-10 Beans of the World; and LEGUMES, Table L-2 Legumes of the World.)

TERRAMYCIN AS PRESERVATIVE

Terramycin is a brand name for the broad-spectrum antibiotic oxytetracycline. Although low levels of antibiotics such as Terramycin effectively extend the shelf life of food, the direct addition of antibiotics to foods is not permitted in the United States. After some initial studies and limited usage of antibiotics as food preservatives, the FDA withdrew their approval because of concern that repeated exposure of the consumer to low concentrations of antibiotics could lead to the development of antibiotic-resistant strains of bacteria. Furthermore, there was wariness lest antibiotics provided a substitute for good sanitary practices.

(Also see BACTERIA IN FOOD, section headed "Bacterial Control Methods"; and ANTIBIOTICS, section headed "Antibiotics in Foods.")

TESTOSTERONE

The male sex hormone, secreted by the leydig cells in the testicles, which controls the male secondary sex characteristics.

TETANY

Spontaneous muscular spasms in the wrists and ankles, resulting when the parathyroid secretion is deficient, causing the amount of calcium in the blood to drop and the phosphorus to increase.

TEXTURE

Food is accepted or rejected on the basis of its chemical and physical properties as perceived by the senses—sight, sound, touch, smell, and taste. Therefore, the texture of a food is important. Texture is a physical quality of food perceived by the sense of touch in the mouth—mouth feel. It is described by such adjectives as chewy, tacky, stringy, hard, soft, rough, smooth, gritty, firm, crisp, coarse, etc. Through experience, people learn the customary texture of foods in their diet, and when the texture is different than expected, the food is judged to be of lower quality. Often, unacceptable foods feel slimy, stringy, and greasy, or unacceptable foods contain unchewable parts, grit, or spicules.

THEINE

This is an alternative name for caffeine.

THERAPEUTIC

Pertaining to the medical treatment of disease.

THERAPEUTIC DIETS

Diets designed to treat a disease or metabolic disorder. They are diets adapted or modified to meet special needs of specific diseases. Some common examples of diseases requiring therapeutic or modified diets are diabetes mellitus, phenylketonuria, kidney diseases, and galactosemia. Depending upon the disorder, these diets may be modified in energy content, in consistency or bulk, or in the kinds and amounts of nutrients such as vitamins, minerals, fats, proteins, or fluids. Despite the modification, the therapeutic diet should remain nutritionally adequate.

(Also see MODIFIED DIETS; and SPECIAL DIETS.)

THERAPY

The medical treatment of disease.

THERMAL

Refers to heat.

THERMODURIC

A term used to describe microorganisms (bacteria) that are heat tolerant. Thermodurics survive for short periods of time at high temperatures, but they do not grow at high temperatures. For example, thermodurics survive pasteurization of milk for short periods of time.

THERMOGENESIS

The production of heat, especially within the body.

THERMOPHILES

Bacteria that are "heat lovers." These bacteria grow at temperatures of 131°F (55°C) to as high as 167°F (75°C). They are somewhat of a curiosity, since many of the proteins of other organisms would coagulate at these high temperatures. Thermophiles are commonly found in hot springs and compost heaps, and do not pose any real health problems. However, thermophiles are responsible for the "flat sour" which occurs in some home-canned food.

(Also see FLAT SOUR; and PRESERVATION OF FOOD.)

THI- (THIO-)

Prefix meaning sulfur containing.

THIAMIN (VITAMIN B-1)

Contents	Page

Thiamin (vitamin B-1)—the antiberiberi, or antineuritic, or antipolyneuritis vitamin—was the first of the B complex vitamins to be obtained in pure form; hence, the name B-1, a name proposed by the British in 1927. Various other names were used for short periods along the way, including antineuritic factor, antiberiberi factor, water-soluble B, aneurin, and simply vitamin B.

The mystery of beriberi, an ancient disease among rice eating peoples in the East, was eventually unraveled as a deficiency disease caused by a lack of thiamin.

Thiamin is required by all species of animals. They must have a dietary source, unless it is synthesized for them by microorganisms in the digestive tract, as in the case of ruminants.

A patient with wet beriberi—lying in bed breathless, water-logged, and apparently dying—may recover in 1 or 2 hours after being given an injection of thiamin; this is perhaps the most dramatic cure in medicine.

HISTORY. The history of thiamin begins with a study of the age-old disease beriberi.

Beriberi, which affects the nervous system, was known to the Chinese as early as 2600 B.C. The word *beriberi* means "I cannot," referring to the fact that persons with the disease cannot move easily. But the cause of beriberi in man, and of polyneuritis—the counterpart in poultry, remained elusive for centuries.

Recognition of the cause of beriberi, and its possible cure by better diet, is a landmark in the history of nutrition, a chronological record of which follows:

In 1873, Van Lent was the first to conclude that the type of diet had something to do with the origin of beriberi, based on reducing the ration of rice in the diet of sailors in the Dutch navy.

In 1882, Kanehiro Takaki, a Japanese medical officer, cured beriberi in sailors of the Japanese navy by giving them less rice and more meat, and milk.

In 1897, Christiaan Eijkman, a Dutch physician, working in a military hospital in the East Indies, produced polyneuritis, a condition resembling beriberi, in chickens, pigeons, and ducks by feeding polished rice; which he wrongfully attributed to too much starch.

In 1901, G. Grijns, another Dutch physician, who continued the work of Eijkman at the same hospital, concluded that beriberi in birds and man resulted from the lack in the diet of an essential nutrient.

In 1912, Casimir Funk, working at the Lister Institute

THIAMIN (vitamin B-1) HELPS THE BODY CELLS CONVERT
CARBOHYDRATES (STARCHES AND SUGARS) OF FOOD TO ENERGY, AND KEEPS THE
NERVOUS SYSTEM, APPETITE, MUSCLE TONE AND ATTITUDE BUOYANT.

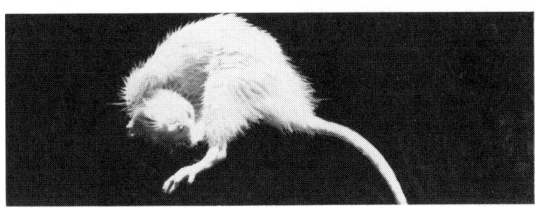 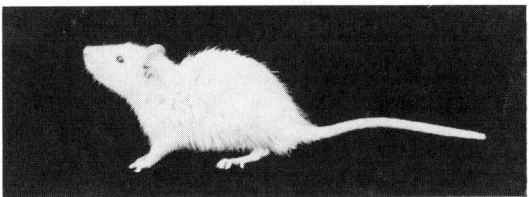

ONE OF THE MOST DRAMATIC CURES IN MEDICINE! SAME RAT BEFORE (LEFT) AND AFTER (RIGHT). <u>LEFT</u>: THIS RAT, 24 WEEKS
OLD, HAD PRACTICALLY NO THIAMIN. IT LOST THE ABILITY TO COORDINATE ITS MUSCLES. <u>RIGHT</u>: THE SAME RAT 24 HOURS
LATER, AFTER RECEIVING FOOD RICH IN THIAMIN — FULLY RECOVERED. (COURTESY, USDA)

TOP FOOD SOURCES

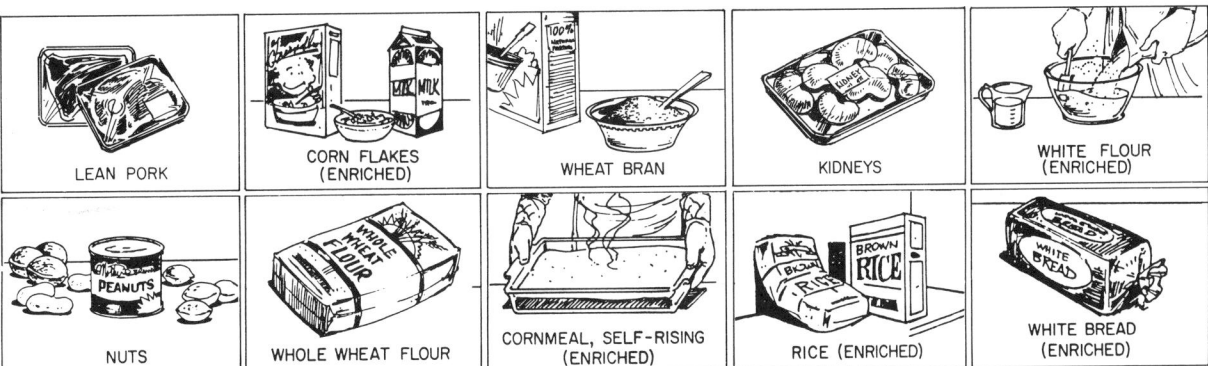

Fig. T-9. The thiamin (vitamin B-1) story.

in London, coined the term *vitamine* and applied it to the antiberiberi substance.

In 1916, Elmer V. McCollum of the University of Wisconsin, designated the concentrate that cured beriberi as "water-soluble B."

In 1926, B. C. P. Jansen and W. P. Donath, in Holland, isolated the antiberiberi vitamin, which, at first, was called aneurin because of its specific action on the nervous system.

In 1936, Robert R. Williams, an American, determined the structure, synthesized it, and gave it the name *thiamine* because it contains sulfur (from *thio*, meaning sulfur-containing) and an amine group. Subsequently, the "e" was dropped and the spelling *thiamin* came to be preferred.

CHEMISTRY, METABOLISM, PROPERTIES.

• **Chemistry**—Thiamin is made up of carbon, hydrogen, oxygen, nitrogen, and sulfur (see Fig. T-10). It consists of a molecule of pyrimidine and a molecule of thiazole linked by a methylene bridge.

THIAMIN

PYRIMIDINE RING   **THIAZOLE RING**

Fig. T-10. Structure of thiamin hydrochloride, the white, crystalline, stable form in which thiamin is usually marketed.

• **Metabolism**—The thiamin ingested in food is available (1) in the free form, or (2) bound as thiamin pyrophosphate (also called thiamin diphosphate), or (3) in a protein-phosphate complex. The bound forms are split in the digestive tract, following which absorption takes place principally in the upper part of the small intestine where the reaction is acid. It is noteworthy, however, that the absorption of thiamin is impaired in alcoholics with folate deficiency.

Following absorption, thiamin is transported to the liver where it is phosphorylated under the action of ATP to form the coenzyme thiamin diphosphate (formerly called thiamin pyrophosphate or cocarboxylase), (see Fig. T-11); although this phosphorylation occurs rapidly in the liver, it is noteworthy that all nucleated cells appear to be capable of bringing about this conversion.

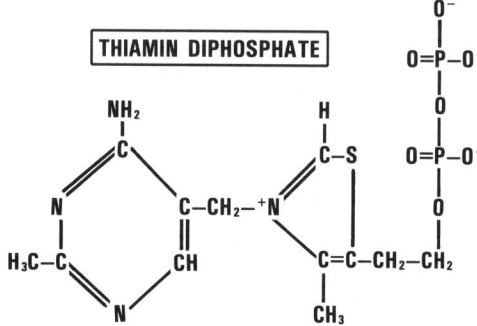

Fig. T-11.   Structure of thiamin diphosphate.

Thiamin is the least stored of all the vitamins. The adult human body contains approximately 30 mg. Of the thiamin stored in the body, about 80% is thiamin pyrophosphate, about 10% is thiamin triphosphate, and the remainder is thiamin monophosphate. The liver, kidneys, heart, brain, and skeletal muscles have somewhat higher concentrations than the blood. If the diet is deficient, tissues are depleted of their normal content of the vitamin in I to 2 weeks, so fresh supplies are needed regularly to provide for maintenance of tissue levels. Body tissues take up only as much thiamin as they need; with the need increased by metabolic demand (fever, increased muscular activity, pregnancy, and lactation) or by composition of the diet (carbohydrate increases the need for thiamin, while fat and protein spare thiamin). Because thiamin is water soluble, most of the vitamin not required for day-to-day use is excreted in the urine. This means that the body needs a regular supply, and that unneeded intakes are wasted. With a well-balanced diet, approximately 0.1 mg is normally excreted every 24 hours. However, the amount excreted in the urine decreases as the intake becomes inadequate and increases as the intake exceeds body needs; because of this, the most widely used biochemical method to assess thiamin status in individuals is the measurement of the vitamin in the urine.

• **Properties**—Synthetic thiamin is usually marketed as thiamin hydrochloride, which is more stable than the free vitamin. It is a crystalline white powder, with a faint yeastlike odor and a salty nutlike taste. It is stable when dry but readily soluble in water, slightly soluble in alcohol, and insoluble in fat solvents. Heating in solutions at 248°F (120°C) in an acid medium (pH 5.0 or less) has little destructive effect. But cooking foods in neutral or alkaline reaction is very destructive. Also, autoclaving and ultraviolet light destroy thiamin.

Thiamin mononitrate is more stable in heat than thiamin hydrochloride; for which reason it is often used for the thiamin fortification of cereal products that have to be cooked. Derivatives of thiamin, thiamin propyl disulfide and thiamin tetrahydrofurfural disulfide, have been synthesized. These products are recommended for oral administration when there is evidence of thiamin deficiency, because they are absorbed more rapidly than thiamin hydrochloride.

MEASUREMENT/ASSAY. The thiamin content of foods is expressed in milligrams or micrograms. It is usually determined by rapid chemical or microbiological methods, which have largely replaced the older bioassay methods in which pigeons, rats, and chicks were used.

FUNCTIONS. Thiamin is essential as a coenzyme (or cofactor) in energy metabolism, as a coenzyme in the conversion of glucose to fat, in the functioning of the peripheral nerves, and in such indirect functions as appetite, muscle tone, and a healthy mental attitude. A discussion of each of these functions follows:

• **As a coenzyme in energy metabolism**—Without thiamin, there could be no energy.

The major functioning form of thiamin is as thiamin diphosphate (formerly called thiamin pyrophosphate or cocarboxylase)—thiamin combined with two phosphate groups, in which it serves as a coenzyme in a number of enzyme systems.

In the metabolism of carbohydrates, thiamin diphosphate is needed in the conversion of pyruvic acid and the subsequent formation of acetyl coenzyme A, which in turn enters the Krebs cycle and produces vital energy. This is one of the most complex and important reactions in carbohydrate metabolism. In addition to thiamin diphosphate, it also requires the following cofactors: coenzyme A, which contains pantothenic acid, nicotinamide adenine dinucleotide (NAD), which contains niacin; magnesium ions; and lipoic acid.

Oxidative decarboxylation (removal of CO_2) in carbohydrate metabolism is also involved in the Krebs cycle in the conversion of alpha-ketoglutaric acid to succinic acid. Because fats and amino acids, as well as carbohydrates, can contribute to alpha-ketoglutaric acid, it follows that thiamin is involved in the metabolism of all three energy producing units.

In thiamin deficiency, pyruvic and alpha-ketoglutaric acids tend to accumulate in the body; sometimes they are measured as a means of determining thiamin status.

• **As a coenzyme in the conversion of glucose to fats— the process called transketolation (keto-carrying)**—Thiamin diphosphate is also a coenzyme with the enzyme transketolase in the important reaction which provides active glyceraldehyde through the pentose shunt. This is a key link providing activated glycerol for lipogenesis for the conversion of glucose to fat. Thiamin diphosphate is the key activator which provides the high energy phosphate bond. Ionized magnesium (Mg $^{++}$) is another cofactor present.

• **In the functioning of peripheral nerves**—Thiamin is involved in the functioning of the peripheral nerves. In this role, it has value in the treatment of alcoholic neuritis, the neuritis of pregnancy, and beriberi.

• **In indirect functions**—Because of its primary role in carbohydrate metabolism, thiamin appears to have several indirect functions in the body; among them, the maintenance of normal appetite, the tone of the muscles, and a healthy mental attitude.

DEFICIENCY SYMPTOMS. The numerous symptoms of thiamin deficiency vary with the severity and duration of the deprivation of the vitamin.

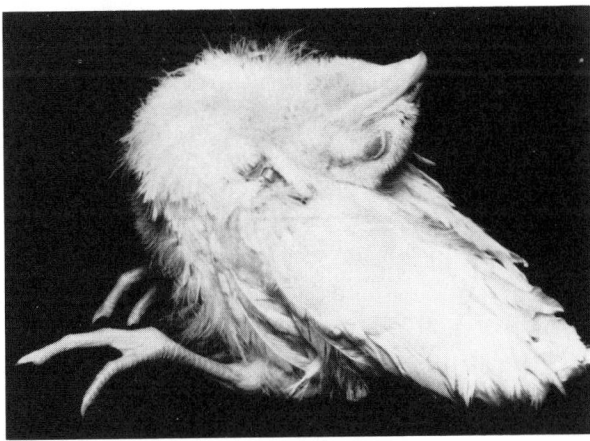

Fig. T-12. Polyneuritis (inflammation of the nerves) in the chick, the counterpart of beriberi in man, caused by thiamin (B-1) deficiency. Note the characteristic head retraction. (Courtesy, H. R. Bird, Department of Poultry Science, University of Wisconsin)

Moderate symptoms may be caused by poor diet, liver damage, or alcoholism. (In many cases, the latter is due to impaired absorption of thiamin caused in part by a deficiency of folacin.) Other persons at risk are kidney patients who are undergoing long-term dialysis treatment, patients fed intravenously for long periods of time, and patients with chronic febrile infections. Individuals consuming large amounts of tea, which contains a thiamin antagonist, or large amounts of raw fish, which contains thiaminase, an enzyme which inactivates the thiamin molecule by splitting it into two parts, may also run increased risk of developing a deficiency.

Symptoms of moderate thiamin deficiency include fatigue; apathy (lack of interest in affairs); loss of appetite; nausea; moodiness; irritability; depression; retarded growth; a sensation of numbness in the legs; and abnormalities of the electrocardiogram.

Clinical Effects of Thiamin Deficiency. If a deficiency of thiamin is not corrected (if thiamin is not present in sufficient amounts to provide the key energizing coenzyme factor in the cells), the clinical effects will be reflected in the gastrointestinal system, the nervous system, and the cardiovascular system. Severe thiamin deficiency of long duration will culminate in beriberi, the symptoms of which are polyneuritis (inflammation of the nerves), emaciation and/or edema, and disturbances of heart function.

• **Gastrointestinal system symptoms**—The gastrointestinal symptoms of a thiamin deficiency are loss of appetite, indigestion, severe constipation, gastric atony (lack of tone), and decreased hydrochloric acid secretion. These manifestations likely result from insufficient energy from glucose being available for the smooth muscles and the glands of the intestinal tract to do their work of digestion.

• **Nervous system symptoms**—The central nervous system depends solely upon glucose for its energy. So, without thiamin to provide this need, neuronal activity is impaired, alertness and reflex responses are diminished, and fatigue and apathy (lack of interest) follow. If thiamin deficiency persists, degeneration of myelin sheaths of nerve fibers in the central nervous system and the peripheral nerves occurs, resulting in nerve irritation, which produces pain and prickly or deadening sensations. Unchecked progressive degeneration of the nervous system may cause paralysis and muscle atrophy (wasting).

• **Cardiovascular system symptoms**—If the thiamin deficiency persists, the heart muscles weaken and heart failure may result. Also, the smooth muscles of the vascular system may be involved, causing peripheral vasodilation. As a result of cardiac failure, peripheral edema may be observed in the extremeties.

• **Beriberi**—The various forms and symptoms of beriberi follow:

1. **Dry beriberi (wasting of tissues).** In humans, this form is characterized by numbness or tingling in the feet and toes, stiffness of ankles, soreness in and wasting (atrophy) of the muscles of the legs, a decrease in the reflex of the knee, a drop in the muscles that support the toes and foot, and difficulty in walking. As the disorder advances, the arms and the other parts of the body are affected because there is nerve degeneration and lack of muscle coordination.

2. **Wet beriberi (collection of fluid in the tissues).** The presence of edema, especially of the legs, distinguishes this form from dry beriberi. Other symptoms are loss of appetite, breathlessness, and disorders of the heart.

3. **Infantile beriberi.** This acute disorder is common between the second and fifth months of life in children who are being suckled by mothers subsisting on beriberi-producing diets. Symptoms of the disease are weakness of voice during bawling (complete lack of sound in severe cases), lack of appetite, vomiting, diarrhea, rapid pulse, cyanosis (dark blue coloration of the skin and mucous membrane), and sudden death.

(Also see BERIBERI.)

• **Other clinical symptoms of thiamin deficiency**—Additional symptoms of thiamin deficiency include, low excretion of thiamin in the urine; electrocardiogram changes; reduced transketolase activity of the red blood cells; and an increase of pyruvic acid in the blood.

RECOMMENDED DAILY ALLOWANCE OF THIAMIN.

The Food and Nutrition Board (FNB) of the National Research Council (NRC) recommended daily allowances of thiamin are given in Table T-3.

TABLE T–3
RECOMMENDED DAILY THIAMIN ALLOWANCES[1]

Group	Age	Weight		Height		Calories	Thiamin
	(yr)	(lb)	*(kg)*	(in.)	*(cm)*	(kcal)	(mg)
Infants	.0–.5	13	*6*	24	*60*	650	0.3
	.5–1.0	20	*9*	28	*71*	850	0.4
Children	1–3	29	*13*	35	*90*	1,300	0.7
	4–6	44	*20*	44	*112*	1,800	0.9
	7–10	62	*28*	52	*132*	2,000	1.0
Males	11–14	99	*45*	62	*157*	2,500	1.3
	15–18	145	*66*	69	*176*	3,000	1.5
	19–24	154	*72*	70	*177*	2,900	1.5
	25–50	154	*79*	70	*176*	2,900	1.5
	51+	154	*77*	68	*173*	2,300	1.2
Females	11–14	101	*46*	62	*157*	2,200	1.1
	15–18	120	*55*	64	*163*	2,200	1.1
	19–24	128	*58*	65	*164*	2,200	1.1
	25–50	138	*63*	64	*163*	2,200	1.1
	51+	143	*65*	63	*160*	1,900	1.0
Pregnant						+300	1.5
Lactating						+500	1.6

[1]*Recommended Dietary Allowances*, 10th ed., NRC–National Academy of Sciences, 1989, p. 285.

In general, the recommended allowances are based (1) on assessments of the effects of varying levels of dietary thiamin on the occurrence of clinical signs of deficiency, (2) on the excretion of thiamin or its metabolites, and (3) on erythrocyte transketolase activity. Most studies have been conducted on subjects fed diets with ratios of carbohydrate and fat similar to those commonly consumed in the United States. There is evidence that dietary fat "spares" thiamin to some extent.

Because thiamin is essential for key reactions in energy metabolism, particularly carbohydrate metabolism, the requirement for thiamin has usually been related to energy intake. For this reason, Table T-3 has been adapted to show the correlations of thiamin with calories.

• **Allowances for infants, children, and adolescents—** As shown in Table T-3, during the growth periods of infancy, childhood, and especially adolescence, thiamin needs are increased.

• **Allowances for adults—**The National Research Council recommended a minimum thiamin intake of 1.22 mg/day for men and 1.03 mg/day for women.

• **Allowance for pregnant and lactating women—**Increased thiamin needs accompany gestation and pregnancy. On the basis of an increased energy intake of 300 kcal/day during pregnancy and an adult allowance of 0.5 mg of thiamin per 1,000 kcal, an additional 0.4 mg/day is recommended throughout pregnancy to accommodate maternal and fetal growth and increased maternal caloric intake.

Thiamin requirements also increase during lactation. The lactating woman secretes approximately 0.2 mg of thiamin/day in milk (Nail et al., 1980). To account for both the thiamin loss in milk and increased energy consumption during lactation, an increment of 0.5 mg is recommended throughout lactation.

Increased thiamin needs exist (1) during times of stress, fevers, infections, chronic illness, or surgery; (2) in old age; (3) with increased muscular work; and (4) in chronic alcoholism (due to high intake of energy in the form of alcohol and to reduced thiamin absorption).

• **Thiamin intake in average U.S. diet—**According to the U.S. Department of Agriculture, in 1990 there was sufficient thiamin in foods available for consumption in the United States to provide an average intake of 2.2 mg per person per day. Of this total, the contribution of food groups was as follows: meats, poultry and fish, 25.4%; dairy products, 8.3%; and flour and cereal products, 42.8%.

TOXICITY.

There are no known toxic effects from thiamin.

THIAMIN LOSSES DURING PROCESSING, COOKING, AND STORAGE.

The thiamin content of foods is influenced by the practices employed in harvesting, handling, processing, cooking, and storing. Factors contributing to thiamin losses are pH, heat, oxidation, inorganic bases, enzymes, metal complexes, and radiation. The bond between the pyrimidine and thiazole rings is weak with the result that the vitamin is easily destroyed, particularly in an alkaline medium or by heat in the presence of moisture. Thiamin is sensitive to both oxidation and reduction. Sulfur dioxide, sulfites, etc., easily break the bond and vitamin activity is lost.

Pertinent facts about thiamin processing and cooking losses follow:

• **Parboiled ("converted") rice—**Rice that is soaked and parboiled ("converted") contains much more thiamin than rice that is milled from the raw state. The parboiling causes the thiamin and other water soluble nutrients to move from the outer layers to the inner layers of the rice kernel. As a result, fewer of them are removed in the milling process.

(Also see RICE.)

• **Processing losses—**Canning causes thiamin losses because of the solubility of the vitamin in the canning fluid; hence, the more canning fluid drained away, the greater the loss.

Drying (dehydrating) food, except fruit, results in only small losses. (Thiamin is destroyed rapidly by sulfite, a fact which may explain the loss of thiamin in dried fruits, such as apricots and peaches, treated with sulfur.)

Fresh frozen vegetables maintain in storage the thiamin content that is present following blanching to destroy the enzyme activity.

Irradiation destroys thiamin. Thus, the thiamin content of pork is virtually depleted by irradiation in food preservation.

• **Normal cooking losses**—Normal cooking of an ordinary mixed diet results in the loss of about 25% of the thiamin.

• **Moist heat**—Boiling for not more than an hour causes little destruction of this vitamin. But, because thiamin is soluble in water, as much as one-third of the original thiamin content may be lost if cooking water is liberal and is discarded.

• **Dry heating**—High dry-heat temperatures, as in toasting bread, can cause considerable loss.

• **Cooking breakfast cereals**—Little thiamin is lost in the cooking of breakfast cereals since they are cooked at moderate temperatures and the cooking water is absorbed.

• **Alkali medium**—Thiamin is readily destroyed in an alkali medium. Hence, the practice of adding baking soda (an alkali) to cooking water to preserve the color of green vegetables is not recommended.

• **Meat losses**—Generally, the thiamin losses in cooking meats are greater than in cooking other foods, ranging from 30 to 50% of the raw value; with the least loss occurring in frying.

• **Bread baking losses**—In baking bread, 15 to 20% of the original thiamin content is lost.

• **The same principles apply to both ascorbic acid and thiamin**—When the principles for the retention of ascorbic acid are observed in food processing and cooking, the maximum thiamin content will be preserved, also.

There is little destruction of thiamin from exposure to air at ordinary temperatures. Hence, storage losses of thiamin in foods are minimal.

ANTITHIAMIN FACTORS IN FOOD.

Certain raw fish and seafood—particularly carp, herring, clams, and shrimp—contain the enzyme thiaminase, which inactivates the thiamin molecule by splitting it into two parts. This effect has been seen in mink and fox fed 10 to 25% levels of certain raw fish, giving rise to a thiamin deficiency disease known as Chastek paralysis. This action can be prevented by cooking the fish prior to feeding, thereby destroying the thiaminase. Of course, humans seldom eat sufficient thiaminase-containing raw fish or seafood to produce a thiamin deficiency.

Other agents known to affect thiamin levels in the body are: a large amount of live yeast in the diet of man, which reduces the amount of thiamin absorbed from the intestine; drinking large amounts of tea or chewing fermented tea leaves, a common practice in some parts of Asia; or imbibing alcohol in excess, which contains an antithiamin substance. Also, it is noteworthy that thiamin-splitting bacteria have been found in the intestinal tract of some Japanese with symptoms of beriberi, but the significance of this is not known at present.

SOURCES OF THIAMIN.

Some thiamin is found in a large variety of animal and vegetable products but is abundant in few. Therefore, a deficiency of thiamin is a distinct possibility in the average diet, especially when calories are curtailed.

In addition to food sources, synthetic thiamin is also available; mostly as thiamin hydrochloride, although thiamin mononitrate is often used for the thiamin fortification of cereal products that have to be cooked.

The thiamin content of sources varies according to food and may be affected by harvesting, processing, enrichment, and storage. A grouping and ranking of foods according to normal thiamin content follows:

• **Rich sources**—Lean pork (fresh and cured), sunflower seed, corn flakes (enriched), peanuts, cottonseed flour, safflower flour, soybean flour.

• **Good sources**—Wheat bran, kidney, wheat flour (enriched), rye flour, nuts (except peanuts, which are a rich source), whole wheat flour, cornmeal (enriched), rice (enriched), white bread (enriched), soybean sprouts.

• **Fair sources**—Egg yolk, peas, turkey (hamloaf), beef liver, luncheon meat, crab, mackerel, salmon steak, roe (cod, herring), lima beans, refried beans, lentils.

• **Negligible sources**—Most fruits, most vegetables, polished rice, white sugar, animal and vegetable fats and oils, milk, butter, margarine, eggs, alcoholic beverages.

• **Supplemental sources**—Thiamin hydrochloride, thiamin mononitrate, yeast (brewers', torula), rice bran, wheat germ, and rice polish.

For additional sources and more precise values of thiamin, see Food Composition Table F-36.

Whole grains and enriched grain products are the best daily sources of thiamin. A quart of milk each day contributes 0.29 mg of the thiamim intake.

Foods lacking in thiamin are man-made—refined rice and cereal flours (from which almost all the natural store of the vitamin has been removed by the millers), refined sugar, separated animal and vegetable oils and fats, and alcoholic beverages. None of the thiamin in yeast used for fermentation is present in beers, wines, and spirits that enter normal commerce, although home-brewed beers and country wines may contain significant amounts. Indeed, there are communities in Africa and Latin America which derive the major part of their thiamin from native beers.

Enrichment of flour (bread) and cereals, with thiamin, riboflavin, niacin, and iron (with calcium enrichment optional), which was initiated in 1941, has been of special significance in improving the dietary level in the United States. On the basis of the average per capita consumption of flour and bread in the United States, slightly more than 40% of the daily thiamin requirement is now supplied by these foods.

Rice enrichment has been practiced for years in some of the rice-eating countries; for example, much of the rice used in Japan is enriched.

NOTE WELL: The thiamin requirements are usually met if the diet does not contain disproportionate amounts of the following:
1. Refined, unfortified cereal
2. White sugar
3. Alcohol

Since these three foods are usually matters of personal choice, nutrition education is important.

(Also see WHEAT, section on "Enriched Flour"; and RICE.)

TOP FOOD SOURCES OF THIAMIN. The top food sources of thiamin are listed in Table T-4.

NOTE WELL: This table lists (1) the top food sources without regard to the amount normally eaten (note that yeast and wheat germ are rich natural sources of thiamin, but they are eaten only in relatively small amounts); (2) the rich sources of commonly consumed foods; and (3) the caloric content of each food.

(Also see VITAMIN[S], Table V-9.)

TABLE T-4
TOP SOURCES OF THIAMIN AND THEIR CALORIC CONTENT[1]

Top Sources[2]	Thiamin (mg/100 g)	Energy (kcal/100 g)	Top Food Sources	Thiamin (mg/100 g)	Energy (kcal/100 g)
Yeast, brewers', debittered	15.61	283	Corn flakes, w/added nutrients	1.20	380
Yeast, torula	14.01	277	Peanuts, raw w/skins	1.14	570
Yeast, brewers'	12.12	—	Pork, fresh, loin, lean, boiled	1.13	300
Sunflower seed, flour, partially defatted	3.60	339	Sesame seed	0.98	563
Yeast, baker's, dry	2.33	282	Bacon, Canadian, broiled or fried, drained	0.92	277
Rice bran	2.26	275	Sausage, links or bulk, cooked	0.79	365
Wheat-soy blend (WSB)/straight grade, wheat flour	2.02	365	Wheat bran	0.72	353
Wheat germ	2.01	391	Kidneys, beef, braised	0.67	252
Sunflower seed kernels, dry, hulled	1.96	560	Wheat flour, all-purpose, enriched	0.64	365
Rice polish	1.84	265	Rye flour, dark	0.61	350
Wheat germ, toasted	1.65	391	Nuts, mixed, shelled	0.59	626
Wheat-soy blend (WSB)/bulgur, flour	1.49	360	Wheat flour, whole (from hard wheats)	0.55	361
Pinenuts, pinon	1.28	593	Pork, cured, canned, ham	0.53	193
Coriander leaf, dried	1.25	279	Cornmeal, degermed, enriched	0.44	362
Cottonseed flour	1.21	356	Rice, white, enriched, raw	0.44	363
Peanuts, raw w/skins	1.14	570	Bread, white, enriched	0.40	270
Pork, fresh, loin, lean, boiled	1.13	300	Soybean sprouts, cooked	0.42	105
Safflower seed, flour, partially defatted	1.12	388	Peas, green, immature, boiled, drained	0.28	71
Soybean flour, defatted	1.09	326	Turkey, hamloaf	0.27	247
Alfalfa seeds	1.08	389	Beef liver	0.25	222
			Luncheon meat, salami, cooked	0.25	261

[1]These listings are based on the data in Food Composition Table F-36. Some top or rich sources may have been overlooked since some of the foods in Table F-36 lack values for thiamin.

Whenever possible, foods are on an "as used" basis, without regard to moisture content; hence, certain high-moisture foods may be disadvantaged when ranked on the basis of thiamin content per 100 g (approximately 3½ oz) without regard to moisture content.

[2]Listed without regard to the amount normally eaten.

THIAMIN DIPHOSPHATE (TDP)

The activating coenzyme necessary for the transketolation reaction in the hexose monophosphate shunt (glucose oxidation) by which active glyceraldehyde is formed for synthesis of fats.

THIRST

Thirst (in humans) is the conscious desire for water. It is the primary means of regulating water intake, and generally, the thirst sensation ensures that water intake meets or exceeds the body's requirement for water. The sensation of thirst is caused by nerve centers in the hypothalamus of the brain which monitor the concentration of sodium (osmolarity) in the blood. When the sodium concentration of the blood increases above the normal 310 to 340 mg/100 ml (*136 to 145 mEq/1*), cells in the thirst center shrink. This shrinking causes more nervous impulses to be generated in the thirst center, thereby creating the sensation of thirst. An increase of only 1% in the osmolarity of the blood is sufficient to evoke the sensation of thirst. Increased osmolarity of the blood is primarily associated with water loss from the extracellular fluid—blood—through low cardiac output, hemorrhage, or intracellular dehydration may stimulate the thirst sensation. As water is lost, the sodium concentration of the remaining fluid increases. When the individual drinks, the sensation disappears.

Increased osmolarity of the blood simultaneously stimulates other nerve centers in the hypothalamus causing the release of antidiuretic hormone (ADH) from the posterior pituitary. ADH release results in the formation of less urine by the kidneys; hence, conserving body water. Thus, drinking water and excreting water are controlled by centers in the hypothalamus which maintains the water balance of the body within narrow limits.

Constant thirst is a classical symptom of diabetes mellitus.

(Also see ENDOCRINE GLANDS; WATER; and WATER AND ELECTROLYTES.)

THREONINE

One of the essential amino acids.
(Also see AMINO ACID[S].)

THROMBIN

An enzyme that facilitates the clotting of blood by promoting the conversion of fibrinogen to fibrin.

THROMBOSIS

The obstruction of a blood vessel by the formation of a blood clot.

(Also see ATHEROSCLEROSIS; and HEART DISEASE, section headed "Coronary Occlusion [Coronary Thrombosis]".)

THYMINE

One of the four nitrogenous bases in nucleic acid.
(Also see NUCLEIC ACID.)

THYROCALCITONIN

Another name for calcitonin, the hormone secreted by the thyroid gland which acts to lower blood calcium levels.

(Also see CALCITONIN; and ENDOCRINE GLANDS.)

THYROID GLAND

An endocrine gland which is located in the neck on top of the windpipe. It secretes the iodine-containing hormones thyroxine (T_4) and triiodothyronine (T_3), and the calcium regulating hormone calcitonin. The thyroid gland may grow to enormous proportions in the condition of goiter.

(Also see ENDOCRINE GLANDS; GOITER; and IODINE.)

THYROIDITIS

Inflammation of the thyroid gland.

THYROID-STIMULATING HORMONE (TSH)

A hormone secreted by the anterior pituitary gland that regulates uptake of iodine and synthesis of thyroxin by the thyroid gland.

THYROTOXICOSIS

Overactivity of the thyroid gland, causing exophthalmic goiter, which is characterized by nervousness, rapid pulse, bulging eyes, high basal metabolism, and loss of weight.

THYROXIN (T_4)

One of the two iodine-containing hormones secreted by the thyroid gland. It contains four iodine atoms per molecule. Hence, it is often called T_4. Thyroxin is less active than its counterpart triiodothyronine. Thyroxin's actions include increased metabolic rate, increased nervous system activity, stimulated protein synthesis, and increased motility and secretion of the gastrointestinal tract.

(Also see ENDOCRINE GLANDS.)

TIMBALE

• A creamy mixture of chicken, lobster, cheese, or fish cooked in individual molds or cups.

• A small pastry shell fried with a timbale iron and filled with a cooked timbale mixture, or served with fruit sauce, or dusted with powdered sugar.

TIN (Sn)

A silvery-white metal, with no known biological function, which has been used by mankind for thousands of years. Nowadays, most tin cans are made of steel covered with a thin coat of tin. This may be a potential hazard when the acids in such foods as citrus fruits and tomato products leach ·tin from the inside of the can. When this tin is ingested, it goes through a methylation process in the digestive tract. Methylated tin is a neurotoxin—a toxin that attacks the central nervous system. Currently, not much is known about the amount of tin in the human diet, indicating the need for more experimental work in this area. A deficiency of tin has been produced in experimental animals, and tin may prove to be a necessary trace element of human nutrition.

(Also see MINERAL[S]; and POISONS; Table P-11 Some Potentially Poisonous [Toxic] Substances.)

TISSUE

A collection of cells, usually of a particular kind which form a definite structure, such as connective tissue, epithelium, muscle, and nerve.

(Also see BODY TISSUE.)

TISSUES OF THE BODY

Tissues are an aggregate of similar cells together with their intercellular substances. In turn tissues combine to form the organs of the body. The major tissues of the body are (1) nervous tissue, (2) muscles, (3) skin, (4) blood cells, (5) fat or adipose, and (6) bone.

(Also see BODY TISSUE.)

TOASTED

Brown, dried, or parched by exposure to a fire, or to a gas or electric heat.

TOCOPHEROL

Any of four different forms of an alcohol. Also known as vitamin E.

(Also see VITAMIN E.)

TOCOTERIENOL

Compounds found in nature that have vitamin E activity, but which are less potent than alpha-tocopherol.

(Also see VITAMIN E.)

TOLBUTAMIDE

An oral drug, a derivative of sulfonylurea, capable of lowering blood glucose (sugar) when a functioning pancreas is still present. Since it acts by stimulating the release of insulin, it may be used in the treatment of diabetes when there is still some residual function of the pancreas.

(Also see DIABETES MELLITUS, section headed "Oral Drugs"; and ORINASE.)

TOMATO *Lycopersicon esculentum*

The fruit of this plant, which was once thought to be poisonous, is now one of the leading vegetable crops of the world. It is a member of the Nightshade family (*Solanaceae*), which also claims as members capsicum peppers, eggplant, and Irish potatoes.

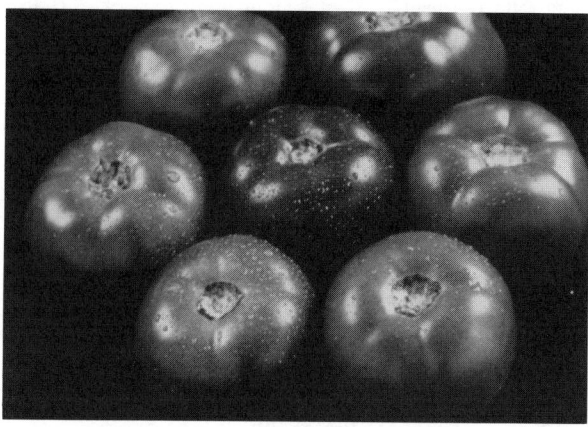

Fig. T-13. The tomato, a leading vegetable in the United States and the rest of the world. (Courtesy, USDA)

ORIGIN AND HISTORY. The modern tomato appears to have been developed from a primitive ancestor, the cherry tomato (*Lycopersicum cerasiforme*), which originated in the Peru-Ecuador area and spread like a weed throughout Latin America. Ironically, the plant was first domesticated in Mexico rather than in South America, because it bore a close resemblance to the tomatillo (*Physalis ixocarpa*), which had long been used as a food by the Mexican Indians.

In the years which followed the discovery of the Americas by Columbus, the Spanish conquistadors vanquished the Aztec Indians of Mexico and took tomato seeds back to Europe with them. However, many Europeans regarded the tomato as poisonous because they recognized it as a member of the Nightshade family, which also included other plants that contained poisonous substances. Also, some of the French thought that the fruit stimulated romantic desire. Hence, they called it the "love-apple" or *pomme d'amour*.

The tomato was brought back to the New World by the English colonists who settled in Virginia. Thomas Jefferson is thought to have been one of the first distinguished Americans to eat tomatoes. Nevertheless, the vegetable did not become popular in the United States until the latter part of the 19th century. The tomato rose steadily in prominence during the 20th century, when many new varieties were bred to grow under a wide variety of climatic conditions. One of the latest developments is the breeding of new varieties with qualities that make them harvestable by machine; they ripen simultaneously and have a tough skin and a squarish shape. Also, there is a naturally-occurring species of tomato (*L. cheesmanii*) which is very tolerant of salt water.

PRODUCTION. Fig. T-14 shows the countries which contribute most of the world's tomato production.

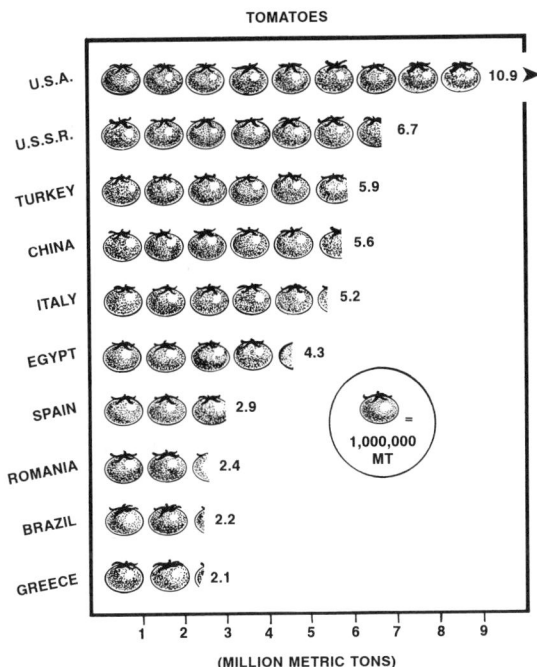

Fig. T-14. The leading tomato-producing countries of the world. (Based upon data from *FAO Production Yearbook*, 1990, FAO/UN, Rome, Italy, Vol. 44, p. 131, Table 52)

About 75% of the total U.S. tomato crop is grown for processing, much of it in California where the regular occurrence of cool night temperatures favors the setting of the fruit. Florida leads in the production of fresh tomatoes.

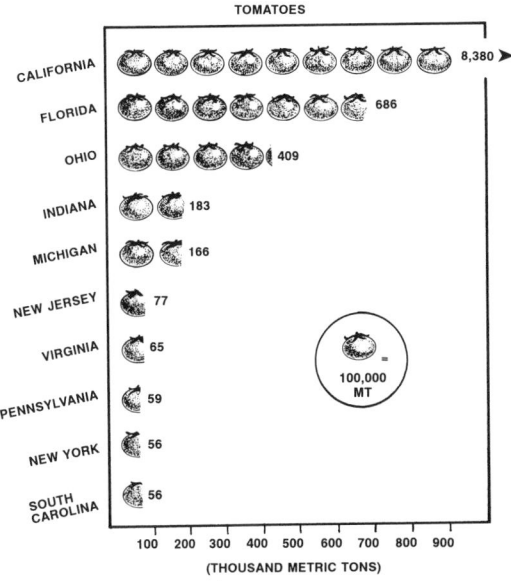

Fig. T-15. The leading tomato-producing states including both for the fresh market and for processing. (Based upon data from *Agricultural Statistics 1991*, USDA, pp. 165 and 166, Tables 240 and 241)

Growing In The Field. Tomatoes require a warm, mild climate; the plant does not thrive in cold weather, nor does it produce fruit when the weather is too hot. The maximum setting of fruit occurs when the night temperature ranges between 59° and 68°F (*15° and 20°C*). Hence, the crop is grown in Florida and other hot areas during the winter, and in the cooler areas during the period extending from spring to fall. The most efficient utilization of the growing season is achieved by starting the young plants from seed in greenhouses or hot beds, then transplanting them in the field when the weather is favorable.

The soil should be fertile and well-drained. Overly acid soil may require the addition of lime. Also, many growers use a fertilizer which supplies nitrogen, phosphorus, and potassium. However, excessive fertilization may overstimulate the growth of foliage at the expense of fruit production. Irrigation is needed in many areas because the combined stresses of water shortages and high temperatures cause the blossoms to drop off before the setting of fruit occurs. When sufficient water is provided, the plants grow better in dry areas than in the humid areas where the disease organisms thrive.

Much of the tomato crop grown for the fresh market is shipped considerable distances and is likely to be damaged, or to spoil, if picked when fully ripe. Therefore, the fruit is harvested at the "mature green" stage or when the color is just beginning to change. (Tomatoes which are not mature will not ripen later.) Green tomatoes will store well for several months at 50 to 60°F (*10 to 16°C*). They may be ripened in a warm, enclosed room. (Tomatoes produce ethylene gas during their normal respiration at room temperature. The ethylene brings about ripening.) Sometimes, ripening is hastened artificially by the use of either additional ethylene, or by treatment with the chemical ethepon, which releases ethylene.

Tomatoes grown for processing are usually picked when red-ripe, since the processors are located near the fields. In California, almost all of this crop is harvested mechanically.

The worldwide average yield of tomatoes per acre is about 17,800 lb (*19,936 kg/ha*), but yields as high as 190,000 lb (*212,800 kg/ha*) have been obtained in Denmark. However, the average U.S. yield of tomatoes per acre is about 44,900 lb (*50,288 kg/ha*), which is approximately equal to yields obtained in California, where much of the crop is produced.

Greenhouse Culture And Hydroponics. The ever-increasing cost of shipping tomatoes long distances during the winter to meet the needs of northern cities may soon make it economically feasible to grow more of this crop in greenhouses located near the urban areas. At the present time, greenhouses are used mainly for producing young tomato plants for transplantation, and to a very limited extent only for growing ready-to-eat tomatoes. A major factor limiting greenhouse production of vegetables is the cost of the electricity and fuel required to operate the facility. However, shipping tomatoes long distances in refrigerated trucks also consumes considerable energy.

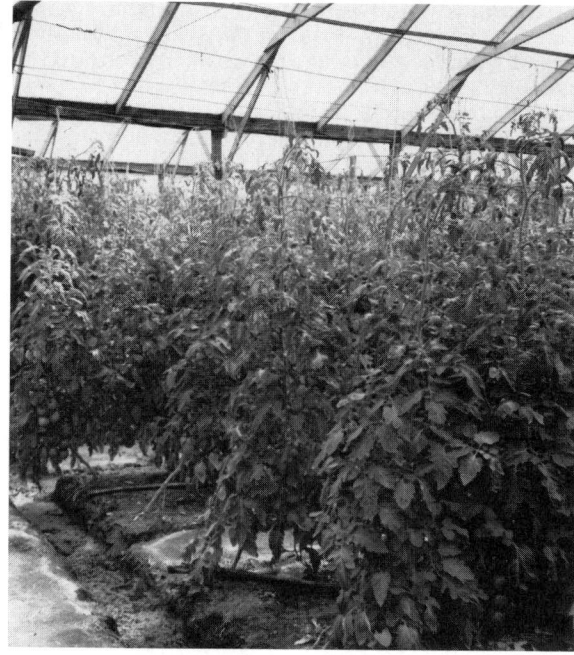

Fig. T-16.   The production of tomatoes in a greenhouse. (Courtesy, Union Pacific Railroad Company, Omaha, Neb.)

Recently, the science of growing plants without soil (hydroponics) has been utilized in greenhouses in order to eliminate some of the problems due to soil structure and soil pests. In hydroponic culture, soil is replaced by an inert porous bed of gravel, sand, or a similar material through which special nutrient solutions are circulated. This type of system is commonly used in commercial greenhouses. It is claimed that the totally controlled environment dispenses with need for the agricultural chemicals used in field production. Hence, hydroponically grown tomatoes may be considered to be "organically grown" and therefore, they may bring a premium price. Furthermore, this type of culture uses water very efficiently, because the nutrient solutions are filtered and recycled. The first major hydroponic facilities for growing vegetables were built in places such as Alaska, the Arabian peninsula, and certain Pacific Islands where the enviromental conditions were unfavorable for field production. Later, other facilities were developed in Arizona and Minnesota. At the present time, only a small fraction of the U.S. tomato crop is produced hydroponically, but this situation may change.

PROCESSING.   About 75% of the U.S. tomato crop is processed; still, the demand for tomato products can hardly be met, as evidenced by the various tomato extenders that are used in certain products. Brief descriptions of some popular products follow:

• **Canned tomatoes**—Washed, deskinned, cooked tomatoes are often canned whole with tomato juice or a similar fluid, salt, spices, and traces (not more than 0.07%) of calcium salts (used to keep the fruit firm). The canned vegetable may also consist of pieces, diced fruit, slices, or wedges.

• **Catsup (ketchup)**—This product is usually made from a concentrated tomato pulp which is strained to remove seeds and skin, then is cooked with a mixture of sugar, water, vinegar, and seasonings such as salt, onion powder, red pepper, garlic powder, cinnamon, celery seed, cloves, and mace. Some or all of the sugar (sucrose) may be replaced by dextrose (glucose) or various derivatives of corn syrup.

• **Chili sauce**—The predominant vegetable ingredient of the mild flavored sauces of this type is usually a tomato puree which has seeds present. Hence, the correct name for these products is "tomato chili sauce." The other ingredients are usually vinegar, water, and seasonings such as salt, peppers, and other spices. It is noteworthy that in items called "hot chili sauce" the major vegetable ingredient is the pulp from chili peppers.

• **Juice**—High quality tomato juice is expected to have a thick consistency and literally to "plop" when poured from the bottle or can. However, it consists of the unconcentrated liquid which has been strained after expression from red tomatoes. Hence, the thickness is achieved by (1) heating the tomatoes before expression of the juice, and/or (2) neutralizing some of the acidity by the addition of a little alkali. Both treatments block the action of the naturally occurring enzyme pectinase which thins the juice by breaking down the pectins. Tomato juice may contain added vitamin C (ascorbic acid) to bring the level of the vitamin up to 10 milligrams per fluid ounce. "Yellow tomato juice" is essentially the same as "tomato juice", except that it is expressed from mature tomatoes of yellow varieties.

• **Juice crystals**—This item is the most concentrated tomato product because it contains 99% solids (about 15 times the solids content of tomato juice). It is usually made by removing the water from tomato juice by a process such as vacuum-puff drying, in which a high vacuum puffs the juice up to a greatly expanded volume so that it may be dried rapidly. The crystals are convenient for food service establishments in that a 1-lb (0.45 kg) portion may be mixed with sufficient water to yield approximately 1 ¾ gal (6.7 liter) of juice (about 14 ½ lb of juice).

• **Paste**—Tomato pulp is strained to remove seeds and skin, then it is concentrated by heating to yield a product that contains at least 24% solids (almost four times the solids content of tomato juice). Sometimes, salt and other seasonings are added. Also, part of the acid of the tomatoes may be neutralized by the addition of baking soda.

• **Powder**—Tomato juice is dried to a powder by a process such as foam-mat drying in which the juice is foamed, then spread on a mat and dried. The powder is much in demand for the production of pizza mixes, powdered spaghetti sauce mixes, and dry soup mixes. Some types of tomato powder may be extended with cheaper ingredients such as beet powder, paprika, red dye, food acids (usually adipic, citric, and/or malic), sugar, vegetable gums, powdered seed hulls, and starches.

• **Puree**—This product, like tomato paste, is made from a strained tomato pulp that is concentrated by heating.

However, it is more watery than paste in that it contains from 8 to 24% solids. Salt is often added for flavoring.

• **Salad dressings**—Tomato products are used in various dressings such as French, Russian, and Thousand Island. There is even a dietetic dressing which is made from tomato juice, flavorings and vegetable gum (for thickening).

• **Sauces**—Many sauces contain some form of tomatoes. For example, barbeque sauce is made from tomato pulp, soy base, vinegar, and spices. However, the most popular tomato sauces are those used in the various pasta dishes.

• **Soups**—The nation's leading producer of canned condensed soups is also one of the leading utilizers of tomatoes. Furthermore, tomato soup is one of the best sellers in the soup company's line.

• **Vegetable juice cocktails**—These products usually contain tomato juice as a major ingredient. Other ingredients may be clam juice, lemon juice, other vegetable juices, and/or seasonings.

SELECTION. Good quality tomatoes are well formed and plump, of uniform red color, free from bruise marks and not overripe or soft. Scars, roughness, slight deformities, irregularity of shape, and well healed growth cracks are typical of the many possible defects of tomatoes which are objectionable only from the standpoint of appearance or the waste involved in preparation for use. Ripe tomatoes are particularly susceptible to damage by bruising from dropping, pinching or other rough handling.

Tomatoes that have been damaged by worms are usually very undesirable. Those having unhealed growth cracks may be satisfactory for immediate consumption, but will seldom keep for more than a very limited time. Puffy tomatoes may have a poor flavor and involve excessive waste in preparation. Puffiness can usually be distinguished by light weight and angular shape. Decay is usually indicated by mold growth, but may appear as soft discolored areas.

PREPARATION. Fresh tomatoes and canned tomato products are very convenient foods for the busy homemaker because (1) the raw vegetable lends itself well to cold soups, relishes, and salads; (2) only a few minutes of simmering is needed to cook the raw vegetable; (3) canned tomato juice may be used to make a wide variety of molded gelatin salads, (4) canned tomato paste or puree may be used when concentrated sauces are desired, and (5) the flavor and color of the tomato blends well with those of many other ingredients. Some examples of easy-to-prepare tomato dishes and a few gourmet-type preparations follow:

• **Aspic**—This type of appetizer or side dish is usually made from tomato juice, flavored or unflavored gelatin, and seasonings such as lemon juice, sugar, salt, pepper, and Worcestershire sauce.

• **Chinese stir-fried dishes**—Tomatoes may be added near the end of the cooking period to stir-fried dishes such as the one shown in Fig. T-17.

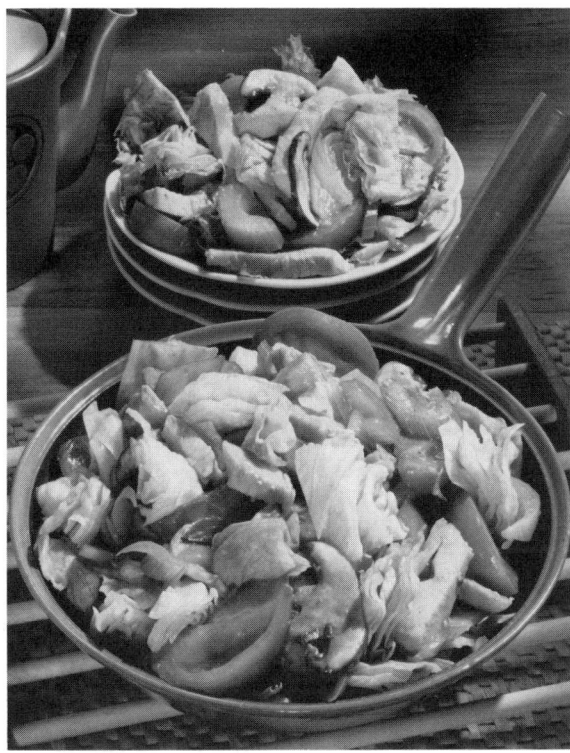

Fig. T-17. Turkey Stir Fry Salad. Tomato wedges and lettuce chunks are added to this dish during the last few minutes of cooking. The other ingredients are turkey strips, fresh mushrooms, sliced celery, onion wedges, vinegar, vegetable oil, soy sauce, cornstarch, brown sugar, curry powder, garlic powder, and a chicken bouillon cube. (Courtesy, California Iceberg Lettuce Commission, San Rafael, Calif.)

• **Eastern European tomato salad**—In Serbia (a region of Yugoslavia) this type of salad is made from tomatoes, raw onions, chili peppers, goat cheese and baked sweet peppers.

• **Gazpacho soup**—This chilled tomato soup, which originated in Spain, contains small pieces of peeled and seeded tomatoes, other vegetables that have been finely chopped or pureed, olive oil, wine vinegar, and various seasonings.

• **Green tomato pie**—Although this dessert is very similar to apple pie with respect to ingredients and preparation, it differs in that deskinned, green tomato wedges are substituted for sliced apples.

• **Guacamole**—Deskinned, deseeded, chopped tomatoes are mixed with mashed avocado pulp, chopped onions, hot green chili peppers, coriander leaves or parsley, and a pinch of salt to make this popular Mexican sauce.

• **Italian pasta dishes**—Many of these items are served with a rich tomato sauce that is easily prepared if one starts with a canned tomato product such as tomato paste or tomato sauce.

• **Lobster with tomato sauce**—Peeled and chopped tomatoes are simmered with white wine, fish stock, brandy, butter, chopped shallots, crushed garlic, parsley, Cayenne pepper, salt, and black pepper to make a delectable French sauce for lobster.

• **Piccalilli**—This popular relish is commonly made from green tomatoes, green peppers, red chili peppers, vinegar, sugar, salt, horseradish, ground mustard, cinnamon, and ginger.

• **Spanish rice**—Quick-cooking types of rice and canned tomato sauce make it possible to prepare this dish in less than one-half hour. Other ingredients are ground beef, chopped onion, chopped green pepper, chili sauce, butter or margarine, salt, Worchestershire sauce, and black pepper.

• **Stuffed tomato**—Fillings such as bread crumbs, cheese, chopped egg, crumbled bacon, fish or seafood, legumes, meats, nuts, poultry, and/or cooked rice may be used to stuff tomatoes. However, the fillings should be cooked first, so that the stuffed tomato shells will require only a few minutes of simmering in a sauce.

• **Tomato chutney**—Chutneys are condiments or relishes that appear to have spread to the rest of the world from India and Indonesia. A typical tomato chutney may contain chopped peeled tomatoes plus chili pepper, chopped dried fruit, vegetable oil, salt, and other seasonings.

CAUTION: A recent research report suggests that the consumption of vegetables of the Nightshade family (capsicum peppers, eggplant, the Irish potato, and the tomato) may aggravate arthritis in susceptible people. Furthermore, some nonarthritic people may be allergic to tomatoes. Therefore, it is suggested that arthritis sufferers and others who are unaccustomed to the heavy consumption of tomatoes and/or the other Nightshade vegetables try eating only small amounts of each vegetable alone until it is certain that there is no sensitivity to one or more of these otherwise nutritious foods.

NUTRITIONAL VALUE. The nutrient compositions of various forms of tomatoes are given in Food Composition Table F-36.

Some noteworthy observations regarding the nutrient composition of tomatoes follow:

1. Fresh tomatoes and tomato juice are high in water content (about 94%) and low in calories. Both items are good sources of vitamins A and C, except that the unfortified juice has only about two-thirds the vitamin C content of raw, ripe tomatoes. However, tomato juice may be fortified to bring the level of the vitamin up to 10 milligrams per fluid ounce (*30 ml*).

2. Ripe (red) tomatoes contain from 3 to 4 times as much vitamin A as mature green tomatoes. Otherwise, green and red tomatoes are about equal in nutritional value.

3. Canned tomatoes contain only about three-fourths the vitamin C content of fresh ripe tomatoes.

4. Tomato puree and plain types of tomato sauce (those without added ingredients such as cheese, meat, mushrooms, etc.) have about twice the solids content and about double the nutritional value of fresh tomatoes and tomato juice.

5. Tomato paste, which has about four times the solids content of fresh tomatoes, is a concentrated source of nutrients. Table T-5 compares the composition of this product with canned corn.

TABLE T-5
NUTRIENT COMPOSITIONS OF TOMATO PASTE AND CANNED CORN[1]

Nutrient or Other Constituent	Tomato Paste	Canned Corn[2]
Water content .... (%)	75	76
Calories .... (kcal)	82	83
Protein .... (g)	3.4	2.5
Phosphorus .... (mg)	70	73
Potassium .... (mg)	888	97
Iron .... (mg)	3.5	0.5
Vitamin A .... (IU)	3,300	350
Vitamin C .... (mg)	49	5
Thiamin .... (mg)	0.20	0.03
Riboflavin .... (mg)	0.12	0.06
Niacin .... (mg)	3.10	1.10

[1]Nutrients per 3½ oz (*100 g*) portion.
[2]Yellow sweet corn, vacuum packed, solids and liquid.

Table T-5 shows that tomato paste provides considerably greater amounts of nutrients per calorie than canned corn. A similar nutritional superiority is noted when the paste is compared to other grains and cereal products. Therefore, this product may make a valuable contribution when it is used in the preparation of pastas, pizzas, and other dishes.

6. Catsup and chili sauce are about equal in nutritional value, since each item is made with similar ingredients and contains about 32% solids (about 5 times the content of fresh tomatoes and tomato juice). However, the nutrients provided per calorie by these products are significantly less than those furnished by tomato paste, because the solids contents and caloric values of the two condiments are boosted by added salt and sugar.

(Also see VEGETABLE[S], Table V-6 Vegetables of the World.)

TOMATO JUICE

The juice extracted from tomatoes that is produced by chopping fresh fruit which may or may not have been preheated, pressing the fruit pulp through a series of screens, adding back some of the pulp to the screened juice, canning, and pasteurization.

The nutrient composition of various forms of tomato juice are given in Food Composition Table F-36.

Some noteworthy observations regarding the nutrient composition of tomato juice follow:

1. 1-cup (*250 g*) of bottled or canned tomato juice provides only 38 Calories (kcal), and is a good source of potassium, iron, vitamin A, and vitamin C. Most juice products often contain added sodium (about 400 mg per cup), but low sodium products are also available.

2. Frozen tomato juice concentrate contains about 4 times the caloric and nutrient contents of the single strength canned juice. Hence, it will make a significant nutritional contribution when added undiluted to dishes such as sauces and soups.

(Also see TOMATO.)

-TOMY

Suffix meaning to cut into; e.g., gastrectomy.

TONIC

• A drug or agent said to improve the health or vigor of an organ, or of the body.

• When referring to muscles, it can mean the state of muscular tension or continuous muscular contraction.

• A bottled quinine water used to make the drink "Gin & Tonic." This drink originated in the tropics where it was used to alleviate fevers, either real or imagined.

TOPHUS

Sodium urate deposits in the fibrous tissues near the joints or in the cartilage of the external ear; present in gout.

TORULARODIN

Carotenoid pigment in *Torula ruba* and *Rhodotorula mucilaginosa* yeasts, with vitamin A activity.

TORULA YEAST

Torula yeast (*Torulopsis utilis*) is a hardy type of yeast that can be propagated on a variety of substrates, such as press liquor obtained during the manufacture of dried citrus pulp, molasses, sulphite waste liquor from the paper industry, saccharified wood (both hexoses and pentoses can be used), and fruit wastes such as coffee beans, apples, etc. While brewers' yeast is truly a by-product food, torula yeast is cultured specifically as a foodstuff for man and animals.

Dried torula yeast is an excellent source of high-quality protein (50 to 62% crude protein) minerals, B vitamins (including vitamin B-12), unidentified factors, and of vitamin D if irradiated. Unlike the bitter-tasting brewers' yeast, torula yeast is tasteless, thereby facilitating its use as a palatable foodstuff.

Torula yeast is available in powder and tablets.

TOTAL CRUDE PROTEIN

The equivalent amounts of crude protein in the food represented by the total nitrogen present.
(Also see ANALYSIS OF FOODS.)

TOTAL MILK SOLIDS

Primarily milk fat, proteins, lactose, and minerals.
(Also see MILK AND MILK PRODUCTS.)

TOTAL PARENTERAL (INTRAVENOUS) NUTRITION (TPN) (CENTRAL INTRAVENOUS NUTRITION)

This nutritional procedure can provide all or most of a patient's nutrient requirements by intravenous means. Total parenteral nutrition is used when the patient cannot be fed through the gastrointestinal tract because of the danger of aggravating an abnormal condition, or because some part of the tract is functioning poorly. Usually, it involves infusion of nutrients by means of a catheter that is passed through a large vein into the vena cava, as is shown in Fig. T-18.

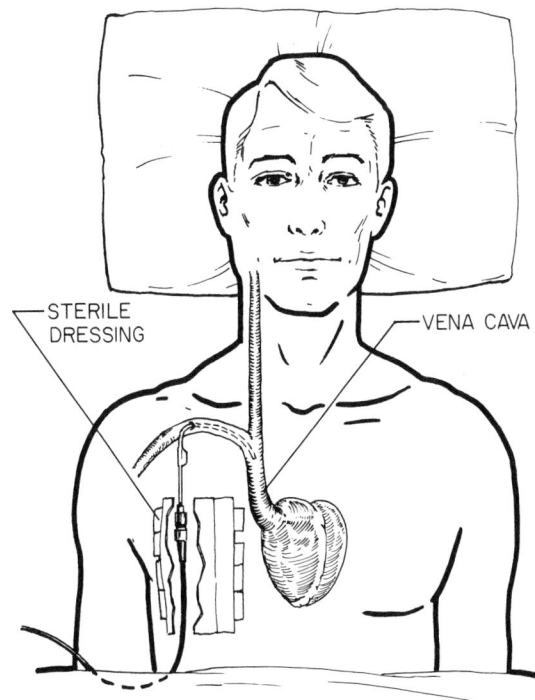

STERILE DRESSING

VENA CAVA

Fig. T-18. Total parenteral (intravenous) nutrition. The concentrated solution of nutrients flows through a sterile tubing attached to a catheter passed through the subclavian vein into the vena cava. This procedure results in rapid mixing of the nutrients with blood returning to the heart, which then pumps the nutrient-rich blood throughout the body.

It is noteworthy that the solutions used in total parenteral nutrition have much higher solute contents than those used in ordinary intravenous feedings (about

30% solute in TPN vs 5% solute in an IV) because (1) nutrient needs cannot be met completely by the latter, and (2) the means by which the former is administered (into a large central vein where rapid mixing with the blood occurs) is sufficiently safe, whereas concentrated (hypertonic) solutions cannot be infused safely into the peripheral veins. Phlebitis and clots are more likely to result from the injection of hypertonic solutions into peripheral veins because the flow of blood in them is slow. Therefore, TPN is sometimes referred to as "central intravenous nutrition" in order to distinguish it from peripheral IVs.

HISTORY. In the early 1940s there were reports of various attempts to provide nutritional support by the infusion of concentrated nutrient solutions into the peripheral veins of patients, but the procedures usually resulted in phlebitis and clots. During the 1950s intravenous fat emulsions were tried because they were much less irritating to the veins than sugars and amino acids. Nevertheless, there were often side effects such as asthma, chills, fever, liver disorders, low back pain, rashes, and various abnormalities of blood clotting. Hence, the use of these emulsions was discontinued until the safer preparations that are now available were developed.

Another procedure which was initiated in the 1950s was the administration of a concentrated solution of glucose via a central vein to patients in kidney failure. This therapy helped to reduce the wasting of their tissues from lack of calories. Use of this procedure declined after improved means of dialysis were developed.

By the late 1950s and early 1960s, a few physicians were successfully infusing hypertonic mixtures of glucose and protein hydrolysates into the central veins of patients who required more nutritional support than the common type of intravenous feeding supplied. However, the major breakthroughs in this technique were made in the mid-1960s by Dr. Stanley Dudrick and his co-workers at the University of Pennsylvania School of Medicine. These medical researchers tested their techniques on puppies and showed that the ones which received only total parenteral nutrition grew as well as their paired littermates which were given regular dog food. The next step was the use of the intravenous procedure on some selected patients who were desperately ill and had no chance of recovery on glucose IVs because they could not be fed orally. There were some dramatic recoveries which demonstrated that the beneficial effects of providing adequate nutrition were far beyond what most doctors believed were possible. For example, ugly oozing fistulas healed themselves without the need for surgical repair, an event that was almost unheard of before the development of this special procedure.

INDICATIONS FOR TPN. The foremost types of conditions requiring total parenteral nutrition are those in which the patient's nutritive needs are high, and cannot be met by more commonly used procedures such as oral, tube, or peripheral intravenous feeding. However, it may also be indicated even when some food can be taken orally or through a nasogastric tube because the nutritional requirements may be so high that they cannot be met via the digestive tract alone. Some of the most common indications for TPN follow:

- **Burns over large areas of the body**—Some badly burned patients may require as much as 7,000 to 10,000 Calories (kcal) per day plus high levels of amino acids to meet the needs for healing. Furthermore, the replacement of body fluids and mineral salts (electrolytes) is usually needed, also. The severe stress accompanying this type of injury usually impairs the appetite considerably, so that only small amounts of food can be taken orally. Also, tube feeding may be dangerous because the concentrated solutions have a tendency to draw fluids into the digestive tract and cause dehydration. Only a fraction of the patient's needs can be met by conventional IVs as evidenced by the fact that prior to the use of TPN, it was common for the patients to lose from 30 to 50 lb (*13.5 to 23 kg*) during the early stages of recovery.

- **Cancer**—People with this type of disease are likely to be somewhat malnourished and run down because (1) the malignant growth may have interfered with the utilization of nutrients and other normal physiological functions; (2) surgery to remove the cancer was probably very stressful in terms of blood, fluid, and tissue losses; (3) chemotherapy and radiation treatments often cause nausea, vomiting, diarrhea, and loss of appetite; and (4) certain types of gastrointestinal cancer may make oral or tube feeding unsuitable. It is noteworthy that patients who are in moderately good condition after the surgery and other anticancer treatments may live many more years. Many doctors now give their cancer patients TPN in order to maintain their strength during the very stressful treatments.

- **Chronic diarrhea**—This condition is a leading killer of infants and young children because it saps all of their vitality and resistance to infection. Furthermore, certain harmful strains of microorganisms may become so well established in the digestive tract that any attempts to provide nutrients orally or by tube feeding may only promote microbial growth and aggravate the diarrhea. The considerable losses of fluids and electrolytes may be replaced by continuous infusion of these substances into a peripheral vein, but the required calories and proteins cannot be provided in this manner. Therefore, TPN is a better means of providing nourishment while allowing the intestines to rest and the germs to starve.

- **Fistulas of the digestive tract**—A fistula is a channel or tunnel through tissue that leads from the inside of the body to the surface of the skin and allows body fluids to seep out while making the internal tissues very susceptible to infection. This undesirable condition may develop during the healing of a surgical or other type of wound. Normally, additional surgery has been needed to close fistulas. However, some patients with fistulas have had remarkable healing without surgery after being given TPN.

• **Inflammatory bowel disease**—Crohn's disease (regional enteritis) and other inflammatory disorders of the intestines are difficult to treat because (1) many of the anti-inflammatory drugs have hazardous side effects when used for extended periods of time, (2) removal of the abnormal part(s) of the small intestine reduces the capacity for absorbing nutrients and does not necessarily prevent the remaining normal parts from developing an inflammatory disease, (3) attempts to feed the patient orally may often aggravate the inflammation, and (4) the malabsorption that is associated with the inflammatory process(es) may result in malnutrition which retards healing. Furthermore, these disorders occur in children and adolescents, as well as in young and old adults. Therefore, it is noteworthy that a group of teenagers who were treated for inflammatory bowel disease and the accompanying malnutrition by TPN alone had extended periods of remission of their bowel problems and significant improvements in nutritional status.

• **Kidney failure**—Patients with acute or chronic kidney failure may become very malnourished and have extensive wasting of tissues due to the severe reduction in appetite caused by the toxicity of the accumulated wastes and/or the various medical treatments for the condition. For example, hemodialysis results in the loss of amino acids, electrolytes, vitamins, and other essential small molecules from the blood, whereas peritoneal dialysis depletes significant amounts of the same nutrients, plus proteins which are not lost in hemodialysis. Therefore, doctors have long given nutrients intravenously to these patients in order to retard the progressive depletion of nutrients and wasting of body tissues. However, TPN provides an opportunity to infuse more concentrated solutions than ordinary peripheral intravenous feeding. Nevertheless, the use of TPN in kidney failure requires very thorough monitoring of the patient's status by frequent blood tests and other diagnostic measures because too little or too much of certain nutrients may cause serious complications.

• **Liver failure**—Normally, the liver, as well as the kidneys, regulates the levels of nutrients and other substances in the blood. The failure of the liver to function occurs frequently in advanced cases of cirrhosis and in a few cases of hepatitis. Mental confusion and/or coma may result from the accumulation of excessive levels of substances that interfere with metabolism in the brain. For example, excesses of the amino acids methionine, phenylalanine, tryptophan, and tyrosine are believed to be responsible for some of the cerebral disorders observed in liver failure. (A healthy liver metabolizes excesses of amino acids to harmless substances.) There is also the possibility that certain toxic substances produced in the intestines are absorbed and built up to high levels in the blood when liver functions are depressed significantly. TPN offers an opportunity to correct these abnormalities by (1) providing required amounts of amino acids that are lacking, while supplying minimal amounts of the potential offenders, and (2) bypassing the digestive tract.

• **Refusal to eat**—People with psychiatric disorders such as anorexia nervosa or those on "hunger strikes" may starve themselves to death unless some means of providing nutrition is instituted. Tube feeding may be unsatisfactory because the patient may regurgitate it. Even TPN should be used cautiously because some patients may try to remove the catheter. Admission of air to the catheter tubing could result in a potentially fatal air embolism.
(Also see ANOREXIA NERVOSA; and STARVATION.)

• **Surgery on the digestive tract**—Normally healthy adults who have had gastrointestinal surgery may be maintained on peripheral intravenous infusions for a few days, then they may be given elemental diets that are well absorbed and yield little or no residue. However, infants, children, and malnourished adults should be given their full nutritional requirements within a few days of the surgery in order to prevent debilitation and the wasting of tissues. If oral or tube feeding is inadvisable because of the condition of the patient, TPN infusions should be started promptly. Other indications for TPN in postsurgical patients are delayed healing, infection, obstruction, inflammation, and immobility of one or more parts of the digestive tract.

• **Undernourished and very-low-birth-weight infants**—Some newborn infants get off to a bad start because of digestive or other problems that interfere with their nutrition, or, they may have a very low birthweight, but be otherwise normal. The nutritional needs of this group are very high in proportion to their size and it is often difficult to meet these requirements by oral feeding alone. Hence, TPN has been used experimentally in such cases, but it must be emphasized that it is *not* a routine procedure.

Use Of TPN At Home. The success of TPN in hospital settings led to the development of techniques and equipment that could be used at home so that patients requiring this therapy would not have to be kept in a hospital. Generally, the most likely candidates for home TPN are patients with reasonable chances of benefiting from it because their major nutritional problems are due to gastrointestinal disorders such as (1) a loss of considerable amounts of small intestine, (2) inflammatory bowel disease, and (3) digestive disorders resulting from chemotherapy and/or radiation treatments.

Home TPN is rather expensive because it requires a special pump or a gas pressure device, sterile tubing, special valves, and the nutrient solutions. It is noteworthy that the valves permit patients to be disconnected from the apparatus for 8 to 14 hours so that many normal activities may be carried out. Hundreds of patients have been placed on home TPN, and some have received this therapy for 5 years or more. It is expected that the cost will be reduced as the number of people on home TPN increases. At any rate, it is usually less expensive than receiving care in an institution.

Composition of Infusions. The TPN solutions that were first used on an experimental basis by Dr. Dudrick and his co-workers at the University of Pennsylvania School of Medicine contained approximately 20% dextrose (glucose), 5% protein, and 5% minerals and vitamins. Hence, the total solute concentration was about 6 times that of an ordinary 5% dextrose (glucose) intravenous feeding. Since then, many modifications of Dudrick's original TPN solutions have been made to accommodate the particular needs of individual patients. However, the commercial TPN preparations that are available in the United States do not always contain essential fatty acids. Therefore, it is noteworthy that deficiencies of these nutrients have been observed in patients receiving parenteral nutrition. This risk is reduced to zero if fat emulsions are infused on a regular basis (1 to 2 times per week). No doubt there are other essential nutrients that should be provided by supplemental means when patients are on TPN for long periods of time.

BENEFITS. Some of the recoveries that were brought about by TPN have been so remarkable that one eminent physician has ranked the development of this procedure on a par with other great medical innovations such as anesthesia, antiseptics, and antibiotics. What TPN has done is to demonstrate very dramatically the pivotal role played by nutrition in healing. Typical benefits of TPN follow:

1. The need to search all over the body for intact veins through which to make peripheral intravenous infusions is eliminated by TPN because an indwelling catheter may remain in place for long periods of time when the proper safeguards are observed.

2. Wasting of tissues after burns, injury, surgery, or other extremely stressful occurrences is minimized by TPN, which provides the high levels of nutrients needed for healing.

3. Bypassing of the digestive tract does away with the needs to cope with diarrhea, flatulence, nausea, vomiting, and other gastrointestinal reactions that interfere with nourishment. Hence, the tract may be rested and allowed to heal without disturbance.

4. Nutrient patterns may be tailormade to suit the needs of the patient because the infusions are made directly into a major blood vessel for delivery to the tissues of the body by the pumping of the heart.

HAZARDS AND PRECAUTIONS. TPN is not a routine nutritional procedure because special precautions must be taken in its administration to prevent undesirable consequences. The main hazards and precautions of TPN are:

• **Aggravation of disorders of metabolism**—When people obtain their nourishment via the digestive tract the absorbed nutrients are conveyed by the portal system of blood vessels to the liver, where excess sugars are converted into fats and glycogen (a complex carbohydrate that is stored in the liver and muscles), fats are combined with proteins for safe transport in the blood, and amino acids are converted into proteins and waste products such as urea.

However, in TPN the regulation of the blood levels of nutrients by the liver is bypassed to a great extent because the infused substances flow to the heart, where they are pumped through the arteries to the body tissues. The latter situation may be dangerous to diabetics because they utilize nutrients more slowly than normal people. Hence, they may develop excessively high blood levels of nutrients, which can lead to (1) loss of excessive amounts of nutrients and water through urination (osmotic diuresis), (2) dehydration (due to excessive loss of water), and/or (3) coma. On the other hand, people with some types of kidney disease may fail to excrete a normal amount of water and consequently become waterlogged (overhydrated) to the point of developing congestive heart failure.

Finally, some people who have been on TPN for 5 months or longer have developed bone demineralization and bone pain. Therefore, patients receiving TPN for the first time should be monitored carefully by blood chemistries, blood gas analyses, urine collection and analyses, and other laboratory tests for metabolism so that the appropriate therapies may be administered for any abnormal conditions that may develop.

• **Injuries resulting from the procedure**—The experts who have used TPN on a regular basis consider the placement of the catheter to be a serious surgical procedure and proceed accordingly. Failure to observe certain precautions may result in mishaps such as puncturing of the vein and passage of the catheter into neighboring blood vessels or organs such as the heart and lungs, and consequences such as bleeding, production of irregular heartbeats, the introduction of air or fluids into the lungs, or inflammation of the catheterized vein so that a spasm occurs or a clot is formed. Therefore, it is best to place the patient in an inclined position with the head downward (15% Trendelenburg position) so that the subclavian vein sticks out and is more easily entered. Also, an x ray should be taken after the catheter has been placed and before it is used to make certain that its location is correct for the patient. It is noteworthy that complications are rare when these precautions are observed strictly.

• **Microbiological contamination**—Infectious microorganisms may get into the body via (1) the point where the vein is punctured, (2) the surface of the catheter, (3) the inside of the tubing and/or the catheter. Also, inside the vena cava the tip of the catheter may serve as a place for bloodborne bacteria to lodge and multiply, then detach themselves and spread through the bloodstream to susceptible body tissues. Therefore, a sudden unexplainable rise in the body temperature of a patient should lead the attending doctors and nurses to suspect a catheter-induced infection, and/or any of the other sources of infection that are likely under the circumstances.

Some of the antiseptic precautions that are commonly used to prevent a catheter-induced infection of the patient consist of (1) shaving the hair from the chest and defatting of the skin with ether or acetone; (2) washing of the shaved and defatted area with sterile gauze sponges wetted with iodine solution; (3) handling of the catheterization assembly with sterile gloves while making sure that it does not come into contact with nonsterile items; (4) application of an antibiotic ointment and a sterile dressing on the area of catheterization, followed by the application of tincture of benzoin around the dressing; (5) periodic changing of the dressing and inspection of the catheter site for redness, infection, leakage, or other problems (ideally, the same nurse should perform this function so that she will readily recognize any changes); and (6) taking care that the solutions are changed under strictly aseptic conditions. These measures ensure a continued sterility of the catheter for months, or even years. The longevity of the preparation is important because there are only four sites (right and left subclavian veins, and right and left jugular veins) that are highly suited for this procedure as it is normally carried out. (Other means of central venous infusion are more complicated and dangerous.)

• **Nutritional deficiencies**—Recent reports in the medical literature have indicated that certain nutritional deficiencies may result from the long-term use of some proprietary brands of TPN infusions, unless the nutrients not present in the solutions are provided by other means. The deficiencies reported up to now have been those of essential fatty acids, the essential minerals chromium and selenium, and the vitamin biotin. Normally, biotin is synthesized by intestinal bacteria, but the administration of broad spectrum antibiotics in the case reported eliminated that source of the vitamin.

It is the responsibility of the doctor who orders the TPN procedure to make certain that all of the essential nutrients are provided to the patient. This may be done readily by adding the required substances to the TPN infusion.

• **Psychological impact**—Many patients may be quite apprehensive of being put on TPN because (1) they may not have known anyone else who received this type of therapy, (2) the providing of nutrients parenterally for more than a few weeks may cause concern over whether normal eating will ever be resumed, and (3) their lives may depend upon the apparatus functioning properly. Therefore, it may be necessary for the doctor, nurse, a knowledgeable member of the family, or a trusted friend to give the patient repeated assurances about the efficacy of the procedure and the possibility of eventually resuming many normal activities, even though it should be necessary to continue TPN for a long time at home.

The expression of anger, disbelief, grief, and/or depression is common for patients dependent upon complex treatments delivered by the medical care team, who may sometimes deliberately or inadvertently create a mystique about their procedures. Some type of psychiatric consultation may be required to help the patient cope with the situation and cooperate in the healing process.

CONTRAINDICATIONS. TPN carries some risks, and should not be used when (1) it is possible to meet all or most of a patient's nutritional needs by oral or tube feeding (some supplementation may be given by peripheral intravenous feeding); (2) the patient is moderately healthy and will be required to abstain from eating for only a few days; (3) there is little hope for improvement of the patient, and (4) certain disorders (cardiovascular, metabolic, or organ disfunctions) are present that are likely to be aggravated by TPN. In the latter cases, it may be possible to use TPN after the patient's condition has been stabilized.

SUMMARY. Total parenteral nutrition is a recently developed procedure that carries some risks, but may help to get seriously ill patients back on their feet, provided that the proper precautions are observed.

TOX-

Prefix meaning poison.

TOXEMIA

A condition produced by the presence of poisons (toxins) in the blood.

TOXEMIA OF PREGNANCY (PREECLAMPSIA AND ECLAMPSIA)

A cardinal indication of toxemia of pregnancy is a sudden weight gain sometime during the last trimester. It is a serious disorder of uncertain origin involving decreased kidney function. Numerous factors including endocrine, metabolic, and nutritional may be responsible for the disorder, and not a toxic substance as the name implies. Other features of the condition consist of high blood pressure, blurred vision, protein in the urine, and puffy neck, ankles, and face—edema. It is most often observed in (1) first pregnancies before the age of 30 years; (2) twin pregnancies; (3) economically underprivileged segments of the population—the malnourished; and (4) women with prior kidney or vascular disease. Preeclampsia and eclampsia are two stages of toxemia of pregnancy. Preeclampsia is characterized by those items mentioned above, while eclampsia indicates that the symptoms have intensified—circulatory failure, convulsions, and coma—possibly resulting in the death of the mother and the baby.

The most effective treatment is delivery of the baby. However, during the course of pregnancy, routine urine analysis and blood pressure checks by a doctor indicate the onset of toxemia. Once the onset of toxemia is noted, control measures such as sodium restriction, diuretics, sedatives, and bed rest may be initiated. Nevertheless, toxemia becomes increasingly difficult to manage the last month of pregnancy, and delivery may be induced slightly before term to prevent harmful effects to both the mother and the child.

Interestingly, pregnant sheep often develop a condition called pregnancy disease or ketosis. Pregnancy disease, like toxemia of pregnancy, is associated with undernourishment, and occurs more frequently in late pregnancy, and in sheep carrying twins or triplets. Some of the symptoms are similar to toxemia of pregnancy in humans. Pregnancy disease is known to be a disturbance in carbohydrate metabolism. As in humans with toxemia, the symptoms rapidly reverse following delivery.

Although the involvement of dietary factors in the development of toxemia is not clear, three points deserve mention. First, a vitamin B-6 deficiency during pregnancy may have a role in the development of toxemia. Second, while sodium restriction and diuretics are traditional approaches to the control of toxemia, there is also an increased demand for sodium during pregnancy; moreover, the Committee on Maternal Nutrition discourages the routine use of salt restriction and diuretics during pregnancy. Third, well-balanced diets provide the best protection against the development of complications during the course of pregnancy.

(Also see PREGNANCY AND LACTATION NUTRITION.)

TOXINS

The poisons produced by certain microorganisms. They are products of cell metabolism. The symptoms of bacterial diseases, such as diptheria, tetanus, botulism, and staphylococcal food poisoning, are caused by toxins.

(Also see FOODBORNE DISEASE; and FOOD POISONING.)

TOXINS, BACTERIAL, FOODBORNE

Food poisoning is caused by the ingestion of bacterial toxins that have been produced in the food by the growth of specific kinds of bacteria before the food is eaten. The powerful toxins are ingested directly, and the symptoms of food poisoning develop rapidly, usually within 1 to 6 hours after the food is eaten. Two common bacteria that produce toxins in food are *Clostridium botulinum* (botulism) and *Staphylococcus aureus* (staphylococcus food poisoning). Each type is quite different in growth habits and in the symptoms of poisoning.

(Also see BACTERIA IN FOOD, Table B-6 Food Poisonings [Bacterial Toxins].)

TRACE ELEMENTS

Minerals which are required in minute quantities, ranging from millionths of a gram (micrograms) to thousandths of a gram (milligrams) per day. The term trace elements does not imply any lesser role for these minerals than for the macro minerals; rather, it represents quantity designations based on the amounts needed. The trace elements known to be essential for humans are chromium, cobalt, copper, fluorine, iodine, iron, manganese, molybdenum, selenium, silicon, and zinc. It seems likely that arsenic, vanadium, tin, and nickel may soon be added to this list.

(Also see MINERAL[S].)

TRANSAMINATION

A metabolic process involving the transfer of an amino group (NH_2) from one compound to another. This is one process which makes possible the synthesis of a limited number of amino acids—nonessential amino acids. Carbon skeletons for this process are produced through various intermediates of carbohydrate metabolism. A new amino acid can be produced when an amino group (NH_2) is transferred from an amino acid to the carbon skeleton. The deaminated molecule—past amino acid—can be used as an energy source.

(Also see METABOLISM; and PROTEIN[S].)

TRANS FATTY ACIDS

The hardening of vegetable oils by hydrogenation (the chemical addition of hydrogen) converts the naturally-occurring *cis* fatty acids to *trans* fatty acids. Generally speaking, it follows that the more an oil has been hardened, the higher the content of trans fatty acids.

The prefixes *cis* and *trans* refer to the orientation of the atoms around the double bond. The *trans* form of essential fatty acids does *not* function as an essential fatty acid in the body.

Trans fatty acids are present in most margarines, salad oils and cooking oils, now being consumed in increasing amounts because of their high level of polyunsaturates and public fear that saturated fats (usually animal fats) are associated with coronary heart disease. The trans fatty acids are formed when vegetable oils are processed for human use.

A growing number of medical and scientific experts are voicing concern over the high consumption of trans fatty acids; among them, Dr. Germain J. Brisson, Professor of Nutrition, University of Laval in Quebec, who has recorded his thinking in a new book entitled, *Lipids in Human Nutrition*.

Usually extolled as "cholesterol free," consumers buy these products (margarines, salad oils and cooking oils) to lower cholesterol intake, theoretically reducing the risk of heart disease. However, the concerns are: (1) that during processing trans fatty acids are produced in relatively large amounts, and (2) that the effects of these large quantities of trans fatty acids ingested by humans have unknown consequences. Because of the highly sophisticated chemical nature of these acids and the way they behave in the human body, there is need for further research to determine the wholesomeness and safety of the products, particularly since fatty acids represent 95% of the fats and oils in our diets.

From the above, it may be concluded that before people drastically change their diets to conform to new theories, more research should be done, particularly on the polyunsaturated fats.

(Also see FATS AND OTHER LIPIDS, section headed "Fatty Acids"; and OILS, VEGETABLE, section headed "Antinutritional and/or Toxic Factors,")

TRANSFERASE

Any of various enzymes that promote a transfer reaction; for example, transaminase.

TRANSFERRIN (SIDEROPHILIN)

Iron-binding protein for transport of iron in the blood. (Also see IRON.)

TRANSKETOLASE

The enzyme is a transketolase and the process is called transketolation (keto-carrying). Transketolase uses thiamin diphosphate as a coenzyme to bring about the transfer of a 2-carbon unit from one sugar (a 2-keto sugar) to aldoses (monosaccharides with the characteristic aldehyde group [-CHO]).

TRAUMA

• A wound or injury.

• A psychological or emotional stress.

TREE TOMATO *Cyphomandra betacea*

The fruit of a small tree (of the family *Solanaceae*) that is native to Peru and is now grown throughout the tropics.

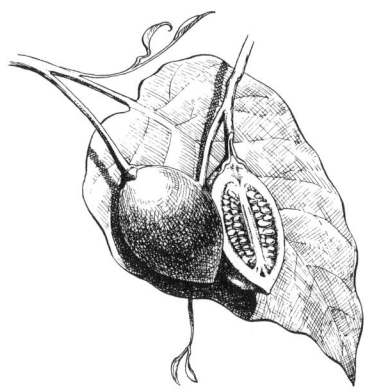

Fig. T-19. The tree tomato.

Tree tomatoes resemble the plum type of common tomato (*Lycopersicum esculentum*) in many respects in that they are usually yellow to red in color, 2 to 3 in. (*5 to 7.5 cm*) long, and contain many seeds. They may be eaten raw, stewed, or when made into jam, jelly, or juice.

The fruit ranges from low to moderately high in calories (50 kcal per 100) and carbohydrates (10%). It is a good source of fiber and vitamin C, and a fair source of iron.

TRICHINOSIS

This disease, caused by the parasitic worm *Trichinella spiralis*, is most common as a human parasite under conditions where raw or inadequately cooked pork is consumed by man. People have also acquired trichinosis from consuming infected bear and walrus meats. In addition to man and hogs, rats, dogs, cats, whales, and many other mammals are susceptile to infection.

The worm was first discovered by Peacock at a human autopsy in London, in 1828, and was first obtained from hog's flesh by Joseph Leidy of Philadelphia in 1846. Today, trichinosis is recognized as a widely disseminated, clinically important disease in the United States and parts of Latin America, with epidemic outbreaks in small or moderate-sized groups of the population.

Infected pork contains the encysted *Trichinella* larvae. When the pork is eaten raw or inadequately processed, the larvae are liberated in the stomach, become encysted in the duodenum and invade the duodenal and jejunal mucosa, where in 3 to 5 days they develop into sexually mature adults, which mate. At this stage, the threadlike worms are hardly visible to the unaided eye. Males are about .06 in. (*1.5 mm*) long and the females, which are somewhat larger, are .14 in. (*3.5 mm*) long. After fertilization, the females invade the tissues of the intestinal wall more deeply and begin to deposit living young, many of which burrow into the mesenteric vessels and are carried to skeletal muscles, where they are filtered out and soon become encysted. The heaviest infection occurs in muscles poor in glycogen.

The common methods of exposure to trichinosis in the United States are diagramatically illustrated in Fig. T-20.

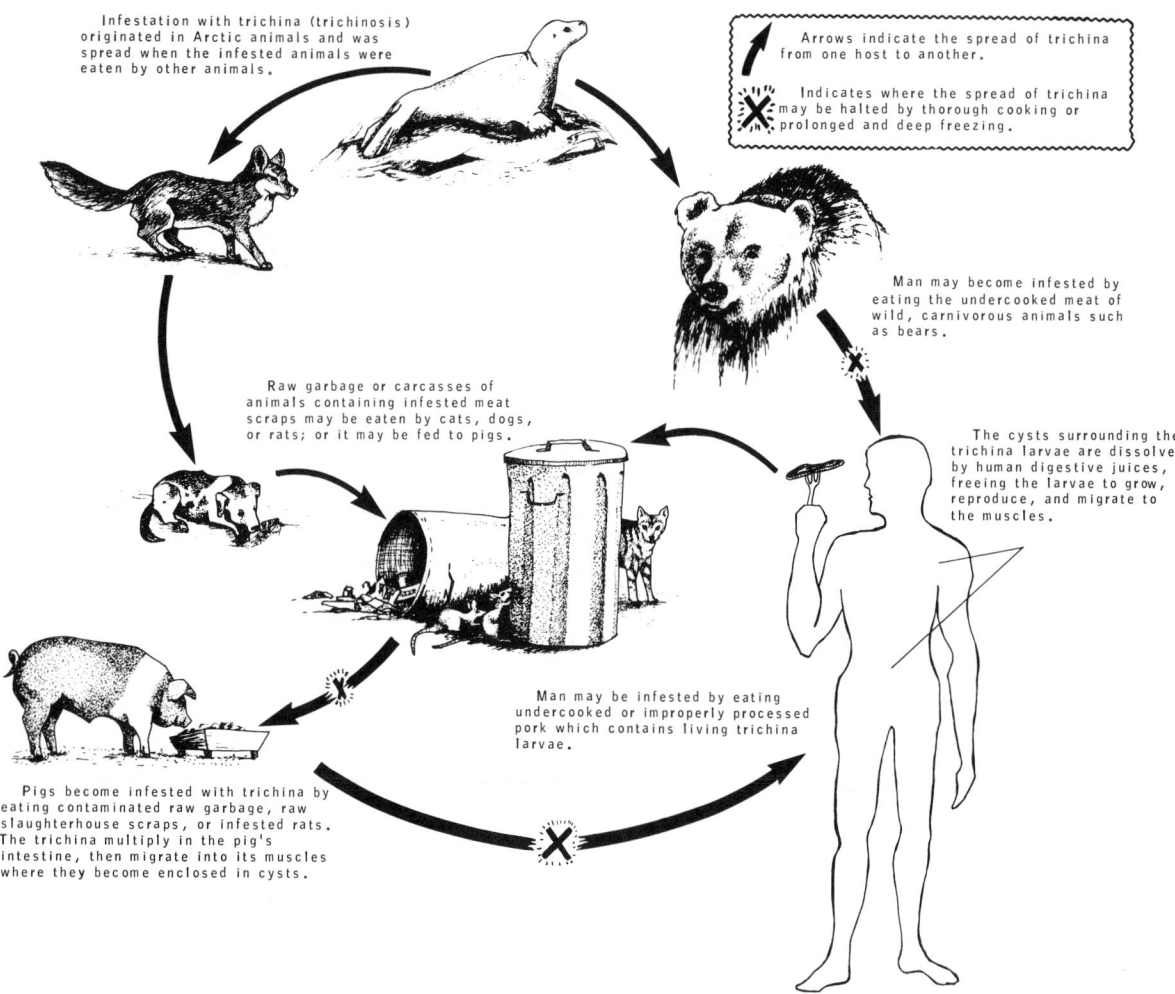

Infestation with trichina (trichinosis) originated in Arctic animals and was spread when the infested animals were eaten by other animals.

Arrows indicate the spread of trichina from one host to another.

Indicates where the spread of trichina may be halted by thorough cooking or prolonged and deep freezing.

Man may become infested by eating the undercooked meat of wild, carnivorous animals such as bears.

Raw garbage or carcasses of animals containing infested meat scraps may be eaten by cats, dogs, or rats; or it may be fed to pigs.

The cysts surrounding the trichina larvae are dissolved by human digestive juices, freeing the larvae to grow, reproduce, and migrate to the muscles.

Man may be infested by eating undercooked or improperly processed pork which contains living trichina larvae.

Pigs become infested with trichina by eating contaminated raw garbage, raw slaughterhouse scraps, or infested rats. The trichina multiply in the pig's intestine, then migrate into its muscles where they become enclosed in cysts.

Fig. T-20.   Diagram illustrating the common methods of exposure to trichinosis in the United States.

In man, the disease may be accompanied by a fever, digestive disturbances, swelling of infected muscles, and severe muscular pain (in the breathing muscles as well as others). Sometimes, no detectable symptoms are produced. In severe epidemics, 0.5 to 30% of the patients succumb, with an average of about 3.0%. No specific symptoms are seen in infected hogs, even when the parasite is present in the muscle tissue, its usual abode.

Diagnosis of trichinosis may be suggested by the patient's history and a high eosinophilia (the abnormal increase of white blood cells), and is confirmed by recovery of the larvae from centrifugalized specimens of blood or from digests of biopsied samples of biceps muscle, as well as by immunologic tests. The most common immunologic test is the intradermal reaction developed by Bachman.

Infected humans should be under the care of a physician. No specific therapeutic is known; only symptomatic treatment (treatment to ease the accompanying pain) is used.

Trichinosis in swine may be lessened by (1) destruction of all rats on the farm, (2) proper carcass disposal of hogs and other animals that die on the farm, and (3) cooking all garbage and offal from slaughter houses. Today, only about 1% of U.S. hogs are garbage fed, and all states have laws requiring that garbage be cooked prior to feeding.

Microscopic examination of pork is the only way to detect the presence of trichinae, but such a method is regarded as impractical in U.S. meat inspection procedure. So, prevention of trichinosis in man is best achieved by (1) cooking all pork thoroughly at a temperature of 137°F (58°C) before it is consumed, or (2) freezing pork for a continuous period of not less than 20 days at a temperature not higher than 5°F (-15°C), or for 24 hours at 2°F (-17°C). The same precautions apply to bear meat. Smoking, salting, or drying do not necessarily kill the larvae.

(Also see DISEASES, Table D-13 Infections and Parasitic Diseases Which May Be Transmitted by Contaminated Foods and Water.)

TRIGLYCERIDES

Chemical compounds which contain three (tri-) molecules of fatty acid combined with one molecule of glycerol. Triglycerides differ from each other because the types of fatty acids linked to the glycerol vary. Fig. T-21 illustrates the formation of a triglyceride. The R in Fig. T-21 indicates a carbon chain which varies according to the fatty acid, while the COOH in Fig. T-21 is the acid portion of the fatty acid. When fatty acids combine with glycerol water (H_2O) is formed.

(Also see FATS AND OTHER LIPIDS; FATTY ACIDS; and OILS, VEGETABLE.)

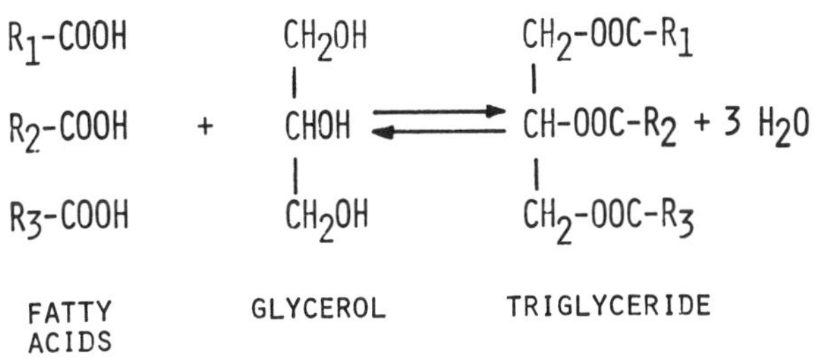

$$R_1-COOH \qquad CH_2OH \qquad CH_2-OOC-R_1$$
$$R_2-COOH \quad + \quad CHOH \rightleftarrows CH-OOC-R_2 + 3\ H_2O$$
$$R_3-COOH \qquad CH_2OH \qquad CH_2-OOC-R_3$$

FATTY ACIDS   GLYCEROL   TRIGLYCERIDE

Fig. T-21. The formation of a triglyceride.

TRIIODOTHYRONINE

One of two iodine containing hormones secreted from the thyroid gland. It is, however, secreted in lesser quantities than its counterpart thyroxin. Triiodothyronine has three iodine atoms per molecule, and it is sometimes called T_3. It is more active than thyroxin. Triiodothyronine's actions include stepping up the metabolic rate, increasing the nervous system activity, increased heart performance, stimulation of protein synthesis, and increased motility and secretion of the gastrointestinal tract.

(Also see ENDOCRINE GLANDS.)

TRIPE

Most tripe is made from the first and second (rumen and reticulum) stomachs of cattle by: washing thoroughly; removing the stomach lining by scalding and scraping; and either (1) pickling in a 60°F (*16°C*) salt brine, or (2) cooking and pickling in a weak salt and vinegar brine.

TRIPEPTIDES

These are three amino acids chemically joined together by peptide bonds. They may be a step in the synthesis of new protein, or a step in the breakdown of dietary protein.

(Also see DIGESTION AND ABSORPTION; and PROTEIN[S].)

TRISTEARIN

A triglyceride of stearic acid.

TRITICALE *Triticum X Secale*

This is a hybrid cereal derived from a cross between wheat (*Triticum*) and rye (*Secale*), followed by doubling

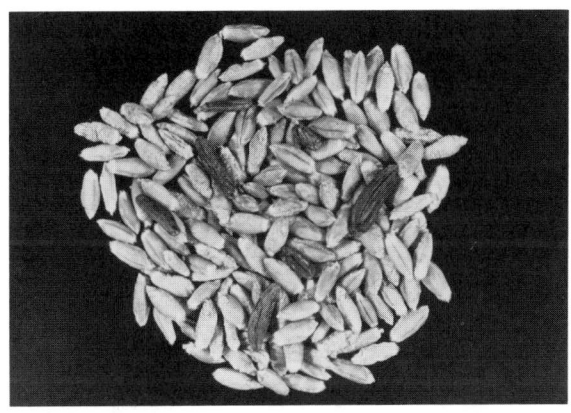

Fig. T-22. Triticale grains. (Photo by International Development Research Center, Ottowa, Canada)

the chromosomes in the hybrid. The objective of the cross: to combine the grain quality, productivity, and disease resistance of wheat with the vigor and hardiness of rye. The first such crosses were made in 1875 when the Scottish botanist Stephen Wilson dusted pollen from a rye plant onto the stigma of a wheat plant. Only a few seeds developed and germinated; and the hybrids were found to be sterile. In 1937, the French botanist Pierre Givaudon produced some fertile wheat-rye hybrids with the ability to reproduce. Intensive experimental work to improve triticale was undertaken at the University of Manitoba, beginning in 1954.

To date, none of the triticale crosses have been entirely satisfactory, due to low yields, excessive shriveled kernels, susceptibility to lodging, low tillering capacity, and lack of adaptability. But there is promise that further breeding will improve these shortcomings.

In comparison with wheat, triticale (1) has a larger grain, but there are fewer of them in each head (spike), (2) has a higher protein content, with a slightly better balanced amino acid composition and more lysine, and (3) is more winter hardy. Nutritional information on triticale flour is presented in the Food Composition Table F-36.

Earlier varieties of triticale did not offer much promise for milling and baking; they resembled their rye parent more than their wheat parent. However, bread of good quality has been made from more recent triticale selections. So far, the main use for triticale has been as a feed grain, pasture, green chop, and silage crop for animals.

(Also see CEREAL GRAINS, Table C-18 Cereal Grains of the World.)

TROPICAL SPRUE

A malabsorption syndrome, particularly of fats, but also of sugar and vitamins. It occurs chiefly in the West Indies, Central America, and the Far East.

The standard treatment is a diet low in fat, high in protein and vitamins, and rich in bananas.

(Also see SPRUE, TROPICAL.)

TRUFFLE *Tuber* spp

The truffle is a pungent wild fungus that grows underground, which is highly prized as a food. The fungus is believed to have a symbiotic relationship with the roots of oak and beech trees, near which it is usually found. Agronomists have not been successful in cultivating truffles. Depending on the species, they vary from white to brown or black in color. They range from 1/4 to 4 in. *(0.6 to 10 cm)* in diameter; and they grow in clusters 3 to 12 in. *(7.7 to 30 cm)* below the ground. They resemble an acorn, a walnut, or a potato in shape. Most culinary truffles are found in western Europe. *Tuber melanosporum* is the famed black truffle of France, while *Tuber magnatum* is the more pungent and odoriferous white truffle that grows in the Italian Piedmont. Also, North Africa produces a truffle (*Terfezios*) in some quantity and they are occasionally found along the Pacific Coast in the United States. Trained dogs or pigs are usually used to sniff out the location of truffles. From 300 to 500 tons are harvested annually.

(Also see MUSHROOMS.)

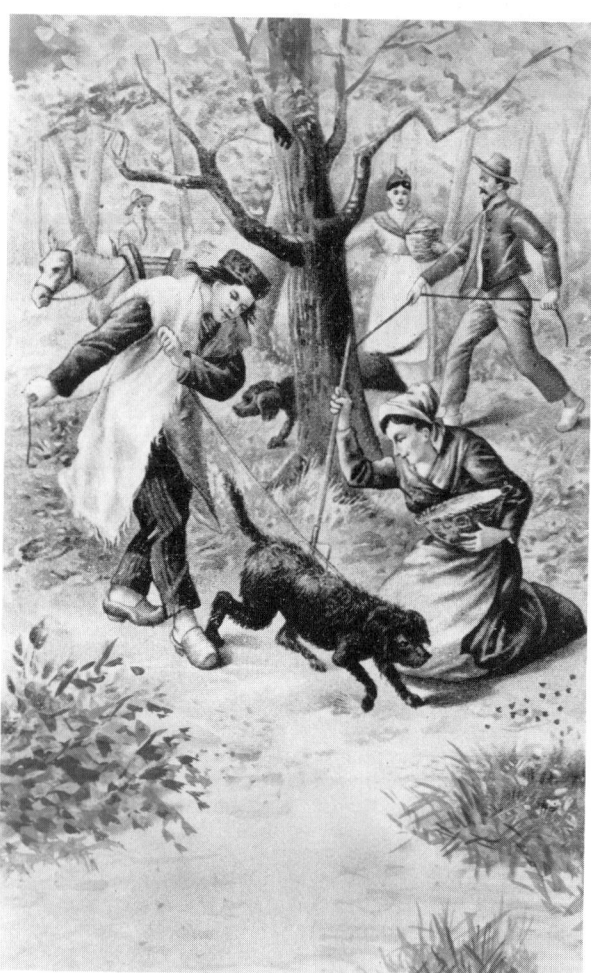

Fig. T-23.   Hunting for truffles in France. (Courtesy, The Bettman Archive)

TRYPSIN

A digestive enzyme formed in the small intestine when another enzyme, enterokinase, acts on trypsinogen, an inactive secretion of the pancreas. Trypsin cleaves polypeptides or proteins at peptide bonds adjacent to the amino acids arginine or lysine.

(Also see DIGESTION AND ABSORPTION.)

TRYPSINOGEN

Inactive form of trypsin.

TRYPTOPHAN

One of the essential amino acids.
(Also see AMINO ACID[S].)

TUBE FEEDING

Among the circumstances which may necessitate tube feeding are surgery of the head and neck, esophageal obstruction, severe burns, gastrointestinal surgery, anorexia nervosa, and coma. Three types of tube feeding may be employed depending upon the situation: (1) a nasogastric tube (from the nose to the stomach) or a nasoduodenal tube (from the nose to the duodenum); (2) a surgically formed opening (stoma) in the stomach; or (3) a surgically formed opening (stoma) in the small intestine. Obviously, the nasogastric tube or the nasoduodenal tube is the method of choice but instances may arise when it is impossible to pass a tube from the nose to the stomach or the duodenum, or when there is gross disease of the stomach or the duodenum. All three types of tube placements are capable of supplying all types of adequate nutrients in a liquid form. Since the nasogastric tube or the nasoduodenal tube is the most common, it will serve to illustrate the principles of tube feeding.

As the name implies, the tube is passed down the nose through the esophagus, and then to the stomach or duodenum. Extreme caution must be exercised in ensuring that the tube is in the stomach or duodenum, and not in the lungs. Also, in precoma or in comatose patients, the danger of aspiration pneumonia as a result of regurgitation of digestive juices must be kept in mind. Because there is less hazard of aspiration from nasoduodenal tube feeding than from nasogastric tube feeding, it is the method of choice of most physicians.

In order for tube feeding to be effective, it must meet several criteria. It must be: (1) nutritionally adequate; (2) easily digested without reactions such as diarrhea or constipation; (3) simply prepared; (4) well tolerated without inducing vomiting; and (5) low cost. There are three tube feedings which meet these criteria and are commonly used: (1) milk-base; (2) milk-base with suspended solids from strained or blenderized foods; and (3) synthetic low-residue formulas. Recipes are available for home preparation of these types of tube feedings. Commercial preparations are also available. All tube feedings generally contain 1/2 to 1 1/2 kcal/ml.

Foods introduced into the tube are generally warmed to body temperature, and flow into the tube by gravity, or by the use of a food pump. The first tube feedings should be frequent and in small volumes, then if tolerated the volume of feedings may be gradually increased. Two liters per day is a common volume.

Several potential hazards of tube feedings are apparent: (1) tube feeding is dangerous when the patient is vomiting; (2) contaminated food leads to gastrointestinal infections; (3) concentrated feeding (high sodium or high protein) may lead to diarrhea, dehydration, and elevated blood urea; and (4) high concentrations of sugar, particularly lactose, are apt to produce diarrhea.

TUBER

A short, thickened, fleshy stem, or terminal portion of a stem or rhizome that is usually formed underground, bears minute leaves each with a bud capable under suitable conditions of developing into a new plant, and constitutes the resting stage of various plants such as the potato and Jerusalem artichoke.

(Also see VEGETABLE[S].)

TUBERCULOSIS (TB)

Even the Pharaohs of ancient Egypt could not escape this disease; studies of mummies have shown that it was active in the earliest Egyptian civilizations. As recently as 100 years ago, tuberculosis was the chief cause of death throughout the world. The decline in the incidence of tuberculosis can be attributed to an improved standard of living, and prompt recognition and treatment. In the Western world where bovine tuberculosis is controlled, the main mode of transmission is airborne droplets discharged during the coughing or sneezing of infected persons. Symptoms of tuberculosis consist of chronic coughing, extreme fatigue, loss of weight, and possibly coughing up blood. Good preventative measures include (1) avoiding infected persons, (2) disposal of tubercular animals, (3) an adequate and nutritious diet, (4) comfortable living quarters, and (5) sufficient daily rest. Successful treatment depends upon early detection by skin test or x ray. Once the diagnosis is established, an antibiotic will likely be prescribed.

During the acute stage of the disease, a high-protein, high-calorie fluid diet, and eventually progressing to a regular diet is beneficial. If the appetite is poor, more than three meals during the day may be required. Some of the drugs used to treat tuberculosis have adverse effects on certain of the B-complex vitamins; hence, supplements should be provided.

(Also see BACTERIA IN FOOD, Table B-5 Food Infections [Bacterial]; and DISEASES, Table D-13 Infectious and Parasitic Diseases Which May Be Transmitted by Contaminated Foods and Water.)

TUBERIN

A globulin constituting the principal protein of the potato tuber.

TULAREMIA

The foodborne disease which is sometimes called rabbit fever, and named after Tulare, California where it was first described. Tularemia is caused by infection with *Fracisella tularensis*. An ulcerous sore breaks out at the location where the germs enter the skin. Other symptoms include headache, chills, drenching sweats, vomiting, and irregular fever. Recovery begins in 3 to 4 weeks, however, the mortality rate is about 6%. Most cases of the disease come from eating undercooked meat from wild rabbit. However, the hunter or the cook may get the disease from handling an infected rabbit. Thoroughly cooking the meat at 130°F (*54°C*) kills the organism. It is also a good practice to wear rubber gloves when handling wild game. Antibiotics are effective for the cure of tularemia. However, some cases may be complicated by pneumonia and require hospitalization, intravenous feeding, and blood transfusions.

(Also see BACTERIA IN FOOD, Table B-5 Food Infections [Bacterial]; and DISEASES, Table D-13 Infectious and Parasitic Diseases Which May Be Transmitted by Contaminated Foods and Water.)

TUN

Liquids, especially wine, ale, or beer, may be stored in a large cask or barrel called a *tun*. At one time, wine, liquor, and some other liquids were measured in terms of a tun, which equals 252 gallons (*958 liter*).

TURBINADO SUGAR

Sometimes this sugar is viewed erroneously as a raw sugar (sucrose), but turbinado sugar goes through a refining process to remove impurities and most of the molasses. It is produced by separating raw sugar crystals and washing them with steam. If produced under proper conditions, it is edible.

(Also see RAW SUGAR; and SUGAR.)

TURNIP *Brassica rapa*

This plant, which is a member of the mustard family (*Cruciferae*), provides a leafy vegetable and a root vegetable. Fig. T-24 shows a typical turnip.

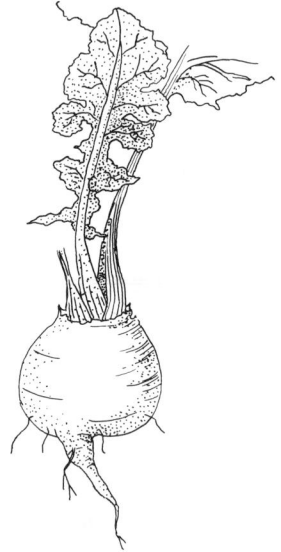

Fig. T-24.   The turnip, a plant that has edible leaves and an edible root.

It is noteworthy that there are several major types of turnip root—(1) carrot-shaped, (2) spindle-shaped, (3) round, and (4) flat and broad.

ORIGIN AND HISTORY. It seems likely that the leaves and roots of wild turnips were used as food before the dawn of agriculture. One type of the plant appears to have originated in southern Europe near the Mediterrean, while the other came from central Asia. Turnips were first cultivated about 4,000 years ago in the Near East.

The ancient Greeks and Romans grew turnips and developed some of the many varieties. At that time many peasants lived on meager diets and depended upon turnips to help alleviate the pangs of hunger. It appears that this vegetable was taken by the Romans to various parts of northern Europe, where it was grown for both human food and fodder for cattle and sheep.

Beginning in the 17th century, turnips helped to increase food production significantly because they were part of the Norfolk four-course system of crop rotation which was first established in Norfolk County, England. (The system was developed from a seven-course system that had been in use in Holland.) The basic principles of the Norfolk system were (1) wheat was grown the first year, (2) turnips were grown the second year, (3) barley, clover, and ryegrass the third year, and (4) cattle and sheep were allowed to graze the grain and grasses during the fourth year. Turnips were an important part of this system because they kept well in outdoor storage over the winter. Hence, they enabled farmers to keep a larger number of animals over the winter when other feeds were scarce.

The use of turnips as food began to decline with the use and popularity of the potato in northern Europe during the 18th century. Since then, the turnip has also been replaced to some extent by its close relative, the rutabaga, which is higher in nutritional value. Nevertheless, the former vegetable has an advantage over the latter one in that it grows to maturity in about one-half the time.

PRODUCTION.   Statistics on turnip production are not readily available. However, the U.S. Department of Agriculture reported that approximately 10 million pounds (*9 thousand metric tons*) of rutabagas and turnips are shipped within the United States.[4] Also, 17.8 million pounds of turnip greens and 19.6 million pounds of turnip greens and turnips were frozen in 1990.[5] Most of the U.S. crop is produced in the southern states.

Turnips do not grow well when the temperature exceeds 75°F (*24°C*). Hence, they are usually planted in the early spring or late summer, or during the fall and winter in the southern states. Fertilizer containing nitrogen, phosphorus, and potassium is often applied to promote optimal growth, although turnips are less demanding in this respect than many of the other vegetables. Furthermore, the varieties which produce large roots require considerable space to grow. Hence, they are usually thinned after the foliage has developed sufficiently to be marketable as turnip greens.

Most types of turnips are ready for harvesting within 30 to 60 days after planting. (The growing period for rutabagas is about 90 days.) In some places, turnips planted in the fall are left in the ground until the following spring, when they produce a crop of fresh greens. Wax or paraffin may be applied to prevent the roots from withering if they are to be stored for a time.

PROCESSING.   Although fresh greens and roots are still marketed, much of the crop is now frozen. The combined production of frozen turnip greens and turnip greens with turnips increased by 16% from 1981 to 1990.[6]

[4]*Agricultural Statistics 1991*, USDA, p. 169, Table 244.

[5]Ibid., p. 172, Table 248.

[6]Ibid., p. 172, Table 248.

Also, the share of this total contributed by turnip greens with turnips rose from 34 to 64% during this period. Turnip roots are diced when they are frozen together with turnip greens.

SELECTION AND PREPARATION. High-quality turnip greens are fresh, young, tender, and green. Leaves which show insect injury, coarse stems, dry or yellowing, excessive dirt, or poor development are usually lacking in quality and may cause excessive waste.

Turnip roots are of high quality if they are heavy in relation to size, and if they are smooth and firm, with few leaf scars around the crown, and with very few fibrous roots at the base. Shriveled or soft turnips may be tough when cooked. Large, coarse, overgrown turnips, which are light in weight in relation to size, are likely to be tough, woody, hollow, and/or strong in flavor.

Southern cooks prepare turnip greens as a hot vegetable mixed with bacon or pork. They are also good in casseroles, soups, and stews; or when served with a cheese sauce, hollandaise dressing, or white sauce.

The most common way of preparing turnip roots is to (1) cut off the peel, (2) dice or slice the pared root, (3) cook the pieces in lightly salted boiling water for 12 to 15 minutes, and (4) mash and serve with butter and seasonings. Sometimes, very small turnips are cooked whole like beets, in which case a half-hour or more of cooking is required. Turnip roots are also good when (1) mashed together with boiled potatoes, (2) served with various sauces, or (3) cooked in casseroles, soups, and stews.

CAUTION: Turnips and other vegetables of the mustard family *(Cruciferae)* contain small amounts of substances called goitrogens that interfere with the utilization of iodine by the thyroid gland. Hence, people who eat very large amounts of these vegetables while on an iodine-deficient diet may develop an enlargement of the thyroid, commonly called a goiter. The best insurance against this potentially harmful effect is the consumption of ample amounts of dietary iodine. This element is abundantly present in iodized salt, ocean fish, seafood, and edible seaweeds.

NUTRITIONAL VALUE. The nutrient compositions of turnip greens and turnip roots are given in Food Composition Table F-36.

Some noteworthy observations regarding the nutrient composition of turnips follow:

1. Turnip greens and turnip roots have a high water content (90 to 94%) and a low calorie content (29 to 53 kcal per cup).

2. Although turnip roots are often considered to be a starchy vegetable, they supply only about one-third as many calories as equal amounts of potatoes.

3. The protein content of the greens is about triple that of the roots. A cup of the greens contains from 3.2 to 4.1 g of protein, which is about the same as that furnished by similar amounts of cooked cereals. However, the cereals supply about four times as many calories.

4. A l-cup *(240 ml)* serving of turnip greens supplies about ¾ as much calcium as a cup of milk. Furthermore, the level of phosphorus is only about ⅓ that of calcium. Hence, the greens are complementary to the many other foods that are low in calcium, but rich in phosphorus (eggs, fish, legumes, meats, nuts, and poultry). The greens are also a good source of iron.

5. Almost all of the vitamin A content of turnips is in the greens, which are one of the leading vegetable sources of this vitamin.

6. The vitamin C content of raw turnip greens is much higher than that of either the cooked greens, or the raw or cooked roots. Hence, the greens should be cooked as briefly as possible in order to retain this vitamin at a high level.

(Also see VEGETABLE[S], Table V-6 Vegetables of the World.)

TURTLE

Reptiles with bodies encased in a bony shell. Both land turtles and water turtles are eaten, but it is the water turtle that is made into the famous turtle soup. The English hold turtle soup in high esteem; it is often served at their great diplomatic dinners and ceremonial repasts.

TWADDELL

This is a hydrometer used for measuring density (specific gravity), of industrial liquids which are greater than one. Measures of specific gravity between 1 and 2 are divided into 200 equal parts, and each division is 1 degree. The specific gravity of a solution equals the number of degrees on the Twaddell scale multiplied by 5 and divided by 1,000. The Twaddell is named for its inventor.

TYPHOID FEVER

A disease transmitted by water or food contaminated with the bacteria *Salmonella typhi* or *Salmonella paratyphi*. Foods or water become contaminated by sewage, flies, infected persons, or symptomless carriers (Typhoid Mary) of the disease. Symptoms consist mainly of fever, nausea, headache, and loss of appetite. Prevention includes (1) protection and disinfection of drinking water, (2) adequate cooking of foods, (3) finding and curing carriers, and (4) sanitary food handling. Fortunately, typhoid fever responds to antibiotics, and it is not as serious as it was at one time. A high protein, high energy, but low fiber diet will support convalescence.

(Also see DISEASES, Table D-13 Infectious and Parasitic Diseases Which May Be Transmitted by Contaminated Foods and Water; and MODIFIED DIETS.)

TYRAMINE

A pressor amine that has action similar to epinephrine; found in mistletoe, certain cheeses, some wines, and ergot, and also obtained from tyrosine by strong heating or by bacterial action.

TYROSINASE

A copper-containing enzyme responsible for the conversion of tyrosine to the dark pigment, melanin. Skin color depends, in part, upon the concentration of melanin. A genetic absence of tyrosinase results in albinism. Tyrosinase is also the enzyme responsible for the browning of cut surfaces of certain fruits and vegetables; as such, it is described by the generic term phenolase.

(Also see PHENOL OXIDASES.)

TYROSINE

One of the nonessential amino acids.
(Also see AMINO ACID[S].)

TYROSINOSIS

A hereditary disorder in the metabolism of the amino acid tyrosine which is characterized by elevated blood levels of tyrosine, liver damage, and kidney damage. Rickets and mental retardation are also associated with tyrosinosis. It results from the lack of the enzyme para-hydroxyphenylpyruvic acid oxidase which normally converts tyrosine to homogentisic acid. The necessary dietary modification is, of course, a diet low in tyrosine and phenylalanine. This can be accomplished by using a casein hydrolysate as the source of protein and calories.

(Also see INBORN ERRORS OF METABOLISM; and MODIFIED DIETS.)

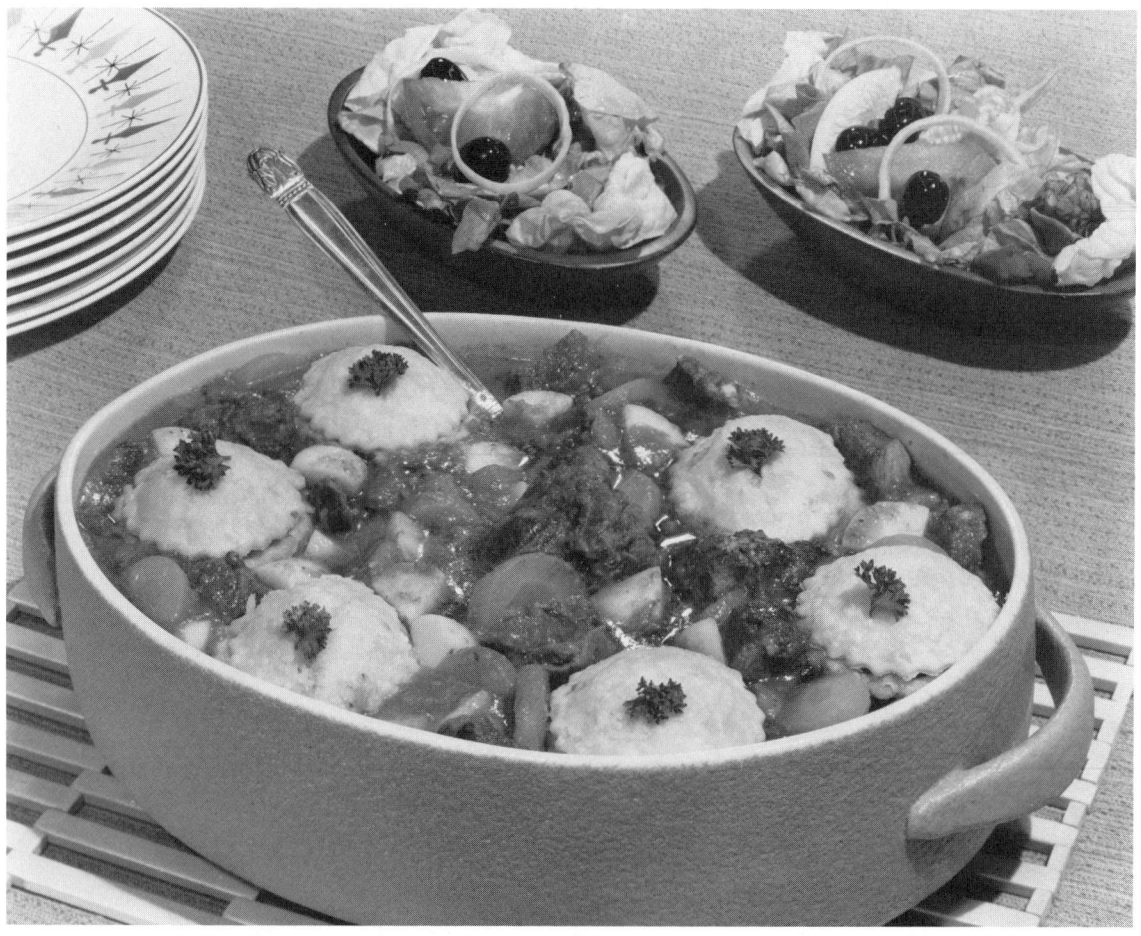

Well-planned, attractively-served meals should be an important event each day, whether serving one or 100. (Courtesy, National Food Processors Assn., Washington, D.C.)

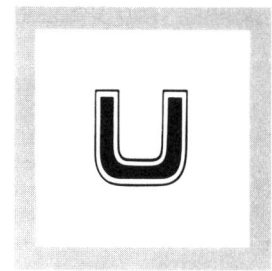

UDO

A Japanese plant grown for its tender young shoots which are eaten as a vegetable and in salads.

ULCERS, PEPTIC

An ulcer is any open sore, other than a wound. Peptic ulcers are open sores or erosions of the surface lining of the digestive tract, usually in the stomach or duodenum. Their appearance is roughly comparable to that of canker sores of the mouth—for those unfortunate sufferers familiar with the appearance of canker sores. The term peptic ulcer is employed since it appears that these ulcers develop from the lessened ability of the lining of the digestive tract to withstand the digestive action of pepsin and hydrochloric acid (HCl). Ulcers can occur in any area of the digestive tract which is exposed to the action of these two substances. However, a vast majority of ulcers occur in two locations: (1) the first part of the small intestine, or duodenum, before the point of entry of the alkaline secretions of the pancreas; and (2) the stomach or gastric portion of the digestive tract, usually along the lesser curvature near the pylorus—opening from the stomach into the duodenum.

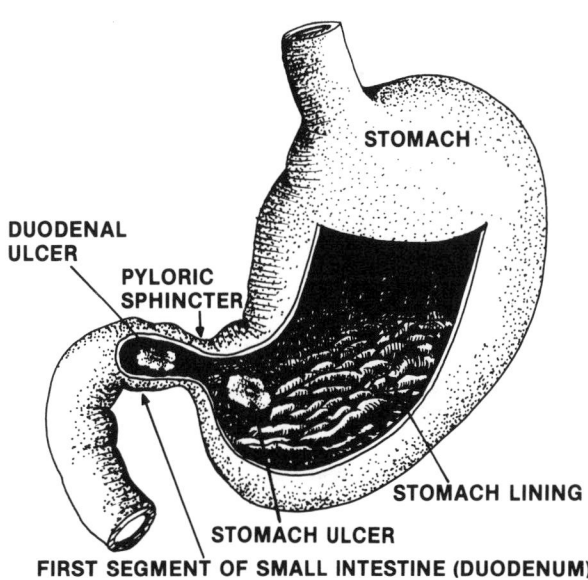

Fig. U-1. The two major sites where peptic ulcers occur.

OCCURRENCE. Overall, peptic ulcers occur in about 10% of all Americans at some time of their lives. Between the two locations, duodenal ulcers are far more common than gastric ulcers. Unfortunately, both are characterized by high recurrence rates.

Duodenal. About 80% of all peptic ulcers are duodenal ulcers. These occur most often in men between the ages of 20 and 50. Thus, after puberty and before menopause the ratio of affected males to females varies from 3:1 to 10:1. For some unexplained reasons, duodenal ulcers are now less common than they were 20 years ago.

Gastric. Again, more males than females are affected by a ratio of about 3.5:1, and, as indicated, gastric ulcers occur less frequently than duodenal ulcers—the ratio being about 1:4. Interestingly, about 20% of the gastric ulcers occur in individuals who have, or who had, a duodenal ulcer.

CAUSES. The basic causes of peptic ulcers remain obscure. It is known that physiologically there is a distrubance in the acid-pepsin secretion and the tissue resistance of the digestive tract lining. Other factors, such as chemicals, heredity and emotions also seem involved in some cases. Hence, peptic ulcers are likely to be caused by multiple factors.

Physiological Factors. Gastric secretion is controlled by release of the hormone gastrin, and stimulation of the vagus nerve. Hence, any physiological factor stimulating gastrin release or the vagus nerve, increases the gastric secretions. Oversecretion of stomach acid and pepsin, hypersecretion, does seem to be a factor, but it is not a clear-cut cause. Some ulcer victims secrete normal amounts of acid, while other individuals exhibit hypersecretion but never develop ulcers. It is true, however, that duodenal ulcers *never* develop in the complete absence of acid. Another factor is the ability of the digestive tract tissue to resist the digestive action of pepsin and acid. At least three factors influence tissue resistance: (1) blood supply to the digestive tract lining; (2) integrity and regeneration of the cells lining the digestive tract, the mucosa; and (3) protection of the mucosa by the mucoprotein, mucin which adheres to the mucosa. Impairment of any of these factors can lead to a breakdown in the normal barrier to diffusion of hydrochloric acid into the mucosa.

The role of endocrine gland secretions is illustrated by (1) the development of ulcers by individuals on corticosteroid (adrenal cortex hormone) therapy, and (2) the ulcerations which occur in individuals suffering from the Zollinger-Ellison syndrome in which a gastrin secreting tumor forms in the pancreas.

Other Contributing Factors. Along with the concept of altered tissue resistance of the mucosa, irritants such as aspirin, alcohol, caffeine, adrenal cortex steroids, and bile acids may damage the protective nature of the cells lining the digestive tract and predispose an individual to ulcer development. Furthermore, hereditary and psychological factors also play a role in predisposing an individual to the development of ulcers.

HEREDITARY. In some cases there is a striking tendency for relatives of individuals with duodenal ulcers to develop duodenal ulcers, while relatives of individuals with gastric ulcers will tend to develop gastric ulcers. Also, individuals with the blood group O—an inherited

characteristic—tend to develop duodenal ulcers more frequently than individuals with the blood type A, B, or AB.

PSYCHOLOGICAL. Emotions, no doubt, alter gastrointestinal functions profoundly. Since the brain is the center of our emotions, gastric secretion can be altered directly through vagus nerve stimulation and/or endocrine control which is ultimately controlled by the integrative features of the brain. Although emotions are known to exist, being able to measure and describe their effects is often very difficult. No two people respond exactly the same to similar environment. Anxiety, worry and strain may cause hypersecretion, altered tissue resistance, increased motility, and ulcers as shown in Fig. U-2.

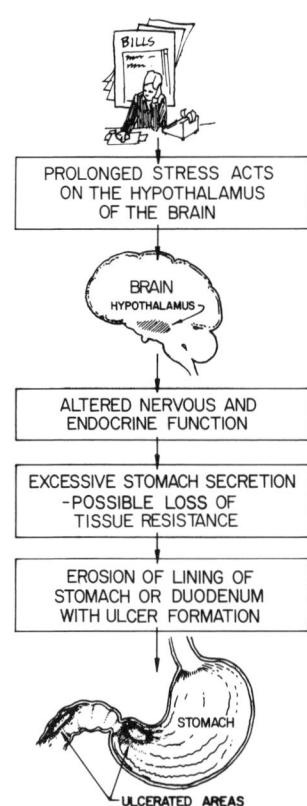

Fig. U-2. Sequence of events in peptic ulcer development due to emotional factors.

SYMPTOMS. The hallmark of peptic ulcers is the sequence of pain-food-relief—the upper abdominal pain associated with ulcers when the stomach is empty, which is relieved by ingesting food or bland liquids. Thus, pain usually relates to eating patterns, and usually occurs several hours after eating and between midnight and 2:00

a.m. Interestingly, this pain is not present before breakfast. Occurrence of the pain relative to eating habits is an important point of differential diagnosis, as persons suffering from gallbladder diseases experience pain that is triggered by eating, rather than relieved. The pain experienced by ulcer sufferers is described as a steady, gnawing, burning, aching, or hungerlike discomfort. However, some victims have no pain even before serious complications develop, and, in some cases, gastric ulcer symptoms may be worsened by eating. A good rule is to have any persistent abdominal pain checked by a physician.

Ulcers that bleed slowly cause the stool to be black and may produce anemia. Other ulcers may bleed more profusely and lead to vomiting of dark brown blood.

DIAGNOSIS. Once a physician suspects an ulcer, x rays are taken after barium is swallowed. These x rays outline the stomach and small intestine and will clearly demonstrate a "crater" in most ulcer victims. This x ray procedure is commonly called an "upper GI series." In most duodenal ulcers, an "upper GI series" is all that is required. Gastric ulcers, however, require some further tests since a small percentage of gastric ulcers are cancers that look like ulcers by x ray. Hence, gastric ulcer patients will probably be subjected to gastroscopy in an effort to rule out malignant disease. This involves passing a flexible lighted tube into the stomach for the direct visual inspection of the ulcer. The miracle of fiber optics makes this feat possible. Furthermore, tissue and washing samples are obtained during the gastroscopy. These also aid differential diagnosis.

COMPLICATIONS. Of course, an ulcer that turns out to be cancerous is a major complication. Other common complications of peptic ulcers include hemorrhage (bleeding), perforation (ulcer breaks through the wall of the stomach or duodenum), and obstruction (due to scar tissue formation). Hemorrhage is the most common complication, and in a minority of patients therapy for hemorrhage includes surgery. Surgery is the mainstay for the treatment of perforation, while obstruction of the stomach outlet may or may not require surgery.

TREATMENT. Treatment, of course, varies with each individual; however, there are some general practices and recommendations which deserve mention. The facets of treatment involve tangible or physical approaches and intangible or psychological approaches.

Physical. Since psychological factors such as emotions and personality can have a large role in development of ulcers, treatment should stress individualized attention to the whole person and not just the ulcer. Nevertheless, some physical manipulations have proven helpful in the treatment of ulcers. These include diet, drugs, and surgery.

DIET. Various dietary regimes have been described for the treatment of ulcer patients. Some have advocated an empty stomach. Others have advocated hourly feedings of milk interspersed with an antacid. Still, the value of strict dietary control is not settled. However, some recommendations can be made on the basis of patient comfort and symptomatic relief.

• **Taboo foods**—Certain substances are gastric stimulants—gastric secretogogues. These known stimulants of gastric secretion should be avoided. Gastric stimulants include caffeine and/or theobromine containing beverages—coffee, tea, chocolate, and various carbonated drinks; and alcoholic beverages. Furthermore, certain foods and drugs are known to be direct mucosal—stomach lining—irritants which should be eliminated. These items include black pepper, chili, vinegar, mustard pickles, alcohol, and aspirin. In addition, different individuals may have some specific food intolerances.

• **Frequent small feedings**—This provides a consistent buffering effect and avoids the distention stimulus which causes stomach acid secretion. Feedings may be given every 1 to 2 hours in the acute stage of some peptic ulcers. Other feeding schedules range from 3 to 6 small meals a day, with between-meal snacks.

• **Carbohydrates, fats, and proteins**—Carbohydrates and fats do not stimulate gastric acid secretion. In fact, fat inhibits gastric secretion. However, they possess the least neutralizing or buffering abilities. While proteins are effective neutralizing agents, there is a catch. Proteins are also major stimulators of gastric secretion. Overall, the diet should provide sufficient carbohydrates to provide an adequate energy intake, unless the picture is complicated by obesity. Fat intake should be moderate and some fatty foods should be avoided altogether. Also, a high-fat diet has been implicated in causing a higher incidence of atherosclerosis in ulcer patients. For this reason most physicians avoid long-term use of milk and cream diets such as the Sippy Diet. Although proteins stimulate gastric acid secretion, protein-containing foods are included in the diet of peptic ulcer patients.

• **Specific restrictive diets**—Long term use of dietary regimens full of regulations are not recommended. Furthermore, rigid dietary regimens have not been shown to promote more rapid ulcer healing nor prevent recurrences. Nevertheless, treatment is individualized. During the acute stages of a bleeding peptic ulcer, hourly feedings of 3 oz (*90 ml*) of milk, milk and cream, half and half, or skim milk supplemented with small servings of bland foods may be prescribed purely to relieve symptoms. Caloric inadequacy for 7 to 10 days during the management of the acute stage presents no real nutritional deficiency or dietary problem. As soon as the pain is relieved, the diet is gradually liberalized, naturally avoiding any particular food or drink that is upsetting. Table U-1 provides some general guidelines from which various diet plans may be derived for each individual during convalescence from a peptic ulcer.

TABLE U-1
GUIDELINES FOR SELECTING FOODS FOR PERSONS WITH PEPTIC ULCERS

Food Category[1]	Foods to Use	Foods to Avoid
Bakery products	Enriched white bread; toast; soda crackers; zwieback; melba toast; hard rolls; sponge cakes; other plain cakes; sugar cookies.	Whole wheat and other whole grain breads; hot bread; graham or coarse crackers; cakes and pastries containing dried fruit or nuts; spice cakes.
Beverages	Postum; decaffeinated coffee.	Alcohol; carbonated drinks; coffee; tea; chocolate.
Cereals and flours	Refined cereals; all ready-to-eat cereals; rice; oatmeal; macaroni; spaghetti; noodles.	Whole grain cereals; cereals containing bran; shredded wheat.
Desserts and sweets	Plain custard; rennet; plain puddings; gelatin desserts; clear plain jelly; honey; moderate amounts of sugar.	Excesses or concentrated sources like candies.
Eggs and substitutes	Boiled; poached; coddled; or scrambled; plain omelets.	Fried eggs.
Fats and oils	Margarine	All fried foods.
Fish and seafoods	Fresh or frozen; boiled; broiled; or baked; scalded canned tuna or salmon; oysters fresh or canned.	Smoked, preserved or pickled fish, crab, lobster, or sardines; other salted fish or fatty fish such as herring or mackerel.
Flavorings and seasonings	Salt	Most all, such as pepper, horseradish, catsup, mustard, vinegar, spices.
Fruits	Applesauce, baked apples without peel; ripe bananas; stewed or canned pears, peaches, apricots—all without peel.	All raw and unripe fruits; dried fruits, skins and peel of all fruits; raisins.
Gravies and sauces	Creamed sauces.	Gravies made from meat extracts.
Juices	Most all, but dilute half and half with water or drink after eating other foods.	
Meats	Tender cuts of beef, lamb, and veal; sliced chicken; liver; crisp bacon.	Fried, smoked, pickled, or cured meats; fat; sausages; ham; salami; weiners.
Milk and Milk products	Buttermilk; cream; milk; plain ice cream; plain milk shakes; cottage cheese; mild cheeses; butter; sour cream; yogurt.	Chocolate; strong cheeses.
Nuts and seeds		All nuts and seeds.
Pickles and relishes		All pickles and relishes.
Soups and chowders	Cream soups using such vegetables as asparagus, beets, carrots, peas, green beans, potatoes, tomatoes, and spinach.	All meat soups, soups from any other vegetables; all canned soups; dehydrated soups; broths; bouillon.
Vegetables	Well-cooked or canned asparagus, carrots, peas, beets, peeled tomatoes, squash, spinach, green beans, mashed or baked potatoes without skins; sweet potatoes without skins; mushrooms.	All raw vegetables; all gas-forming vegetables which include cabbage, cauliflower, Brussels sprouts, broccoli, cucumbers, onions, radishes, turnips; salad, coleslaw.

[1]Food categories are those listed in the Food Composition Table F-36 of this book.

Some nutritionists advocate a liberal diet which consists of the patient's usual dietary practices providing his choices yield an adequate nutrient intake. Even with a liberal diet, moderate use of coffee, tea, and alcohol is encouraged. Of course, the energy content of the diet should maintain weight, and in the case of obese individuals it should promote weight reduction. Obesity represents an added risk factor should complications develop and/or surgery become necessary.

ANTACIDS AND DRUGS. Antacids provide symptomatic relief—not accelerated healing. The most effective and safest antacids are magnesium hydroxide and aluminum hydroxide. These are most effective when taken 1 hour after a meal; liquid preparations are more effective than tablets. Calcium-containing antacid should be avoided.

Anticholinergic drugs—drugs that block cholinergic nerves, and hence block acid secretion by the stomach—have been used in the treatment of peptic ulcers. However, these drugs produce some adverse side effects such as blurred vision, dry mouth, rapid heartbeat, retention of urine, and constipation.

A new drug, cimetidine—an antihistamine—specifically blocks all forms of gastric secretion. Cimetidine is now widely employed in the treatment of peptic ulcers.

SURGERY. Most ulcer victims recover without surgery. However, about 15% of all peptic ulcer patients will develop complications requiring surgery. Complications consist of those mentioned above—bleeding, perforation, obstruction, and cancer—plus those cases where there is continued pain even after extensive treatment. Naturally, careful consideration must be given to all factors before surgery is recommended.

Psychological. Many ulcer patients improve within 24 to 48 hours with a change in environment; hence, the psychological side of treatment cannot be ignored. Both physical and psychological rest promote the healing of peptic ulcers. To this end sedatives may be prescribed. Often victims are urged to curtail their business and social responsibilities. Furthermore, those treating peptic ulcer patients need to demonstrate support and reassurance.

PREVENTION. Peptic ulcers tend to recur. Those that recur and do not respond to treatment, or that recur frequently, may require surgery. Of course, at the first inkling of recurrent symptoms active therapy should be initiated. Continued antacid therapy is not recommended as a means of prevention.

A peptic ulcer provides one more reason for giving up smoking, since it appears to aggravate and contribute.

Being able to relax—although difficult to determine for each individual—would seem to offer some prevention due to the implication of emotions and personality type in the development of peptic ulcers. Each individual should determine the best form of relaxation based on needs and experiences.

(Also see ANTACIDS; DIGESTION AND ABSORPTION; MODIFIED DIETS; and STRESS.)

ULTRAHIGH TEMPERATURE STERILIZATION (UHT STERILIZATION)

Rapid heating of a food to temperature in the range of 205° to 307°F *(96° to 153°C)*, then holding at these temperatures for three seconds or less. In combination with aseptic packaging, this process is designed for the manufacture of products with improved keeping qualities.
(Also see PRESERVATION OF FOOD).

ULTRASONIC HOMOGENIZER

The use of high-frequency—over 20,000 vibrations per second—pressure waves of the same nature as sound waves to disintegrate fat globules or break up particles. This process is employed in a variety of food emulsifications, such as fruit and vegetable purees, milk homogenization, and peanut butter.

ULTRAVIOLET LIGHT (ULTRAVIOLET RADIATION)[1]

Light is a form of radiant energy. It travels in vibrations or waves. Each color of light vibrates with a different wavelength and carries a specific amount of energy.

The range of these wavelengths is measured in nanometers (nm), a unit of length equal to:

$$\frac{1}{100,000,000} \text{ mm}$$

The range of electromagnetic waves of some radiations follows:

Radiation	Approximate Wavelength nanometer (nm)
X ray	50.0
Ultraviolet	300.0
Visible light	600.0
Infrared rays	1,000.0

Other forms of energy-carrying radiation are similar to light, though they are invisible to us; only visible light can be seen. These other forms of radiant energy include radio waves, infrared, ultraviolet and x rays (see Fig. U-3). Note that ultraviolet light has wavelengths shorter than visible light but longer than x rays. Because it cannot be seen by the human eye, ultraviolet light is also known as invisible light or black light.

[1]This section was authoritatively reviewed by, and helpful suggestions were received from, Stephen A. Book, Ph.D., California Environmental Protection Agency, State of California, Sacramento.

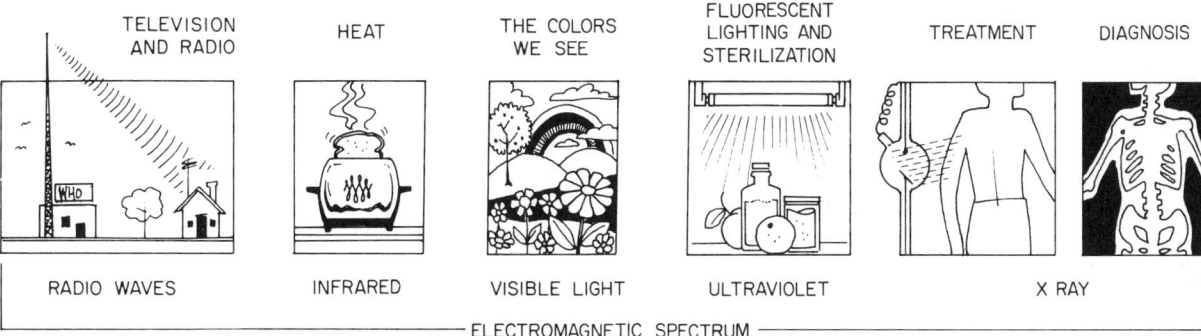

Fig. U-3. Electronic spectrum. "Visible light" covers only a small part of the range.

All radiations are important, but the discussion that follows will be limited to ultraviolet light because of its importance in human health and nutrition.

Ultraviolet light is generally divided into the near (400 to 300 nm), the far (300 to 200 nm), and the vacuum (200 to 4 nm) ultraviolet regions. The last wavelengths, which are particularly harmful to life, are strongly absorbed by the earth's atmosphere.

Ultraviolet light is created by the same processes that generate visible light—transitions in atoms in which an electron in high-energy state returns to a less energetic state.

USES OF ULTRAVIOLET LIGHT. Ultraviolet light serves mankind in numerous ways; among them, the following:

1. **Manufacture of vitamin D in the skin.** If the skin is exposed to the sun or to a sunlamp, the ultraviolet rays act on the provitamin 7-dehydrocholesterol in the skin and transform it into vitamin D_3.

(Also see VITAMIN D.)

2. **Formation of vitamin D in plant foods.** If ergosterol (the provitamin found in plants) is irradiated with ultraviolet light, vitamin D_2 is produced. This is the well known Steenbock Irradiation Process, which was patented by Dr. Harry Steenbock of the University of Wisconsin.

3. **Sterilization.** Certain ranges of ultraviolet rays can kill bacteria. This property is used in sterilizing water, milk and other foodstuffs, and medicinal facilities and equipment. Also, modern food and drug plants often use germicidal lamps to disinfect their products and the containers.

4. **Industrial uses.** Ultraviolet rays have many important industrial uses, including use in fluorescent lamps and sun lamps, in testing materials, in identifying ores in mining, and in lighting the instrument panels of aircraft. Scholars use the fluorescent effect of ultraviolet rays to examine old documents.

Ultraviolet rays, within moderation, are believed to have an invigorating effect upon the human body. But excessive exposure may be harmful, especially to the eyes and skin. Fair skinned people and those who sunburn easily and do not tan are especially susceptible to ultraviolet light induced cancer of the skin.

NOTE WELL: Para-aminobenzoic acid (PABA) may be used for protection against sunburn; usually about 5% PABA is incorporated in an ointment, to be applied over exposed parts of the body. Currently, some dermatologists are recommending other sunscreen lotions; so, for protection against sunburn, see your dermatologist.

(Also see PARA-AMINOBENZOIC ACID.)

CAUTION: Today, tan can be secured from bottled pills, sold under different brand names. All presumably contain the same active ingredients—beta-carotene and canthaxanthin, both of which are food coloring agents—in approximately the proportions of 36 mg of canthaxanthin to 4 mg of beta-carotene. Directions are given on the package. One possible danger in taking such pills is that the artificial tan may lull the user into thinking that he or she is protected from sunburn. But the artificial tan does not protect the skin from burning the way natural tan does.

UMBLES

The entrails of an animal used as a food.

UNDERWEIGHT

This term means different things to different people. To some, it refers to mere slenderness, whereas to others it signifies undernourishment to the extent that a risk to health may be present. This article considers underweight to be a body weight that is notably low for a person's age, height, sex, and other personal characteristics. It is also considered to be an indication that the body contents of fat and lean tissue may be too low to ensure optimal responses to stresses such as chilling, diseases, fasting, injuries, prolonged and/or strenuous physical activities, and surgery.

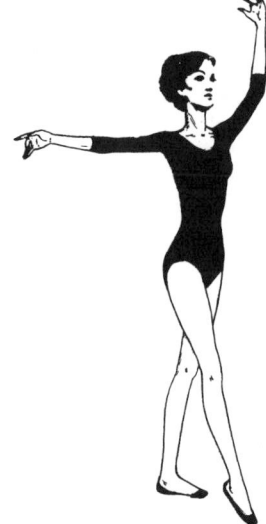

Fig. U-4. Slenderness is considered attractive, but being too thin may be hazardous to health.

EFFECTS ON HEALTH. The desirable or undesirable effects of underweight on the health of different people depend somewhat upon factors such as their life-styles (active or sedentary), their overall states of physical fitness, and the presence or absence of certain other health conditions. This means that some people are likely to be healthiest when they are moderately underweight, whereas others might be fittest for the important activities of their lives when they are average weight, or a little overweight. Therefore, the various effects of underweight are noteworthy.

Beneficial Effects.   The people who may benefit the most from being moderately underweight are those who engage in predominantly intellectual work (artists, office workers, students, teachers, writers, etc.) and live otherwise sedentary lives because it is generally believed that slender people are less likely to become sleepy and tired when physical activity is limited. Runners and other athletes whose sports require the ability to maintain a rapid pace may also benefit from being a little underweight. Finally, people living in tropical climates or those troubled with one or more of the conditions in Table U-2 may be better off underweight than overweight.

TABLE U-2
HEALTH CONDITIONS WHICH MAY BE LESSENED IN SEVERITY
BY A MODERATE DEGREE OF UNDERWEIGHT

Condition	Description	Benefits Conferred by Underweight
Adult onset diabetes	The insulin secreted by the pancreas is ineffective in lowering the blood sugar. This condition is made worse by obesity.	Resistance of the tissues to insulin is lessened by weight reduction and is less likely to occur in underweight people. (Sometimes, this condition is due mainly to a chromium deficiency, rather than to overweight.)
Angina pectoris	A sharp pain in the chest which regularly accompanies physical exertion and is often due to a lack of sufficient circulation of blood in the heart muscle.	This condition is only about 1/2 as likely to occur in underweight and normal weight men as it is in the obese. Furthermore, the nonobese are less likely to have a heart attack.
Atherosclerosis	Certain vital arteries of the body are plugged with deposits of cholesterol and fibrous matter.	The development of atherosclerosis usually proceeds more slowly in slender people because they are less likely to have high blood levels of fats and sugar.
Breathing difficulties	Shortness of breath occurs after only moderate physical exertion.	Physical activity is less taxing to the underweight because (1) less weight has to be moved, and (2) less tissue has to be oxygenated by respiration.
Chronic tiredness	Fatigue occurs too readily, even though what would normally be sufficient rest is obtained. Blood sugar control may be erratic.	A lower body weight requires a lower expenditure of energy. Also, the blood sugar level may be maintained more readily in slender people, provided that the diet is adequate. However, some overly thin people may tire easily.
Congestive heart failure	When the heart is overtaxed the lungs and other tissues become congested with accumulated fluid.	The heart is less likely to be overtaxed when the body weight is normal or subnormal.
Coronary heart disease	Blockage of the coronary arteries by atherosclerotic deposits and/or clots reduces blood flow to the heart muscle.	Slender people are less likely to have a heart attack, and if they have one, they are more likely to survive.
Enlargement of the heart	The heart muscle may become enlarged when it has a heavy workload.	Reduction of the body weight reduces the workload of the heart for a given level of physical activity.
Excessive numbers of red blood cells (polycythemia)	Tissue shortages of oxygen may stimulate the production of excessive red cells. This condition, which is more common in males than females, is dangerous because blood clots may form readily.	Polycythemia is less common in slender males than in obese ones.
Gallstones	These "stones" are usually formed from the cholesterol and other substances present in the bile.	Gallstones occur more frequently in females than in males, and afflict the obese more than slender people.

(Continued)

TABLE U-2 (*Continued*)

Condition	Description	Benefits Conferred by Underweight
Gout and/or high blood levels of uric acid	Excessively high levels of urates in the blood may result in deposits of uric acid in the soft tissues of the body.	Heavy people are more prone to high blood levels of urates than lightweight people. However, the tendency to develop gout is hereditary.
Heat sensitivity	The layer of body fat under the skin acts as insulation which slows the loss of heat from the body.	Slender people lose heat more readily and keep cooler than heavy people. Hence, the former are less vulnerable to heat exhaustion.
Hernia	A loop of the intestine may become herniated through a weak spot in the abdominal muscles, particularly when there are large amounts of fatty tissue.	Hernias are less common in underweight people than heavy people. However, a heavier muscled person may be able to lift a greater weight without the risk of a hernia than a weak and flabby thin person.
High blood fats	Excessively high blood levels of cholesterol and triglycerides may increase the risk of cardiovascular diseases.	Underweight people usually have lower levels of blood fats than heavier ones, and loss of weight is often accompanied by decreases in blood cholesterol and triglycerides.
High blood pressure	Systolic blood pressure tends to rise in proportion to excess body weight.	An elevated blood pressure may often be lowered somewhat by loss of weight.
Kidney diseases	Excess weight appears to confer susceptibility to kidney diseases, although it may not be the direct cause of these disorders.	The death rate from kidney diseases is considerably lower in people who are normal weight or underweight.
Low blood sugar (hypoglycemia)	Obese people have a higher-than-average incidence of blood sugar disorders.	Slender people are less likely to have blood sugar problems. (Except when they have lost weight as a result of diabetes.)
Troubles with the legs and feet	Problems with arthritis and other joint problems, sore feet, varicose veins, and weak leg muscles are aggravated by increased body weight.	A low body weight puts less strain on the lower limbs.

Potentially Harmful Effects. In the early 1900s, underweight people were charged higher life insurance premiums than other policy holders because they were more susceptible to tuberculosis, which at that time was often fatal. Today, tuberculosis is rare, except in certain poverty-stricken areas, and leanness is extolled as a virtue. (Now, some obese policyholders may be charged higher premiums.) Nevertheless, there are certain other potentially harmful effects of a pronounced underweight, which may sometimes be the result of chronic undernutrition. Some of the more common undesirable effects follow:

• **Cessation or irregularity of menstrual periods in females**—It appears that females must have a certain minimum of body fat for the maintenance of a normal menstrual cycle. Overly slender female athletes and others who are notably underweight may have cessation of their periods until they put on additional body fat.

• **Growth retardation in growing infants and children**—Underweight infants, children, and adolescents may not grow well because (1) their caloric intake may be too low, and (2) too much of the dietary protein is used for energy instead of promoting the growth of tissues. Furthermore,

these children may have underdeveloped and flabby muscles, which indicates that they may have a mild form of protein-energy malnutrition.

(Also see MALNUTRITION; and PROTEIN AS ENERGY SOURCE.)

• **Increased susceptibility to chilling and infections**—Thin people are likely to become chilled in cool environments because they lack the normal amounts of body fat which acts as (1) insulation to prevent the escape of body heat, and (2) sources of stored energy that may be drawn upon when needed. Chilling may reduce the resistance to various infectious diseases because it slows the movements of the hairlike projections (cilia) which line the respiratory tract. The movements of the cilia literally "sweep" invasive microorganisms away. Finally, people who are notably underweight may become even thinner if they develop a fever. The metabolism of nutrients is stepped up greatly by fevers. Lack of stored fat may result in the "burning" of tissue protein to provide energy.

• **Lack of vigor, endurance, and sexual drive**—Chronic undernutrition appears to sap the physical drive as a result of the body's effort to spare its tissues from being utilized for energy. This type of adaptation to undernutrition appears to be the result of reductions in the secretion of the hormones which prepare the body for vigorous activities.

• **Low resistance to certain stresses**—Stresses such as chilling, emotional upsets, fasting, injury, prolonged physical activity, and surgery normally stimulate great increases in the secretion of hormones which mobilize body fat and protein to cope with the stress. However, chronic undernutrition may reduce these hormonal responses so that the body handles the stresses poorly. For example, underfed people cannot tolerate food deprivation to the same extent that well-fed people can.

• **Slow healing of injuries and surgical wounds**—People without much flesh on their bones have only minimal body reserves for providing the large quantities of calories and protein which are required for healing. It is not always possible to provide all of the nutrient requirements in the diet when the healing of large areas of the body is taking place. Hence, the healing proceeds more slowly in the people who lack tissue reserves.

• **Tendencies to be apathetic, irritable, listless, mentally depressed, nervous, restless, and sleepless**—The reductions in metabolism which accompany chronic undernutrition may have behavioral as well as physical effects because the brain and nervous system are very sensitive to changes in the body chemistry.

• **Weak muscles**—Sometimes, notably underweight people have been sustained by the metabolism of protein in their muscles for energy since the lack of body fat reserves makes the protein-rich tissues the sole sources of calories when the diet is inadequate to meet the body's needs. Hence, their muscles are likely to be small and weak.

FACTORS THAT MAY BE RESPONSIBLE FOR UNDERWEIGHT.

Lack of sufficient dietary calories is only one of the causes of underweight. Hence, attempts to bring about a gain in weight by merely increasing the caloric content of the diet may fail when there are other contributing factors that are unrecognized. Therefore, some of the major causes of underweight are noteworthy.

Dietary Practices. Many people would like to be able to eat more food without gaining weight, yet there are some who appear to have difficulty eating enough to maintain a normal body weight. Furthermore, the problem of consuming sufficient calories is more common in infancy, childhood, and adolescence than it is in adulthood because much more food energy per pound of body weight is required during growth, as is shown in the section which follows.

CALORIE REQUIREMENTS. Fig. U-5 shows how caloric requirements per pound of body weight decrease steadily throughout the life cycle.

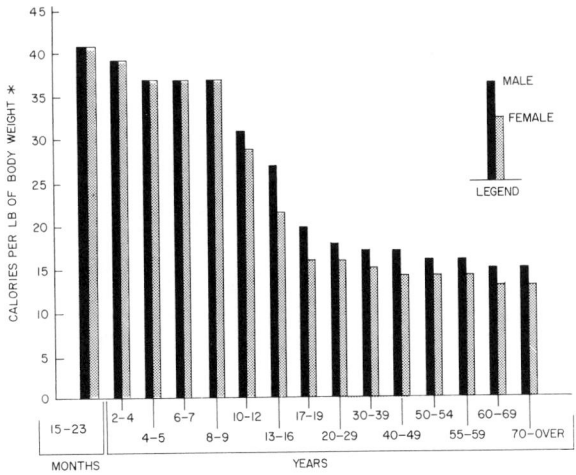

* TO CONVERT TO CALORIES PER KG, MULTIPLY BY 2.2

Fig. U-5. Caloric requirements according to sex and age groups.

It may be noted from Fig. U-5 that children up to age 9 require about twice as many calories per pound of body weight as adults. Therefore, underweight is more likely to be found in the former group who have to eat much more in proportion to their size.

OTHER ASPECTS OF THE DIET. Some of the other reasons why some people may find it difficult to consume sufficient calories follow:

1. The diet may contain too much fibrous vegetable matter, which is very filling. Distention of the small intestine with bulky food curbs the appetite in many people. It is noteworthy that on the average, vegetarians tend to be more slender than meat eaters.

2. Excessive amounts of fluids may be taken with meals. Hence, filling occurs before sufficient solid food is consumed. A similar effect occurs when the foods themselves are very high in water content, as in the cases of gelatin desserts or salads, thin soups and stews, and various vegetable dishes.

3. Oversalted foods may cause feelings of fullness in some people because the salt draws fluid from the intestinal wall into the intestinal contents, thereby producing a bulking effect.

4. Too much fat may be consumed. Fatty foods delay the emptying of the stomach and may make some people lose their appetites.

Finally, the diets of some underweight people may be lacking in the minerals and vitamins that promote hearty appetites. For example, a deficiency of the essential trace mineral zinc leads to loss of taste, and, an insufficient amount of the vitamin thiamin can lead to loss of appetite.

Other Factors. Even when adequate amounts of calories are consumed, various factors that alter the normal utilization of food by the body may prevent the gaining of weight; among them, the following:

• **Digestive disturbances**—The most common digestive disorders which interfere with the utilization of the nutrients in foods are diarrhea, insufficient secretion of digestive juices (mainly gastric juice, bile, and pancreatic juice), malabsorption syndromes, and vomiting. Other less common digestive disorders are celiac disease (malabsorption due to an intolerance of the cereal protein gluten), colitis, and cystic fibrosis.

• **Febrile illnesses**—Each °F of fever raises the metabolic rate by about 7%. Hence, a person with a body temperature of 103°F (39°C) will have a metabolic rate that is almost one-third higher than normal. The calculation is:

103°F − 98.6°F = 4.4°F
4.4°F × 7% per °F = +30.8%.

Unfortunately, the appetite usually declines during a fever, while the need for calories is increased greatly. Many children and a few adults have frequent low-grade febrile illnesses.

• **Glandular disorders**—In diabetes, the energy-yielding nutrients are utilized poorly as a result of the insufficiency and/or the ineffectiveness of the hormone insulin which is secreted by the pancreas. The action of insulin is required for the entry of the nutrients into the cells. On the other hand, in hyperthyroidism there is an overproduction of thyroid hormones, which results in the production of excessive amounts of heat energy from carbohydrates, fats, and proteins. The latter condition brings about the breakdown of body tissues to supply the energy-yielding nutrients.

• **Parasitic infestations**—People who harbor certain intestinal parasites such as hookworms and tapeworms have to share some of their nutrients with these unwelcome guests. Also, the parasitic invaders may cause inflammation of the digestive tract which makes it unpleasant to eat.

• **Unusually great amounts of physical activity**—Habitual exercising to exhaustion may result in leanness because fatigue may depress both the appetite and the optimal functioning of the digestive tract. This effect is often worsened by warm environments which further stress the body. It is noteworthy that some hyperactive children are very lean because of their continual activity.

ASSESSMENT OF WEIGHT STATUS. It may not always be easy to determine when a person is sufficiently underweight to require that remedial measures be taken because there is considerable variation in body weights among people of equal heights and the same sex.

Body Weight for Height, Age, and Sex. One procedure for assessing the weights of adults is to consider that the ranges of normal weights for males or females extend from the 10th to the 90th percentiles of the average weights for selected heights of persons aged 25 to 34. The young adult group is taken as a standard because it is widely believed that weight gained after the attainment of maturity is a detriment rather than a benefit to health. These data are given in Table U-3.

TABLE U-3
AVERAGE WEIGHTS (without clothing) FOR PERSONS AGED 25 to 35 YEARS[1] [2]

Height (without) shoes			Men						Women					
			Light[3] (10th percentile)		Average		Heavy[4] (90th percentile)		Light[3] (10th percentile)		Average		Heavy[4] (90th percentile)	
(ft)	(in.)	(cm)	(lb)	(kg)	(lb)	(kg)	(lb)	(kg)	(lb)	(kg)	(lb)	(kg)	(lb)	(kg)
4	10	147	—	—	—	—	—	—	97	44	119	54	147	67
4	11	150	—	—	—	—	—	—	97	44	126	57	151	69
5	0	152	—	—	—	—	—	—	97	44	125	57	171	78
5	1	155	—	—	—	—	—	—	103	47	130	59	172	78
5	2	157	—	—	—	—	—	—	107	49	135	62	172	78
5	3	160	110	50	151	69	196	89	109	50	138	63	178	81
5	4	163	126	57	151	69	195	89	110	50	141	64	188	86
5	5	165	128	58	155	71	194	88	115	52	143	65	187	85
5	6	167	134	61	160	73	191	87	118	54	146	67	190	86
5	7	170	136	62	168	77	199	91	123	56	153	70	191	87
5	8	173	140	64	166	76	196	89	129	59	162	74	217	99
5	9	175	148	68	176	80	225	102	124	56	153	70	177	81
5	10	178	148	68	185	84	215	98	—	—	—	—	—	—
5	11	180	142	65	178	81	212	96	—	—	—	—	—	—
6	0	183	157	72	190	86	224	102	—	—	—	—	—	—
6	1	185	165	75	195	89	224	102	—	—	—	—	—	—
6	2	188	158	72	191	87	226	103	—	—	—	—	—	—

[1] Adapted by the authors from *Weight by Height and Age for Adults 18-74 Years: United States 1971-74*, U.S. Dept. of Health, Education, and Welfare, 1979, pp. 18, 21, Tables 2, 3.
[2] *Note:* These weights are not what are commonly called "ideal" or "desirable" weights because recent studies have cast doubt upon the basis for the latter.
[3] Most people who weigh less than this amount are likely to be underweight.
[4] Most people who weigh more than this amount are likely to be obese.

The problem with the data in Table U-3 is that there is no specification of body build. Hence, an adult with a large frame might be underweight with a weight falling between the 10th percentile and the average weight. Therefore, some other measures of the "fleshiness" of a person are needed.

NOTE: Weight norms for infants, children, and adolescents are given elsewhere.

(Also see CHILDHOOD AND ADOLESCENT NUTRITION; and INFANT DIET AND NUTRITION.)

Skinfold Thicknesses. About one-half of the body fat content is distributed under the skin. Therefore, the thicknesses of various skinfolds are measures of body fatness. For example, it is generally considered that a triceps skinfold (which is usually measured at a point about halfway between the shoulder and the elbow) smaller than 1/2 in. (*12.5 mm*) for men or less than 5/8 in. (*16 mm*) for women is indicative of insufficient subcutaneous fat or underweight condition.

Midarm Muscle Circumference. This calculated value gives an approximate estimate of the muscle mass, which is useful in determining whether an underweight person is lacking fat alone (measured by skinfold thickness) or is short on both fat and muscle. The value for the midarm muscle circumference (MAMC) is derived from measurements of the triceps skinfold (TSF) and the midarm circumference (MAC) by the following formula:

$$MAMC = MAC - (3.14 \times TSF)$$

For example, a man who has a midarm circumference (measured by placing a tape measure around the upper arm where the triceps skinfold is measured) of 11 in. (*279 mm*), and a skinfold thickness of ½ in. (*12.5 mm*) would have a midarm muscle circumference of 9 7/16 in. (*240 mm*). These measurements would indicate that while he has just enough subcutaneous fat, he is lacking some muscle since the standard values for muscle circumferences are 10 in. (*254 mm*) for males and 9 in. (*232 mm*) for females.

MEASURES FOR GAINING WEIGHT. The selection of the measures to be used for gaining weight should take into account whether additional fat alone is needed, or a combination of extra muscle and fat is required. A diet high in calories will be suitable for the former objective, but the latter objective requires a diet that is high in both calories and protein.

Some suggestions for using high-calorie foods to gain weight are given in Table U-4.

Suggestions for using high-protein foods as sources of additional calories and protein are given in Table U-5.

TABLE U-4
USING HIGH-CALORIE FOODS
FOR GAINING WEIGHT[1]

Food(s)	Suggestions
Butter and margarine	Add to soup, mashed and baked potatoes, hot cereal, grits, rice, noodles, and cooked vegetables; stir into sauces and gravies; combine with herbs and seasonings and spread on cooked meats, hamburgers and fish; use melted butter as a dip for raw vegetables, and seafoods such as shrimp, scallops, crab, or lobster.
Whipped cream and imitation whipped toppings	Use unsweetened cream in soups and sweetened cream or toppings on cocoa, desserts, gelatin, pudding, fruits, pancakes, waffles; fold unsweetened cream into mashed potatoes or vegetable purees.
Table cream	Use in soups, sauces, egg dishes, batters, puddings, and custards; put on cereal; mix with pasta and rice; add to mashed potatoes; pour on chicken and fish while baking; use as binder in hamburgers, meatloaf, and croquettes; substitute for milk in recipes. Make cocoa with cream, add marshmallows.
Sour cream	Add to soups, baked potatoes, vegetables, sauces, salad dressings, stews, baked meat and fish dishes, gelatin desserts, bread and muffin batter.
Mayonnaise	Add to salad dressing; spread on sandwiches and crackers; combine with meat, fish, or vegetable salads; use as binder in croquettes; use in sauces and gelatin dishes.
Honey	Add to cereal, milk drinks; fruit desserts; glaze for meats such as chicken and ham; add to yogurt as dessert.
Granola	Use in cookie, muffin, bread batters; sprinkle on vegetables, yogurt, ice cream, pudding, custard, fruit; layer with fruits and bake; mix with dry fruits and nuts for a snack; substitute for bread or rice in pudding recipes.
Dried fruits	Cook and serve for breakfast or as dessert; add to muffins, cookies, breads, cakes, rice and grain dishes, cereals and puddings, stuffings; bake in pies and turnovers; combine with cooked vegetables such as carrots, sweet potatoes, yams, acorn and butternut squash, combine with nuts or granola for a finger snack.

[1]Source: *Diet and Nutrition*, NIH Publication Number 80-2038, U.S. Dept. HEW, 1979, p. 36.

TABLE U-5
USING HIGH-PROTEIN FOODS TO INCREASE DIETARY PROTEIN AND CALORIES[1]

Food(s)	Suggestions
Cheese	Melt on sandwiches, hamburgers, hot dogs, other meats or fish, vegetables, eggs, desserts like stewed fruit or pies; grate and add to sauces, casseroles, vegetable dishes, mashed potatoes, rice, noodles, meatloaf, breads, or muffins.
Cottage cheese	Mix with or use to stuff fruits or vegetables; add to casseroles or egg dishes like quiche, scrambled eggs, souffles; add to spaghetti or noodles; use in gelatin, pudding-type desserts, or cheesecake; add to pancake batter, stuff crepes and pastalike shells or manicotti.
Cream cheese	Spread on sandwiches, fruit slices, and crackers; add to egg or vegetables; roll into balls and coat with chopped nuts, wheat germ, and/or granola.
Milk or cream	Add to water used in cooking, or use in place of water in preparing foods such as hot cereal, soups. Serve cream sauces with vegetables and other appropriate dishes.
High-protein milk	Blend whole milk with dry skim milk powder using 1 cup dry powder for each quart of milk; substitute for regular milk in beverages and in cooking whenever possible; substitute for water in soups, cocoa, and pudding mixes; use on cereals, jello, and stewed fruits.
Powdered milk	Add to regular milk and milk drinks such as eggnog and milk shakes; use in casseroles; add to meatloaf, breads, muffins, sauces, cream soups, pudding and custards, and milk-based gelatin salads or desserts.
Plain or sweetened yogurt	Add to fruits and desserts; use to top cereal, pancakes, waffles, fill crepes; add to milk-based beverages and gelatin dishes.
Ice cream	Use in beverages such as sodas, milk shakes, or other milk drinks; add to cereals, fruits, gelatin desserts, and pies; blend or whip with bananas and soft or cooked fruits; sandwich between enriched cake slices, cookies, or graham crackers.
Egg	Add chopped, hardcooked eggs to salads and dressings, vegetables, casseroles, creamed meats; beat eggs into mashed potatoes or vegetable purees; add an extra egg to French toast and pancake batter, or milk shakes.

Food(s)	Suggestions
Egg yolks	Beat into sauces; add extra yolks to quiche, scrambled eggs, custards, puddings, pancake and French toast batter; a rich boiled custard made with egg yolks, high-protein milk and sugar is a good source of calories and protein. Add extra hardcooked yolk to deviled egg filling and sandwich spreads.
Peanut butter	Spread on sandwiches, toast, muffins, crackers, waffles, pancakes, fruit slices; use as a dip for raw vegetables like carrots, cauliflower, celery; add to meatloaf, appropriately flavored soups and sauces, cookies, breads, muffins; blend with milk drinks and beverages; swirl through soft ice cream and yogurt; top cookies and cakes.
Nuts	Serve as snacks; add chopped or ground nuts to ice cream, yogurt, puddings, breads, muffins, pancakes, waffles, cookies, meatloaf and hamburgers, vegetable dishes, salads, sandwiches; blend with parsley or spinach, herbs and cream for a noodle, pasta or vegetable sauce; roll a banana in chopped nuts.
Fish, meat, or poultry	Add small pieces of any cooked meat or fish to vegetables, salads, casseroles, soups and biscuit ingredients; use in omelets, souffles, quiches, sandwich fillings, chicken and turkey stuffings; wrap in pie crust or biscuit dough as turnovers; add to stuffed baked potatoes. Liver is an especially good source of protein and other nutrients if accepted.
Textured vegetable protein	Add to hamburgers, meatloaf, meatballs, spaghetti sauce, and ground or chopped meat dishes, casseroles, and sandwich fillings.
Legumes	Dry peas, beans, and bean curd (tofu) can be cooked and made into soup or added to casseroles, pastas, and grain dishes which also contain cheese or meat. Mash with cheese and milk.
Wheat germ	Add to casserole, meat, bread, muffin, and pancake or waffle recipes; sprinkle on fruit, cereal, ice cream, or yogurt; sprinkle on top of vegetables and toast to add a crunchy topping; use in place of breadcrumbs.

[1]Source: *Diet and Nutrition*, NIH Publication Number 80-2038, U.S. Dept. HEW, 1979, pp. 35-36.

SUMMARY. Ideal body weights for different people vary according to age, sex, body build, life-style, and other factors. Hence, some feel better when slender, whereas others may benefit from a little extra weight. Therefore, a doctor should be consulted before one attempts to gain or lose a considerable amount of weight.

UNESCO

United Nations Educational, Scientific, and Cultural Organization, with headquarters in Paris, France.

UNIDENTIFIED FACTORS

In addition to the vitamins as such, certain unidentified or unknown factors are important in nutrition. They are referred to as "unidentified" or "unknown" because they have not yet been isolated or synthesized in the laboratory. Nevertheless, rich sources of these factors and their effects have been well established. A diet that supplies the specific levels of all the known nutrients but which does not supply the unidentified factors may be inadequate for best performance. There is evidence that these factors exist in dried whey, marine and animal products, distillers' solubles, antibiotic fermentation residues, yeasts, alfalfa meal, and certain green leafy vegetables.

UNSATURATED FAT

A fat having one or more double bonds; not completely hydrogenated.
(Also see FATS AND OTHER LIPIDS.)

UNSATURATED FATTY ACID

Any one of several fatty acids containing one or more double bonds, such as oleic, linoleic, linolenic, and arachidonic acids.
(Also see FATS AND OTHER LIPIDS.)

UREA (NH$_2$CONH$_2$)

Before amino acids (protein) can enter energy metabolic pathways, the amino group (NH$_2$) must first be removed. This is accomplished by a process called deamination which produces a carbon skeleton that can be used for energy, and ammonia (NH$_3$). To facilitate elimination from the body, this ammonia is converted to urea in the urea cycle in the liver. Urea circulates in the blood, and is removed from the blood by the kidneys. It is the main nitrogenous constituent of urine. Normally 20 to 35 g of urea are excreted in the urine every 24 hours.
(Also see METABOLISM; PROTEIN[S]; and UREA CYCLE.)

UREA CYCLE (KREBS-HENSELEIT CYCLE)

Most of the ammonia (NH$_3$) produced through deamination—removal of amino groups (NH$_2$) from amino acids—is converted to urea in the liver for excretion by the kidneys. To facilitate elimination, 1 mole of ammonia (NH$_3$) combines with 1 mole of carbon dioxide (CO$_2$), another metabolic waste product. This compound is then phosphorylated to produce carbamyl phosphate. Carbamyl phosphate then combines with ornithine to form citrulline—an intermediate in the urea cycle. The amino acid, aspartic acid, contributes another amino group (NH$_2$), and citrulline is then converted to the amino acid arginine. Urea splits off from arginine forming ornithine, and the cycle is completed. Fig. U-6 illustrates the urea cycle.
(Also see METABOLISM; PROTEIN[S]; and UREA.)

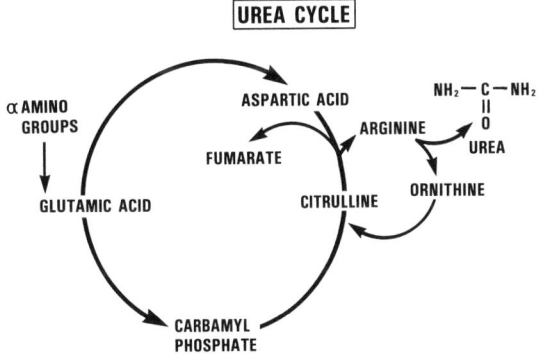

Fig. U-6. Urea cycle (nitrogen excretion).

UREASE

An enzyme which acts on urea to produce carbon dioxide and ammonia. It is found in the human digestive tract where it acts on the urea in the digestive secretions.
(Also see DIGESTION AND ABSORPTION; and ENZYME.)

UREMIA

A toxic accumulation of urinary constituents in the blood.
(Also see DISEASES.)

URIC ACID

The main end product of purine—adenine, guanine and xanthine—metabolism in birds, reptiles, and man, which is excreted in the urine. Uric acid is formed from purines consumed in the diet, and from body purines derived from the breakdown of nucleic acids. Mammals other than man further metabolize uric acid to allantoin, which is excreted in the urine. However, man lacks the enzyme, urate oxidase, necessary for this conversion. Therefore, about 0.5 to 1.0 g of uric acid is lost in the urine each day. A high level of uric acid in the blood is associated with the development of gout. In addition, uric acid may form kidney stones, especially in individuals suffering from gout.

(Also see ARTHRITIS, section headed "Gout [gouty arthritis]"; METABOLISM; and URIC ACID KIDNEY STONES.)

URIC ACID KIDNEY STONES

Kidney stones formed from uric acid—the excretory product of purines in humans. Stones develop when (1) blood levels of uric acid are elevated, (2) urinary uric acid excretion is high, and (3) an acid urine is produced. Individuals suffering from gout are a thousand fold more likely to develop uric acid kidney stones than the general population. Formation of uric acid kidney stones may be minimized by keeping the urine alkaline, increasing the fluid intake, and reducing the purine intake. Most fruits and vegetables contribute to the formation of an alkaline urine, while meat, fish and poultry contribute to the formation of an acid urine. A purine-restricted diet begins with the elimination of foods with high purine content such as anchovies, asparagus, brains, kidneys, liver, meat extracts, mincemeat, sardines, and sweetbreads.

(Also see ARTHRITIS, section headed "Gout [gouty arthritis]"; CALCIUM, section headed "Calcium Related Diseases"; MODIFIED DIETS; and KIDNEY STONES.)

URICASE (URATE OXIDASE)

A copper-containing enzyme which all mammals possess with the exception of man and other primates. It is responsible for the conversion of uric acid to allantoin.

(Also see URIC ACID.)

URINARY CALCULI (WATER BELLY, KIDNEY STONES, UROLITHIASIS)

Mineral deposits which occur in the urinary tract. These deposits may block the flow of urine, followed by rupture of the urinary bladder and death. In severe cases of some duration, watery swellings (edema) of the lower abdomen may develop.

(Also see CALCIUM, section headed "Calcium Related Diseases"; KIDNEY STONES; MODIFIED DIETS; and URIC ACID KIDNEY STONES.)

URINARY SYSTEM

The organs engaged in the excretion of urine. They consist of the kidneys, the ureters, the bladder, and the urethra.

URINE

Liquid or semisolid matter produced in the kidneys and discharged through the urinary organs. Normally, it is a clear, transparent, amber-colored, slightly acid fluid.

(Also see KIDNEYS; UREA; and UREA CYCLE.)

USDA

The abbreviation commonly used for the United States Department of Agriculture.

(Also see U.S. DEPARTMENT OF AGRICULTURE.)

U.S. DEPARTMENT OF AGRICULTURE (USDA)

In 1796, President George Washington recommended the creation of a national board of agriculture, which eventually developed into the United States Department of Agriculture. The USDA and the FDA (Food and Drug Administration) share the responsibility for assuring the safety of the nation's food supply. Meat and meat products, and poultry and poultry products are the main food concerns of the USDA, operating under the authority of the Federal Meat Inspection Act (FMIA) and the Poultry Products Inspection Act (PPIA). Also, the USDA is involved in research, educational, nutritional, and health programs. The following eight divisions of the USDA have primary responsibilities in the areas of human health and nutrition: (1) the Agriculture Research Service; (2) the Animal and Plant Health Inspection Service; (3) the Consumer and Marketing Service; (4) the Cooperative State Research Service; (5) the Federal Extension Service; (6) the Food and Nutrition Service; (7) the Labeling and Registration Section; and (8) the Veterinary Services Division.

(Also see DISEASES, section headed "U.S. Department of Agriculture.")

U.S. DEPARTMENT OF HEALTH AND HUMAN SERVICES (FORMERLY, HEALTH, EDUCATION, AND WELFARE)

An agency of the federal government with rsponsibility for public health in its broadest aspects. This agency is under the jurisdiction of the U.S. Public Health Service (USPHS) and includes the following: (1) Alcohol, Drug Abuse and Mental Health Administration; (2) Center for Disease Control (CDC); (3) Food and Drug Administration (FDA); (4) Health Resources Administration; (5) Health Services Administration; and (6) National Institutes of Health (NIH).

(Also see DISEASES, section headed "U.S. Department of Health and Human Services.")

USP (UNITED STATES PHARMACOPIA)

A unit of measurement or potency of biologicals that usually coincides with an international unit. (Also see IU.)

U.S. PUBLIC HEALTH SERVICE (USPHS)

This service is in the U.S. Department of Health and Human Services and is concerned with the prevention and treatment of disease. It works in the areas of vector control, pollution control, and control of communicable diseases of man. In addition to its own research program, the USPHS provides grants for health-related research at many universities and research institutes in the United States.

A part of this important complex is the National Institute of Health (NIH), which was formed in 1930, and is composed of the following nine sister institutes:

The National Cancer Institute
The National Heart Institute
The National Institute of Allergy and Infectious Diseases
The National Institute of Arthritis and Metabolic Diseases
The National Institute of Dental Research
The National Institute of Mental Health
The National Institute of Neurological Diseases and Blindness (including multiple sclerosis, epilepsy, cerebral palsy, and blindness)
The National Institute of Child Health and Human Development
The National Institute of General Medical Science

U.S. RECOMMENDED DAILY ALLOWANCES (U.S. RDA)

These allowances are guides to the amounts of vitamins and minerals an individual needs each day to stay healthy. They were set by the Food and Drug Administration (FDA) as nutritional standards for labeling purposes. The U.S. RDAs are *based* on the Recommended Dietary Allowances established by the Food and Nutrition Research Council, and they replace the Minimum Daily Requirements (MDR) which were used for years as guidelines for labeling products. For practical purposes, the many categories of dietary allowances for males and females of different ages were condensed to as few as nutritionally possible for labeling. Generally, the highest values for the ages combined in a U.S. RDA were used. For example, the U.S. RDAs for adults and children over 4 years are representative, generally, of the dietary allowances recommended for a teen-age boy.

There are four groupings of the U.S. RDAs, shown in Table U-6. The best known, and the one that will be used on most nutrition information panels and most vitamin and mineral supplements, is for adults and children over 4 years of age. The second is for infants up to 1 year, and the third is for children under 4 years. The latter two are to be used on infant formulas, baby foods, and other foods appropriate for these ages, as well as vitamin-mineral supplements intended for their use. The fourth

TABLE U–6
U.S. RECOMMENDED DAILY ALLOWANCES
(U.S. RDA)[1]

Nutrient	Adults & Children 4 Years or Older	Infants from Birth to 1 Year	Children Under 4 Years	Pregnant or Lactating Women
Required on labels:				
Protein . . . . g	50–63	13–14	16	60/65
Vitamin A . . . . mcg RE	500–1000	375	400	800/1,300
Vitamin C mg	60	30–35	40	70/95
Thiamin . . .mg	1.5	0.3–0.4	0.7	1.5/1.6
Riboflavin mg	1.7	0.4	0.8	1.8
Niacin mg NE	20	5–6	9	17–20
Calcium . . .mg	1,200	600	800	1,200
Iron . . . . . .mg	15	6–10	10	30/15
Optional on labels:				
Vitamin D . . . . .mcg	10	7.5–10	10	10
Vitamin E IU	30	3–4	6	10–12
Vitamin B-6 . . . . .mg	2	0.3–0.6	1	2.2
Folate . . .mcg	200	25–35	50	400/280
Vitamin B-12 . . . . . . .mcg	2	0.3–0.5	0.7	2.2/2.6
Phosphorus . . . . .mg	1,200	400–600	800	1,200
Iodine . . .mcg	150	40–50	70	175/200
Magnesium . . . . .mg	350	40–60	80	320/355
Zinc . . . . . .mg	15	5	10	15/19
Copper . . .mg	2	0.6	1	2
Biotin . . . .mcg	30–100	10–15	20	30/100
Pantothenic acid . . . . .mg	4–7	2–3	3	4–7

[1]*Recommended Dietary Allowances*, NRC, 1989, pp. 284–285.

is for pregnant women or women who are nursing their babies.

• **Labels and U.S. RDA**—Whenever a food product is labeled "enriched," or a product has added nutrients, or a nutritional claim is made for a product, the FDA requires that the nutritional content be listed on the label. In addition, many manufacturers put nutrition information on products when not required to do so. The lower part of the nutrition label must give the percentages of the U.S. Recommended Daily Allowances (U.S. RDA) of protein and of seven vitamins and minerals in a serving of the product, in the following order: protein, vitamin A, vitamin C, thiamin, riboflavin, niacin, calcium, and iron. As shown in Table U-6, listing is optional relative to the percentage of 12 other vitamins and minerals. Likewise, listing of cholesterol, fatty acid, and sodium content is optional—for now. Nutrients present at levels less than 2% of the U.S. RDA may be indicated by a zero or an asterisk which refers to the statement, "contains less than 2% of the U.S. RDA of these nutrients." Nutrition labels also list how many calories and how much protein, carbohydrate, and fat are in a serving of the product.

Unfortunately, some confusion has arisen since the National Research Council's *Recommended Dietary Allowances* have for years been called the RDAs; hence, U.S. RDA should always refer to the U.S. Recommended *Daily* Allowances used for labeling purposes.

(Also see ENRICHMENT [Fortification, Nutrification, Restoration]; LABELS, FOOD; and RDA [Recommended Dietary Allowances].)

UTERUS (WOMB)

The organ that receives the fertilized egg from the fallopian tube and holds it during the 9 months of its growth until the infant is expelled at childbirth. It is situated deep in the pelvic cavity between the bladder and the rectum.

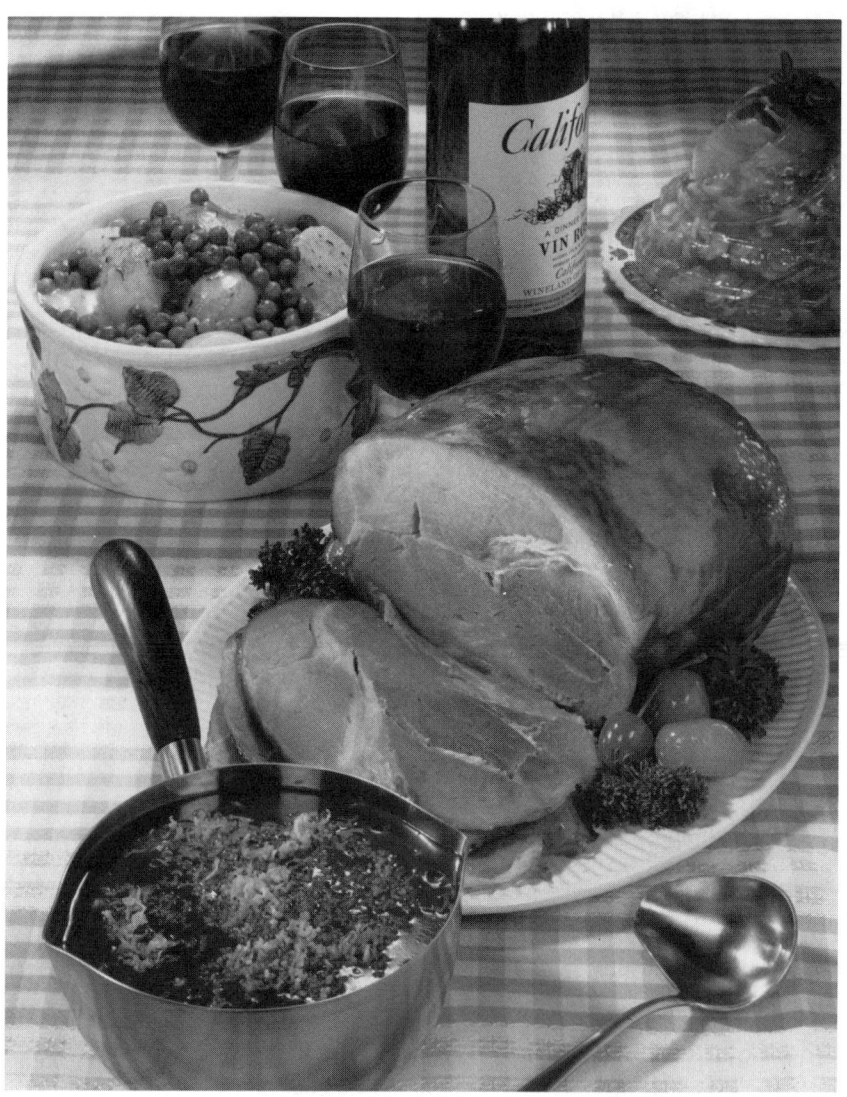

The first wine was made in the Middle East 6,000 to 7,000 years ago. Also, it is noteworthy that Noah raised grapes and made wine (Genesis 9:20-21). Today, wine is being used to enhance more and more meals. (Courtesy, Wine Institute, San Francisco, Calif.)

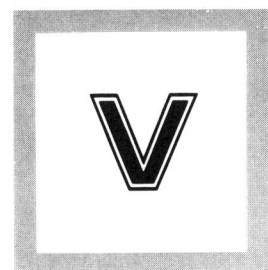

VACUUM COOLING

A means of rapidly cooling fruits and vegetables to prevent deterioration. Produce is sprayed with water, then while still wet it is subjected to a vacuum which causes the water to evaporate; thereby rapidly chilling the produce. Some vacuum coolers are railroad car size.
(Also see HYDROCOOLING.)

VACUUM-DEHYDRATED

Freed of moisture after removal of surrounding air while in an airtight enclosure.

VACUUMIZATION (VACREATION)

In milk processing, the subjection of heated milk to vacuum for the purpose of removing volatile off-flavors and odors and/or moisture. (Also see DEAERATION.)

VALENCE

The power of an element or radical to combine with (or to replace) other elements or radicals. The valence number of an element is the number of atoms of hydrogen with which one atom of the element can combine.

VALINE

One of the essential amino acids.
(Also see AMINO ACID[S].)

VANADIUM (V)

Vanadium was first identified in 1831 by Sefstrom, of Sweden, who named it after the Norse goddess of beauty, Vanadis (because of the beautiful color of its compounds). However, it was not obtained in pure form until 1927. It has many industrial uses, especially in Vanadium steel.

In 1970, Dr. Klaus Schwarz demonstrated that the trace element Vanadium (V) is needed by higher animals. Vanadium-deficient diets resulted in retarded growth, impaired reproduction, increased packed blood cell volume and iron in the blood and bone of rats, and increased hematocrit in chicks.

VANASPATI

This is a term applied in India to hydrogenated fat made from vegetable oils. It is a butter substitute, like margarine in the United States.

VASCULAR

Pertaining to the blood vessels of the body.

VASOPRESSIN

The antidiuretic hormone secreted by the pituitary gland.

VEGANS

A vegan is an individual who is a strict vegetarian. All foods of animal origin—meat, poultry, fish, eggs, and dairy products—are excluded from the diet of vegans. In addition, vegans share a philosophy and life-style. (Also see VEGETARIAN DIETS.)

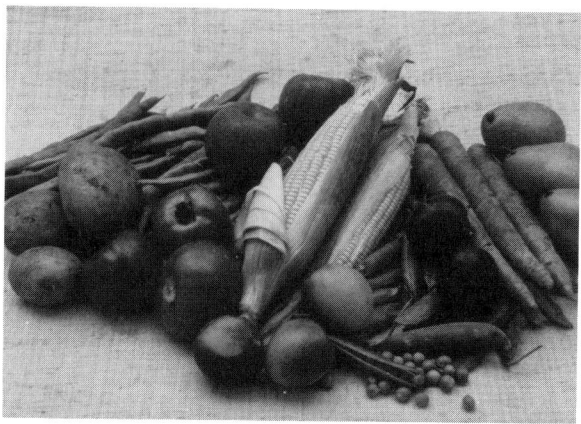

Fig. V-1.   Vegetables. (Courtesy, USDA)

VEGETABLE(S)

In the phrase "the vegetable kingdom," the word *vegetable* refers to the entire world of plants. In an 1893 decision, the U.S. supreme court held, in effect, that a plant or plant part generally eaten as part of the main course of the meal is a vegetable, while a plant part which is generally eaten as an appetizer, as a dessert, or out of hand is a fruit. As used herein, the term refers to the edible part of a plant that is consumed in raw or cooked form with the main course of a meal. Some typical parts of plants used as vegetables are: bulbs (garlic, onions), flowers (broccoli, cauliflower), fruits (pumpkins, squashes, tomatoes), leaves (lettuce, spinach), roots (beets, carrots), seeds (beans, corn, peas), stalks (celery), stems (asparagus), and tubers (Irish potatoes, yams). Although green land plants provide most of the vegetables for human diets, certain fungi and algae may also be used for vegetables. The different types of vegetables are shown in Fig. V-2.

It is noteworthy that the only grain commonly used as a vegetable in the United States is sweet corn, whereas several types of legumes are so utilized. Therefore, this

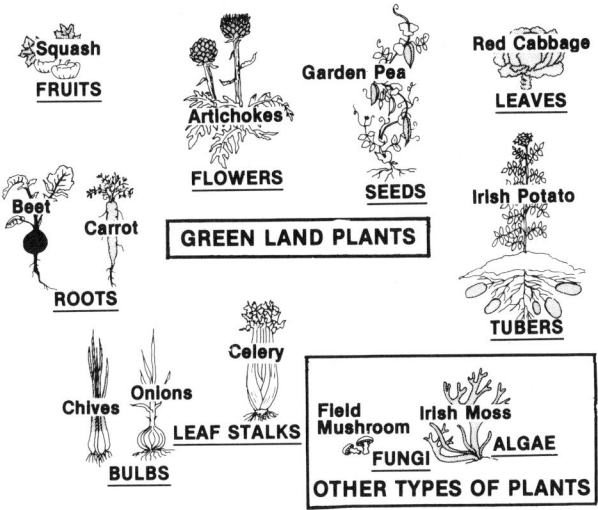

Fig. V-2. Common types of vegetables.

article will cover only the items that Americans usually serve as vegetables.

HISTORY. It has been difficult for archaeologists, botanists, geographers and other researchers to trace the history of all of the vegetables people have used over the ages because (1) few remains of the more succulent parts of plants have been found at archaeological excavations since these parts decay very readily; (2) most of the identifiable plant fragments have been found in relatively dry areas, while evidence of vegetables used in the humid tropics is scarce; and (3) some of the vegetables that were once consumed by man may have become extinct, and others may have evolved into forms that bear little resemblance to the ancestral species. Nevertheless, enough evidence has been found to support some tentative conclusions about the first cultivation of the important vegetable crops.

Long before the development of the first agricultural societies some 10,000 to 12,000 years ago, most people lived in nomadic bands that obtained their food by fishing, hunting, and gathering wild plants. This period of human history apparently lasted for 2 million years or so. It is not known why some of the nomads eventually settled in certain areas, but this change appears to have been accompanied by (1) the herding of animals and (2) a regular pattern of harvesting wild plants. The first cultivation of local plants appears to have occurred in the regions where systematic gathering had long been practiced. In many cases, the first long-term settlements were made in places where diverse geographical features such as mountains, foothills, valleys, and rivers were in close proximity. Hence, the varied habitats favorerd the growth of numerous plant species. A wide variety of plant foods would have been needed to form a nutritious diet when fish and game became scarce, or the early settlers would have succumbed to malnutrition. Figs. V-3 and V-4 show the locations of the regions where many of the important vegetables were first cultivated.

It is uncertain how people learned to plant crops. Some researchers have suggested that the planting of seeds and the techniques of vegetative propagation (the use of vegetative parts from a parent plant to propagate new plants) might have been discovered when it was observed that new plants grew from seeds and other parts of plants thrown on rubbish heaps. Apparently, propagation of plants by seeds became the most important means of vegetable production in the temperate regions, whereas the vegetative propagation of root and tuber crops was utilized to a large extent in subtropical and tropical areas. Certain plants are adapted to the former climatic zones because their seeds reach maturity in the fall, remain dormant over the winter and germinate in the spring, whereas many roots and tubers are adapted to alternating wet and dry seasons in the tropics.

Once people had learned to plant crops, it would have been natural for them to move their fields to areas which appeared to be more favorable. For example, the early farmers in the foothills of the Zagros mountains (located near the border between present day Iraq and Iran) soon moved down into the valley between the Tigris and Euphrates rivers (the site of ancient Mesopotamia). Some of the crops became hybridized by cross pollination with other species in the new environment, and new types of plants resulted from the accidental crossing. (It is suspected that the modern type of corn resulted from the accidental crossing of a primitive corn with teosinte in the Tehucan valley of Mexico about 3,000 years ago.) No doubt many other accidental crosses and other changes resulted when explorers and traders brought plants to distant lands. Plants adapt genetically to new environments over successive generations.

Sometime in the early days of agriculture it was noted that crops could be improved greatly by sowing only the seeds from the plants with outstanding characteristics. However, some of the most dramatic improvements in certain vegetables have been made only recently, after the principles of genetics were clarified in the late 19th and the early 20th centuries.

The modern era of genetics was ushered in by the publication of *The Origin of Species* by the English naturalist Charles Darwin in 1859. This monumental work provided an explanation for the development of new species from pre-existing ones. Shortly thereafter, in 1866, the Austrian monk Mendel suggested some of the basic principles of hereditary transmission in his reports of the breeding experiments he conducted with garden peas. Unfortunately, his findings were ignored until 34 years later, when three European biologists independently duplicated his findings.

After the writings of Darwin and Mendel became more fully accepted in the early 1900s, plant breeders set out to improve the most important crops. Most of the development of hybrid corn was done in the United States during the first half of the 20th century. Soon, the production of vegetable seeds became a major industry and many species were bred for characteristics such as high yields, size, color, taste, and texture. Lately, suitability for mechanical harvesting has become a major objective of plant breeders since it is often difficult to obtain enough workers to pick certain crops by hand. A typical vegetable that has been adapted in this way is the to-

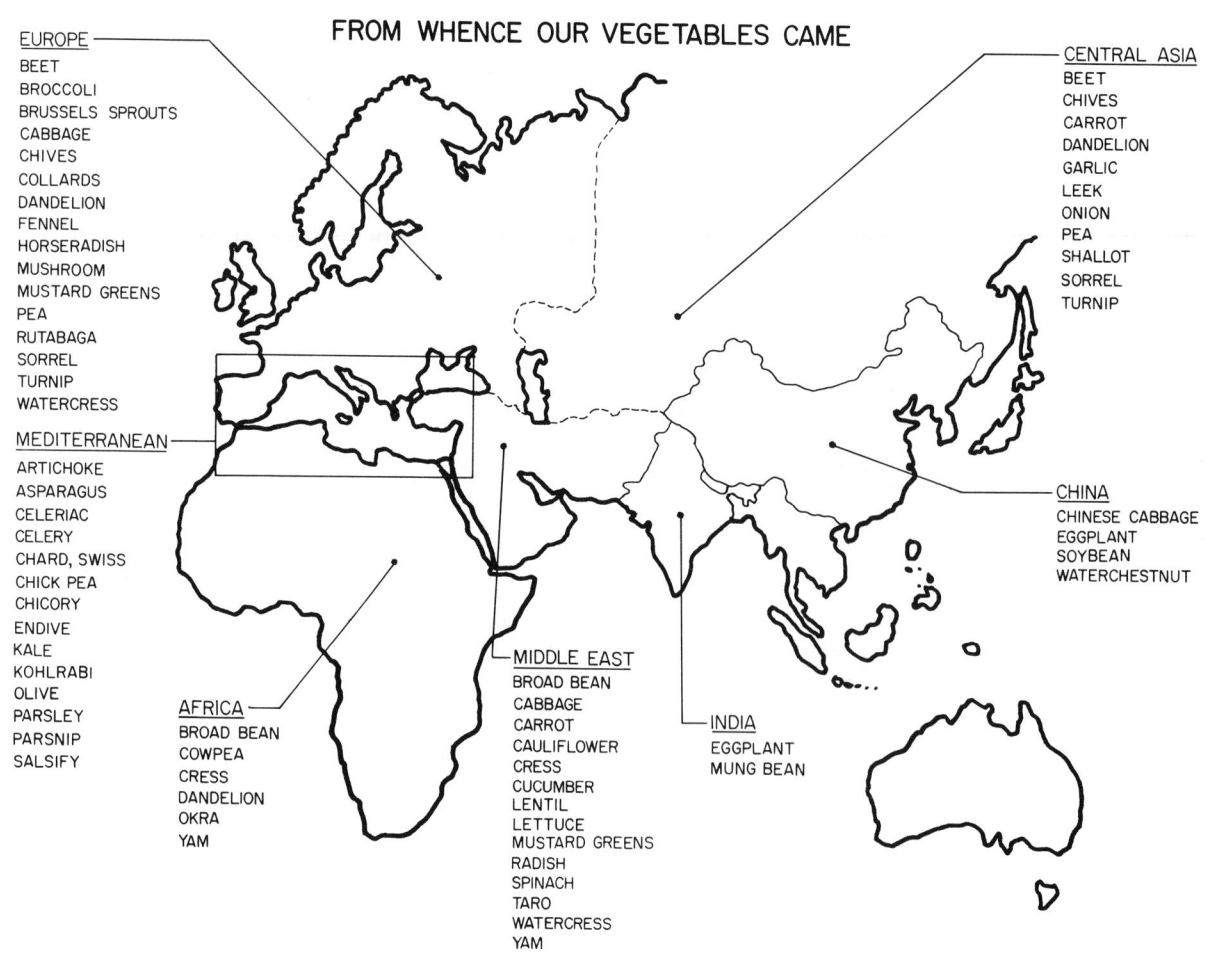

FROM WHENCE OUR VEGETABLES CAME

EUROPE
BEET
BROCCOLI
BRUSSELS SPROUTS
CABBAGE
CHIVES
COLLARDS
DANDELION
FENNEL
HORSERADISH
MUSHROOM
MUSTARD GREENS
PEA
RUTABAGA
SORREL
TURNIP
WATERCRESS

MEDITERRANEAN
ARTICHOKE
ASPARAGUS
CELERIAC
CELERY
CHARD, SWISS
CHICK PEA
CHICORY
ENDIVE
KALE
KOHLRABI
OLIVE
PARSLEY
PARSNIP
SALSIFY

AFRICA
BROAD BEAN
COWPEA
CRESS
DANDELION
OKRA
YAM

MIDDLE EAST
BROAD BEAN
CABBAGE
CARROT
CAULIFLOWER
CRESS
CUCUMBER
LENTIL
LETTUCE
MUSTARD GREENS
RADISH
SPINACH
TARO
WATERCRESS
YAM

INDIA
EGGPLANT
MUNG BEAN

CENTRAL ASIA
BEET
CHIVES
CARROT
DANDELION
GARLIC
LEEK
ONION
PEA
SHALLOT
SORREL
TURNIP

CHINA
CHINESE CABBAGE
EGGPLANT
SOYBEAN
WATERCHESTNUT

Fig. V-3.   Places of origin and/or domestication of vegetables in the Old World.

FROM WHENCE OUR VEGETABLES CAME

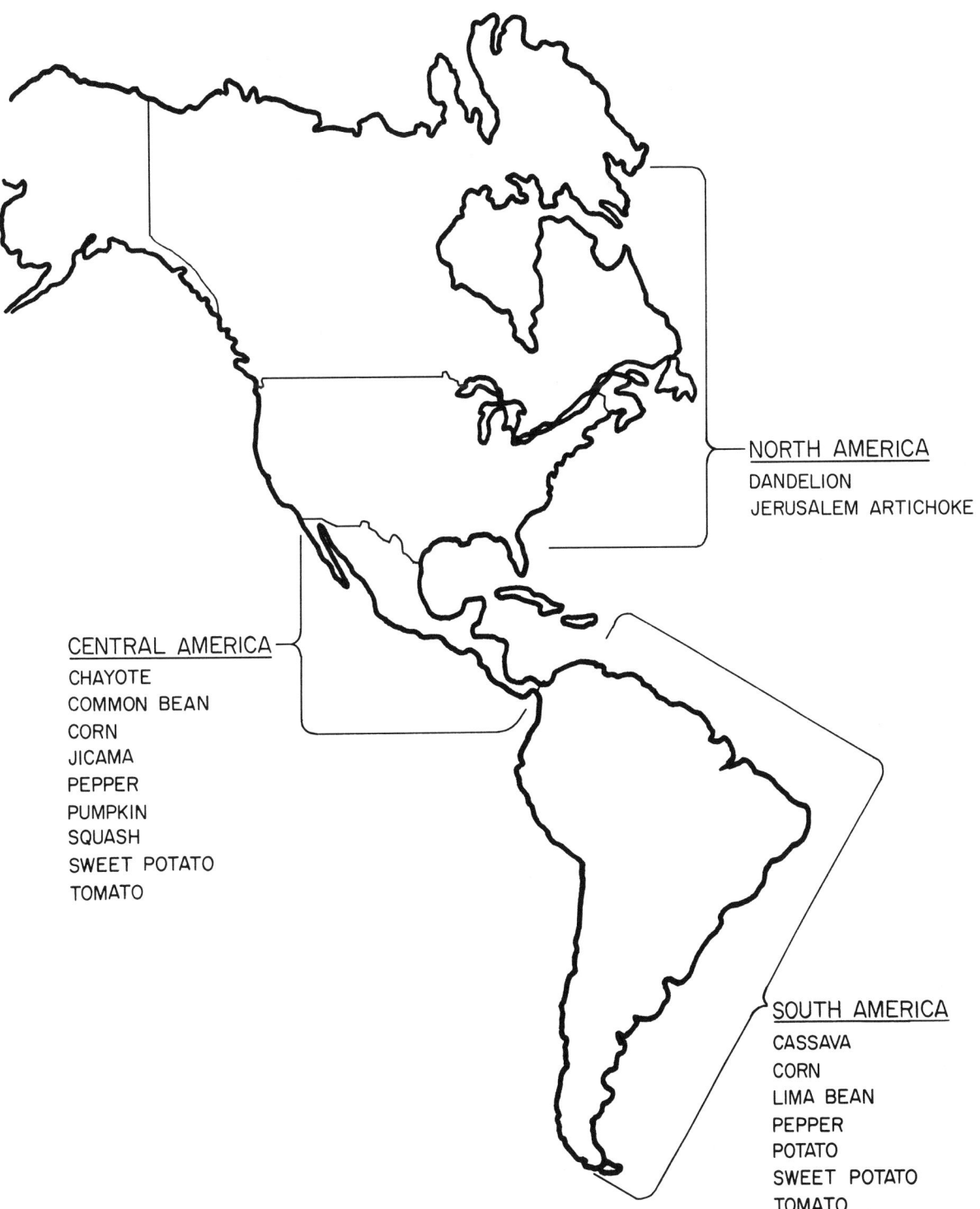

NORTH AMERICA
DANDELION
JERUSALEM ARTICHOKE

CENTRAL AMERICA
CHAYOTE
COMMON BEAN
CORN
JICAMA
PEPPER
PUMPKIN
SQUASH
SWEET POTATO
TOMATO

SOUTH AMERICA
CASSAVA
CORN
LIMA BEAN
PEPPER
POTATO
SWEET POTATO
TOMATO

Fig. V-4.   Places of origin and/or domestication of vegetables in the New World.

mato, which has been made firmer so that it will not be damaged by the picking machine.

Details on the history of individual vegetables are given in Table V-6 of this article, and in the separate articles covering each of the leading vegetable crops.

PRODUCTION AND PROCESSING.

The production of vegetables is an important part of the American agricultural scene. Market gardeners live near centers of population. Truck farmers live farther away; they grow vegetables and ship them in refrigerated trucks or cars to all parts of the nation. Home gardeners are everywhere; their vegetables provide cheap food and the maximum freshness and nourishment from crops that lose some of their goodness after harvesting; plus healthful exercise.

Commercial vegetable production in the United States doubled between 1910 and 1976.[1] During the period 1910 to 1976, the consumption of almost all vegetables except cabbage increased markedly. But, between 1976 and 1990, there was a slight drop in per capita consumption from 228 lb to 210 lb. The present consumption of cabbage is about 8.2 lb (*3.7 kg*) per person per year, or about one-third of what it was in 1910. The data for vegetable production in the world and in the United States are shown in Figs. V-5, V-6, and V-7.

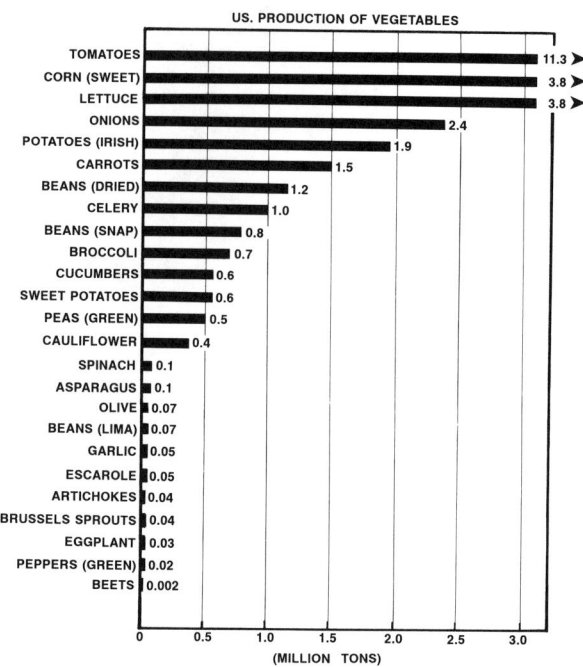

Fig. V-6.   U.S. production of vegetable crops. (Source: *Statistical Abstract of the United States*, U.S. Dept. of Commerce, 1991, p. 669, Table 1167, and *Agricultural Statistics, 1991*)

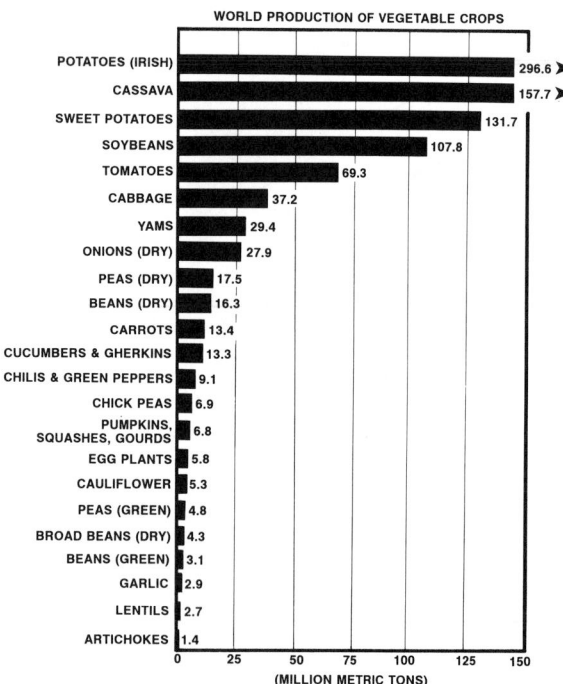

Fig. V-5.   World production of vegetable crops. (Source: *FAO Production Yearbook*, 1990, FAO/UN, Rome, Italy, Vol. 44)

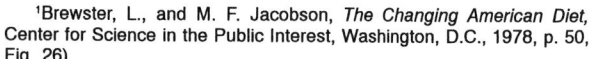

[1]Brewster, L., and M. F. Jacobson, *The Changing American Diet*, Center for Science in the Public Interest, Washington, D.C., 1978, p. 50, Fig. 26)

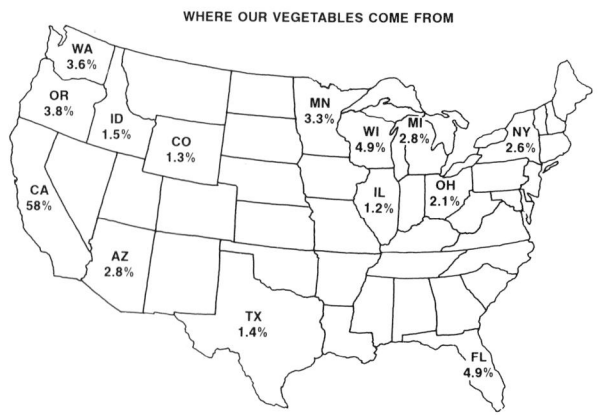

Fig. V-7.   The leading vegetable-producing states in the United States. (Source: *Agricultural Statistics 1991*, USDA, p. 144, Table 199)

Fig. V-5 shows that starchy roots and tubers (Irish potatoes, sweet potatoes, and cassava) are by far the leading vegetable crops of the world, followed by various legumes. These two types of vegetables complement each other in that the former are rich in calories, while the latter are excellent sources of protein.

Fig. V-6 does not show soybeans, which are by far the leading vegetable crop in the United States, because this legume is little used as a vegetable in this country. Rather, the crop is grown mainly for oil production, livestock feeding, and export. Therefore, the leading crop that is eaten as a vegetable in the United States is the Irish potato, which accounts for almost one-half of the per capita vegetable consumption. Fig. V-8 shows the trends in U.S. vegetable consumption which have occurred during the past three decades.

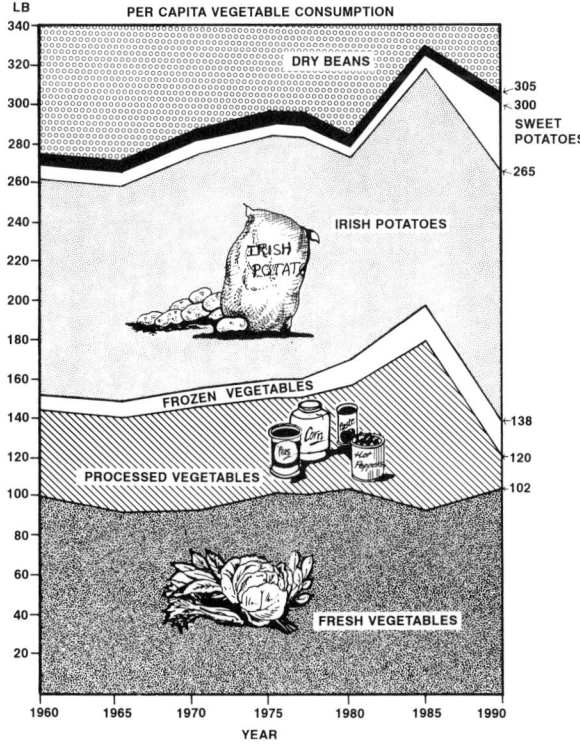

Fig. V-8.   Recent trends in U.S. vegetable consumption. (Source: *Statistical Abstract of the United States*, U.S. Dept. of Commerce, 1980, p. 131, Table No. 211; 1988, p. 115; and 1991, p. 127)

Propagation and Growing.   Most of the leading vegetable crops are grown from seeds. Hence, samples of commercial lots of vegetable seeds are usually tested to determine the percentage of seed that germinates under optimal conditions. Certain infectious diseases of plants may be controlled by treating seeds with fungicides which (1) eliminate disease from the seed itself and/or (2) protect the seeds against infected soil.

Some of the common vegetables are propagated from the vegetative tissues of parent plants rather than from seeds. Therefore, the following plant parts which are ordinarily used for vegetative (asexual) propagation are noteworthy:

• **Bulbs**—These tissues are modified underground stems that are enclosed by fleshy leaf scales. Garlic and onions are grown from bulbs.

• **Corms**—Although corms resemble bulbs in both shape and botanical characteristics, they differ in that they are (1) often much larger, and (2) made up mainly of stem material. They are used in the propagation of dasheen, taro, and similar tropical plants that are rich in starch.

• **Root crowns**—Crowns are the uppermost portions of roots, which are usually found near the surface of the soil. Both asparagus and rhubarb are grown from root crowns.

• **Root cuttings**—Side roots that are trimmed from the main root are used to propagate horseradish.

• **Stem cuttings**—Pieces of cassava stems are inserted in the ground to propagate this starchy tropical vegetable.

• **Stem tubers**—Tubers are portions of underground stems or rhizomes that are greatly enlarged in diameter due to their functioning as food storage organs. The leading exmple of a vegetable tuber is the Irish potato, which is allowed to develop bud clusters called "eyes," which are cut into eye-bearing pieces called "seed potatoes."

• **Suckers**—This term usually refers to the offshoots from root crowns, which are used to propagate plants such as the artichoke.

• **Tuberous roots**—The roots of the sweet potato and similar plants have greatly swollen portions that may be utilized in the propagation of the plant.

The use of plant parts other than seeds is called cloning, because the new plants which are produced have the same genetic makeup as the parent plant (unless, one or more mutations occur in the clones). Therefore, vegetative propagation insures that desired characteristics are retained in certain crops. However, vegetative tissues remain viable for only a few months to a year after being removed from the parent plant, whereas seeds retain their viability for 1 to 5 years or more.

Although seeds or other parts of plants may grow when placed in or on soil and left unattended thereafter, the best yields are likely to be obtained only when certain agricultural practices are followed. Furthermore, new methods of vegetable culture have been developed in recent times. The ways in which these techniques are utilized around the world may mean the difference between the adequate feeding of all the hungry or widespread malnutrition and disruption of the social order.

PRODUCTION IN FIELDS.
It seems likely that most of the vegetables used around the world will continue to be grown outdoors in fields because indoor or enclosed culture is profitable only in certain limited circumstances. Therefore, some of the most important practices associated with outdoor production follow.

Preparation of the Soil for Planting. Plowing the soil is one of the most important means of preparation because it (1) loosens the soil so that the plants grow readily; (2) mixes in animal manure, chemical fertilizer, and/or green manure; (3) uproots weeds and other unwanted vegetation so that they may be removed by raking; and (4) incorporates air into the soil.

Some of the other important soil preparation measures are (1) treatment with biological and/or chemical agents to destroy disease organisms, weeds, and plant-attacking pests such as nematodes; (2) drainage of water-logged soils; (3) leveling, terracing, or contour plowing to minimize soil erosion; and (4) adjustment of the soil acidity or alkalinity to suit the particular vegetable crop(s).

Planting. After the soil has been prepared, seeds or vegetative tissues (bulbs, cuttings, tubers, etc.) are planted by hand or by machine. Most vegetable crops remain in the same field from planting to harvesting. However, some vegetables are nurtured in special beds during their early stages of growth, after which they are transplanted to the fields where the remainder of the growth occurs. The special culturing of young plants under protected environments such as cold frames and greenhouses allows the grower to get a head start on the production of the crop during the optimal growing period. These measures are very important in areas where the growing season is short, because early frosts may kill the crop before it is ready to be harvested. Additionally, horticulturists are constantly seeking varieties of vegetables with short growing periods. The use of these varieties sometimes makes it possible to raise an additional crop during the growing season.

Cultivation. Loosening of the soil between rows of plants helps to eliminate weeds before they become well established. Many of the common weeds grow more vigorously than the crops, so the war on weeds is an unending struggle. Cultivation is also used to heap the soil around the plants that require this treatment at certain stages of growth.

Weed Eradication. Crops may be sprayed with chemical weed killers at various stages of their growth. This treatment may be needed in addition to the weed eradication performed during soil preparation and cultivation.

Application of Fertilizers. Normally, most of the required fertilizer(s) is added during soil preparation. However, some growing crops benefit from "side dressings" of fertilizer(s)

Irrigation. California contains less than 2% of the arable farm land of the United States, yet this state contributes over 10% of the total farm value of American crops, even though only minimal amounts of rain fall during the peak growing season. The unusually high agricultural productivity of California is due mainly to the judicious use of irrigation. Fig. V-9 shows a typical irrigation system. However, the overwatering of certain soils

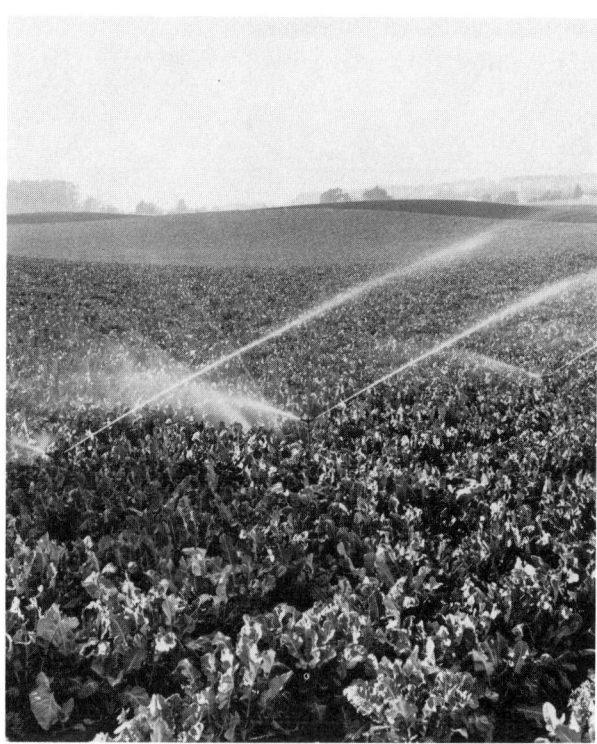

Fig. V-9.   Irrigation of broccoli on a farm near the coast of California. (Photo by J. C. Allen & Son, West Lafayette, Ind.)

is as bad or worse than underwatering them, because the former practice may bring toxic levels of salts to the surface of the soils. The salting of soils due to excessive irrigation once made it impossible to grow wheat in ancient Mesopotamia. Unfortunately, a similar salting of the soil occurred in a wheat-growing area of California in the 20th century.

GREENHOUSE CULTURE.
The production of vegetables in greenhouses when outdoor climatic conditions are unfavorable is called forcing. Greenhouses are usually constructed of a metal and/or a wood framework covered with glass or plastic which admits light. Also, they are likely to be heated so that the temperature inside is optimal for plant growth. The forcing of young plants is a means of extending short growing seasons,

since the plants may be transplanted out of doors when they are well along in their growth. Hence, they may reach maturity before crops that were planted outdoors from seed.

Greenhouses are expensive to operate, so they are used for the most valuable crops. Therefore, flowers and ornamental plants have been given priority over vegetable crops in greenhouses. Nevertheless, this method of vegetable production may be profitable when there is a great demand for out-of-season items, such as may occur in the densely populated areas of the northern states. Recently, greenhouse culture has utilized hydroponics in order to eliminate some of the problems due to soil structure and soil pests.

HYDROPONICS.   This term refers to the growing of plants without soil, but on an inert porous bed of gravel, sand, or a similar material through which nutrients and water are circulated. Hydroponics is most commonly used in commercial greenhouses such as the one shown in Fig. V-10.

However, hydroponic culture requires a considerable investment in housing, environmental control systems, special pumps, filters, culture beds, and energy to run the various components. Therefore, it does not seem likely that this method of raising vegetables will supplant field crops in any areas other than those in which arable soil and a favorable environment are lacking. For example, hydroponics has been used to produce vegetables in places such as Alaska, the Arabian peninsula, and certain islands in the Pacific. It is noteworthy that hydroponic culture makes very efficient use of water, because

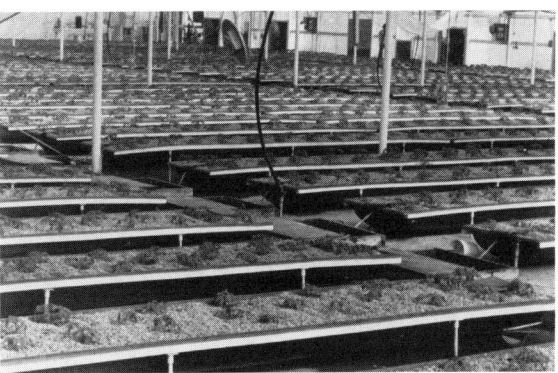

Fig. V-10.   Tomato-growing facility of a 7-acre hydroponic farm in Provo, Utah. (Courtesy, Techni-Culture, Inc., Scottsdale, Ariz.)

the nutrient solutions can be recycled after filtration to remove impurities.

Harvesting.   The mechanization of vegetable harvesting has proceeded slowly because it is difficult to design devices that handle these tender crops without causing blemishes and other injuries that reduce their market value. Therefore, various combinations of hand labor and mechanized procedures are utilized on the large commercial vegetable farms. Figs. V-11 and V-12 show some typical harvesting operations.

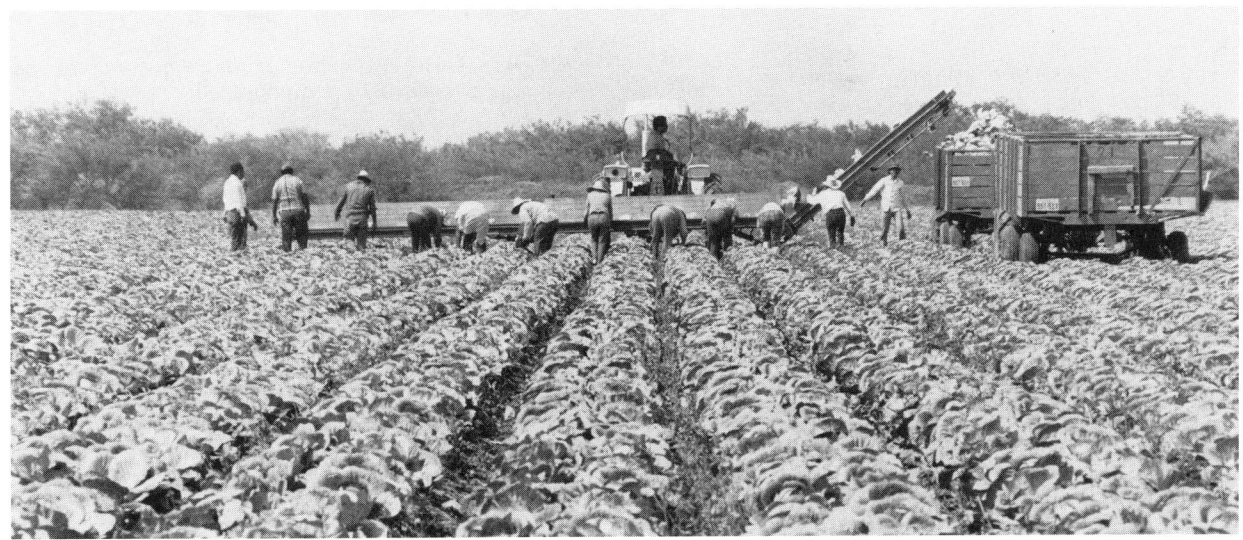

Fig. V-11.   Harvesting cabbage on a farm near San Juan, Texas. Workers cut the mature cabbage heads and drop them onto a conveyor belt which carries them to a wagon. Immature heads may never be picked, because it won't pay to go over the field again. (Courtesy, USDA)

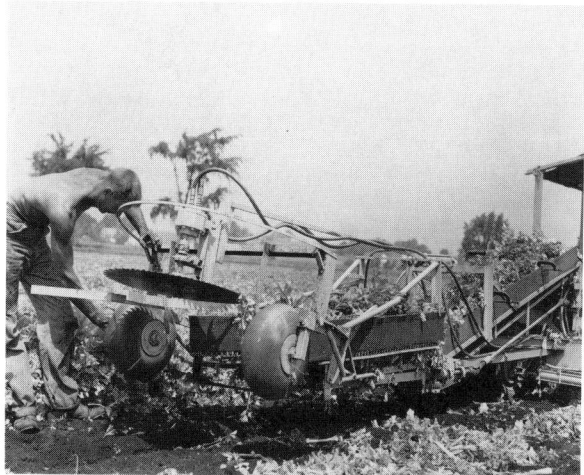

Fig. V-12.   Harvesting celery in Michigan. (Photo by J. C. Allen & Son, West Lafayette, Ind.)

It may be noted from Fig. V-12 that certain harvesting operations leave part of the vegetable crops in the field. Therefore, some communities have gleaners that volunteer to collect the unharvested vegetables for distribution to the needy.

Marketing Fresh Vegetables.   Today, the United States leads the world in the marketing of fresh vegetables transported over long distances, thanks to the utilization of modern means of transportation and refrigeration. Hand in hand with these developments, came significant changes in vegetable farming throughout the country. In earlier times, many small farms produced a variety of vegetables which were (1) sold locally, and (2) consumed fresh or following preservation and storage for a few months. Today, many large farms produce only one type of vegetable, which is often sold to brokers or wholesalers who arrange for storage, transportation, and sale to the wholesale or retail market. As a result of these changes in agriculture, the number of roadside markets in the United States has dwindled. Nevertheless, some may still be found in areas where there is a sufficient demand for a locally-grown produce. Fig. V-13 shows a typical roadside vegetable market.

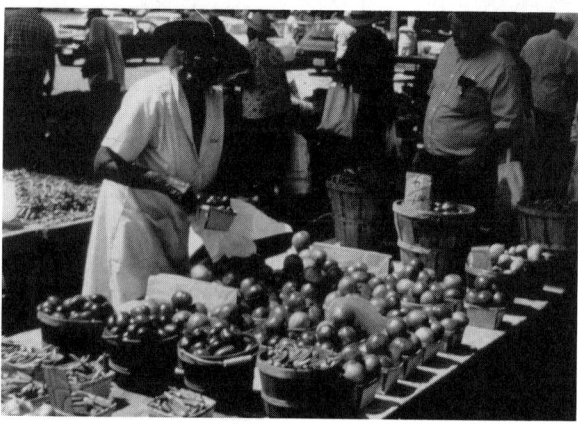

Fig. V-13.   A farmer's market. (Courtesy, USDA)

Vegetables which are to be shipped long distances must often be harvested before they reach their full maturity, then cooled by water sprays or other means so that (1) they will be less susceptible to damage during shipping, and (2) excessive maturation and deterioration are avoided. Therefore, immature produce may require artificial ripening in order to have maximum appeal to consumers. A common method of ripening fruits and vegetables artificially is to place them in sealed chambers filled with ethylene gas. Ethylene is produced by certain fruits and vegetables during their natural ripening. For example, tomatoes produce abundant amounts of this gas. Hence, they may be ripened at home by merely enclosing them in a plastic bag at room temperature. It is noteworthy that refrigeration reduces the production of ethylene gas by fruits and vegetables.

U.S. DEPARTMENT OF AGRICULTURE GRADE STANDARDS.   The middlemen in the marketing chain between the farmer and the consumer rarely have the opportunity to inspect the produce before committing themselves to the price they are willing to pay. Therefore, the USDA has established voluntary grade standards for fruits and vegetables in order to provide (1) a common basis for wholesale trading, and (2) a means by which prices may be determined. One or more of the parties to a wholesale vegetable transaction may request and pay for grading of the shipment by an inspector licensed by the USDA. The official USDA grades for fresh vegetables are as follows:[2]

• **U.S. Fancy**—Premium quality; covers only the top quality range produced.

• **U.S. No. 1**—The chief trading grade; represents good average quality that is practical to pack under commercial conditions; covers the bulk of the quality range produced.

• **U.S. No. 2**— Intermediate quality between U.S. No. 1 and U.S. No. 3; noticeably superior to U.S. No. 3.

• **U.S. No. 3**—The lowest merchantable quality practical to pack under normal conditions.

Most grading is visual. Internal as well as external quality of many products is examined. Models, color guides, and color photographs are available for graders to check samples for shape, degree of coloring, and degree of defects or damage. Products may be graded in the area where they are produced; at assembly, packaging, or processing plants; at terminal markets; or in a railcar or a receiver's warehouse or store.

Some of the other functions of the grade standards are: (1) to help establish loan values for produce in storage; (2) to assure that products purchased by the military services and various governmental agencies are of acceptable quality; (3) to provide purchasing specifications that may be used by restaurants, shipping lines, and other food establishments; and (4) to establish a basis for the trading of vegetable crops on the futures market.

---

[2]*Uniform Grade Nomenclature Policy for United States Standards for Grades of Fresh Fruit, Vegetables, Nuts and Other Special Products,* USDA, 1976.

Storage. The increased yields which have been brought about by modern agricultural technology may be wasted in part if there is considerable deterioration of vegetables due to lack of adequate storage. Even in the United States, about 25% of the produce spoils.[3] These losses may exceed 60% in the areas of the world where refrigeration and other storage facilities are lacking. Also, much of the vegetable crop is harvested in the summer and in the fall, and little in the winter or spring. Hence, before commercial refrigeration was developed in the latter half of the 19th century, there was a large supply of many vegetables right after harvest, but a small supply about 6 months later. The great fluctuations in the supplies of fresh vegetables in the northern countries led to a rise of severe vitamin C deficiency (scurvy) in the late winter and early spring of each year. Although outbreaks of scurvy occurred through the centuries, they were less severe in rural areas where fruits and vegetables were stored at home over the winter. Table V-1 gives storage information for selected vegetables.

TABLE V-1
RECOMMENDED STORAGE CONDITIONS AND STORAGE PERIODS FOR SELECTED VEGETABLES[1]

| Vegetable | Place to Store | Storage Conditions | | Length of Storage Periods |
		Temperature[2]	Humidity	
		(°F)		
Beans and peas, dry	Any cool, dry place.	32° to 40°	Dry	As long as desired.
Cabbage, late	Pit, trench, or outdoor cellar.	Near 32° as possible	Moderately moist	Through late fall and winter.
Cauliflower	Storage cellar.	Near 32° as possible	Moderately moist	6 to 8 weeks.
Celery, late	Pit or trench; roots in soil.	Near 32° as possible	Moderately moist	Through late fall and winter.
Endive	Roots in soil in storage cellar.	Near 32° as possible	Moderately moist.	2 to 3 months.
Onions	Any cool, dry place.	Near 32° as possible	Dry	Through fall and winter.
Parsnips	Where they grew, or in storage cellar.	Near 32° as possible	Moist	Through fall and winter.
Peppers	Unheated basement or room.	45° to 50°	Moderately moist	2 to 3 weeks.
Potatoes	Pit or in storage cellar.	35° to 40°	Moderately moist	Through fall and winter.
Pumpkins and squashes ..	Home cellar or basement.	55°	Moderately moist	Through fall and winter.
Root crops (miscellaneous)	Pit or in storage cellar.	Near 32° as possible	Moist	Through fall and winter.
Sweet potatoes	Home cellar or basement.	55° to 60°	Moderately dry	Through fall and winter.
Tomatoes (mature green)	Home cellar or basement.	55° to 70°	Moderately dry	4 to 6 weeks.

[1]Adapted by the authors from Wott, J. A., *Storing Vegetables & Fruits at Home*, Bull. HO-125, Purdue University Cooperative Extension Service, p. 4.
[2]To convert to centrigrade, subtract 32 and multiply by 5/9.

The storage conditions and conditions given in Table V-1 were used during the winter months prior to the development of modern refrigeration and freezing. Also, they are still used by some home gardeners and families on small farms in the northern United States. Today, most people either limit their storage of fresh vegetables to the small amounts that may be kept in a refrigerator and/or in a freezer; or utilize large commercial lockers for cold storage. Fortunately, most supermarkets carry a variety of fresh vegetables throughout the year, thanks to (1) large refrigerated warehouses which may even be equipped with ripening chambers that utilize ethylene gas, and (2) fast transportation systems, that are usually refrigerated, which bring fresh produce from warmer areas where it is grown without interruption.

At the present time it is uncertain how the ever increasing cost of electrical energy and other fuels will affect the refrigerated storage of produce. Perhaps, it will stimulate an increased utilization of food processing measures which reduce the need for storing vegetables.

[3]Wu, M. T., and D. K. Salunkhe, "The Use of Certain Chemicals to Increase Nutritional Value and to Extend Quality in Economic Plants," *Storage, Processing, and Nutritional Quality of Fruits and Vegetables,* edited by D. K. Salunkhe, CRC Press, Inc., Cleveland, Ohio, 1974, p. 80.

Processing. Various methods of processing vegetables have been used since early times. For example, the Indians living in the mountainous areas of Peru have long prepared chuno (a crude freeze-dried product) from potatoes by tramping out the water with their feet between alternate periods of freezing and thawing. Some of the more commonly used methods of processing vegetables follow.

CANNING. In this process, vegetables in metal or glass containers are heated sufficiently to kill the microorganisms that cause spoilage. After heating, the containers are fitted with airtight closures. Canning was developed by the fresh food technologist Appert at the beginning of the 19th century. Since then, it has become one of the major means of processing vegetables. Also, about one out of three American families can fruit and vegetables at home.[4] However, many people are using questionable procedures for home canning, which may result in spoilage and illness due to food poisoning. It is noteworthy that since 1925 fewer than a dozen deaths have been reported from the consumption of hundreds of billions of cans of commercially processed foods, whereas hundreds of deaths have resulted from eating items that were improperly canned at home.[5] Therefore, it is extremely important that only reliable procedures be used in canning, such as those given in U.S. Department of Agriculture publications. For example, acidic items such as tomato products and various types of pickled vegetables may be canned in a boiling water bath, whereas all other vegetables are on the alkaline side of neutrality and require pressure steaming to make them safe. Few harmful bacteria grow well in an acid medium, so they are easily destroyed by moderate heating of acidic foods. On the other hand, deadly organisms such as *Clostridium botulinum* grow readily in anaerobic (without air) alkaline mediums. Table V-2 gives some directions for canning alkaline vegetables.

[4]"USDA Survey Reveals Canning Practices," *Research News,* USDA, September 1976, p. 1.

[5]Tope, N. F., "Pressure Canners, Vital for Low-Acid Foods," *Gardening for Food and Fun: The Yearbook of Agriculture 1977,* USDA, p. 323.

TABLE V-2
DIRECTIONS FOR CANNING SELECTED VEGETABLES[1]

Vegetable		Preparation	Process @ 10 lb Pressure	
			Pint	Quart
			(minutes)	
Asparagus	(raw)	Wash, trim, cut in 1-in. pieces. Pack as tightly as possible without crushing to ½ in. of top of jar. Add salt.[3] Cover with boiling water, leaving ½-in. space at top of jar. Place jars in pressure cooker.	25	30
	(hot)	Wash, trim, cut in 1-in. pieces. Cover with boiling water. Boil 2 or 3 minutes. Pack hot to ½ in. of top. Add salt.[3] Cover with boiling water. Leave ½-in. space at top of jar. Place jars in pressure cooker.	25	30
Beans Lima	(raw)	Can only young tender beans. Shell and wash beans. *Small beans:* fill to 1 in. of top for pint jars, 1½ in. for quarts. *Large beans:* fill to 3/4 in. of top for pints, 1¼ in. for quarts. Do *not* press or shake beans down. Add salt.[3] Cover with boiling water, or leave ½-in. space at top of jar. Place jars in pressure cooker.	40	50
	(hot)	Shell beans, cover with boiling water and bring to boil. Pack hot beans loosely to 1 in. of top. Add salt.[3] Cover with boiling water, leaving 1-in. space at top of jar. Place jars in pressure cooker.	40	50
Beans Snap-green or wax	(raw)	Wash, trim, and cut in 1-in. pieces. Pack tightly to ½ in. of top. Add salt.[3] Cover with boiling water, leaving ½-in. space at top of jar. Place jars in pressure cooker.	20	25
	(hot)	Wash, trim, and cut in 1-in. pieces. Cover with boiling water, boil 5 minutes. Pack hot beans loosely to ½ in. of top. Add salt.[3] Cover with boiling hot cooking liquid, leaving ½-in. space at top of jar. Place jars in pressure cooker.	20	25

Footnotes at end of table

(Continued)

TABLE V-2   *(Continued)*

Vegetable	Preparation	Process @ 10 lb Pressure	
		Pint	Quart
		(minutes)	
Beets (hot)	Cut off tops, leave an inch of stem. Leave roots. Wash beets. Cover with boiling water. Boil until skins slip easily (15 to 25 minutes). Skin and trim. Leave small beets whole; cut larger beets into ½-in. cubes or slices. Pack hot beets to ½ in. of top. Add salt.[3] Cover with boiling water, leaving ½-in. space at top of jar. Place jars in pressure cooker.	30	35
Corn (raw) Cream style	Husk, remove silks, wash. Cut corn from cob at center of kernel, scrape cobs. Use pint jar only. Pack to 1½ in. of top. Do not shake or press down. Add salt.[3] Fill to ½ in. of top with boiling water. Place jars in pressure cooker.	95	—
(hot)	Prepare as for raw pack. To each quart measure of corn add 1 pt. boiling water. Heat to boiling. Use pint jars only. Pack hot corn to 1 in. of top. Add salt.[3] Place jars in pressure cooker.	85	—
Corn Whole kernel (raw)	Husk, remove silk, wash. Cut from cob about 2/3 depth of kernel. Pack corn to 1 in. of top. Do not shake or press down. Add salt.[3] Fill to ½ in. of top with boiling water. Place jars in pressure cooker.	55	86
(hot)	Prepare as for raw pack. To each quart measure of corn add 1 pt. boiling water. Heat to boiling. Pack hot corn to 1 in. of top, cover with boiling hot liquid, leaving 1 in. at top of jar. Add salt.[3] Place jars in pressure cooker.	55	85
Greens (beets, chard, spinach, etc.)	Can only freshly picked, tender greens. Pick over, wash thoroughly, remove tough stems and midribs. Place about 2½ lb greens in cheesecloth bag, steam 10 minutes or until well wilted. Pack hot greens loosely to ½ in. of top. Add ¼ tsp salt/pint, ½ tsp salt/quart. Cover with boiling water, leaving ½ in. at top of jar. Place jars in pressure cooker.	70	90
Peas (raw) Fresh green	Shell, wash. Pack to 1 in. of top. Do not shake or press down. Add salt.[3] Cover with boiling water, leaving 1½ in. space at top of jar. Place jars in pressure cooker.	40	40
(hot)	Shell, wash. Cover with boiling water. Bring to boil. Pack hot peas loosely to 1 in. of top. Add salt.[3] Cover with boiling water, leaving 1-in. space at top of jar. Place jars in pressure cooker.	40	40
Squash Summer (raw)	Wash, do not pare, trim ends. Cut in ½-in. slices; then halve or quarter if necessary to make pieces uniform in size. Pack pieces tightly to 1 in. of top of jar. Add salt.[3] Cover with boiling water, leaving 1½ in. space at top of jar. Place jars in pressure cooker.	25	30
(hot)	Prepare as for raw pack. Add just enough water to cover. Bring to boil. Pack hot squash loosely to ½ in. of top. Add salt.[3] Cover with boiling hot cooking liquid to ½ in. of top of jar.	30	40

[1]VanZandt, D. P., *Preserving Foods: Home Canning of Low-Acid Vegetables*, University of Maryland Cooperative Extension Service Fact Sheet 277, pp. 4–6. To convert to metric, see WEIGHTS AND MEASURES.
[2]Processing time *after* the pressure reaches 10 lb (240° F). The pressure should be kept constant by regulating the heat under the canner.
[3]Unless stated otherwise, add 1/2 tsp salt per pint and 1 tsp per quart. Salt may be omitted if desired.
(Additional information on the home canning of vegetables may be obtained from the local county agricultural extension office.)

DRYING. The preservation of food by drying it in the sun is about 5,000 years old. Dried vegetables keep well because the water content is so low that spoilage microorganisms cannot grow. Drying must be done as fast as possible at a temperature that does not seriously affect the flavor, texture, and color of the vegetables. If the temperature is too low, the food may undergo spoilage before it has been dried adequately. A drying temperature that is too high may cause (1) the water-filled cells of the vegetable to expand and burst, or (2) hardening of the surfaces of the vegetables so that moisture does not escape readily.

Vegetables contain enzymes that may cause color and flavor changes during drying unless enzyme activity is retarded or stopped by (1) treatment with an antioxidant such as ascorbic acid (vitamin C), (2) blanching, and/or (3) sulfuring. Table V-3 gives directions for drying selected vegetables.

TABLE V-3
DIRECTIONS FOR DRYING SELECTED VEGETABLES[1]

Vegetable	Preparation	Pretreatment	Drying Procedure[2]	Dryness Test
Beans Green lima	Shell, and wash.	Steam 15 to 20 minutes, or until tender but firm. Place in boiling water 5 minutes. Drain.	Spread on tray in a single layer 1/8"-1/4" deep. Place tray in cold oven, heat gradually to 160°F. Stir frequently. Allow 6-16 hours in oven or home constructed dryer.	Shatter when hit with a hammer.
Beans Snap (green or wax)	Wash, trim and slice lengthwise or cut in 1-in. pieces.	Steam about 20 minutes or until tender but firm; or Place in boiling water 5 minutes. Drain.	Same as for lima beans.	Brittle, dark green to brownish.
Beets	Cut top from beets, leaving 1½ in. stem. Retain roots. Wash.	Boil whole 30 to 60 minutes depending on size. Cool and peel. Cut in ¼-in. cubes, or slice 1/8 in. thick.	Same as for lima beans.	Brittle, dark red.
Carrots	Top, wash, and scrape. Dice into ¼-in. cubes or slice 1/8-in. thick.	Blanch in boiling water 3-4 minutes. Drain well; or Steam 15 minutes or until tender. Drain.	Spread in single layer on trays. Place tray in cold oven. Heat gradually to 160°F. Reduce heat when nearly dry. Stir frequently to prevent clumping. Average drying time 6-10 hours.	Brittle, deep orange color.
Corn Tender, sweet	Husk, trim, and wash. Sort ears on basis of maturity because immature corn requires less blanching time. Cut from cob after blanching and cooling enough to handle.	Steam on the cob 10-15 minutes, or until milk is set. Boil 6-8 minutes in large volume of water.	Spread kernels ½-in. deep on trays. Dry as suggested for carrots.	Hard and brittle.
Herbs (for seasoning) Basil, celery leaves, chives, parsley, thyme, others	Gather when leaves are mature but before flowers develop. Wash thoroughly; remove excess water.	No treatment necessary.	Place leaves on a cookie sheet in a warm oven, 160°F; or Hang small bundles of stems in warm, dry, airy place (may be enclosed in large brown paper or nylon net bag).	Brittle and crumble easily.

Footnotes at end of table

(Continued)

TABLE V-3 *(Continued)*

Vegetable	Preparation	Pretreatment	Drying Procedure[2]	Dryness Test
Mushrooms (young, firm)	Peel, large mushrooms if desired. Wash and remove base of stem. Dry small mushrooms whole cut or slice large ones. If stems are tender, slice ⅛ in. thick before drying.	Blanch 4 minutes for small or medium whole, or 3 minutes for sliced mushrooms. To prevent darkening, add 1 tsp citric acid or 3 tsp lemon juice or ½ tsp ascorbic acid to each quart of water.	Mushrooms may be dried either artificially or in the sun.	Leathery to brittle.
Onions	Peel. Remove outer discolored layers. Cut uniform slices ⅛-in. to ¼-in. thick.	No treatment.	Same as carrots, but use temperature 140°-150°F to prevent scorching.	Brittle and cream colored. Crush in blender for onion powder.
Peas Green (young tender)	Shell peas, and rinse in cool water.	Steam shelled peas 15 minutes, until tender but firm; or Blanch in boiling water 1½ minutes. Drain.	Same as carrots.	Shatter when hit with a hammer.
Peppers (sweet, bell)	Wash. Cut out stem ends and remove seeds of green peppers. Slice or dice.	Blanch in hot water 2 minutes. Drain.	Same as carrots.	Pliable
Peppers, chili (red)	Select mature pods. Wipe clean with damp cloth. String whole pods together with needle and cord or suspend plants in bunches root side up, where air can get to them.	Blanching not necessary.	Drying at room temperature several weeks. Oven method 6-16 hours.	Shrunken, dark red, flexible.
Pimentos	Wash.	Place in 400°F oven for 3 or 4 minutes until peel is charred. Cool and peel.	Same as carrots.	Pliable
Potatoes	Scrub thoroughly, trim off blemishes and remove eyes.	Boil in jackets until only crisp, tender. Cool and peel if desired. Shred on metal vegetable grater; or Peel and cut into shoestring thickness. Rinse well. Steam 5 minutes. Chill and dry.	Spread on tray in single layer ⅛-in. deep. Place in cold oven on drying trays. Gradually heat to 160°F. Toss with fork for even drying. Allow 6-10 hours.	Brittle, creamy white color.
Pumpkin	Cut in half, remove seeds and stringy portion. Cut into thin strips and peel. Slice strips into ⅛-in. slices.	Steam blanch until tender 6-8 minutes.	Same as carrots.	Leathery
Squash Firm, winter varieties	See pumpkin.	See pumpkin.		Leathery

[1]Miller, E.L. *Drying Foods*, Publication C-536, Kansas State University Cooperative Extension Service, 1976, pp. 20-27. To convert to metric, see WEIGHTS AND MEASURES.
[2]If suggested temperature ranges are not possible to control, maintain the drying temperature at 160°F or as low as possible.

FREEZING. The art of freezing vegetables has been developed so that most items retain essentially all of the quality of fresh vegetables after as much as 8 to 12 months of frozen storage. Nevertheless, there may be drastic reductions in the colors, flavors, nutritive values, and textures of frozen vegetables unless recommended practices are followed. Details of these practices follow:

• **Washing, peeling, trimming, and cutting into pieces—** Vegetables that are to be frozen and consumed at a later date require much the same careful preparation that would normally be accorded in preparing them for serving at the next meal. Also, bruised, damaged, or otherwise unwholesome pieces should be rejected because it makes little sense to invest labor and freezer space in poor quality food.

• **Blanching—**This procedure consists of heating the vegetables briefly in boiling water, steam, or hot fat in order to stop or slow the actions of enzymes which cause changes in color, flavor, and texture.

• **Cooling—**The vegetables should be cooled rapidly after blanching and before freezing so that (1) cooking stops, and (2) freezing occurs as rapidly as possible. Excessively slow freezing results in the formation of large knifelike ice crystals which rupture the cell walls of the plant tissue and cause the vegetable to be somewhat mushy when thawed.

Rapid cooling is best achieved by immersing the blanched vegetables in either cold running water or iced water containing about equal weights of ice and the hot vegetable.

• **Packing, in freezer containers—**The vegetables should be drained well before packing into containers. Headspace is left in the containers because the vegetables will expand a little when they are frozen. The packages of vegetables should be sealed, labeled, and dated.

• **Freezing—**Quick freezing is achieved by limiting the amount of vegetables placed in the freezer to that which may be frozen within 24 hours—approximately 2 to 3 lb of vegetables per cubic foot of freezer space. The freezer temperature should be maintained at 0°F (-18°C) or lower.

Table V-4 gives directions for freezing selected vegetables.

TABLE V-4
DIRECTIONS FOR FREEZING SELECTED VEGETABLES[1]

Vegetable	Preparation	Blanching Time (Boiling water unless otherwise specified)	Headspace
		(minutes)	(in.)
Asparagus 1. Small stalks 2. Medium stalks 3. Large stalks	Wash thoroughly, sort by size, cut in 2-in. lengths if desired. Blanch and chill. Alternate tips and stem ends when packaging whole.	 2 3 4	 None
Beans (snap, green, or wax)	Wash, remove ends, cut in 1- or 2-in. pieces. Blanch and chill.	3	1/2
Broccoli 1. Water 2. Steam	Wash and trim. If insects are present, soak ½ hour in solution of 4 tsp salt to 1 gal of cold water. Separate stalks so flowerets are no more than 1½ in. across. Blanch and chill.	 3 5	 None
Corn (on the cob) 1. Small ears (1¼ in. or less in diameter) 2. Medium ears (1¼-1½ in. diameter) 3. Large ears (over 1½ in. in diameter)	Husk ears, remove silk, wash corn, sort according to size. Blanch and chill.	7 9 11	None
Corn (cream style)	Same as for on the cob. Blanch and chill. Cut kernels from cob at 1/2 depth of kernel. Scrape cob with back of knife to remove juice.	4 (Before cutting kernels from cob)	1/2
Corn (whole kernel)	Same as for cream style. Blanch and chill. Cut kernels from cob at 2/3 depth of kernel.	4 (Before cutting kernels from cob)	1/2

Footnotes at end of table

(Continued)

TABLE V-4   *(Continued)*

Vegetable	Preparation	Blanching Time (Boiling water unless otherwise specified)	Headspace
		(minutes)	(in.)
Greens (beets, chard, collards, kale, spinach, turnip, etc.) 1. Beet greens, kale, chard, mustard and turnip greens. 2. Collards 3. Spinach 4. Very tender leaves.	Wash thoroughly, remove tough stems and bruised leaves, cut chard leaves in pieces. Blanch and chill.	2 3 2 1½	1/2
Mushrooms 1. Whole (not over 1 in. across) 2. Quarters or buttons 3. Slices	Sort by size, wash thoroughly in cold water, trim stem ends, slice or quarter mushrooms larger than 1 in. in diameter. Pan fry until almost done or steam. Cool. (Before steaming to prevent darkening, soak 5 minutes in solution of tsp lemon juice to 1 pt of water.)	5 3½ 3	1/2
Peas (green)	Shell, blanch and chill.	1½	1/2
Pepper (sweet or hot) 1. Halves 2. Slices	*Sweet:* Wash, remove stems, cut in half or in slices, remove seeds. *Hot:* Wash and stem. Pack in small containers.	3 2 For use in uncooked foods—blanching not necessary.	1/2 for blanched peppers. No headspace if not blanched.
Squash (summer or winter) 1. Summer 2. Winter	*Summer:* Wash, cut into 1/2-in. slices. *Winter* Wash, cut into pieces and remove seeds.	3 Cook pieces until soft. Remove pulp from rind and mash.	1/2 1/2

¹VanZandt, D. P., *Preserving Foods: Freezing Vegetables,* University of Maryland Cooperative Extension Service Fact Sheet 278, 1979, pp. 2-3, Table 1. To convert to metric, see WEIGHTS AND MEASURES.

PICKLING. This type of processing preserves vegetables in vinegar or a salt solution (brine) or a combination of the two. Other ingredients may be added to alter the flavor and/or the texture of the pickles. The major types of vegetable pickles follow:

• **Brined pickles**—These pickles are produced by a fermentation process carried out for several weeks in a salt solution. Salt tolerant bacteria promote the fermentation, while the growth of spoilage microorganisms is inhibited by the salt solution. Dilled cucumbers, olives, sauerkraut, and certain other vegetables are preserved this way.

• **Fresh pack pickles**—This process is also called the quick process because (1) the fermentation step is eliminated, and (2) the vegetables are just mixed with the pickling ingredients and canned.

• **Relishes**—Some or all of the chopped vegetable ingredients of these mixtures may be pickled. The flavorings may be hot, spicy, sweet, or sour. Corn relish, chili sauce, catsup, chowchow, and chutney are among the more commonly used relishes.

All pickle products require heat treatment to (1) destroy organisms that cause spoilage, (2) inactivate enzymes within the vegetables that cause spoilage, and (3) inactivate enzymes within the vegetables that alter color, flavor, and texture. Hence, most pickled vegetables are heat treated and canned by a process similar to that used for acid fruits and tomatoes.

It is noteworthy that the canning of pickled nonacid vegetables is a much safer way of preserving them than canning them in the nonpickled form because the use of an acid medium is an excellent way to prevent the growth of food spoilage microorganisms. (Directions for making vegetable pickles at home may be obtained from the county agricultural extension agent.)

**FEDERAL STANDARDS FOR PROCESSED VEGE-
TABLE PRODUCTS.** All over the United States, canned
spinach and tomato paste are essentially the same
because food standards set by the Federal Government
stipulate the requirements which these products must
meet if they move in interstate commerce. There are four
major sets of standards which apply to various processed
vegetable products. These follow:

• **U.S. Department of Agriculture Grade Standards**—
These standards, like those for fresh produce, are voluntary. They cover canned, frozen, and dried fruits and vegetables, and related products such as preserves; and rice,
dry beans, and peas.

USDA provides official grading services for a fee, often
in cooperation with State departments of agriculture, to
packers, processors, distributors, or others who wish
official certification of the grade of a product. Also, the
grade standards are often used by packers and processors as guidelines for their quality control.

• **Food and Drug Administration Standards of Identity**—
These mandatory standards establish what a given food
product *is*—for example, what a food must be to be labeled "catsup." They also provide for the use of optional
ingredients in addition to the mandatory ingredients.

Vegetable products for which standards of identity
have been formulated are canned vegetables, tomato
paste, tomato puree, catsup, vegetable juices, and frozen
vegetables.

• **Food and Drug Administration Minimum Standards of
Quality**—FDA standards of quality are mandatory, as opposed to USDA grade standards of quality which are
voluntary. They have been set for a number of canned
vegetables to supplement standards of identity, by speci-
fying the minimum acceptable characteristics for such
factors as tenderness, color, and freedom from defects.

• **Food and Drug Administration Standards of Fill of Container**—These mandatory standards tell the packer how
full a container must be to avoid deception. They prevent
the selling of air or water in place of food.

**RECENT DEVELOPMENTS IN VEGETABLE PROC-
ESSING.**   The canning and drying of vegetables are convenient means of preservation because the products of
these processes may be stored for long periods of time
without refrigeration, whereas frozen vegetables require
continuous storage in a freezer that must be run by one
or more forms of energy. However, canned and dried
items often retain only the appearances of the fresh produce because (1) the original crisp texture has been either
softened or toughened excessively, (2) much of the
mineral and vitamin content has been lost, (3) flavors have
deteriorated, and (4) long soaking and cooking is required
to restore the original water content of dried items.
Therefore, food technologists have long been at work
seeking ways to overcome these problems, while providing economical products. Some recent developments
follow:

• **Artificial vegetables**—These products utilize constituents of sea plants to simulate the textural characteristics of land plants. A typical item may be made from
(1) alginates (gums extracted from marine algae), (2) calcium and/or magnesium salts, (3) water, (4) minerals and
vitamins, and (5) coloring and flavoring agents. Certain
other substances such as gum tragacanth, pectin, or
starch paste may be added to modify the consistency and
texture of the product, which varies from that of cooked
turnips to that of crisp, raw cucumbers. Hence, this process has been used to make imitation cucumbers, potatoes, turnips, and water chestnuts. These products may
be useful for people on special diets in which certain
nutrients are restricted greatly, because the nutrient content of the artificial items may be controlled within very
narrow limits.

• **Crispy canned goods**—The textures of fresh, raw vegetables may be obtained in canned items by coating the
fresh vegetable pieces with a mixture of carboxymethyl
cellulose gum (a chemically altered form of cellulose) and
another gum prior to processing in the conventional
manner.

• **Instantly-rehydratable dried vegetables**—Rehydration
times for these products may be shortened greatly by
compressing the vegetable pieces during drying. Apparently, thin, flat flakelike pieces regain their water content much more rapidly than thicker pieces. Some of
these products, such as dried and chopped carrots, celery, and green peppers may be merely soaked in cold
water and used in salads.

• **Nonstarchy thickeners for "creamed" vegetable mixtures**—Canned cream style corn, chow mein, chop suey,
and similar products often contain a starchy thickening
agent such as cornstarch or wheat flour. The starchy ingredient tends to mask the flavors of the vegetables,
thereby making the mixture taste bland and insipid. However, from 15 to 85% of the starch may be eliminated by
using alginate gums extracted from marine algae as
thickeners. This substitution results in a reduction of the
caloric content of the vegetable products, since alginates
are not metabolized by the body.

• **Precooked beans**—Many busy homemakers are reluctant to prepare beans because of the long cooking time.
These products, which have usually been soaked in a
tenderizing solution and steamed or pressure cooked, require only about 35 minutes of cooking time in an open
pot, or only 5 to 10 minutes in a pressure cooker.

• **Quick-cooking dried peas**—This convenience food is
prepared by soaking the peas in an enzyme solution,
followed by steaming and drying. Normally, dried split
peas require at least 25 mintues cooking time, but quick-
cooking dried peas require only about half as much time.

NUTRITIVE VALUES. "Eat your vegetables" is the
admonition of mothers and doctors alike; and with reason. They know that vegetables are good—and good for

us. They give bulk to the diet, which aids the digestive process; and they are rich sources of certain essential minerals and vitamins.

Vegetables are high in water content; hence, they are considerably lower in calories and proteins than most of the grains and legumes. However, most vegetables are fair to excellent sources of fiber (poorly digested car-

bohydrate which stimulates movements of the digestive tract), various essential macrominerals and microminerals, vitamins, and vitaminlike factors. The nutrient composition of the commonly used vegetables is given in Food Composition Table F-36. Table V-5 groups vegetables according to the amounts of vitamins A and C that they supply.

TABLE V-5
AMOUNTS OF VITAMIN A, VITAMIN C, AND CALORIES
FURNISHED BY 100 G OF SELECTED VEGETABLES[1, 2]

Nutritional Group	Vegetable	Vitamin Content		Food Energy
		A	C	
		(IU)	(mg)	(kcal)
High in vitamins A and C	Parsley (raw)	8,500	172	44
	Spinach	8,100	28	23
	Collards	7,800	76	33
	Kale	7,400	62	28
	Turnip Greens	6,300	69	20
	Mustard Greens	5,800	48	23
	Cantaloupes	3,400	33	30
	Broccoli	2,500	90	26
High in vitamin A	Carrots (raw)	11,000	8	42
	Carrots (cooked)	10,500	6	31
	Sweet potatoes	8,100	22	141
	Swiss Chard	5,400	16	18
	Winter Squash	4,200	13	63
	Green Onions	2,000	32	36
High in vitamin C	Peppers (immature green)	420	128	22
	Brussels Sprouts	520	87	36
	Cauliflower	60	55	22
	Kohlrabi	20	43	24
	Cabbage	130	33	20
	Chinese Cabbage	150	25	14
	Asparagus	900	26	20
	Rutabaga	550	26	35
	Radishes (raw)	322	26	17
	Tomatoes (ripe, raw)	900	23	22
	Tomatoes (ripe, cooked)	1,000	24	26
Other green vegetables	Beans, green	540	12	25
	Celery	240	9	17
	Lettuce (leaf)	1,900	18	18
	Lettuce (head)	330	6	13
	Okra	490	20	29
	Peas (garden)	540	20	71
	Beans, lima	280	17	111
Starchy vegetables	Corn, sweet (yellow)	400	9	91
	Onions (dry)	40	10	38
	Peas (field, southern)	350	17	108
	Potatoes (baked in skin)	Trace	20	93
Other vegetables	Beets	20	6	32
	Cucumbers	250	11	15
	Eggplants	10	3	19
	Pumpkins	1,600	9	26
	Rhubarb	80	6	141
	Summer Squash	440	11	15
	Turnips (roots)	Trace	22	23

[1]Data from the Food Composition Table F-36.
[2]Figures are for amounts of vitamins and calories per 100 g sample of cooked vegetables (unless normally eaten raw). 100 g are equal to about 1/2 cup. Vitamin C values are generally higher if the vegetable is eaten raw; for example, 100 g of cabbage contain 33 mg of vitamin C when cooked, but 47 mg when raw.

Neither Food Composition Table F-36 nor Table V-5 show the bioflavonoid content of the vegetables because this information is not readily available. *Bioflavonoids are vitaminlike substances that have actions similar to those of vitamin C, such as the strengthening of capillary walls against breakage or leakage of fluid.*[6] They might also act as antioxidants,[7] thereby sparing other nutrients that have similar functions or are prone to oxidation, such as selenium and vitamins A, C, and E.

It is noteworthy that bioflavonoids are members of a large family of compounds called flavonoids, which include (1) purple, blue, and red anthocyanin pigments in beets, eggplant, radishes, red cabbage, and red-skinned potatoes; (2) yellow anthoxanthin pigments in cauliflower, onions, and potatoes; and (3) various colorless substances. It is not certain which of the flavonoids act as bioflavonoids. However, broccoli, garlic, green peppers, onions, and tomatoes are believed to be among the richest sources of bioflavonoids.

Effects of Processing and Preparation.   The maximum amounts of essential nutrients are supplied by raw, fresh vegetables that are harvested at just the right stage of maturity. However, many people find some vegetables unappealing when raw, and it is not practical to use only fresh vegetables, which are available only at certain times of the year. Furthermore, raw vegetables contain more undigestible carbohydrates (fiber) than cooked vegetables, and might have a strong laxative effect on people unaccustomed to so much fiber. Therefore, the effects of the various processing and preparation procedures have to be taken into account when planning menus that furnish all of the required nutrients.

NOTE: The information which follows is based on relatively few studies and may not be valid in all cases because (1) different vegetables are affected in different ways; (2) the effects depend partly upon the condition of the vegetables—whether immature or mature, fresh or taken from long storage, whole or in pieces, and untreated or treated; and (3) information is lacking on some of the effects of commonly used procedures. Nevertheless, pertinent information pertaining to nutrient losses in processing and preparation follow:

• **Artificial ripening**—Most commercially grown tomatoes are picked before full maturity in order to avoid excessive softness and oversusceptibility to damage and spoilage. However, one study showed that tomatoes ripened on the vine contained up to one-third more ascorbic acid than those allowed to ripen after picking.[8]

• **Baking**—Various studies of baked Irish potatoes and baked sweet potatoes have shown that baking results in vitamin losses as follows: carotene (provitamin A), 24%; thiamin, 24%; riboflavin, 11%; niacin, 18%; pantothenic acid, 23%; pyridoxine (vitamin B-6), 20%; and ascorbic acid (vitamin C), 20%.[9] Much lower losses of these vitamins were observed when the potatoes were boiled instead of baked.

• **Blanching**—This procedure is used to stop enzyme action in vegetables prior to canning, drying, or freezing. There are considerable losses (up to 80%) of water soluble minerals and vitamins when the vegetables are blanched in boiling water, then cooled by immersion in cold water.[10] Apparently, the nutrients are leached out into the water. These losses may be reduced greatly by (1) blanching with steam instead of boiling water, (2) cooking with air instead of water, or (3) blanching with microwaves. It is noteworthy that the vitamin losses from unblanched vegetables during frozen storage are from 2 to 3 times as great as those from blanched vegetables.

• **Boiling**—The losses of minerals and water-soluble vitamins increase as the amount of cooking water increases. Hence, greater mineral and vitamin retention results in steaming and waterless cooking.

• **Canning**—Blanching, plus the strong heat treatments applied to nonacid vegetables, appears to be responsible for the large vitamin losses in canning, because much less loss occurs in the more mildly processed tomato products. The nutrient losses may be reduced or offset by (1) utilization of newer procedures, such as microwave blanching, and (2) restoration of nutrients lost during processing (enrichment or fortification).

• **Chopping, dicing, grating, mashing, mincing, or slicing**—Any process which breaks many vegetable cells is likely to be responsible for significant losses of certain vitamins. The longer the broken pieces of vegetables are held, the greater the losses. Therefore, vitamins may be conserved by (1) cutting up vegetables just prior to serving, and (2) using a plastic knife for cutting, because metals speed up the destruction of vitamin C.

• **Drying**—Moderate amounts of carotene (provitamin A) and vitamin C may be destroyed in the process, unless the vegetables are sulfured before drying. However, sul-

[6]Kuhnau, J., "The Flavonoids. A Class of Semi-Essential Food Components: Their Role in Human Nutrition," *World Review of Nutrition and Dietetics*, Vol. 24, edited by G. H. Bourne, published by S. Karger, Basel, Switzerland, 1976, p. 175.

[7]Charley, H., "Fruits and Vegetables," *Food Theory and Applications*, edited by P. C. Paul and H. H. Palmer, John Wiley & Sons, Inc., New York, N.Y., 1972, p. 291.

[8]Pantos, C. E., and P. Markakis, "Ascorbic Acid Content of Artificially Ripened Tomatoes," *Journal of Food Science*, Vol. 38, 1973, p. 550.

[9]Lachance, P. A., "Effects of Food Preparation Procedures on Nutrient Retention with Emphasis on Food Service Practices," *Nutritional Evaluation of Food Processing*, 2nd ed., edited by R. S. Harris and E. Karmas, The Avi Publishing Company, Inc., Westport, Conn., 1975, pp. 508-509.

[10]Fennema, O., "Effects of Freeze-Preservation on Nutrients," *Nutritional Evaluation of Food Processing*, 2nd ed., edited by R. S. Harris and E. Karmas, The Avi Publishing Company, Inc., Westport, Conn., 1975, pp. 246-247.

furing destroys most of the thiamin content. Vitamin losses are greater during slow processes, such as sun drying, than they are for more rapid processes like freeze drying.

• **Fermenting and/or pickling**—Pickles, olives, and sauerkraut are the only fermented and pickled vegetables used to any extent in the United States. Vitamin losses in these products may vary widely as a result of factors such as heat developed during fermentation, volume of pickling solution, and temperatures under which the pickles are canned and stored.

• **Freezing**—Most of the losses of vitamins in frozen vegetables occur during blanching, since freezing itself is responsible for only small losses. The vitamin losses during frozen storage may be considerably greater when blanching is omitted prior to freezing. The use of less drastic blanching procedures may help to prevent vitamin losses in frozen vegetables.

• **Frying**—Vitamin losses during the frying of vegetables vary greatly as a result of factors such as (1) time and temperature of frying, (2) type of frying (shallow fat, deep fat, or stir frying), and (3) fat or oil that is used (those which break down during frying may increase the rate of vitamin destruction).

• **Holding on a steam table**—Losses of vitamin C, thiamin, and riboflavin appear to increase with the length of time that vegetables are kept warm on a steam table.

• **Microwave cooking**—The vitamin losses during this procedure are small, and are comparable to those which occur when vegetables are cooked with little or no water.

• **Peeling, scraping, and/or trimming**—Removal of the outer leaves, peels,and/or skins of certain vegetables may result in disproportionately high losses of nutrients because the outer layers are often richer in minerals and vitamins than the inner layers. Therefore, these measures, which are often performed mainly for cosmetic reasons, should be used only to the extent that is absolutely necessary.

• **Pressure cooking**—This method of cooking vegetables results in a greater retention of minerals and vitamins than boiling in a saucepan. However, best results are obtained when the vegetables are placed on a rack above the water so that they are cooked only by steam.

• **Steaming**—Vegetables cooked with steam, but not in contact with water, have better nutrient retention than those cooked in boiling water.

• **Sulfuring**—This process, which consists of either exposing vegetables to fumes from burning sulfur, or dipping them in a sulfite solution, is used to prevent discoloration and spoilage. It is generally utilized before vegetables are to be dried. Sulfuring helps to prevent the losses of both carotene (provitamin A) and vitamin C, but it destroys thiamin. Fortunately, vegetables are utilized more as sources of the first two vitamins, than as a source of thiamin.

VEGETABLES OF THE WORLD. A few dozen or so species of vegetable plants account for most of the world's vegetable production. Pertinent information relative to vegetable crops is presented in Table V-6, Vegetables of the World.

TABLE V-6
VEGETABLES OF THE WORLD

Popular and Scientific Name(s); Origin and History	Importance; Principal Areas; Growing Conditions	Processing; Preparation; Uses	Nutritive Value[1]
Artichoke, Globe— *Cynara scolymus* **Origin and History:** Native to the Mediterranean region. An important crop of ancient Greece and ancient Rome. (Also see ARTICHOKE GLOBE.)	**Importance:** Ranks among the top 2 dozen vegetable crops in the world and in the U.S. About 1.3 milion metric tons are produced worldwide each year. **Principal Areas:** European countries and California. **Growing conditions:** Requires a mild, temperate climate and a fertile well-drained soil. Propagated by suckers from the root crown of the parent plant, which is productive for up to 4 years but is killed by hard frosts.	**Processing:** The flower buds are harvested when they first reach maturity, and while they are still tender. Then, they are graded by size, since the large buds are most favored. The entire buds and the hearts of the buds are sold fresh or canned, and very immature buds are preserved in oil. **Preparation:** Boiled, baked, or fried (after dipping in a batter). Cooked buds may be canned or preserved with spices and oil. **Uses:** Appetizer, vegetable dish. Sometimes the young shoots (suckers) of the plant are blanched and eaten raw.	Caloric content varies considerably because most of the carbohydrate consists of inulin, which is not used by the body. However, inulin is converted to available carbohydrate during storage. Hence, fresh artichokes contain about 9 kcal/100 g, whereas stored ones contain up to 47 kcal/100 g. Moderately high fiber (2.4%). Long thought to have diuretic and laxative effects.[2]

Footnotes at end of table

(Continued)

TABLE V-6 *(Continued)*

Popular and Scientific Name(s); Origin and History	Importance; Principal Areas; Growing Conditions	Processing; Preparation; Uses	Nutritive Value[1]
Asparagus *Asparagus officinalis* **Origin and History:** Originated around the eastern Mediterranean. First used as a medicinal plant. (Also see ASPARAGUS.)	**Importance:** Among the top 2 dozen vegetable crops in the U.S.A., where about 110 thousand metric tons are produced annually. **Principal Areas:** Europe and the U.S.A. **Growing Conditions:** Temperate climate and well-drained soil. Propagated by suckers from the root crown of the parent plant, which may have originally been grown from seed.	**Processing:** The first spears are usually harvested after the root crowns have had 2 years to become established in their bed. During the harvesting season, shoots may be cut every day. The freshly cut spears are washed, bunched, and packed. Much of the crop is canned or frozen. **Preparation:** Poached in water. Usually served with butter, sauce, or in an omelet. Slices may be stir-fried. **Uses:** Vegetable dish, entree (when served with a sauce and chopped hard boiled eggs on toast)	High in water (94%), low in calories (20 kcal per 100 g), and a good source of vitamin A. Also, it is a fair source of thiamin, riboflavin, and niacin. Herbal lore has it that asparagus juice eases the discomforts of arthritis, neuritis, and rheumatism.[2]
Bean, Common (French bean, kidney bean, navy bean, snap bean) *Phaseolus vulgaris* **Origin and History:** Originated in Mexico and in Peru; and domesticated independently in each area from a common wild ancestor. Its cultivation was spread northward and southward by American Indians, and it was taken to Europe and beyond by Spanish explorers. (Also see BEAN, COMMON.)	**Importance:** One of the world's leading vegetable crops. Globally, about 16.3 million metric tons of dried common beans and dried lima beans are produced annually (over 80% of the crop is common beans). **Principal Areas:** India, China, Brazil, and various other countries of Asia, the Americas, Africa, and Europe. **Growing Conditions:** Temperate climate and moderately warm, well-drained soil. Generally, this crop is grown during the warm season in the cooler parts of the temperate zone, and during the cool seasons in the subtropics and tropics (where it is often grown at high altitudes).	**Processing:** May be picked when immature for green pods and seeds (usually called snap beans or green beans), or when mature for seeds only. Fresh immature beans and dried mature beans are marketed fresh, canned, or frozen. **Preparation:** Boiled, baked with pork and/or molasses, or previously boiled beans may be fried (refried beans in Mexico). Fresh green beans may be cooked briefly and served with butter and seasonings. **Uses:** Vegetable dish, and in casseroles, soups, and stews.	3½ oz (*100 g*) of cooked mature beans supply about 118 kcal and about 7 g protein (about as much as 1 oz of lean meat). Beans are also a good source of phosphorus and iron. Immature (green) pods and seeds are high in water content (92%), low in calories (25 kcal per 100 g), and fair sources of vitamins A and C. Mature beans have a mild laxative effect and cause gas pains in some people.
Bean, Lima (butter bean) *Phaseolus lunatus* **Origin and History:** First cultivated in Peru between 7 and 8 thousand years ago. Spread throughout the Americas by the Indians. Brought to Europe and Asia by the Spanish. (Also see LIMA BEAN.)	**Importance:** Among the top 2 dozen vegetable crops in the U.S., where about 112 thousand metric tons are produced annually. **Principal Areas:** Temperate, subtropical, and tropical areas around the world. **Growing Conditions:** Large-seeded types require at least 4 months without frost and a considerable amount of warm weather. Other types tolerate a wider range of temperatures.	**Processing:** May be picked when immature (baby or green limas), or when fully mature. Fresh immature beans and dried mature beans are marketed fresh, canned, or frozen. **Preparation:** Boiled or baked. **Uses:** Vegetable dish, casseroles, soups, stews.	3½ oz (*100 g*) of cooked mature beans supply 138 kcal and about 8 g of protein. Lima beans are also a good source of phosphorus and iron. Immature (baby or green) limas contain more water than the mature beans. Hence, the former supply only about 3/4 as much energy (calories) and protein as the latter.

Footnotes at end of table

TABLE V-6 (Continued)

Popular and Scientific Name(s); Origin and History	Importance; Principal Areas; Growing Conditions	Processing; Preparation; Uses	Nutritive Value[1]
Bean, Mung (golden gram, green gram) *Phaseolus aureus* **Origin and History:** Originated in India. (Also see MUNG BEAN.)	**Importance:** Major food in India. Used mainly for sprouting in China and in U.S. **Principal Areas:** India and Pakistan. **Growing Conditions:** Subtropical or tropical climate.	**Processing:** Picked when fully mature. Sprouted by suppliers of Chinese food in the U.S. **Preparation:** Boiled or sprouted. **Uses:** Cooked beans as a vegetable dish. Sprouts in egg rolls, salads, sandwiches, soups. In Chinese cooking, the sprouts may be stir-fried with green onions and seasoned with soy sauce.	3½ oz (*100 g*) of the raw, sprouted beans supply 35 kcal, 4 g of protein, and 19 mg of vitamin C.
Beet *Beta* spp. **Origin and History:** One of the vegetables derived in pre-Christian times from the wild beet that is native to Europe and Asia. (Also see BEET.)	**Importance:** Among the top 2 dozen vegetable crops in the U.S.A. **Principal Areas:** U.S.A. and European countries. **Growing Conditions:** Temperate climate.	**Processing:** When ripe, they are pulled from the ground by hand or by machine, and the tops are removed. Most of the beet roots are canned or pickled, while the greens are sold fresh. **Preparation:** Roots are usually boiled. Tops may be eaten raw. **Uses:** Roots—vegetable dish, pickles, baby foods, beet soup (Borsch). Greens—ingredient of salads and soups.	High in water content (91%) and low in calories (32 kcal per 100 g). The heavy consumption of beets may lead to the passage of red-colored urine (beeturia), a condition generally regarded as harmless. Beets and beet juice have long been used as herbal remedies for a wide variety of ailments.[2]
Broad bean (fava bean) *Vicia faba* **Origin and History:** Native to northern Africa and the Near East. The Chinese used it for food almost 5,000 years ago. Also, it was cultivated by the Hebrews in Biblical times. (Also see BROAD BEAN.)	**Importance:** One of the leading vegetables grown in the temperate areas of the world. About 4.3 million metric tons are produced annually. **Principal Areas:** China, Egypt, Italy, U.K., Morocco, Spain, Denmark, and Brazil. **Growing Conditions:** Temperate climate. Withstands drought.	**Processing:** Immature pods and seeds may be picked, or mature seeds harvested, shelled, and dried. The dried beans may be sold fresh, canned, or frozen. **Preparation:** Boiled, steamed, or baked. Immature pods may be cooked whole or after slicing. **Uses:** Vegetable dish, ingredient of casseroles, soups, and stews.	Similar in nutritional value to the common bean. Some people have an inherited susceptibility to a hemolytic anemia that may be brought on by the eating of these beans (the condition called favism).

Footnotes at end of table

(Continued)

TABLE V-6 (Continued)

Popular and Scientific Name(s); Origin and History	Importance; Principal Areas; Growing Conditions	Processing; Preparation; Uses	Nutritive Value[1]
Broccoli *Brassica oleracea* **Origin and History:** Developed from the wild cabbage that was native to coastal Europe, which had spread through the Near East to the Orient at an early date. (Also see BROCCOLI.)	**Importance:** Among the top 2 dozen vegetable crops in the U.S.A., where about 556 thousand metric tons are produced annually. **Principal Areas:** U.S.A. and European countries. **Growing Conditions:** Temperate climate. Yield is increased by nitrogenous fertilizer.	**Processing:** The stalks and flower heads are harvested before the flower buds open. A large part of the crop is frozen. **Preparation:** Boiled briefly until tender, but still crisp. May be served with a wide variety of seasonings, dressings, and sauces. **Uses:** Vegetable dish, entree (such as broccoli au gratin with sliced hard boiled eggs on toast).	High in water (91%), low in calories (26 kcal per 100 g), an excellent source of vitamin A, and a good source of protein (3.6%), calcium, and phosphorus.
Brussels Sprouts *Brassica oleracea* **Origin and History:** Believed to have first been developed from wild cabbage sometime around the 15th century in the area that is now Belgium.	**Importance:** Among the top 2 dozen vegetable crops in the U.S.A. **Principal Areas:** U.S.A. and European countries. **Growing Conditions:** Mild, temperate climate. Benefits from nitrogenous fertilizers.	**Processing:** The lower sprouts are usually picked first. Some of the crop is sold fresh, while the rest is frozen. **Preparation:** Boiled briefly until tender, but crisp. May be served with butter or a special sauce. **Uses:** Vegetable dish.	High in water (88%), low in calories (36 kcal per 100 g), a good source of vitamin C and protein (4.9%), and a fair source of vitamin A.
Cabbage *Brassica oleracea capitata* **Origin and History:** May have been used in eastern Asia as early as 8,000 years ago. It is believed that Celtic peoples brought domesticated forms to Europe. (Also see CABBAGE.)	**Importance:** One of the leading vegetable crops of the U.S.A. and of the world, with a worldwide production of about 37 million metric tons annually. **Principal Areas:** China, Japan, Poland, and U.S.A. (Enormous heads grow in Alaska during the summer.) Requires nitrogenous fertilizer.	**Processing:** Early cabbage may be harvested while still immature, but late cabbage is usually allowed to become fully mature. Most of the crop is marketed fresh, fermented into sauerkraut, or made into cole slaw. **Preparation:** Boiled very briefly; stuffed with chopped meats, rice, other vegetables, and seasonings. Raw cabbage may be chopped and added to salads; or stir-fried to make Chinese dishes. **Uses:** Vegetable dish, ingredient of casseroles, salads, soups, and stews.	High in water (94%), low in calories (20 kcal per 100 g), and a good source of vitamin C. (Raw cabbage contains about 50% more vitamin C than cooked cabbage.) It is claimed that cabbage is of value in the prevention and treatment of ulcers and various cancers of the digestive tract.[2]

Footnotes at end of table

(Continued)

TABLE V-6 (Continued)

Popular and Scientific Name(s); Origin and History	Importance; Principal Areas; Growing Conditions	Processing; Preparation; Uses	Nutritive Value[1]
Carrot *Dacus carota* **Origin and History:** Believed to have originated in the Near East and central Asia, where they were cultivated for thousands of years as medicinal plants. Some of the early varieties were black or purple. (Also see CARROT.)	**Importance:** One of the major vegetable crops of the U.S.A and of the world, with a worldwide production of about 14 million metric tons annually. **Principal Areas:** China, U.S.A., and European countries. **Growing Conditions:** Cool, temperate climate. Requires well-drained light soil.	**Processing:** Mature carrots are usually loosened in the soil by a special carrot lifter, then pulled out by hand or machine. Removal of the tops increases keeping qualities. Some of the crop is sold fresh (carrots keep very well in cold storage), while the rest is canned or frozen. **Preparation:** Boiled, fried (usually after dipping in batter). Raw carrots may be shredded or chopped for salads. **Uses:** Vegetable dish, carrot cake, juices, puddings, souffles, salads.	High in water (88%), low in calories (40 kcal per 100 g), and an excellent source of vitamin A. Cooked carrots are more digestible than raw carrots. It is not certain whether the medicinal benefits long attributed to the consumption of carrots and/or carrot juice are due to the vitamin A content or unidentified factors.[2]
Cassava (manioc, yucca) *Manihot esculenta* **Origin and History:** Thought to have originated in eastern Brazil. Taken to Africa in the 16th century by the Portuguese. (Also see CASSAVA.)	**Importance:** The third leading vegetable crop in the world, with an annual production of about 158 million metric tons. **Principal Areas:** Indonesia, Brazil, Nigeria, Zaire, and Tanzania. **Growing Conditions:** Moist, tropical climate. Propagated by stem cuttings inserted in the soil. Very resistant to attack by insects and most plant diseases.	**Processing:** Harvesting is done by (1) cutting the stems about 6 in. *(15 cm)* above the soil, (2) digging to loosen the root, and (3) pulling up the root by the stub of the stem. Many varieties contain toxic cyanides which must be destroyed by boiling, expression of the juice, and/or fermentation. Tapioca is made by gentle heating of cassava starch to cause clumping. Flour or meal may be made from the dried roots. **Preparation:** Roots—boiled, baked; Flour or meal—making of doughs for baking; Tapioca-cooked with milk or water to make puddings. **Uses:** Starchy vegetable, flour, tapioca (puddings, thickenings).	Provides mainly water and starch, plus moderate amounts of fiber and iron. Certain varieties require processing to remove toxic substances.
Cauliflower *Brassica oleracea* **Origin and History:** Native to Asia Minor. Brought to Europe by Italian traders (via Crete and Malta). (Also see CAULIFLOWER.)	**Importance:** Among the top 2 dozen vegetable crops in the world and in the U.S.A. About 5 million metric tons are produced worldwide each year. **Principal Areas:** U.S.A. and European countries. **Growing Conditions:** Cool, moist, temperate climate. Does not tolerate frost or hot weather.	**Processing:** The flower heads are harvested by cutting the stem with a knife. Usually, leaves are left around the heads to protect them from damage during shipping. The crop may be sold fresh, frozen, canned, or pickled. **Preparation:** Boiled, steamed, or served raw in relish trays and salads. **Uses:** Vegetable dish, entree (with cheese sauce on toast).	Low in calories (25 kcal per 100 g) due to its high water content (93%). Good source of vitamin C (Raw cauliflower contains about 50% more of the vitamin than the cooked vegetable, but the latter is more digestible.

Footnotes at end of table

(Continued)

TABLE V-6 *(Continued)*

Popular and Scientific Name(s); Origin and History	Importance; Principal Areas; Growing Conditions	Processing; Preparation; Uses	Nutritive Value[1]
Celeriac (turnip-rooted celery) *Apium graveolens* **Origin and History:** Native to the Mediterranean region. (Also see CELERIAC.)	**Importance:** A minor vegetable that is popular in certain European countries. Little used elsewhere. **Principal Areas:** European countries. **Growing Conditions:** Moist, temperate climate. Plants are started from seed in greenhouses or hotbeds, then transplanted when the weather is suitable for growth in a field.	**Processing:** The plant is harvested by pulling it up when mature. The root is the edible portion. **Preparation:** Steamed, then served whole, diced, or pureed. (Europeans often mix it with hot, mashed potatoes and serve it with butter or a cream sacue.) **Uses:** Vegetable dish; ingredient of salads, soups, and stews.	Low in calories (40 kcal per 100 g) due to its high water content (88%). Also contains about twice as much protein (1.8%) and fiber (1.3%) as ordinary celery.
Celery *Apium graveolens* **Origin and History:** Native to the Mediterranean region. Thought to have been domesticated in either France or Italy. (Also see CELERY.)	**Importance:** One of the top 10 vegetable crops in the U.S.A. where about 891 thousand metric tons are produced annually. **Principal Areas:** U.S.A. and European countries. **Growing Conditions:** Cool, moist, temperate climate. Usually, plants are started from seed in cold frames, greenhouses, or hotbeds. The young plants are transplanted in a field when the weather is sufficiently warm.	**Processing:** The stalks of the growing plant may be blanched (whitened) by covering them with paper or soil. Harvesting, washing, and packing are now highly mechanized in areas where large crops are grown. **Preparation:** Served raw; or baked, boiled, braised, or fried. **Uses:** Vegetable dish; ingredient of salads, soups, and stews. Celery seed is used as a flavoring, but it is rather bitter.	Very high in water content (94%) and low in calories (16 kcal per 100 g). Long believed to help rid the body of excessive water.[2]
Chard; Swiss (seakale beet) *Beta vulgaris* **Origin and History:** One of the vegetables derived in pre-Christian times from the wild beet that is native to the shores of the Mediterranean. (Also see SWISS CHARD.)	**Importance:** A minor, but popular, vegetable in Europe and the U.S. **Principal Areas:** Europe and the U.S. **Growing Conditions:** Temperate climate. May be started from seed in a greenhouse or a hotbed, then transplanted when the danger of hard frost is over.	**Processing:** Leaves may be picked from the plants until fall frost occurs. The leaves, but not the stems, may be frozen for later use. **Preparation:** Served raw; or leaves and stems cooked (usually boiled or fried) separately, since the stems require longer cooking. **Uses:** Vegetable dish; entree (with cheese sauce and hard boiled eggs on toast); ingredient of salads, soups, and mixed dishes (such as chard fried with meat and onions or garlic).	Very high in water (91%) and low in calories (25 kcal per 100 g). A good source of iron and vitamin C, and an excellent source of vitamin A. Has a high oxalic acid content which may reduce the utilization of calcium, iron, and other essential minerals.

Footnotes at end of table

(Continued)

TABLE V-6 *(Continued)*

Popular and Scientific Name(s); Origin and History	Importance; Principal Areas; Growing Conditions	Processing; Preparation; Uses	Nutritive Value[1]
Chayote *Sechium edule* **Origin and History:** Native to southern Mexico and Central America. Spread throughout Caribbean by local Indians. (Also see CHAYOTE.)	**Importance:** A minor, but popular, vegetable in the tropical areas of the New World. **Principal Areas:** Mexico, Central America, and West Indies. **Growing Conditions:** Subtropical or tropical climate (freezing kills the plant); requires large amounts of water.	**Processing:** Usually, the fruits are picked when ripe and used immediately. Some of the fruit may be preserved by pickling. The large tuberous roots may also be harveted for food use. **Preparation:** Boiled, steamed, baked (after stuffing), or dipped in batter and fried. **Uses:** Vegetable dish (served with butter or cream sauce), ingredient in salads, and relish (when pickled).	Resembles squashes in water content (92%) and caloric value (28 kcal per 100 g). However, the mineral and vitamin content of this vegetable is low (it is a fair source of vitamin C).
Chickpea (garbanzo bean) *Cicer arietinum* **Origin and History:** Probably native to Asia Minor. It is suspected that the Aryans brought it westward to the Mediterranean region and eastward to the Indian subcontinent. (Also see CHICKPEA.)	**Importance:** Among the leading vegetable crops of the world, with an annual production of about 7 million metric tons. **Principal Areas:** Over 87% of the crop is grown in India and Pakistan. Most of the rest comes from Mexico, Turkey, and Ethiopia. **Growing Conditions:** Warm season in temperate climate, or cool season in the subtropics and tropics (where it may be grown at high elevations).	**Processing:** After harvesting, the seeds are dehulled and dried. In India, the dried seeds are sometimes ground into a flour. **Preparation:** Boiled, fried, or roasted. **Uses:** Snack, vegetable dish, and ingredient of salads, soups, and stews. In India, the flour is used to make certain confections.	Similar to the various beans in nutritional value. Hence, chickpeas are a good source of calories and protein (100 g or about 1/2 cup of cooked beans supplies about 7 g of protein, the amount in 1 oz of lean meat). They are also a good source of phosphorus and iron.
Chicory *Chicorium intybus* **Origin and History:** Thought to have originated in the Mediterranean region. Certain varieties have been developed as green leafy vegetables, while others have been selected mainly for their roots. (Also see CHICORY.)	**Importance:** A minor, but popular vegetable in various European countries and in the U.S. **Principal Areas:** Europe and the U.S. **Growing Conditions:** Temperate climate. It is often grown in greenhouses or on heated beds in cellars. (Growing in the dark produces light colored leaves).	**Processing:** Blanching (the production of light colored leaves) may be done in the field by tying the outer leaves together around the head of each plant so that light is excluded. The darker outer leaves may be removed after harvesting. Roots may be chopped, roasted until brown, and ground into a powder which resembles finely ground coffee. **Preparation:** Greens—served raw or boiled briefly. Roots—boiled. **Uses:** Greens—vegetable dish, ingredient of salads, soups, and stews. Roots—vegetable dish; extender or substitute for coffee (when roasted).	The leaves are high in water (93%) and low in calories (20 kcal per 100 g). Unblanched (green) chicory is an excellent source of vitamin A, but the blanched forms contain only traces of this vitamin. Sometimes used as a tonic for the digestive system, and to treat disorders of the skin. (In the skin treatment, the juice of the leaves is mixed with a little vinegar and applied externally.)[2]

Footnotes at end of table

(Continued)

TABLE V-6 (*Continued*)

Popular and Scientific Name(s); Origin and History	Importance; Principal Areas; Growing Conditions	Processing; Preparation; Uses	Nutritive Value[1]
Chinese Cabbage *Brassica chinensis and Brassica pekinensis* **Origin and History:** Thought to have originated in Asia Minor and to have been brought to China, where it was developed over thousands of years. (Also see CHINESE CABBAGES.)	**Importance:** Major vegetable crops in eastern Asia, where about one-half of the world's crop of various cabbages is produced. **Principal Areas:** China and Japan. **Growing Conditions:** Cool temperate climate. It is usually grown in southern China during the winter, and elsewhere in China during the fall.	**Processing:** In China, the mature heads are harvested when winter approaches. After removal of loose outer leaves, the heads are stored in a cold cellar. Some of the crop is preserved by pickling. **Preparation:** Boiled briefly, or minced and stir fried with other vegetables, meats, poultry, and/or seafoods. **Uses:** Vegetable dish; ingredient of salads, soups, and various Chinese dishes.	Very high in water (95%) and low in calories (14 kcal per 100 g). Green types are good to excellent sources of vitamin A and fair sources of vitamin C.
Chives *Allium schoenoprasum* **Origin and History:** Native to the temperate zones of Asia and Europe. (Also see CHIVES.)	**Importance:** Commercial production is limited to that utilized by a few processors. Very popular among home gardeners. **Principal Areas:** Temperate zones of Asia, Europe, and North America. **Growing Conditions:** Cool temperate climate. Propagated by bulbs or by seeds.	**Processing:** The long, slender leaves are cut from the plant with a knife. Finely chopped leaves are often frozen. **Preparation:** Chopped and added to various dishes. **Uses:** Decorative flavoring or garnish for cottage cheese, cream cheese, omelets, salads, sandwich fillings, and soups.	Low in calories (28 kcal per 100 g) due to high water content. An excellent source of vitamin A and a fair source of vitamin C.
Collards *Brassica oleracea acephala* **Origin and History:** Believed to have been developed from the primitive leafy, nonheading cabbage of Europe. (Collards and kale are very closely related.) (Also see COLLARDS.)	**Importance:** A minor vegetable crop. **Principal Areas:** Southeastern U.S. **Growing Conditions:** Temperate climate. One of the hardiest of the cabbage vegetables, in that it is quite resistant to cold and heat.	**Processing:** Small, young heads or large, mature heads may be harvested. Much of the crop is chopped and frozen. **Preparation:** Boiled with salt pork; stir-fried chopped greens with bits of bacon and chopped onions. **Uses:** Vegetable dish; ingredient of casseroles, salads, soups, and stews.	Like other greens in high water content (90%) and low caloric content (33 kcal per 100 g), but contains about twice as much protein (about 4%). Also a good source of calcium, an excellent source of vitamin A, and a very good source of vitamin C.

Footnotes at end of table

(Continued)

TABLE V-6 *(Continued)*

Popular and Scientific Name(s); Origin and History	Importance; Principal Areas; Growing Conditions	Processing; Preparation; Uses	Nutritive Value[1]
Corn, Sweet *Zea mays saccharata* **Origin and History:** Probably developed from older varieties of corn indigenous to Mexico and South America. (Also see CORN.)	**Importance:** One of the leading vegetable crops in the U.S., where about 3 million metric tons are produced annually. **Principal Areas:** U.S., and Mexico, and Canada. **Growing Conditions:** Mild temperate climate with a hot, humid summer. Usually requires the application of fertilizers containing nitrogen, phosphorus, and potassium.	**Processing:** Once sweet corn reaches its flavor peak, it must be harvested, husked, and processed rapidly to avoid excessive loss of its sweetness. Hence, the fresh ears cannot be stored for long. Much of the crop is canned and frozen. **Preparation:** Boiled, steamed with husk on but with silk removed, or roasted. **Uses:** Vegetable dish; ingredient of casseroles, fritters, salads, soups, stews, and succotash.	The cooked fresh vegetable has a high water content (77%) and a moderate caloric content (83 kcal per 100 g) and protein content (3.2%). Yellow corn is a fair source of vitamin A.
Cowpea (black-eyed pea) *Vigna unguiculata* **Origin and History:** Native to Central Africa. Brought to the West Indies and the southeastern U.S. by African slaves. Also spread to the Mediterranean, India, and China. (Also see COWPEA.)	**Importance:** A valuable crop in the subtropical and tropical areas of the world. **Principal Areas:** Africa, India, China, West Indies, and southeastern U.S. **Growing Conditions:** Subtropical climate for production of mature beans. Immature pods and seeds may be produced in cool, temperate climates.	**Processing:** Immature pods and seeds are often harvested in China; whereas, mature dried seeds are preferred in the U.S. The former are usually sold fresh or frozen, and the latter as dried, canned, or frozen. **Preparation:** Boiled or baked mature, dried beans. Immature pods and seeds may be chopped and stir fried with meats and other foods. **Uses:** Vegetable dish; entree (when cooked with pork); and ingredient of casseroles, salads, soups, and stews.	3½ oz (*100 g*, or about 2/3 cup) of the cooked, mature beans supply 76 kcal and 5 g of protein. Compared with cooked, mature beans, the cooked immature seeds contain more calories (108 kcal per 100 g), protein (8%), iron (50% more), and vitamins A and C (a fair source of each). While the cooked green pods and seeds are low in both calories (34 kcal per 100 g) and protein (2.6%), they are a very good source of vitamin A and a fair to good source of vitamin C.
Cress *Lepidium sativum* **Origin and History:** Appears to have originated in Western Asia and/or Ethiopia. Cultivated for many centuries in various European countries. (Also see CRESS.)	**Importance:** A minor vegetable crop that is grown mainly by home gardeners. **Principal Areas:** All over the world. **Growing Conditions:** Cool, temperate climate. Seeds germinate quickly when exposed to light.	**Processing:** May be harvested within a few weeks after sowing, and should be picked before the arrival of hot weather, when it quickly goes to seed. **Preparation:** No cooking is required, but it may be added to various hot dishes. **Uses:** Ingredient of salads, sandwiches, and soups.	High in water (89%) and low in calories (32 kcal per 100 g). An excellent source of vitamin A and a good source of vitamin C.

Footnotes at end of table

(Continued)

TABLE V-6 (Continued)

Popular and Scientific Name(s); Origin and History	Importance; Principal Areas; Growing Conditions	Processing; Preparation; Uses	Nutritive Value[1]
Cucumber *Cucumis sativa* **Origin and History:** Believed to be native to southeastern Asia. (Also see CUCUMBER AND GHERKIN.)	**Importance:** A leading vegetable crop with an annual worldwide production of cucumbers and gherkins of about 13 million metric tons. **Principal Areas:** China, Japan, U.S.A., and Poland. **Growing Conditions:** Mild temperate climate.	**Processing:** All of the fruits should be picked before they ripen in order to limit the draining of nutrients from the vine. Much of the crop is made into various types of pickles. **Preparation:** Cooking is not required. However, raw slices may be dipped in batter and fried, or stuffed and baked. **Uses:** Vegetable dish; ingredient of relishes, salads, sandwiches, and soups.	Largely water (95%). Very low in calories (15 kcal per 100 g). An old wives' tale has it that cucumber juice will aid the growth of the hair and nails.[2]
Dandelion *Taraxacum officinale* **Origin and History:** There are many related species native to various parts of the world, including Europe, North Africa, Central Asia, and North America. (Also see DANDELION.)	**Importance:** A very common wild plant or weed that is cultivated on a small scale. **Principal Areas:** U.S. and European countries. **Growing Conditions:** Temperate climate. Plants may be started from seed in a greenhouse, then transplanted in the field when the weather is mild enough.	**Processing:** The leaves should be picked while they are still young and tender (before flowers appear). Roots are harvested by digging up the entire plant. **Preparation:** The leaves need not be cooked, but the roots should be boiled or roasted (roasted roots may be ground to make an extender or substitute for coffee). **Uses:** Greens—vegetable dish, ingredient of salads and soups. Roots—vegetable dish and coffee substitute.	High in water (86%) and low in calories (45 kcal per 100 g). A fair to good source of calcium and iron, and an excellent source of vitamin A. Through the years, dandelion greens have been used by some advocates as a laxative, a tonic for digestion, and to help rid the body of excessive water.[2]
Eggplant (aubergine) *Solanum melongena* **Origin and History:** Believed to have originated in India. However, it may also have been domesticated independently in China. (Also see EGGPLANT.)	**Importance:** Ranks among the top 2 dozen vegetable crops in the world and in the U.S.A. The annual worldwide production is about 5.8 million metric tons. **Principal Areas:** China, Japan, Turkey, Italy, and Egypt. **Growing Conditions:** Warm temperate climate. Requires 5 months of frost-free weather.	**Processing:** The maximum production is brought about by picking the fruits before they reach full size. (Fruit that is between 1/3 and 2/3 full size has the best eating quality.) **Preparation:** Baked or fried (after dipping in a batter). The fruit may also be stuffed with various combinations of bread crumbs, ground meat, cheese, and/or vegetables before being baked. **Uses:** Vegetable dish, entree, ingredient of various mixed dishes.	Contains mainly water (94%) and is low in calories (only 19 kcal per 100 g). However, some Italian cooks press out much of the water so that the resulting product becomes twice as rich in calories and protein as the unpressed vegetable. It is suspected that the unripe fruits may contain high levels of solanine.

Footnotes at end of table

(Continued)

TABLE V-6 (Continued)

Popular and Scientific Name(s); Origin and History	Importance; Principal Areas; Growing Conditions	Processing; Preparation; Uses	Nutritive Value[1]
Endive (escarole) *Cichorium endivia* **Origin and History:** Native to the eastern Mediterranean region. (Also see ENDIVE.)	**Importance:** Among the top 2 dozen vegetable crops in the U.S.A. **Principal Areas:** U.S.A. and European countries. **Growing Conditions:** Mild temperate climate. May be started from seed in a hot-bed or a greenhouse, then transplanted when there is no danger of frost.	**Processing:** The leaves are harvested by cutting them off near the surface of the soil. **Preparation:** May be served raw, stuffed or baked, or tossed in hot bacon drippings or melted butter. **Uses:** Vegetable dish, ingredient of salads and sandwiches.	Similar to other greens in high water content (93%), and low caloric content (20 kcal per 100 g). Also, it is a fair to good source of iron and an excellent source of vitamin A. The bitter flavor is believed to stimulate the flow of digestive juices.[2]
Fennel *Foeniculum vulgare* **Origin and History:** Originated in southern Europe. The variety with the fleshy leaf stalks (Florence fennel) was developed in Italy. (Also see FLORENCE FENNEL.)	**Importance:** A minor vegetable used mainly as a flavoring agent and a medicinal plant. **Principal Areas:** European countries and U.S. **Growing Conditions:** Mild, temperate climate. It is often planted in the summer for harvesting in the fall.	**Processing:** The plant should be pulled from the ground when the leaf stalks are between 3 and 6 in. (8 to 15 cm) long. **Preparation:** Leaves and stalks may be served raw, boiled, or parboiled with butter, cheese, and seasonings. **Uses:** Leaves and stalks—vegetable dish; ingredient of casseroles, salads, soups, and stews. Oil is extracted from the seeds and used as a flavoring agent.	Contains 90% water and 28 kcal per 100 g. An excellent source of vitamin A. Long used as a medicinal plant since it is believed to stimulate the digestive processes. The ancient Greeks believed that it increased the fitness of their athletes.[2]
Garlic *Allium sativm* **Origin and History:** Believed to have originated in central Asia, and to have been brought westward thousands of years ago. The Egyptians used it as early as 3200 B.C. It is also mentioned in the Old Testament. (Also see GARLIC.)	**Importance:** Among the top 2 dozen vegetable crops in the world, and in the U.S. The annual worldwide production is about 2.4 million metric tons. **Principal Areas:** India, Spain, and Egypt. **Growing Conditions:** Requires a temperate climate where there is little or no frost early in the year, when the bulbs are planted.	**Processing:** Garlic is harvested by loosening the bulbs with a cutter bar, then pulling them from the ground. Usually, they are dried in small bunches in windows for 1 or more weeks. Much of the U.S. crop is made into garlic powder and garlic salt. **Preparation:** Raw bulbs are peeled, then minced or crushed, after which they are added to raw salads or cooked with other items. **Uses:** Flavoring for salads, relishes, meat, poultry, seafood, soups, sauces, dressings, and other nonsweet dishes.	Lower in water content (61%) and higher in calories (137 kcal per 100 g) and protein (6%) than many of the other vegetables. Since ancient times, used to prevent or treat a wide variety of ailments.[2] (Recent research has shown it to be a diuretic and a mild germicide, and an aid in preventing blood clots.)

Footnotes at end of table

(Continued)

TABLE V-6 (Continued)

Popular and Scientific Name(s); Origin and History	Importance; Principal Areas; Growing Conditions	Processing; Preparation; Uses	Nutritive Value[1]
Horseradish *Amoracia rusticana* **Origin and History:** Native to eastern Europe.	**Importance:** A minor vegetable crop used mainly as a seasoning agent. **Principal Areas:** Temperate regions around the world. **Growing Conditions:** Temperate climate. Requires a rich, moist, fertile soil. Propagated by root cuttings (usually those that are trimmed from the sides of the main root).	**Processing:** The highest quality horseradish is obtained by stripping the smaller side roots from the main root during the growing period. When the roots are harvested, the leaves and side roots are trimmed off. Fresh horseradish should be grated as soon as possible. **Preparation:** Grated horseradish is usually mixed with vinegar or beet juice, but it may also be mixed with sweet or sour cream. **Uses:** Condiment (one of the 5 bitter herbs of the Jewish Passover).	The raw root has a moderately high water content and caloric content (87 kcal per 100 g). Also, it is a good source of vitamin C. However, the pungent flavor limits the amount which may be eaten. When eaten, the pungency is thought to help clear out congested breathing passages.[2] Used externally as a counter-irritant.
Jerusalem Artichoke *Helianthus tuberosis* **Origin and History:** Native to North America. Taken to France in the 17th century. Spread throughout Europe and Asia. (Also see JERUSALEM ARTICHOKE.)	**Importance:** Grows wild throughout North America, but there is a small cultivated crop called "sun-chokes." **Principal Areas:** U.S. and European countries. **Growing Conditions:** Adapted to a wide variety of conditions in temperate climates. Propagated by pieces of tubers.	**Processing:** The long, woody stems must be cut off before the tubers can be harvested. Sometimes, tubers are left in the soil until needed. **Preparation:** May be served unpeeled, and raw, cooked with other vegetables, pureed and served like mashed potatoes, or fried (after dipping the cooked vegetable in a batter). **Uses:** Vegetable dish and substitute for Irish potatoes.	Composed mainly of water (80%) and carbohydrates (17%). Most of the latter consists of inulin, a substance not utilized by the body. Hence, the caloric value of the fresh vegetable is negligible. However, the inulin is slowly converted into fructose (fruit sugar) when the tubers are left in the ground. This conversion tends to raise the caloric value.
Jicama *Exogonium bracteatum* **Origin and History:** Originated in Mexico. (Also see JICAMA.)	**Importance:** A minor vegetable crop that is much appreciated where it is available. **Principal Areas:** Mexico, California, and China. **Growing Conditions:** Subtropical climate. Requires rich, moist soil. Propagated by tubers.	**Processing:** The tubers are harvested after the vine has flowered by digging around the base of the vine. **Preparation:** Peeled and served raw, or pan fried like potatoes. **Uses:** Appetizer, ingredient of raw salads and other mixed dishes.	High in water content (88%) and low in calories (45 kcal per 100 g) and protein (1.2%).

Footnotes at end of table

(Continued)

TABLE V-6 *(Continued)*

Popular and Scientific Name(s); Origin and History	Importance; Principal Areas; Growing Conditions	Processing; Preparation; Uses	Nutritive Value[1]
Kale *Brassica oleracea acephala* **Origin and History:** Believed to have been developed from the wild cabbage that is native to the Mediterranean region. (Kale and collards are very closely related, except that kale has curly-edged leaves.) (Also see KALE.) 	**Importance:** A minor vegetable crop. **Principal Areas:** U.S. and European countries. **Growing Conditions:** Cool, temperate climate (Kale differs from collards, in that it does not tolerate hot weather.) Requires well-drained fertile soil.	**Processing:** In commercial production, the leaves are harvested by cutting the plant off at soil level with a large knife. Much of the crop is frozen, but some is canned. **Preparation:** Boiled and stir fried (in the preparation of Chinese dishes). Often served with butter or a cheese sauce. **Uses:** Vegetable dish, ingredient of various mixed dishes.	Very similar to collards (to which it is very closely related) in water content (88%), caloric value (39 kcal per 100 g), protein content (about 4%), and vitamin value (an excellent source of vitamin A, and a good source of iron and vitamin C). The eating of moderately large quantities of this vegetable may give some people gas pains.
Kohlrabi *Brassica oleracea caulorapo* **Origin and History:** Developed from wild cabbage by unidentified people of the Mediterranean region in pre-Christian times. (Also see KOHLRABI.) 	**Importance:** A minor vegetable crop which is more appreciated in Europe (especially Germany) than in the U.S. **Principal Areas:** European countries and U.S. **Growing Conditions:** Cool temperate climate. Requires a rich soil, or one to which fertilizer has been added.	**Processing:** Kohlrabi is usually harvested when the swollen stem is 2 to 3 in. *(5 to 8 cm)* in diameter. The root is cut off after harvesting. **Preparation:** May be eaten raw, or after steaming. Eastern European cooks scoop out the center and stuff the hollow with various mixtures of bread crumbs, meat, seasonings, etc. **Uses:** Vegetable dish; ingredient of salads, soups, and stews.	Similar to the other vegetables of the cabbage species in water content (92%), caloric value (24 kcal per 100 g), protein content (2%), and vitamin C content (a good source).
Leek *Allium porrum* **Origin and History:** Native to Central Asia. (Also see LEEK.) 	**Importance:** Grown to a much greater extent in European market gardens than in the U.S. **Principal Areas:** Northwestern European countries. **Growing Conditions:** Temperate climate. May be transplanted from greenhouse or hotbed.	**Processing:** Often blanched (lightened in color) during growth by the banking of soil around the plants. (Some growers wrap the stems with cardboard before piling up the soil.) **Preparation:** Boiled, braised, cooked in mixed dishes similar to those which utilize asparagus, or used raw as relishes. **Uses:** Appetizer; ingredient of quiches, salads, soups, and stews.	Like most other vegetables in water content (85%), caloric value (52 kcal per 100 g), and protein content (2.2%).

Footnotes at end of table

(Continued)

TABLE V-6 (Continued)

Popular and Scientific Name(s); Origin and History	Importance; Principal Areas; Growing Conditions	Processing; Preparation; Uses	Nutritive Value[1]
Lentil *Lens esculenta* **Origin and History:** May have been cultivated as early as 7000 B.C. at various sites in the Near East. (Also see LENTIL[S].)	**Importance:** Among the top 2 dozen vegetable crops of the world. An estimated 2.7 million metric tons are produced annually. **Principal Areas:** India, Syria, Turkey, Ethiopia, U.S.S.R., Spain, Iran, and Bangladesh. **Growing Conditions:** Temperate climate. May be grown during the cool season in the subtropics and the tropics.	**Processing:** Seeds are picked when fully mature. They may or may not be dehulled prior to drying. Sometimes, the dried seeds are ground into a flour. **Preparation:** Boiled or stewed. **Uses:** Vegetable dish; ingredient of casseroles, soups, and stews. Lentil flour may be mixed with one or more cereal flours to make protein-fortified foods for infants and children.	Has a nutritive value that is about the same as the other cooked mature legumes (106 kcal per 100 g and 8% protein). Also, it is a good source of iron.
Lettuce *Lactuca sativa* **Origin and History:** It appears that lettuce was first cultivated by the Egyptians in 4500 B.C. Later, the ancient Greeks and ancient Romans spread it throughout Europe. (Also see LETTUCE.)	**Importance:** One of the leading vegetable crops in the U.S.A., with an annual production of about 3.3 million metric tons. **Principal Areas:** U.S.A., Europe, and Africa. **Growing Conditions:** Cool, temperate climate. (Warm temperatures may cause lettuce to go to seed before it is ready for harvesting.) Requires well-drained, but moist soil. Fertilization with sources of nitrogen, phosphorus and potassium may be needed for certain soils.	**Processing:** Leaf lettuce may be harvested at any time, but head lettuce is usually allowed to develop full size heads. Lettuce that is to be shipped for long distances is crated, vacuum cooled, and loaded into refrigerator railroad cars or trucks. **Preparation:** Washed and served raw in salads; braised; or steamed. **Uses:** Ingredient of salads (lettuce is by far the most commonly used salad green in the U.S.) and soups.	A little higher in water content (95%) and lower in caloric value (about 16 kcal per 100 g) than many of the other leafy vegetables. The vitamin A value increases with the greenness of the leaves (it ranges from a fair to a good source of the vitamin).
Mushroom, Common Cultivated *Agricus bisporus* **Origin and History:** Many of the world's ancient civilizations depicted one or more types of mushrooms in their art. However, it appears that the common cultivated mushroom was first grown commercially in France around 1700. (Also see MUSHROOMS.)	**Importance:** The annual U.S. mushroom crop is 337 thousand metric tons or more. **Principal Areas:** U.S.A. and European countries. **Growing Conditions:** Commercial production usually involves the planting of specially grown spores in a bed of compost inside a growing shed where the temperature and humidity may be controlled.	**Processing:** Young mushrooms are usually plucked from the bed shortly after they have emerged and while they are still in the button stage. Much of the crop is canned, but some is sold fresh. **Preparation:** May be sliced and served raw, stuffed and baked, fried or stewed alone or with other items, or cooked in sauces. **Uses:** Vegetable dish; ingredient of casseroles, quiches, salads, soups, and stews.	High in water content (over 90%) and low in caloric value (around 20 kcal per 100 g). Contains between 2% and 3% protein.

Footnotes at end of table

(Continued)

TABLE V-6 (Continued)

Popular and Scientific Name(s); Origin and History	Importance; Principal Areas; Growing Conditions	Processing; Preparation; Uses	Nutritive Value[1]
Mustard Greens (Indian Mustard) *Brassica juncea* **Origin and History:** Thought to be native to Ethiopia. Used in Egypt for many centuries. Brought to Louisiana from France. (Also seen MUSTARD GREENS.) 	**Importance:** A minor vegetable crop that is much appreciated in the southeastern U.S. **Principal Areas:** Southeastern U.S., central and southern Europe, North Africa, and western Asia. **Growing Conditions:** Temperate climate. Must be planted at the beginning of spring, or in the fall, because high temperatures make the crop go to seed.	**Processing:** Leaves may be harvested anytime from when they emerge to just before the seedstalks develop. Much of the crop is sold fresh. **Preparation:** Boiled with salt pork or stir-fried chopped greens with bits of bacon and chopped onions. **Uses:** Vegetable dish; ingredient of casseroles, salads, soups, and stews.	Has a nutritional value like that of most greens (92% water; 23 kcal per 100 g; and 2% to 3% protein). Also, this vegetable is an excellent source of vitamin C. (Raw mustard greens contain about twice as much vitamin C as cooked greens.)
Okra *Hibiscus esculentus* **Origin and History:** Thought to be native to Ethiopia. Used in Egypt for many centuries. Brought to Louisiana from France. (Also see OKRA.) 	**Importance:** A minor vegetable crop. **Principal Areas:** Southern U.S., Europe, Africa, and Asia. **Growing Conditions:** Warm temperate climate. The fruit develops during the summer.	**Processing:** Continuous harvesting of the young pods insures maximum yield. (Old pods are virtually inedible.) **Preparation:** May be dipped in egg and cornmeal, then fried; boiled or stewed, alone or with other items. **Uses:** Vegetable dish; ingredient of soups and stews.	Contains about 90% water and around 30 kcal per 100 g. A fair source of vitamin A. The mucilaginous material from cooked okra has been used to soothe irritations throughout the digestive tract.[2]
Olive *Olea europaea* **Origin and History:** Originated in the Mediterranean area. The limestone hills of Attica, the Greek peninsula, were the seat of its first cultivation. (Also see OLIVE.) 	**Importance:** One of the world's leading crops. About 9.2 million metric tons of olives and 1.8 million metric tons of olive oil are produced annually. **Principal Areas:** Greece, Spain, and Italy. **Growing Conditions:** Subtropical or tropical climate. The tree is propagated by grafting cuttings onto seedlings.	**Processing:** In some areas, the fruit is knocked down from the tree by mechanical shakers onto cloths spread on the ground. Table olives require long soaking in a weak salt solution to remove a bitter component. **Preparation:** Processed olives are ready to eat. **Uses:** Relish; ingredient of salads and other mixed dishes such as pizza.	The oil content (ranges from 13% to 36%) contributes calories (from 93 to 338 kcal per 100 g) and monounsaturated fats that are less susceptible to rancidity than the polyundaturated fats. Some products may have a high sodium content (as much as 3300 mg per 100 g).

Footnotes at end of table

(Continued)

TABLE V-6 (Continued)

Popular and Scientific Name(s); Origin and History	Importance; Principal Areas; Growing Conditions	Processing; Preparation; Uses	Nutritive Value[1]
Onion *Allium cepa* **Origin and History:** Native to Central Asia, where it has been used for thousands of years. (Also see ONION.) 	**Importance**: A leading vegetable crop in the world and in the U.S.A. The annual world-wide production of dry onions is about 28 million metric tons per year. **Principal Areas:** China, India, U.S.A., Japan, and the European countries. **Growing Conditions:** Cool, temperate climate. Propagated by seeds or by sets (small bulbs).	**Processing:** The bulbs are usually harvested when the tops start to turn yellow and fall over. Usually, the fresh onions are dried right after harvesting. Much of the crop is sold fresh (dried), while the rest is frozen and canned. **Preparation:** Served raw in salads; or baked, boiled, or fried—alone or with other items. **Uses:** Vegetable dish; ingredient of casseroles, quiches, salads, soups, and stews.	Contains mainly water (about 90%), but few calories (30 or so per 100 g). Through the ages, used as a mild disinfectant in wounds and to drive parasites from the digestive tract. Recent research has shown that onions may help to prevent excessive clotting of the blood.[2]
Parsley *Petroselinum crispum* **Origin and History:** Originated in the Mediterranean area. (Also see PARSLEY.) 	**Importance**: A minor vegetable crop. **Principal Areas:** European countries and U.S. **Growing Conditions:** Cool, temperate climate. However, the seeds need warmth to germinate. Hence, it is often transplanted from greenhouses and hotbeds.	**Processing:** Usually, the outer leaves of the plant are harvested when large enough. Some of the crop may be dried, and some is sold fresh. **Preparation:** Served raw, stir fried with other items or boiled briefly in mixed dishes. **Uses:** Ingredient of casseroles, quiches, relishes, salads, soups, and stews.	Similar to other greens in nutritional value (85% water; 44 kcal per 100 g), and an excellent source of vitamin A. However, parsley surpasses most of the other green, leafy vegetables in protein content (almost 4%), calcium, iron, and vitamin C.
Parsnip *Pastinaca sativa* **Origin and History:** Believed to be native to the Mediterranean area, where it was cultivated by the ancient Greeks and Romans. (Also see PARSNIP.) 	**Importance**: A minor vegetable crop. **Principal Areas:** European countries and U.S. **Growing Conditions:** Requires a rich, moist soil, that does not pack down too readily. Usually planted in the early spring.	**Processing:** Harvested in the late fall by digging carefully with a spading fork, and/or loosening them by plowing the ground around them. Eating quality is improved by storage at 34° F (1° C) for 2 weeks. **Preparation:** Parboiled or steamed. Cooked parsnips may be mashed, formed into cakes, and fried. **Uses:** Vegetable dish; ingredient of soups and stews.	A typical root vegetable in water content (82%), and caloric value (66 kcal per 100 g).

Footnotes at end of table

(Continued)

TABLE V-6 (*Continued*)

Popular and Scientific Name(s); Origin and History	Importance; Principal Areas; Growing Conditions	Processing; Preparation; Uses	Nutritive Value[1]
Pea, Garden (English pea, green pea) *Pisum sativum* **Origin and History:** Thought to have originated in Central Asia and Europe, with possibly secondary developments in the Near East and North Africa. It appears that the Chinese were the first to eat the immature pods and seeds. Later, Louis XIV popularized the eating of green peas in France. (Also see PEA, GARDEN.)	**Importance:** Accounts for the greater part of the worldwide production of all types of peas, for which there is an annual production of about 4.8 million metric tons. **Principal Areas:** The U.S.A. and the U.K. are the two top producers of the garden pea. **Growing Conditions:** Cool, temperate climate. Usually planted in the early spring, or in the winter in areas with mild climates.	**Processing:** Usually picked when immature by special machines called viners. The green pods and seeds may be marketed fresh, frozen, or cooked and canned. Mature seeds are usually dried whole or after splitting. **Preparation:** Boiled briefly (immature pods and seeds), pressure cooked (dried mature seeds). **Uses:** Vegetable dish; ingredient of casseroles, soups, and stews.	Cooked mature peas are similar in nutritive value to the various types of mature beans (70% water, 115 kcal per 100 g, and 8% protein). In comparison with mature peas, cooked immature (green) peas contain more water (82%) and fewer calories (71 kcal per 100 g) and less protein (5%). However, they are a better source of vitamins A and C.
Pepper, Chili *Capsicum frutescens* **Origin and History:** Native to Central America and South America. (Also see PEPPERS.)	**Importance:** Together, chili peppers and sweet peppers (which are closely related) rank among the top 2 dozen vegetables of the world, with an annual production of about 9 million metric tons. **Principal Areas:** India, Thailand, African countries, and Spain. **Growing Conditions:** Tropical climate.	**Processing:** Usually harvested when ripe, then dried in the sun. Marketed as dried, canned, or pickled. **Preparation:** Minced and added to various cold or hot dishes. **Uses:** Seasoning; appetizer; vegetable dish; and ingredient of casseroles, pizza, salads, sandwiches, soups, and stews.	The immature (green) chilis which contain about 89% water and 37 kcal per 100 g, are fair sources of vitamin A and excellent sources of vitamin C. Mature (red) chilis which contain about (80%) water and 65 kcal per 100 g, are exceptionally rich in vitamin A (21,600 IU per 100 g) and supply about 50% more vitamin C than green chilis.
Pepper, Sweet *Capsicum annum* **Origin and History:** Native to Central America and South America. (Also see PEPPERS.)	**Importance:** The annual worldwide production of both sweet peppers and chili peppers is about 9 million metric tons. **Principal Areas:** China, European countries, North America, and South America. **Growing Conditions:** Requires hot summers, and is killed by frost.	**Processing:** Often picked while still green. However, some fruits are left on the plant until they have ripened fully and have turned red, orange, or yellow. **Preparation:** Chopped and served raw in salads; fried; or stuffed with bread crumbs, chopped meat, rice, spices, and baked. **Uses:** Entrees (when stuffed and baked); vegetable dishes, and ingredient of casseroles, salads, sandwiches, soups, and stews.	The immature (green) and the mature (red) peppers contain 91 to 94% water, and about 20 to 30 kcal per 100 g. However, red peppers contain about ten times as much vitamin A and twice as much vitamin C as green peppers.

Footnotes at end of table

(Continued)

TABLE V-6 (*Continued*)

Popular and Scientific Name(s); Origin and History	Importance; Principal Areas; Growing Conditions	Processing; Preparation; Uses	Nutritive Value[1]
Potato (Irish Potato) *Solanum tuberosum* **Origin and History:** Native to the mountainous areas near the west coast of South America. (Also see POTATO.)	**Importance:** One of the leading vegetable crops in the world and in the U.S. About 284 million metric tons are produced worldwide each year. **Principal Areas:** Soviet Union, China, and Poland. **Growing Conditions:** Cool, temperate climate. Grown at high altitudes in subtropical and tropical areas. The size of the tubers increases with the light received by the plant.	**Processing:** The crop must be harvested before hard freezes occur. Usually, the potatoes are dug with a combination digger and combine. A large part of the crop is stored under cool, humid conditions, while the rest is canned, dehydrated, or frozen. **Preparation:** Baked, boiled, fried, roasted, or stewed. **Uses:** Vegetable dish; ingredient of casseroles, salads, soups, and stews.	Boiled potatoes contain about 80% water, 76 kcal per 100 g, and 2% protein. They are also fair sources of vitamin C. It is noteworthy that the protein-to-calorie ratio of potatoes is such that if sufficient amounts of the vegetable are consumed, both the protein and calorie requirements may be met. (Most adults would have to eat about 4½ lb of potatoes per day to meet their requirements.)
Pumpkin *Cucurbita maxima, C. mixta, C. moschata, and C. pepo* **Origin and History:** Most species are believed to have originated in Mexico and Central America. (Also see PUMPKIN.)	**Importance:** Pumpkins, squashes, and related gourds rank among the top 2 dozen vegetables of the world, with an annual production of about 6.8 million metric tons. **Principal Areas:** Yugoslavia, China, Romania, Egypt, Italy, Turkey, and the Americas. **Growing Conditions:** Cool, temperate climate. Usually planted in the spring after the soil has warmed up and there is no danger of frost.	**Processing:** Harvested when fully mature by cutting from the vine, following which they are usually left in piles in the fields for a week or two to harden the shell. Some of the crop may be stored for up to several months, while the rest may be canned. **Preparation:** Cooked as a vegetable or baked in a pie. **Uses:** Vegetable dish; ingredient of pumpkin cakes, custards, and pies.	Similar in nutritive value to most other squashes (92% water, 26 kcal per 100 g, 1% protein, and a good to excellent source of vitamin A).
Radish *Raphanus sativus* **Origin and History:** Believed to have originated in western Asia. Cultivated by the Babylonians and the Egyptians 4,000 years ago. (Also see RADISH.)	**Importance:** A minor, but popular, vegetable. Often grown in home gardens and kept for family use. **Principal Areas:** Temperate and sub-tropical areas of the world. **Growing Conditions:** Requires warm, light, well-drained soils that are highly fertile.	**Processing:** The roots are harvested when they reach marketable size. (Those left in the ground too long become pithy.) Winter varieties may be stored for several months, but other types are usually marketed as they become available. **Preparation:** Served raw in salads, or steamed with other ingredients and seasonings. **Uses:** Appetizer; ingredient of mixed vegetable dishes, relishes, and salads.	High in water (94%) and low in calories (17 kcal per 100 g) and protein (1%). Long used to stimulate digestive processes and to help rid the body of excessive water.[2]

Footnotes at end of table

(*Continued*)

TABLE V-6 (*Continued*)

Popular and Scientific Name(s); Origin and History	Importance; Principal Areas; Growing Conditions	Processing; Preparation; Uses	Nutritive Value[1]
Rutabaga (Swede) *Brassica napobrassica* **Origin and History:** A hybrid of grape and the turnip, which originated in Europe in the Middle Ages. (Also see RUTABAGA.)	**Importance:** A minor vegetable for human consumption, but an important feed and forage crop for livestock. **Principal Areas:** Europe and North America. **Growing Conditions:** Cool, temperate climate. Low temperatures make the plant go to seed.	**Processing:** Usually, the roots are harvested in the fall by pulling them up by hand. Then some of the crop is stored in a cold, damp environment. The roots keep better if they are covered with a thin layer of wax before storage. **Preparation:** Boiled and mashed, or cooked with other items in mixed dishes. **Uses:** Vegetable dish; ingredient of soups and stews; and feed for livestock.	Similar in nutritive value to other root vegetables (90% water, 35 kcal per 100 g, and 1% protein). It is noteworthy that a mashed mixture of rutabaga and potatoes is lower in calories than mashed potatoes alone.
Salsify (Oysterplant) *Tragopogon porrifolius* **Origin and History:** Native to the Mediterranean countries. (Also see SALSIFY.)	**Importance:** A minor vegetable crop. **Principal Areas:** Soviet Union and other European countries. **Growing Conditions:** Temperate climate. Requires a well-drained, crumbly soil.	**Processing:** Roots may be harvested in the fall and winter. Some of the crop is usually stored. **Preparation:** Boiled; sauteed (after breading); served raw; or roasted to make a coffee substitute. **Uses:** Vegetable dish; ingredient of salads, soups, and stews; and low-carbohydrate substitute for starchy vegetables. (Most of the carbohydrate in salsify is inulin, which is not metabolized by the body.)	Very similar to the Jerusalem artichoke in water content (78%) and carbohydrates (18%). Most of the latter consists of inulin, a substance not utilized by the body. Hence, the caloric value of the fresh vegetable is negligible. However, the caloric value increases when some of the inulin is converted into fructose after long storage of the roots in the ground.
Shallot *Allium cepa* **Origin and History:** Believed to have originated in Central Asia as a modification of the ordinary type of onion. (Onions produce larger and fewer bulbs.) (Also see SHALLOT.)	**Importance:** Of little commercial importance. Grown mainly in home gardens. **Principal Areas:** European countries and the U.S. **Growing Conditions:** Temperate climate. Grown in the winter for green onions, and in the summer for dry, mature onions.	**Processing:** Usually harvested from late fall to early spring. The "green onions" are trimmed and skinned, whereas the dry bulbs are treated like ordinary onions. **Preparation:** Chopped and served raw; sauteed; or boiled. **Uses:** Appetizer; ingredient of relishes, salads, and soups.	Like other members of the onion family in water content (80%) and caloric value (72 kcal per 100 g).

Footnotes at end of table

(*Continued*)

TABLE V-6 (Continued)

Popular and Scientific Name(s); Origin and History	Importance; Principal Areas; Growing Conditions	Processing; Preparation; Uses	Nutritive Value[1]
Sorrel (Dock) *Rumex acetosa* **Origin and History:** Native to Asia and Europe. Cultivated in France and Italy since the 14th century. (Also see SORRELS.)	**Importance:** A minor vegetable crop. **Principal Areas:** North America, Europe, and Asia. **Growing Conditions:** Temperate climate. Requires rich, moist soil and abundant sunshine.	**Processing:** Flowering shoots are cut off as they appear in order to encourage leaf development. Leaves and stems may be harvested as desired. Sometimes the leaves are dried for storage. **Preparation:** Served raw, or boiled briefly. **Uses:** Seasoning; and ingredient of casseroles, salads, soups, and other mixed dishes.	Similar in nutritional value to other green leafy vegetables (91% water, 28 kcal per 100 g, 2% protein, an excellent source of vitamin A, and a good source of vitamin C).
Soybean *Glycine max* **Origin and History:** Native to northeast China where it has been used for at least 3,000 years. Brought to the U.S. from Europe in the 19th century. It became a very important American crop in the 20th century. (Also see SOYBEAN.)	**Importance:** One of the world's leading legume and vegetable crops with an annual production of about 108 million metric tons. Rarely used as a vegetable in the U.S.A., although much of the crop comes from this country. **Principal Areas:** U.S.A., China, and Brazil. **Growing Conditions:** Temperate climate. Requires warm weather for high yields. Susceptible to damage by frost.	**Processing:** May be picked while still immature or when fully mature. Immature seeds may be sold fresh or canned. Mature seeds may be roasted and salted like peanuts. Oil is extracted from much of the American crop. **Preparation:** Boiled immature or mature seeds. The latter require soaking and cooking to eliminate various harmful substances. Asians often ferment soybean cakes. **Uses:** Vegetable dish; entree; protein supplement; and ingredient of baked goods, casseroles, meat substitutes, salads, soups, and stews.	Cooked mature soybeans exceed the nutritional values of the other types of beans in caloric value (130 kcal per 100 g) and protein content (11%). Cooked immature soybeans contain fewer calories (118 kcal per 100 g) and less protein (10%), but are fair sources of vitamin A and C.
Spinach *Spinacia oleracea* **Origin and History:** Native to southwestern Asia (believed to have originated in Persia). (Also see SPINACH.)	**Importance:** One of the top 2 dozen vegetable crops grown in the U.S., with an annual production of about 175 thousand metric tons. **Principal Areas:** U.S. and European countries. **Growing Conditions:** Cool, temperate climate (goes to seed readily in hot weather).	**Processing:** Leaves may be harvested as soon as they are large enough. Much of the crop is canned and frozen. **Preparation:** Cooked briefly in as little water as possible; served raw in salads; baked in casseroles and quiches. **Uses:** Vegetable dish; main dish (when served with chopped eggs and/or a cheese sauce on toast); and ingredient of casseroles, quiches, salads, and soups.	Like other greens in water content (91%), caloric value (26 kcal per 100 g), protein content (3%), and vitamins (an excellent source of vitamin A and a fair to good source of vitamin C). Also, it contains about twice as much iron as other greens.

Footnotes at end of table

(Continued)

TABLE V-6 (*Continued*)

Popular and Scientific Name(s); Origin and History	Importance; Principal Areas; Growing Conditions	Processing; Preparation; Uses	Nutritive Value[1]
Squash, Summer *Cucurbita pepo* **Origin and History:** Appears to have originated in Mexico and Guatemala, and to have spread throughout North America before the European explorers arrived. (Also see SQUASHES.)	**Importance:** Together, pumpkins, squashes, and related gourds rank among the top 2 dozen vegetable crops of the world, with an annual production of about 6.8 million metric tons. **Principal Areas:** Yugoslavia, China, Romania, Egypt, Italy, Turkey, and the Americas. **Growing Conditions:** Temperate climate. Requires warm, well-drained soil.	**Processing:** The immature squashes are picked before the rinds have hardened. Summer squashes do not keep as well as winter squashes. Hence, the former are usually sold fresh, canned, or frozen. **Preparation:** Baked; boiled; or fried (after dipping in beaten egg and flour). **Uses:** Vegetable dish; main dish (after stuffing with bread crumbs, cheese, meat, and/or seasonings); ingredient of casseroles, and other mixed dishes.	Differs from pumpkins and winter squashes in containing more water (94%), but lesser amounts of food energy (around 20 kcal per 100 g), protein (1%) and vitamin A (only a fair source).
Squash, Winter *Cucurbita maxima, C. mixta, C. moschata,* and *C. pepo* **Origin and History:** Most species are believed to have originated in Mexico and Central America.	**Importance:** Pumpkins, squashes, and related gourds rank among the top 2 dozen vegetables of the world, with an annual production of about 6.8 million metric tons. **Principal Areas:** Yugoslavia, China, Romania, Egypt, Italy, Turkey, and the Americas. **Growing Conditions:** Cool, temperate climate. Usually planted in the spring after the soil has warmed up and there is no danger of frost.	**Processing:** Harvested only when fully ripe. Then, they may be left in small piles in the field for a week or two to harden the shell. Some of the crop may be stored for up to several months, and some may be canned or frozen. **Preparation:** Baked or broiled. **Uses:** Vegetable dish; may be used instead of pumpkin to make custards and pies.	The different varieties, when boiled and mashed, have an average composition of 90% water, 40 kcal per 100 g, and 1% protein. A deep orange or yellow color indicates the types which are excellent sources of vitamin A.
Sweet Potato *Ipomoea batatas* **Origin and History:** Appears to have originated in Mexico, Central America, and South America. (Also see SWEET POTATO.)	**Importance:** One of the leading vegetable crops of the world, with an annual production of about 132 million metric tons. **Principal Areas:** China (produces about 85% of the world's crop), and other countries in Asia, Africa, and the Americas. **Growing Conditions:** Warm, temperate to tropical climate.	**Processing:** Although immature roots may be harvested, only the mature ones are suitable for storage. Those to be stored are usually cured in the sun to toughen the skin and to heal wounds. Much of the crop is canned. **Preparation:** Baked, boiled, or fried. Cooked, mashed sweet potatoes may be baked into biscuits, bread, cakes, and pies. **Uses:** Vegetable dish; ingredient of baked goods, casseroles, and other mixed dishes.	The uncandied cooked vegetable contains about 70% water, 125 kcal per 100 g, and 2% protein. It is also an excellent source of vitamin A and a fair source of vitamin C.

Footnotes at end of table

(*Continued*)

TABLE V-6 (*Continued*)

Popular and Scientific Name(s); Origin and History	Importance; Principal Areas; Growing Conditions	Processing; Preparation; Uses	Nutritive Value[1]
Taro *Colocasia esculenta* **Origin and History:** Native to southeastern Asia. Spread throughout the Pacific Basin by the ancestors of the Polynesians. (Also see TARO.)	**Importance:** Among the leading tuberous plants grown and consumed in the tropics. **Principal Areas:** Moist, tropical areas around the world. **Growing Conditions:** Warm, moist climate. Requires a highly fertile soil.	**Processing:** Harvested after the leaves begin to turn yellow. Small tubers may be stored more successfully than large ones. **Preparation:** Baked, boiled, or fried (like potato chips). **Uses:** Starchy vegetable; used to make "poi" in Hawaii.	Taro tubers are similar in nutritional value to other root and tuber vegetables (73% water, 98 kcal per 100 g, and 2% protein).
Tomato *Lycopersicon esculentum* **Origin and History:** Originated in South America and spread as a weed to Mexico, where it was first domesticated. (Also see TOMATO.)	**Importance:** One of the leading vegetable crops in the world, and in the U.S.A. The annual worldwide production is about 69 million metric tons. **Principal Areas:** U.S.A., U.S.S.R., China, Italy, Turkey, Egypt, and Spain. **Growing Conditions:** Temperate to tropical climate. Requires more than 3 months without frost, but also needs night temperatures around 59°F (*15°C*) for development of fruits.	**Processing:** Much of the crop is picked when mature, but still green. Then, the fruits may be ripened in special rooms under controlled temperature and humidity. Some of the crop is sold fresh, while the rest is canned or made into other products. **Preparation:** Served raw in salads; broiled; stewed; stuffed and baked; or cooked in sauces. **Uses:** Vegetable dish; ingredient of catsup, juices, relishes, salads, soups, stews, and other mixed dishes.	Cooked ripe tomatoes are high in water content (93%), low in calories (22 kcal per 100 g) and in protein (1%). Also, they are a good source of vitamin A and a fair source of vitamin C.
Turnip *Brassica rapa* **Origin and History:** One type is native to Europe, while another is native to central Asia. (Also see TURNIP.)	**Importance:** A minor vegetable crop that is more important in Europe than in the U.S. **Principal Areas:** European countries. **Growing Conditions:** Cool, temperate climate. Grows best during the spring and early fall since it does not do well in hot weather.	**Processing:** The roots are harvested before they become tough and fibrous. Dipping the roots in hot paraffin lengthens the time they may be stored without deterioration. **Preparation:** Boiled and mashed, or cooked with other items in mixed dishes. **Uses:** Vegetable dish; ingredient of salads, soups, and stews; and feed for livestock.	Cooked turnip roots have a high water content (94%) and are low in calories (23 kcal per 100 g) and protein (1%). They are a fair source of vitamin C. Compared to the roots, the cooked greens contain about the same amounts of water and calories, but twice as much protein, iron, and vitamin C, and many times as much vitamin A (of which they are an excellent source).

Footnotes at end of table

(*Continued*)

TABLE V-6 (*Continued*)

Popular and Scientific Name(s); Origin and History	Importance; Principal Areas; Growing Conditions	Processing; Preparation; Uses	Nutritive Value[1]
Waterchestnut, Chinese (Ma-tai, Pi-tsi) *Elocharis tuberosa,* and *Elocharis dulcis* **Origin and History:** Native to southern China. (Also see WATERCHESTNUT.)	**Importance:** Minor, but much appreciated vegetable. **Principal Areas:** China, Japan, and East Indies. **Growing Conditions:** Temperate climate. Grows wild in shallow water near the shores of lakes, and in marshes. Cultivated in China (grown in rice paddies).	**Processing:** The corms are dug from the mud by hand after the rice paddies have been drained. Starch may be extracted from the grated corms. **Preparation:** Boiled briefly (after peeling). **Uses:** Ingredient of mixed Oriental dishes, salads, and soups.	Has a nutritional value like that of the other tuberous vegetables (78% water, 79 kcal per 100 g, and 1.4% protein).
Watercress *Nasturtium officinale* **Origin and History:** Appears to be a cross (hybrid) between plants native to western Asia and Europe. Used as a medicinal plant since the 1st century. (Also see WATERCRESS.)	**Importance:** Minor crop, which also grows wild. **Principal Areas:** Germany, France, and the United Kingdom. **Growing Conditions:** Temperate climate. Requires an abundant supply of running water which is alkaline and contains nitrates.	**Processing:** Usually cultivated and harvested by hand. **Preparation:** Served raw in salads, or cooked with other vegetables to add flavor. **Uses:** Ingredient of salads, sandwiches, and soups.	Very similar to other greens in nutrient composition (93% water, 19 kcal per 100 g, and 2.2% protein). A good source of calcium, iron, and vitamin C, and an excellent source of vitamin A. Herbal remedy for minor disorders (lack of appetite, mild depression, and waterlogging).[2]
Yam (Asiatic Yam) *Dioscorea alata* **Origin and History:** Originated in southeast Asia and in Africa. (Also see YAM.)	**Importance:** Worldwide production of yams is about 29 million metric tons per year. **Principal Areas:** Moist, tropical areas of Asia, Africa, and the Americas. **Growing Conditions:** Warm, moist climate. Do not grow well below 68°F (20°C). Require fertile soils and at least 40 in. (*250 cm*) of rainfall during the 8 months growing season.	**Processing:** Usually cultivated and harvested by hand. In some parts of the world the newly harvested tubers are stored on special racks in the shade. Some of the crop is made into flour, which stores better than the whole tubers. **Preparation:** Baked; boiled and mashed; or fried (after slicing). **Uses:** Staple food, starchy vegetable, and ingredient of soups and stews.	Somewhat like the potato in nutritional value (74% water, 101 kcal per 100 g, and 2.1% protein).

[1]See Food Composition Table F-36 for additional details.
[2]No medical claims are made for any of the vegetables listed in this table. The various beliefs regarding the beneficial effects of certain items are presented (1) for historical and informational purposes, and/or (2) to stimulate further investigation of the claimed merits.

VEGETABLE BUTTERS

Due to their fatty acid composition, the lipids extracted from some plants are solid—fats—at room temperature and, hence, exhibit the consistency of butter and even the yellow color. Most lipids extracted from plants are liquids—oils—at room temperature. Two familiar vegetable butters are cocoa butter and coconut butter.

• **Cocoa butter**—The fat pressed from the roasted cacao bean is known as cocoa butter. It is yellow and possesses a slight chocolate smell and flavor. Cocoa butter is mainly used in drugs and cosmetics. As a food it is pleasant to the taste and easily digestible.

• **Coconut butter**—This is derived by pressing the dried coconut meats or copra, and then after bleaching and various other processes the oil is transformed into a product of firm consistency that looks like butter. Coconut butter is common in France.

Other less known vegetable butters include Shea butter from the African plant *Butyrospermum parkii*, Mowrah fat or illipe butter from the Indian plant *Bassia longifolia*, and nutmeg butter. By broadening the definition of butter to include foods that are spread like butter, peanut butter, hazelnut butter, and walnut butter are included as vegetable butters.

VEGETABLE MARROW

This is a variety of summer squash. It can (1) be cylindrical or oval in shape, (2) have a smooth skin, and (3) be white to dark green or mottled in color.
(Also see SQUASHES.)

VEGETABLE OILS

These oils are pressed or extracted from a variety of plant seeds. Of primary importance as sources of edible oil on a world basis are soybeans, cottonseed, peanuts, corn germ, olives, coconut, rapeseed, sesame, sunflower, safflower, cocoa beans, and various oil palms.
(Also see OILS, VEGETABLE; and FATS AND OTHER LIPIDS, section headed "Animal and Vegetable.")

VEGETARIAN DIETS

In its purest form, a vegetarian diet consists of only foods of plant origin—no meat, fish, or other animal products are allowed. Most vegetarian diets allow vegetables, fruits, cereals and breads (often whole grain), yeast, dry beans, peas and lentils, nuts and peanut butter, seeds, vegetable oils, sugars and syrups, and possibly some rather unusual foods. Often a vegetarian diet is assumed to mean only no meat in the diet. For some types of vegetarianism this may be true.

TYPES OF VEGETARIANS. Persons following vegetarian patterns fall into one of the four basic types of vegetarianism.

1. *Ovolactovegetarians.* These individuals consume a diet of plant origin supplemented with milk, milk products, and eggs.

2. *Lactovegetarians.* These individuals eat a diet of plant origin supplemented with milk and milk products only.

3. *Pure vegetarians or vegans.* These individuals eat all foods of plant origin, and no animal-originating foods, dairy products, or eggs. In addition, the term vegan may embody a philosophy which discourages the use of anything that even indirectly requires the taking of animal life.

4. *Fruitarians.* These individuals consume diets consisting of raw or dried fruits, nuts, honey, and olive oil. Some may supplement with grains and legumes.

Each type of vegetarianism may run some risk of dietary inadequacy—some more so than others.

PREVALENCE OF VEGETARIANISM. The practice of vegetarianism is not new. Throughout history there have been various individuals, groups or cults that have subscribed to a vegetarian diet. Of the five major religions of the world—Christianity, Judaism, Islam, Hinduism, and Buddhism—all place restrictions on some food of animal origin. Because of the belief in the transmigration of souls, the preservation of animal life is a basic tenet of Hinduism, Brahmanism, Buddhism, and Jainism.

Buddhism developed in India during the 6th century B.C. Buddha stressed a kinship between all forms of life and taught that no creature should be killed. Buddhism gradually spread into China and Japan.

Among the Greeks, the mathematician Pythagoras is generally considered the founder of the vegetarian movement in the 6th century B.C.

Among the Christian religions, there have been many advocators of vegetarianism. Plutarch of Chaironeia (46-120 A.D.) encouraged people not to kill for gluttony. Then, about a century later, Porphyry (223-304 A.D.) wrote on abstaining from animal foods. Just before the fall of the Roman Empire, Clement of Alexandria, a church father, discouraged flesh-eating. During the Dark Ages, the vegetarian way of life virtually disappeared, except in some orders of the Catholic church, such as the Cistercian monks. With the Renaissance, the ancient teachings of vegetarianism were restudied and new concepts developed which led to the development of modern vegetarianism. Luigo Cornaro (1467-1566 A.D.) encouraged moderation in the diet. The idea of friendliness to animals for humane reasons was championed by Michel of Montaigne who lived between 1533 and 1592 A.D. Famous persons such as Milton, Pope, Voltaire, Rousseau, Linnaeus, and Cuvier encouraged a return to nature. Also, during this time the Pythagorian way of life was promoted.

The spread of vegetarianism into the Western World began in 1809 in Manchester, England when members of the Bible Christian Church under the leadership of William Cowherd pledged to abstain from alcoholic drinks and flesh foods. Also, in 1809, a British physician, William Lambe, published "Reports of the Effects of a Peculiar Regimen in Scirrhous Tumors and Cancerous Ulcers." His "peculiar regimen" was abstinence from all flesh foods and the free use of water. Following this, John Frank Newton adopted the "peculiar regimen," recovered his health, and, in 1811, wrote a book called *The Return to Nature.*

Gradually, the vegetarian movement spread into the European countries. Eduard Baltzer founded the first German Vegetarian Society in 1867, which the Nazis liquidated in 1934. In France, the first vegetarian society was not founded until 1899.

Organized vegetarianism was brought to the United States by the Reverend William Metcalfe and 41 members of his church, who landed in Philadelphia in 1817. Their numbers grew, and their cause was furthered by the influence of several prominent men who became convinced of the advantages of the fleshless diet. Among these were Reuben D. Mussey (1780-1866), fourth president of the American Medical Association and Edward Hitchcock (1793-1864), professor of Science and then president of Amherst College, whose "Lectures on Diet, Regimen, and Employment" were published in 1831. Also, contributing to the vegetarian movement in 1829 was Sylvester Graham, a young Presbyterian who believed he had regained his health on a vegetarian diet, and who began writing and speaking on moderation in eating. Graham is best remembered for advocating the use of unbolted "graham" flour and the "graham" cracker. In 1858, Dr. James Caleb Jackson opened Our Home Hygienic Institute in Danville, New York, which emphasized, among other things, the Graham-type diet. Mother Ellen Harmon White, spiritual leader of the Seventh-day Adventist church, founded the Western Health Reform Institute at Battle Creek, Michigan, in 1866. Later, Dr. John Harvey Kellogg was hired as superintendent, and the name was changed to the Battle Creek Sanitarium or "San" where, in an effort to provide a wholesome, palatable nonflesh diet for the sanitarium patrons, Dr. Kellogg and his brother, W. K. Kellogg, developed cereal foods. From this vegetarian movement sprang two breakfast cereal businesses—Kelloggs of Battle Creek and General Foods Corporation. C. W. Post, the founder of General Foods, had been a patient-guest at the "San."

While the history of vegetarian movements can be traced, it is important to remember that in much of the world, adherence to a vegetarian diet is not by choice but by economics and availability. For centuries large populations of the world have survived on vegetarian diets of one type or another out of necessity.

Vegetarianism has more or less always existed. However, in the United States, there is a renewed movement toward vegetarianism—some for religious convictions, and some for personal convictions as an attitude of the future. In recent years, various religious cults such as Zen Buddhism, Hare Krishnas, and some yogic groups, which promote vegetarianism, have gained popularity in the

United States. As a movement of the future, vegetarianism seems to have roots in various other movements; for example, ecology, counterculture, environmental pollution, and population studies suggesting increased heart disease, cancer, and various other ills with increased meat consumption. Many animal products have been promoted as unhealthy due to additives, preservatives, cholesterol, fat, and lack of fiber. Hardest hit has been the eggs, cured meats, and red meats. Moreover, proponents of animal rights make animal production methods seem inhumane; hence, eating animal products becomes an inhumane activity. Still other individuals say cereal grains could be better used to feed the hungry world than to feed cattle and pigs. So, much of the move toward vegetarianism may actually be a move toward what many feel is a more healthful diet—at least based upon popularized theories, or a move toward some feeling of a right action.

PROBLEMS OF VEGETARIANISM. Whatever the reason for choosing a vegetarian life-style, some nutritional problems are inherent unless the person practicing possesses a sound knowledge of nutrition. Furthermore, the level of vegetarianism is important. Those at the greatest risk are the vegans or pure vegetarians and fruitarians, and among these individuals their dietary practices are the most hazardous to pregnant or lactating women, infants, growing children, adolescents, and people who are ill or recovering from disease. Dietary concerns for fruitarians and vegans include energy, protein, calcium, iron, zinc, vitamin D, riboflavin, and vitamin B-12, a discussion of each of which follows:

• **Energy**—Among adults, energy (calories) is not likely to be a problem. However, infants and growing children may not be able to meet the energy demands for their body due to the high bulk—fiber—and low energy content of the diet. When energy needs are not met, protein is used for energy. Indeed, slow-growing children have been noted in some pure vegetarian groups—even a few cases of protein-calorie malnutrition.

(Also see ENERGY UTILIZATION BY THE BODY.)

• **Protein**—The requirement for protein is not for protein *per se*, but rather a requirement for the essential amino acids. Foods of plant origin have a lower digestibility and their essential amino acid patterns are not as well balanced as foods of animal origin. However, if adequate calories—energy—is provided by the diet, then combinations of foods of plant origin can satisfactorily meet the essential amino acid requirements. Combinations of foods from different plant sources complement each other. That is, the weakness of one in terms of amino acid content is strengthened by the addition of another. For vegetarian diets, complementary protein sources are generally combinations of whole grains and legumes. Vegetarian diets based on only one cereal grain should be avoided, especially in feeding young children.

(Also see PROTEIN[S].)

• **Calcium**—Since milk provides a large share of the calcium in the normal diet, calcium may be marginal in vegetarian diets. The most reliable and practical source of calcium for the pure vegetarian is fortified soybean milk.

(Also see CALCIUM.)

• **Iron**—Problems with iron nutrition are not entirely limited to vegetarians. However, the absorption of iron from foods of plant origin is lower than that of foods of animal origin. Moreover, the concentration of iron in foods of plant origin is lower. Vegetarians should choose good food sources of iron and include a food high in ascorbic acid (vitamin C) to enhance the absorption of iron. Supplemental iron is advisable.

(Also see IRON.)

• **Zinc**—The grains are good sources of zinc, but the zinc absorption may be decreased by the presence of phytic acid. Yeast fermentation of whole wheat flours lowers the phytic acid and increases the availability of zinc and other trace minerals.

(Also see ZINC.)

• **Vitamin D**—Top sources of vitamin D are fatty fish, egg yolks, liver, and dairy products, all of which are deleted from a vegetarian or fruitarian diet. Exposure to sunlight may fulfill the requirement for vitamin D. However, supplemental vitamin D may be necessary.

(Also see VITAMIN D.)

• **Riboflavin**—Major sources of riboflavin are meats, milk, and dairy products. However, vegetarians obtain significant amounts of riboflavin from legumes and whole grains. Moreover, a number of cereal products are enriched with riboflavin.

(Also see RIBOFLAVIN.)

• **Vitamin B-12 (cobalamins)**—Lack of vitamin B-12 is one of the major problems of vegetarian diets. There are no practical plant sources of vitamin B-12, and once a deficiency has occurred, its effects on the nerves are not always reversible. Nursing vegetarian mothers place their babies at the peril of developing a B-12 deficiency. Vitamin B-12 should be provided by a supplement, by fortified foods such as soybean milk or meat analog (substitutes), or by yeast grown on a B-12-enriched media. The amount of B-12 provided by seaweeds, fermented soy, or algae may or may not be adequate. There is no way of being certain unless laboratory analyses have been performed.

The time required to develop signs of a vitamin B-12 deficiency varies dramatically from individual to individual. Some vegetarians may ingest low levels for years and appear in good health, while others develop signs in a much shorter time.

(Also see VITAMIN B-12.)

HEALTHFUL VEGETARIAN DIETS. Planning nutritious total vegetarian diets requires care and knowledge of the strengths and weaknesses of the various foods. By combining the information contained in Table V-7 and using the following guidelines, healthful vegetarian diets may be planned:

1. Reduce substantially all high calorie, low nutrient density foods (empty-calories). Instead, use unrefined foods as far as practical, which, on a caloric basis, supply their share of nutrients.

2. Replace meat by the protein-rich group of legumes, seeds and nuts.

3. Increase intake of whole grain breads and cereals, legumes, nuts, and seeds to maintain energy intake.

4. Use a variety of legumes and whole grains, with some seeds and/or nuts, in meals each day to achieve good protein complementation; for example, beans with corn or rice, cereals with legumes and green, leafy vegetables, and peanuts with wheat.

5. Use a variety of fruits and vegetables, but be sure to include food high in ascorbic acid *in each meal* to enhance iron absorption.

6. Replace the nutrients lost by deleting milk and dairy products by (a) taking a modest amount of nutritional yeast (brewers' or torula), (b) eating dried fruits, (c) providing supplemental vitamin D by daily exposure to the sun, and (d) providing supplemental vitamin B-12.

7. Secure added food energy (calories) from such foods as sweeteners (sugar and syrups), margarine, oils, and shortenings; used either as ingredients in recipes, or at the table.

8. Eat sufficient amounts to maintain ideal weight for age and height. Larger servings and additional foods such as nuts or margarine may be necessary.

9. Consult the Food Composition Table F-36 when planning vegetarian diets to ensure the selection of nutritious foods.

10. Make use of a number of good vegetarian cookbooks for preparing tasty and nutritious dishes.

NOTE WELL: Pure vegetarian diets are not recommended for infants and small children. Also, pure vegetarian diets for pregnant or lactating women should be planned with great care.

(Also see INFANT DIET AND NUTRITION; and PREGNANCY AND LACTATION NUTRITION.)

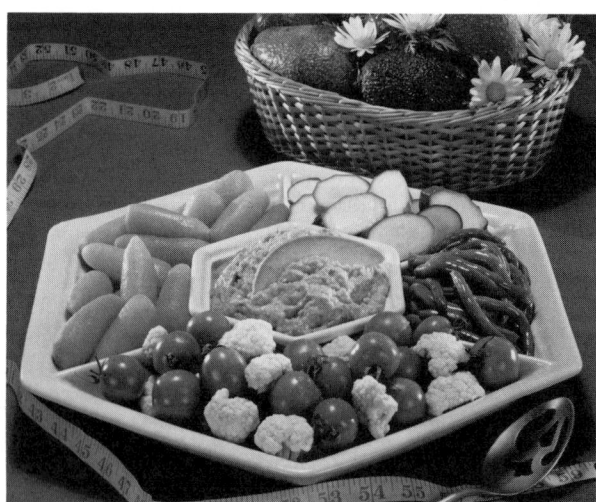

Fig. V-14. Vegetables are an important part of the diet, but a balanced diet is even more important. (Courtesy, Harshe-Rotman & Druck, Inc., Public Relations, Los Angeles, Calif.)

TABLE V-7
THE VEGETARIAN FOUR FOOD GROUPS—THE BASIC FOUR[1]

Group	Foods Included	Amount Recommended	Contribution to the Diet	Comments
Protein rich	Dry beans, dry peas, soybeans, lentils, nuts, including peanuts and peanut butter; meat analogs.	Choose five servings every day. Count as a serving: 1/2 c. of cooked dry beans, dry peas, soybeans, or lentils; 2 Tbsp peanut butter; 1/4 to 1/2 c. nuts, sesame or sunflower seeds. Count one serving as equivalent to 1 oz of lean meat, poultry, or fish.	Foods in this group are valued for their protein. They also provide iron, thiamin, riboflavin, niacin, and phosphorus.	Commercially prepared plant protein products are not essential for a well balanced vegetarian diet. However, when changing from a nonvegetarian to a vegetarian diet, meat analogs are helpful because they replace the accustomed entree without further changes in the menu being necessary. They are convenience-type foods. Labels should be checked for nutritional data. Nuts are concentrated foods contributing flavor and unsaturated fat to the diet.
Milk and cheeses	Fortified soy milk and soy cheese (tofu).	Some milk every day for everyone. Recommended amounts are given below in terms of 8-oz cups: (8-oz cup) Children under 9 ....2 to 3 Children 9 to 12 ....3 or more Teenagers ....4 or more Adults.................2 or more Pregnant women ....3 or more Nursing mothers ....4 or more	Provides calcium, and vitamin B-12.	Children in particular need fortified soybean milk. Large servings of greens like collards, kale, mustard greens, turnip greens, and dandelion greens contribute to meeting the calcium requirement. Vitamin D normally obtained from milk should be supplemented by daily exposure to sunlight. Vitamin B-12 must be provided in fortified foods such as soy milk or yeast grown on B-12-enriched media; or provided as a supplement. Nursing mothers need supplemental vitamin D and B-12.

Footnote at end of table

(Continued)

TABLE V-7 (*Continued*)

Group	Foods Included	Amount Recommended	Contribution to the Diet	Comments
Vegetables and fruits	All vegetables and fruits including dried fruits; with emphasis on those that are valuable sources of vitamin C and vitamin A.	Choose four or more servings every day, including: 1 serving of a good source of vitamin C or two servings of a fair source; one serving, at least every other day, of a good source of vitamin A. If the food chosen for vitamin C is also a good source of vitamin A, the additional serving of a vitamin A food may be omitted. The remaining 1 to 3 or more servings may be of any vegetable or fruit, including those that are valuable for vitamin C and vitamin A. Count as one serving: 1/2 c. of vegetable or fruit; or a portion as ordinarily served, such as one medium apple, banana, orange, or potato, half a medium grapefruit or cantaloupe or the juice of one lemon.	Fruits and vegetables are valuable chiefly because of the vitamins and minerals they contain. In this plan, this group is counted on to supply nearly all the vitamin C needed and over half of the vitamin A. In addition, some members of this group supply fiber. Dark-green and deep-yellow vegetables are good sources of vitamin A. Most dark-green vegetables, if not overcooked, are also reliable sources of vitamin C, as are citrus fruits. Dark-green vegetables are valued for riboflavin, folacin, iron, and magnesium as well. Nearly all vegetables and fruits are low in fat, and none contain cholesterol. Unpeeled fruits and vegetables and those with edible seeds supply fiber. Dried fruits are good sources of iron.	A food high in vitamin C (ascorbic acid) at each meal enhances iron absorption. For sweetening cereals use raisins, dates, or sliced bananas. Avocados supply some fat. Dried fruits concentrate the mineral content.
Breads and cereals	All breads and cereals should be whole-grain or enriched products; whole grains include: wheat, oats, corn, rye, millet, barley, rice, wild rice.	Choose five or more servings daily; or if no cereals are chosen, have an extra serving of breads or baked goods, which will make at least five servings from this group daily. Count as one serving: 1 slice of bread; 1 oz ready-to-eat cereal; 1/2 to 3/4 c. cooked cereal, cornmeal, grits, macaroni, noodles, rice, spaghetti, etc.	Foods in this group furnish worthwhile amounts of protein, iron, several of the B vitamins, and food energy. Whole-grain products also contribute magnesium, folacin, and fiber. Yeast fermentation of whole grain flours, such as in bread-making, lowers the phytates and significantly increases the availability of zinc.	Includes all products made with whole-grains or enriched flour, or meal. Example: bread, biscuits, muffins, waffles, pancakes, cooked or ready-to-eat cereals, cornmeal, flour, grits, macaroni and spaghetti, noodles, rice, rolled oats, barley, and bulgur. Most breakfast cereals are fortified at nutrient levels higher than those occurring in the natural grain. Use whole grains to complement protein-rich group.

[1] In ovolactovegetarian or lactovegetarian diets, eggs and/or milk and milk products are used in place of some of the servings of food from the protein rich group. Milk recommendations follow those set forth in the milk and cheese group. To convert to metric, see WEIGHTS AND MEASURES.

MEAT SUBSTITUTES. Vegetarians can have their meat and eat it too! There is a whole line of products developed primarily from plant proteins that look like meat and taste like meat. Similar to the vegetarian movement of the late 1800s which spawned the development of Kelloggs and General Foods, the vegetarian movement of the late 1900s has created a market for meat analogs or substitutes. These are manufactured by two companies, primarily—Loma Linda Foods and Worthington

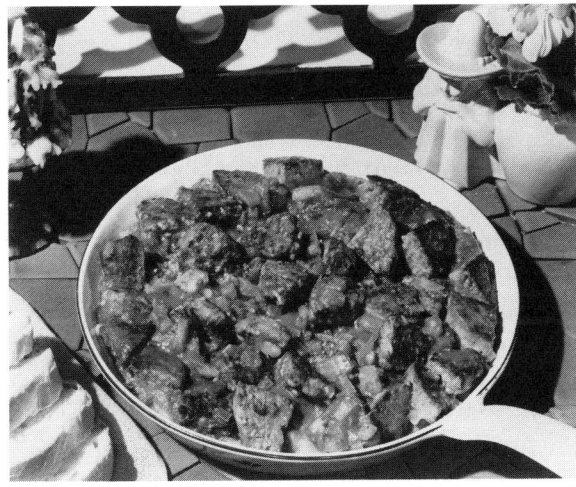

Fig. V-15. Recipe featuring Worthington Foods' Prostage® (1 lb frozen rolls). (Courtesy, Worthington Foods, Division of Miles Laboratories, Inc., U.S.A., Worthington, Ohio)

Foods. Although these products are not necessary for a well balanced vegetarian diet, they do help when an individual is shifting from a nonvegetarian diet to a vegetarian diet. Furthermore, meat analogs add variety to a vegetarian diet. They can be produced to simulate the appearance, texture, and flavor of meat, poultry and fish; and they can be made to meet the known nutrients in animal sources. Individuals purchasing these meat analogs should realize that they are convenience foods. Also, nutritional information on the labels must be checked to determine their adequacy.

(Also see MEAT[S], section headed "Meat Substitutes.")

POSSIBLE HEALTH BENEFITS OF VEGETARIANISM.
Vegetarianism has been credited with minimizing a variety of diseases including obesity, cancer, coronary heart disease, dental caries, diabetes, and diverticular disease of the colon. However, in many cases, lack of complete data prohibits sound conclusions. Nevertheless, the following generalizations about the health of vegetarians can be made:

• **Obesity**—Those vegetarians who abstain from all animal food, generally, have lower weights for their heights than nonvegetarians. Vegetarians consume less food energy (calories) because the digestive tract becomes full sooner.

• **Cancer**—Epidemiologic data (studies of populations) indicates a possible association between risks of colon and breast cancers and the Western world diet which is generally low in dietary fiber and high in animal protein (especially beef), saturated and total fat as well as refined carbohydrates. Seventh-day Adventists, who consume a vegetarian rather than a typical Western diet, exhibit lower death rates than the general population for cancers of the lung, mouth, and some other areas. Diet may not be the only factor or the contributing factor in cancer incidence; other factors also must be considered. The Seventh-day Adventists, for example, also abstain from tobacco, alcohol, and coffee. Moreover, Mormons, who do not abstain from meat, also demonstrate lower cancer rates than the general population.

(Also see CANCER.)

• **Coronary heart disease**—There are some studies that suggest a possible association between vegetarianism and a lower level of coronary heart disease. Compared to the general population, Seventh-day Adventists exhibit lower incidence of atherosclerosis and later occurrence of the first heart attack. Western European populations subjected to World War I and II rationing demonstrated decreased incidence of circulatory diseases. Their diets were essentially lactovegetarian. Also, blood pressure does appear to be substantially *reduced* among vegetarians.

Pure vegetarians who consume no animal food generally exhibit the lowest serum cholesterol levels when compared to nonvegetarians, ovolactovegetarians, and lactovegetarians. They have lower low-density lipoprotein cholesterol (LDL) coupled with higher high-density lipoprotein cholesterol (HDL) levels. Vegetarians also show lower levels of serum triglycerides.

Other dietary as well as nondiet-related risks must also be considered, however. For example, the vegetarian diet typically includes high-fiber content from legumes. It is low in animal protein and includes a high level of complex carbohydrates and phytosterols. In addition, diabetes mellitus, high blood pressure, obesity, and smoking may have been lower among the vegetarian groups studied. Regardless of the potential preventative benefits, persons known to be at the risk of developing coronary heart disease may benefit by adopting a vegetarian-type diet.

(Also see HEART DISEASE.)

• **Dental caries**—No conclusive evidence is yet available on the dental health status of vegetarians as opposed to nonvegetarians. On regimens such as vegetarian diets that encourage the use of coarse foods which might cleanse the teeth, and which discourage the consumption of sugar, particularly sticky sweets and high-sugar snack foods, one might anticipate reduction in dental caries risk. However, dental caries is also related to (1) bacterial flora of the mouth, (2) oral hygiene, (3) fluoridation of water supplies, and (4) resistance of the teeth due to genetic influences and adequate dietary amounts of protein, calcium, phosphorus, and vitamins A, C, and D.

• **Diabetes**—Diabetes mellitus has been reported to improve with diets of high-fiber and low-concentrated carbohydrates, such as vegetarianism encourages.
(Also see DIABETES MELLITUS.)

• **Diverticular disease**—High-fiber diets such as those encouraged by vegetarianism will relieve the symptoms of diverticular disease. Moreover, high-fiber diets relieve constipation, which when chronic is believed to cause this disease.

Severely restrictive vegetarian diets, such as fruitarian and Zen macrobiotic diets, increase the risk of malnutrition and deficiency diseases. Well balanced and planned vegetarian diets may have some benefits over the diets of the general population, and some groups who have practiced vegetarianism on a long-term basis have demonstrated excellent health. The health risks of vegetarianism can be avoided and the benefits maximized when dietary planning is based on accurate, up-to-date nutritional information.
(Also see CHOLESTEROL; FIBER; FOOD GROUPS; MEAT; WORLD FOOD; and ZEN MACROBIOTIC DIET.)

VENISON

The name venison comes from the Latin *venatio*, meaning "game" or "hunting." Presently, the term connotes the flesh of any antlered animal.

Venison should be aged before eating or freezing. This may be accomplished by hanging the carcass in a walk-in cooler at 34° to 36°F (*1° to 2°C*); aging young deer for 1 week, and older deer for 2 to 3 weeks.

Many freezer locker stores have power saws and capable meat cutters who will cut, trim off the fat, wrap, and label venison for a few cents per pound. Unless the hunter has meat cutting expertise, it is usually best to use this service.

Venison lends itself well to corning (corned venison); to curing, drying, and smoking (dried venison); to sausage making, when mixed with 50% or more of fat pork trimmings, and prepared as summer or smoked sausage; and to freezing. The most widely used method of preservation is by freezing at 0°F (*-18°C*) or lower. Ground meat may be stored in the freezer for 2 to 3 months, and roasts and steaks for 8 to 12 months.

Venison may be cooked like beef—steaks and chops broiled or sauteed, legs roasted, and the less tender cuts pot-roasted. The best tenderizer for game is a tasty marinade. Any fat should be cut off and replaced with other fat, such as bacon or salt pork. Salt pork is excellent for larding large pieces of meat; smaller pieces may be wrapped in bacon. Venison, like beef, may be served rare, medium, or well done.

VERJUICE

The two different meanings of this term are as follows:

• The juice extracted from either unripe apples or unripe grapes, which was once used to make various drinks, but is now used mainly to impart a tart flavor to various sauces in European cuisine.

• Any tart juice, such as that expressed from cress, crabapples, gooseberries, or sorrel, which may be either fermented or unfermented.

VERMICELLI

It refers to a pasta that is much like spaghetti—only thinner.
(Also see MACARONI AND NOODLE PRODUCTS.)

VERMOUTH

A white wine flavored with wormwood or other herbs such as anise, cinnamon, bitter orange peel, cloves, and elderberries. There are two types: (1) a dark or reddish, richly flavored (sweet) Italian variety; and (2) a pale yellow or light, dry French variety. Vermouth can be used as a liqueur or in cocktails.
(Also see WINE.)

VETCH

The name applied to several different legumes (pulses) some of which are used for food. The starchy root of the tuber-vetch is roasted, while the chick-vetch is prepared in the same manner as chick peas.
(Also see VEGETABLE[S]; and LEGUMES.)

VICILIN

A globulin (simple protein) associated with a legume, such as peas, lentils, and broad beans.

VIENNA BREAD

A bread that is eaten in France mainly as toast or croutons, or in sandwiches. It has a very thin crust; and it is baked in square pans.
(Also see BREADS AND BAKING.)

VILLI

Small threadlike projections attached to the interior side of the wall of the small intestine.
(Also see DIGESTION AND ABSORPTION.)

VILLIKININ

A hormone produced by glands in the upper intestinal mucosa, which is released in response to the presence of chyme entering the intestine. Villikinin stimulates alternating contractions and extensions of the villi, which stirs and mixes the chyme and exposes additional nutrient material for absorption.

VINEGAR

The word vinegar is derived from the French word *vinaigre*, literally meaning sour wine. Indeed, sour wine was the original source of vinegar. Vinegar was a by-product of wine makers and brewers until about the 17th century when vinegar making became a separate industry in France.

Throughout much of recorded history, vinegar has been used in foods, in preservation, and as a medicine. In the Old Testament (Ruth 2:14), it is recorded that Ruth dipped bread in vinegar. The Greeks and Romans of old always had vinegar vessels on the dining table for dipping bread. The ancient Chinese and the Babylonians used pickling solutions containing salt, sugar, and vinegar. Hippocrates prescribed vinegar for his patients.

By definition, vinegar is a sour liquid containing 4 to 12% acetic acid. Any product that will yield alcoholic fermentaion—apples, grapes, pears, peaches, plums, figs, oranges, berries, honey, sugar, syrups, hydrolyzed starchy materials, beers and wines—is acceptable for the production of vinegar. However, wine and cider are the best raw materials for vinegar production. In addition to the acetic acid, other organic acids and esters are present in vinegar giving it a flavor and aroma characteristic of the material from which it was derived. Thus, there are a variety of vinegars: wine vinegar, apple-cider vinegar, beer vinegar, and malt vinegar.

In 1864, Louis Pasteur demonstrated that bacteria caused the conversion of alcohol to acetic acid. Hence, vinegar making is dependent upon the action of yeast and bacteria on the raw product. Fig. V-16 illustrates the chemical reactions involved in the production of vinegar.

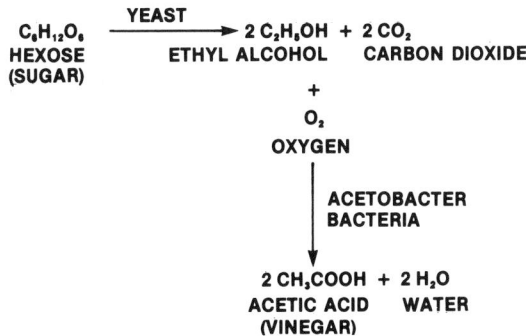

Fig. V-16.   Biochemical changes of vinegar making.

Cider and wine are the best raw materials for vinegar production. In the United States, cider is most frequently used. Basically, apples are mechanically crushed and pressed, and adjusted to contain not less than 8%, and not more than 20%, fermentable sugar. Following fermentation by yeast, the sugar content should preferably be below 0.3%. Next, this alcohol-containing substrate is subjected to the action of acetobacter organisms until the alcohol is converted to acetic acid, following which the vinegar is usually clarified, possibly pasteurized, then bottled.

METHODS OF PRODUCTION.

All methods of producing vinegar rely on the biochemical actions of yeast and acetobacter bacterin. However, several methods are employed to take advantage of these microorganisms, of which the following are noteworthy:

• **Home production**—By allowing barrels of cider or wine to ferment spontaneously, vinegar—although not always of high quality—can be produced at home. However, it must be remembered that provision should be made for the entrance of air into the barrel. The acetic acid bacteria form a thin film on the top of the solution, and this film eventually becomes thick and gelatinous—mother of vinegar. Home production is slow and costly, and demands much attention.

• **Orleans process**—There are several slow methods for the production of vinegar. However, most of them are some modification of the Orleans process, or French method, which is the best of the slow methods. Briefly, this process is carried out in 53 gal (*200 liter*) barrels which are filled with 65 to 70 liter of vinegar and 10 to 15 liter of wine. Then, at weekly intervals, 10 to 15 liter of vinegar are withdrawn, and 10 to 15 liter of wine are added for about 4 weeks. The process is slow but continuous.

• **German process or quick vinegar method**—An apparatus called a generator is employed to help the microorganisms work at a rapid pace. The generator is an upright tank filled with something like beachwood shavings. Acetobacter bacteria live on the beachwood and the alcoholic solution is allowed to trickle down through the shavings where the bacteria act on the alcohol. The tank is not allowed to fill, and air continually rises through the generator. Large amounts of heat are produced, which must be closely monitored. This process is one of the commercial methods for vinegar production. It reduces production time from months to days.

• **Fringe method or continuous process**—This is a commercial process developed in Germany, which produces vinegar by submerged fermentation. The system is patterned after successful antibiotic production by a similar process. This system depends on heavy stirring and the continuous bubbling of air through the tank containing the alcohol. The Fringe method greatly increases the efficiency and speed of conversion of alcohol to acetic acid; a 2,500 gal (*9,500 liter*) batch of mix containing 10.5% alcohol requires only 3 to 5 days to become 10.5% acetic acid.

• **Synthetic acetic acid**—Acetic acid for commercial purposes may also be manufactured by the destructive distillation—decomposition by heat in the absence of air—of certain hardwoods. No microorganisms are involved in this type of acetic acid production. This is purely a chemical process.

ELIMINATING VINEGAR-MAKING PROBLEMS.

Among the problems encountered when producing vinegar from alcohol are vinegar eels or nematode worms, mites, vinegar flies, wine flowers, and darkening of the vinegar. Sanitary practices during all stages of production help control vinegar eels, mites, and vinegar flies.

Wine flowers are yeastlike organisms which form a whitish film on the alcohol and break down alcohol to carbon dioxide and water. They can be controlled by storing alcohol in filled closed containers or by adding one part vinegar to three parts alcohol.

Darkening of vinegar is caused by iron, tannin, or an oxidase. Darkening due to tannin or iron can be removed by aeration, while pasteurization prevents darkening due to an oxidase.

USES OF VINEGAR. In the home, vinegar is used for baking, candies, pickling, production of sour milk, salad dressings, and sweet-and-sour sauces.

Commercially, vinegar is used for mayonnaise, mustard, pickled foods, salad dressings, and tomato products.

(Also see PRESERVATION.)

VIRAL INFECTIONS, FOODBORNE

Infectious hepatitis is the most common foodborne viral disease. The virus is found in excreted stools and blood of infected persons. It may be spread by poorly handled food or seafood taken from sewage contaminated water. In addition to hepatitis, there is some suggestion that the viruses responsible for epidemic diarrhea of the newborn, intestinal flu, and poliomyelitis may be transmitted in contaminated foods.

(Also see DISEASES, Table D-13 Infectious and Parasitic Diseases Which May Be Transmitted By Contaminated Foods and Water.)

VIRUS

A disease-producing agent that (1) is so small that it cannot be seen through an ordinary microscope (it can be seen by using an electron microscope), (2) is capable of passing through the pores of special filters which retain ordinary bacteria, and (3) propagates only in living tissues.

VISCOSITY

A term which indicates the condition or the property of being thick like syrup or glue. Viscous fluids resist flow or motion.

VISUAL PURPLE (RHODOPSIN)

Photosensitive vitamin A-containing pigment found in the rods of the retina.

(Also see VITAMIN A, section headed "Functions.")

VITAMERS

A substance structurally related to a certain vitamin, which possesses some biological activity—although usually less than the true vitamin, and which may relieve a particular vitamin deficiency.

VITAMIN(S)

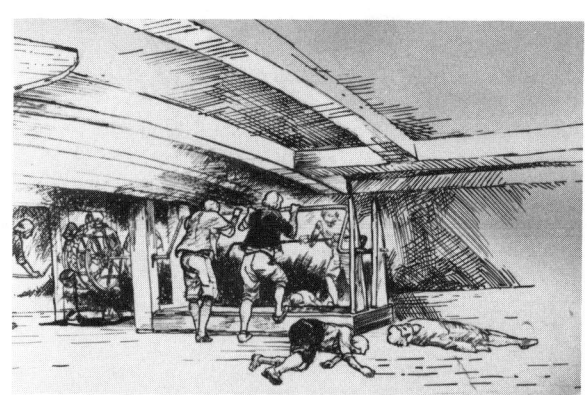

Fig. V-17. This shows an artist's dramatic impression of how British sailors, who ate little except salt meat and biscuits when on long voyages 200 years ago, suddenly collapsed and died of scurvy. (Reproduced with permission of *Nutrition Today*, P. O. Box 1829, Annapolis, MD 21404, ©, 1979)

For proper physiological function, the human body requires some 40 to 50 dietary essentials, of which 14 are vitamins.

Throughout history, vitamin deficiencies have been a major cause of disease, morbidity, and death. Pellagra, scurvy, and beriberi decimated armies, ships' crews, and nations; they even reshaped the course of history. The importance of dietary factors in the genesis of diseases became recognized in the 18th century. But the significance of these observations was not fully understood until early in the 20th century, when scientists found it desirable in many types of investigations to use the biological approach—the use of laboratory animals (largely white, albino rats and mice; guinea pigs; and chicks) fed on purified diets using pure protein such as casein or albumen, pure fat such as lard, and pure carbohydrate such as dextrin, plus minerals to supplement chemical analyses in measuring the value of food. These diets were made up of relatively pure nutrients (proteins, carbohydrates, fats, and minerals) from which the unidentified factors were largely excluded. With these purified diets, all researchers shared a common experience—the animals not only failed to thrive, but they even failed to survive if the investigations were continued for any length of time. At first, many investigators explained such failures on the basis of unpalatability and monotony of diets. Finally, it was realized that these purified diets were lacking in certain factors, minute in amounts, the identities of which were unknown to science. These factors were essential for the efficient utilization of the main ingredients of the food and for the maintenance of health and life itself. The discovery, synthesis, and commercial production of vitamins followed. With these developments, the vitamin era of science was ushered in and the modern approach to nutrition was born.

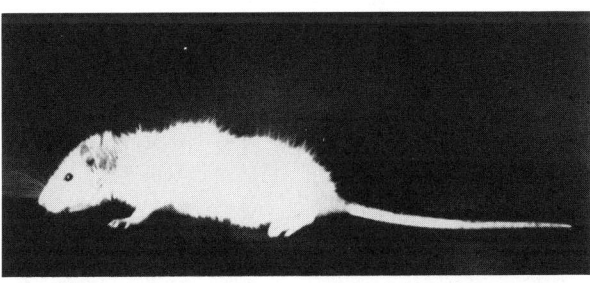

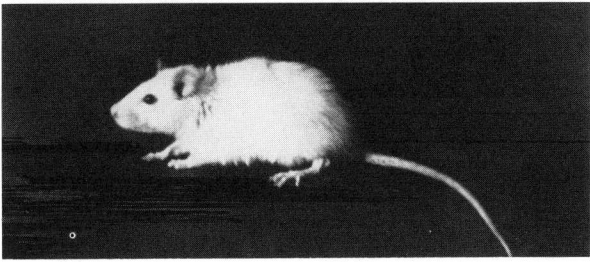

Fig. V-18. The belief that certain factors in very minute amounts are needed by people and animals was difficult to conceive and hold in the early 1900s. Like many episodes of science, it was a mystery story. Yet, finally it was solved by the biological approach—the use of laboratory animals in controlled feeding experiments.
In 1909, Thomas B. Osborne and Lafayette B. Mendel of the Connecticut Agricultural Experiment Station (New Haven), began investigations with purified foodstuffs. (Although different mixtures were used, the basic ingredients of their purified diets were: casein, starch, sugar, and lard.)
The two white rats pictured above were the result of pioneering vitamin studies conducted by Osborne and Mendel during the years 1913 to 1917. *Top*: Rat on a diet deficient in B vitamins; note the rough, scraggly coat, and the emaciation. *Bottom*: The same rat after 12 days on a diet that included B vitamins; note the marked changes in the coat. (Courtesy, The Connecticut Agricultural Experiment Station, New Haven, Conn.)

HISTORY/DISCOVERY OF VITAMINS. Until the early 1900s, if a diet contained proteins, fats, carbohydrates, minerals, and water, it was considered to be a complete diet. True enough, the disease known as beriberi made its appearance in the rice-eating districts of the Orient when milling machinery was introduced from the West, having been known to the Chinese as early as 2600 B.C.; and scurvy was long known to occur among sailors fed on salt meat and biscuits. However, for centuries these diseases were thought to be due to toxic substances in the digestive tract caused by pathogenic organisms, rather than food deficiencies; and more time elapsed before the discovery of vitamins.

Largely through the trial-and-error method, it was discovered that specific foods were helpful in the treatment of certain of these maladies. Hippocrates (460-377 B.C.), the Greek, known as the father of medicine, advocated liver as a cure for night blindness 400 years before the birth of Christ. At a very early date, the Chinese also used a concoction rich in vitamin A as a remedy for night blindness; and cod-liver oil was used in treating or preventing rickets long before anything was known about the cause of the disease. In 1747, James Lind, a British naval surgeon, in a study involving 12 sailors with scurvy on board the "Salisbury," showed that the juice of citrus fruits was a cure for the disease. Nicholas Lunin, as early as 1881, while a student of von Bunge at the University of Dorpat, had come to the conclusion that certain foods, such as milk, contain, beside the principal ingredients, small quantities of unknown substances essential to life. In 1882, Kanehiro Takaki, Director-General of the Japanese Navy, greatly reduced the number of beriberi cases among naval crews by adding meat and evaporated milk to their diet of rice. In 1897, Christiaan Eijkman, a Dutch medical officer, working in Java, had satisfied himself that the disease beriberi was due to the continued consumption of a diet of polished rice.

Credit for the discovery of vitamins cannot be given to any one person. Rather, a number of scientists, working independently in several countries, had the curiosity to study why diets composed of purified food ingredients were not able to support the life of experimental animals. A chronology of the experimenters and experiments which led to the discovery of vitamins and ushered in a new era in nutrition follows.(Also see Table V-8 Chronology of the Discovery/Isolation and Synthesis of Vitamins.)

1. In *1901*, the Dutch physician, G. Grijns, reported that the water and alcohol extract of the outer layer of rice contained an unknown substance which prevented beriberi in man and polyneuritis in fowls.

2. In *1905*, another Dutchman, Pekelharing, at the University of Utrecht, observed that a diet of casein, egg albumen, rice flour, lard, and salts kept mice alive for only 4 weeks. When he added milk to the mixture, however, the mice remained healthy.

3. In *1906*, Sir Frederick G. Hopkins of Cambridge University in England, the most advanced thinker in nutrition of his time, determined by careful experiments that rats became sick and died on a diet consisting of pure

protein, carbohydrate, fat, and all the known necessary minerals. But by supplementing each animal's diet with less than one-third of a teaspoonful of milk per day, they lived. The addition to the diet of an alcoholic extract of milk solids or of certain dried vegetables also enabled the animals to live and grow; however, the ash of either milk or vegetables was ineffective. Thus, Hopkins showed that the essential unknowns which existed in certain foods were organic in nature (rather than inorganic) and could be dissolved in alcohol. He called these substances "accessory food factors." For his work in establishing the existence of the substances we now call vitamins, Hopkins was the recipient of the Nobel Prize in physiology in 1929.

4. In *1907*, Holst and Frolich of Oslo, Norway, conducted the first experimental test with guinea pigs. On a cereal diet, they produced a disease in guinea pigs identical to human scurvy.

5. In *1907*, Elmer V. McCollum, at the University of Wisconsin, although aware that animals could not survive on purified rations of protein, fat, carbohydrate, and mineral salts, believed (together with many others of his time) that the failure to survive was due to the unpalatability of the mixture and the consequent refusal to eat a sufficient amount of the diet. Therefore, he tried to improve the appeal by adding sugar and various flavors, but the animals still died. Even though this experiment appeared to be a failure, it led to the subsequent discovery by McCollum and Davis of a factor which later became known as vitamin A. (It is noteworthy that Miss Marguerite Davis, a young biologist who had just obtained her bachelor's degree from the University of California, volunteered to do the rat work for McCollum without salary.)

6. In *1909-1911*, Osborne and Mendel, at the Connecticut Experiment Station, were able to keep rats alive and growing by including in their purified diet small amounts of milk powder from which both fat and protein had been removed (whey). The ash of this product, however, was totally ineffective.

7. In *1912*, Dr. Casimir Funk, a 28-year-old Polish biochemist working in London, coined the word *vitamine*. Funk postulated, as others had before him, that beriberi, scurvy, pellagra, and possibly rickets, were caused by a lack in the diet of "special substances which are of the nature of organic bases, which we will call vitamines." Presumably, the name vitamines alluded to the fact that they were vital to life, and that they were chemically of the nature of amines (nitrogen-containing). The name caught the popular fancy and persisted, despite the fact that the chemical assumption was later proved incorrect, with the result that the "e" was dropped in 1920; hence, the word *vitamin*. In 1922, Funk's book entitled *The Vitamins* was published.

8. In *1913*, working independently, McCollum and Davis (of the University of Wisconsin) and Osborne and Mendel (of the Connecticut Experiment Station) demonstrated the presence of an essential dietary substance in fatty foods. McCollum and Davis found it in butterfat and egg yolk; Osborne and Mendel discovered it in cod-liver oil. These researchers believed that only one factor, which they called fat-soluble vitamin A, was needed to supplement the purified diets.

Within 2 years of the discovery of the essentiality of the factor called fat-soluble A in 1913, it was recognized that two factors (not one) were lacking in the purified diets for normal growth—one factor was soluble in fat, the other was soluble in water. This finding aroused great interest among nutrition researchers and led to the identification of several fat-soluble and water-soluble factors. Also, through the years, methods for the laboratory synthesis of various vitamins were developed. So, today, most of the vitamins are available in pure crystalline form.

A chronological summary of the discovery/isolation and synthesis of the various vitamins is given in Table V-8.

TABLE V–8
CHRONOLOGY OF THE DISCOVERY/ISOLATION AND SYNTHESIS OF VITAMINS

Year	Discovery/Isolation	Synthesis
1849[1]	Choline	
1866–67		Choline
1913	Vitamin A[2]	
1926	Thiamin (B-1)	
1929	Vitamin K[3]	
1931	Vitamin A[2]	
1932	Vitamin C (Ascorbic Acid) Vitamin D₂	
1933	Riboflavin (B-2)	Vitamin C (Ascorbic Acid)
1935		Riboflavin (B-2)
1936	Biotin Vitamin E	Thiamin (B-1)
1937	Niacin (Nicotinic acid)	
1938	Vitamin B-6 (pyridoxine)	Vitamin E
1939	Pantothenic acid (B-3) Vitamin K[3]	Vitamin B-6 (pyridoxine) Vitamin K[3]
1940		Pantothenic acid (B-3)
1943		Biotin
1945	Folacin (Folic acid)	Folacin (Folic acid)
1947		Vitamin A[2]
1948	Vitamin B-12	
1952		Vitamin D₃
1955		Vitamin B-12

[1]In 1844 and 1846, Gobley isolated a substance from egg yolk, which he called lecithin. In 1849, Strecker isolated a compound from hog bile, to which he subsequently (in 1862) applied the name choline.

[2]A more detailed chronology of vitamin A is: in 1913, it was discovered, independently, by McCollum and Davis of the University of Wisconsin, and Osborne and Mendel of the Connecticut Experiment Station; in 1931, its chemical formula was determined by P. Karrer, a Swiss researcher; and, in 1947, it was synthesized by Isler, working in Switzerland.

[3]Vitamin K was discovered in 1929, isolated in 1939, and synthesized in 1939.

The actual existence of vitamins, therefore, has been known only since 1912, and it was much later before it was possible to see or touch any of them in a pure form. Previously, they were merely mysterious invisible "little things" known only by their effects. In fact, most of the present fundamental knowledge relative to the vitamin content of both human foods and animal feeds was obtained through measuring their potency in promoting growth or in curing certain disease conditions in animals —a most difficult and tedious method. For the most part, small laboratory animals were used, especially rats, guinea pigs, pigeons, and chicks.

Today, there are 14 known vitamins. Additionally, there are at least nine other vitaminlike substances that have been proposed as a result of various experiments, but it is unlikely that all of them are distinct essentials. Yet, the probability that there are still undiscovered vitamins is recognized. Each of the vitamins and vitaminlike substances is alphabetically listed and discussed in a separate section of this encyclopedia.

DEFINITION. *Vitamins are organic substances that are essential in small amounts for the health, growth, reproduction, and maintenance of one or more animal species, which must be included in the diet since they either cannot be synthesized at all or in sufficient quantities in the body.*

Each vitamin performs a specific function; hence, one cannot replace, or act for, another. In general, the human body cannot synthesize them, at least in large enough amounts to meet its needs. However, vitamin D is an exception; when a person is exposed to ultraviolet rays, this vitamin is synthesized from its precursor, which is found in the skin. Some of the vitamin needs of animals can be supplied by microorganisms growing in the digestive tract, especially in animals with a rumen (cow, sheep, goat) or a large cecum (horse, rabbit).

NOMENCLATURE AND CLASSIFICATION. The earliest classification of vitamins, proposed by E. V. McCollum and M. Davis in 1913; listed two groups of vitamins—"fat-soluble A" and "water-soluble B." Classification by solubility in fat or water is still in use.

In 1920, before scientists had determined the chemical composition of any of the vitamins, they were generally designated by a letter of the alphabet, either by order of their discovery or by the initial letter of a word suggesting their role in nutrition. For example, in order of discovery, there were the fat-soluble vitamins A, D, and E and the water-soluble B-1, B-2, and C. Vitamin K, however, was named by its Danish discoverer after its antihemorrhagic function from the Danish term "Koagulation Faktor."

In the 1920s, it became clear that vitamin B was in reality a mixture of several vitamins; hence, the term *vitamin B complex* was devised. This term is still used to describe, collectively, the nine water-soluble vitamins other than vitamin C. All the B-complex vitamins are soluble in water, all are present in large amounts in the liver, and all are nitrogen-containing.

As the chemical structure of vitamins became known, chemically descriptive names were given to many of them. In 1920, Sir Jack Cecil Drummond of England proposed the use of simple alphabetical letters (A, B, C, D, etc.) in place of the cumbersome "fat-soluble A" and "water-soluble B," etc. As a result, some of the letter designations were dropped. In other cases, they persisted. In still other cases, both the letter and name became established.

Presently, there is no universal agreement on the nomenclature of the vitamins. But the modern tendency is to use the chemical name, particularly in describing members of the B complex. In this encyclopedia, the most common designations are used.

Today, vitamins are generally classed as (1) fat-soluble vs water-soluble vitamins, (2) vitamin B complex, and (3) vitaminlike substances.

Fat-Soluble vs Water-Soluble Vitamins. Many phenomena of vitamin nutrition are related to solubility— vitamins are soluble in either fat or water. Consequently, it is important that both nutritionists and consumers be well informed about solubility differences in vitamins and make use of such differences in programs and practices. Based on solubility, vitamins may be grouped as follows:

The Fat-Soluble Vitamins	The Water-Soluble Vitamins
Vitamin A	Biotin
	Choline
Vitamin D	Folacin (folic acid)
	Niacin (nicotinic acid; nicotin amide)
Vitamin E	Pantothenic acid (vitamin B-3)
	Riboflavin (B-2)
Vitamin K	Thiamin (vitamin B-1)
	Vitamin B-6 (pyridoxine; pyridoxal; pyridoxamine)
	Vitamin B-12 (cobalamins)
	Vitamin C (ascorbic acid; dehydroascorbic acid)

It is noteworthy that vitamin C is the only member of the water-soluble group that is not a member of the B family.

The two groups of vitamins exhibit the following several differences that distinguish them both chemically and biologically:

• **Chemical composition**—The fat-soluble vitamins contain only carbon, hydrogen, and oxygen, whereas the water-soluble B vitamins contain these three elements plus nitrogen.

• **Occurrence**—Vitamins originate primarily in plant tissues; with the exceptions of vitamins C and D, they are present in animal tissues only if an animal consumes foods containing them or harbors microorganisms that synthesize them. Fat-soluble vitamins can occur in plant tissue in the form of a provitamin (or precursor of a vitamin), which can be converted into a vitamin in the animal body. But no provitamins are known for any water-soluble vitamin. Also, the B vitamins are universally distributed in all living tissues, whereas the fat-soluble vitamins are completely absent from some.

• **Absorption**—Fat-soluble vitamins are absorbed from the intestinal tract in the presence of fat. It follows that any factor that increases the absorption of fat, such as small particle size or the presence of bile, will also increase the absorption of fat-soluble vitamins. Generally speaking, the absorption of the water-soluble vitamins is a simpler process because there is constant absorption of water from the intestine into the bloodstream.

• **Storage**—The fat-soluble vitamins are stored in appreciable quantities in the body, whereas the water-soluble vitamins are not. Any of the fat-soluble vitamins can be stored wherever fat is deposited; and the greater the intake, the greater the storage. By contrast, the water-soluble B vitamins are not stored in any appreciable amount. Moreover, the large amounts of water which pass through the body daily tend to carry out the water-soluble vitamins, thereby depleting the supply. Hence, they should be suppied in the diet on a daily basis. However, because all living cells contain all the B vitamins, and because the body conserves nutrients that are in short supply by using them only in vital reactions, deficiency symptoms do not appear immediately following their removal from the diet.

• **Excretion**—The fat-soluble vitamins are excreted exclusively in the feces via the bile. The water-soluble vitamins are excreted primarily in the urine, although limited amounts may be present in the feces. This difference in pathway of excretion reflects the difference in solubility.

• **Physiological action**—The fat-soluble vitamins are required for the regulation of the metabolism of structural units, and each vitamin appears to have one or more specific roles. Collectively, the water-soluble B vitamins are primarily concerned with the transfer of energy.

• **Deficiency symptoms**—The absence of one or more vitamins in the diet may lead to failure in growth or reproduction, or to characteristic disorders known as deficiency diseases. In severe cases, death may follow.

The sign of a fat-soluble vitamin deficiency can sometimes be related to the function of the vitamin. For example, vitamin D is required for calcium metabolism and a deficiency results in bone abnormalities. On the other hand, the signs of a B-vitamin deficiency are much less specific and are difficult to relate to function in most cases. Most B-vitamin deficiencies result in dermatitis, rough hair, and poor growth. Deficiencies of some produce loss of pigment in the hair, whereas deficiencies of others cause anemia. It is noteworthy, too, that not all animals suffer from the same deficiency diseases. Thus, man, the monkey, and the guinea pig get scurvy on diets that provide no vitamin C in the diet, whereas rats, fowl, and ruminants make this vitamin in their bodies and do not need it in their food.

The short supply of a vitamin may be more serious than a short supply of food. However, such vitamin deficiencies are less widespread throughout the world than hunger itself, for starvation has always stalked across much of the world, being referred to as famine only when the numbers dying approach the millions.

• **Toxicity**—Excesses of fat-soluble vitamins A and D can cause serious problems, whereas the water-soluble vitamins are relatively nontoxic.

Vitamin B Complex.   With the exception of vitamin C, all of the water-soluble vitamins can be grouped together under the vitamin B complex, of which there are the following nine:

Biotin
Choline
Folacin (folic acid)
Niacin (nicotinic acid; nicotin amide)
Pantothenic acid (vitamin B-3)
Riboflavin (vitamin B-2)
Thiamin (vitamin B-1)
Vitamin B-6 (pyridoxine; pyridoxal; pyridoxamine)
Vitamin B-12 (cobalamins)

The story of the B vitamins began with the study of the age-old disease beriberi. In 1873, Van Lent was apparently the first to conclude that the type of diet had something to do with the origin of beriberi. By reducing the ration of rice in the diet of the sailors in the Dutch navy, he was able to eradicate beriberi almost entirely.

Others followed with studies linking rice to beriberi; among them: Kanehiro Takaki, a Japanese naval medical officer, in 1882; Christiaan Eijkman, a Dutch physician working in the East Indies, in 1897; G. Grijns, another Dutch physician who continued the work of Eijkman in the East Indies, in 1901; and Casimir Funk working in London, in 1912.

In 1916, Dr. Elmer V. McCollum of the University of Wisconsin designated the concentrate that cured beriberi as "water-soluble B," to distinguish it from the antinightblindness factor (called vitamin A) which had been found in carrots and butterfat of milk. At that time, McCollum thought that the antiberiberi substance was one factor only.

Finally, in 1926, B. C. P. Jansen and W. P. Donath, in Holland, isolated the antiberiberi vitamin, and in 1936 Robert R. Williams, an American, determined the structure and synthesized it.

As research continued (1919-1922), it was found that vitamin B was not a single substance, that it actually consisted of several factors. Collectively, they came to be known as the *vitamin B complex*, but each factor was given a separate designation. Some members of the group came to be referred to by subscript numbers as vitamins B_1, B_2, etc.; others became known by their chemical names; still others received both a number and a chemical designation.

These vitamins differ in both chemical structure and specific functions. Yet, there are similarities. All of them are water-soluble; all of them are abundant in liver and yeast, and they often occur together in the same foodstuffs; each of them contains carbon, hydrogen, oxygen, and nitrogen; some of them contain mineral elements in their molecules (thiamin and biotin contain sulfur, and vitamin B-12 contains cobalt and phosphorus); most of them are part of a coenzyme molecule concerned with the breakdown of carbohydrate, protein, and fat in the body; the actions of many of them are interrelated; few of them are stored in large amounts in the body, so they must be provided daily; certain organs, particularly the liver, contain higher concentrations of them than others; and they are excreted from the body by way of the kidneys.

Another noteworthy characteristic of the B vitamins

is that they are synthesized by microbial fermentation in the digestive tract, especially by ruminants (cattle and sheep) and herbivorous nonruminants (horse and rabbit). Some animals eat their own feces (coprophagy), thus recycling the vitamins synthesized in the microbial fermentation in the large intestine and cecum; rabbits, in particular, are known to do this on a routine basis. Unlike ruminants and herbivorous nonruminants, however, man, pigs, and poultry have only one stomach and no large cecum like the horse and rabbit. As a result, they do not synthesize enough of most B vitamins. Consequently, for man and other monogastrics, the B vitamins must be provided regularly in the diet in adequate amounts if deficiencies are to be averted.

A lack of the B-complex vitamins is one of the forms of malnutrition that occurs often throughout the world. Because the B vitamins are usually found together in the same foodstuffs, a deficiency of several factors is usually observed rather than a deficiency of a single factor.

Many physiologic and pathologic stresses influence the need for the B vitamins. Larger amounts are needed during growth and in pregnancy and lactation than in maintenance of health in adult life. The requirement may be increased by diseases that elevate metabolism and by conditions associated with poor absorption, improper utilization, or increased excretion. Administration of antibiotics may lead to vitamin deficiency in some circumstances; in others, antibiotics spare vitamin requirements.

(Also see VITAMIN B COMPLEX.)

Vitaminlike Substances. Certain substances, although not considered true vitamins, closely resemble vitamins in their activity, and are sometimes classed with the B-complex vitamins. They're commonly refered to as "vitaminlike substances." When listed in vitamin preparations, usually the names of these substances are followed by an asterisk, which is tied in with another asterisk at the bottom of the label reading: "Need in human nutrition has not been established."

The nutritional status and biological role(s) of each of the vitaminlike substances require further clarification; indeed, some of them are very controversial. In the meantime, the authors discuss each of them for two primary purposes: (1) historical and informational, and (2) stimulation of research. Additionally, cognizance is taken of the fact that there is usually a considerable time lag between the scientific validation and the acceptance of a vitamin, essential nutrient, and/or medical treatment. A list of the vitaminlike substances follows:

Bioflavonoids
Carnitine (vitamin B-T)
Coenzyme Q (ubiquinone)
Inositol
Laetrile (vitamin B-17), amygdalin, nitrilosides)
Lipoic acid
Pangamic acid (vitamin B-15)
Para-aminobenzoic acid (PABA)
Vitamin B-13 (orotic acid)

Each of these vitaminlike substances is alphabetically listed and discussed in this encyclopedia.

DETERMINATION OF THE VITAMINS IN FOOD.
The potency, or vitamin content, of foods may be determined by biological, microbiological, chemical, physical methods, and/or human assay.

Biological (Animal) Assay. Before the chemical nature of vitamins was known, their potency could be measured by their ability to promote growth or cure a deficiency when test doses were fed to experimental animals—usually rats, mice, guinea pigs, pigeons, or chicks. Such measurement is known as "biological assay" or "bioassay" and is expressed in terms of units. Vitamins A, D, and E are still measured in international units (I.U.). (Also, vitamin A values are given in RE [mcg retinol equivalent]; vitamin D is given in micrograms of cholecalciferol; and vitamin E is given in milligrams of alpha-tocopherol equivalents.)

In most common methods of bioassay, laboratory animals are first depleted of the particular vitamin being studied by being fed a diet lacking in it. Then some of the depleted animals are divided into different groups and fed graded doses of the known vitamin, with each group receiving one of the doses in the series. The response of the animals to the intake, in growth and/or other appropriate criteria, is measured and recorded in a standard response curve. Simultaneously, a second set of depleted animals is divided into different groups, with each group fed increasing amounts of the food being assayed; and the responses of each of these groups is recorded. Then, the vitamin potency of the product being tested is estimated by comparing the responses of the second set of animals with the standard response curve of the first group.

Biological assays are laborious, time-consuming, and costly. Large numbers of samples are needed to produce statistically reliable results; the animals should be of approximately the same age, sex, and weight; it takes time to produce nutrient-deficient animals; and quite often the data obtained are highly variable. In addition, data from one species are not always relevant to another species.

The fundamental value of the biological assay is that it gives positive proof of biological activity. It is still the basis of comparison or standardization for newer microbiological or chemical methods.

Microbiological Assay. This assay is a measure of the ability of a vitamin to promote the growth of a microorganism. A microorganism is selected that is known to require the vitamin, or other nutrient, in question. Therefore, if the vitamin is not present, the selected microorganism will not grow. Actually, the procedure is the same as the biological assay; the only difference is that some suitable microorganism is used in place of rats or other animals. Growth media is prepared so that it is nutritionally complete except for the vitamin to be tested. Graded levels of the vitamin are then added to the media and a growth response curve is prepared. Then, the sample to be assayed can be tested and compared to the growth response curve to determine the concentration of the nutrient. The B vitamins may be assayed in this manner.

The microbiological assay requires less time than the biological assay. Its main disadvantage is that the vitamin being tested must first be extracted from the foodstuff before being added to the growth medium used for the microorganism.

Chemical Assay. Today, foods may be analyzed by highly sophisticated chemical procedures, with the vitamin content expressed in units of weight—milligrams (mg) or micrograms (mcg).

Chemical assays are much faster than biological assays, but, at intervals, they must be compared with bioassays in order to rule out the possibility of assaying as a vitamin some substance that does not function as a vitamin in the body.

Physical Assay. Each of the vitamins may now be determined by physical methods—measurement of absorption spectra, chromatography, fluorescence, turbidity, etc.

Human Assay. Actually, this is a special biological type of assay designed for humans. Experiments with people are very costly and difficult to control. Besides, it is necessary to protect the health and rights of the subjects, and to avoid psychic factors in interpreting the results. The use (1) of *placebos* as controls (pills that, unknown to the subject, contain an inactive substance such as sugar), and (2) of double blind tests (in which none of the participants—the subjects, the investigator, the person giving the diets or supplements, and the diagnostician—know the composition of the dietary variables) is standard procedure in human nutrition studies. In such studies, a code may be used for various test groups, the disclosure of which is not revealed until all tests are completed.

FACTORS INFLUENCING THE UTILIZATION OF VITAMINS.
Vitamin deficiency is usually caused by an insufficiency of the nutrient in the diet being consumed. However, the utilization of vitamins may be influenced by availability, antivitamins, provitamins, synthesis in the gut, and interactions of nutrients.

Availability. Not all the vitamins in foods are in absorbable form. For example, (1) niacin in many cereals is bound to a protein and cannot be absorbed through the intestinal wall, unless the food is treated with an alkali to release the vitamin from the inaccessible complex; (2) fat-soluble vitamins may fail to be absorbed if the digestion of fat is impaired; and (3) vitamin B-12 requires a factor produced in the stomach (the intrinsic factor) for its absorption.

Antivitamins (Vitamin Antagonists, or Pseudovitamins). Antivitamins, which are present in some natural foods, are compounds that do not function as vitamins even though they are chemically related to them. As a result, they may cause vitamin deficiencies if the body (1) is unable to distinguish between them and true vitamins, and (2) incorporates them into essential body compounds.

Provitamins. These are nonvitamin substances that occur in foods which can be converted into vitamins

in the body. Well known examples of provitamins are: (1) beta-carotene, which is converted to vitamin A in the intestinal wall; (2) 7-dehydrocholesterol in the skin, which is converted to vitamin D_3 by ultraviolet light (sunlight); (3) ergosterol of plants, which is converted to vitamin D_2 by ultraviolet light; and (4) the amino acid tryptophan, which can be converted to niacin. (Because of the poor efficiency—60 mg of tryptophan required to produce 1 mg of niacin—tryptophan is not utilized for its provitamin value.)

Synthesis In The Gut. Although some species of bacteria can synthesize vitamins, other species compete with the host for the vitamins ingested in food and retain them until they are excreted in the feces.

In health, the small intestine of man is usually sterile. The large intestine carries a heavy load of bacteria, but usually absorption from the large intestine is limited to water and salts. It is unlikely, therefore, that bacterial synthesis in the gut affects the amounts of most vitamins available to the healthy human body.

When an intestinal disorder is present, especially if there is diarrhea, the small intestine may harbor large numbers of bacteria. These are likely to reduce, rather than increase, the amounts of available vitamins.

Interaction Of Nutrients. Several vitamins are closely linked to other nutrients. For example, (1) if the diet is rich in carbohydrates or alcohol, more thiamin is needed for metabolism; and (2) if the intake of polyunsaturated fats is high, more vitamin E is required. There are several other similar interactions. For this reason, the nutritive value of a diet in respect to a given vitamin may differ from the chemical analysis of its vitamin content. For this reason, too, the diet should supply a well balanced mixture of all the nutrients, including the vitamins, such as is provided by eating a wide variety of traditional foods—meat, milk, eggs, fruits (including citrus fruits), vegetables (including green leafy vegetables), whole grain cereals and bread, and butter or fortified margarine.

VITAMIN CONTENT OF FOODS. The vitamin content of foods is given in Food Composition Table F-36. However, in selecting foods to furnish vitamins in the diet, it is well to keep in mind the following:

1. The vitamin losses of vegetables due to storage tend to parallel the degree of wilting. Such losses are progressive in the long storage of fresh vegetables and fruits.

2. The effects of processing and preparation of foods on vitamin retention must be clearly understood. For example, the fat-soluble vitamins (A, D, E, and K) are not easily lost by ordinary cooking methods, and they do not dissolve out in the cooking water. On the other hand, the water-soluble vitamins (B complex and C) are dissolved easily in cooking water, and a portion of the vitamins may be destroyed by heating; therefore, cooking food only until tender and in as little water as possible is, in general, the best procedure.

3. It is important to determine (a) how often any given food will be included in the diet, and (b) the size serving that will normally be eaten.

4. Economic factors such as availability and cost must be considered.

VITAMIN SUPPLEMENTATION OF THE DIET.

Ideally, there should be enough of all the vitamins in the natural dietary selected on the basis of the Six Food Groups to prevent disease and promote health. When we get our vitamins from such a diet, we usually also obtain the various other nutrients essential to health. Also, when vitamins are consumed in ordinary foods, they are never at a toxic level. The rule, therefore, is: Eat *enough* of *proper* foods *consistently* and chances are you'll get your full complement of needed vitamins. But for many Americans these three words—*enough, proper,* and *consistently*—are the catch. In the first place, lots of folks don't know what constitutes a good diet; and, worse yet, altogether too many people neglect or ignore the rules even if they know them. In either case, the net result is always the same: We shortchange ourselves on the right amounts of good, nutritious food, including vitamins. As a result, more and more doctors and nutritionists are recommending vitamin preparations as supplements. Additional arguments advanced in favor of judicious vitamin supplementation are:

1. **The vitamin content of animal and plant species and parts differ.** The vitamin content of foods varies widely; it's affected by species (for example, pork, is higher in thiamin than beef), and by parts (leaf, stalk, and seed of plants; and organ meats vs muscle meats of animals).

2. **Vitamin losses occur in processing, cooking, and storing.** Unfortunately, many of the vitamins naturally present in foods are destroyed by sunlight, oxidation, mold growth, and heat, to which they are subjected in processing, cooking, and storing. So, by the time they reach the table much of their vitamin value has disappeared. By contrast, during olden times, for the most part man ate whole or natural foods which were subjected to little processing except for field preparation prior to consumption. Then came the food processing and refinement era, followed by the convenience, fabricated, and fast-food era.

Although it is apparent that raw foods supply adequate amounts of vitamins and other micronutrients, it's unlikely that today's processed, cooked, and stored foods provide adequate amounts of certain vitamins and other trace nutrients, especially for certain critical periods of life, unless they are enriched or supplemented.

One authoritative study revealed the following losses of vitamins from the processing and preservation of foods:[11]

a. The losses in seven vitamins from milling wheat and making flour ranged from 50 to 86.3%. Half of the pantothenic acid, 71.8% of the vitamin B-6, 86.3% of the alphatocopherol, and two-thirds of the folacin were removed.

b. The average losses by food groups in vitamin B-6 and pantothenic acid from canning and freezing were as shown in the unnumbered table:

[11]Schroeder, Henry A., M.D., Losses of Vitamins and Trace Minerals Resulting From Processing and Preservation of Foods, *The American Journal of Chemical Nutrition*, Vol. 24, May 1971, pp. 562-573.

| Food Group | Frozen | | Canned | |
	Vitamin B-6	Pantothenic Acid	Vitamin B-6	Pantothenic Acid
	(%loss)	(%loss)	(%loss)	(%loss)
Fish and seafood	17.3	20.8	48.9	19.9
Meat and poultry		70.2	42.6	26.2
Vegetables, roots		36.8	63.1	46.1
Vegetables, legumes ...	55.6	57.1	77.4	77.8
Vegetables, green	36.7	48.2	57.1	56.4
Fruit and fruit juices .	15.4	7.2	37.6	50.5

The appalling processing and preservation losses revealed above underscore the dietary need for whole grains and unprocessed foods of many varieties. They also suggest that the vitamin enrichment and/or supplementation of certain refined and processed foods may be necessary in order to meet the recommended allowances of certain vitamins.

3. **Poor eating habits are commonplace.** Although there is an abundance of good food available, strange as it may seem many folks have fallen into poor eating habits like some typical Americans herewith described:

a. The sizeable group that skips breakfast entirely or settles for a sweet roll and a cup of coffee at the office, or the smaller group that skips lunch.

b. Those whose hustle and bustle causes them to "eat and run" or just "grab a bite," with the result that they do not eat a balanced diet.

c. Those who take time for a good breakfast of fruit, eggs, and perhaps bacon or ham, *only* on a leisurely Sunday morning.

d. The teenagers who virtually live on "snacks" at home, and on a diet of hamburgers, hot dogs, and soft drinks when they're out with the gang.

e. The mothers who breakfast on coffee and a piece of toast after the family has gone its way, and who nibble on leftovers for lunch.

f. Those who avoid milk because they have gotten out of the habit as they have grown older.

g. Those who don't like green leafy vegetables, either raw or cooked.

h. The thousands of people who have personal food prejudices; they don't like fish, or liver, or salads, for example.

i. Those who automatically and routinely order a sandwich instead of a salad, a soft drink instead of milk or fruit juice, and a sweet roll for breakfast instead of cereal and/or eggs.

j. The calorie counters and weight watchers add millions more to the number of folks who regularly shortchange themselves on the essential vitamins.

k. Then there are the thousands of bachelors and bachelor girls, who live alone and complain that "it's no fun to cook for just oneself."

l. The growing number of the elderly, many of whom suffer from poor appetites and poor teeth and may not eat enough or eat the right foods.

Think for a moment of all the people who have fallen into one or more of the above poor eating habits! Of course, it's easier to think of those who have good eating habits, because there are fewer of them. But for the millions of Americans with poor eating habits supplemental vitamins are in the nature of "diet insurance"—they're a way of making sure that they are getting enough vitamins each day. That's the reason many of today's doctors and nutritionists recommend vitamin supplementation of the food we eat.

4. **Several vitamins are not stored.** Several of the vitamins cannot be accumulated and stored in the body for any considerable period of time; they are used up quickly and therefore must be constantly replaced or renewed with a continuing supply from the outside.

5. **Fewer calories usually mean fewer vitamins.** With increased mechanization and decreased manual labor, fewer calories are consumed—and with it fewer vitamins.

6. **More vitamins required for growth, pregnancy, and lactation.** Vitamin intakes need to be increased during the critical periods of growth, pregnancy, and lactation. Babies are given supplemental vitamins from the time they are born until they are at least a year old and sometimes longer. Also, vitamin intakes are usually increased during pregnancy and lactation.

7. **Increased vitamins may be needed for therapeutic reasons.** Vitamin supplementation may be needed when a person is unable to consume an adequate diet due to illness, allergies, or emotional upsets. Likewise, vitamin supplementation may be prescribed when a serious dietary deficiency has occurred because of ignorance or poor eating habits; however, such supplementation should never replace the correction of factors leading to the dietary inadequacy. At such times, vitamin supplementation should be taken on the recommendation of physicians to help control particular conditions diagnosed by them.

8. **More vitamins needed during stress.** There are times when vitamin intakes may need to be increased, such as during infections; chronic disease; heavy drinking and/or smoking; regular use of birth control pills; restrictive dieting; environmental stress; and regular use of drugs which interfere with vitamin function. In these situations, professional advice should be sought relative to the given need, and proper adjustment should be made in the dietary pattern or the diet should be supplemented with a vitamin or a vitamin-mineral preparation.

9. **Lack of vitamins not easily recognizable.** "Too much" or "too little" of some food nutrients may soon show up on the bathroom scale as a pound or two gained or lost. But a lack of a vitamin(s) isn't so immediately recognizable.

Initially, it was thought that each vitamin was primarily a protective substance, which prevented a specific disease. While it is true that a specific disease can result from lack of a specific vitamin, specific deficiencies of a single vitamin are comparatively rare today. Instead, it is recognized that vitamins are interdependent of each other and on other nutrients for buoyant good health; hence, people are likely to have a deficiency of a group of vitamins, some consequences of which may be: a tired, run-down feeling; not quite up to par; insomnia; easily irritated; or lowered resistance to minor infection. Such signs and illnesses do not necessarily indicate vitamin deficiency, but, of course, the physician should be consulted. Also, everyone should understand the essential role of vitamins in maintaining health.

10. **Vitamin needs vary with individuals.** Vitamin needs vary according to age, kind of work, and general physical condition. Moreover, different individuals have different needs for different vitamins.

11. **We can learn from animals.** Much of the research on vitamins has been done with laboratory animals—rats, mice, guinea pigs, chicks, monkeys, dogs, etc. This makes sense when one realizes that many generations of white mice, for example, can be studied over a period of a few months or years, whereas if such clinical research were limited to humans, it would take 50 years or longer to make comparable tests with successive generations. Therefore, many conclusions concerning the role of vitamins in nutrition have been reached through basic research with animals.

Perhaps we can also learn from larger animals, especially the monogastrics (such as pigs which have one stomach like people), in still another way—their vitamin supplementation program. First, the following things relative to their foods are important.

a. Animals get more vitamins in natural foods than people. Generally speaking, animals consume less refined foods than people; for example, they usually consume processed whole cereals, rather than flour. Not only that, they are usually fed the more nutritious by-products of milling—the outer coats and the germ of seeds.

b. Formerly, a wide variety of feed ingredients were added to livestock rations for their vitamin content, much like the recommendation still made in human diets as evidenced by the opening sentence of this section reading as follows:

"Ideally, there should be enough of all the vitamins in the natural dietary selected on the basis of the Six Food Groups to prevent disease and promote health."

In the case of animals, the concept of getting all the vitamins through food ingredients was abandoned many years ago, for much the same reasons detailed in the first ten points of this section. So, today animal nutritionists rely on vitamin supplements. In modern feed formulation, premixes (comparable to mixed vitamin supplements for humans) often represent the commonsense approach to providing vitamins.

Commercial livestock producers recognize that subacute deficiencies of vitamins can exist, although actual deficiency symptoms do not appear. Yet, such borderline deficiencies may result in poor and expensive gains, impaired reproduction, and/or depressed production. Moreover, the cost for vitamin supplementation constitutes a very small fraction of the total feed bill. Also, and most important, it is noteworthy that animals have never fallen into the poor eating habits common to people. Who ever heard of a pig or a chicken drinking coffee, cokes, or alcohol; eating sweets or snacks; or having food prejudices?

So, today, more and more physicians and nutritionists rely on vitamin supplements, which in many cases are chemically pure sources that need to be taken only in very minute amounts, and which cost only a small fraction of the total food bill. Also, informed physicians and nutritionists no longer prescribe vitamins merely to prevent deficiency symptoms, or to meet minimum requirements, but, rather, to impart buoyant good health.

Undoubtedly, the use of vitamin supplements far exceeds the need for them in many cases. The potency of preparations on the market varies widely, and the number of nutrients present differs from one product to another. Moreover, the consumer may be unable to interpret the label informatioin in terms of his own requirements.

Although water-soluble vitamins in excess of body needs will be excreted in the urine—with no harm done, except to the pocketbook, excessive intakes of vitamins A and D may be toxic. So, large amounts of vitamins should be taken under the direction of a physician or nutritionist.

VITAMIN TABLE. Table V-9 is a summary of each of the 14 known vitamins and of the 9 vitaminlike sub-

stances, totaling 23. Note that the 23 factors are divided into 3 appropriate groups—(1) fat-soluble vitamins, (2) water-soluble vitamins, and (3) vitaminlike substances—with the members within each group listed alphabetically. Note, too, that information relative to each of the 23 substances is given under the following headings: functions; deficiency and toxicity symptoms; recommended daily allowances; sources; and comments.

Additionally, a separate and more complete presentation relative to each vitamin and vitaminlike substance appears alphabetically in the encyclopedia under its respective name.

TABLE V-9
VITAMIN TABLE

Functions	Deficiency and Toxicity Symptoms	Recommended Daily Allowance				Sources	Comments
		Age Group	Years	Vitamin			
FAT-SOLUBLE VITAMINS **Vitamin A** Helps maintain normal vision in dim light—prevents night blindness. Prevents xerophthalmia, an eye condition which may lead to blindness in extreme vitamin A deficiency. Essential for body growth. Necessary for normal bone growth. Necessary for normal tooth development. Helps keep the epithelial tissues of the skin, and of the lining of the nose, throat, respiratory and digestive systems, and genitourinary tract, healthy and free of infection. May help prevent miscarriage of women during the first three months of pregnancy. New information suggests that vitamin A (1) acts	**Deficiency symptoms—** Night blindness (nyctalopia) xerosis, and xerophthalmia. Stunted growth of children. Slowed bone growth, abnormal bone shape, and paralysis. Unsound teeth, characterized by abnormal enamel, pits, and decay. Rough, dry, scaly skin—a condition known as follicular hyperkeratosis (it looks like "gooseflesh"); increased sinus, sore throat, and abscesses in ears, mouth, or salivary glands; increased diarrhea and kidney and bladder stones. Reproductive disorders, including poor conception, abnormal embryonic growth, placental injury, and death of the fetus. **Toxicity**—Toxicity of vitamin A is characterized by loss of appetite, headache, blurred vision, excessive irritability, loss of hair, dryness and flaking of the skin (with itching), swelling over the long bones, drowsiness, diarrhea, nausea, and enlargement of the liver and spleen.			*Vitamin A*[1] (mcg RE)	(IU)	**Rich sources**—Liver and carrots. **Good sources**— Dark-green leafy vegetables: beet greens, collards, dandelion greens, kale, mustard greens, spinach, Swiss chard, turnip greens. Yellow vegetables: pumpkins, sweet potatoes, squash (winter). Yellow fruits: apricots, peaches. Some seafoods: crab, halibut, oysters, salmon, swordfish, whale meat. **Fair sources**— Butter (regular salted), cantaloupe, cheese, cream, egg yolk, lettuce, margarine (fortified), tomatoes, whole milk. **Negligible sources**— Breads and cereals (except yellow corn), chicken, cottage cheese (not creamed), dry beans, muscle meats, potatoes, skim milk. **Supplemental sources**— Synthetic vitamin A, cod and other fish liver oils. For additional sources and more precise values of vitamin A see Food Composition Table F-36.	The forms of vitamin A are: alcohol (retinol), ester (retinyl palmitate), aldehyde (retinal or retinene), and acid (retinoic acid). Retinol, retinyl palmitate, and retinal are readily converted from one form to another, but retinoic acid cannot be converted to other forms. Retinoic acid fulfills some of the functions of vitamin A, but it does not function in the visual cycle.
		Infants	0.0–0.5	375	1,250		
			0.5–1.0	375	1,250		
		Children	1–3	400	1,333		
			4–6	500	1,667		
			7–10	700	2,333		
		Males	11–14	1,000	3,333		
			15–18	1,000	3,333		
			19–24	1,000	3,333		
			25–50	1,000	3,333		
			51+	1,000	3,333		
		Females	11–14	800	2,667		
			15–18	800	2,667		
			19–24	800	2,667		
			25–50	800	2,667		
			51+	800	2,667		
		Pregnant		800	2,667		
		Lactating		1,200	4,000		

in a coenzyme role, as for instance in the form of intermediates in glycoprotein synthesis; and (2) functions like steroid hormones, with a role in the cell nuclei, leading to tissue differentiation. Other functions of vitamin A: necessary for (1) thyroxine formation and prevention of goiter; (2) protein synthesis; and (3) synthesis of corticosterone from cholesterol, and the normal synthesis of glycogen. (Also see VITAMIN A.)

[1]*Recommended Dietary Allowances*, 10th ed., NRC–National Academy of Sciences, 1989, p. 285.

The recommended daily allowances (RDA) are given in both International Units (IU) and Retinol Equivalents (RE). An International Unit (IU) of vitamin A is defined on the basis of rat studies as equal to 0.344 mcg of crystalline retinylacetate (which is equivalent to 0.3 mcg of retinol, or to 0.6 mcg of beta-carotene). These standards are based on experiments which show that in rats only about 50% of the beta-carotene is converted to vitamin A.

TABLE V-9 (Continued)

Functions	Deficiency and Toxicity Symptoms	Recommended Daily Allowance				Sources	Comments
		Age Group	Years	Vitamin			

| | | | | *Vitamin D*[1] | | | |
| | | | | (mcg) | (IU) | | |

Vitamin D
Increases calcium absorption from the small intestine.
Promotes growth and mineralization of the bones.
Promotes sound teeth.
Increases absorption of phosphorus through the intestinal wall, and increases resorption of phosphates from the kidney tubules.
Maintains normal level of citrate in the blood.
Protects against the loss of amino acids through the kidneys.
(Also see VITAMIN D.)

Deficiency symptoms— Rickets in infants and children, characterized by enlarged joints, bowed legs, knocked knees, outward projection of the sternum (pigeon breast), a row of beadlike projections on each side of the chest at the juncture of the rib bones and joining (costal) cartilage (called rachitic rosary), bulging forehead, pot belly, and delayed eruption of temporary teeth and unsound permanent teeth.
Osteomalacia in adults, in which the bones soften, become distorted, and fracture easily.
Tetany, characterized by muscle twitching, convulsions, and low serum calcium.
Toxicity— Excessive vitamin D may cause hypercalcemia (increased intestinal absorption, leading to elevated blood calcium levels), characterized by loss of appetite, excessive thirst, nausea, vomiting, irritability, weakness, constipation alternating with bouts of diarrhea, retarded growth in infants and children, and weight loss in adults.

Age Group	Years	(mcg)	(IU)
Infants	0.0–0.5	7.5	300
	0.5–1.0	10	400
Children	1–3	10	400
	4–6	10	400
	7–10	10	400
Males	11–14	10	400
	15–18	10	400
	19–24	10	400
	25–50	5	200
	51+	5	200
Females	11–14	10	400
	15–18	10	400
	19–24	10	400
	25–50	5	200
	51+	5	200
Pregnant		10	400
Lactating		10	400

[1]*Recommended Dietary Allowances*, 10th ed., NRC–National Academy of Sciences, 1989, p. 285.
400 IU of vitamin D = 10 mcg cholecalciferol.

Sources

Vitamin D is more sparse in foods than any other vitamin.
Rich sources—Fatty fish (bloater, herring, kipper, mackerel, pilchard, salmon, sardines, tuna) and fish roe.
Fair sources—Liver, egg yolk, cream, butter, cheese.
Negligible sources— Muscle meats, milk (unfortified), fruits, nuts, vegetables, grains.
D-fortified foods— Milk (400 IU/qt) and infant formulas.
Other foods to which vitamin D is often added include: breakfast and infant cereals, breads, margarines, milk flavorings, fruit and chocolate beverages, and cocoa.
Supplemental sources— Fish liver oils (from cod, halibut, or swordfish); irradiated ergosterol or 7-dehydro-cholesterol such as viosterol.
Exposure to sunlight or sunlamp— Manufacture in the skin.
For additional sources and more precise values of vitamin D, see Food Composition Table F-36.

Comments

Vitamin D includes both—D_2 (ergocalciferol, calciferol, or viosterol) and D_3 (cholecalciferol).
Vitamin D is unique among vitamins in three respects: (1) it occurs naturally in only a few common foods (mainly in fish oils and a little in eggs and milk), (2) it can be formed in the body and in certain foods by exposure to ultraviolet rays, and (3) the active compound of vitamin D (1, 25-$(OH)_2$-D_3) functions as a hormone.

TABLE V-9 (Continued)

Functions	Deficiency and Toxicity Symptoms	Recommended Daily Allowance			Sources	Comments
		Age Group	Years	Vitamin		

Functions	Deficiency and Toxicity Symptoms	Age Group	Years	Vitamin E[1] (mg αTE)	Vitamin E[1] (IU)	Sources	Comments
Vitamin E (Tocopherols) As an antioxidant which (a) retards rancidification of fats in plant sources and in the digestive tracts of animals, and (b) protects body cells from toxic sustances formed from the oxidation of unsaturated fatty acids. As a powerful antioxidant, vitamin E readily oxidizes itself (it combines with oxygen), thereby minimizing the destruction by oxidation of unsaturated fatty acids and vitamin A in the intestinal tract and in the tissues. As an essential factor for the integrity of red blood cells. As an agent essential to cellular respiration, primarily in heart and skeletal muscle tissues. As a regulator in the synthesis of DNA, vitamin C, and coenzyme Q. As a protector of lung tissue from air pollution (smog). As a sometimes replacement for selenium. (Also see VITAMIN E.)	**Deficiency symptoms—** Innumerable vitamin E deficiency symptoms have been demonstrated in animals; and they are highly variable from species to species. But vitamin E deficiency symptoms as such rarely occur in humans. Newborn infants (especially the premature), suffering from a deficiency of vitamin E (caused by shortened life span of red blood cells), characterized by edema, skin lesions, and blood abnormalities. Patients unable to absorb fat (like those suffering from sprue or from fibro-cystic disease of the pancreas) have low blood and tissue tocopherol levels, increased red blood fragility and shortened red blood cell life span, and increased urinary excretion of creatine. **Toxicity—**Vitamin E is relatively nontoxic. Some persons consuming daily doses of more than 300 IU of vitamin E have complained of nausea and intestinal distress. Excess intake of vitamin E appears to be excreted in the feces.	Infants	0.0–0.5	3	4.47	**Rich sources—** Salad and cooking oils (except coconut oil), alfalfa seeds, margarine, nuts, (almonds, Brazil nuts, filberts, peanuts, pecans), sunflower seed kernels. **Good sources—** Asparagus, avocados, beef and organ meats, blackberries, butter, eggs, green leafy vegetables, oatmeal, potato chips, rye, seafoods (lobster, salmon, shrimp, tuna), tomatoes. **Fair sources—** Apples, beans, carrots, celery, cheese, chicken, liver, peas. **Negligible sources—** Most fruits, sugar, white bread. **Supplemental sources—** Synthetic dl-alpha-tocopherol acetate, wheat germ, wheat germ oil. Most of the commerical vitamin E is synthetic dl-alpha-tocopherol acetate. It is the least expensive source of the vitamin, but, unlike natural food sources, it provides no other essential nutrient. For additional sources and more precise values of vitamin E (alpha-tocopherol), see Food Composition Table F-36.	There are 8 tocopherols and tocotrienols, of which alpha-tocopherol has the greatest vitamin E activity.
			0.5–1.0	4	5.96		
		Children	1–3	6	8.94		
			4–6	7	10.43		
			7–10	7	10.43		
		Males	11–14	10	14.90		
			15–18	10	14.90		
			19–24	10	14.90		
			25–50	10	14.90		
			51+	10	14.90		
		Females	11–14	8	11.92		
			15–18	8	11.92		
			19–24	8	11.92		
			25–50	8	11.92		
			51+	8	11.92		
		Pregnant		10	14.90		
		Lactating		12	16.39		

[1]*Recommended Dietary Allowances*, 10th ed., NRC–National Academy of Sciences, 1989, p. 285.

The recommended daily allowances (RDA) are given in both International Units (IU) and alpha-tocopherol equivalents. 1 mg d-tocopherol = 1 alpha-TE. See section on Vitamin E. (tocopherols) for variation in allowances and calculation of vitamin E activity of the diet as alpha-tocopherol equivalents.

(Continued)

TABLE V-9 *(Continued)*

Functions	Deficiency and Toxicity Symptoms	Recommended Daily Allowance			Sources	Comments
		Age Group	Years	Vitamin		
Vitamin K Vitamin K controls blood coagulation; recent research suggests that it acts in some way to convert precursor proteins to the active blood clotting factors. Vitamin K is essential for the synthesis in the liver of four blood-clotting proteins: 1. Factor II, prothrombin. 2. Factor VII, proconvertin. 3. Factor IX, Christmas factor. 4. Factor X, Stuart-Power. (Also see VITAMIN K.)	**Deficiency symptoms—** 1. Delayed blood clotting. 2. Hemorrhagic disease of newborn. Vitamin K deficiency symptoms are likely in— 1. Newborn infants, especially if premature and breast-fed. 2. Infants born to mothers receiving anti-coagulants. 3. Obstructive jaundice (lack of bile). 4. Fat absorption defects (celiac disease, sprue). 5. Anticoagulant therapy or toxicity. **Toxicity—**The natural forms of vitamins K_1 and K_2 have not produced toxicity even when given in large amounts. However, synthetic menadione and its various derivatives have produced toxic symptoms in rats and jaundice in human infants when given in amounts of more than 5 mg daily.			*Vitamin K*[1] (mcg)	Vitamin K is fairly widely distributed in foods and is available synthetically. **Rich sources**—Tea (green), turnip greens, broccoli, lettuce, cabbage, beef liver, spinach. **Good sources**— Asparagus, watercress, bacon, coffee, cheese, butter, pork liver, oats. **Fair sources**—Peas (green), wheat (whole), beef fat, ham, beans (green), eggs, pork tenderloin, peaches, ground beef, chicken liver, raisins. **Negligible sources**— Applesauce, bananas, bread, cola, corn, corn oil, milk (cow's), oranges, potatoes, pumpkin, tomatoes, wheat flour. **Supplemental sources**— Chiefly synthetic menadione. The vitamin K values of some common foods is given in Table V-25.	There are two naturally occurring forms of vitamin K: K_1 (phylloquinone, or phytylmenaquinone), and K_2 (menaquinones), multiprenyl-menaquinones. Vitamin K_1 occurs only in green plants. Vitamin K_2 is synthesized by many microorganisms, including bacteria in the intestinal tracts of human beings and other species. There are several synthetic compounds, the best known of which is menadione, formerly known as K_3.
		Infants	0.0–0.5	5		
			0.5–1.0	10		
		Children	1–3	15		
			4–6	20		
			7–10	30		
		Males	11–14	45		
			15–18	65		
			19–24	70		
			25–50	80		
			51+	80		
		Females	11–14	45		
			15–18	55		
			19–24	60		
			25–50	65		
			51+	65		
		Pregnant		65		
		Lactating		65		

[1]*Note well:* The vitamin K values are "Estimated Safe and Adequate Daily Intakes," and not RDA; from *Recommended Dietary Allowances*, 10th ed., NRC–National Academy of Sciences, 1989, p. 285.

Except for newborn babies, no recommended allowances are made for this vitamin because of the synthesis of vitamin K by intestinal bacteria in healthy persons.

The intake suggested for young infants is based on 1 mcg/kg, assuming no intestinal synthesis. Thus, the amount provided by current formulas of 4 mcg/100 kcal should be ample for normal infants. The suggested intake of 10 mcg/day is also in the range supplied by breast milk (15 mg/liter)

(Continued)

TABLE V-9 *(Continued)*

Functions	Deficiency and Toxicity Symptoms	Recommended Daily Allowance			Sources	Comments
		Age Group	Years	Vitamin		
WATER-SOLUBLE VITAMINS: **Biotin** Biotin is required for many reactions in the metabolism of carbohydrates, fats, and proteins. It functions as a coenzyme mainly in decarboxyla-tion-carboxylation and in deamination. Biotin serves as a coenzyme for transferring CO_2 from one compound to another (for decarboxylation—the removal of carbon dioxide; and for carbo-xylation—the addition of carbon dioxide). Numerous decarboxylation and carboxylation reactions are involved in carbohydrate, fat, and protein metabolism; among them, the following:	**Deficiency symptoms**—The deficiency symptoms in man include: a dry scaly dermatitis, loss of appetite, nausea, vomiting, muscle pains, glossitis (inflammation of the tongue), pallor of skin, mental depression, a decrease in hemoglobin and red blood cells, a high cholesterol level, and a low excretion of biotin; all of which respond to biotin administration. There is now substantial evidence that seborrheic dermatitis (an abnormally oily skin, which results in chronic scaly inflammation) of infants under 6 months of age is due to nutritional biotin deficiency. **Toxicity**—There are no known toxic effects.			*Biotin*[1] (mcg)	**Rich sources**— Cheese (processed), kidney, liver, soybean flour. **Good sources**— Cauliflower, chocolate, eggs, mushrooms, nuts, peanut butter, sardines and salmon, wheat bran. **Fair sources**— Cheese (natural), chicken, oysters, pork, spinach, sweet corn, whole wheat flour. **Negligible sources**—Refined cereal products; most fruits and root crops. **Supplemental sources**— Synthetic biotin, yeast (brewers', torula), alfalfa leaf meal (dehydrated). Considerable biotin is synthesized by the micro-organisms in the intestinal tract; and much of it is absorbed, as evidenced by the fact that 3 to 6 times more biotin is excreted in the urine and feces than is ingested. For additional sources and more precise values of biotin, see Food Composition Table F-36.	Biotin is closely related meta-bolically to folacin, pantothenic acid, and vitamin B-12. It is noteworthy that the amount of avidin in raw egg white exceeds the amount of biotin in the whole egg. But, since avidin is destroyed by cooking, the usual diet includes little of the biotin-interfering substance.
		Infants	0.0–0.5	10		
			0.5–1.0	15		
		Children and adolescents	1–3	20		
			4–6	25		
			7–10	30		
			11+	30–100		
		Adults		30–100		

[1]*Note well:* the biotin values are "Estimated Safe and Adequate Daily Intakes," and *not* RDA; from *Recommended Dietary Allowances*, 10th ed., NRC–National Academy of Sciences, 1989, p. 284.

1. Interconversion of pyruvate and oxaloacetate. The formation of oxaloacetate is important because it is the starting point of the tricarboxylic acid cycle (TCA), known also as the Krebs cycle, in which the potential energy of nutrients (ATP) is released for use by the body.
2. Interconversion of succinate and propionate.
3. Conversion of malate to pyruvate.
4. Conversion of acetyl CoA to malonyl CoA, the first step in the formation of long chain fatty acids (fat synthesis).
5. Formation of purines, essential part of DNA and RNA, and for protein synthesis.
6. Conversion of ornithine to citrulline, an important reaction in the formation of urea.

Biotin also serves as a coenzyme for deamination (removal of $-NH_2$) reactions that are necessary for the production of energy from certain amino acids (at least of aspartic acid, serine, threonine); for amino acids to be used as a source of energy, they must first be deaminated—the amino group must be split off.
(Also see BIOTIN.)

(Continued)

TABLE V-9 *(Continued)*

Functions	Deficiency and Toxicity Symptoms	Recommended Daily Allowance			Sources	Comments
		Age Group	Years	Vitamin		
Choline Choline has several important functions; it is vital for the prevention of fatty livers, the transmitting of nerve impulses, and the metabolism of fat. 1. It prevents fatty livers through the transport and metabolism of fats. Without choline, fatty deposits build up inside the liver, blocking its function and throwing the whole body into a state of ill health. 2. It is needed for nerve transmission. Choline combines with acetate to form acetyl-choline, a substance which is needed to jump the gap between nerve cells so that impulses can be transmitted. 3. By a phenomenon known as transmethylation, it serves as a source of labile methyl groups, which facilitate metabolism. (Also see CHOLINE.)	**Deficiency symptoms**—Poor growth and fatty livers are the deficiency symptoms in most species except chickens and turkeys. Chickens and turkeys develop slipped tendons (perosis). In young rats, choline deficiency produces hemorrhagic lesions in the kidneys and other organs. **Toxicity**—No toxic effects have been observed.	The Food and Nutrition Board of the National Research Council does not recommend any human allowance for choline because of lack of evidence of need. The Committee of the American Academy of Pediatrics recommends that choline be added to infant formulas in amounts equivalent to breast milk. Human milk contains about 145 mg of choline per liter, nearly 0.1% of total solids. It is estimated that the average mixed diet for adults in the U.S. contains 400 to 900 mg per day of choline and betaine, or about 0.1 to 0.18% of the diet.			**Rich sources**—Egg yolk, eggs, liver (beef, pork, lamb). **Good sources**—Soybeans, potatoes (dehydrated), cabbage, wheat bran, navy beans, alfalfa leaf meal, dried buttermilk and dried skimmed milk, rice polish, rice bran, whole grains (barley, corn, oats, rice, sorghum, wheat), hominy, turnips, wheat flour, blackstrap molasses. **Negligible sources**—Fruit, fruit juices, milk, vegetables. **Supplemental sources**—Yeast (brewers', torula), wheat germ, soybean lecithin, egg yolk lecithin, and synthetic choline and choline derivatives. Also, the body manufactures choline from methionine, with the aid of folacin and vitamin B-12. So, the needs for choline can be supplied in two ways: (1) by dietary choline, and/or (2) by body synthesis through transmethylation.	It is noteworthy that choline has been known for a very long time. It was isolated in 1849, named in 1862, and synthesized in 1866-67. But the compound did not attract the attention of nutrition investigators at the time. The classification of choline as a vitamin is debated because it does not meet all the criteria for vitamins, especially those of the B vitamins.

(Continued)

TABLE V-9 *(Continued)*

Functions	Deficiency and Toxicity Symptoms	Recommended Daily Allowance			Sources	Comments
		Age Group	Years	Vitamin		
				Folate[1] (mcg)		
Folacin/Folate (Folic acid) In the body, folic acid is changed to at least five active enzyme forms, the parent form of which is tetra-hydrofolic acid. Folacin coenzymes are responsible for the following important functions: 1. The formation of purines and pyrimidines which, in turn, are needed for the synthesis of the nucleic acids DNA and RNA, vital to all cell nuclei. This explains the important role of folacin in cell division and reproduction.	**Deficiency symptoms—** Megaloblastic anemia (of infancy), also called macrocytic anemia (of pregnancy), in which the red blood cells are larger and fewer than normal, and also immature. The anemia is due to inadequate formation of nucleo-proteins, causing failure of the megaloblasts (young red blood cells) in the bone marrow to mature. The hemoglobin level is low because of the reduced number of red blood cells. Also, the white blood cell, blood platelet, and serum folate levels are low. Other symptoms include a sore, red, smooth tongue (glossitis), disturbances of the digestive tract (diarrhea), and poor growth. **Toxicity**—Normally, no toxicity.	Infants	0.0–0.5	25	**Rich sources**—Liver and kidney. **Good sources**— Avocados, beans, beets, celery, chickpeas, eggs, fish, green leafy vegetables (such as asparagus, broccoli, Brussels sprouts, cabbage, cauliflower, endive, lettuce, parsley, spinach, turnip greens), nuts, oranges, orange juice, soybeans, and whole wheat products. **Fair sources**— Bananas, brown rice, carrots, cheese (Cheddar), cod, halibut, rice, and sweet potatoes. **Poor sources**— Chicken, dried milk, milk, most fruits, muscle meats (beef, pork, lamb), products made from highly refined cereals (including white flour), and most root vegetables (including Irish potatoes). **No folacin**—Fats and oils, and sugar supply no folacin. **Supplemental sources**— Yeast, wheat germ, and commercially synthesized folic acid (pteroyl-glutamic acid, or PGA) Intestinal bacterial synthesis of folacin may be important in man, but the amount produced and absorbed has not been determined. For additional sources and more precise values of folacin (folic acid), see Food Compo-sition Table F-36.	There is no single vitamin compound with the name *folacin*; rather, the term folacin is used to designate folic acid and a group of closely related substances which are essential for all vertebrates, including man. Ascorbic acid, vitamin B-12, and vitamin B-6 are essential for the activity of the folacin coenzymes in many of their metabolic processes; again and again pointing up to interdepen-dence of various vitamins. Folacin deficiencies are thought to be a health problem in the U.S. and throughout the world. Infants, adolescents, and pregnant women are particularly vulnerable. The folacin requirement is increased by tropical sprue, certain genetic disturbances, cancer, parasitic infection, alcoholism, and oral contra-ceptives. Raw vegetables stored at room temperature for 2 to 3 days lose as much as 50 to 70% of their folate content. Between 50 and 95% of food folate is destroyed in cooking.
			0.5–1.0	35		
		Children	1–3	50		
			4–6	75		
			7–10	100		
		Males	11–14	150		
			15–18	200		
			19–24	200		
			25–50	200		
			51+	200		
		Females	11–14	150		
			15–18	180		
			19–24	180		
			25–50	180		
			51+	180		
		Pregnant		400		
		Lactating		280		

[1]*Recommended Dietary Allowances*, 10th ed., NRC–National Academy of Sciences, 1989, p. 285.

The RDA are expressed in terms of "total" folacin; that is, the amount of folic acid activity available from all food folates.

2. The formation of heme, the iron-containing protein in hemoglobin.
3. The interconversion of the three-carbon amino acid serine from the two-carbon amino acid glycine.
4. The formation of the amino acids tyrosine from phenylalanine and glutamic acid from histidine.
5. The formation of the amino acid methionine from homocysteine.
6. The synthesis of choline from ethanolamine.
7. The conversion of nicotinamide to N-methylnicotinamide, one of the metabolites of niacin that is excreted in the urine.

(Also see FOLACIN.)

(Continued)

TABLE V-9 *(Continued)*

Functions	Deficiencies and Toxicity Symptoms	Recommended Daily Allowance					Sources	Comments
		Age Group	Years	Calories	Protein	Niacin[1]		
				(kcal)	(g)	(mg NE)		

Niacin (Nicotinic acid; nicotinamide) The principal role of niacin is as a constituent of two important coenzymes in the body: nicotinamide adenine and dinucleotide (NAD) and nicotinamide adenine dinucleotide phosphate (NADP). These coenzymes function in many important enzyme systems that are necessary for cell respiration. They are involved in the release of energy from carbohydrates, fats, and protein. NAD and NADP are also involved in the synthesis of fatty acids, protein, and DNA. Also, niacin is thought to (1) have a specific effect on growth, (2) reduce the levels of cholesterol, and (3) protect to some degree against nonfatal myocardial infarction. However, because of possible undesirable side effects, massive doses should be under the direction of a physician. (Also see NIACIN.)

Deficiency symptoms—A deficiency of niacin results in pellagra, the symptoms of which are: dermatitis, particularly of areas of skin which are exposed to light or injury; inflammation of mucous membranes, including the entire gastrointestinal tract, which results in a red, swollen, sore tongue and mouth, diarrhea, and rectal irritation; and psychic changes, such as irritability, anxiety, depression, and in advanced cases, delirium, hallucinations, confusion, disorientation, and stupor. **Toxicity**—Only large doses of niacin, sometimes given to an individual with mental illness, are known to be toxic. However, ingestion of large amounts may result in vascular dilation, or "flushing" of the skin, itching, liver damage, elevated blood glucose, elevated blood enzymes, and/or peptic ulcer.

Age Group	Years	Calories (kcal)	Protein (g)	Niacin[1] (mg NE)
Infants	0–.5	650	13	5
	.5–1	850	14	6
Children	1–3	1,300	16	9
	4–6	1,800	24	12
	7–10	2,000	28	13
Males	11–14	2,500	45	17
	15–18	3,000	59	20
	19–24	2,900	58	19
	25–50	2,900	63	19
	51+	2,300	63	15
Females	11–14	2,200	46	15
	15–18	2,200	44	15
	19–24	2,200	46	15
	25–50	2,200	50	15
	51+	1,900	50	13
Pregnant		+300	60	17
Lactating		+500	65	20

[1]*Recommended Dietary Allowances*, 10th ed., NRC–National Academy of Sciences, 1989, p. 285. Calorie values from p. 33, Table 3–5 of the same report.
On the average, 1 mg of niacin is derived from each 60 mg of dietary tryptophan.

Sources: Generally speaking, niacin is found in animal tissues as nicotinamide and in plant tissues as nicotinic acid. Both forms are of equal niacin activity. **Rich sources**—The best food sources of niacin are liver, kidney, lean meats, poultry, fish, rabbit, corn flakes (enriched), nuts, peanut butter. **Good sources**—Milk, cheese, and eggs, although low in niacin content, are good antipellagra foods, because of their high tryptophan content, and because their niacin is in available form. Other good sources are: bran flakes, sesame seed, sunflower seed. Also, enriched cereal flours and products are good sources of niacin. **Negligible sources**—Cereals (corn, wheat, oats, rice, rye) tend to be low in niacin. Moreover, 80 to 90% of the niacin is in the bran layer (outer seed coat) and removed in milling; and the niacin may be present in bound form (i.e. niacytin) and unavailable. Fruits, roots, vegetables (other than mushrooms and legumes), butter, and sugar (white) are insignificant sources of niacin. **Supplemental sources**—Both synthetic nicotinamide and nicotinic acid are commercially available. For pharmaceutical use, nicotinamide is usually used; for food nutrification, nicotinic acid is usually used. Also, yeast is a rich natural source of niacin. For additional sources and more precise values of niacin, see Food Composition Table F-36.

Comments: Although nicotinic acid was prepared and named in 1867, it took another 70 years before it was known that it would cure blacktongue in dogs and pellagra in humans. An average mixed diet in the U.S. provides about 1% protein as tryptophan. Thus, a diet supplying 60 g of protein contains about 600 mg of tryptophan, which will yield about 10 mg of niacin (on the average, 1 mg of niacin is derived from each 60 mg of dietary tryptophan). Niacin is the most stable of the B-complex vitamins. Cooking losses of a mixed diet usually do not amount to more than 15 to 25%. Born of centuries of experience, (1) in Mexico, corn has long been treated with lime water before making tortillas; and (2) the Hopi Indians of Arizona have long roasted sweet corn in hot ashes. Both practices liberate the nicotinic acid in corn.

(Continued)

TABLE V-9 *(Continued)*

Functions	Deficiency and Toxicity Symptoms	Recommended Daily Allowance			Sources	Comments
		Age Group	Years	Vitamin		
Pantothenic acid (Vitamin B-3) Pantothenic acid functions in the body as part of two enzymes— coenzyme A (CoA) and acyl carrier protein (ACP). CoA functions in the following important reactions: 1. The metabolic processes by which carbo- hydrates, fats, and proteins are broken down and energy is released. 2. The formation of acetyl- choline, a sub- stance of importance in transmitting nerve impulses. 3. The synthesis of porphyrin, a precursor of heme, of importance in hemoglobin synthesis. 4. The synthesis of cholesterol and other sterols. 5. The steroid hormones formed by the adrenal and sex glands. 6. The mainten- ance of normal blood sugar, and the forma- tion of anti- bodies. 7. The excretion of sulfonamide drugs. ACP, along with CoA, required by the cells in the biosynthesis (the building up) of fatty acids. (CoA, without ACP, is involved in the breakdown of fatty acids.) (Also see PANTOTHENIC ACID.)	**Deficiency symptoms**— Pantothenic acid defi- ciency has been produced in human volunteers by either (1) feeding semi- synthetic diets low in pantothenic acid, or (2) adding a pantothenic antagonist to the diet. The symptoms: irritableness and restlessness; loss of appetite, indigestion, abdominal pains, nausea; headache; sullenness, mental depression; fatigue, weakness; numbness and tingling of hands and feet, muscle cramps in the arms and legs; burning sensation in the feet; insomnia; respiratory infections; rapid pulse; and a staggering gait. Also, in these subjects there was increased reaction to stress; increased sensitivity to insulin, resulting in low blood sugar levels; increased sedimentation rate for erythrocytes; decreased gastric secretions; and marked decrease in antibody production. **Toxicity**—Pantothenic acid is relatively nontoxic. However, doses of 10 to 20 g per day may result in occasional diarrhea and water retention.			*Pantothenic Acid*[1] (mg)	**Rich sources**— Organ meat (liver, kidney, and heart), cottonseed flour, wheat bran, rice bran, rice polish. **Good sources**— Nuts, mushrooms, soybean flour, salmon, blue cheese, eggs, buckwheat flour, brown rice, lobster, sunflower seeds. **Fair sources**— Chicken, broccoli, sweet peppers, whole wheat flour, avocados. **Negligible sources**— Butter, corn flakes, white flour, fats and oils, mar- garine, precooked rice, sugar. **Supplemental sources**— Synthetic calcium pantothenate is widely used as a vitamin supple- ment. Yeast is a rich natural supplement. Intestinal bacteria synthesize pantothenic acid, but the amount and availability is unknown. For additional sources and more precise values of pantothenic acid, see Food Compo- sition Table F-36.	Coenzyme A, of which pantothenic acid is a part, is one of the most important substances in body metabolism. The following two facts indicate that there may be need for dietary supplementation of pantothenic acid for buoyant good health: 1. Losses of up to 50%, and even more, of the pantothenic content of foods may occur from production to consumption. 2. Deficiencies of pantothenic acid occur in farm animals fed natural rations (which are much less refined than human foods); hence, panto- thenic acid is commonly added to com- mercial poultry and swine rations.
		Infants	.0– 0.5	2		
			.5– 1.0	3		
		Children and adolescents	1.0– 3.0	3		
			4.0– 6.0	3-4		
			7.0–10.0	4-5		
			11.0+	4-7		
		Adults		4-7		

[1]*Note well:* The pantothenic acid values are "Estimated Safe and Adequate Daily Intakes," and *not* RDA; from *Recommended Dietary Allow- ances,* 10th ed., NRC–National Academy of Sciences, 1989, p. 284.

TABLE V-9 *(Continued)*

Functions	Deficiency and Toxicity Symptoms	Recommended Daily Allowance			Sources	Comments
		Age Group	Years	Vitamin		
				Riboflavin[1] (mg)		
Riboflavin (Vitamin B-2) Riboflavin has an essential role in the oxidative reductions in all body cells by which energy is released. Thus, riboflavin functions in the metabolism of amino acids, fatty acids, and carbohydrates. Riboflavin, through its role in activating pyridoxine (vitamin B-6), is necessary for the formation of niacin from the amino acid tryptophan. Riboflavin is thought to be (1) a component of the retinal pigment of the eye; (2) involved in the functioning of the adrenal gland; and (3) required for the production of corti-costeroids in the adrenal cortex. (Also see RIBOFLAVIN.)	**Deficiency symptoms**— Unlike all the other vitamins, riboflavin deficiency is not the cause of any severe or major disease of man. Rather, riboflavin often contributes to other disorders and disabilities such as beriberi, pellagra, scurvy, keratomalacia, and nutritional megaloblastic anemia. Riboflavin deficiency symptoms are: sores at the angles of the mouth (angular stomatitis); sore, swollen, and chapped lips (cheilosis); swollen, fissured, and painful tongue (glossitis); redness and congestion at the edges of the cornea of the eye; and oily, crusty, scaly skin (seborrheic dermatitis). **Toxicity**—There is no known toxicity of riboflavin.	Infants	0.0–0.5	0.4	**Rich sources**— Organ meats (liver, kidney, heart). **Good sources**— Corn flakes (enriched), almonds, cheese, eggs, lean meat (beef, pork, lamb), mushrooms (raw), wheat flour (enriched), turnip greens, wheat bran, soybean flour, bacon, cornmeal (enriched). **Fair sources**— Chicken (dark meat), white bread (enriched), rye flour, milk, mackerel and sardines, green leafy vegetables, beer. **Negligible sources**—Fruits (raw), roots and tubers, white sugar, fats and oils (butter, margarine, salad oil, shortening). **Supplemental sources**—Yeast (brewers', torula). Riboflavin is the only vitamin present in significant amounts in beer. For additional sources and more precise value of riboflavin (B-2), see Food Composition Table F-36.	Body storage of riboflavin is very limited; so, day-to-day needs must be supplied in the diet. Two properties of riboflavin may account for major losses: (1) it is destroyed by light; and (2) it is destroyed by heat in an alkaline solution. Because riboflavin is heat stable in neutral or acid solutions and only slightly soluble in water, little of it is lost in home cooking or commercial canning.
			0.5–1.0	0.5		
		Children	1–3	0.8		
			4–6	1.1		
			7–10	1.2		
		Males	11–14	1.5		
			15–18	1.8		
			19–24	1.7		
			25–50	1.7		
			51+	1.4		
		Females	11–14	1.3		
			15–18	1.3		
			19–24	1.3		
			25–50	1.3		
			51+	1.2		
		Pregnant		1.6		
		Lactating		1.8		

[1]*Recommended Dietary Allowances*, 10th ed., NRC–National Academy of Sciences, 1989, p. 285.

(Continued)

TABLE V-9 *(Continued)*

Functions	Deficiency and Toxicity Symptoms	Recommended Daily Allowance				Sources	Comments
		Age Group	Years	Vitamin			
				Cal-ories (kcal)	*Thia-min* [1] (mg)		
Thiamin (Vitamin B-1) As a coenzyme in energy metabolism. Without thiamin, there could be no energy. As a coenzyme in the conversion of glucose to fats— the process called transketolation (Keto-carrying). In the functioning of the peripheral nerves. In this role, it has value in the treatment of alcoholic neuritis, the neuritis of pregnancy, and beriberi. In direct functions in the body, including (1) main-tenance of normal appetite, (2) the tone of the muscles, and (3) a healthy mental attitude. (Also see THIAMIN.)	**Deficiency symptoms**— Moderate thiamin deficiency symptoms include fatigue; apathy (lack of interest); loss of appetite; nausea; moodiness; irritability; depression; retarded growth; a sensation of numbness in the legs; and abnormalities of the electro-cardiogram. More advanced thiamin deficiency is reflected in the gastrointestinal system, the nervous system, and the cardio-vascular system. Severe thiamin deficiency of long duration culminates in beriberi, the symptoms of which are polyneuritis (inflammation of the nerves), emaciation and/or edema, and disturbances of heart function. Additional symptoms of thiamin deficiency include low excretion of thiamin in the urine; electro-cardiogram measurement; reduced transketolase activity of the red blood cells; and increase of pyruvic acid in the blood. **Toxicity**—None, for there are no known toxic effects from thiamin.	Infants	0.0–0.5	650	0.3	Thiamin is found in a large variety of animal and vege-table products but is abundant in few. **Rich sources**—Lean pork (fresh and cured), sunflower seed, corn flakes (enriched), peanuts, cottonseed flour, safflower flour, soybean flour. **Good sources**— Wheat bran, kidney, wheat flour (enriched), rye flour, nuts (except peanuts, which are a rich source), whole wheat flour, cornmeal (enriched), rice (enriched), white bread (enriched), soybean sprouts. **Fair sources**—Egg yolk, peas, turkey (hamloaf), beef liver, luncheon meat, crab, mackerel (fried), salmon steak (broiled), roe (cod, herring), lima beans, refried beans, lentils. **Negligible sources**—Most fruits, most vegetables, polished rice, white sugar, animal and vegetable fats and oils, milk, butter, margarine, eggs, alcoholic beverages. **Supplemental sources**—Thiamin hydrochloride, thiamin mononitrate, yeast (brewers', torula), rice bran, wheat germ, and rice polish. Enriched flour (bread) and cereal which was initiated in 1941, has been of special significance in improving the dietary level of thiamin in the U.S. For additional sources and more precise values of thiamin, see Food Composition Table F-36.	A patient with wet beriberi—lying in bed breathless, water-logged, and apparently dying— may recover in one to two hours after being given an injection of thiamin. This is perhaps the most dramatic cure in medicine. Synthetic thiamin is usually marketed as thiamin hydro-chloride or thiamin mononitrate. Antithiamin factors are present in certain raw fish and seafood, live yeast, tea and fermented tea leaves, and alcohol.
			0.5–1.0	850	0.4		
		Children	1–3	1,300	0.7		
			4–6	1,800	0.9		
			7–10	2,000	1.0		
		Males	11–14	2,500	1.3		
			15–18	3,000	1.5		
			19–24	2,900	1.5		
			25–50	2,900	1.5		
			51+	2,300	1.2		
		Females	11–14	2,200	1.1		
			15–18	2,200	1.1		
			19–24	2,200	1.1		
			25–50	2,200	1.1		
			51+	1,900	1.0		
		Pregnant		+300	1.5		
		Lactating		+500	1.6		

[1]*Recommended Dietary Allowances*, 10th ed., NRC–National Academy of Sciences, 1989, p. 285.
1 kcal = 4.184 kj (kilojoules)
1,000 kj = 1 mj (megajoules)
Because the principal functions of thiamin are concerned in energy metabolism, its requirement by the body bears a direct relation to the energy intake.

(Continued)

TABLE V-9 *(Continued)*

Functions	Deficiency and Toxicity Symptoms	Recommended Daily Allowance			Sources	Comments
		Age Group	Years	Vitamin		
Vitamin B-6 (Pyridoxine; pyridoxal; pyridoxamine) Vitamin B-6, in its coenzyme forms, usually as pyridoxal phosphate but sometimes as pyridoxamine phosphate, is involved in a large number of physiologic functions, particularly: 1. In protein (nitrogen) metabolism, including— a. Transamination b. Decarboxylation c. Deamination d. Transsulfuration e. Tryptophan conversion to nicotinic acid. f. Hemoglobin formation. g. Absorption of amino acids. 2. In carbohydrate and fat metabolism, including— a. The conversion of glycogen to glucose-1-phosphate. b. The conversion of linoleic acid to arachidonic acid. 3. In clinical problems, including— a. Central nervous system disturbances. b. Autism, a mental and emotional affliction in children. c. Anemia that is iron-resistant. d. Kidney stones. e. Tuberculosis, in countering the antagonistic drug isonicotinic acid used in its treatment. f. Physiologic demands in pregnancy. g. Oral contraceptives. (Also see VITAMIN B-6).	**Deficiency symptoms**—In adults, the deficiency symptoms are: greasy scaliness (seborrheic dermatitis) in the skin around the eyes, nose, and mouth, which subsequently spread to other parts of the body; a smooth, red tongue; loss of weight; muscular weakness; irritability; mental depression. In infants, the deficiency symptoms are: irritability, muscular twitchings, and convulsions. **Toxicity**—B-6 is relatively nontoxic. But large doses may result in sleepiness and be habit-forming when taken over an extended period.			*Vitamin B-6*[1] (mg)	**Rich sources**—Rice bran, wheat bran, sunflower seed. **Good sources**—Avocados, bananas, corn, fish, kidney, lean meat, liver, nuts, poultry, rice (brown), soybeans, whole grain. **Fair sources**—Eggs, fruits (except bananas and avocados, which are good sources), milk, vegetables. **Negligible sources**—Cheese (Cheddar, cottage), fat, milk, sugar, white bread. **Supplemental sources**—Pyridoxine hydrochloride is the most commonly available synthetic form; and yeast (torula, brewers'), rice polish, and wheat germ are used as natural source supplements. For additional sources and more precise values of vitamin B-6 (pyridoxine), see Food Composition Table F-36.	In rats, the three forms of vitamin B-6 have equal activity; and it is assumed that the same applies to man. Processing or cooking foods may destroy up to 50% of the B-6. Because vitamin B-6 is limited in many foods, supplemental B-6 with synthetic pyridoxine hydrochloride may be indicated, especially for infants and during pregnancy and lactation.
		Infants	0.0–0.5 0.5–1.0	0.3 0.6		
		Children	1–3 4–6 7–10	1.0 1.1 1.4		
		Males	11–14 15–18 19–24 25–50 51+	1.7 2.0 2.0 2.0 2.0		
		Females	11–14 15–18 19–24 25–50 51+	1.4 1.5 1.6 1.6 1.6		
		Pregnant		2.2		
		Lactating		2.1		

[1]*Recommended Dietary Allowances*, 10th ed., NRC–National Academy of Sciences, 1989, p. 285.

(Continued)

TABLE V-9 *(Continued)*

Functions	Deficiency and Toxicity Symptoms	Recommended Daily Allowance			Sources	Comments
		Age Group	Years	Vitamin		
Vitamin B-12 (Cobalamins) In the body, vitamin B-12 functions in two coenzyme forms: coenzyme B-12, and methyl B-12. Vitamin B-12 coenzymes perform the following physiological roles at the cellular level, especially in the cells of the bone marrow, nervous tissue, and gastrointestinal tract: 1. Red blood cell formation and control of pernicious anemia. 2. Maintenance of nerve tissue. 3. Carbohydrate, fat, and protein metabolism. 4. Synthesis or transfer of single carbon units. 5. Biosynthesis of methyl groups (-CH3), and in reduction reactions such as the conversion of disulfide (S-S) to the sulfhydryl group (-SH). In the following therapeutic uses: 1. The control of pernicious anemia. 2. In the treatment of sprue. (Also see VITAMIN B-12.)	**Deficiency symptoms—** Vitamin B-12 deficiency in man may occur as a result of (1) dietary lack, which sometimes occurs among vegetarians who consume no animal food; or (2) deficiency of intrinsic factor due to pernicious anemia, total or partial removal of the stomach by surgery, or infestation with parasites such as the fish tapeworm. The common symptoms of a dietary deficiency of vitamin B-12 are: sore tongue, weakness, loss of weight, back pains, tingling of the extremities, apathy, and mental and other nervous abnormalities. Anemia is rarely seen in dietary deficiency of B-12. In pernicious anemia, the characteristic symptoms are: abnormally large red blood cells, lemon-yellow pallor, anorexia, dyspnea, prolonged bleeding time, abdominal discomfort, loss of weight, glossitis, an unsteady gait, and neurological disturbances, including stiffness of the limbs, irritability, and mental depression. Without treatment death follows. **Toxicity—**No toxic effects of vitamin B-12 are known.			*Vitamin B-12*[1] (mcg)	**Rich sources**—Liver and other organ meats—kidney, heart. **Good sources—** Muscle meats, fish, shellfish, eggs, and cheese. **Fair sources—**Milk, poultry, yogurt. **Negligible sources—** Bread (both whole wheat and white), cereal grains, fruits, legumes, vegetables. **Supplemental sources—** Cobalamin, of which there are at least three active forms, produced by microbial growth; available at the corner drugstore. Some B-12 is synthesized in the intestinal tract of human beings. However, little of it may be absorbed. For additional sources and more precise values of vitamin B-12, see Food Composition Table F-36.	Plants cannot manufacture vitamin B-12. Hence, little is found in vegetables, grains, legumes, and fruits. Vitamin B-12, like so many other members of the B complex, is not a single substance; rather, it consists of several closely related compounds with similar activity. Vitamin B-12 is the largest and the most complex of all vitamin molecules. It is noteworthy (1) that vitamin B-12 is the only vitamin that requires a specific gastrointestinal tract secretion for its absorption (intrinsic factor); and (2) that the absorption of vitamin B-12 in the small intestine requires about 3 hours (compared to seconds for most of the other water-soluble vitamins).
		Infants	0.0–0.5	0.3[2]		
			0.5–1.0	0.5		
		Children	1–3	0.7		
			4–6	1.0		
			7–10	1.4		
		Males	11–14	2.0		
			15–18	2.0		
			19–24	2.0		
			25–50	2.0		
			51+	2.0		
		Females	11–14	2.0		
			15–18	2.0		
			19–24	2.0		
			25–50	2.0		
			51+	2.0		
		Pregnant		2.2		
		Lactating		2.6		

[1]*Recommended Dietary Allowances*, 10th ed., NRC–National Academy of Sciences, 1989, p. 285.
[2]The recommended dietary allowance for vitamin B-12 in infants is based on average concentration of the vitamin in human milk. The allowances after weaning are based on energy intake (as recommended by the American Academy of Pediatrics) and consideration of other factors, such as intestinal absorption.

(Continued)

TABLE V-9 *(Continued)*

Functions	Deficiency and Toxicity Symptoms	Recommended Daily Allowance			Sources	Comments
		Age Group	**Years**	**Vitamin**		

Functions	Deficiency and Toxicity Symptoms	Age Group	Years	Vitamin C[1] (mg)	Sources	Comments
Vitamin C (Ascorbic acid) Formation and maintenance of collagen, the substance that binds body cells together. So, vitamin C makes for more rapid and sound healing of wounds and burns. Metabolism of the amino acids tyrosine and tryptophan. Absorption and movement of iron. Metabolism of fats and lipids, and cholesterol control. Sound teeth and bones. Strong capillary walls and healthy blood vessels. Metabolism of folic acid. (Also see VITAMIN C.)	**Deficiency symptoms— Early symptoms, called latent scurvy:** loss in weight, listlessness, fatigue, fleeting pains in the joints and muscles, irritability, shortness of breath, sore and bleeding gums, small hemorrhages under the skin, bones that fracture easily, and poor wound healing. **Scurvy:** swollen, bleeding, and ulcerated gums; loose teeth; malformed and weak bones, fragility of the capillaries with resulting hemorrhages throughout the body; large bruises; big joints, such as the knees and hips, due to bleeding into the joint cavity; anemia; degeneration of muscle fibers; including those of the heart; and tendency of old wounds to become red and break open. Sudden death from severe internal hemorrhage and heart failure is always a danger. **Toxicity**—Adverse effects reported of intakes in excess of 8 g per day (more than 100 times the recommended allowance) include: nausea, abdominal cramps, and diarrhea; absorption of excessive amounts of iron; destruction of red blood cells; increased mobilization of bone minerals; interference with anticoagulant therapy; formation of kidney and bladder stones; inactivation of vitamin B-12; rise in plasma cholesterol; and possible dependence upon large doses of vitamin C.	Infants	0.0–0.5	30	Natural sources of vitamin C occur primarily in foods of plant origin— fruits (especially citrus fruits) and leafy vegetables. **Richest natural sources**—Acerola cherry, *camu-camu,* and rose hips. **Excellent sources** —Raw, frozen, or canned citrus fruit or juice: oranges, grapefruit, lemons, and limes. Guavas, peppers (green, hot), black currants, parsley, turnip greens, poke greens, and mustard greens. **Good sources**— Green leafy vegetables: broccoli, Brussels sprouts, cabbage (red), cauliflower, collards, kale, lamb's-quarter, spinach, Swiss chard, and watercress. Also, cantaloupe, papaya, strawberries, and tomatoes and tomato juice (fresh or canned). **Fair sources**—Apples, asparagus, bananas, blackberries, blueberries, Irish potatoes, lima beans, liver, peaches, pears, sweet potatoes. **Negligible sources**—Cereal grains and their by-products, cow's milk, eggs, fats, fish, meat, nuts, poultry, sugar. **Supplemental sources**—Vitamin C (ascorbic acid) is available wherever vitamins are sold. For additional sources and more precise values of vitamin C, see Food Composition Table F-36.	Actually, several compounds have vitamin C activity. So, the term vitamin C is a combined name for all of them. The terms ascorbic acid and dehydro-ascorbic acid should be used when specific reference is made to them. All animal species appear to require vitamin C, but dietary need is limited to humans, guinea pigs, monkeys, fruit-eating bats, red-vented bulbul birds, certain fish, and perhaps certain reptiles. Of all the vitamins, ascorbic acid is the most unstable. It is easily destroyed during storage, processing, and cooking; it is water-soluble, easily oxidized, and attacked by enzymes.
			0.5–1.0	35		
		Children	1–3	40		
			4–6	45		
			7–10	45		
		Males	11–14	50		
			15–18	60		
			19–24	60		
			25–50	60		
			51+	60		
		Females	11–14	50		
			15–18	60		
			19–24	60		
			25–50	60		
			51+	60		
		Pregnant		70		
		Lactating		95		

[1]*Recommended Dietary Allowances*, 10th ed., NRC–National Academy of Sciences, 1989, p. 285.
0.05 mg of ascorbic acid = 1 IU of vitamin C.

(Continued)

TABLE V-9 *(Continued)*

Functions	Deficiency and Toxicity Symptoms	Recommended Daily Allowance			Sources	Comments
		Age Group	Years	Vitamin		
VITAMINLIKE SUBSTANCES: **Bioflavonoids** (Vitamin P) Bioflavonoids function as follows: 1. They influence capillary fragility and permeability, perhaps together with vitamin C; increasing the strength of the capillaries and regulating their permeability. These actions help prevent hemorrhages and ruptures in the capillaries and connective tissues and build a protective barrier against infection.	**Deficiency symptoms**—The symptoms of bioflavonoid deficiency are closely related to those of a vitamin C deficiency. The tendency to bleed (hemorrhage) or bruise easily are especially noted. **Toxicity**—Bioflavonoids are nontoxic.	There are no NRC-National Academy of Sciences recommended daily allowances (RDA) of bioflavonoids. The average daily intake of flavonoids in the American diet amounts to about 1 g, of which one-half (0.5 g) is absorbed from the gut. The label on a rather typical vitamin C-bioflavonoid supplement reads as follows: *Each tablet contains:* *(mg)* Rose hip powder . . . . .500 Vitamin C . . . . .500 Lemon bioflavonoid . . . . .500 Rutin (buckwheat) . . . . 50 *Note:* Need in human nutrition not established			**Rich sources**— Citrus peel (especially orange and lemon peel), white pulp of citrus fruits, tangerine juice, rose hips, buckwheat leaves. **Good sources**— Onions with colored skins, leafy vegetables, fruit, coffee, tea, cocoa, red wine, beer. **Poor sources**— Frozen orange juice, most root vegetables.	Bioflavonoids are a group of natural pigments in vegetables, fruits, flowers, and grains. They appear as companions of natural vitamin C, but they are not present in synthetic vitamin C. Bioflavonoids do not fill the two prerequisites of a vitamin; they are not essential food constituents, and deficiency symptoms which can be cured by their administration are unknown. *At this time, no evidence exists that bioflavonoids serve any useful role in human nutrition or in the prevention or treatment of disease in humans; hence, this presentation is for two purposes (1) informational, and (2) stimulation of research.*

2. They are active antioxidant compounds in food, ranking second only to the fat-soluble tocopherols in this regard.
3. They possess metal-chelating capacity; and they affect the activity of the enzymes and membranes.
4. They have a synergistic effect on ascorbic acid, and they appear to stabilize ascorbic acid in human tissues.
5. They possess a bacteriostatic and/or antibiotic effect, which is sufficiently high to account for the measurable antiinfectious properties of normal daily food.
6. They possess anticarcinogenic activity in two ways; a cytostatic effect against malignant cells and a biochemical protection of the cell from damage by carcinogenic substances.

(Also see BIOFLAVONOIDS.)

(Continued)

TABLE V-9 *(Continued)*

Functions	Deficiency and Toxicity Symptoms	Recommended Daily Allowance			Sources	Comments
		Age Group	Years	Vitamin		
Carnitine (Vitamin B-T) Carnitine plays an important role in fat metabolism and energy production in mammals. It functions as follows: 1. *Transport and oxidation of fatty acids.* Carnitine plays an important role in the oxidation of fatty acids by facilitating their transport across the mitochondrial membrane.	**Deficiency symptoms—** If the body's supply of carnitine is low, the cells cannot get the fatty acids they need for energy production and growth. This is rare, but life-threatening! The symptoms of carnitine deficiency include muscle weakness, failure to thrive, poor growth, recurrent infections, cardiomyopathy, and hypoglycemia. **Toxicity—**Not known.	Under normal conditions, there is no dietary requirement for carnitine. However, where a metabolic abnormality exists which inhibits synthesis, interferes with use, or increases catabolism of carnitine, illness may follow, which is sometimes relieved by dietary supplement. There is need for further research on the dietary role of carnitine in human health and disease.			Generally speaking, carnitine is high in animal foods and low in plant foods. Few foods have been assayed for carnitine, but based on available data, the following evaluation of dietary sources of carnitine may be helpful. **Rich sources—** Muscle meat, liver, heart, yeast (torula and brewers'), chicken, rabbit, milk, whey. **Good sources—** Avocado, casein, wheat germ. **Poor sources—** Cabbage, cauliflower, peanuts, wheat. **Negligible sources—** Barley, corn, egg, orange juice, spinach.	Carnitine, a vital conenzyme in animal tissues and involved in fat metabolism, is another vitaminlike substance that has received much attention recently. It is similar to a vitamin with the exception that under normal conditions higher animals synthesize their total needs within their bodies; hence, no need appears to exist to supply this substance in food on a daily basis. The lower level of carnitine in plant foods in comparison with animal foods is explainable on the basis that plant materials are most likely deficient in the essential amino acids, lysine and methionine, precursors of carnitine. Thus, a vegetarian diet will likely be low in carnitine, in both preformed carnitine and the amino acid precursors of carnitine.

Carnitine is part of the shuttle mechanism whereby long-chain fatty acids are made into acyl carnitine derivatives and transported across the mitochondrial membrane, which is impermeable to long-chain fatty acids *per se* and to their coenzyme A esters. Once across the membrane, the acyl carnitines are reconverted to their fatty acid CoA form and undergo B-oxidation to liberate energy.
2. *Fat synthesis.* Although this role is controversial, carnitine appears to be involved in transporting acetyl groups back to the cytoplasm for fatty acid synthesis.
3. *Ketone body utilization.* Carnitine stimulates acetoacetate oxidation; thus, it may play a role in ketone body utilization.
(Also see CARNITINE.)

(Continued)

TABLE V-9 *(Continued)*

Functions	Deficiency and Toxicity Symptoms	Recommended Daily Allowance			Sources	Comments
		Age Group	Years	Vitamin		
Coenzyme Q (Ubiquinone) Coenzyme Q functions in the respiratory chain in which energy is released from the energy-yielding nutrients as ATP. There is evidence that specific ubiquinones function in the remission (prevention) of some of the symptoms of vitamin E deficiency. (Also see COENZYME Q.)	**Deficiency symptoms**—Nonspecific. **Toxicity**—Unknown.	Coenzyme Q is synthesized in the body. So, dietary allowance seems unimportant.			Quinones occur widely in aerobic organisms, from bacteria to higher plants and animals. Because they are synthesized in the body, they cannot be considered a true vitamin. The entire series of ubiquinones has been prepared synthetically.	Coenzyme Q, or ubiquinone, is a collective name for a number of ubiquinones— lipidlike compounds that are chemically somewhat similar to vitamin E. The importance of coenzyme Q as a catalyst for respiration imparts status as an essential metabolite. It may have other significant roles. For man and other higher animals a simple precursor substance with an aromatic ring may have vitaminlike status, but dietary ubiquinone seems, on the whole, to be unimportant unless it provides the aromatic nucleus for endogenous (body) synthesis.
Inositol The functions of inositol are not completely understood, but the following roles have been suggested: 1. It has a lipo-tropic effect (an affinity for fat, like choline). In this role, inositol aids in the metabolism of fats and helps reduce blood cholesterol. 2. In combination with choline, inositol pre-vents the fatty hardening of arteries and protects the heart.	**Deficiency symptoms**—Myo-inositol is a "growth factor" for certain yeasts and bacteria, and for several lower organisms up to and including several species of fish. Earlier experiments indicated that a deficiency of inositol caused retarded growth and loss of hair in young mice, and loss of hair around the eyes (spectacled-eyes) in rats. But these symptoms are now being questioned because the experimental diets used were partially deficient in certain other vitamins. **Toxicity**—There is no known toxicity of inositol.	Need for inositol in human nutrition has not been established. So, no recommended daily allowance is given. Most authorities feel that people should consume about the same amount of inositol as choline. Therapeutic doses, which should be under the supervision of a physician, range from 500 to 1,000 mg daily.			Inositol is abundantly present in nature. **Rich sources**— Kidney, brain, liver, yeast, heart, wheat germ, citrus fruits, and blackstrap molasses **Good sources**— Muscle meat, fruits, whole grains, bran of cereal grains, nuts, legumes, milk, and vegetables. In animal cells, inositol occurs as a component of phospholipids. In plant cells, it is found as phytic acid, an organic acid that binds calcium, iron, and zinc in an insoluble complex and interferes with their absorption.	There is no evidence that humans cannot synthesize all the inositol needed by the body. So, its classification as a vitamin is disputed. More properly perhaps, it should be classified as an essential nutrient, rather than a vitamin, for certain species of bacteria and animals.

3. It appears to be a precursor of the phosphoinosities, which are found in various body tissues, especially in the brain. (Also see INOSITOL.)

TABLE V-9 *(Continued)*

Functions	Deficiency and Toxicity Symptoms	Recommended Daily Allowance			Sources	Comments
		Age Group	Years	Vitamin		

Laetrile
(Vitamin B-17, amygdalin, nitrilosides)
According to its advocates, Laetrile or amygdaline is a highly selective substance that attacks only the cancerous cells. They explain this phenomenon as follows: Upon being absorbed by normal body cells, the enzyme rhodanese detoxifies the cyanide, which is then excreted through the urine. But cancer cells are completely deficient in rhodanese; instead, they are surrounded by another enzyme, beta-glucosidase, which releases the bound cyanide from the Laetrile at the site of the malignancy. So, Laetrile is believed to attack only the malignant cells.

Deficiency symptoms—The advocates claim that prolonged deficiency of amygdalin may lead to lowered resistance to malignancies.
Toxicity—None reported. But not more than 1.0 g should be taken at one time because of the hazard of hydrogen cyanide poisoning.

The usual dosage is 0.25 to 1.0 g taken at meals. Cumulative daily amounts of more than 3.0 g are sometimes taken, *but more than 1.0 g should never be taken at any one time.*
According to the advocates, 5 to 30 apricot kernels eaten through the day may be effective as a preventive of cancer, but they should not be eaten all at one time.

A concentration of 2 to 3% Laetrile is found in the whole kernels of most fruits, including apricots, apples, cherries, peaches, plums, and nectarines.

Note well: Laetrile has no known value for humans. The authors present this section relative to the controversial compound for informational purposes only. Further, it is listed with the vitaminlike substances because it is sometimes erroneously designated as vitamin B-17. Both the pros and cons relative to Laetrile are given, then the reader may make a judgment.

Regardless of the validity of the claims and counter claims pertaining to Laetrile, it is noteworthy that more and more medical authorities are accepting the nutrition approach in the prevention and treatment of cancer. Although the results of such nutrients as Laetrile, vitamin A (carotene), folic acid, and vitamin C, along with a general supplemental program of minerals and vitamins are significant for cancer treatment, perhaps even more important in the long run is the apparent success of nutrients of many kinds in strengthening the body's immune system.

Those who oppose Laetrile, submit evidence that it is not effective as a treatment.
Those who support the use of Laetrile do so primarily on the basis that it is a preventive of cancer, rather than as a treatment of cancer.
(Also see LAETRILE.)

Lipoic acid
Lipoic acid functions as a coezyme. It is essential, together with the thiamin-containing enzyme, pyrophosphatase

Deficiency symptoms—No characteristic deficiency symptoms have been produced.
Toxicity—Not known.

Because the body can synthesize the needed lipoic acid, no dietary requirement for humans and animals has been established.

Yeast and liver.

Lipoic acid is not a true vitamin because it can be synthesized in the body and is not necessary in the diet of animals. However, it functions in the same manner as many of the B-complex vitamins.

(TPP), for reactions in carbohydrate metabolism which convert pyruvic acid to acetyl-coenzyme A. Lipoic acid, which has two sulfur bonds of high-energy potential, combines with TPP to reduce pyruvate to active acetate, thereby sending it into the final energy cycle. It joins the intermediary products of protein and fat metabolism in the Krebs cycle in the reactions involved in producing energy from these nutrients. A metal ion (magnesium or calcium) is involved in this oxidative decarboxylation, along with lipoic acid and four vitamins: thiamin, pantothenic acid, niacin, and riboflavin.
(Also see LIPOIC ACID.)

(Continued)

TABLE V-9 (*Continued*)

Functions	Deficiency and Toxicity Symptoms	Recommended Daily Allowance			Sources	Comments
		Age Group Years		Vitamin		
Pangamic acid (Vitamin B-15) Numerous functions have been attributed to pangamic acid; among them, the following: 1. Stimulation of transmethylation reactions. 2. Stimulation of oxygen uptake. 3. Inhibition of fatty liver formation. 4. Adaptation to increased physical activity. 5. Control of blood cholesterol levels. (Also see PANGAMIC ACID.)	**Deficiency symptoms—** There is indication that a deficiency of pangamic acid may cause fatigue (a tired feeling), hypoxia (an insufficient supply of oxygen in blood cells), heart disease, and glandular and nervous disorders. **Toxicity—**The so-called "Russian formula" appears to be relatively free of toxicity.	No NRC-National Academy of Sciences recommended daily allowances (RDA) have been established. But the usual dosage of pangamic acid is from 150 to 300 mg daily.			**Rich sources—**All cereals and cereal products, with corn and rice particularly rich. Also, apricot kernels and brewers' yeast. **Good sources—** Wherever B-complex vitamins are found in natural foods.	*The authors make this presentation for two primary purposes: (1) informational, and (2) stimulation of research. The nutritional status and biological role(s) of pangamic acid await clarification. Its stimulation of such fundamental processes as*

transmethylation, cellular respiration, etc. may have physiological application. Certainly, there is sufficient indication of the value of pangamic acid as a therapeutic agent to warrant further study. In the meantime, pangamic acid should not be taken unless prescribed by a physician.
Pangamic acid is a vitaminlike substance, rather than a vitamin.
FDA classifies it as a food additive.
It has been widely studied and accepted in the U.S.S.R. as a necessary food factor (with important physiological actions.) The Russians have used pangamic acid in treating cardiovascular disorders associated with insufficiency of oxidative metabolism, and in the treatment of liver disorders, a number of skin diseases, and some toxicoses.

Functions	Deficiency and Toxicity Symptoms	Recommended Daily Allowance	Sources	Comments
Para-aminobenzoic acid (PABA) For man and other higher animals, PABA functions as an essential part of the folacin molecule. **Human pharmaceutical uses—** PABA is sometimes used as a human pharmaceutical, not as a vitamin, in the following: as an antirickettsial; to counteract the bacteriostatic action of sulfonamides; and as a protective agent against sunburn.	**Deficiency symptoms—** Sulfa drugs may induce a deficiency of not only PABA, but of folic acid as well. The symptoms: fatigue, irritability, depression, nervousness, headache, constipation, and other digestive disorders **Toxicity—**PABA is not known to be toxic to man. But continued high doses may result in nausea and vomiting.	The need for PABA has not been established; hence, it follows that there is no recommended daily allowance.	Food composition tables do not list PABA, but the following foods are generally recognized as the richest sources: brewers' yeast, fish, soybeans, peanuts, beef liver, eggs, wheat germ, lecithin, molasses.	In addition to having activity as a growth factor for certain bacteria, PABA has considerable folacin activity when fed to deficient animals in which intestinal synthesis of folacin takes place. For example, in rats and mice, it can completely replace the dietary source of folacin. This explains why para-amino-benzoic acid was once considered to be a vitamin in its own right. For man and other higher animals, PABA has no vitamin activity in animals receiving ample folacin, and it is not required in the diet; hence, it can no longer be considered a vitamin.

1. **Antirickettsial.** PABA is sometimes used in the treatment of certain rickettsial diseases—diseases in man and animals caused by microscopically small parasites of the genus *Rickettsia*, notably thypus and Rocky Mountain spotted fever.
2. **Sulfonamide antagonist.** PABA has the ability to reverse the bacteriostatic effects of sulfonamides, thereby counter-acting their action. This is an antimetabolite action, explainable on the basis of similarity of structures. According to this theory, sulfonamides suppress bacterial growth by replacing their chemical analog PABA in bacterial enzyme systems; PABA in excess reverses the effect.
3. **Sunscreen agent.** PABA is used for protection against sunburn; usually about 5% PABA is incorporated in an ointment, to be applied over exposed parts of the body.
(Also see FOLACIN; and PARA-AMINOBENZOIC ACID.)

(*Continued*)

TABLE V-9 *(Continued)*

Functions	Deficiency and Toxicity Symptoms	Recommended Daily Allowance			Sources	Comments
		Age Group	Years	Vitamin		
Vitamin B-13 (Orotic acid) Vitamin B-13 has been found to stimulate the growth of rats, chicks, and pigs under certain conditions. Orotic acid is utilized by the body in the metabolism of folic acid and vitamin B-12. Also, it appears to aid the replacement or restoration of some cells. There is indication that vitamin B-13 may be helpful in the treatment of multiple sclerosis. (Also see VITAMIN B-13.)	**Deficiency symptoms—** Deficiency symptoms have not been proven. But it is believed that a deficiency may lead to liver disorders, cell degeneration, and premature aging; and to degenerative symptoms in multiple sclerosis victims. **Toxicity**—Not reported.	Dietary requirements are not known.			Vitamin B-13 is found in such natural sources as distillers' solubles, whey, soured or curdled milk, and root vegetables. Also, this nutrient is available in supplemental form as calcium orotate.	It is highly possible that the so-called vitamin B-13 is a growth promotant and a preventive of certain disorders. At this time, however, it is not known whether it plays an essential role in an otherwise adequate diet.

VITAMIN A

Contents

Vitamin A is probably the most important of all vitamins, if any vitamin can be singled out and ranked. More than any other vitamin, deficiencies of vitamin A are still widespread throughout most developing countries of the world and involve millions of people, especially children.

Vitamin A is required by man and all other animals. It is strictly a product of animal metabolism—present in all species of mammals, birds, and fish, no vitamin A being found in plants. The counterpart in plants is known as carotene, which is the precursor of vitamin A. Because the animal body can transform carotene into vitamin A, this compound is often spoken of as *provitamin A.*

Carotene, which derives its name from the carrot, from which it was first isolated over 100 years ago, is the yellow-colored, fat-soluble substance that gives the characteristic color to carrots and many other vegetables and to several fruits.

Thus, the ultimate source of all vitamin A is the carotenes which are synthesized by plants. Man and other animals convert a considerable proportion of the foods they eat into vitamin A.

VITAMIN A . . .

needed for growth, healthy eyes, skin and other tissues

TWO RATS FROM SAME LITTER, 11 WEEKS OLD

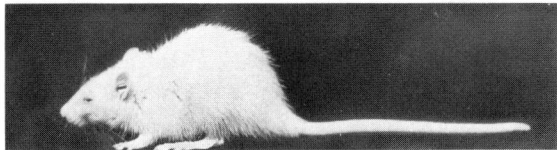

THIS RAT HAD NO VITAMIN A. NOTE THE INFECTED EYE, ROUGH FUR, AND SICK APPEARANCE. IT WEIGHED ONLY 53 g.

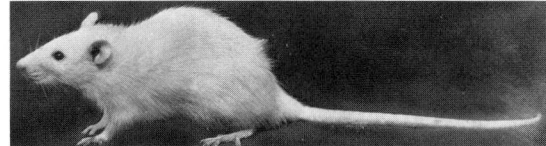

THIS RAT HAD PLENTY OF VITAMIN A. IT HAS BRIGHT EYES, SLEEK FUR, AND APPEARS ALERT AND VIGOROUS. IT WEIGHED 123 g.

TOP FOOD SOURCES

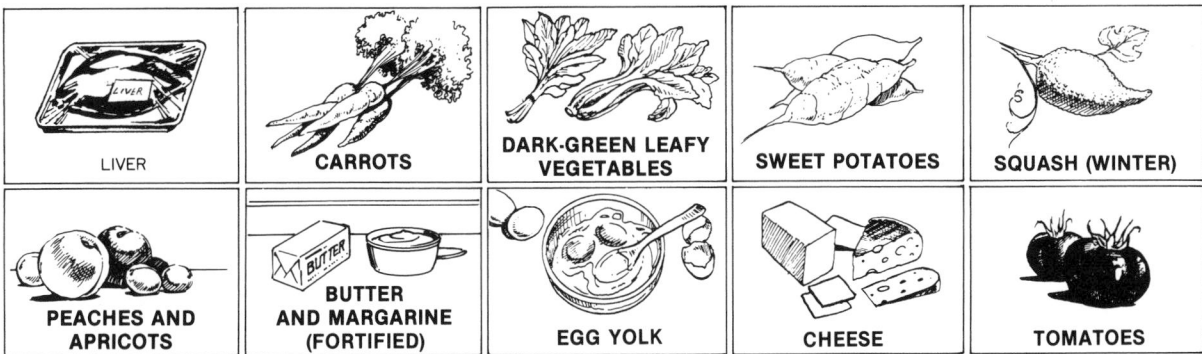

LIVER | CARROTS | DARK-GREEN LEAFY VEGETABLES | SWEET POTATOES | SQUASH (WINTER)

PEACHES AND APRICOTS | BUTTER AND MARGARINE (FORTIFIED) | EGG YOLK | CHEESE | TOMATOES

Fig. V-19.   Vitamin A made the difference! *Left:* Rat on vitamin A- deficient diet. *Right:* Rat that received plenty of vitamin A. (Adapted from USDA sources) Note, too, ten top food sources of vitamin A.

HISTORY. At a very early date, the Chinese used a concoction rich in vitamin A as a remedy for night blindness; and, in ancient Greece, Hippocrates prescribed various forms of liver, a good source of preformed vitamin A, as a treatment for night blindness. But it remained for laboratory experiments conducted in the early 1900s to identify vitamin A as a distinct nutrient.

In 1913, vitamin A was discovered by Elmer V. McCollum and Marguerite Davis of the University of Wisconsin, and by Thomas B. Osborne and Lafayette B. Mendel of the Connecticut Experiment Station. Working independently, each research team demonstrated the presence of an essential dietary substance in fatty foods. McCollum and Davis found it in butterfat and egg yolks; Osborne and Mendel discovered it in cod-liver oil. These researchers believed that only one factor, which they called fat-soluble A, was needed to supplement purified diets. They described the condition as the "type of nutritive deficiency exemplified in the form of an infectious eye disease prevalent in animals inappropriately fed." In 1915, McCollum and Davis also noted that a deficiency of fat-soluble A caused night blindness.

In 1919, Steenbock and co-workers at the University of Wisconsin noted that an unknown substance, present in sweet potatoes, carrots, and corn, later to be identified as carotene, would support normal growth and reproduction.

In 1920, the English scientist Drummond proposed that this compound be called vitamin A.

In 1930, Moore, of England, demonstrated that this pro-vitamin A activity was beta-carotene.

In 1931, P. Karrer, a Swiss researcher, isolated the active substance in halibut-liver oil and determined the chemical formula for vitamin A—the first vitamin to have its chemical structure determined. For this, and for his work with riboflavin, he received the Nobel Prize. However, vitamin A was not produced (by Karrer) in crystalline form from fish liver oils until 1937, and it did not become available in synthetic form (by Isler working in Switzerland) until 1947. Today, pure, inexpensive synthetic forms of vitamin A are readily available.

CHEMISTRY, METABOLISM, PROPERTIES.

• **Chemistry**—*Vitamin A* may be a misleading term because it sounds as if only one chemical compound has vitamin A activity. Actually, several forms of vitamin A exist, with each possessing different degrees of activity.

There are two forms of vitamin A as such, retinol and dehydroretinol. Retinol (formerly called vitamin A), which is found as an ester (retinyl palmitate) in ocean fish oils and fats, and in liver, butterfat, and egg yolk, is biologically active as an alcohol, an aldehyde, and an acid. The alcohol, the most common form (see Fig. V-20 for formula), is usually referred to as retinol, the aldehyde as retinal or retinene, and the acid as retinoic acid.

Dehydroretinol, or vitamin A_2, differs from retinol in that (1) it has an extra double bond, and (2) it has about 40% the biological value (activity). It is found only in freshwater fish and in birds that eat these fish; hence, it is of limited interest.

Today, the general term *vitamin A* is used for both *retinol* and *dehydroretinol.*

In addition to the actual forms of vitamin A, related compounds, known as *carotenes,* are found in several fruits and vegetables. Carotene is also called (1) provitamin A, because it can be converted to vitamin A in the body; and (2) precursor of vitamin A, because it precedes vitamin A. At least 10 of the carotenoids found in plants can be converted with varying efficiencies into vitamin A. Four of these carotenoids—alpha-carotene, beta-carotene, gamma-carotene, and cryptoxanthine (the main carotenoid of corn)—are of particular importance due to their provitamin A activity. Of the four, *beta-carotene* (see Fig. V-21) has the highest vitamin A activity and provides about two-thirds of the vitamin A necessary for human nutrition.

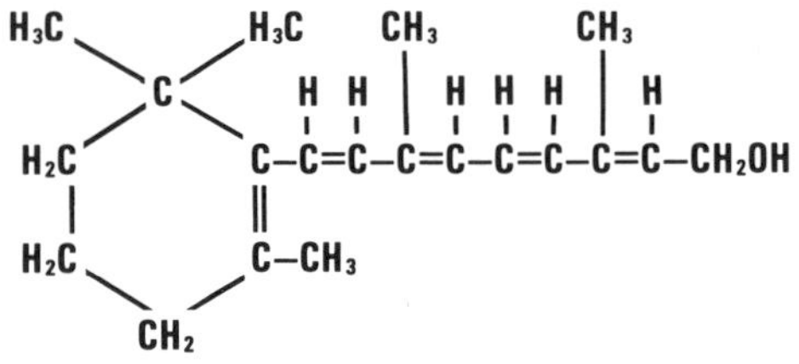

Fig. V-20.   The structure of vitamin A (retinol).

• **Metabolism**—Foods supply vitamin A in the form of vitamin A, vitamin A esters, and carotenes. Almost no absorption of vitamin A occurs in the stomach. In the small intestine, vitamin A and beta-carotene are emulsified with bile salts and products of fat digestion and absorbed in the intestinal mucosa. Here, much of the conversion of beta-carotene to vitamin A (retinol) takes place. There are wide differences in species and individuals as to how well they utilize the carotenoids. Their absorption is affected by several factors, including the presence in the small intestine of bile, dietary fat, and antioxidants. Bile aids emulsificatiion; fat must be absorbed simultaneously; and antioxidants, such as alpha-tocopherol and lecithin, decrease the oxidation of carotene. Also, the presence of enough protein of good quality enhances the conversion of carotene to vitamin A—a matter of great importance in developing countries where protein is limited in both quantity and quality.

The absorption of vitamin A is adversely affected by the presence of mineral oil in the intestinal tract. Since mineral oil is not absorbed, and since it holds carotene and vitamin A in solution, carotene and vitamin A are lost through excretion. Therefore, mineral oil should never be used as a substitute for regular fats in food preparation (for example, as a salad dressing); neither should it be taken at mealtime when it is used as a laxative. It is noteworthy, too, that intestinal parasites adversely affect the absorption of vitamin A and carotene and the conversion of carotene to vitamin A—a factor of importance in tropical regions where intestinal parasite infections are common.

In the blood, vitamin A esters are transported in association with a retinol-binding protein, whereas the carotenoids are associated with the lipid-bearing protein. Storage of vitamin A is largely in the liver, but small amounts are also stored in the lungs, body fat, and kidneys. The amount of body storage of vitamin A tends to increase with age, but of course this depends on the quantity in the diet and the amount absorbed. It is estimated that a normal adult may store sufficient vitamin A in his liver to meet his needs for 4 to 12 months. Infants and children do not build up such reserves; hence, they are much more susceptible to deficiencies.

From the liver, vitamin A enters the bloodstream as a free alcohol, whereupon it travels to the tissues for use.

No vitamin A is excreted in the urine because it is not water-soluble, but considerable unabsorbed carotene is normally found in the feces.

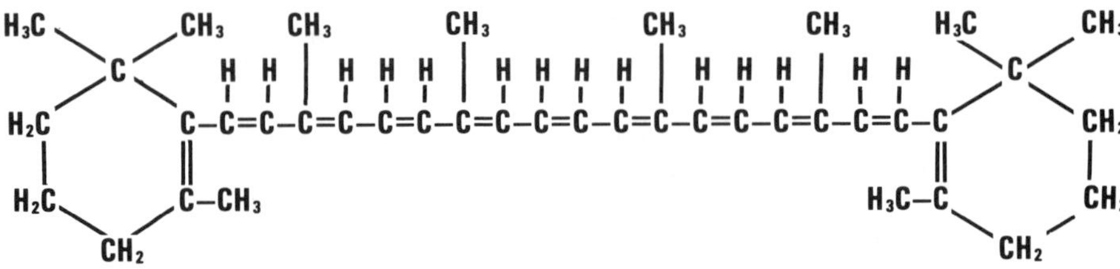

Fig. V-21.   The structure of beta-carotene.

• **Properties**—Vitamin A (retinol) is an almost colorless (pale yellow) fat-soluble substance. It is insoluble in water; hence, there is no loss by extraction from cooking. Although the esters of vitamin A are relatively stable compounds, the alcohol, aldehyde, and acid forms are rapidly destroyed by oxidation when they are exposed to air and light. Since vitamin A occurs in the stable form (the ester) in most foods, normal preparation procedures do not destroy much vitamin A activity. However, fats that undergo oxidative rancidity, can lose their vitamin A rapidly. We depend mainly on storage in a cool, dark place (refrigeration) and on added antioxidants, such as vitamin E, to protect fats and oils from vitamin A loss.

The carotenoid pigments (which are referred to as carotene in this discussion) are deep red color, but in solution they are bright yellow or orange yellow. They impart the color to many fruits and vegetables, including apricots, peaches, carrots, sweet potatoes, squash, pumpkins, and yellow corn. As a general rule of thumb, the more intense the pigmentation in these foods, the higher the provitamin A content. Green vegetables, particularly dark green and leafy ones, are also rich in provitamin A. They contain carotenoids, although their color is masked by that of the green pigment, chlorophyll. The properties of solubility and stability of carotene and carotenoid pigments are similar to those of vitamin A.

The yellow color of beta-carotene is so intense that it is widely used as a coloring agent by the food industry. For such purposes, beta-carotene is valued more for its aesthetic contribution than its nutritive value, although the potential vitamin A value of the food it colors is also increased.

MEASUREMENT/ASSAY.

The assay of vitamin A is accomplished by two basic methods: biological, or chemical. The bioassay procedure is based on a biological response such as growth of rats or chicks deficient in vitamin A. It measures the total vitamin A, including provitamin A, present. But, because of the difficulties and time factor in bioassays, chemical assays are usually used.

Until recently, dietary allowances of vitamin A were stated in terms of either International Units (IU) or United States Pharmacopeia (USP) units, which are equal. An International Unit (IU) of vitamin A is defined on the basis of rat studies as equal to 0.344 mcg of crystalline retinylacetate (which is equivalent to 0.300 mcg of retinol, or to 0.60 mcg of beta-carotene). These standards were based on experiments that showed that in rats only about 50% of the beta-carotene is converted to vitamin A. In man, however, beta-carotene is not as available as in the rat, due to poorer absorption in the intestines and other factors, with the result that various factors have been used to compensate for this when vitamin A activity of foods and diets have been expressed in IU.

In order to quantify vitamin A values for humans within the metric system, therefore, international agencies have now introduced the biological equivalent of 1 microgram (1 mcg) of retinol as the standard. In 1967, the FAO/WHO proposed that vitamin A allowances be expressed as the equivalent weight of retinol, and that the use of IU be discontinued. The United Kingdom adopted this change and coined the term "Retinol Equivalent" (RE). The U.S. Food and Nutrition Board (National Academy of Science,

National Research Council) and Canada followed suit. The RE system of measurement takes into account the amount of absorption of the carotenes as well as the degree of conversion to vitamin A; hence, it is more precise than the IU system.

In terms of International Units, beta-carotene (by weight) is ½ as active, and the other provitamin A carotenoids are ¼ as active, as retinol. Also, retinol is completely absorbed by the intestine, but only about ⅓ of the intake of provitamin A carotenoids is absorbed. Of the absorbed carotenoids, only ½ of the beta-carotene and ¼ of the other provitamin A carotenoids are converted to retinol. It follows that beta-carotene is only 1/6 as active, and the other carotenoids 1/12 as active, as retinol.

The vitamin A values in the food composition tables of this book are in International Units.[12]

But the recommended daily allowances (RDA) are expressed in both IU and RE.

The relationships and equivalents between International Units, Retinol Equivalents, beta-carotene, and the other provitamin A carotenoids are detailed in the rest of this section.[13]

International Units can be converted to micrograms as follows:

1 IU (or 1 USP unit) of vitamin A
 = 0.3 mcg retinol
 = 0.344 mcg retinyl acetate
 = 0.6 mcg beta-carotene
 = 1.2 mcg other mixed carotene with vitamin A activity

Vitamin A values can be converted to Retinol Equivalents as follows:

1 Retinol Equivalent of vitamin A
 = 1 mcg retinol
 = 6 mcg beta-carotene
 = 12 mcg other provitamin A carotenoids
 = 3.33 IU retinol
 = 10 IU beta-carotene

To calculate the Retinol Equivalents in a diet or foodstuff, one of the following equations should be used:

1. If retinol and beta-carotene are given in mcg, then:

$$\text{mcg retinol} + \frac{\text{mcg beta-carotene}}{6} = \text{Retinol Equivalents}$$

EXAMPLE: A diet contains 500 mcg retinol and 1,800 mcg beta-carotene—

$$500 + \frac{1,800}{6} = 800 \text{ Retinol Equivalents}$$

---

[12]Both the FAO/WHO and the FNB recommend that, in the future, foods be analyzed separately for (1) retinol, (2) beta-carotene, and (3) other provitamin A carotenoids, for inclusion in food composition tables, and that (4) total RE, as micrograms, also be listed in the tables. Until this information is available, we will primarily employ the still widely used IU values.

[13]These relationships and equivalencies were derived from studies on rats; and it has been assumed that they apply to human beings.

2. If both retinol and beta-carotene are given in IU, then:

$$\frac{\text{IU of retinol}}{3.33} = \frac{\text{IU of beta-carotene}}{10} = \text{Retinol Equivalents}$$

EXAMPLE: A diet contains 1,666 IU of retinol and 3,000 IU of beta-carotene—

$$\frac{1,666}{3.33} + \frac{3,000}{10} = 800 \text{ Retinol Equivalents}$$

3. If beta-carotene and other provitamin A carotenoids are given in mcg, then:

$$\frac{\text{mcg beta-carotene}}{6} + \frac{\text{mcg other carotenoids}}{12} = \text{Retinol Equivalents}$$

EXAMPLE: A 100-g sample of sweet potatoes contains 2,400 mcg beta-carotene and 480 mcg of other provitamin A carotenoids—

$$\frac{2,400}{6} + \frac{480}{12} = 440 \text{ Retinol Equivalents}$$

This method of evaluating the vitamin A content of foods is recommended because the vitamin A requirement depends on the proportion of vitamin A (retinol) to provitamin A (carotene) in the diet.

FUNCTIONS. Vitamin A is essential for a number of physiological processes; among them, (1) vision, (2) growth, (3) bone development, (4) tooth development, (5) maintenance of healthy epithelial tissues, (6) protective effect against cancer, (7) reproduction, and (8) coenzyme and hormone roles.

It is noteworthy that the basic physiological functions of vitamin A are, in general, common to man and all other animals. These follow:

• **Vision**—The best understood function of vitamin A is related to the maintenance of normal vision in dim light —the prevention of night blindness. The retina of the eye —the light-sensitive inside layer at the back of the eye which may be likened to the film of a camera—contains two kinds of light receptors: the rods for vision in dim light, and the cones for vision in bright light and color vision. (The terms "rods" and "cones" are derived from the shape of the cells.) *Rhodopsin* (*visual purple*) is the pigment in the rods that contains vitamin A; iodopsin is the main pigment in the cones that contains vitamin A. All of the pigments are composed of the same vitamin A fraction (retinol) but of different proteins. Opsin is the protein of rhodopsin.

The visual cycle proceeds as follows: When light strikes the normal retina, this pigment—called rhodopsin (visual purple)—is bleached to another pigment known as retinaldehyde (visual yellow). As a result of this change, images are transmitted to the brain through the optic nerve. Rhodopsin is rebuilt in the dark, but some vitamin A is lost in the reactions, and rod vision is impaired unless sufficient vitamin A is supplied by the blood from the diet or body stores to replace it. The ability of the eyes to adjust to changes from bright light to dim light is reduced. This condition is known as *night blindness*, or nyctalopia. Fig. V-22 shows, in simplified form, the role of vitamin A in vision.

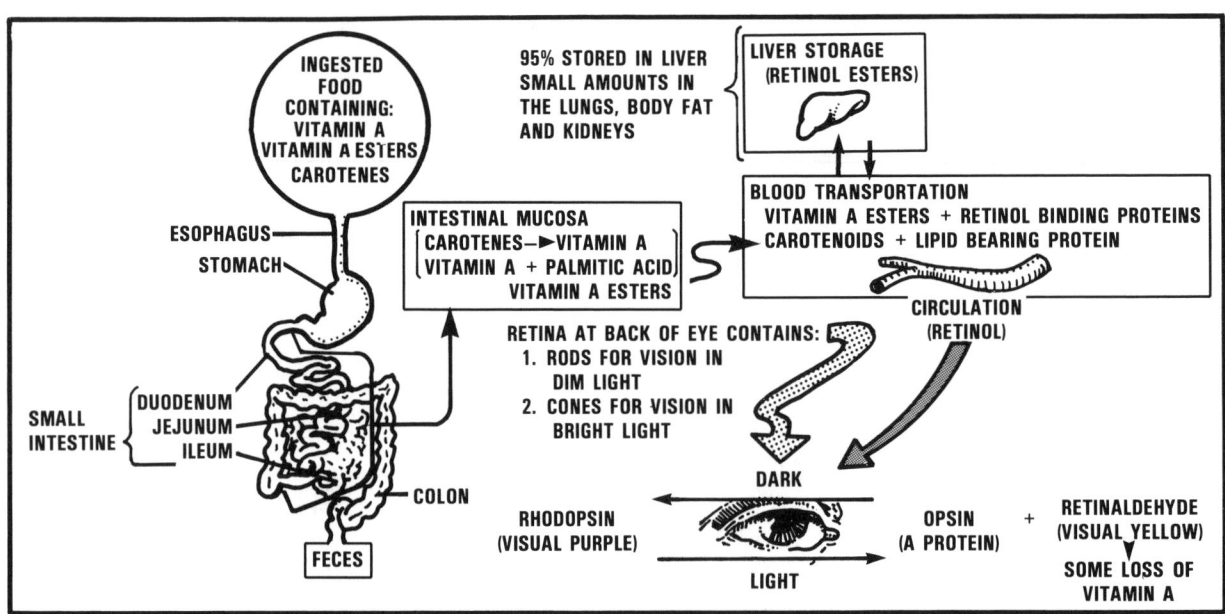

Fig. V-22. Metabolism of vitamin A and its role in vision in dim light.

The cones are not as sensitive to changes in the amount of vitamin A as the rods. Thus, vision in bright light and color vision are not affected to any extent in the early stages of vitamin A deficiency.

Night blindness is the earliest symptom of vitamin A deficiency in humans. It first manifests itself as a slow, dark adaptation, thence it progresses to total night blindness. In man, the "dark adaptation test," which measures the eyes' ability to recover visual activity in dim light, is used as a means of determining vitamin A status. However, night blindness or dark adaptation tests are not always reliable in diagnosing a deficiency. Measurements of serum vitamin A and carotene values in comparison with known standards are most useful. Serum levels of 10 to 19 mcg of vitamin A, or of 20 to 39 mcg of carotene, per 100 ml are considered low.

Night blindness can usually be cured in a half hour or so by the injection of vitamin A. It is noteworthy that both retinol and retinaldehyde are effective in the visual process, but retinoic acid has no visual function; if retinoic acid is the only form of vitamin A fed to experimental animals, blindness results.

In 1967, the Nobel Prize in Medicine was awarded to Dr. George Wald of Harvard University, who clarified the role of vitamin A in vision, which, to that time, had been an extremely complicated picture.

Night blindness has a long medical history, associated with diet. It is common in Newfoundland among fishermen working in open boats in bright sunshine with their eyes exposed to the glare on the water. There, it is said that if a man cannot see at night his vision will be restored by the next night if he eats the liver of a codfish or of a sea gull.

Vision can also be impaired because of *xerophthalmia* (from the *Latin* words for *dry* and *eye*), another manifestation of a vitamin A deficiency. In this condition, the conjunctiva (the covering of the eye) dries out, the cornea becomes inflamed, and the eyes become ulcerated. It may progress to blindness in extreme deficiency of vitamin A. Xerophthalmia is a very common disease in infants and undernourished children in those parts of the world where the deficiency is prevalent; but it may be prevented by including in the diet a good source of vitamin A.

• **Growth**—Vitamin A aids in the building and growth of body cells; hence, it is essential for body growth. Because of this, prior to the time that vitamin A was isolated and its chemical formula determined, its potency in food was measured by growth rate. Since animals on a vitamin A-free diet stop growing when their bodies are depleted of its stores, foods to be assessed were fed to these animals in known amounts for a prescribed period of time and their growth response noted. Better growth meant a higher vitamin A content in the food. Also, it has long been known that vitamin A is essential for the growth of children and for the normal development of babies before birth.

Although the relationship of vitamin A to growth was the first function studied, its role in the growth process is poorly understood. Experimental animals on vitamin A-deficient diets lose their appetites and fail to grow. The loss of appetite is attributed to the loss of the sense of taste because of keratinization (drying out) of the taste buds. When supplements of retinol or of retinoic acid are given in amounts to bring about growth, sense of taste returns to normal.

• **Bone development**—Vitamin A is especially needed for bone growth. If the intake is not sufficient, the bones will stop growth before the soft tissues are affected. Thus, if the brain and spinal cord grow too fast for the stunted skull and spinal column, injury of brain and nerves may occur and paralysis and various other neurological signs may result. In some cases, there is a constriction of the bone canal through which the optic nerve passes, thereby resulting in blindness. It is noteworthy, however, that a deficiency of vitamin A may cause degeneration of the nervous tissue without causing bone malformation.

• **Tooth development**—Vitamin A is essential for normal tooth development. Like other epithelia, the enamel-forming cells are affected by lack of vitamin A; instead of an even protective layer of enamel, fissures and pits will be present and the teeth will tend to decay. Also, when there is a shortage of vitamin A, the odontoblasts which form dentine become atrophied.

• **Maintenance of healthy epithelial tissues**—Epithelial tissues are of two kinds: (1) those that cover the outer surface of the body—the resistant, protective skin (epidermis); and (2) those that line all the tubular system—the secretory mucous membranes. Without vitamin A, the epithelial cells become dry and flat, and gradually harden to form scales that slough off. This process is known as keratinization. The skin may become rough, dry and scaly; and the membranes lining the nose, throat, and other air passages, and the gastrointestinal and genitourinary tracts, may become keratinized. Whenever these tissue changes occur, the natural mechanism for protection against bacterial invasion is impaired and the tissue may become infected easily. It follows that vitamin A deficiency commonly manifests itself in those parts that are particularly susceptible to infections. Vitamin A is also necessary for the health of the membranes lining the stomach and intestinal wall, and for the health of the sex glands, uterus, and the membranes that line the bladder and urinary passages. Renal calculi (kidney stones) may be related to the keratinization of the urinary tract.

Although adequate vitamin A is necessary to maintain healthy epithelial tissues, excessive intakes will not increase resistance to infections which enter through the epithelium.

• **Protective effects against cancer**—Vitamin A, either as retinol or carotene, appears to play an important nutritional role in keeping the body free of certain kinds of cancer, especially cancers of epithelial tissue (the skin and various membranes that line the mouth, internal passages, and hollow organs). This does not call for megadoses of vitamin A; rather, it indicates that getting sufficient vitamin A in the daily diet is likely a very important anticancer measure.

• **Reproduction**—In most animals, the absence of vitamin A in the diet will dramatically reduce reproductive ability. In the male rat, spermatogenesis stops; in the female, there may be an abnormal estrus cycle, fetal resorption, or congenital malformations. In rabbits, there is a reduction in fertility and an increase of abortion in pregnant does. Hatchability is significantly reduced when hens are fed a vitamin A-deficient ration. Lack of vitamin A in the diet of pregnant women during the first trimester (the first 3 months) may cause miscarriage.

Quite often, retinoic acid, the acid form of vitamin A, is used to study the effects of vitamin A deficiency on reproduction, because it can be substituted freely for retinol and retinaldehyde (the aldehyde form of vitamin A) for all physiological functions except reproduction and vision.

• **Coenzyme and hormone roles**—New information suggests that vitamin A (1) acts in a coenzyme role, as for instance in the form of intermediates in glycoprotein synthesis; and (2) functions like steroid hormones, with a role in the cell nuclei, leading to tissue differentiation.

• **Other functions of vitamin A**—Studies have indicated that vitamin A deficiency reduces the rate of thyroxine formation and increases the incidence of goiter in people. Also, protein synthesis is adversely affected by vitamin A deficiency. Animal studies indicate that vitamin A functions in the synthesis of corticosterone from cholesterol, resulting in a decrease in the body's capacity to synthesize glycogen.

DEFICIENCY SYMPTOMS. A deficiency of vitamin A may be due to a dietary lack of vitamin A and/or provitamin A, or to poor absorption. A diet that contains an insufficiency of vitamin A activity will, in due time, cause night blindness, xerosis, or xerophthalmia, stunted growth; slowed bone growth; unsound teeth; rough, dry, scaly skin; increased sinus trouble, sore throat, and abscesses in the ears, mouth, or salivary glands; and increased diarrhea and kidney and bladder stones.

It is noteworthy that vitamin A deficiency symptoms, and their prominence, vary from one species to another, as is true for other vitamins. Common deficiency symptoms follow:

• **Night blindness, xerosis, and xerophthalmia**—The earliest symptom of a vitamin A deficiency is the inability to see in dim light—the condition known as night blindness (nyctalopia). Night driving—facing the bright lights of oncoming vehicles—is difficult, and even dangerous, for persons whose eyes are slow to adjust.

The next symptom (following night blindness) to appear is usually xerosis (dryness) of the conjunctiva (the delicate membrane that lines the eyelids and covers the exposed surface of the eyeball), in which there may be (1) wrinkling, pigmentation, and accumulation of debris, and (2) loss of transparency.

When associated with generalized xerosis in children, Bitot's spots (named for the French physician who first discovered them)—which appear as small plaques of silvery gray, usually with a foamy surface, on the conjunctiva—are usually caused by a deficiency of vitamin A. However, in adults these spots may have another cause.

Extreme vitamin A deficiency over a long period of time may cause xerophthalmia, characterized by the following stages: (1) the cornea (the transparent membrane that coats the outer surface of the eye) becomes dry, then inflamed and edematous; (2) the eyes become cloudy and infected, which leads to ulceration; and (3) keratomalacia, a softening and keratinizing of the cornea, culminating in permanent blindness if the disease is not arrested. Xerophalmia occurs most frequently in undernourished infants and children in India, the Middle East, Southeast Asia, and parts of Africa and South America. It has been estimated that throughout the world (exclusive of China) about 80,000 children become blind each year from vitamin A deficiency, and that about one-half of these die.

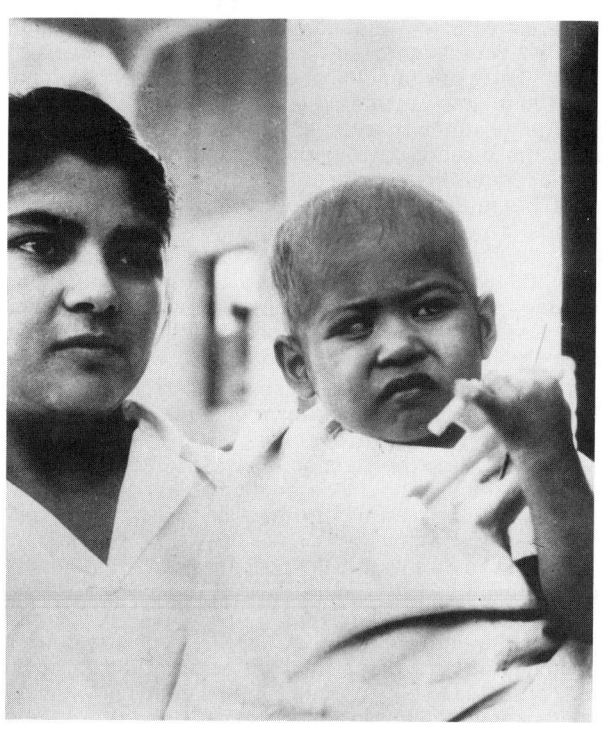

Fig. V-23.   Keratomalacia, characterized by softening and ulceration of the cornea of the eye, due to a vitamin A deficiency. Unless vitamin A or carotene is provided, blindness may follow. (Courtesy, FAO, Rome, Italy)

• **Stunted growth**—A deficiency of vitamin A results in stunted growth of children.

• **Slowed bone growth**—When young animals are deprived of vitamin A, the bones fail to lengthen, and the remodeling processes necessary for the formation of compact bone cease to operate. Abnormalities in bone shape result. Bone growth in the cranium and spine slows, while nerve tissue continues to grow; sometimes this results in overcrowding of the skull and spine, and mechanical compression damage to nerve tissue with paralysis and degeneration.

• **Unsound teeth**—If a child gets too little vitamin A when his teeth are developing, the enamel forming cells become abnormal and pits are formed. Such pits may harbor food deposits, which may ferment and form acids that etch the enamel and lead to decay.

• **Rough, dry, scaly skin; increased sinus trouble, sore throat, and abscesses in ears, mouth, or salivary gland; increased diarrhea and kidney and bladder stones**—A deficiency of vitamin A injures the epithelial tissues throughout the body, and leads to a peculiar type of horny degeneration called keratinization. The epithelial cells form the outer layer of the skin and the mucous membranes that line the mouth and digestive, respiratory, and genitourinary tracts. Instead of being soft and moist, they become hard and dry. As a result, (1) the skin, especially in the areas of the arms, legs, shoulders, and lower abdomen, may become rough, dry, and scaly—a condition known as follicular hyperkeratosis or phrynoderma (it looks like "gooseflesh"); and (2) bacteria have easy access to the mucous membranes, with the result that there is increased susceptibility to infections such as sinus trouble, sore throat, and abscesses in the ears, mouth, or salivary glands. Also, certain other troubles, noninfective in character, increase as a result of the damaged epithelium, including diarrhea and the formation of kidney and bladder stones.

• **Reproductive disorders**—Deficient animals of all species studied—rat, fowl, pig, cow, sheep, dog, guinea pig, and others—show the following reproductive disorders: poor conception, abnormal embryonic growth, placental injury; and, in severe deficiency, death of the fetus. The same deficiency symptoms have been described in humans.

RECOMMENDED DAILY ALLOWANCE OF VITAMIN A.

The Food and Nutrition Board (FNB) of the National Research Council (NRC) recommended daily allowances of vitamin A are given in Table V-10.

TABLE V–10
RECOMMENDED DAILY VITAMIN A ALLOWANCES[1]

Group	Age	Weight		Height		RDA[2]	
	(years)	(lb)	*(kg)*	(in.)	*(cm)*	(mcg RE)	(IU)
Infants	0.0–0.5	13	*6*	24	*60*	375	1,250
	0.5–1.0	20	*9*	28	*71*	375	1,250
Children	1–3	29	*13*	35	*90*	400	1,333
	4–6	44	*20*	44	*112*	500	1,667
	7–10	62	*28*	52	*132*	700	2,333
Males	11–14	99	*45*	62	*157*	1,000	3,333
	15–18	145	*66*	69	*176*	1,000	3,333
	19–24	160	*72*	70	*177*	1,000	3,333
	25–50	174	*79*	70	*176*	1,000	3,333
	51+	170	*77*	62	*173*	1,000	3,333
Females	11–14	101	*46*	64	*157*	800	2,667
	15–18	120	*55*	64	*163*	800	2,667
	19–24	128	*58*	65	*164*	800	2,667
	25–50	138	*63*	64	*163*	800	2,667
	51+	143	*65*	63	*160*	800	2,667
Pregnant						800	2,667
Lactating						1,200	4,000

[1]*Recommended Dietary Allowances*, 10th ed., NRC–National Academy of Sciences, 1989, p. 285.

[2]The recommended daily allowances (RDA) are given in both International Units (IU) and Retinol Equivalents (RE). An International Unit (IU) of vitamin A is defined on the basis of rat studies as equal to 0.344 mcg of crystalline retinylacetate (which is equivalent to 0.3 mcg of retinol, or to 0.6 mcg of beta-carotene). These standards are based on experiments which show that in rats only about 50% of the beta-carotene is converted to vitamin A.

The estimated requirements of vitamin A are based on two kinds of studies: (1) nutritional status studies on various population groups throughout the world, and (2) controlled depletion experiments carried out on man and other animals. But the FNB-NRC recommended allowances given in Table V-10 are considerably in excess of the estimated requirements because (1) animal studies have shown that little vitamin A is stored at intakes minimal to growth, and (2) human surveys of liver stores have found low reserves in 20 to 30% of the populations studied. A discussion of vitamin A allowances follows:

• **Infants and children**—The daily allowance for infants from birth to 6 months is based on the average retinol content of human milk, which is about 49 mcg per 100 ml. Thus, an infant consuming 850 ml of breast milk would receive approximaely 420 mcg (420 RE) of retinol. The allowance for infants from 6 months to 1 year of age, who are fed solid foods in addition to milk, is reduced to 400 RE (300 as retinol, 100 as beta-carotene).

Since little information is available regarding the actual requirements of children and adolescents, the FNB-NRC recommended daily allowances were interpolated from the infant and the adult allowance and based on body weight and growth needs.

• **Adults**—The FNB-NRC recommended daily allowance of vitamin A for adult men is set at 1,000 mcg RE (3,333 IU),

In order to quantify vitamin A values within the metric system, international agencies have introduced the biological equivalent of 1 microgram (1 mcg = 1/1000 milligram) of retinol as the standard. This is known as the *Retinol Equivalent* (RE). The RE system of measurement takes into account the amount of absorption of the carotenes as well as the degree of conversion to vitamin A; hence, it is more precise than the IU system.

Because the body size of women is usually smaller than that of men, the RDA of vitamin A for adult women is set at 80% of that of men, or 800 mcg RE (2,667 IU).

• **Pregnancy and lactation**—During pregnancy, the RDA of vitamin A is not increased. During lactation, the RDA is increased to 4,000 IU (1,200 RE) to compensate for the vitamin A secreted in breast milk.

• **Therapeutic uses**—Retinol is valuable in the treatment of night blindness and xerophthalmia, malabsorption syndrome or obstructive jaundice, and malnourished people who show Bitot's spots or follicular keratosis.

For the prevention of blindness in vitamin A-deficient children, massive doses of vitamin A (200,000 IU) by mouth at 6-month intervals have been effective.

• **Vitamin A intake in average U.S. diet**—In 1990, the vitamin A value of foods available in the United States amounted to about 1,630 RE per person per day: 35.4% of which was from fruits and vegetables; 29.2% from fats, oils, and dairy products; 30.9% from meat, fish, and eggs; and 4.3% from miscellaneous foods. This does not account for subsequent losses in processing, cooking, and storage.

Vegetarians will need to increase their intake of pro-vitamin A carotenoids in order to meet the recommended allowances.

Vitamin A is efficiently stored in the liver, and well-nourished persons have several months' supply that the body can utilize.

TOXICITY (Hypervitaminosis A). Excessive intake of preformed vitamin A, called hypervitaminosis A, may cause serious injury to health. However, massive intakes of carotene are not harmful because they are not converted to vitamin A rapidly enough to cause toxicity. The excess carotene will merely produce a yellow coloration of the skin, which disappears when the intake is reduced.

Symptoms of vitamin A toxicity are: loss of appetite, headache, blurred vision, excessive irritability, loss of hair, drying and flaking of the skin (with itching), swelling over the long bones, drowsiness, diarrhea, nausea, and enlargement of the liver and spleen. The most direct and positive diagnosis of hypervitaminosis A is the determination of the vitamin A concentration in the plasma or serum from a fasting blood sample. Values higher than 100 mcg per 100 ml (normal 20 to 60 mcg/100 ml) can be considered suspect, whereas values greater than this indicate toxicity.

Poisoning of men and dogs from eating polar bear liver has been reported in the Arctic since 1596. Polar bear liver contains 13,000 to 18,000 IU of vitamin A per gram. It is estimated that a hungry Arctic explorer may eat about 500 g of liver per day, containing about 9,000,000 IU of vitamin A.

Chronic toxic symptoms (hypervitaminosis A) may occur in adults who receive doses of vitamin A in excess of 50,000 IU daily over a prolonged period. Lesser doses will produce symptoms in children; infants who receive 18,500 IU daily may show signs of toxicity within 12 weeks. Acute toxicity occurs in adults who are given massive doses of 2 to 5 million IU daily, and in infants from doses as low as 75,000 to 300,000 IU daily. Vitamin C can help prevent the harmful effects of vitamin A toxicity. When excess intake of vitamin A is discontinued, recovery is usually rapid and complete; in some cases, the toxicity symptoms disappear within 72 hours.

On the basis of the evidence presently available, prolonged daily doses of vitamin A to adults in excess of 50,000 IU, and to infants in excess of 18,500 IU, should be under the supervision of a qualified physician or nutritionist.

VITAMIN A LOSSES DURING PROCESSING, COOKING, AND STORAGE. The carotene losses of vegetables following harvest tend to parallel the degree of wilting. In order to conserve their maximum carotene value, they should be stored at low temperatures or be quick frozen.

Freezing and freeze-drying causes little loss. But drying of eggs, vegetables or fruits, with exposure to air, sunlight, or high temperatures, may cause serious loss of vitamin A value.

Because vitamin A and the carotenes are insoluble in water and stable to heat at ordinary cooking temperatures, it was once thought that little vitamin A activity was lost from foods in cooking and processing, *unless* they were exposed to air. However, cooking or canning vegetables produces a rearrangement of atoms in the carotene molecule, resulting in carotenes of substantially lower vitamin A value. It is estimated that, on the average, the vitamin A value of cooked green vegetables is decreased by 15 to 20% and the value of yellow vegetables by 30 to 35%.

Both vitamin A and the carotenoids are easily oxidized and rapidly destroyed on exposure to ultraviolet light, with the rate of destruction influenced by the associated substances and the temperature and moisture conditions. Butter exposed in thin layers in air at 122°F (*50°C*) loses all of its vitamin A potency in 6 hours, but in the absence of air there is little destruction at 248°F (*120°C*) over the same period. Yellow corn has been reported to lose as much as 60% of its carotene in 7 months' storage.

Animal fats should be kept in a cold, dark place; and fish liver oils should be protected from light by being kept in dark bottles. Rancid fat destroys both vitamin A and carotene. Also, minerals such as iron oxide, charcoal, sulfur, ground limestone, bone meal, manganese, and iodine, contribute to the destruction of vitamin A in foods.

SOURCES OF VITAMIN A. Grouping by rank of common sources of vitamin A follows:

• **Rich sources**—Liver and carrots.

• **Good sources**—Dark-green leafy vegetables: beet greens, collards, dandelion greens, kale, mustard greens, spinach, Swiss chard, turnip greens; yellow vegetables: pumpkins, sweet potatoes, squash (winter); yellow fruits: apricots, peaches; some seafoods: crab, halibut, oysters, salmon, swordfish, whale meat.

• **Fair sources**—Butter (regular salted), cantaloupe, cheese, cream, egg yolk, lettuce, margarine (fortified), tomatoes, whole milk.

• **Negligible sources**—Breads and cereals (except yellow corn), chicken, cottage cheese (not creamed), dry beans, muscle meats, potatoes, skim milk.

• **Supplemental sources**—Synthetic vitamin A, cod and other fish liver oils.

For additional sources and more precise values of vitamin A, see Food Composition Table F-36.

Only animal foods contain vitamin A as such. Although they are usually classed as food supplements rather than foods, the fish liver oils are the richest natural sources. Fish eat smaller fish or crustaceans, which, in turn, have fed on marine plants that contain provitamins A. Herbivorous animals eat green plants and convert these substances into the vitamin itself in their bodies. Carnivorous animals get the vitamin from feeding on plant-eating animals. The cow and the hen are efficient in converting the provitamins A in plant foods into the vitamin A in milk fat and eggs, respectively; and into the vitamin A in their body tissues. But some provitamin A in the diet escapes their conversion, with the result that milk fat, egg yolk, and other animal products contain a mixture of vitamin A and its plant precursors. The proportion of each depends partly on the animal species, or even the breed, and partly on the feed consumed. For example, the "golden" color of Guernsey milk is due to the high content of provitamin A, while whiter Holstein milk contains a higher proportion of vitamin A. But both milks have about the same amount of total vitamin A activity.

Also, the vitamin A value of animal foods varies widely according to the vitamin A value of the feed of the animals that produced them. For example, livers from older animals and from animals on green grass are higher in vitamin A than the livers of younger animals on dry, bleached feeds; and the butterfat in milk is usually yellower and of higher vitamin A value when the cows are grazing on green pastures than when they are confined to a corral.

The principal source of vitamin A in the diet is likely to be from the carotenes, which are widespread in those plant foods that have high green or yellow colorings.

There is a direct correlation between the greenness of a leaf and its carotene content; dark-green leaves, such as beet greens, collards, dandelion greens, kale, mustard greens, spinach, Swiss chard, and turnip greens, are rich in carotene, but pale leaves, like cabbage and lettuce, are insignificant sources. The yellow vegetables and fruits, such as carrots, apricots, cantaloupe, peaches, pumpkins, squash (winter), sweet potatoes, and yellow corn, are rich in provitamin A carotenoids.

• **Synthetic vitamin A**—Today, synthetic forms of vitamin A are the most potent and inexpensive sources. They are just as effective and safe as the natural forms, but it must be remembered that they contain no other nutrients.

TOP FOOD SOURCES OF VITAMIN A. The top food sources of vitamin A are listed in Table V-11.

NOTE WELL: This table lists (1) the top sources, without regard to the amount normally eaten (left column), and (2) the top food sources (right column); and the caloric (energy) content of each food.
(Also see VITAMIN[S], Table V-9.)

TABLE V-11
TOP SOURCES OF VITAMIN A AND THEIR CALORIC CONTENT

Top Sources[2]	Vitamin A		Energy	Top Food Sources	Vitamin A		Energy
	(IU/ 100 g)	(RE/100 g)[3]	(kcal/ 100 g)		(IU/ 100 g)	(RE/100 g)[3]	(kcal/ 100 g)
Carrots, dehydrated	100,000	10,000	341	Liver, beef, fried	53,400	16,036	222
Cod-liver oil	85,000	25,526	899	Liver, calf, fried	32,700	9,820	261
Peppers, hot chili, mature, red, dried, pods	77,000	7,700	321	Liver, chicken broilers/fryers, simmered	16,375	4,917	165
Liver, lamb, broiled	74,500	22,372	261	Liver, hog, fried in margarine	14,900	4,474	241
Paprika, domestic	60,604	6,060	289	Dandelions greens, raw	14,000	1,400	45
Liver, beef, fried	53,400	16,036	222	Carrots, raw	11,000	1,100	42
Sweet potato, dehydrated, flakes, dry	47,000	4,700	379	Mustard greens (tendergreen), raw	9,900	990	22
Pepper, red	41,610	4,161	318	Spinach, raw	8,100	810	26
Chili powder	34,927	3,493	314	Sweet potato, baked in skin	8,100	810	141
Liver, calf, fried	32,700	9,820	261	Collards, cooked in water	7,800	780	33
Pumpkin, canned	27,383	2,738	33	Turnip greens, raw	7,600	760	28
Parsley, dried	23,340	2,334	276	Chard, Swiss, raw	6,500	650	25
Alfalfa leaf meal, dehydrated	22,940	2,294	215	Squash, winter, butternut, baked	6,400	640	68
Peppers, hot chili, mature, red, raw, pods	21,600	2,160	80	Peaches, dehydrated, sulfured, uncooked	5,000	500	340
Liver, turkey, simmered	17,500	5,255	174	Cantaloupe, raw	3,400	340	30
Liver, chicken broilers/fryers, simmered	16,375	4,917	165	Margarine	3,307	993	719
				Butter, regular, salted	3,058	754	717
Carrots, canned, drained, solids	15,000	1,500	23	Apricots, raw	2,700	270	51
Liver, hog, fried in margarine	14,900	4,474	241	Lettuce (dark green and white Paris)	1,900	190	18
Apricots, dehydrated, sulfured, uncooked	14,100	1,410	332	Eggs, chicken, raw, yolk, fresh	1,839	552	369
Dandelion greens, raw	14,000	1,400	45	Nectarine, raw	1,650	165	64
				Tomatoes, ripe, boiled	1,000	100	26

[1]These listings are based on the data in Food Composition Table F-36. Some top or rich sources may have been overlooked since some of the foods in Table F-36 lack values for vitamin A.

Whenever possible, foods are on an "as used" basis, without regard to moisture content; hence, certain high-moisture foods may be disadvantaged when ranked on the basis of vitamin A content per 100 g (approximately 3½ oz) without regard to moisture content.

[2]Listed without regard to the amount normally eaten.

[3]In converting International Units (IU) to Retinol Equivalents (RE), it was assumed that the vitamin A activity of foods from plants is due to beta-carotene and the vitamin A activity of foods from animals is due to retinol. Butter is an exception. Butter values are from USDA Handbook No. 8-4.

VITAMIN A DEFICIENCY

This refers to an insufficiency of vitamin A, which may be due to either (1) a dietary lack of vitamin A and/or pro-vitamin A, or (2) poor absorption.

(Also see VITAMIN A, sections headed "Deficiency Symptoms;" and "Blindness Due to Vitamin A Deficiency.")

VITAMIN ANTAGONIST

A substance so similar in structure to the vitamin that the body accepts it in place of the vitamin is known as a vitamin antagonist. But the antagonist is unable to perform the functions of the true vitamin.

VITAMIN B-6 (PYRIDOXINE; PYRIDOXAL; PYRIDOXAMINE)

VITAMIN B-6

PROMOTES GROWTH AND FEATHERING IN CHICKS.

IT'S ESSENTIAL FOR HUMANS, TOO.

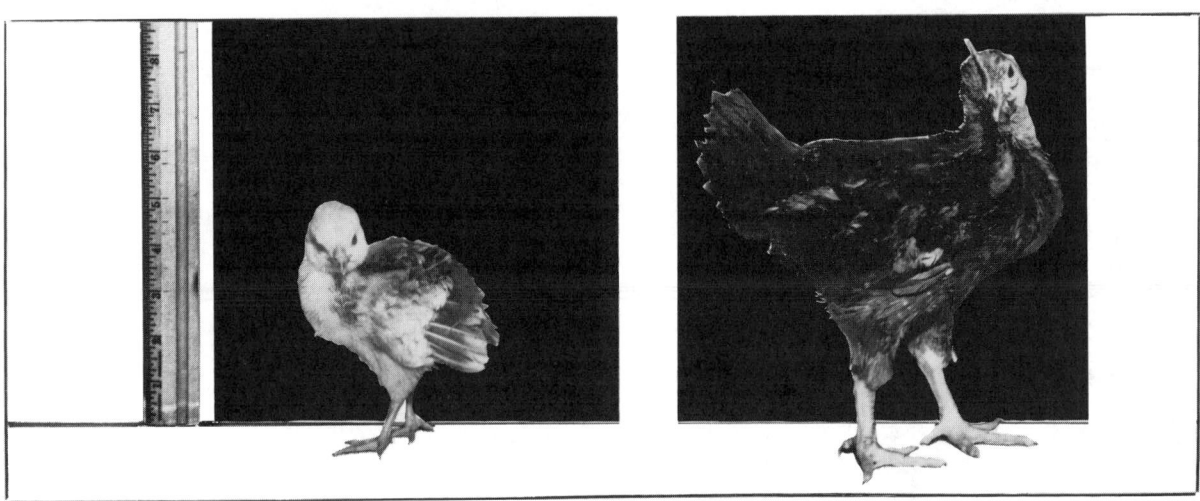

VITAMIN B-6 MADE THE DIFFERENCE! <u>LEFT:</u> CHICK SHOWS RETARDED GROWTH AND ABNORMAL FEATHERING DUE TO VITAMIN B-6 DEFICIENCY. <u>RIGHT:</u> NORMAL, CONTROL CHICK. (COURTESY, G.F. COMBS, UNIVERSITY OF GEORGIA)

TOP FOOD SOURCES

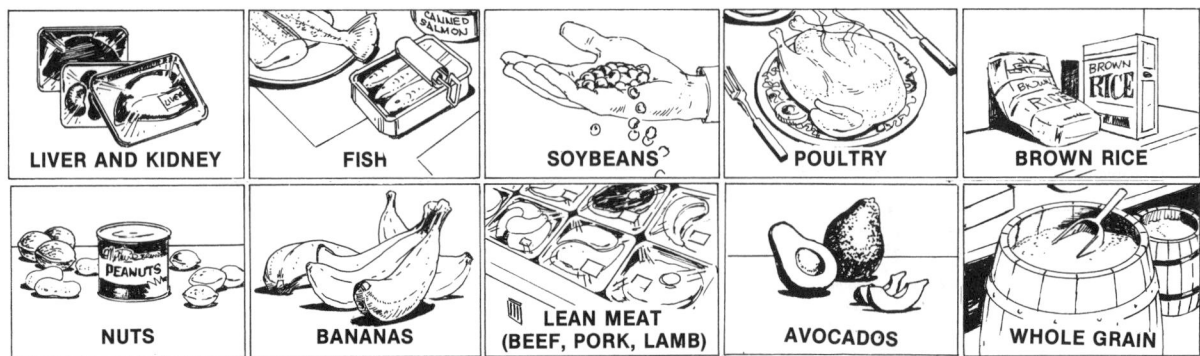

Fig. V-24.   The vitamin B-6 story.

By official action of the Society of Biological Chemists and the American Institute of Nutrition, vitamin B-6 is now the approved collective name for three closely related naturally occurring compounds with potential vitamin B-6 activity: pyridoxine, pyridoxal, and pyridoxamine. Pyridoxine is found largely in vegetable products, whereas the pyridoxal and pyridoxamine forms occur primarily in animal products. There is no information on the relative biological activity of the three compounds in man, but in rats they are equally active if given parenterally (injected intramuscularly or intravenously).

The need for vitamin B-6 was first demonstrated in rats, but it is now established that it is also a dietary essential for the human, pig, chick, dog, and other species, including microorganisms.

HISTORY.

In 1926, Goldberger and Lillie conducted an experiment designed to produce pellagra in rats. A severe dermatitis resulted, which was believed to be analogous to pellagra. In 1934, the Hungarian scientist, Gyorgy, produced a cure for this condition with an extract from yeast; but the curative compound of the extract was neither thiamin, niacin, nor riboflavin, but a substance which he called *vitamin B-6*. In 1938, five different laboratories, working independently, isolated the vitamin in crystalline form, but credit for obtaining the first crystals is generally given to Lepkovsky of the University of California. In 1939, Stiller *et al.*, of Merck and Co., established the chemical structure of the vitamin; and Harris and Folkers, of Merck, along with Kuhn, the German scientist, synthesized the compound.

When the vitamin was first isolated, the German biochemists gave it the name of adermin, while American researchers called it pyridoxine. Because the compound has a pyridine ring (five carbon and one nitrogen) and three hydroxy groups, Gyorgy, the Hungarian, expressed preference for the name pyridoxine, which became widely adopted.

In 1942, Snell discovered the vitamin B-6 activity of two closely related substances in natural products, which he named pyridoxal and pyridoxamine. Umbreit followed in 1945 with a report of the coenzyme functions of the vitamin in phosphate forms.

CHEMISTRY, METABOLISM, PROPERTIES.

• **Chemistry**—Vitamin B-6 is found in foods in three forms which are readily interconvertible—pyridoxine, pyridoxal, and pyridoxamine. Also vitamin B-6 is found in physiological systems in the forms of pyridoxal phosphate and pyridoxamine phosphate. The structural formulas of the three naturally occurring free forms of these compounds are given in Fig. V-25.

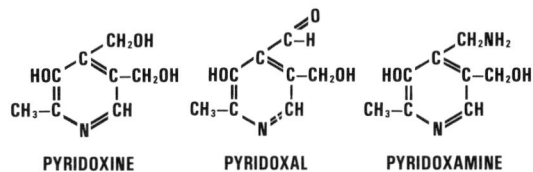

Fig. V-25. Structures of pyridoxine, pyridoxal, and pyridoxamine.

• **Metabolism**—In the free form, vitamin B-6 is absorbed rapidly from the upper part of the small intestine, thence it enters the body by the portal vein. It is present in most body tissues, with a high concentration in the liver. It is secreted into milk and excreted primarily via the urine. Measurement of B-6 in the urine is the assay method used in nutrition surveys.

• **Properties**—Vitamin B-6 is readily soluble in water, quite stable to heat and acid, but easily destroyed by oxidation and exposure to alkali and ultraviolet light. All three forms are white crystalline substances.

Of the three forms, pyridoxine is more resistant to food processing and storage conditions and probably represents the principal form in food products.

MEASUREMENT/ASSAY.

No international standard or unit system of vitamin B-6 is in current usage. Analytical results are expressed in weight units of pyridoxine hydrochloride. One milligram of pyridoxine hydrochloride is equivalent to 0.82 mg pyridoxine or 0.81 mg pyridoxal, or 0.82 mg pyridoxamine.

The vitamin B-6 content in foods and tissues is determined by microbiological assay, chemical methods, and animal bioassays. The animal bioassays, using either the rat or chick, are time consuming, expensive, and variable; therefore, they have been generally replaced by microbiological and chemical methods.

FUNCTIONS.

Vitamin B-6, in its coenzyme forms, usually as pyridoxal phosphate but sometimes as pyridoxamine phosphate, is involved in a large number of physiologic functions, particularly in protein (nitrogen) metabolism, and to a lesser extent in carbohydrate and fat metabolism. Also, it appears to hold a key role in a number of chemical problems. Discussion follows:

• **Vitamin B-6 in protein metabolism**—Vitamin B-6 in its phosphorylated forms is active metabolically in the following types of reactions in amino acid metabolism:

1. **Transamination.** It is involved in shifting an amino group (NH_2) from a donor amino acid to an acceptor acid to form another amino acid. This reaction is important in the formation of nonessential amino acids. Transamination is illustrated in Fig. V-26.

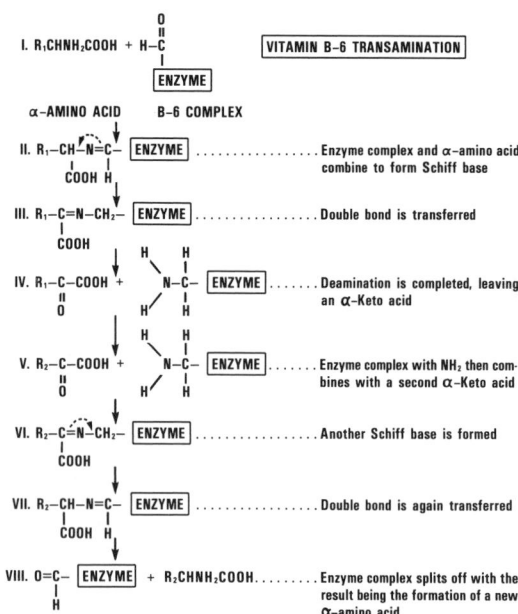

Fig. V-26.   Vitamin B-6 in transamination.

2. **Decarboxylation.** It is active in the removal of the carboxyl groups (COOH) from certain amino acids to form another compound. Decarboxylation is necessary for the synthesis of serotonin, norephinephrine, and histamine from tryptophan, tyrosine, and histidine, respectively.

3. **Deamination.** It aids in deamination. By removing amino groups (NH_2) from amino acids not needed for growth, it helps to render carbon residues available for energy.

4. **Transulfuration.** It aids in the transfer of sulfhydryl-group (HS) from the amino acid methionine to another amino acid (serine) to form the amino acid cysteine.

5. **Tryptophan conversion to niacin (nicotinic acid).** It assists in forming niacin (nicotinic acid) from tryptophan, thereby playing a role in the niacin supply.

6. **Hemoglobin formation.** It is necessary for the formation of a precursor of prophyrin compounds which is part of the hemoglobin molecule.

7. **Absorption of amino acids.** Vitamin B-6 is believed to play a role in the absorption of amino acids from the intestine.

• **Vitamin B-6 in carbohydrate and fat metabolism**—Vitamin B-6 in its phospohorylated forms also plays a role in carbohydrate and fat metabolism, although this role is less important than protein metabolism:

1. **Catabolism of glycogen.** It is an essential part of phosphorylase, the enzyme that brings about the conversion of glycogen to glucose-1-phosphate in muscle and liver.

2. **Fatty acid metabolism.** It takes part in fat metabolism, although the exact mode of action is unknown; for example, it is believed to be involved in the conversion

of the essential unsaturated fatty acid, linoleic acid, to another fatty acid, arachidonic acid.

• **Clinical problems of pyridoxine deficiency**—It seems apparent that vitamin B-6 is also involved in a number of clinical problems; among them, the following:

1. **Central nervous system disturbances.** It assists in energy transformation in brain and nerve tissue; hence, the functioning of the central nervous system. When vitamin B-6 is lacking, convulsive seizures occur in both human infants and experimental animals.

2. **Autism.** This is a severe disturbance of mental and emotional development in young children, characterized chiefly by withdrawal from reality and lack of responsiveness or interest in other people in the normal activities of childhood. Although more experimental work is needed, nine studies reported in the world literature show that megadoses of vitamin B-6 are helpful in treating autism.[14]

3. **Anemia.** In studies on human subjects, vitamin B-6 has been effective in treating anemia that does not respond to iron—so-called iron-resistant anemia.

4. **Kidney stones.** It has been reported that a deficiency of vitamin B-6 causes increased urinary excretion of oxalates; thus, a lack of the vitamin may result in the formation of kidney stones.

5. **Tuberculosis.** The drug isoniazid (isonicotinic acid hydrazide, INH), which is used as a chemotherapeutic agent in treating tuberculosis, has been shown to be an antagonist to pyridoxine, causing a side effect of neuritis in some patients. Treatment with large doses (50 to 100 mg daily) of pyridoxine prevents this effect.

6. **Physiologic demands in pregnancy.** Pyridoxine deficiencies during pregnancy have been demonstrated and subsequently corrected by supplementation with vitamin B-6.

7. **Oral contraceptives.** Some women on estrogen-progesterone oral contraceptives appear to require additional vitamin B-6.

• **Other functions**—It appears from experimental studies that vitamin B-6 is involved in—

1. Antibody formation, for protection against infectious diseases, although this role is unproved.
2. Messenger RNA synthesis.
3. Nucleic acid metabolism.
4. Endocrine gland functions.
5. Biosynthesis of coenzyme A.

DEFICIENCY SYMPTOMS. It is difficult to produce a dietary deficiency of vitamin B-6 in human beings because it is so widely distributed in foods. The characteristic symptoms are: skin lesions—especially at the tip of the nose, anemia, convulsive seizures, and reduced antibody production. In adults, there may also be depression and confusion. If the vitamin B-6 deficiency is prolonged, the symptoms may include dizziness, nausea, vomiting, and kidney stones.

---

[14]Rimland, Bernard, Ph.D., Letters (to the editor), *Science News*, Vol. 119, No. 16, April 18, 1981, p. 243.

Experimentally, vitamin B-6 deficiency in adults has been produced by using a low vitamin B-6 diet along with one of the antagonists of the vitamin—desoxypyridoxine. After 2 to 3 weeks, the following symptoms were noted: greasy scaliness (seborrheic dermatitis) in the skin around the eyes, nose, and mouth, which subsequently spread to other parts of the body; a smooth, red tongue; loss of weight; muscular weakness; irritability; and mental depression. Administration of as little as 5 mg of pyridoxine, pyridoxal, or pyridoxamine daily corrected all the abnormalities in a few days.

The effects of vitamin B-6 deprivation appear to be more dramatic in infants than in adults. In 1951, vitamin B-6 deficiency symptoms suddenly occurred in infants 6 weeks to 6 months old in various parts of the United States who were fed on a commercially canned, liquid-milk formula which, unknowingly at the time, was deficient in vitamin B-6. The most telling symptoms: irritability, muscular twitchings, and convulsions. Also, there was a loss of weight, abdominal distress, and vomiting. The similarity of the convulsive seizures to those observed in rats on a diet deficient in vitamin B-6 suggested that the disturbance might be due to a lack of the vitamin. Intramuscular injection of pyridoxine hydrochloride relieved the symptoms in 5 minutes. It was later found that most of the vitamin B-6 in the formula had been destroyed by heat during the canning process. Since then, the manufacturer has added a heat-stable form of vitamin B-6 to the product.

RECOMMENDED DAILY ALLOWANCE OF VITAMIN B-6.
The Food and Nutrition Board (FNB) of the National Research Council (NRC) recommended daily allowances of vitamin B-6 are given in Table V-12.

TABLE V–12
RECOMMENDED DAILY
VITAMIN B-6 ALLOWANCES[1]

Group	Age	Weight		Height		Vitamin B-6
	(years)	(lb)	(kg)	(in.)	(cm)	(mg)
Infants	0.0–0.5	13	6	24	60	0.3
	0.5–1.0	20	9	28	71	0.6
Children	1–3	29	13	35	90	1.0
	4–6	44	20	44	112	1.1
	7–10	62	28	52	132	1.4
Males	11–14	99	45	62	157	1.7
	15–18	145	66	69	176	2.0
	19–24	160	72	70	177	2.0
	25–50	174	79	70	176	2.0
	51+	170	77	68	173	2.0
Females	11–14	101	46	62	157	1.4
	15–18	120	55	64	163	1.5
	19–24	128	58	65	164	1.6
	25–50	138	63	64	163	1.6
	51+	143	65	63	160	1.6
Pregnant						2.2
Lactating						2.1

[1]*Recommended Dietary Allowances*, 10th ed., NRC–National Academy of Sciences, 1989, p. 285.

The establishment of allowances for vitamin B-6 is complicated by the following facts: (1) the requirement varies with dietary protein intake—there is increased need for vitamin B-6 with increased intakes of protein; (2) the uncertainty of the availability of the vitamin in the diet; and (3) the uncertainty as to the extent of intestinal bacterial synthesis of the vitamin, and the degree to which it is utilized by the body. Also, there is evidence of increased need of the vitamin in pregnancy and lactation, in the elderly, in various pathologic and genetic disturbances, and in persons receiving certain drugs (such as isoniazid, commonly used in the treatment of tuberculosis; or penicillamine, a metabolite of penicillin). Nevertheless, the NRC has set recommended allowances to assure a safety margin and to make a deficiency unlikely under most circumstances. Discussion follows:

• **Recommended allowance for infants**—Although based on limited information, a recommended dietary allowance of 0.3 mg of vitamin B-6 per day is considered adequate for the young infant. For older infants (0.5 to 1.0 year of age) consuming a mixed diet, a daily allowance of 0.6 mg of vitamin B-6 is recommended.

• **Recommended allowance for children and adolescents**—The recommended allowances for children range from 1.0 mg to 1.4 mg per day, depending on age.

• **Recommended allowance for pregnancy**—Theoretically, several factors imply an increased need for vitamin B-6 in pregnancy: (1) because vitamin B-6 requirements increase with increasing protein in the diet, the extra protein allowance for the pregnant woman necessitates a modest increase in intake of the vitamin; (2) all forms of vitamin B-6 cross the placenta readily and are concentrated in the fetal blood; and (3) estrogens apparently increase tryptophan oxygenase activity, which will result in need for additional vitamin B-6.

An additional allowance of 0.6 mg of vitamin B-6 per day (for a total allowance of 2.6 mg/day) is recommended during gestation.

• **Recommended allowance for lactation**—The content of vitamin B-6 in milk appears to reflect the nutritional state of the mother with respect to the vitamin.

An additional allowance of 0.6 mg of vitamin B-6/day (for a total allowance of 2.2 mg/day) is recommended during lactation.

• **Vitamin B-6 and oral contraceptive agents**—Recent studies indicate that the vitamin B-6 requirement for most oral contraceptive users is approximately the same as that for nonusers; thus, the current evidence does not appear to justify the routine supplementation of the dietary vitamin B-6 with pyridoxine. However, some women report that depression occurs when they are taking oral contraceptives, probably as a result of the failure to convert tryptophan to serotonin, a neurotransmitter in the brain. When this problem occurs, the physician may suggest higher levels of vitamin B-6 (about 30 mg daily) in order to normalize tryptophan metabolism.

• **Vitamin B-6 intake in average U.S. diets**—In 1988, according to the U.S. Department of Agriculture, the overall average per capita availability of vitamin B-6 per day in the United States was only 2.2 mg, not including waste or cooking losses. Also, it is noteworthy that 40% of the available vitamin B-6 was provided by meat, poultry, and fish.

TOXICITY. Although vitamin B-6 is relatively non-toxic, side effects, such as sleepiness, may follow injection of large doses. Also, it may be habit-forming when taken in large doses over an extended period; a vitamin B-6 dependency has been induced in normal human adults given a supplement of 200 mg of pyridoxine daily for 33 days while on a normal diet.

VITAMIN LOSSES DURING PROCESSING, COOKING, AND STORAGE. More than 75% of the vitamin B-6 content of wheat is lost in milling white flour. Although vitamin B-6 is not added in white flour enrichment programs, perhaps it should be.

Canning and freezing result in considerable losses of vitamin B-6 with the losses being smaller in frozen foods. Freeze-dehydration and subsequent storage appear to have no adverse effect on the vitamin B-6 content of meat and poultry.

Considerable losses of vitamin B-6 occur during cooking. Beef loses 25 to 50% of its raw vitamin B-6 content in cooking, with the losses higher from oven braising than from oven roasting. Home cooking of fruits and vegetables results in a loss of about 50% of the vitamin B-6.

Storage losses appear to be minimal. Studies have shown that the storage of potatoes for as long as 6 months at 40°F (*4.4°C*) results in no loss of the vitamin.

Henry A. Schroeder, M.D., of the Dartmouth Medical School, conducted an extensive survey of the B-6 content in hundreds of common foods, and found that modern processing was causing massive losses of the vitamin. His studies showed B-6 losses as follows: From milling wheat and making all-purpose flour, 82.3%; from canning vegetables, 57 to 77%; from freezing vegetables, 37 to 56%; from canning meat and poultry, 42.6%; and from canning seafood, 48.9%.[15]

---

[15]Schroeder, Henry A., M.D., Losses of Vitamins and Trace Minerals Resulting From Processing and Preservation of Foods, *The American Journal of Chemical Nutrition*, Vol. 24, May 1971, pp. 562-573.

SOURCES OF VITAMIN B-6. In animal tissues and yeast, vitamin B-6 occurs mainly as pyridoxal and pyridoxamine. In plants, all three members of the vitamin are found, but pyridoxine predominates. The occurrence of vitamin B-6 in various forms has complicated the task of determining the content of the vitamin in foods.

Although vitamin B-6 is widely distributed in foods, many sources provide very small amounts. Thus, there is concern, as well as ever-increasing evidence, that in more that a few instances normal diets may be borderline or low in this vitamin.

Groupings by rank of common food sources of vitamin B-6 follow:

• **Rich sources**—Rice bran, wheat bran, sunflower seed.

• **Good sources**—Avocados, bananas, corn, fish, kidney, lean meat, liver, nuts, poultry, brown rice, soybeans, whole grain.

• **Fair sources**—Eggs, fruits (except bananas and avocados, which are good sources), vegetables.

• **Negligible sources**—Cheese (Cheddar, cottage), fat, milk, sugar, white bread.

• **Supplemental sources**—Pyridoxine hydrochloride is the most commonly available synthetic form; and yeast (torula, brewers'), rice polish, and wheat germ are used as natural source supplements.

For additional sources and more precise values of vitamin B-6 (pyridoxine), see Food Composition Table F-36.

Fat and sugar, which supply over one-third of the energy intake of the average American, are devoid of vitamin B-6. Generally speaking, processed or refined foods are much lower in vitamin B-6 than the original food; thus, white bread, rice, noodles, macaroni, and spaghetti are all quite low in vitamin B-6.

There is evidence that intestinal bacteria produce vitamin B-6. But the extent of this source, and the degree to which the bacterial-synthesized vitamin is utilized by the body, are undetermined.

Because vitamin B-6 is important for buoyant good health, and because it is limited in many foods, supplemental vitamin B-6 may be indicated, especially for infants and during pregnancy and lactation.

TOP FOOD SOURCES OF VITAMIN B-6.

The top food sources of vitamin B-6 are listed in Table V-13.

NOTE WELL: This table lists (1) the top sources without regard to the amount normally eaten (left column), and (2) the top food sources (right column); and the caloric (energy) content of each food.

(Also see VITAMIN[S], Table V-9.)

TABLE V-13
TOP SOURCES OF VITAMIN B-6 (PYRIDOXINE) AND THEIR CALORIC CONTENT[1]

Top Sources[2]	Vitamin B-6 (Pyridoxine)	Energy	Top Food Sources	Vitamin B-6 (Pyridoxine)	Energy
	(mg/100 g)	(kcal/100 g)		(mg/100 g)	(kcal/100 g)
Yeast, torula	3.00	277	Tuna, raw, Bluefin and Yellowfin	.90	141
Rice bran	2.50	276	Beef liver, fried	.84	222
Yeast, brewers', debittered	2.50	—	Walnuts, Persian or English	.73	694
Rice, polish	2.00	265	Salmon, smoked	.70	176
Yeast, baker's dry (active)	2.00	282	Mackerel, cooked	.68	230
Wheat bran, crude	1.38	353	Rice, brown, cooked	.62	119
Sunflower seed kernels, dry hulled	1.25	560	Chicken giblets, fried	.61	252
Wheat germ, toasted	1.15	391	Liver, chicken, broiler/fryer, simmered	.58	165
Parsley, dried	1.00	276	Cereal, whole wheat, cooked	.53	45
Cottonseed flour	.98	356	Banana, yellow, raw	.51	85
Tuna, raw, Bluefin and Yellowfin	.90	141	Beef, round cuts, cooked	.50	250
Beef liver, fried	.84	222	Pork, fresh loin, cooked, roasted or boiled	.48	300
Walnuts, Persian or English	.73	694	Corn, raw, sweet, white or yellow	.47	96
Soybean flour, defatted	.72	326	Beef kidney, raw	.43	113
Salmon, smoked	.70	176	Halibut, raw	.43	97
Mackerel, cooked	.68	230	Tuna, canned in water or oil, salt or no salt	.43	200
Soybean flour, low-fat	.68	356	Avocados	.42	167
Wheat-soy blend (WSB)/straight grade, wheat flour	.67	365	Chicken, broiler or fryer, roasted or fried	.41	225
Hog liver, fried in margarine	.65	241	Peanuts, roasted and salted	.40	585
Chicken, fryer, light meat, no skin, fried	.63	197	Wheat flour, whole (from hard wheats)	.34	361
Rice, brown, cooked	.62	119			
Whey, acid dry	.62	339			

[1] These listings are based on the data in Food Composition Table F-36. Some top or rich sources may have been overlooked since some of the foods in Table F-36 lack values for vitamin B-6.

Whenever possible, foods are on an "as used" basis, without regard to moisture content; hence, certain high-moisture foods may be disadvantaged when ranked on the basis of vitamin B-6 content per 100 g (approximately 3½ oz) without regard to moisture content.

[2] Listed without regard to the amount normally eaten.

VITAMIN B-12 (COBALAMINS)

Contents · Page

Vitamin B-12, like so many other members of the B complex, is not a single substance; rather, it consists of several closely related compounds with similar activity.

The term "cobalamins" is applied to this group of substances because all of them contain cobalt. Vitamin B-12, which is the most active member, is cyanocobalamin, named after the cyanide ion in the molecule. Other chemically related compounds known to have vitamin B-12 activity include hydroxocobalamin, nitritocobalamin, and thiocyanate cobalamin.

The most distinguishing characteristics of vitamin B-12 are: (1) unlike any other vitamin, the inability of higher plants to synthesize it (although it can be synthesized by animals); and (2) its most important deficiency state—Addisonian pernicious anemia, named after Thomas Addison, a physician working in London, who first described the malady in 1849. The anemia progressed slowly and ended with the death of the patient in 2 to 5 years. So feared and fatal was its course that it became known as pernicious anemia.

VITAMIN B-12

IT'S ESSENTIAL FOR HUMANS, TOO!

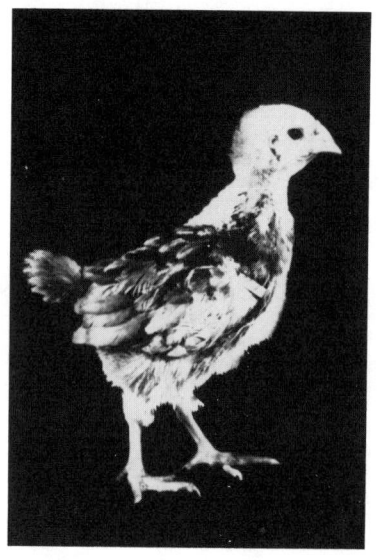 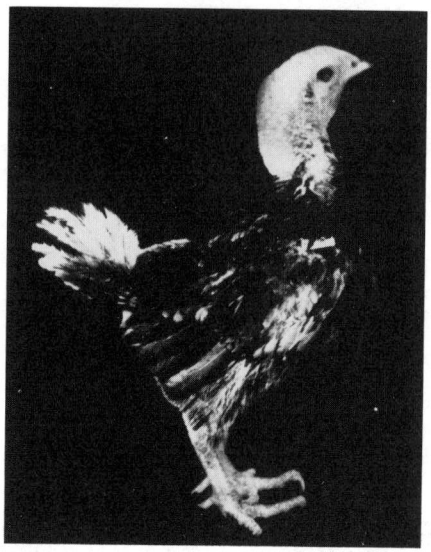

VITAMIN B-12 MADE THE DIFFERENCE! THE BIGGER CHICK AT THE RIGHT AND HIS SMALLER COMPANION ARE BOTH 3½ WEEKS OLD. LEFT: THE SMALL CHICK, FED A RATION DEFICIENT IN VITAMIN B-12, WEIGHED 157 g. RIGHT: THE LARGER CHICK, FED THE SAME RATION PLUS VITAMIN B-12, WEIGHED 280 g. (COURTESY, MERCK AND COMPANY, RAHWAY, N.J.)

TOP FOOD SOURCES

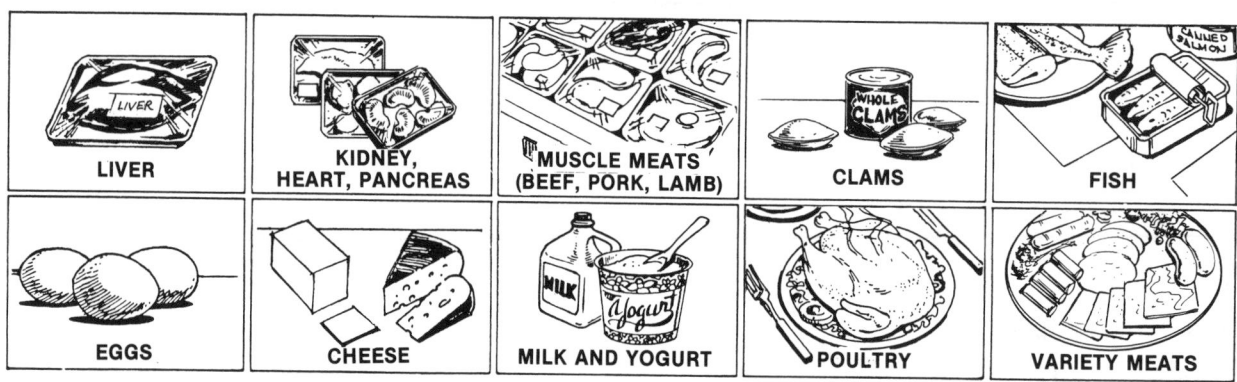

Fig. V-27.   The vitamin B-12 (cobalamins) story.

HISTORY.   For 77 years (from 1849 to 1926) following the description of pernicious anemia by Thomas Addison of England, there was no hope for victims of the disease. Finally, step by step, scientists evolved with the treatment for Addisonian pernicious anemia and the discovery of vitamin B-12, a chronological record of which follows:

1.   In 1925, George Hoyt Whipple, the Dean of the School of Medicine and Dentistry, University of Rochester, from 1921 to 1953, showed that liver was a great benefit in blood regeneration in dogs rendered anemic by bleeding.

2.   In 1926, Minot and Murphy of the Harvard Medical School reported that feeding large amounts of raw liver (1/4 to 1/2 lb per day) restored the normal level of red blood cells in cases of pernicious anemia. For this discovery, they shared a Nobel Prize with Whipple.

Following the report of Minot and Murphy, liver concentrates were developed, alleviating the necessity of eating large quantities of this food; and biochemists began a long series of studies to isolate the active component present in liver, which, at the time, was called the "antipernicious anemia factor."

3. In 1929, W. B. Castle of Harvard showed that pernicious anemia could be controlled by feeding patients beef muscle incubated in normal gastric juice, although neither beef muscle nor gastric juice was effective alone. This finding led him to postulate that two factors were involved: one an "extrinsic factor" in food, and the other an "intrinsic factor" in normal gastric secretion; which, given together, caused red blood cell formation in pernicious anemia.

4. In 1948, two groups of researchers working independently, Rickes and co-workers of Merck and Co., Inc. of New Jersey, and Smith and Parker of England, isolated from a liver concentrate a crystalline, red pigment, which they called vitamin B-12.

5. In 1948, R. West, of Columbia University, New York, showed that injections of vitamin B-12 induced a dramatic beneficial response in patients with pernicious anemia.

6. In 1955, the structure of vitamin B-12 (cyanocobalamin) was determined by Dorothy Hodgkin and co-workers, at Oxford. Later (1964), Hodgkin was awarded the Nobel Prize.

7. In 1955, Woodward's group at Harvard synthesized vitamin B-12 using a very complicated and expensive procedure. Fortunately, soon thereafter, it was found that highly active vitamin B-12 concentrates can be produced from cultures of certain bacteria and fungi grown in large tanks containing special media; and this remains the main method of commercial production.

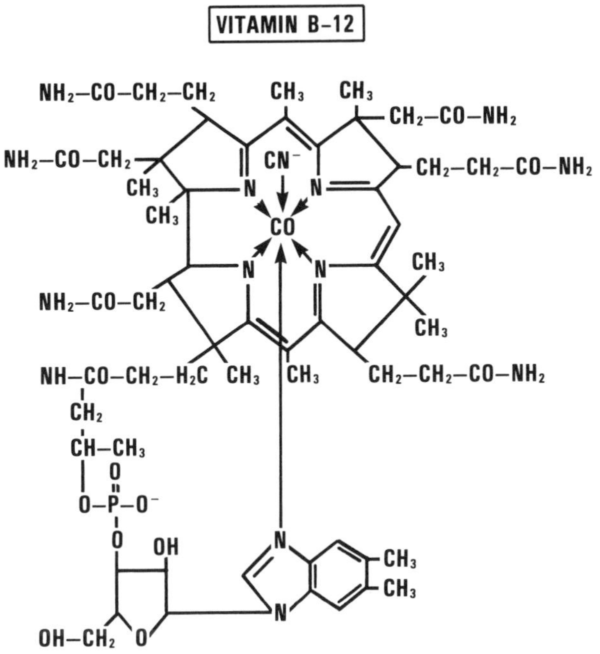

Fig. V-28. Structure of vitamin B-12.

CHEMISTRY, METABOLISM, PROPERTIES.

• **Chemistry**—Vitamin B-12 is the largest and the most complex of all vitamin molecules. The main part of the molecule consists of a porphyrin ring containing cobalt as the central element. A cyanide (-CN) group may be attached to the cobalt, in which case the compound is called cyanocobalamin (or vitamin B-12); the commercially available form of the vitamin, little of which occurs naturally. The cyanide group attachment to the cobalt can be replaced by a hydroxy group (-OH), giving hydroxocobalamin, the common naturally occurring form of the vitamin; or it can be replaced by a nitrite group (-NO$_2$), giving nitritocobalamin, a form found in certain bacteria.

A coenzyme form of vitamin B-12 contains an adenosine (a nucleoside, which consists of a purine [adenine] combined with a pentose sugar, ribose) molecule in place of the cyanide and is thought to be the most common form in foods. Methylcobalamin is another form of the vitamin with a coenzyme role. All these forms have approximately equal vitamin B-12 activity in the diet.

The structure of vitamin B-12 (C$_{63}$ H$_{90}$ O$_{14}$ N$_{14}$ PCo) is shown in Fig. V-28.

Vitamin B-12 occurs as a protein complex in animal proteins. The ultimate source, however, is the microorganisms in the gastrointestinal tract of herbivorous animals. Such microorganisms are found in large amounts in the rumen (the first stomach) of cows and sheep. Apparently, some synthesis occurs in the intestinal bacteria of man, also; but the amount supplied from this source is small and unknown.

• **Metabolism**—It is noteworthy (1) that vitamin B-12 is the only vitamin that requires a specific gastrointestinal tract secretion for its absorption (*intrinsic factor*); and (2) that the absorption of vitamin B-12 in the small intestine requires about 3 hours (compared to seconds for most other water-soluble vitamins). The absorption of vitamin B-12 involves the following five steps:

1. First, vitamin B-12 is released from the protein (the peptide bonds) to which it is linked in foods by the action of hydrochloric acid and intestinal enzymes.

2. Next, vitamin B-12 is bound to a highly specific glycoprotein, Castle's intrinsic factor, which is secreted in the stomach.

3. The vitamin B-12 intrinsic factor forms a complex with calcium and passes through the upper part of the small intestine to receptor sites in the ileum through which absorption of vitamin B-12 takes place.

4. In crossing the intestinal mucosa, vitamin B-12 is freed from the complex (the B-12-intrinsic factor-calcium complex).

5. In the intestinal cells, vitamin B-12 is transferred to a plasma transport protein known as transcobalamin II, for transport in the blood circulation.

In normal persons, from 30 to 70% of the vitamin B-12 is absorbed as outlined above, in comparison with 1 to 3% absorbed by simple diffusion. Pernicious anemia results from a complete failure to absorb the vitamin, a condition caused by gastric abnormality (usually lack of intrinsic factor). Hence, therapeutic doses of B-12 given to pernicious anemia patients usually must be administered intramuscularly.

Intrinsic factor regulates the amount of absorption of vitamin B-12 to about 1.5 to 3.0 mcg daily. Absorption decreases with age (it drops to about 5% in the elderly), and with iron and vitamin B-6 deficiencies; and it increases with pregnancy. Infant levels are approximately twice that of the mother. Also, absorption is greater if the vitamin is provided in three meals than if all of it is provided in a single meal.

The liver is the principal site of storage of vitamin B-12; normally, it contains 2,000 to 5,000 mcg, sufficient to take care of the body needs for 3 to 5 years. Small amounts of vitamin B-12 are stored in the kidneys, muscle, lungs, and spleen. Storage in the bone marrow is limited, amounting to only 1 to 2% of that in the liver.

Vitamin B-12 is excreted by way of the kidneys and in the bile.

The most useful measurement for the detection of a vitamin B-12 deficiency is the serum vitamin B-12 level. Normal serum levels of vitamin B-12 range from 200 to 700 picograms (l pg = 10^{-12} g per milliliter).

• **Properties**—The deep-red needlelike crystals are slightly soluble in water, stable to heat, but destroyed by light and by strong acid or alkaline solutions. There is little loss (only about 30%) of the vitamin by ordinary cooking procedures.

Vitamin B-12 is remarkably potent. It has a biologic activity 11,000 times that of the standard liver concentrate formerly used in the treatment of pernicious anemia.

MEASUREMENT/ASSAY.   No International Units have been defined for the biological activity of vitamin B-12. However, pure cobalamin can be used as a standard substance. Vitamin B-12 is measured in micrograms or picograms (pg, micromicrograms).

High potency preparations of vitamin B-12 are usually assayed by spectrophotometry. Also, vitamin B-12 may be assayed colorimetrically or fluorometrically. Some assays involve measurement of cobalt. However, food sources are usually assayed for vitamin B-12 by either (1) the microbiological method, or (2) the biological method, using chicks or rats.

FUNCTIONS.   In the human body, vitamin B-12 is converted to a coenzyme form, if it is not already in such form. There are two active coenzyme forms: Coenzyme B-12 (adenosylcobalamin), and methyl B-12 (methylcobalamin). Coenzyme B-12 has an adenosine ribonucleoside attached to the cobalt atom in the vitamin B-12 molecule in place of the cyanide group, whereas methyl B-12 contains a methyl group in place of the cyanide group. The conversion of vitamin B-12 to coenzyme forms requires many nutrients, including riboflavin, niacin, and magnesium.

Vitamin B-12 coenzymes perform the following physiological roles at the cellular level, especially in the cells of the bone marrow, nervous tissue, and gastrointestinal tract:

1. **Red blood cell formation and control of pernicious anemia**. Vitamin B-12 is essential for the blood-forming organs of the bone marrow to function properly. Without sufficient B-12 coenzymes, the red blood cells do not mature normally, with the result that large, immature cells (megaloblasts) form and are released into the blood, causing megaloblastic anemia.

2. **Maintenance of nerve tissue**. Vitamin B-12 is essential to the health of the nervous system. Vitamin B-12 coenzymes are necessary for the synthesis of myelin, a lipoprotein, in the nervous tissue; but it is not known whether the vitamin is involved in the synthesis of the lipid of the protein part of myelin.

3. **Carbohydrate, fat, and protein metabolism**. Since coenzyme B-12 is necessary for the conversion of methylmalonate to succinate, it is required for normal carbohydrate and fat metabolism. It is also involved in protein metabolism, since the requirement for B-12 increases as protein intake increases.

4. **Synthesis or transfer of single carbon units**. Vitamin B-12 is thought to be required for the synthesis of single carbon units, whereas folacin participates in their transfer. It follows that B-12 takes part in most of the same reactions as folacin, including—
   a.   The interconversion of serine and glycine
   b.   The formation of methionine from homocysteine
   c.   The formation of choline from ethanolamine
5. **Other functions**. Vitamin B-12 also serves as a coenzyme in the biosynthesis of methyl groups ($-CH_3$), and in reduction reactions such as the conversion of disulfide (S-S) to the sulfhydryl group (-SH).

• **Therapeutic uses of vitamin B-12**—Vitamin B-12 is being used in the treatment of the following maladies:

1. **Pernicious anemia**. The discovery that B-12 would control pernicious anemia was a great clinical breakthrough. Now a patient can be given intramuscular injections of 15 to 30 mcg of B-12 daily during a relapse, then maintained afterward by an injection of about 30 mcg every 30 days.
2. **Sprue**. Vitamin B-12 is effective in the treatment of sprue, especially if used in conjunction with folic acid. Actually, the role of B-12 may be indirect—to facilitate the action of folic acid.

DEFICIENCY SYMPTOMS.   Vitamin B-12 deficiency in man may occur as a result of (1) dietary lack, which sometimes occurs among vegetarians who consume no animal foods; or (2) deficiency of intrinsic factor, due to pernicious anemia, total or partial removal of the stomach by surgery, or infestation with parasites such as the fish tapeworm.

The common symptoms of a dietary deficiency of vitamin B-12 are: sore tongue, weakness, loss of weight, back pains, tingling of the extremities, apathy, and mental and other nervous abnormalities. Anemia is rarely seen in dietary deficiency of B-12.

In pernicious anemia, the characteristic symptoms are: abnormally large red blood cells (macrocytes), lemon-yellow pallor, anorexia, dyspnea (short of breath), prolonged bleeding time, abdominal discomfort, loss of weight, glossitis (inflammation of the tongue), an unsteady gait, and neurological disturbances, including stiffness of the limbs, irritability, and mental depression. Without treatment, death follows. Only injections of vitamin B-12 can alleviate efficiently the symptoms of pernicious anemia.

• **Dietary deficiencies**—Dietary deficiencies of vitamin B-12 may occur under the following circumstances:

1. **Among vegans and ovolactovegans.** People who live exclusively on plant foods (vegans) may be seriously deficient in vitamin B-12. Vegetarianism is, for religious reasons, common among Hindus in India and elsewhere, but most of them are ovolactovegetarians. (They consume animal products other than flesh foods.) Yet, for large numbers of Hindus the intake of animal foods, and therefore of vitamin B-12, falls far short of the recommended allowances.

2. **In some developing countries.** Vitamin B-12 deficiencies are not uncommon in developing countries where foods of plant origin predominate, especially among pregnant and lactating women. For example, very low intakes of the vitamin have been reported in Peru and in parts of Africa.

3. **Where consumption of animal products by mothers is low.** In areas of the world where intakes of animal products by mothers is low, vitamin B-12 deficiency in infants may occur.

When and where animal foods are in short supply, vitamin B-12 now makes it possible to rectify the above situations, and to use plant and cereal foods much more wisely in the human diet.

RECOMMENDED DAILY ALLOWANCE OF VITAMIN B-12.
The Food and Nutrition Board (FNB) of the National Research Council (NRC) recommended daily allowances (RDA) of vitamin B-12 are given in Table V-14.

TABLE V–14
RECOMMENDED DAILY
VITAMIN B-12 ALLOWANCES[1]

Group	Age	Weight		Height		Vitamin B-12
	(years)	(lb)	(kg)	(in.)	(cm)	(mcg)
Infants	0.0–0.5	13	6	24	60	0.3[2]
	0.5–1.0	20	9	28	71	0.5
Children	1–3	29	13	35	90	0.7
	4–6	44	20	44	112	1.0
	7–10	62	28	52	132	1.4
Males	11–14	99	45	62	157	2.0
	15–18	145	66	69	176	2.0
	19–24	160	72	70	177	2.0
	25–50	174	79	70	176	2.0
	51+	170	77	68	173	2.0
Females	11–14	101	46	62	157	2.0
	15–18	120	55	64	163	2.0
	19–24	128	58	65	164	2.0
	25–50	138	63	64	163	2.0
	51+	143	65	63	160	2.0
Pregnant						2.2
Lactating						2.6

[1]*Recommended Dietary Allowances*, 10th ed., NRC–National Academy of Sciences, 1989, p. 285.

These recommended daily allowances provide for a margin of safety to cover variance in individual needs, absorption, and body stores. However, in using this table as a nutritional guide, the following facts should be noted: (1) exact daily human requirements of vitamin B-12 cannot be given because it is synthesized by intestinal flora; (2) in the absence of intrinsic factor (e.g., pernicious anemia), the vitamin is not absorbed; and (3) it is assumed that at least 50% of the vitamin B-12 in food is absorbed.

• **Infants and children**—The recommended allowance for infants up to 6 months of age is 0.3 mcg per day. This is based on the average concentration of the vitamin in human milk. For infants receiving commercial formulas, the Committee of Nutrition of the American Academy of Pediatrics recommends a daily vitamin B-12 intake of 0.15 mcg/100 kcal; thus, a 1-year-old child weighing 10 kg and receiving 1,000 kcal should receive 1.5 mcg of vitamin B-12 per day. The recommended daily allowances given in Table V-14 for older infants and preadolescent children have been calculated on the basis of average energy intakes by using the latter formula.

• **Adults**—The recommended daily allowance for both males and females over 10 years of age is 2.0 mcg of vitamin B-12. This value will maintain adequate vitamin B-12 nutrition and a substantial reserve body pool in most normal persons.

• **Pregnancy and lactation**—The recommended dietary allowance for pregnant and lactating women is 2.2 mcg and 2.6 mcg, respectively.

Only the effects of gross deficiency of vitamin B-12 are known; hence, it is possible that a minor degree of deficiency, especially if of long duration, may prevent buoyant good health, even in well fed populations.

• **Vitamin B-12 intake in average U.S. diet**—The U.S. Department of Agriculture reported that, in 1988, the amount of vitamin B-12 in the U.S. food supply averaged 9.1 mg per person per day. (But the intake may have ranged from a low of 1 to a high of 100 mg per day.) Meat, fish, and poultry contributed 77% of the 9.1 mg of vitamin B-12 available in the typical U.S. daily diet; dairy products contributed 17.5%; eggs, 3.8%; and 1.0% was derived from other sources.

TOXICITY. No toxic effects of vitamin B-12 are known.

VITAMIN B-12 LOSSES DURING PROCESSING, COOKING, AND STORAGE.
About 30% of the vitamin B-12 activity of foods is lost during ordinary cooking.

Although only about 10% of the vitamin B-12 activity in milk is lost by pasteurization, from 40 to 90% of the B-12 is destroyed by evaporating milk.

It is noteworthy that in the presence of ascorbic acid vitamin B-12 withstands less heat.

Vitamin B-12 is destroyed by light.

SOURCES OF VITAMIN B-12. The sole source of vitamin B-12 in nature is synthesis by microorganisms. It is synthesized by the many microorganisms in the rumen and intestine of herbivorous animals. The vitamin B-12 bound to a protein in animal foods results from such synthesis. This explains why vitamin B-12 is found in all foods of animal origin.

Plants cannot manufacture vitamin B-12; hence, except for trace amounts absorbed from the soil (because of the bacteria, soil is a good source of B-12) by the growing plant, very little is found in plant foods—in vegetables, grains, legumes, fruits, etc.

A classification of the B-12 content of food sources follows:

• **Rich sources**—Liver and other organ meats—kidney, heart.

• **Good sources**—Muscle meats, fish, shellfish, eggs, and cheese.

• **Fair sources**—Milk, poultry, yogurt.

• **Negligible sources**—Bread (both whole wheat and white), cereal grains, fruits, legumes, vegetables.

• **Supplemental sources**—Cobalamin, of which there are at least three active forms, produced by microbial growth; available at the corner drugstore.

For additional sources and more precise values of vitamin B-12, see Food Composition Table F-36.

Some vitamin B-12 is formed by microorganisms in the intestinal tract of human beings. However, the synthesis is so far down in the colon that little of it may be absorbed.

The story of vitamin B-12 lends support to all developing country programs designed to improve animal production and to increase the supply and consumption of animal protein. Also, it is recognized that vitamin B-12 deficiency is not an uncommon consequence of many diseases and of surgical operations on the stomach and small intestine.

TOP FOOD SOURCES OF VITAMIN B-12.

NOTE WELL: This table lists (1) the top sources without regard to the amount normally eaten (left column), and (2) the top food sources (right column); and the caloric (energy) content of each food.

(Also see VITAMIN[S], Table V-9.)

TABLE V-15
TOP SOURCES OF VITAMIN B-12 AND THEIR CALORIC CONTENT[1]

Top Sources[2]	Vitamin B-12 (mcg/100 g)	Energy (kcal/100 g)	Top Food Sources	Vitamin B-12 (mcg/100 g)	Energy (kcal/100 g)
Liver, beef, fried	111.3	222	Liver, beef, fried	111.3	222
Clams, raw, soft meat and liquid	98.0	54	Liver, chicken, cooked, simmered	19.4	165
Kidneys, lamb, raw	63.0	105	Oysters, raw	15.0	73
Liver, turkey, cooked, simmered	47.5	174	Luncheon meat, liverwurst, fresh	13.9	496
Kidneys, calf, raw	25.0	113	Mackerel, salted	12.0	305
Liver, chicken, cooked, simmered	19.4	165	Crab (Blue, Dungeness, Rock, King), steamed	10.0	93
Pancreas beef (medium fat), raw	16.3	283	Sardines, Atlantic, canned in oil	10.0	200
Roe (Cod, Haddock, Herring), canned, solid/liquid	15.0	118	Cheese, natural Mozzarella, low moisture	8.0	318
Oysters, raw	15.0	73	Salmon, Atlantic, canned, solids/liquid	6.9	124
Luncheon meat, liverwurst, fresh	13.9	496	Pork, fresh, loin separable, lean, cooked, broiled	3.0	270
Mackerel, salted	12.0	305	Catfish, freshwater, raw	2.2	103
Cod, dehydrated, lightly salted	10.0	375	Tuna, canned in oil, drained, solids	2.2	197
Crab (Blue, Dungeness, Rock, King), steamed	10.0	93	Lamb, composite of cuts	2.1	273
Eggs, chicken, dried, whole	10.0	593	Frankfurter, raw, nonfat dry milk	1.7	300
Sardines, Atlantic, canned in oil	10.0	200	Cheese, natural, Swiss (domestic)	1.7	372
Kidneys, hog, raw	9.5	106	Beef, all cuts, including hamburger, broiled or roasted	1.6	314
Cheese, natural Mozzarella, low moisture	8.0	318	Sausage, smoked, link	1.6	313
Herring, canned, solids/liquid, plain	8.0	202	Halibut, Greenland, raw	1.5	174
Eggs, chicken, dried, yolk	7.1	687	Eggs, chicken, fried	1.4	210
Salmon, Atlantic, canned, solids/liquid	6.9	124	Bologna	1.3	316

[1]These listings are based on the data in Food Composition Table F-36. Some top or rich sources may have been overlooked since some of the foods in Table F-36 lack values for vitamin B-12.

Whenever possible, foods are on an "as used" basis, without regard to moisture content; hence, certain high-moisture foods may be disadvantaged when ranked on the basis of vitamin B-12 content per 100 g (approximately 3½ oz) without regard to moisture content.

[2]Listed without regard to the amount normally eaten.

VITAMIN B-13 (OROTIC ACID)

It is highly possible that the so-called vitamin B-13 is a growth promotant and a preventative of certain disorders. At this time, however, it is not known whether it plays an essential role in an otherwise adequate diet; hence, this presentation is for two purposes; (1) informational, and (2) stimulation of research.

HISTORY. This compound, called B-13, was first obtained from distillers' solubles. Subsequently, one of its constituents, orotic acid, has been synthesized in Europe and used to treat multiple sclerosis.

CHEMISTRY. Vitamin B-13 is a compound of unknown structure which appears either to contain orotic acid or to yield it on decomposition (see Fig. V-29).

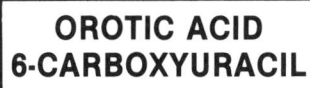

OROTIC ACID
6-CARBOXYURACIL

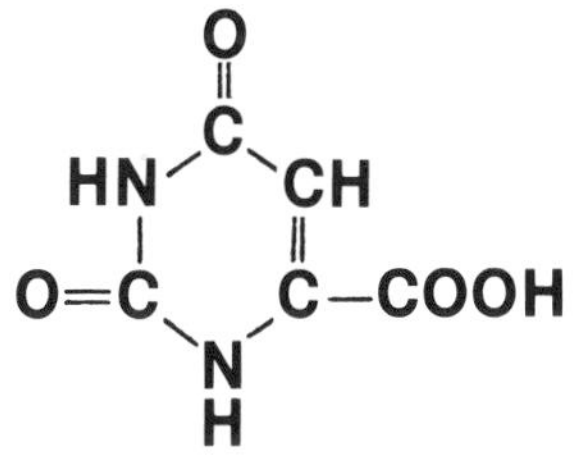

Fig. V-29. Orotic acid.

FUNCTIONS. Vitamin B-13 has been found to stimulate the growth of rats, chicks, and pigs under certain conditions.

Orotic acid is utilized by the body in the metabolism of folic acid and vitamin B-12. Also, it appears to aid the replacement or restoration of some cells.

There is indication that vitamin B-13 may be helpful in the treatment of multiple sclerosis.

DEFICIENCY SYMPTOMS. Deficiency symptoms have not been proved. But it is believed that a deficiency may lead to liver disorders, cell degeneration, and premature aging; and to degenerative symptoms in multiple sclerosis victims.

RECOMMENDED DAILY ALLOWANCE OF VITAMIN B-13. Dietary requirements are not known.

SOURCES OF VITAMIN B-13. Vitamin B-13 is found in such natural sources as distillers' solubles, whey, soured or curdled milk, and root vegetables. Also, this nutrient is available in supplemental form as calcium orotate.

(Also see VITAMIN[S], Table V-9.)

VITAMIN B-15

The designation that is sometimes erroneously given to "pangamic acid." In 1951, Krebs *et al.* reported the presence of a water-soluble factor in apricot kernels, which they subsequently isolated in crystalline form from rice bran and polish. The name pangamic acid (*pan*, meaning universal; *gamic*, meaning seed) was applied to the substance to connote its seeming universal presence in seeds; and it was assigned the fifteenth position in the vitamin B series by its discoverers. Subsequently, the designation as vitamin B-15 was dropped because the substance does not meet the classical definition of a vitamin.

(Also see PANGAMIC ACID; and VITAMIN[S], Table V-9.)

VITAMIN B COMPLEX

With the exception of vitamin C, all of the water-soluble vitamins can be grouped together under the vitamin B complex.

The story of the B vitamins begins with the study of the age-old disease beriberi.

In 1873, Van Lent was apparently the first to conclude that the type of diet had something to do with the origin of beriberi. By reducing the ration of rice in the diet of the sailors in the Dutch navy, he was able to eradicate beriberi almost entirely.

In 1882, Kanehiro Takaki, a Japanese Naval medical officer, reported that he had cured beriberi in sailors of the Japanese Navy by giving them less rice and more meat, milk, and vegetables. Takaki attributed the cure to the protein content of the diet.

Fifteen years later (1897), Christiaan Eijkman, a Dutch physician assigned to a prison hospital in the East Indies, observed beriberi among the inmates and sought the answer through experiments with chickens. To save money, he fed the birds scraps—mostly polished rice—from the patients' meals. The chickens unexpectedly developed a bad nerve ailment, which resulted in paralysis.

Later, the unsympathetic director of the hospital withheld permission to use scraps, and Dr. Eijkman had to buy natural (unmilled) rice for the chickens he used in his experiment. The ailing birds improved after they began eating the natural rice.

Dr. Eijkman then began a series of experiments that led to the first clear concept of disease due to nutritional deficiency. He fed polished white rice to chickens, pigeons, and ducks. They developed the paralysis that he had observed previously, then recovered when he fed them natural (unmilled) rice. Birds fed whole rice remained well.

Eijkman noted that the disease in birds which resulted from a polished rice diet resembled beriberi in man. He theorized that rice contained too much starch, which poisoned nerve cells, and that the outer layers, removed from the grain in milling, were an antidote.

Another Dutch physician, Dr. G. Grijns, continued the

work of Eijkman. But he interpreted Eijkman's findings differently. In 1901, he concluded that beriberi in birds and man was due to a deficiency or absence of an essential nutrient from the diet.

From then on, chemists in many countries tried to concentrate the substance in rice that prevented beriberi in order to obtain it in pure form. Among them was Casimir Funk, of the Lister Institute, London, who, in 1912, coined the term ''vitamine'' and applied it to the antiberiberi substance.

In 1916, Dr. Elmer V. McCollum of the University of Wisconsin designated the concentrate that cured beriberi as ''water-soluble B,'' to distinguish it from the antinightblindness factor (called vitamin A) which had been found in carrots and butterfat of milk. At that time, McCollum though that the antiberiberi substance was one factor only.

In 1926, B. C. P. Jansen and W. P. Donath, in Holland, isolated the antiberiberi vitamin, and in 1936 Robert R. Williams, an American, determined the structure and synthesized it.

As research continued (1919-1922), it was found that vitamin B was not a single substance, that it actually consisted of several factors. Collectively, they came to be known as the *vitamin B complex*, but each factor was given a separate designation. Some members of the group came to be referred to by subscript numbers as vitamins B_1, B_2, etc.; others became known by their chemical names; still others received both a number and a chemical designation. These vitamins differ in both chemical structure and specific functions. Yet, there are similarities. All of them are water-soluble; all of them are abundant in liver and yeast, and they often occur together in the same foodstuffs; each of them contains carbon, hydrogen, oxygen, and nitrogen; some of them contain mineral elements in their molecules (thiamin and biotin contain sulfur, and vitamin B-12 contains cobalt and phosphorus); most of them are part of a coenzyme molecule concerned with the breakdown of carbohydrate, protein, and fat in the body; the actions of many of them are interrelated; few of them are stored in large amounts in the body, so they must be provided daily; certain organs, particularly the liver, contain higher concentrations of them than others; and they are excreted from the body by way of the kidneys.

Another noteworthy characteristic of the B vitamins is that they are synthesized by microbial fermentation in the digestive tract, especially by ruminants (cattle and sheep) and herbivorous nonruminants (horse and rabbit). Some animals eat their own feces (coprophagy), thus recycling the vitamins synthesized in the microbial fermentation in the large intestine and cecum; rabbits, in particular, are known to do this on a routine basis. Unlike ruminants and herbivorous nonruminants, however, man, pigs, and poultry have only one stomach and no large cecum like the horse and rabbit. As a result, they do not synthesize enough of most B vitamins. Consequently, for man and other monogastrics, the B vitamins must be provided regularly in the diet in adequate amounts if deficiencies are to be averted.

At the present time, 9 fractions of the vitamin B complex are generally recognized, and others are postulated. Those discussed in this book (alphabetically under their name designations) are: biotin, choline, folacin (folic acid), niacin (nicotinic acid; nicotinamide), pantothenic acid (vitamin B-3), riboflavin (vitamin B-2), thiamin (vitamin B-1), vitamin B-6 (pyridoxine, pyridoxal; pyridoxamine), and vitamin B-12 (cobalamins).

A lack of B-complex vitamins is one of the forms of malnutrition that occur often throughout the world. Because the B vitamins are usually found in the same foodstuffs, a deficiency of several factors is usually observed rather than a deficiency of a single factor.

Many physiologic and pathologic stresses influence the need for the B vitamins. Larger amounts are needed during growth and in pregnancy and lactation than in maintenance of health in adult life. The requirement may be increased by diseases that elevate metabolism and by conditions associated with poor absorption, improper utilization, or increased excretion. Administration of antibiotics may lead to vitamin deficiency in some circumstances; in others, antibiotics spare vitamin requirements.

(Also see BERIBERI; and VITAMIN[S].)

VITAMIN B-T

In 1947, Fraenkel found that the meal worm, *Tenebrio molitor*, required a growth factor present in yeast. Fraenkel called the factor *Vitamin B-T*; vitamin B because of its water-soluble property, and T for *Tenebrio*. Because of not being recognized as a vitamin, the name was subsequently changed to carnitine.

(Also see CARNITINE; and VITAMIN[S].)

VITAMIN C (ASCORBIC ACID; DEHYDRO-ASCORBIC ACID)

Contents

Vitamin C—also called *ascorbic acid, dehydroascorbic acid, hexuronic acid*, and the *antiscorbutic vitamin*—is the very important substance, first found in citrus fruits, which prevents scurvy, one of the oldest scourges of mankind. All animal species appear to require vitamin C, but a *dietary need* is limited to humans, guinea pigs, monkeys, bats, certain fish, and perhaps certain reptiles. These species lack the enzyme L-gulonolactone oxidase which is necessary for vitamin C synthesis from 6 carbon sugars.

VITAMIN C
helps to build healthy gums, teeth, and bones
TWO GUINEA PIGS OF SAME AGE

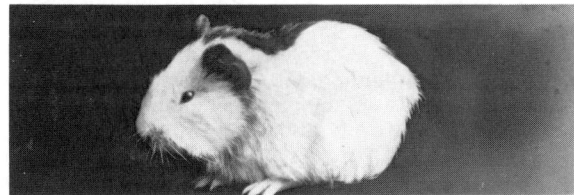 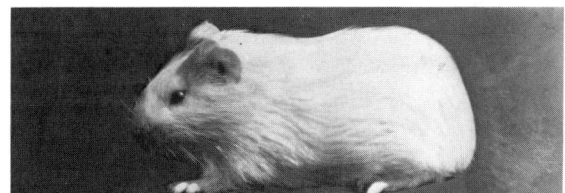

THIS GUINEA PIG HAD NO ASCORBIC ACID AND DEVELOPED SCURVY. NOTE CROUCHED POSITION DUE TO SORE JOINTS.

THIS GUINEA PIG HAD PLENTY OF ASCORBIC ACID. IT IS HEALTHY AND ALERT; ITS FUR IS SLEEK AND FINE.

TOP FOOD SOURCES

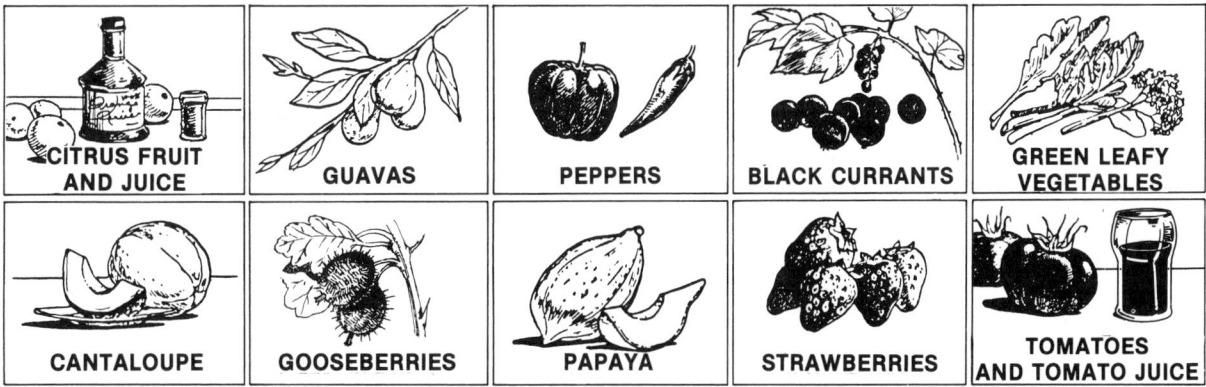

Fig. V-30. Vitamin C (ascorbic acid) made the difference! *Left:* Guinea pig on vitamin C-deficient diet. *Right:* Guinea pig that received plenty of vitamin C. Note, too, top sources of vitamin C. (Adapted from USDA sources.)

HISTORY. Scurvy, now known to be caused by a severe deficiency of vitamin C, has been a dread disease since ancient times. It was once common among sailors who ate little except bread and salt meat while on long voyages.

The historical incidence and conquest of scurvy constitute one of the most thrilling chapters in the development of nutrition as a science. A chronological summary of the saga of scurvy and vitamin C follows:

As early as 1550 B.C., scurvy was described by the Egyptians on medical papyrus rolls (man's first writing paper, made by the Egyptians from the papyrus plant as early as 2400 B.C.), discovered in Thebes by George Moritz Ebers, a German Egyptologist and novelist, who, in 1874, edited it in a romantic historical novel on medicine which he titled *Papyrus Ebers*).

In the Old Testament (which was written over a long period of time, thought to be from 1100 B.C. to 500 B.C.), reference is made to this disease.

About 450 B.C., Hippocrates, the Greek "father of medicine" described the symptoms of the malady—gangrene of the gums, loss of teeth, and painful legs in soldiers.

In 1248-54, Jean Sire de Joinville, the French chronicler, accompanied Louis IX of France to Cyprus and Egypt. In 1309, he completed in final form the *History of Saint Louis*, an account of the Crusade, in which he told of a disease (scurvy) "which attacked the mouth and the legs."

In 1497, when Vasco da Gama, Portuguese navigator, sailed around the Cape of Good Hope and established the first European trading colony on the coast of Malabar in India, 100 of his crew of 160 men perished of scurvy on the voyage.

During the winter of 1535 in Canada, Jacques Cartier, the daring explorer who laid claim to Canada for France, recorded in his log that the lives of many of his men dying of scurvy were saved "almost overnight," when they learned from the Indians that drinking a brew made from the growing tips of pine or spruce trees cured and prevented the malady. (It is now known that the "brew" contained vitamin C.)

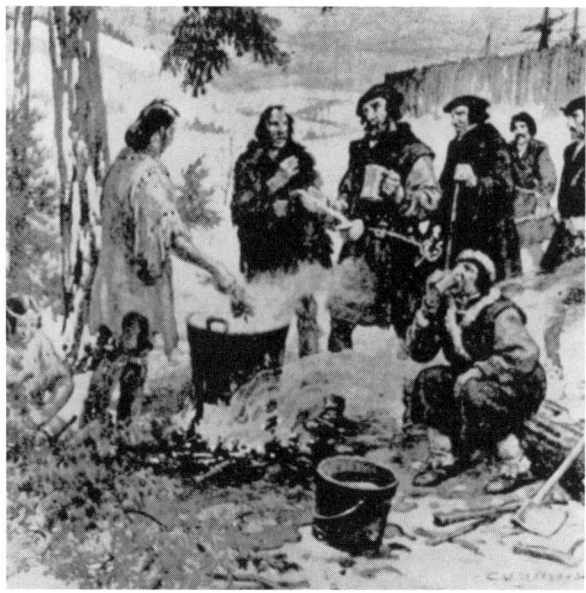

Fig. V-31. Friendly Huron-Iroquois Indians shown in Quebec in 1535, (1) making a broth from pine branches, and (2) serving it to Jacques Cartier and his men to cure scurvy. (Reproduced with permission of *Nutrition Today*, P. O. Box 1829, Annapolis, MD 21404, ©, 1979)

In the 15th and 16th centuries, scurvy was a scourge throughout Europe, so much so that medical men wondered if all diseases might stem from it. It was particularly prevalent and severe on long voyages of sailing ships, in cities, and in times of crop failures. During this period, there was also a tendency to associate scurvy and venereal disease; some authorities of the day believed that both diseases were brought from abroad by sailors. Mercury was sometimes used as a treatment, with disastrous results.

In 1600-1603, Captain James Lancaster, English navigator, recorded that on the long voyage to the East Indies he kept his crew hearty merely by the addition of a mandatory "three spoonfuls of lemon juice every morning."

In 1747, James Lind, an English naval surgeon, tested six remedies on 12 sailors who had scurvy and found that oranges and lemons were curative. His classical studies, the results of which were published in 1753, are generally credited as being the first experiments to show that an essential food element can prevent a deficiency disease. But another 50 years elapsed before the British Navy required rations of lemons or limes on sailing vessels.

On two historic voyages, each of three-years duration, from 1768 to 1771 and from 1772 to 1775, British Captain James Cook, avoided scurvy—hitherto the scourge of

long sea voyages. He had his ship stocked with concentrated slabs of thick brown vegetable soup and barrels of sauerkraut. Of the sauerkraut he said: "It is not only a wholesome vegetable food, but, in my judgment, highly antiscorbutic, and spoils not by keeping." In addition, he sent seamen ashore at every port visited to gather all sorts of fresh fruits and green vegetables (including grasses), which the crew prepared, served, and ate. As a result, not one of the crew died from scurvy.

In 1795 (one year after Lind's death), by Admiralty Order, the British Royal Navy began providing 1 oz of lime juice daily in every sailor's food ration; from this date forward, British sailors were stuck with the nickname "limeys."

In 1907, Holst and Frolich, of Norway, produced scurvy experimentally in guinea pigs by feeding them a diet deficient in foods containing ascorbic acid.

In 1928, Szent-Gyorgy, a Hungarian scientist, working in Hopkins' laboratory at Cambridge University, in England, isolated a substance from the ox adrenal glands, oranges, and cabbage leaves, which he called hexuronic acid; but he did not test it for antiscorbutic effect.

In 1932, Charles Glen King and W. A. Waugh, at the University of Pittsburg, isolated from lemon juice a crystalline material that possessed antiscorbutic activity in guinea pigs; this marked the discovery of *vitamin C*, a deficiency of which caused the centuries-old scourge of scurvy.

In 1933, vitamin C was synthesized by Reichstein, a Swiss scientist.

In 1938, *ascorbic acid* was officially accepted as the chemical name for vitamin C.

CHEMISTRY, METABOLISM, PROPERTIES.

• **Chemistry**—Ascorbic acid is a compound of relatively simple structure, closely related to the monosaccharide sugars. It is synthesized from glucose and other simple sugars by plants and by most animal species (see Fig. V-32).

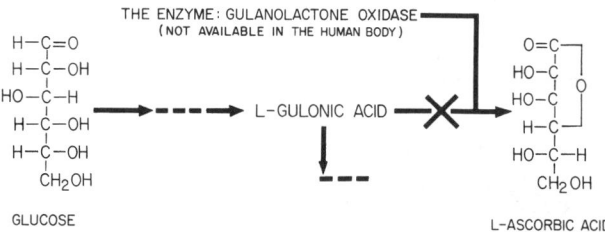

Fig. V-32. Metabolic relation of glucose to ascorbic acid. In man, the absence of oxidase prevents this reaction, making the intake of preformed ascorbic acid in food necessary.

Man, monkeys, guinea pigs, fruit-eating bats, and red-vented bulbul birds (the latter two are native to India), cannot make the conversion from glucose to ascorbic acid, because these species lack the necessary enzyme (oxidase). Scurvy, then, in man can really be classed as a disease of distant genetic origin—an inherited metabolic error; a defect in carbohydrate metabolism due to the lack of an enzyme, which, in turn, results from the lack of a specific gene.

Two forms of vitamin C occur in nature: ascorbic acid (the reduced form), and dehydroascorbic acid (the oxidized form).[18] Their structural formulas are shown in Fig. V-33.

Although most of the vitamin C exists as ascorbic acid, both forms appear to be utilized similarly by the human. Also, the body efficiently utilizes either synthetic L-ascorbic acid or the vitamin in its natural form as in orange juice.

Ascorbic acid is easily oxidized to dehydroascorbic acid, which is just as easily reduced back to ascorbic acid. However, dehydroascorbic acid may be irreversibly oxidized, particularly in the presence of alkali, to diketo-gulonic acid, which has no antiscorbutic activity (see Fig. V-34.)

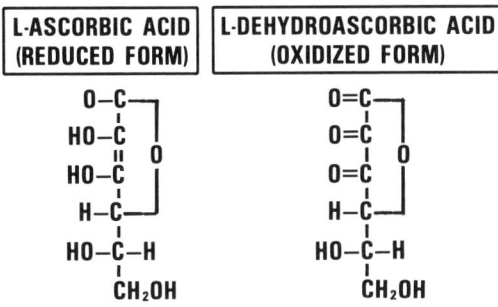

Fig. V-33. Structural formulas of vitamin C.

Certain derivatives of vitamin C (for example, erythrobic acid and ascorbyl palmitate) are used as antioxidants in food products to prevent rancidity, to prevent browning of fruit, and to cure meat. Erythrobic acid (D-araboascorbic acid) is poorly absorbed and has little antiscorbutic activity.

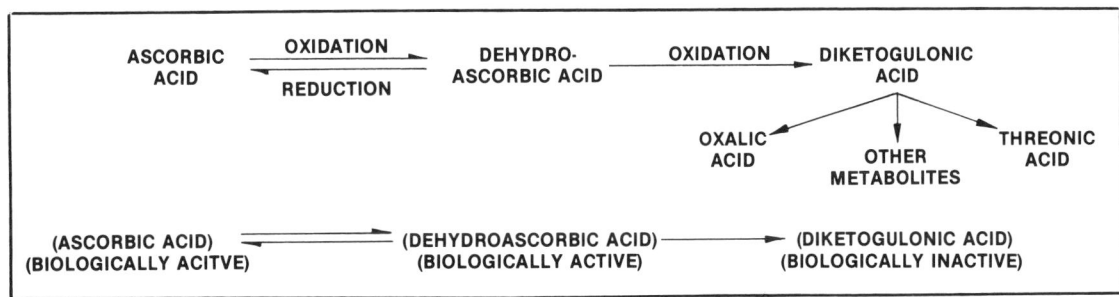

Fig. V-34. Relationship of ascorbic, dehydroascorbic, and diketogulonic acids.

- **Metabolism**—Pertinent facts about the absorption, storage, and excretion of vitamin C follow:

1. **Absorption**. Vitamin C is readily and rapidly absorbed from the upper part of the small intestine into the circulatory system. Thence, it is taken up unevenly by the tissues; the adrenal gland and the retina of the eye contain an especially high concentration of vitamin C, but the liver, spleen, intestine, bone marrow, pancreas, thymus, pituitary, brain, and kidney also contain appreciable amounts. Blood cells contain more than blood serum.

2. **Storage**. Unlike the majority of the water-soluble vitamins, limited stores of vitamin C are held in the body. Thus, the signs of scurvy do not appear for some weeks in humans receiving no vitamin C.

A plasma level of 0.6 mg ascorbic acid per 100 ml (1) indicates tissue saturation, and (2) a body storage equivalent to 1,500 mg in the healthy adult. Adequate vitamin C nutrition is indicated when plasma concentra-

tions range between 0.40 and 0.59 mg per 100 ml, representing a body pool of 600 to 1,499 mg. On a vitamin C-deficient diet, body stores (1) are used at an average rate of 3% of the existing reserve body pool per day, and (2) will supply the body with vitamin C for a period of about 3 months. When the body pool falls below 300 mg, signs of scurvy begin to appear.

3. **Excretion**. Vitamin C is largely excreted in the urine, with the amount excreted controlled by the kidney tubules. When the tissues are saturated, a large amount is excreted; but when the tissue reserves are depleted, only a small amount is excreted. Some vitamin C is always excreted by the kidneys even when the tissues are severely depleted.

- **Properties**—Ascorbic acid is a white, odorless crystalline powder, which is quite stable when dry.

Of all the vitamins, ascorbic acid is the most unstable when in solution. It is highly soluble in water, but not in fat. The oxidation (destruction) of ascorbic acid is accelerated by air, heat, light, alkalies, oxidative enzymes, and traces of copper and iron. It is markedly destroyed by cooking, particularly where the pH is alkaline. Cooking losses also result because of its solubility. The

---

[18]Actually, several chemical compounds have vitamin C activity. So, it is now recommended that the term *vitamin C* be used as the combined name of all compounds having the biological activity of ascorbic acid, and that the terms *ascorbic acid* and *dehydroascorbic acid* be used only when specific reference to them is made.

destruction of ascorbic acid is slowed down by foods that are acidic, by refrigeration, and by protection from exposure to air.

MEASUREMENT/ASSAY. The concentration of ascorbic acid in tissues and foods is expressed in milligrams. One I.U. is the activity of 0.05 mg of ascorbic acid.

Ascorbic acid is generally determined by chemical assay, accomplished by taking advantage of its reducing properties.

For bioassay work, guinea pigs are the preferred experimental animals because of their susceptibility to a deficiency of vitamin C. Thus, they are still used for demonstration of deficiency of the vitamin and to make comparative assays.

FUNCTIONS. The specific biochemical functions of vitamin C are not clearly understood. Nevertheless, it is established as a very important substance for body welfare because of being implicated in the following roles: (1) formation and maintenance of collagen, which makes for more rapid and sound healing of wounds and burns; (2) metabolism of the amino acids tyrosine and tryptophan; (3) absorption and movement of iron; (4) metabolism of fats and lipids, and cholesterol control; (5) as an antioxidant in the protection of vitamins A and E and the polyunsaturated fatty acids; (6) sound teeth and bones; (7) strong capillary walls and healthy blood vessels; (8) metabolism of folic acid; and perhaps in a number of other roles. Details follow:

• **Collagen formation**—The most clearly established functional role of vitamin C is the formation and maintenance of collagen, the substance that binds body cells together in much the same manner as mortar binds bricks.

Collagen is a fibrous protein that contains large amounts of the amino acids proline and hydroxyproline. Postulation is that vitamin C is essential for making hydroxyproline in the body as follows: Vitamin C activates the enzyme prolyl hydroxylase, which, in turn, effects the conversion of proline (by the addition of an "OH" group) to hydroxyproline in the formation of collagen.

Vitamin C is also required for the conversion of lysine to hydroxylysine, another amino acid that is an essential part of collagen. The reaction is brought about by the enzyme lysine hydroxylase. The role of vitamin C in the formation of hydroxylysine is thought to be similar to its role in the formation of hydroxyproline.

Both of the above reactions require vitamin C, and both are essential for collagen formation. In turn, failure to synthesize collagen results in delayed healing of wounds and burns. So, the administration of vitamin C makes for more rapid and sound healing of wounds.

• **Metabolism of tyrosine and tryptophan**—Vitamin C is necessary in the metabolism of the amino acids tyrosine and tryptophan.

In the metabolism of tyrosine, a deficiency of vitamin C will result in the build-up and excretion of the intermediary product, P-hydroxyphenylpyruvate, as a result of inactivating the enzyme P-hydroxyphenylpyruvic acid oxidase. When large amounts of tyrosine are being metabolized, vitamin C protects the enzyme P-hydroxyphenylpyruvic acid oxidase from inactivation (rather than activates as was formerly thought), and enhances the synthesis of norepinephrine, a neurotransmitter, from tyrosine.

Also, vitamin C is required for the conversion of tryptophan to 5-hydroxytryptophan, the first step in the formation of the serotonin, a compound that raises blood pressure through vasoconstrictor action.

• **Iron utilization**—When the two nutrients are ingested simultaneously, dietary vitamin C increases the absorption of iron by converting ferric iron to the more readily absorbed ferrous form. Vitamin C is also necessary for the movement of transferritin (a combination of ferric iron and the protein transferrin) to the liver, and for the formation of the iron-protein compound ferritin for storage in the liver, spleen, and bone marrow. (Also see Iron.)

• **Metabolism of fats and lipids**—There is some evidence that vitamin C affects fat and lipid metabolism as follows:

1. Vitamin C serves as a cofactor, along with ATP and magnesium ions, in the inactivation of the enzyme *adipose tissue lipase*, the enzyme that mobilizes the free fatty acids from adipose tissue to meet the energy demands of the body. When the body's energy needs have been met, vitamin C (along with the other two controlling agents—ATP and magnesium ions) inactivates the adipose tissue lipase.

2. Vitamin C may have a role in the metabolism of cholesterol. The levels of cholesterol in the liver and blood serum appear to rise during a deficiency of the vitamin, and to fall with the administration of the vitamin. The increased accumulation of cholesterol appears to be due to a decrease in the rate of conversion of cholesterol to bile acids when vitamin C intake is inadequate.

Vitamin C also appears to be involved in the metabolism of cholesterol in another way. Through its sulfated metabolite, *ascorbic acid sulfate*, it appears to bring about the formation of cholesterol sulfate, a water-soluble compound that is excreted in the urine. By this means, cholesterol may be mobilized from the body tissues, with the result that there is a lowering of blood cholesterol levels.

• **Antioxidant in the protection of vitamins A and E and the polyunsaturated fatty acids**—Ascorbic acid is an important antioxidant; thus, it has a role in the protection of vitamins A and E and the polyunsaturated fatty acids from excessive oxidation.

• **Sound teeth and bones**—Vitamin C is required for the normal development of odontoblasts, a layer of cells that forms dentin in teeth. It follows that a deficiency of vitamin C may cause defects in tooth dentin, especially during the critical period of tooth formation.

Also, vitamin C is necessary for the proper calcification and soundness of bone.

• **Strength of capillary walls and blood vessels**—Vitamin C is necessary for maintaining strength of capillary walls, especially of the small blood vessels. Shortages of the vitamin result in weakened and inelastic capillary walls, which may rupture and hemorrhage, evidenced by easy bruising, pinpoint peripheral hemorrhages, bone and joint hemorrhages, easy bone fracture, fragile bleeding gums with loosened teeth, and poor wound healing.

• **Metabolism of folic acid (folacin)**—Vitamin C is required for the conversion of the inactive form of the vitamin, folic acid (folacin), to its active form, folinic acid. When there is an insufficiency of vitamin C in the diet, the metabolism of folic acid (folacin) is impaired and the megaloblastic anemia that occurs in scurvy, and sometimes in infancy, may result.

In addition to the above functions of vitamin C, investigators have suggested a number of other roles for vitamin C. Although the evidence for most of these functions is not conclusive, a brief summary of each of them follows in the hope that it will stimulate further research:

• **Synthesis or release of the steroid hormones; stress**— It has been observed (1) that the normally high concentration of ascorbic acid in the adrenal glands is depleted with the synthesis of steroid hormones, and (2) that there is an increased requirement of vitamin C in all forms of stress—extremely high or low temperature, shock, fatigue, injury, burns, surgery, cigarette smoking, toxic levels of heavy metals (such as lead, mercury, and cadmium, etc.). Hence, it has been theorized that vitamin C is involved with either the synthesis or release of the steroid hormones by the adrenal glands; and that the greater the stress, the higher the vitamin C requirement.

Dr. James Cason, Professor of Chemistry, University of California, Berkeley, cites the following item in support of the role of ascorbic acid in resisting stress: A 150-lb goat makes about 13 g of ascorbic acid daily under ordinary circumstances, but if a goat is put under stress it will produce up to twice this amount.[17] It seems reasonable, therefore, that ascorbic acid would help man to resist stress, too.

• **Protection in infection and fever**—There are decreased tissue and blood levels of ascorbic acid during infections and fever, indicating either increased need for this vitamin or increased destruction of it. Thus, higher than normal intakes of vitamin C may be needed to provide maximum protection against infections and fevers.

• **Prevention and cure of colds and flu**—There is much controversy concerning the effectiveness of massive doses of vitamin C in the prevention and cure of the common cold and flu. Linus Pauling, a respected chemist with the rare distinction of receiving two Nobel Prizes—one for science and the other for peace, is the most enthusiastic advocate of using vitamin C as a drug. His book *Vitamin C and the Common Cold and the Flu*, published in 1970, has had great influence. As a result of his advocacy, many people throughout the world began taking tablets of ascorbic acid. Nevertheless, as a result of studies on thousands of people, the only reasonable conclusion that can be drawn is that vitamin C has no effect on the number of colds people get, but in some people it lessens the severity of cold symptoms.

There should be an awareness that large doses of vitamin C are known to increase (1) the urinary output of oxalic acid and uric acid, and (2) the intestinal absorption of iron. Thus, massive doses of vitamin C may be hazardous to those with a liability to kidney stones or iron-storage disease.

• **Phagocyte activity and formation of antibodies**— Ascorbic acid may have a stimulating effect on the phagocytic activity, and on the formation of antibodies.

• **Reducing the requirements for certain vitamins**— Ascorbic acid (the reduced form of vitamin C) lessens animal requirements for thiamin, riboflavin, pantothenic acid, folacin, vitamin A, and vitamin E; likely, it has a similar role in man.

• **Smoking**—Recent research confirms the long-time claim that smoking lowers the blood level of vitamin C, although it is not known whether this is due to actual destruction or reduced availability of ascorbic acid. But there is no evidence that heavy smokers need more vitamin C than that supplied by the recommended dietary allowances.

• **Cancer**—Dr. Linus Pauling declares that vitamin C is beneficial to cancer victims, according to Dr. James Cason, Professor of Chemistry, University of California, Berkeley, who reported on the following cancer-vitamin C study in which Dr. Pauling was involved.[18]

In 1976, Cameron and Pauling published the results of an ongoing investigation of cancer therapy with vitamin C at a hospital in Scotland, where Dr. Cameron is physician in residence. The study involved 1,100 cancer victims who had been diagnosed as "terminal." One hundred of these (matched for sex, age, and type of cancer for comparison with a control group) were given massive doses of 10 g/day of vitamin C in double blind placebo procedure, and the remaining 1,000 were the comparison group. The vitamin C-treated patients lived an average of four times longer than the comparison group. At the time of publication in 1976, all the comparison group were dead, while 16 of the 100 who received vitamin C were alive. Moreover, 1 year after publishing the results, Dr. Pauling reported, "13 of these 'hopeless' patients are still alive, some as long as 5 years after having been pronounced untreatable, and most of them are in such good apparent health as to suggest that they now have normal life expectancy."

But a controlled study by Dr. Edward T. Creagan, Mayo Clinic, showed no anticancer effect or improved survival as a result of megadoses of vitamin C. Likewise, Drs. J. Roberto Moran and Henry L. Greene, researchers at Vanderbilt University School of Medicine, concluded from a study of the benefits

---

[17]Cason, James, Ascorbic Acid, Amygdalin and Carcinoma, *The Vortex*, June 1978, pp. 9-23.

[18]*Ibid.*

and risks of vitamin C megadoses that "at present no strong evidence can be found to support the routine prophylactic (preventive) use of ascorbic acid in well-nourished people."

• **Removal of ammonia in the deamination of proteins and peptides**—Vitamin C appears to accelerate the deamination of proteins and peptides and the conversion of ammonia (HN_3) to urea for excretion. Some have even conjectured that these processes (the oxidative deamination and the urea cycle) affect aging and longevity.

• **Antihistamine**—Ascorbic acid is an antihistamine; hence, it may be effective in treating respiratory infections due to a histamine.

• **Detoxifying drugs**—Vitamin C appears to be involved in a set of biochemical reactions responsible for detoxifying drugs, and for eliminating them from the body. Specifically, the vitamin may facilitate steps in which iron is introduced into the heme groups that subsequently become part of the proteins that carry out the detoxification reactions.

• **Longevity**—In 1992, the UCLA School of Public Health reported in the *Journal of Epidemiology* that (1) daily intake of 300 mg of vitamin C from food and supplements may increase life expectancy in men by 6 years, and (2) daily intake of 150 mg vitamin C from food, without supplements, may increase life expectancy in men by 2 years. The study focused on 11,000 adults, 25 to 74 years of age.

DETERMINING VITAMIN C STATUS. Vitamin C status in people may be determined by clinical signs and by blood levels of the vitamin. Evidence of capillary bleeding in the skin (perifolliculosis) and in the gums are clinical signs that may indicate a vitamin C deficiency.

Different investigators have employed a variety of tests for estimating the vitamin C nutrition of man and animals. The simplest of these is measurement of the L-ascorbic acid content of serum or plasma. Approximate values of L-ascorbic acid of man which may be used for guide purposes follow:

Nutritional Status	Serum or Plasma Concentration (mg/100 ml)
Well nourished	over 0.60
Adequate	0.40–0.59
Low	0.10–0.39
Deficient	under 0.10

In a study of the ascorbic acid level per 100 ml of blood plasma of 48 women and 41 men, the senior author of this encyclopedia, Audrey H. Ensminger, found 14 subjects, or 15.7%, at the scurvy level.

DEFICIENCY SYMPTOMS. When deprived of a dietary source of vitamin C for a sufficient length of time, man, along with other primates and several other species, develops scurvy, a potentially fatal disease.

• **Early symptoms, called latent scurvy**—Early symptoms of vitamin C deficiency, called latent scurvy, include: loss of weight, listlessness, fatigue, fleeting pains in the joints and muscles, irritability, shortness of breath, sore and/or bleeding gums, small hemorrhages under the skin, bones that fracture easily, and poor wound healing.

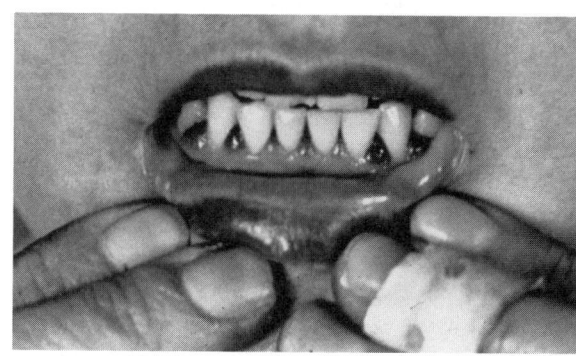

Fig. V-35.   Scorbutic gums. (Reproduced with permission of *Nutrition Today*, P. O. Box 1829, Annapolis, MD 21404, ©, 1979.)

• **Scurvy**—A severe deficiency of vitamin C results in acute scurvy, characterized by: swollen, bleeding, and ulcerated gums; loose teeth; malformed and weak bones; fragility of the capillaries with resulting hemorrhages throughout the body; large bruises; big joints, such as the knee and hip, due to bleeding into the joint cavity; anemia; degeneration of muscle fibers, including those of the heart; and tendency of old wounds to become red and break open. Sudden death from severe internal hemorrhage and heart failure is always a danger.

RECOMMENDED DAILY ALLOWANCE OF VITAMIN C. Many studies have been conducted to determine the human vitamin C requirements. Consideration has been given to the effect of age, environment, physical exertion, infections, and fevers. Also, various measurements for determining the adequacy of vitamin C have been devised, including: (1) the daily intake of vitamin C necessary to prevent the symptoms of scurvy; (2) the amount of vitamin C required to saturate whole blood, blood plasma, white blood cells, or body tissue; and (3) the intake of vitamin C necessary to maintain blood and urinary ascorbic acid levels within normal range. The results of these studies vary widely.

A daily intake of 10 mg of ascorbic acid will prevent scurvy. But this should be regarded as a minimum level. In order to provide for individual differences and margins of safety, the Food and Nutrition Board of the National Academy of Sciences recommends the following allowances: 30 mg for infants, 40 mg for children, 60 mg for males and females over 14 years, 70 mg for pregnancy, and 95 mg for lactation (see Table V-16).

TABLE V–16
RECOMMENDED DAILY VITAMIN C ALLOWANCES[1]

Group	Age	Weight		Height		Vitamin C
	(years)	(lb)	(kg)	(in.)	(cm)	(mg)[2]
Infants	0.0–0.5	13	6	24	60	30
	0.5–1.0	20	9	28	71	35
Children	1–3	29	13	35	90	40
	4–6	44	20	44	112	45
	7–10	62	28	52	132	45
Males	11–14	99	45	62	157	50
	15–18	145	66	69	176	60
	19–24	160	70	70	177	60
	25–50	174	70	70	178	60
	51+	170	70	70	178	60
Females	11–14	101	46	62	157	50
	15–18	120	55	64	163	60
	19–24	128	58	65	164	60
	25–50	138	63	64	163	60
	51+	143	65	63	160	60
Pregnant						70
Lactating						95

[1]*Recommended Dietary Allowances*, 10th ed., NRC–National Academy of Sciences, 1989, p. 285.
[2]0.05 mg of ascorbic acid = 1 IU of vitamin C.

It is noteworthy that the joint FAO/WHO Expert Committee makes somewhat lower recommendations than those given in Table V-16: 20 mg for infants and children up to 13 years of age, 30 mg for adults (males and females over 13 years), and 50 mg during pregnancy and lactation.

It is recognized, however, that these allowances are not necessarily adequate to meet the additional requirements of persons depleted by disease, traumatic stress, or prior dietary inadequacies. Also, the recommended levels given in Table V-16 may not be sufficient to assure vigorous good health.

● **Recommended allowances for infants, children, and adolescents**—A dietary allowance of 30 mg per day is recommended for infants. This is based on the fact that (1) human milk contains 30 to 55 mg/liter of vitamin C, although it varies with the mother's dietary intake of the vitamin; and (2) the breast-fed infant receives approximately 850 ml of milk per day. However, newborn infants, especially if they are premature, may have an increased requirement for the metabolism of tyrosine during the first week of life. To protect against possible adverse effects of the transient tyrosinemia, an intake of 100 mg/day of ascorbic acid is recommended during this period.

For children up to the age of 11 years, an allowance of 45 mg/day of vitamin C is recommended. For older children, an allowance of up to 60 mg/day is recommended as adequate to meet individual needs and to provide a margin of safety. Allowances, dosages, and intakes follow:

● **Recommended allowance for adults**—A dietary allowance of 60 mg of vitamin C per day is recommended for adults of both sexes. This will maintain an ascorbate body pool of 1,500 mg—a body pool of sufficient magnitude to protect against signs of scurvy in the adult male for a period of 30 to 45 days, and allow for an ascorbate catabolism rate of 3 to 4% and an average ascorbate absorption efficiency of approximately 85%.

● **Recommended allowances for pregnancy and lactation**—During pregnancy, plasma vitamin C levels fall. It is not known whether this is due to a physiological response of pregnancy and/or to increased demands of pregnancy. It is known that the placenta normally transmits sufficient ascorbic acid from mother to fetus to result in fetal levels 50% greater than maternal levels at birth. To provide for this fetal need, an additional allowance of 10 mg of ascorbic acid per day is recommended for pregnant women, particularly during the second and third trimester of pregnancy.

Human milk from well-nourished women is relatively high in ascorbic acid, but it varies with the mother's dietary intake of the nutrient. During lactation, a daily loss of 25 to 45 mg of vitamin C may occur in the secretion of 850 ml of milk. So, for lactating women, an additional allowance of 35 mg/day of vitamin C is recommended in order to assure a satisfactory level of the vitamin in breast milk.

● **Massive doses of ascorbic acid**—Intakes of ascorbic acid in excess of 1,000 mg/day (1 g/day) or more have been reported to have some effect in reducing the frequency and severity of symptoms of colds and flu. To date, the results of research work have generally shown that the benefits of large doses of vitamin C are too small to justify recommending routine intake of large amounts. But further studies are needed.

Large doses of ascorbic acid have been reported to lower serum cholesterol in some hypercholesterolemic subjects, but not in others.

Ascorbic acid supplements can prevent the reduced platelet and plasma concentrations of ascorbic acid observed in aspirin-treated rheumatoid-arthritis patients.

The use of massive doses of vitamin C to improve the performance of athletes has long been a controversial issue. Present findings indicate that the vitamin is ineffective for this purpose, and that large doses may have a negative effect on athletic performance by disturbing the equilibrium between oxygen transport and oxygen utilization.

Large doses of ascorbic acid have generally been considered nontoxic, except for gastrointestinal symptoms experienced by some people. However, a number of adverse effects of excessive intakes of ascorbic acid have been reported, such as acid-induced uricosuria, absorption of excessive amounts of food iron, and impaired bactericidal activity of leucocytes.

Since many of the claims of significant beneficial effects of large intakes of ascorbic acid have not been sufficiently substantiated, and since excessive intakes may have some adverse effects, routine consumption of large intakes of ascorbic acid is not recommended without medical advice.

● **Vitamin C intake in average U.S. diet**—In 1988, the U.S. Department of Agriculture reported that the foods available for civilian consumption in the United States provided 118 mg of vitamin C per person per day. Of this amount, fruits (especially citrus fruits) and vegetables provided 89.8% of the total.

TOXICITY.   Doses of up to 2 g per day (which is more than 30 times the recommended daily allowance) of ascorbic acid are nontoxic to adults. However, in amounts of 2 to 8 g per day, caution should be exercised; and there is clear evidence that intakes in excess of 8 g per day (more than 100 times the recommended daily allowance) may be distinctly harmful.

A number of adverse effects of excessive intakes of vitamin C have been reported, such as: nausea; abdominal cramps, and diarrhea; absorption of excessive amounts of food iron; destruction of red blood cells; increased mobilization of bone minerals; interference with anticoagulant therapy; formation of kidney and bladder stones; the inactivation of vitamin B-12; a rise in plasma cholesterol; and possible dependence upon large doses of vitamin C (small doses no longer meet nutritional needs). It is also noteworthy that undesirable side effects may be greater in certain physiological states (e.g., pregnancy).

Since excessive intakes of vitamin C may be hazardous, routine consumption of large amounts (above 2 g daily by adults) of the vitamin is not recommended without medical advice.

LOSSES OF VITAMIN C DURING PROCESSING, COOKING, AND STORAGE.

Of all the vitamins, ascorbic acid is the most unstable. It is easily destroyed during harvesting, processing, cooking, and storage, because it is water-soluble, easily oxidized, and attacked by enzymes. Thus, a warm environment, exposure to air, solubility in water, heat, alkalinity, and dehydration are detrimental to the retention of ascorbic acid in foods. Also, cutting of vegetables releases an enzyme and increases the leaching by water. Hence, foods may lose much of their original vitamin C content from the time they are harvested until they are eaten. Details follow:

• **Processing Losses**—The method of preparing fruits and vegetables affects the amount of the vitamin. Much vitamin C is lost when the products are washed slowly, cut up into small pieces, and soaked after peeling. In preparing foods for quick freezing, canning, or drying, a brief blanching with steam favors retention of vitamin C, because this process destroys the enzymes that hasten destruction of the vitamin in raw foods. The least loss of vitamin C occurs when foods are preserved by quick freezing; the most loss occurs when foods are preserved by drying, especially if they are exposed to sunlight. Losses of vitamin C from drying may be lessened by sulfuring before drying and by rapid dehydration (away from sunlight). Manufacturers of canned and frozen fruits and vegetables should take special care to use products of high quality, then process them quickly. If this precaution is taken—if the products reach the cannery fresh from nearby fields and are heated quickly in vacuum-sealed cans—commercially canned fruits and vegetables may compare favorably in vitamin C content with home-cooked products. The vitamin C content of canned fruit juices varies considerably, unless they are specially protected in processing or fortified with vitamin C.

• **Cooking losses**—There is a great deal of variation in the amount of vitamin C lost in home cooking, depending on the nature of the food, the reaction (acid or alkaline), the length of time and the degree of heating, and the extent to which the food is exposed to water and air in the cooking process.

To retain a maximum of the ascorbic acid, frozen fruits should be used promptly, and frozen vegetables should be plunged directly into boiling water for immediate cooking.

Losses may be minimized by cooking with peel left on or with the product in large pieces, by cooking with as much exclusion of air as possible (e.g., using a tightly covered vessel or pressure cooker); by boiling the cooking water for a minute before adding the food; by shortening the boiling time; by using a small amount of water; and by consuming the cooking water.

Increased cooking losses of vitamin C result from cooking in copper or iron utensils (the ions of which inactivate the vitamin); from adding baking soda to vegetables to retain the green color (as an alkaline medium facilitates oxidation); from mashing the food and leaving it in a hot place or exposed to air; or from holding cooked foods warm for prolonged periods of time, such as on hot plates or on steam tables in cafeterias.

• **Storage losses**—Losses of vitamin C occur during prolonged storage, whether at home or in a market, especially if the product is damaged or is in a warm place. New potatoes, which contain about 30 mg/100 g of ascorbic acid, may lose 75% of the vitamin during 9 months of storage. Leafy vegetables (with large surface areas) lose more vitamin C in storage than do roots and tubers. Refrigeration during storage reduces losses. In markets, more of the vitamin of vegetables is retained when they are kept in crushed ice than when they are kept in a refrigerator.

Citrus fruit juices stored in the refrigerator lose negligible amounts of the vitamin; the acid content of the juice helps preserve vitamin C.

HOW TO CONSERVE VITAMIN C IN FOODS IN THE HOME.

Since vitamin C is essential for health, its maximum value should be conserved in foods. Losses may be minimized by keeping in mind that vitamin C is water-soluble and easily destroyed by oxidation, and that heat, alkalinity, and exposure to air hasten its destruction.

Practical suggestions for conserving vitamin C in foods in the home follow:

• Buy fresh fruits and vegetables in small quantities so that they will be used promptly. Store them in the refrigerator.

• Prepare foods immediately before they are to be served raw or cooked; do a minimum of chopping and cutting, and cook with the skins left on when possible; and do not allow foods to be exposed to air or stand in water before cooking.

• Use frozen foods promptly.

• Do not thaw frozen vegetables before cooking; keep them in the refrigerator until ready to cook, then, in their frozen state, plunge them directly into a limited amount of boiling water for immediate cooking.

• Cook in a small quantity of water, for as short a period of time as feasible, in a tightly covered cooking vessel; cook by steaming or broiling (instead of boiling).

• Never cook in copper or iron pans, and do not add soda in cooking; copper, iron, and soda hasten vitamin C destruction.

• Serve vegetables as soon after cooking as possible.

• Prepare fresh fruit juices immediately before serving. It is noteworthy, however, that acid juices (orange, grapefruit, tomato) may be left in a covered glass container in the refrigerator for several days with little loss in vitamin C.

SOURCES OF VITAMIN C.
Vitamin C occurs primarily in foods of plant origin—fruits (especially citrus fruits) and vegetables; those that may be eaten fresh, uncooked, or previously frozen are the best sources.

It is noteworthy that the vitamin content of plant foods varies greatly, depending on such factors as variety, climate, amount of sunshine, stage of maturity, part of plant (little is found in dry seeds), and length of storage. In general, the more sunshine to which a plant is exposed, the higher the vitamin C content; and the more mature the plant, the lower the vitamin C content.
A good rule to follow in order to assure sufficient vitamin C in the diet is to include a daily serving of citrus fruit or juice.
Groupings by rank of foods according to vitamin C values follow:

• **Richest natural sources**—The richest natural sources of vitamin C are the acerola cherry, *camu-camu*, and rose hips. Rose hips, which form the base of the rose bloom, are not eaten as such; rather, they are either made into a syrup (or extract) or brewed as a tea. During World War II food rationing in England, rose hip syrup was issued by the British Ministry of Food to help fortify the vitamin C intake of the English people. The acerola cherry, commonly called the Barbados cherry or West Indian cherry, which is grown in Florida, Hawaii, and Puerto Rico, has the highest ascorbic acid content of any known food. The *camu-camu* is native to the jungles of Peru. Also, pine needles, which are rich in vitamin C, have long been extracted (brewed) and used to prevent scurvy by the Indians of Canada and the northern Russians.

• **Excellent sources**—Raw, frozen, or canned citrus fruit or juice—oranges, grapefruit, lemons, and limes—are excellent sources of vitamin C; so much so that they have become virtually synonymous with the vitamin in the United States. Guavas, peppers (green or hot), black currants, parsley, turnip greens, poke greens, and mustard greens are also excellent sources.

• **Good sources**—Green leafy vegetables: broccoli, Brussels sprouts, red cabbage, cauliflower, collards, kale, lamb's-quarter, spinach, Swiss chard, and watercress. Also, cantaloupe, gooseberries, papaya, strawberries, and tomatoes and tomato juice (fresh or canned). Contrary to common opinion, it takes 3 times as much tomato juice as citrus juice to supply the same amount of vitamin C.

• **Fair sources**—Apples, asparagus, bananas, blackberries, blueberries, Irish potatoes, lima beans, liver, peaches, pears, and sweet potatoes are fair sources of ascorbic acid. However, where large amounts of any of these foods are eaten, they may provide considerable intake of the vitamin.

• **Negligible sources**—Cereal grains and their by-products, cow's milk (especially after pasteurization), eggs, fats, fish, meat, nuts, poultry, and sugar are practically devoid of vitamin C. If the mother's diet has contained sufficient vitamin C, human milk will contain 4 to 6 times as much ascorbic acid as cow's milk and will protect the infant from scurvy.

• **Synthetic ascorbic acid**—Pure ascorbic acid is available wherever vitamins are sold, at a cost as little ½¢ or less per 100 mg (which is more than the recommended daily allowance). It is less expensive than an equivalent amount in natural foods, but natural foods also supply a variety of minerals and other vitamins; hence, vitamin C supplements should be used to augment, rather than replace, natural food sources. Also, the satiety derived from eating fresh strawberries is not experienced when swallowing a tablet or a capsule. Nevertheless, the body utilizes synthetic vitamin C as effectively as it does the vitamin C in foods.

For additional sources and more precise values of vitamin C, see Food Composition Table F-36.

CAUTION: Isoascorbic acid (erythroascorbic acid), which is often used as a preservative in foods, has little vitamin C biological value for humans. Commonly used analytical procedures do not distinguish this compound from ascorbic acid.

TOP FOOD SOURCES OF VITAMIN C.
The top food sources of vitamin C are given in Table V-17.
NOTE WELL: This table lists (1) the top sources without regard to the amount normally eaten (left column), and (2) the top food sources (right column); and the caloric (energy) content of each food.

(Also see ADDITIVES, Table A-3; and VITAMIN[S], Table V-9.)

TABLE V-17
TOP SOURCES OF VITAMIN C (ASCORBIC ACID) AND THEIR CALORIC CONTENT[1]

Top Sources[2]	Vitamin C (Ascorbic Acid)	Energy	Top Food Sources	Vitamin C (Ascorbic Acid)	Energy
	(mg/100 g)	(kcal/100 g)		(mg/100 g)	(kcal/100 g)
Acerola[3]	1,743	27	Lemon juice, frozen, unsweetened, concentrate	230	116
Coriander, leaf, dried	567	279	Orange juice, canned, concentrated, unsweetened, undiluted	229	223
Peppers, hot, chili, mature, red, raw, pods	369	80	Parsley, raw	172	44
Orange juice, dehydrated	359	380	Orange juice frozen, concentrate, unsweetened, undiluted	158	158
Grapefruit juice, dehydrated	350	378	Turnip greens, raw	139	28
Guavas, whole, raw, common	242	62	Grapefruit juice, frozen, unsweetened, undiluted	138	145
Tomato juice, dehydrated	239	21	Mustard greens	130	22
Peppers, hot, chili, immature, green, pods, raw	235	31	Kale, boiled, drained, leaves	93	39
Lemon juice, frozen, unsweetened, concentrate	230	116	Broccoli, cooked, spears	90	26
Orange juice, canned, concentrated, unsweetened, undiluted	229	223	Brussels sprouts, cooked	87	36
Cabbage, common, dehydrated, unsulfited	211	308	Lamb's-quarter, raw	80	43
			Watercress leaves and stems, raw	79	19
Peppers, sweet, mature, red, raw	204	31	Cauliflower, raw	78	27
Currants, raw, black, European	200	54	Collards, cooked in small amount of water	76	33
Parsley, raw	172	44	Cabbage, red, raw	61	31
Orange juice frozen, concentrate, unsweetened, undiluted	158	158	Strawberries, raw	59	37
Grapefruit and orange juice frozen, unsweetened, undiluted	144	157	Papaya	56	39
Turnip greens, raw	139	28	Spinach	51	26
Grapefruit juice, frozen, unsweetened, undiluted	138	145	Oranges, raw, peeled, all varieties	50	49
Orange peel, raw	136	—	Grapefruit	40	40
Pokeberry (poke) shoots, raw	136	23			

[1]These listings are based on the data in Food Composition Table F-36. Some top or rich sources may have been overlooked since some of the foods in Table F-36 lack values for vitamin C.

Whenever possible, foods are on an "as used" basis, without regard to moisture content; hence, certain high-moisture foods may be disadvantaged when ranked on the basis of vitamin C content per 100 g (approximately 3½ oz) without regard to moisture content.

[2]Listed without regard to the amount normally eaten.

[3]Average value for whole, pitted, raw juice, and raw pulp and skin.

VITAMIN D

Contents

The importance of vitamin D—the sunshine vitamin—in human nutrition lies in the role of regulating calcium and phosphorus metabolism. Vitamin D promotes intestinal absorption of calcium and phosphorus and influences the process of bone mineralization. In the absence of vitamin D, mineralization of bone matrix is impaired, resulting in rickets in children and osteomalacia in adults. Although rickets is rare in the United States, it is still prevalent in many countries.

A bone disorder, which we now call rickets, has been known since 500 B.C. But the disease was first properly described in London about 300 years ago. The word *rickets* is derived from the Old English word *wrikken*, meaning to bend or twist.

Vitamin D is unique among the vitamins in two respects: (1) it occurs naturally in only a few common foods (mainly in fish oils, and a little in liver, eggs, and milk), and (2) it can be formed in the body by exposure of the skin to ultraviolet rays of the sun—light of short wavelength and high frequency; hence, it is known as the "sunshine vitamin."

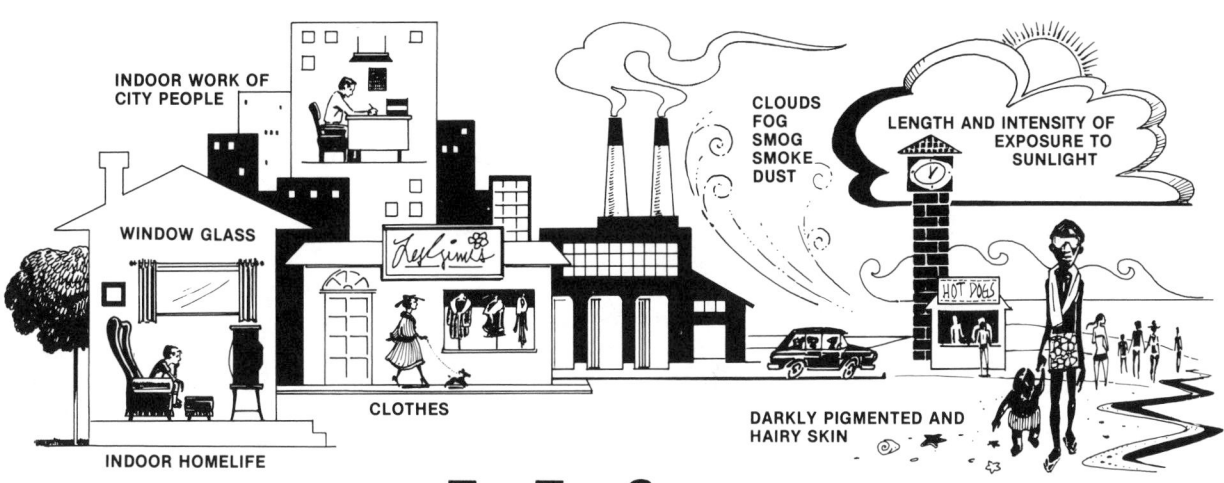

Ten Top Sources

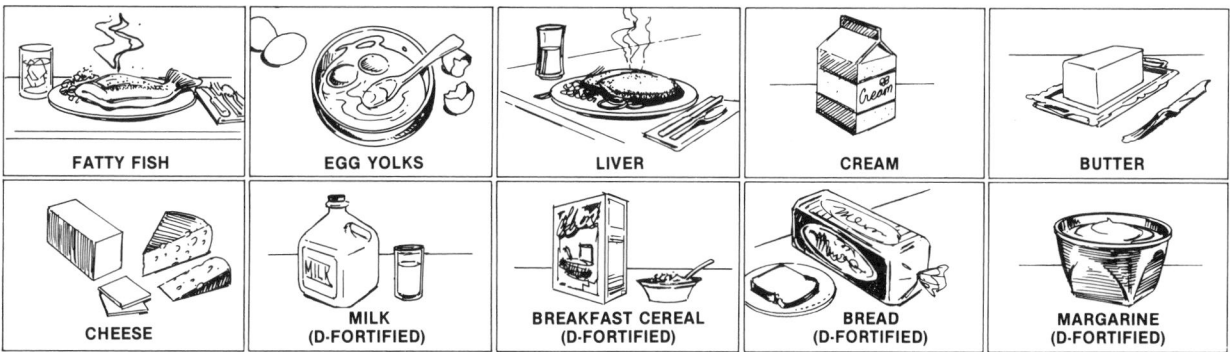

FATTY FISH	EGG YOLKS	LIVER	CREAM	BUTTER
CHEESE	MILK (D-FORTIFIED)	BREAKFAST CEREAL (D-FORTIFIED)	BREAD (D-FORTIFIED)	MARGARINE (D-FORTIFIED)

Fig. V-36. Factors that inhibit the sunshine vitamin—that screen out light and prevent the formation of vitamin D. Note, too, top food sources of vitamin D.

HISTORY. The history of rickets as a deficiency disease is much older than our knowledge of how to prevent it. During the Industrial Revolution in England in the 1600s, the disease became very prevalent in children in the crowded slums. Industrial smoke and high tenement buildings shut out the sunlight; so, as industrial cities grew, rickets spread. But no one blamed lack of sunshine (vitamin D) for the crippling disease. Instead, it was attributed to bad home environment and hygiene, and it became known as "a disease of poverty and darkness."

In 1824, cod-liver oil, long known as a folk medicine, was found to be important in the treatment of rickets. But the remedy lost favor with the medical profession because physicians could not explain its action.

As early as 1890, Palm, an English physician, observed that where sunshine was abundant, rickets was rare, but where the sun seldom shone, rickets was common.

In 1918, Sir Edward Mellanby of England demonstrated that rickets was a nutritional deficiency disease. He pro-duced rickets in puppies, then cured it by giving them cod-liver oil. But Mellanby incorrectly attributed the cure to the newly discovered fat-soluble vitamin A.

In 1922, McCollum at Johns Hopkins University found that, after destruction of all the vitamin A in cod-liver oil, (oxidation, by passing heated air through cod-liver oil) it still retained its ricket-preventing potency. This proved the existence of a second fat-soluble vitamin, carried in liver oils and certain other fats, which he called "calcium-depositing vitamin." It is of interest to note that, though McCollum discovered the existence of vitamin D, he did not call it by this name until after this designation was in common use by others.

In 1924, the mystery of how sunlight could prevent rickets was partially solved. Dr. Harry Steenbock of the University of Wisconsin and Dr. A. Hess of Columbia University, working independently, showed that the anti-rachitic activity could be produced in foods and in ani-mals by ultraviolet light. The process, known as the

Steenbock Irradiation Process was patented by Steenbock, with the royalties assigned to the Wisconsin Alumni Research Foundation of the University of Wisconsin. Subsequent research disclosed that it was certain sterols in foods and animal tissues that acquired antirachitic activity upon being irradiated. Before irradiation, the sterols were not protective against rickets.

By the late 1920s, it had been established that rickets could be prevented and cured by exposure to direct sunlight (ever since, vitamin D has been popularly called "the sunshine vitamin"), by irradiation with ultraviolet light, by feeding irradiated food, or by feeding cod-liver oil. Later, the natural vitamin D of fish liver oils was identified as the same substance that is produced in the skin by irradiation.

In 1932, crystals of pure vitamin D_2 (ergocalciferol) were isolated from irradiated ergosterol by Windaus of Germany and Askew of England; and in 1936, crystals of pure vitamin D_3 (cholecalciferol) were isolated from tuna liver oil by Brockmann of Germany.

In 1952, the first total synthesis of a form of vitamin D (in this case vitamin D_3) was accomplished by R. B. Woodward of Harvard. He was awarded the Nobel Prize in Chemistry in 1965 for this and other similar achievements.

CHEMISTRY, METABOLISM, PROPERTIES.

Although about 10 sterol compounds with vitamin D activity have been identified, only two of these, known as provitamins D or precursors, are of practical importance today from the standpoint of their occurrence in foods—ergocalciferol (vitamin D_2, calciferol, or viosterol) and cholecalciferol (vitamin D_3); the name cholecalciferol of the latter is a reflection of its cholesterol precursor. Because these substances are closely related chemically, the term vitamin D is used collectively to indicate the group of substances that show this vitamin activity.

• **Chemistry**—Fig. V-37 shows the structures of vitamins D_2 and D_3.

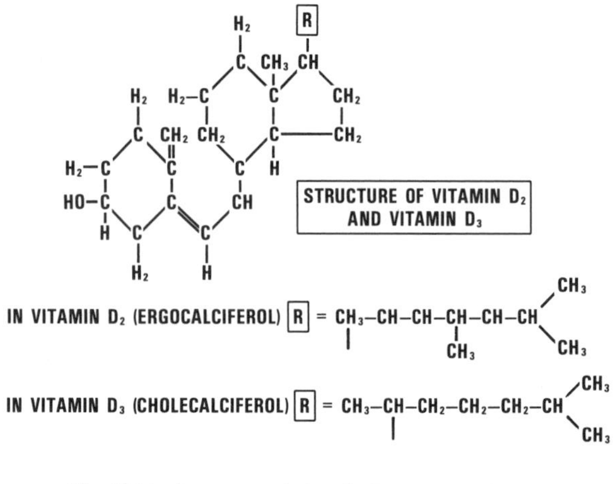

IN VITAMIN D_2 (ERGOCALCIFEROL) [R] = CH_3–CH–CH–CH–CH–CH

IN VITAMIN D_3 (CHOLECALCIFEROL) [R] = CH_3–CH–CH_2–CH_2–CH_2–CH

Fig. V-37.   Structure of vitamin D_2 and vitamin D_3.

Ultraviolet irradiation of the two provitamins—ergosterol and 7-dehydrocholesterol—will produce vitamins D_2 and D_3, respectively. Ergosterol is found in plants (in yeasts and fungi), whereas 7-dehydrocholesterol is found in fish liver oils and in the skin of man and other animals. Therefore, people or animals that are exposed to sunlight for extended periods of time do not need dietary supplementation of vitamin D. Both forms of vitamin D, D_2 and D_3, have equal activity for people and most other mammalian species. But chickens, turkeys, and other birds are exceptions—they utilize vitamin D_3 more efficiently than vitamin D_2.

• **Metabolism**—Vitamin D is unique in that man and animals normally obtain it from two sources; formation in the skin, and by mouth. The steps involved in the metabolism of vitamin D follow:

1. **Formation of vitamin D_3 in the skin and its movement into the circulation.** The unique mechanism for the synthesis, storage, and slow, steady release of vitamin D_3 from the skin into the circulation is shown in Fig. V-38.

When the skin is exposed to the ultraviolet radiation of sunlight, part of the store of 7-dehydrocholesterol undergoes a photochemical reaction in the epidermis and the dermis and forms previtamin D_3. Once previtamin D_3 is formed in the skin, it undergoes a slow temperature-dependent transformation to vitamin D_3, which takes at least 3 days to complete. Then, the vitamin D-binding protein transports D_3 from the skin into the circulation.

2. **Absorption.** Vitamin D taken by mouth is absorbed with fats from the small intestine (from the jejunum and ileum), with the aid of bile. Vitamin D formed in the skin by irradiation of the provitamin present there is absorbed directly into the circulatory system.

3. **Utilization.** Cholecalciferol—obtained either from the diet or from the irradiation of the skin—is transported by a specific vitamin D carrier protein (a globulin) to the liver where it is converted to 25-hydroxycholecalciferol (25-OH-D_3).[19] From the liver 25-OH-D_3 is transported to the kidneys where it is converted to l,25-$(OH)_2$-D_3, the most active form of vitamin D in increasing calcium absorption, bone calcium mobilization, and increased intestinal phosphate absorption. The active compound l,25-$(OH)_2$-D_3 functions as a hormone, since it is a vital substance made in the body tissues (the kidneys) and transported in the blood to cells within target tissues. This physiological active form of vitamin D_3 is then either transported to its various sites of action or converted to its metabolite forms of 24,25-dihydroxycholecalciferol or l,24,25-trihydroxycholecalciferol (see Fig. V-39).

Although most of the research on vitamin D metabolism has been conducted on cholecalciferol, studies by DeLuca on ergocalciferol indicate that it is metabolized similarly to cholecalciferol; that it is changed to a similar active metabolite in the liver—25-hydroxyergocalciferol (25-OH-D_2).

---

[19]Identified by DeLuca and co-workers of the University of Wisconsin. First reported in *Proc. Nat. Acad. Sci.,* **61:1503, 1968.**

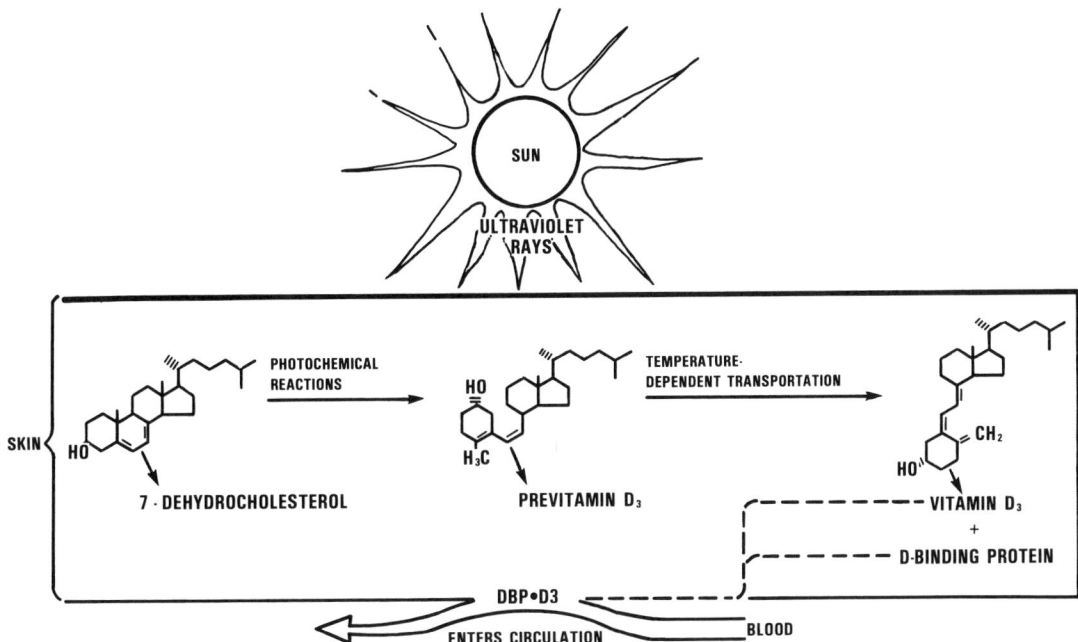

Fig. V-38. Diagram showing the sequence of steps in the formation of vitamin D-3 in the skin and its transport into the circulation.

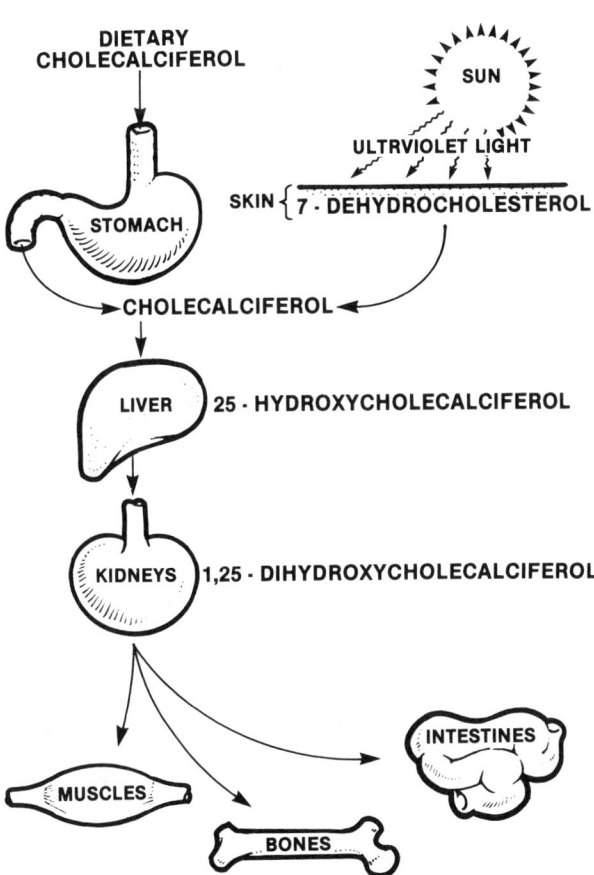

Fig. V-39. Fate of cholecalciferol in the body.

4. **Storage**. The major storage sites of vitamin D are the fatty tissues and skeletal muscle. Some of it is also found in the liver, brain, lungs, spleen, bones, and skin. But body storage of vitamin D is much more limited than the storage of vitamin A.

5. **Excretion**. The main pathway of excretion of vitamin D is by way of the bile into the small intestine, thence the feces. Less than 4% of the intake is excreted in the urine.

• **Properties**—Pure vitamins D are white, crystalline, odorless substances that are soluble in both fats and fat solvents (such as ether, choloroform, acetone, and alcohol). They are insoluble in water, and they are resistant to heat, oxidation, acid, and alkali.

Although the precursors are activated by ultraviolet light, excessive irradiation results in the formation of slightly toxic compounds that have no antirachitic activity.

MEASUREMENT/ASSAY. Vitamin D potency is expressed in International Units (IU) and United States Pharmacopeia Units (USP), which are equal. One IU, or one USP, of vitamin D is defined as the activity of 0.025 mcg of pure crystalline vitamin D_3 (cholecalciferol).

The ultraviolet light absorption property of vitamin D may be used for the assay of pure preparations free of irrelevant absorption. But it does not distinguish between vitamin D_2 and D_3.

Both vitamin D_2 and D_3 give a yellow-orange color with antimony trichloride. This color reaction forms the basis of the USP XVIII method for vitamin D. Since color reactions are subject to interferences from many sources, they should be limited to high potency pharmaceutical preparations or fortified foods. Combinations of column and thin-layer chromatographic purification steps with the antimony trichloride reaction have been successfully used.

Gas-liquid chromatography provides a means of combining qualitative and quantitative assays.

Food and feed samples, which contain vitamin D in very low concentrations, are not usually assayed by chemical methods. For these substances, bioassays are the only means available for the assessment of vitamin D activity. Rats and chicks are used as test animals; rats respond equally well to D_2 and D_3, whereas chicks respond only to D_3. The assays measure the alleviation (curative test) or the development (prophylactic test) of vitamin D deficiency in terms of the degree of rickets produced.

A bioassay method, known as the *line test*, uses stained longitudinal sections of the distal end of radius bones to evaluate calcification. Usually the test animal is the rat, although the chick must be used if the vitamin D activity of a sample intended for poultry nutrition is to be determined. Young rats from mothers having a deficient supply of vitamin D are kept on a rachitogenic diet so that no calcification occurs in the ends of the long bones. When a test material is fed to these vitamin D-deficient rats, its value as a source of vitamin D is measured by the amount that must be fed for 7 to 10 days to produce a good calcium line (line test) in the ends of the long bones. Standard cod-liver oil is fed to a similar group of animals and is used as a basis of comparison.

FUNCTIONS.   Vitamin D is primarily associated with calcium and phosphorus. It influences the absorption of these minerals and their deposit in bone tissue. Research is continuing to unfold the relationship of vitamin D to calcium and phosphorus metabolism. Although there are many gaps in our knowledge relative to the exact mechanism by which vitamin D carries out its various physiological functions, the current thinking is as follows:

• **Calcium absorption**—It has been clearly established that vitamin D increases calcium absorption from the small intestine, and that a vitamin D deficiency produces large calcium losses in the feces.

• **Phosphate level**—Adequate vitamin D enhances the levels of phosphates in the body, because of (1) improved absorption of phosphorus through the intestinal wall, independent of calcium absorption; and (2) increased resorption of phosphates from the kidney tubules. When sufficient vitamin D is not available, urinary excretion of phosphate increases and the blood level drops.

Maintenance of a satisfactory phosphate level, and of the vital balance between calcium and phosphorus in the blood, is essential (1) to the process of bone calcification and (2) to the prevention of tetany.

• **Bone and teeth metabolism**—The growth and proper mineralization of the bones and teeth require vitamin D.

Lack of vitamin D or lack of exposure to sunlight of children results in weak bones and overgrowth of the softer tissues (cartilage) at the ends of the bones. The joints enlarge, and bowed legs, knock knees, beaded ribs, and skull deformities may result. Lack of vitamin D in adults may result in osteomalacia, in which changes occur in the shafts of bones and bone structure softens. Adequate vitamin D is also important during reproduction and lactation. Extreme deficiencies may result in congenital malformations of the newborn and injury to the skeleton of the mother.

With lack of vitamin D, the enamel and the dentin of the teeth, which are composed almost entirely of calcium and phosphorus, may not develop normally. Thus the teeth of rachitic children and animals have thin, poorly calcified enamel, with pits and fissures, and are especially prone to decay.

The withdrawal of calcium and phosphorus storage from bone (resorption) is stimulated by the action of vitamin D. In this way, vitamin D helps to maintain the blood levels of the two minerals.

• **Citrate metabolism**—The level of citrate in the blood decreases in a vitamin D deficiency. Citrate is an important organic acid involved in many metabolic functions, including mobilization of minerals from bone tissue and removal of calcium from the blood.

The effect on citrate metabolism is thought to be due to changes in mineral metabolism brought about by the absence or presence of vitamin D rather than to a direct action of the vitamin on the formation of citrate.

• **Amino acid levels in the blood**—Vitamin D is involved in the amino acid levels in the blood, by protecting against the loss of amino acids through the kidneys. When there is a deficiency of vitamin D, the excretion of amino acids in the urine is increased.

DEFICIENCY SYMPTOMS.

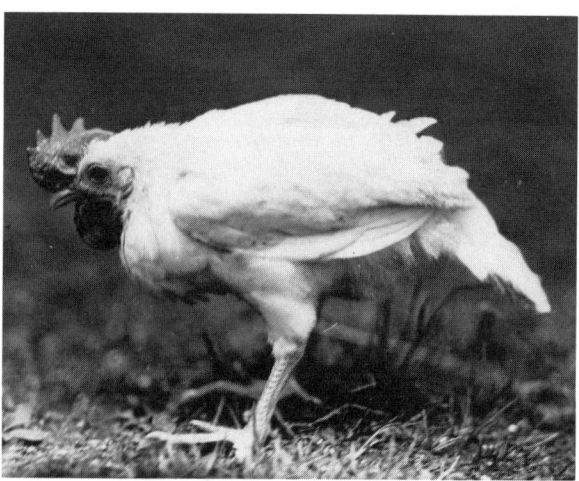

Fig. V-40.   A chick deficient in vitamin D, showing ungainly way of balancing the body. The beak is also soft and rubbery. (Courtesy, Department of Poultry Science, Cornell University)

A deficiency of vitamin D leads to inadequate absorption of calcium and phosphorus from the intestinal tract and to faulty mineralization of the bones and teeth, followed by skeletal malformations. The major deficiency symptoms follow:

• **Rickets**—Lack of vitamin D will cause rickets in infants and children, even though the diet is adequate in calcium and phosphorus. (Rickets may also be caused by lack of either calcium or phosphorus, or an incorrect ratio of the two minerals.) This disease, is caused from failure of the bones to calcify normally (meaning that the deposition of calcium and phosphorus salts is not normal). As a result, they are soft and pliable and become deformed. The weight of the body causes the ends of the long bones of the legs to flatten and mushroom outward, giving the appearance of enlarged knee and ankle joints. Other bone

changes occurring in rickets include enlarged wrist joints; bowed legs; knocked knees; outward projection of the sternum ("pigeon breast"); a row of beadlike projections on each side of the chest at the juncture of the rib bones and joining (costal) cartilage (called "rachitic rosary"); delayed closure of the fontanel of the skull, causing a bulging of the forehead; narrowing of the pelvis so as to make childbirth difficult in subsequent years; and spinal curvature.

Sometimes muscles are poorly developed. Often rickets is associated with protrusion of the abdomen, or "pot belly," due to weakness of the abdominal muscles.

Eruption of the temporary teeth is delayed; and the permanent teeth may be thin, pitted, and grooved, with the result that they decay easily.

Since the 1930s, the incidence of rickets in the United States has declined, largely because of the addition of vitamin D supplements to breast-fed infants and of the fortification of infant formulas and fluid and evaporated milk with vitamin D. Since 1968, nonfat dry milk for use in various food programs has also been fortified with vitamin D (and vitamin A).

The best protection against rickets and the most favorable bone growth are secured when calcium and phosphorus are supplied in approximately equal amounts (as in milk) and when liberal quantities of vitamin D are available.

When preventive measures are not taken, rickets occurs in northern regions, especially in dark, crowded cities during the winter months, where the ultraviolet rays of sunshine cannot penetrate through the fog, smoke, and soot. Dark-skinned children are more susceptible to rickets than those of the white race; and premature infants are more susceptible than full-term infants, because of the additional demands for vitamin D imposed by increased growth rate and calcification of the bones.

Rickets is still a serious problem in many tropical and semitropical countries and among the poor in overcrowded sections of large cities. In Africa, rickets may be caused by the custom of not exposing babies to sunlight, little vitamin D or calcium in the diet, intestinal parasites, and recurrent diarrhea.

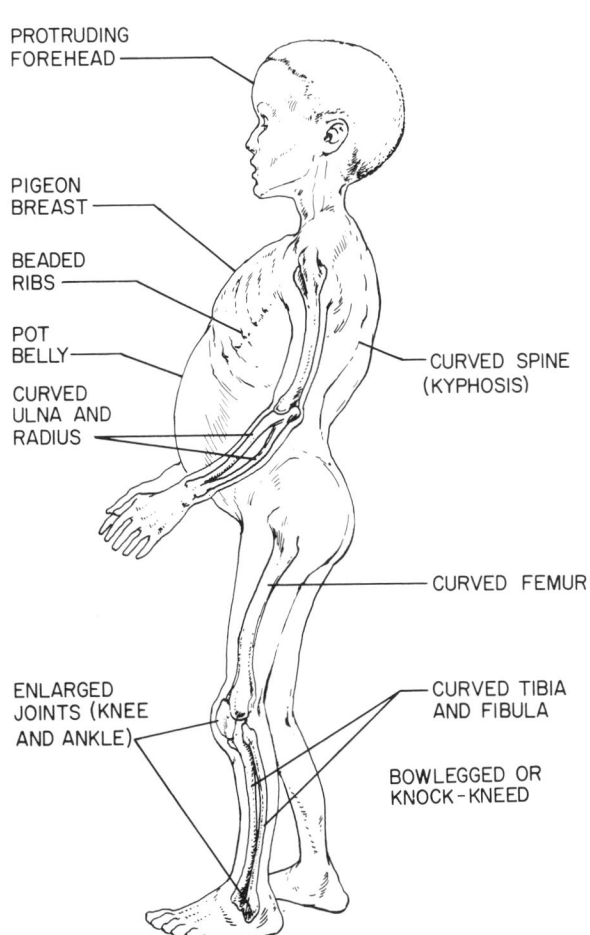

PROTRUDING FOREHEAD
PIGEON BREAST
BEADED RIBS
POT BELLY
CURVED ULNA AND RADIUS
CURVED SPINE (KYPHOSIS)
CURVED FEMUR
ENLARGED JOINTS (KNEE AND ANKLE)
CURVED TIBIA AND FIBULA
BOWLEGGED OR KNOCK-KNEED

Fig. V-41. Symptoms of severe rickets.

• **Tetany**—A deficiency of vitamin D may cause tetany, though it is not the only cause. Tetany may also result from insufficient absorption of calcium or from a disturbance of the parathyroid gland. Tetany is characterized by muscle twitching, cramps, convulsions, and low serum calcium—less than 7 mg per 100 ml.

• **Osteomalacia**—This is the adult form of rickets, caused by depletion of the bone stores of calcium and phosphorus, as a result of a lack of vitamin D or exposure to sunlight, or lack of either calcium or phosphorus. It is most common during pregnancy, lactation, and old age. Since longitudinal bone growth has stopped in adults, only the shafts on long and flat bones, such as the pelvis, are affected. The bones soften, become distorted, and fracture easily. Also, osteomalacia generally causes rheumatic-type pain in the bones of the legs and lower back.

RECOMMENDED DAILY ALLOWANCE OF VITAMIN D.

The minimum vitamin D requirements are not known, mainly because information on the amount of cholecalciferol formed by the action of sunlight on the skin is not available. The amount formed varies with the length and intensity of exposure to sunlight; the color of skin (dark-pigmented skin can prevent as much as 95% of the sun's ultraviolet light from penetrating into the skin and forming cholecalciferol); the amount of window glass and clothing, which prevent ultraviolet rays from reaching the skin; the season (sunlight is usually scarce during the winter months, when there are cloudy and foggy days); and the amount of atmospheric pollution ("smog," smoke, dust).

The Food and Nutrition Board (FNB) of the National Research Council (NRC) recommended dietary allowances of vitamin D are given in Table V-18.

TABLE V–18
RECOMMENDED DAILY VITAMIN D ALLOWANCES[1]

Group	Age	Weight		Height		Mcg/IU[2]	
	(years)	(lb)	(kg)	(in.)	(cm)	(mcg)	(IU)
Infants	0.0–0.5	13	6	24	60	7.5	300
	0.5–1.0	20	9	28	71	10	400
Children	1–3	29	13	35	90	10	400
	4–6	44	20	44	112	10	400
	7–10	62	28	52	132	10	400
Males	11–14	99	45	62	157	10	400
	15–18	145	66	69	176	10	400
	19–24	160	72	70	177	10	400
	25–50	174	79	70	176	5	200
	51+	170	77	68	173	5	200
Females	11–14	101	46	62	157	10	400
	15–18	120	55	64	163	10	400
	19–24	128	58	65	164	10	400
	25–50	138	63	64	163	5	200
	51+	143	65	63	160	5	200
Pregnant						10	400
Lactating						10	400

[1]*Recommended Dietary Allowances,* 10th ed., NRC–National Academy of Sciences, 1989, p. 285.
[2]400 IU of vitamin D = 10 mcg cholecalciferol.

As shown in Table V-18, the recommended daily allowance of vitamin D for infants, children, and adolescents (from birth to 18 years of age) is 10 mcg (400 IU). Allowances and intakes follow:

• **Infants and children**—The vitamin D content of human milk has long been regarded as inadequate for infant needs. Thus, an allowance of 10 mcg (400 IU) should be provided to both breast-fed and bottle-fed infants, either as an oral supplement or included in the formula, particularly since exposure to sunlight of infants is often inadequate.

• **Adults**—With the cessation of skeletal growth, calcium needs decrease, and, with it, the need for vitamin D. So, the recommended allowance for vitamin D is reduced to 5 mcg (200 IU) after the age of 25 years. Actually, the requirements for the normal adult can usually be met by adequate exposure to sunlight. However, solar radiation may be inadequate under certain climatic conditions or because of chronic air pollution, under which circumstances a dietary source may be necessary.

• **Pregnancy and lactation**—Calcium needs increase during gestation. Moreover, vitamin D and its active metabolites cross the placenta readily. Therefore, the allowance for the pregnant woman is increased by the addition of 5 mcg (200 IU) to her nonpregnant allowance. Because of the increased calcium needs during lactation, an additional allowance of 5 mcg (200 IU) is also recommended during lactation.

Because vitamin D is a potentially toxic substance, and because there is lack of evidence that amounts above the recommended allowance confer health benefits, intakes should closely approximate the recommended allowances. Only individuals with diseases affecting vitamin D absorption or metabolism should take vitamin D in excess of the recommended allowances; even then, such treatment should be on the recommendation, and under the supervision, of a physician or a nutritionist.

• **Vitamin D intake in the United States**—It is difficult to estimate the average daily intake of vitamin D per person in the United States because there is no way in which to determine the amount manufactured in the body by the action of sunlight. However, because of the widespread use of fortified milk and other foods, intakes of at least 400 IU daily per person appear probable.

TOXIC (HYPERVITAMINOSIS D).

There is wide individual difference in the tolerance to vitamin D; hence, it is impossible to give the level at which vitamin D intake becomes toxic. But, generally speaking, the intake of vitamin D should not exceed a total of 10 mcg (400 IU) per day. Excessive amounts of vitamin D (above 50 mcg [2,000 IU]/day) can lead to hypercalcemia (toxicity caused by elevated blood levels of calcium) as a result of increased intestinal absorption of calcium. Symptoms of mild toxicity include loss of appetite, excessive thirst, nausea, vomiting, irritability, weakness, constipation (which may alternate with bouts of diarrhea), retarded growth in infants and children, and weight loss in adults. Chronic hypercalcemia results in abnormal deposition of calcium in the soft tissues (including the heart, blood vessels, lungs, and tubules of the kidneys), with particular damage to the kidneys. If massive doses of vitamin D are continued, widespread calcification of the soft tissues may ultimately prove fatal.

Excessive intakes of vitamin D during pregnancy and early infancy may cause idiopathic hypercalcemia, or the hypercalcemic syndrome, a condition characterized by narrowing of the aortic valve of the heart, a peculiar facial appearance, and mental retardation.

The ingestion of excess vitamin D is due mainly to the use of dietary supplements that contain large amounts of the vitamin. Because of the vitamin D added to milk and infant formulas, as well as the vitamin D produced by exposure to sunlight, parents should consider all these sources before giving their children vitamin D supplements.

Adults should also be warned about taking massive doses of vitamin D (as well as about taking massive doses of vitamin A) over a long period of time *unless* it is under the supervision of a physician or nutritionist. Even moderate overdosage of vitamin D is not wise for the elderly.

The concurrent administration of large quantities of vitamin A with potentially toxic levels of vitamin D will reduce the toxicity of the latter.

VITAMIN D LOSSES DURING PROCESSING, COOKING, AND STORAGE.

Vitamin D in foods and food supplements is remarkably stable. Processing does not affect its activity; and because vitamin D is stable to heat and insoluble in water, there is little loss in cooking foods. Foods containing vitamin D can be stored for long periods of time with little deterioration.

The commercial forms of vitamin D_2 and D_3 supplements, which come in either oily solutions or powders, are destroyed relatively rapidly by light, oxygen, and acids. Therefore, they must be stored in opaque, hermetically-sealed containers from which the air is displaced by an inert gas, such as nitrogen. The crystalline compounds are relatively stable to heat.

SOURCES OF VITAMIN D.

Vitamin D is found in foods more sparsely than any other vitamin. But, fortunately, nature ordained that man could generate some of his supply of vitamin D by sunlight.

Groupings by rank of common sources of vitamin D follow:

• **Rich sources**—Fatty fish (bloater, herring, kipper, mackerel, pilchard, salmon, sardines, tuna) and fish roe.

• **Fair sources**—Liver, egg yolk, cream, butter, cheese.

• **Negligible sources**—Muscle meats, milk (unfortified), fruits, nuts, vegetables, grains.

• **D-fortified foods**—Milk (400 IU/qt [*242 IU/liter*]) and infant formulas. Other foods to which vitamin D is often added include: breakfast and infant cereals, breads, margarines, milk flavorings, fruit and chocolate beverages, and cocoa.

• **Supplemental sources**—Fish liver oils (from cod, halibut, or swordfish); irradiated ergosterol or 7-dehydrocholesterol, such as viosterol.

• **Exposure to sunlight or sunlamp**—Manufactured in the skin.

For additional sources and more precise values of vitamin D, see Food Composition Table F-36. However, few vitamin D values are available, because foods do not lend themselves well to chemical analysis for this vitamin. For foods, costly and time-consuming bioassays with rats or chicks are the only means available for the assessment of vitamin D activity.

Among animal foods, fatty fish are rich sources of vitamin D. They obtain the vitamin by feeding on plankton which live near the surface of the sea exposed to sunlight. Liver, egg yolk, and butter contain useful amounts of vitamin D, but the potency of these foods varies widely according to the extent to which the animals have been exposed to sunlight or ultraviolet light and to the feeds given them. Muscle meats contain only traces. Both human milk and cow milk are a poor source of vitamin D.

Vegetables, grains and their products, and fruits have little or no vitamin D activity. Although it is usually assumed that living plants do not contain vitamin D activity, an important exception is certain tropical and subtropical shrubs and plants of the *Solanum* family,[20] native to the West Indies, recently found to contain such large amounts of the vitamin D hormone as to be extremely toxic to animals and cause extensive economic losses.

Vitamin D is added to most commercial milk and infant formulas. These two foods are considered most suitable for vitamin D fortification because of their calcium and phosphorus content and the role of vitamin D in the absorption and utilization of the two minerals. Also, milk is consumed in large quantities by the young, who especially need vitamin D for skeletal development.

Practically all whole, low-fat, and nonfat fluid milks on the market today are fortified with 400 IU of vitamin D per quart. Either vitamin D_2 (ergosterol) or D_3 (irradiated cholecalciferol) is added, with the form of the added vitamin listed on the label. Evaporated milk is required by federal law to be fortified with sufficient vitamin D to provide 400 IU per quart when it is reconstituted. Although the fortification of nonfat dry milk is optional, most of it is fortified at a level that supplies 400 IU per reconstituted quart.

Although milk is the only food for which vitamin D fortification is recommended by the Food and Nutrition Board of the National Research Council and the Council of Foods and Nutrition of the American Medical Association, other foods to which vitamin D is added include breakfast cereals, infant cereals, breads, margarine, milk flavorings, fruit and chocolate beverages, and cocoa. Concern has been expressed about the possibility of over-consumption of vitamin D as a result of widespread fortification of foods with the vitamin. Obviously, when vitamin D-enriched milk is used in the amount of 1 qt daily, no other source of vitamin D is required.

All fish liver oils (cod-liver, halibut, and swordfish liver oils) are rich sources of vitamin D, but they are not part

---

[20]Potatoes and eggplant belong to the *Solanum* family, but they are not known to be a source of vitamin D activity. The *Solanum*-toxic plant known as day-blooming jessamine, wild jessamine, or King-of-the-Day has been introduced into the United States and cultivated for ornamental purposes.

of the usual American diet. Preparations containing them are available for use as supplementary sources of vitamin D, particularly for infants. Other vitamin D concentrates are made by irradiating pure ergosterol or 7-dehydrocholesterol; these are available in liquid and tablet form. Viosterol, which is a solution of irradiated ergosterol dissolved in neutral oil, is an example. Such preparations are labeled with the units per dose or tablet and are prescribed accordingly.

The alternative to oral sources of vitamin D is its manufacture in the skin. The vitamin can be produced in the skin if it is exposed to the short wavelengths of the sun's rays (or to a sunlamp), the ultraviolet rays, which act on the provitamin 7-dehydrocholesterol in the skin and transform it into vitamin D_3. But the amount of these rays that act on the skin is affected by atmospheric clouds, smoke, fog, dust, window glass, clothing, skin pigmentation, and season; hence, it is highly variable and cannot either be determined or relied upon. So, some other source of vitamin D is usually needed.

TOP FOOD SOURCES OF VITAMIN D. Table V-19, Top Food Sources of Vitamin D and Their Caloric Content, contains data on the vitamin D content of the richest sources of vitamin D.

(Also see VITAMIN[S], Table V-9.)

TABLE V-19
TOP FOOD SOURCES OF VITAMIN D
AND THEIR CALORIC CONTENT[1]

Food	Vitamin D	Energy
	(IU/100 g)	(kcal/100 g)
Cod-liver oil	8,500	899
Herring, Atlantic, raw	900	176
Salmon, Sockeye (Red), canned	500	167
Sardines, canned in oil, drained solids	300	200
Tuna, canned in oil	232	288
Whipping cream, heavy 37.6% fat	100	345
Milk, cow's, canned, evaporated, skimmed	88	78
Liver, chicken, simmered	67	165
Liver, hog, fried, in margarine	51	241
Whipping cream, light 31.3% fat	50	195
Chicken eggs, fried, hard cooked or poached	49	174
Milk, cow's, 1%, 2%, 3.25%, 3.3%, or 3.7% fat	41	56
Liver, lamb, broiled	23	261
Liver, beef, fried	19	222
Luncheon meat, liverwurst, fresh	15	496
Liver, calf, fried	14	261

[1]These listings are based on the data in Food Composition Table F-36. Some top sources may have been overlooked since many of the foods in Table F-36 lack values for vitamin D.

Whenever possible, foods are on an "as used" basis, without regard to moisture content; hence, certain high-moisture foods may be disadvantaged when ranked on the basis of vitamin D content per 100 g (approximately 3½ oz) without regard to moisture content.

VITAMIN E (TOCOPHEROLS)

Contents | Page

For many years, vitamin E was known as the *antisterility* vitamin, a name taken from early work with rats, in which species a dramatic improvement in fertility was observed when vitamin E was added to a diet deficient in the substance.

Today, vitamin E is recognized as an essential nutrient for higher animals, including man. In humans, however, sexual potency has never been linked with vitamin E.

HISTORY. In 1922, Evans and Bishop, of the University of California, discovered that a fat-soluble dietary factor (then called *factor X*) in lettuce and wheat germ was essential for successful reproduction in rats. In 1924, Sure, of the University of Arkansas, named the factor vitamin E. In 1936, Evans and co-workers isolated crystalline vitamin E from wheat germ oil and named it tocopherol, from the Greek words *tokos* (offspring) and *pherein* (to bear), meaning "to bear offspring." In 1938, the vitamin was first synthesized by the Swiss chemist, Karrer.

CHEMISTRY, METABOLISM, PROPERTIES.

• **Chemistry**—Eight tocopherols and tocotrienols with vitamin E activity, collectively called vitamin E, have been identified. Differing from each other in the number and position of the methyl (CH_3) groups around the ring of the molecule, they are: alpha- (see Fig. V-43), beta-, gamma-, and delta-tocopherol; and alpha-, beta-, gamma-, and delta-tocotrienol. Alpha-tocopherol has by far the greatest vitamin E activity; the other tocopherols have biological activities ranging from 1 to 50% that of alpha-tocopherol. Nevertheless, the nonalpha-tocopherol compounds in foods normally consumed contribute vitamin E activity equivalent to about 20% of the indicated alpha-tocopherol content of a mixed diet.

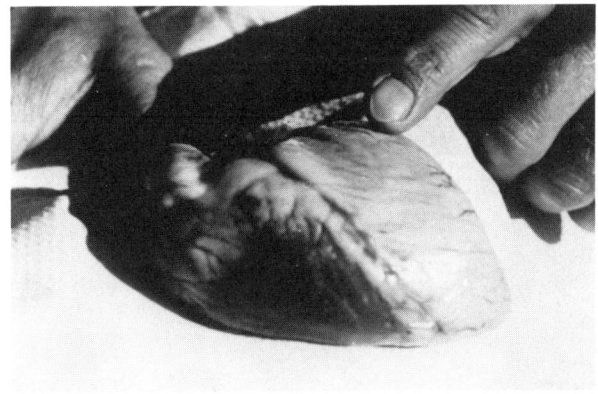
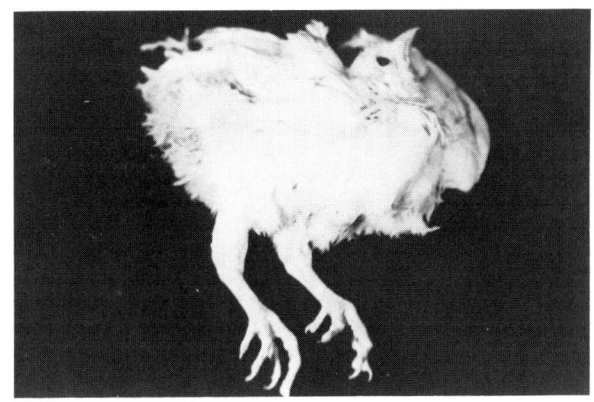

TOP FOOD SOURCES

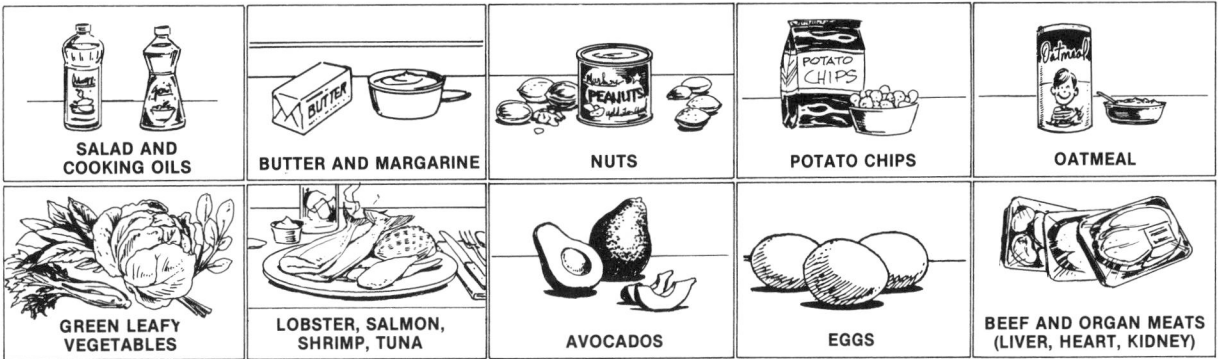

SALAD AND COOKING OILS	BUTTER AND MARGARINE	NUTS	POTATO CHIPS	OATMEAL
GREEN LEAFY VEGETABLES	LOBSTER, SALMON, SHRIMP, TUNA	AVOCADOS	EGGS	BEEF AND ORGAN MEATS (LIVER, HEART, KIDNEY)

Fig. V-42. *Left:* White muscle disease in a calf, showing characteristic whitish areas or streaks in the heart. (Courtesy, Oregon State University) *Right:* A chick with nutritional encephalomalacia (crazy chick disease), due to a lack of vitamin E. Note head retraction and loss of control of legs. (Courtesy, Department of Poultry Science, Cornell University) Note, too, top food source of vitamin E.

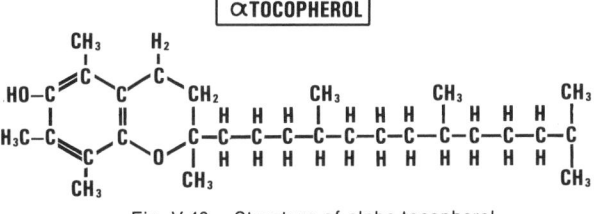

Fig. V-43.   Structure of alpha-tocopherol.

• **Metabolism**—A discussion of the absorption, transportation, storage, and excretion of vitamin E follows.

1. **Absorption.** As with other fat-soluble vitamins, the presence of both bile and fat are required for the proper absorption of vitamin E. Absorption takes place in the small intestine, where 20 to 30% of the intake passes through the intestinal wall into the lymph.

2. **Transportation.** Once absorbed, vitamin E is transported attached to the beta-lipoprotein fraction of the blood. In normal adults in the United States, the total tocopherol content of the plasma ranges from 0.5 to 1.2 mg/100 ml. A level below 0.5 mg is considered undesirable. The ratio of total tocopherol to the total lipids in the plasma appears to be more important than the actual tocopherol level; a ratio of 0.8 mg of total tocopherol to 1 g of total lipids in the plasma is accepted as an indication of adequate vitamin E nutritional status. The predominant form of vitamin E in both the plasma and red cells is alpha-tocopherol, which accounts for 83% of the total tocopherol; gamma-tocopherol accounts for most of the remainder.

3. **Storage**. Adipose (fatty) tissue, liver, and muscle are the major storage sites, although small amounts of vitamin E are stored in most body tissues. Relatively high amounts are found in the adrenal and pituitary glands, heart, lungs, testes, and uterus. Vitamin E is deposited in the fat of tissues and is mobilized from them with fat.

There is little transfer of vitamin E across the placenta to the fetus; hence, newborn infants have low tissue stores.

4. **Excretion.** The major pathway of excretion of vitamin E is by way of the feces, although a small amount is excreted in the urine.

• **Properties**—The tocopherols and tocotrienols are light yellow, viscous oils, soluble in alcohol and fat solvents, but insoluble in water. They are stable to acids and heat, but they are destroyed upon exposure to oxygen, ultraviolet light, alkali, and iron and lead salts. Their ability to take up oxygen gives them important antioxidant properties. Vitamin E is not destroyed to any great extent by normal cooking temperatures, but there are appreciable losses of vitamin E activity in oils heated long periods of time at high temperature, such as in deep fat frying, because rancidity develops.

Currently, the bulk of commercial vitamin E is synthetic dl-alpha-tocopherol acetate, an ester of alpha-tocopherol, a form more stable to heat and oxidation than the free alcohol form, but with the same vitamin E activity. This stable form of alpha-tocopherol is added to vitamin preparations, various medicinal products, foods, and animals feeds.

MEASUREMENT/ASSAY. By agreement of international committees, it is now preferred to use "milligrams of alpha-tocopherol equivalents" as a summation term for all vitamin E activity. In this encyclopedia, however, both International Units (IU) and alpha-tocopherol equivalents will be used because (1) food composition tables generally give values in IU, and (2) IU is still used for labeling most food products. Table V-20 shows the relationship between milligrams of alpha-tocopherol equivalents and IU.

TABLE V-20
RELATIONSHIP BETWEEN ALPHA-TOCOPHEROL EQUIVALENTS AND INTERNATIONAL UNITS (IU)

Compound (1 mg)	Alpha-tocopherol Equivalents in 1 mg	IU Activity in 1 mg
	(mg)	(IU)
d-alpha-tocopherol[1]	1.0	1.49
d-alpha-tocopheryl acetate	0.91	1.36
d-alpha-tocopheryl acid succinate	0.81	1.21
dl-alpha-tocopherol	0.74	1.10
dl-alpha-tocopheryl acetate[2]	0.67	1.00
d-gamma-tocopherol[3]	0.10	0.15

[1]The natural form in foods and the standard for "alpha-tocopherol equivalents," usually just called alpha-tocopherol.

[2]The common commercial form of vitamin E—a synthetic and stable form. Naturally occurring dl-alpha-tocopheryl acetate is considered to have the same potency as the synthetic product. This is the standard for International Units.

[3]The most abundant form in food oils.

For purposes of calculating the total vitamin E activity of mixed diets, the milligrams of beta-tocopherol should be multiplied by 0.5, those of gamma-tocopherol by 0.1, and those of alpha-tocotrienol by 0.3. (These are the only vitamins with significant activity that may be present in U. S. diets.) When these are added to the milligrams of alpha-tocopherol, the sum is the total milligrams of alpha-tocopherol equivalents. If only alpha-tocopoherol in a mixed diet is reported, the value in milligrams should be increased by 20% (multiply by 1.2) to account for the other tocopherols that are present, thus giving an approx-

imation of the total vitamin E activity as milligrams of alpha-tocopherol equivalents.

A colorimetric method is the most commonly used assay method for estimating vitamin E activity. Additionally, spectrofluorometric and gas-liquid chromatographic methods are sometimes used. Animal tests are available, but are now rarely used.

FUNCTIONS. The primary function of vitamin E (tocopoherols) is to help protect the integrity of cellular and intracellular structures and to prevent destruction of certain enzymes and intracellular components. But there is much controversy as to how this function is carried out.

The authors of this encyclopedia are of the opinion that vitamin E is more important in human nutrition than is now known; based on current evidence, they subscribe to the following thinking relative to the functions of vitamin E:

1. **As an antioxidant which (a) retards the rancidification of fats in foods and in the digestive tract, and (b) protects cells from toxic substances formed from the oxidation of unsaturated fatty acids.** As a powerful antioxidant, vitamin E readily oxidizes itself (it combines with oxygen), thereby minimizing the destruction by oxidation of unsaturated fatty acids and vitamin A in the intestinal tract and in the tissues.

As an antioxidant, vitamin E prevents rancidity of fats in plant sources and in the animal's digestive tract. But the primary biological role of vitamin E is as an antioxidant inhibiting the oxidation of polyunsaturated fatty acids in tissue membranes, especially at the cellular level—in the membranes that surround the cells, the subcellular particles, and the erythrocytes. It stabilizes the lipid (fat) parts of cells and protects them from damage from toxic free radicals formed from the oxidation of polyunsaturated fatty acids; it reacts with the peroxides, converting them to forms that are not harmful to the cells. By functioning as a natural inhibitor of the destruction of cells, and by protecting tissue from breaking down, vitamin E may have a role in preventing a number of degenerative disorders—including aging.

In its antioxidant role, vitamin E also protects vitamin A (and carotene), vitamin C, sulfur-containing enzymes, and ATP from being oxidized, thereby enabling these essential nutrients to perform their specific functions in the body.

It is noteworthy that when fat is added to the diet it will destroy the vitamin E in both the diet and the digestive tract if rancidity occurs. For this reason, the quantitative relationship between vitamin E and the amount and kind of dietary fat is of practical importance; the higher the consumption of polyunsaturated fats, the higher the vitamin E requirement.

2. **As an essential factor for the integrity of red blood cells.** Evidence has been accumulating that vitamin E functions in the body in maintaining the integrity of the red blood cells. Thus, it is noteworthy that hemolytic anemia, an abnormality of the red blood cells in premature babies, may be corrected with vitamin E. Also, full-term babies with this same abnormality make a more rapid and complete recovery when fed with human milk (rather than cow's milk); and laboratory tests show that

human milk contains from 2 to 4 times as much vitamin E as cow's milk.

3. **As an agent essential to cellular respiration.** Alpha-tocopherol appears to be necessary in cellular respiration, primarily in heart and skeletal muscle tissues. Thus, muscular dystrophy has been produced experimentally in various animals on E-deficient rations; however, vitamin E supplements have not been effective in treating people with muscular dystrophy.

4. **As a regulator in the synthesis of body compounds.** The tocopherols appear to be involved in the biosynthesis of DNA, probably by regulating the incorporation of pyrimidines into the nucleic acid structures.

Vitamin E also appears to act as a cofactor in the synthesis of vitamin C, and in the synthesis of coenzyme Q—a factor that is essential in the respiratory mechanism of cells that releases energy from carbohydrates and fats.

5. **As a protector of lung tissue from air pollution.** Recent studies on rats have shown that vitamin E may protect lung tissue from smog—from damage by such oxidant components of air pollution as nitrogen dioxide (NO_2) and ozone. At the present time, it is not known whether or not vitamin E protects human lungs from damage by air pollution.

6. **As a sometimes replacement for selenium.** Both vitamin E and selenium are antioxidants, although each takes a different approach. Nevertheless, vitamin E has a sparing or replacement effect on selenium.

The belief among some people that vitamin E is "the sex vitamin" and will reduce sterility and increase potency in man is not based on scientific fact; it is one of the falsities of nutrition information which is given wide publicity.

INTERRELATIONSHIP OF VITAMIN E AND SELENIUM.

During the 1950s, an interrelationship between vitamin E and the element selenium was established. It was found that selenium prevented exudative diathesis (a hemorrhagic disease) in vitamin E-deficient chicks and liver necrosis in vitamin E-deficient rats. Subsequent research demonstrated that both selenium and vitamin E protect the cell from the detrimental effects of peroxidation, but each takes a distinctly different approach to the problem. Vitamin E is present in the membrane components of the cell and prevents free-radical formation, while selenium functions throughout the cytoplasm to destroy peroxides. This explains why selenium will correct some deficiency symptoms of vitamin E, but not others.

There is also some indication that vitamin E and selenium work together to protect cell membranes, cell nuclei, and chromosomes from carcinogens—substances that can cause cancer. But much more experimental work is needed on this subject.

DEFICIENCY SYMPTOMS.

Innumerable symptoms of vitamin E deficiency have been demonstrated in animals; and they are highly variable from species to species. A deficiency of vitamin E may produce changes in the reproductive, nervous, and circulatory systems; in the muscles, liver, and alimentary tract; and in fat deposits. Some species manifest only a single symptom,

whereas others react with a wide range of pathologies. All are preventable with alpha-tocopherol; some may be prevented by selenium or antioxidants. Table V-21 lists some of the vitamin E deficiency symptoms that have been demonstrated in different animal species.

TABLE V-21
SUMMARY OF VITAMIN E DEFICIENCY SYMPTOMS IN DIFFERENT ANIMAL SPECIES

Specie	Symptoms of Deficiency
Calf	Muscular dystrophy (white muscle disease), heart muscle abnormalities.
Chick	Encephalomalacia (crazy chick disease), exudative diathesis (a hemorrhagic disease), muscular dystrophy, poor hatchability, degeneration of the liver, heart muscle abnormalities.
Dogs	Infertility, liver damage.
Guinea pigs	Infertility, muscular dystrophy.
Hamsters	Infertility, muscular dystrophy.
Lamb	Muscular dystrophy (stiff lamb disease), heart muscle abnormalities.
Mink	Skeletal and heart muscle abnormalities.
Monkey	Anemia, infertility, heart muscle abnormalities.
Mouse	Degeneration of the heart, liver, and muscles; infertility.
Rabbit	Muscular dystrophy, infertility, heart muscle abnormalities.
Rat	Males become permanently sterile and females are unable to carry their young to full term, degeneration of the liver, muscular dystrophy in weanling rats, exudative diathesis (a hemorrhagic disease), heart muscle abnormalities.
Swine	Degeneration of the liver, infertility, muscular dystrophy, exudative diathesis (a hemorrhagic disease).

Many dietary factors seem to contribute to the development of vitamin E deficiency symptoms; among them, total fat, unsaturated fats, cod-liver oil (which is high in unsaturated acids), amount of protein, choline, cystine, inositol, cholesterol, vitamin A, and minerals have been implicated, at one time or another, as causing or aggravating deficiency symptoms.

Vitamin E deficiency symptoms as such rarely occur in humans because vitamin E (1) is widely distributed in foods, (2) is stored in almost all body tissues, and (3) is retained in the body for relatively long periods. However, clinical evidence of deficiency has been observed in infants, especially those born prematurely and formula-fed. Also, vitamin E deficiency occurs in individuals suffering from kwashiorkor (a protein deficiency), and in children and adults who have impaired fat absorption.

Newborn infants (especially the premature) have low plasma levels of vitamin E (the vitamin E concentration in full term newborn infants is about one-third that of adults, and that of premature infants is even lower), because transfer of vitamin through the placenta to the fetus is limited. As a result, hemolytic anemia (caused by shortened life span of red cells) may occur in the early weeks of life. In this condition, the membranes of the red blood cells are weakened by the action on them of the products of peroxidation of polyunsaturated fats and the cells rupture easily, producing a condition characterized by edema, skin lesions, and blood abnormalities. Supplements of vitamin E bring about increases in blood levels of the vitamin, decreases in red blood cell hemolysis, and a return to normal hemoglobin levels.

Individuals suffering from kwashiorkor, due to a severe protein deficiency, have very little tocopherol in their serum; the fragility of their red blood cells is greater than normal, and they frequently suffer from an accompanying anemia.

The symptoms of vitamin E deficiency produced by artificial diets high in unsaturated fatty acids or observed in patients unable to absorb fat (sprue, fibrocystic disease of the pancreas) include low blood and tissue tocopherol levels, increased red blood cell fragility and shortened red blood cell life-span, and increased urinary excretion of creatine (the latter is indicative of muscle damage). Marked improvement in these conditions is noted following administration of alpha-tocopherol.

RECOMMENDED DAILY ALLOWANCE OF VITAMIN E.
The Food and Nutrition Board (FNB) of the National Research Council (NRC) recommended daily allowances of vitamin E are given in Table V-22.

The requirements of vitamin E for humans is known to vary with other ingredients in the diet; for example, the presence of large amounts of polyunsaturated fatty acids (PUFA), such as linoleic acid, markedly increases the requirement. This is important in today's diets, in which large amounts of vegetable oils are used. So, individuals consuming diets high in PUFA need more vitamin E than the amounts listed in Table V-22; those whose diets are low in PUFA need less. Also, the presence of rancid fats, oxidizing substances, and selenium modify the requirements for vitamin E.

TABLE V–22
RECOMMENDED DAILY VITAMIN E ALLOWANCES[1]

Group	Age	Weight		Height		RDA[2]	
	(years)	(lb)	(kg)	(in.)	(cm)	(mg α-TE)	(IU)
Infants	0.0–0.5	13	6	24	60	3	4.47
	0.5–1.0	20	9	28	71	4	5.96
Children	1–3	29	13	35	90	6	8.94
	4–6	44	20	44	112	7	10.43
	7–10	62	28	52	132	7	10.43
Males	11–14	99	45	62	157	10	14.90
	15–18	145	66	69	176	10	14.90
	19–24	160	72	70	177	10	14.90
	25–50	174	79	70	176	10	14.90
	51+	170	77	68	173	10	14.90
Females	11–14	101	46	62	157	8	11.92
	15–18	120	55	64	163	8	11.92
	19–24	128	58	65	164	8	11.92
	25–50	138	63	64	163	8	11.92
	51+	143	65	63	160	8	11.92
Pregnant						10	14.90
Lactating						12	16.39

[1]*Recommended Dietary Allowances*, 10th ed., NRC–National Academy of Sciences, 1989, p. 285.
[2]The recommended daily allowances (RDA) are given in both International Units (IU) and alpha-tocopherol equivalents. 1 mg d-alpha-tocopherol = 1 alpha-TE. See narrative for variation in allowances and calculation of vitamin E activity of the diet as alpha-tocopherol equivalents.

• **Infants**—The vitamin E content of human milk, 2 to 5 IU (1.3 to 3.3 mg d-alpha-tocopherol equivalent) per liter (1.06 qt), is considered to be adequate for full-term infants. An intake in this range should be provided in a mixed diet of solid foods and milk up to the age of 1 year (about 20 lb [*9.1 kg*] body weight).

From the standpoint of vitamin E, cow's milk differs from human milk in two ways: (1) it contains only 1/10 to 1/2 as much vitamin E, varying with the feed consumed by the cow; and (2) it is much lower in polyunsaturated fats, containing about 1/2 as much.

Increased vitamin E is required for both premature and full-term infants fed commercial formulas made from vegetable oils that are high in polyunsaturated fats, like linoleic acid. According to the Committee on Nutrition of the Academy of Pediatrics, full-term infants require at least 0.7 IU (about 0.47 mg) of vitamin E per gram of linoleic acid in a formula preparation.

• **Children**—Little is known about the vitamin E requirement of children. It is assumed that the requirements for vitamin E will increase with increasing body weight to maturity, but not at so rapid a rate as during the early growth period.

• **Adults**—Present knowledge indicates that a dietary intake of vitamin E that maintains a blood concentration of total tocopherols above 0.5 mg/100 ml will also ensure an adequate concentration in all tissues. A range of 10 to 20 IU (7 to 13 mg d-alpha-tocopherol equivalent) can be expected to balance diets supplying 1,800 to 3,000 kcal, whereas some high fat diets may contain over 25 IU (17 mg).

• **Pregnancy and lactation**—During pregnancy and lactation, the Food and Nutrition Board recommends that the daily allowance of vitamin E be increased to compensate for the amount deposited in the fetus and secreted in the milk; that the RDA be increased by 2.98 IU (2 mg alpha-tocopherol) during pregnancy, and 4.47 IU (3 mg alpha-tocopherol) during lactation. (See Table V-22.)

• **Vitamin E intake in average U.S. diet**—Limited reports on the vitamin E intake in the U.S. diet show a daily intake of 16.7 mg of alpha-tocopherol. To this must be added the additional forms of vitamin E other than alpha-tocopherol, particularly gamma-tocopherol from soybean oil, which provide significant amounts of vitamin E activity in usual diets in the United States. Generally, non-alpha-tocopherol forms of vitamin E in a mixed diet are considered to supply about 20% of the total vitamin E activity. For the latter reason, calculations based only on alpha-tocopherol underestimate the amount of dietary vitamin E activity.

TOXICITY. Compared with vitamins A and D, vitamin E is relatively nontoxic. Excess intakes of vitamin E are excreted in the feces.

VITAMIN E LOSSES DURING PROCESSING, COOKING, AND STORAGE.

Food processing, storage, and packaging cause considerable loss of vitamin E. The tocopherols are subject to destruction by oxygen; and oxidation is accelerated by exposure to light, heat, alkali, and the presence of certain trace minerals such as iron (Fe^{+++}) and copper (Cu^{++}).

The milling of grains removes about 80% of the vitamin E; for example, in converting whole wheat to white flour, and in processing corn, oats, and rice.

Various methods of processing cause considerable destruction of vitamin E. Dehydration causes 36 to 45% loss of alpha-tocopherol in chicken and beef, but little or none in pork. Canning causes losses of 4l to 65% of the alpha-tocopherol content of meats and vegetables. An 80% destruction occurs during the roasting of nuts.

Deep-fat frying of foods causes vitamin E losses of 32 to 75%. However, normal home baking or cooking in water do not involve large losses of tocopherol. Also, being insoluble in water, tocopherols are not drained off with water.

There is a great loss of tocopherol in the storage of potato chips and french fried potatoes. One study showed after-manufacture losses of tocopherol in potato chips stored at 73°F (*23°C*) of 71% in 1 month and 77% in 2 months. When the chips were frozen at 10°F (− *12°C*), the losses were 63% in 1 month and 68% in 2 months. The after-manufacture losses of french fries stored at 10°F (− *12°C*) were 68% in 1 month and 74% in 2 months.

SOURCES OF VITAMIN E. Vitamin E (the tocopherols) occurs mainly in a variety of plant materials, especially oil seed crops (vegetable oils), some grains, nuts, and green leafy vegetables. The amount in plant foods is affected by species, variety, stage of maturity, season, time and manner of harvesting, processing procedures, and storage time. Animal tissues and animal products are usually low to poor sources of vitamin E and are influenced by the dietary consumption of tocopherols by the animal.

Groupings by rank of common food sources of vitamin E follow:

• **Rich sources**—Salad and cooking oils (except coconut oil), alfalfa seeds, margarine, nuts (almonds, Brazil nuts, filberts, peanuts, pecans), sunflower seed kernels.

• **Good sources**—Asparagus, avocados, beef and organ meats, blackberries, butter, eggs, green leafy vegetables, oatmeal, potato chips, rye, seafoods (lobster, salmon, shrimp, tuna), tomatoes.

• **Fair sources**—Apples, beans, carrots, celery, cheese, chicken, peas.

• **Negligible sources**—Most fruits, sugar, white bread.

• **Supplemental sources**—Synthetic dl-alpha-tocopherol acetate, wheat germ, wheat germ oil. Most of the commercial vitamin E is synthetic dl-alpha-tocopherol acetate. It is the least expensive source of the vitamin, but, unlike natural food sources, it provides no other essential nutrient.

For additional sources and more precise values of vitamin E (alpha-tocopherol), see Food Composition Table F-36.

Wheat germ and wheat germ oil, which are used as supplements, are the richest natural sources of vitamin E, followed by the vegetable oils (almond, corn, cottonseed, olive, palm, peanut, rapeseed, safflower, soybean, and sunflower—coconut oil is a poor source of vitamin E). It follows that margarine and cooking and salad oils are major sources in the diet; fortunately, the hydrogenation process used in their manufacture has little, if any, effect on the vitamin E content.

Refined grain products contain little vitamin E—most of the vitamin is removed in the milling process.

Human milk contains 2 to 4 times as much vitamin E as cow's milk.

TOP FOOD SOURCES OF VITAMIN E. The top food sources of vitamin E are listed in Table V-23. *Note well:* This table lists (1) the top sources without regard to the amount normally eaten (left column), and (2) the top food sources (right column); and the caloric (energy) content of each food.

(Also see ADDITIVES, Table A-3; and VITAMIN[S], Table V-9.)

TABLE V-23
TOP SOURCES OF VITAMIN E (ALPHA-TOCOPHEROL) AND THEIR CALORIC CONTENT[1]

Top Sources[2]	Vitamin E (alpha-tocopherol)	Energy	Top Food Sources	Vitamin E (alpha-tocopherol)	Energy
	(mg/100 g)	(kcal/100 g)		(mg/100 g)	(kcal/100 g)
Wheat germ oil	149.4	884	Margarine, salted, liquid oil	28.4	720
Sunflower seed oil, 60% and over			Almonds, dried, shelled, whole	27.9	598
linoleic acid	44.9	884	Peanuts, roasted w/skins, whole and		
Almond oil	39.2	884	salted	9.7	584
Cottonseed oil	35.3	884	Potato chips	6.4	568
Safflower oil, over 70% linoleic acid	34.1	884	Tuna, canned in oil	6.3	289
Alfalfa seeds	33.0	389	Blackberries, raw	3.5	29
Rice bran oil	32.3	884	Asparagus, boiled	2.5	18
Margarine, salted, liquid oil	28.4	720	Oatmeal or rolled oats, cooked	2.3	52
Almonds, dried, shelled, whole	27.9	598	Turnip greens, raw	2.2	28
Filberts (hazelnuts), whole, shelled	21.0	700	Shrimp, French fried, dipped in egg		
Cod-liver oil	20.0	899	breadcrumbs, flour	1.9	225
Palm oil	19.1	884	Avocados, raw, California, halved fruit		
Corn oil	14.3	884	served w/skin	1.7	168
Sunflower seed kernels, dry, hulled	13.0	560	Rye, whole grain	1.7	362
Olive oil	11.9	884	Butter, regular, salted	1.6	717
Peanut oil	11.6	884	Egg, fried	1.6	232
Soybean oil	11.0	884	Lobster, boiled	1.5	119
Fat, vegetable shortening	9.9	884	Salmon, Atlantic, canned, solids/liquid	1.4	124
Peanuts, roasted w/skins, whole and			Broccoli, raw	1.3	23
salted	9.7	584	Pecans, unsalted	1.2	739
Wheat, soy blend w/straight grade			Tomatoes, raw	1.2	17
wheat flour	7.0	365	Beef, hindshank, flank or chuck rib,		
			lean, cooked	.9	203

[1]These listings are based on the data in Food Composition Table F-36. Some top or rich sources may have been overlooked since some of the foods in Table F-36 lack values for vitamin E (alpha-tocopherol).

Whenever possible, foods are on an "as used" basis, without regard to moisture content; hence, certain high-moisture foods may be disadvantaged when ranked on the basis of vitamin E content per 100 g (approximately 3½ oz) without regard to moisture content.

[2]Listed without regard to the amount normally eaten.

VITAMIN F

A now discredited term, which was once given to the unsaturated fatty acids, linoleic acid, linolenic acid, and arachidonic acid, found to be essential for laboratory rats. There is no evidence that lack of these fatty acids in the diet will result in clinical manifestations in adult humans (although they may be required for babies). Also, the use of unsaturated fatty acids is sometimes recommended for the treatment of atherosclerosis.

VITAMIN K

Contents   Page

Vitamin K, known as the *antihemorrhagic vitamin*, is necessary for the synthesis of prothrombin and other blood clotting factors in the liver. Presently, the term vitamin K is used to describe a chemical group of quinone compounds, rather than a single entity, which have characteristic antihemorrhagic effects.

Defective blood coagulation is the only well-established symptom of vitamin K deficiency. Deficiencies are rare in humans, but considerable use is made of synthetic substances that act as antagonists of vitamin K (such as dicoumarol, an anticoagulant) to prevent clotting of blood in patients with certain circulatory disorders.

HISTORY. In 1929, Professor Carl Peter Hendrik Dam, biochemist at the University of Copenhagen, Denmark, observed that certain experimental diets produced fatal hemorrhages in chicks. Bleeding could be prevented by giving a variety of foodstuffs, especially alfalfa (lucerne) and fishmeal. Further, it was found that the active principle in these materials could be extracted with ether; thus, a new fat-soluble factor was *discovered*. In 1935, Dam named it the Koagulation vitamin (the Danish word for coagulation), from which the shortened term vitamin K (from the first letter of Koagulation) was derived. In 1939, Dam and Karrer isolated vitamin K in pure form; and, that same year, Almquist and Klose *synthesized* vitamin K. In 1943, Dam received the Nobel Prize in physiology and medicine for his brilliant work.

In 1941, Link and coworkers at the University of Wisconsin discovered dicoumarol—an antimetabolite of vitamin K.

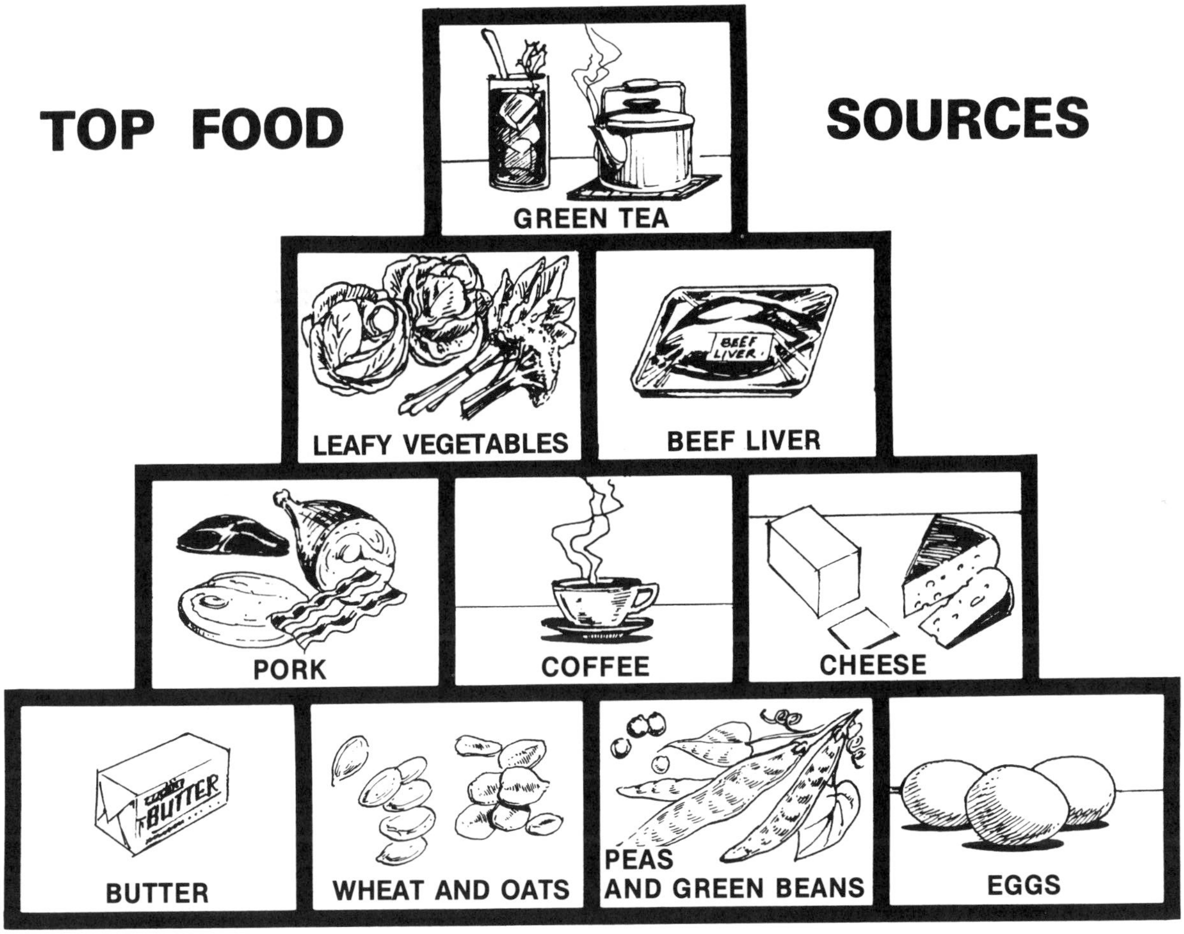

TOP FOOD 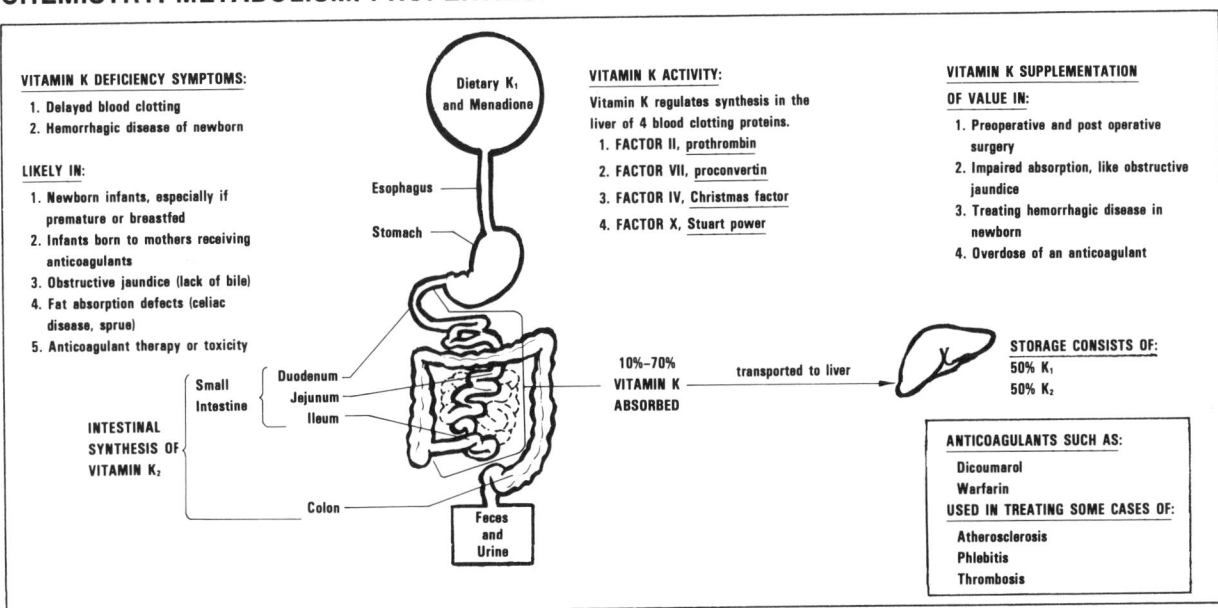 SOURCES

GREEN TEA

LEAFY VEGETABLES

BEEF LIVER

PORK

COFFEE

CHEESE

BUTTER

WHEAT AND OATS

PEAS AND GREEN BEANS

EGGS

Fig. V-44. Top sources of vitamin K for common foods.

CHEMISTRY. METABOLISM. PROPERTIES.

VITAMIN K DEFICIENCY SYMPTOMS:

1. Delayed blood clotting
2. Hemorrhagic disease of newborn

LIKELY IN:

1. Newborn infants, especially if premature or breastfed
2. Infants born to mothers receiving anticoagulants
3. Obstructive jaundice (lack of bile)
4. Fat absorption defects (celiac disease, sprue)
5. Anticoagulant therapy or toxicity

INTESTINAL SYNTHESIS OF VITAMIN K₂

Dietary K₁ and Menadione

Esophagus

Stomach

Small Intestine

Duodenum
Jejunum
Ileum

Colon

Feces and Urine

VITAMIN K ACTIVITY:

Vitamin K regulates synthesis in the liver of 4 blood clotting proteins.

1. FACTOR II, prothrombin
2. FACTOR VII, proconvertin
3. FACTOR IV, Christmas factor
4. FACTOR X, Stuart power

10%–70%
VITAMIN K ABSORBED

transported to liver

VITAMIN K SUPPLEMENTATION

OF VALUE IN:

1. Preoperative and post operative surgery
2. Impaired absorption, like obstructive jaundice
3. Treating hemorrhagic disease in newborn
4. Overdose of an anticoagulant

STORAGE CONSISTS OF:
50% K₁
50% K₂

ANTICOAGULANTS SUCH AS:

Dicoumarol
Warfarin

USED IN TREATING SOME CASES OF:

Atherosclerosis
Phlebitis
Thrombosis

Fig. V-45. Vitamin K utilization.

• **Chemistry**—A number of chemical compounds possessing vitamin K activity have been isolated or synthesized. There are two naturally occurring forms of vitamin K; vitamin K_1 (phylloquinone or phytylmenaquinone) which occurs only in green plants, and K_2 (menaquinones or multiprenyl-menaquinones), which is synthesized by many microorganisms, including bacteria in the intestinal tracts of human beings and other species. Additionally, several synthetic compounds have been prepared that possess vitamin K activity, the best known of which is menadione (2-methyl, 1, 4-naphthoquinone), formerly known as K_3. Menadione, which is converted to vitamin K_2 in the body, is 2 to 3 times as potent as K_1 and K_2. The structural formulas of K_1, K_2 and menadione, all of which are called vitamin K are shown in Fig. V-46.

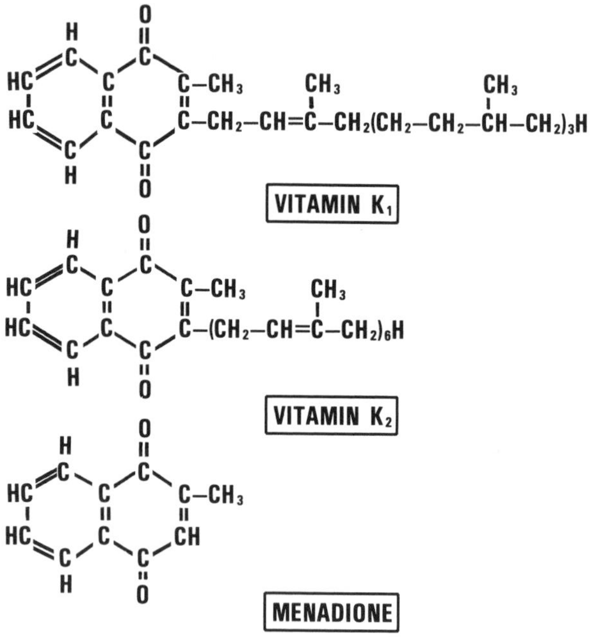

Fig. V-46.   Structures of vitamin K_1, vitamin K_2, and menadione.

• **Metabolism**—Normally, vitamin K_1 is taken into the body in the diet, vitamin K_2 is synthesized in the intestine, and menadione is taken as a vitamin supplement.

1. **Intestinal synthesis.** Vitamin K_2 is synthesized by the normal bacteria in the small intestine and the colon; hence, an adequate supply is generally present. Since the intestine of a newborn infant is sterile at birth, however, the supply of vitamin K is inadequate until normal bacterial flora of the intestine develops on about the third or fourth day of life.

The intestinal synthesis of vitamin K reduces the food dietary requirements for the vitamin in man and other mammals (but not birds; birds have such a short intestinal tract and harbor so few microorganisms that they require a dietary source of vitamin K), although it appears that

little of the vitamin K produced in the lower gut is absorbed. It is noteworthy, however, that animals that practice coprophagy, such as the rabbit, can utilize much of the vitamin K that is eliminated in the feces.

2. **Absorption.** Since the natural vitamins K (K_1 and K_2) are fat soluble, they require bile and pancreatic juice in the intestine for maximum absorption. Thus, anything that interferes with the normal absorption of fat, interferes with the absorption of natural vitamin Ks. By contrast, some of the synthetic vitamin K compounds are water soluble and more easily absorbed. Absorption takes place mainly in the upper part of the small intestine. Normally, 10 to 70% of the vitamin K in the intestines is absorbed. However, there is uncertainty as to how much of the vitamin K_2 that is synthesized in the colon is absorbed, based on the fact that absorption of nutrients in general from the large intestine appears to be limited because of the nature of the epithelial lining.

3. **Transportation.** Vitamin K passes unchanged from the small intestine into the lymph system. Thence, it is carried to the thoracic duct, where it enters the bloodstream. In the blood, it is attached to beta-lipoproteins and transported to the liver and other tissues.

4. **Metabolism.** Whether the vitamin Ks' functions are unchanged or are transformed to other metabolically active forms has not been determined. It is known that menadione must be converted to K_2 in the bodies of both animals and humans for it to be biologically active.

5. **Storage.** Vitamin K is stored only in small amounts. Modest amounts are stored in the liver, with the skin and muscle following in concentration. About 50% of the vitamin K found in the human liver is K_1 from the diet; the other 50% is K_2 from bacterial synthesis in the intestine.

6. **Excretion.** Excess vitamin K is excreted in the feces and urine.

• **Properties**—The naturally occurring forms of vitamin K are yellow oils; the synthetic forms are yellow crystalline powders. All K vitamins are resistant to heat and moisture, but they are destroyed on exposure to acid, alkali, oxidizing agents, and light—particularly ultraviolet light. Since natural vitamin K is stable to heat and not water soluble, little of it is lost in normal cooking processes. However, some of the synthetic forms of vitamin K are soluble in water.

MEASUREMENT/ASSAY. Vitamin K can be measured in micrograms of the pure synthetic compound (menadione), and the vitamin K activity of other substances can be expressed in similar terms.

The potency of low concentration samples, such as occurs in most foods, is commonly determined by bioassay, using young chicks, and is based on the minimum dose that will maintain the normal coagulation of the blood at the end of 1 month. In pure solutions, vitamin K may be assayed by U.V. spectrophotometry or colorimetric methods. Other accepted techniques are the oxidimetric assay after catalytic reduction to the hydroquinone and the polarographic determination.

FUNCTIONS. Vitamin K is essential for the synthesis by the liver of four blood clotting proteins—factor II, or prothrombin; factor VII, or proconvertin; factor IX,

Christmas factor; and factor X, Stuart-Power factor. The exact way in which vitamin K functions in the synthesis of these proteins is unknown. Recent research suggests that vitamin K acts in some way to convert precursor proteins to the active blood clotting factors. Without vitamin K, or when an antagonist is given, the level of the blood clotting proteins in the blood is reduced and clotting time is prolonged.

At this time, there is no evidence that vitamin K has any functions in humans or animals other than in the blood coagulation process, although vitamin K-dependent proteins have been identified in the bone, kidney, and liver.

VITAMIN K ANTAGONISTS (ANTICOAGU-LANTS).

The discovery of vitamin K antagonists stemmed primarily from investigations into a disorder in cattle known as "sweet clover disease," in which there is a loss of clotting power of the blood. As a result, blood forms soft swellings beneath the skin on different parts of the body, and serious or fatal bleeding may occur at the time of dehorning, castration, calving, or following injury. The causative agent of "sweet clover disease" was identified by Campbell, *et al.*, (1941) of the University of Wisconsin, as dicoumarol, an oxidative product of coumarin, found in sweet clover hay that had undergone spoilage during harvesting or storage.

The discovery of the cause of "sweet clover disease" opened up an entirely new field. The synthesis of several dicoumarol derivatives followed. These antivitamins, or antagonists, decrease the ability of the blood to clot by inhibiting the synthesis of prothrombin and the other K-dependent blood clotting factors. They are used medically to reduce clotting of the blood in patients with certain circulatory disorders, especially some forms of atherosclerosis, phlebitis, and thrombosis. It is noteworthy that Warfarin, a commercial product similar in structure to dicoumarol, is a very potent rat poison; it kills rats by causing them to bleed to death internally.

DEFICIENCY SYMPTOMS.

The symptoms of vitamin K deficiency are increased clotting times and hemorrhaging. Two laboratory tests are commonly used to assess vitamin K status: (1) the *prothrombin time*—the measurement in a plasma sample of the speed of conversion of prothrombin to thrombin; and (2) the *blood clotting time*—the placing of freshly drawn blood in a clean test tube, tilting it once each minute, and determining the time required for the clot to form (for normal blood the clotting time is about 10 minutes).

Fowl are very susceptible to vitamin K deficiency. When vitamin K is absent, they develop delayed blood clotting, causing hemorrhages under the skin and serious internal bleeding, followed by death if not corrected. Deficiencies have also been produced in cattle, pigs, rats, dogs, and all other species studied.

Although a hemorrhagic syndrome, due to a vitamin K deficiency, is rare in adult humans, it can be caused by the following:

1. Some defect in the absorption as in obstructive jaundice, or in malabsorption due to celiac disease or sprue.

2. Sterilization of the bowels by an antibiotic or a sulfa drug, thereby reducing the synthesis of vitamin K.

3. Anticoagulant therapy for certain circulatory disorders.

Hemorrhagic disease, due to a vitamin K deficiency, may occur in newborn babies—particularly those born prematurely and breast fed, those on unfortified soy formulas, or those whose mothers have been taking anticoagulants—between the second and fifth days of life; causing bleeding either in the skin, nervous system, peritoneal cavity, or alimentary tract. Because human milk provides less vitamin K than cow's milk, vitamin K deficiency is more common in breast fed than in formula-fed babies. Hemorrhagic disease due to a vitamin K deficiency can be prevented by giving a dose of 1 mg of vitamin K_1 intramuscularly immediately after birth. It is noteworthy, however, that vitamin K deficiency is not always the cause of hemorrhagic disease; injury at birth is undoubtedly responsible in some cases.

Vitamin K has proved ineffective in treating hemophilia, an inherited condition causing abnormal hemorrhaging in man.

RECOMMENDED DAILY ALLOWANCE OF VITAMIN K.

The Food and Nutrition Board (FNB) of the National Research Council (NRC) recommended daily allowances of vitamin K are given in Table V-24.

TABLE V-24
ESTIMATED SAFE AND ADEQUATE
DAILY DIETARY INTAKES OF VITAMIN K[1]

Group	Age	Vitamin K
	(years)	(mcg)
Infants	0.0–0.5	5
	0.5–1.0	10
Children	1–3	15
	4–6	20
	7–10	30
Males	11–14	45
	15–18	65
	19–24	70
	25–50	80
	51+	80
Females	11–14	45
	15–18	55
	19–24	60
	25–50	65
	51+	65
Pregnant		65
Lactating		65

[1]*Recommended Dietary Allowances*, 10th ed., NRC–National Academy of Sciences, 1989, p. 285.

The major criterion for assessing the adequacy of vitamin K status in adult humans is the maintenance of plasma prothrombin concentrations in the normal range, i.e., from 80 to 120 mcg/ml.

In 1976, the Committee on Nutrition of the American Academy of Pediatrics recommended that infant formulas include a minimum of 4 mcg per 100 kcal of vitamin K for milkbase formulas and 8 mcg per 100 kcal for soy isolate and other milk substitute formulas. Vitamin K hypoprothrombinemia (due to K deficiency) occurs in infants fed certain soy protein isolates, meat base formula, or formula containing hydrolyzed casein. Such diets may be low in vitamin K.

The intake suggested for young infants is based on 2 mcg/kg, assuming no intestinal synthesis. Therefore, the amount provided by current formulas of 4 mcg/100 kcal should be ample for normal infants. The suggested intake of 12 mcg/day is also in the range supplied by breast milk (15 mcg/liter).

• **Vitamin K intake in average U.S. diet**—The average mixed diet in the United States supplies 300 to 500 mcg of vitamin K per day; hence, there is little danger of insufficiency under normal conditions.

TOXICITY (HYPERVITAMINOSIS K).
The natural forms of vitamins K_1 and K_2 have not produced toxicity even when given in large amounts. However, synthetic menadione and its various derivatives (formerly called K_3) have produced toxic symptoms in rats and jaundice in human infants when given in amounts of more than 5 mg daily. Consequently, the U.S. Food and Drug Administration does not allow any menadione in any food supplements, including prenatal vitamin capsules.

Vitamin K_1 preparations are preferred for the treatment of such medical conditions as liver disease, severe malabsorption syndromes, and anticoagulant overdosage.

VITAMIN K LOSSES DURING PROCESSING, COOKING, AND STORAGE.
For maximum vitamin K, food should be fresh. Frozen foods tend to be deficient in vitamin K. Ordinary cooking processes destroy very little natural vitamin K, since the vitamin is stable to heat and not water soluble. However, some of the synthetic compounds are soluble in water and subject to greater loss in cooking. Sunlight destroys vitamin K_1; and all vitamin K compounds tend to be unstable to alkali.

SOURCES OF VITAMIN K.
Vitamin K is fairly widely distributed in foods.

Also, synthesis in the intestine is an important source of vitamin K_2; and vitamin K supplements (chiefly the synthetic menadione) are available.

Groupings by rank of common sources of vitamin K follow:

• **Rich sources**—Green tea, turnip greens, broccoli, lettuce, cabbage, beef liver, spinach.

• **Good sources**—Asparagus, watercress, bacon, coffee, cheese, butter, pork liver, oats.

• **Fair sources**—Green peas, whole wheat, beef fat, ham, green beans, eggs, pork tenderloin, peaches, ground beef, chicken liver, raisins.

• **Negligible sources**—Applesauce, bananas, bread, cola, corn, corn oil, cow's milk, oranges, potatoes, pumpkin, tomatoes, wheat flour.

• **Supplemental sources**—Chiefly synthetic menadione.

No vitamin K values are listed in Food Composition Table F-36, for the reason that few foods have been assayed for this vitamin.

TOP FOOD SOURCES OF VITAMIN K.
The vitamin K content of some common foods is given in Table F-25.

(Also see VITAMIN[S], Table V-9.)

TABLE V-25
VITAMIN K AND CALORIE CONTENT
OF SOME COMMON FOODS[1]

Food	Vitamin K	Energy
	(mcg/100 g)	(kcal/100 g)
Tea, green	712	1
Turnip greens	650	28
Broccoli	200	26
Lettuce	129	15
Cabbage	125	24
Beef liver	92	222
Spinach	89	26
Asparagus	57	20
Watercress	57	19
Bacon	46	300
Coffee	38	3
Cheese	35	402
Butter	30	717
Pork liver	25	241
Oats	20	390
Peas, green	19	71
Wheat, whole	17	357
Beef fat	15	902
Ham	15	350
Beans, green	14	24
Eggs	11	157
Pork tenderloin	11	254
Peaches, raw	8	38
Ground beef	7	301
Chicken liver	7	165
Raisins	6	289

[1]Adapted from Goodhart, Robert S. and Maurice E. Shils, *Modern Nutrition in Health and Disease,* 6th ed., Lea & Febiger, 1980, p. 172, Table 6C-1; data taken from the studies of Dam and Glavind, Richardson, Doisy and Matschiner and Doisy.

VITAMIN L

Factors L_1 and L_2, which are found in yeast, are said to be necessary for lactation. However, they have not become established as vitamins; hence, there is no such thing as vitamin L at this time.

VITAMIN P

The designation first given to bioflavonoids—a group of natural pigments in vegetables, fruits, flowers, and grains. Although the flavonoids display a synergistic action toward ascorbic acid, the initial claim, made in 1936, that some or all of the flavonoids are indispensable food components equivalent to vitamins was not substantiated. As a result, in 1950 the Joint Committee of Biochemical Nomenclature of the American Society of Biological Chemists and the American Institute of Nutrition recommended that the term "vitamin P" be dropped. Following this, the name bioflavonoids came into use except in France and the U.S.S.R., where the term vitamin P persists.

(Also see BIOFLAVONOIDS.)

VITAMIN SUPPLEMENTS

Rich synthetic or natural food sources of one or more of the complex organic compounds, called vitamins, that are required in minute amounts by people and animals for normal growth, production, reproduction, and/or health.

(Also see VITAMIN[S].)

VOLATILE OILS

These are obtained from flowers, stems, leaves, and often the entire plant, and they are used for perfumery and flavorings. Often these are called essential oils. They vaporize quickly.

(Also see ESSENTIAL OILS.)

VOMITING

The forcible expulsion of the contents of the stomach through the mouth.

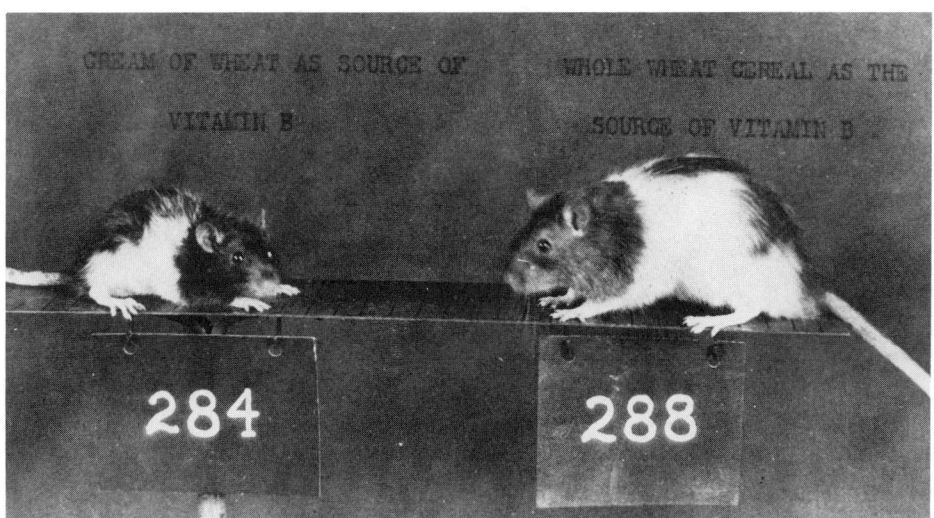

B vitamins made the difference! Experiment conducted in the early 1930s by Osborne and Mendel at the Connecticut Agricultural Experiment Station. Rat on left received B vitamins obtained from a breakfast cereal. The other rat was supplied B vitamins from whole wheat. Today, most cereals are enriched with vitamins. (Courtesy, The Connecticut Agricultural Experiment Station, New Haven, Conn.)

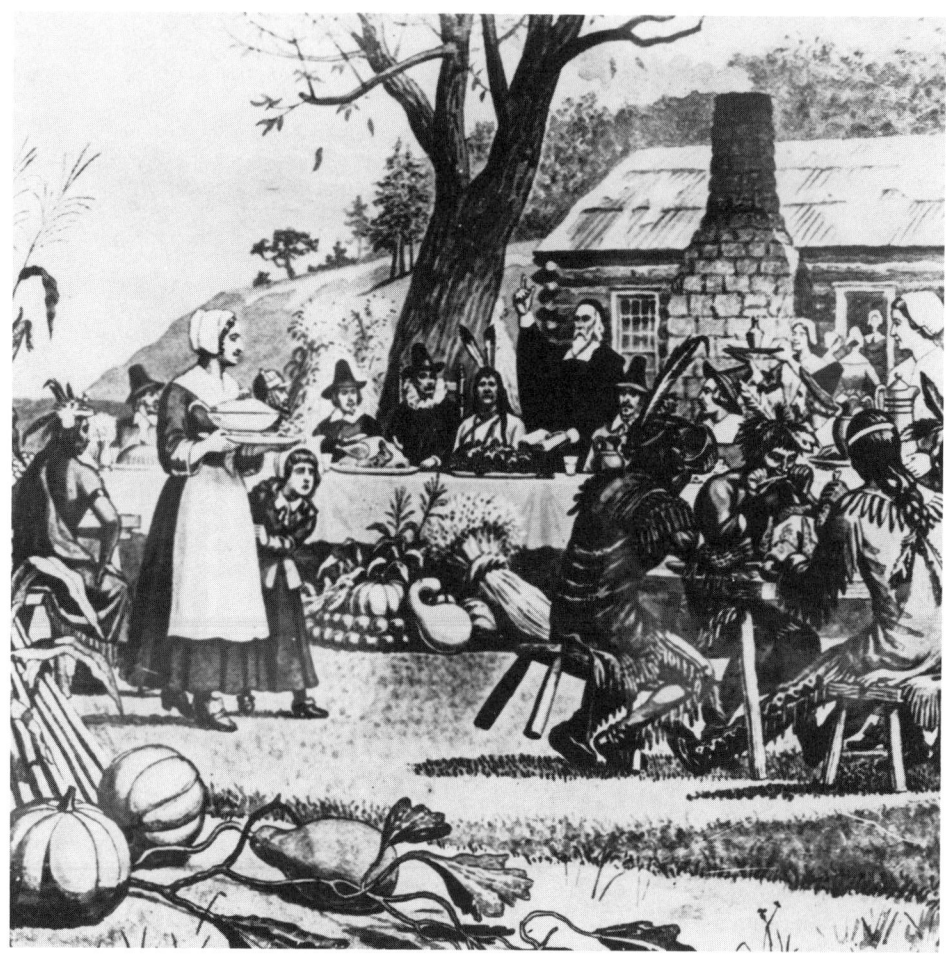

The first American Thanksgiving. In olden times, people ate whole or natural foods which were subjected to little processing from garden to table. (Courtesy, The Bettmann Archive, New York, NY)

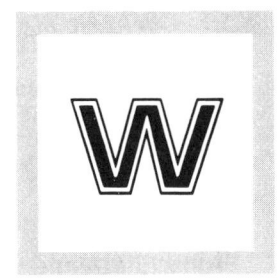

WALNUT (BLACK WALNUT; ENGLISH WALNUT) *Juglans* **spp**

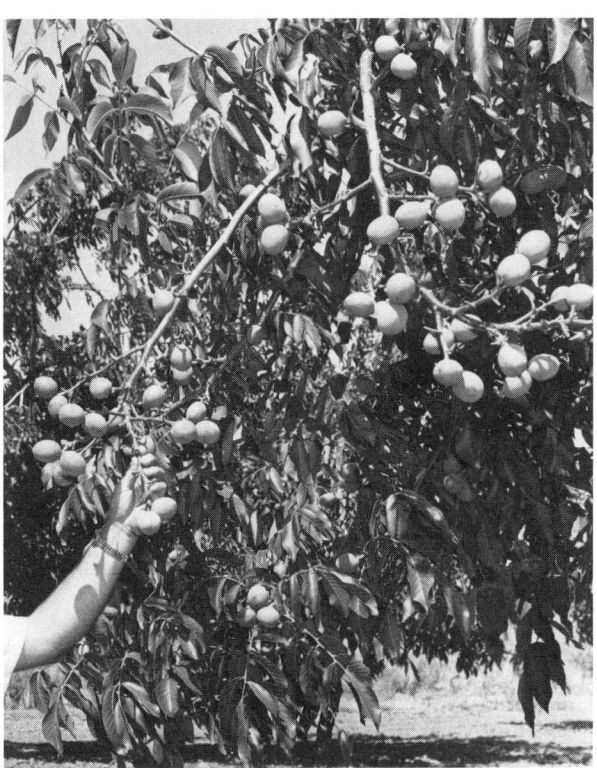

Fig. W-1. English walnuts approaching maturity. (Courtesy, Sun-Diamond Growers of California, Stockton, Calif.)

The term walnut refers to several varieties of nuts. Two are of commercial importance: (1) the English walnut (Persian walnut), *Juglans regia*; and (2) the black walnut, *Juglans nigra*. Of these two, the English walnut tree bears walnuts that are the most valuable commercially.

Walnut trees are large, long living trees which can grow to heights of 70 to 150 ft (*21 to 46 m*). Leaves of the walnut are spaced alternately along the branches and each is divided into an odd number of small leaflets, usually from 7 to 23. Male flowers of the tree are borne in long unbranched, drooping catkins, while the female flowers are borne singly or in short spikes. Walnut trees self-pollinate and cross-pollinate. The drupelike fruit—the nut—is borne singly or in clusters of two or three. Nuts are 1 ½ to 2 ½ in. (*3.8 to 6.4 cm*) in diameter, and oblong to round in shape. Nuts are composed of an outer, leathery husk and an inner, hard, furrowed shell which surrounds the "meat." Besides providing food, walnut trees are also a popular ornamental and shade tree and their wood is esteemed for its rich beauty.

ORIGIN AND HISTORY. Black walnuts are native to the Central Mississippi Valley and the Appalachian region of North America. However, they have been planted beyond their natural range and they grow over a wide area on good agricultural soils. Black walnuts were an important source of food for the American Indians and early settlers.

English, or Persian walnuts, as they are also called, are a native of southeastern Europe and western Asia—not England as the name suggests. Perhaps, it gained the name English walnut because it was brought to America on English ships. The name Persian walnut is descriptive of its origin. Since Roman times, the English walnut has been cultivated commercially in Europe. In the New World, English walnuts for commercial production grow best from central California to Oregon. They do not grow well in the southern states. Other areas are suited for English walnut growth for local consumption.

PRODUCTION. Worldwide, commercial production of English walnuts amounts to about 946,626 metric tons each year, in those countries for which there are reliable statistics. The United States produces 21% of this amount—all in California. The California crop of English walnuts is valued at about $230 million. Other leading walnut-producing countries, by rank, are: Turkey, China, Romania, Iran, France, and Yugoslavia. Only Turkey and China produce over 100,000 metric tons each year, while the other countries listed, produce 30,000–50,000 metric tons each year.

Production in most areas of the world is rather incidental, but in California, English walnut production is a well-developed agricultural concern.

Black walnut production is limited to trees in forests and farmsteads. In some areas, these are collected, shelled, and sold. No reliable production figures are available.

Propagation and Growing.

English walnuts are commercially produced in orchards of grafted trees, instead of from seedling trees. Rootstocks used in California are *Juglans hindsii* and Paradox (a cross of *Juglans hindsii* and *Juglans regia*) and in the East, eastern black walnut *Juglans nigra*. Nurserymen or local nut growers know the best variety for a given location.

Franquette is the standard old variety. It is a late leafing and harvesting variety, with small nuts of high quality. Yields are moderate and requirements for cultural care minimal. Hartley is the preferred variety for the inshell trade, and important for export.

Walnuts are planted at least 60 ft (*18 m*) apart. They require good-textured, deep, well-drained, fertile soils for optimal growth and production. Extensive root development can occur to 15 ft (*5 m*) in deep soils. The climate should be cold enough in the winter to break dormancy of the trees, yet trees can be damaged by winter temperatures as low as 14°F (*-10°C*), especially when followed by a warm period. Two hundred or more frost-free days are required for commercial production.

Harvesting.

Walnuts are mature and ready for harvest as soon as the tissue between the kernel and the inner lining of the shell turns brown. Shortly after that time, nuts can easily be shaken from the tree. Any harvest delay will result in a darker colored kernel, and also allow time for mold and entrance of the navel orange worm.

The homeowner can easily harvest walnuts as they fall from the tree. Harvesting in many countries is done with local hand labor. However, economic farming enterprises must, with the present labor market, harvest mechanically. Special equipment required for harvest includes a tree shaker, a windrower or sweeping device to pile the nuts into a neat, long row, and a pickup machine. Nuts are shaken to the ground, windrowed, picked up, and transported in bulk.

Once harvested, nuts are taken to the huller, where the remaining hulls are mechanically removed and the shells brushed clean. From there, the nuts go into a drying facility and are treated with forced air at 109°F (*43°C*) for 24 to 36 hours.

The husk of black walnuts does not separate readily from the shell and it is usually allowed to rot away. Also, the shell is hard to crack and the meat is difficult to remove.

PROCESSING.

At packing houses, those English walnuts to be marketed in the shells (about 40%) are sized, bleached, and bagged for shipment. Others are machine-shelled, and the kernels are graded for color and size, and packaged for the retail trade. Some of the poorer grades may be used to make walnut oil and shell flour.

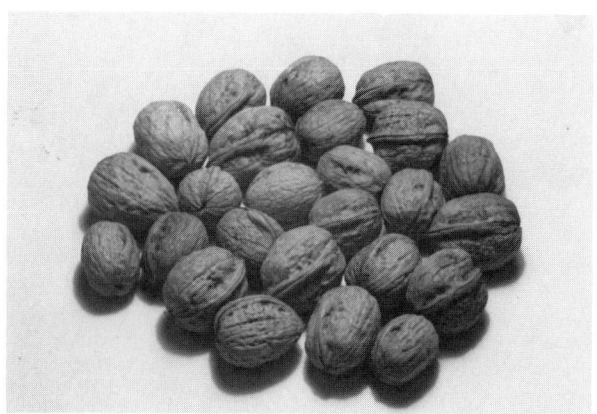

Fig. W-2.   English walnuts with their husks removed are ready for selling or cracking. (Courtesy, Sun-Diamond Growers of California, Stockton, Calif.)

SELECTION.

Walnuts in shells should be free from splits, cracks, stains, or holes. Moldy nuts may not be safe to eat. Nutmeat should be plump and fairly uniform in color and size. Limp, rubbery, dark, or shriveled kernels are likely stale. If antioxidants are added to delay the onset of rancidity, thus extending the shelf life of packaged nut meat, they are listed on the package.

PREPARATION.

Walnuts (kernels) are eaten alone as a snack, or they are used in endless ways in baking and confectionery.

The dried nuts will store for at least a year under fairly variable conditions, up to 2 years if the storage temperature is kept below 40°F (*4.8°C*).

The few black walnuts that are available can be used in baked goods, candy, and ice cream.

NUTRITIONAL VALUE.

Walnuts—English and black—are extremely nutritious. They contain only 3 to 4% water and they are "supercharged" with 678 to 694 Calories (kcal) for each 100 g (about 3 1/2 oz). Walnuts are high in calories primarily because they are about 60% fat (oil). Additionally, each 100 g also provides 15 to 20 g of protein, 3 mg of iron and zinc, and only 2 mg of sodium. More complete information regarding the nutritional value of walnuts is provided in Food Composition Table F-36.

(Also see NUT[S], Table N-8 Nuts of the World.)

WARBURG'S YELLOW ENZYME

A protein isolated in 1932 by two German scientists, Warburg and Christian. It played a role in the discovery of the vitamin riboflavin.

(Also see RIBOFLAVIN.)

WATER (H₂O)

Contents

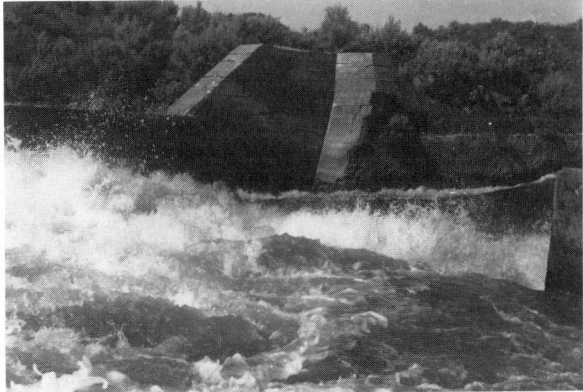

Fig. W-3. Plenty of cool, fresh, clean water, Lake Walcott canal, Minidoka County, Idaho. (Photo by Jayne Parker)

Chemically, water is the combination of two gases—hydrogen (H) and oxygen (O)—which are joined in the ratio of two hydrogen atoms to one oxygen. Thus, the chemical formula for water is H_2O. It is the most abundant chemical, and it performs endless functions in one of its three forms—liquid, solid, gas.

IMPORTANCE OF WATER TO LIFE.

Water is a nutrient. It is one of the most vital of all nutrients. In fact, water is the only substance necessary to all life. Many organisms can live without air, but none can live without water. Humans and animals can survive for a longer period without food than without water. Only oxygen is more important to human life. Fortunately, water is usually provided in abundance and at little cost. In most U.S. cities it can be delivered to the kitchen for about 15¢ per ton.

Water is the most abundant body constituent. The younger the individual the more water the body contains. It accounts for about 98% of the embryo, for about 75% of infants, and for about 50 to 65% of the body weight of adults. In general, as the fat content of the body increases, the water content decreases.

In the body, water performs the following important functions:

1. It is necessary to the life and shape of every cell, and a constituent of every body fluid.

2. It acts as a carrier for various substances, serving as a medium in which nourishment is carried to the cells and waste products are removed therefrom.

3. It assists with temperature regulation in the body, cooling the individual by evaporation from the skin as perspiration.

4. It is necessary for many important chemical reactions of digestion and metabolism.

5. It lubricates the joints, as a constituent of the synovial fluid; it acts as a water cushion for the nervous system, in the cerebrospinal fluid; it transports sound, in the perilymph in the ear; and it is concerned with sight and provides a lubricant for the eye.

6. It acts as a solvent for a number of chemicals which can subsequently be detected by taste buds.

7. It aids in gas exchange in respiration by keeping the alveoli of the lungs moist.

The total body water involved in all of these functions is contained in two major compartments in the body: (1) the extracellular or water outside the cells (about 20% of the body weight), and (2) the intracellular or the water inside each cell (about 45% of the body weight).

Deficits or excesses of more than a few percent of the total body water are incompatible with health, and large deficits, of about 20% of the body weight lead to death. Under normal circumstances, thirst ensures that water intake meets or exceeds the requirement for water. Surplus water is excreted from the body, principally in the urine, and to a lesser extent in the perspiration, feces, and water vapor from the lungs.

Water Balance. In healthy individuals, total body water remains reasonably constant. An increase or decrease in water intake brings about an appropriate increase or decrease in water output to maintain the balance. Water enters the body as a liquid, and as a component of the food—including metabolic water derived from the breakdown of food. Water is lost from the body (1) by the skin as perspiration, (2) by the lungs as water vapor in expired air, (3) by the kidneys as urine, and (4) by the intestine in the feces. Therefore, under normal conditions the intake of water from the various sources is approximately equal to output of water by the various routes. For example, if a large volume of water is drunk, then the volume of urine excreted increases, or if water drinking is severely limited then the volume of urine formed is drastically reduced.

Water intake for a normal adult during a 24-hour period averages about 2.1 to 2.9 qt (*2 to 2.7 liter*) and water output via all four routes averages the same, assuming light activity and no visible perspiring, as Table W-1 shows.

TABLE W-1
DAILY WATER LEDGER

Water In		Water Out	
Source	**Amount**	**Source**	**Amount**
	(ml)		(ml)
Fluids	1,500	Skin	700
Water in foods	850	Lungs	350
Metabolic water	250	Kidneys	1,400
		Feces	150
Total	2,600	Total	2,600

The body is equipped with a number of mechanisms for regulating body water within narrow limits. Important among these mechanisms are nerve centers in the hypothalamus of the brain which control the sensation of thirst and water output by the kidneys. Stimulation of the thirst center in the hypothalamus results when water loss amounts to about 1% of the body weight, and creates the conscious desire for water. If water is not drunk, discomfort increases—heart rate increases, body temperature rises, and working and thinking abilities deteriorate. Heat exhaustion is certain if physical work is attempted when water loss is 10% of the body weight. Stimulation of other nerve centers in the hypothalamus causes the release of antidiuretic hormone (ADH) from the posterior pituitary. Release of ADH results in the formation of less urine, thereby conserving body water. The urine formed appears more concentrated, dark, and cloudy than when water intake is adequate. Despite the controls to maintain water balance, several factors can influence water balance and the requirement for water.

Requirement for Water.   The requirement for water to maintain the water balance can be influenced by age,

physical activity, heat, diet, illness, and injury. In general, the requirement for water can best be taken care of by allowing free access to plenty of clean, fresh water at all times. A discusion of each of the factors influencing the requirement for water follows:

• **Age**—Water needs for infants and children are proportionately higher than those for adults. The normal turnover rate of water per day is about 6% of the total body water in the adult and about 15% in the young infant. The turnover is so high in infants because (1) the water loss from the skin is largely due to the greater surface area in relation to body weight, and (2) the ability of the kidneys to concentrate urine is much less than that of adults.

The multitude of factors determining water loss precludes the setting of a general value for minimal water requirement.

Under ordinary circumstances, a reasonable allowance is 1 ml/kcal for adults and 1.5 ml/kcal for infants. Table W-2 presents daily water allowances in terms of the recommended dietary allowances for energy.

TABLE W-2
DAILY WATER ALLOWANCE FOR INFANTS AND ADULTS[1]

Category	Age	Weight		Energy Needs	Water Needs		
	(years)	(lb)	(kg)	(kcal)	(ml/kcal)	(ml)	(8 oz cups)
Infants	0.0–0.5	13	6	650	1.5	975	4.1
	0.5–1.0	20	9	850	1.5	1,275	5.4
Males	25–50	174	79	2,900	1.0	2,900	12.3
Females	25–50	138	63	2,200	1.0	2,200	9.4
Pregnancy				2,500	+30 ml	2,530	10.8
Lactating				2,700	+750 ml	3,450	14.7

[1]Based on *Recommended Dietary Allowances,* 10th ed., 1989, National Academy of Sciences/National Research Council, pp. 247–250.

• **Physical activity**—Even in a comfortable environment, physical activity increases the loss of water from the body through perspiration and water vapor from the lungs. Although considerable amounts of sodium are lost in the perspiration, the loss of water significantly exceeds that of sodium. Hence, water depletion is the major problem. If water loss is not replenished then physical performance begins to deteriorate when the water deficit exceeds 3% of the body weight. Despite this fact, extremely ill-advised practices—withholding water, wearing rubberized apparel, and inducing vomiting—are sometimes used to meet weight ranges in competitive sports such as wrestling.

Sir Edmund Hillary, the first person to climb Mt. Everest, attributed the success of his expedition during the last few days of the climb to an adequate supply of water. Other expeditions attempting the climb had evidently failed to drink or carry sufficient water.

• **Heat**—The combination of high temperature and increased physical activity may increase water losses from the skin and lungs threefold to tenfold. These increased water losses must be covered by increased intake, and

free access to water is essential. Water needs for individuals living in hot dry climates are increased as losses from the lungs and skin are elevated 50 to 100%. Failure to replace water losses arising from prolonged sweating may result in heat exhaustion. Furthermore, providing salt (sodim chloride) without free access to water may lead to the development of significant hypernatremia—elevated blood sodium. Symptoms of acute water lack during hard work in a hot environment appear rapidly, and recovery following water ingestion is even more rapid.

(Also see HEAT EXHAUSTION; and MINERS' CRAMPS.)

• **Diet**—High-protein diets require extra water for excretion of urea. Special attention must be given to the water needs of infants on high-protein formulas, since the concentrating ability of the infant's kidney is not well developed.

• **Illness**—In persistent vomiting large amounts of water are lost. Prolonged diarrhea also results in excessive loss of water. Fever accelerates the loss of body water through increased perspiration and the excretion of body waste. Illnesses in which a fever, vomiting, and/or diarrhea are present, can rapidly result in dehydration especially in infants, children, and older individuals.

In the opposite direction, some conditions are associated with excessive retention of water or edema. Often edema is noted in the following diseases: congestive heart failure, cirrhosis of the liver, nephritis, and nephrosis. In all of these diseases there is a reduction in sodium excretion which promotes the retention of water.

• **Injury**—During the postoperative period adequate fluid is essential since large fluid losses may occur due to vomiting, hemorrhage, exudates, diuresis, or fever. Abnormal loss of water also occurs from burns.

When water losses are not replaced, dehydration occurs and persons suffer a series of changes which may be summarized as follows:
1. Sensation of thirst when water loss amounts to about 1% of body weight.
2. Thirst accompanied by vague discomfort and loss of appetite.
3. Tingling and numbness in arms and hands.
4. Increase in pulse rate, respiratory rate, and body temperature.
5. Weakness, spastic muscles, and mental confusion.
6. Increase in concentration of the blood (hemoconcentration), decreased blood volume, and difficult circulation.
7. Cracked skin and cessation of urine formation.
8. Death when dehydration weight loss becomes greater than 20% of the initial weight.

Water Sources. The water required to replace body losses is available from three sources: (1) drinking water and other beverages, (2) water contained in solid foods, and (3) metabolic water resulting from the breakdown (catabolism) of fats, carbohydrates, and proteins.

DRINKING WATER. Nearly three-fourths of the earth's surface is covered with water, but only about 3% of this is "fresh" water—fit drinking water. Drinking water comes from a variety of sources. In ancient times water supply stopped when it failed to rain and springs and streams dried up. Primitive man lived near springs, rivers, and lakes because he had only the crudest vessels for hauling and storing water. Later, man discovered ways of getting water by artificial means. With this discovery he no longer needed to live close to natural supplies. The first system of an artificial water supply was probably a well. Two famous wells of Biblical history are Jacob's well and Joseph's well. Then, imitating the rivers of nature, man caused water to flow through ditches, followed by the development of pipelines, dams, and reservoirs. Roman aqueducts still survive, proving the remarkable vastness of early man-made waterworks. Our drinking water today comes from underground wells and reservoirs. Some is transported through miles of pipelines in huge quantities to move water to places where the demand is greatest.

• **Pollution**—Water which is altered in composition or condition rendering it unsuitable for any or all of its functions is considered polluted. Therefore, despite the source of drinking water, the most important requisite is that it be free from disease-causing organisms and toxic chemicals which may arise from sewage, and from other liquid waste from domestic, industrial or agricultural use of water. In 75% of the world—Canada, United States, and much of Europe excluded—water sanitation is so poor that 10 million people die each year. Many diseases are waterborne, but cholera and typhoid are the classical examples. Industrialized nations face the problem of water pollution due to many new chemicals added to the environment. More than 1,700 compounds have been found in water. Some of these chemicals enter the water supply through industrial and agricultural practices; and they represent either a direct health hazard to man, or an indirect hazard by encouraging the rapid growth of undesirable microorganisms causing stagnation, bad odors, and discolored water. In the United States, water quality is monitored by the Environmental Protection Agency (EPA) and the Public Health Service. In the rivers and streams the EPA monitors (1) fecal coliform bacteria, an indication of sewage; (2) dissolved oxygen, an indicator of microorganism overgrowth; and (3) phosphorus, which encourages microorganism overgrowth. The Public Health Service checks public water supplies for contaminants.

Worldwide, there have been instances of water contaminated with arsenic, cadmium, copper, mercury, lead, and nitrates. The World Health Organization set the safe limits shown in Table W-3 on the water levels of these and other possible toxic substances.

(Also see MINERAL[S], section headed "Contamination of Drinking Water, Foods, or Air with Toxic Minerals"; NITRATES AND NITRITES; and POISONS.)

TABLE W-3
TENTATIVE LIMITS FOR TOXIC SUBSTANCES THAT MAY AFFECT HEALTH[1]

Substance	Upper Limit of Concentration
	(mg/liter)
Arsenic	.05
Cadmium	.01
Cyanide	.05
Lead	.10
Mercury	.001
Selenium	.01
Nitrates[2]	45.0
Polycyclic hydrocarbons[3]	.0002

[1]*Health Hazards of the Human Environment*, 1972, World Health Organization, p. 67, Table 4.
[2]The U.S. Public Health Service recommends 10 mg/liter.
[3]This includes benzopyrene, benzoperylene, fluoranthene, benzacephenanthrylene, benzofluoranthene, and indenopyrene.

• **Hard water**—Hard water contains the bicarbonate and sulfate salts, principally of calcium and magnesium. Water hardness due to calcium and magnesium bicarbonate is known as temporary or bicarbonate hardness since boiling the water results in the decomposition of the bicarbonates and the precipitation of calcium and magnesium carbonate. Boiling produces no change in a solution of sulfates; hence, the hardness caused by sulfates is known as permanent or noncarbonate hardness. Some hard waters contain enough calcium to contribute significantly to the body's requirement for calcium.

(Also see WATER HARDNESS.)

• **Soft water**—When hard water is subjected to a process—an ion exchange reaction—in which calcium and magnesium are replaced by sodium, it is said to be softened. Sodium sulfates and sodium carbonates are soluble and do not prevent the action of soap as do the calcium and magnesium salts which increase the quantity of soap for cleaning purposes. Some waters are naturally soft. Soft water has been associated with a higher mortality rate from cardiovascular diseases. However, the data is not sufficient to allow more than speculation. Water with a sodium content above 20 mg/liter may make a significant contribution to the daily sodium intake for persons on sodium restricted diets.

• **Demineralized or deionized water**—By passing water through two ion exchange resins, all mineral salts can be removed—both anions (negatively charged elements) and cations (positively charged elements). This is demineralized water. It is as pure as water can be. Frequently, demineralized water is utilized in scientific investigation to prevent the introduction of interfering substances during sensitive analyses of minute quantities.

• **Distilled water**—This type of water is produced by converting water to steam, and cooling the steam in a clean collecting system. Dissolved materials remain behind so distilled water contains only the substances taken up from the storage containers. This water may be sold as distilled water, or in some cases standard amounts of minerals are added back to the distilled water and it is sold commercially as bottled water for use in homes and offices.

• **Mineral water**—Waters from some natural springs possess a strong odor or taste. Over the years mystical powers have been attributed to mineral waters. Mineral waters contain small quantities of sodium chloride, sodium carbonate, sodium bicarbonate, salts of calcium and magnesium, and sometimes iron or hydrogen sulphide. Many of these waters are naturally aerated with carbon dioxide. Perrier, Contrexeville, Vichy, Apollinaris, and Evian waters are bottled on a large scale and sold worldwide.

• **Soda water**—Water which has been charged with carbon dioxide to make it bubble and fizz is called soda water.

• **Chlorinated water**—Chlorination of drinking water was one of the major health advances of this century. During the purification of water for public use, chlorine is initially added to water to kill bacteria and destroy objectionable organic matter. Later, in a final purification step, water is checked to make certain that there is a proper level of chlorine which will guard against contamination in the distribution system. The chlorine added at the beginning of the purification process may have been depleted during the processing, and more chlorine will be needed.

In emergencies, household bleach, which contains chlorine, can be used to purify water by adding 8 to 16 drops of bleach to 1 gal (2 to 4 drops/liter) of the water (8 drops per gallon to clear water and 16 drops per gallon to cloudy water), mixing and allowing to stand for 30 minutes. If after standing the water does not have the distinct smell or taste of chlorine, another dose of chlorine should be added, and the water allowed to stand for another 15 minutes after mixing. The taste or smell of chlorine in water is a sign of safety. Water purification tablets that release chlorine can be purchased at sporting goods stores and drugstores.

• **Fluoridated water**—Some communities practice the addition of trace amounts—0.5 to 1.0 ppm—of fluoride, usually as the sodium salt, to their drinking water. Many reports indicate that the fluoridation of water reduces dental caries. Some water sources are naturally fluoridated—some at such high levels as to cause fluorosis.

(Also see FLUORINE OR FLUORIDE.)

• **Sea water**—Water from the sea cannot be used for drinking. Sea water is much more concentrated than the body fluids, and the kidneys are unable to handle the excess sodium and chloride. Records of castaways during World War II show that drinking large amounts of sea water was usually fatal. Still, fresh water supplies are dependent upon the continuous solar distillation of the seas.

Aside from the ingestion of drinking water, numerous liquids which are 88 to 92% water contribute to our daily water needs; for example, coffee, tea, soft drinks, and alcoholic beverages. However, pure cool water satisfies the thirst sensation without contributing calories.

FOODS. Many solid foods contain a high water content, and contribute to meeting our water requirement. Even such "dry" foods as crackers, ready-to-eat cereals, and nuts provide some water, while some fruits and vegetables contain over 90% water. Table W-4 illustrates, over a wide range, the water content of foods.

TABLE W-4
WATER CONTENT OF FOODS[1]

Foods	Water
	(%)
Fruits and vegetables	70-95
Milk	87
Cooked cereals	80-88
Fish and shellfish................	60-86
Cheese, cottage	79
Meat and poultry	40-75
Eggs	74
Cooked beans	69
Cheese, Cheddar	39
Bread	36
Butter	16
Crackers	2-6
Nuts	2-5

[1]Approximate values from Food Composition Table F-36.

METABOLIC WATER.   Metabolic water is produced from the catabolism—breakdown—of nutrients. When 100 g of carbohydrates are oxidized, 60 g of water are produced. The oxidation of proteins yields 42 g of water for every 100 g of protein. Fats can be said to be "wetter than water." For every 100 g of fat that are oxidized, close to 110 g of water are produced. However, there are some losses of water in the oxidation of both proteins and fats. Water must be used to excrete nitrogen in the deamination process of protein—thus lowering the net availability of water. In fact, it requires more water to excrete nitrogen as urea than is formed in the deamination process. The oxidation of fats requires increased respiration. Water is lost from the lungs during this increased respiration, and the net yield of water produced from fat is less than that from the oxidation of carbohydrates.

On the average, 13 g of metabolic water are formed for every 100 Calories (kcal) of metabolizable energy in the typical human diet.

WATER SUPPLY AND USE.   The total quantity of fresh water on the earth exceeds all possible present and future needs. However, much of the fresh water is inaccessible, or unevenly distributed from place to place or season to season. Global reserves of fresh water add up to enough to fill the Mediterranean ten times over, but more than three-fourths of this water is bound up in glaciers and polar ice where it is beyond the reach of our current technology. Hence, the main sources of supply are the waters of the lakes, rivers and water vapor in the atmosphere—the water cycle shown in Fig. W-4. These sources make up less than 1% of the total fresh water. The ultimate source of all fresh water is, of course, the continuous distillation of the oceans by solar radiation.

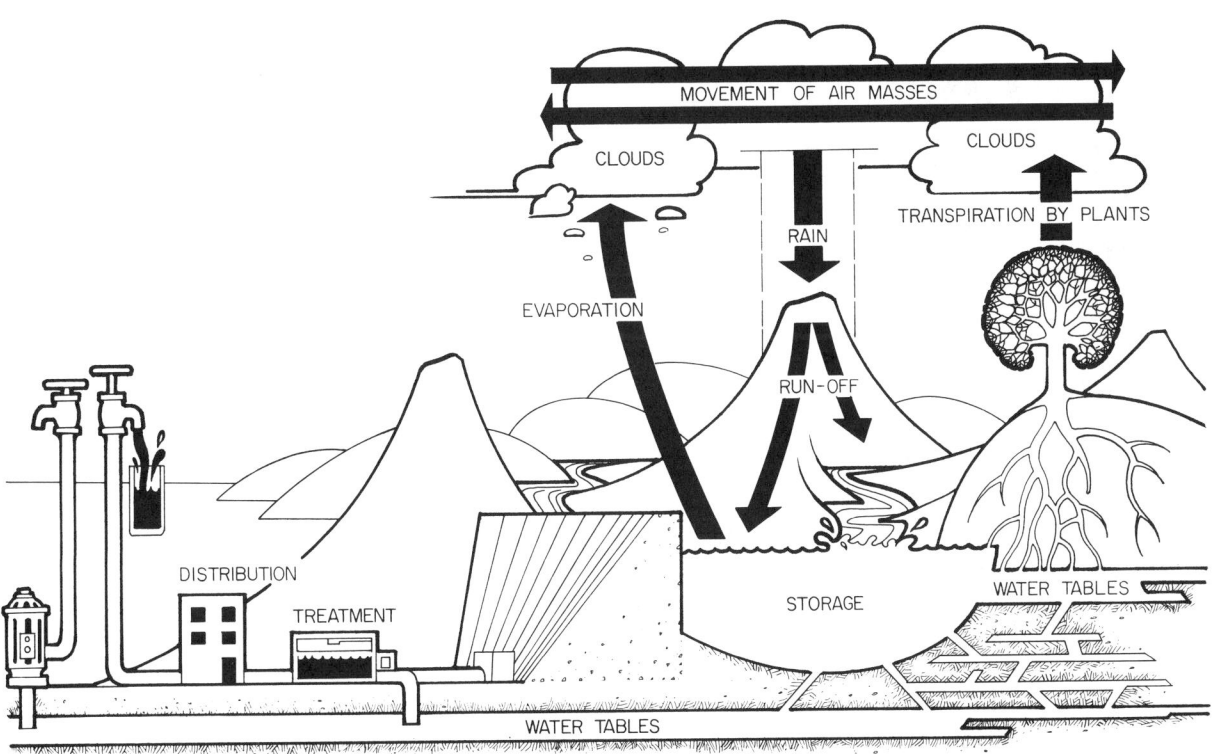

Fig. W-4.   Our dependence on the water cycle.

Personal use of water is a small part of civilization's use of water, even when considering our daily use of 24 gal (*91 liter*) for flushing the toilet; 32 gal (*121 liter*) for bathing, laundry and dishwashing; and 25 gal (*95 liter*) for swimming pools and watering the lawn. In the United States, domestic use of water amounts to about 10% of the total consumption.

In the United States, the use of water by industry and agriculture is about equally split. Both require 45% of the total water consumption. Of the industrial use, some two-thirds can be accounted for by the following industries: metal, chemical, petroleum refining, pulp and paper manufacturing, and food processing. Water in agriculture is used for the irrigation of crops, and for livestock, which, like humans, need drinking water. Traced back through their creation, two breakfast eggs require 240 gal (*910 liter*) of water, a dinner steak requires 3,500 gal (*13,265 liter*), and the family car requires 60,000 gal (*227,400 liter*) to manufacture.

Considering the staggering use of water, it would seem

we are running low, but not so. For the most part, ensuring an adequate supply of water lies in the proper management of water use by individuals, industries, and agriculture.

(Also see MINERAL[S]; THIRST; WATER AND ELECTROLYTES; and WATER BALANCE.)

WATER, AERATED

Municipal water works may aerate water by spraying into the air to remove disagreeable tastes and odors. Also, well water can be improved by aeration, particularly if it contains carbon dioxide, hydrogen sulfide or iron. The term aerated water is synonymous to mineral water in British usage. However, mineral water in Britian is water that has been aerated or charged with carbon dioxide—soda water or soft drink.

WATER AND ELECTROLYTES

Thoughts of constant, never ending motion are almost inseparable from thoughts of water—the water of the sea, of the rivers, and even household water. The water of our bodies is no different. It is constantly in motion—entering the body, leaving the body, and moving in and around the cells of the body. Life depends upon the movement of water and substances dissolved in the water which bathes the cells. Water is one of a few inorganic chemicals which exists as a liquid at the temperature of life processes. It is the chemical of life. Among the many important properties of water is its ability to act as a solvent for a variety of organic and inorganic chemicals. Of the inorganic chemicals, some of these—for example, acids, alkalis, and salts—will separate into ions when dissolved in water. Ions are atoms or molecules that carry an electrical charge—positive or negative. Such compounds which separate into positive and negative ions in solutions are called electrolytes. Those with a positive charge are cations, while those with a negative charge are anions.

Table W-5 lists ions which are found dissolved in the water of the body. Sodium, potassium, and chloride, are the primary electrolytes which are most often discussed due to their important relationships in body fluids.

TABLE W-5
IMPORTANT IONS OF THE BODY

Cations			Anions		
Name	Formula	Charge	Name	Formula	Charge
Sodium	Na^+	+1	Chloride	Cl^-	−1
Potassium	K^+	+1	Bicarbonate	HCO_3^-	−1
Calcium	Ca^{++}	+2	Phosphate	$HPO_4^=$	−2
Magnesium	Mg^{++}	+2	Sulfate	$SO_4^=$	−2

Hence, electrolytes become chemical compounds such as sodium chloride (table salt), potassium chloride, calcium phosphate, magnesium sulfate, sodium bicarbonate, and so on.

Electrolytes may be dissolved in water at different concentrations. This introduces another concept. Electrolytes are measured according to the total number of particles in solution, not their total weight. Thus, the unit of measure for electrolytes is milliequivalents, which is abbreviated as mEq. It refers to the number of ions—cations and anions—in solution in a given volume, generally one liter. Hence, milliequivalents are expressed as mEq/liter. The concentration of electrolytes in the compartments of the body determines the flow of water within the body.

BODY FLUID COMPARTMENTS. Fluids—water, electrolytes, and other dissolved substances—are contained in two major compartments within the body. In order to gain this concept of body compartments, all the cells of the body must be thought of as a whole. Then, all fluid outside of the cells is termed extracellular fluid, while all fluid within the cells is termed intracellular fluid. Fluids in each compartment differ in composition.

• **Extracellular fluid**—The extracellular fluid, the "internal sea" that bathes the cells, is further subdivided. The blood plasma which represents about 5%—about 3 qt (2.8 liter)—of the body weight is one division, and the fluid which is contained in the small spaces between all cells is the other division. This division is called the interstitial (between cells) fluid and it represents about 15% of the body weight or about 9.5 qt (9.0 liter).

Sodium (Na^+) is the main cation in the extracellular fluids—representing 90% of all ions. Hence, sodium concentration exerts a great controlling force in the body fluid balances. It is sodium which provides the force to maintain the extracellular water volume vital to the cells of the body. Other cations in the extracellular fluid include potassium (K^+), calcium (Ca^{++}), and magnesium (Mg^{++}). The amounts of these in the extracellular fluid are relatively small when compared to sodium, but still their presence is vital.

The main anion of the extracellular fluid is chlorine (Cl^-). As such, it provides most of the negative ions to balance the positive ions of sodium. Other anions of the extracellular fluid include bicarbonate (HCO_3^-), phosphate ($HPO_4^=$), sulfate ($SO_4^=$), and some protein and organic acids such as lactic and pyruvic acid.

It is the extracellular fluid that supplies cells with nutrients and other needed substances, and it removes the wastes generated by the cells.

(Also see SODIUM; and CHLORINE OR CHLORIDE.)

• **Intracellular fluid**—Inside each cell of the body, the main cation is potassium (K^+). Hence, it provides the force to maintain the water volume within the cells. Intracellular fluid represents about 40% of the body weight or about 25 qt (*23.7 liter*). Sodium (Na^+) is low within the cells. About one-third of the potassium inside a cell is bound to protein. This is an important concept when trying to understand some of the changes that occur when there is extensive tissue breakdown during illness or injury. The main anion of the intracellular fluid is phosphate ($HPO_4^=$). Besides providing negatiave charges, the phosphate ion is important in the energy-producing reactions of the cell. Energy-storing compounds are phosphate compounds such as adenosine triphosphate (ATP). There is also a high concentration of protein within the cell. These proteins contribute to the negative—anion—charges of the intracellular fluid.

It is the balance of the electrolytes—their concentration in terms of mEq/liter—in the water outside and inside cells that help to maintain the status quo of the body. This balance between electrolytes within each fluid compartment is called electrical neutrality. This neutrality must be maintained. Shifts or losses of electrolytes result in counteracting shifts which return electroneutrality. Fig. W-5 demonstrates the balance of cation and anion concentrations in terms of mEq/liter which exists inside and outside of cells.

(Also see POTASSIUM; and PHOSPHORUS.)

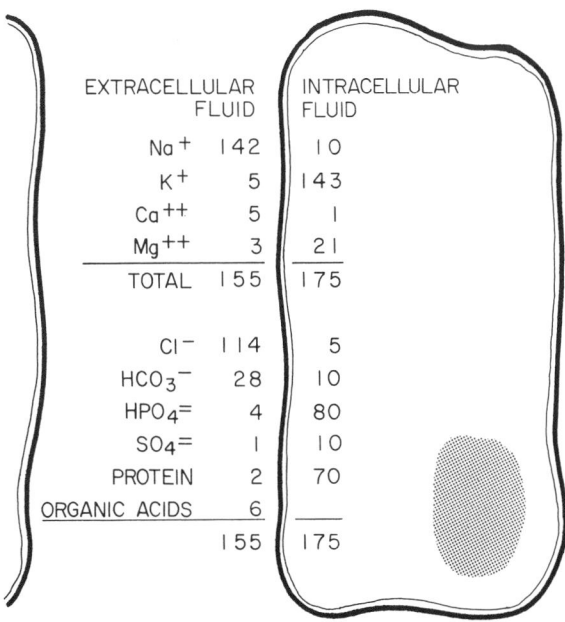

	EXTRACELLULAR FLUID	INTRACELLULAR FLUID
Na^+	142	10
K^+	5	143
Ca^{++}	5	1
Mg^{++}	3	21
TOTAL	155	175
Cl^-	114	5
HCO_3^-	28	10
$HPO_4^=$	4	80
$SO_4^=$	1	10
PROTEIN	2	70
ORGANIC ACIDS	6	
	155	175

Fig. W-5. The balance of electrolytes in the intracellular fluid and the extracellular fluid. Values are mEq/liter.

REGULATION OF WATER AND ELECTROLYTE BALANCE.

Basically, water (1) enters the body via the digestive tract as liquid or food, (2) moves into the blood and tissue, and (3) leaves via the kidneys, skin, lungs, or feces. Water entering and leaving the body is under rigid control, and under normal conditions water leaving the body equals the water entering the body—a condition of water balance. Moreover, the shifts of water between various body compartments and water balance are controlled by the concentration and distribution of the electrolytes.

Movement of Water and Electrolytes. In the body, water and electrolytes are moved across cell membranes by one or more of five processes: (1) osmosis, (2) diffusion, (3) active transport, (4) filtration, and (5) pinocytosis. Discussion of each of these follows:

1. **Osmosis.** Osmosis is the movement of water based upon a concentration difference. When two volumes of water containing different concentrations of dissolved substances are separated by a membrane which allows the passage of water, the water will move from the more dilute solution to the more dense solution. Sometimes this is also expressed as the movement of water from an area of high water concentration (dilute solution) to an area of lower water concentration (dense solution). Therefore, when two solutions of differing concentration are separated by a membrane permeable to water, this pulling or pushing force which moves the water is called the osmotic pressure. Osmolarity is the measure of osmotic pressure. The eventual outcome of the process of osmosis is the equalization of the concentration differences through a change in volume. Osmosis is an important process controlling the movement of water in the body. It is the osmotic pressure of sodium that maintains the extracellular water volume. The concept of osmosis is illustrated in Fig. W-6.

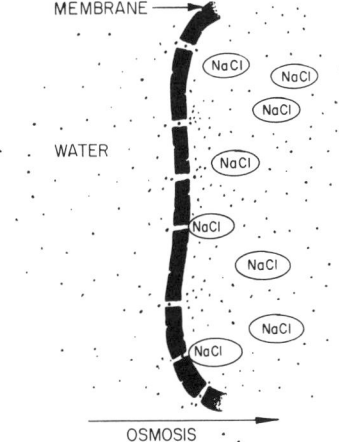

Fig. W-6. The process of osmosis. The left side of the membrane has a higher water concentration since it does not contain sodium chloride (NaCl). The right side of the membrane is a dense solution of NaCl but a lower concentration of water.

2. **Diffusion.** This process is the random movement of molecules. The particles move from the area of highest concentration to an area of lowest concentration until

concentration is uniform. Diffusion occurs because all molecules are constantly in motion and colliding into each other. It may or may not occur across a membrane. Diffusion is an important process for transporting substances in body fluids.

3. **Active transport.** Sometimes substances in the body must be moved from an area where the concentration is low to an area where it is high. Neither osmosis nor diffusion can accomplish this task since they follow a natural downhill tendency. Active transport is an uphill process. It requires energy. Depending upon the area of the body, sodium, potassium, calcium, iron, hydrogen, chloride, sugars, and amino acids may all be moved by active transport. The concept is much like an air compressor. Energy drives a piston which pulls air from an area of low concentration, and then forces the air into a container where the air is already more concentrated. Active transport maintains the low sodium ion (Na^+) and high potassium ion (K^+) level inside the cell which has already been discussed.

4. **Filtration.** When the pressure applied to a fluid is lower on one side of a membrane than on the other, fluid is forced through the membrane. This process may be visualized by imagining a strainer full of water. The weight of the water forces the water to flow through the holes of the strainer. Filtration is the process whereby fluids of the capillaries are delivered to the interstitial (between) cell spaces. Moreover, it is an important process in the kidneys.

5. **Pinocytosis.** This process moves substances into cells, but the substances do not pass through the membrane. Rather, they become attached to the outside of the cell membrane and then the membrane surrounds these substances forming a small capsule—so called pinocytic vesicle. This capsule breaks away from the cell membrane and moves deep into the cell where the capsule is dissolved and the substance within the capsule is released. Pinocytosis allows large molecules such as proteins, dissolved in water, to be transported into the cell.

Putting these five processes into perspective requires the realization that the body is a dynamic system. Adjustments are constantly taking place. Water and electrolyte balance is no different. Water enters the body as a liquid, and as a component of the food—including metabolic water derived from the breakdown of food. In the digestive tract water and the many substances dissolved in water—including electrolytes—are transported across the membrane lining the digestive tract into the blood. Then the blood plasma—a water solution—transports nutrients and other substances to the cells, and picks up the waste products from the cells. The kidneys act to regulate the composition of the body fluids by conserving some substances and excreting others into the urine. Furthermore, the kidneys regulate water loss from the body. Additional water is lost from the body by the skin, the lungs, and the feces. As water and the substances dissolved in it move through the body, some or all five of these processes—osmosis, diffusion, active transport, filtration, and pinocytosis—are at work maintaining balance within the body. In order to maintain the composition of the extracellular fluid and the intracellular fluid, the volume of water intake is very nearly equal to the volume of water lost. Whenever body fluids become too concentrated, water moves into this area and dilutes the body fluid. However, a number of factors act to regulate the movement of water.

(Also see DIGESTION AND ABSORPTION.)

BODY FLUID COMPARTMENTS

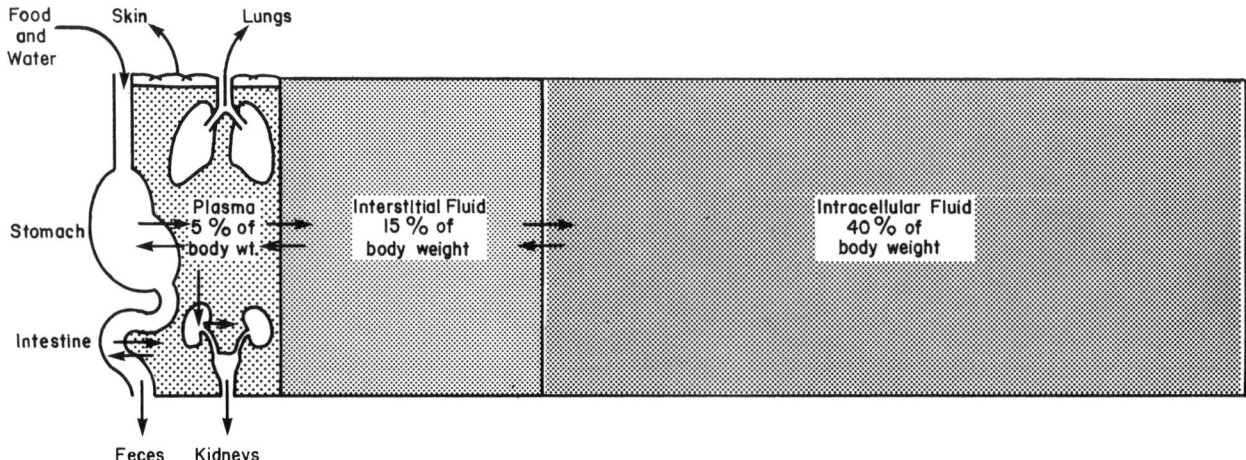

Fig. W-7.   The body fluid compartments, the routes of exchange—the digestive system, skin, lungs, and kidneys, and the constant movement between compartments as indicated by the arrows.

Factors Regulating Movement. The body requires water. To ensure that this requirement is fulfilled, the sensation of thirst creates a conscious desire for water. The sensation of thirst is caused by nerve centers in the hypothalamus of the brain which monitors the concentration primarily of sodium in the blood. When the sodium concentration, and hence the osmolarity of the blood, increases above the normal 310 to 340 mg/100 ml (*136 to 145 mEq/liter*), cells in the thirst center shrink. They shrink because the increased osmotic pressure of the blood pulls water out of their cytoplasm. This shrinking causes more nervous impulses to be generated in the thirst center, thus creating the sensation of thirst. Increased osmolarity of the blood is primarily associated with water loss from the extracellular fluid. As water is lost the sodium concentration of the remaining fluid increases. When water is drunk, it moves across the membrane lining the gut into the blood thereby decreasing the sodium concentration—osmolarity—of the blood. In turn, the cells of the hypothalamus take on water and return to their normal size. This time water moves back into these cells via osmosis in the opposite direction.

Increased osmolarity of the blood simultaneously stimulates other nerve centers in the hypothalamus causing the release of antidiuretic hormone (ADH) from the posterior pituitary. This hormone makes a portion of the kidney permeable to water. Thus, water originally destined to be urine moves, by osmosis, back into circulation. ADH release results in the formation of less urine by the kidneys; hence, conserving body water and helping dilute the body fluids and decrease the sodium ion concentration. Thus, drinking water and excreting water are controlled by centers in the brain which help maintain body water within appropriate ranges, and in turn control the extracellular sodium ion concentration. While many changes in the body fluids are compensated for by shifting water, electrolytes are also regulated to some degree.

Sodium and potassium, the major electrolytes of the extracellular and intracellular fluid, respectively, are controlled by the hormone aldosterone which comes from the cortex (outside layer) of the adrenal gland. Of prime importance is the regulation of the potassium ion in the extracellular fluid since both nerve and muscle function are dependent on its close regulation. Aldosterone also acts to conserve sodium. Secretion of the hormone aldosterone is controlled by a chain of events called the renin-angiotensin system. Briefly, renin is released from the kidney in response to (1) changes in blood pressure, (2) blood levels of potassium, or (3) nervous stimulation. It then converts angiotensinogen, a protein in the blood, to angiotensin which stimulates the secretion of aldosterone. Aldosterone causes the reabsorption of sodium from the urine and the loss of potassium in the urine. Potassium is exchanged for sodium. This conservation also causes water to be reabsorbed via osmosis. Under some stressful situations such as surgery, the release of adrenocorticotropin hormone (ACTH) from the anterior pituitary may cause the secretion of aldosterone.

It is evident that a marvelous organ, the kidney, is largely responsible for regulating the water and electrolyte balance of the body. Each kidney contains about one million minute functional units called nephrons. As the blood passes through, these nephrons, they select, re-ject, conserve, and eliminate water, electrolytes and other substances in order to maintain the volume and the composition of the extracellular fluid. Each day they rejuvenate about 50 gal (*190 liter*) of blood. Moreover, they function to regulate red blood cell production, aldosterone secretion, blood pressure, and calcium metabolism. So important is their function that without it death results in 8 to 14 days.

IMBALANCES OF WATER AND ELECTROLYTES. When the day-to-day and individual-to-individual variations in water and electrolyte intake are considered, maintaining the consistent water and electrolyte levels of the body is truly an amazing feat. However, there are times when the controlling mechanisms are disrupted and excesses or deficiencies result. Of prime concern are water and the major electrolytes, sodium, potassium, and chlorine. So intimate are the relationships between water and the major electrolytes that separation is often difficult.

Water Depletion. Life without water is short. When water is unavailable, or when water is lost faster than it can be replaced, events occur in the following order:

1. Sensation of thirst, when water loss amounts to about 1% of body weight.

2. Thirst accompanied by vague discomfort and loss of appetite.

3. Tingling and numbness in arms and hands.

4. Increase in pulse rate, respiratory rate, and body temperature.

5. Weakness, spastic muscles, and mental confusion.

6. Increase in concentration of the blood (hemoconcentration), decreased blood volume, and difficult circulation.

7. Cracked skin and cessation of urine formation.

8. Death when dehydration weight loss becomes greater than 20% of the initial weight.

Various stages of the above may occur when losses of water are incurred by (1) evaporation, (2) vomiting and diarrhea, (3) hemorrhage, or (4) burns.

1. **Evaporation.** Increased physical activity and/or a hot environment can dramatically increase the loss of water occuring through the skin as perspiration. Moreover, a hot and/or dry environment also increases the water vapor lost in expired air. Losses from the lungs are exaggerated by physical activity. Failure to replace these water losses leads to decreased physical performance or heat exhaustion. Fever during an illness also increases water loss due to evaporation. (Also see HEAT EXHAUSTION.)

2. **Vomiting and diarrhea.** Daily secretions into the digestive tract amount to 8,000 to 10,000 ml per day. (The total blood volume is only about 5,000 to 6,000 ml.) These secretions include saliva, stomach juices, bile, and pancreatic and intestinal juices. Fortunately, under normal circumstances, most of this large volume is reabsorbed in the digestive tract and only 100 to 200 ml of water are lost in the feces. However, vomiting and/or diarrhea allow large water losses to occur, and can result in rapid and dangerous losses of water, especially in infants or elderly individuals.

3. **Hemorrhage**. This represents a rather obvious loss of fluid from the body. In order to restore the blood volume several important water and electrolyte related adjustments take place. Fluid moves from the interstitial space which eventually becomes dehydrated. Then fluid moves out of the cells. Aldosterone secretion is stimulated via the renin-angiotensin system and the secretion of ACTH. The secretion of ADH is stimulated, as is the sensation of thirst.

4. **Burns**. The skin protects the body from drying out. However, following a serious burn, there is a loss of water and electrolytes, mainly sodium, at the burn site. At first the water lost is from the extracellular spaces, but eventually water is drawn from the intracellular compartment, which also brings potassium out of the cell causing blood levels of potassium to rise. Immediate intravenous fluid therapy seeks to replace electrolytes and water. The amounts given depend upon the extent of the burns. Three to five days after the burn, electrolyte and water balance should be reestablished.

Water Excess. Sometimes excessive water accumulates in the tissues, specifically the interstitial compartment. Outwardly, this condition is noted as swelling and it may occur in any area of the body. It is called *edema*, though some may still call it *dropsy*. In general, there are four causes of edema: (1) elevated fluid pressure in the capillaries as in heart failure; (2) low osmotic pressure in the blood due to decreased blood protein in such conditions as liver cirrhosis, kidney disease, severe burns, and starvation; (3) blockage of the lymph vessels as caused by the parasitic worm, filariae, in the disease elephantiasis; or (4) increased capillary permeability due to the release of histamine in allergic reactions. Edema may require the restriction of dietary sodium and/or diuretics.

• **Diuretics**—These are drugs which act to increase the output of sodium and water in the urine, and are often used to treat disorders of the heart, kidneys, or liver which cause edema. A majority of the diuretics act upon the kidneys by depressing the sodium reabsorbed. Thus, sodium remaining in the urine carries more water out of the body with it. Diuretics include thiazides, furosemide, and ethacrynic acid. Xanthine diuretics are mild diuretics but they are used by many people—perhaps unknowingly—since they are the caffeine, theophylline and theobromine present in tea, coffee, cola and other soft drinks, cocoa, and many over-the-counter pain relievers. Moreover, water and ethyl alcohol (alcoholic beverages) can act as diuretics by inhibiting the release of ADH.

• **Water intoxication**—When water intake is more rapid than urine formation, the extracellular compartment fluid is diluted and water moves into the cells—cellular edema. Swelling of the cells of the brain causes drowsiness and weakness, convulsions, and coma. Water intoxication may be observed in (1) patients given excessive amounts of intravenous glucose and water, (2) individuals who absorb water from the colon during enemas or colon irrigations, (3) individuals who absorb water from wounds or burns treated with wet dressings, or (4) individuals who have impaired antidiuretic hormone.

Sodium Depletion. Sodium is the major positively charged ion—cation—in the extracellular fluid. Depletion is rare. Urinary output reflects the dietary intake. However, strict vegetarian diets without salt, heavy prolonged sweating, diarrhea, and vomiting or adrenal cortical insufficiency—lack of aldosterone—may result in sodium depletion. Continued depletion results in loss of appetite, muscle cramps, mental apathy, loss of body water, headache, and reduced milk production in lactating mothers. Sodium depletion heat exhaustion occurs most frequently in persons unacclimatized to working in a hot environment who replace water losses but fail to replace electrolyte losses. It is characterized by fatigue, nausea, giddiness, vomiting, and exhaustion. The blood volume decreases, kidney blood flow is impaired, and cellular edema occurs. The chain of events is illustrated in Fig. W-8.

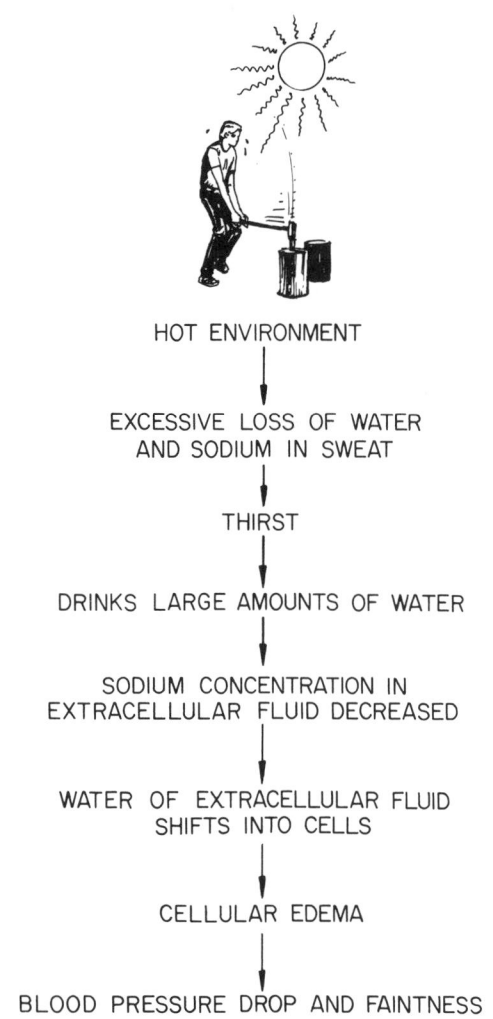

HOT ENVIRONMENT

↓

EXCESSIVE LOSS OF WATER
AND SODIUM IN SWEAT

↓

THIRST

↓

DRINKS LARGE AMOUNTS OF WATER

↓

SODIUM CONCENTRATION IN
EXTRACELLULAR FLUID DECREASED

↓

WATER OF EXTRACELLULAR FLUID
SHIFTS INTO CELLS

↓

CELLULAR EDEMA

↓

BLOOD PRESSURE DROP AND FAINTNESS

Fig. W-8.   Development of cellular edema.

Sodium Excess. Most of the sodium ingested is excessive, and for the most part it is excreted by the kidneys in combination with bicarbonate or phosphate.

However, under some circumstances sodium accumulates in the extracellular fluid and causes edema since the retention of sodium is accompanied by water retention. Such conditions include (1) cardiac or renal failure, (2) adrenal tumors which secrete excessive cortical hormones, and (3) adrenocorticotropic hormone (ACTH) or steroid hormone therapy. In these conditions, individuals benefit from sodium restricted diets.

Excessive sodium may be harmful (1) when ingested in large quantities, especially with a low water intake; (2) when the body has been depleted by a salt-free vegetarian diet or excess sweating, followed by gorging on salt; (3) when large amounts are fed to infants or individuals afflicted with kidney diseases, whose kidneys cannot excrete the excess in the urine; or (4) when the body is adapted to a chronic low-salt diet, followed by ingesting large amounts of salt. A dramatic example of excessive sodium (salt) is provided by imagining a sailor lost at sea who decides to drink sea water. The sea water is a much more concentrated salt solution than the extracellular fluids. Drinking sea water would only worsen a stranded sailor's condition as shown in Fig. W-9.

(Also see SALT; and SODIUM.)

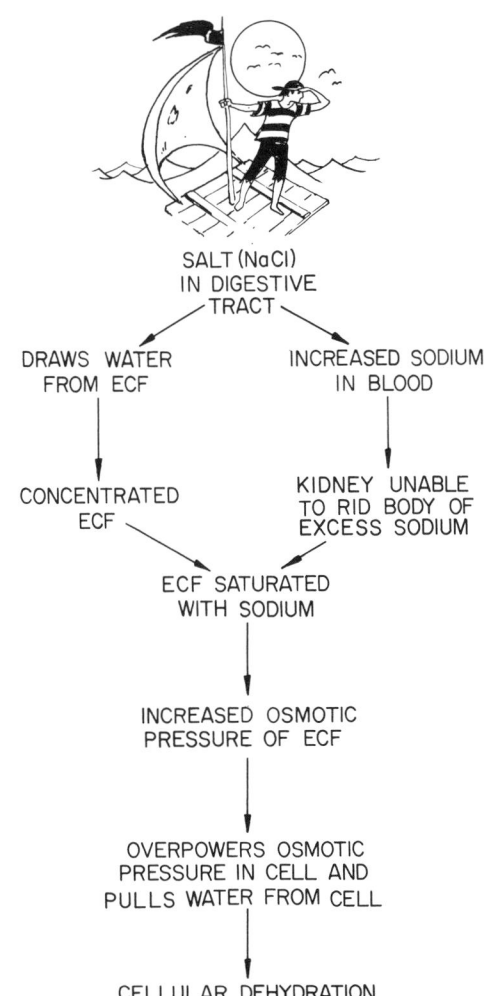

SALT (NaCl)
IN DIGESTIVE
TRACT

DRAWS WATER
FROM ECF

INCREASED SODIUM
IN BLOOD

CONCENTRATED
ECF

KIDNEY UNABLE
TO RID BODY OF
EXCESS SODIUM

ECF SATURATED
WITH SODIUM

INCREASED OSMOTIC
PRESSURE OF ECF

OVERPOWERS OSMOTIC
PRESSURE IN CELL AND
PULLS WATER FROM CELL

CELLULAR DEHYDRATION

Fig. W-9. Cellular dehydration from drinking sea water. ECF stands for extracellular fluid.

Potassium Depletion. Deficiencies of potassium rarely result from dietary lack of the mineral. Potassium is lost whenever muscle is broken down owing to starvation, malnutrition, or injury since it is tied to protein inside cells. Crash diets, diarrhea, vomiting, gastric suction, diabetic acidosis, and burns also induce potassium loss from the body. Also lean tissue growth increases the need for potassium. A potassium-depleted individual may display irregular heart function, muscle weakness, irritability, paralysis, nausea, vomiting, diarrhea, and swollen abdomen.

(Also see MALNUTRITION, PROTEIN-ENERGY; and STARVATION.)

Potassium Excess. The kidneys provide the major regulatory mechanism for maintaining potassium balance. Hence, a potassium buildup in the blood—hyperkalemia—is the frequent complication of kidney failure. Other causes of potassium excess include adrenal insufficiency, severe dehydration, or shock after injury wherein the potassium in the cells leaks into the blood. Symptoms of an excess are muscular weakness, mental apathy, and irregular heart action. Both an excess and depletion of potassium affect the heart muscle. Indeed, if either becomes severe enough the heart will stop. Although, it would be nearly impossible to ingest enough potassium-containing foods to create an excess, ill advised individuals who take a supplemental source such as potassium chloride run the risk of increasing potassium to dangerous levels.

(Also see POTASSIUM.)

Chloride. Excess chlorine in the diet is excreted via the urine accompanied by excess sodium or potassium and sometimes ammonia. Loss of chloride generally parallels that of sodium. However, deficiencies of chloride may develop from vomiting, diarrhea, stomach pumping, injudicious use of diuretic drugs, or strict vegetarian diets used without salt. A deficiency of chloride causes an increase in the pH of the body. This condition is called alkalosis and it is characterized by slow and shallow breathing, listlessness, muscle cramps, lack of appetite, and sometimes convulsions.

(Also see CHLORINE OR CHLORIDE.)

ACID-BASE BALANCE. Aside from their involvement in body fluid distribution, water and electrolytes are involved in the acid-base balance of the body. This is important since the body tolerates only very minor shifts in this balance which refers to the hydrogen ion concentration of the body fluids. An acid is a chemical that can release hydrogen ions, whereas a base, or alkali, is a chemical that can accept hydrogen ions. The degree of acidity is expressed in terms of pH. A pH of 7 is the neutral point between an acid and alkaline (base). Substances with a lower pH than 7 are acid, while substances with a pH above 7 are alkaline. The normal pH of the extracellular fluids of the body is 7.4, with a range of 7.35 to 7.45. Maintenance of the pH within this narrow range is necessary to sustain the life of cells. The extremes between which life is possible are 7.0 to 7.8. To help maintain this narrow range the body has other chemicals called buffers. A buffer protects the acid-base balance of a solution by rapidly offsetting changes in its ionized hydrogen concentration—a chemical sponge. It protects against added acid or base. The three most important chemical buffers are the bicarbonate buffer, phosphate buffers, and hemoglobin and protein buffers.

1. **Bicarbonate buffer.** This buffer, which is present in all body fluids, is a mixture of carbonic acid (H_2CO_3) and sodium bicarbonate ($NaHCO_3$). When a strong acid is added to this mixture, it combines immediately with the bicarbonate ion to form carbonic acid—an extremely weak acid. Thus, this buffer system changes a strong acid to a weak acid and keeps the fluids from becoming strongly acid. However, when a strong base is added to this mixture, the base immediately combines with the carbonic acid to form water and a neutral bicarbonate salt. These reactions are shown in Fig. W-10. The lungs and kidneys can easily adjust ratios of carbonic acid and sodium bicarbonate.

HCl	+	NaHCO₃	→	H₂CO₃	+	NaCl
HYDROCHLORIC ACID		SODIUM BICARBONATE		CARBONIC ACID		SODIUM CHLORIDE
(STRONG ACID)		(BASE-BUFFER)		(WEAKER ACID)		(SALT)

NaOH	+	H₂CO₃	→	NaHCO₃	+	H₂O
SODIUM HYDROXIDE		CARBONIC ACID		SODIUM BICARBONATE		WATER
(STRONG BASE)		(ACID-BUFFER)		(WEAKER BASE)	

Fig. W-10.   Buffering action of the carbonic acid-sodium bicarbonate system.

2. **Phosphate buffers.** These chemical buffers are especially important for maintaining normal hydrogen ion concentration in the intracellular fluids, because their concentration inside the cells is many times greater than the concentration of the bicarbonate buffer.

3. **Hemoglobin and protein buffers.** Hemoglobin and plasma proteins act as buffers. Proteins are also important buffers within the cells.

The lungs and kidneys also have an important role in maintaining the acid-base balance. The extent to which they are involved depends upon the amount of adjustment necessary.

• **Lungs**—Carbon dioxide combines with water and electrolytes in the extracellular fluid to form carbonic acid in accordance with the following reaction:

$$CO_2 + H_2O \rightarrow H_2CO_3$$

Ultimately, the lungs control the body's supply of carbonic acid. This is so because, normally, respiration removes carbon dioxide at the same rate that it is formed by all cells of the body as one of the end products of metabolism. However, if respiration decreases below normal, carbon dioxide will not be excreted normally; instead, it will accumulate in the body fluids, causing an increase in the concentration of carbonic acid. As a result, the hydrogen ion concentration rises. On the other hand, if the respiration rate rises above normal, the opposite effect occurs; carbon dioxide is blown off at a more rapid rate than it is formed, thereby decreasing the carbon dioxide and carbonic acid concentrations. Complete lack of breathing for a minute will reduce the pH of the extracellular fluid from the normal of 7.4 down to about 7.1, while over-breathing can increase it to about 7.7 in a minute. Thus, the acid-base balance of the body

can be changed greatly by under- or over-ventilation of the lungs. Conversely, the level of hydrogen ion in the blood controls respiration, when for some reason the pH of the extracellular fluid rises—hydrogen ion decreases—the breathing rate is depressed. Furthermore, the system works in the other direction. When the pH drops—hydrogen ion concentration increases—the breathing rate speeds up. Thus, acidosis greatly increases both the depth and rate of respiration, while alkalosis lessens the depth and rate of respiration. This respiratory mechanism is so effective in regulating the acid-base balance that it usually returns the pH of the body fluids to normal within a few minutes after an acid or alkali has been administered.

• **Kidneys (renal)**—In addition to carbonic acid, a number of other acids are continually being formed by the metabolic process of the cells, including phosphoric, sulfuric, uric, and keto acids. On entering the extracellular fluids, all of these can cause acidosis. Normally, the kidneys rid the body of these excess acids as rapidly as they are formed, preventing an excessive build up of hydrogen ions.

Occasionally, too many basic compounds enter the body fluids, rather than too many acidic compounds. This may occur when basic compounds are injected intravenously or when large quantities of alkaline food or drugs are consumed.

The kidneys regulate acid-base balance by (1) excreting hydrogen ions into the urine when the extracellular fluids are too acidic, and (2) excreting basic substances, particularly sodium bicarbonate ($NaHCO_3$), into the urine when the extracellular fluids become too alkaline.

The kidneys also conserve base by eliminating extra hydrogen ions (H^+) through the production and excretion of ammonia (NH_4):

$$NH_3 \text{ (from deamination of amino acids)} + H^+ \rightarrow NH_4$$

If the normal amounts of buffers are present in the blood, and if the lungs and kidneys are normal, one can recover promptly from the effects of severe muscular exercise, intake of acid or base, unbalanced diets (so far as acids and bases are concerned), short periods of starvation, short bouts of vomiting, and other adverse conditions. Disorders of the kidney and respiratory system also lead to a serious derangement of the acid-base balance. When the failure is due to the lungs it is called respiratory acidosis or respiratory alkalosis. If the failure is mainly related to the accumulation of the products of metabolism or excessive loss of acid or base from the body, it is called metabolic acidosis or metabolic alkalosis. Since metabolic acidosis or alkalosis relates more directly to water and electrolytes, some examples follow:

• **Metabolic acidosis**—Conditions which may result in metabolic acidosis include: (1) uncontrolled diabetes mellitus wherein there is production of keto acids; (2) prolonged vomiting which causes the loss of alkali from the intestine; (3) severe diarrhea causing large amounts of sodium bicarbonate ($NaHCO_3$) to be lost; (4) kidney diseases preventing the kidneys from excreting even normal amounts of acids formed by the metabolic processes; and (5) other conditions such as starvation and thyrotoxicosis which cause the production of keto acids.

• **Metabolic alkalosis**—included are (1) initial vomiting (stomach contents only), resulting in loss of ionized hydrogen and chlorine; (2) potassium depletion caused by insufficient potassium intake, gastrointestinal loss of potassium, or ACTH therapy, inducing alkalosis as ionized hydrogen and sodium move into the cells to replace the lost potassium; and (3) excess intake of alkali powders of sodium bicarbonate, as in long-term ulcer therapy.

Food plays a role—though not as important as those above—in the acid-base balance of the body. For years it was known that the rabbit's urine is normally alkaline while the dog's urine is acid. In general, the urine of vegetarians is neutral, that of omnivorous animals is slightly acid, and that of carnivors is strongly acid.

Certain foods, depending upon their electroyte composition, form acids or bases in the body. Testing a solution of the mineral residue of a food—the ash—will give an acid, alkaline (basic), or neutral reaction, depending upon the relative proportions of acid-forming elements— chlorine, phosphorus, and sulfur, and of alkali-forming elements—potassium, sodium, calcium, and magnesium. The type of reaction of the food ash in water is important because it gives an indication of the contribution of the food to the acidity, alkalinity, or neutrality of the body fluids, and, ultimately, to the urine. Only highly refined foods—fats, sugars, and starches—do not yield an ash.

• **Acid foods**—The acid-forming elements predominate over the alkaline-forming mineral elements in foods containing moderate to large amounts of protein with the exception of milk and some of the other dairy products which contain sufficient calcium to give an alkaline reaction. Whole grains give an acid reaction disproportionate to their protein content due to the extra phosphorus present in the form of phytates. Although most fruits have an alkaline ash, others like prunes, plums, and cranberries make a net contribution of acid to the body since they contain organic acids that are not metabolized by the body, but which pass unchanged into the urine.

• **Alkaline foods**—Fruits and vegetables generally contain higher proportions of alkali-forming mineral elements than the acid-forming elements since their protein content is usually low. Corn and lentils, however, are acid forming. Surprising as it may seem, because of their pronounced acid taste, an alkaline residue is formed from tomatoes, citrus fruit, and rhubarb, due to their organic acids (citric, ascorbic, oxalic, and others) being completely metabolized in the body to carbon dioxide, water, and energy. Coconuts, almonds, and chestnuts yield an alkaline ash, while peanuts and walnuts yield an acid.

Water and electrolytes are maintained in an equilibrium in the body. The primary electrolytes are sodium, potassium, and chlorine. Besides controlling extracellular and intracellular water volume, these electrolytes are also involved in electrical neutrality of body fluids and the acid-base balance of the body. Minor electrolytes such as calcium, magnesium, phosphate, and sulfate are vital to survival. However, their functions are more thoroughly discussed under the appropriate sections of this book.

(Also see ACID-BASE BALANCE; and ACID FOODS AND ALKALINE FOODS.)

WATER BALANCE

Water is the major constituent of the body; it accounts for 50 to 75% of the body weight. Next to oxygen, it is the most important constituent for life itself. A person can live for several weeks without food but for only a few days without water. Dehydration (water loss) will kill far quicker than starvation.

Large deficits or excesses in the body water are reason for concern. In healthy individuals, the total amount of body water remains reasonably constant. Therefore, an increase or decrease in water intake brings about an appropriate increase or decrease in water output to maintain the balance. Fig. W-11 illustrates the intake of water, the routes of water output, and the movement of fluid between the compartments of the body. Water enters the

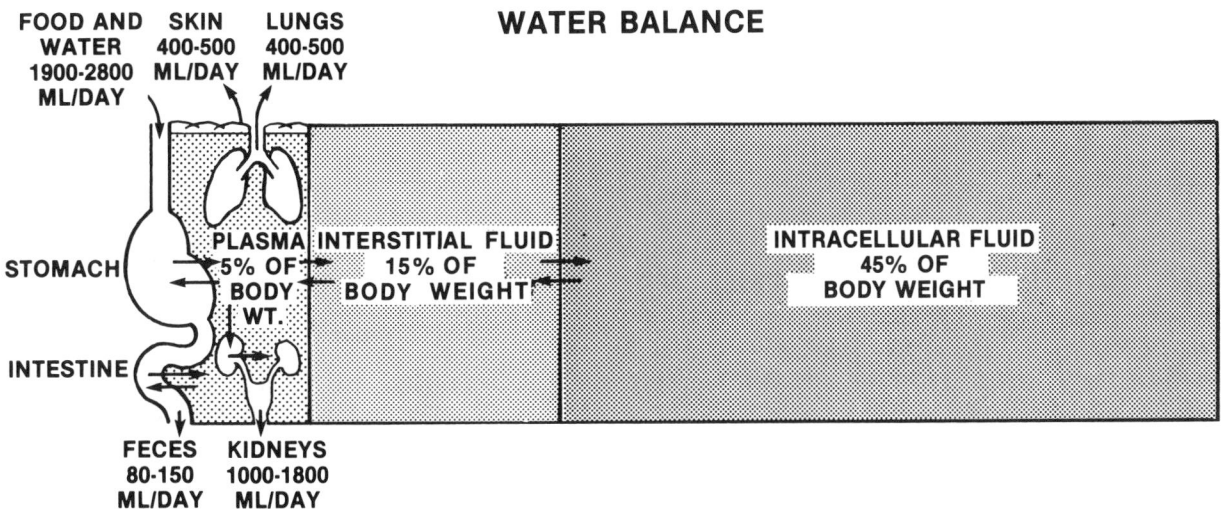

Fig. W-11. Water balance in humans, showing the daily amount of water input and output by the various routes, and the compartments of the body which contain water. Arrows represent fluid movement.

body as a liquid, and as a component of the food—including metabolic water derived from the breakdown of food. Water is lost from the body by (1) the skin as perspiration, (2) the lungs as water vapor in expired air, (3) the kidneys as urine, and (4) the intestines in the feces. As Fig. W-11 shows, under normal conditions total water intake is approximately equal to total water output by the various routes.

The body is equipped with a number of mechanisms for regulating body water within narrow limits. Important among these mechanisms are nerve centers in the hypothalamus which control the sensation of thirst and water output by the kidneys. Stimulation of the thirst center in the hypothalamus creates the desire for water, while stimulation of other nerve centers in the hypothalamus causes the release of antidiuretic hormone (ADH) from the posterior pituitary. Release of ADH results in the formation of less urine; hence, conserving the body water. Water needs of the body are disrupted by fever, high protein diets, dry hot climates, high altitudes, vomiting, diarrhea, and injury.

(Also see BODY FLUIDS; ENDOCRINE GLANDS; METABOLISM; METABOLIC WATER; and WATER AND ELECTROLYTES.)

WATERBORNE DISEASES

Many of the same diseases that are transmitted by contaminated food may also be transmitted by contaminated water. Important among these diseases are amebic dysentery, bacillary dysentery, cholera, intestinal flu, infectious hepatitis, poliomyelitis, salmonellosis, and typhoid fever. In addition, certain parasitic diseases, including beef tapeworms, fish tapeworms, liver flukes, and round worms, may be spread to man, either directly or indirectly, through contaminated water.

Because of the importance of water to the normal function of the body, it is imperative that our water supplies be safeguarded. Large cities sterilize water by the addition of chlorine, while questionable water in the home may be boiled vigorously for 1 to 3 minutes. However, chlorine or boiling does not eliminate toxic levels of industrial chemicals or metals that find their way into water supplies.

(Also see DISEASES, Table D-13 Infectious and Parasitic Diseases Which May Be Transmitted By Contaminated Foods and Water; and WATER.)

WATERCHESTNUT CHINESE (MA-TAI; KUROKUWAI) *Elocharis tuberosa, E. dulcis*

This aquatic plant, which has edible tubers, is a member of the Sedge family (*Cyperaceae*). The Chinese call it *ma-tai*, and the Japanese call it *kurokuwai*. The Chinese waterchestnut is not related to the waterchesnut (*Tropa natans*) which is grown in certain parts of Asis and Europe. Fig. W-12 shows a typical Chinese waterchestnut.

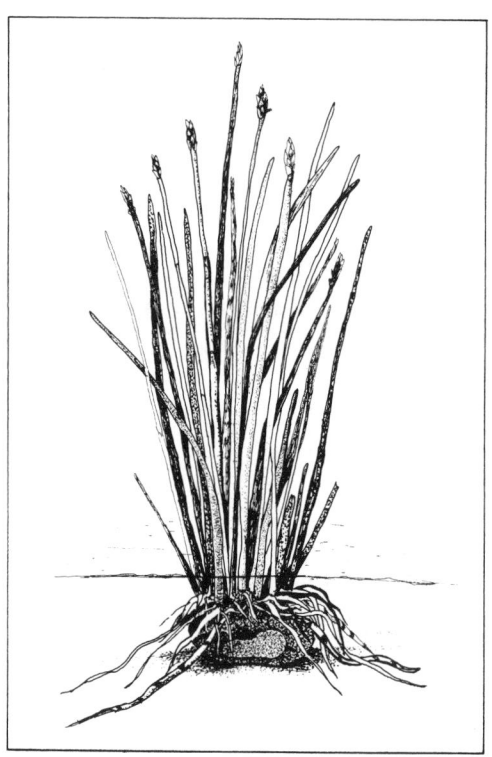

Fig. W-12. The Chinese waterchestnut, an appetizing ingredient of certain Oriental dishes.

ORIGIN AND HISTORY. The Chinese waterchestnut is believed to be native to southern China, where it has long been cultivated. However, it spread extensively throughout the Old World tropics so that it now grows wild in a large area extending southward to the East Indies and the other islands of the southwestern Pacific, and westward to Madagascar. It is also cultivated in many of these places.

PRODUCTION. China is the leading producer and exporter of this vegetable, but small amounts are grown elsewhere in the Old World. Recently, the growing market for the crop led to its cultivation in Florida. Production statistics are not available.

The plant is propagated by planting tubers near the surface of soil that is submerged under an inch or so of water. In China, sprouted tubers are planted in rice paddies in the spring, and the mature tubers are harvested manually after the paddies are drained in the fall. Yields of up to 30,000 lb per acre (*33,600 kg/ha*) are obtained under optimal conditions.

PROCESSING. Much of the Chinese crop is canned for export. Sometimes, starch is extracted by washing grated raw tubers on a fine screen.

PREPARATION. Although most Americans use canned Chinese water chestnuts, a few people may grow their own. In the latter case, the tubers should be peeled before using them. Usually, the vegetable is diced or sliced, then boiled briefly. The cooked pieces retain their crispness and are good in salads, soups, and stir-fried mixed dishes.

NUTRITIONAL VALUE. The nutrient compositions of various forms of Chinese waterchestnuts are given in Food Composition Table F-36.

Some noteworthy observations regarding the nutrient composition of Chinese waterchestnuts follow:

1. Compared to Irish potatoes, Chinese waterchestnuts contain about the same amount of calories, but only 2/3 the protein, and only 1/5 the vitamin C.

2. Chinese waterchestnuts are deficient in minerals and vitamins. Hence, they should be consumed with foods rich in these nutrients. Chinese mixed dishes are usually nutritious combinations of a variety of complementary foods.

(Also see VEGETABLE[S], Table V-6 Vegetables of the World.)

WATERCRESS *Nasturtium officinale*

This green leafy vegetable, which is a member of the mustard family (*Cruciferae*), has long been considered to have exceptional medicinal and nutritional values. As indicated by its name, watercress, which is the best known of the three cress plants (the other two are: garden cress and Swedish cress), grows in water. Fig. W-13 shows watercress leaves and stems.

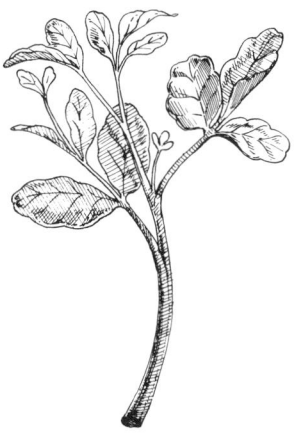

Fig. W-13. Watercress, a nutritious vegetable used mainly in salads and sandwiches.

ORIGIN AND HISTORY. Watercress is known to have been used as a medicinal plant as early as the 1st century A.D. because it is described in the writings of the Greek naturalist and physician Dioscorides, who lived at that time. However, it was not cultivated for many centuries because an abundant supply could not be found growing wild in many of the shallow streams throughout Europe and western Asia. Furthermore, con-

siderable experimentation was required to determine its special requirements for growth.

The first large scale cultivation of watercress is believed to have been carried out in Germany during the latter half of the 18th century. Shortly thereafter, farms for its production were established in the vicinities of London and Paris.

Watercress was brought to various parts of the world by European immigrants. As a result, the plant has escaped from cultivation in areas such as New Zealand, where it is a weed in many of the streams.

PRODUCTION. The considerable amount of labor and the special conditions that are required for the production of watercress has limited its commercial production to areas where it is profitable, although it is grown elsewhere on a small scale. Hence, no statistics on its production are available.

Usually, watercress is grown in shallow running spring water that is slightly alkaline and which contains sufficient nitrates to ensure the growth of the plant. Also, the water must be cool and uncontaminated. The tops of the plants are cut when they are only a few inches tall. Properly maintained beds may yield up to ten cuttings per year, and as much as 24,000 lb per acre (*26,880 kg/ha*).

Freshly harvested watercress must be kept under refrigeration if it is to be shipped a considerable distance.

PROCESSING. None of the crop is processed; all of it is sold fresh.

SELECTION AND PREPARATION. High-quality watercress is fresh, young, crisp, tender, rich medium-green in color, and free from dirt or yellowed leaves. Wilting, yellowing, or other discoloration of leaves indicates overage, lack of desirable freshness, or other damage.

This vegetable is most commonly served raw in salads and sandwiches, and as a garnish for cooked meats. However, it may be tossed briefly in hot butter or boiling cream.

CAUTION: Watercress and other vegetables of the mustard family (*Cruciferae*) contain small amounts of goiter-causing (goitrogenic) substances that interfere with the utilization of the essential mineral iodine by the thyroid gland. Hence, people who eat very large amounts of these vegetables while on an iodine-deficient diet may develop an enlargement of the thyroid, commonly called a goiter. The best insurance against this potentially harmful effect is the consumption of ample amounts of dietary iodine. This element is abundantly present in iodized salt, ocean fish, seafood, and edible seaweeds.

NUTRITIONAL VALUE. The nutrient composition of watercress is given in Food Composition Table F-36.

Some noteworthy observations regarding the nutrient composition of watercress follow:

1. Watercress has a high water content (93%) and a very low calorie content (24 kcal per cup).

2. A 1-cup (*240 ml*) serving of watercress supplies about 2/3 as much calcium as a cup of milk. Furthermore, the level of phosphorus is only about 1/3 that of calcium. Hence, this vegetable is complementary to the many

other foods that are low in calcium, but rich in phosphorus (eggs, fish, legumes, meats, nuts, and poultry). It is also a good source of iron.

3. Watercress is an excellent source of vitamins A and C.

(Also see VEGETABLE[S], Table V-6 Vegetables of the World.)

WATER, DEMINERALIZED (DEIONIZED WATER)

By passing water through two ion exchange resins, all mineral salts can be removed—both anions (negatively charged elements) and cations (positively charged elements). This is demineralized water. It is as pure as water can be. Frequently, demineralized water is utilized in scientific investigation to prevent the introduction of interfering substances during sensitive analyses of minute quantities.

(Also see WATER.)

WATER, EXTRACELLULAR

That water in the body which is found outside of the cells of the body. The blood plasma and interstitial fluid make up the extracullular water.

(Also see BODY FLUIDS; and WATER BALANCE.)

WATER GLASS

This is the common term for the chemical, *sodium silicate*, a solution of which may be used to preserve eggs by sealing the pores in the shell. Other uses include fireproofing of fabrics, waterproofing, a detergent in soaps, and adhesives.

WATER HARDNESS

Hard water contains the bicarbonate (HCO_3) and sulfate (SO_4) salts principally of calcium (Ca) and magnesium (Mg) leeched from mineral deposits in the earth, though aluminum and iron salts are sometimes involved. Water hardness due to calcium and magnesium bicarbonate is known as temporary or bicarbonate hardness since boiling the water results in the decomposition of the bicarbonates and the precipitation of calcium and magnesium carbonate (CO_3) or hydroxide (OH). Boiling produces no change in water containing calcium and magnesium sulfate. Hence, the hardness caused by sulfates is known as permanent or noncarbonate hardness.

Following a chemical analysis, water hardness is expressed in parts per million (ppm) of an equivalent amount of calcium carbonate. This method is used for expressing the amount of magnesium as well as the amount of calcium, and for expressing the noncarbonate as well as the carbonate hardness. Total hardness of water varies with locality and source. A water with a total hardness of less than 100 ppm of calcium carbonate is generally considered soft, while a water with a total hardness above 300 ppm is considered very hard.

Hard water requires more soap because of the formation of insoluble salts of calcium and magnesium with soap. Furthermore, hard water leaves deposits in pipes and appliances. Some municipal water supplies have reported 2,000 ppm and some are known to be as high as 4,400 ppm.

(Also see WATER.)

WATER, INTRACELLULAR

That water in the body which is contained within the cells of the body. It represents about 45% of the body weight.

(Also see BODY FLUIDS; and WATER BALANCE.)

WATER LEMON (YELLOW GRANADILLA)
Passiflora laurifolio

This type of passion fruit (of the family *Passifloraceae*) grows wild in the hot, humid lowlands of the West Indies and northeastern South America. The fruits of this vine have an orange-yellow peel and a seedy, white pulp. They may be eaten fresh or made into confections, ice cream, ices, jams, jellies, juices, and sherbets. Its excellent flavor has made it popular throughout the tropical areas of the world.

(Also see FRUIT[S], Table F-47 Fruits of the World—"Passion Fruit.")

WATERMELON *Citrullus vulgaris*

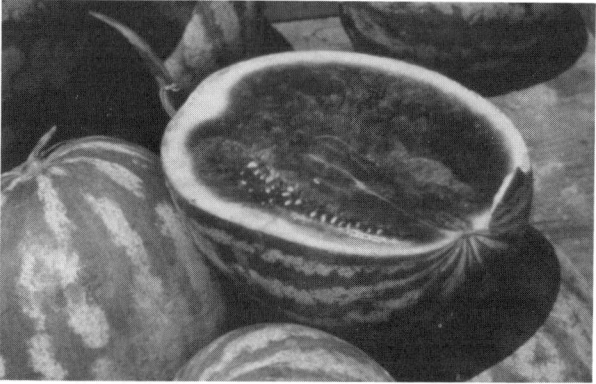

Fig. W-14. Refreshing, cool, crisp, and juicy watermelon. (Courtesy, USDA)

Watermelons are the fruit of an annual prostrate vine with multiple stems, branching out 12 to 15 ft (*4 to 5 m*). They may weigh 5 to 85 lb (*2.3 to 38.3 kg*), and vary in shape from round to oval to oblong-cylindrical. On the outside the hard rind of watermelons may be very light to very dark green with stripes or mottling, while the inside edible flesh (pulp) is red, pink, orange, yellow or white. Red is the most familiar color in the United States. Most watermelons contain white, brown, or black seeds, but there are seedless watermelons.

The pumpkin, squash, muskmelon, and cucumber are relatives of the watermelon.

ORIGIN AND HISTORY.
Watermelons originated in Africa, where they still occur in the wild. From Africa, they spread to southern Asia. Since ancient times, watermelons have been cultivated in the Mediterranean region and Egypt. Although they spread to India before recorded history, it seems that watermelons did not reach China until the 10th or 11th century A.D. Watermelons were introduced into the New World soon after its discovery. Today, watermelons are grown worldwide in tropical, semitropical and in many temperate climates.

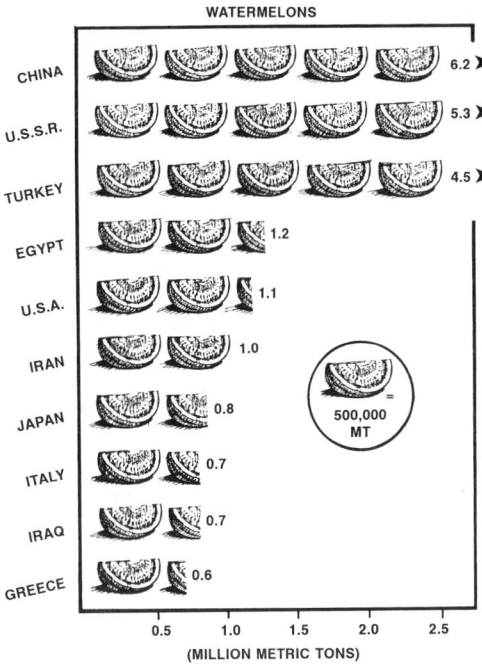

Fig. W-16. Leading watermelon-producing countries of the world. (Based on data from *FAO Production Yearbook*, 1990, FAO/UN, Rome, Italy, Vol. 44, p. 162, Table 54)

Although watermelons can grow as far north as Canada, those produced for interstate shipment are primarily produced in the southern states where Texas and Florida are the leading producers.

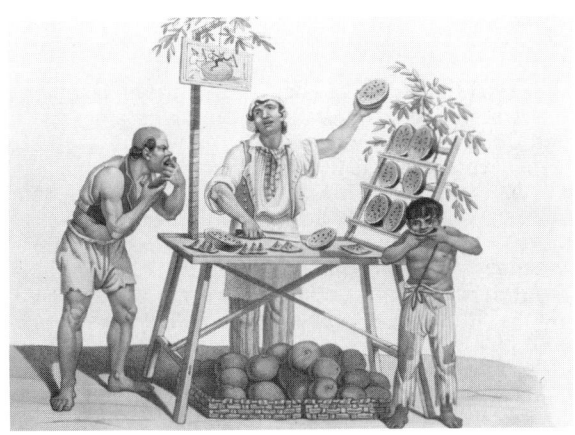

Fig. W-15. A watermelon salesman. Watermelon has been popular down through the ages. (Photo courtesy of the Bettmann Archive, Inc., New York, N.Y., after a colored lithograph by Muller.)

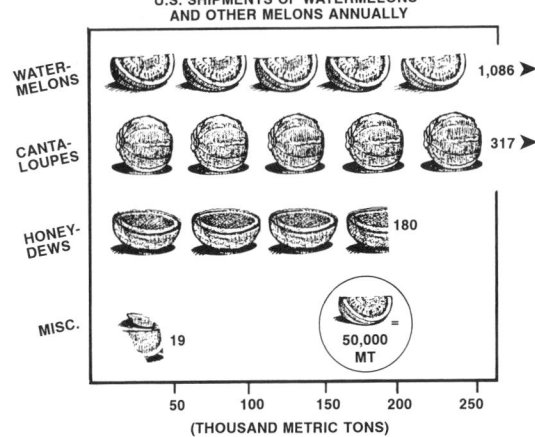

Fig. W-17. Total reported melon domestic rail, truck, and air shipments, 1990. (Data from *Agricultural Statistics 1991*, USDA, p. 169, Table 244)

PRODUCTION.
Watermelons grow best on fertile sandy soil, in the hot drier areas of the world where there is plenty of sunshine. They are fairly drought-resistant, but killed by frost. The leading watermelon-producing countries of the world are shown in Fig. W-16; as noted, the United States is among them.

Propagation and Growing. Watermelons are grown from seeds which are sown directly into the field or planted first in a nursery and then transplanted to the field or garden when temperatures are certain to remain above 55°F (*13°C*) at night and 80°F (*27°C*) during the day.

A large number of watermelon cultivars are available. Small watermelons include: the New Hampshire Midget, Sugar Baby, and You Sweet Thing Hybrid, while the large watermelons include: Charleston Gray and Crimson Sweet. The seedless watermelons, which sometimes have a few white seeds, include the Burpee Hybrid Seedless and Triple Sweet Seedless.

Watermelons are usually planted in hills which have two plants, and which are spaced 8 to 10 ft (*2.4 to 3 m*) apart. In the United States, each acre of commercially grown watermelons yields 500 to 600, 20-lb (*9.1 kg*) melons. Depending upon the variety, watermelons require 70 to 90 days from planting to harvest.

Harvesting. The pulp of the watermelon colors as it ripens, but outwardly ripe watermelons can be recognized by yielding a dull thud when they are tapped, and by the withering of the tendrils. Also, ripe fruit turns light yellow where it contacts the ground. Watermelons are best when vine ripened. They are removed from the vine with a sharp knife, and then handled very carefully. Once harvested watermelons can only be stored for 2 to 3 weeks. However, with modern transportation and storage, watermelon can be enjoyed in many areas.

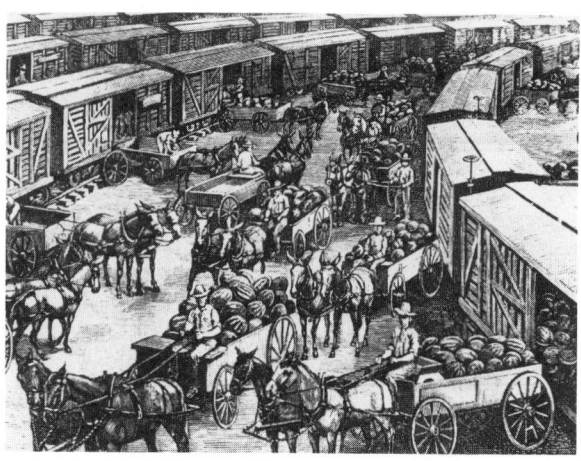

Fig. W-18. Early-day shipping of watermelons by rail from Atlanta, Georgia. (Photo courtesy of the Bettmann Archive, Inc., New York, N.Y.)

PROCESSING AND PREPARATION. Almost all watermelons are consumed fresh after being chilled, sliced and served with a fork or spoon. Some people prefer a little salt to enhance the sweetness. Also, the seeds can be removed from fresh watermelon, following which it can then be used in fruit dishes and desserts.

• **"Watermelon bust"**—In some areas, a favorite summertime activity during or following a long hot day is a "watermelon bust." People get together and enjoy cool, crisp melons. Cooling the melons in a mountain stream adds atmosphere to the event. But, cooled by any method, participants eat their fill—generally without the aid of a spoon, fork or plate.

Other uses of watermelon are not very popular. Sometimes, the rinds of watermelons are pickled or candied. In Russia, a fermented drink is made from the juice. Sometimes, Orientals preserve chunks of watermelon in brine.

In some countries of the Middle East and in China, the seeds are also eaten. They are roasted and eaten like popcorn, or preserved in salt.

SELECTION. Judging the quality of a watermelon is very difficult unless it is cut in half or quartered. When cut, indicators of a good watermelon include firm, juicy flesh with good red color, free from white streaks, and seeds which are dark brown or black. Poor quality melons are usually immature or overmature. Immature melons have pale colored flesh and white streaks or "white heart," while overmaturity or aging after harvest is indicated by dry mealy flesh or watery stringy flesh.

When selecting an uncut watermelon a few appearance factors are helpful, though not totally reliable. The watermelon surface should be relatively smooth; the rind should have a slight dullness (neither shiny nor dull); the ends of the melon should be filled out and rounded; and the underside, or "belly," of the melon should have a creamy color.

NUTRITIONAL VALUE. The nutritional values of fresh watermelon and watermelon seeds are listed in Food Composition Table F-36.

Fresh watermelon is true to its name. It contains about 93% water, and only 26 Calories (kcal) per 100 g (about 3 1/2 oz). The calories are primarily derived from the naturally-occurring sugar which gives watermelon its sweetness. Watermelons contain 6 to 12% sugar (carbohydrate) depending upon the variety and growing conditions. Vitamin A is present in significant amounts—about 590 IU/100 g.

The nutritional composition of watermelon seeds is typical of many other seeds and nuts—high in protein, fat, carbohydrates, and calories. Each 100 g of seeds contains about 25 g protein, 40 g of fat and 30 g of carbohydrate for a whopping 536 Calories (kcal) per 100 g.

(Also see FRUIT[S], Table F-47 Fruits of the World.)

WATER-SOLUBLE VITAMINS

The large amounts of water which pass through most animals daily tend to carry out the water-soluble vitamins of the body, thereby depleting the supply. Thus, they must be supplied in the diet on a day-to-day basis. The water-soluble vitamins are: vitamin C (ascorbic acid), B-1 (thiamin), B-2 (riboflavin), B-6 (pyridoxine), niacin (nicotinic acid), pantothenic acid, biotin, folic acid (folacin), choline, B-12, and inositol.

(Also see VITAMIN[S].)

WAX, APPLE

The waxy material present in apple skin which is sometimes removed by dewaxing with hot isopropyl alcohol vapor in order to reduce the amount of peel lost during the processing of apples into canned slices or juice. Dewaxing of apples makes it possible to remove the peel with a lye solution.

(Also see APPLE.)

WAX BEANS

(See BEAN, COMMON.)

WAX GOURD (CHINESE PRESERVING MELON) *Benincasa hispida*

The fruit of a vine (of the family *Cucurbitaceae*) that is native to Malaysia, but is now grown throughout the tropics of Asia.

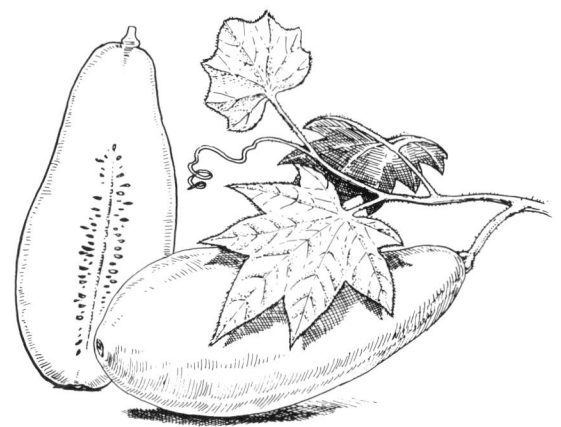

Fig. W-19. The wax gourd, an Asian fruit that has an edible flesh and edible seeds.

Wax gourds are large, heavy, oblong fruits that range from 6 to 8 in. (*15 to 20 cm*) in diameter, and from 8 to 14 in. (*20 to 35 cm*) long. The fruits may be boiled or candied, and the seeds fried. Also, the young leaves and flower buds are eaten as vegetables.

The nutrient composition of the wax gourd is given in Food Composition Table F-36.

Some noteworthy observations regarding the nutrient composition of the wax gourd follow:

1. The raw fruit has a very high water content (96%) and is very low in calories (13 kcal per 100 g) and carbohydrates (3%).

2. Wax gourds are a fair to good source of potassium and vitamin C.

WEANING

The process whereby feeding an infant from the breast or bottle is replaced by cup feeding. Weaning is usually accomplished by substituting a cup feeding for the breast or bottle feeding one period daily. Infants learn fast and only 4 to 5 days are required for babies to become accustomed to a cup. Gradually, a second cup feeding daily may be offered. By the time an infant is 7 to 9 months old, he should know how to drink out of a cup. Eventually, the infant will be drinking homogenized milk and eating a variety of solid foods, and the proportion of calories derived from breast or bottle milk decreases. Weaning usually requires 2 to 3 weeks, depending upon the diligence of the mother.

(Also see BREAST FEEDING; and INFANT DIET AND NUTRITION.)

WEIGHT AND HEIGHT-AGE PERCENTILE STANDARDS

Charts or tables used to determine deviations in growth patterns—weight and height—from normal growth patterns. They are based on careful measurements of selected populations of children over a period of years, and they are expressed in percentiles—distribution of ranked values for weight and height divided into hundreths. Thus, the 50th percentile on the table or chart represents the median, or in other words the central tendency of all children. These weight and height-age percentile standards or growth charts may be used to spot undernutrition or over nutrition in children or adolescents.

WEIGHTS AND MEASURES

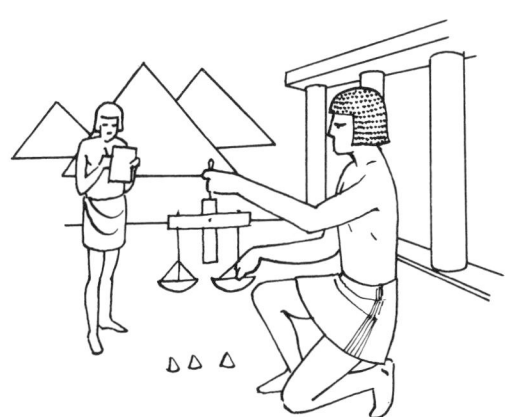

Fig. W-20. Scales were developed by ancient Egyptians to weigh grains.

Weights and measures are the standard employed in arriving at weights, quantities, and volumes. Even among primitive people, such standards were necessary; and with the growing complexity of life, they became of greater and greater importance.

HISTORY. Systems of weights and measures evolved gradually and were subject to many influences.

Counting was probably the earliest form of measure. In prehistoric times, the principal product of each tribe was often used as a unit of barter. For example, a tiller of the soil might trade 20 handfuls of grain to a shepherd for a lamb. The development and application of linear measure followed between 10,000 and 8000 B.C., and preceded the development of measures of weight and capacity. The units of measure in these early systems were based on natural objects. For example, the Egyptians used the *cubit* as the unit of linear measure, which they defined as the distance between the elbow and the tip of the middle finger.

Primitive people also learned that there was a uniformity of weight among similar seeds and grains, so some of these were used as standards of weight. For example, the *carat*, used by modern jewelers as the unit for weighing precious stones, was derived from the carob seed; and the *grain*, which is still used as a unit of weight, was originally the weight of a grain of wheat or barley. Other arbitrary measures that were used included cupped hands, hollow gourds, pots, and baskets.

All these methods of measurement depended on units that varied greatly. As primitive societies became more sophisticated, the need arose for a standardized system of weights and measures.

ENGLISH SYSTEM. In about 1300, London merchants adopted a weight system called *avoirdupois* (from the old French term, *aveir-de-peis*), meaning "goods of weight." This system, which was used to weigh bulky goods, is based on a pound of 7,000 grains or 16 oz. It is still used in many English-speaking countries.

U.S. CUSTOMARY SYSTEM. The weights and measures in common use in the American colonies at the time of the American Revolution were all of English origin. Since the system of weights and measures in Great Britain at that time were neither scientific nor uniform, the same weaknesses were reflected in the units used in the colonies. The need for changing the standards was recognized by the framers of the Articles of Confederation and of the Constitution. The subject was often discussed, but no official action was taken for many years. On May 29, 1830, the Senate passed a resolution directing the Secretary of the Treasury to make a comparison of the weights and measures in use in the principal customhouses. The study was made, followed by real progress toward the unification of weights and measures in the United States through the subsequent distribution of uniform standards to the customhouses based on the following: (1) the yard of 36 in.; (2) the avoirdupois pound of 7,000 grains; (3) the wine gallon of 231 cu. in.; and (4) the Winchester bushel of 2,150.42 cu.in. These units are still in use in the United States.

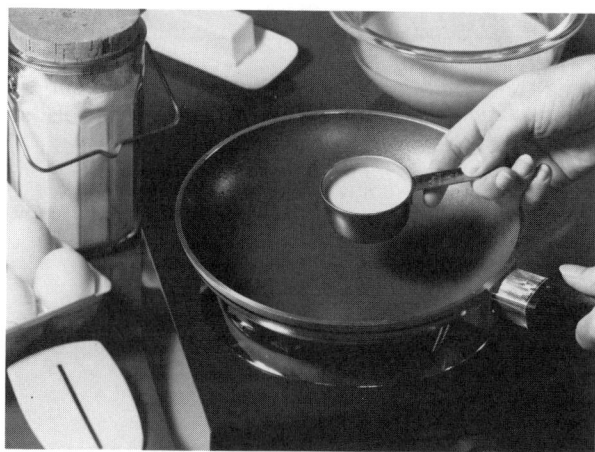

Fig. W-21.   Accurate measurements make for a successful cook. (Courtesy, American Egg Board, Park Ridge, Ill.)

METRIC SYSTEM.   In 1790, the National Assembly of France asked the French Academy of Science to create a standard system of weights and measures. A commission appointed by the academy proposed a system that was both simple and scientific. This system became known as the *Metric System*, and France officially adopted it in 1795. But the government did not require the French people to use the new units of measurement until 1840.

The original measurement standards of the metric unit have been replaced by more accurate ones, and others have been added to the system. Also, whenever necessary, an international group of scientists holds a General Conference of Weights and Measures to revise the system.

By the mid-1970s, almost every country in the world had either converted to the Metric System or planned to do so. The United States is the only major power that lags behind the rest of the world in accepting the Metric System, but it is in the process of converting from the "U.S. Customary," or English System, to the Metric System. As the need for international uniformity increases, it seems probable that the Metric System will replace the U.S. Customary system almost entirely. So, everyone should have a working knowledge of it.

The Metric System is a decimal system based on multiples of ten.

The basic metric units are the *meter* (length/distance), the *gram* (weight), and the *liter* (capacity). The units are then expanded in multiples of 10 or made smaller by 1/10. The prefixes, which are used in the same way with all basic metric units, follow:

"milli-"	=	1/1,000
"centi-"	=	1/100
"deci-"	=	1/10
"deca-"	=	10
"hecto-"	=	100
"kilo-"	=	1,000

COMMON FOOD WEIGHTS AND MEASURES. In preparing foods, it is often more convenient for the cook to measure the ingredients, rather than weigh them. Table W-6 Common Food Weights and Measures will serve as a useful guide when preparing foods by measure.

TABLE W-6
COMMON FOOD WEIGHTS AND MEASURES
(All measurements are level)

ABBREVIATIONS COMMONLY USED

tsp	= teaspoon		oz	= ounce or ounces
Tbsp	= tablespoon		lb	= pound or pounds
c	= cup		sq	= square
pt	= pint		min	= minute or minutes
qt	= quart		hr	= hour or hours
gal	= gallon		mod.	= moderate or
pk	= peck			moderately
bu	= bushel		doz	= dozen

MEASUREMENTS

3 tsp = 1 Tbsp	1 c = ½ pt
4 Tbsp = ¼ c	2 c = 1 lb
5⅓ Tbsp = ⅓ c	2 c = 1 pt
8 Tbsp = ½ c	2 pt (4 c) = 1 qt
16 Tbsp = 1 c	4 qt (liquid) = 1 gal
1 oz = 2 Tbsp	8 qt (solid) = 1 pk
1 gill = ½ cup	4 pk = 1 bu
8 oz = 1 c	
16 oz = 1 lb	

BUTTER OR MARGARINE

2 Tbsp = 1 oz
½ c = ¼ lb = 1 stick
2 c = 1 lb

CEREALS

Rice	1 c = ½ lb
Rice	1 c raw precooked = 2 c cooked
Rice	1 c raw converted = 3 to 4 c cooked
Rice	1 c raw long-grain = 4 c cooked
Noodles	1 c = 1¼ c cooked
Macaroni	1 c = 2¼ c cooked

COFFEE, GROUND

1 lb = 80 Tbsp or 5 c
½ c makes 10 c beverage

EGGS

5 eggs = about 1 c
8 to 10 egg whites = 1 c
12 to 15 egg yolks = 1 c

FLOUR

All-purpose	4 c sifted = 1 lb
Cake	1 c sifted = 1 c all-purpose flour less 2 Tbsp
Cornmeal	3 c = 1 lb
Potato flour . . . . . . (for thickening)	1 Tbsp = 2 Tbsp flour
Cornstarch . . . . . (for thickening)	1 Tbsp = 2 Tbsp flour
Arrowroot . . . . (for thickening)	2 tsp = 5 tsp flour

FRUITS

Apples	1 lb = 3 med. or 3 c sliced
Candied fruit	1 lb = 1½ c
Lemon (whole) . . .	1 = 2 to 3 Tbsp juice
Lemon . . . . (grated rind)	1 = about 1½ to 2 tsp
Orange (whole) . . .	1 = 6 to 8 Tbsp or ⅓ to ½ c juice
Orange . . . . (grated rind)	1 = about 1 Tbsp
Raisins	1 lb = 3 c

MARSHMALLOWS

¼ lb = 16

MILK AND CHEESE

Milk	1 c = ½ c evaporated milk + ½ cup water
Milk	1 cup = 4 Tbsp powdered whole milk + 1 cup water
Cream	1 c = 2 c whipped cream
Cheese (grated) . .	4 to 5 c = 1 lb
Cottage cheese . .	1 c = ½ lb
Cream cheese	3-oz package = 7 Tbsp

NUTS

Unshelled	1 lb = 2 c nut meats
Shelled	1 lb = 3 to 4 c nut meats

SUGAR

Granulated	1 lb = 2 c
Brown	1 lb = 2¼ c
Confectioners	1 lb = 3½ c
Powdered	1 lb = 2⅓ c

CONTENTS OF CANS

Size (No.)	Weight	Measure (c)
¼	4 to 4.5 oz	½
½	7.5 to 8 oz	1
Picnic		1¼
No. 1 short . . . . or No. 300	10 to 13 oz	1¾
No. 1 tall . . . . or No. 303	1 lb	2
No. 2	1 lb 4 oz	2½
No. 2½	1 lb 14 to 15 oz	3½
No. 3	2 lb to 2 lb 1 oz	4
No. 10	6 lb 8 oz to 8 lb 12 oz	12 to 13

TEMPERATURES

	Fahrenheit (°F)	Centigrade (°C)
Simmering point	180	82
Boiling point of water at sea level	212	100
Ovens:		
Very slow	200 - 250	93 - 121
Slow	300	149
Moderately slow	325	163
Moderate	350	177
Moderately hot	375	191
Hot	400	204
Very hot	450 - 500	232 - 260
Extremely hot	over 500	260

CONVERSIONS OF U.S. CUSTOMARY AND METRIC.

A comparison of U.S. Customary and Metric Systems is shown in Figs. W-22 and W-23.

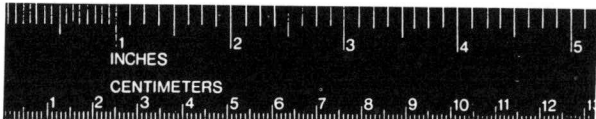

Fig. W-22.   Inches-centimeter scale for direct conversion and reading.

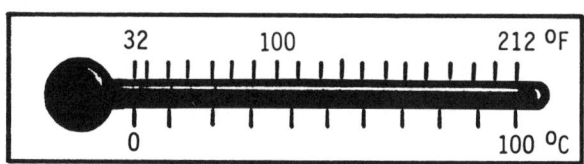

Fig. W-23.   Fahrenheit-Celsius (Centigrade) scale for direct conversion and reading.

The following tables will facilitate conversion from U.S. Customary to Metric units, and vice versa:

Table W- 7 Weight Equivalents
Table W- 8 Weight-Unit Conversion Factors
Table W- 9 Conversion Factors, U.S. Customary to Metric
Table W-10 Conversion Factors, Metric to U.S. Customary

TABLE W-7
WEIGHT EQUIVALENTS

1 lb	= 453.6 g	= .4536 kg = 16 oz
1 oz	= 28.35 g	
1 kg	= 1,000 g	= 2.2046 lb
1 g	= 1,000 mg	
1 mg	= 1,000 mcg	= .001 g
1 mcg	= .001 mg	= .000001 g

1 mcg per g or 1 mg per kg is the same as ppm

TABLE W-8
WEIGHT-UNIT CONVERSION FACTORS

Units Given	Units Wanted	For Conversion Multiply By	Units Given	Units Wanted	For Conversion Multiply By
lb	g	453.6	kcal/kg	kcal/lb	0.4536
lb	kg	0.4536	kcal/lb	kcal/kg	2.2046
oz	g	28.35			
kg	lb	2.2046	ppm	mcg/g	1.
kg	mg	1,000,000.	ppm	mg/kg	1.
kg	g	1,000.	ppm	mg/lb	0.4536
g	mg	1,000.	mg/kg	%	0.0001
g	mcg	1,000,000.	ppm	%	0.0001
mg	mcg	1,000.	mg/g	%	0.1
			g/kg	%	0.1
mg/g	mg/lb	453.6			
mg/kg	mg/lb	0.4536			
mcg/kg	mcg/lb	0.4536			
Mcal	kcal	1,000.			

TABLE W-9
CONVERSION FACTORS
U.S. CUSTOMARY TO METRIC

Symbol	When You Know	Multiply By	To Find	Symbol
U.S. Customary				*Metric*
LENGTH				
in.	inches	**2.5**	*centimeters*	*cm*
ft	feet	**30**	*centimeters*	*cm*
yd	yards	**0.9**	*meters*	*m*
mi	miles	**1.6**	*kilometers*	*km*
AREA				
in.²	square inches	**6.5**	*square centimeters*	*cm²*
ft²	square feet	**0.09**	*square meters*	*m²*
yd²	square yards	**0.8**	*square meters*	*m²*
mi²	square miles	**2.6**	*square kilometers*	*km²*
	acres	**0.4**	*hectares*	*ha*
MASS (weight)				
oz	ounces	**28**	*grams*	*g*
lb	pounds	**0.45**	*kilograms*	*kg*
	short tons (2000 lb)	**0.9**	*metric ton*	*t*
VOLUME				
tsp	teaspoons	**5**	*milliliters*	*ml*
Tbsp	*tablespoons*	**15**	*milliliters*	*ml*
in.³	cubic inches	**16**	*milliliters*	*ml*
fl oz	fluid ounces	**30**	*milliliters*	*ml*
c	cups	**0.24**	*liters*	*liter*
pt	pints	**0.47**	*liters*	*liter*
qt	quarts	**0.95**	*liters*	*liter*
gal	gallons	**3.8**	*liters*	*liter*
ft³	cubic feet	**0.03**	*cubic meters*	*m³*
yd³	cubic yards	**0.76**	*cubic meters*	*m³*
TEMPERATURE (exact)				
°F	degrees Fahrenheit	**5/9** (after subtracting 32)	*degrees Celsius*	*°C (Centigrade)*

TABLE W-10
CONVERSION FACTORS
METRIC TO U.S. CUSTOMARY

Sym-bol	When You Know	Multiply By	To Find	Sym-bol
Metric			*U.S. Customary*	
LENGTH				
mm	*millimeters*	0.04	inches	in.
cm	*centimeters*	0.4	inches	in.
m	*meters*	3.3	feet	ft
m	*meters*	1.1	yards	yd
km	*kilometers*	0.6	miles	mi
AREA				
cm²	*square centimeters*	0.16	square inches	in.²
m²	*square meters*	1.2	square yards	yd²
km²	*square kilometers*	0.4	square miles	mi²
ha	*hectares* (10,000 m²)	2.5	acres	
MASS (weight)				
g	*grams*	0.035	ounces	oz
kg	*kilograms*	2.2	pounds	lb
t	*metric ton* (1000 kg)	1.1	short tons	
VOLUME				
ml	*milliliters*	0.03	fluid ounces	fl oz
ml	*milliliters*	0.06	cubic inches	in.³
liter	*liters*	2.1	pints	pt
liter	*liters*	1.06	quarts	qt
liter	*liters*	0.26	gallons	gal
m³	*cubic meters*	35	cubic feet	ft³
m³	*cubic meters*	1.3	cubic yards	yd³
TEMPERATURE (exact)				
°C	*degrees Celsius* (Centigrade)	9/5 (then add 32)	degrees Fahrenheit	°F

WEY

A British unit of measure varying according to the commodity and locality. For example, a wey of oats is 48 bushels, while a wey of corn or salt is 40 bushels.

WHALE OIL

A yellowish brown oil made by (1) boiling the blubber of whales, and (2) skimming off the oil. After hardening by hydrogenation some of it is used for making margarine and soap.

WHEAT, family *Gramineae;* genus *Triticum*

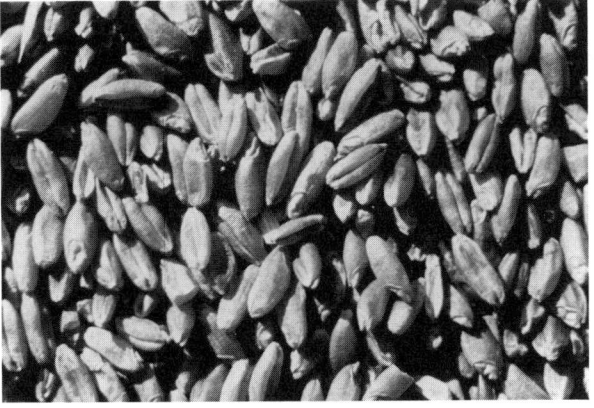

Fig. W-24. Wheat kernels. (Courtesy, USDA)

WERNICKE'S DISEASE (SYNDROME OR ENCEPHALOPATHY)

A nutritional disorder of the nervous system which is mainly associated with a thiamin deficiency. Wernicke's syndrome is often noted in chronic alcoholics, dry beriberi, and semistarvation. Some of the typical symptoms consists of double vision, poor balance, apathy, uncoordinated walk, rapid eye movements, confusion, and delusions. It is closely associated with Korsakoff's psychosis (syndrome); hence, it is often referred to in combination as the Wernicke-Korsakoff syndrome. Wernicke's disease represents a medical emergency; once recognized, it should be treated immediately with thiamin—possibly massive doses. If the disease is not too advanced, vitamin therapy will rapidly restore the afflicted individual to one who is attentive, alert, and responsive.

(Also see BERIBERI, section headed "Dry Beriberi"; and DEFICIENCY DISEASES, Table D-1 Major Dietary Deficiency Diseases—"Wernicke's encephalopathy.")

Wheat, the most important of the grains, provides more nourishment for more people throughout the world than any other food; indeed, it is the staff of life. While rice is the common food in the Orient, wheat is basic to the diet of Europe, Africa, North and South America, Australia, and a large part of Asia. One-third of the world's population depends on wheat as its main staple. Total world production of wheat is about 112 g per day per person, enough to supply 408 Calories (kcal) and 12 g of protein daily if it were evenly distributed and unrefined. In many developing countries, wheat supplies 40 to 60% of the available energy and protein.

More than 70% of the world's croplands is devoted to the production of grains. Wheat accounts for the largest area—more than 22%. Every month of the year, a crop of wheat is being harvested somewhere in the world. It flourishes in many different climates and elevations, and under varied soil conditions.

Wheaten foods provide generously of carbohydrates, protein, and certain minerals and vitamins. Of all the cereals, wheat alone could meet minimum protein requirements if used as the sole cereal product, with the exception of infants and young growing children (who need supplemental lysine when fed wheat-based diets) and possibly pregnant and lactating females. A diet with large amounts of wheat and only small amounts of protein from animal sources provides adequate quantity and quality protein.

(Also see Cereal Grains.)

ORIGIN AND HISTORY. The development and progress of civilization can be linked to the history of wheat. Prior to recorded history, man cultivated wheat.

No one knows where the wheat plant originated, although it was cultivated where modern man is supposed to have first appeared—in southwestern Asia. The common ancestor of all wheats is believed to be a species called wild einkorn (meaning "one seed"), found in excavated ruins in the upper reaches of the Tigris-Euphrates basin in Southwestern Asia—called the "Fertile Crescent," the presumed birthplace of our civilization. The 14- and 21-chromosome species of wheats are believed to have developed as natural hybrids of the original einkorn.

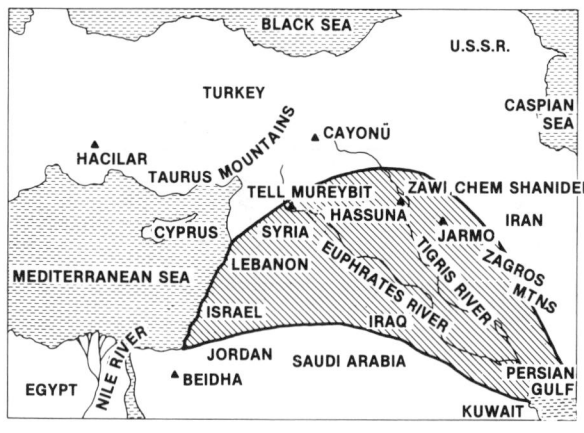

Fig. W-25.   The fertile crescent.

Man probably used wheat as food 10,000 to 15,000 years before Christ. In 1948, archaeologists from the University of Chicago found kernels of wheat, believed to be about 6,700 years old, preserved in the ruins of an ancient village in Iraq.

The first wheat food was probably the grain itself, stripped of its husk, or glumes, and chewed, a way in which it is still eaten in many parts of the world. But a form of bread was found in the remains of a Stone Age village of Swiss lake dwellers.

Bronze tablets dating from the 9th century before Christ depict the grinding of wheat and the making of bread in Assyria. In the 5th century B.C., the Greek historian, Herodotus, wrote of Egyptian bread baking. Tombs along the Nile River contain 5000 B.C. murals showing the planting and harvesting of wheat, the grinding of flour, and the making of bread. Some tombs were even stocked with wheat and bread. The Egyptians sifted their meal to make white flour and bread. Also, Egypt is generally recognized as the place where leavened bread originated.

Ancient Chinese writings describe the growing of wheat 2,700 years before Christ. Even today, wheat is considered a sacred crop in some parts of China.

In 300 B.C., Theophrastos, a Greek philosopher, wrote of the many different kinds of wheat grown along the Mediterranean Sea. Written records, works of art, and the excavations of ancient cities depict the progressive improvement of the art of milling and baking in Greece and Rome through the Middle Ages. Baking and brewing were developed together as man gained arts and skills.

Man even clothed wheat with religious significance and made it the object of primitive worship. The Greeks invested a "bread goddess," Demeter, with the rule of agriculture and explained the changing seasons with the story of her daughter, Persephone. According to the whimsical story, Persephone was kidnapped and made to live in Hades, the underworld, during the autumn and winter of each year. Demeter's Roman counterpart was Ceres, for whom cereal grains were named. Beginning with the Book of Genesis, the Bible refers to the sowing, harvesting, milling, and uses of wheat. According to the Book of Revelation, the Hebrews exchanged "a measure of wheat for a penny." Samson, the man of great strength, was a miller and was made to mill wheat into flour when he was imprisoned.

The reverence in which people held wheat and bread through the ages still lives in the Lord's Prayer: "Give us this day, our daily bread." In the Hebrew faith, the eating of unleavened matzoth during the Passover also marks the significance of bread in religion. In Europe, bread is commonly referred to as "the staff of life."

In wars, battles were sometimes postponed until the harvest had been gathered in, and the well-fed armies usually defeated the hungry ones. The fall of Napolean can be attributed to lack of grain. His armies advanced so rapidly into Russia that food supplies were left far behind. Likewise, the Civil War has been described by some American historians as a victory of bread over cotton; the North raised enough wheat to feed itself, whereas the South could not eat its principal product—cotton. Again, wheat figured in the allied victory of World War I; the balance of power was tipped against Germany when America began supplying food to the allies. Former President Herber Hoover once said:

"The first word in war is spoken by guns but the last word has always been spoken by bread."

Even today, in the struggle for peace, America's abundant wheat is a powerful weapon—more powerful than bullets.

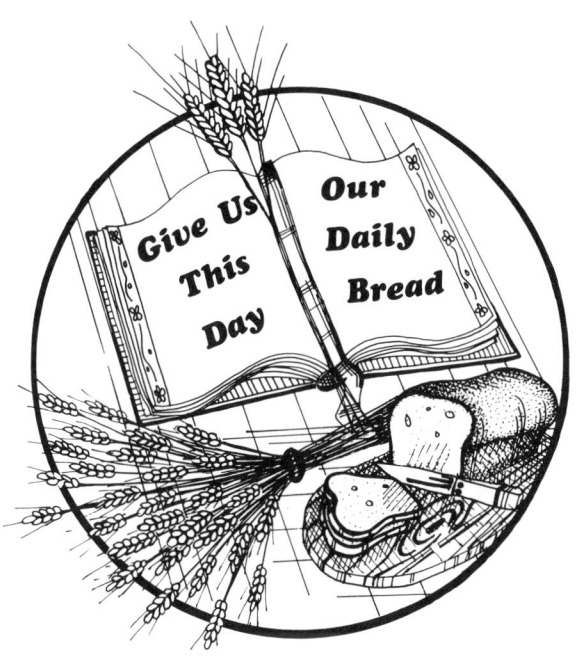

Fig. W-26. Throughout the ages, wheat and bread have lived in the Lord's Prayer.

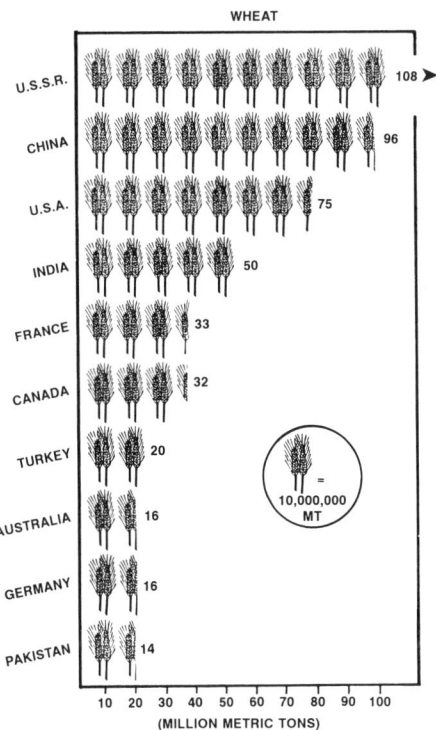

Fig. W-27. Ten leading wheat-producing countries of the world. (Source: *FAO Production Yearbook*, 1990, FAO/UN, Rome, Italy, Vol. 44, p. 70, Table 16)

Columbus brought wheat to the western hemisphere when he returned to the West Indies in 1493. Cortez took wheat from Spain to Mexico in 1519; and the missionaries took it from there into what are now Arizona and California.

WORLD AND U.S. PRODUCTION.

Farmers of the world grow approximately 595 million metric tons of wheat each year. The Soviet Union, which produces about 18% of the world crop, is the leading wheat-producing nation of the world. But the U.S.S.R. does not grow enough wheat for its own needs. The black soil in the southern part of the country, extending over 1,500 miles (*2,410 km*) from the Ural Mountains on the northeast into the Danube River Basin on the southwest, is well suited to wheat. This prairie land, with a deep, fertile soil, has a climate similar to the Great Plains area of the United States, though the winters are much colder and there is less rainfall.

The United States ranks third among the wheat-producing countries of the world. Ten leading wheat-producing countries of the globe and their production are shown in Fig. W-27.

Wheat yields vary considerably among countries, and are related primarily to water supply and intensity of cultivation. Also, yields are affected by type of wheat sown; winter wheat, with a longer growing season, is normally higher yielding than spring wheat. Recently, the five high-yielding wheat countries of the world, by rank, and the number of bushels each of them produced per acre, were: Ireland, 119 (*8,149 kg/ha*); Netherlands, 113 (*7,716 kg/ha*); Denmark, 112 (*7,651 kg/ha*); United Kingdom, 101 (*6,905 kg/ha*); and Belgium-Luxembourg, 99 (*6,749 kg/ha*). The United States, with an average yield of 39 bu per acre (*2,656 kg/ha*), ranked thirty-second.

In the United States, wheat ranks second only to corn in total acreage and production. Wheat is grown in every state of continental United States, although production in New England is minor. The greatest acreage is in the Central Plains and north central states.

The types and varieties grown vary by location. In the southern Great Plains—Oklahoma, Texas, Kansas, Colorado, and Nebraska—hard red winter wheats are grown. In the northern Great Plains (Minnesota, North Dakota, South Dakota, and Montana), the winters are often too severe for winter wheat; so, hard red spring wheat is grown. In eastern United States, in the valleys of the Ohio and Potomac Rivers, soft red winter wheat is widely grown. Hard and soft types of white wheats are grown in the Columbia River Basin, and on the rolling Palouse lands of Washington, Oregon, and Idaho. In the light rainfall areas of the Western Great Plains and the Pacific Northwest where irrigation is impractical, wheat is often planted every other year on acreage kept free from weeds and tilled to conserve and store up moisture—a practice called summer fallowing.

The ten leading wheat-producing states of the United States, by rank, are: Kansas, Oklahoma, Washington, Texas, Illinois, Montana, Nebraska, Colorado, Ohio, and Idaho (see Fig. W-28).

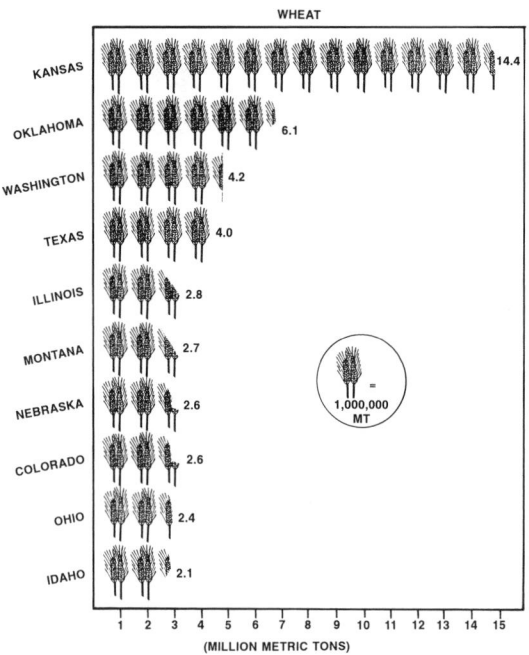

Fig. W-28. Ten leading wheat-producing states of the United States in bushels of wheat (1 bu equals 60 lb or *27 kg*). (Source: *Agricultural Statistics 1991*, USDA, p. 6, Table 8)

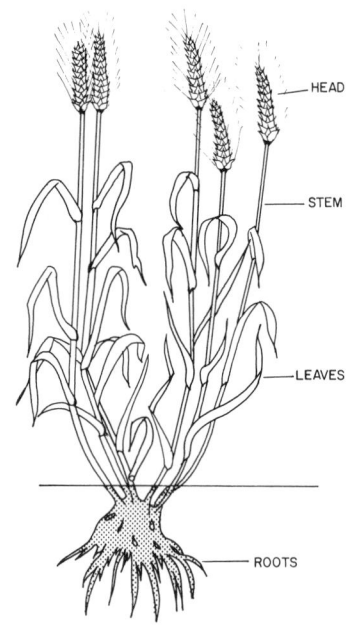

Fig. W-29. Parts of the wheat plant.

The Green Revolution.

In the 1960s, scientists achieved remarkable success in developing new high-yielding varieties of wheat and rice. They produced plants that have short, strong stalks, which enable them to stand upright under the great weight of the higher yields. When these "shorty" varieties are properly fertilized and irrigated, yields are often doubled. The rapid spread of these new varieties to the developing countries, particularly in Asia, is referred to as the Green Revolution.

Because of these new varieties, wheat production in Mexico, India, Pakistan, the Philippines, Sri Lanka, and Thailand has greatly increased; and the threat of massive famine in these countries has been delayed. In 1970, Norman E. Borlaug, an American agricultural scientist on the staff of the Rockefeller Foundation, was awarded the Nobel peace prize for his wheat research that led to the development of the high-yielding varieties and the Green Revolution.

(Also see GREEN REVOLUTION.)

THE WHEAT PLANT.

Although cultivated wheat varieties differ greatly in their growth habits and physical characteristics, all are annuals of the grass family, *Gramineae*, and of the genus *Triticum*. The principal parts are the roots, stem (column), leaves, and head (spike) (see Fig. W-29).

When growing, wheat is a bright green color and looks like grass. It usually grows 24 to 48 in. (*61 to 122 cm*) tall, depending on variety, moisture, fertility, and length of daylight. When mature, it turns to a golden brown. Most of the root system is in the top 12 in. (*30 cm*) of soil, although roots may extend down 3 to 8 ft. (*1.0 to 2.4 m*) in loose ground. The leaves are long and slender. The wheat head that holds the kernels is at the top of the main center stem. Many varieties of wheat have coarse, prickly hairs called beards on the husk of the wheat kernel. Each kernel contains a germ and serves as a seed. As in all plants, the single kernel of wheat develops in a flower. A healthy plant produces an average of 50 kernels of wheat. The clusters of kernels cling tightly to the stem until they are fully ripe. When threshed, the grains are beaten free from the other parts of the plant and separated from the straw and chaff. The grains of wheat are white, red, yellow, or purple.

KINDS OF WHEAT.

Wheat is classified according to climatic adaptation, color of kernel, relative hardness of kernel, species, and varieties.

• **Winter wheat vs spring wheat**—There are two broad kinds of wheat, winter wheat and spring wheat. Winter wheats are planted in mild climates, whereas spring wheats are planted where the winters are extremely cold. Each group includes varieties of both hard and soft wheat.

Winter wheats, which are adapted to the Middle Great Plains, are planted in the fall and harvested in the following June and July. They get a start before cold weather, become dormant during the winter, and continue growth again in the spring. Frost affects the young plants adversely, but a covering of snow protects them and promotes tillering.

Spring wheats are planted in the spring after the threat of frost is over and the ground is dry enough to work, and they ripen in the summer of the same year, usually a few weeks after winter wheat.

● **Color of kernel**—Both winter and spring wheat produce grain that is red or white, with various shades of yellows or amber.

● **Texture of the ripened grain**—Wheat is classed as hard or soft. Hard wheats tend to be higher in protein content than soft wheats, and are primarily used in bread flour. Durham wheats are also hard wheats, used for macaroni production. Softer wheats are lower in protein and are chiefly milled into flour for cakes, cookies, pastries, and crackers.

● **Species of wheat**—All the wheats grown throughout the world belong to one of 14 species, but only the following seven are of commercial importance in the United States:
1. Common wheat
    a. Hard red spring
    b. Hard red winter
    c. Soft red winter
    d. White
2. Club wheat
3. Polish wheat
4. Spelt
5. Durum wheat
    a. Durum
    b. Red durum
6. Poulard wheat
7. Emmer

Approximately 95% of the wheat grown in the United States is of the common type. The remaining acreage is made up largely of club and durum wheats. Minor acreages of poulard, emmer, spelt, and Polish wheats are grown for livestock feed.

Of the 14 species of wheat, only three—common, club, and durum—account for 90% of all wheat grown in the world today.

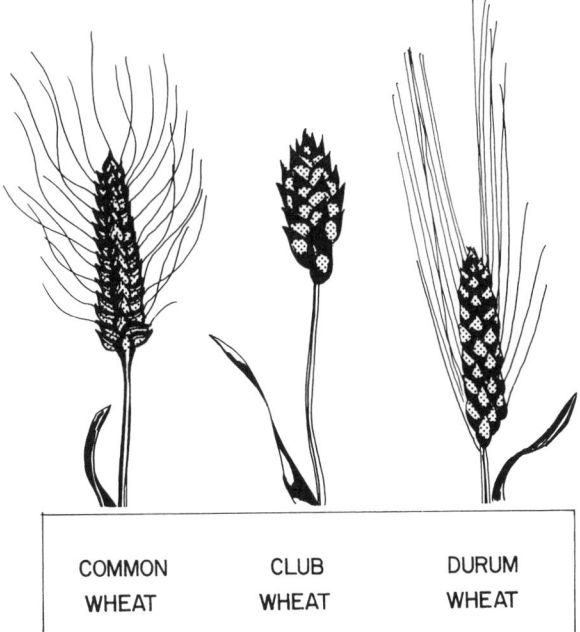

COMMON WHEAT	CLUB WHEAT	DURUM WHEAT

Fig. W-30. Heads of three most common types of wheat.

Common wheat is bread wheat. It probably originated in Turkey and southern U.S.S.R. Over 200 varieties of common wheat have been described, of which about 100 are now cultivated. They may be either red or white, hard or soft, and spring or winter type. The most important common wheat states are Kansas, Texas, Nebraska, Oklahoma, Colorado, North Dakota, South Dakota, Montana, and Minnesota.

Club wheat is grown primarily for flour, in the Pacific Northwest. It may be either winter or spring type.

Durum wheat is grown for spaghetti, macaroni, and noodles. The kernels are white or red. The varieties of this species grown in North America are all spring wheats, grown in North Dakota, South Dakota, Montana, Minnesota, and parts of Canada.

● **Varieties of wheat**—Each species of wheat is divided into many varieties. About 30,000 varieties of wheat are grown in various parts of the world; more than 200 of these are grown in the United States. Each variety is different from the others in some way.

Hybrid Wheats. Hybrids are developed by crossing varieties of wheat selected for desirable traits—greater yield, resistance to diseases and insects, a shorter growing season, better milling and baking qualities, and shorter straw to lessen lodging. For example, one variety may be desirable because it is rust resistant, whereas another variety may rate high for its bread-baking qualities. So, the plant breeder crosses the two in an attempt to get a good, rust-resistant wheat. Under favorable conditions, hybrid wheats have generally shown yield increases of 20 to 40% over the parent varieties.

To establish a new variety, the scientist selects the parents with the characteristics that he desires. From one head, he removes the full-grown, but not-yet-ripe, anthers, which produce pollen. He then covers the wheat head to prevent natural cross pollination. A few days later when the stigmas are ready to receive pollen, he removes the cover, pollinates the head from the ripe anthers of the other selected plant. The seed of the hybrid is then planted for several generations, with the plant breeder selecting wheat at each step that possesses the characteristics that he desires. Finally, the new variety is standardized and planted again and again until there is enough seed for commercial use.

As the knowledge of genetics increased, it was found that certain genes in the chromosome arrangement of reproductive cells control specific characteristics of a plant—like length of straw, plumpness and quality of kernel, yield, and other similar attributes. Further, it was found that the genetic makeup of the wheat plant could be artificially modified by the use of chemicals and irradiation, thereby making it possible to produce mutations at will. This genetic knowledge was used in the development of improved strains of wheat through hybridization of selected plants, followed by seed increase of true breeding strains from these matings. However, at this point and period of time, the genetic phenomenon of hybrid vigor, so well known in hybrid corn, could not be utilized in wheat because of its flower arrangement; in wheat, the flower contained within the glumes of the head is both male and female and crossed seed can be produced only by first removing the male part of each flower by hand and then transferring pollen from another plant to the undisturbed female parts of these flowers. But geneticists sought and found some strains of wheat having flowers with normal female parts but sterile male parts (male sterile) and others having the genetic ability to overcome this male sterility (male fertility restoration). So, the phenomenon of male sterility in wheat served the same purpose in wheat seed production as detasseling did in the production of seed for hybrid corn. But in hybrid wheat the male sterile plant must be crossed again with plants that restore male fertility so that the resulting hybrid seed will grow plants that produce kernels.

WHEAT CULTURE—PAST AND PRESENT.

Archaeologists date the first tools of ancient man as early as 250,000 years ago. But it was only 10,000 to 15,000 years ago that man began to turn his tool-making skill to the production of agricultural implements. The transition from hunting food to cultivating food marked the beginning of civilization.

A good wheat crop depends upon (1) good climate—cool, with moderate rainfall; (2) good soil; and (3) good culture—proper seedbed preparation, seeding, harvesting, and threshing.

• **Seedbed preparation**—The first step in planting wheat is seedbed preparation—the breaking up of the soil. The most primitive implement for this purpose was a sharp digging stick, much like those still in use in Central Africa. Subsequently, ingenious man improved his tools and adapted them to his own needs. But the greatest changes in farming came with the development of iron and steel, about 150 years ago. In 1819, Jethro Wood, a New York farmer, patented a cast iron plow. Iron was soon replaced by steel; and the gang plow, consisting of a series of plow shares attached to a single frame, followed.

Today, tractors pull a number of plows joined together. Then the farmer pulverizes the soil, reducing the earth to smaller fragments, by discing, harrowing, and/or cultivating. Fertilizers are usually added to the soil before the wheat is seeded. However, nitrogen fertilizer may be added after the wheat is up and growing.

• **Seeding**—The Egyptians scattered seed wheat directly into the mud left by the retreat of the annual flood waters along the Nile. Then, they drove cattle and sheep over the fields to trample the seed into the ground. But, for thousands of years, broadcasting has been the most common method of seeding wheat—scattering the seeds evenly by hand; a procedure still used in many parts of the world.

It is noteworthy that radio and television stations have adopted the word, "broadcast"—suggesting the sowing of words as seeds of thought across the nation.

The modern farmer seeds ¾ to 2 bu of wheat per acre (50 to 133 kg/ha) with a machine called a drill. Wheat for planting is contained in the hopper at the top, from which it is funneled evenly down into the earth and covered lightly with soil. With a large drill, one man can plant more than 100 acres (40 ha) per day.

After the seed is in the ground, the farmer cannot do a great deal for his crop until harvest. Sometimes he

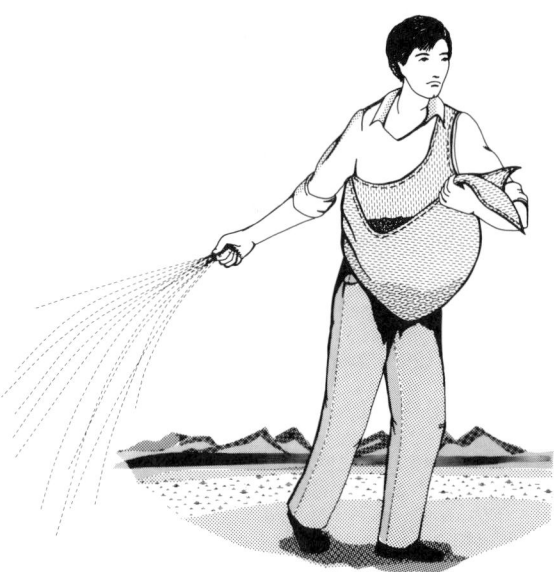

Fig. W-31.   Broadcasting wheat—how it used to be done. Working in this manner, a skilled man can seed 1 acre of wheat in 60 minutes.

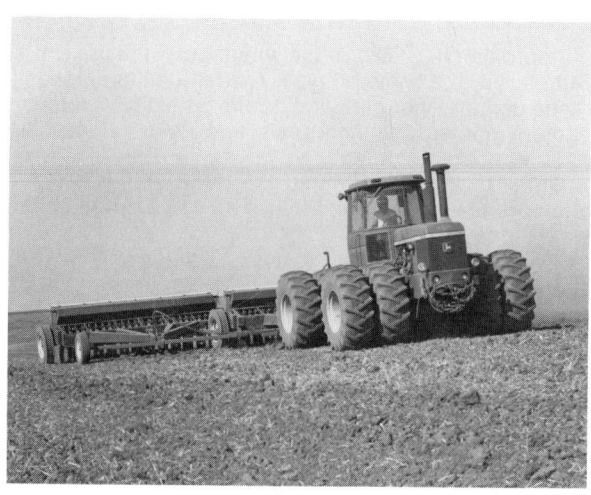

Fig. W-32.   Seeding winter wheat in the famed Palouse wheat area of eastern Washington, showing a John Deere wheel tractor pulling three 12 ft International drills. With this equipment, 20 acres per hour can be seeded. (Photo by Henry Fisher, Oakesdale, Wash.)

sprays chemicals on weeds to kill them and keep them from robbing the wheat plants of moisture and nourishment.

• **Harvesting**—When wheat is ripe, it must be harvested as soon as possible; otherwise, bad weather may ruin the crop. Wheat is ready for harvest when it is dry and hard—when the moisture content is down to 13%. In olden times, the farmer rubbed a head of wheat in his hands, blew away the chaff, and sampled the grain. If the kernels cracked easily between his teeth and chewed into a gum, the crop was ready to cut. Modern farmers usually check the moisture content of wheat by instrument, to determine whether or not it is ready for harvest and can be safely stored.

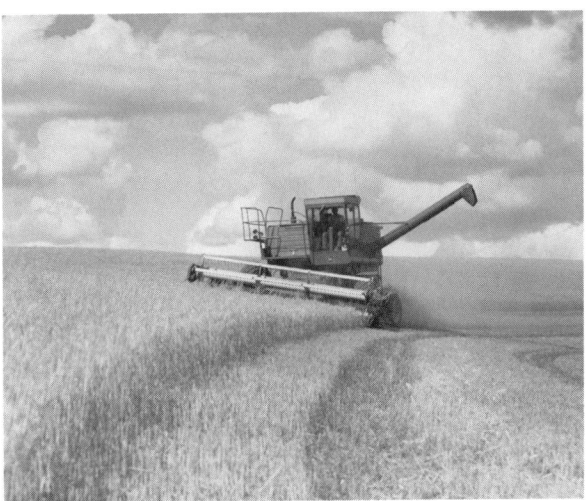

Fig. W-33.   Harvesting wheat in eastern Washington with a John Deere combine. This machine, which is operated by one man, cuts a swath 18 ft wide and is capable of harvesting over 300 bushels of wheat per hour. (Photo by Henry Fisher, Oakesdale, Wash.)

The first wheat reapers were saw-toothed stones fitted into a wood or bone handle, or skillfully crafted sickles inlaid with a cutting edge of flint. Next came the adaptation of iron and steel to the sickle, making for a balanced tool, easy to swing.

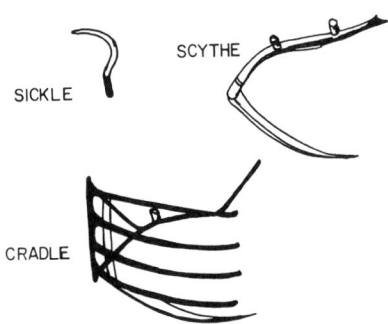

SICKLE

SCYTHE

CRADLE

Fig. W-34.   Primitive wheat harvesting tools.

Even after 4,000 years, sickles are still widely used in the developing countries. They are light enough for work by women and children, and they permit the cutting of the straw at any height. The importance of the sickle in the history of man has been symbolized; it has been perpetuated in many works of art, and in the Russian hammer and sickle.

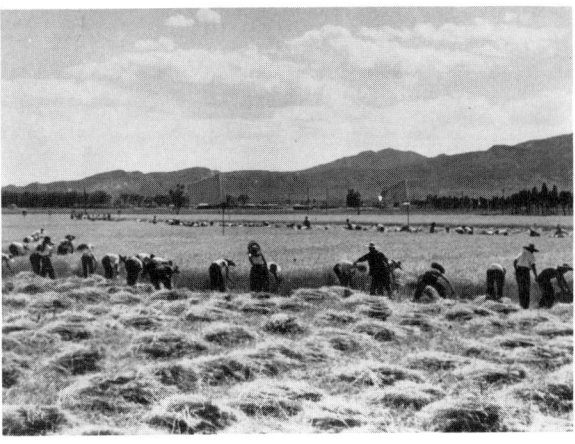

Fig. W-35.   Harvesting wheat with sickles in China. (Courtesy, *China Pictorial*)

The sickle was followed by the scythe—a longer blade with only a slight curve, fastened at right angles to a long wooden handle. Wheat could be cut faster with the scythe, and the worker could stand upright. As men scythed their way through a field, others followed in the swath and collected the bunches of grain and bound them into sheaves. In time, the curved fingers of the cradle were added, to catch the grain as it was cut and leave it bunched and easier to gather and bundle into a sheaf.

In America, sheaves of wheat were once piled in a small stack called a shock, arranged to shed water when it rained; then allowed to dry until ready for threshing. At other times, the sheaves were gathered from the field and stacked in some convenient spot, often in a circular bell shape or beehive arrangement. Even today, in damp climates cut wheat is sometimes hung from a large rack and allowed to dry.

With the use of iron and steel, better and more efficient methods of cutting wheat engaged the attention of many men. Among them was a prosperous and talented Virginian, Robert McCormick. Besides farming, he was a weaver, and he operated a saw mill, grist mill, a smelter, and a blacksmith shop. He tried to construct a machine to cut his grain. His son, Cyrus McCormick, continued work on the invention until 1831, when, at age 22, he first demonstrated a mechanical reaper, which he subsequently patented in 1834. McCormick's invention was a crude machine mounted on two wheels. The main wheel, to which the gearing was attached, was made of cast iron and had projections on its outer rim to keep it from slipping. The cutting part consisted of a horizontal steel bar (called the cutter bar) to which triangular knives were attached, which slid back and forth in a groove, pro-

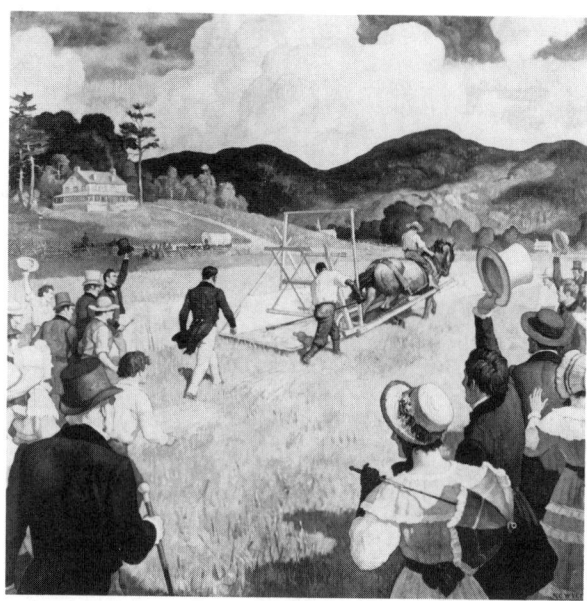

Fig. W-36. Cyrus McCormick's first reaper. This photograph, reproduction of a famous painting, shows the young inventor striding behind his masterpiece, the world's first reaper. A boy is riding the horse, and Jo Anderson, a slave, is raking the cut grain from the platform. Friends and neighbors are gathered in the field to witness the important test. In the distance are the Blue Ridge Mountains. The building on the left is Steele's Tavern. (Courtesy, International Harvester, Chicago, III.)

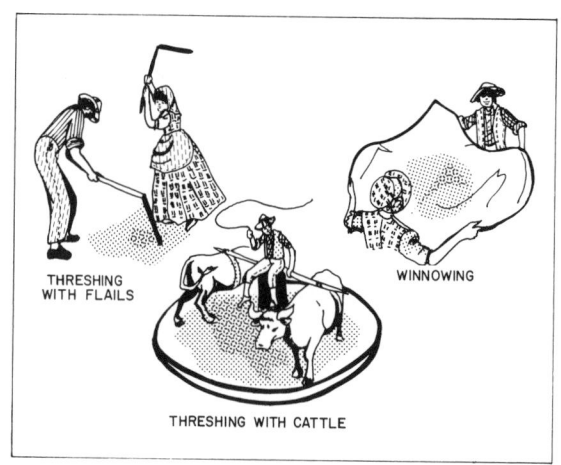

Fig. W-37. Primitive threshing.

tected by pointed guards. A reel swept the stalks back against the knives and picked up the stalks that were bent or lodged. As the grain was cut, it fell back on the platform. In the first models, a man walked beside the reaper and raked the cut stalks together by hand. Later a moving belt was added to collect the grain in a box. Men riding on a platform attached to the machine took it from this box and bound it. Then came the knotting device, a clever gadget which tied the sheaves before they were dropped to the ground.

At this point and period of time, harvesting was a two-phased operation; harvesting machines (binders) cut the wheat, then stationary threshing machines separated the stems and chaff from the kernels of grain.

Today, virtually all wheat is combined by machines that reap and thresh in one operation as they move across the field.

• **Threshing**—A number of primitive methods have been used, and are still used, in developing countries to thresh the cut grain and remove the wheat from the glumes. For thousands of years, wheat heads were spread on a plot of bare, hard ground, known as a threshing floor. Then cattle or horses were driven around and around on it, treading the wheat from the chaff. Separation was completed by winnowing—tossing the mixture into the air, with the wind blowing away the lighter chaff and heavier kernels dropping to the floor.

Also, a hand tool called a flail is still used in some of the developing countries. It consists of a short stick or club fastened by a leather strap to a long wooden handle. Farmers beat the grain from the straw with this crude implement. Then they toss the mixture of grain and straw into the air to be separated by the wind or by fanning it with a large sheet.

The Romans used a device called a tribulum for threshing. A series of small flints were set into a board. The board was turned face down, weighted with stones, and dragged across the grain. Such equipment and methods of threshing are still used today.

The need and ingenuity that led to the development of the reaper also led to the invention of the threshing machine. The first threshing machine used fans to separate the chaff from the grain. It was powered by a steam engine to which it was connected by means of a belt. "Threshing rigs," consisting of the threshing machine and the steam engine, were expensive. Often they were owned by companies of 10 to 25 farmers, or by independent businessmen. Moreover, it took a sizable crew of 20 to 30 people to operate a threshing rig. Usually, sufficient manpower was mobilized by the neighbors "swapping" help. The threshed grain was usually hauled from the fields in horse- or mule-drawn "bundle wagons" and fed into the threshing machine by means of a pitchfork. Sometimes, it was fed from a stack. Chaff and straw were blown into a stack; and clean grain was collected in a wagon or in bags.

The coming of the combine, which cut and threshed wheat in one operation, drove the threshing machine, powered by a steam engine, into oblivion. The grain from a combine goes into a truck drawn alongside the machine, or is collected in a bin mounted on the combine, and dumped when filled. The threshed straw is usually dropped from the rear of the machine. At first, combines were drawn by horses or tractors; today, most of them are self-powered. A wheat producer may own his own combine; may contract with a professional combine crew; or may join with neighboring farmers to harvest his own and nearby fields cooperatively.

FEDERAL GRADES OF WHEAT.

Based on the way that the grain is used, the following seven classes of wheat are recognized in the official grain standards of the United States:

1. Hard red spring wheat
2. Durum wheat
3. Red durum wheat
4. Hard red winter wheat
5. Soft red winter wheat
6. White wheat
7. Mixed wheat

In general, the criteria for grading wheat are: (1) test weight per bushel, (2) moisture content, (3) heat-damaged kernels, (4) damaged kernels, (5) foreign material, (6) shrunken and broken kernels, and (7) defects. The highest grade is U.S. No. 1 and the lowest is U.S. Sample grade.

Table W-11 gives the standards by which wheat is graded.

TABLE W-11
WHEAT GRADES AND GRADE REQUIREMENTS

Grade	Minimum Test Weight Per Bushel[2]		Maximum Limits of—					Wheat of Other Classes[1]	
			Defects						
	Hard Red Spring Wheat or White Club Wheat	All other classes and sub-classes	Heat damaged kernels	Dam-aged kernels (total)	Foreign material	Shrunken and broken kernels	Defects (total)	Con-trasting classes	Wheat of other classes (total)
	(lb)	(lb)	(%)	(%)	(%)	(%)	(%)	(%)	(%)
U.S. No. 1	58.0	60.0	.1	2.0	.5	3.0	3.0	1.0	3.0
U.S. No. 2	57.0	58.0	.2	4.0	1.0	5.0	5.0	2.0	5.0
U.S. No. 3	55.0	56.0	.5	7.0	2.0	8.0	8.0	3.0	10.0
U.S. No. 4	53.0	54.0	1.0	10.0	3.0	12.0	12.0	10.0	10.0
U.S. No. 5	50.0	51.0	3.0	15.0	5.0	20.0	20.0	10.0	10.0
U.S. Sample grade	U.S. Sample grade shall be wheat which does not meet the requirements for any of the grades from U.S. No. 1 to U.S. No. 5, inclusive; or which contains more than two crotalaria seeds (*Crotalaria spp.*) in 1,000g of grain, or contains castor beans (*Ricinus communis*), stones, broken glass, animal filth, an unknown foreign substance(s), or a commonly recognized harmful or toxic substance(s); or which is musty, sour, or heating; or which has any commercially objectionable foreign odor except of smut or garlic; or which contains a quantity of smut so great that any one or more of the grade requirements cannot be applied accurately; or which is otherwise of distinctly low quality.								

[1]Red durum wheat of any grade may contain not more than 10.0% of wheat of other classes.
[2]Divide by 2.2 to convert to kg.

MILLING WHEAT.

The main parts of the wheat grain are:

1. **The endosperm**, which constitutes about 83% of the kernel and is the source of white flour.

2. **The coat** (bran or coarse bran; and aleurone or fine bran), which constitutes about 14.5% of the kernel and is the source of bran, used primarily for animal feed.

3. **The germ**, which constitutes 2.5% of the kernel and is the source of wheat meal and wheat germ oil, used for human food or animal feed.

On threshing, the husk is removed and the grain is made naked. The wheat endosperm is covered with two kinds of fibrous coatings; the coarsest outer layer is called bran, and the less fibrous layer is the aleurone. At the base of the kernel is the germ. The objective of milling is to separate the starchy endosperm from the other parts of the grain. Whole wheat yields about 72% white flour, and 28% by-products, consisting of bran and germ. (By contrast, in China, by official ruling, the minimum extraction rate permissible for wheat flour is

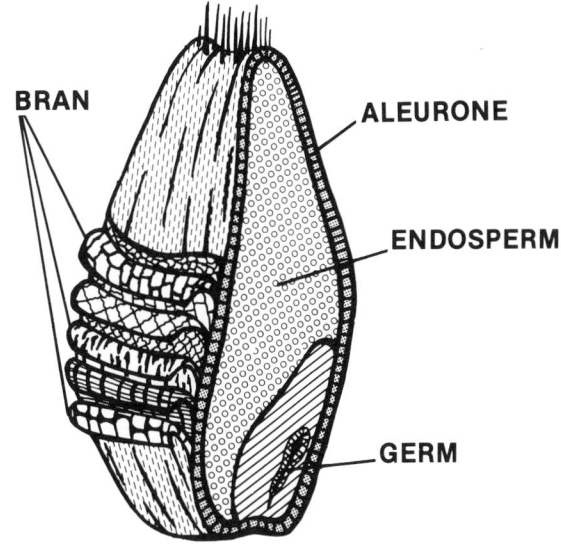

Fig. W-38. Structure of the wheat grain.

81%; hence, the wheat flour of China is less refined than in the United States.) Since an average bushel of wheat weighs 60 lb (*27 kg*), this means that approximately 2.3 bu of wheat are required to produce 100 lb (*45 kg*) of flour and 38 lb (*17 kg*) of millfeed.

Whole wheat flour, as the name would indicate, contains the finely ground endosperm, bran, and germ. In comparison with products made from white flour, whole wheat products have a distinctive flavor and a coarser texture, and, because of the higher fat content of the germ, they are more difficult to keep and sometimes become rancid.

Since prehistoric times, the goal of milling has been the separation of the bran and germ from the endosperm, to make white flour.

• **Primitive milling**—Pairs of stones, one for pounding or rubbing against the other, are found at the sites of ancient settlements in almost all parts of the world. Although crude, the pounding or rubbing of the whole wheat effectively reduced it to flour or meal. With an accompanying shuffling action, some of the bran was pushed to one side to leave a portion of the flour whiter than the rest. In some excavations, the pairs of stones suggest the beginning of the mortar and pestle; in others the two stones suggest saddlestones; and in still others the rotary action of two stones suggests a quern.

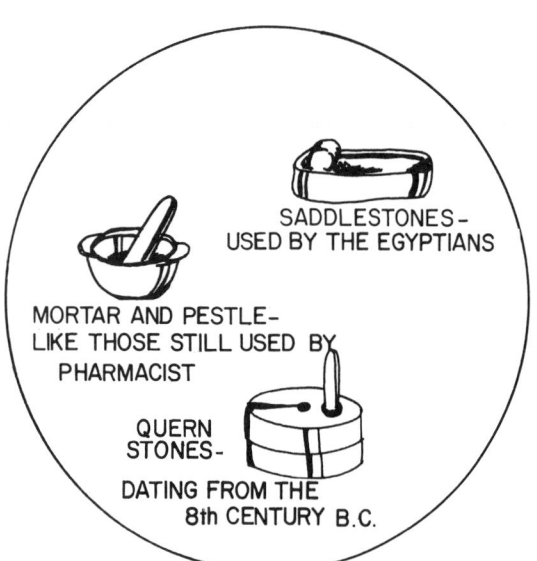

Fig. W-39.   Millstones—the first flour mills.

The addition of levers to millstones gave millers more power and increased output, and the extension of the top stone of the quern made a hopper. But, for thousands of years, flour for bread was produced by mills employing exactly the same principle—two stones, geared so that one turned against the other; powered by men, horses, oxen, water, or wind.

• **Milling in early America**—Oliver Evans, an ingenious American millwright, introduced screw conveyors and bucket elevators and developed a continuous system for milling flour as a single, uninterrupted operation. Evans granted a license to Thomas Jefferson in 1808, permitting him to use his improved technology. It is noteworthy, too, that George Washington was both a wheat farmer and a miller, and that his flour was known for its quality.

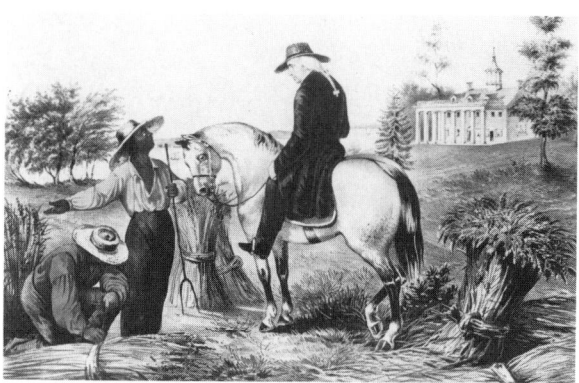

Fig. W-40.   George Washington, wheat farmer, at Mount Vernon. (From a Currier and Ives lithograph, obtained from The Bettmann Archive)

The invention of the steam engine by James Watt in 1769, the introduction of the roller mill system, and the application of the middlings purifier, combined to make modern milling.

The steam engine could be geared directly to the turning of millstones or employed to raise water in reservoirs, freeing the miller from his dependence on natural sources of power.

Corrugated rollers eliminated the cost of dressing millstones and produced a larger amount of better grade flour from a given amount of wheat.

The middlings purifier improved the yield and grade of flour through better separation of the outer bran and germ from the floury, inner endosperm.

• **Modern milling**—In modern milling, wheat passes through about 2 dozen processes before it is made into table flour. Fig. W-4I is a simplified diagram showing what happens in milling.

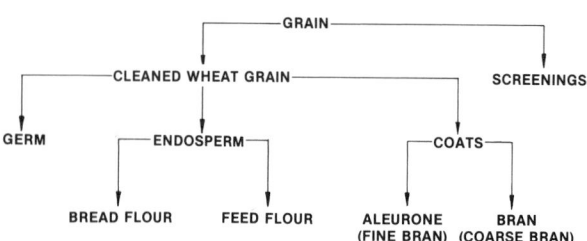

Fig. W-41.   A simplified flow diagram of wheat milling.

No two flour mills are ever quite alike—in the exact sequence, placement of identity of machinery. Nevertheless, the flow chart in Fig. W-42 shows the basic steps in processing wheat into flour.

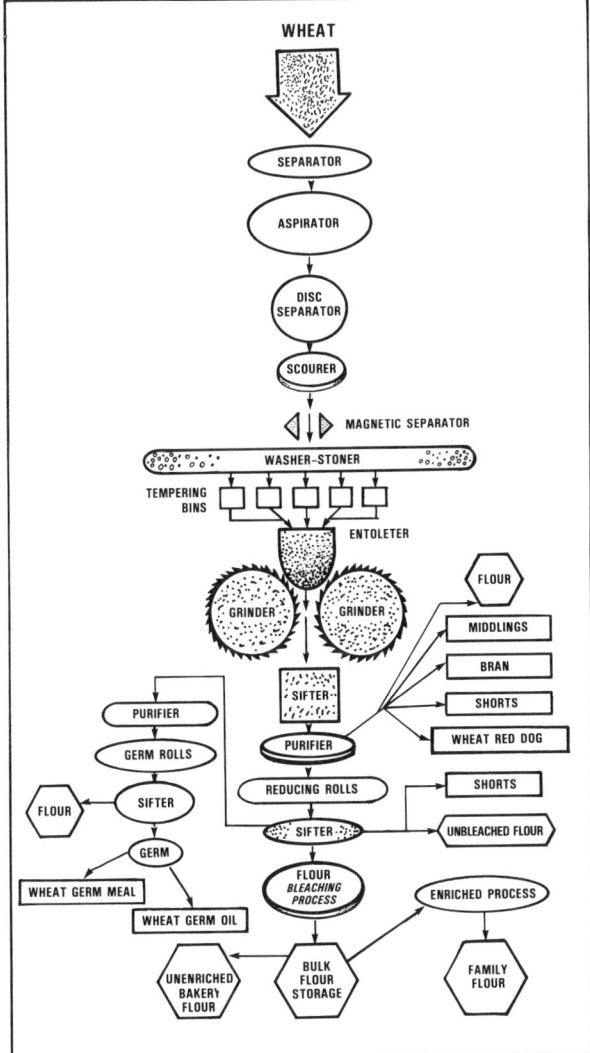

Fig. W-42. Mill flow diagram. The hexagonals show products for human consumption; the rectangles show products for livestock.

A brief explanation of the mill flow diagram follows:

1. **Cleaning the wheat.** At the very beginning of the milling process, there are a number of pieces of equipment and steps for separating wheat from other seeds and foreign material, and for cleaning and scouring each small kernel. In Fig. W-42, the cleaning process begins with a separator and extends to the "tempering bins."

2. **Conditioning the wheat for grinding.** The modern miller conditions or "tempers" wheat before grinding; a process in which moisture is added (up to approximately 16% properly dispersed in the grains). Tempering facilitates the separation of the bran from the endosperm and helps provide a constant, controlled amount of moisture and temperature throughout the milling process.

3. **Grinding wheat.** From the Entoleter machines, the wheat is fed in a continuous, metered stream into the grinder. The "first break" rolls of a mill are corrugated, rather than smooth like the reduction rolls that reduce the particles of endosperm further along in the process. From here on the process is repeated over and over again—sifters, purifiers, reducing rolls—until the maximum amount of flour is separated, consisting of at least 72% of the wheat. The other 28% of the kernel is classified as millfeed.

Toward the end of the line in the millstream, the finished flour flows through a device which releases a bleaching-maturing agent in measured amounts.

If intended for packing as family flour, the enrichment ingredients—a combination of thiamin, niacin, riboflavin, and iron—are added in a mixing machine as the flour flows to the packing room. If intended for bakery customers, the flour is not enriched, since most bakers add their own form of enrichment formula to dough. If the flour is self-rising, a leavening agent and salt are added at this stage, to both family and bakery flour.

Flour may be packed in standard 2, 5, 10, 25, 50, or 100 lb bags; or it may be shipped in 3,000 lb (1,361 kg) metal containers ("tote bins"), or 45,000 lb (20,408 kg) bulk trucks, or 100,000 lb (45,351 kg) bulk hopper railway cars.

• **New milling developments**—Since plump wheat is about 83% endosperm and 17% bran and germ, ideal milling would remove all the floury inner portion, because flour is more valuable than feed. Generally speaking, millers have not been able to remove more than 72% acceptable white flour, leaving the balance mixed with various millfeeds. Nevertheless, some mills are more efficient than others, with the result that they are able to mill more flour of a better grade from a given shipment of wheat than their competitors.

Machines, developed in the early 1960s, grind flour finer than the usual roller mill, following which air classifiers separate the larger, heavier granules containing more carbohydrate from the smaller, lighter particles containing more protein (15 to 22%). The high-carbohydrate flour is suitable for cakes, cookies, and pastries. The high-protein flour may be used alone or to fortify and blend with other flours. Blending permits a miller to tailor a flour of exact protein value to a buyer's specifications.

Another development in milling technology has come with the construction of an improved type of "compact mill," approaching a push button level of automation.

Flour. Different grades and kinds of wheat are required for milling into the several grades and kinds of flours.

GRADES OF FLOUR; TEST BAKING. The highest quality flour is known as "patent flour."

The percentage of protein in a flour generally serves as one standard of quality. The protein of wheat and flour is composed of *gliadin* and *glutenin*, which, when mixed with liquid, form *gluten*. The elastic gluten developed by kneading the dough entraps the carbon dioxide formed by the fermentation of sugar and starches by yeast, or released by chemical leavening or air beaten into the mixture. The result is the unique "rising" or expansion characteristics of wheat flour doughs.

The mineral or ash content of flour is also used as an index of flour quality or grade; the lower the ash, or the lesser the residue, the whiter or more refined the flour.

Small quantities of wheat are usually milled for test baking. Various flours are checked by different baking

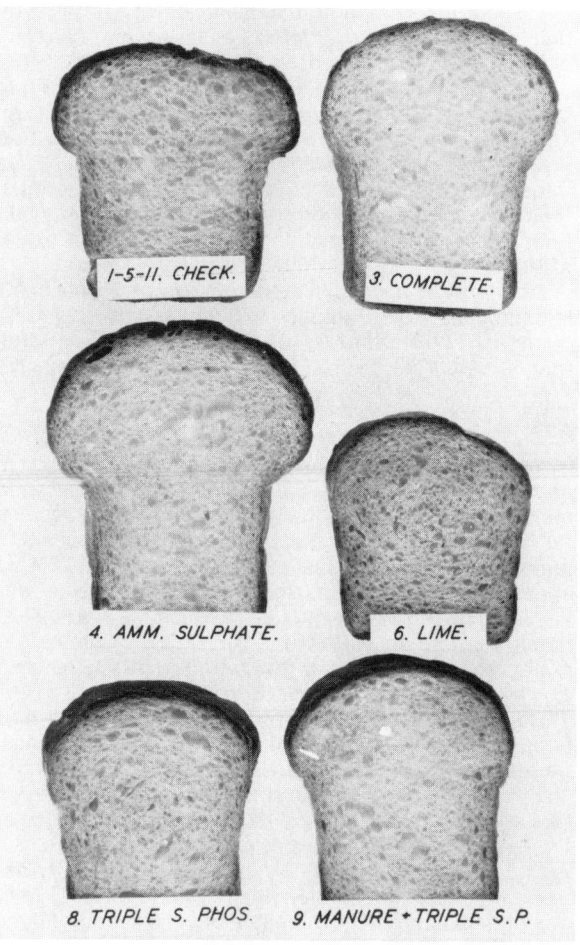

1-5-11. CHECK. *3. COMPLETE.*

4. AMM. SULPHATE. *6. LIME.*

8. TRIPLE S. PHOS. *9. MANURE + TRIPLE S.P.*

Fig. W-43. Baking tests reveal important differences in the quality of the bread (as indicated by the appearance of the loaves) made from wheat produced by different fertilizer treatments. (Courtesy, The University of Alberta, Edmonton, Canada)

procedures according to end use. For hard wheat, test loaves are baked to determine the mixing time and tolerance of doughs, the degree to which the flour will absorb liquid, potential loaf volume, texture, crumb, color, and flavor. For soft wheat, similar determinations are made with test cakes, cookies, or crackers.

KINDS OF FLOURS. There are many kinds of flours, each designed and best suited for a specific purpose, the main ones of which are discussed in the sections that follow:

• **Bakery flour**—Bakery bread wheat doughs are usually processed by machinery; therefore, the dough must have machine tolerance, or strength, in order to withstand the beating action of mechanical kneading and handling. This calls for "stronger" wheat—higher in the proteins, gliadin and glutenin, which form gluten—resulting in stronger doughs.

During the 1950s, the separate steps in the dough mixing method were consolidated into machines that process dough continuously. Continuous mixing machines require flours with critical requirements on almost every point, including granulation.

• **Family flour**—The decreasing production and sale of family flour reflects the decline in home baking.

Bread doughs worked by hand require strong arms, somewhat limiting the market to flour made from mellow gluten wheats that produce doughs that can be hand manipulated. There has been a trend away from the use of very strong wheats because the average homemaker does not have the strength or the patience to knead the dough long enough to develop the strong gluten.

The problems of the family flour requirements were partially solved with the making of "all-purpose" flours—mixed flours suited for both (1) good cakes, biscuits, and pastries, and (2) good bread.

Another innovation of family flour developed in the early 1960s was a granular or more dispersible type of flour. From the standpoint of the family, this flour offers the following advantages in comparison with regular flour: free-pouring—like salt; dust-free; alleviating the need for sifting; and dispersing in cold liquid, rather than balling or lumping.

Special soft wheat cake flours, and whole wheat flours are also available to homemakers. Graham flour is a whole wheat product made from 11.5% protein hard red winter wheat.

• **Specialty flours**—For the bakery trade, millers make a wide variety of different flours designed for different products, such as Italian and French breads and rolls.

Small retail shops usually keep a supply of several different kinds of flour, including: hard wheat flour for breads; soft wheat or cake flour for cookies, cakes, doughnuts, and cakelike products; and in-between flour for certain rolls, coffee cakes, and other pastries.

Special soft wheat flours are milled for cookie, cracker,

and pretzel bakers; and other special flours are prepared for canners who make soups, gravies, desserts requiring thickening, and flour-based sauces.

• **Durum wheat flour**—The milling of durum wheat flour for making macaroni requires additional purifiers to separate the branny material from the desired semolina, a coarse granulation of the endosperm. By federal definition, semolina cannot contain more than 3% flour.

Durum millers also make "granulars," or a coarse product with greater amounts of flour; or they grind the wheat into flour for special use in macaroni products, particularly in noodles.

• **Bleached flour**—At one time, it was necessary to age flour; by storing it in a warehouse for a considerable time and turning it so as to expose it to the oxidizing action of the air. The stored flour lost some of its creamy color and baked better. But the process necessitated storage facilities, took time, and required labor; and the results were variable. Today, the same end result is achieved, more quickly and better, by the use of additives. In either case, the proteins are slightly oxidized. In storage, they're oxidized from the air; in bleaching, they're oxidized from the maturing agent. The oxidation of flour makes gluten stronger, or more elastic, and produces better baking results. Some oxidizing agents, such as those in which a calcium or phosphorus compound is used as a carrier, also improve the nutritive value of the flour. Only cookie, pie crust, and cracker flours are more satisfactory without bleach.

Today, flour must be plainly marked "bleached" if one of several government approved oxidizing-maturing agents has been added.

• **Phosphated flour**—Phosphated flour is popular in certain areas, particularly where biscuits are commonly made with sour milk and buttermilk. Since the acid content of sour milk varies, phosphated flour provides greater assurance of leavening action from baking soda. The amount of calcium phosphate permitted in the flour is very small, not less than 0.25% and not more than 0.75%. Nevertheless, this low level of phosphation constitutes a significant nutritional enhancement, because a cup (*115 g*) of sifted phosphated flour supplies from 68 mg to 165 mg of calcium, and from 176 to 328 mg of phosphorus—compared to only 18 mg of calcium and 100 mg of phosphorus in unphosphated flour.

• **Self-rising flour**—Calcium phosphate is an ingredient of baking powder as well as in the leavening agents of self-rising flour, which also contains salt and soda. A typical self-rising flour contains 305 mg of calcium and 536 mg of phosphorus per cup (*115 g*).

In chemically-leavened flour, in the presence of liquid, the acid of the phosphate reacts with baking soda to produce a leavening gas, carbon dioxide—the same as the yeast organisms produce in yeast-raised products. Addi-

tionally, the calcium and phosphorus improve the nutritive qualities of the flour.

• **Whole wheat, cracked wheat, farina**—Whole wheat (or graham flour) is made from the entire wheat kernel.

Cracked or crushed wheat refers to wheat that has been broken into fragments.

Farina is purified middlings; it is the glandular endosperm that contains no bran and no more than 3% flour. Farina is most commonly used as a cooked breakfast cereal.

(Also see FLOUR, Table F-25 Major Flours.)

Enriched Flour. Since 1941, millers and bakers have followed the practice of enriching their products. Earlier surveys had indicated that the levels of certain nutrients were inadequate in the national diet; among them, the B vitamins, iron, iodine, and vitamin D. Since public need was demonstrated, the American Medical Association, leading nutritionists, government agencies, millers, and bakers worked together to develop an enrichment program with widely used, available, and inexpensive foods, like bread, to serve as carriers.

Originally, the FDA differentiated between enrichment and fortification, but now the two programs are used interchangeably. Nevertheless, the following vocabulary for and definition of food improvement persist:

• **Enriched**[1]—Refers to the addition of specific nutrients to a food *as established in a federal standard of identity and quality* (for example: enriched bread). The amounts added generally are moderate and include those commonly present at even lower levels.

• **Fortified**[2]—Refers to the addition to foods of specific nutrients. The amounts added are usually in excess of those normally found in the food because of the importance of providing additional amounts of the nutrients to the diet. Some foods are selected for fortification because they are an appropriate carrier for the nutrient. *Example*: Milk is frequently fortified with vitamin D.

• **Restored**—The replacement of nutrients lost in processing food.

Although the principle followed with white flour is basically enrichment, rather than restoration, and although the quantity of the nutrients in the enrichment formula were established on the basis of dietary need, they also happen to restore to white flour the approximate amounts of those same nutrients as were present in whole wheat (see Table W-12).

---

[1]"Nutrition Labeling—Terms You Should Know," *FDA Consumer Memo*, DHEW Publication No. 74-2010, 1974, pp. 2-3.

[2]*Ibid.*

TABLE W-12

COMPARISON OF NUTRIENTS IN WHEAT FLOUR AND WHEAT BREAD[1]

(Minimum and maximum enrichment levels for the three B vitamins —
thiamin, riboflavin, and niacin — and iron are given in the table below)

One Pound[2]	Protein	Fat	Calcium	Iron	Thiamin	Riboflavin	Niacin
	(g)	(g)	(mg)	(mg)	(mg)	(mg)	(mg)
Flour							
Whole Wheat	60.3	9.1	186	15.0	2.49	.54	19.7
Unenriched (all purpose)	47.6	4.5	73	3.6	.28	.21	4.1
Enriched (all purpose)	47.6	4.5	73-960[3]	13.-16.5[3]	2.90[3]	1.80[3]	24.0[3]
Bread							
Whole Wheat (2% nonfat dry milk)	47.6	13.6	449	10.4	1.17	.56	12.9
Unenriched (white) (3 to 4% nonfat dry milk)	39.5	14.5	381	3.2	.31	.39	5.0
Enriched (white) (3 to 4% nonfat dry milk)	39.5	14.5	381-600[4]	8.-12.5[4]	1.80[4]	1.10[4]	15.04

[1]The source of this data is *From Wheat to Flour*, published by Wheat Flour Institute, Chicago, Ill., 1976, p. 68; except where noted otherwise.
[2]Multiply by 2.2 to obtain the amount per kg.
[3]*Code of Federal Regulations*, Title 21, Revised 4/1/78, Section 137.165 provides that enriched flour must contain the specified amounts of iron, thiamin, riboflavin, and niacin; but that the addition of calcium is optional. However, no claim for calcium on the label may be made if the flour contains less than 960 mg per lb.
[4]*Code of Federal Regulations*, Title 21, Revised 4/1/78, Section 136.115 provides that enriched bread, buns, and rolls must contain the specified amounts of iron, thiamin, riboflavin, and niacin; but that the addition of calcium is optional. However, no claim for calcium on the label may be made if the bread contains less than 600 mg per lb.

Tables W-13, W-14, W-15, and W-16 show the standards for enriching flour, self-rising flour, macaroni products, and enriched bread, buns, and rolls. Calcium and vitamin D are permitted as optional additions to flour and bread, in the amounts specified. At about the same time that the flour enrichment program got underway (1941), iodine was added to table salt to prevent goiter, and vitamin D was added to milk to prevent rickets (Since most milk is now fortified with vitamin D, it is seldom added to bakery foods).

TABLE W-13

STANDARD FOR ENRICHED FLOUR[1]

Required Ingredients per Pound of Flour[2]	
Thiamin	2.9 mg
Riboflavin	1.8 mg
Niacin	24.0 mg
Iron	13.0-16.5 mg
Optional Ingredient	
Calcium	960 mg

[1]*Code of Federal Regulations*, Title 21, Revised 4/1/78, Section 137.165.
[2]Multiply by 2.2 to obtain the amount per kg.

TABLE W-14

STANDARD FOR ENRICHED SELF-RISING FLOUR[1]

Required Ingredients per Pound of Flour[2]	
Thiamin	2.9 mg
Riboflavin	1.8 mg
Niacin	24.0 mg
Iron	13.0-16.5 mg
Optional Ingredient	
Calcium	960 mg

[1]*Code of Federal Regulations*, Title 21, Revised 4/1/78, Section 137.185.
[2]Multiply by 2.2 to obtain the amount per kg.

TABLE W-15

STANDARD FOR ENRICHED MACARONI PRODUCTS[1]

Required Ingredients per Pound of Flour[2]		
	(minimum)	(maximum)
Thiamin	4.0 mg	5.0 mg
Riboflavin	1.7 mg	2.2 mg
Niacin	27.0 mg	34.0 mg
Iron	13.0 mg	16.5 mg
Optional Ingredients		
Calcium	500.0 mg	625.0 mg
Vitamin D	250 U.S.P. units	1000 U.S.P. units

[1]*Code of Federal Regulations*, Title 21, Revised 4/1/78, Section 139.115.
[2]Multiply by 2.2 to obtain the amount per kg.

TABLE W-16

STANDARD FOR ENRICHED BREAD, BUNS, AND ROLLS[1]

Required Ingredients per Pound of Flour[2]	
Thiamin	1.8 mg
Riboflavin	1.1 mg
Niacin	15.0 mg
Iron	8.0-12.5 mg
Optional Ingredient	
Calcium	600.0 mg

[1]*Code of Federal Regulations*, Title 21, Revised 4/1/78, Section 136.115.
[2]Multiply by 2.2 to obtain the amount per kg.

Since the start of the enrichment program in 1941, the available supplies of the B vitamins—thiamin, riboflavin, and niacin—and of iron in the national diet have increased. The enrichment program has played a significant role in the practical elimination of the vitamin deficiency diseases ariboflavinosis, beriberi, and pellagra, and of simple iron-deficiency anemia.

Today, enrichment is required in 34 states and Puerto Rico. In practice, however, all family flour is enriched, and about 90% of all commercially baked standard white bread is enriched.

As shown in Table W-12, whole wheat and enriched flour and breads contribute almost equal amounts of a number of those nutrients considered essential for optimum nutrition. But because less than 2% of wheat used for food is eaten in whole wheat form, enriched products are by far the more important in American diets.

It is noteworthy that England, Canada, and a few other countries have enrichment programs somewhat similar to the United States, but that France forbids enrichment.

NUTRITIONAL VALUE OF WHEAT. Whole wheat flour is made by grinding the entire kernel of wheat. Thus, it contains nutrients found in all three parts—the bran, endosperm, and germ. To produce white flour which

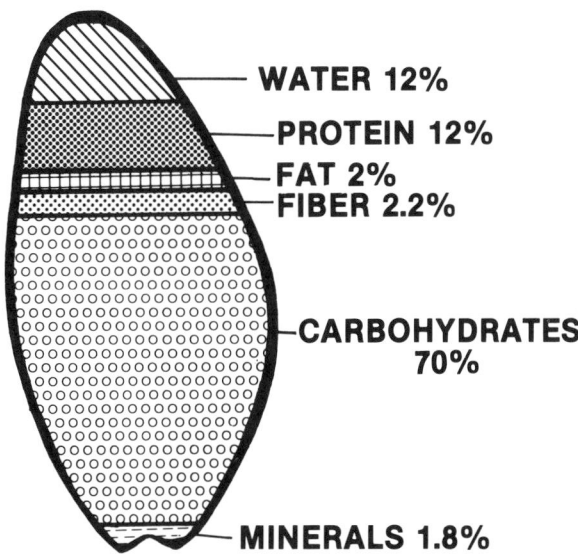

WATER 12%

PROTEIN 12%

FAT 2%

FIBER 2.2%

CARBOHYDRATES 70%

MINERALS 1.8%

Fig. W-44. Proximate analysis of whole wheat.

has better keeping qualities than whole wheat flour, millers remove the bran and germ and use only the endosperm. Some of the B vitamins, calcium, and iron are lost. The processing of white flour removes additional nutrients.

Wheat is high in carbohydrates; hence, it is a high energy source. Its contribution to the available food energy of the following countries is noteworthy: Israel, 35%; France, 30%; Australia, 25%; England, 20%; and United States, Canada, and West Germany, 18%. As a

source of energy in the United States, wheat ranks on a par with three other major sources of energy: meats, processed fats, and processed sugar. Together, these four foods comprise three-fourths of the food energy available in the United States.

Wheat has the highest protein value of any of the cereals. Still, the protein is of poor quality. Table W-17 compares the essential amino acids in whole wheat, white flour, and wheat germ to high-quality proteins. Like rice and corn and their products wheat is particularly deficient in lysine; hence, it should be eaten with a complementary protein source such as a legume. Although not indicated in Table W-17, wheat germ contains about 23% protein, whole wheat contains about 12% protein and white flour contains about 11% protein. Interestingly, the protein in wheat germ is extra rich in lysine, the amino acid that is deficient in the rest of the wheat grain.

TABLE W–17
PROFILE OF ESSENTIAL AMINO ACIDS IN WHOLE WHEAT, WHITE FLOUR, AND WHEAT GERM COMPARED TO MILK— A HIGH-QUALITY PROTEIN[1,2]

Amino Acid	Whole Wheat	White Flour	Wheat Germ	Cow's Milk
	← (mg/g protein) →			
Histidine	19	20	27	27
Isoleucine	32	46	36	47
Leucine	58	77	64	95
Lysine	25	22	63	78
Methionine and cystine	33	33	37	33
Phenylalanine and tyrosine	68	89	68	102
Threonine	26	29	40	44
Tryptophan	11	12	12	14
Valine	38	43	48	64

[1]Additional information about the essential amino acid content of wheat and flour products may be found in Table P-37, Proteins and Amino Acids in Selected Foods.
[2]*Recommended Dietary Allowances*, 10th ed., 1989, National Academy of Sciences, p. 67, Table 6–5. The essential amino acid requirements of infants can be met by supplying 0.79 g of a high-quality protein per pound of body weight (1.73 g/kg body weight) per day.

The nutritive value of the many different forms of wheat and wheat products is given in Food Composition Table F-36.

(Also see BREADS AND BAKING, sections headed "Nutritive Values of Breads and Related Items," and "Improving the Nutritive Values of Breads and Baked Goods"; MINERAL[S]; PROTEIN[S]; and VITAMIN[S].)

For some individuals, the consumption of wheat creates health problems. If supplementary foods are inadequate, excessive amounts of wheat products can lead to kwashiorkor or beriberi. However, persons to whom wheat products are available are usually able to obtain a wider variety of foods, and deficiency diseases have not been directly attributed to overdependence on wheat products. Celiac disease, however, is apparently due to a genetically-determined intolerance to wheat gluten or an acquired defect in the intestinal lining. Also, the use of refined flour in wheat products, especially those of a sticky nature such as biscuits, is believed to be a major factor predisposing to dental caries.

WHEAT PRODUCTS AND USES. The most common use of wheat is for food made from flour. Breakfast foods and beer or other alcoholic fermentations also take considerable quantities of wheat.

Breads date back thousands of years, in war and in peace, in famine and in plenty, to the discovery of wheat, the invention of milling, and the development of baking.

Wheat is not normally fed to animals because of its high cost and greater value for human food. However, surplus or damaged wheat and the by-products of milling find important use as livestock feeds and, eventually, enter the human diet as meat, milk, and eggs. Some wheat products are also used for industrial purposes.

Table W-18 presents in summary form the story of wheat products and uses.

(Also see BREADS AND BAKING; CEREAL GRAINS, Table C-18 Cereal Grains of the World; and BREAKFAST CEREALS.)

TABLE W-18
WHEAT PRODUCTS AND USES

Product	Description	Uses	Comments
HUMAN FOODS			
Flour	White flour is the finely ground endosperm of wheat. Whole wheat flour contains the finely ground endosperm, bran, and germ.	Wheat flours are used for many purposes, such as bread, pastries, cakes, cookies, crackers, macaroni, puddings, and soups. (Also see BREADS AND BAKING, section headed "Types of Breads and Baked Doughs.")	For each purpose, a flour of particular properties is required. Additives, such as maturing agents, bleaching agents, and self-rising ingredients, are frequently blended into wheat flours at the mill. Family flour is enriched at the mill, while flour being shipped to the baker is enriched at the bakery.
Bulgur	A partly debranned, parboiled wheat product, used either whole or cracked.	Bulgur is used as a substitute for rice; e.g., in pilaf, an eastern European dish consisting of wheat, meat, oil, and herbs cooked together.	Bulgur is exported in large quantities, especially to the Far East. Bulgur provides a cheap food that is acceptable to rice-eating people because it can be cooked in the same way as rice, and it resembles rice superficially.
Fermented minchin	A product made by putting wheat gluten in a tightly covered container for 2 to 3 weeks and allowing it to be overgrown with both molds and bacteria. Then 10% salt is added and the mixture allowed to age for 2 weeks.	Aged fermented minchin is cut into thin strips and used as a condiment with other foods.	
Wheat germ	The germ is the embryo or sprouting part of the wheat seed.	As an ingredient of specialty breads.	Wheat germ is available for human food, but it is usually added to animal feeds.
Wheat gluten	Wheat gluten is a mixture of two proteins, gliadin and glutenin. When mixed with water, they impart the characteristic stickiness to dough.	For making monosodium glutamate which imparts a meatlike flavor to foods. For adding to white flour to make a high-gluten bread.	Some people may develop an intolerance to gluten.
Wheat starch	A white, odorless, tasteless granular or powdery material.	Wheat starch is used as a thickener in soup where its lower gelatinization temperature and shorter gel temperature range is an advantage. Syrup and sugar.	

(Continued)

TABLE W-18 *(Continued)*

Product	Description	Uses	Comments
		HUMAN FOODS *(Continued)*	
Wheat tempeh	Fermented cake of cooked wheat grains.	Vegetarian main dish when sliced and baked or fried, topping and/or an ingredient of salads, sandwiches, soups, sauces, casseroles, and spreads.	An experimental food developed by USDA scientists who utilized the mold *Rhizopus oligosporus* in a procedure similar to that used by Asians to make soybean tempeh. The nutritional value of the original grain is enhanced by the mold fermentation in that (1) proteins are partially digested, and (2) certain B vitamins are synthesized. It is noteworthy that the mold synthesizes vitamin B-12, which makes tempeh one of the few vegetable foods that contain the vitamin.
Breakfast foods, ready-to-eat: Bran flakes	Tan colored, paper thin flakes.	Ready-to-eat breakfast food.	
Puffed wheat	Whole wheat depericarped (the outer covering removed), cooked, puffed by extruding through a machine, then dried-toasted.	Ready-to-eat breakfast food.	(Also see BREAKFAST CEREALS.)
Shredded wheat	Whole wheat is cooked with water to gelatinize starch, cooled, shredded by machine, cut to shape, baked, then dried and cooled.	Ready-to-eat breakfast food.	Shredded wheat has a protein content considerably lower than puffed wheat.
Wheat flakes	Whole wheat, that has been rolled, cooked, flavored, then dried.	Ready-to-eat breakfast food.	
Breakfast foods, to be cooked: Whole wheat grains	Unground whole wheat.	Cooked cereals, starchy vegetable, puddings such as frumenty.	Cook 40-50 minutes in an open pot or a pressure cooker after soaking overnight in water. Frumenty is cooked grains which have been reheated with milk and served with cream, butter, sugar, and/or jam.
Cracked wheat	Whole grains broken into small pieces.	Cooked cereals, breads, soups, casseroles, starchy vegetable.	Cracked wheat has a nutlike flavor and texture, and cooks much faster than whole kernels of the grain. Only limited amounts can be used in breads because the sharp edges on the particles cut the strands of gluten which make the dough elastic.
Farina (Cream of Wheat)	This is granulated endosperm that contains no bran and no more than 3% flour; it's similar to semolina except that the wheat is not a durum variety.	A hot breakfast cereal.	Enriched farina is popularly known as "Cream of Wheat", a product made famous by Nabisco.
Malted cereals	Cracked wheat and malted barley, mixed.	Cooked cereals, baked items.	May also be used to make muffins and other quick breads.
Rolled wheat	Whole grains rolled into flat pieces (flakes) after steaming.	Cooked cereals, cookies, filler in meatloaf.	Can be substituted for rolled oats in most recipes.
Wheat meal	Ground wheat from which the bran has been removed.	Cooked wheat breakfast foods.	

(Continued)

TABLE W-18 (*Continued*)

Product	Description	Uses	Comments
FORTIFIED FOODS, BASED ON WHEAT PRODUCTS, FOR DEVELOPING COUNTRIES			
Bal Ahar	Coarsely ground mixture of bulgur wheat, peanut flour, skim milk powder, minerals and vitamins. Contains 22% protein.	Infant cereal, suitable for mixing with water.	Produced by the government of India The protein quality is on a par with that of milk.
Bread fortified with lowfat cottonseed flour	Bread made from a mixture of 90% wheat flour and 10% cottonseed flour.	High protein bread.	Developed at Universidad Agraria La Molina in Lima, Peru. The special cottonseed flour (Protal) raises the protein level of wheat bread from 9% to 11%.
Cereal products fortified with fish protein concentrate (FPC)	Products made from wheat flour fortified with dried, defatted, whole fish powder.	Breads, crackers, and noodles.	Developed at Universidad Agraria La Molina in Lima, Peru.
Fortified atta	Whole wheat flour mixed with peanut flour, minerals and vitamins.	Baked goods commonly used by people in India.	Produced by flour mills that are subsidized by the Indian government. Breads resemble unleavened breads in consistency, and contain about 13.5% protein.
Fortified couscous	Coarsely ground wheat mixed with high protein wheat fractions.	Cereals, casseroles, soups, and other traditional dishes prepared by people in Algeria and neighboring countries.	Developed by International Milling for U.S. Agency for International Development (AID). High protein wheat fractions are obtained by special milling procedures. Fortified couscous has higher quantity and quality of protein than ordinary couscous.
Laubina	Finely ground mixture of cooked bulgur wheat, cooked chickpeas, skim milk powder, sugar, minerals, and vitamins.	Infant cereal.	Developed at the American University of Beirut in Lebanon. Promoted prompt recovery of hospitalized infants suffering from severe protein-energy malnutrition, but was not effective in curing anemia.
Leche alim	Mixture of toasted wheat flour, fish protein concentrate (FPC), sunflower meal, and skim milk powder. Contains 27% protein.	High protein infant cereal suitable for mixing with water.	Produced by the Pediatrics Laboratory of the University of Chile in Santiago.
Rolled wheat and soy flake mixture	Mixture of 85% rolled wheat and 15% soy flakes.	Cereal	Developed by USDA and test marketed by AID.
Superamine	Finely ground mixture of wheat flour, chickpea flour, lentil flour, skim milk powder, sugar, minerals, vitamins, and flavoring. Contains 21% protein.	High protein powder which may be mixed with water and cooked briefly (2 to 4 minutes).	Developed as a cooperative project between FAO, WHO, UNICEF, and the Algerian government.
Vitalia macaroni	Pasta made from semolina, wheat, soy, corn, and rice derivatives. Contains 18% protein.	High protein macaroni product.	Produced by Instituto de Investigaciones Tecnoligicas, in Bogota, Colombia.
Wheat protein beverage powder	A finely ground mixture of wheat protein concentrate, skim milk powder, sugar, vegetable oil, minerals, vitamins, and flavoring.	Powder suitable for mixing with water to make a high protein beverage.	Experimental products developed by USDA scientists, who devised means of producing a partially digested, low starch, high protein concentrate from wheat flour. Protein quality is intermediate between milk and egg proteins.

(*Continued*)

TABLE W-18 *(Continued)*

Product	Description	Uses	Comments
FERMENTATION BEVERAGES			
Wheat grain	Cleaned, whole wheat.	Canadian whiskey	Canadian whiskey is produced from any one of the cereal grains; hence, corn, rye, or barley may also be used.
Wheat starch	Malt converts wheat starch to sugar, which is fermented by yeast to ethyl alcohol and carbon dioxide.	1. Ethyl alcohol, used largely for alcoholic beverages. 2. Denatured alcohol for industrial purposes. 3. Gasohol (10% anhydrous ethanol, 90% gasoline) — a motor fuel.	(Also see CORN, section headed "Distilling and Fermentation.")
LIVESTOCK FEEDS			
Wheat grain	The wheat grain, un-processed or pro-cessed.	All classes of livestock.	Whole wheat can be used for mature poultry, but the grain should be processed (generally it's cracked or coarsely ground) for most animals. Finely ground wheat forms a pasty mass in the mouth and is unpalatable. It is usually best that wheat not exceed 50% of the concentrate mix. Most of the wheat fed to livestock is in the form of mill by-products. Under the column headed "Description," wheat millfeeds as defined by the American Feed Control Officials are given.
Flour, feed	The finely ground en-dosperm of wheat.	Fed chiefly to young pigs, young calves, and poultry.	
Wheat bran	This is the coarse outer covering layer of the wheat kernel. It con-tains most of the vitamins and protein of the wheat grain. Bran is a bulky feed, with a slightly laxative effect.	Wheat bran is fed to all classes of livestock. Its bulk and laxative qualities make it a favorite (1) horse feed, (2) feed for animals just before and after parturition, and (3) for starting animals on feed. Because of the popularity of high-energy poultry rations, wheat bran is now less used in poultry rations than formerly.	
Wheat germ meal	This product consists chiefly of wheat germ together with some bran and middlings or shorts. Wheat germ meal is low in fiber, high in protein (minimum of 25% crude protein) and fat (minimum of 7%), and rich in vitamin E.	Used chiefly in dog foods, mink feeds, and feeds for laboratory animals.	
Wheat germ meal, defatted	This is the product that remains after removal of part of the oil or fat from wheat germ meal. It must contain not less than 30% crude protein.	Fed to all classes of livestock.	Much lower than wheat germ meal in fat and vitamin E.
Wheat germ oil	The oil extracted from wheat germ meal.	As a rich source of Vitamin E.	

(Continued)

Product	Description	Uses	Comments
		LIVESTOCK FEEDS (Continued)	
Wheat middlings	This is a mixture of fine particles of wheat bran, wheat shorts, wheat germ, and wheat flour; generally derived from milling spring wheat. It is the most common by-product from flour mills. Wheat middlings must not contain more than 9.5% crude fiber.	Used chiefly for swine, calves, and poultry, although they may be fed to other stock.	
Wheat red dog	This consists of the "tail of the mill" together with fine particles of wheat bran, wheat germ, and wheat flour. It must not contain more than 4% crude fiber.	Fed chiefly to swine, especially to young pigs, young calves, and poultry.	
Wheat screenings	This is the product obtained from the initial cleaning of wheat, consisting of small and shrunken kernels and weed seeds. It is usually finely ground and mixed with other wheat by-products. The declaration "Ground Wheat Screenings" must be included in the name of the product to which it is added, for example, "wheat shorts with ground wheat screenings."	All classes of livestock.	The composition is quite variable, and weed seeds are a hazard — unless screenings are finely ground.
Wheat shorts	This is a mixture of the fine particles of wheat bran, wheat germ, and wheat flour; generally derived from milling winter wheat. It must not contain more than 7% crude fiber.	Used chiefly for swine, calves, and poultry, although they may be fed to other stock.	
Forages: Wheat silage	Wheat cut for silage when the grain is in the milk to soft dough stage.	For ruminants.	Wheat for silage should be packed well.
Wheat straw	The straw of wheat following threshing.	Roughage for cattle.	Of the cereal straws, wheat ranks third in nutritive value — behind oat straw and barley straw. Highest and best use is for dry cows.
Wheat, hay	Wheat cut for hay when the stems and leaves are still green and the grain is in the milk to soft dough stage.	As a forage, primarily for cattle.	Wheat hay is about 70% as valuable as alfalfa hay for mature ruminants.
Wheat pasture	Usually, wheat pasture consists of winter wheat grown for grain, pastured lightly in the fall and early spring before the stems begin to elongate.	For cattle, sheep, and swine.	In the South and Southwest, wheat is often used as winter pasture, when most other pasture crops are dormant.

(Continued)

TABLE W-18 (*Continued*)

Product	Description	Uses	Comments
OTHER USES			
Wheat gluten	Wheat gluten is a mixture of the two proteins, gliadin and glutenin.	Adhesives, emulsifiers, polishes	
Wheat starch	A white powder, insoluble in alcohol and cold water.	Coating paper and paperboard, and as sizes in the manufacture of textiles	Corn starches are the dominant starches in the U.S. Wheat starch is used when some specific property is sought.
Wheat straw	The wheat stalk following threshing.	Stuffing or weaving material, as a soil mulch, and for livestock bedding.	

WHEAT FEED FLOUR

A wheat product consisting of wheat flour together with fine particles of wheat bran, wheat germ, and the offal from the "tail of the mill."

WHEAT GERM

Wheat germ is the embryo or sprouting part of the wheat seed. A kernel of wheat is composed of three principal parts: The starchy endosperm, which constitutes about 83% of the kernel and is the source of white flour; the coat, which constitutes about 14.5% of the kernel and is the source of bran; and the germ, which constitutes 2.5% of the kernel and is the source of wheat germ meal and wheat germ oil. Wheat germ meal is used chiefly as a livestock feed, although some of it is now used as a human nutritional supplement. Wheat germ oil is used primarily as a rich vitamin E supplement for man and animals.

Wheat germ meal consists chiefly of wheat germ together with some bran and middlings or shorts. It is low in fiber, good in protein (minimum 25% crude protein), high in fat (7%), and rich in vitamin E. Defatted wheat germ meal is the product that remains after removal of part of the oil or fat from wheat germ meal. It must not contain less than 30% crude protein; and it is much lower than wheat germ meal in vitamin E.

Flour millers use the endosperm to make white flour and discard the bran and germ. In discarding the bran and germ, they are losing 77% of the thiamin, 80% of the riboflavin, 81% of the niacin, 72% of the vitamin B-6, 50% of the pantothenic acid, 67% of the folacin, 86% of the alpha-tocopherol, and 29% of the choline.[3]

Thus, wheat germ is a rich source of the nutrients that are discarded from the flour in milling. However, the oil of wheat germ decomposes readily after the germ is removed from the kernel, causing short shelf life and problems in marketing raw wheat germ. Thus, the product is usually defatted when offered for sale. The label will show whether the germ is defatted.

Wheat germ is added to many kinds of foods, such as bread, cookies, cereals, and milkshakes. Wheat germ oil may be taken to restore nutrients lost in defatting the germs.

(Also see WHEAT.)

WHEATMEAL, NATIONAL

The name given to 85% extraction wheat flour when intoduced into the United Kingdom in 1941 (as distinct from whole wheat meal, which is 100% extraction). Later, the name was changed to "national flour."

WHEY

The water and solids of milk that remain after the curd is removed (e.g., in the manufacture of cheese). It contains about 93.5% water and 6.5% lactose, protein, minerals, enzymes, water-soluble vitamins, and traces of fat.

(Also see MILK AND MILK PRODUCTS.)

WHIPPLE'S DISEASE (INTESTINAL LIPODYSTROPHY)

A relatively rare, and previously considered fatal, disease of predominantly middle-age men. It is characterized by adominal pain, diarrhea progressing to steatorrhea (fatty diarrhea), marked weight loss, anemia, arthritis, fever, and impaired intestinal absorption—a malabsorption syndrome. Whipple's disease produces structural changes in the lymphatics and intestinal mucosa which seem responsible for the malabsorption. Usually there is evidence of the malabsorption of fat with the loss of fat soluble vitamins, vitamin B-12, and xylose. Furthermore, the victim demonstrates low blood levels of calcium, magnesium and potassium—hypocalcemia, hypomagnesemia, and hypokalemia, respectively. Ex-

---

[3]Schroeder, Henry A., M.D., "Losses of Vitamins and Trace Minerals Resulting from Processing and Preserving Foods," *The American Journal of Clinical Nutrition*, Vol. 24, May 1971, pp. 562-573, Table 3.

cessive loss of albumin into the intestine results in low circulating levels of albumin in the blood—hypoalbuminemia. Evidence from intestinal biopsies suggests that it is due to a microorganism. Moreover, antibiotic therapy brings about dramatic improvement, but it is required on a long-term (10 to 12 months) basis.

Diet and replacement therapy are based on the nutritional deficiencies evident, on-going needs, and specific absorptive defects.

(Also see MODIFIED DIETS; and MALABSORPTION SYNDROME.)

WHITE BLOOD CELLS (LEUKOCYTES)

The colorless blood cells, generally called white blood cells or corpuscles.

WHOLE WHEAT MEAL

Meal that is made by grinding the entire wheat kernel.

WILD EDIBLE PLANTS

In the beginning, all plants were wild. Then, through the ages man collected, selected, and cultivated those plants which fitted his needs, while the others remained in the wild. As man started to travel more widely, he carried plants with him to introduce to new locations. Occasionally, these would escape his cultivation and fare so well in their new environment that they eventually became a wild plant—sometimes a weed. Still others, came as weeds, but they came from other countries with crop seeds or on animals or birds.

Often what is called a wild plant, and an unfamiliar food source to most, was however, very familiar to the natives of a land. When colonists arrived in the New World, very few Indians had gardens or cultivated crops. Instead, most of them supplemented their diets by collecting edible wild plants with which they were familiar. Instead of the potatoes, carrots, radishes, parsnips, beets, and turnips known today, Indians relied on wild roots and tubers. They also collected various nuts, fruits, greens, and seeds. In some areas, natives still depend upon edible wild plants for food, and at times a distinction between wild and domesticated is difficult.

Perhaps, the future of edible wild plants lies ahead, as some wild plants may represent forgotten or undiscovered food sources. Wild edible indigenous plants, if exploited, could offer alternative food sources in some areas of the world. In addition, there are other plants which could be exploited for fiber, energy, and medicine.

TYPES OF WILD FOODS AVAILABLE. In the wild a knowledgeable person may find the selection of foods as varied as that in the supermarket. Wild greens for use in salads or for cooking as a potherb include dandelions, chickweed, clover, chicory, miner's lettuce, mint, purslane, lamb's quarter, and watercress. Roots and tubers, or potatolike wild foods include the arrowhead, bulrush, cattail, and water lily. Shoots and stems that can be used as a vegetable include asparagus, burdock, bracken fern, and thistle. There is an endless array of wild nuts and berries available. Many plants produce seeds which can be ground and used like meal or flour. Nature even provides substitutes for coffee and tea. Many leaves can be brewed green or dried for tealike beverages; for example, wintergreen, catnip, colt's foot, Labrador tea, and cassina (holly). Caffeineless coffee substitutes can be made from roasted roots of chicory, chufa, dandelions, or salsify. Such examples of edible wild plants continue on and on.

STALKING WILD EDIBLE PLANTS. In the United States, people just buy their plants in the supermarkets in cans, or frozen, or fresh, so why should anyone be interested in what grows wild and what may have an unfamiliar flavor? There are several reasons:

• **Outdoor groups**—Groups such as the Boy Scouts, Girl Scouts, garden clubs, nature study groups, and campers and hikers always have a natural curiosity about the plants they observe, and often wish to know or need to know the identity of edible plants.

• **Hobby**—For many people, identifying and collecting wild edible plants represents a satisfying hobby. By starting with a few familiar plants, they gradually branch out to identifying more and more plants as they acquire new knowledge and sharpen their techniques of identification. To these individuals, the "weeds" in the garden, in the lawn, and along the roads take on new meaning. Collecting and eating wild greens, potherbs, berries, nuts, roots and tubes, is an enjoyable adventure. Also, foods of the wild are tasty and can be preserved for future use by drying, freezing, canning, or use in jams. It is doubtful, however, that collecting wild edible plants would ever result in saving money. Gathering wild plants requires much time and often travel, and some must be hulled, or soaked, or prepared in some time-consuming way.

• **Survival**—Some individuals have experienced a time when life depended on being able to identify wild edible plants. Experienced outdoorsmen have stated: "If you starve to death in the wilderness it is because you are just plain tired of living." Indeed, manuals for training members of the United States Armed Forces contain sections on the identification, collection, and preparation of edible wild plants in areas throughout the world. Each year, campers, fishermen, and hunters become lost and many suffer needlessly because of their lack of knowledge of edible wild plants.

There are many more examples of the role of wild plants in the survival of people. When the Forty-Niners stampeded California's streams, deserts, and mountains in search of gold, the scarcity of fresh food brought scurvy to the camps. The Indians and Spanish introduced the Forty-Niners to what is now called miner's lettuce. To combat scurvy in the northern portions of this continent, frontiersmen, explorers, and gold diggers learned to identify and use a plant now called scurvy grass. When rations were low on the Lewis and Clark expedition, the sweet yellow fruit of the papaw was eaten. During World War II, the people of England and Scandinavia collected vitamin C-rich rose hips from wild roses.

While stalking the wild plants can spell fun, adventure, and survival, it may also spell danger. Before eating a wild plant it should be positively identified. For most plants, this requires knowledge, skill, and experience. Some poisonous plants are easily confused with edible plants. Some edible plants are poisonous at certain stages of development, or certain parts of the plant are poisonous. However, in times of *survival emergencies* the following advice is often given:

1.   Never eat large quantities of a strange plant food without first testing it. (A disagreeable taste in a food item, which is otherwise safe to eat, may sometimes be removed. If cooking is possible, boiling in one or more changes of water may remove the unpleasant taste.)

2.   Take a teaspoonful of the plant food, prepared in the way it will be used (raw, boiled, baked, etc.), hold it in your mouth for about 5 minutes. If, by this time no burning sensation, or other unpleasant effect, has occurred, swallow it.

3.   Wait 8 hours. If no ill effects such as nausea, cramps, or diarrhea occur, eat a handful and wait 8 hours. If no ill effects are noted at the end of this time, the plant may be considered edible.

4.   If serious ill effects develop, induce vomiting.

5.   Even foods deemed safe should be eaten with restraint until you become used to them.

6.   Remember that olives are bitter and grapefruit is sour, so an unpleasant taste does not, in itself, mean poison. But a burning, nauseating, or bitter taste is a warning of danger. A small quantity of even poisonous food is not likely to prove fatal or even dangerous, whereas a large quantity may be. This, however, does not apply to mushrooms, which are best avoided in any case.

7.   In general, it is safe to try foods that you observe being eaten by birds and mammals, but there are some exceptions.

Enthusiasts who are unable to escape completely into the wilds and must do their foraging near civilization, should be somewhat cautious. Vacant lots and roadsides where wild plants may be found, may get sprayed with herbicides. Also, plants along busy roads have been known to contain high levels of lead, due to the lead in some gasolines burned in cars. Plants should be gathered at least 100 ft (*31 m*) away from a busy road.

EDIBLE WILD PLANTS OF NORTH AMERICA.
In North America, there are hundreds of edible wild plants, and worldwide there are hundreds more. Therefore, a complete listing is not within the scope of this book. However, Table W-19 provides descriptions of a few of the edible wild plants of North America. Also, some edible wild plants appear as individual entries in this book. Table W-19 is for interest and information only. It is not meant to serve as a guide for collecting wild plants. For those who have further interest, there are numerous excellent books on this subject, and many are specific for locations. Foragers of wild plants should completely familiarize themselves with the identification of edible and poisonous wild plants in an area. Moreover, beginners would do well to take lessons from persons with experience in stalking the wild life.

(Also see FRUIT[S]; MEDICINAL PLANTS; POISONOUS PLANTS; and VEGETABLE[S].)

TABLE W-19
EDIBLE WILD PLANTS OF NORTH AMERICA

Common and Scientific Name	Description	Geographical Distribution	Preparation and Uses	Comments
Acorn (oak) *Quercus* sp 	Nut or seed from all species of oak; leaves of oak simple and alternate; leaves deciduous in the north, evergreen on some southern oaks, nuts in a scaly cup.	Grows throughout southern Canada and the United States in various soil types and at various altitudes, with the exception of the northern prairies.	Roasted and used like any other nut; dried and ground into a fine meal to use in combination with cornmeal or wheat flour; roasted and ground as a coffee substitute; may be boiled and dried to leach bitterness.	There are about 85 species of oak. All acorns are good to eat, but some are less sweet than others. Acorns were a wild food relied upon by the Indians, and acorns helped the Pilgrims survive their first winters in the New World.

(Continued)

TABLE W-19 (Continued)

Common and Scientific Name	Description	Geographical Distribution	Preparation and Uses	Comments
Amaranth (pigweed, redroot, wild beet) *Amaranthus sp*	Annual herb, veiny, alternate leaves, bears seeds which are black and grow in terminal clusters.	Common weed in cultivated ground, waste places, and along roadsides from southern Canada to New England and south.	Seeds make suitable raw or cooked cereal, seeds may be added to soups, stews, and bread; young leaves serve as a spinachlike green.	Amaranth is known as America's forgotten cereal grain. Some research is underway to stimulate interest in commercial production. Food Composition Table F-36 provides information on the nutritional value of amaranth seeds and leaves. The seeds contain about 13% protein, are high in energy (calories) and are good sources of most minerals and vitamins. The leaves are a good source of calcium, iron, and vitamin A.
Arrowhead (wapatoo) *Sagittaria latifolia*	Deep green arrowhead-shaped leaves that protrude from the water or lie flat like a lily pad; stalk a single stem that bears fruit which grows from lateral spikes in the form of round heads containing seeds; fibrous root system grows into the shallow mud forming small tubers in the late fall.	Along the edges of lakes, ponds, and swamp areas throughout most of the United States and southern Canada.	Tubers harvested in late fall, winter, and early spring; roasted, boiled and served like potatoes.	Lewis and Clark wrote about Indian women collecting arrowhead tubers by freeing them from the mud with their toes. Freed tubers float to the surface.
Asparagus *Asparagus officinalis* (Also see ASPARAGUS.)	Young shoots thick and spear-shaped in the early spring; later become tall and branching with delicate, feathery leaves and red berries.	Moist ground near civilization, river banks, and ditches; throughout the United States and many areas of the world.	Same as for commercially grown asparagus; young shoots eaten raw or boiled.	Asparagus is cultivated and sold in most grocery stores as a fresh, canned, or frozen product. In some areas, sufficient asparagus grows wild that it can be picked in the spring and preserved by home canning or freezing.
Beechnuts (American beech) *Fagus grandiflora*	Usually grows 50 to 80 ft *(15 to 24 m)* high; crown symmetrically conical and thick; buds slender, cone-shaped, and sharply tipped; stiff elliptic to egg-shaped leaves with straight veins and sawtoothed edges; leaves emerald green above and yellow beneath; seed capsule a soft 4-part burr containing 2 triangular nuts (beechnuts).	From the Maritime Provinces of Canada to Ontario and Wisconsin, south to Texas and Florida in fertile, moist, cool, shady areas.	Roasted or raw like any other nut; roast and grind as a coffee substitute.	In the spring young leaves of the beech tree may be cooked and used as a green. As an emergency food the inner bark of the tree can be dried and pulverized for a flour. The nutritive value of beechnuts is indicated in Food Composition Table F-36.

(Continued)

TABLE W-19 (*Continued*)

Common and Scientific Name	Description	Geographical Distribution	Preparation and Uses	Comments
Bitterroot *Lewisia rediviva*	A low and somewhat fleshy plant, narrow and spoon-shaped, oblong leaves which sprout when snows recede; white to pink flower appearing after the leaves wither; prominent, white, large, fleshy, starchy root.	Grows on dry, open, often stony ground in Montana, British Columbia, south to Colorado, Utah, and northern California.	Roots collected in springtime when frost is barely out of the ground; peeled to expose white starchy somewhat mucilaginous core; then boiled to a jellylike consistency.	The bitterroot is the state flower of Montana. It was collected by the Lewis and Clark Expedition and carried back to Washington, D.C. Indians used the bitterroot to thicken soups.
Bulrush *Scirpus* sp	Often grows taller than a man; stems round to triangular; flowers in heads, spikes, umbels, or solitary spikelets.	Along streams and marshes throughout the West.	Edible parts include young shoots just protruding from the mud and rootstalks; eaten raw, baked, dried, or ground into a flour; young shoots yield a sweet syrup when boiled.	Indians also used the long leaves for weaving mats. Young shoots are thirst-quenching when eaten raw.
Burdock *Arctium minus* and *Arctium lappa*	Some reach heights of 3 ft *(1m)* or more; large alternate, egg-shaped, dark green leaves which may be over a foot long; purple to white, rounded flowers producing a soft burr.	Moist soil in southern Canada and much of the United States, with the exception of a southern stretch from California eastward.	Leaves and shoots edible and cooked as greens; first year roots peeled, and then boiled, fried, or roasted.	Every farmer is familiar with this bothersome weed. The adhesiveness of the burr provides for its wide distribution.
Cattail *Typha* sp	Grows to a height of 2 to 10 ft *(0.6 to 3m)*; light green, long slender leaves; jointless stem terminating in a sausage-shaped seed head.	Wet places throughout North America except in far north areas.	Edible roots, young shoots, seed heads and pollen; peeled roots eaten raw, roasted, baked, boiled, or dried and pounded into a flour; young shoots eaten raw or boiled; seed heads prepared like corn on the cob when cut as young flower heads; pollen collected and used as a flour substitute.	All four native American cattail species were regularly used by Indians and early settlers. Cattails are a neglected source of food and fiber for man.

(Continued)

TABLE W-19 (Continued)

Common and Scientific Name	Description	Geographical Distribution	Preparation and Uses	Comments
Chokecherry *Prunus virginiana*	Tree or shrub with reddish-gray bark; recognized in the fall by clusters of red or black cherries; dull, dark green leaves on top and paler below; pea-sized cherries grow in clusters, and each contains one big hard stone.	From Mexico to the Arctic Ocean and from the Atlantic to the Pacific; prefers to grow in rich moist areas.	Berries sought for wine and jelly; very tart for eating fresh.	The leaves and stones should be avoided, but the Indians used to crush the berries—stone and all—to form cakes which were dried and then eaten or used to flavor pemmican (dried beef, buffalo, or venison).
Chufa (earth almond, nut grass, zula nuts) *Cyperus esculentus* and *Cyperus rotundus*	Light green, grasslike leaves; central flower stalk; shorter leaves surround flower cluster; roots with long horizontal runners terminating in nutlike tubers.	Alaska to Mexico and coast to coast; grows in rich, moist soil; troublesome weed in some areas.	Nutlike tubers eaten raw, cooked like any vegetable or dried, ground to a powder and mixed with other flour; roasted, ground tubers make coffee substitute.	Chufa is widely distributed throughout the world and is cultivated in Europe. Ancient Egyptians held chufa in such esteem that they placed it in their tombs.
Chickweed *Stellaria media*	An annual with weak and reclining stems tufted with hair; opposite oval, sharp pointed leaves; small, white flowers borne in terminal clusters.	Common in shady areas and waste ground, cultivated ground, woods, meadows, and lawns throughout the United States and in the north from Alaska to Greenland.	Young growing tips good in salads or as a potherb; resembles spinach flavor.	Chickweed is a robust plant that can survive frost, snow, and even ice. It often takes over gardens before anything else comes to life in the spring.
Cranberry *Vaccinium* sp (Also see CRANBERRY; and FRUIT(S), Table F-47 Fruits of the World.)	Low, creeping evergreen shrub; oval to oblong leaves; white to pink flowers; juicy red berries.	Three wild species, from Alaska to Newfoundland, south to Virginia, North Carolina, and Oregon.	Berries unappetizing raw; usually cooked and sugared to taste; may be dried for preservation then soaked, cooked, and sugared; can be substituted for the uses of store bought varieties.	This plant is familiar to many people because of its similarity to those of the Thanksgiving tradition. Wild cranberries cling to the stems and are kept fresh all winter long by snow.

(Continued)

TABLE W-19 (*Continued*)

Common and Scientific Name	Description	Geographical Distribution	Preparation and Uses	Comments
Currants and Gooseberries *Ribes* sp (Also see CURRANT; FRUIT[S], Table F-47 Fruits of the World; and GOOSEBERRY.)	About 75 species of currants and gooseberries; maplelike leaves with 3 to 5 sawtoothed lobes; spicily fragrant golden blossoms; berries range from yellow to reddish to dark black; thorne on gooseberries; no thorns on currants.	Range from the Gulf of Alaska to the Gulf of Mexico and from the Pacific to the Atlantic; distributed in part due to escape from domestication.	Fruit enjoyed raw, but more palatable when cooked; makes delicious pies, tarts, sauces, jams, jellies, and wine.	The golden currant is native to North America. It was discovered on the headwaters of the Missouri and Columbia Rivers during the Lewis and Clark Expedition.
Dandelion *Taraxacum officinale* (Also see DANDELION; and VEGETABLE[S], Table V-6 Vegetables of the World.)	Leaves in rosettes directly from the roots, either upright or close to the ground; leaves green and deeply indented forming large teeth; yellow flowers on long hollow stalks.	Almost every inhabited corner of North America.	Leaves eaten raw or cooked as greens; roots scraped, sliced, and boiled or roasted and ground for use as coffee substitute; white crowns cooked like a vegetable.	Changing the water used for boiling the greens will remove the bitter taste. Flower heads have been used to make a wine.
Dock *Rumex* sp	Stout plants, bulky with mainly basal leaves; grooved stems, simple or branched; tapering or heart-shaped leaves a few inches to a foot long with wavy or curly edges; flower in tall, batonlike whorled clusters of tiny green blossoms; reddish-brown seed.	Throughout North America.	Leaves mixed with other greens in a salad; bitter dock leaves boiled in several changes of water eaten as a potherb.	Some docks may be poisonous if not prepared properly. Dock is a close relative of domestic buckwheat. Some Indians ground the seed to use in preparing flour and meal.

(*Continued*)

TABLE W-19 (Continued)

Common and Scientific Name	Description	Geographical Distribution	Preparation and Uses	Comments
Elderberry *Sambusus* sp (Also see FRUIT[S], Table F-47 Fruits of the World.)	May be shrubs of 5 ft *(1.5 m)* to treelike of 30 ft *(9.2 m)* or more in height; large, pithy, brown colored stem bearing opposite compound leaves; clusters of minute creamy blossoms turning to clusters of berries which are black, deep purple to red when ripe.	Prefer rich, moist soil from Alaska to Newfoundland south throughout most of the United States.	Berries not usually appetizing raw; berries best dried, cooked, or used in jellies; elderberry wines famous; flowers dipped in batter and fried or crushed into stew for flavor.	The green leaves, stems, and pith are said to be poisonous. For some individuals eating raw fruits may cause nausea. In some areas, the red fruited varieties are reported to be poisonous.
Evening primrose *Oenothera* sp	Either a low-growing plant with large white flowers or a taller plant with yellow flowers; flowers open at dusk; stems erect and simple or branched at the base; leaves wavy, margined, and toothed.	Grow from British Columbia to Newfoundland, and south throughout most of the United States; found on dry, stony slopes; sandy, gravelly areas, and arid ridges up to 1½ miles *(2.4 km)* above sea level.	Young shoots and leaves like asparagus or used in salads; dry or green leaves for tea; first year roots boiled or placed in stews; pith also used in stews.	Primrose was one of the first North American edibles to be introduced into the Old World.
Glasswort (Samphire) *Salicornia* sp	Apparently leafless stem usually branching near the base forming a clawlike appearance; a small light green plant.	Found in saline (salt) bogs and marshes from Alaska and Labrador southward down the Pacific and Atlantic seaboards as well as around the Gulf of Mexico.	Salty-tasting plants used in salad; pickling in any pickle mix after boiling young shoots and branches; cooked as a potherb.	When added to a stew, glasswort may provide all of the necessary salting. Pickled, the glasswort becomes a conversation piece when served as hors d'oeuvres.
Ground cherry *Physalis* sp	Low, trailing plant seldom rising more than 1 ft *(30 cm)* high; dark green leaves toothed, or unevenly fissured and usually oblong or ovate and bluntly pointed; yellow flowers eventually form balloonlike husks surrounding a pea-sized tomatolike fruit.	Grow in moist to dry medium, open ground in southern Canada and throughout the United States with the exception of Alaska.	Fruits contained in balloonlike husk eaten raw or cooked; makes good preserves and pies; can be ingredient of stew.	Actually, they are closely related to the tomato and not even remotely related to cherries. Some species have been commercially cultivated for their berries. Fully ripened fruit is best and safe.

(Continued)

TABLE W-19 *(Continued)*

Common and Scientific Name	Description	Geographical Distribution	Preparation and Uses	Comments
Groundnut (Indian potatoes) *Apios americana*	A climbing and twining perennial legume with alternate compound leaves which are made up of 3 to 7 or 9 broadly oval, sharply pointed, roundly based, 1 to 3 in. *(3 to 8 cm)* long leaflets on either side of a common leafstalk; fragrant maroon to chocolate blossoms which are pealike; beanlike pod for fruit; tuberous lemonsized enlargements on rootstalk which lay in strings just beneath the surface.	All of the eastern and much of the midwestern United States, from the Gulf of the St. Lawrence to the Gulf of Mexico, in areas of damp soil.	Seeds inside pods cooked and used like peas; tubers prepared like potatoes — boiled in salty water, mashed with butter and served.	Indians esteemed the groundnut. Wampanoags shared it with the Pilgrims who depended on groundnuts their first rugged winter. In the 1580s, Sir Walter Raleigh's colonists collected these tubers on North Carolina's Roanoke Island and sent them home to Queen Elizabeth. Groundnuts are considered one of America's forgotten crops, which may hold some hope for the future if rediscovered.
Hazelnut (filbert) *Corylus* sp (Also see NUTS, Table N-8 Nuts of the World.)	Multibranched shrub or small tree; husk covering and nuts vary between three native species; toothed leaves	Three species native to Canada and United States, distributed from Newfoundland to British Columbia south to Georgia, and Tennessee; and west of the Cascade Mountains.	Nuts eaten raw, used in cookies, candies, or other foods; delicious ground into a meal and made into bread.	Nuts ripen in the fall and are similar to commercial hazelnuts.
Hickory *Carya* sp	Slow growing tree sometimes reaching the age of 250 years, and a height of 180 ft *(55 m)* or more; fragrant leaves when crushed; leaves to 14 in. *(36 cm)* long composed of 5 to 7 leaflets which are toothed on the edges and lighter color underneath, thick-husked, egg-shaped nut (hickory nut) with whitish nut shell over $1/8$ in. *(3.2 mm)* thick.	A typically North American tree. The shagbark hickory (Carya ovata) grows from Quebec, Canada south to Texas and Florida; and the shellbark hickory *(Carya lacinosa)* grows from New York and Nebraska south to North Carolina, Alabama, Mississippi, and Oklahoma.	Collected, shelled, and eaten raw; used like any other nut.	The crushed green nutshells can be used to poison fish in a pond — when survival is at stake. Both the Indians and colonists relied on hickory nuts as a food. Food Composition Table F-36 gives the nutritive value of hickory nuts. Hickory wood may be used to smoke tasty hams and bacon.

(Continued)

TABLE W-19 *(Continued)*

Common and Scientific Name	Description	Geographical Distribution	Preparation and Uses	Comments
Jerusalem artichoke *Helianthus tuberosus* (Also see JERUSALEM ARTICHOKE; and VEGETABLE[S], Table V-6 Vegetables of the World.)	Large perennial sunflower; slender and branched growing 6 to 10 ft *(1.8 to 3.1 m)* high; narrower and more sharply tipped leaves than other wild sunflower; 2 to 3 in. *(5 to 8 cm)* in diameter; leaves thick, broadly based, rough and hard; slender flattish potatolike tubers underground.	Prefers damp ground along roads, ditches, streams, paths, and other waste lands from Saskatchewan to Ontario, Canada and south to Kansas and Georgia.	Tubers simmered in their skins with small amount of water, peeled, salted, and buttered; or peeled, oiled, and roasted; used as pickles and in pies; eaten raw.	Once these plants were cultivated by the Indians and settlers of the eastern United States. Jerusalem artichokes grow wild where they have escaped from cultivation. They do not have any connection to the city of Jerusalem.
Jojoba *Simmondsia chinensis*	Highly branched evergreen shrub; entire, simple, thick, leathery, opposite leaves; small, greenish-yellow flowers borne in axillary clusters; brown acornlike fruit or nut.	Dry slopes and along washes in southern Arizona, southern California and south into Sonora and Baja California.	Nuts eaten raw, roasted, or parched, but rather bitter; Indian coffee substitute prepared by roasting and grinding nuts.	The jojoba bean or nut is high in oil. Jojoba oil duplicates the oil of the sperm whale, only it is purer. It holds great potential in the future as a replacement for petroleum derivatives. It could improve the economy in areas where the land is useless for conventional crops.
Kinnikinic *Arctostaphylos* sp	Vinelike evergreen with reddish bark; egg-shaped, veiny, thick, small, tough leaves with a shine on top; pink to white flowers; reddish berries on the plant throughout winter.	Grows on poor soil in the Arctic, Canada, and southward in the United States to California and Virginia; common in dry, sunny woods, in the mountains and even above the tree line.	Raw berries rather tasteless but nutritious; better cooked and mixed with other berries.	Sometimes these are called bearberries because they are sought by the bears upon emerging from hibernation. Dried, pulverized leaves of the kinnikinic have been used as a tobacco substitute and extender. The leaves can be dried and used to make a tea.
Lamb's Quarter (Goosefoot) *Chenopodium* sp	Bunching annual growing from 1 to 6 ft *(30 to 183 cm)* high; leaves greyish-green or bluish-green and floury white particularly underneath; leaves from 1 to 4 in. *(3 to 10 cm)* long and goosefoot-shaped; inconspicuous green flowers; tiny black seeds.	Common weed of wasteland and stream banks throughout Canada, and United States; found primarily in and around areas once cultivated.	Entire young plant edible as a green or cooked like spinach; seeds also edible ground into a meal or cooked whole and used like a hot breakfast cereal.	Of all the wild greens, lamb's quarter is preferred by many because it has no harsh flavor. A native of Europe and Asia; also, a relative of beets and spinach.

(Continued)

TABLE W-19 *(Continued)*

Common and Scientific Name	Description	Geographical Distribution	Preparation and Uses	Comments
Maple (Sugar maple) *Acer saccharum* (Also see MAPLE SYRUP.)	Native North American tree growing 60 to 100 ft *(18 to 31 m)* high; 5-lobed leaf which is sparsely and irregularly toothed and from 3 to 5 in.*(8 to 13 cm)* long; leaves turn golden yellow with some scarlet and crimson; winged seeds.	From Newfoundland to Ontario, Canada, to Minnesota and south as far as Georgia and Louisiana; prefers moist areas.	Sap collected in the early spring, boiled down to delicious maple syrup and maple sugar; young leaves, seeds, and inner bark eaten by some.	The maple leaf is the emblem of Canada. Indians introduced the colonists to the collection of sap and the formation of syrup and sugar.
Miner's Lettuce *Montia* sp	Small succulent plant with rounded, fleshy leaves; some leaves join to form a rounded disk or cup; stalk continues through middle of cup developing an elongated flower cluster; stem on each white to pink flower; shiny black seeds.	Prefers shaded, moist areas from British Columbia, Canada across to North Dakota and south to California and Arizona.	Stems and leaves eaten raw or boiled; used in salads like lettuce; boiled roots edible and have flavor of chestnuts.	California 49'er prospectors learned to use miner's lettuce to prevent scurvy. Miner's lettuce has been introduced into Europe where it is cultivated and called winter purslane.
Mountain Sorrel (Scurvy grass) *Oxyria digyna*	Succulent plant with long-stemmed round or kidney-shaped leaves arising from the stalk close to the root; inconspicuous greenish or crimson flower in clusters on long full, branching stalk; reddish fruits with a flatly encircling wing.	Circles the North Pole, from Alaska to Greenland; throughout British Columbia, Canada at higher elevations; White Mountains in New Hampshire and higher mountains in new Mexico and southern California.	Eaten raw in salads, purees, or on sandwiches as young plants; mature plants simmered and enjoyed as a potherb.	Eskimos collect Mountain Sorrel and ferment it as a sauerkraut. Used as a source of vitamin C in the far north regions; hence, the name scurvy grass.
Mulberry (Red Mulberry) *Morus rubra* (Also see FRUIT[S], Table F-47 Fruits of the World.)	Small tree generally 20 to 30 ft *(6 to 9 m)* high; dark green, sharply tipped, sawtoothed leaves; branches form dense, broad, round domes; bark greyish-brown to reddish-brown; berries composed of many 1-seeded drupes and dark purple when mature.	Native from New England to the Dakotas and south to Texas and Florida, especially abundant in Mississippi and Ohio valleys.	Berries popular raw or for pie, jellies, and juice.	Fruit can be easily gathered in quantity by spreading a tarpaulin underneath a heavily laden branch and then shaking it. Birds love mulberries.

(Continued)

TABLE W-19 *(Continued)*

Common and Scientific Name	Description	Geographical Distribution	Preparation and Uses	Comments
Nettles (Stinging Nettle) *Urtica* sp	Single stemmed perennials; growing from a few inches to several feet tall depending upon conditions; egg-shaped to oblong leaves with heartlike bases and tapered tips; stalks, leafstems, and the underneath of leaves are fuzzy with fine stinging bristles; green flowers between leaves and stalk.	From Alaska across Canada and throughout much of the United States.	Boiled, short, tender, young plants first appearing in spring or boiled, tender, new leaves appearing on the plant later on; bristles quelled by boiling in water.	Worldwide nettles are considered protein rich, versatile, and potentially valuable. In some parts of the world nettles are used for cloth, paper, fish line, and beer, in addition to food.
Pinon Pine *Pinus monophylla* and *Pinus edulis*	Evergreen tree with needlelike leaves; flowers in the spring; woody scaled cones reach maturity in 2 to 3 years.	Throughout the United States and Canada with the exception of the central plains, the tundras and the deserts for pines in general.	Cone picked just before ripening and then roasted, yielding flavorful pine nuts in their shells from inside the cone; in dire need, inner bark can be eaten raw or cooked.	Numerous animals depend upon pine nuts as part of their food supply, hence, human gatherers compete with an army of animals. Infusions made from needles contain vitamin C.
Plantain *Plantago* sp	A short stemless perennial; strongly ribbed, spadelike green leaves growing directly from the root; tiny greenish or drab bronze flowers on central spikes which are leafless.	From Alaska to Labrador and south throughout Canada and the United States.	Young leaves eaten raw; older leaves cooked like spinach, or pureed, sieved, in a cream sauce; infusions made from leaves.	Most people recognize plantain but few realize it is edible and contains vitamins A and C. It is such a sturdy persistent plant that it may be found poking through the sidewalks in big cities like Boston, San Francisco, or New York.
Pokeweed (Poke) *Phytolacca* sp	Tall, stout perennial growing from a large fleshy taproot; large alternate petioled, oblong to lanceolate leaves; small white or greenish tassels of flowers between the leaves; berries rich, lush purple in fall.	Throughout the South and eastern half of the United States and west to Texas.	Only the small tender shoots edible when no more than 8 in. tall; leaves used as greens and stems served like asparagus.	The bitter roots and the mature stalk are poisonous. Civil War soldiers used ink made from the juice of ripe poke berries. Some people grow poke sprouts in their cellars.
Poplar *Populus* sp	Trees with a variety of characteristics; leaves generally triangular with 3 to 5 major veins meetng at the base; slim, long stems on leaves; brittle branches.	From Alaska through the Hudson Bay area to Newfoundland, Canada; south to Pennsylvania, along the mountains to Kentucky; west through the Rockies to Mexico and California.	Inner bark eaten fresh, brewed into a tea, cooked like noodles, or dried and ground into a flour.	There are many names and many species of poplar. Many a frontiersman relied on them for nutrition.

(Continued)

TABLE W-19 (*Continued*)

Common and Scientific Name	Description	Geographical Distribution	Preparation and Uses	Comments
Prairie Turnip (Bread root) *Psoralea* sp	Thick roots giving rise to flowering stems and 3 to 5 leaflets clustered at the end of the petiole; flowers purplish-blue and become tiny seed pods.	Thrives on the high plains and prairies from Manitoba, Canada, and Wisconsin to New Mexico, Texas, and west to the Rockies.	Roots edible raw, roasted, or pounded into a meal.	The prairie turnip was an important vegetable for the Sioux and Cree Indians. John Colter, who escaped from the Indians and returned to his friends to tell about what is now Yellowstone Park, is reported to have lived for a week on prairie turnips.
Prickly Pear (Indian fig) *Opuntia* sp	A cactus with pear-shaped pads and fruits; solitary flowers appearing in spring and early summer which develop into thorny little knobs about the size of prunes — the fruit.	Desert areas throughout the West; and in the East from New England to Florida.	Pulp scooped from the fruit eaten raw, boiled, fried, stewed, or dried for future use; newer; tender pads which are despined, sliced, and then boiled or roasted.	The fruits of some of the larger species are especially sweet and were enjoyed by many Indians and early pioneers. A bitterish and slightly sticky juice, squeezed from the insides of prickly pears makes an emergency water source.
Purslane *Portulaca oleracea*	Fleshy prostrate herb with alternate paddle-shaped leaves growing in rosettes about a tiny yellow flower; minute round seed vessels.	Prevalent in fertile, sandy soil from the warmer regions of Canada to the southern states.	Entire herb good to eat raw in a salad or cooked; gives body to soups or stews; young shoots good pickled; may be stored frozen.	Purslane is a native of India and Persia (Iran) which was introduced into North America in colonial times. The use of purslane as food has been recorded for several thousand years.
Salsify (Oyster plant) *Tragopogon* sp (Also see VEGETABLE[S], Table V-6 Vegetables of the World.)	Milky, juiced plants growing from about 1 to 4 ft *(30 to 122 cm)* high; long grasslike alternate leaves clasped to a smooth stem contain a single large flower; mature seed heads resemble a giant dandelion top; long white tapering root.	From coast to coast in the northern United States and southern Canada.	Roots collected and cooked before flowering stem develops; very young raw roots sliced into salads; tender young leaves also edible.	Salsify is grown commercially in this country and in Europe. Cooked salsify tastes like oysters to some people; hence, the name oyster plant.

(*Continued*)

TABLE W-19 (*Continued*)

Common and Scientific Name	Description	Geographical Distribution	Preparation and Uses	Comments
Tepary Bean *Phaseolus acutifolius*	Herbaceous plants with long, trailing stems; pinnately trifoliate leaves, axillary flowers which may vary in color.	Dry, hot areas of Arizona, Texas, New Mexico, and northern Mexico; domesticated but common in the wild.	Similar to common beans.	The tepary bean is a very drought- and heat-adapted food crop. It is high in protein and mild tasting. Only a handful of Indians still use the tepary bean. It is considered one of America's forgotten crops.
Thistle *Cirsium* sp	Many species but generally succulent plant with spines on leaves and stems; perennial or biennial plants; often large flower-heads which are pink, purple, red, yellow, or white.	In Canada and United States, from east to west.	Root of many species eaten raw, boiled, or roasted, nutritious but bland; peeled stems cooked as greens.	The peeled cooked spiny stem is said to taste like an artichoke.
Water Cress *Nasturtium officianale* (Also see VEGETABLE[S], Table V-6 Vegetables of the World.)	Prostrate, green, and leafy, growing in mats or clumps; innumerable white threadlike roots; leaves with 3 to 9 segments; minute, white flowers; needlelike seedpods.	Common in Canada and United States, growing in every state; thrives in cold water and wet places.	Salad plant used as raw greens; adds zest to other edible greens; also good simmered.	This pungent, tasty green will stimulate the appetite, and enliven hors d'oeuvres.
Water Lily (Yellow water lily) *Nuphar* sp	Bright golden, waxy flowers and broad, green leaves floating on ponds, shallow lake rims, and other quiet waters; blossom during summer; flowers develop many large seeds resembling kernels of popcorn; large scaly, yellowish roots deep enough to be below frost line.	Found in waters from Alaska to Labrador, south to California and the Gulf of Mexico.	Starchy roots roasted or boiled and then peeled; sweetish interiors used in soups and stews; roots dried and ground to a flour; seeds gathered in the autumn fried, shelled, cooked, buttered and salted, or eaten like a breakfast cereal.	Indian squaws used to gather roots from the homes of beavers and muskrats, or they would dive to collect the roots.

(*Continued*)

TABLE W-19 (*Continued*)

Common and Scientific Name	Description	Geographical Distribution	Preparation and Uses	Comments
Wild Rose *Rosa* sp 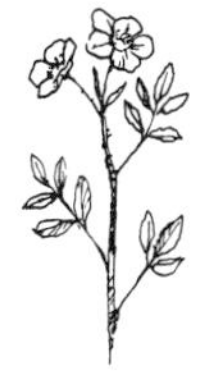	Thorny bush similar to domestic rose; reddish colored stems from several feet to a dozen feet tall with branched, brambled stems; usually a pinkish flower 1 to 3 in. *(3 to 8 cm)* in diameter; flowers form red seed pods called hips which often cling throughout the winter.	From the Aleutian Islands, across Alaska and across Canada to the northern Atlantic coast, south throughout Canada and the United States wherever moisture is sufficient.	Rose hips eaten raw, cooked, stewed, candied, or made into preserves; pulpier fruits best.	According to some reports, each pound *(0.45 kg)* of raw pulp from wild rose hips contains 4,000 to 7,000 mg of vitamin C. The taste of rose hips is said to be a delicate applelike flavor.

WILD RICE *Zizania aquatica*

Wild rice (*Indian rice, water oats*), which is native to the Great Lakes Region—especially in what is now Minnesota, Wisconsin, and Manitoba, is the only native cereal crop to be domesticated in the United States; all other cereal grains were cultivated elsewhere and brought to America.

"Taming" wild rice was not easy. It ripened at different stages, and, as it ripened, the grain fell off the stalk, making harvest difficult. As a result, it was formerly harvested by Indians in canoes. However, in the 1960s, the University of Minnesota developed an improved variety of wild rice that ripened more uniformly without shattering, adapted to harvest with combines—just like wheat or barley. Today, 75% of the annual U.S. wild rice crop of 3 to 4 million lb (*1.4 to 1.8 mil kg*) is grown in the marshy areas of northern Minnesota (the remaining 25% of the supply comes from Canada, Wisconsin, Michigan, and California); and, today, 90% of Minnesota's wild rice is grown in paddies and harvested by combine, and only 10% is grown in lakes and harvested by canoes.

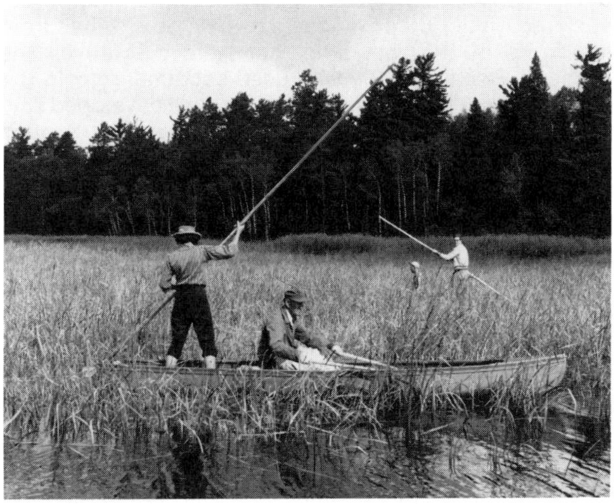

Wild rice can be cooked by the same methods as regular rice. Cooking times vary, depending on the size, color, and processing; generally, the larger the kernel and the darker the color, the longer it takes to cook. When properly cooked, the slender, round, purplish black, starchy grain is excellent food, highly esteemed by gourmets and others familiar with the taste. Wild rice is usually high in protein content and low in fat compared to other cereals. (For the composition of wild rice, see Food Composition Table F-36.) Normally, it sells at 2 to 3 times the price of cultivated rice.

(Also see CEREAL GRAINS, Table C-18 Cereal Grains of the World; and RICE, section headed "Wild Rice.")

Fig. W-45. Harvesting wild rice in the Chippewa National Forest, Minnesota. One person "poles" the boat, and the other person harvests the rice by means of two sticks—he pulls a batch of ripe rice stalks over the boat with one stick, then knocks the rice into the bottom of the boat with the other stick. (Courtesy, USDA)

WINDBERRY (BILBERRY) *Vaccinium myrtillus*

A fruit of a low shrub (of the family *Ericaceae*) that is native to Eruope and northern Asia. It is closely related to blueberries and huckleberries. Windberries are used fresh or in confections, jams, and pies.

(Also see BLUEBERRY; FRUIT[S], Table F-47 Fruits Of The World—"Blueberry"; "Huckleberry.")

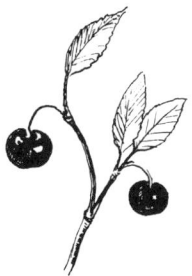

Fig. W-46. The windberry.

WINE

Contents

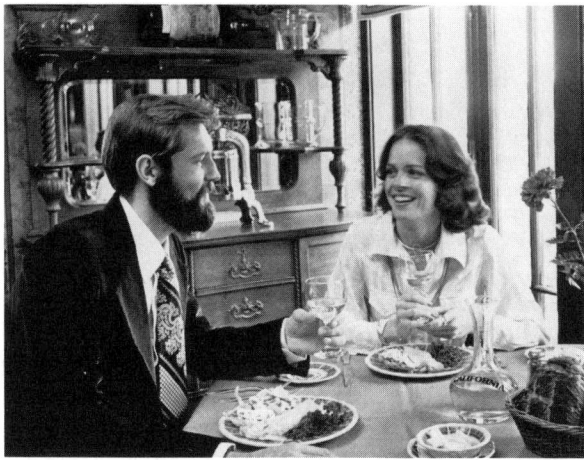

Fig. W-47. Many young couples are now enjoying table wine with their meals. (Courtesy, Wine Institute, San Francisco, Calif.)

This term refers to the fermented juice of the grape. If other fruit juices are used to make wine, the name of the fruit must precede the word *wine*. Wine is believed to have been one of the oldest medicines in the world and has long been used as a base for many tonics. However, most people drink wine for enjoyment. Recently, Americans increased their consumption of this beverage at the expense of other alcoholic drinks, as evidenced by the fact that the per capita sales of all types of wine in the United States doubled in the period between 1956 and 1976.[4] Since 1976, the per capita consumption of wine has not changed much; it has gone from 2.7 gal to 3.0 gal.

By comparison, the per capita wine consumption in Portugal is 23 gal; in Italy, 21 gal; and in France, 20 gal.

---

[4]Folwell, R. J., and J. L. Baritelle, *The U.S. Wine Market*, Agri. Economic report No. 417, USDA, 1978.

HISTORY OF WINE MAKING. Some historians suspect that certain cave dwelling, primitive peoples of the Eurasian continent may have enjoyed fermented juices from spoiled wild fruit long before grapes were first cultivated some 7,000 years ago in the region around the Caspian Sea. (Grapes naturally contain the vital ingredients for fermentation because they are rich in sugar and have a waxy outer coating that collects wild airborne yeast cells.)

Archaeologists have found 6,000 to 7,000 year old pottery wine jars that suggest that the first wines were made in the Middle East from grapes, figs, and dates. Apparently the art of grape growing (viticulture) was spread westward by migratory peoples, such as the Jews, since the *Bible* mentions that Noah raised grapes and made wine (Genesis 9:20-21). It is noteworthy that Egyptian accounts of winemaking date back to about 2500 B.C. They also stored jars of wine in special wine cellars dug out of the earth, because they apparently realized that this highly esteemed drink kept better when it was stored in a cool environment. The ancient Minoan, Greek, and Etruscan civilizations also produced wine for their own use and trading, as evidenced by the airtight clay pots they used as containers. Later, the Greeks originated symposiums, which were gatherings of people who drank wine together, engaged in intellectual discussions, and played simple games. (The symposia may have represented a refinement of the earlier dionysian orgies that often ended in drunkenness and violence.)

Roman wine festivals, or bacchanalia (named after Bacchus, the god of wine), were characterized by drinking to intoxication and resembled the dionysian orgies, except that the Romans did not allow women to drink wine. The Romans were the first to retard the spoilage of wine by storing it in their smoke houses. They also became experts in vine growing and helped to spread this art throughout their European colonies.

By the early Christian era, the Gauls in France rivaled the Romans in their wine-making skills. When Rome fell, each region of Europe made its own types of wines from the fruits of the vineyards that were planted by the Romans. Because wine was used sacramentally in the celebration of the Mass, the monasteries developed special recipes for making local wines. Later, some groups of monks (such as the Benedictines) took winemaking a step further and made special distilled liqueurs by processes that were kept secret to insure their livelihood.

The European colonists of North America found fields of wild grapes when they arrived. However, the first wines made from the American species (*Vitis labrusca*) were inferior to those made from Old World grapes (*V. vinifera*). Nevertheless, the wild species were much hardier in the climate of eastern N. America than the Old World species. (There is some evidence that the Vikings who landed in eastern Canada found grapes there, also). Finally, in 1769 the Old World varieties were successfully introduced into California by the Spanish priest Father Junipero Serra who founded a string of missions with vineyards.

By the 19th century, many European varieties of wine grapes were brought to western United States, where they grew well in the mild climate. A better native American grape was developed after the Concord grape was first grown by E. W. Bull of Concord, Massachusetts in 1852.

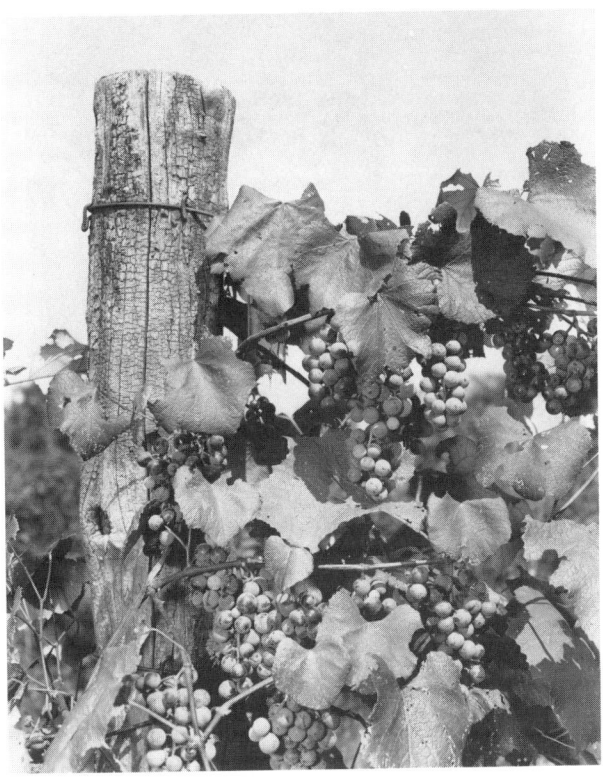

Fig. W-48. Concord grapes, a native American variety that produces rich, full-bodied wine. (Courtesy, J. C. Allen & Son, West Lafayette, Ind.)

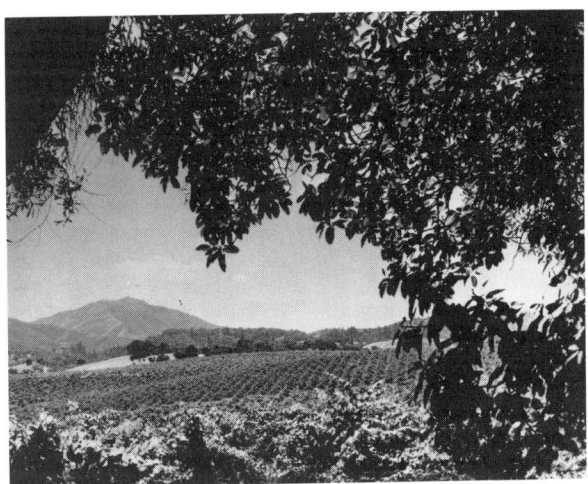

Fig. W-49. Vineyard landscape in the California wine country. (Courtesy, Wine Institute, San Francisco, Calif.)

The hardiness of the American vines led to their introduction into European vineyards to which they carried the plant louse, *phylloxera*. This parasite caused massive destruction of vines throughout Europe until it was found that resistant vineyards could be produced by grafting European vines onto the louse-resistant American rootstocks. Eventually, most of the vineyards of Europe were reestablished, but many years were required for the production of the mature vines that yield the best wine grapes. Another important development of the 19th century was the discovery by the French microbiologist Pasteur that the heating of wines destroyed the undesirable bacteria that caused spoilage.

The growth of the American wine industry during the 20th century was interrupted by Prohibition, which lasted from 1919 to 1933. However, the consumption of wine has risen steadily since 1933; and there have been many innovations and improvements in the production of wines as a result of research programs in viticulture and enology. What were formerly the trade secrets jealously guarded by a few winemakers have now been formulated into scientific practices of the entire industry. As a result, many high quality American wines are available at very reasonable prices.

BASIC PRINCIPLES OF WINE PRODUCTION.

Actual production practices vary somewhat from winery to winery, since the grapes used and the wines produced are distinctively different for each growing region. For example, the high acid and low to moderate alcoholic content of the European-type table wines are produced from the grapes grown in the cooler areas of northern California, Oregon, and Washington, whereas the dessert wines are made from the high sugar content grapes grown in the hot Central Valley of California. (A long, hot growing season is needed to produce grapes that are very rich in sugars.) Only the basic principles that are utilized in most wineries will be presented here.

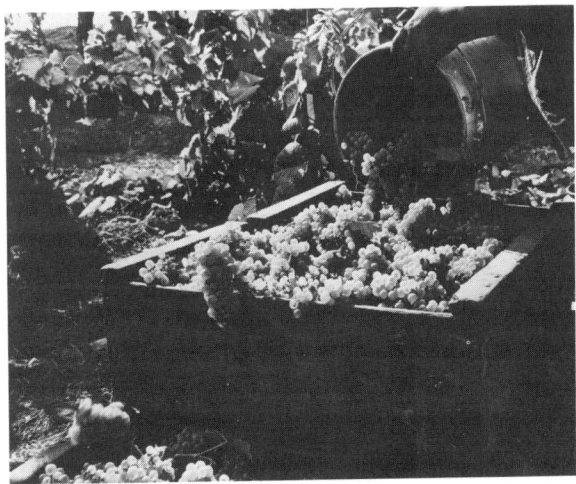

Fig. W-50. Buckets of fresh grapes on the way to becoming California wines. (Courtesy, Wine Institute, San Francisco, Calif.)

Fermentation. The juice from the crushed grapes is usually fermented by pure cultures of certain strains of yeasts, by processing steps like those that follow:

1. **Preparation of the must.** The must, juice, to be fermented is extracted by passing the fresh grapes through a "stemmer-crusher," after which the juice is treated with sulfur dioxide to kill any undesirable wild yeasts. *Note well:* Because sulfites trigger severe reactions among some people, since June 1978, the Bureau of Alcohol, Tobacco, and Firearms, has required that all wines containing more than 10 parts per million of sulfites carry the phrase "Contains sulfites" on the neck, back, or side panels of containers.

2. **Fermentation.** A culture of the most suitable strain of yeast is added to the must in fermentation tanks. In most cases, the juice contains sufficient sugar to produce the desirable alcoholic content. However, some of the grapes grown in cool climates are too low in sugar and require additional sugar for complete fermentation. Large fermentation tanks may be equipped with cooling coils to prevent the temperature from rising too high, since the yeast cells may be killed by too much heat. The dark-colored wines are produced by fermenting the grape pulp with the skins present, whereas the lighter-colored wines are fermented with only minimal contact with the skins.

Clarification. Newly fermented wines contain considerable sediment which is usually removed by (1) fining, in which an agent such as gelatin or egg white is added to bring certain materials out of solution or suspension; (2) settling out of suspended materials; (3) filtration of the wine through special filter pads; and (4) centrifugation, when the wines are not fully clarified by the preceding processes.

Aging. Some wines are intended for consumption right after their production but others must be mellowed by aging for a few years to remove the harsh flavors and allow the more desirable ones to develop. This process has long been carried out in wooden barrels that contribute flavors of their own, while absorbing some of the astringent constituents. However, many of the less expensive wines are held in redwood, concrete, or lined wine tanks for periods ranging from a few months to 2 years or so.

After aging, the wines are filtered, treated with sulfur dioxide to prevent spoilage; and bottled.

A little more aging may occur in the bottle, as the sulfur dioxide content decreases gradually. Corked bottles of wine are stored with the cork end inclined downward so that the cork is kept wet and the admission of air is prevented. *Note well:* In 1991, the Food and Drug Administration issued a temporary standard for wine prohibiting the sale of wine with more than 300 parts per billion of lead as a temporary measure until a permanent standard can be set. Also, FDA has said that it will soon propose a ban on lead foil wrappers to cover corks in wine bottles.

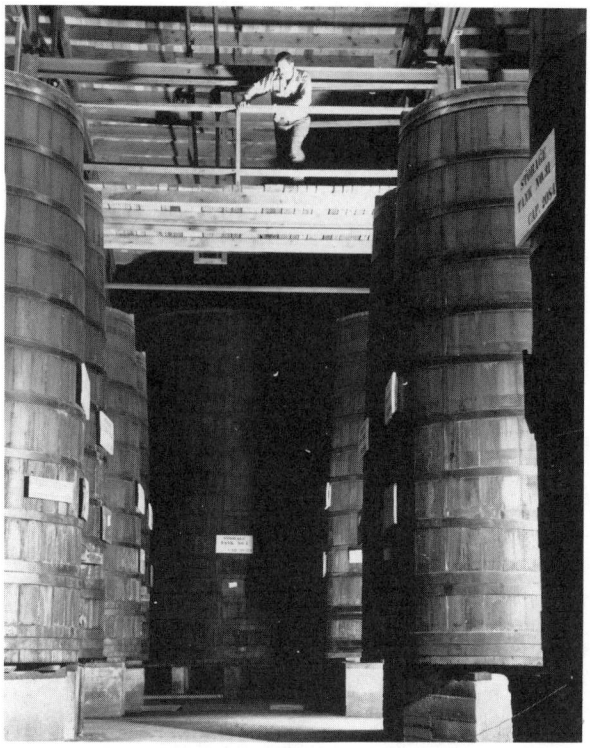

Fig. W-51. These great wooden tanks, filled with aging wines, are in a cool winery in a California valley. (Courtesy, Wine Institute, San Francisco, Calif.)

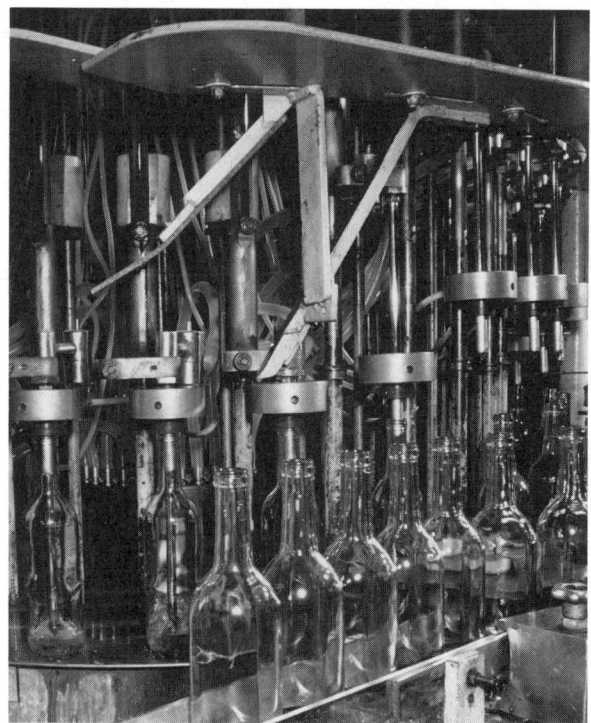

Fig. W-52. Bottles are mechanically filled with wine. (Courtesy, Wine Institute, San Francisco, Calif.)

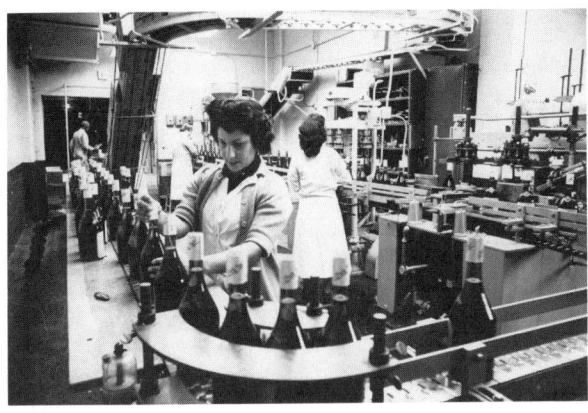

Fig. W-53. Lines of California wine, already corked and aged, are labeled and packaged, which is the last step in the production of California's fine wines. (Courtesy, Wine Institute, San Francisco, Calif.)

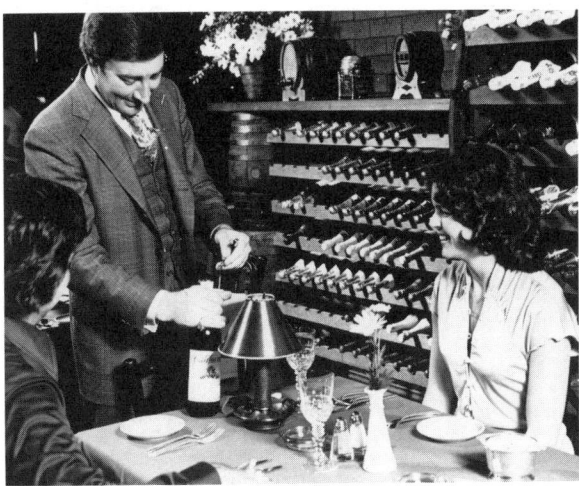

Fig. W-54. The opening and tasting of a bottle of wine is a pleasant ritual that is performed in many highclass restaurants. (Courtesy, Wine Institute, San Francisco, Calif.)

TYPES OF WINES AND RELATED PRODUCTS.

The names listed on the labels of European wines are confusing to all but the experts in the field because they give vineyards and regions of production that are unfamiliar to most consumers. Furthermore, the quality of these wines varies from year to year because the climates of the grape producing regions are quite variable. Therefore, highclass restaurants allow the customers to taste imported wines before they are served.

The years in which good wines were produced in a region are called "vintage years." However, wines produced in the more predictable climate of California vary little from year to year. Some of the common types of wines are presented in Table W-20.

TABLE W-20
TYPES OF WINES AND RELATED PRODUCTS

Product	Description	Uses	Comments
Apple wine *(hard cider)*	Apple cider or juice that has been allowed to ferment.	Served cold or hot as a beverage. Distilled to make apple brandies such as applejack (an American product) or Calvados (from Normandy, France).	Some people increase the alcoholic content of this drink by allowing it to remain at subfreezing temperatures, then decanting the unfrozen concentrated liquid.
Aromatic wine	A fortified wine flavored with one or more aromatic plant parts such as bark, flowers, leaves, roots, etc.	An aperitif (drink served before a meal to stimulate the appetite) that is best when poured over ice. Mixer for cocktails and similar drinks.	Vermouth is one of the best known types of aromatic wines.
Bordeaux	A wine produced in the Bordeaux region of France. May be red, white, or rose.	During meals or with the dessert. Good when chilled slightly and served in elongated Bordeaux glasses.	The best Bordeaux wines come from the districts of Graves, Medoc, Pomerol, St.-Emilion, and Sauternes.
Brandy	Distillate from a wine (Hence, the characteristics of each product stem from those of the original wine, the type of distillation and the aging process).	After dinner drink. In desserts and other dishes.	Brandy improves when aged in wooden casks, but not when held in a glass bottle.

(Continued)

Product	Description	Uses	Comments
Burgundy	A wine produced in the Burgundy region of France. May be red, white, or sparkling.	During meals or with the dessert. Good when chilled slightly.	The best Burgundy wines come from the northern section called "Cote d'Or".
Cabernet	Wine made from the Cabernet Sauvignon grape, which was brought from Bordeaux, France to California.	After dinner drink.	Cabernet Sauvignon is reputed to be one of the best California wines.
Chablis	An excellent dry white wine (with a green-gold tint) from the French town of Chablis. However, the name is sometimes applied to similar dry, white wines made elsewhere.	With fish, hors d'oeuvre, seafood, and shellfish.	The best wine for serving with oysters.
Champagne	A sparkling wine that is made by allowing wine from Pinot grapes to undergo a second fermentation after a small amount of sugar has been added to the bottle.	An aperitif that is served chilled. However, it may also be served at any time during any meal. A tulip-shaped glass helps to retain the bubbles.	In France, the name Champagne is limited to the sparkling wines produced in the Province of Champagne. Also made in California and New York.
Chianti	Red wine from the Tuscany region of Italy that is often sold in a round-bottom flask placed in a straw basket. However, the best wine comes in tall bottles that can be binned for aging.	With meals, particularly when Italian meat or pasta dishes are served.	The best known Italian wine. Some types of Chianti (such as those sold in the straw-covered flasks) deteriorate after about 2 years.
Claret	A dry, red Bordeaux wine made from Cabernet Sauvignon grapes.	With or after a meal.	The name "Claret" is an English term for this type of wine. (Elsewhere, it may be called a red Bourdeaux wine.)
Cognac	Brandy that is double distilled from wine made in the Charente district of France.	After dinner drink.	Cognac is best after it has been long aged in Limousin oak barrels.
Cold Duck	A sparkling wine that is similar to champagne.	An aperitif or with meals.	Among the sparkling wines, it is second in popularity to champagne and accounts for about one-third of the sales of this type of wine.
Concord wine	A strong-flavored, dark red wine made from Concord grapes (a native American variety).	With and after dinner.	Most of this wine is produced in New York.
Crackling wines	Wines that are less carbonated than sparkling wines.	An aperitif or with dinner.	Crackling Burgundy is usually much appreciated, but not always easy to find.
Cream sherry	A heavy, dark-colored, sweetened sherry that is made by a process similar to the one developed in Jerez de la Frontera, Spain.	With dessert or after dinner.	Cream sherries from California rival those from Spain.
Dessert wines	Fortified (with additional alcohol in the form of a brandy) wine that contains from 15 to 20% alcohol by volume.	With dessert or after dinner.	Should be served in small, narrow glasses.
Dry wines	A wine that is *not* sweet or or sweetened. (In other words, all or most of the natural sugar content has been converted to alcohol.)	With or after a meal.	People who have a tendency to develop low blood sugar after eating sweets should stick to dry wines.

(Continued)

Product	Description	Uses	Comments
Fortified wines	Wines that have had their natural alcohol content increased by the addition of a brandy.	With dessert or after dinner.	Should be served in small, narrow glasses.
Honey wine (mead)	An ancient type of wine that was made from fermented honey flavored with herbs.	With meals.	The use of mead may predate that of the grape wines.
Light wines	A wine that has a low alcoholic content.	With meals.	These wines have enjoyed a recent surge in popularity. A wine containing only 8% alcohol is now being made in California.
Madeira	One of the wines made on the island of Madeira, which is located 500 miles (800 km) southeast of the coast of Portugal. (The wines range from light and dry to heavy and rich.)	Depending upon the type of wine, it may be served at various parts of the meal.	Madeira wines are the longest-lived (they keep for many years without deterioration) of any of the wines.
May wine	A light, white Rhine wine that is flavored with the herb woodruff.	Served chilled in a punch bowl with pieces of fresh fruit floating on top.	Good for serving at garden parties or other outdoor types of receptions
Moselle wines	Light wines (the alcohol content is usually about 10% or less) made in the valley of the Moselle River in Germany which lies to the west of the Rhine.	With lunch or dinner.	The most renowned Moselle wine is Bernkasteler Doktor, because it is reputed to have cured an ailing archbishop.
Mulled wine	Heated, sweetened, spiced wine served in a cup.	Served during the winter holidays.	Drinking a cup of mulled wine is a quick way to warm up after coming in from the cold.
Muscatel	A sweet fortified wine made from Muscat grapes.	Served with dessert.	Should be served in small, narrow glasses.
Perry (pear wine)	Light wine made from pear juice.	With meals	Among the least expensive wines.
Pinot	Wine made from Pinot grapes.	Starting material for making champagne. Served with meals.	California Pinot wines rival those of France.
Port	The type of fortified wine that originated in the town of Oporto in Portugal.	With dessert or after dinner.	Port wines are now made in countries other than Portugal. Hence, the Epicurean consumer should check the label carefully. Tawny port is aged longer than other port wines.
Pulque	Fermented juice of the agave plant that grows in Mexico and in southwestern U.S.	Used to make a distilled liquor, or used shortly after its preparation because it does not keep well.	A common drink in Mexico.
Red wines	Wines produced from dark-colored grapes that are fermented together with their skins (which contain most of the color pigments).	Served at meals featuring beef or lamb dishes, other than stews flavored with wine. (In the latter cases, wine is served after the meal.)	Usually, red wines have a higher iron content than lighter colored wines. Hence, they are the best for building up the blood of anemic persons.
Resinated (Greek) wines	Greek wines that contain a resin which imparts a pinelike flavor.	Best when served with mild-flavored main dishes made from fish, pork, or poultry.	Unresinated wines of high quality are also made in Greece.
Rice wine (sake)	A Japanese wine made from fermented white rice.	With meals at Japanese restaurants. May be served hot.	Although some people consider sake to be a beer (because it is made from a grain), it has an alcoholic content like that of wines.

(*Continued*)

TABLE W-20 (*Continued*)

Product	Description	Uses	Comments
Riesling	White wine made from the Riesling grape, which is considered to be the finest wine grape grown in Germany.	With meals.	Some California Riesling wines rival those of Germany.
Rhine wines	Wines vary from grapes grown in the Rhine River Valley of Germany. (The wines range from dry and light to rich and sweet.)	Depends upon the characteristics of the wine.	The best Rhine wines are those made from Riesling grapes.
Rose wines	Rose-colored wines produced by fermenting dark-colored grapes without the skins present, or from lighter grapes in the presence of their skins.	With cold foods and light meals, or when either a red or white wine might be used.	The best rose wines are made from grenache grapes.
Sauternes	Wines made in the Sauternes district of Bordeaux, France from grapes withered somewhat by a *Botrytis* mold that is also called "noble rot".	Should be served cold at the end of a meal; preferably, at which no other wine has been served.	Serve in small, narrow glasses. California Sauterne is quite different from French Sauternes.
Sherry	A fortified wine made by a process similar to the one developed in Jerez de la Frontera, Spain. (Sherries range from pale-colored dry wines to rich, sweet ones.)	Depends upon the characteristics of the particular wine.	Dry Spanish sherries are difficult to duplicate elsewhere, but the sweeter types made in California may rival the Spanish ones.
Sparkling wines	Wines that are bubbly with carbon dioxide gas by virtue of having undergone a second fermentation initiated by the addition of a small amount of sugar.	Accompaniments to any part(s) of a meal.	The consumption of these wines has risen considerably in the United States during the past 2 decades.
Sweet wines	Fortified wines that contain considerable amounts of unfermented sugars. (The addition of extra alcohol prevents the fermentation of the sugars which are present.)	Served as dessert.	Should be served in a small, narrow glass and consumed cautiously. (Some people become intoxicated more readily on sweet wines than on dry wines.)
Table wines	Unfortified wines of low to moderate alcoholic content. (They usually contain 14% or less of alcohol.)	Served with meals.	A 4 oz *(120 ml)* glass of a table wine contains about ½ oz *(15 ml)* of pure alcohol, which is about the amount that the body of a medium size man can metabolize in an hour.
Tokay	A rich white dessert wine made in Hungary that comes in dry and sweet varieties.	At meals or with desserts, depending upon whether the dry or sweet variety is served.	The sweeter the Tokay, the more expensive it is.
Vermouth	A fortified wine that is flavored with a variety of aromatic herbs and comes in dry and sweet varieties.	Preparation of Martinis or other cocktails. Sweet Italian vermouth is often served on ice as an aperitif.	Vermouth mixes well with soda water and/or small amounts of sweet liqueurs.
White wines	Made by fermenting grapes separated from their skins in order to keep the content of colored pigments low.	Served at meals featuring fish, pork, poultry, seafood, shellfish, or other bland-flavored items.	If two or more different types of wine are to be served, the white wine should be served before a red wine.
Zinfandel	A red wine made from Zinfandel grapes grown in California.	At meals featuring beef or lamb dishes other than stews that contain wine.	Zinfandel grapes are the variety most widely grown in California.

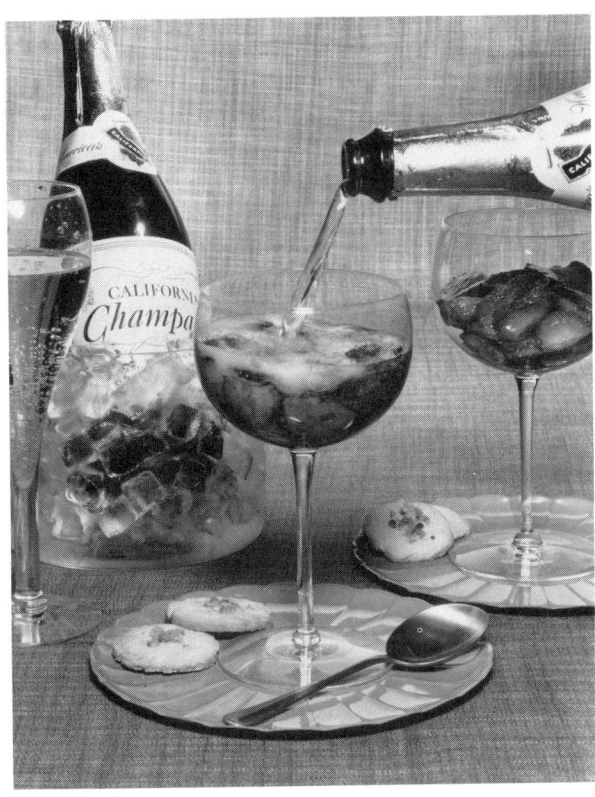

Fig. W-55. Champagne poured over fresh strawberries may be served as an appetizer or desert. (Courtesy, Wine Institute, San Francisco, Calif.)

MEDICINAL AND NUTRITIONAL EFFECTS.
Many curative powers have been attributed to wine, since it has been used medicinally from the time of the ancient Greek physician, (460 to 370 B.C.) Hippocrates. However, the observations made in the early days of medicine were often clouded by unidentified factors that may have helped to alleviate or worsen diseases. Therefore, some of the beneficial effects ascribed to wine in a recent article are noteworthy:[5]

1. Wine contains many constituents other than alcohol that tend to slow the rate at which the alcoholic content is absorbed. (Earlier studies showed that wine consumed with a meal produced a peak blood alcohol level that was only about one-quarter of that resulting from the same amount of alcohol taken in the form of gin or vodka.) Hence, intoxication is less likely to occur when moderate amounts of wine are consumed.

2. The anthocyanins (colored pigments) and tannins (astringent substances) in wines have greater antiviral effects than unfermented grape juice. However, these experiments were conducted in laboratory vessels, rather than in animal or human subjects.

3. Two 4 oz (120 ml) glasses of wine taken daily alter the blood patterns of cholesterol and other fats so that the likelihood of atherosclerotic heart disease is reduced by a small, but significant, amount.

4. Wine has a relaxing effect that may be due in part to ingredients other than alcohol.

5. The aroma and taste of good wines stimulate the appetite.

6. Substances present in both normal wine and dealcoholized wine promote better absorption of the essential minerals calcium, phosphorus, magnesium, and zinc than pure alcohol or deionized water. (It has long been thought that the absorption of iron is improved by wine. Hence, an old time remedy for iron deficiency anemia was "beef, iron, and wine.")

DANGERS OF DRINKING TOO MUCH WINE.
Intoxication and other serious threats to health may result from the overconsumption of any of the alcoholic beverages. Experiments have shown that the body of a medium size man can metabolize about ½ oz (15 ml) of pure alcohol per hour. This is equivalent to the amount of alcohol present in a 4 oz (120 ml) glass of most table wines. It is noteworthy that four 8 oz (250 ml) portions of California Zinfandel wine were consumed with meals at 4 hour intervals (between 9 A.M. and 9 P.M.) by young male volunteers who showed no signs of intoxication.[6] However, the consumption of similar amounts of wine without food has been shown to produce blood alcohol levels that are twice as high as those resulting from the consumption of wine with food. Therefore, it seems best to restrict the consumption of table wines to not more than 1 pt (480 ml) per day in order to allow for differences in the rates of alcohol absorption under various conditions of drinking.
(Also see ALCOHOLISM.)

[5]McDonald, J. B., "Not by Alcohol Alone," *Nutrition Today*, Vol. 14, January/February, 1979, pp. 14-19.

[6]*Ibid*, p. 18.

SUMMARY. People have used wine moderately and immoderately for many centuries, yet there are still many unanswered questions about the medicinal and nutritional effects of this beverage. Nevertheless, normal healthy people can enjoy the benefits of a moderate amount of wine per day while our researchers continue their efforts to learn the answers to these questions.

WINEBERRY *Rubus phoenicolasius*

The fruit of an oriental type of raspberry (fruit of the family *Rosaceae*).

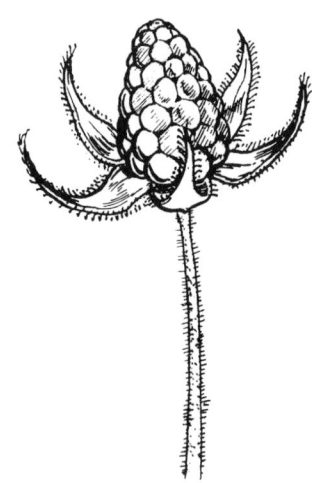

Fig. W-56.   The wineberry.

Wineberries are orange-colored and originated in northern China and Japan. They may be eaten fresh or made into jam, jelly, juice, pies, and wine.

(Also see FRUIT[S], Table F-47 Fruits Of The World—"Raspberry"; and RASPBERRY.)

WINTERIZATION

Some oils solidify or crystallize and become cloudy at refrigerator temperatures, due to the presence of triglycerides containing saturated fatty acids which have a higher melting point. The process of winterization filters out these triglycerides from a chilled oil thus improving consumer acceptability by providing an oil that remains clear. The higher melting triglycerides removed from the oil may be used in margarines and shortening.

(Also see OILS, VEGETABLE.)

WITCHES' MILK

Secretion from the mammary glands of the newborn of both sexes thought to be due to placental permeability to the lactation-producing hormones of the mother.

WOOD ALCOHOL (METHANOL; METHYL ALCOHOL; CH₃OH)

Originally, this product was obtained from the destructive distillation of wood; hence, it was termed wood alcohol. It is extremely poisonous (causes blindness).

(Also see METHYL ALCOHOL.)

WOODCOCK

Many hunters consider the woodcock to be the best winged game bird; and many gourmets consider it one of the most succulent morsels. It is full of glory when roasted before the hunter who shot it.

WORK, MUSCULAR; ENERGY REQUIREMENTS

Work is accomplished when a force acts to move an object some distance. Muscles are capable of creating a force and of performing work. However, for muscles to create a force they require chemical energy. Thus, anytime muscular work is performed the energy demands of the body increase. In fact, muscular activity is the most powerful stimulus for increasing the metabolic rate—the rate at which the body utilizes energy. Short bursts of strenuous exercise can increase the metabolic rate forty times that of the resting state. From day to day, a person engaged in sedentary work may require only 2,500 Calories (kcal) or less per day, while a person doing hard manual labor may require 5,000 Calories (kcal) or more per day.

(Also see CALORIC [ENERGY] EXPENDITURE; and METABOLIC RATE.)

WORLD FOOD

Contents   Page

In 1798, an English clergyman named Thomas Robert Malthus predicted part of the world food problem. He

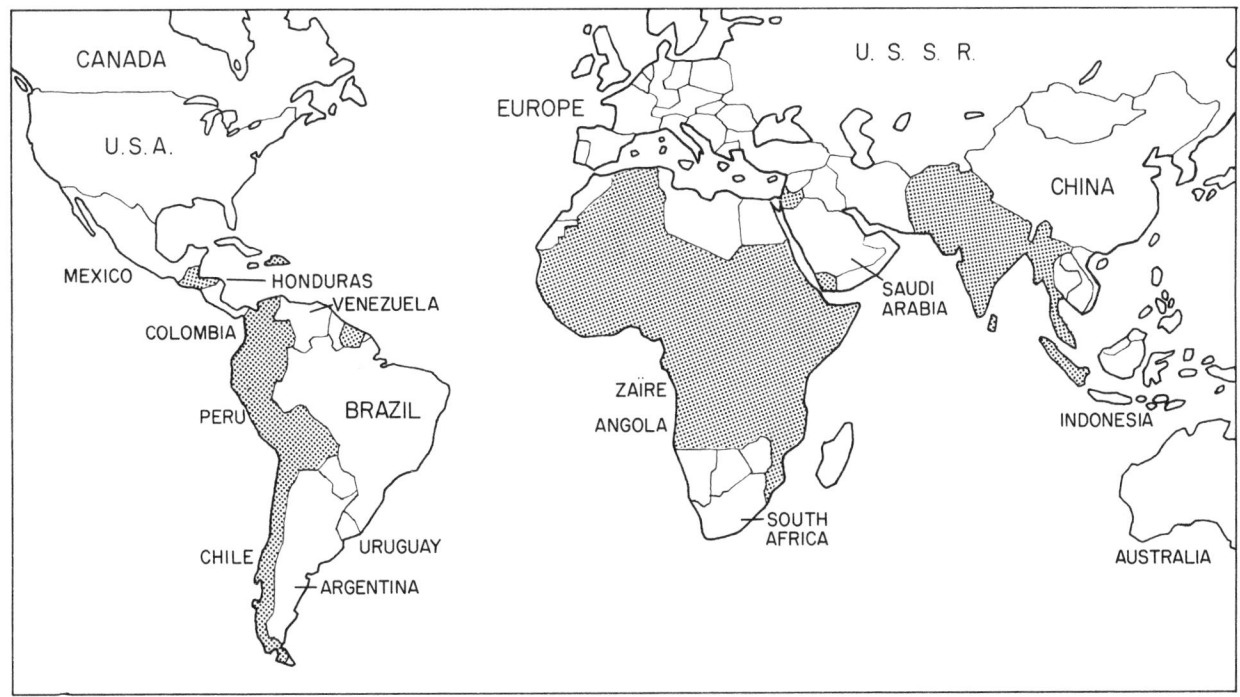

Fig. W-57. The geography of world food problems. The darkened areas are countries where the undernourished population exceeded 15%.

stated, "The power of population is infinitely greater than the power of the earth to provide subsistence for man." Malthus, however, failed to see the many changes of the future. For almost 200 years, we proved Malthus wrong because, as the population increased, new land was brought under cultivation; and machinery, chemicals, new crops and varieties, and irrigation were added to step up the yields. Now, science has given us the miracle of better health and longer life; and world population is increasing at the rate of about 240,000 people a day. At this rate, world population will double by the year 2045. To meet the needs of a more sophisticated and demanding world population of this size, world food production needs to increase at an average rate of about 2.5% per year.

World food problems are more complex than just too many people and too little food. Thus, during the 25-year period 1961–63 to 1983–85, people as a whole were better fed than previously. On the average, the food available per capita rose from 2,320 calories to 2,660 calories. But the exceptions were many! In the low income countries as a group, apart from China and India, per capita food supplies in 1983–85 were no higher than 15 years earlier. More disturbing yet, about 75% of the people in the world live in the developing countries where only 40% of the world's food is produced. Also, this is where most of the world's increase in population is occurring. Their rapid population growth causes severe economic strains on food production, processing and distribution. Finally, there is the problem of money. Countries

able to produce sufficient food for their needs could supply food to the developing countries where production does not meet the needs. However, these developing countries generally lack the money necessary to purchase food from other countries. Therefore, the world food problems are related to (1) population, (2) production and distribution, and (3) wealth.

(Also see MALTHUS.)

POPULATION, PRODUCTION, AND WEALTH AROUND THE WORLD.
Around the world, population, food production, and wealth are unequally distributed, and will remain so in the future.

● **Population**—The world population is about 5.3 billion and by the year 2000 it will be 6.2 billion. Assuming all 6.2 billion people stood shoulder to shoulder and occupied an average width of 2 ft, 6.2 billion people would circle the world 91 times, or reach to the moon and back nearly five times!

Numbers are, however, only part of the problem. As Table W-21 shows, there is and will be dramatic unequal distribution of the people of the world. Only 21% of the population will be in developed regions of the world by the year 2000. Africa, Asia, and Oceania, will have 70% of the population. Among the individual nations the United States will have only 4% of the world's population, compared to 21% in the People's Republic of China, or 16% in India.

TABLE W-21
POPULATION PROJECTIONS FOR WORLD, MAJOR REGIONS, AND SELECTED COUNTRIES[1]

Area	Year 1975	Year 2000	Percent of World Population in 2000
	(millions)		(%)
World	4,090	6,351	100
More developed regions	1,131	1,323	21
Less developed regions	2,959	5,028	79
Major regions			
Africa	399	814	13
Asia and Oceania	2,274	3,630	57
Latin America	325	637	10
U.S.S.R. and Eastern Europe	384	460	7
North America, Western Europe, Japan, Australia, and New Zealand	708	809	13
Selected countries and regions			
People's Republic of China	935	1,329	21
India	618	1,021	16
Indonesia	135	226	4
Bangladesh	79	159	2
Pakistan	71	149	2
Philippines	43	73	1
Thailand	42	75	1
South Korea	37	57	1
Egypt	37	65	1
Nigeria	63	135	2
Brazil	109	226	4
Mexico	60	131	2
United States	214	248	4
U.S.S.R.	254	309	5
Japan	112	133	2
Eastern Europe	130	152	2
Western Europe	344	378	6

[1]*Global 2000 Report to the President,* Entering the Twenty-First Century, p. 9, Table 1.

TABLE W-22
PER CAPITA GRAIN PRODUCTION, CONSUMPTION, AND TRADE, ACTUAL AND PROJECTED, AND PERCENT INCREASE IN PER CAPITA TOTAL FOOD PRODUCTION AND CONSUMPTION[1]

Area	Grain 1969-71	Grain 1973-75	Grain 2000	Food (Percent increase over the 1970-2000 period)
	(kilograms per capita)			(%)
United States				
Production	1,018.6	1,079.3	1,640.3	51.1
Consumption	824.9	748.0	1,111.5	28.3
Trade[2]	+ 194.7	+ 344.0	+ 528.8	
Western Europe				
Production	364.9	388.4	394.0	1.0
Consumption	432.4	443.3	548.8	15.5
Trade	− 65.4	− 57.6	− 154.8	
Japan				
Production	121.7	108.5	135.4	6.1
Consumption	267.5	274.4	452.3	54.2
Trade	− 138.1	− 175.9	− 316.7	
U.S.S.R.				
Production	697.6	711.2	903.2	28.1
Consumption	663.1	796.1	949.9	41.4
Trade	+ 16.1	− 42.0	− 46.7	
People's Republic of China				
Production	216.3	217.6	259.0	17.4
Consumption	220.2	222.4	267.8	19.1
Trade	− 4.0	− 4.8	− 8.8	
Latin America				
Production	236.1	241.0	311.4	33.7
Consumption	226.5	238.3	278.1	25.1
Trade	+ 11.8	+ 2.7	+ 33.3	
North Africa/Middle East				
Production	217.1	214.6	222.5	− 1.8
Consumption	276.2	273.8	292.8	2.2
Trade	− 50.8	− 69.8	− 70.3	
South Asia				
Production	161.6	162.4	170.0	4.6
Consumption	170.0	171.8	181.0	5.8
Trade	− 8.4	− 11.8	− 11.0	
Southeast Asia				
Production	244.7	214.5	316.5	35.9
Consumption	207.2	182.6	228.5	14.6
Trade	+ 37.5	+ 31.9	+ 87.5	
East Asia				
Production	137.3	136.0	163.5	22.8
Consumption	176.2	171.5	217.3	27.3
Trade	− 40.4	− 38.8	− 53.8	

[1]*Global 2000 Report to the President,* Entering the Twenty-First Century, pp. 20 and 21, Table 6.
[2]In trade figures, a plus sign indicates export, while a minus sign indicates import.

• **Production**—Food production depends upon a number of factors, among which are (1) the availability and use of land, (2) farming methods, (3) soil fertility, (4) water, (5) weather and climatic conditions, (6) civil order, and (7) incentives to producers. Therefore, the ability of countries to produce sufficient food for their need varies as shown in Table W-22.

Several important observations can be made from Table W-22. As far as past and future grain production is concerned, only three areas listed produce more grain than is consumed; thus leaving grain for export to other countries. Of the three—United States, Latin America, and Southeast Asia—the United States has the greatest excess for export. In terms of the percent increase in production and consumption of food between now and the year 2000, only the United States, Latin America, and Southeast Asia will significantly increase the percentage of food produced over that consumed. Most areas of the world will consume more food than they produce.

• **Wealth**—Living standards have risen during the 20th century, but wealth remains unequally distributed. In many countries the economic development lags; hence, they are unable to purchase food or apply technology to increase food production within their country. By comparing the per capita income some idea may be gained of the economic well-being of the countries and of the citizens' ability to purchase a nutritious diet. Table W-23 presents some of the countries with the highest incomes, and some of the lowest incomes.

TABLE W-23
PER CAPITA INCOME FOR SELECTED COUNTRIES[1]

Country	Per Capita Income
Highest:	(U.S. $)
Qatar	27,000
Switzerland	26,309
Iceland	21,660
Denmark and West Germany	19,750
U.S.A.	**16,490**
Japan	15,030
Australia	14,458
Norway	13,790
Luxumbourg	13,380
United Kingdom	13,329
Netherlands	13,065
France	13,046
Austria	12,521
United Arab Emirates and Finland	11,900
Lowest:	
Niger	310
Zambia	304
India	300
Somalia	290
Zimbabwe	275
Tanzania and China	258
Togo	240
Uganda and Afghanistan	220
Myanmar (Burma)	210
Vietnam	180
Nepal	160
Ethiopia	121
Bangladesh	113

[1]*The World Almanac and Book of Facts 1991*, pp. 684–771.

Several crucial observations can be made from the information in Table W-23. There is a wide gap between the highest per capita income countries and the lowest per capita income countries, and the gap will widen by 2000. In general, areas with the greatest population have the lowest per capita income.

In most low income countries, consumers spend ½ or more of their income for food; whereas, in the higher income countries, the proportion drops to less than ⅕.

For example, consumers in different countries spend the following proportion of their income for food: U.S.A., 10.3%; Canada, 11.3%; United Kingdom, 12.8%; Netherlands, 14.2%; Australia, 15%; Denmark, 15.7%; France, 16.4%; West Germany, 16.6%; Sweden, 17%; and Austria, 17.4%. Moreover, among the people of all countries, food takes a larger chunk of the income of the poor than it does of the rich, e.g., India where they spend 53% on food; the Philippines, 51%; and South Korea, 36%. The great disparities of wealth within countries can also be expected to widen by the year 2000.

(Also see INCOME, PROPORTION SPENT FOR FOOD.)

TYPE OF DIET. A country's staple food is its primary source of carbohydrate, and for much of the poor population it must also serve as the principle source of protein. The degree to which this generally low-quality protein is supplemented by a more valuable or complementary source of protein (animal or legume protein) depends on income. The developing countries where wheat and rice are the principal crops have been the most successful in meeting food demand. In countries where corn is the chief crop, about 15% of the population is undernourished. In countries where the people subsist on millet and sorghum or root and tubers (much of Africa), some degree of malnutrition is virtually universal.

Worldwide, those individuals at the lowest income level receive calories in the diet from the country's main food, usually a cereal grain, which contains small amounts of vegetable fats and proteins plus carbohydrates. As income rises, calories from the main food are replaced by animal fat, animal protein, and sugar. Also, as income rises, the total caloric intake rises sharply.

OUTLOOK AND OPTIONS RELATIVE TO WORLD FOOD. While the inclusion of animal products into a country's diet ensures better nutrition, it is inevitable that during periods of food scarcity some individuals will suggest that cereal grains be diverted from livestock and poultry feeding—that they will challenge the efficiency of animals in converting feed to food and the place of animals in the economical production of human food. Animal agriculture will be on trial. Increasingly, the charge will be made that much of the world goes hungry because of the substitution of meat, milk, and eggs for direct grain consumption. The goal is to feed the world a nutritious diet by the most efficient methods. Before deciding, individuals in both camps—(1) feed the grain to people, or (2) feed the grain to animals—should possess a sound knowledge of the options rather than moral indignation. When this is done, the outlook for the future may be brighter. To this end the important sections that follow are presented.

Who Shall Eat? Cereal grain is the most important single component of the world's food supply, accounting for between 30 and 70% of the food produced in all world regions. It is the major, and sometimes almost exclusive, source of food for many of the world's poorest people, supplying 60 to 75% of the total calories many of them consume. However, in many developed countries, more grain is fed to animals than is consumed directly by humans. Under such circumstances, sporadic food shortages and famine in different parts of the world give rise to the following recurring questions:

1.   Who should eat grain—people or animals? Shall we have food or feed?

2.   Can we have both food and feed?

FAVORING BREAD ALONE.   Historically, the people of new and sparsely populated countries have been meat eaters, whereas the people of the older and more densely populated areas have been vegetarians. The latter group has been forced to eliminate most animals and to consume plants and grains directly in an effort to avoid famine.

Among the arguments sometimes advanced by those who favor bread alone—the direct human consumption of grain—are the following:

1.   **More people can be fed.**   About 2,000 lb (*907 kg*) of grain must be supplied to livestock in order to produce enough meat and other livestock products to support a man for a year, whereas 400 lb (*181 kg*) of grain (corn, wheat, rice, soybeans, etc.) eaten directly will support a man for the same period of time. Thus, a given quantity of grain eaten directly will feed five times as many people as it will if it is first fed to livestock and then is eaten indirectly by humans in the form of livestock products. This is precisely the reason why the people of the Orient have become vegetarians.

2.   **On a feed, calorie, or protein conversion basis, it is not efficient to feed grain to animals and then to consume the livestock products.** This fact is pointed up in Figs. W-58 through W-60.

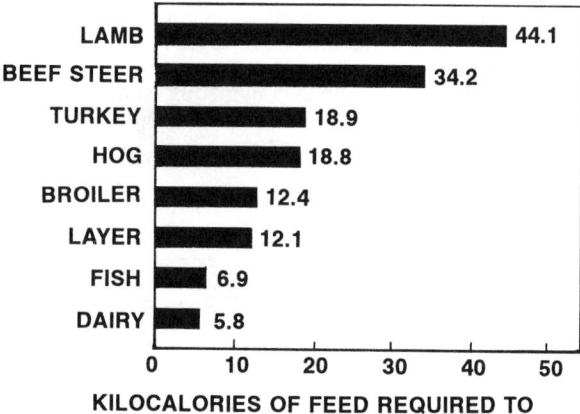

KILOCALORIES OF FEED REQUIRED TO PRODUCE ONE KILOCALORIE OF PRODUCT

Fig. W-59.   Kilocalories in feed required to produce 1 kcal of product. This shows that it takes 44.1 kcal in feed to produce 1 kcal in lamb, whereas only 5.8 kcal in feed will produce 1 kcal in milk.

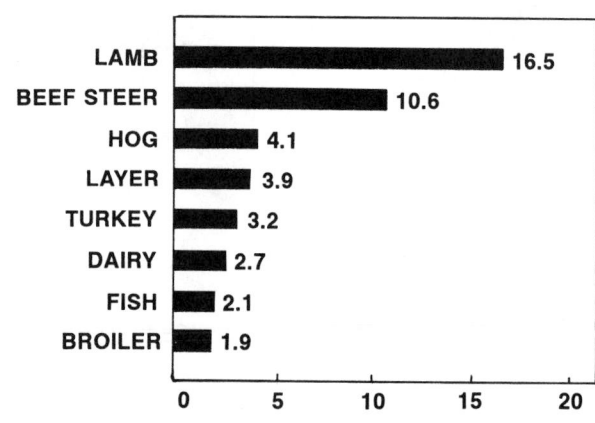

POUNDS OF FEED PROTEIN REQUIRED TO PRODUCE ONE POUND OF PRODUCT PROTEIN

Fig. W-60.   Pounds of feed protein required to produce 1.0 lb of product protein. This shows that it takes 16.5 lb of feed protein to produce 1.0 lb of lamb protein, whereas only 1.9 lb of feed protein will produce 1.0 lb of broiler protein. (One lb equals *0.45 kg*.)

Thus, in the developing countries, where the population explosion is greatest, virtually all grain is eaten directly by people; precious little of it is converted to animal products.

As people become more affluent, they actually use more grain, but most of it is converted into animal products, for they consume more meat, milk, and eggs. It is noteworthy, too, that no nation appears to have reached such a level of affluency that its per capita grain requirement has stopped rising.

FAVORING ANIMALS.   Practicality dictates that a hungry world should consider the following facts in favor of sharing grain with animals, then consuming the animal products:

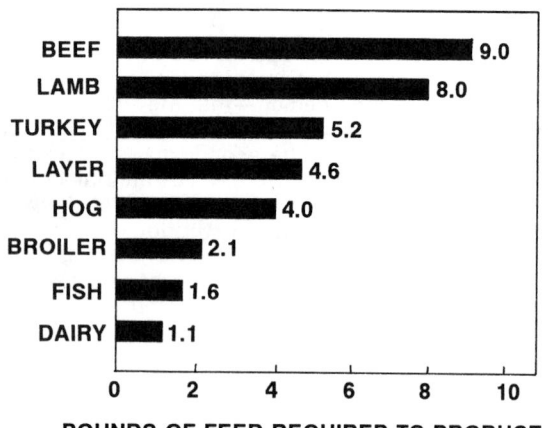

POUNDS OF FEED REQUIRED TO PRODUCE ONE POUND OF PRODUCT

Fig. W-58.   Pounds of feed required to produce 1 lb of product. This shows that it takes 9 lb of feed to produce 1 lb of on-foot beef, whereas it takes only 1.1 lb of feed to produce 1 lb of milk. (One lb equals *0.45 kg*.)

1. **Animals provide needed power.** In the developing nations, cattle, water buffalo, and horses still provide much of the agricultural power. Such draft animals are a part of the agricultural scene of Asia, Africa, the Near East, Latin America, and parts of Europe; areas characterized by small farms, low incomes, abundance of manpower, and lack of capital. They can be fueled on roughages to produce power, a most important consideration in times of energy shortage; and both cattle and water buffalo may be used for work, milk, and meat.

Although the general trend in the world is toward more and more mechanization, animals will continue to provide most of the agricultural power for the small/farm food/crop agriculture in many of the developing countries.

If the entire world were suddenly to adopt American farming and food processing methods, increasing the diets of all 5.3 billion people to the American level, the energy consumed would exhaust the world's known petroleum reserves in 13 years.

Modern, mechanized feed and food production requires an extra input of fuel, which is mostly of fossil origin. This auxiliary energy is expended in endless ways to improve agricultural productivity; it is used for drainage and irrigation, clearing of forest land, seedbed preparation, weed and pest control, fertilization, and efficient harvesting. In addition to production as such, there are two other important steps in the feed-food line as it moves from the producer to the consumer; namely, processing and marketing, both of which require higher energy inputs than to produce the food on the farm. In 1990, U.S. farms expended an average of 2.8 Calories (kcal) on the farm per calorie of food grown. By contrast, the Chinese wet rice peasant, using animal power (water buffalo), expends only 1 Calorie (kcal) of energy to produce each 50 Calories (kcal) of food.

(Also see ENERGY REQUIRED FOR FOOD PRODUCTION.)

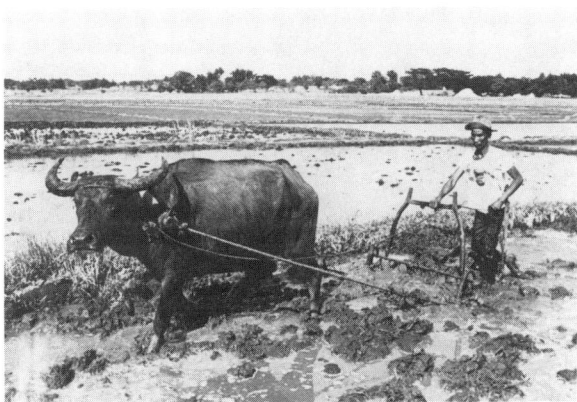

Fig. W-61. An Oriental wet rice peasant, using animal power (water buffalo), expends only 1 Calorie (kcal) of energy to produce each 50 Calories (kcal) of food. By comparison, the average U.S. farmer, using mechanical power (tractors), expends 2.8 Calories (kcal) of fuel energy to produce 1 Calorie (kcal) for food. (Courtesy, International Bank for Reconstruction and Development, Washington, D.C.)

2. **Animals provide needed nutrients.** Animal products provide all the essential amino acids (including lysine and methionine in which vegetable sources are deficient), plus minerals and vitamins, along with palatability and digestibility.

Foods of animal origin (meat, milk, and their various by-products) are especially important in the American diet; they provide ⅔ of the total protein, about ⅓ of the total energy, ⅘ of the calcium, ⅔ of the phosphorus, and significant amounts of the other minerals and vitamins needed in the human diet.

In addition, meat, dairy products, and eggs are a rich source of vitamin B-12, which does not occur in plant foods—only in animal sources and fermentation products. Also, it is noteworthy that the availability of iron in beef is twice as high as in plants.

About ⅔ of the world's protein supply is provided from plant sources, ⅓ from animal sources. Since the Food and Agriculture Organization of the United Nations reports that the world's diet needs animal protein in amounts equivalent to ⅓ of the total protein requirements, there should be ample animal protein, *provided* it were equally distributed. But it isn't. The people in the developed countries have five times as much high-quality animal protein per person as the people living in the developing countries (Table W-24). The gap between total protein (animal and plant combined) is not as wide (106.2 g vs 58.3 g per person per day in the developed and developing countries, respectively).

TABLE W-24
WORLD PROTEIN PER PERSON PER DAY IN GEOGRAPHIC AREAS OR COUNTRY[1]

Area or Country	Total Protein	Source	
		Animal	Plant
	←	(g/day)	→
U.S.S.R.	106.2	56.1	50.1
Europe	102.0	59.6	42.4
North-Central America	95.6	56.7	38.9
Oceania	88.9	56.8	32.1
South America	65.0	29.5	35.5
Asia	61.0	13.2	47.8
Africa	58.3	12.5	45.8
World Total	70.4	24.7	45.7

[1]*FAO Production Yearbook 1991*, FAO/UN, Rome, Italy, p. 239.

The most important role of animal protein is to correct the amino acid deficiencies of the cereal proteins, which supply about two-thirds of the total protein intake, and which are notably deficient in the amino acid, lysine. The latter deficiency can also be filled by soybean meal, fish, protein concentrates and isolates, synthetic lysine, or high-lysine corn. But such products have neither the natural balance in amino acids nor the appetite appeal of animal protein.

(Also see PROTEIN[S], section headed "Protein for the World.")

3. **Much of the world's land is not cultivated.** Vast acreages throughout the world—including arid and semiarid grazing lands; and brush, forest, cutover, and swamplands—are unsuited to the production of bread grains or any other type of farming; their highest and best use is, and will remain, for grazing and forest.

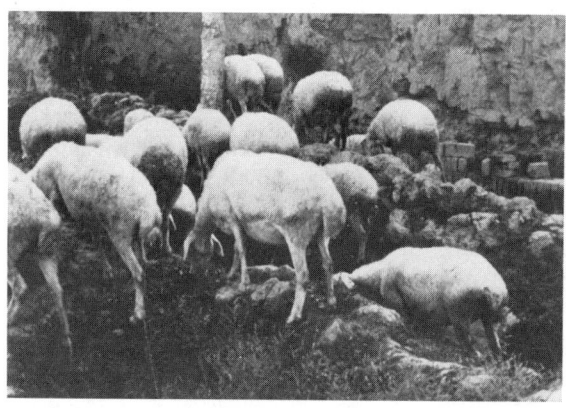

Fig. W-62. Vast areas throughout the world, such as this rough terrain, are not suited to cultivation. Hence, their only use is for grazing or forest.

In the United States, only 21% of the land area of the 50 states is cultivated. About 900 million acres, or 46.8%, of the land area, exclusive of Alaska and Hawaii, is pasture and grazing land.

In China, only 10.0% of the land is cultivated. North of China's Great Wall, life centers on pastoral areas; large flocks and herds of cattle, sheep, and horses roam these vast grasslands.

4. **Forages provide most of the feed for livestock.** Pastures and other roughages—feeds not suitable for human consumption—provide most of the feed for livestock, especially for ruminants (four-stomached animals such as cattle, sheep, goats, buffalo, and certain wild species including deer, antelope, and elk), throughout the world. Fortunately, the uniqueness of the ruminant's stomach permits it to consume forages, and, through bacterial synthesis, to convert such inedible (to humans) roughages into high-quality proteins—meat and milk. Hence, cattle and sheep manufacture human food from nonedible forage crops. Additionally, they serve as the primary means of storing (on the hoof, without refrigeration) such forage from one season to the next.

Despite grains being relatively plentiful in the United States, forages provide the bulk of animal feeds; pastures and other roughages account for 93.8% of the total feed of sheep, 84.5% of the feed of beef cattle, 58.7% of the feed of dairy cattle, and 61.7% of the feed of all livestock.

5. **Food and feed grains are not synonymous.** Animals do not compete to any appreciable extent with the hungry people of the world for food grains, such as rice or wheat. Instead, they eat feed grains and by-product feeds—like field corn, grain sorghum, barley, oats, milling by-products, distillery wastes, and fruit and vegetable wastes—for which there is little or no demand for human use in most countries, plus forages and grasses—fibrous stuff that man cannot eat. For example, in the United States only 3% of the corn—the major animal feed grain—is used for human food. Also, it is noteworthy that the feed grains which the United States ships overseas are used almost entirely for livestock and poultry production abroad.

6. **Ruminants utilize low-quality roughages.** Cattle, sheep, and goats efficiently utilize large quantities of coarse, high-cellulose roughages, including crop residues, straw, and coarse low-grade hays. Such products are indigestible to humans, but from 30 to 80% of the cellulose material is digested by ruminants.

Of all U.S. crop residues, the residue of corn (cornstalks and husklage) is produced in the greatest abundance and offers the greatest potential for expansion in cow numbers. In 1990, 66,952,000 acres of corn, yielding 118.5 bushels per acre, were harvested in this country.

Normally, over and above the grain, corn produces over 200 million tons of corn residue each year. That's more than 200 million tons of potential cow feed, enough to winter more than 150 million pregnant cows. Mature cows are physiologically well adapted to utilizing such roughage. Moreover, when corn residue is used to the maximum as cow feed, acreage which would otherwise be used to pasture the herd is liberated to produce more corn and other crops. Also, there are many other crop residues which, if properly utilized, could increase the 150 million head figure given above.

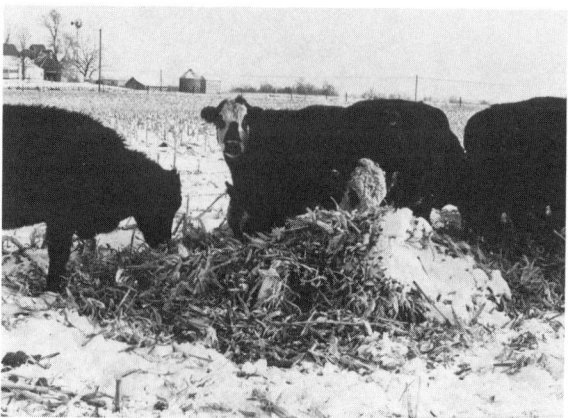

Fig. W-63. Cattle can utilize efficiently large quantities of coarse, humanly inedible roughages, like cornstalks. This shows cows feeding on corn residue which had been harvested by mechanical means. (Courtesy, Iowa State University)

7. **Animals utilize by-products.** Animals provide a practical outlet for a host of by-product feeds derived from plants and animals, which are not suited for human consumption. Some of these residues (or wastes) have been used for animal feeds for so long, and so extensively, that they are commonly classed as feed ingredients, along with such things as the cereal grains, without reference to their by-product origin. Most of these processing residues have little or no value as a source of nutrients for human consumption. Among such by-products are corncobs, cottonseed hulls, gin trash, oilseed meals, beet pulp, citrus pulp, molasses (cane, beet, citrus, and wood), wood by-products, rice bran and hulls, wheat milling by-products, and fruit, nut, and vegetable refuse. It is estimated that each year ruminants convert more than 9 million tons of by-products into human food.

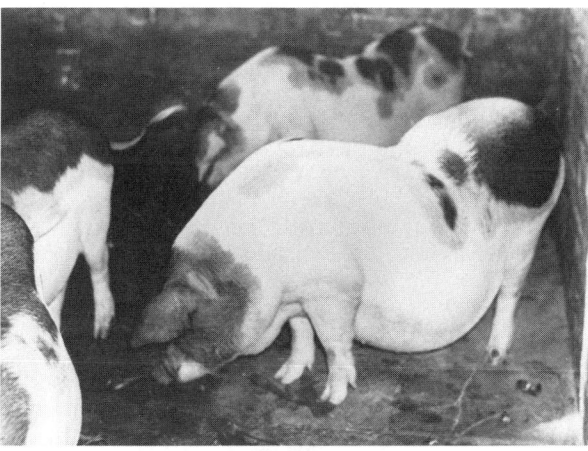

Fig. W-64. Chinese hogs in Kwang Tung Province, in China. Their ration consisted of two by-products—rice millfeed and bagasse (the pitch of sugarcane), along with water hyacinth—all of which the pigs ate with relish. In China, swine utilize millions of tons of otherwise wasted crop residues and by-products. (Photo by A. H. Ensminger)

8. **Animals provide elasticity and stability to grain production.** Livestock feeding provides a large and flexible outlet for the year-to-year changes in grain supplies. When there is a large production of grain, more can be fed to livestock, with the animals carried to heavier weights and higher finish. On the other hand, when grain supplies are low, herds and flocks can be maintained by reducing the grain that is fed and by increasing the grasses and roughages in the ration. Thus, when grains are in short supply, fewer slaughter cattle are grain fed— more are grass finished. In the years ahead, depending on future grain supplies and prices, it is predicted that less than two-thirds of the U.S. domestic beef supply will come from feedlot cattle, in comparison with the 77% of U.S. slaughter cattle that were grain fed in 1973. Also, during periods of high-priced grains, heavier feeder cattle will go into feedlots, and they will be fed for a shorter period on less grain and more roughage than when grains are more abundant and cheaper.

In the future, animals will increasingly be "roughage burners," with the proportion of grain to roughage determined by grain supplies and prices.

Beef cattlemen, dairymen, and sheepmen will more and more rely upon the ability of the ruminant to convert coarse forage, grass, and by-product feeds, along with a minimum of grain, into palatable and nutritious food for human consumption, thereby competing less for humanly edible grains. The longtime trend in animal feeding will be back to roughages; increasingly, all flesh will be grass.

9. **Animals step up the protein content and quality of foods.** Grains, such as corn, are much lower in protein content in cereal form than after conversion into meat, milk, or eggs. On a dry basis, the protein contents of selected products are corn, 10.45%; beef (Choice grade, total edible, trimmed to retail level, raw), 30.7%; milk, 26.4%; and eggs, 47.0%. Also, animals increase the quality (e.g., biological value) of the protein—a higher proportion of the protein is assimilated by the body. (Also see PROTEIN[S].)

10. **Ruminants convert nonprotein nitrogen to protein.** Ruminant animals (cattle, sheep, and goats) can use nonprotein nitrogen, like urea, to produce protein for humans in the form of meat and milk.

11. **Animals provide medicinal and other products.** Animals are not processed for meat alone. They are the source of hundreds of important by-products, including some 100 medicines such as insulin, epinephrine, and heparin, without which the lifestyle and health of many people would be altered.

Besides medicines, many familiar products are derived from animals, including leather, shoe polish, photographic film, soap, lubricants, candles, glue, buttons, and bone china, to name a few.

12. **Animals maintain soil fertility.** Animals provide manure for the fields, a fact which was often forgotten during the era when chemical fertilizers were relatively abundant and cheap. One ton (907 kg) of average manure contains 18 lb (8.2 kg) of nitrogen, 9 lb (4.1 kg) of phosphorus, and 13 lb (5.9 kg) of potassium.

The energy crisis prompted concern that farmers would not have sufficient chemical fertilizers at reasonable prices in the years ahead. Since nitrogenous fertilizers are oil- and petroleum-based, there is cause for concern. As a result, a growing number of American farmers are returning to organic farming; they are using more manure—the unwanted barnyard centerpiece of the past 30 years, and they are discovering that they are just as good reapers of the land and far better stewards of the soil.

(Also see ORGANICALLY GROWN FOOD.)

Meeting The Feeds Vs Foods Dilemma. Life on earth is dependent upon *photosynthesis*. Without it, there would be no oxygen, no plants, no feed, no food, no animals, and no people.

As fossil fuels (coal, oil, shale, and petroleum)—the stored photosynthates of previous millenia—become exhausted, the biblical statement, "all flesh is grass" (Isaiah 40:6), comes alive again. The focus is on photosynthesis. Plants, using solar energy, are by far the most important, and the only renewable, energy-producing method; the only basic food-manufacturing process in the world; and the only major source of oxygen in the earth's atmosphere. Even the chemical and electrical energy used in the brain cells of man is the product of sunlight and the chlorophyll of green plants. Thus, in an era of world food shortages, it is inevitable that the entrapment of solar energy through photosynthesis will, in the long run, prove more valuable than all the underground fossil fuels—for when the latter are gone, they are gone forever.

(Also see PHOTOSYNTHESIS.)

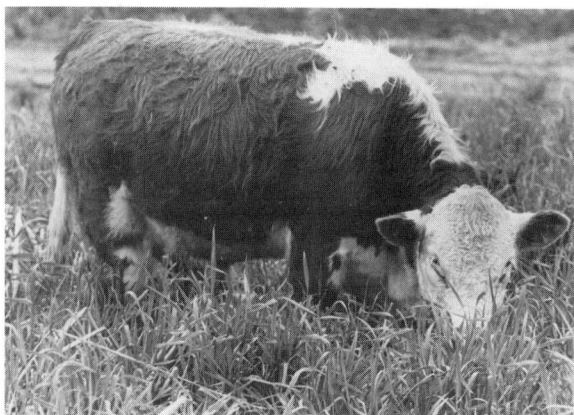

Fig. W-65. Ruminants—cattle, sheep, and goats—convert the photosynthetic energy derived from solar energy and stored in grass into food for humans. (Courtesy, *Progressive Farmer,* Birmingham, Ala.)

Practicality dictates that a hungry world should, and will, proceed in about the following order in meeting the feeds vs foods dilemma:

1. Consume a higher proportion of humanly edible grains and seeds, and their by-products, directly—without putting them through animals, simply because approximately five times more people can be fed by doing it this way.

2. Utilize a higher proportion of roughages to concentrates in animal rations as increasing quantities of cereal grains are needed for human consumption.

3. Retain more of those species that can utilize a maximum of humanly inedible feeds and a minimum of products suitable for human consumption. This would favor cows, sheep, and goats, provided they are fed a maximum of pasture and other roughages. Both poultry and swine may compete with man for grains. Nevertheless, it is expected that further increases in poultry will come, primarily because of their efficiency as converters of protein from feed to food, and their adaptability to small-scale production. Also, it is expected that there will be further increases in swine, especially in China, where pigs are scavengers and manure producers par excellence.

4. Propagate the most efficient feed to food species converters (see Figs. W-58, W-59 and W-60). This means dairy cows, fish, and poultry. Because beef cattle and sheep are at the bottom of the totem pole when it comes to feed efficiency, the pressure will be to eliminate them, except as roughage consumers. Although not mentioned yet, rabbits are also efficient converters of feed to food, and can utilize roughages to some extent. Moreover, rabbits are easily adapted to small-scale agriculture.

5. Increase the within-species efficiency of all animals and eliminate the inefficient ones. This calls for more careful selection and more rigid culling than ever before.

6. Improve pastures and ranges. Good pasture will produce 200 to 400 lb (*91 to 181 kg*) of beef or lamb per acre annually (in weight of young weaned, or in added weight of older animals); superior pastures will do much better.

Improving The World Food Situation.

The world food situation can be improved provided major problems are solved, many of which are not self-correcting. Among the most pressing are curbing population growth, transferring food from the developed food-exporting countries to the developing food-deficit countries, providing for emergency disaster and famine relief, achieving an acceptable degree of stability of world food prices, and finding the proper combination of techniques and policies to bring about a substantial improvement in food production in developing countries. On a longtime basis, the world food situation can best be improved by a massive infusion of education, science, and technology—by self-help programs—so that they can produce more of their own food.

• **Population control**—Members of the animal kingdom other than man have their numbers held in check by the many factors encompassed in the term "balance of nature." Man is different! His strong propensity is to overpopulate the earth and to create conditions which threaten his very existence—his food supply, the water he drinks, the environment in which he lives, and the very air he breathes.

Without doubt, people will continue to live longer. Hence, curbing population growth will be required to maintain the balance between production and demand for food. It will be necessary to bring the number of people and their supply of food into proper balance. Alternate methods of population control are starvation, disease, and/or war.

• **Fair prices and profits**—People do those things which are most profitable to them; and farmers are people. The American farmer, and farmers in certain other countries of the world, can produce more, but higher prices than have existed in the past will be necessary to assure this.

Farmers, like any businessmen, have always demonstrated their willingness to respond to incentives—prices and profits.

• **Increase cultivable land**—Ever since man stopped living a nomadic life, he has been hunting for arable (cultivable) land. Fortunately, there is still much of it to be had. Studies show that about twice as much of the world's land is suitable for crops as is presently used. More than half of the potential, but presently unused, arable land is in the tropics, and about a sixth of it is in the humid tropics—the largest areas being in Africa and South America.

• **More irrigation**—The value of irrigation for increasing crop yields is generally known. Yet, a study of the world's 20 major irrigating countries, in areas irrigated, showed that only 15% of their total cultivated area was irrigated. Thus, the potential to increase crop yields through irrigation is very great.

• **Improve crop yields**—While the amount of land that could be brought into production is perhaps double that currently used, all recent studies of world food production conclude that, outside of Africa and Latin America, yield-increasing techniques—irrigation, fertilizer, new seeds, and improved technology—will be the primary source of future food increases.

In addition to irrigation, fertilizer is a key factor in yield increases, although it must be combined with improved varieties of seeds and improved cultural practices if it is to have much impact on yields. As evidence of the soundness of the fertilizer approach, it is noteworthy that almost half of the 50% gain in crop output per acre in the United States since 1940 is attributed to the increased use of fertilizers. From this, it may be concluded that increased use of fertilizer could increase world food output by 50% in the years ahead.

• **Full use of pastures and ranges**—Some sparsely populated areas of the world, such as Australia, New Zealand, Argentina's pampas area, and the western range areas of the United States and Canada, are now important sources of livestock products. But there are still vast areas of sparsely settled grasslands where the production of livestock products is small; among them, large portions of Africa, the highlands of central Asia, some portions of the Andean area of South America, and the nomadic grazing areas of the Near East. In these areas, subsistence is the goal and animal numbers are generally regarded as being more important than the yield of salable products. Nevertheless, the potential for increased production in these areas is considerable. Also, and most important, the only practical way of harvesting human food from many of these areas is through livestock. So, grass—the world's largest crop—should no longer be taken for granted. In an era of world food shortages, the contribution of properly managed grazing lands in terms of food and fiber production needs to be pursued. No other program offers so much potential to increase the world's food production capacity quickly and at so little cost; this is especially true of the grasslands in the tropics and subtropics.

• **Produce leaner beef**—Leaner beef is higher in protein content than fat beef. On a carcass basis, trimmed to retail level, Standard grade runs 19.4% protein vs 17.4% for Choice grade—that's 2% higher. Besides, leaner beef can be produced with much less grain.

Consumer preferences and costs of production underlie the relative prices of fat and lean beef, but changes in U.S. grading standards help consumers adjust their consumption patterns. For this reason, when grain prices are high, producers exert pressure to have the beef-grading system changed so as to reduce the amount of grain fed.

• **Select efficient animals**—Improved genetics, along with improved feeding and management, have made for more meat, milk, and eggs. Yet, further improvements are possible and needed, especially in the developing countries. Although 60% of the animals of the world are raised in the developing countries, primarily in Africa and Asia, these nations produce less than 30% of the world's meat, milk, and eggs. This low productivity is largely due to the failure to utilize the scientific principles of husbandry and disease control.

• **Feed roughage and by-products**—In the future, cattle and sheep will increasingly be "roughage burners." Stockmen will rely upon the ability of the ruminant to convert coarse forage, grass, and by-product feeds, along with a minimum of concentrate, into palatable and nutritious food for human consumption, thereby competing less for humanly edible grains.

Ruminants can make the transition to more roughage with ease. For them, it is merely a "return to nature," for they evolved as consumers of forage.

• **Control disease and parasites**—Diseases in farm animals reduce the supply of meat and other animal products by an unknown, but large, quantity, and add substantially to the cost of food and fiber. The cost of animal diseases to U.S. producers and consumers is estimated to be somewhere between $10 and $12 billion annually.

Deaths of animals take a tremendous toll. Even greater economic losses—hidden losses—result from failure to reproduce living young, and from losses due to retarded growth and poor feed efficiency, carcass condemnations and decreases in meat quality, and labor and drug costs. Also, considerable cost is involved in keeping out diseases that do not exist in a country, such as keeping foot-and-mouth disease out of the United States. Quarantine of a diseased area may cause depreciation of land values or even restrict whole agricultural programs. Additionally, and most importantly, it is recognized that some 200 different types of infectious and parasitic diseases can be transmitted from animals to human beings; among them, such dreaded diseases as brucellosis (undulant fever), leptospirosis, anthrax, Q fever, rabies, trichinosis, tuberculosis, and tularemia. Thus, rigid meat and milk inspection is necessary for the protection of human health. This is added expense which the producer, processor, and consumer must share.

Thus, the potential throughout the world of providing more food through animal disease and parasite control is very great. The level of animal health attained in the advanced countries shows that tremendous scope exists for improvement in most developing areas. It is estimated that if the tsetse fly of the high rainfall belt of tropical Africa were brought under control, the savannah pastures could carry a cattle population of 120 million head, approximately equal to the total cattle population of the United States.

• **Create new and improved protein sources**—It is generally recognized that diet customs are somewhat emotional in character—that many people will put synthetic clothes on their backs long before they will put synthetic food in their stomachs. Yet, when people are hungry or suffering from malnutrition, they are not finicky about the "pedigree" of their food.

Researchers are attempting to bolster traditional protein sources and to develop entirely new proteins, with their efforts centered around the following approaches and protein sources: (1) improvement of traditional sources through genetic manipulation, (2) fortification with synthetic nutrients, or addition of protein concentrates from fish, oilseeds, and other foods, (3) use of the versatile soybean, and (4) development of single cell protein technology.

(Also see SINGLE-CELL PROTEIN; and SOYBEAN.)

• **Improve small-scale farming methods**—The United States and other developed countries are well known for agriculture that is large in scale and high in capital investments, substituting machinery for human labor. Although it has made the United States the world's largest exporter of food, the technology for large-scale agriculture has been difficult to implement abroad.

Subsistence farming is the principal agricultural practice internationally, especially in the developing countries. Unlike the large U.S. operations, subsistence farms are small in scale and low in capital investments, requiring intensive labor of the approximately one billion farmers who operate them. About 40% of the world's farmers have fewer than 11 acres (*4.5 ha*) of land; 35% have fewer than 2.5 acres (*1 ha*). These farms feed a majority of the world population. To provide effective technical assistance to these farmers, scientists must understand the problems of small-scale agriculture.

Although leading scientists have recently identified small-scale agriculture as a priority for research and several international agricultural research centers have initiated mixed cropping and homestead farming studies, research is still lacking on integrated small-scale agriculture, including crop production, methodology, vegetable crops, small animal production, and energy generation.

History shows that world food production has never been immune from shortfalls. These food shortages become more likely as world population increases. As food prices increase because of higher energy costs, the needy will depend on diets made up of the cheapest, most-accessible food without regard for nutrition.

One way to increase the food base and income is for farmers in densely populated agrarian regions to increase the agricultural production on their small land holdings. These farmers would then have the incentive to remain on the farm, avoiding the social problems that result when farmers migrate to the city. Appropriate small-scale agriculture could integrate crops and small animals (poultry, rabbits, milking goats, and sheep) into a system that would meet the nutritional requirements of the family, improving the quality as well as the quantity of food. This integrated approach could make a significant contribution to national health, wealth, and stability.

• **Farm the sea**—The ocean, which covers 70.73% of the earth's surface and, therefore, receives a proportionate amount of all the solar energy reaching this planet, is one of the most promising potentials for providing added food for the world's spiraling human population. It is an immense reservoir of food which man has only lightly tapped. Hence, there is growing interest in the sea as a source of food supply, including both fish and vegetables.

• **Eliminate waste**—Waste of food supplies will increasingly nag the consciences and pocketbooks of all people—producers and consumers alike.

Pests cause an estimated 30% annual loss in the worldwide potential production of crops, livestock, and forests. Every part of our food, feed, and fiber supply—including marine life, wild and domestic animals, field crops, horticultural crops, and wild plants—is vulnerable to pest attack. Obviously, if these losses could be prevented, or reduced, world food supplies would be increased by nearly one-third. The problems are complex, but the stakes are high.

This worldwide annual loss of 30% potential food productivity occurs despite the use of advanced farming technology and mechanized agriculture. Furthermore, in many of the developing countries losses greatly exceed this figure.

Pests of many kinds attack plants during all stages of their growth, and they attack food and food products after harvest—in storage, during transportation to market, in warehouses, in elevators, in ships, in supermarkets, and in homes after purchase. A few notable pest losses include: plant diseases, insects, weeds, rats, and birds.

Why Be Your Brother's Keeper? Famine and starvation are not new to the people of the world, but what is new are the electronic means of communication which are shrinking the size of the world and increasing our awareness. People can sit in their living rooms and watch others starve in some other area, or people in a remote village can become aware that there is another world where people have enough of life's essentials. There are numerous reasons to worry enough to take action, but the three major ones follow:

1. **Humanitarian.** Developing countries need help and many developed countries have the knowledge and resources to help. The challenge of a difficult task and the moral uplift that comes only from doing for others can serve to temper and balance the affluence of American life as exemplified in the late Albert Schweitzer's dictum: "It is only giving that stimulates."

2. **Security.** By the year 2000, there will be four times as many people in the developing countries as in the developed countries. Developed countries cannot afford to be too little and too late with their assistance. The idea that security is more than military might is not new. Seneca, nearly 2,000 years ago, warned the Roman Senate: "A hungry people listens not to reason nor is its demand turned aside by prayers."

The expectations of the poor are demanding fulfillment. Hopefully, some measure of their ambitions can be realized by peaceful means.

3. **Economic.** An important way to expand our own economy in the future will be the creation of additional markets for U.S. goods and products. This aim is not entirely self-serving, because achievement of sustained economic growth by the hungry countries will depend upon their participation in world markets on a competitive basis.

While people of the world do not share a common history, they do share a common future. By sharing and applying know-how, the whole world will have a brighter tomorrow. Dreams will come true—faster and more abundantly, with more food and animals in the future.

(Also see CEREAL GRAINS, sections headed "Feeds for Livestock" and "Future Prospects for the Cereal Grains"; ENERGY REQUIRED FOR FOOD PRODUCTION; GREEN REVOLUTION; HUNGER, WORLD; MALNUTRITION, PROTEIN-ENERGY; MALTHUS; NUCLEIC ACIDS, section headed "Genetic Engineering"; PHOTOSYNTHESIS; and POPULATION, WORLD.)

WORLD HEALTH ORGANIZATION (WHO)

A specialized agency of the United Nations founded in 1948 to further international cooperation for improved health conditions—physical, mental, and social well-being. The main offices are located in Geneva, Switzerland; and there are six regional offices around the world. Primarily, member governments, on the basis of their relative ability, finance the WHO with yearly contributions. About 130 countries are members. The World Health Assembly, the policy-making body; the Executive Board, a board of health specialists; and the Secretariat, the regional offices and field staff, are the principle organs through which the WHO operates.

The WHO is involved in three distinct health-related areas:

1. It provides a research service and sets standards of international sanitary regulations. The WHO keeps member countries informed on the most recent developments in the use of vaccines, control of drug addiction, nutritional discoveries, cancer research, and health hazards of nuclear radiation. It also standardizes quarantine measures with minimal interference of international trade and air travel.

2. It encourages member nations to enlarge and strengthen their health programs. To do this, the WHO, on request, provides (a) technical advice to governments, (b) sends out international teams of experts, (c) helps set up health centers, and (d) offers aid for the training of medical and nursing personnel.

3. It helps control epidemic and endemic diseases by promoting mass campaigns involving nationwide vaccination programs, clinics for early diagnosis and prevention of diseases, pure water supplies, good sanitation systems, health education, and antibiotic and insecticide use. It has been effective with campaigns against tuberculosis, malaria, and smallpox.

Besides its own programs, the WHO often works closely with the FAO (Food and Agriculture Organization).

(Also see FOOD AND AGRICULTURE ORGANIZATION OF THE UNITED NATIONS; and DISEASES, section headed "International and Voluntary Organizations Engaged in Health and/or Nutrition Activities.")

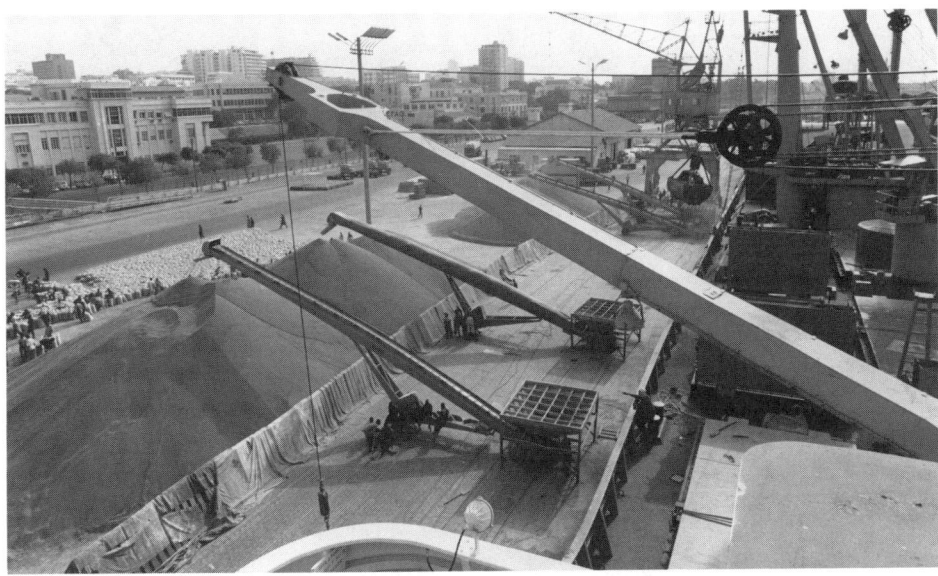

Improving the world food situation involves both short-run and long-run arrangements. The short-run: grain reserves for droughts, floods, and similar emergencies. The long-run: population control and self-help programs through the application of science and technology.

The above picture shows U.S. sorghum grain unloaded at the docks in Dakar (Africa). (Courtesy, Agency for International Development, Washington, D.C.)

PRODUCING THE NATION'S FOOD

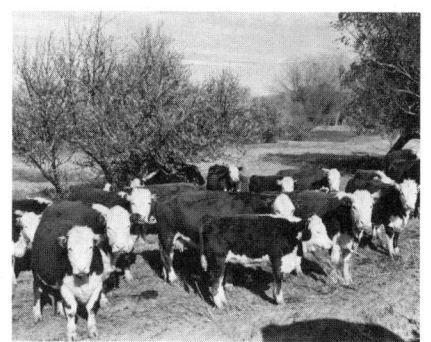

BEEF ON THE HOOF

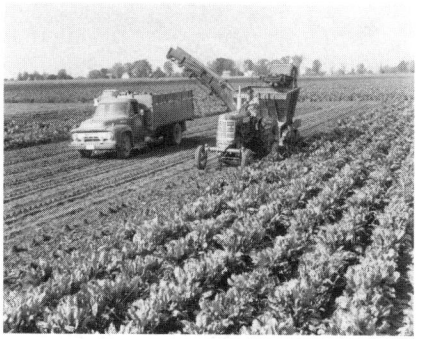

HARVESTING SUGAR BEETS

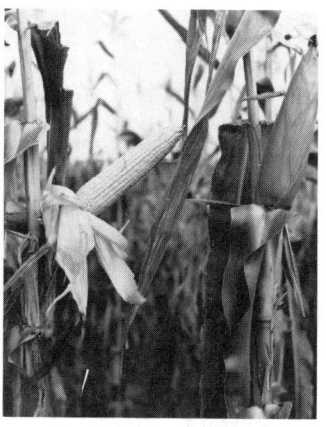

GROWING CORN

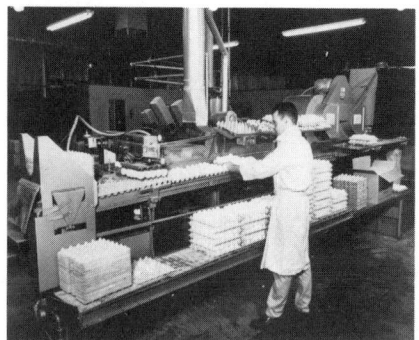

HANDLING EGGS

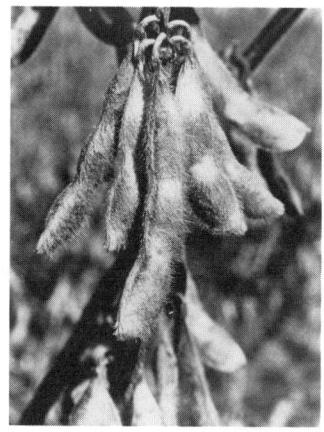

SOYBEAN CULTURE

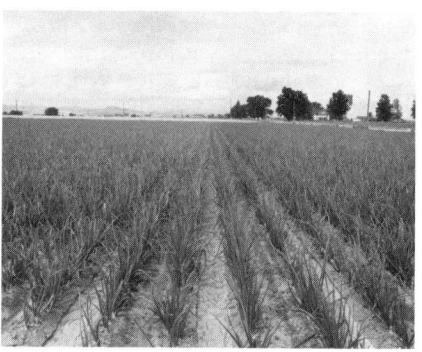

FIELD OF ONIONS

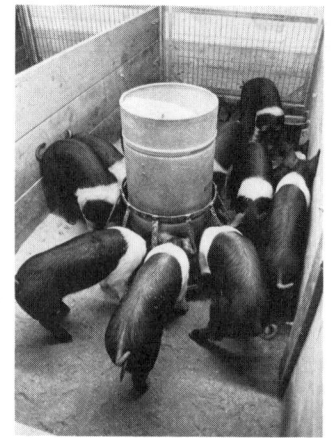

PIGS TO PORK

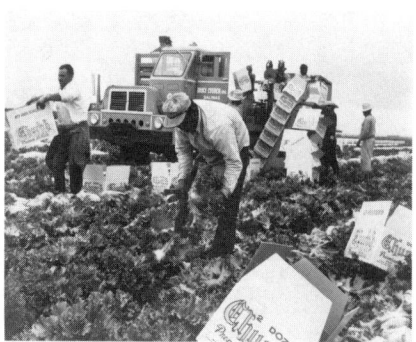

PACKING LETTUCE

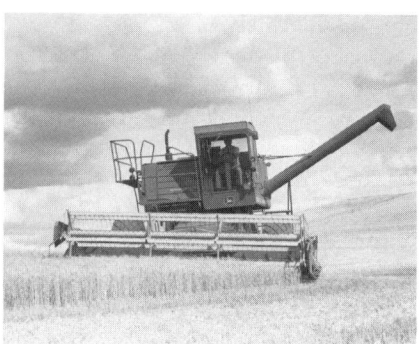

CUTTING WHEAT

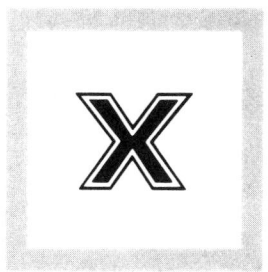

XANTHINE

An intermediate in the metabolism of purines. It was first isolated from gallstones. It occurs in animal organs, yeast, potatoes, coffee, and tea.

XANTHOMA

A benign flat yellow tumor, containing a deposit of fatty substance, commonly located on the inner side of the lower eyelid.

XANTHOPHYLL

While it is one of the most widespread naturally occurring carotenoid alcohols, it does not possess any vitamin A activity. Xanthophyll is a yellow pigment, which can be (1) isolated from certain natural products, and (2) produced synthetically.

Feeds that contain large amounts of xanthophylls produce a deep yellow color in the beak, skin, and shank of yellow-skinned breeds of chickens. The consumer associates this pigmentation with quality and, in many cases, is willing to pay a premium price for a bird of this type. Also, processors of egg yolks are frequently interested in producing dark-colored yolks to maximize coloration of egg noodles and other food products. The latter can be accomplished by adding about 60 mg of xanthophyll per kilogram of diet. In recognition of these consumer preferences, many producers add ingredients that contain xanthophylls to poultry rations.

Rich natural sources of xanthophyll follow:

Feedstuff	Xanthophyll Content
	(mg/kg)
Marigold petal meal	7,000
Algae, common, dried	2,000
Alfalfa juice protein, 40% protein	800
Alfalfa meal, 20% protein	240

(Also see ZEAXANTHIN.)

XEROPHTHALMIA

The term describing keratinization and cloudiness of the cornea caused by a vitamin A deficiency. Xerophthalmia occurs most frequently in undernourished infants and children in India, the Middle East, Southeast Asia, and parts of Africa and South America, in areas where the diet is lacking in whole milk, butter, and green or yellow vegetables. Vitamin A should be administered immediately to persons with xerophthalmia in order to arrest the disease and prevent the loss of sight.

(Also see BLINDNESS DUE TO VITAMIN A DEFICIENCY; DEFICIENCY DISEASES, Table D-1 Major Dietary Deficiency Diseases; and VITAMIN A, section headed "Deficiency Symptoms.")

XEROSIS

Abnormal dryness of the skin or front of the eye.

XYLITOL ($C_5H_{12}O_5$)

Xylitol is a sugar alcohol. The aldehyde group ($C = O$) of the pentose sugar—5-carbon sugar—xylose is replaced by a hydroxyl group (OH). It can be made from birchwood chips, berries, leaves and mushrooms. Xylitol is commercially produced in Finland from birchwood chips hydrolyzed by acid to xylose. In the body, xylitol is formed as an intermediate during the formation of xyluose. Ingested xylitol is also converted to xyluose. Xyluose then enters the pentose-phosphate cycle of carbohydrate metabolism.

Xylitol tastes almost as sweet as sucrose, table sugar; additionally, it has a cool taste when dissolved in the mouth due to its negative heat of solution. Furthermore, xylitol cannot be metabolized by the acid producing bacteria of the mouth which cause tooth decay. Indeed, some clinical trials have demonstrated a marked reduction in tooth decay through the use of xylitol. Xylitol is approved by the FDA for use in special dietary foods, and some chewing gums are sweetened, in part, with it. However, a British study suggested that xylitol causes cancer in laboratory animals. This places the future use of xylitol in foods in question.

Xylitol is absorbed slowly from the intestine. Hence, the consumption of large quantities may cause an osmotic diarrhea.

(Also see ADDITIVES, Table A-3; CARBOHYDRATE[S], section headed "Derivatives of Monosaccharides"; and SWEETENING AGENTS.)

XYLOSE (WOOD SUGAR; $C_5H_{10}O_5$)

A 5-carbon—pentose—sugar widely distributed in plant material such as maple wood, cherry wood, straw, cotton seed hulls, corncobs, and peanut shells. It is one of the most abundant plant sugars in the world. However, it is of little or no importance as an energy source for the body. Xylose is not found in its free state in nature but rather as xylan—a polysaccharide built from numerous units of xylose. The sweet-tasting alcohol of xylose, known as xylitol, has been approved by the FDA for use in special dietary foods. Also xylose is employed as a diagnostic aid for the detection of malabsorption. Urinary excretion of less than 4.5 g in 5 hours following ingestion of a 25 g load suggests decreased absorptive capacity.

(Also see CARBOHYDRATE[S], Table C-14 Classification of Carbohydrates and section headed "Monosaccharides.")

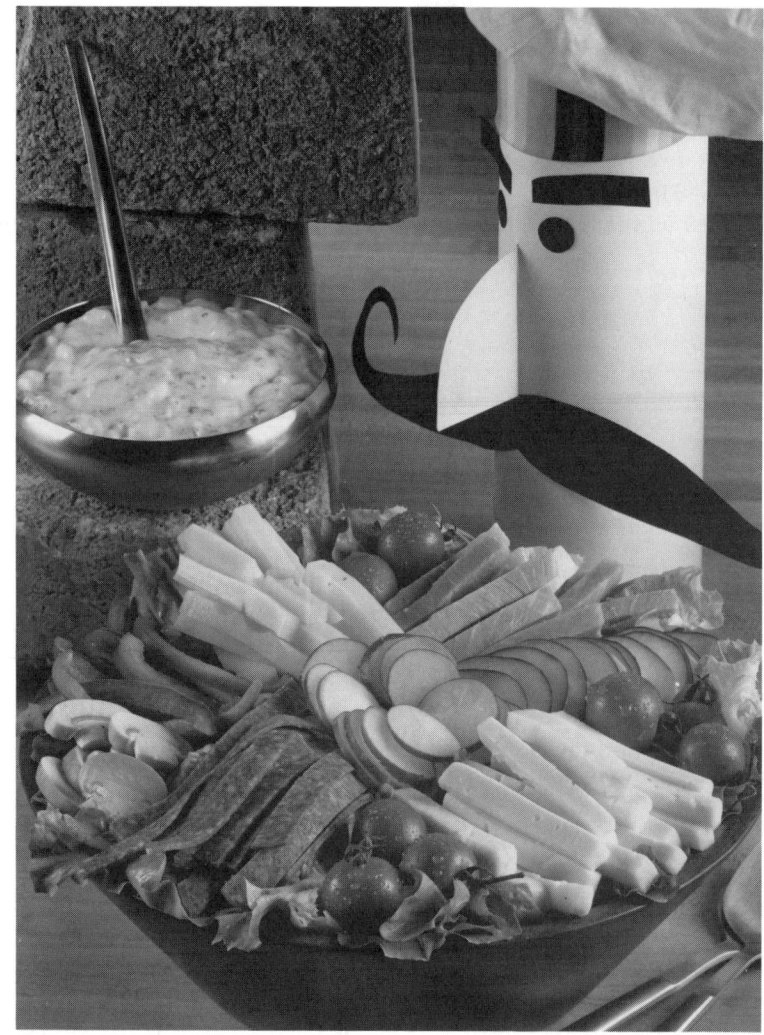

Buffet salad platter. (Courtesy, United Dairy Industry Association, Rosemont, Ill.)

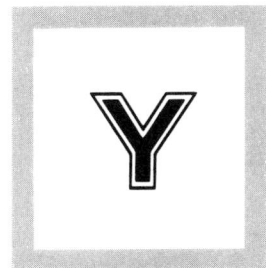

YAM *Dioscorea* spp

The starchy tubers of these tropical plants are consumed by millions of people living in the tropical belt extending around the world. Yams belong to the family *Dioscoreaceae* and the genus *Discorea*, which are named after Dioscorides, a Greek physician and naturalist who lived in the 1st century A.D. They are not related to the sweet potato, although the rich, sweet varieties of the latter are sometimes erroneously called "yams," which they closely resemble. Fig. Y-1 shows a typical yam.

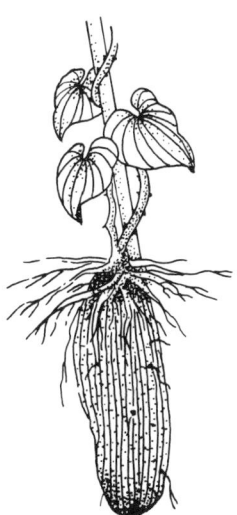

Fig. Y-1. The yam, a tuberous plant that is nutritionally similar to the Irish potato.

ORIGIN AND HISTORY. Yams apparently evolved from a very ancient family of flowering plants that existed long before man appeared on the earth. However, it is not certain how the wild species of yams came to be distributed in both the Old World and the New World since only a few other families of plants are native to both hemispheres.

Archaeological evidence suggests that yams were first cultivated in Africa about 11,000 years ago, and in Southeast Asia by at least 10,000 years ago. The first growing of the tubers by South American Indians appears to have occurred much later because cassava was a more important crop in tropical America.

Yams, like many other crops, were taken from the original sites of their cultivation to neighboring regions. Hence, the Southeast Asian tubers were spread westward to India and northeastward to southern China. Similarly, those grown in northern South America came to be important crops throughout the Caribbean. Finally, the native African yams were spread throughout a tropical belt between 15° north and south latitudes on the Dark Continent.

The oceanic transport of yams appears to have first occurred about 3,500 years ago, when Southeast Asians took them on their migrations to Polynesia. Two thousand years later, Malaysians took some yams to East Africa. Still more recently (about 500 years ago), the Portuguese and Spanish explorers and slave traders stocked their ships with yams from the various ports of call. Hence, they were instrumental in bringing Asian yams to the Americas and West Africa, and African yams to the Caribbean. The Spanish also took the South American white potato to Europe, where it served well as a food until the 1840s, when it was wiped out by a blight. Hence, it is noteworthy that the cold tolerant Chinese yam (*D. opposita*) was grown experimentally in Europe with the aim of replacing the stricken potato. However, potatoes with more resistance to blight were bred from Peruvian stock and the yam never became part of the European diet.

In recent times, the use of yams has declined somewhat due to the lower labor requirements for producing cassava and sweet potatoes. However, certain wild species of yams have been found to contain substances that are valuable raw materials for the production of birth control pills and other medicinal agents.

PRODUCTION.   The estimated worldwide production of yams is about 20 million metric tons per year, much of which comes from the area between the Ivory Coast and Cameroun in West Africa. Other important yam-producing regions are Southeast Asia, tropical islands in the western Pacific, and the Caribbean. Fig. Y-2 shows these areas. Few yams are grown for food in the United States, because the weather is too cold and the growing season too short.

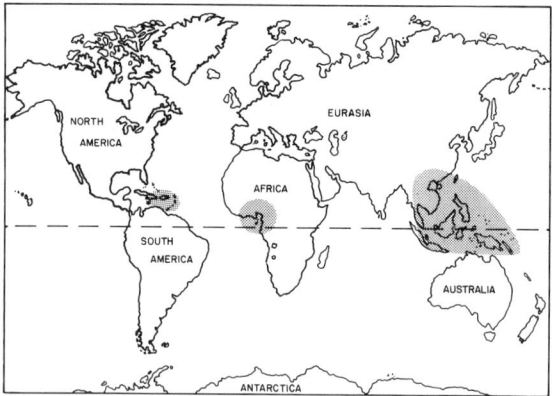

Fig. Y-2.   Important yam-producing areas of the world.

Most species of yams require a growing period of 7 to 8 months in which the temperature ranges between 77° and 86°F (25° and 30°C). Also, they do best in regions which have at least 40 in. (100 cm) of rainfall per year. Finally, yams cannot tolerate a dry season that persists for more than 4 months.

The plants are propagated vegetatively by planting crowns of tubers, whole small tubers, or pieces of large tubers. However, cut pieces of tubers should be dried in the sun for a few hours prior to planting in order to prevent rotting of the pieces. The soil should be well cultivated to encourage optimal growth of the tubers. Sometimes the soil is piled up in ridges, but this is not necessary if it is adequately drained and aerated. Many soils may need supplemental nitrogen, phosphorus, and potassium because high yields of tubers result in the removal of substantial amounts of these minerals from the soil. The maximum yields are obtained when the yam vines are supported on stakes or trellises.

Harvesting of yams must be done carefully to avoid injuring the tubers which may be stored for several months if they have no bruises or cuts. When the growing conditions are optimal, yields as high as 24,300 lb of tubers per acre (27,216 kg/ha) are obtained in the West Indies.

PROCESSING.   In Africa, yams may be sliced, dried, and ground into a flour. Toxic varieties must be soaked or boiled in water to remove the harmful substances. Some types of yams are processed to make drugs that are used in oral contraceptives and in the treatment of arthritis.

PREPARATION.   Yams may be baked, boiled, fried, or roasted like Irish potatoes. The smaller tubers may be peeled or unpeeled, then cooked whole, whereas the larger tubers are usually cut up to save time in cooking. *Fufu* is a West African dish that is prepared by (1) boiling pieces of peeled tubers, then (2) mashing them to make a sticky dough. Usually, *fufu* is served as an accompaniment to soups and stews. Also, pieces of yam or yam flour may be added directly to various hot dishes.

CAUTION: A tropane alkaloid, *dioscorine*, has been isolated from some varieties of yams, especially from *Dioscorea hispida* and from a type of yam native to Nigeria. It is not clear from the literature whether yams contain toxic quantities of this alkaloid even if eaten in large amounts. However, if the toxicity in man is similar to that in the mouse, it would appear that it is unlikely that one could consume lethal amounts of the drug in yams.[1]

NUTRITIONAL VALUE.   The nutrient compositions of various forms of yams are given in Food Composition Table F-36.

Some noteworthy observations regarding the nutrient composition of yams follow:

1.   Compared to potatoes, yam tubers contain about 50% more calories, but about the same amount of protein. However, yams furnish only half as much vitamin C.

2.   Yams are a fair to good source of calcium, phosphorus, and iron, but they contain almost no carotene.

3.   Yam leaves are an excellent source of carotene, and a fair to good source of calcium, iron, and vitamin C. Hence, the leaves complement the tubers in nutritional value.

YAMS OF THE WORLD.   There is considerable variation among the major types and varieties of yams with regard to characteristics such as color, shape, and palatability. Table Y-1 provides data on the leading food yams of the world.

(Also see VEGETABLE[S], Table V-6 Vegetables of the World.)

---

[1]Strong, Frank M., Chairman, Subcommittee on *Naturally Occurring Toxicants in Foods*, National Academy of Sciences, 1973, p. 180.

TABLE Y-1
YAMS OF THE WORLD

Name(s)	Description	Place of Origin, Geographical Adaptation, Cultural Characteristics	Importance—Use	Comments
African Bitter Yam; Cluster Yam (*Dioscorea dumetorum*)	Tubers may be single or in clusters. Raw tubers have a bitter taste due to the content on the toxic alkaloid dihydrodioscorine.	Indigenous to humid tropics of Africa between 15° N and S latitudes. Both cultivated and wild plants are used as food.	Used as food in times of scarcity after tubers have been detoxified by soaking and boiling in water	Some of the cultivated forms have ben selected so as to have a minimal content of the toxic alkaloid.
Asiatic Bitter Yam (*Dioscorea hispida*)	The bulky tubers grow near the surface of the soil and may be lobed or compound. A tropane alkaloid, dioscorine, was isolated from this variety of yams in 1951.	Grows wild from India to Southeast Asia and the islands of the western Pacific.	Source of poison for hunting game or killing people. May be eaten during famines Grated or sliced tuber is detoxified by long soaking and/or boiling with several changes of water.	The tubers are easily harvested.
Chinese Yam; Cinnamon Yam (*Dioscorea opposita, Dioscorea batatas*)	Spindle-shaped tubers may reach 39 in. (*1 m*) in length. Flowers have a cinnamonlike odor.	Cultivated in China, Japan, Korea, and Taiwan because it is more tolerant of cold than any other yam.	A medicinal plant in China Was grown experimentally in Europe as a potato substitute after the latter crop was destroyed by blight in the 1840s	Difficult to harvest because the tubers descend vertically.
Cush-Cush Yam (*Dioscorea trifida*)	Small tubers are from 6 to 8 in. (*15 to 20 cm*) long and may have a white, yellow, pink, or purple flesh.	Native to northern South America and grown throughout the Caribbean (It is the only yam indigenous to the Americas.)	One of the four most important food yams of the world	Very edible and flavorful.
Greater Yam; Asiatic Yam (*Dioscorea alata*)	Cylindrical tubers usually weigh from 11 to 22 lb (*5 to 10 kg*), and the color of their flesh ranges from white to reddish purple.	First cultivated in Southeast Asia, now widely grown throughout the humid tropics Requires at least 60 in. (*1,500 mm*) of annual rainfall.	One of the four most important food yams of the world, and the most important one in Asia	Keeps well for 5 to 6 months after digging. Very popular in the Caribbean region. The highest yielding yam crop.
Lesser Yam (*Dioscorea esculenta*)	Potatolike tubers are 6 to 8 in. (*15 to 20 cm*) long and grow in clusters. Slightly sweet and soft in texture.	Originated in Thailand Grown in China from about 300 A.D.	Production is limited to Southeast Asia and the islands of the western Pacific	Highly palatable and almost free of fibrous material. Does not keep as well as certain other yams.
Potato Yam; Aerial Yam (*Dioscorea bulbifera*)	The aerial tubers (bulbils) weigh from 1 to 4 lb (*0.5 to 2 kg*) and may contain a toxic principle. Underground tubers are hard and bitter.	Grows wild in both Africa and Asia. Asiatic varieties are less toxic than African varieties.	Requires detoxification by boiling and/or soaking. Not used as much as other more edible yams.	May be consumed during famines. Hence, people should be advised of the need for detoxification.

(Continued)

Name(s)	Description	Place of Origin, Geographical Adaptation, Cultural Characteristics	Importance—Use	Comments
White Guinea Yam; White Yam (*Dioscorea rotunda*)	Cylindrical tubers with rounded or pointed ends, and a white mealy flesh. Palatability varies according to variety.	Originated in West Africa, where it is grown in a region extending from the Ivory Coast to Cameroun Tubers are produced in about 8 months.	One of the four most important food yams of the world, and the most important one in West Africa where it is considered to be the best yam for making *fufu*.	Stores much better than the yellow Guinea yam. The plant tolerates the long dry season typical of the savannas of West Africa.
Yellow Guinea Yams; Yellow Yam (*Dioscorea cayensis*)	The flesh of the tubers is pale yellow.	Indigenous to the forest zone of West Africa, which has a short dry season. Requires about 12 months to reach maturity.	One of the four most important food yams of the world. Produced in Africa and the West Indies.	Not as popular as the white Guinea yam. Does not store well.

YAM BEAN (MANIOC BEAN; POTATO BEAN; TURNIP BEAN) *Pachyrrhizus erosus; P. tuberosus*

These climbing vines, which are tropical legumes, are grown mainly for their edible tubers. Hence, the various common names contain both the word bean and the names of other more popular tuberous plants. The major characteristics of *P. erosus* and *P. tuberosus* are very similar, except that the bean pods of the latter are not eaten because they have irritating hairs. Therefore, the name yam bean will be the sole designation used in the rest of this article. Fig. Y-3 shows a typical yam bean.

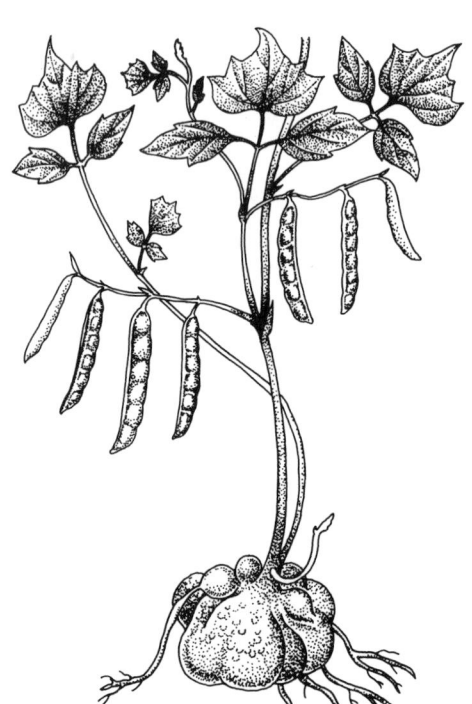

Fig. Y-3. The yam bean, a leguminous plant which has an edible tuber.

ORIGIN AND HISTORY. Various species of yam beans are native to a wide area extending from northern South America to Mexico. The Spanish took these plants to the Philippines during the 16th century. Since then, they have been adopted as crops throughout the tropics of the world.

PRODUCTION. Most of the crop comes from the humid tropical areas of western Pacific and Southeast Asia. Statistics on production are not available.

Yam beans, unlike many other tropical tubers, are grown from seeds. In the Orient, the young plants are trained to climb bamboo trellises. About 10 months are required for the production of mature tubers, which are harvested by plowing or pulling them from the ground. The average yield of tubers is about 8,000 lb per acre (*8,960 kg/ha*).

PROCESSING. The tubers of the plant are rarely processed, although starch is sometimes extracted by washing the grated tubers on a screen.

PREPARATION. Raw yam bean tubers have a crisp texture and are good when served diced or sliced in a salad. The tubers may also be boiled, fried, or roasted. The immature pods of *P. erosus* may be cooked and eaten like snap beans.

CAUTION: The mature seeds and leaves of yam beans should not be consumed, because they contain a harmful agent that is not known to be destroyed by cooking.

NUTRITIONAL VALUE. The nutrient compositions of various forms of yam bean are given in Food Composition Table F-36.

Some noteworthy observations regarding the nutrient composition of yam bean follow:

1. Compared to Irish potatoes, yam bean tubers have a higher water content and are lower in calories, protein and vitamin C. However, the protein-to-calorie ratios are about the same (2.8 g per 100 kcal) for both tubers. This means that yam bean tubers may be a fair source of pro-

tein for adults, providing that sufficient quantities are consumed.

2. Yam bean tubers are low in minerals and vitamins. Hence, they should be eaten with foods that supply these essential nutrients.

YARD-LONG BEAN (ASPARAGUS BEAN)
Vigna sesquipedalis; Dolichos sesquipedalis

The name of this bean denotes the unusually long bean pods, which are utilized like snap beans. It is also called the asparagus bean, and it is very closely related to the cowpea (black-eyed pea). The Latin term *sesquipedalis* means a foot and a half long, which is a much more accurate description of the length of the bean pods than the term "yard-long." Fig. Y-4 shows the long slender pods of this legume.

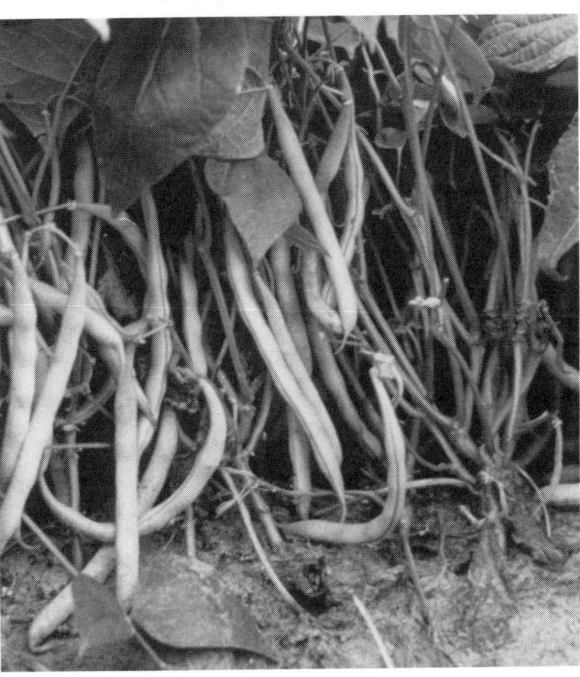

Fig. Y-4. The yard-long bean (asparagus bean). (Courtesy USDA)

ORIGIN AND HISTORY. It was originally believed that the yard-long bean was native to the tropics of Asia, where it has long been grown for the immature pods and seeds. However, it is now fairly certain that the wild ancestors of all types of cowpeas and their close relatives came from Central Africa over 5,000 years ago. From Africa, the ancestral species were apparently spread eastward to India and China, northward to the Mediterranean and Europe, and westward to the West Indies and the Americas. Furthermore, it seems that the peoples of Southeastern Asia selected the plants to obtain extra long pods.

PRODUCTION. Most of this crop is grown in the Far East, but some is also grown in Africa, the West Indies, Hawaii, and California. The seeds cannot be planted until warm weather has arrived, since the plant grows best when the temperature ranges between 68°F *(20°C)* and 95°F *(35°C)*. Irrigation may be required if the rainfall is inadequate. Poles should be provided as support for the climbing vines.

The immature (green) pods and seeds are usually ready for picking within 6 to 8 weeks after planting, and the plants may continue to bear pods for an additional 2 months.

PROCESSING. Statistics relative to the quantity of beans processed are not readily available. However, it appears that much of the crop is sold as a fresh vegetable, but that some is also canned or frozen.

SELECTION AND PREPARATION. Yard-long beans may be prepared and served in the same ways as snap beans. For example, the fibrous ends of the beans may be cut off, the pods cut into strips about 1 in. *(2.5 cm)* long, and stir fried with a little fat or oil plus pieces of fish, meat, poultry, or seafood. Chinese dishes often include thin slices of water chestnuts.

NUTRITIONAL VALUE. The nutrient composition of yard-long beans is given in Food Composition Table F-36.

Yard-long bean pods contain about the same amount of calories, protein, minerals, and vitamins as snap beans. However, the raw green leaves of the plant, which are consumed in Africa, provide about ten times as much carotene as the pods. This has prompted the development of equipment for extracting, coagulating and drying the juice from crushed leafy material. All that is needed is a market for the product.

(Also see BEAN[S], Table B-10, Beans of the World; and LEGUMES, Table L-2 Legumes of the World.)

YAUPON (CASSINA)

The leaves of the yaupon are used as a tea substitute. It is a holly (*Ilex cassine*) which grows in the southern United States. The Indians attributed many virtues to the tea, and allowed only men to drink it. Yaupon tea contains caffeine.

YEAST

Fungi, of which three types are used commercially in the food industry: *Brewers' yeast*, a by-product from the brewing of beer and ale; *dried yeast*, used in leavened breads; and *torula yeast*, cultured as a foodstuff for man and animals, as a source of protein, minerals, B vitamins, and unidentified factors.

(Also see BREADS AND BAKING, section headed "Breads Leavened with Yeast and Other Microorganisms"; BREWERS' YEAST; and TORULA YEAST.)

YEAST EXTRACT

A preparation of the water-soluble fraction of autolysed (self-digested) yeast, valuable both as a rich source of the B vitamins and for its strong savory flavor. Yeast is allowed to autolyse, extracted with hot water, and concentrated by evaporation.

YEAST FERMENTATION, BOTTOM

This refers to fermentation during the manufacture of beer with a yeast that sinks to the bottom of the tank. Most beers are produced this way. Ale, porter, and stout are the principal beers produced by top fermentation.

YOGURT

A fermented milk product prepared from lowfat milk, skim milk, or whole milk. After fermentation, the yogurt may be mixed with other ingredients such as nonfat dry milk solids, vegetable gums, flavoring, or fruit preserves. (Also see MILK AND MILK PRODUCTS.)

YOLK INDEX

This is an expression of egg quality—freshness—in terms of the spherical nature of the yolk. It is derived by measuring the height and width of the yolk. As the egg deteriorates, the index decreases.

(Also see EGGS, section headed, "Physical Characteristics of the Egg and Grading.")

YORKSHIRE PUDDING

This is a quick bread made with flour, milk and eggs, and either cooked in the pan underneath the roast of beef, or in separate muffin tins, with the meat drippings poured into the cups first. It is a first cousin to the popover.

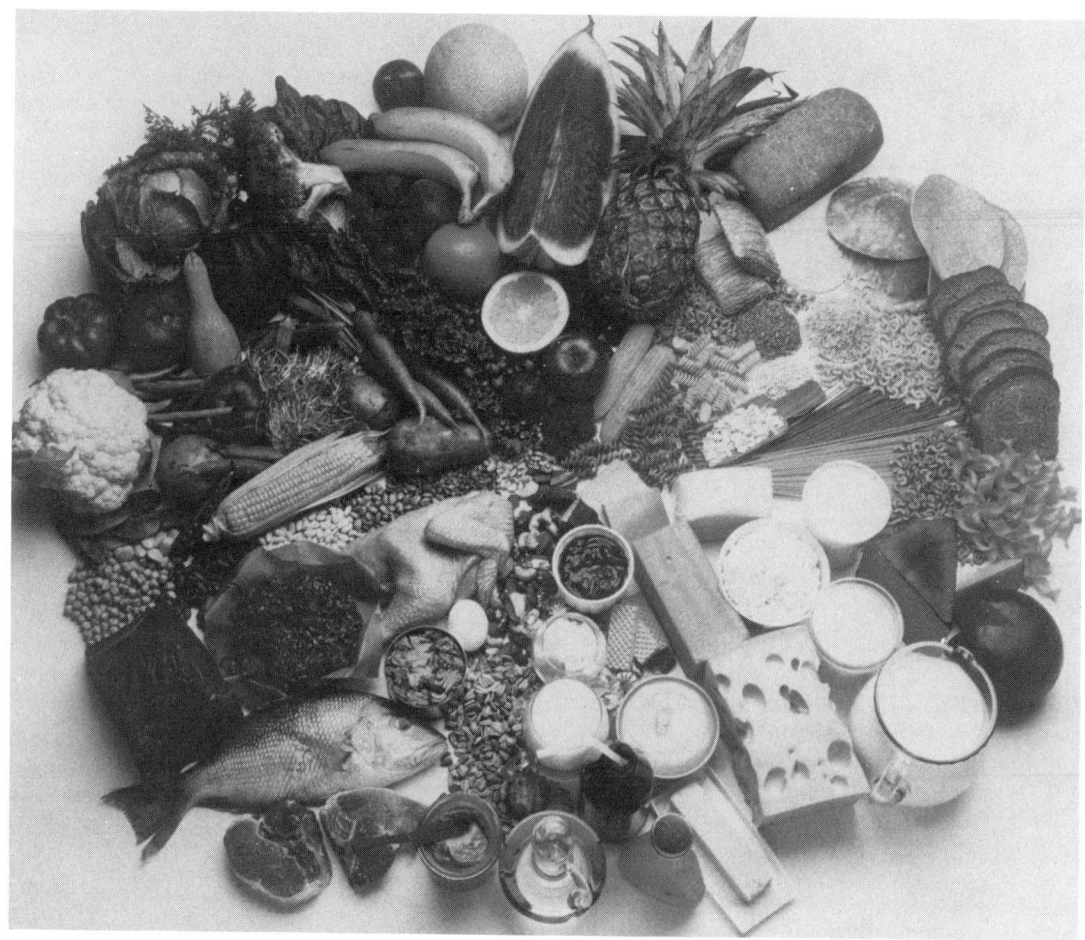

Foods for buoyant good health. (Courtesy, CAST and USDA)

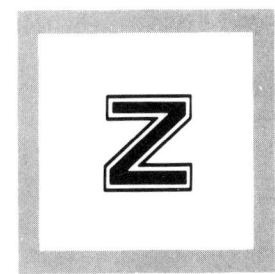

ZANTE CURRANT

This fruit is not a currant, but is actually a raisin; it is made from black Corinth grapes that are only about one-quarter of the size of an ordinary raisin and look like a dried blackcurrant. The name *Zante* was given to the raisin because it was first produced on a large scale on the island of Zante in the southeastern part of Greece. Now, they are also produced in Australia.

Zante currants have a tart, tangy flavor and are commonly used in baked products such as coffee cakes and hot cross buns.

(Also see GRAPE; and RAISIN.)

ZEAXANTHIN

It is a carotenoid alcohol, and the pigment of yellow corn. However, it possesses no vitamin A activity. Zeaxanthin is widespread in nature and occurs together with xanthophyll.

(Also see XANTHOPHYLL.)

ZEDOARY ROOT

An aromatic root from one of two plants of the East Indies which belongs to the ginger family. Zedoary is a GRAS (generally recognized as safe) natural flavor additive.

(Also see ADDITIVES.)

ZEIN

A protein derived from corn. It lacks the essential amino acids lysine and tryptophan. Commercially, zein is extracted from corn gluten meal with alcohol. In the food industry, its prime use is as an edible coating for foodstuffs such as nut meats and candy. In manufacturing, it has a variety of uses: plastics, paper coatings, adhesives, shellac substitute, printing, laminated board, and microencapsulation.

(Also see CORN; and PROTEIN[S].)

ZEN MACROBIOTIC DIET

This phrase encompasses both a diet and a philosophy of life. Zen refers to meditation, and macrobiotic suggests a tendency to prolong life. The Zen philosophy is hundreds of years old; its beginnings may be traced back to India around 470 A.D. From India, the Zen philosophy moved to China in about 520 A.D., but it was not introduced into Japan until the 1100s and 1200s. Zen seeks to discipline the mind so that an individual comes into touch with the inner workings of his body—a "larger awareness" that cannot be taught. In the United States, the Zen philosophy and the Zen cooking—claimed traditional for the ancient Zen Japanese—was popularized by a Japanese named Georges Ohsawa, who coined the term macrobiotic.

According to the macrobiotic plan, there are ten diets or stages of the same diet. In order to live a happy, harmonious life, the follower progresses from the lowest dietary stage, −3, to the highest or +7. As the macrobiotic follower progresses, desserts, fruits and salads, animal foods, soup, and vegetables, in that order, are eliminated and replaced by increased amounts of cereal grains in the diet. Therefore, only certain stages are pure vegetarian diets, though meat is considered undesirable. All dietary stages encourage the restriction of fluid intake. Furthermore, fluid restriction is encouraged if an individual perspires. Table Z-1 lists the ten stages of the Zen macrobiotic diet and the percentage of food from the different sources.

TABLE Z-1
TEN STAGES OF THE ZEN MACROBIOTIC DIET,[1]
FROM LOWEST TO HIGHEST

Stage No.	Cereal Grains	Vegetables	Soup	Animal	Fruits and Salads	Desserts
			(%)			
− 3	10	30	10	30	15	5
− 2	20	30	10	25	10	5
− 1	30	30	10	20	10	
+ 1	40	30	10	20		
+ 2	50	30	10	10		
+ 3	60	30	10			
+ 4	70	20	10			
+ 5	80	20				
+ 6	90	10				
+ 7	100					

[1]All ten stages encourage the sparing use of drinking liquid.

The foods used at the different stages seek to establish a balance between foods classified as yang (the male principle) foods, and yin (the female principle) foods. The proper balance is 5 parts yin to 1 part yang. Such things as color, direction of growth, sodium and potassium level, water content, climate, taste, season, source (plant or animal), weight, and vitamin content are said to classify a food as more yang or more yin. For example, progressing from yang foods to yin foods, the following order would be observed: meat, eggs, fish, grains, vegetables, fruits, dairy products, sugar, alcohol, drugs, and chemicals. Brown rice is considered to contain a perfect balance of yang and yin. Hence, brown rice is the principal food of the diet, and the ultimate diet consists solely of brown rice. Brown rice contains no vitamin A, C, or B-12; low levels of other vitamins; low levels of calcium, iron, and other minerals; and a low-quality protein. Moreover, 2.2 lb (*1 kg*) of cooked brown rice would provide only 1,190 Calories (kcal) of energy—filling, but hardly adequate.

It is the overzealous individuals who persist in following the more rigid diet—high level of brown rice—who are in danger of developing serious nutritional deficiencies. Infants, children, and nursing or pregnant mothers are in particular peril. There have been reports of scurvy, anemia, hypoproteinemia (low blood protein), hypocalcemia (low blood calcium), slowed growth, rickets, loss of kidney function due to low fluid intake, and a few deaths attributed to the followers of the Zen macrobiotic diet.

(Also see VEGETARIAN DIETS.)

ZEST

The colored, oily outer layer of the peel on citrus fruits, which is also called the flavedo. It may be green due to the predominance of the pigment chlorophyll, or yellow to orange when ample amounts of carotene and xanthophyll pigments are present. The color of the zest is *not* always a good indicator of ripeness because some species of citrus fruits require cool nights for the development of the yellow and orange pigments in the peel. However, the color change from green to yellow, or from green to orange, may be induced artificially by exposing the fruit to ethylene gas in a warm room. It is noteworthy that the zest is the part of the peel that is grated and added to enhance various dishes.

(Also see CITRUS FRUITS; and FLAVEDO.)

ZINC (Zn)

Contents

Contrary to what many people think, zinc is needed for more than covering pipes, coating wire fences, and galvanizing buckets. It is an essential element for man.

Zinc is widely distributed throughout the body, but the highest concentrations are found in the skin (the skin contains 20% of the total body zinc), hair, nails, eyes, and prostate gland. Traces occur in the liver, bones, and blood. Also, it is a constituent of enzymes involved in most major pathways. In total, the human body contains about 2.2 g of zinc—more than any other trace element except iron.

HISTORY. Zinc was first shown to be biologically important more than 100 years ago when it was found to be needed for the growth of certain bacteria. In the 1920s, it was demonstrated to be required for the growth of experimental rats. But, it wasn't until the early 1960s that zinc was shown to be an essential nutrient of man.

ABSORPTION, METABOLISM, EXCRETION. Zinc is poorly absorbed; less than 10% of dietary zinc is taken into the body, primarily in the duodenum. It appears that metallic zinc and zinc in its carbonate, sulfate, and oxide forms are all absorbed equally well. Large amounts of calcium, phytic acid, or copper inhibit zinc absorption. Cadmium appears to be a zinc antimetabolite.

After zinc is absorbed in the small intestine, it combines with plasma proteins for transport to the tissues. Relatively large amounts of zinc are deposited in bones, but these stores do not move into rapid equilibrium with the rest of the organism. The body pool of biologically available zinc appears to be small and to have a rapid turnover, as evidenced by the prompt appearance of deficiency signs in experimental animals.

Most of the zinc derived from metabolic processes is excreted in the intestine—in pancreatic, intestinal, and bile secretions. Only small amounts are excreted in the urine.

FUNCTIONS OF ZINC. Zinc is needed for normal skin, bones, and hair. (It imparts "bloom" to the hair.) It is a component of several different enzyme systems which are involved in digestion and respiration. Also, zinc is required for the transfer of carbon dioxide in red blood cells; for proper calcification of bones; for the synthesis and metabolism of proteins and nucleic acids; for the development and functioning of reproductive organs; for wound and burn healing; for the functioning of insulin; and for normal taste acuity (the ability to taste accurately).

DEFICIENCY SYMPTOMS. The most common cause of zinc deficiency is an unbalanced diet, although other factors may be responsible. For example, the consumption of alcohol may precipitate a zinc deficiency by flushing stored zinc out of the liver and into the urine.

Lack of zinc in the human diet has been studied in detail in Egypt and Iran, where the major constituent of the diet is an unleavened bread prepared from low extraction wheat flour. The phytate present in the flour limits the availability of zinc in these diets, with the result

TOP FOOD   SOURCES

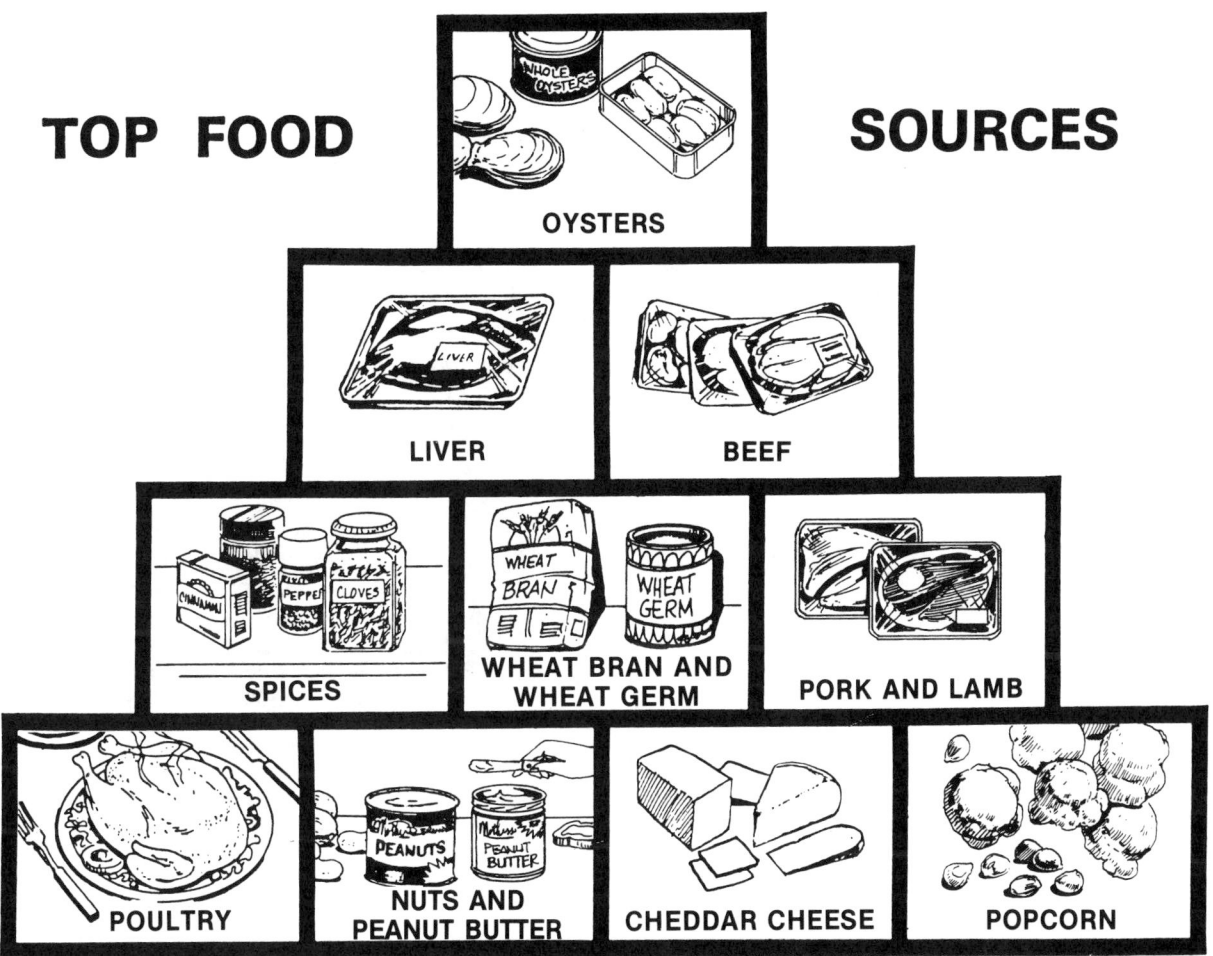

Fig. Z-1. Top food sources of zinc.

that the requirements for the element are not satisfied. Zinc-response has also been observed in young children from middle-class homes in the United States who consume less than an ounce (*28 g*) of meat per day.

Zinc deficiency is characterized by loss of appetite, stunted growth in children, skin changes, small sex glands in boys, loss of taste sensitivity, lightened pigment in hair (dull hair), white spots on the fingernails, and delayed healing of wounds. In the Middle East, pronounced zinc deficiency in man has resulted in hypogonadism and dwarfism. In pregnant animals, experimental zinc deficiency has resulted in malformation and behavioral disturbances in the offspring—a finding which suggests that the same thing may happen to human fetuses.

INTERRELATIONSHIPS. Zinc is involved in many relationships: in the metabolism of carbohydrates, fats, proteins, and nucleic acids; in interference with the utilization of copper, iron, and other trace minerals, when there are excess dietary levels of zinc; in protection against the toxic effects of cadmium, when there is ample dietary zinc; in reduced absorption, when there are high dietary levels of calcium, phosphorus, and copper.

RECOMMENDED ALLOWANCE OF ZINC. Studies have shown that, in healthy adults, equilibrium or positive balance is obtained with intakes of 12.5 mg of zinc per day when this intake is derived from a mixed diet. This has been accepted as a minimum requirement, as the balance studies did not take into account sweat and skin losses.

The National Academy of Sciences, National Research Council, recommended daily zinc allowances are given in Table Z-2.

TABLE Z-2
RECOMMENDED DAILY ZINC ALLOWANCES[1]

Group	Age	Weight		Height		Zinc
	(year)	(lb)	(kg)	(in.)	(cm)	(mg)
Infants	0.0–0.5	13	6	24	60	5
	0.5–1.0	20	9	28	71	5
Children	1–3	29	13	35	90	10
	4–6	44	20	44	112	10
	7–10	62	28	52	132	10
Males	11–14	99	45	62	157	15
	15–18	145	66	69	176	15
	19–24	160	72	70	177	15
	25–50	174	79	70	176	15
	51+	170	77	68	173	15
Females	11–14	101	46	62	157	12
	15–18	120	55	64	163	12
	19–24	128	58	65	164	12
	25–50	138	63	64	163	12
	51+	143	65	63	160	12
Pregnant						15
Lactating: 1st 6 mo.–19 mg; 2nd 6 mo.–16 mg						19/16

[1]*Recommended Dietary Allowances*, 10th ed., 1989, NRC–National Academy of Sciences, p. 285.

The Table Z-2 recommended daily allowances are predicated on the consumption of a mixed diet containing animal products. Diets that supply sufficient animal protein usually also furnish enough zinc, but vegetarian diets may be somewhat low.

The zinc requirement of preadolescent children has been estimated at 6 mg/day. In view of recent information showing that dermal loss is greater than had been suspected, and to allow for variation in availability of zinc, an allowance of 10 mg is recommended for this age group. The NRC recommended allowance for the first 6 months of life is 5 mg/day. The NRC recommends an intake of 15 mg of dietary zinc per day for adults and during pregnancy.

• **Zinc intake in average U.S. diet**—The average zinc content of mixed diets consumed by the American adult has been reported to be between 10 and 15 mg/day, but vegetarian and low-protein diets may provide less.

TOXICITY.   Toxicity of zinc in man occurs with the ingestion of 2 g or more. Zinc sulfate, taken in these amounts, produces acute gastrointestinal irritation and vomiting. However, zinc has been administered to patients in tenfold excess of the dietary allowances for months and years without adverse reactions. But there is evidence that excessive intakes of zinc may aggravate marginal copper deficiency. For the latter reason, the continuous taking of zinc supplements of more than 15 mg/day, in addition to the dietary intake, should not be done without medical supervision.

Toxicity of zinc is characterized by anemia, depressed growth, stiffness, hemorrhages in bone joints, bone resorption, depraved appetite, and in severe cases, death.

The anemia appears to result from an interference with iron and copper utilization because addition of these two elements can overcome the anemia caused by excessive zinc.

Zinc poisoning may result from eating foods that have been stored in galvanized containers.

SOURCES OF ZINC.   Human colostrum (the first secretion of a woman after childbirth) is a good source of zinc.

The zinc content of most municipal drinking water is negligible.

Groupings by rank of common food sources of zinc follow:

• **Rich sources**—Beef, liver, oysters, spices, wheat bran.

• **Good sources**—Cheddar cheese, crab, granola, lamb, peanut butter, peanuts, popcorn, pork, poultry.

• **Fair sources**—Beans, clams, eggs, fish, sausages and luncheon meats, turnip greens, wheat cereals, whole grain products (wheat, rye, oats, rice, barley).

• **Negligible sources**—Beverages, fats and oils, fruits and vegetables, milk, sugar, white bread.

• **Supplemental sources**—Wheat germ, yeast (torula), zinc carbonate, zinc gluconate, zinc sulfate. (Zinc carbonate or zinc sulfate are commonly used where zinc supplementation is necessary.)

For additional sources and more precise values of zinc, see Food Composition Table F-36.

NOTE WELL: The biological availability of zinc in different foods varies widely; meats and seafoods are much better sources of available zinc than vegetables. Zinc availability is adversely affected by phytates (found in whole grains and beans), high calcium, oxalates (in rhubarb and spinach), high fiber, copper (from drinking water conveyed in copper piping), and EDTA (an additive used in certain canned foods).

TOP ZINC SOURCES.   The top sources are listed in Table Z-3.

NOTE WELL: This table lists (1) the top sources without regard to the amount normally eaten (left column), and (2) the top food sources (right column); and the caloric (energy) content of each food.

(Also see MINERAL[S], Table M-67.)

TABLE Z-3
TOP ZINC SOURCES[1]

Top Sources[2]	Zinc (mg/100 g)	Energy (kcal/100g)	Top Food Sources	Zinc (mg/100 g)	Energy (kcal/100g)
Oysters, raw meat only, Pacific and Eastern	148.6	86	Oysters, raw meat only, Pacific and Eastern	148.6	86
Wheat germ, toasted	15.4	391	Wheat germ, toasted	15.4	391
Sesame seeds, decorticated	10.3	588	Wheat bran, crude	9.8	353
Poppy seeds	10.2	533	Liver, calf, fried	6.1	261
Wheat bran, crude	9.8	353	Beef, variety of cuts, separable lean, cooked, broiled, roasted	6.0	220
Yeast, torula	9.9	277	Beef, ground, not less than 77% lean, cooked	4.4	301
Chervil, dried	8.8	237	Lamb, variety of cuts, separable lean, cooked, broiled, roasted	4.3	185
Liver, hog, fried in margarine	8.3	241	Turkey, all classes, dark meat w/skin, cooked, roasted	4.2	221
Cardamon	7.5	311	Popcorn, popped	4.1	386
Alfalfa seeds	6.9	389	Cheese, natural, cheddar	4.0	402
Celery seeds	6.9	392	Pork, trimmed lean cuts, separable lean, cooked, roasted	3.8	240
Chicken eggs, dried yolks	6.2	687	Peanut butter	2.9	593
Thyme, ground	6.2	276	Chicken, broilers or fryers, dark meat w/skin, cooked, roasted	2.8	176
Liver, calf, fried	6.1	261	Whole wheat flour (from hard wheats)	2.4	361
Beef, variety of cuts, separable lean, cooked, broiled, roasted	6.0	220	Granola	2.1	429
Basil, dried	5.8	251	Turnip greens, raw	1.9	28
Mustard seeds, yellow	5.7	469	Frankfurters, all meat, cooked	1.6	248
Caraway seeds	5.5	333	Chicken eggs, fried or hard cooked	1.5	183
Chicken eggs, dried, whole	5.4	593	Bologna	1.5	316
Tea bag, orange pekoe	5.4	1	Tuna, canned in oil, drained solids	1.1	197

[1]These listings are based on the data in Food Composition Table F-36. Some top or rich sources may have been overlooked since many of the foods in Table F-36 lack values for zinc.

Whenever possible, foods are on an "as used" basis, without regard to moisture content; hence, certain high-moisture foods may be disadvantaged when ranked on the basis of zinc content per 100 g (approximately 3½ oz) without regard to moisture content.

[2]Listed without regard to the amount normally eaten.

ZIZANIA AGUATICA (WILD RICE; INDIAN RICE)

A food crop native to eastern North America, found in the Great Lakes region. Although wild rice is cultivated, the Indians still collect the grain for their own use and as a cash crop.

(Also see RICE, section headed "Wild Rice"; and WILD RICE.)

ZOLLINGER-ELLISON SYNDROME

Frequently, this disease produces malabsorption. It is caused by the development of a gastrin-secreting tumor in the pancreas or duodenal wall, which stimulates excessive, continued gastric secretion. This over secretion by the stomach acidifies and dilutes the intestinal contents, leading to major disturbances in fat digestion and absorption, primarily due to the inactivation of the enzyme, pancreatic lipase. Other factors contributing to malabsorption include (1) alteration in the chemical nature of bile salts, reducing their effectiveness; (2) structural and function changes in the intestinal lining; and (3) hypermotility. Eventually, multiple peptic ulcers develop due to the excessive secretion of the hormone, gastrin. Total gastrectomy seems to be the therapy of choice.

ZWITTERION

The term used to describe the property of amino acids, when ionized in solution, to behave either as an acid or a base depending on the need of the solution in which they are present. This capacity makes amino acids good buffer substances.

ZYMASE

The name which is sometimes applied to the mixture of enzymes in yeast that change sugar to alcohol during fermentation.

ZYMOGENS

These are inactive forms of enzymes—proenzymes. Zymogens convert to active enzymes under the influence of various agents such as pH changes or other enzymes. Examples of zymogens are some of the enzymes involved in the digestion of protein. Typsinogen and pepsinogen are both zymogens secreted into the intestine by the pancreas where they are converted to the active enzymes trypsin and pepsin, respectively.

ZYMOMETER

An instrument which is employed to measure the degree of fermentation of a fermenting liquid.

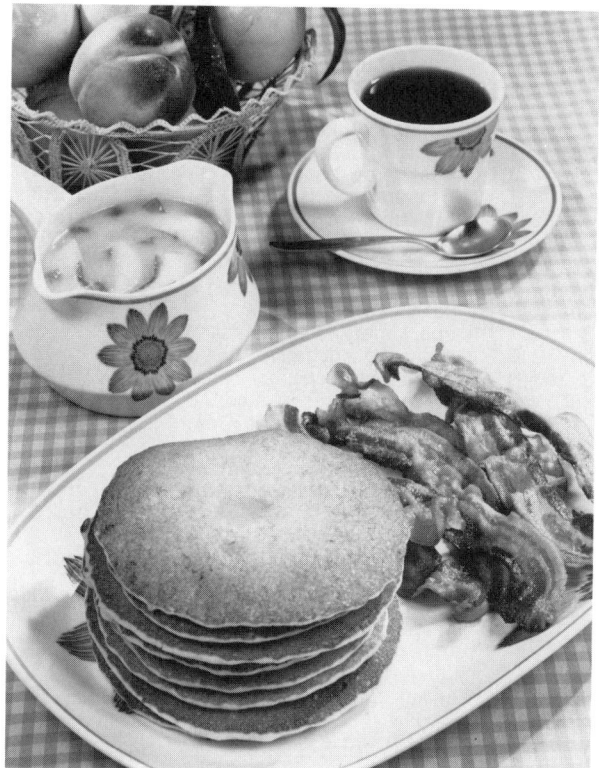

A good breakfast increases the speed of mental response and improves the performance of work. (Courtesy, The California Peach Commodity Committee, Sacramento, Calif.)

The consumption of meat by man antedates recorded history. Primitive man recognized that a meat-rich diet was far more concentrated than leaves, shoots, and fruits.

Meat is an excellent source of high-quality protein, of certain minerals, especially iron, and of the B-complex vitamins. It supplies nutrients which contribute significantly to the dietary balance of meals, and it is easily digested. (Courtesy, American Meat Institute)

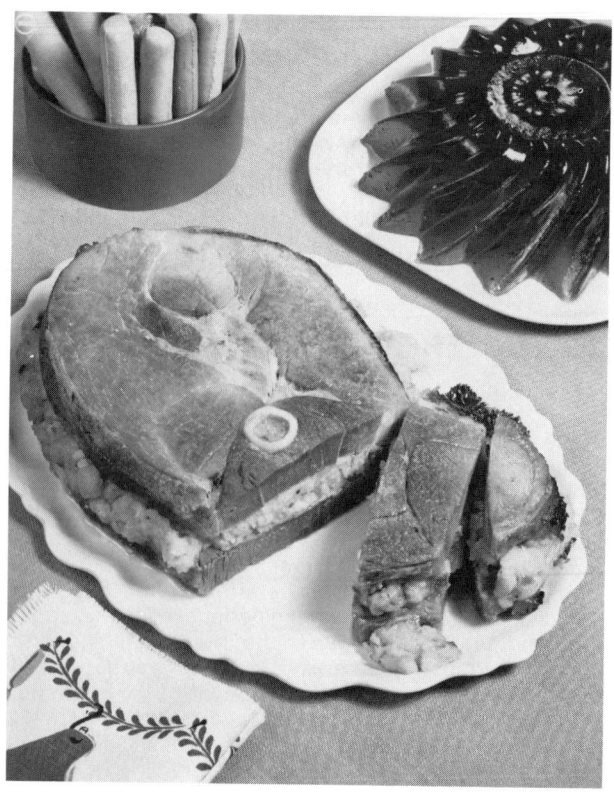

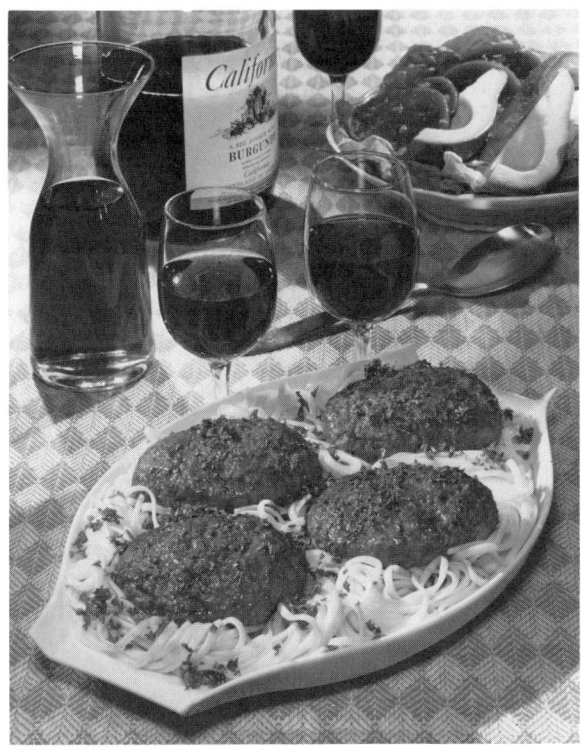

Wine was first made from grapes in the Middle East 6,000 to 7,000 years ago. Hippocrates, the ancient Greek physician (460 to 370 B.C.), prescribed it as a medicine.

When used in moderation, wine has a relaxing effect, stimulates the appetite, and promotes better absorption of essential minerals. (Courtesy, Wine Institute, San Francisco, Calif.)

Meals should be nutritious, attractive, palatable, and reasonable in cost. (Courtesy, California Beef Council, Burlingame, Calif.)

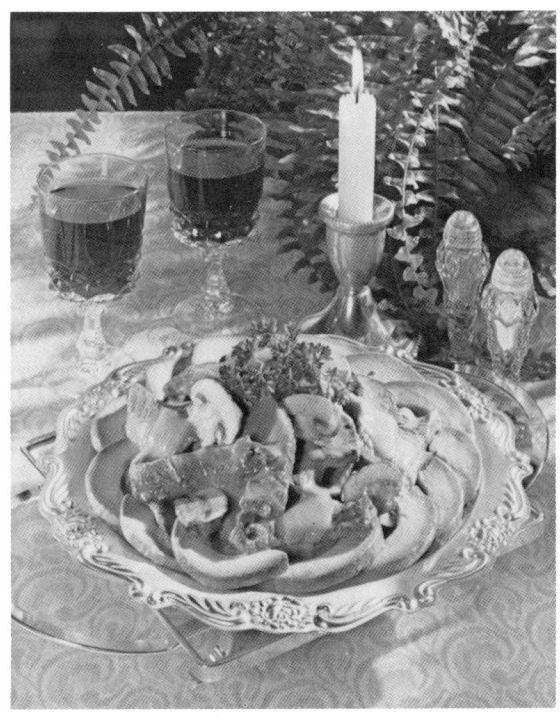

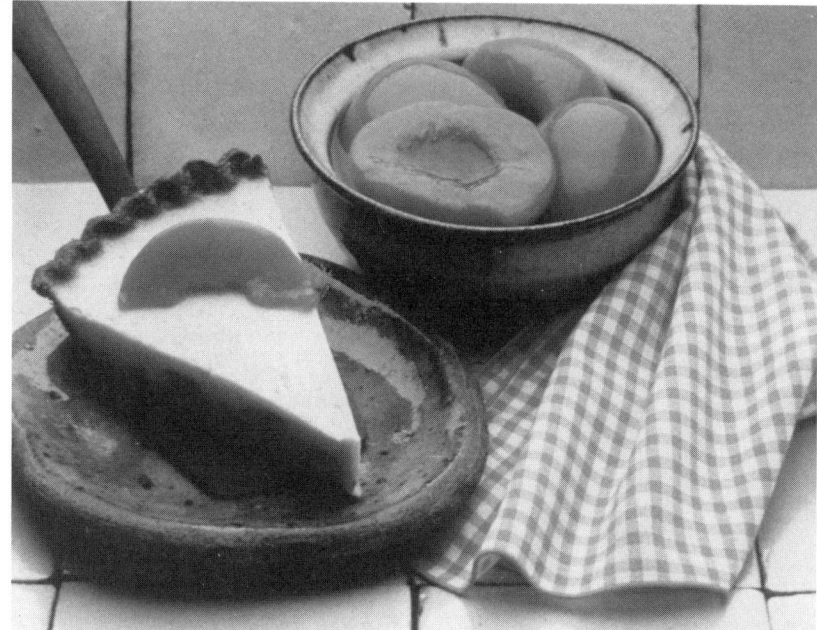

Fruits are fair to excellent sources of calories, fiber, various essential macrominerals and microminerals, and vitamins. (Courtesy, USDA)

Desserts, like this chilled pie, may be a delightful and romantic conclusion to a meal—and an aid to digestion. (Courtesy, Hershey Foods Corp., Hershey, Penn.)

B

D

I

Y

Z

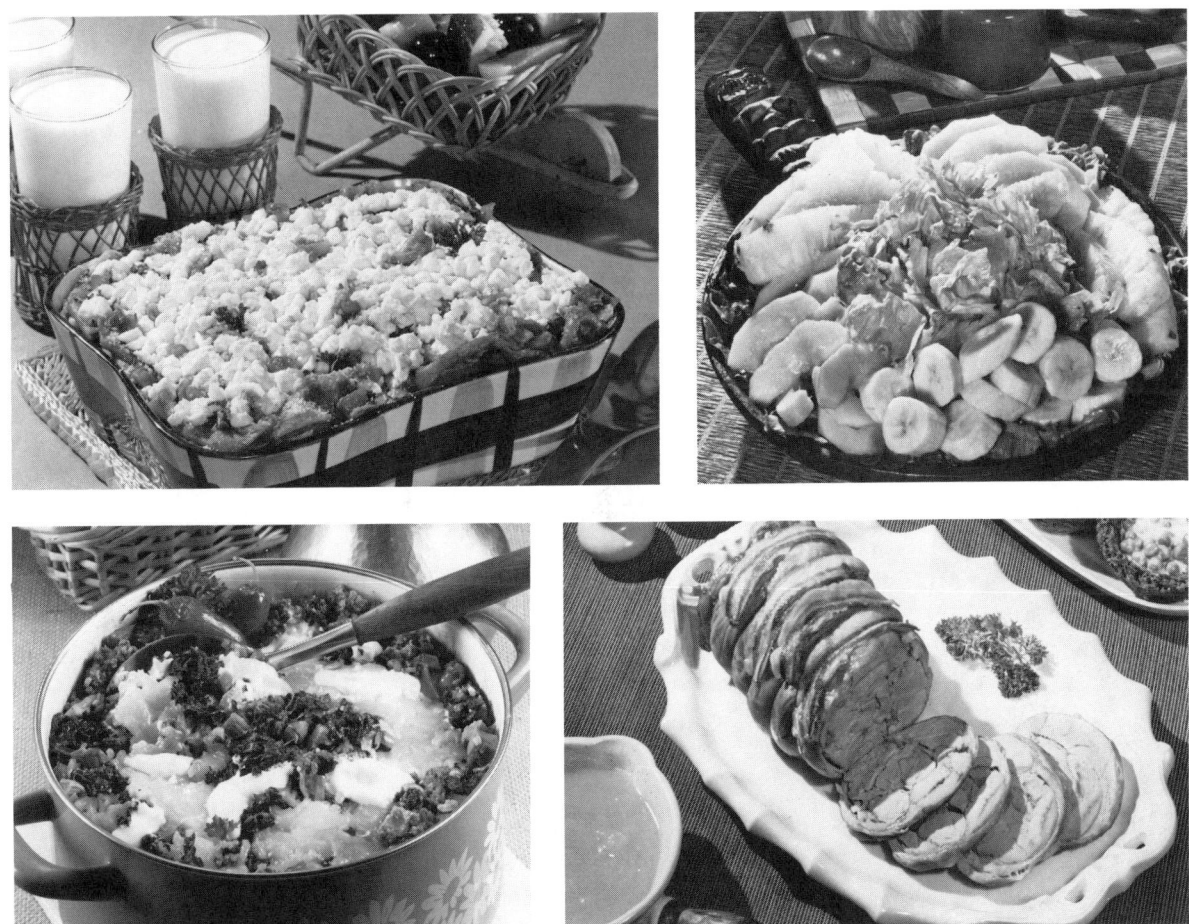

To ensure nutritional adequacy, the daily diet should include definite amounts of foods from each of the Food Groups.